The SHOULDER

Volume 2

The SHOULDER

SECOND EDITION

EDITORS

CHARLES A. ROCKWOOD, Jr., M.D.
Professor and Chairman Emeritus
Department of Orthopaedics
The University of Texas
Health Science Center at San Antonio
San Antonio, Texas

FREDERICK A. MATSEN III, M.D.
Professor and Chairman
Department of Orthopaedics
University of Washington
School of Medicine
Seattle, Washington

ASSOCIATE EDITORS

MICHAEL A. WIRTH, M.D.
Associate Professor
Department of Orthopaedics
The University of Texas
Health Science Center at San Antonio
San Antonio, Texas

DOUGLAS T. HARRYMAN II, M.D.
Associate Professor of Orthopaedics
Department of Orthopaedics
University of Washington
School of Medicine
Seattle, Washington

W.B. SAUNDERS COMPANY
A Division of Harcourt Brace & Company
Philadelphia London Toronto Montreal Sydney Tokyo

W.B. SAUNDERS COMPANY
A Division of Harcourt Brace & Company

The Curtis Center
Independence Square West
Philadelphia, Pennsylvania 19106

Library of Congress Cataloging-in-Publication Data

The shoulder / [edited by] Charles A. Rockwood, Jr., Frederick A. Matsen III.—2nd ed.

p. cm.

Includes bibliographical references and index.

ISBN 0–7216–8134–4

1. Shoulder—Diseases. 2. Shoulder—Surgery. I. Rockwood, Charles A. II. Matsen, Frederick A.

[DNLM: 1. Shoulder. 2. Shoulder Joint. WE 810 S55861 1998]

RC939.S484 1998 617.5′72—dc21

DNLM/DLC 97-33313

ISBN 0–7216–8134–4—Set
ISBN 0–7216–8135–2—Vol. 1
ISBN 0–7216–8136–0—Vol. 2

THE SHOULDER

Printed in the United States of America

Last digit is the print number: 9 8 7 6 5 4 3 2

We dedicate these volumes to Anne, Patsy, and our children, who have supported us so fully during our careers as shoulder surgeons. We also dedicate these volumes to the millions of individuals who suffer with disorders of the shoulder and to the clinicians and investigators who seek to improve their comfort and function.

Contributors

ANSWORTH A. ALLEN, M.D.
Instructor in Orthopaedic Surgery, Cornell University Medical College, New York Hospital; Assistant Attending Orthopaedic Surgeon, The Hospital for Special Surgery, New York, New York

DAVID W. ALTCHEK, M.D.
Associate Professor of Orthopaedics, Cornell University Medical College, Hospital for Special Surgery, New York, New York

KAI-NAN AN, Ph.D.
Professor of Bioengineering and John and Posy Krehbiel Professor of Orthopedics, Mayo Medical School; Chair, Division of Orthopedic Research, Mayo Clinic, Rochester, Minnesota

MICHEL A. ARCAND, M.D.
Attending Surgeon, Oklahoma Orthopedic Institute, Norman, Oklahoma

STEVEN P. ARNOCZKY, D.V.M.
Professor of Veterinary Medicine and Wade O. Brinker Chair of Veterinary Surgery, Michigan State University, East Lansing, Michigan

CRAIG T. ARNTZ, M.D.
Associate Clinical Professor, Department of Orthopedics, University of Washington School of Medicine, Seattle, Washington; Active Staff, Valley Medical Center, Renton, Washington

LOUIS U. BIGLIANI, M.D.
Professor of Orthopaedic Surgery, Columbia University College of Physicians and Surgeons; Chief, The Shoulder Service, and Vice-Chairman, Department of Orthopaedic Surgery, New York Orthopaedic Hospital, Columbia-Presbyterian Medical Center, New York, New York

DESMOND J. BOKOR, M.B., B.S., F.R.A.C.S.
Consultant Orthopedic Surgeon, Western Sydney Orthopaedic Associates; Honorary Orthopaedic Surgeon, University of Sydney and Westmead Hospital, Sydney, Australia

ERNEST M. BURGESS, M.D., Ph.D.
Clinical Professor, Department of Orthopaedics, University of Washington; Endowed Chair of Orthopaedic Research, University of Washington School of Medicine; Attending Physician, University of Washington Affiliated Hospitals; Senior Scientist, Prosthetics Research Study, Seattle, Washington

W.Z. BURKHEAD, Jr., M.D.
Clinical Associate Professor, University of Texas Southwestern Medical School; Attending Physician, W.B. Carrell Memorial Clinic, Dallas, Texas

KENNETH P. BUTTERS, M.D.
Clinical Instructor, University of Oregon Health Sciences University, Eugene, Oregon

MICHAEL A. CAUGHEY, M.B., Ch.B., F.R.A.C.S.
Clinical Lecturer, University of Auckland School of Medicine; Consultant Orthopaedic Surgeon, Middlemore Hospital, Auckland, New Zealand

ERNEST U. CONRAD III, M.D.
Professor of Orthopaedics, University of Washington School of Medicine; Director of Sarcoma Service, Director of Division of Orthopaedics, and Director of Bone Tumor Clinic—Children's Hospital, University of Washington, Children's Hospital and Medical Center, Seattle, Washington

EDWARD V. CRAIG, M.D.
Professor of Clinical Surgery, Cornell University Medical College; Attending Surgeon, Hospital for Special Surgery, New York, New York

FRANCES CUOMO, M.D.
Assistant Professor of Orthopaedic Surgery, New York University School of Medicine; Associate Chief, Shoulder Service, Hospital for Joint Diseases, New York, New York

STEPHEN FEALY, M.D.
Orthopaedic Resident, Hospital for Special Surgery, Cornell University Medical Center, New York, New York

EVAN L. FLATOW, M.D.
Associate Professor of Orthopaedic Surgery, Columbia University; Associate Chief, Shoulder Service, New York Orthopaedic Hospital, Columbia-Presbyterian Medical Center, New York, New York

MAUREEN A. GALLAGHER, Ph.D.
Associate Director, Shoulder Institute, Hospital for Joint Diseases, New York, New York

PETER HABERMEYER, M.D.
Assistant Professor, University of Munich, Stuttgart, Germany

DOUGLAS T. HARRYMAN II, M.D.
Associate Professor of Orthopaedics and Co-Director, Shoulder and Elbow Service, Department of Orthopaedics, University of Washington School of Medicine, Seattle, Washington

RICHARD J. HAWKINS, B.A., M.D., F.A.C.S., F.R.C.S.(C.)
Clinical Professor, University of Colorado; Clinical Professor, University of Dallas, Southwestern Medical School; Consultant, Vail Valley Medical Center and Steadman Hawkins Clinic, Vail, Colorado

EIJI ITOI, M.D., Ph.D.
Assistant Professor of Orthopedic Surgery, Akita University School of Medicine, Akita, Japan

KIRK L. JENSEN, M.D.
Assistant Clinical Professor, Department of Orthopaedic Surgery, University of California, San Francisco; Staff, San Francisco General Hospital, San Francisco; Staff Orthopaedic Surgery, Summit Medical Center, Oakland, California

CHRISTOPHER M. JOBE, M.D.
Associate Professor, Department of Orthopaedic Surgery, Loma Linda University School of Medicine; Active Staff Member, Loma Linda University Medical Center; Consulting Staff, Jerry L. Pettis Memorial Veterans' Administration Hospital, Loma Linda, California

FRANK W. JOBE, M.D.
Clinical Professor, Department of Orthopaedics, University of Southern California School of Medicine, Los Angeles; Orthopaedic Consultant, Los Angeles Dodgers, PGA Tour, and Senior PGA Tour; President, Kerlan-Jobe Orthopaedic Clinic, Inglewood, California

RONALD S. KVITNE, M.D.
Assistant Clinical Professor, Department of Orthopaedics, University of Southern California, Los Angeles, California; Senior Staff Member, Centinela Hospital Medical Center, Inglewood, California

MARK D. LAZARUS, M.D.
Clinical Assistant Professor of Orthopaedic Surgery, Temple University School of Medicine; Director of Shoulder and Elbow Surgery, Department of Orthopaedic Surgery, Albert Einstein Medical Center, Philadelphia, Pennsylvania

ROBERT D. LEFFERT, M.D.
Professor of Orthopaedic Surgery, Harvard Medical School; Chief, Surgical-Upper Extremity Rehabilitation Unit, and Visiting Orthopaedic Surgeon, Massachusetts General Hospital, Boston, Massachusetts

STEVEN B. LIPPITT, M.D.
Assistant Professor of Orthopaedic Surgery, Northeast Ohio Universities College of Medicine, Akron, Ohio

JOACHIM F. LOEHR, M.D.
Associate Professor, University of Zurich; Attending Staff Physician, W. Schulthess Klinik, Zurich, Switzerland

LEONARD J. MARCHINSKI, M.D.
Staff Surgeon, Reading Hospital and Medical Center, West Reading, Pennsylvania

FREDERICK A. MATSEN III, M.D.
Professor and Chairman, Department of Orthopaedics, University of Washington School of Medicine, Seattle, Washington

BERNARD F. MORREY, M.D.
Professor of Orthopedics, Mayo Medical School; Chair, Department of Orthopedics, Mayo Clinic, Rochester, Minnesota

STEPHEN J. O'BRIEN, M.D.
Associate Professor of Orthopaedic Surgery, Hospital for Special Surgery, Cornell University Medical College; Assistant Scientist; Associate Attending Orthopaedic Surgeon, New York Hospital, New York, New York

CHARLES A. PETERSON II, M.D.
Physician, Ventura Orthopaedic, Hand and Sports Medicine Group, Oxnard, California

MARILYN M. PINK, Ph.D., P.T.
Director of Biomechanic Laboratory, Centinela Hospital Medical Center, Inglewood, California

ROGER G. POLLOCK, M.D.
Assistant Professor of Orthopaedic Surgery, Columbia University; Attending Physician, Shoulder Service, New York Orthopaedic Hospital, Columbia-Presbyterian Medical Center, New York, New York

L. BRIAN READY, M.D., F.R.C.P.C.
Professor, Department of Anesthesiology, University of Washington School of Medicine; Director, UWMC Pain Service, University of Washington Medical Center, Seattle, Washington

ROBIN R. RICHARDS, M.D., F.R.C.S.(C.)
Associate Professor, Division of Orthopaedic Surgery, Department of Surgery, University of Toronto; Head, Division of Orthopaedic Surgery, Department of Surgery, St. Michael's Hospital, Toronto, Ontario, Canada

CHARLES A. ROCKWOOD, Jr., M.D.
Professor and Chairman Emeritus, Department of Orthopaedics, The University of Texas Health Science Center at San Antonio, San Antonio, Texas

SCOTT A. RODEO, M.D.
Assistant Professor of Orthopaedic Surgery, Cornell University Medical College; Assistant Attending Orthopaedic Surgeon, Hospital for Special Surgery, Cornell University Medical Center, New York Hospital, New York, New York

ANDREW S. ROKITO, M.D.
Assistant Professor of Orthopaedic Surgery, New York University School of Medicine; Assistant Chief, Shoulder Service, and Associate Director, Sports Medicine Service, Hospital for Joint Diseases, New York, New York

ROBERT L. ROMANO, M.D.
Clinical Professor, Department of Orthopaedics, University of Washington School of Medicine; Staff Physician, Providence Medical Center, Seattle, Washington

RICHARD ROZENCWAIG, M.D.
Chief Resident in Orthopaedics, Ochsner Clinic, New Orleans, Louisiana

JAMES O. SANDERS, M.D.
Chief of Staff, Shriners Hospital for Children, Erie, Pennsylvania

DOUGLAS G. SMITH, M.D.
Associate Professor of Orthopaedic Surgery, University of Washington; Co-Principal Investigator, Prosthetics Research Study, Seattle, Washington

KEVIN L. SMITH, M.D.
Assistant Professor, University of Washington School of Medicine; Staff, Shoulder and Elbow Service, University of Washington Medical Center, Seattle, Washington

KIT M. SONG, M.D.
Assistant Professor of Orthopaedics, University of Washington School of Medicine; Assistant Director, Department of Orthopedics, Children's Hospital and Medical Center, Seattle, Washington

STEVEN C. THOMAS, M.D.
Private Practice, Las Vegas, Nevada

JAMES E. TIBONE, M.D.
Professor, Department of Orthopedics, University of Southern California, Los Angeles; Associate, Kerlan-Jobe Orthopaedic Clinic, Inglewood, California

HANS K. UHTHOFF, M.D.
Professor Emeritus, University of Ottawa; Attending Physician, Ottawa General Hospital, Ottawa, Ontario, Canada

GILLES WALCH, M.D.
Ancien Assistant des Hôpitaux de Lyon, Université de Médécine de Lyon; Chirurgien Orthopediste, Clinique E de Vialar, Lyon, France

RUSSELL F. WARREN, M.D.
Professor of Orthopaedics, Cornell University Medical College; Surgeon and Chief of Hospital for Special Surgery, New York, New York

PETER WELSH, M.B.Ch.B., F.R.C.S.C.
Associate Professor, Department of Surgery, University of Toronto; Chief of Staff and Chief of Surgery, Orthopaedic and Arthritic Hospital, Toronto, Ontario, Canada

GERALD R. WILLIAMS, Jr., M.D.
Assistant Professor, Department of Orthopaedic Surgery, University of Pennsylvania School of Medicine, Philadelphia, Pennsylvania

MICHAEL A. WIRTH, M.D.
Associate Professor, Department of Orthopaedics, The University of Texas Health Science Center at San Antonio; Chief, Orthopaedic Shoulder Service, Audie Murphy Veterans' Hospital, San Antonio, Texas

VIRCHEL E. WOOD, M.D.
Professor, Orthopaedic Surgery, Loma Linda University School of Medicine; Chief, Hand Surgery Service, Loma Linda University Medical Center, Loma Linda, California

D. CHRISTOPHER YOUNG, M.D.
Assistant Clinical Professor of Orthopaedic Surgery, Medical College of Virginia; Orthopaedic Surgeon, West End Orthopaedic Clinic, Richmond, Virginia

CRAIG ZEMAN, M.D.
Physician, Ventura Orthopaedic, Hand and Sports Medical Group, Oxnard, California

JOSEPH D. ZUCKERMAN, M.D.
Associate Professor of Orthopaedic Surgery, New York University School of Medicine; Chairman, Department of Orthopaedic Surgery, and Chief, Shoulder Service, Hospital for Joint Diseases, New York, New York

Foreword
to the First Edition

It is a privilege to write the Foreword for *The Shoulder* by Drs. Charles A. Rockwood, Jr., and Frederick A. Matsen III. Their objective when they began this work was an all-inclusive text on the shoulder that would also include all references on the subject in the English literature. Forty-six authors have contributed to this text.

The editors of *The Shoulder* are two of the leading shoulder surgeons in the United States. Dr. Rockwood was the fourth President of the American Shoulder and Elbow Surgeons, has organized the Instructional Course Lectures on the Shoulder for the Annual Meeting of the American Academy of Orthopaedic Surgeons for many years, and is a most experienced and dedicated teacher. Dr. Matsen is President-Elect of the American Shoulder and Elbow Surgeons and is an unusually talented teacher and leader. These two men, with their academic know-how and the help of their contributing authors, have organized a monumental text for surgeons in training and in practice, as well as one that can serve as an extensive reference source. They are to be commended for this superior book.

CHARLES S. NEER II, M.D.
Professor Emeritus, Orthopaedic Surgery,
Columbia University; Chief, Shoulder Service,
Columbia-Presbyterian Medical Center, New York

Preface
to the Second Edition

It is with great pleasure that we present the second edition of *The Shoulder.* We have been most gratified with the interest shown in this comprehensive work on what must surely be the most complex and remarkable joint in the human body.

The need for such a book seems even greater today than 8 years ago when the first edition was published. While the number of publications concerning the shoulder rises at an almost exponential rate, there has been a parallel increase in the difficulty in synthesizing this information in a way that is useful in our evaluation and management of individuals with shoulder problems. Thus, we have tried to temper the fascination with new data, new procedures, and new devices with a renewed focus on the patient. We do shoulder surgery to make a difference in the well-being of our patients. Knowing whether we have made a difference requires us to document not only the "outcome" (the status of the patient after treatment) but also the "ingo" (the status of the patient before treatment). Through these pages we have tried to indicate practical approaches to the evaluation of the patient and of the effectiveness of treatment. We hope that the reader will be encouraged to continue asking the questions suggested by Codman almost 90 years ago: Did the treatment make the patient better and if not, why not?

Each of the chapters in this book has been completely revised from the first edition, and for these revisions we express our gratitude to the leading shoulder surgeons who have authored these chapters and to our associate editors, Douglas T. Harryman II, M.D., and Michael A. Wirth, M.D. We also express our sincere appreciation to Susan DeBartolo at the University of Washington and to Kay Stevenson at the University of Texas in San Antonio for their terrific dedication to making this book excellent.

Finally, we offer the reader a CD-ROM in which we have attempted to share in a dynamic way some of the critical steps of the important shoulder operations. This was a new adventure for us. We were stimulated to undertake this project because it is so difficult to communicate the essence of surgery in words and still photographs. We hope that you will find this feature an exciting and useful addition to *The Shoulder.*

We conclude by thanking all of the readers of the first edition who have given us encouragement and suggestions for making this book even better.

CHARLES A. ROCKWOOD, JR., M.D.
FREDERICK A. MATSEN III, M.D.

Contents

C H A P T E R

14

FREDERICK A. MATSEN III, M.D.
STEVEN C. THOMAS, M.D.
CHARLES A. ROCKWOOD, JR., M.D.
MICHAEL A. WIRTH, M.D.

Glenohumeral Instability

"It deserves to be known how a shoulder which is subject to frequent dislocations should be treated. For many persons owing to this accident have been obliged to abandon gymnastic exercises, though otherwise well qualified for them; and from the same misfortune have become inept in warlike practices, and have thus perished. And this subject deserves to be noticed, because I have never known any physician [to] treat the case properly; some abandon the attempt altogether, and others hold opinions and practice the very reverse of what is proper."

HIPPOCRATES, 2400 YEARS AGO.

"In every case the anterior margin of the glenoid cavity will be found to be smooth, rounded, and free of any attachments, and a blunt instrument can be passed freely inwards over the bare bone on the front of the neck of the scapula."

PERTHES, 1906.

"...the only rational treatment is to reattach the glenoid ligament (or the capsule) to the bone from which it has been torn."

BANKART, 1939.[30]

HISTORICAL REVIEW

Early Descriptions

The first report of a shoulder dislocation is found in humankind's oldest book, the Edwin Smith Papyrus (3000 to 2500 BC).[718] Hussein reported that in 1200 BC in the tomb of Upuy, an artist and sculptor to Ramses II, there was a drawing of a scene that was strikingly similar to Kocher's method of reduction[275] (Fig. 14–1).

The most detailed early description of anterior dislocations came from the father of medicine, Hippocrates, who was born in 460 BC on the island of Cos.[2] Hippocrates described the anatomy of the shoulder, the types of dislocations, and the first surgical procedure. In one of his classic procedures for reduction, he emphasized the need for suitably sized leather-covered balls to be placed into the axilla, because without them the heel could not reach the head of the humerus in his reduction maneuver. Other Hippocratic techniques are described by Brockbank and Griffiths (Fig. 14–2).[67]

Hippocrates criticized his contemporaries for improper burning of the shoulder, a treatment popular at the time. In this first description of a surgical procedure for recurrent dislocation of the shoulder, he described how physi-

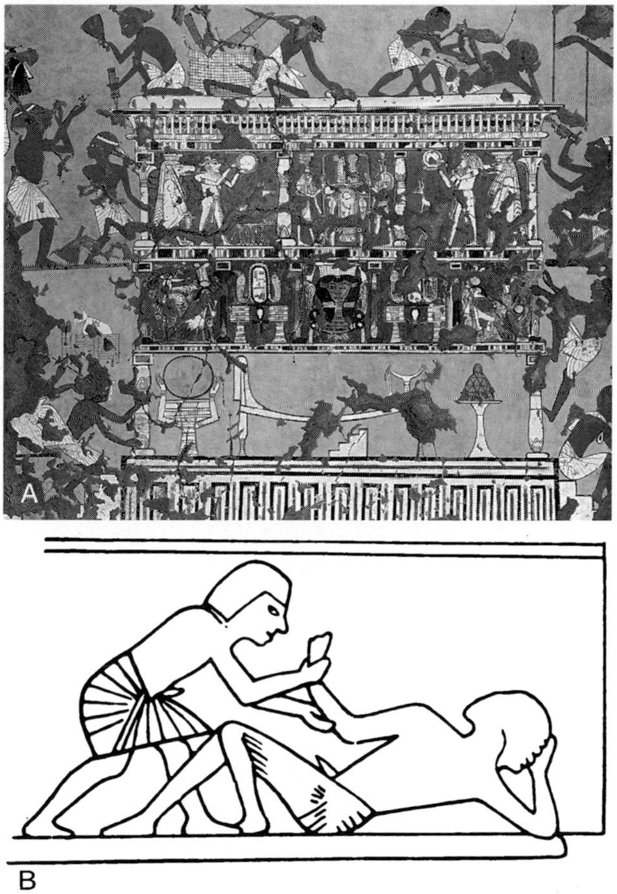

Figure 14–1

The Kocher technique is 3000 years old. *A*, Drawing from the tomb of Upuy in the year 1200 BC. (All rights reserved, The Metropolitan Museum of Art. Egyptian Expedition of the Metropolitan Museum of Art, Rogers Fund, 1930. Photograph © 1978 The Metropolitan Museum of Art.) *B*, Schematic drawing of the picture in the upper right corner of the tomb painting depicting a patient on the ground while a man—possibly a physician—is manipulating a dislocated shoulder in the technique of Kocher. (From Hussein MK: Kocher's method is 3,000 years old. J Bone Joint Surg *50B*:669–671, 1968.)

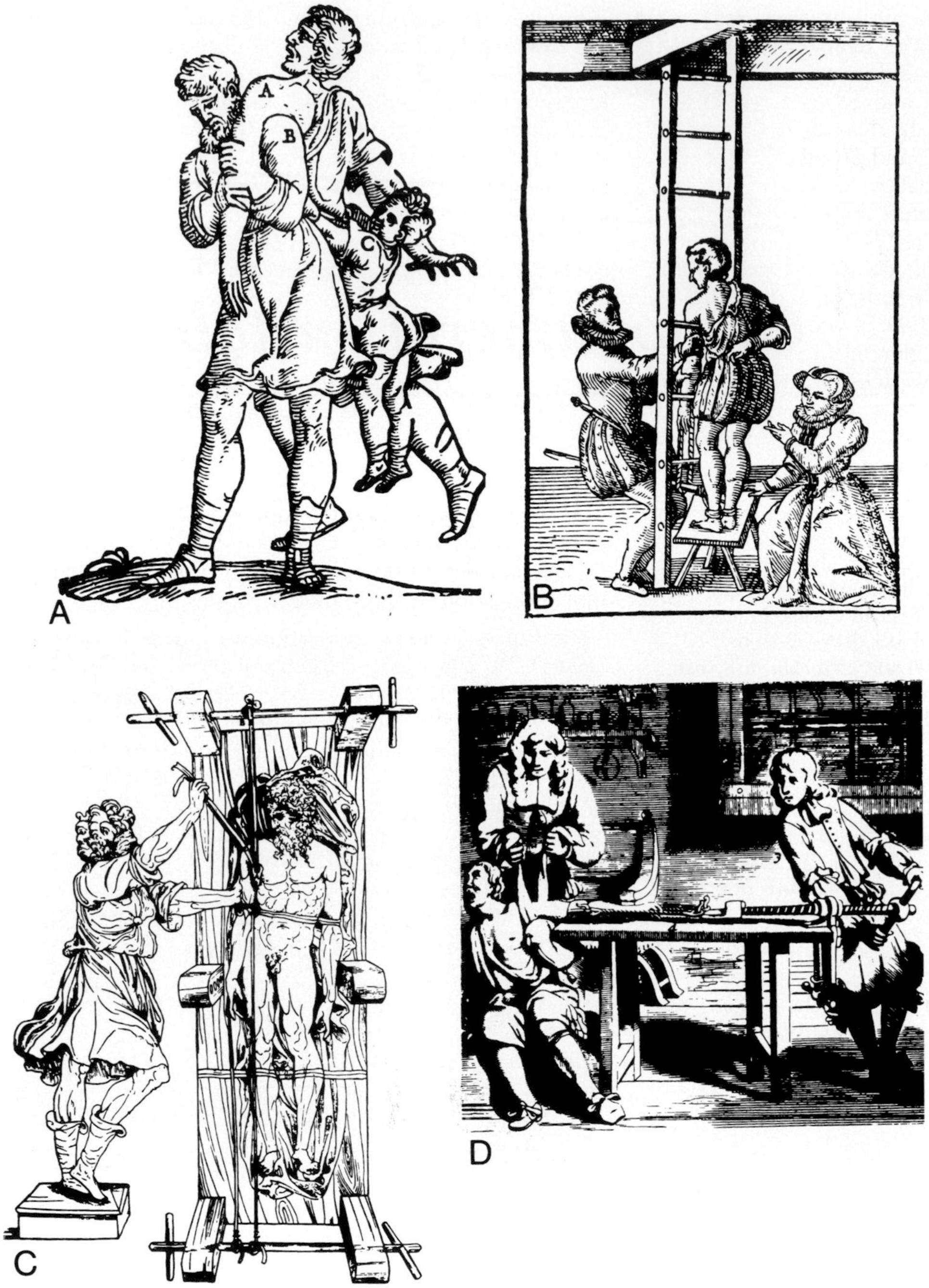

Figure 14–2

Modified techniques of Hippocrates to reduce dislocations of the shoulder. *A,* Reduction over the operator's shoulder. (From the Venice edition of Galen in 1625.) *B,* Reduction over the rung of the ladder. When the stepstool on which the patient is standing is withdrawn, the weight of the patient's body produces a reduction of the dislocation. (From deCruce in 1607.) *C,* Use of the rack to reduce the shoulder dislocation (Vidius). *D,* Reduction of the dislocation by a medieval type of screw traction (From Scultetus in 1693). (From Brockbank W and Griffiths DL: Orthopaedic surgery in the 16th and 17th centuries. J Bone Joint Surg *30B*:365–375, 1948.)

cians had burned the top, anterior, and posterior aspects of the shoulder, which only caused scarring in those areas and promoted the downward dislocation. He advocated the use of cautery in which an oblong, red-hot iron was inserted through the axilla to make eschars, but only in the lower part of the joint. Hippocrates displayed considerable knowledge of the anatomy of the shoulder, and he warned the surgeon not to let the iron come in contact with the major vessels and nerves since this would cause great harm. After the burnings, he bound the arm to the side, day and night for a long time, "for thus more especially will cicatrization take place, and the wide space into which the humerus used to escape will become contracted."

The interested reader is referred to the text by Moseley,[438] which has a particularly good section on the historical aspects of management of shoulder instability.

Humeral Head Defect

In 1861, Flower[169] described the anatomic and pathologic changes found in 41 traumatically dislocated shoulders from specimens in museums in London. He wrote that "where the head of the humerus rests upon the edge of the glenoid fossa absorption occurs, and a groove is evacuated, usually between the articular head and the greater tuberosity." In 1880, Eve[153] reported an autopsy on a patient who died 12 hours after an acute anterior dislocation in which he found the deep groove in the posterolateral aspect of the head. Joessel also observed the defect.[300] According to Hill and Sachs,[253] beginning in 1882 publications appeared by Kuster,[334] Cramer,[106] Löbker,[372] Schüller,[579] Staffel,[610] and Franke[171] that described the finding of a posterolateral defect in humeral heads resected for relief of chronic or recurrent dislocation.

In 1887, Caird[74] of Edinburgh concluded that in the true subcoracoid dislocation there must be an indentation fracture of the humeral head that is produced by the dense, hard anterior lip of the glenoid fossa. In experiments on cadavers, he was able to produce the head defect. He said that the hard, dense glenoid lip would cut into the soft cancellous bone like a knife (Fig. 14–3).

Roentgen's discovery of the x-ray in 1895 ushered in new evaluations and studies on the anatomy of the anterior glenoid and on humeral head defects. The first description of the radiographic changes in the humeral head associated with recurrent instability is attributed to Franke only 3 years after Roentgen's discovery in 1898.[248] Hermodsson demonstrated that the posterolateral humeral head defect is the result of a compression fracture caused by the anterior glenoid rim following the exit of the humeral head from the glenoid fossa.[248] He also observed that: (1) the defect is seen in most cases; (2) the longer the head is dislocated, the larger the defect will be; (3) the defects generally are larger with anteroinferior dislocations than with anterior dislocations; and (4) the defect is usually larger in recurrent anterior dislocations of the shoulder.

In 1925, Pilz reported the first detailed radiographic examination of recurrent dislocation of the shoulder and stated that routine radiographs were of little help. He stressed the need for an angled-beam projection to observe the defect.[511] In 1940, Hill and Sachs published a very clear and concise review of the available information on the humeral head compression fracture defect that now carries their names.[253]

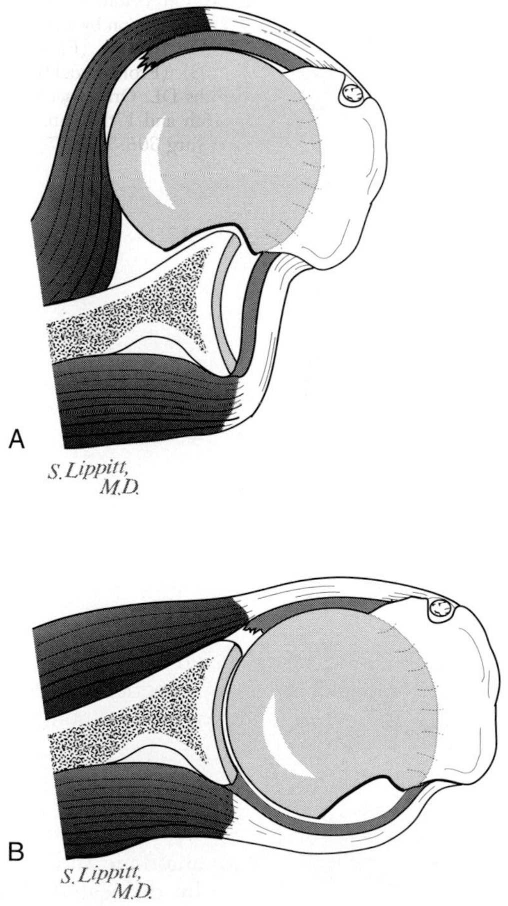

Figure 14–3

A, Anterior dislocation shown in axillary projection with a posterior lateral humeral head defect (Hill-Sachs defect) and a tear of the anterior capsule and labrum from the glenoid lip (Bankart lesion). *B*, The dislocation is reduced; the humeral head and capsular lesions remain.

Anterior Capsule and Muscle Defects

According to the Hunterian lecture given by Reeves in 1967, Roger of Palermo in the 13th century taught that the lesion in an acute dislocation was a capsular rupture. Bankart,[28] following the concepts of Broca and Hartman,[66] Perthes,[509] Flower,[169] and Caird,[74] claimed that the essential lesion was the detachment of the labrum and capsule from the anterior glenoid resulting from forward translation of the humeral head (referred to by subsequent authors as the Bankart lesion) (see Fig. 14–3). Later experimental and clinical work by Reeves[526] and Townley[641] suggested that other lesions may be responsible for recurrent dislocation, such as failure of the initial injury to incite a healing response, detachment of the subscapularis tendon, and variance in the attachment of the inferior glenohumeral ligament.

Moseley and Overgaard[441] found laxity in 25 consecutive cases, and DePalma and associates[125] reported subscapularis laxity, ruptures, and decreased muscle tone in 38 consecutive cases. Several of their cases, and some from Hauser,[230] revealed a definite defect along the anterior or inferior aspect of the subscapularis tendon, as if it had been partially torn from its bone attachment, along with separation of those muscle fibers that insert into the humerus directly below the lesser tuberosity. McLaughlin,[408] DePalma and associates,[125] Jens,[289] and Reeves[528] have noted at the time of surgery prior to arthrotomy that with abduction and external rotation the humeral head would dislocate under the lower edge of the subscapularis tendon. Symeonides[624] biopsied the subscapularis muscle tendon unit at the time of surgery and found microscopic evidence of "healed post-traumatic lesions." He stated that instability results because traumatic lengthening of the subscapularis muscle leads to a loss of the power necessary to stabilize the shoulder.

Rotator Cuff Injuries

In 1880, Joessel[300] reported on his careful postmortem studies of four cases of known recurrent dislocations of the shoulder. In all cases he found a rupture of the posterolateral portion of the rotator cuff from the greater

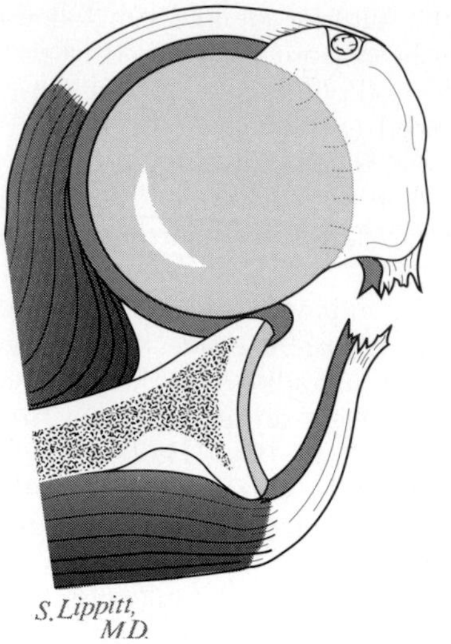

Figure 14–4

An anterior dislocation shown in axillary projection with a tear in the posterior rotator cuff.

tuberosity and a greatly increased shoulder joint capsule volume (Figs. 14–4 and 14–5). He also noted fractures of the humeral head and the anterior glenoid rim (Fig. 14–6). He concluded that cuff disruptions that did not heal predisposed the individual to a recurrence of the problem; that recurrences were facilitated by the enlarged capsule; and that fractures of the glenoid or head of the humerus resulted in a smaller articular surface, which may tend to produce recurrent dislocation. However, his four patients were elderly and may have had the degenerative cuff changes that are so common in older people.

Treatment of Acute Traumatic Dislocations

Hippocrates[257] discussed in detail at least six different techniques to reduce the dislocated shoulder. From century to century the literature has included woodcuts, drawings, and redrawings, illustrating modifications of Hippocrates' teachings by investigators such as Paré, de Cruce, Vidius, and Scultetus. Hippocrates' original technique is still used occasionally.[2] The stockinged foot of the physician is used as countertraction. The heel should not go into the axilla (i.e., between the anterior and posterior axillary folds) but should extend across the folds and against the chest wall. Traction should be slow and gentle; as with all traction techniques, the arm may be gently rotated internally and externally to disengage the head.

In 1870, Kocher,[323] a Nobel prize winner for medicine in 1909, gave a somewhat confusing report of his technique for levering in the anteriorly dislocated shoulder. If Kocher had not been so famous as a thyroid surgeon, his article might have received only scant attention.

In 1938, Milch described a technique for reduction in the supine position in which the arm is abducted and externally rotated, and the thumb is used to gently push the head of the humerus back in place.[421] Lacey modified the technique by performing the maneuver with the patient prone on an examining table.[336] Russell and associates have reported on the ease and success of this technique.[566]

In the Kocher technique, the humeral head is levered on the anterior glenoid and the shaft is levered against the anterior thoracic wall until the reduction is completed. DePalma warned that undue forces used in rotation leverage can damage the soft tissues of the shoulder joint, the vessels, and the brachial plexus.[122] Beattie and co-workers reported a fracture of the humeral neck during a Kocher procedure.[39] Other authors have reported spiral fractures of the upper shaft of the humerus and further damage to the anterior capsular mechanism when the Kocher leverage technique of reduction was used. McMurray[414] reported that of 64 dislocations reduced by the Kocher method, 40% became recurrent, whereas of 112 dislocations reduced by gently lifting the head in place, only 12% became recurrent.

Since 1975, numerous articles have appeared in the literature describing simple techniques to reduce the dislocated shoulder: the forward elevation maneuver,[287, 665] the external rotation method,[361, 427] the scapular manipulation,[9] the modified gravity method,[364] the crutch and chair technique,[497] the chair and pillow technique,[685] and others.[94, 389]

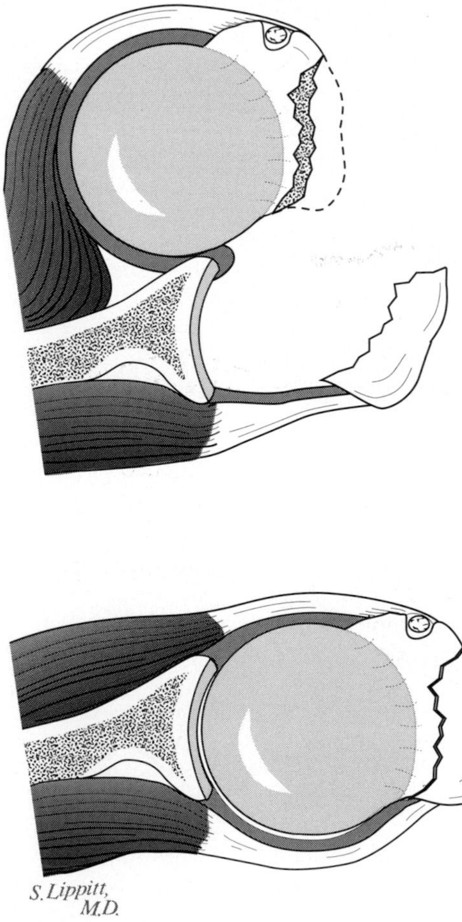

Figure 14–5

This anterior dislocation is shown in the axillary projection with a displaced fracture of the greater tuberosity.

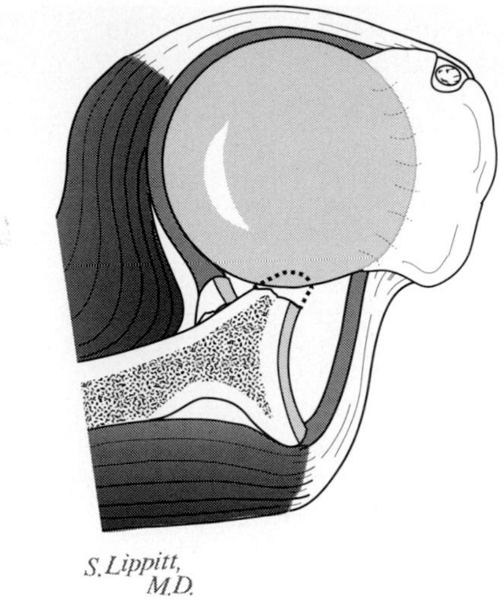

Figure 14–6

This anterior dislocation is shown in the axillary projection with a displaced fracture of the anterior glenoid rim.

Operative Reconstructions for Anterior Instability

Most of the published literature on shoulder dislocations is concerned with the problem of recurrent anterior dislocations. As mentioned previously, Hippocrates[257] described the use of a white-hot poker to scar the anteroinferior capsule. Since then hundreds of operative procedures have been described for the management of recurrent anterior dislocations. The reader who has a yearning for the detailed history should read the classic texts by Moseley[438] and Hermodsson.[248]

Various operative techniques have been based on the posterolateral defect and the soft tissue disruptions on the front of the shoulder. Bardenheuer[32] in 1886 and Thomas[630, 631] from 1909 to 1921 discussed capsular plication or shrinking; in 1888, Albert[7] performed arthrodesis; and in 1901, Hildebrand[252] deepened the glenoid socket.

In 1906, Perthes[509] wrote a classic paper on the operative treatment of recurrent dislocations. He stated that the operation should be directed to a repair of the underlying lesion (i.e., repair of the capsule, the glenoid labrum detachment from the anterior bony rim, and the rotator cuff tear). He repaired the capsule with suture to the anterior glenoid rim through drill holes and, in several cases he used staples to repair the anterior capsular structures. This report gave the first description of repair of the anterior labrum and capsule to the anterior glenoid rim. Two patients were followed for 17 years, one patient for 12 years, two patients for 3 years, and one patient for 1 year and 9 months. All had excellent function with no recurrences.

The muscle-sling myoplasty operation was used in 1913 by Clairmont and Ehrlich.[89] The posterior third of the deltoid, with its innervation left intact, was removed from its insertion on the humerus, passed through the quadrilateral space, and sutured to the coracoid process. When the arm was abducted the deltoid contracted, which held up the humeral head. Finsterer,[165] in a similar but reversed procedure, used the coracobrachialis and the short head of the biceps from the coracoid and transferred them posteriorly. Both operations failed because of high recurrence rates.

In 1923, Bankart[28] first published his operative technique, noting that only two classes of operations were used at that time for recurrent dislocations of the shoulder[1]: those designed to diminish the size of the capsule by plication or pleating,[630, 631] and those designed to give inferior support to the capsule.[2, 89, 92] Bankart condemned both in preference to his procedure. He stated that the essential lesion was the detachment or rupture of the capsule from the glenoid ligament. He recommended repair using interrupted sutures of silkworm gut passed between the free edge of the capsule and the glenoid ligament. At that time he did not repair the lateral capsule to the bone of the anterior glenoid rim. In his 1939 article, Bankart[30] described the essential lesion as a "detachment of the glenoid ligament from the anterior margin of the glenoid cavity" and stated that "the only rational treatment is to reattach the glenoid ligament (or the capsule) to the bone from which it has been torn." He further wrote that "the glenoid ligament may be found lying loose either on the head of the humerus or the margin of the glenoid cavity" and that "in every case the anterior margin of the glenoid cavity will be found to be smooth, rounded, and free of any attachments, and a blunt instrument can be passed freely inwards over the bone on the front of the neck of the scapula." He recommended the repair of the lateral capsule down to the raw bone of the anterior glenoid and held it in place with suture through drill holes made in the anterior glenoid rim with sharp, pointed forceps. Although no references were listed in either article, Bankart must have been greatly influenced by the previously published work of Broca and Hartmann[66] and particularly of Perthes,[509] which described virtually identical pathology and repair.

Beginning in 1929, Nicola[459–463] published a series of articles on management of recurrent dislocations of the shoulder. He used the long head of the biceps tendon and the coracohumeral ligament as a suspension checkrein to the front of the shoulder. Henderson[243, 244] described another checkrein operation that looped half of the peroneus longus tendon through drill holes in the acromion and the greater tuberosity. In 1927, Gallie and LeMesurier[176] described the use of autogenous fascia lata suture in the treatment of recurrent dislocations of the shoulder. This procedure has been modified by Bateman.[37]

Posterior Glenohumeral Instability

In 1839, in a Guy's Hospital report, Cooper described in detail a dislocation of the os humeri upon the dorsum scapulae.[101] This report is a classic, because Cooper presented most of the characteristics associated with posterior dislocations: the dislocation occurred during an epileptic seizure; pain was greater than with the usual anterior dislocation; external rotation of the arm was entirely impeded, and the patient could not elevate the arm from the side; the shoulder had an anterior void or flatness and a posterior fullness; and the patient was "unable to use or move his arm to any extent." In this report of a case in which Cooper had acted as a consultant, a reduction could not be accomplished and the patient never recovered the use of his shoulder. A postmortem examination of the shoulder, performed 7 years later, revealed that the subscapularis tendon was detached and the infraspinatus muscles were stretched posteriorly about the head of the humerus. The report suggested that the detached subscapularis was "the cause of the symptoms." Cooper further described a resorption of the anterior aspect of the humeral head where it was in contact with the posterior glenoid–probably the first description of the so-called reversed Hill-Sachs lesion.

Another classic article on the subject was published in 1855 by Malgaigne,[388] who reported on 37 cases of posterior dislocations of the shoulder. Three cases were his own and 34 cases were reviewed from literature. This series of cases was collected 40 years before the discovery of x-rays, and it points out that with adequate physical examination of the patient the correct diagnosis can be made.

RELEVANT ANATOMY

Skin

Shoulder stabilization surgery can usually be accomplished through cosmetically acceptable incisions in the lines of the skin (see also Chapter 2). Anteriorly the surgeon can identify and mark the prominent anterior axillary crease by adducting the shoulder. An incision placed in the lower part of this crease provides excellent access to the shoulder for anterior repair and yet heals nicely with a subcuticular closure (Figs. 14–7 and 14–8). When cosmesis is a concern, the incision can be made more into the axilla as described by Leslie and Ryan.[355]

Posteriorly, an analogous vertical incision in line with the extended posterior axillary crease (best visualized by extending the shoulder backwards) also heals well (Fig. 14–9). Fortuitously, these creases lie directly over the joint to which the surgeon needs access.

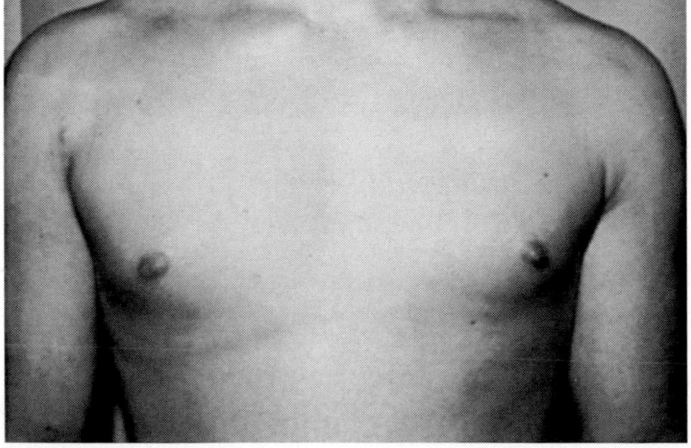

Figure 14–7

A cosmetic anterior approach on the patient's right shoulder. The incision is made in the axillary skin crease.

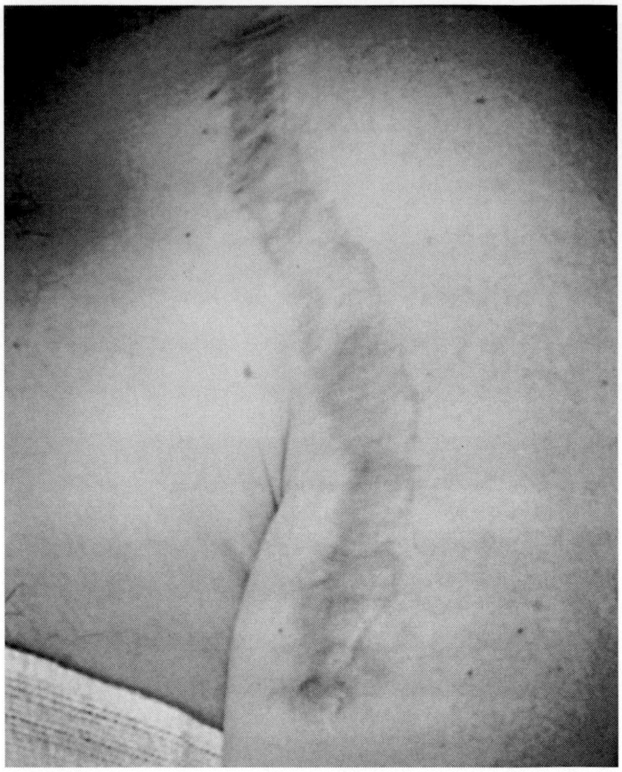

Figure 14–8

A noncosmetic approach across the front of the shoulder.

First Muscle Layer

The shoulder is covered by the deltoid muscle arising from the clavicle, acromion, and scapular spine. The anterior deltoid extends to a line running approximately from the midclavicle to the midlateral humerus. This line passes over the cephalic vein, the anterior venous drainage of the deltoid, and over the coracoid process. The deltoid is innervated by the axillary nerve, whose branches swoop upward as they extend anteriorly (Fig. 14–10). The commonly described "safe zone" 5 cm distal to the acromion does not take into account these anterior branches, which may come as close as 2 cm to the acromion. At the deltopectoral groove, the deltoid meets the clavicular head of the pectoralis major, which assists the anterior deltoid in forward flexion. The medial and lateral pectoral nerves are not in the surgical field of shoulder stabilization. Splitting the deltopectoral interval just medial to the cephalic vein preserves the deltoid's venous drainage and takes the surgeon to the next layer. It is important to note that extension of the shoulder tightens the pectoralis major and the anterior deltoid as well as the coracoid muscles, compromising the exposure. Assistants must therefore be reminded to hold the shoulder in slight flexion to relax these muscles and facilitate access to the joint.

Posteriorly, the medial edge of the deltoid is too medial to provide useful access to the glenohumeral joint. Access must be achieved by splitting the deltoid, which is most done conveniently at the junction of its middle and posterior thirds. This junction is marked by the posterior cor-

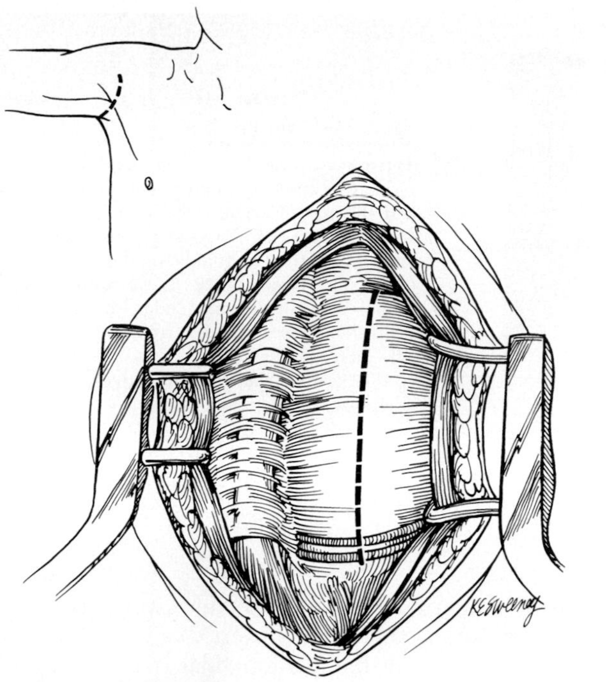

Figure 14–9

A posterior approach for treatment of posterior glenohumeral instability. The incision is centered over the posterior glenoid rim *(inset)*. Note the deltoid-splitting approach to minimize the amount of deltoid origin that must be released. Also note the incision in the infraspinatus and teres minor tendons. (From Matsen FA and Thomas SC: Glenohumeral instability. *In* Evarts CM [ed]: Surgery of the Musculoskeletal System, 2nd ed. New York: Churchill Livingstone, 1989.)

ner of the acromion. The site is favorable for a split because it overlies the joint and also because the axillary nerve exiting the quadrangular space divides into two trunks (its anterior and posterior branches) near the inferior aspect of the split.

Coracoacromial Arch and the Clavipectoral Fascia

The coracoid process is the "lighthouse" of the anterior shoulder, providing a palpable guide to the deltopectoral groove, a locator for the coracoacromial arch, and an anchor for the coracoid muscles (the coracobrachialis and short head of the biceps) that separate the lateral "safe side" from the medial "suicide" where the brachial plexus and major vessels lie. The surgeon comes to full appreciation of the value of such a lighthouse when it is lacking—for example, when re-exploring a shoulder for complications of a coracoid transfer procedure. The clavipectoral fascia covers the floor of the deltopectoral groove. Rotation of the humerus enables the surgeon to identify the subscapularis moving beneath this fascial layer. Incision of the fascia up to but not through the coracoacromial ligament preserves the stabilizing function of the coracoacromial arch.

Humeroscapular Motion Interface

The humeroscapular motion interface (Figs. 14–11 and 14–12) separates the structures that do not move on humeral rotation (the deltoid, coracoid muscles, acromion, and coracoacromial ligament) from those that do (the rotator cuff, long head of the biceps tendon, and humeral tuberosities). During shoulder motion, substantial gliding takes place at this interface (Fig. 14–13). The humeroscapular motion interface provides a convenient plane for medial and lateral retractors and is also the plane in which the principal nerves lie.

The axillary nerve runs in the humeroscapular motion interface, superficial to the humerus and cuff and deep to the deltoid and coracoid muscles (Fig. 14–14; see also Fig. 14–10). Sweeping a finger from superior to inferior

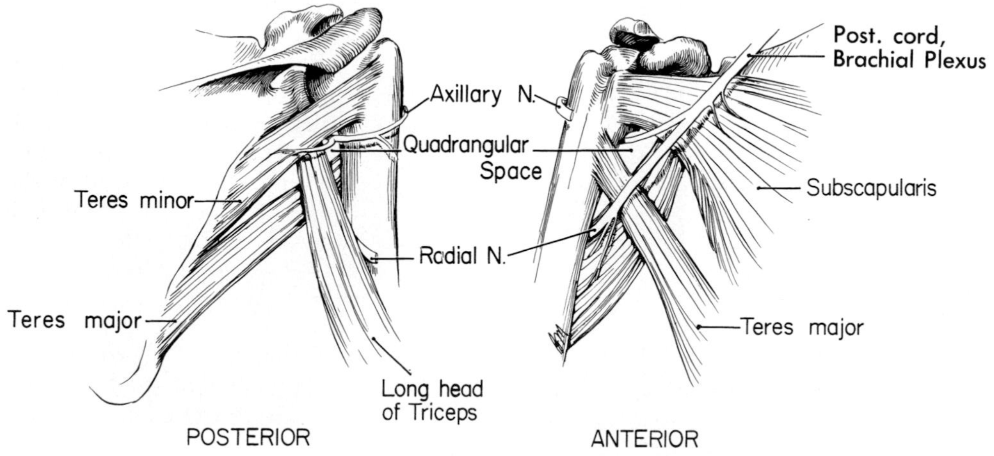

Figure 14–10

Relations of the axillary nerve to the subscapularis muscle, the quadrangular space, and the neck of the humerus. With anterior dislocations, the subscapularis is displaced forward, which creates a traction injury to the axillary nerve. The nerve cannot move out of the way because it is held above by the brachial plexus and below where it wraps around behind the neck of the humerus. (From Rockwood CA and Green DP [eds]: Fractures [3 vols], 2nd ed. Philadelphia: JB Lippincott, 1984.)

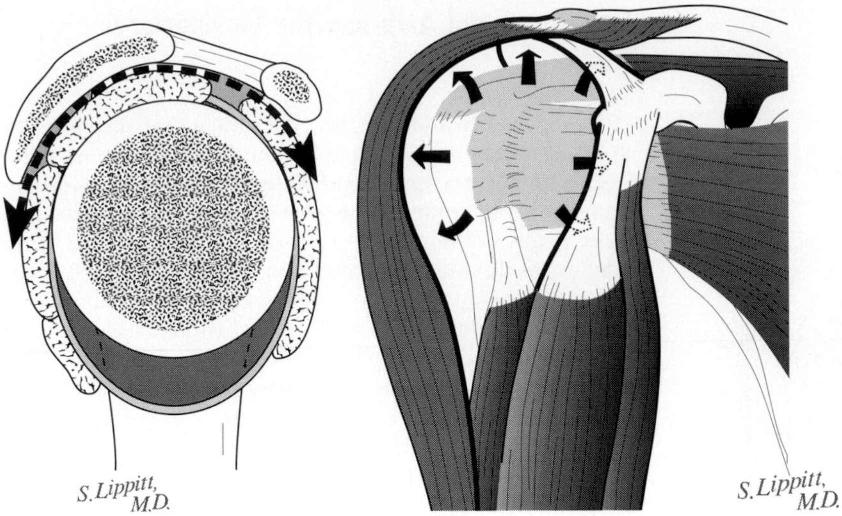

Figures 14–11 and 14–12

The humeroscapular motion interface is an important location of motion between the humerus and the scapula. The deltoid, acromion, coracoacromial ligament, coracoid process, and tendons attaching to the coracoid lie on the superficial side of this interface, whereas the proximal humerus, rotator cuff, and biceps tendon sheath lie on the deep side. (Modified from Matsen FA III, Lippitt SB, Sidles JA, and Harryman DT II: Practical Evaluation and Management of the Shoulder. Philadelphia: WB Saunders, 1994.)

along the anterior aspect of the subscapularis muscle catches the axillary nerve, hanging like a watch chain across the muscle belly. If this nerve is traced proximally and medially, it leads the finger to the bulk of the brachial plexus. If the nerve is traced laterally and posteriorly, it leads the finger beneath the shoulder capsule toward the quadrangular space. From a posterior vantage, the axillary nerve is seen to exit the quadrangular space beneath the teres minor and extend laterally, where it is applied to the deep surface of the deltoid muscle. By virtue of its prominent location in close proximity to the shoulder joint anteriorly, inferiorly, and posteriorly, the axillary nerve is the most frequently injured structure in shoulder surgery.

The musculocutaneous nerve lies on the deep surface of the coracoid muscles and penetrates the coracobrachialis with one or more branches lying a variable distance distal to the coracoid. (The often-described 5 cm "safe zone" for the nerve beneath the process refers only to the average position of the main trunk and not to an area that can be entered recklessly.) The musculocutaneous nerve is vulnerable to injury from retractors placed under the coracoid muscles and to traction injury in coracoid

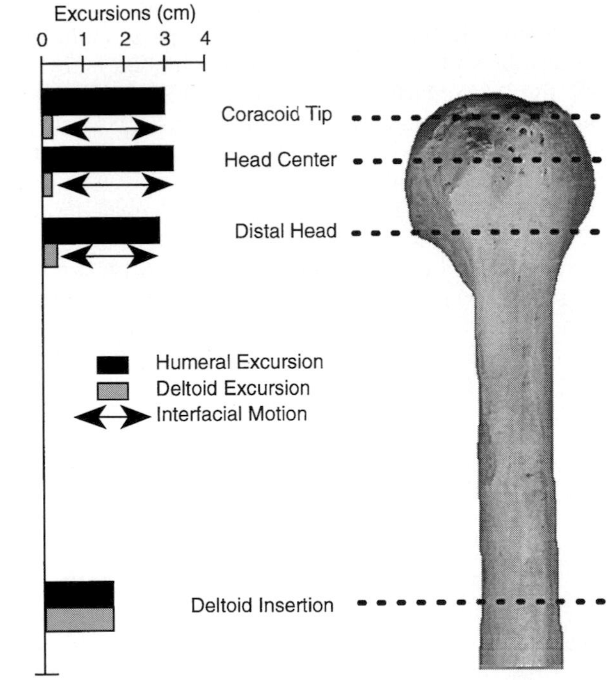

Figure 14–13

Mean humeroscapular interface motion recorded in vivo from five normal subjects using magnetic resonance imaging. The humerus at the right shows the levels at which the motions were measured. The excursion (in centimeters) of the humerus (black) and the deltoid (gray) from maximal internal to maximal external rotation are indicated by the horizontal bars. The magnitudes of motion at the interface between the deltoid and the humerus are indicated by the double-headed arrows. The mean excursions at the humerothoracic motion interface were approximately 3 cm proximally and 0 cm at the deltoid insertion. (From Matsen FA III, Lippitt SB, Sidles JA, and Harryman DT II: Practical Evaluation and Management of the Shoulder. Philadelphia: WB Saunders, 1994.)

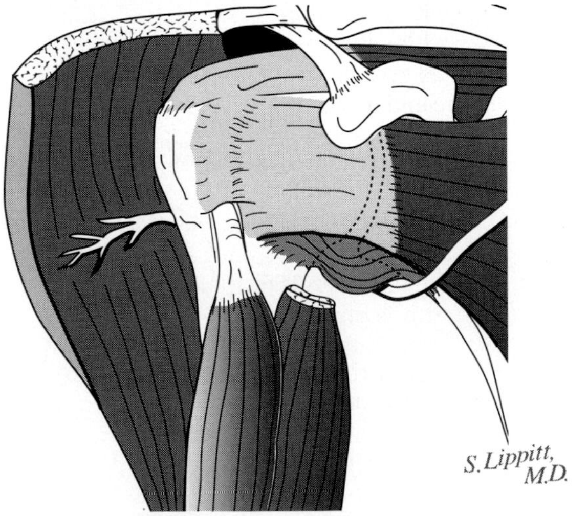

Figure 14–14

The axillary nerve in the humeroscapular motion interface between the cuff and the humerus on the inside and the coracoid muscles and the deltoid on the outside. (From Matsen FA III, Lippitt SB, Sidles JA, and Harryman DT II: Practical Evaluation and Management of the Shoulder. Philadelphia: WB Saunders, 1994.)

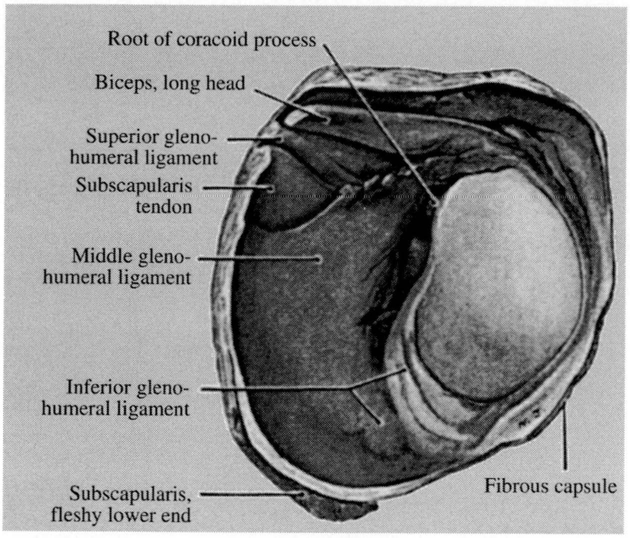

Figure 14–15

Anterior glenohumeral ligaments. This drawing shows the anterosuperior, anterior middle, and anteroinferior glenohumeral ligaments. The middle and inferior anterior glenohumeral ligaments are often avulsed from the glenoid or the glenoid labrum in traumatic anterior instability. (From Grant's Atlas of Anatomy, 4th ed. Baltimore: Williams & Wilkins, 1956.)

transfer. Knowledge of the position of these nerves can make the shoulder surgeon both more comfortable and more effective.

Rotator Cuff

The next layer of the shoulder is the rotator cuff. The tendons of these muscles blend in with the capsule as they insert to the humeral tuberosities.[90] Thus, in reconstructions that require splitting of these muscles from the capsule, this splitting is more easily accomplished medially, before the blending becomes complete. The nerves to these muscles run on their deep surfaces: the upper and lower subscapular to the subscapularis and the suprascapular to the supraspinatus and infraspinatus. Medial dissection on the deep surface of these muscles may jeopardize their nerve supply.[713]

The cuff is relatively thin between the supraspinatus and the subscapularis (the "rotator interval"). This allows the cuff to slide back and forth around the coracoid process as the arm is elevated and lowered. Splitting this interval toward the base of the coracoid may be helpful when mobilization of the subscapularis is needed.

The tendon of the long head of the biceps originates from the supraglenoid tubercle (Figs. 14–15 and 14–16). It runs beneath the cuff in the area of the rotator interval and exits the shoulder beneath the transverse humeral ligament and between the greater and lesser tuberosities. It is subject to injury on incising the upper subscapularis from the lesser tuberosity. In the bicipital groove of the humerus this tendon is endangered by procedures that involve lateral transfer of the subscapularis tendon across the groove (see also Chapters 1 and 2).

Scapulohumeral Ligaments

The glenohumeral joint capsule is normally large, loose, and redundant allowing for the full and free range of motion of the shoulder. By virtue of their mandatory redundancy, the capsule and its ligaments are lax throughout most of the range of joint motion. They can thus exert major stabilizing effects only when they come under tension as the joint approaches the limits of its range of motion.

The three anterior glenohumeral ligaments were first described by Schlemm.[578] Since then, many observers have described their anatomy and their roles in limiting glenohumeral rotation and translation (see Figs. 14–15 and 14–16).[118, 121, 163, 164, 408, 441, 473, 527, 645, 682]

Codman and others pointed out the variability of the ligaments (see Fig. 14–15).[95, 118, 122, 163, 441, 472, 689] These authors also demonstrated a great variation in the size and number of synovial recesses that form in the anterior capsule above, below, and between the glenohumeral ligaments. They observed that if the capsule arises at the labrum, there are few if any synovial recesses (in this situation there is a generalized blending of all three ligaments, which leaves no room for synovial recesses or weaknesses, and hence the anterior glenohumeral capsule

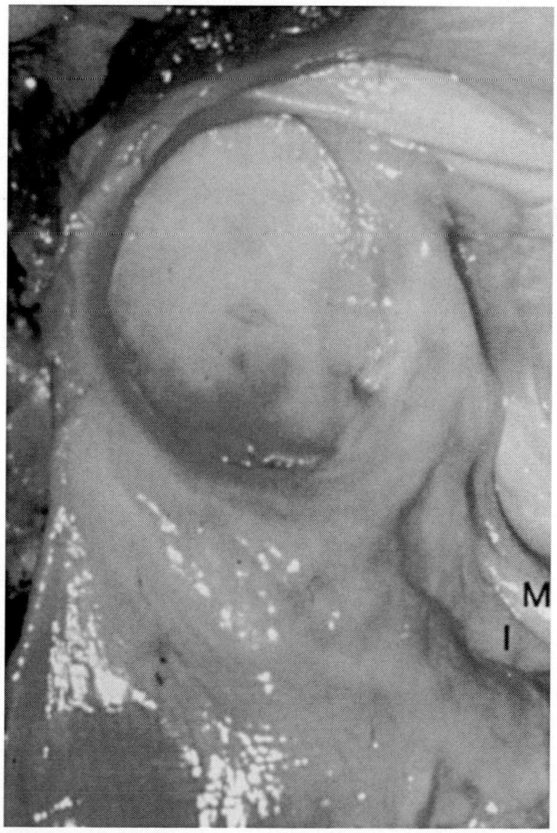

Figure 14–16

Cadaver dissection of the glenoid, biceps tendon insertion, and associated glenohumeral ligaments. This dissection demonstrates the anterior glenohumeral ligaments. Note the relationship of the anterior inferior (I) and the anterior middle (M) glenohumeral ligaments to the anterior rim of the glenoid.

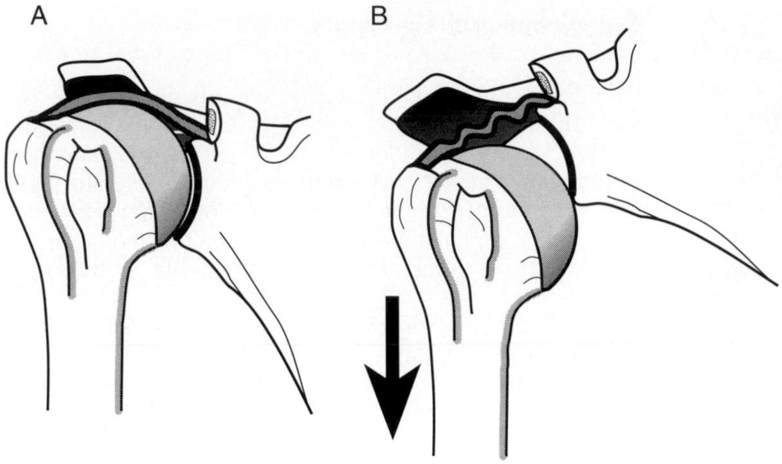

Figure 14–17

Scapular dumping. With the scapula in a normal position (A), the superior capsular mechanism is tight, supporting the head in the glenoid concavity. Drooping of the lateral scapula (B) relaxes the superior capsular structures and rotates the glenoid concavity so that it does not support the head of the humerus. (From Matsen FA III, Lippitt SB, Sidles JA, and Harryman DT II: Practical Evaluation and Management of the Shoulder. Philadelphia: WB Saunders, 1994.)

is stronger). However, the more medially the capsule arises from the glenoid (i.e., from the anterior scapular neck), the larger and more numerous are the synovial recesses. The end result is a thin, weak anterior capsule. Uhthoff and Piscopo[648] demonstrated in an embryologic study that in 52 specimens the anterior capsule inserted into the glenoid labrum in 77% and into the medial neck of the scapula in 23%.

The superior glenohumeral ligament (SGHL) is identified as the most consistent capsular ligament.[124] It crosses the rotator interval capsule lying between the supraspinatus and subscapularis tendons. Another interval capsular structure, the coracohumeral ligament (CHL), originates at the base of the coracoid, blends into the cuff tendons, and inserts into the greater and lesser tuberosities.[91, 225, 293, 330, 487, 614]

Harryman and associates have pointed out that these two ligaments and the rotator interval capsule come under tension with glenohumeral flexion, extension, external rotation, and adduction.[225] When they are under tension, these structures resist posterior and inferior displacement of the humeral head. Clinical and experimental data have shown that releasing or surgically tightening the rotator interval capsule increases or decreases the allowed posterior and inferior translational laxity, respectively.[34, 225, 452, 467, 667]

These ligaments and capsule as well as the inferior glenoid lip provide static restraint against inferior translation.[34] It is of anatomic interest and clinical significance that when the lateral scapula is allowed to droop inferiorly, the resultant passive abduction of the humerus relaxes the rotator interval capsule and the superior ligaments; as a result the humeral head can be "dumped" out of the glenoid fossa (Fig. 14–17).[394] Drooping of the lateral scapula is normally prevented by the postural action of the scapular stabilizers, particularly the trapezius and the serratus. Elevation of the lateral scapula with the arm at the side enhances inferior stability in two ways: the resultant glenohumeral adduction tightens the superior capsule and ligaments and the scapular rotation places more of the inferior glenoid lip beneath the humeral head.[281, 667]

While the SGHL and CHL come under tension with external rotation in adduction, the middle glenohumeral ligament (MGHL) is tensioned by external rotation when the humerus is abducted to 45 degrees.[624, 627, 645] The MGHL originates anterosuperiorly on the glenoid and inserts midway along the anterior humeral articular surface adjacent to the lesser tuberosity. In over one third of shoulders, the MGHL is absent or poorly defined, a situation that may place the shoulder at greater risk for anterior glenohumeral instability.[435]

With greater degrees of shoulder abduction, for example in the "apprehension" position, the inferior glenohumeral ligament (IGHL) and the inferior capsular sling come into play.[474, 627, 645] The IGHL originates below the sigmoid notch and courses obliquely between the anteroinferior glenoid and its humeral capsular insertion.[471] O'Brien and associates have described an anterior thickening of the IGHL, the anterior superior band.[471] The anterior and posterior aspects of the IGHL are said to function as a cruciate construct, alternatively tightening in external or internal rotation.[471, 667, 673]

When the humerus is elevated anteriorly in the sagittal

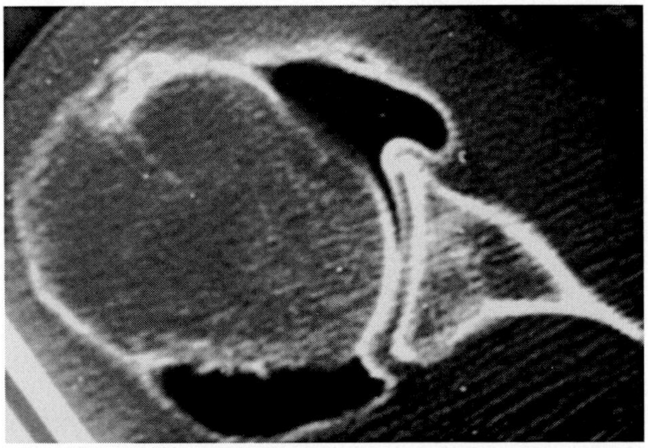

Figure 14–18

A computed tomography arthrogram of the glenohumeral joint. The depth of the bony glenoid is enhanced by contributions of the articular cartilage and the glenoid labrum. This further increases the stability of the glenohumeral joint. Note that in this position the anterior and posterior capsuloligamentous structures are relaxed and cannot contribute to stability.

plane (flexion), the posteroinferior capsular pouch along with the rotator interval capsule come into tension.[224, 225, 471, 532, 667] If the humerus is internally rotated while elevated in the sagittal plane, the interval capsule slackens but the posterior inferior pouch tightens. Posteroinferior capsular tension also limits flexion, internal rotation, and horizontal adduction.[224, 225, 532] Excessive tightness of this portion of the capsule is a well-recognized clinical entity (see Chapter 15 on the rotator cuff).

Glenoid Labrum

The glenoid labrum is a fibrous rim that serves to deepen the glenoid fossa and allow attachment of the glenohumeral ligaments and the biceps tendon to the glenoid (Fig. 14–18; see also Figs. 14–15 and 14–16). Anatomically, it is the interconnection of the periosteum of the glenoid, the glenoid bone, the glenoid articular cartilage, the synovium, and the capsule. While microscopic studies have shown that a small amount of fibrocartilage exists at the junction of the hyaline cartilage of the glenoid and fibrous capsule; the vast majority of the labrum consists of dense fibrous tissue with a few elastic fibers (Fig. 14–19).[180, 441, 641] The posterosuperior labrum is continuous with the long head tendon of the biceps. Anteriorly it is continuous with the inferior glenohumeral ligament (see Fig. 14–16).[203, 437, 440, 643] Hertz and associates outlined the microanatomy of the labrum,[250] while Prodromos and coworkers,[517] DePalma,[122] and Olsson[482] have described the changes in the glenoid labrum with age.

In cadavers, isolated labral deficiency is not usually sufficient to allow glenohumeral dislocation.[492, 526, 528, 641] However, clinical studies reveal a high incidence of labral deficiency in recurrent traumatic instability.[30, 112, 120, 395, 555, 649]

The reader is referred to a review of the gross anatomy of the glenohumeral joint surfaces, ligaments, labrum, and capsule by Warner (see Chapter 1).[393]

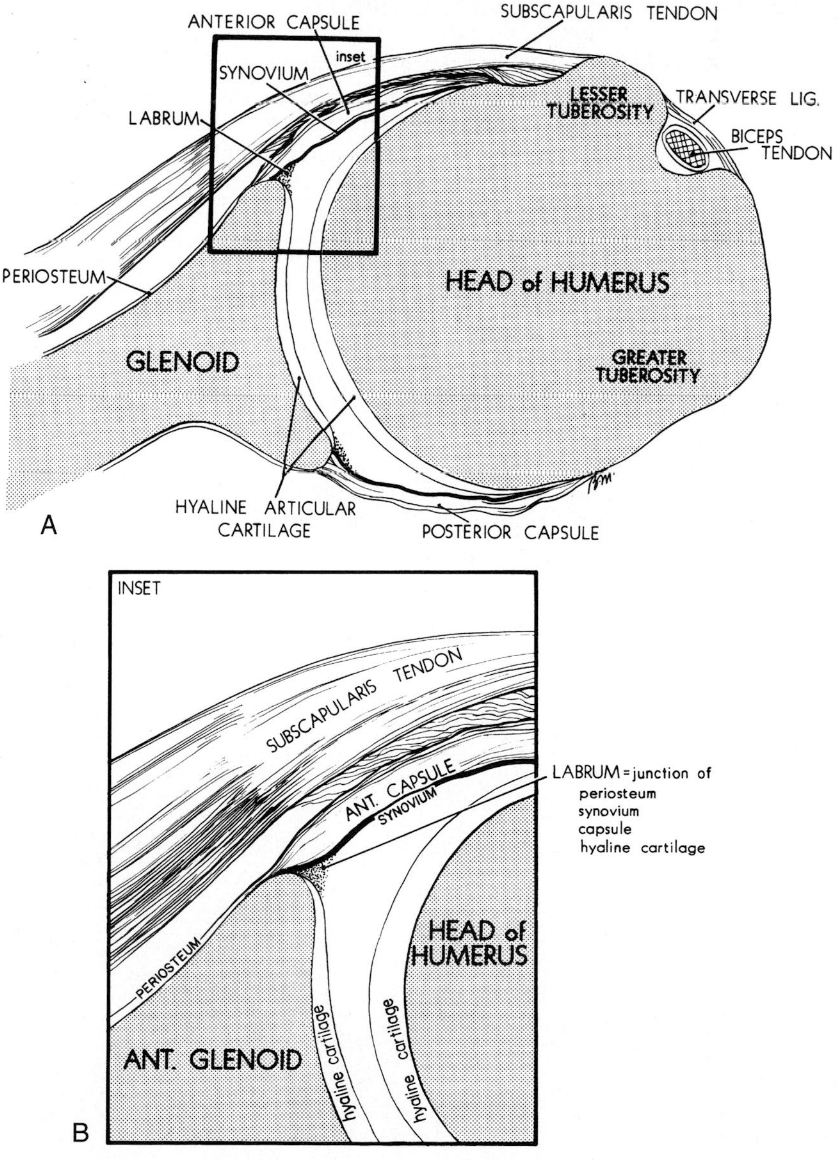

Figure 14–19

Normal shoulder anatomy. *A*, A horizontal section through the middle of the glenohumeral joint demonstrating normal anatomic relationships. Note the close relation of the subscapularis tendon to the anterior capsule. *B*, A close-up view in the area of the labrum. The labrum consists of tissues from the nearby hyaline cartilage, capsule, synovium, and periosteum. (From Rockwood CA and Green DP [eds]: Fractures [3 vols], 2nd ed. Philadelphia: JB Lippincott, 1984.)

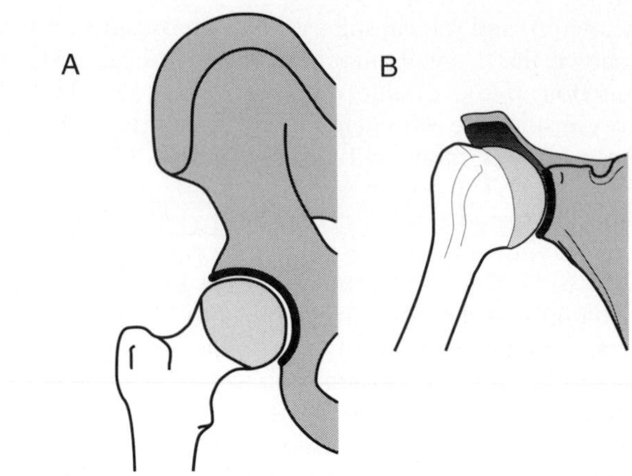

Figure 14–20

In contrast with the hip *(A)*, the shallow glenoid captures relatively little of the articulating ball *(B)*. (From Matsen FA III, Lippitt SB, Sidles JA, and Harryman DT II: Practical Evaluation and Management of the Shoulder. Philadelphia: WB Saunders, 1994.)

MECHANICS OF GLENOHUMERAL STABILITY

The most remarkable feature of the glenohumeral joint is its ability to precisely stabilize the humeral head in the center of the glenoid on one hand and to allow a vast range of motion on the other. This balance of stability and mobility is achieved by a combination of mechanisms particular to this articulation.

- In contrast to the hip joint, the glenohumeral joint does not offer a deep stabilizing socket. An acetabular-like socket would limit motion by contact of the anatomic neck of the humerus with its rim. Instead, the small arc of the glenoid captures relatively little of the humeral articular surface so that neck-rim contact is avoided for a wide range of positions (Fig. 14–20).[115, 387, 394, 569, 645]
- In contrast to hinge-like joints with shallow sockets, such as the knee, interphalangeal joints, elbow, and ankle, the glenohumeral joint does not offer isometric articular ligaments that provide stability as the joint is flexed around a defined anatomic axis. Instead, the glenohumeral ligaments play important stabilizing roles only at the extremes of motion, being lax and relatively ineffectual in most functional positions of the joint (Fig. 14–21).[394, 667]

In spite of its lack of a deep socket or isometric ligaments, the normal shoulder precisely constrains the humeral head to the center of the glenoid cavity throughout most of the arc of movement.[269, 270, 513, 514] It is remarkable that this seemingly unconstrained joint is able to provide this precise centering, resist the gravitational pull on the arm hanging at the side for long periods, remain located during sleep, allow for the lifting of large loads, permit throwing a baseball at speeds approaching 100 mph, and maintain stability during the application of an almost infinite variety of forces of differing magnitude, direction, duration, and abruptness.

The mechanics of glenohumeral stability can be understood most easily in terms of the relationship between the net force acting on the humeral head and the shape of the glenoid fossa. A working familiarity with the mechanics of glenohumeral stability will greatly enhance understanding of the workings of the normal joint, laboratory models of instability, clinical problems of instability, and clinical strategies for managing glenohumeral instability.

The basic laws of glenohumeral stability can be stated as follows:

1. The glenohumeral joint will not dislocate as long as the net humeral joint reaction force* (Fig. 14–22) is directed within the effective glenoid arc† (Figs. 14–23 and 14–24).
2. The humeral head will remain centered in the gle-

*The net humeral joint reaction force is the result of all muscular, ligamentous, inertial, gravitational, and other external forces applied to the head of the humeral head (other than the force applied by the glenoid).

†Recognizing that the rim of the glenoid is deformable under load, the effective glenoid arc is the arc of the glenoid available to support the humeral head under the specified loading conditions.

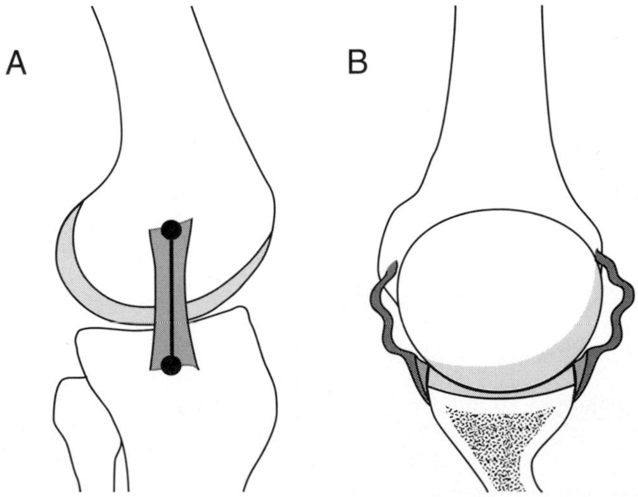

Figure 14–21

In contrast with the knee, where the ligaments remain isometric during joint motion *(A)*, the glenohumeral ligaments must be slack in most of the joint's positions *(B)*. (Modified from Matsen FA III, Lippitt SB, Sidles JA, and Harryman DT II: Practical Evaluation and Management of the Shoulder. Philadelphia: WB Saunders, 1994.)

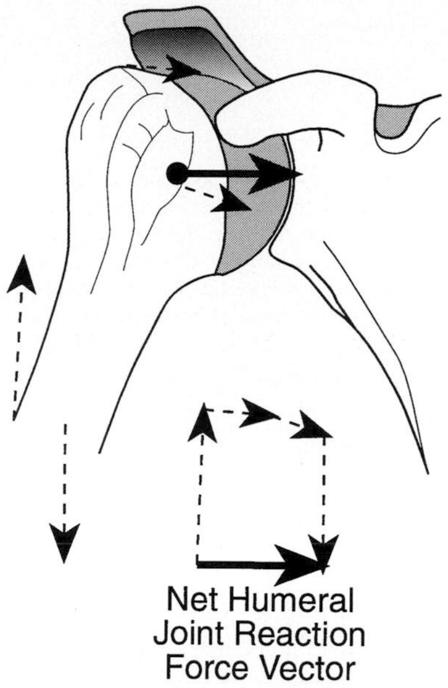

Figure 14–22

The *net humeral joint reaction force* is the vector sum of all forces acting on the head of the humerus relative to the glenoid fossa. (From Matsen FA III, Lippitt SB, Sidles JA, and Harryman DT II: Practical Evaluation and Management of the Shoulder. Philadelphia: WB Saunders, 1994.)

noid fossa if the glenoid and humeral joint surfaces are congruent and if the net humeral joint reaction force is directed within the effective glenoid arc.

The effective shape of the glenoid is revealed by the *glenoidogram*, which, rather than showing how the glenoid *looks*, shows how it *works* (Figs. 14–25 and 14–26).[349, 394] The glenoidogram is the path taken by the center of the humeral head as it is translated away from the center of the glenoid fossa in a specified direction under defined loads. The shape of the glenoidogram indicates the extent of the effective glenoid arc in that direction. If the net humeral joint reaction force passes outside the effective glenoid arc, the joint becomes unstable. The glenoidogram is oriented with respect to the *glenoid center line,* a reference line perpendicular to the center of

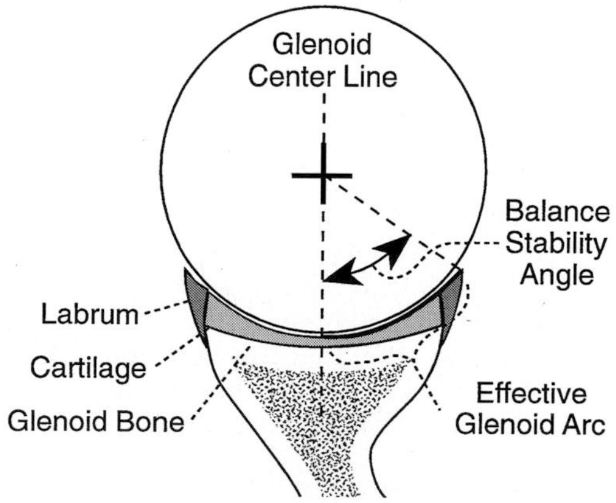

Figure 14–23

The effective glenoid arc is the arc of the glenoid able to support the net humeral joint reaction force. The balance stability angle is the maximal angle that the net humeral joint reaction force can make with the glenoid center line (see Fig. 14–27) before dislocation occurs. The shape of the bone, cartilage, and labrum all contribute to the effective glenoid arc and the balance stability angle.

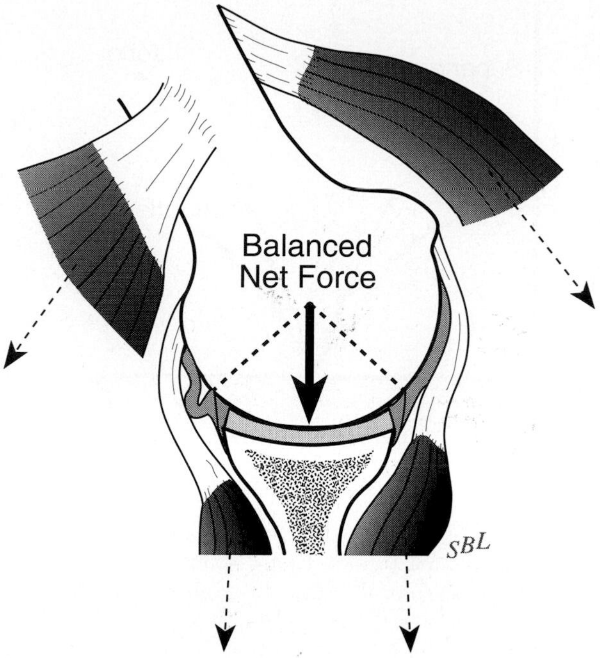

Figure 14–24

The deltoid and cuff muscle forces *(dotted arrows)* maintain the net humeral joint reaction force *(solid arrow)* within the balance stability angles *(dotted lines).* (Modified from Matsen FA III, Lippitt SB, Sidles JA, and Harryman DT II: Practical Evaluation and Management of the Shoulder. Philadelphia: WB Saunders, 1994.)

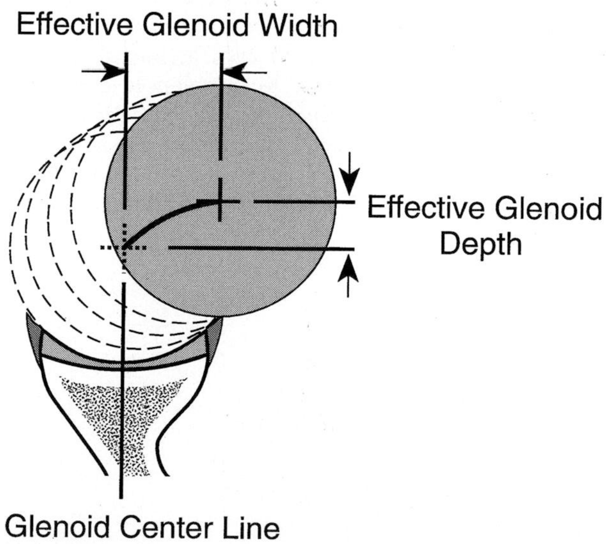

Figure 14–25

The glenoidogram is the path of the humeral head as it translates in a specified direction across the face of the glenoid away from the glenoid center line under defined loads. The glenoidogram shows the effective glenoid depth and width for the specified direction of translation and loading conditions. (Modified from Matsen FA III, Lippitt SB, Sidles JA, and Harryman DT II: Practical Evaluation and Management of the Shoulder. Philadelphia: WB Saunders, 1994.)

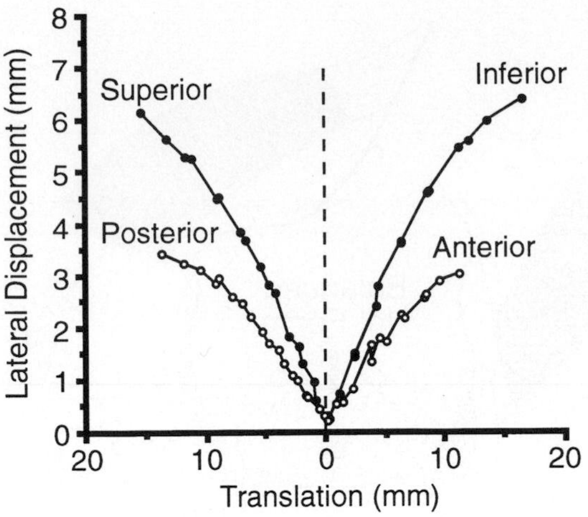

Figure 14–26

Measured glenoidograms for four different directions of translation in a young cadaver shoulder. The dotted vertical line represents the glenoid center line (see Fig. 14–27). The effective glenoid depth in this shoulder was 3.4 mm for translation in the posterior direction, 3.2 mm in the anterior direction, 6.2 mm in the superior direction, and 6.4 mm in the inferior direction. Note the high degree of symmetry about the glenoid center line and the deep valley when the head is exactly centered in the glenoid socket. (From Matsen FA III, Lippitt SB, Sidles JA, and Harryman DT II: Practical Evaluation and Management of the Shoulder. Philadelphia: WB Saunders, 1994.)

the glenoid fossa (Figs. 14–27 and 14–28). The maximal angle that the net humeral joint reaction force can make with the glenoid center line in a given direction is the *balance stability angle* (Fig. 14–29; see also Fig. 14–23). The balance stability angles vary for different directions around the glenoid. The requisite for a stable glenohumeral joint is that the net humeral joint reaction force is maintained within the balance stability angles.

Net Humeral Joint Reaction Force

The direction of the net humeral joint reaction force is controlled actively by the elements of the rotator cuff and by other shoulder muscles. Each active muscle generates a force whose direction is determined by the effective origin and insertion of that muscle (Fig. 14–30). The neural control of the magnitude of these muscle forces provides the mechanism by which the direction of the net humeral joint reaction force is controlled. For example, by increasing the force of contraction of a muscle whose force direction is close to the glenoid center line, the direction of the net humeral joint reaction force can be aligned more closely with the glenoid fossa (Fig. 14–31). The elements of the rotator cuff are well positioned to contribute to this muscle balance.[35, 36, 50, 73, 228, 282, 283, 313, 492, 508, 545, 573, 653, 654, 657, 706]

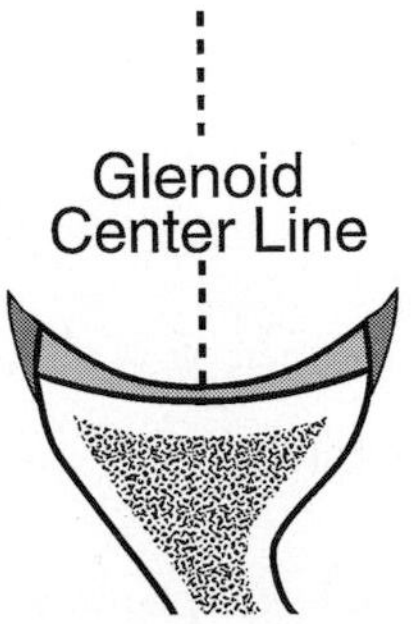

Figure 14–27

The *glenoid center line* is a line perpendicular to the surface of the glenoid fossa at its midpoint. (Modified from Matsen FA III, Lippitt SB, Sidles JA, and Harryman DT II: Practical Evaluation and Management of the Shoulder. Philadelphia: WB Saunders, 1994.)

Strengthening and neuromuscular training help to optimize the neuromuscular control of the net humeral joint reaction force. Conversely, the net humeral joint reaction force is difficult to optimize when muscle control is impaired by injury, disuse, contracture, paralysis, loss of coordination, or tendon defects (Fig. 14–32). Neuromuscular training may be guided by proprioceptors in the labrum and ligaments.[211, 229, 290, 656] Blasier and associates[49] and Kronberg and co-workers[328] showed that individuals with generalized joint laxity have less acute proprioception and altered muscle activation. Zuckerman and associates demonstrated that motion and position sense are compromised in the presence of traumatic anterior instability and restored at 1 year after surgical reconstruction.[721]

The reader is referred to reviews of neuromuscular stabilization of the shoulder by Lieber and Friden (see Chapter 4)[393] and Speer and Garrett (see Chapter 8).[393] In the same references are found reviews of the role of capsular feedback and pattern generators in shoulder kinematics by Grigg (see Chapter 9)[393] and of muscle optimization by Flanders (see Chapter 39).[393]

Balance Stability Angle and the Stability Ratio

The balance stability angle is the maximal angle that the net humeral joint reaction force can make with the glenoid center line before glenohumeral dislocation occurs. The tangent of this balance stability angle is the ratio between its displacing component (perpendicular to the glenoid center line) and its compressive component (parallel to the glenoid center line), which is known as the *stability ratio*. The stability ratio is the maximal displacing force in a given direction that can be stabilized by specified compressive load, assuming that frictional effects are minimal.* The effective glenoid arc, balance stability

*Measured stability ratios may be influenced by the friction of the joint surfaces and by other stabilizing mechanisms such as adhesion/cohesion and the glenoid suction cup (which are discussed later). These effects tend to increase the displacing force necessary to dislocate the humeral head for a given compressive load. It is essential to control for these effects in the laboratory. Specifically, the underlubricated, aged cadaver joints available to the laboratory may have substantially greater coefficients of friction in vitro than the exquisitely lubricated and smooth joint of the young person in vivo.

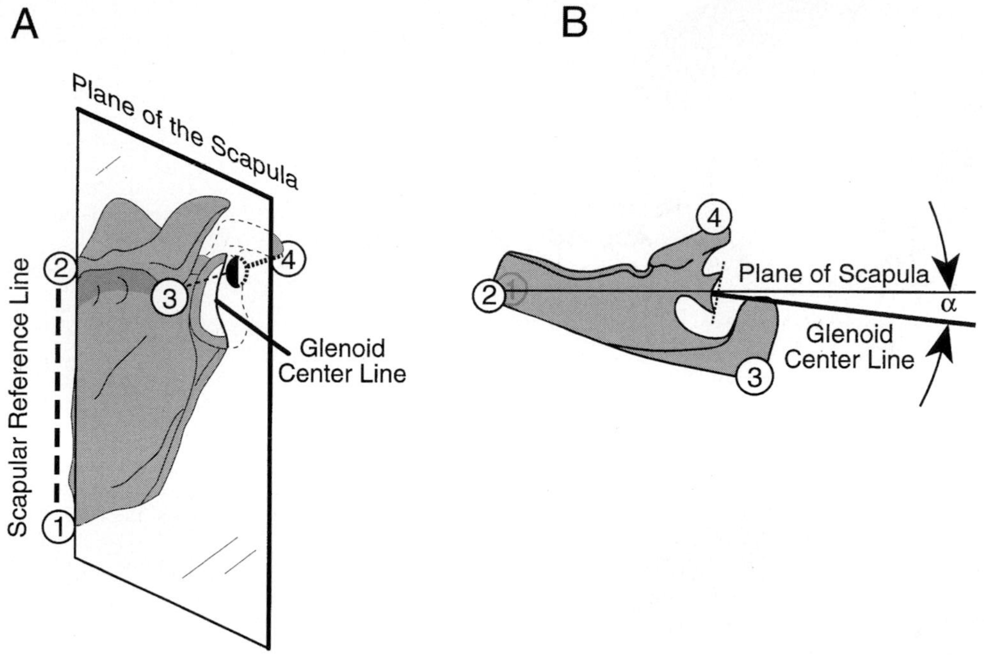

Figure 14–28

The glenoid center line can be related to scapular coordinates and to the plane of the scapula. These reference points are all easily palpated: (1) the inferior pole of the scapula, (2) the medial end of the spine of the scapula, (3) the posterior angle of the acromion, and (4) the coracoid tip. The scapular reference line connects reference points 1 and 2. The plane of the scapula passes through points 1 and 2 and halfway between points 3 and 4. The glenoid center line usually makes a slightly posterior angle (∝) with the plane of the scapula. (Modified from Matsen FA III, Lippitt SB, Sidles JA, and Harryman DT II: Practical Evaluation and Management of the Shoulder. Philadelphia: WB Saunders, 1994.)

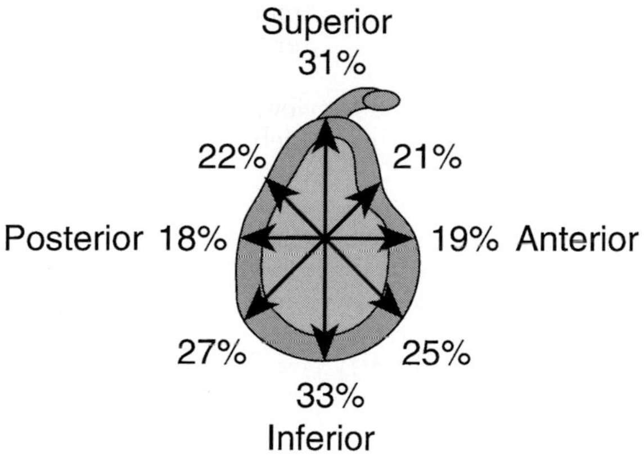

Figure 14–29

The balance stability angle varies around the face of the glenoid. For the normal glenoid, the superior and inferior balance stability angles are greater than the anterior and posterior balance stability angles. This figure shows the balance stability angles measured in eight directions around the face of the glenoid. Values are the means for 10 cadaver shoulders with a compressive load of 50 N. (Modified from Matsen FA III, Lippitt SB, Sidles JA, and Harryman DT II: Practical Evaluation and Management of the Shoulder. Philadelphia: WB Saunders, 1994.)

Figure 14–30

Each active muscle generates a force (F) whose direction is determined by the effective origin and insertion of that muscle. Note that the rotator cuff tendons wrap around the head of the humerus so that their effective point of attachment is on the humeral articular surface. Note also that each muscle force has a compressive (F_c) and a displacing (F_d) component. The product of the force multiplied by the radius (R) is the torque (F × R). (Modified from Matsen FA III, Lippitt SB, Sidles JA, and Harryman DT II: Practical Evaluation and Management of the Shoulder. Philadelphia: WB Saunders, 1994.)

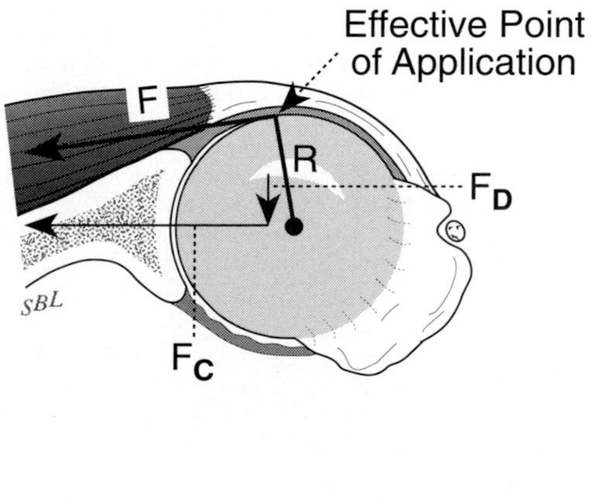

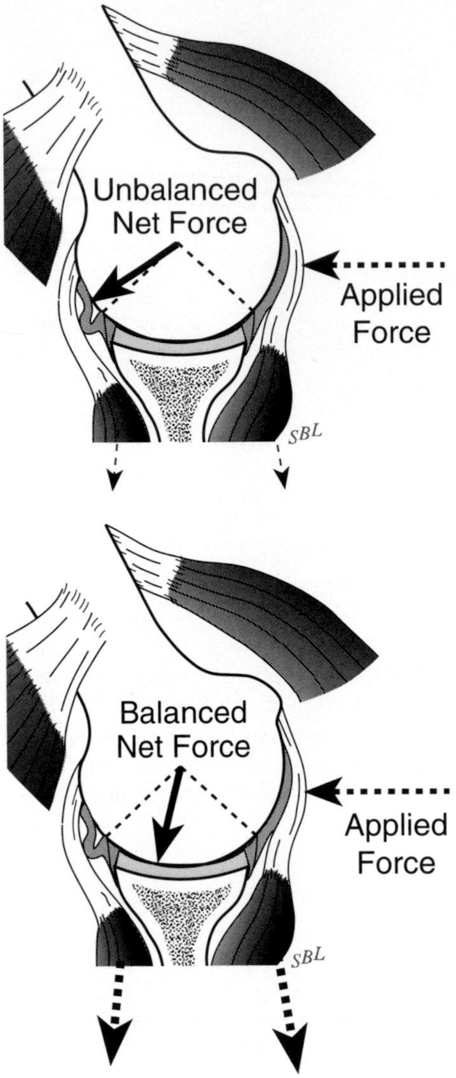

Figure 14–31

Stabilization of the glenohumeral joint against an applied translational force. Strong contraction of the cuff muscles provides an increased compression force into the glenoid concavity. As a result, the net humeral force is balanced within the glenoid concavity.

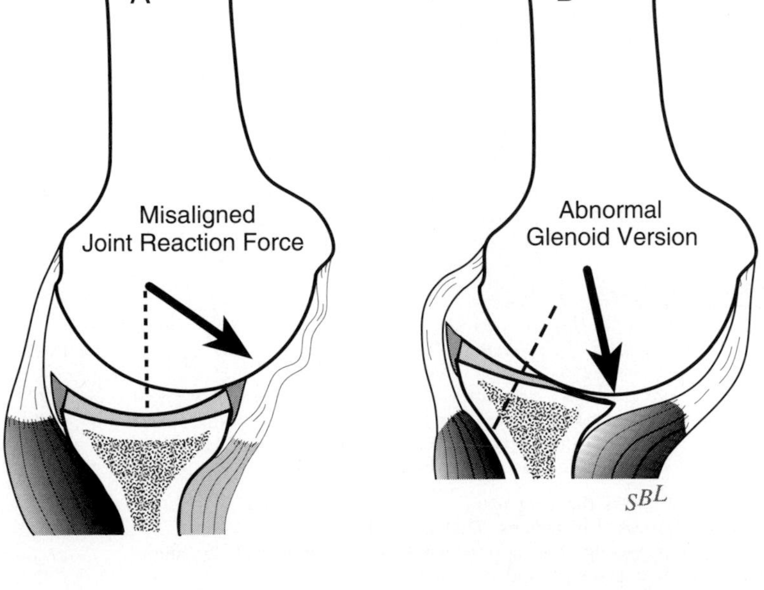

Figure 14–32

A, Stability is compromised by muscle imbalance. In this example, the humerus is aligned with the glenoid center line, but the net humeral joint reaction force is misaligned owing to weakness of the posterior cuff musculature. *B,* Balance stability is compromised with an abnormal glenoid version. In this example, the humerus is aligned with the plane of the scapula, but severe glenoid retroversion results in a posteriorly directed glenoid center line that is divergent from the net humeral joint reaction force. (Modified from Matsen FA III, Lippitt SB, Sidles JA, and Harryman DT II: Practical Evaluation and Management of the Shoulder. Philadelphia: WB Saunders, 1994.)

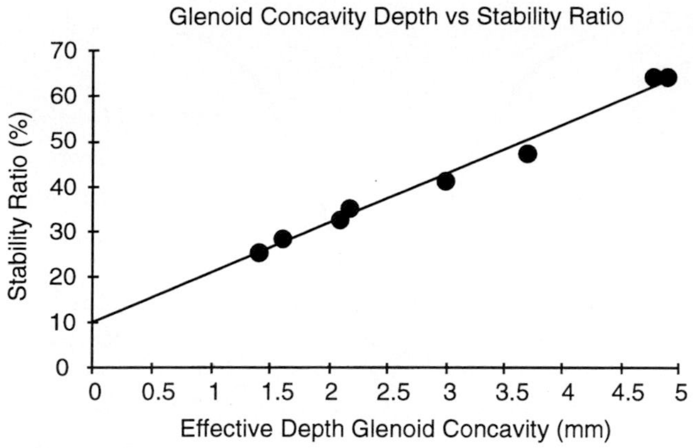

Figure 14–33

A nearly linear relationship exists between the effective depth of the glenoid concavity and the stability ratio with a 50-N compressive load. These data include points representing superior, inferior, anterior, and posterior translations before and after excision of the glenoid labrum. (From Matsen FA III, Lippitt SB, Sidles JA, and Harryman DT II: Practical Evaluation and Management of the Shoulder. Philadelphia: WB Saunders, 1994.)

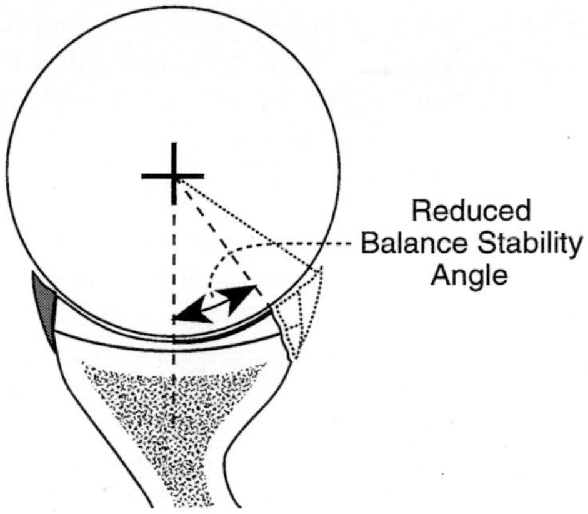

Figure 14–34

The balance stability angle and effective glenoid arc are reduced by a fracture of the glenoid rim. (Modified from Matsen FA III, Lippitt SB, Sidles JA, and Harryman DT II: Practical Evaluation and Management of the Shoulder. Philadelphia: WB Saunders, 1994.)

angle, and stability ratios vary around the perimeter of the glenoid (see Fig. 14–29). It is useful to note that for small angles, the stability ratio can be estimated by dividing the balance stability angle by 57 degrees.*

The stability ratio is frequently used in the laboratory because it is relatively easy to measure: A compressive load is applied and the displacing force is progressively increased until dislocation occurs. For example, Lippitt and associates[369] found that a compressive load of 50 N resisted displacing loads up to 30 N and that the effectiveness of this stabilization mechanism varied with the depth of the glenoid (Fig. 14–33). Investigation of these parameters provides important information on stability mechanics, for example, resection of the labrum has been shown to reduce the stability ratio by 20%.[369] Furthermore, a 3-mm anterior glenoid defect has been shown to reduce the balance stability angle more than 25% from 18 to 13 degrees.[394]

Clinically, the stability ratio can be sensed using the "load and shift" test, wherein the examiner applies a compressive load pressing the humeral head into the glenoid while noting the amount of translating force necessary to move the humeral head from its centered position.[593] This test gives the examiner an indication of the adequacy of the glenoid concavity and is one of the most practical ways to detect deficiencies of the glenoid rim.

Effective Glenoid Arc

The glenoid concavity is formed by a combination of the shape of the underlying bone and the overlying cartilage and labrum (see Figs. 14–23 and 14–25).[269, 604] The effective glenoid arc may be compromised by congenital deficiency (glenoid hypoplasia), excessive compliance, traumatic lesions (rim fractures or Bankart defects) or wear (Fig. 14–34).[8, 26, 29, 102, 111, 269, 300, 349, 369, 394–396, 450, 495, 555, 629] The effective arc may be augmented by anatomic repair of fractures or Bankart lesions (Fig. 14–35), rim augmentation, congruent glenoid bone grafting, and glenoid osteotomy.[349]

*At small angles the tangent of an angle is approximately equal to the angle expressed in radians. Thus the stability ratio (tangent of the balance stability angle) is approximately the balance stability angle divided by 57 degrees per radian.

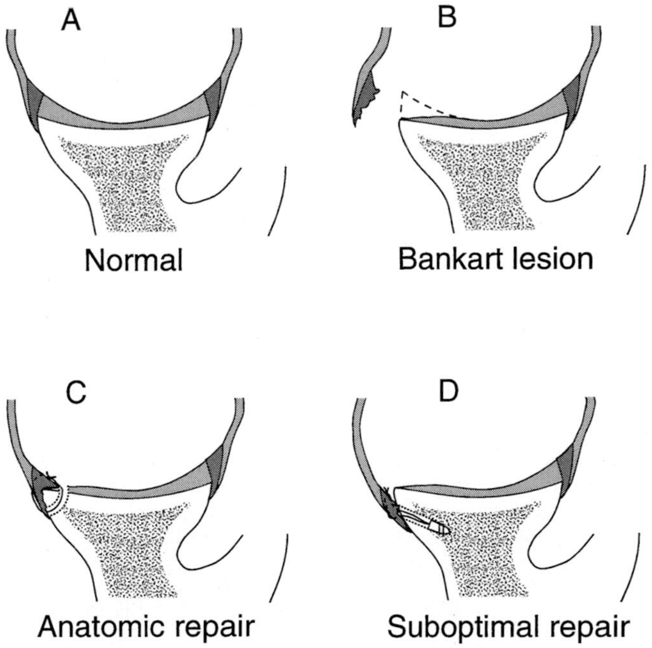

Figure 14–35

Normally the capsule and labrum deepen the effective glenoid fossa *(A)*. This effect is lost in the presence of a Bankart lesion, particularly if the articular cartilage is worn away *(B)*. Anatomic repair of the detached glenoid labrum and glenohumeral ligaments to the glenoid rim helps to restore the effective glenoid arc *(C)*. By contrast, when the labrum and capsule heal to the neck, the effective glenoid arc is not restored *(D)*. (Modified from Matsen FA III, Lippitt SB, Sidles JA, and Harryman DT II: Practical Evaluation and Management of the Shoulder. Philadelphia: WB Saunders, 1994.)

The effective shape of the glenoid is revealed by the glenoidogram. As the humeral head is translated from the center of the glenoid to the rim in a given direction, the center of the humeral head traces the glenoidogram, which has a characteristic "gull-wing" shape. The glenoidogram is different for different directions of translation (see Fig. 14–26, which demonstrates data recorded for the superior, inferior, anterior, and posterior directions in a typical shoulder). The shape of the glenoidogram can be predicted from the humeral radius of curvature, the glenoid radius of curvature, and the balance stability angle.*

Predicted glenoidograms are qualitatively similar to glenoidograms measured experimentally (compare Figs. 14–26 and 14–36). The glenoidogram also reveals another important aspect of shoulder stability: the slope of the glenoidogram at any point is equal to the tangent of the balance stability angle (which is equal to the stability ratio) at that point. For most glenoidograms, it can be seen that the slope is steepest when the humeral head is centered in the glenoid (see Fig. 14–36). Thus the joint has the highly desirable property of being most stable when the head is centered. As the humeral head is moved away from the center, the slope of the glenoidogram and the stability ratio become less. Thus, as the head is displaced from the glenoid center, it becomes progressively more unstable. Once enough force is applied to displace the head from the center, that same amount of force would easily displace the humeral head over the glenoid lip. Note also that when the humeral head is translated to the lip of the glenoid, the stability ratio is, as expected, zero. These observations relate to the "jerk" tests described for anterior[353] and posterior[394] instability: in these tests there is no translation of the humeral head until the point where sudden and substantial translation occurs.[349, 369]

*Glenoidograms can be predicted given the radius of curvature of the humeral head (Rh), the radius of curvature of the glenoid fossa (Rg), the effective glenoid width (W) and depth (D), and the balance stability angle in radians. For each value of x (the distance away from the glenoid center line), the perpendicular distance of the center of the humeral head away from the glenoid bottom, y, is given by D-Rh + SQRT(Rh·Rh-(W-x)·(W-x)). The sample spreadsheet displays the case where Rg = Rh = 25 mm and the BSA = 30 degrees = 0.5236 radians. In this case the effective glenoid width (W) is = Rg·Sin(BSA) and the effective glenoid depth (D) is equal to Rg·(1-cos(BSA)). The results of this prediction are shown in Table 14–1 and in Figure 14–36.

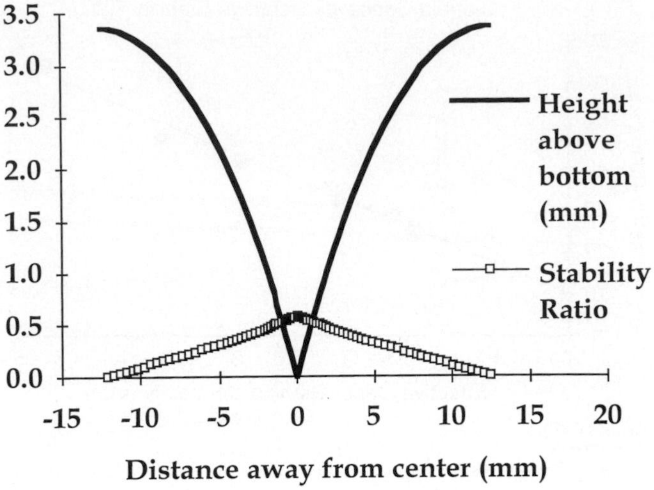

Figure 14–36

The glenoidogram predicted for a shoulder with glenoid and humeral radii (R_g) and (R_h) of 25 mm and a balance stability angle (A) of 30 degrees. For a position x millimeters from the center, the effective glenoid depth (y) was calculated from the formula: $y = R_g \cdot (1\text{-}\cos A) - R_h + (R_h^2 - (R_g \cdot (\sin A) - x)^2)^{1/2}$). Also shown are the local stability ratios (equal to the slope of the glenoidogram) for the different humeral positions along the glenoidogram. Note that the stability ratio is maximum when the humeral head is centered in the glenoid.

Glenoid Version

Glenoid version is the angle that the glenoid center line makes with the plane of the scapula (see Fig. 14–28). The glenoid center line usually points a few degrees posterior to the plane of the scapula (see Fig. 14–28). Changing the version of the glenoid articular surface imposes a corresponding change in the humeroscapular positions in which the net humeral joint reaction force will be contained by the effective glenoid arc. Glenoid version may be altered by glenoid dysplasia (Fig. 14–37),[695] fractures, glenoid osteotomy,[698] and glenoid arthroplasty. Abnormal glenoid version positions the glenoid fossa in an abnormal

Table 14–1 PREDICTED COORDINATES OF GLENOIDOGRAM

EFFECTIVE GLENOID WIDTH (W) *Rg*sin (BSA)*	*EFFECTIVE GLENOID DEPTH (D)* *Rg* (1-cos [BSA])*	*X*	*Y* *D-Rh+ SQRT (Rh*Rh- [W-x] * [W-x])*
12.5	3.35	0	0
12.5	3.35	0.1	0.057428086
12.5	3.35	0.2	0.114245197
12.5	3.35	0.3	0.170456105
12.5	3.35	0.4	0.226065482
12.5	3.35	0.5	0.281077905
12.5	3.35	0.6	0.335497855
12.5	3.35	0.7	0.38932972
12.5	3.35	0.8	0.442577799
12.5	3.35	0.9	0.495246303
12.5	3.35	1.0	0.547339357

BSA, balance stability angle.

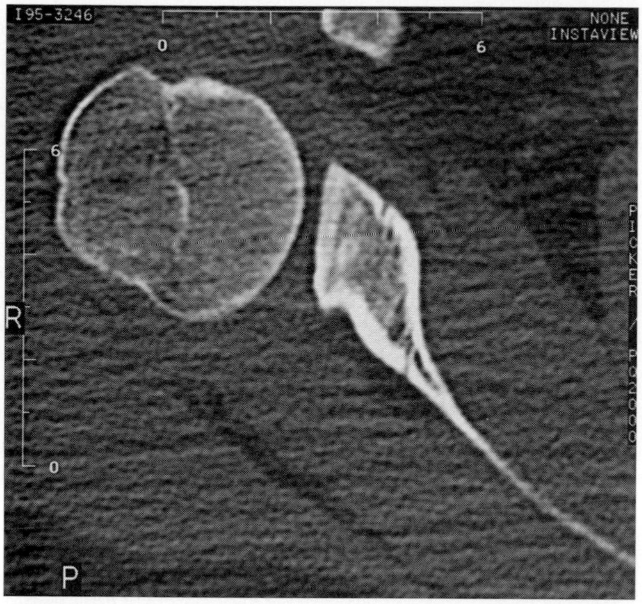

Figure 14–37

A computed tomography scan of a shoulder with glenoid dysplasia resulting in the absence of the posterior glenoid lip and glenoid retroversion.

relationship to the forces generated by the scapulohumeral muscles. Normalization of the abnormal glenoid version is often a critical step in glenohumeral reconstruction.

Apparent changes in glenoid version can arise from loss of part of the glenoid rim (see Figs. 14–32 and 14–34).[64, 274, 524] Dias and associates found no difference in apparent glenoid version between normal subjects and recurrent anterior dislocators.[128] Dowdy and O'Driscoll[135] found only minor variances of radiographic glenoid version among patients with and without recurrence after stabilization surgery. However, Hirschfelder and Kirsten[259] found increased glenoid retroversion in both the symptomatic and unsymptomatic shoulders of individuals with posterior instability; Grasshoff and co-workers[205] found increased anteversion in shoulders with recurrent anterior instability.

Changes in version may be difficult to quantitate on axillary radiographs unless the view is carefully standardized (Fig. 14–38). Even with optimal radiographic technique, the important contributions of the cartilage and labrum to the depth and orientation of the fossa cannot be seen on plain radiographs or computed tomography (CT) scans.[269, 604] When it is important to know the orientation of the cartilaginous joint surface in relation to the scapular body, a double-contrast CT scan is necessary (see Fig. 14–18).

Scapular Positioning

A special feature of the glenohumeral joint is that the glenoid can be positioned on the thorax (in contrast to the fixed acetabulum of the hip). This scapular alignment greatly increases the range of positions in which the criteria for glenohumeral stability can be met (Fig. 14–39). Consider the arm elevated 90 degrees in the sagittal thoracic plane. This position can be achieved with the scapula protracted or retracted. If the scapula is protracted, the humerus is closely aligned with the glenoid center line. When the humerus is in this position, most of the humeroscapular muscles are oriented to compress the humeral head into the glenoid fossa. Alternatively, if the scapula is maximally retracted, the humerus is almost at right angles to the glenoid center line (Fig. 14–40). In this position, the net humeral joint reaction force is directed posteriorly and may not be contained within the balance stability angle.[60, 195, 280, 489, 514, 669]

Which humeroscapular position is used to achieve a given humerothoracic position is a question of habit and

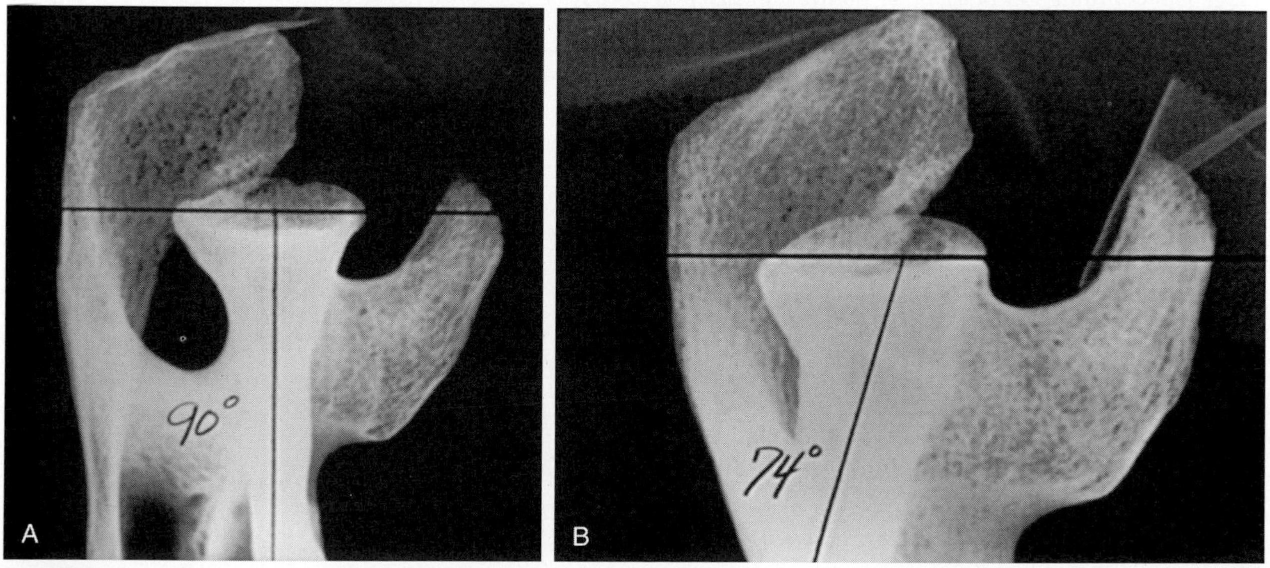

Figure 14–38

Two radiographs of the same cadaver scapula showing the variation in apparent glenoid retroversion depending on the radiographic projection.

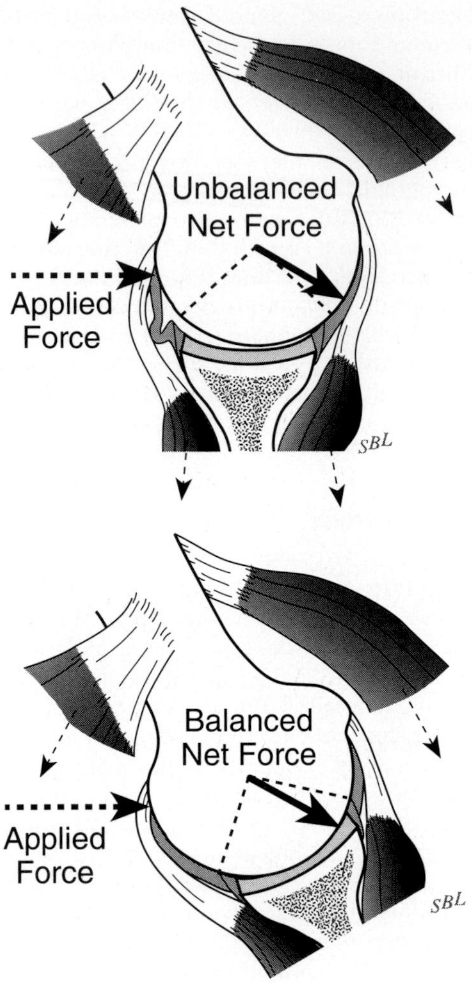

Figure 14–39

Stabilization against an applied translational force by repositioning the glenoid concavity to support the net humeral force.

training. The coordination of scapular position and glenohumeral muscle balance are important elements of the neuromuscular control of glenohumeral stability.

Atwater has documented that in most throwing and striking skills, the shoulder abduction angle is usually 100 degrees.[22] Higher and lower release points are achieved by tilting the trunk rather than by increasing or decreasing the shoulder abduction angle relative to the trunk.

Ligaments

PROPERTIES OF LIGAMENTS

Each glenohumeral ligament has clinically important properties that can be characterized by the relationship of the distance between its origin and insertion and its tension.[170] These properties include:

1. Its resting length (how far can its origin and insertion be separated with minimal force)
2. Its elastic deformability (how much additional separation of the origin and insertion can be achieved by the application of larger forces without permanently changing the ligament's properties)
3. Its plastic deformability (beyond the ligament's elastic limit, how much additional separation between the origin and insertion can be achieved by the application of larger forces which permanently deform the ligament up to the point where the ligament fails)

These properties can be demonstrated as a plot of the ligament's tension versus the distance between the ligament's origin and insertion. The same relationship pertains whether the ligament's origin and insertion are separated by translation of the humeral head or by rotation (Fig. 14–41).

At point "A," the origin and insertion of the ligament are closely approximated. At point "B," the origin and insertion have been separated enough to initiate tension in the ligament. Thus, the resting length of the ligament is shown as A-B. Stefko and associates[612] measured the length of the anterior band of the IGHL to be 37 mm.

Additional separation of the origin and insertion causes increasing ligament tension. Up to point "C," this separation is elastic (i.e., it does not result in permanent change in the ligament). Further separation of the origin and

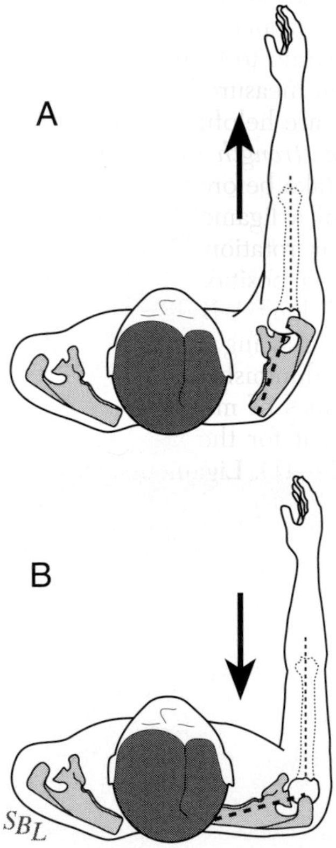

Figure 14–40

Essentially identical humerothoracic positions can be achieved using different humeroscapular positions, which, in turn, have different implications for balancing the net humeral force. *A,* The humerus is elevated so that it is closely aligned with the glenoid center line. This should be the most stable position. *B,* The same humerothoracic position can be achieved with the humerus almost perpendicular to the glenoid center line, challenging the ability of the joint to balance the net humeral force. (From Matsen FA III, Lippitt SB, Sidles JA, and Harryman DT II: Practical Evaluation and Management of the Shoulder. Philadelphia: WB Saunders, 1994.)

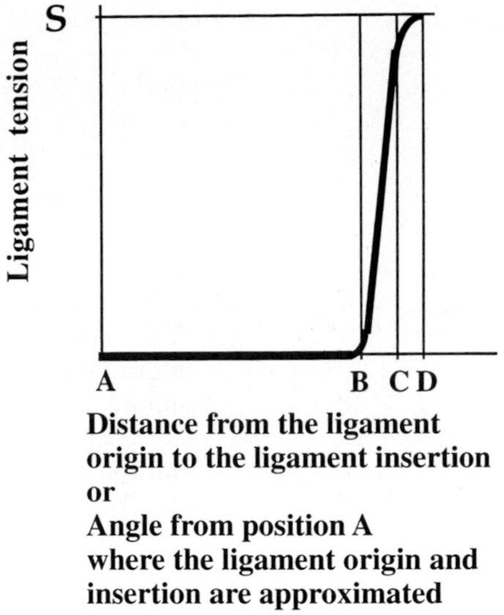

Figure 14–41

The distance from the ligament origin to the ligament insertion or the angle from position A where the ligament origin and insertion are approximated.

insertion plastically deform the ligament up to the point "D" where the ligament fails at a tension of "S." The midsubstance strain to failure of the anterior band of the IGHL has been measured from 7 to 11%.[612]

Such graphs are helpful in describing the properties of ligaments. The *strength* of a ligament is the amount of tension it can take before failure (S).

The *laxity* of a ligament is the amount of translation (Fig. 14–42) or rotation (Fig. 14–43) it allows from a specified starting position when a small load is applied. Ligaments with long A-B distances demonstrate substantial laxity if the starting point for laxity testing is close to "A." Laxity is diminished when the joint is positioned near the extremes of motion (Fig. 14–44); that is, when the starting point for the laxity measurement is close to "B" (see Fig. 14–41). Ligaments with small A-B distances are short or contracted. *Translational and rotational laxity are equivalent*: They both reflect the ability to separate the attachment points of the ligament.

A typical relationship between humeroscapular position and torque (capsular tension × humeral head radius) is shown in (Fig. 14–45).[394] Note that the greatest part of glenohumeral motion and function takes place in the area where there is no tension in the capsule (corresponds with zone A-B in Fig. 14–41). Also note that at the limits of motion (corresponds to zone B-C), the torque increases rapidly with changes in position as suggested by the rapid increase in tension shown in Figure 14–41.

These diagrams help to distinguish laxity from instability. Normally stable shoulders may demonstrate substantial laxity (e.g., consider the very lax but very stable glenohumeral joints of gymnasts). In an important study, Emery and Mullaji[146] found that of 150 asymptomatic shoulders in school children, 50% demonstrated positive signs of "increased laxity."

Some investigators have measured increased laxity in patients with glenohumeral instability.[97, 291, 292, 310, 391] However, evidence indicates that these differences are not always significant.[226, 365, 394] Starting in a neutral position, the translational laxities of eight normal living subjects were found to be 8 ± 4, 8 ± 6, and 11 ± 4 mm, in the anterior, posterior, and inferior directions, respectively. Interestingly, virtually identical laxities were measured in 16 patients who required surgery because of symptomatic recurrent instability (Fig. 14–46), indicating that in these subjects, the measured laxity was not the determinant of glenohumeral stability.[365, 394] Sperber and Wredmark[609] found no differences in joint volume or capsular elasticity between healthy and unstable shoulders. These results indicate that the amount of laxity cannot be used to distinguish clinically stable shoulders from those that are unstable.

The *stretchiness* of a ligament is its elasticity. Ligaments with long B-C distances are stretchy and have "soft" end points on clinical laxity tests (see Fig. 14–41). Ligaments with short B-C distances are stiff and have "firm" endpoints on clinical laxity tests.

Figure 14–42

Glenohumeral translation is the movement of the center of the humeral head with respect to the face of the glenoid. The amount of translation allowed is determined by both the initial position of the joint and the length of the ligament that becomes tight.

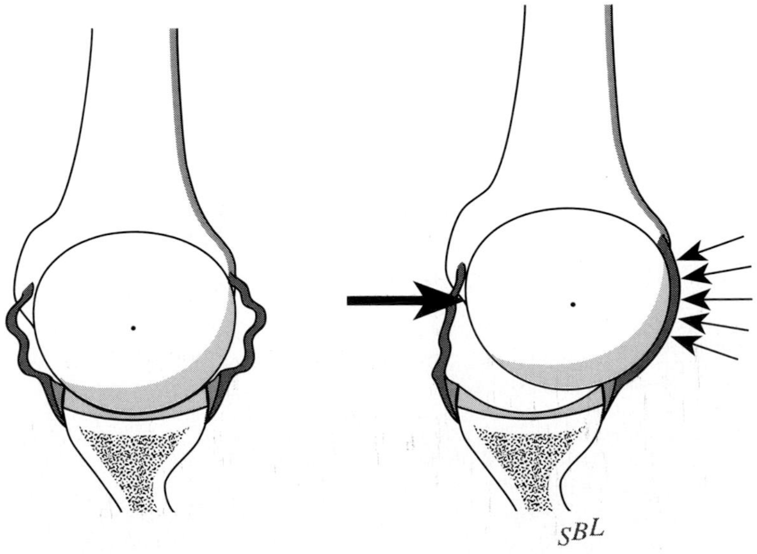

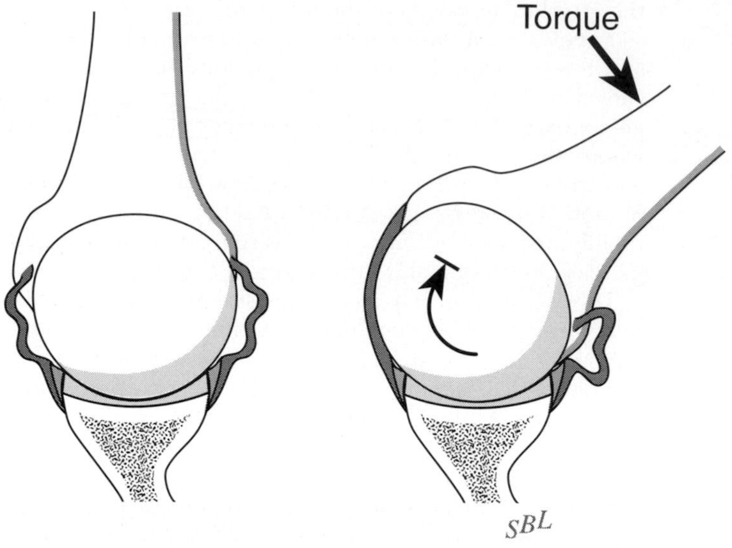

Figure 14–43

Glenohumeral rotation is the movement of the humerus around the center of the humeral head, which remains centered in the glenoid fossa. The amount of rotation allowed is determined by both the initial position of the joint and the length of the ligament that becomes tight.

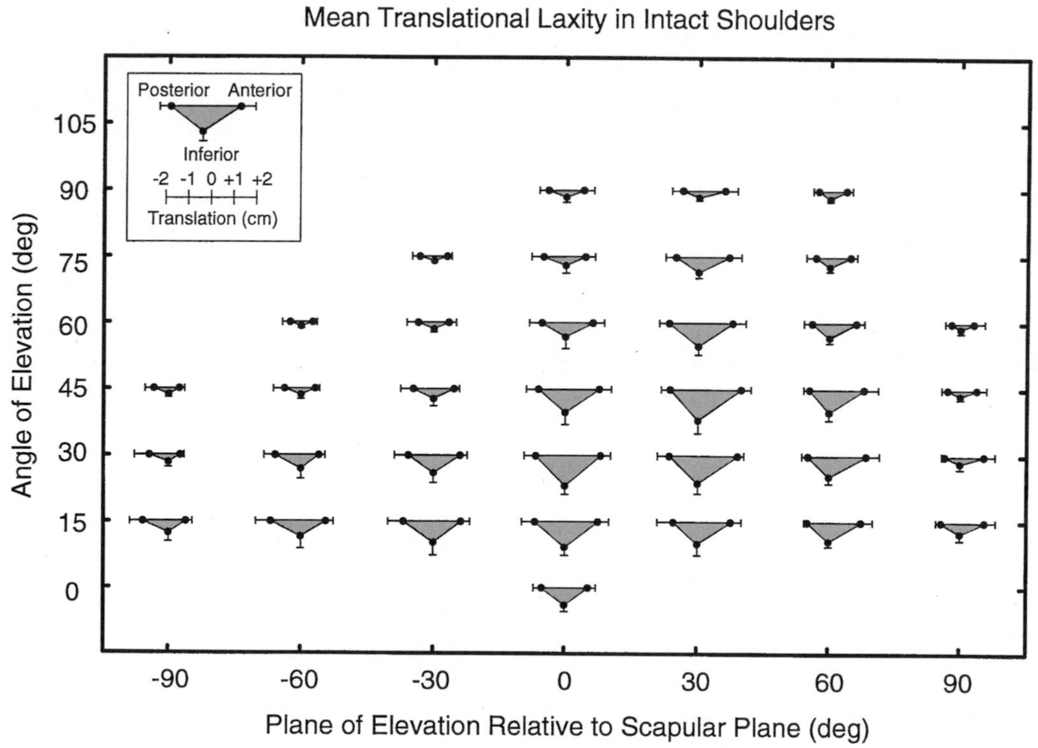

Figure 14–44

Mean translational laxity as measured in eight cadaveric shoulders. The applied translational force was 30 N (approximately 6 lb), and it was applied along each of the following axes anterior, posterior and inferior. The planes of elevation are measured relative to the plane of the scapula (see Fig. 14–28), not the thoracic plane. The angles of elevation are measured relative to the scapular reference line (see Fig. 14–28). Standard deviations are shown at the vertex of each triangle. (From Matsen FA III, Lippitt SB, Sidles JA, and Harryman DT II: Practical Evaluation and Management of the Shoulder. Philadelphia: WB Saunders, 1994.)

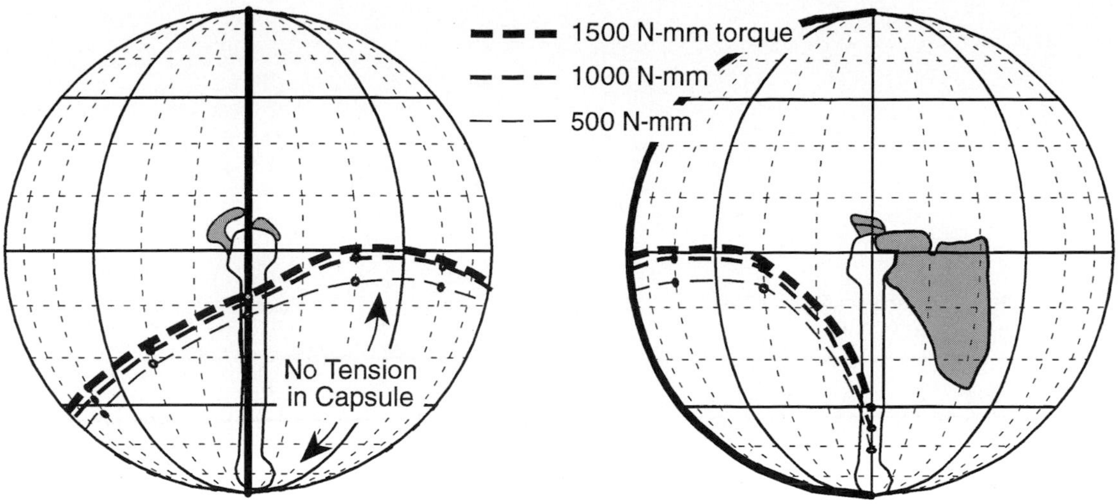

Figure 14–45

The range of humeroscapular elevation with no capsular tension. This global diagram represents data from a cadaver experiment in which the humerus was elevated in various scapular planes, allowing free axial rotation. Elevation was performed until the torque reached 500, 1000, and 1500 N/mm. The positions associated with these torque levels are indicated by the isobars. The area within the inner isobars indicates the range of positions in which there was no tension in the capsuloligamentous structures. (From Matsen FA III, Lippitt SB, Sidles JA, and Harryman DT II: Practical Evaluation and Management of the Shoulder. Philadelphia: WB Saunders, 1994.)

Biochemical composition (e.g., in Ehlers-Danlos syndrome), anatomic variation (anomalies of attachment), use (or disuse), age, disease (e.g., diabetes, frozen shoulder) injury, and surgery (e.g., capsulorrhaphy) can affect the strength, laxity, and stretchiness of glenohumeral ligaments.

The reader is referred to the reviews of the material properties of the inferior glenohumeral ligament by Mow and associates (see Chapter 2)[393] and of the role of ligaments in glenohumeral stability by Lew and co-workers (see Chapter 3).[393]

LIGAMENTOUS STABILIZATION

The glenohumeral ligaments exert two stabilizing effects. The first effect is that they serve as *checkreins*, restricting the range of joint positions to those that can be stabilized by muscle balance. This is important because at extreme glenohumeral positions, the net humeral joint reaction force becomes increasingly difficult to balance within the glenoid (Fig. 14–47). For example, excessive abduction, extension, and external rotation of the shoulder may allow the net humeral joint reaction force to exceed the anterior-inferior balance stability angle. Similarly, excessive posterior capsular laxity allows the net humeral joint reaction force to achieve large angles with the glenoid center line, angles that may exceed the posterior balance stability angle. Furthermore, at the extremes of motion, the muscles tend to be near their maximal extension, a position in which their force-generating capacity is diminished.[360]

The patient can modify the checkrein function by altering the position of the scapula (see Fig. 14–17). Surgeons can modify the checkrein function: capsular tightening moves points B, C, and D closer to point A, reducing laxity (see Fig. 14–41). The checkrein function is inoperant when the ligament is not under tension (i.e., when the humeroscapular position is within the tension-free zone) (see Figs. 14–41 and 14–45).

The second stabilizing effect is that when torque is applied to the humerus so that a ligament comes under tension, this ligament applies a force to the proximal humerus. Because of the attachments of the ligament this *countervailing force* both compresses the humeral head into the glenoid fossa and also resists displacement in the direction of the tight ligament (Fig. 14–48).

An analysis of ligament function* demonstrates the limits of the stability provided by ligaments acting alone. For example, it suggests that if the torque resulting from a force of a modest 10 lb applied to the arm at a distance of 40 inches from the center of a humeral head with a 1-inch radius was resisted only by the tension in the inferior

*The magnitude of the countervailing force is determined by the applied torque and limited by the strength of the ligament. The direction of this force is tangent to the humeral head at the point of its contact with the glenoid rim.

The countervailing force mechanism operates in the arc B-C, where the ligament is elastically deformed. If the ligament behaves perfectly elastically, the tension in the ligament provides a stabilizing force (T) where:

T = (angular position-angle B) * diameter of humeral head * Pi/360 degrees * spring constant of the ligament

This relationship predicts that

- Until angle B is reached, no force is generated by the ligament.
- The larger the angle past position B, the more force is generated (up to the elastic limit).
- Stiffer ligaments generate more force for a given angular displacement.
- Larger humeral heads generate more force for each degree of angular displacement.

Ligament tension results from applied torque. When an externally applied force B acts at a distance E from the center of the humeral head, it creates a torque (Q) that is the product of B and E (see Fig. 14–49). If this torque is resisted by a ligament closely applied to the humeral head (i.e., the effective moment arm equals the head radius [R]), the tension in the ligament (T) is

T = Q/ R = B * E/R

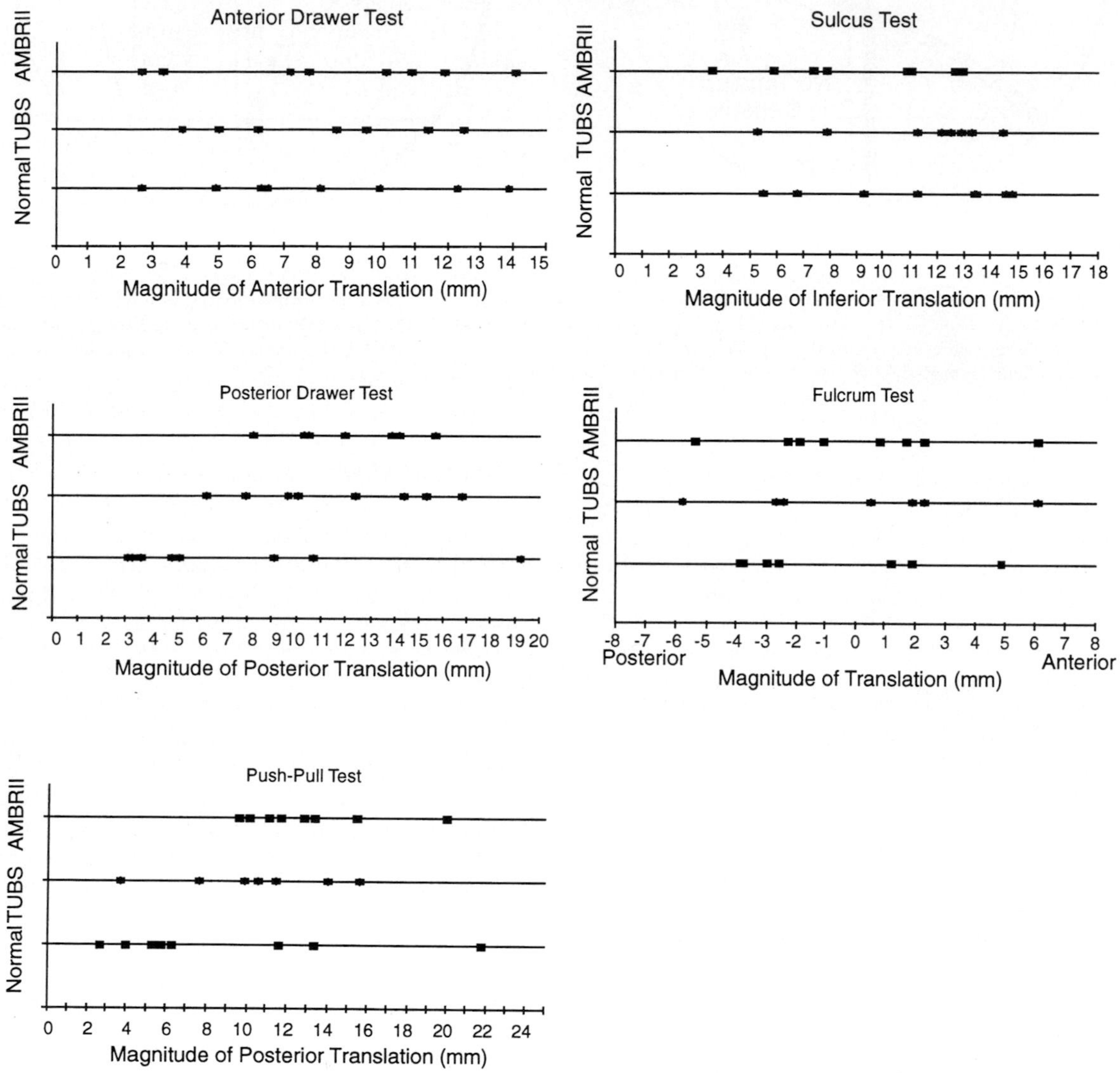

Figure 14–46

The magnitude of translation on laxity tests for three groups of shoulders in vivo: eight normal shoulders, eight shoulders with symptomatic atraumatic instability (AMBRII), and eight shoulders with symptomatic traumatic instability (TUBS). Each shoulder is represented by a mark on the horizontal lines. Note that for each of these laxity tests, the *range* of translations for the normal subjects is essentially the same as the range of translations for subjects with symptomatic instability requiring surgical repair. (From Matsen FA III, Lippitt SB, Sidles JA, and Harryman DT II: Practical Evaluation and Management of the Shoulder. Philadelphia: WB Saunders, 1994.)

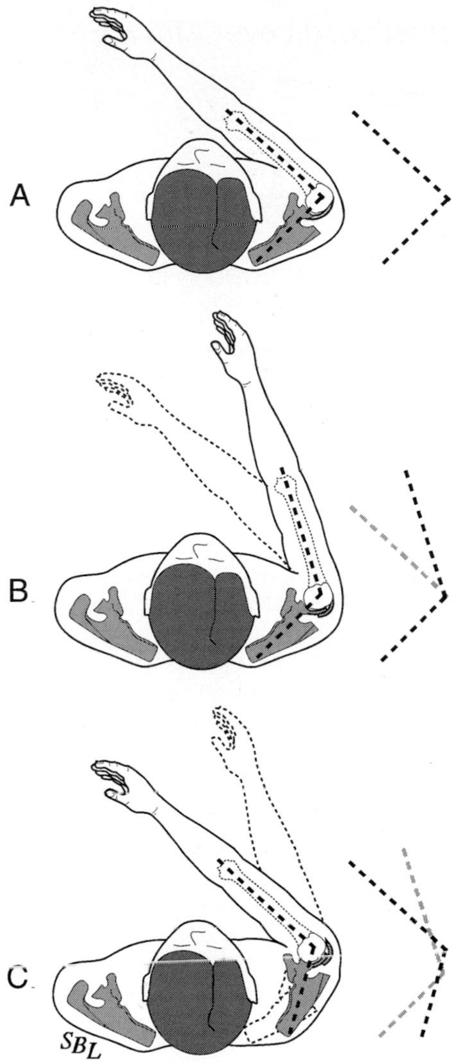

Figure 14–47

A, Excessive posterior capsular laxity allows an excessively small angle between the humerus and the plane of the scapula so that posterior stability is challenged. *B*, Normal tightness appropriately limits the allowed angular position to the range that can be stabilized. *C*, Cross-body adduction is achieved by scapular protraction as well as by humeroscapular angulation.

glenohumeral ligament (IGHL), the IGHL would need to be able to withstand a tension of 400 lb (Fig. 14–49).

If tension in the ligament exceeds the strength of the ligament (S), the ligament breaks. A few investigations have attempted to measure the strength of the glenohumeral capsular ligaments. Kaltsas[311] has studied some of the material properties of the shoulder capsule and found it to be more elastic and stronger than the capsule of the elbow. He noted that the entire glenohumeral capsule ruptured at 2000 N of distraction (450 lb). Stefko and associates[612] found that the average load leading to failure of the entire IGHL was 713 N or 160 lb. Bigliani and coworkers[47] noted in 16 cadaver shoulders that the IGHL could be divided into three anatomic regions: a superior band, an anterior axillary pouch, and a posterior axillary pouch, of which the thickest was the superior band (2.8 mm). With relatively low strain rates, the stress at failure was found to be nearly identical for the three regions of the ligament, averaging 5.5 MPa, which is 5.5 N (1.2 lb)/mm^2. Thus, in order to function as the primary stabilizer for a load of 300 lb, such as in the example earlier, the IGHLs of these cadavers would need to be 250 mm^2 in cross-section. No experimental measurements have demonstrated that the IGHL alone is sufficiently strong to balance the torque resulting from a load of 10 lb applied to the arm at a distance of 30 inches from the center of a humeral head.

Excessive ligament tension can produce obligate translation of the humeral head. Harryman and associates[224] demonstrated that certain passive motions of the glenohumeral joint forced translation of the humeral head away from the center of the joint. This obligate translation occurs when the displacing force generated by ligament tension (quantity "P" in Fig. 14–48) overwhelms the concavity compression stability mechanism (Fig. 14–50). In Harryman's study, anterior humeral translation occurred at the extremes of flexion and cross-body adduction while posterior humeral translation occurred at the extremes of extension and external rotation. Operative tightening of the posterior portion of the capsule increased the anterior translation on flexion and cross-body adduction and caused it to occur earlier in the arc of motion compared with the intact joint. Operative tightening of the posterior part of the capsule also resulted in significant superior translation with flexion of the glenohumeral joint. These data indicate that glenohumeral translation may occur in sports when the joint is forced to the extremes of its motion, such as at the transition between late cocking and early acceleration. Such obligate translations may account for the posterior labral tears and calcifications seen at the posterior glenoid in throwers. In addition, these results point to the hazard of overtightening the glenohumeral capsule, which may result in a form of secondary osteoarthritis known as capsulorrhaphy arthropathy. Hawkins and Angelo[234] pointed to these com-

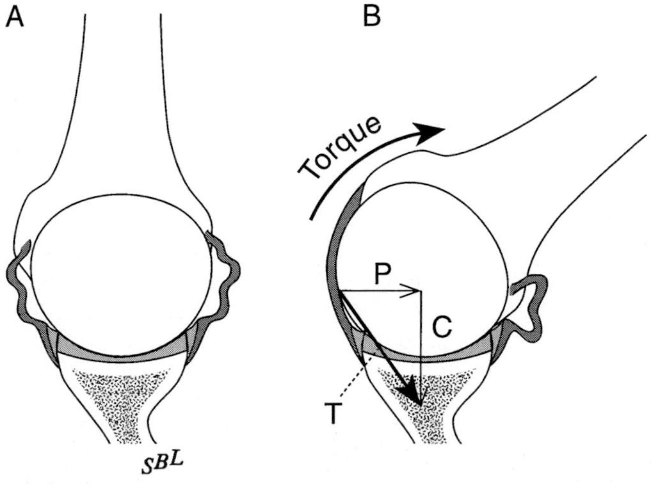

Figure 14–48

A, When the glenohumeral ligaments are slack, they exert no force. *B*, When torque is applied, the ligaments come under tension (T). This ligament tension exerts a compressive force (*C*) directed into the glenoid and a displacing force (P) pushing the humeral head away from the tight ligament.

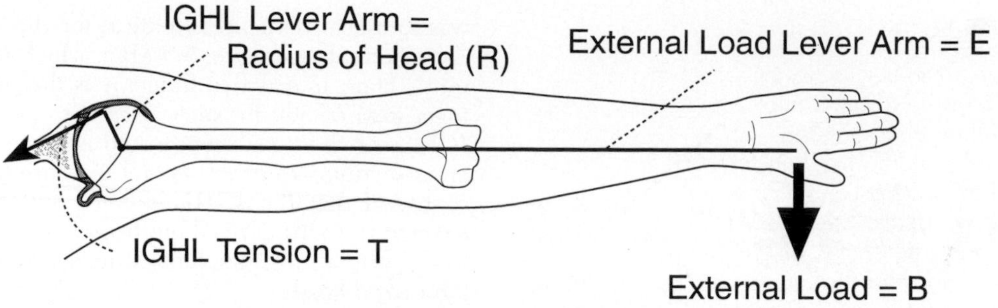

Figure 14–49

Torque balance. In the absence of other forces, the product of the ligament tension (T) and the humeral head radius (R) must equal the product of the external load (B) and its lever arm (E). If the point of application of the external force is 40 inches away from the head center and if the radius of the head is 1 inch, the tension in the ligament must be 40 times the external force. (Modified from Matsen FA III, Lippitt SB, Sidles JA, and Harryman DT II: Practical Evaluation and Management of the Shoulder. Philadelphia: WB Saunders, 1994.)

plications of obligate translation in overtightened capsular repairs.

Stability at Rest

It is apparent that the relaxed glenohumeral joint is held together without either active muscle contraction or ligament tension. The intact shoulder of a fresh anatomic specimen,[332] the anesthetized and paralyzed shoulder of a patient in the operating room, and the arm relaxed at the side[34] all maintain the normal relationships of the glenoid and humeral joint surfaces. This resting stability is due to a group of mechanisms including adhesion-cohesion, the glenoid suction cup, and limited joint volume. These mechanisms save energy as was pointed out by Humphry in 1858[273]: "We have only to remember that this power is in continual operation to appreciate the amount of animal force that is economized."

ADHESION-COHESION

This is a stabilizing mechanism by which joint surfaces wet with joint fluid are held together by the molecular attraction of the fluid to itself and to the joint surfaces. Fluids such as water and joint fluid demonstrate the property of cohesion; that is, they tend to stick together. Some surfaces, such as clean glass or articular cartilage, can be wet with water or synovial fluid, meaning that the fluid adheres to them. When two surfaces with adherent fluid are brought in contact, the adhesion of the fluid to the surfaces and the cohesion of the fluids tend to hold the two surfaces together (like two wetted microscope slides). The amount of stability generated by adhesion-cohesion is related to the adhesive and cohesive properties of the joint fluid, the "wetability" of the joint surfaces, and the area of contact between the glenoid socket and the humerus. Joint fluid has the highly desirable properties of having high tensile strength (difficult to pull apart) and having little shear strength (allows easy sliding of the two joint surfaces on each other with low resistance).[1, 2, 594]

The adhesion-cohesion effect is reduced by any factor that lowers the cohesion of joint fluid (e.g., in inflammatory joint disease), reduces wetability of the joint surfaces (as may occur in degenerative joint disease), or diminishes the glenohumeral contact area (e.g., in a displaced articular surface fracture or a congenitally small glenoid). It is also noteworthy that adhesion-cohesion forces do not stabilize a prosthetic shoulder replacement, because metal and polyethylene are insufficiently compliant to provide the necessary near-perfect congruence and because water does not adhere to their surfaces.

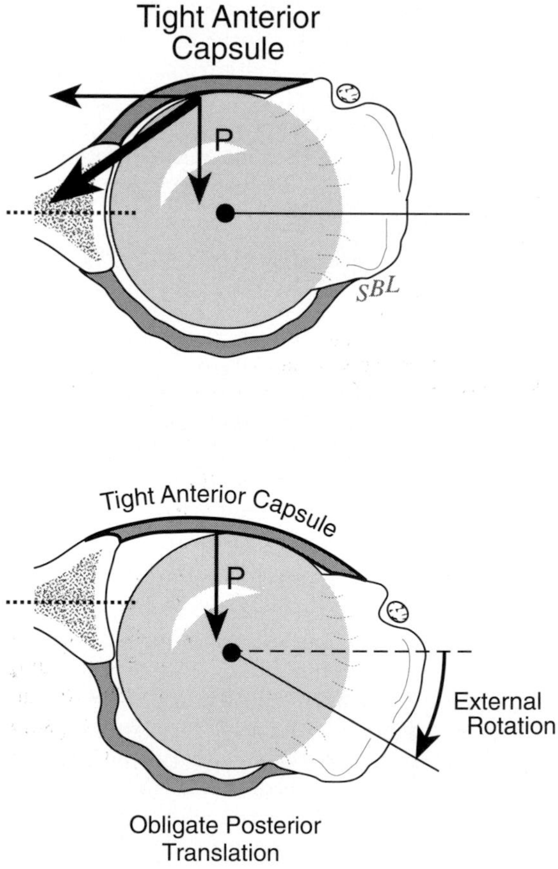

Figure 14–50

If the humerus is rotated beyond the point where the ligaments become tight, the displacing force (P) can push the humeral head out of the glenoid center—a phenomenon known as obligate translation. (Modified from Matsen FA III, Lippitt SB, Sidles JA, and Harryman DT II: Practical Evaluation and Management of the Shoulder. Philadelphia: WB Saunders, 1994.)

GLENOHUMERAL "SUCTION CUP"

This mechanism provides stability by virtue of the seal of the labrum and capsule to the humeral head (Fig. 14–51). A suction cup adheres to a smooth surface by expressing the interposed air or fluid and then forming a seal to the surface. A rubber suction cup is noncompliant in the center but becomes more flexible toward its periphery. In a similar manner, the center of the glenoid is covered with a relatively thin layer of articular cartilage. At greater distances from the center, the articular cartilage becomes thicker, providing greater flexibility. More peripherally, the glenoid labrum and, finally, the capsule provide even more flexibility. This graduated flexibility permits the socket to conform and seal to the smooth humeral articular surface. Compression of the head into the glenoid fossa expels any intervening fluid so that a "suction" is produced that resists distraction.

The glenoid suction cup stabilization mechanism was demonstrated by Harryman and associates.[228] In elderly cadaver shoulders without degenerative changes, the suction cup resisted an average of 20 ± 3 N of lateral traction (about 4 lb). Creation of a defect in the labrum completely eliminated the suction cup effect. No suction cup effect could be demonstrated in the two shoulders with mild degenerative change of the joint surface. It is likely that this effect would be even stronger in younger living shoulders in which the articular cartilage, glenoid labrum, and joint capsule are larger, more hydrated, and more compliant. Like stabilization from adhesion-cohesion, the glenoid suction cup centers the head of the humerus in the glenoid without muscle action and is effective in midrange positions in which the capsule and ligaments are not under tension.

LIMITED JOINT VOLUME

This is a stabilizing mechanism in which the humeral head is held to the glenoid by the relative vacuum created when they are distracted (Figs. 14–52 and 14–53). While it is common to speak of the glenohumeral joint space, there is essentially no space and minimal free fluid within the confines of the articular surfaces and the joint capsule of the normal glenohumeral joint. The scarcity of fluid within the joint can be confirmed on magnetic resonance imaging (MRI) scans of normal joints, on inspection of normal joints, and on attempts to aspirate fluid from normal joints. The appearance of the *potential* joint volume can only be demonstrated after instilling fluids such as air, saline, or contrast materials into the joint. Osmotic action by the synovium removes free fluid, keeping a slightly negative pressure within the normal joint.[357, 443, 594] This negative intra-articular pressure holds the joint together with a force proportional to the joint surface area and the magnitude of the negative intra-articular pressure. For example, if the colloid osmotic pressure of normal synovial fluid is 10 mm Hg and the colloid osmotic

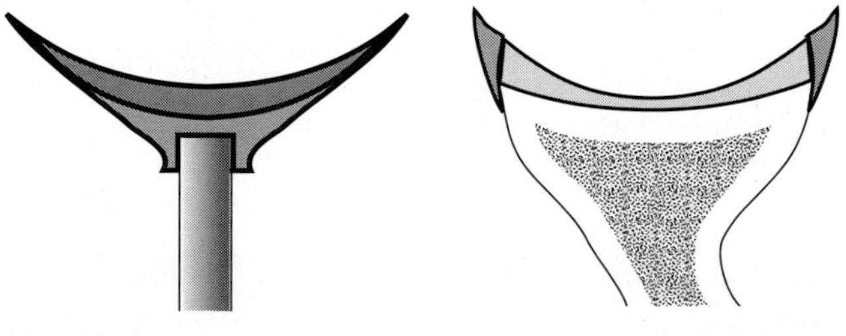

Figure 14–51

In cross-section, the glenoid looks much like a rubber suction cup with respect to its feathered, compliant edges and a more rigid center. (Modified from Matsen FA III, Lippitt SB, Sidles JA, and Harryman DT II: Practical Evaluation and Management of the Shoulder. Philadelphia: WB Saunders, 1994.)

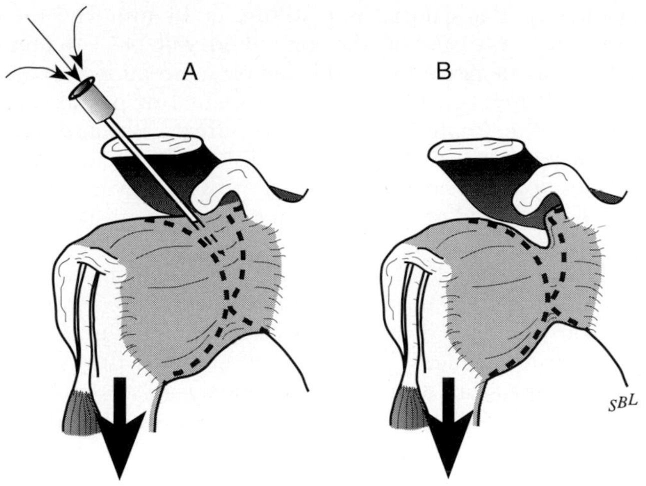

Figure 14–52

Normally, the glenohumeral capsule establishes a limited joint volume so that the distraction of the humeral head produces a relative vacuum within the capsule that resists further displacement. *A,* Venting of the capsule eliminates the limited joint volume effect. *B,* The limited joint volume effect is reduced if the capsule is excessively compliant, allowing its displacement into the joint. (From Matsen FA III, Lippitt SB, Sidles JA, and Harryman DT II: Practical Evaluation and Management of the Shoulder. Philadelphia: WB Saunders, 1994.)

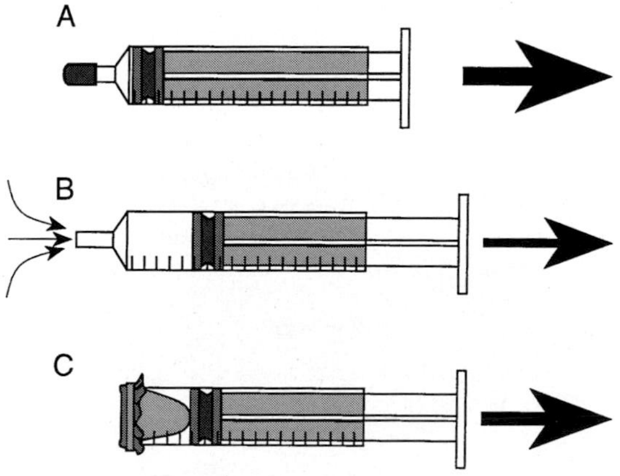

Figure 14–53

Limited joint volume effect demonstrated with a syringe model. Substantial force is required to pull the plunger from a plugged syringe *(A).* This stabilizing effect is lost if the syringe is uncapped *(B)* or if the end of the syringe is covered with a compliant material *(C).* (From Matsen FA III, Lippitt SB, Sidles JA, and Harryman DT II: Practical Evaluation and Management of the Shoulder. Philadelphia: WB Saunders, 1994.)

pressure of the synovial interstitium is 14 mm Hg, the equilibrium pressure in the joint fluid will be −4 mm Hg.[594] This negative intra-articular pressure adds a small amount of resistance to distraction (about 1 oz per square inch) to the limited joint volume effect. Because the normal joint is sealed, attempted distraction of the joint surfaces lowers the intra-articular pressure even more, progressively adding substantial resistance to greater displacement.[228, 286]

The limited joint volume effect is reduced if the joint is vented (opened to the atmosphere) or when the capsular boundaries of the joint are very compliant. Under the latter circumstances, attempted distraction draws the flexible capsule into the joint, producing a "sulcus" (see Figs. 14–52 and 14–53). The decreased stability from venting the joint was initially described by Humphry in 1858[273] and subsequently by others.[104, 158, 333, 449, 487, 488, 592, 632, 633, 706] Gibb and associates[191, 394] found that simply venting the capsule with an 18-gauge needle reduced the force necessary to translate the head of the humerus halfway to the edge of the glenoid by an average of 50%. Wulker found that venting the joint increased the joint displacement with an applied load of 50 N by 50% in all directions.[707]

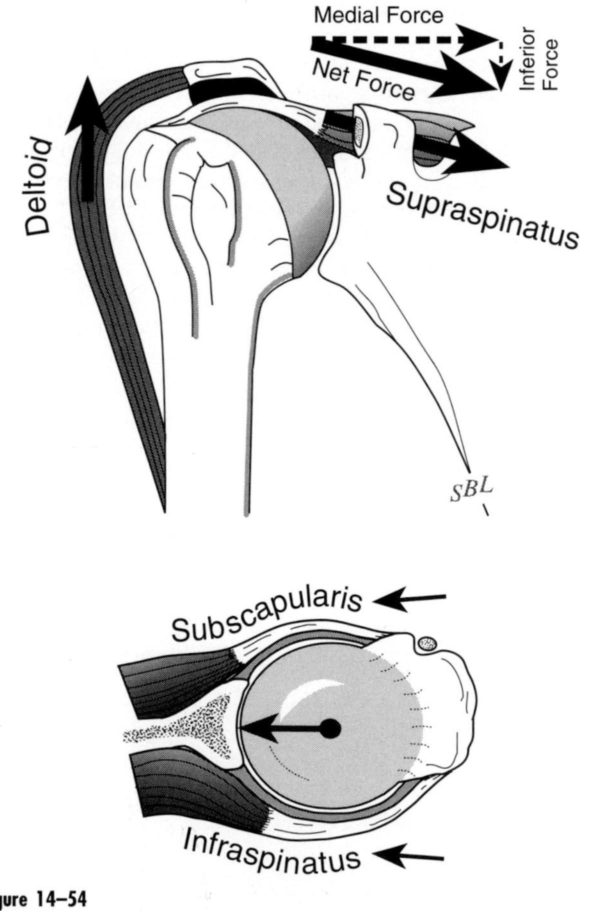

Figure 14–54

The supraspinatus muscle compresses the humeral head into the glenoid, providing stability against displacement by the deltoid force. It is not optimally oriented to depress the head of the humerus, because the inferiorly directed component of its force is small. (From Matsen FA III, Lippitt SB, Sidles JA, and Harryman DT II: Practical Evaluation and Management of the Shoulder. Philadelphia: WB Saunders, 1994.)

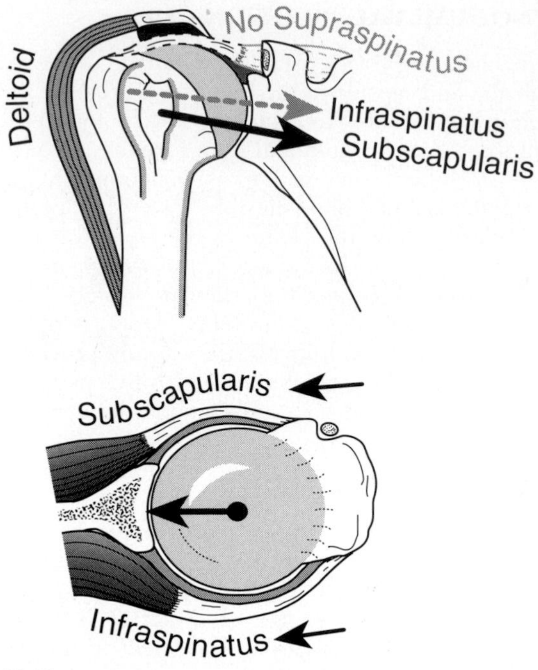

Figure 14–55

Compressive forces from the infraspinatus and subscapularis can stabilize the humeral head in the absence of a supraspinatus, provided the glenoid concavity is intact. (Modified from Matsen FA III, Lippitt SB, Sidles JA, and Harryman DT II: Practical Evaluation and Management of the Shoulder. Philadelphia: WB Saunders, 1994.)

From these results it is expected that glenohumeral stability from limited joint volume is compromised by arthrography, arthroscopy, articular effusions, hemarthrosis, and in other situations in which free fluid is allowed to enter the glenohumeral joint. In a very interesting study, Habermeyer and co-workers[217, 218] found that the mean stabilizing force obtained by atmospheric pressure was 146 N (32 lb). In 15 stable living shoulders, traction on the arm caused negative intra-articular pressure proportionate to the amount of force exerted. In contrast, unstable shoulder joints with a Bankart lesion did not exhibit this phenomenon.

These stabilizing mechanisms may be overwhelmed by the application of traction, such as in the cracking of the metacarpophalangeal joint. A "crack" is produced as the joint cavitates: subatmospheric pressure within the joint releases gas (more than 80% carbon dioxide) from solution in the joint fluid. This is accompanied by a sudden increase in the separation of the joint surfaces. Once a joint has cracked, it cannot be cracked again until about 20 minutes later when all the gas has been reabsorbed.[551, 650]

Superior Stability: The Same Plus a Unique Addition

Superior stability benefits from all the same mechanisms as anterior, posterior, and inferior stability: glenoid orientation, muscle balance, glenoid shape, ligamentous effects, adhesion-cohesion, the suction cup, and limited joint volume. Compression of the humeral head into the glenoid concavity is an important mechanism by which the head of the humerus is centered and stabilized in the glenoid fossa to resist superiorly directed loads (Fig. 14–54). Even when a substantial supraspinatus defect is present, compression from the subscapularis and infraspinatus can hold the humeral head centered in the glenoid (Fig. 14–55). More severe cases of chronic rotator cuff deficiency, however, may be associated with superior subluxation of the head of the humerus and wear on the superior lip of the glenoid fossa (Fig. 14–56). This erosive wear flattens the superior glenoid concavity and thus reduces the effective glenoid depth in that direction. Once the effective superior glenoid depth is lost, repair of the rotator cuff tendons or complex capsular reconstructions cannot completely restore the glenohumeral stability previously provided by concavity compression (see Fig. 14–56).

In addition to the mechanisms that stabilize the shoulder in other directions, there is a unique aspect of superior stability: the ceiling effect provided by the superior cuff tendon interposed between the humeral head and the coracoacromial arch. As every shoulder surgeon has observed, in the normal shoulder in a resting position there is no gap between the humeral head, the superior cuff tendon, and the coracoacromial arch. As a result, the slightest amount of superior translation compresses the cuff tendon between the humeral and the arch. Thus when the humeral head is pressed upwards (e.g., when pushing up from an arm chair or with isometric contraction of the deltoid), further superior displacement is opposed by a downward force exerted by the coracoacromial arch through the cuff tendon to the humeral head. Ziegler and associates[716] demonstrated this stabilizing effect in cadavers by demonstrating acromial deformation when the neutrally positioned humerus was loaded in a superior direction. By attaching strain gauges percutaneously to the acromion they were able to measure its deformation under load. The acromion thus became an in situ load transducer. By applying known loads to the acromion, they were able to derive calibration load-deformation curves that were essentially linear. Superiorly directed loads applied to the humerus were then correlated with resultant acromial loads and with superior humeral displacement. In 10 fresh cadaver specimens with the superior cuff tendon intact but not under tension, superiorly directed loads of 80 N produced only 1.7 mm of superior displacement of the humeral head relative to the acromion. When the cuff tendon was excised, a similar load produced a superior displacement of 5.4 mm ($P < .0001$). In specimens where the cuff tendon was intact, an upward load of 20 N gave rise to an estimated acromial load of 8 N. Greater humeral loads up to 80 N were associated with a linear increase in acromial load up to 55 N when an upward load of 80 N was applied (Fig. 14–57). In a single in vivo experiment where the acromion was instrumented and calibrated as in the cadavers, very similar relationships between upward humeral load and acromial load were noted (see Fig. 14–57). These acromial loads must have been transmitted through the intact cuff tendon. When the tendon was excised, the humeral head rose until it contacted and again loaded the acromial undersurface (Fig. 14–58).

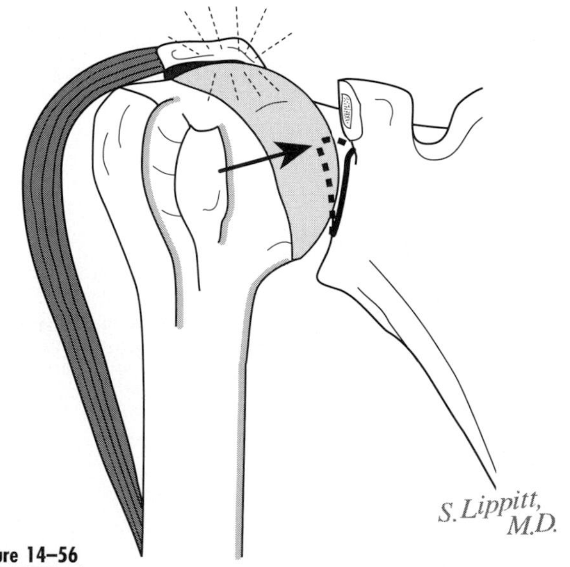

Figure 14–56

Erosion of the superior glenoid concavity compromises the concavity compression stability mechanism, allowing upward translation. (Modified from Matsen FA III, Lippitt SB, Sidles JA, and Harryman DT II: Practical Evaluation and Management of the Shoulder. Philadelphia: WB Saunders, 1994.)

Flatow and associates[168] used a cadaver model to explore the active and passive restraints to superior humeral translation. Whereas Ziegler's study was conducted with the arm in a neutral position with axial loads, Flatow's involved abducting the humerus with simulated deltoid and cuff muscle forces. Both groups noted that the presence of the supraspinatus tendon limited superior translation of the humeral head, even if there was no tension from simulated muscle action.

Both Ziegler and Flatow cautioned that the effectiveness of the cuff tendon as a superior stabilizing mechanism is dependent on an intact coracoacromial arch. Sacrifice of the ceiling of the joint, the coracoacromial ligament, or the undersurface of the acromion can be expected to compromise the resistance to superior displacement of the humeral head.

The reader is referred to a review of the stabilization of the glenohumeral joint surfaces by articular contact and by contact in the subacromial space authored by Soslowsky and associates (see Chapter 5).[393]

TYPES OF GLENOHUMERAL INSTABILITY

Glenohumeral instability is the inability to maintain the humeral head centered in the glenoid fossa.[393, 394] Clinical cases of instability can be characterized according to the circumstances under which they occur, the degree of instability, and the direction of instability.

Circumstances of Instability

Congenital instability may result from local anomalies, such as glenoid dysplasia[695] or systemic conditions such as

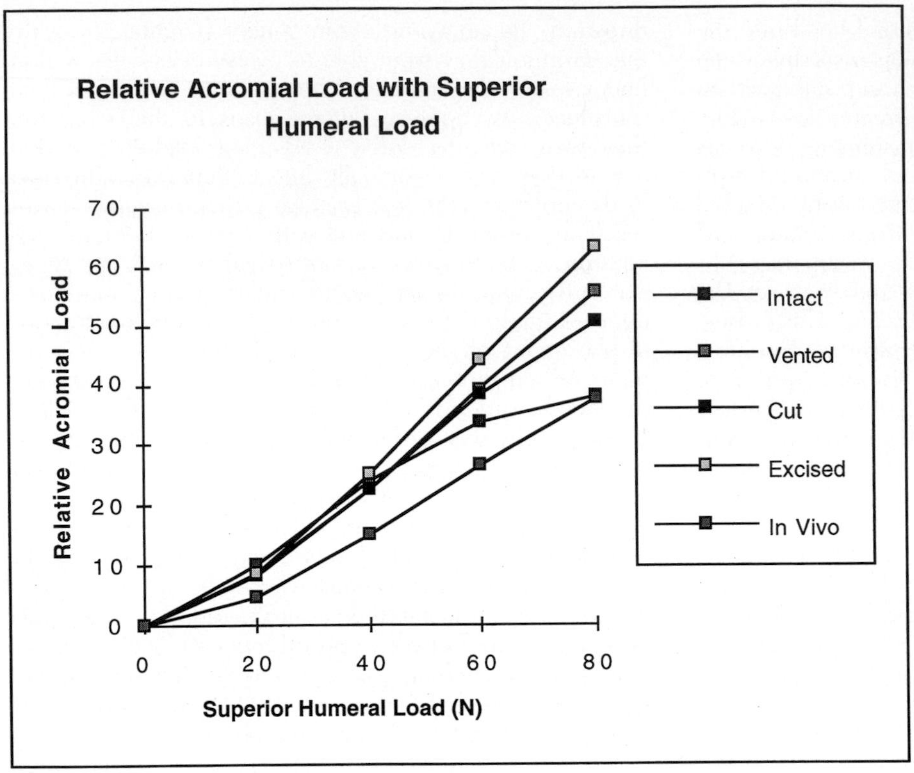

Figure 14–57

Relative acromial load as a function of superiorly directed humeral load. The chart compares loads for (1) intact specimens, (2) after venting of the joint to air, (3) after cutting (but not excising the cuff tendon), and (4) after excising the superior cuff tendon. Also included are the data from (5) a single in vivo experiment done with the identical instrumentation. Note that there is minimal difference in these acromial load—humeral load relationships, even when the cuff tendon has been excised. In this latter case, the humeral head loaded the acromion directly, rather than through the interposed cuff tendon.

Ehlers-Danlos syndrome. Instability is acute if seen within the first days after its onset; otherwise, it is chronic. A dislocation is locked (or fixed) if the humeral head has been impaled on the edge of the glenoid, making reduction of the dislocation difficult. If a glenohumeral joint has been unstable on multiple occasions, the instability is recurrent. Recurrent instability may consist of repeated glenohumeral dislocations, subluxations, or both.

Instability may arise from a traumatic episode in which an injury occurs to the bone, rotator cuff, labrum, capsule, or a combination of ligaments. Recurrent traumatic instability typically produces symptoms when the arm is placed

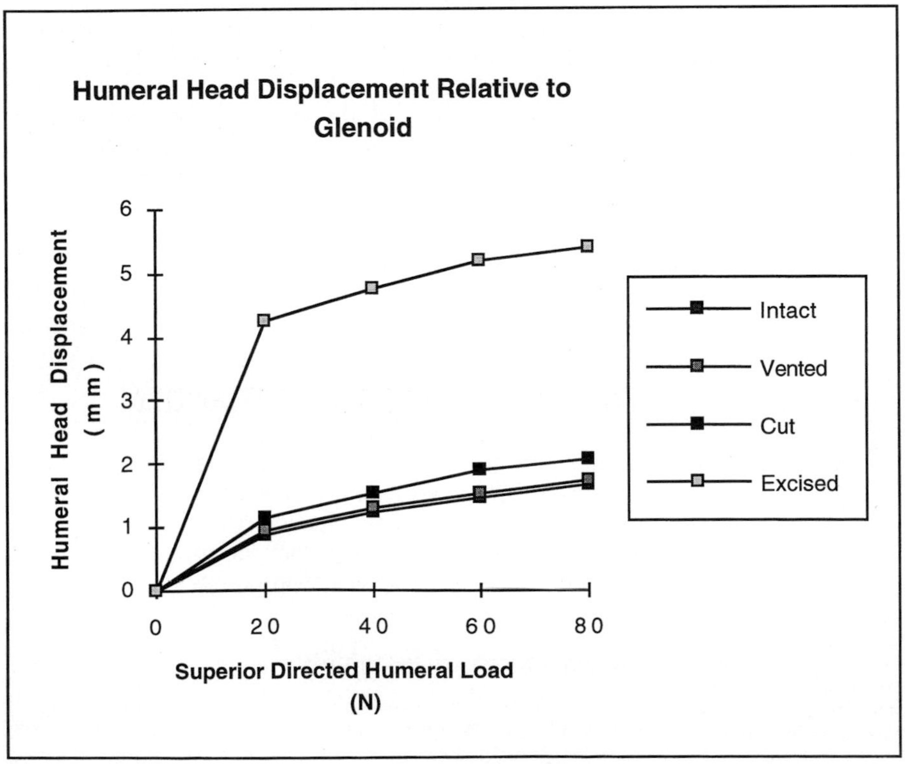

Figure 14–58

Mean superior humeral displacement (relative to the scapula) as a function of superior humerus load. The chart compares displacements for (1) intact specimens, (2) after venting of the joint to air, (3) after cutting (but not excising the cuff tendon), and (4) after excising the superior cuff tendon.

in positions near that of the original injury. Conversely, instability may arise from the atraumatic decompensation of the stabilizing mechanisms. The degree to which the shoulder was "torn loose" as opposed to "born loose" or just "got loose" is critical in determining the best management strategy.

We have found that most patients with recurrent instability fall into one of two groups. On one hand, patients with a *traumatic* etiology usually have *unidirectional* instability; often have obvious pathology, such as a *Bankart* lesion; and often require *surgery* when instability is recurrent, thus the acronym: *TUBS*. On the other hand, patients with *atraumatic* instability often have *multidirectional* laxity, which is frequently *bilateral* and usually responds to a *rehabilitation* program. However, if surgery is performed, the surgeon must pay particular attention to performing an *inferior* capsular shift and closing the rotator *interval*, thus the acronym: *AMBRII*. Rowe[552] carefully analyzed 500 dislocations of the glenohumeral joint and determined that 96% were traumatic (caused by a major injury) and the remaining 4% were atraumatic. DePalma,[123] Rockwood,[540] and Collins and Wilde[98] also recognized the importance of distinguishing between traumatic and atraumatic instability of the shoulder.

Patients with atraumatic instability may have generalized joint laxity. Imazato[278] and Hirakawa[258] demonstrated that patients with "loose" shoulders have relatively immature, more soluble, and less cross-linked collagen fibers in their capsule, muscles, and skin than do controls; presumably, tissues like the glenoid labrum would also contain immature collagen, thus making them more deformable under load. Further evidence of constitutional factors is gained from a number of reports of positive family histories and bilateral involvement among those individuals with shoulder dislocations (Fig. 14–59). O'Driscoll and Evans[478] and Dowdy and O'Driscoll[134] found a family history of shoulder instability in 24% of patients who required surgery for anterior glenohumeral instability. Morrey and Janes[436] reported a positive family history in approximately 15% of patients who were operated on for recurrent anterior shoulder instability. A positive family history was also noted twice as frequently in patients whose postoperative course was complicated by recurrent instability compared with patients with successful surgery. Rowe and colleagues[555] reported a positive family in 27% of 55 patients with anterior shoulder instability who were treated with a Bankart procedure. Bilateral instability was noted in 50% of patients with a positive family history compared with 26% of patients with negative family history, which suggested the possibility of a genetic predisposition.

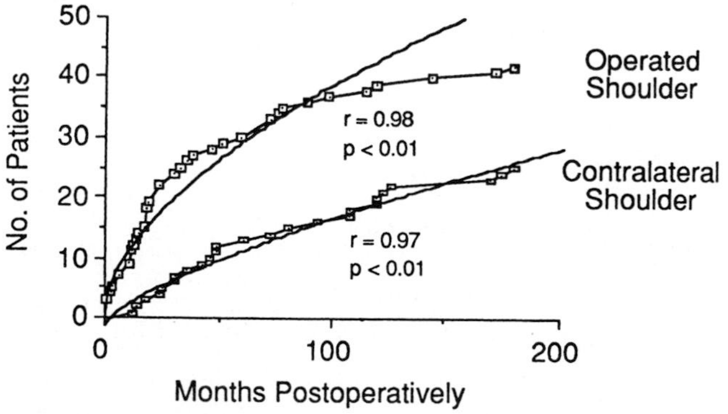

Figure 14–59

Incidence of contralateral shoulder instability from the data of O'Driscoll and Evans. (From O'Driscoll SW and Evans DC: The DuToit Staple Capsulorrhaphy for Recurrent Anterior Dislocation of the Shoulder: Twenty Years of Experience in Six Toronto Hospitals. American Shoulder and Elbow Surgeons 4th Open Meeting, Atlanta, 1988.) Thirteen per cent of the patients with normal contralateral shoulders at the time of surgery developed contralateral instability within the next 15 years.

When instability develops with no or minimal injury,[183, 518, 559] the initial reason for the loss of stability is often unclear. However, it appears that once lost, the factors that maintain stability may be difficult to regain. Certain phenomena may be self-perpetuating: When the humeral head rides up on the glenoid rim, the rim becomes flattened and less effective, allowing easier translation. Furthermore, when normal neuromuscular control is compromised, the feedback systems that maintain head centering fail to provide effective input. Thus, the joint becomes launched on a cycle of instability leading to loss of the effective glenoid concavity and loss of neuromuscular control leading to more instability.

If a patient intentionally subluxates or dislocates his or her shoulder, instability is described as voluntary. If the instability occurs unintentionally, it is involuntary. Voluntary and involuntary instability may coexist. Voluntary anterior dislocation may occur with the arm at the side or in abduction/external rotation. Voluntary posterior dislocation may occur with the arm in flexion, adduction, and internal rotation or with the arm at the side. The association of voluntary dislocations of the shoulder with emotional instability and psychiatric problems has been noted by several authors (Figs. 14–60 and 14–61).[77, 556] The desire to voluntarily dislocate the shoulder cannot be treated surgically. However, the fact that patients can voluntarily demonstrate their instability does not necessarily mean they are emotionally impaired.

Neuromuscular causes of shoulder instability have been reported as well. Percy[506] described a woman who, after an episode of encephalitis, developed a posterior dislocation. Kretzler and Blue[326] have discussed the management of posterior dislocations of the shoulder in children with cerebral palsy. Sever,[586] Fairbank,[157] L'Episcopo,[335] Zachary,[715] and Wickstrom[686] have reported techniques for the management of neurologic dislocation of the shoulder caused by upper brachial plexus birth injuries. Stroke is another important neurologic cause of instability.[720]

Degree of Instability

Recurrent instability may be characterized as dislocation, subluxation, or apprehension. Dislocation of the glenohumeral joint is the complete separation of the articular surfaces; immediate, spontaneous relocation may not occur. Glenohumeral subluxation is defined as symptomatic translation of the humeral head on the glenoid without complete separation of the articular surfaces. Subluxation of the glenohumeral joint is usually transient, with the

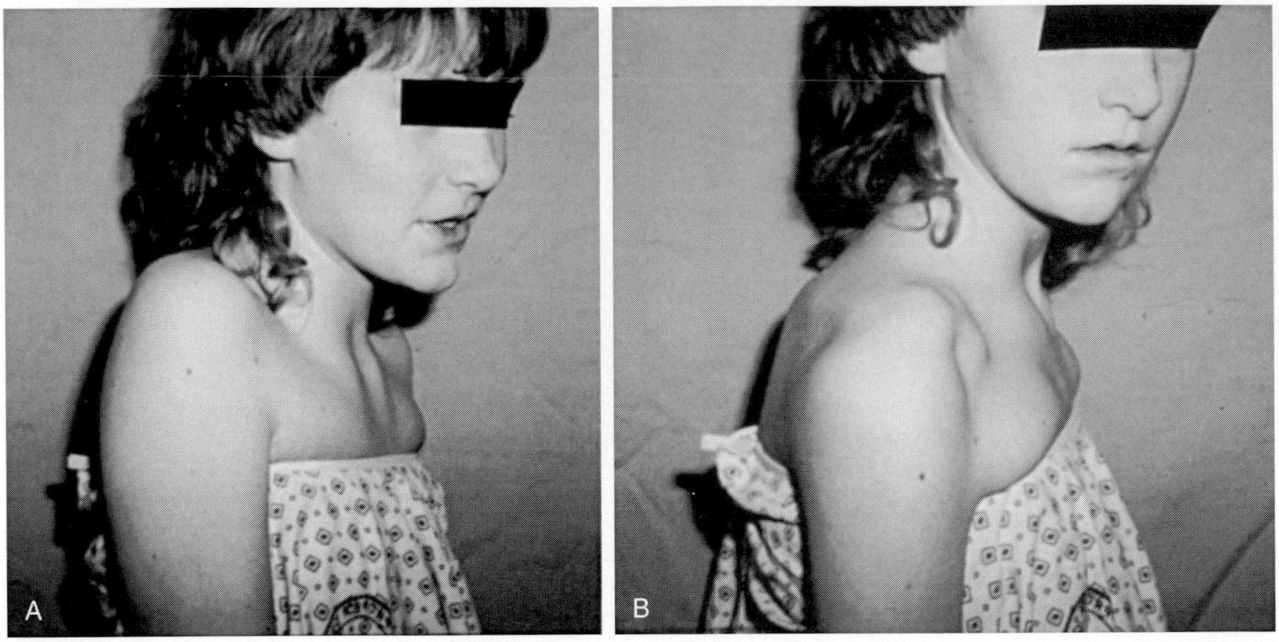

Figure 14–60

Voluntary instability. This patient had no significant history of injury but could voluntarily dislocate her shoulder with minimal discomfort. The patient is shown with the right shoulder reduced *(A)* and posteriorly dislocated *(B)*.

humeral head returning spontaneously to its normal position in the glenoid fossa. In a series of patients with anterior shoulder subluxation reported by Rowe and Zarins,[559] 87% were traumatic and more than 50% were not aware that their shoulders were unstable. Like dislocations, subluxations may be traumatic or atraumatic, anterior, posterior, or inferior, acute, or recurrent, or they may occur after previous surgical repairs that did not achieve complete shoulder stability. Recurrent subluxations may coexist with or be initiated by glenohumeral dislocation. Rowe and Zarins[552, 560] reported seeing a Hill-Sachs compression fracture in 40% of the patients in

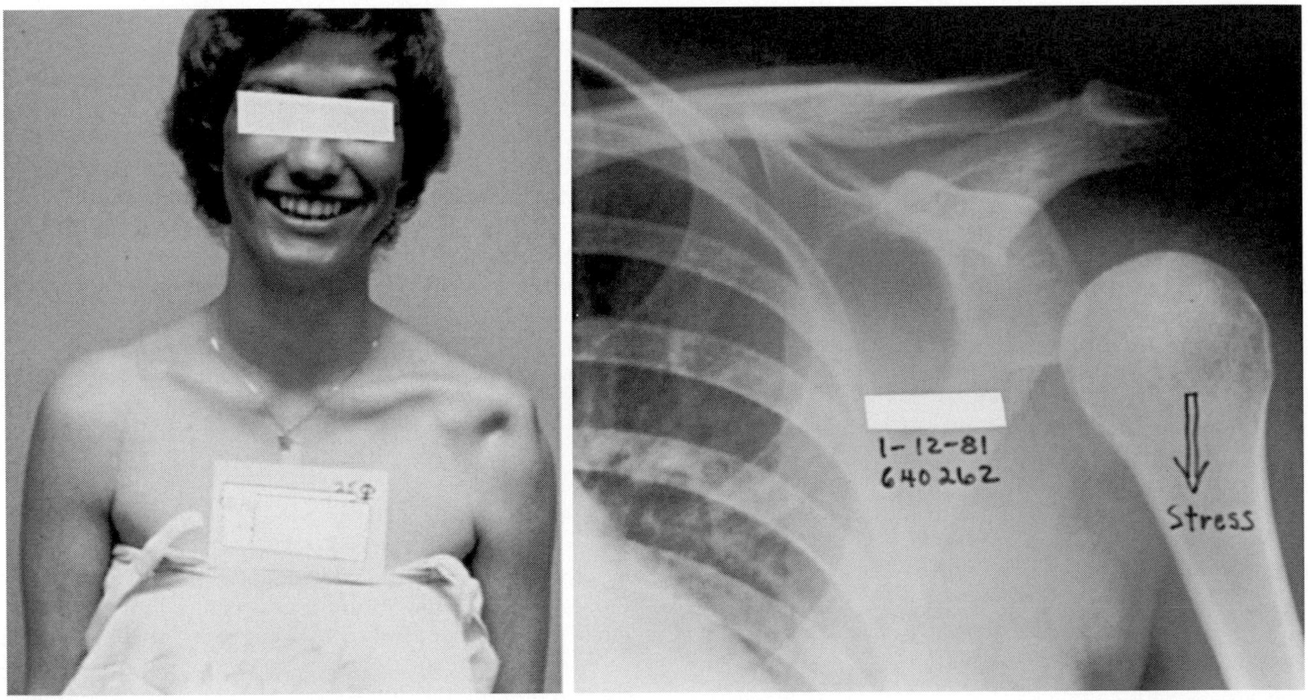

Figure 14–61

A patient with voluntary inferior instability. She performed this maneuver without discomfort. (From Rockwood CA and Green DP [eds]: Fractures [3 vols], 2nd ed. Philadelphia: JB Lippincott, 1984.)

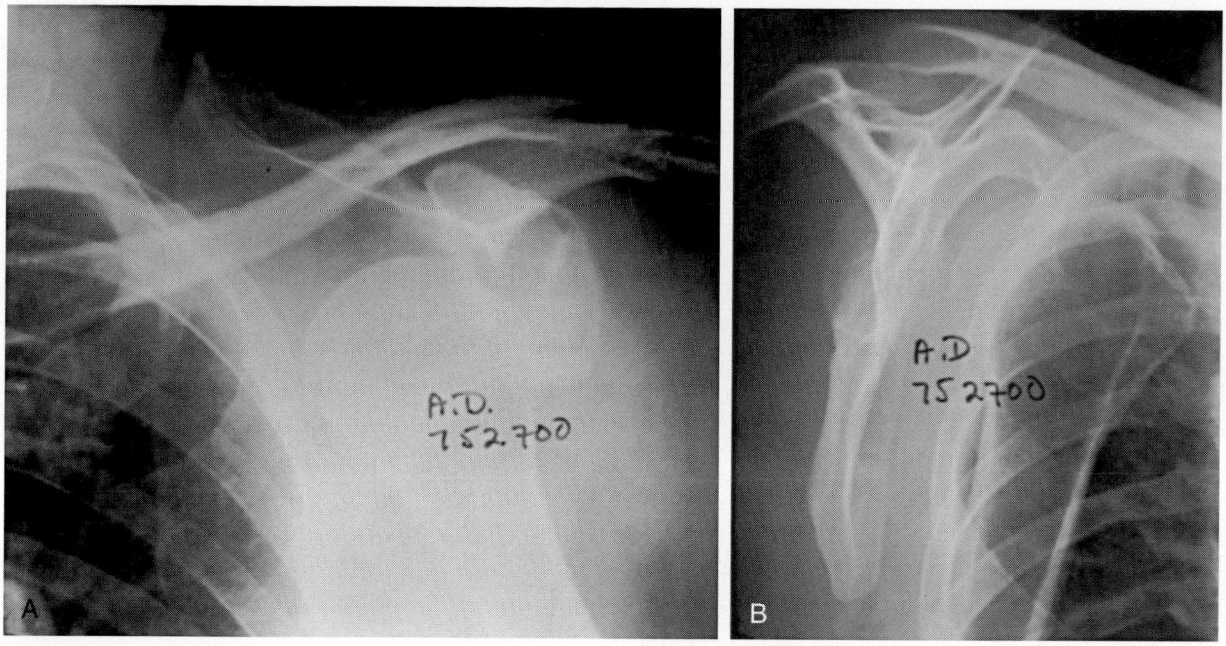

Figure 14–62

Subcoracoid dislocation. *A,* This anteroposterior view reveals that the head is medially displaced away from the glenoid fossa. On this view, it is difficult to be sure whether the head is dislocated anteriorly or posteriorly. *B,* On the true scapular lateral view, the humeral head is completely anterior to the glenoid fossa. (From Rockwood CA and Green DP [eds]: Fractures [3 vols], 2nd ed. Philadelphia: JB Lippincott, 1984.)

their series on subluxation of the shoulder, an observation indicating that at some time these shoulders had been completely dislocated. Apprehension refers to the fear that the shoulder will subluxate or dislocate. This fear may prevent the individual from participating fully in work or sports.

Directions of Instability

Dislocations of the shoulder account for approximately 45% of all dislocations.[315] Of these, almost 85% are anterior glenohumeral dislocations.[85]

ANTERIOR DISLOCATIONS

Subcoracoid dislocation is the most common type of anterior dislocation. The usual mechanism of injury that causes subcoracoid dislocations is a combination of shoulder abduction, extension, and external rotation producing forces that challenge the anterior capsule and ligaments, the glenoid rim, and the rotator cuff mechanism. The head of the humerus is displaced anteriorly with respect to the glenoid and is inferior to the coracoid process (Fig. 14–62). Other types of anterior dislocation include subglenoid (the head of the humerus lies anterior to and below the glenoid fossa), subclavicular (the head of the humerus lies medial to the coracoid process, just inferior to the lower border of the clavicle), intrathoracic (the head of the humerus lies between the ribs and the thoracic cavity) (Fig. 14–63),[193, 439, 503, 576, 683] and retroperitoneal (Figs. 14–64 and 14–65).[694] These rarer types of dislocation are usually associated with severe trauma and have a high incidence of fracture of the greater tuberosity of the humerus and rotator cuff avulsion. Neurologic, pulmonary, and vascular complications can occur, as can subcutaneous emphysema. West[683] reported a case of intrathoracic dislocation in which with reduction the humerus was felt to slip out of the chest cavity with a sensation similar to that of slipping a large cork from a bottle. His patient, who had an avulsion fracture of the

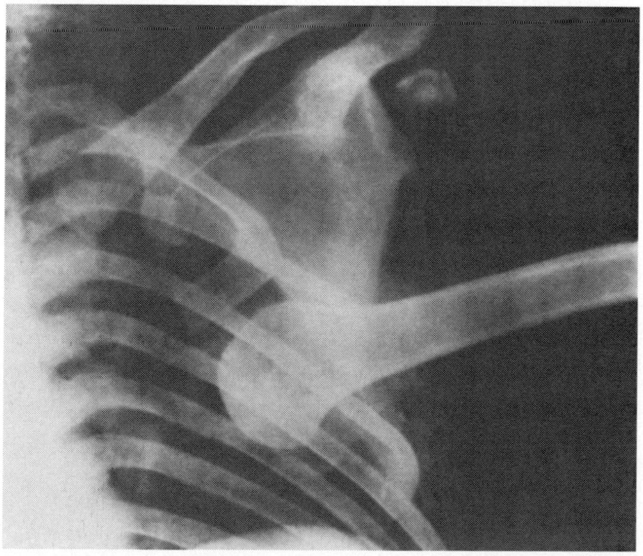

Figure 14–63

An intrathoracic anterior dislocation of the left shoulder. Note the wide interspace laterally between the third and fourth ribs and the avulsion fracture of the greater tuberosity, which remained in the vicinity of the glenoid fossa. (From Rockwood CA Jr, Green DP, and Bucholz RW [eds]: Fractures in Adults. Philadelphia: JB Lippincott, 1991.)

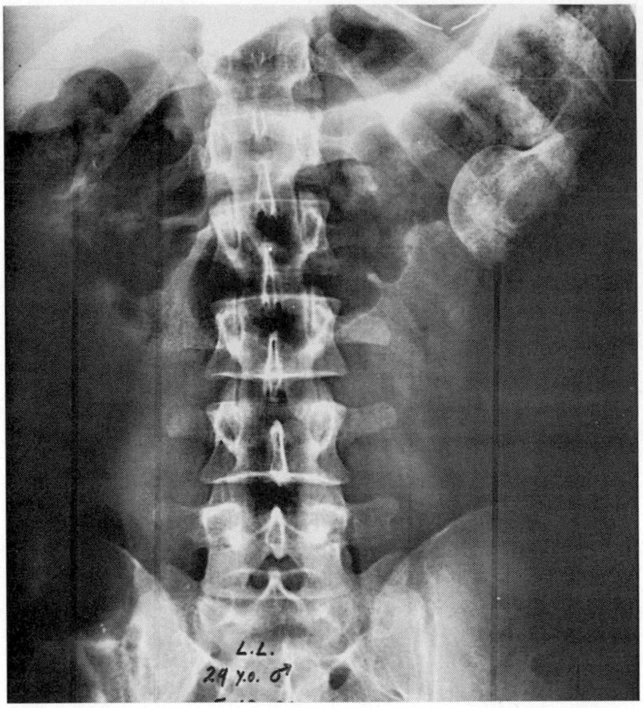

Figure 14–64

An abdominal radiograph revealing the proximal humerus in the left upper quadrant *(arrow).*

greater tuberosity and no neurologic deficit, regained a functional range of motion and returned to his job as a carpenter.

POSTERIOR DISLOCATIONS

Posterior dislocations may leave the humeral head in a subacromial (head behind the glenoid and beneath the acromion), subglenoid (head behind and beneath the glenoid), or subspinous (head medial to acromion and beneath the spine of the scapula) location. The subacromial dislocation is the most common by far (Fig. 14–66). Posterior dislocations are frequently locked. Hawkins and coworkers[238] reviewed 41 such cases related to motor vehicle accidents, surgeries, and electroshock therapy.

The incidence of posterior dislocations is estimated at 2% but is difficult to ascertain because of the frequency with which this diagnosis is missed. Thomas[628] reported seeing only four cases of posterior shoulder dislocation in 6000 x-ray examinations. The literature reflects that the diagnosis of posterior dislocation of the shoulder is missed in more than 60% of cases.[149, 240, 418, 504, 660] A 1982 article by Rowe and Zarins[560] indicates that the diagnosis was missed in 79% of cases! McLaughlin[406] stated that posterior shoulder dislocations are sufficiently uncommon that their occurrence creates a "diagnostic trap."

One of the largest series of posterior dislocations of the shoulder (37 cases) was recorded by Malgaigne[388] in 1855, 40 years before the discovery of x-rays. Malgaigne and colleagues made the diagnosis by performing a proper physical examination! Cooper[101] stated that the physical findings are so classic that he called it "an accident which cannot be mistaken."

Posterior dislocation may result from axial loading of

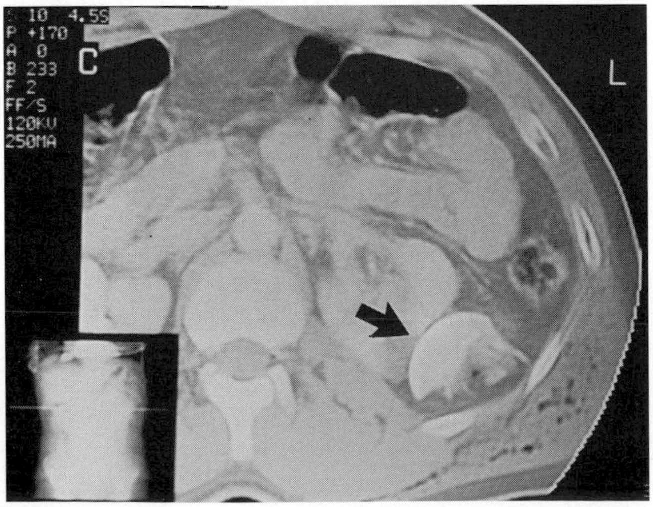

Figure 14–65

An enhanced computed tomography scan of the abdomen. Note the retroperitoneal location of the humeral head posterior to the left kidney *(arrow).*

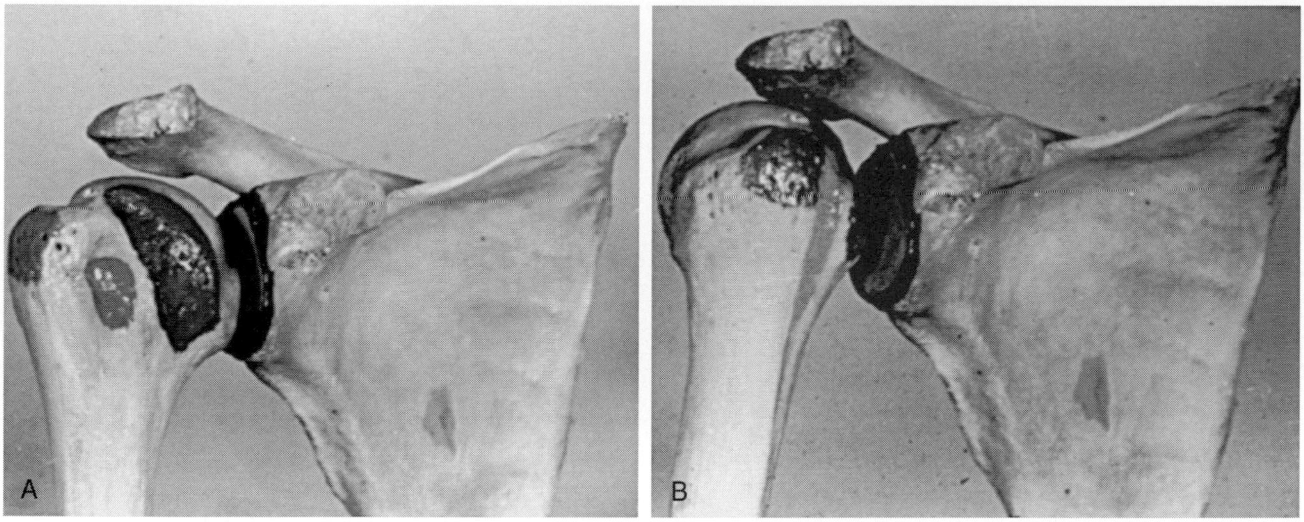

Figure 14–66

The subacromial posterior dislocation can appear deceptively normal on x-rays. *A,* Normal position of the humeral head in the glenoid fossa. *B,* In the subacromial type of posterior shoulder dislocation, the arm is in full internal rotation, and the articular surface of the head is completely posterior, leaving only the lesser tuberosity in the glenoid fossa. This positioning explains why abduction—and particularly external rotation—is blocked in posterior dislocations of the shoulder. (From Rockwood CA and Green DP [eds]: Fractures [3 vols], 2nd ed. Philadelphia: JB Lippincott, 1984.)

the adducted, internally rotated arm[429] or from violent muscle contraction or by electrical shock or convulsive seizures.[5, 77, 166, 232, 363, 400, 423, 483, 518, 584] In the case of involuntary muscle contraction, the combined strength of the internal rotators (latissimus dorsi, pectoralis major, and subscapularis muscles) simply overwhelms the external rotators (infraspinatus and teres minor muscles) (Fig. 14–67). Heller and associates have proposed a classification for posterior shoulder dislocation.[242]

INFERIOR DISLOCATIONS

Inferior dislocation of the glenohumeral joint was first described by Middeldorpf and Scharm[420] in 1859. Lynn[379]

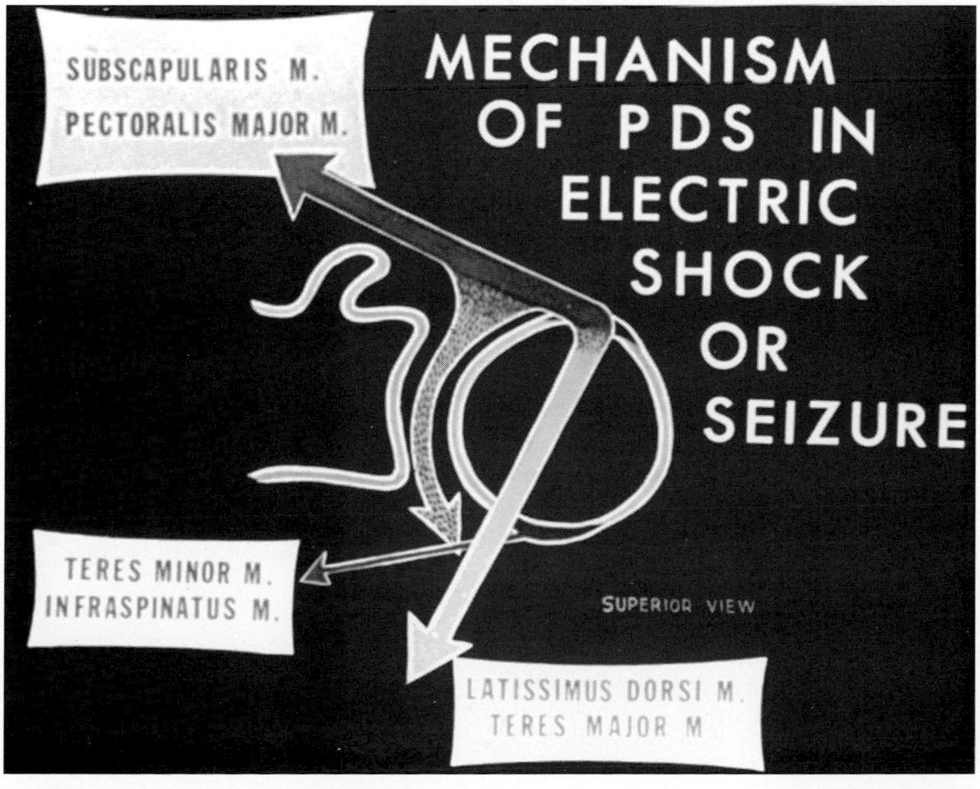

Figure 14–67

Mechanism of posterior dislocation of the shoulder that is caused by an accidental electrical shock or a convulsive seizure. The strong internal rotators simply overpower the weak external rotators.

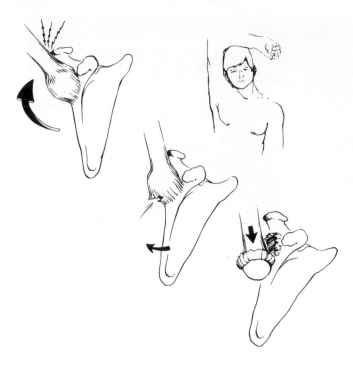

Figure 14–68

Mechanism of luxatio erecta. With hyperabduction of the humerus, the shaft abuts the acromion process, which stresses and then tears the capsule inferiorly and levers the head out inferiorly. The head and neck may be buttonholed through a rent in the inferior capsule, or the entire capsule may be separated. The rotator cuff muscles are always detached, and there may be an associated fracture of the greater tuberosity. (From Rockwood CA Jr, Green DP, and Bucholz RW [eds]: Fractures in Adults. Philadelphia: JB Lippincott, 1991.)

in 1921 carefully reviewed 34 cases, and in 1962 Roca and Ramos-Vertiz[539] reviewed 50 cases from the world literature. Laskin and Sedlin[343] reported a case in an infant. Three bilateral cases have been reported by Murrard,[445] Langfritz,[342] and Peiro and co-workers.[505] Nobel[466] reported a case of subglenoid dislocation in which the acromion-olecranon distance was shortened by 1.5 inches.

Inferior dislocation may be produced by a hyperabduction force that causes abutment of the neck of the humerus against the acromion process, which levers the head out inferiorly (Figs. 14–68 to 14–71). The humerus is then locked with the head below the glenoid fossa and the humeral shaft pointing overhead, a condition called luxatio erecta (Fig. 14–72; see also Fig. 14–68). The clinical picture of a patient with luxatio erecta is so clear that it can hardly be mistaken for any other condition. The humerus is locked in a position somewhere between 110 and 160 degrees of adduction (see Figs. 14–69 and 14–70). Severe soft tissue injury or fractures about the proximal humerus occur with this dislocation (see Figs. 14–69 and 14–72). At the time of surgery or autopsy, various authors have found avulsion of the supraspinatus, pectoralis major, or teres minor muscles and fractures of the greater tuberosity.[329, 343, 379, 420, 445, 539] Neurovascular involvement is common.[179, 356, 379, 416] Lev-El and associates[356] reported a patient who had an injury to the axillary artery and subsequently developed a thrombus that required resection and vein graft. Gardham and Scott[179]

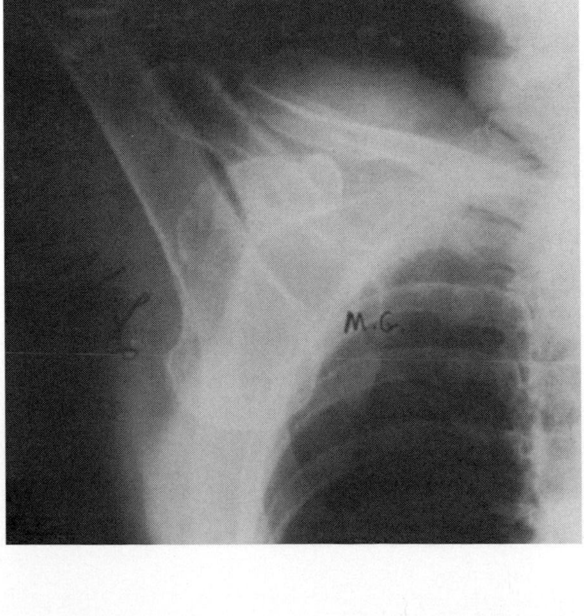

Figure 14–69

Anteroposterior x-ray film of the inferior dislocation reveals that the entire humeral head and surgical neck of the humerus are inferior to the glenoid fossa. (From Rockwood CA Jr, Green DP, and Bucholz RW [eds]: Fractures in Adults. Philadelphia: JB Lippincott, 1991.)

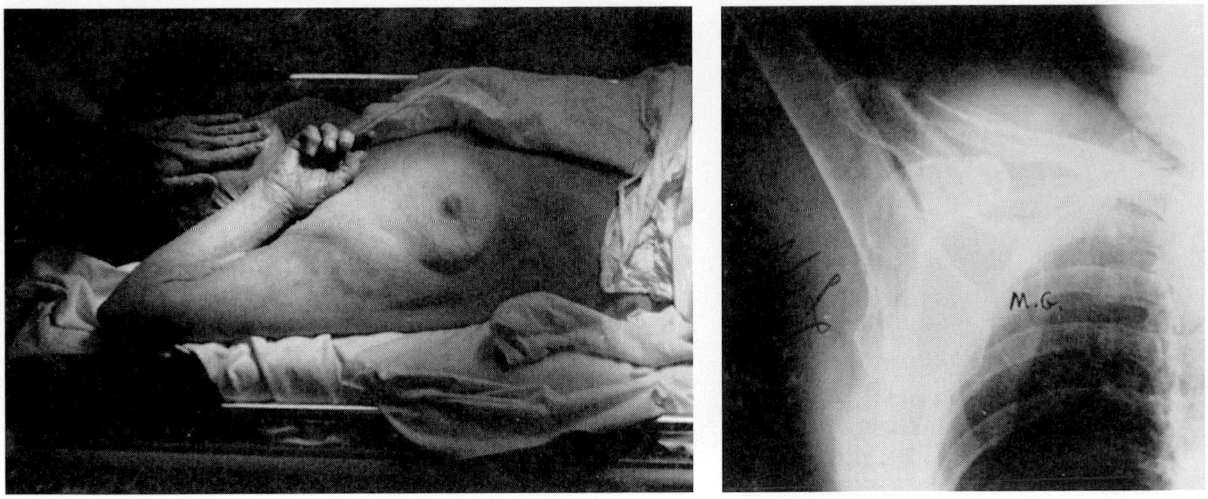

Figure 14–70

Inferior dislocation (luxatio erecta) of the right shoulder in a 75-year-old woman. Note that the arm is directed upward in relationship to the trunk *(left)*. The hand of the flexed elbow is lying on the anterior chest. An anteroposterior x-ray film of the inferior dislocation reveals that the entire humeral head and surgical neck of the humerus are inferior to the glenoid fossa *(right)*. (From Rockwood CA Jr, Green DP, and Bucholz RW [eds]: Fractures in Adults. Philadelphia: JB Lippincott, 1991.)

reported a case in 1980 in which the axillary artery was damaged in its third part and was managed by a bypass graft using the saphenous vein. Rockwood and Wirth found that in 19 patients with this condition, all 19 had a brachial plexus injury and some vascular compromise before reduction. The force may be so great as to force the head out through the soft tissues and the skin. Lucas and Peterson[376] have reported a case of a 16-year-old boy who caught his arm in the power take-off of a tractor and suffered an open luxatio erecta injury. Reduction of an inferior dislocation can often be accomplished by traction and countertraction maneuvers (Fig. 14–73). When closed reduction cannot be accomplished, the buttonhole rent in the inferior capsule must be surgically enlarged before reduction can occur.

SUPERIOR DISLOCATIONS

Speed[605] reported that Langier, in 1834, was the first to record a case of superior dislocation of the glenohumeral joint; Stimson reviewed 14 cases that had been reported in the literature prior to 1912.[618] In current literature little is mentioned about this type of dislocation, but undoubtedly occasional cases do occur. The usual cause is an extreme forward and upward force on the adducted arm. With displacement of the humerus upward, fractures

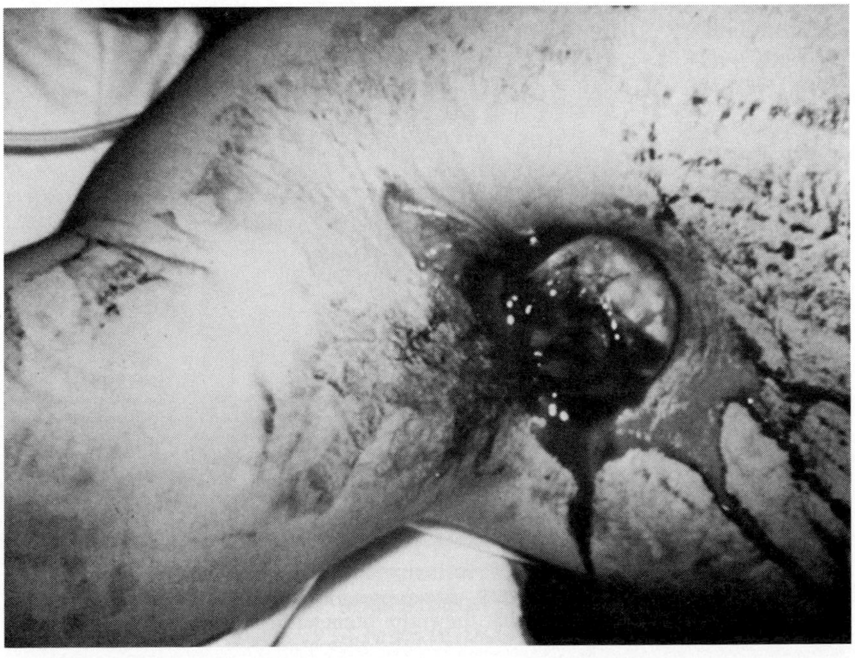

Figure 14–71

Photograph of the right shoulder and axilla of a patient who had an open inferior dislocation of the humeral head out through the axilla. (Courtesy of George Armstrong.) (From Rockwood CA Jr, Green DP, and Bucholz RW [eds]: Fractures in Adults. Philadelphia: JB Lippincott, 1991.)

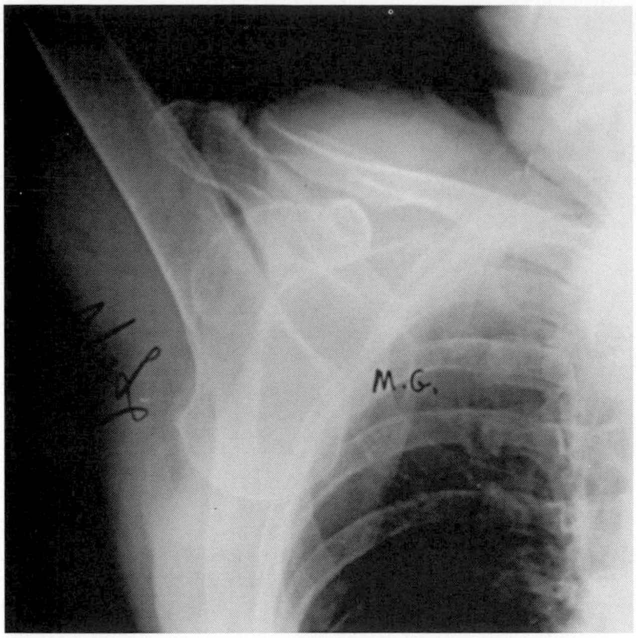

Figure 14–72

This anteroposterior x-ray of the inferior dislocation reveals that the entire humeral head and surgical neck of the humerus are inferior to the glenoid fossa.

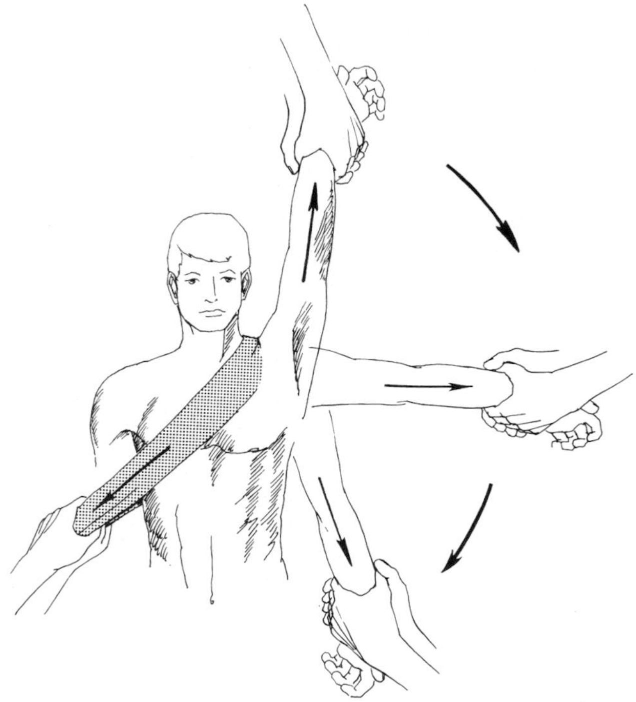

Figure 14–73

Technique of reduction of an inferior dislocation (luxatio erecta) of the glenohumeral joint. Countertraction is applied by an assistant using a folded sheet across the superior aspect of the shoulder and neck. Traction on the arm is first applied upward, and then gradually the arm is brought into less abduction and finally placed at the patient's side as demonstrated. (From Rockwood CA Jr, Green DP, and Bucholz RW [eds]: Fractures in Adults. Philadelphia: JB Lippincott, 1991.)

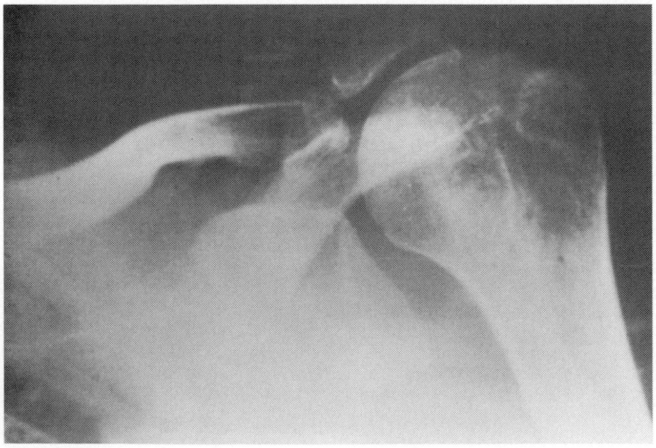

Figure 14–74

Superior dislocation of the left shoulder. Note that the head of the humerus is displaced superiorly from the glenoid fossa and that the fracture of the acromion process has also been displaced upward. (From Rockwood CA Jr, Green DP, and Bucholz RW [eds]: Fractures in Adults. Philadelphia: JB Lippincott, 1991.)

may occur in the acromion, acromioclavicular joint, clavicle, coracoid process, or humeral tuberosities (Fig. 14–74). Extreme soft tissue damage occurs to the capsule rotator cuff, biceps tendon, and surrounding muscles. Clinically, the head rides above the level of the acromion. The arm is short and adducted to the side. Shoulder movement is restricted and quite painful. Neurovascular complications are usually present.

BILATERAL DISLOCATIONS

Mynter[446] first described this condition in 1902; according to Honner,[260] only 20 cases were reported prior to 1969. Bilateral dislocations have been reported by McFie,[400] Yadav,[708] Onabowale and Jaja,[483] Segal and colleagues,[584] and Carew-McColl.[77] Most of these cases were the result of convulsions or violent trauma. Peiro and co-workers[505] reported bilateral erect dislocation of the shoulders in a man caught in a cement mixer. Bilateral dislocation of the shoulder secondary to accidental electrical shock has been reported by Carew-McColl[77] and Fipp.[166] Nicola and co-workers[458] have reported cases of bilateral posterior fracture-dislocation after a convulsive seizure. Ahlgren and associates[5] reported three cases of bilateral posterior fracture-dislocation associated with a convulsion. Lindholm and Elmstedt[363] reported a case of bilateral posterior fracture-dislocation after an epileptic seizure, which was treated by open reduction and internal fixation with screws. Parrish and Skiendzielewski[498] reported a patient with bilateral posterior fracture-dislocations after status epilepticus. The diagnosis was missed for more than 12 hours. Pagden and associates[491] reported two cases of posterior shoulder dislocation after seizures related to regional anesthesia. Costigan and co-workers[103] reported a case of undiagnosed bilateral anterior dislocation of the shoulder in a 74-year-old patient admitted to the hospital for an unrelated problem. The patient had no complaints related to the shoulders and was able to place both hands on her head and behind her back.

CLINICAL PRESENTATION

Dislocation

HISTORY

The history should define the mechanism of the injury, including the position of the arm, the amount of applied force, and the point of force application.[518, 559, 560] Injury with the arm in extension, abduction, and external rotation favors anterior dislocation. Electroshock, seizures, or a fall on the flexed and adducted arm are commonly associated with posterior dislocation. If the instability is recurrent, the history defines the initial injury, the position or action that results in instability, how long the shoulder stays "out," whether radiographs are available with the shoulder out of joint, and what means have been necessary to reduce the shoulder. The history also solicits evidence of neurologic or rotator cuff problems after previous episodes of shoulder instability. Previous treatment for the recurrent instability as well as the effectiveness of this treatment are documented.

PHYSICAL EXAMINATION OF THE DISLOCATED SHOULDER

Anterior Dislocation

The acutely dislocated shoulder is usually very painful. Muscles are in spasm in an attempt to stabilize the joint. The humeral head may be palpable anteriorly. The posterior shoulder shows a hollow beneath the acromion. The arm is held in slight abduction and external rotation. Internal rotation and adduction are usually limited. Because of the frequent association of nerve injuries[116] and, to a lesser extent, vascular injuries,[52] an essential part of the physical examination of the anteriorly dislocated shoulder is the assessment of the neurovascular status of the upper extremity and the charting of the findings before reduction.

Posterior Dislocation

Recognition of a posterior dislocation may be impaired by the lack of a striking deformity of the shoulder and by the fact that the shoulder is held in the traditional sling position of adduction and internal rotation. However, a directed physical examination will reveal the diagnosis. The classical features of a posterior dislocation include:

1. Limited external rotation of the shoulder (often to less than 0 degrees)
2. Limited elevation of the arm (often to less than 90 degrees)
3. Posterior prominence and rounding of the shoulder compared with the normal side
4. Flattening of the anterior aspect of the shoulder
5. Prominence of the coracoid process on the dislocated side

Asymmetry of the shoulder contours can often be best visualized by viewing the shoulders from above while standing behind the patient (Fig. 14–75).

The motion is limited because the head of the humerus is fixed on the posterior glenoid rim by muscle forces, or the head may actually be impaled on the glenoid rim. With the passage of time, the posterior rim of the glenoid may further impact the fracture of the humeral head and produce a deep hatchet-like defect or V-shaped compression fracture, which engages the head even more securely. Patients with old, unreduced posterior dislocations of the shoulder may have 30 to 40 degrees of glenohumeral abduction and some humeral rotation owing to enlargement of the groove. With long-standing disuse of the muscles about the shoulder, atrophy will be present, which accentuates the flattening of the anterior shoulder, the prominence of the coracoid, and the fullness of the posterior shoulder.

A proper physical examination is essential. Rowe and Zarins[560] reported 23 cases of unreduced dislocation of the shoulder, of which 14 were posterior. Hill and McLaughlin[255] reported that in their series the average time from injury to diagnosis was 8 months. In the interval before the diagnosis of posterior dislocation of the shoulder is made, the injury may be misdiagnosed as a "frozen shoulder"[255, 409, 410] for which vigorous therapy may

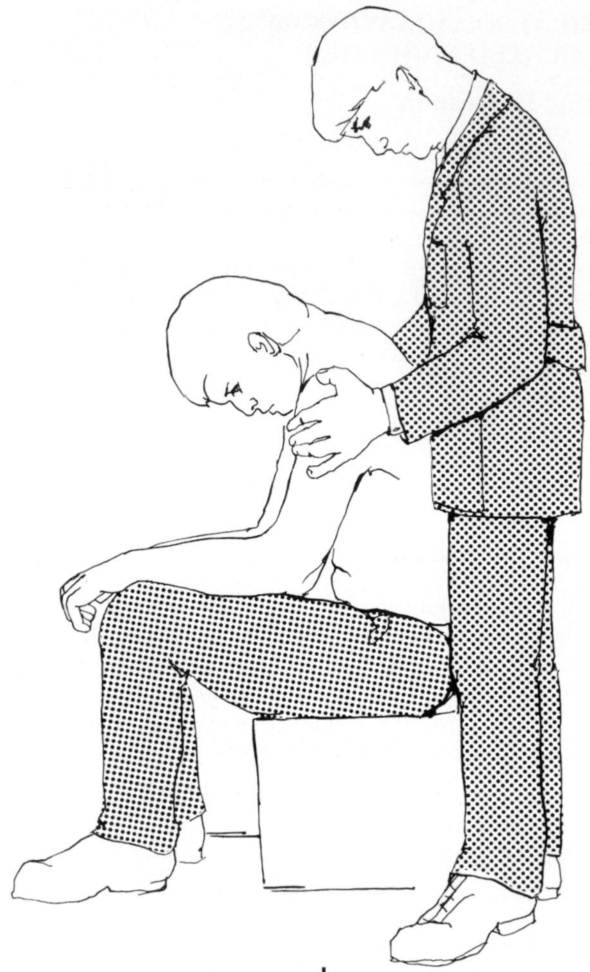

Figure 14–75

Inspection of the anterior and posterior aspects of the shoulders can best be accomplished by having the patient sit on a low stool, with the examiner standing behind him. Then the injured shoulder can easily be compared with the uninjured one. (From Rockwood CA and Green DP [eds]: Fractures [3 vols], 2nd ed. Philadelphia: JB Lippincott, 1984.)

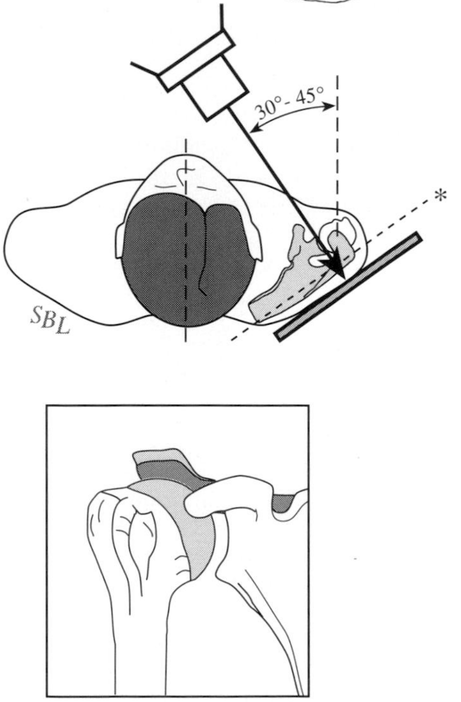

Figure 14–76

The anteroposterior view in the plane of the scapula is obtained by orienting the beam perpendicular to the plane of the scapula (see Fig. 14–28) and centering it on the coracoid tip while the film is parallel to the plane of the scapula. (From Grashey R: Atlas Typischer Rontgenfilder, 1923.)

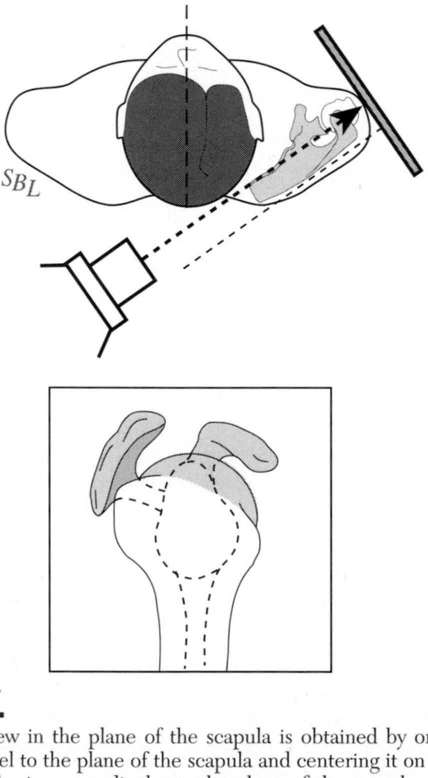

Figure 14–77

A lateral view in the plane of the scapula is obtained by orienting the beam parallel to the plane of the scapula and centering it on the glenoid while the film is perpendicular to the plane of the scapula.

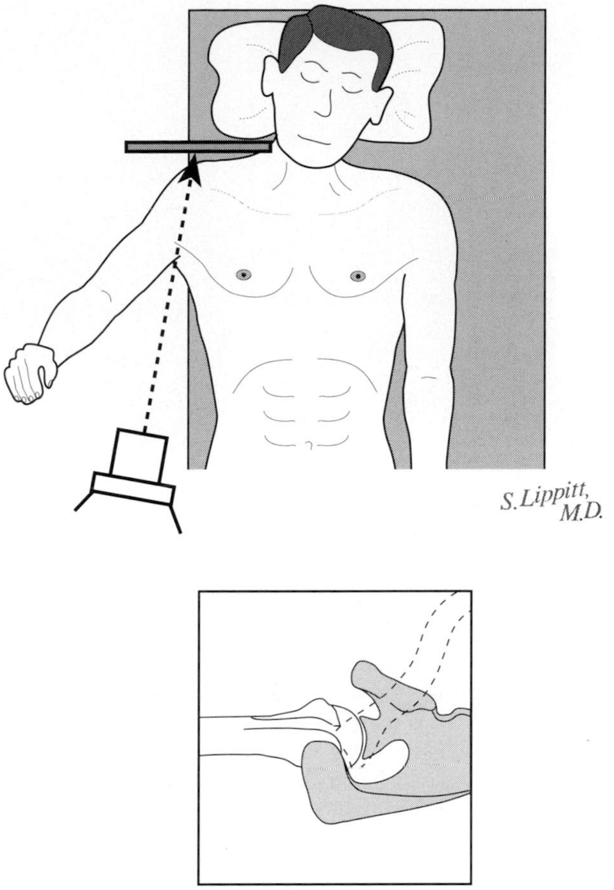

Figure 14–78

The axillary view is obtained by orienting the beam parallel to the scapula and centering it between the coracoid tip and the posterior angle of the acromion.

be mistakenly instituted in an attempt to restore the range of motion.

RADIOGRAPHIC EVALUATION

When a shoulder is dislocated, radiographs need to demonstrate: (1) the direction of the dislocation, (2) the existence of associated fractures (displaced or not), and (3) possible barriers to relocation. The glenohumeral joint is most reliably imaged using three standardized views referred to the plane of the scapula: an anteroposterior view in the plane of the scapula (Fig. 14–76), a scapular lateral (Fig. 14–77), and an axillary view (Fig. 14–78). The complete series of three views oriented to the scapula provide much more information than the commonly obtained view in the plane of the body (Fig. 14–79). McLaughlin has said that the reliance on anteroposterior radiographs will lead the unwary orthopedist into a "diagnostic trap."[406] Dorgan[133] reported that, in addition to obesity, technical factors may prevent accurate identification of the glenohumeral joint in the transthoracic lateral view.

Anteroposterior View in the Plane of the Scapula

In 1923, Grashey[204] recognized that in order to take a true anteroposterior radiograph of the shoulder joint, the

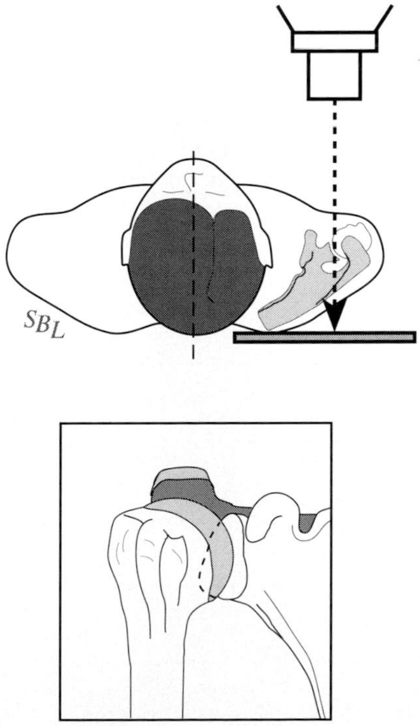

Figure 14–79

The anteroposterior view in the plane of the body presents an overlapping and often confusing view of the glenohumeral joint.

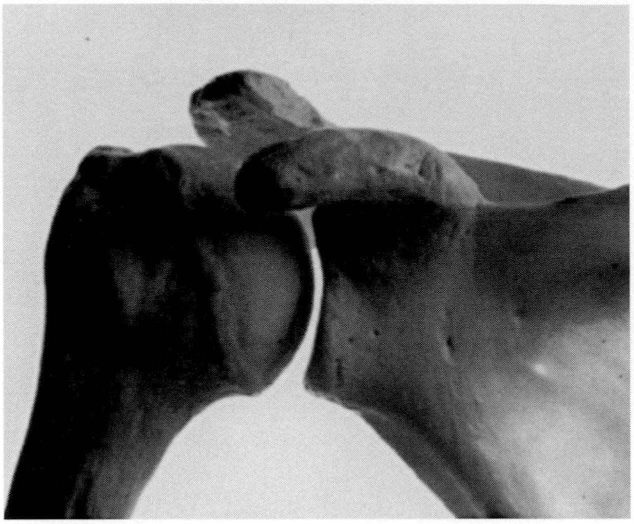

Figure 14–80

A simulated x-ray view of a scapular anteroposterior view using back-lighted skeletal models. This view reveals the radiographic glenohumeral joint space and provides a good opportunity to detect fractures of the humerus or glenoid lip.

direction of the x-ray beam must be perpendicular to the plane of the scapula. This view is most easily accomplished by placing the scapula flat on the cassette (a position that the patient can help to achieve) and passing the x-ray beam at right angles to this plane, centering it on the coracoid process (Fig. 14–80; see also Fig. 14-76). This view can be taken with the arm in a sling; with the body rotated to the desired position (Figs. 14–81 and 14–82). In the normal shoulder this view reveals a clear separation of the humeral subchondral bone from that of the glenoid (see Fig. 14–76).

Lateral View in the Plane of the Scapula

This view is taken at right angles to the anteroposterior in the plane of the scapula (Figs. 14–83 and 14–84; see also Fig. 14–77).[406, 409, 410, 448, 541] Like the anteroposterior view, it can be obtained by positioning the body without moving the dislocated shoulder. The radiographic beam is passed from medial to lateral parallel to the body of the scapula while the cassette is held perpendicular to the beam at the anterolateral aspect of the shoulder (see Figs. 14–77 and 14–84).[541] In this view, the contour of the scapula projects as the letter "Y."[563] The downward stem of the Y is projected by the body of the scapula; the upper forks are projected by the coracoid process anteriorly and by the spine and acromion posteriorly (Figs. 14–85 and 14–86). The glenoid is located at the junction of the stem and the two arms of the Y. In the normal shoulder, the humeral head is at the center of the arms of the Y; that is, in the glenoid fossa. In posterior dislocations the head is seen posterior to the glenoid (see Fig. 14–86); in anterior dislocations the head is anterior to it (see Fig. 14–85).

Axillary View

In this view, first described by Lawrence in 1915,[347, 417] the cassette is placed on the superior aspect of the shoulder. This view requires that the humerus be abducted

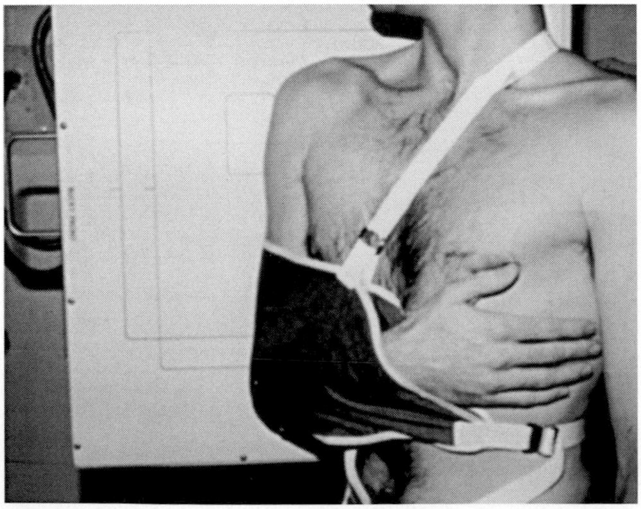

Figure 14–81

Positioning of the patient in a sling for an anteroposterior x-ray in the plane of the scapula. The scapula is placed flat on the cassette. The x-ray beam is positioned at right angles to the cassette and centered on the coracoid process.

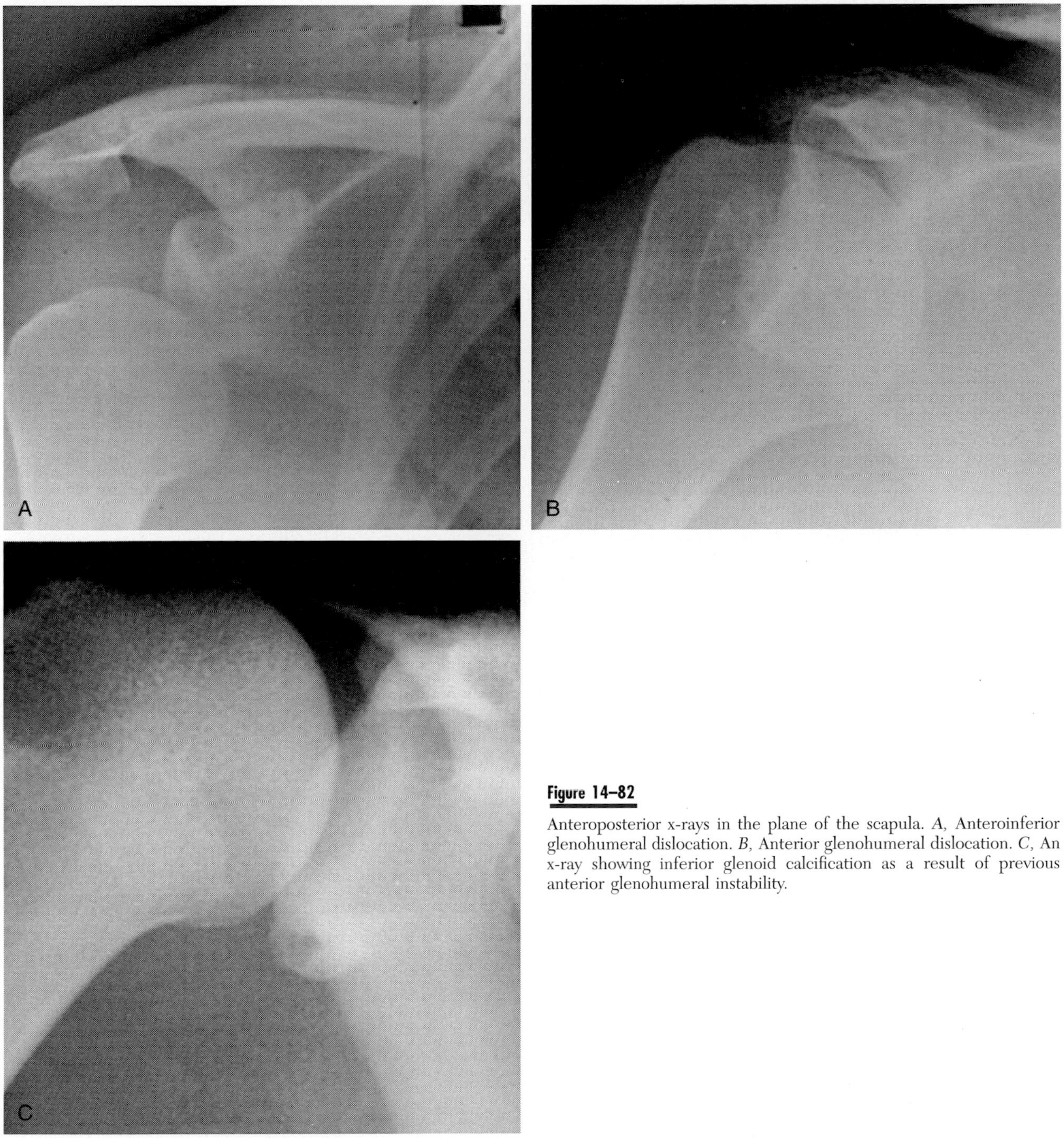

Figure 14–82

Anteroposterior x-rays in the plane of the scapula. *A,* Anteroinferior glenohumeral dislocation. *B,* Anterior glenohumeral dislocation. *C,* An x-ray showing inferior glenoid calcification as a result of previous anterior glenohumeral instability.

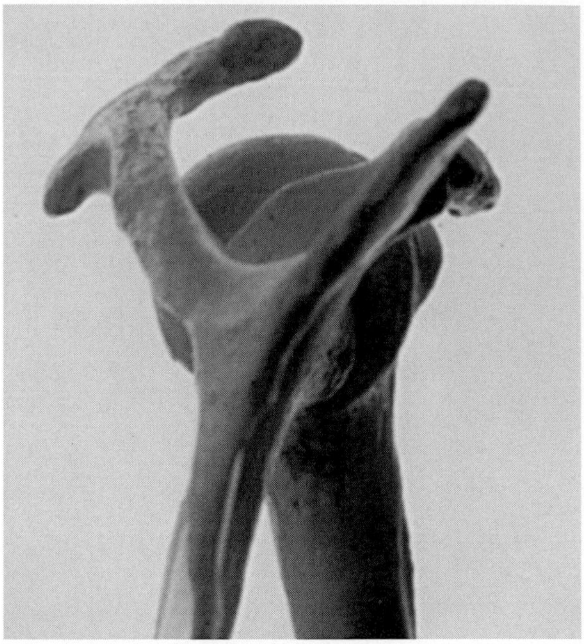

Figure 14–83

Simulated scapular lateral x-ray view with backlighted skeletal models. The x-ray beam is passed parallel to the plane of the scapula and is centered on the scapular spine. The view reveals the anteroposterior relationship of the head of the humerus in the glenoid fossa. The glenoid fossa is identified as the intersection of the spine of the scapula, the coracoid process, and the body of the scapula.

sufficiently to allow the radiographic beam to pass between it and the thorax. Fortunately, sufficient abduction can be achieved by gentle positioning of the dislocated shoulder or by modifications of the technique (Figs. 14–87 to 14–90; see also Fig. 14–78). The axillary radiograph is critical in the evaluation of the dislocated shoulder: It not only reveals unambiguously the direction and magnitude of head displacement relative to the glenoid but also the presence and size of head compression fractures, fractures of the glenoid, and fractures of the humeral tuberosities (Figs. 14–91 to 14–95). The axillary view may also be helpful in judging the bony competence and version of the glenoid fossa, but the projection must be standardized to avoid misinterpretation (see Fig. 14–38).

In his text on radiographic positioning, Jordan demonstrated the various techniques for obtaining axillary lateral views.[309] Cleaves[93, 417] and Teitge and Ciullo[516] have described variations on this view (see Fig. 14–89). Rockwood has pointed out that in the situation when the patient cannot abduct the arm sufficiently, a curved cassette or a rolled cardboard cassette can be placed in the axilla and the radiographic beam passed from a superior position (see Fig. 14–87). Bloom and Obata[53] have modified the axillary technique so that the arm does not have to be abducted (see Fig. 14–88). They call this the Velpeau axillary lateral view. While wearing a sling or Velpeau dressing, the patient leans backward 30 degrees over the cassette on the table. The x-ray tube is placed above the shoulder, and the beam is projected vertically down through the shoulder onto the cassette.

In summary, in the evaluation of a possibly dislocated shoulder or a fracture-dislocated shoulder we recommend the three orthogonal projections of the shoulder (antero-

Text continued on page 660

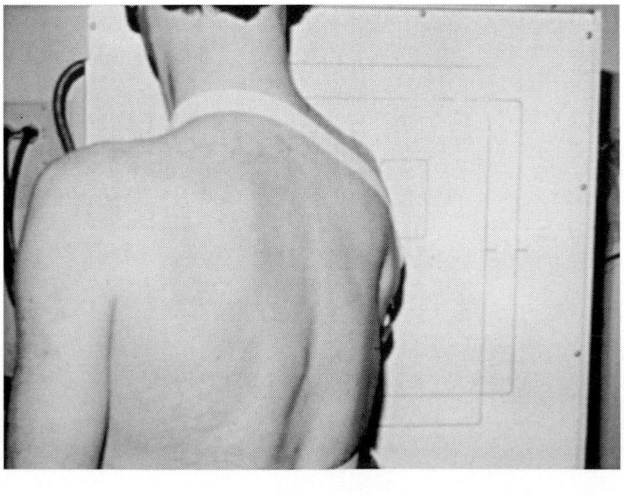

Figure 14–84

Position of the patient in the sling for a scapular lateral x-ray. The scapula is positioned perpendicular to the cassette. The beam should be placed parallel to the spine of the scapula and perpendicular to the cassette.

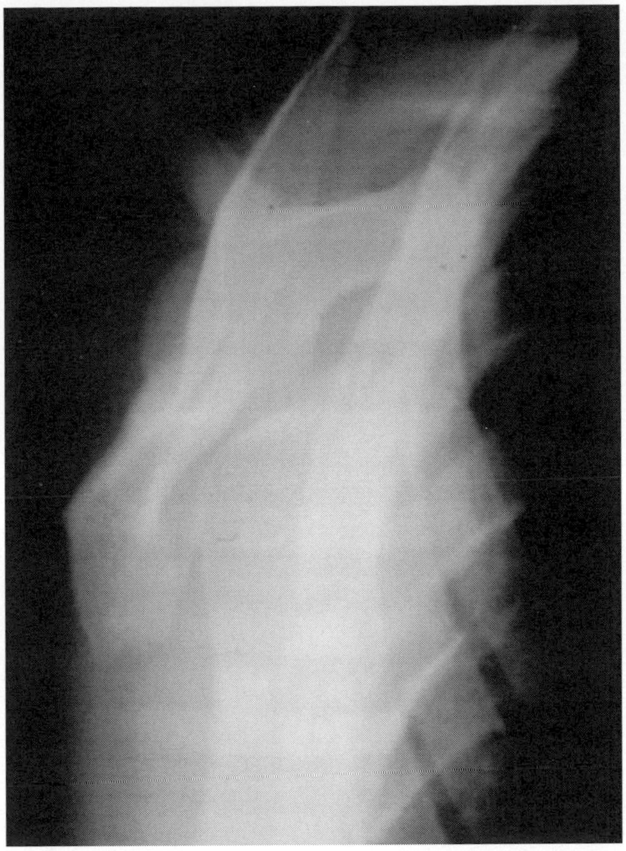

Figure 14–85

Scapular lateral view showing an anterior glenohumeral dislocation. Note that the humerus is no longer centered at the base of the Y.

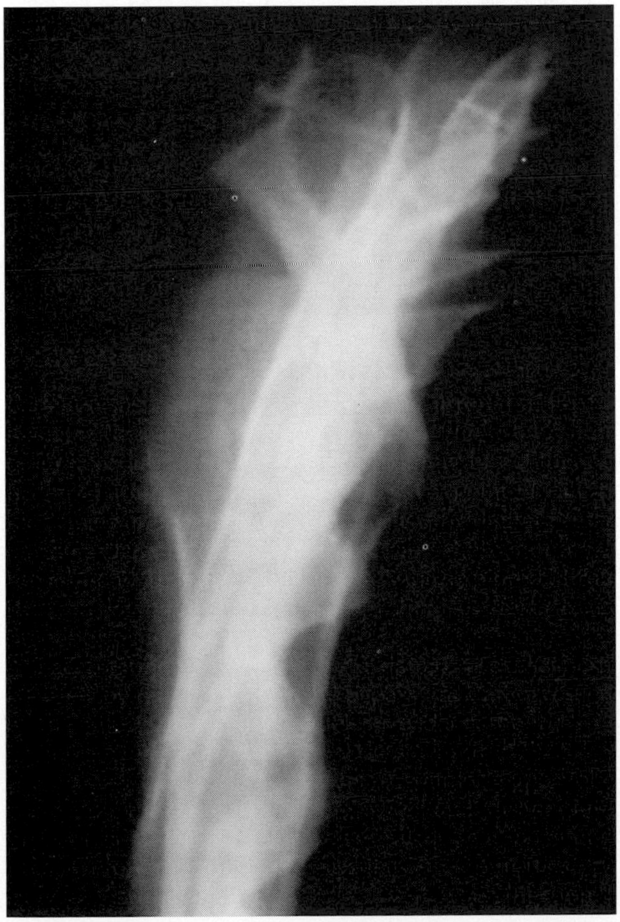

Figure 14–86

A scapular lateral view showing a posterior glenohumeral dislocation. The head of the humerus is dislocated posterior to the glenoid fossa and in this view appears to be sitting directly below the spine of the scapula.

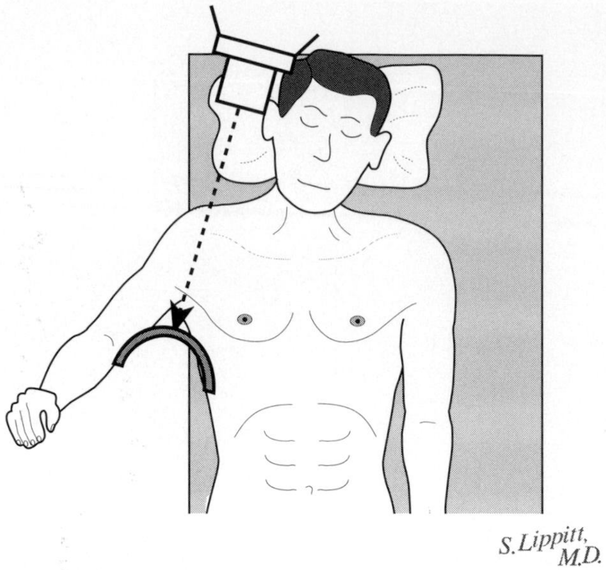

Figure 14–87

The axillary view with a curved cassette, a method that is useful if the arm cannot be adequately abducted for a routine axillary view.

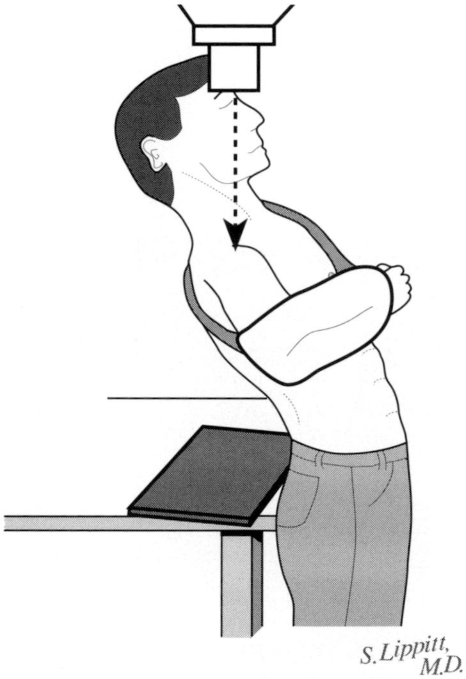

Figure 14–88

The Velpeau axillary lateral x-ray technique. With the arm in a sling, the patient leans backward until the shoulder is over the cassette. (Modified from Bloom MH and Obata WG: Diagnosis of posterior dislocation of the shoulder with use of the Velpeau axillary and angle-up roentgenographic views. J Bone Joint Surg *49A*:943–949, 1967.)

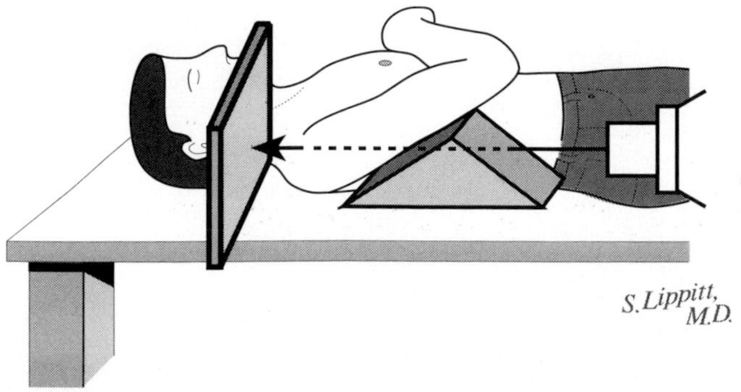

Figure 14–89

A trauma axillary lateral x-ray. This arm is flexed on a foam wedge. (Modified from Tietge RA and Ciullo JV: The CAM axillary x-ray. Orthop Trans *6*:451, 1982.)

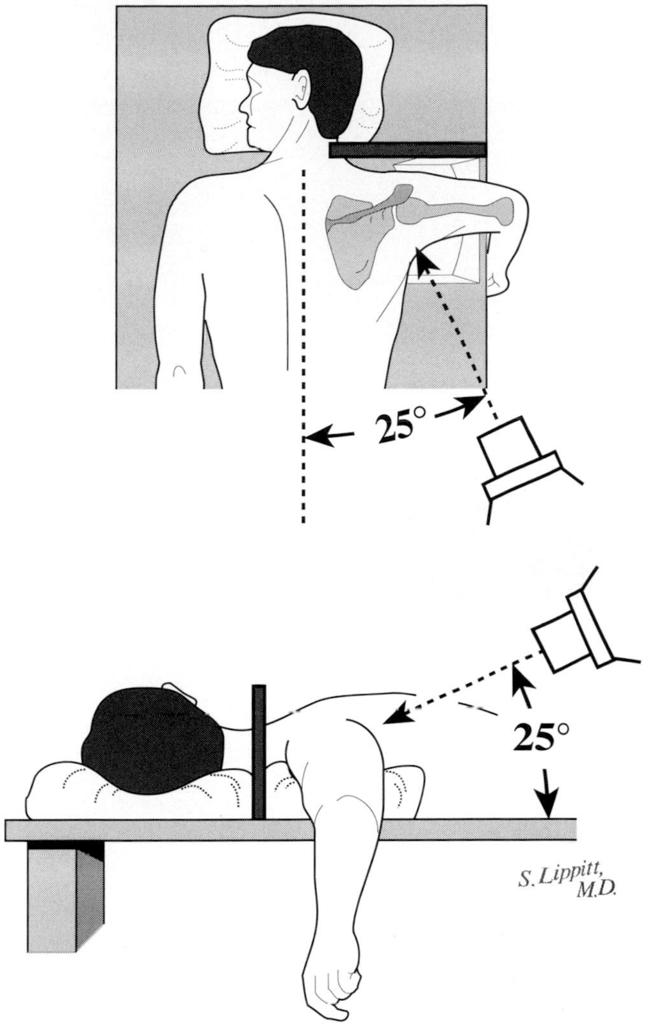

Figure 14–90

The West Point axillary lateral view. The patient is prone with the beam inclined 25 degrees down and 25 degrees medially. (Modified from Rokous JR, Feagin JA, and Abbott HG: Modified axillary roentgenogram. Clin Orthop *82*:84–86, 1972.)

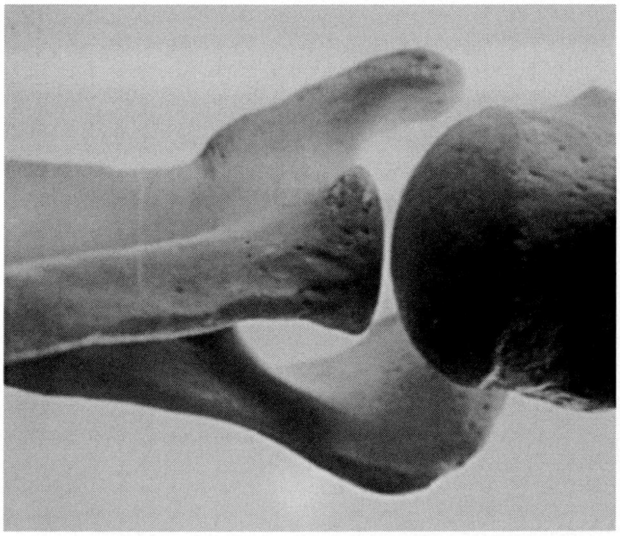

Figure 14–91

Simulated axillary view using a backlighted skeletal model. An x-ray beam is passed up the axilla, projecting the glenoid fossa between the coracoid process anteriorly and the scapular spine posteriorly. This projection reveals the radiographic glenohumeral joint space, the anteroposterior position of the head of the humerus relative to the glenoid, and a view of fractures of the glenoid lip and humerus.

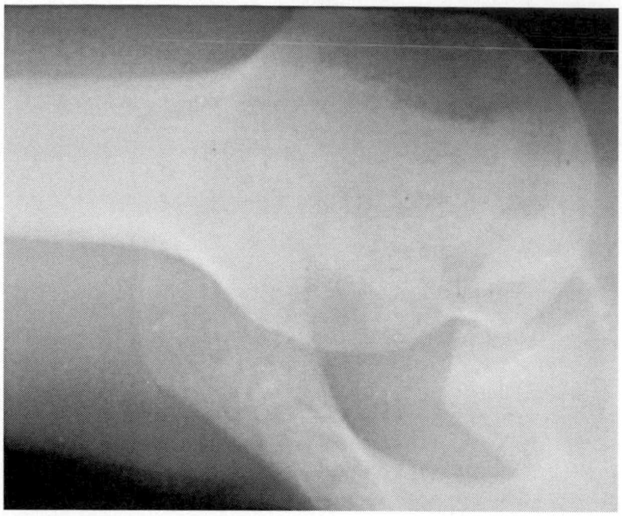

Figure 14–92

An axillary view. Note the posterior humeral head defect (Hill-Sachs lesion), secondary to a previous anterior glenohumeral dislocation.

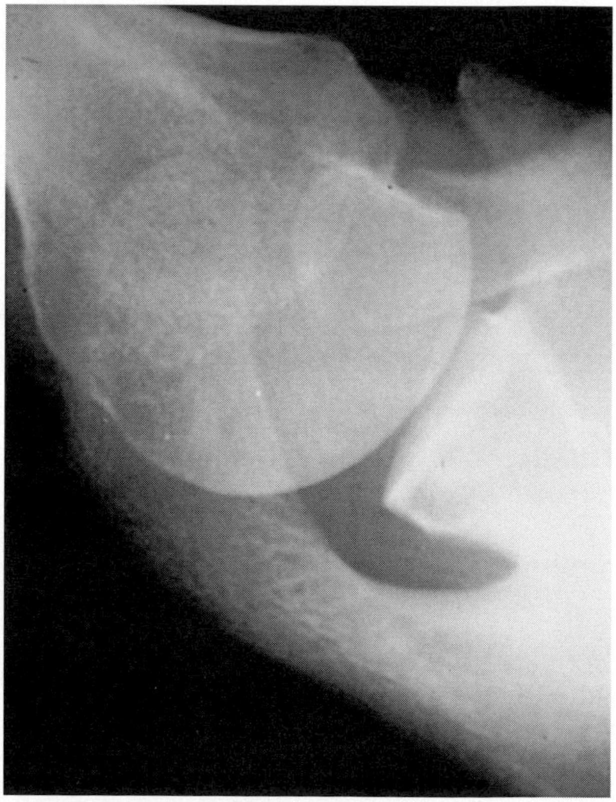

Figure 14–93

An axillary view. This patient has an anterior humeral head defect that occurred as a result of a posterior glenohumeral dislocation.

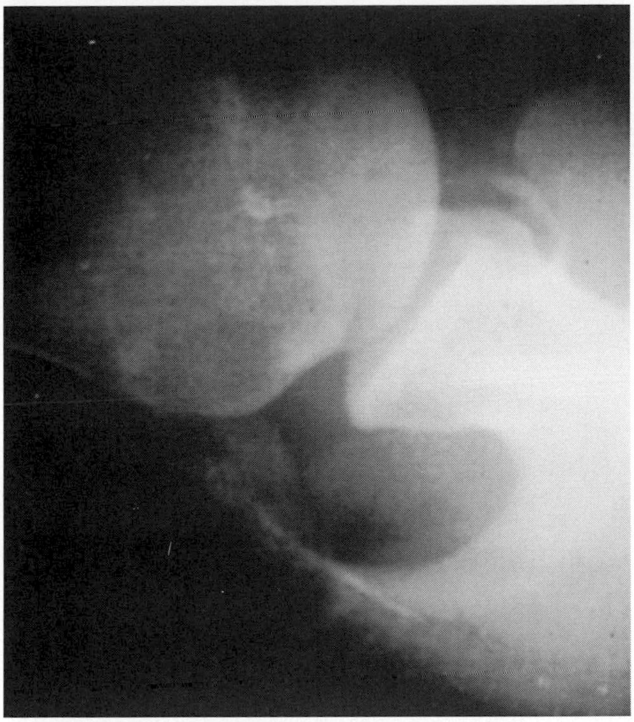

Figure 14–94

An axillary view showing an anterior glenoid defect and calcification as a result of an anterior glenohumeral dislocation. A posterior lateral humeral head defect is also seen.

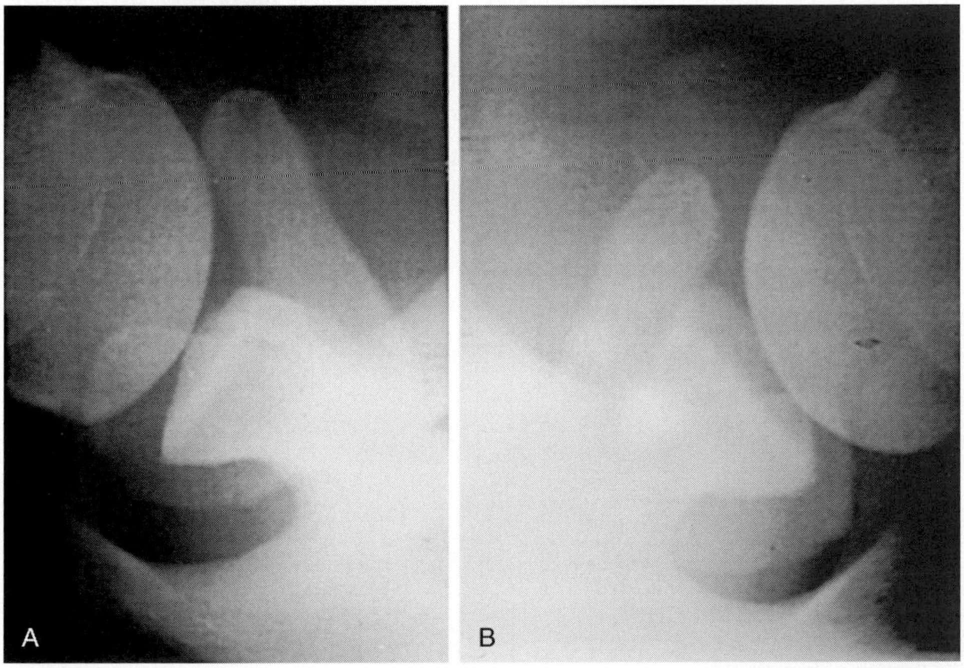

Figure 14–95

Bilateral axillary views. *A*, Rounding of the anterior glenoid rim as a result of recurrent anterior glenohumeral dislocation is evident on this axillary view. *B*, Normal side is shown for comparison.

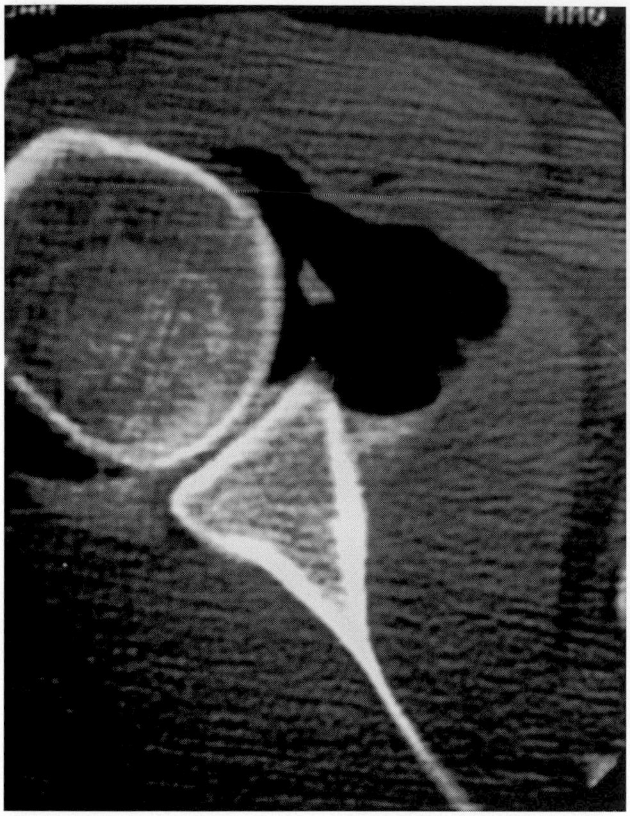

Figure 14–96

A computed tomography scan of the glenohumeral joint with air contrast. This study demonstrates a bony avulsion from the anterior glenoid rim.

posterior and lateral in the plane of the scapula and axillary views), which provide a sensitive assessment of shoulder dislocation. The use of fewer views or other less interpretable projections may obscure significant pathologic processes. If the three views cannot be taken, if there is a question regarding the diagnosis, or if there is a need to define anatomy in greater detail, a CT scan may be of great assistance (Figs. 14–96 to 14–99; see also Fig. 14-18).[319, 533, 591] Using modern methods of three-dimensional reconstruction, anterior inferior glenoid lesions and posterior lateral humeral head lesions can be shown in striking detail (Figs. 14–100 and 14–101). It is noteworthy that the patient whose shoulder is shown in these figures obtained an excellent result from nonoperative treatment despite the damage shown on the reconstructions.

INJURIES ASSOCIATED WITH ANTERIOR DISLOCATIONS

Ligaments and Capsule

A common feature of traumatic anterior dislocations is avulsion of the anterior-inferior glenohumeral ligaments and capsule from the glenoid lip, especially in younger individuals (Figs. 14–102 and 14–103; see also Fig. 14–3). Nonhealing of this avulsion is a major factor in recurrent traumatic instability. Occasionally, the capsule may be avulsed from the anteroinferior humerus, sometimes with a fleck of bone.

Fractures

Fractures of the glenoid (Fig. 14–104; see also Figs. 14–6 and 14–99), humeral head (see Figs. 14–92 and 14–93) and tuberosities (Figs. 14–105 to 14–107; see also Fig. 14–5) may accompany traumatic dislocations. A CT scan may be helpful in determining the degree of posterior displacement of fractures (Figs. 14–108 and 14–109; see also Figs. 14–97 to 14–99).

It is important to seek evidence of a nondisplaced humeral neck fracture on the pre-reduction radiographs, lest this fracture be displaced during attempted closed reduction (see Fig. 14–107).[161]

Other fractures, such as fractures of the coracoid pro-

Text continued on page 665

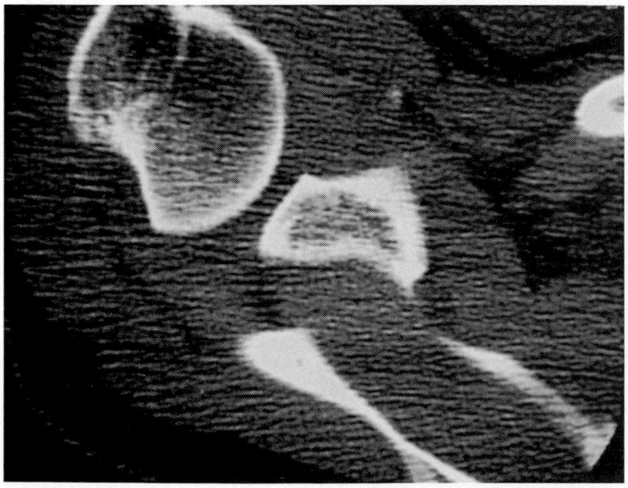

Figure 14–97

A computed tomography scan of the glenohumeral joint. The posterior humeral head defect and the anterior glenoid defect are well demonstrated.

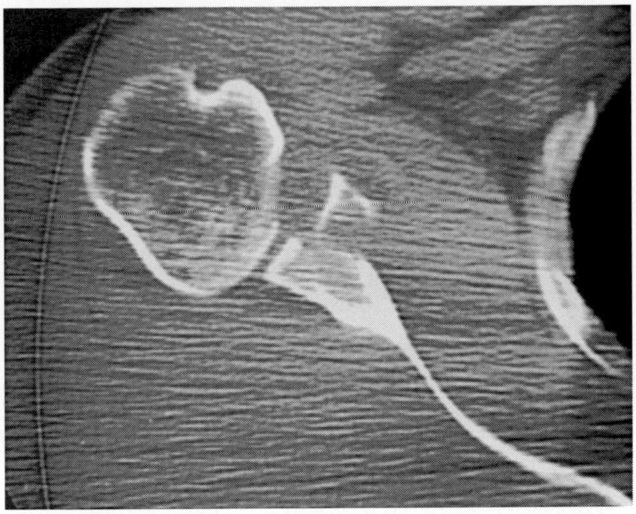

Figure 14–98

A computed tomography scan of the glenohumeral joint. This scan shows a fracture of the anterior glenoid rim secondary to anterior glenohumeral dislocation.

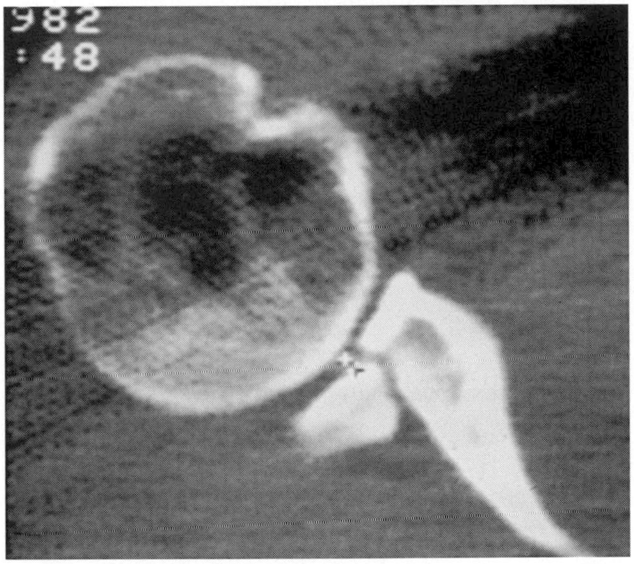

Figure 14–99

A computed tomography scan of the glenohumeral joint demonstrates a fracture of the posterior glenoid rim as a result of posterior dislocation of the glenohumeral joint.

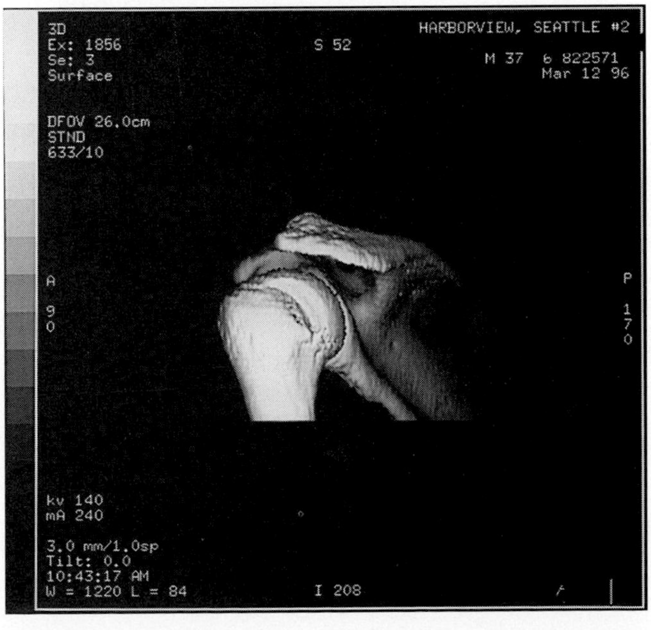

Figure 14–100

A three-dimensional computed tomography reconstruction after reduction of a first-time dislocation showing a posterior lateral humeral head defect.

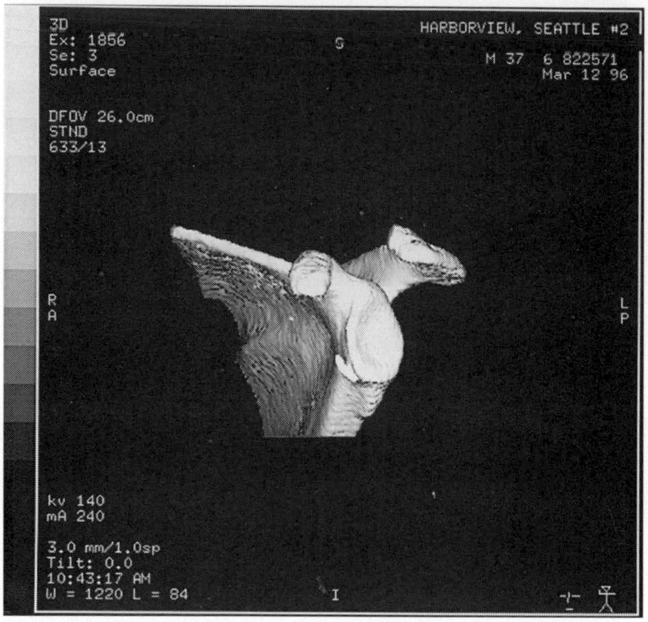

Figure 14–101

A three-dimensional computed tomography reconstruction after reduction of a first-time dislocation showing anterior glenoid avulsion.

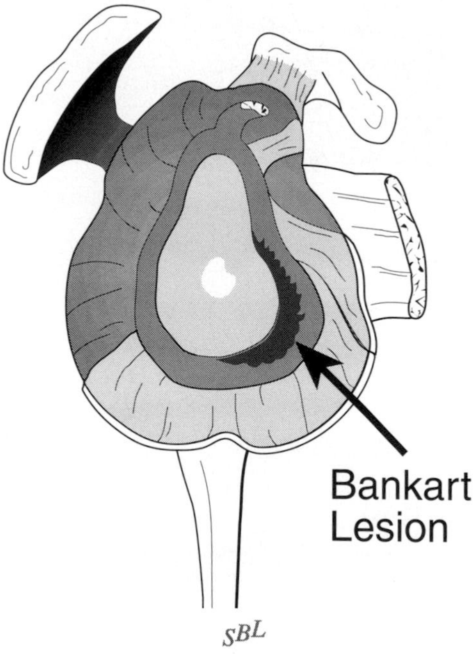

Figure 14–102

The capsulolabral detachment typical of traumatic instability. (Modified from Matsen FA III, Lippitt SB, Sidles JA, and Harryman DT II: Practical Evaluation and Management of the Shoulder. Philadelphia: WB Saunders, 1994.)

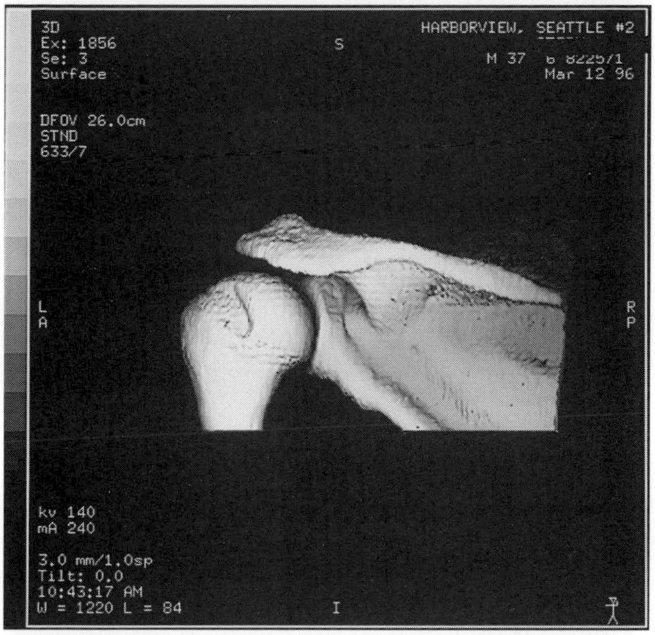

Figure 14–103

A three-dimensional computed tomography reconstruction of the left shoulder of a 37-year-old man 3 days after his first traumatic glenohumeral dislocation. The patient went on to normal shoulder function with nonoperative management.

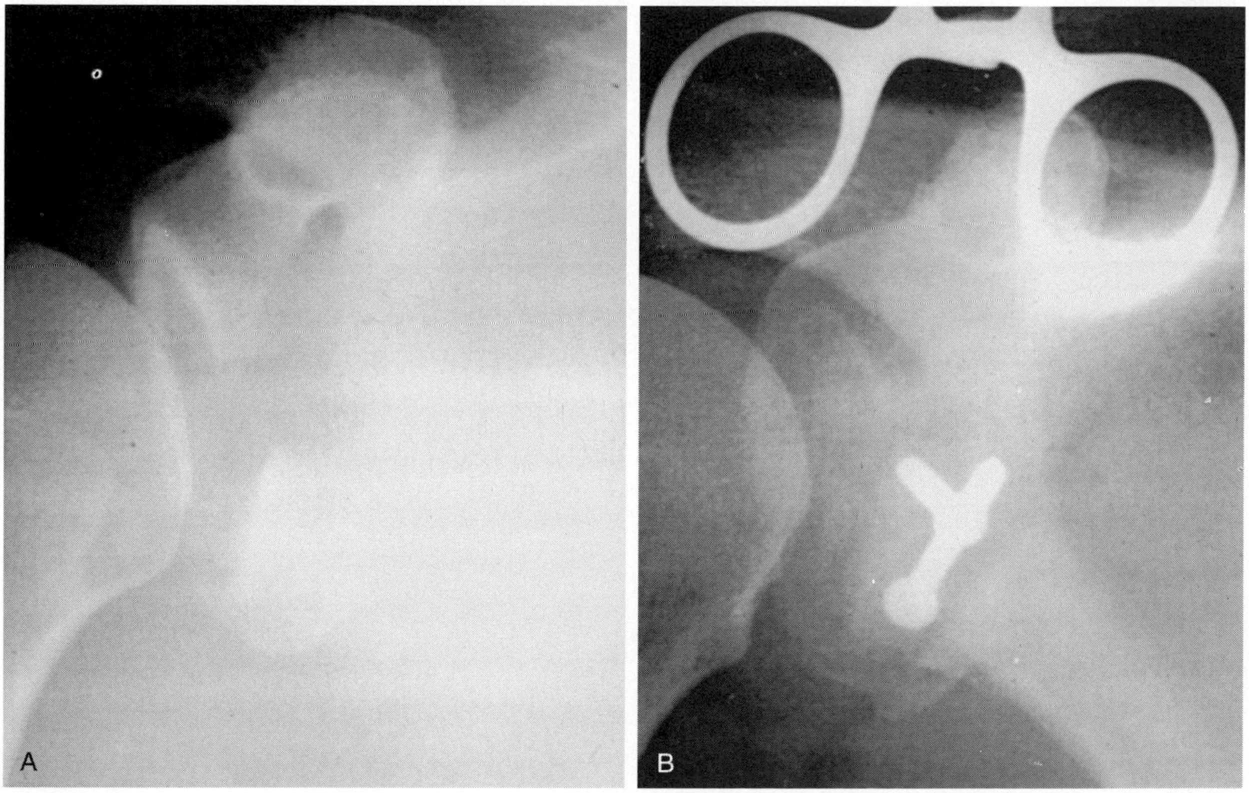

Figure 14–104

An anterior glenoid rim fracture. *A*, An anteroposterior x-ray demonstrates an anterior glenoid rim fracture secondary to traumatic anterior dislocation. *B*, An intraoperative anteroposterior x-ray shows reduction and screw fixation of an anterior glenoid rim fracture.

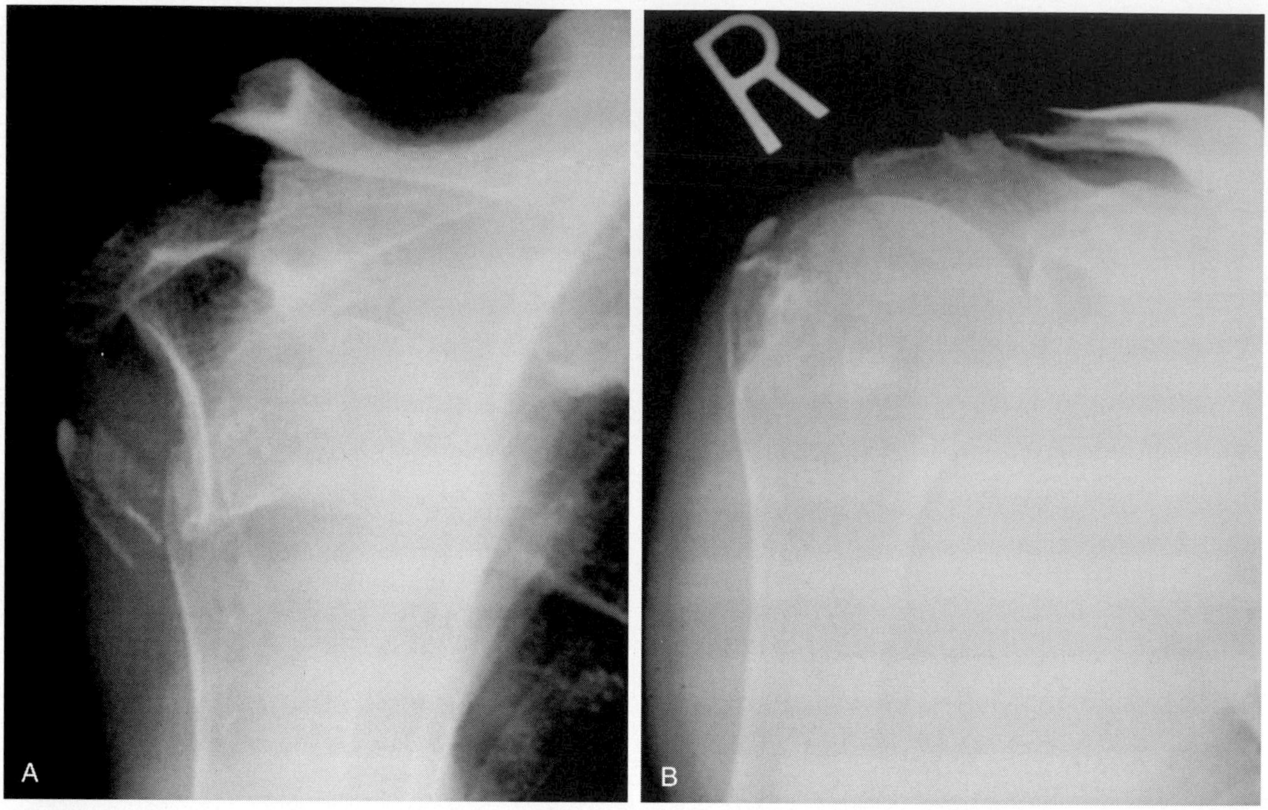

Figure 14–105

Greater tuberosity fracture. *A,* An anteroposterior x-ray prior to reduction showing a fracture of the greater tuberosity. *B,* A postreduction anteroposterior x-ray of a greater tuberosity fracture.

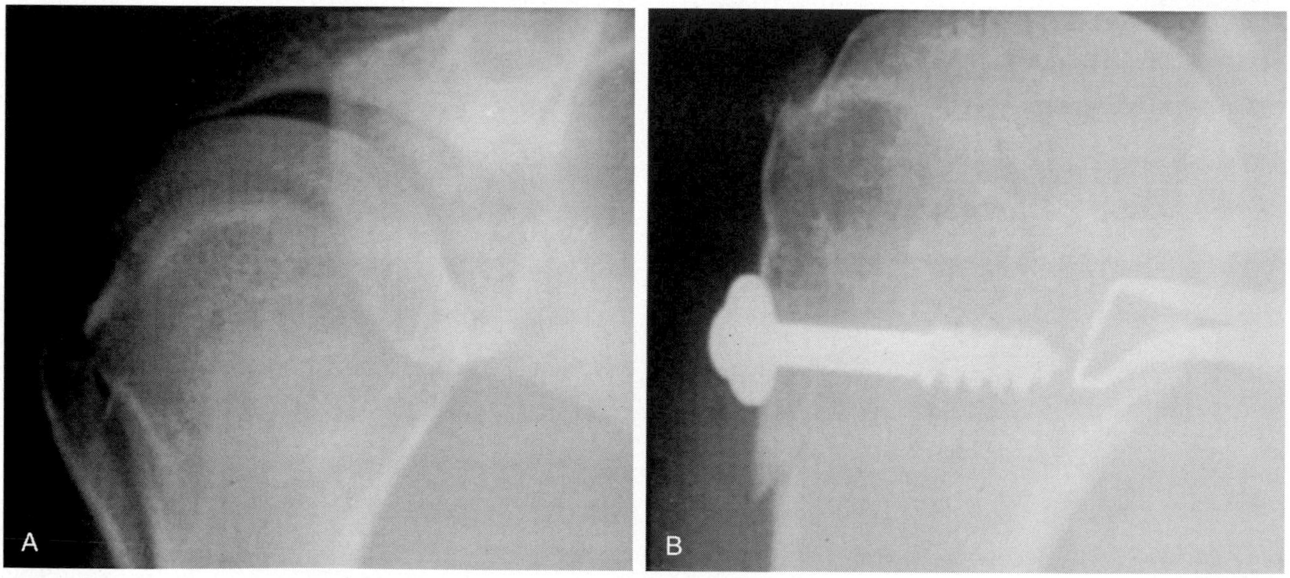

Figure 14–106

A, An x-ray showing a displaced greater tuberosity fracture. *B,* An intraoperative x-ray showing screw fixation of a greater tuberosity fracture.

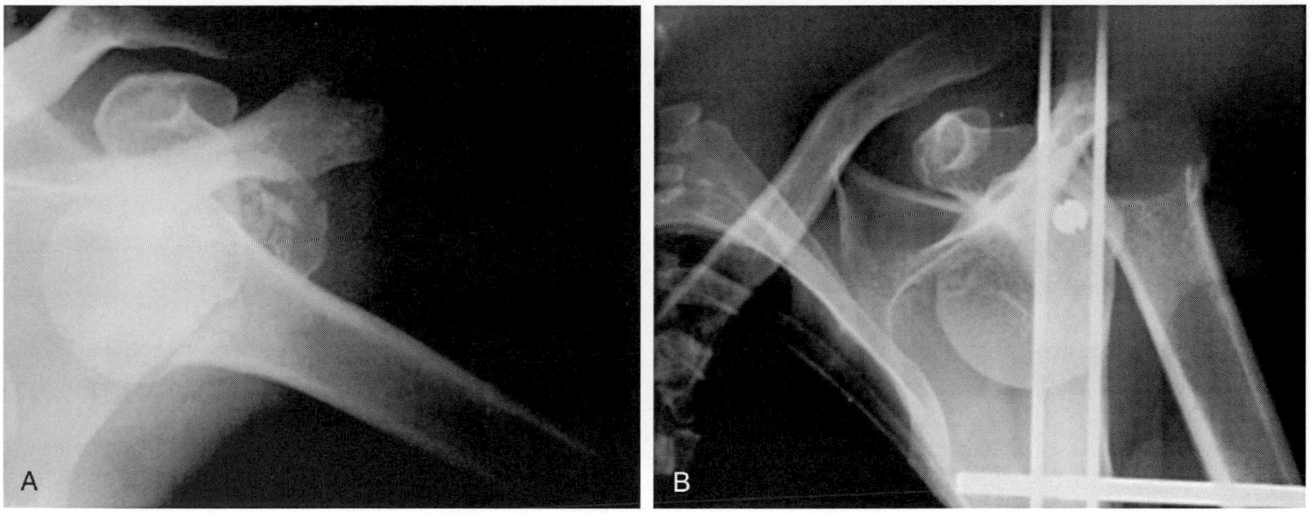

Figure 14–107

A, An anteroposterior view showing an anteroinferior dislocation with an associated greater tuberosity fracture. *B*, An anteroposterior view after a reduction attempt showing displacement of a humeral neck fracture.

cess, may be associated with glenohumeral dislocations.[40, 704]

Cuff Tears

Rotator cuff tears may accompany anterior and inferior glenohumeral dislocations (see Fig. 14–4). The frequency of this complication increases with age: in patients older than 40 years of age, the incidence exceeds 30%; in patients older than 60 years of age, the incidence exceeds 80%.[285, 501, 510, 528, 603, 624, 638]

Rotator cuff tears may present as pain or weakness on external rotation and abduction.[235, 454, 510, 526, 685] Sonnabend reported a series of primary shoulder dislocations in patients older than 40 years of age.[603] Of the 13 patients who had complaints of weakness or pain after 3 weeks, 11 had rotator cuff tears. However, the presence of a rotator cuff tear may be masked by a coexisting axillary nerve palsy.[199, 302]

Shoulder ultrasonography,[381] arthrography, or MRI is considered to evaluate the possibility of an associated cuff tear when shoulder dislocations occur in patients older than 40 years of age, when there has been substantial initial displacement of the humeral head (e.g., in a subglenoid dislocation), and when there is persistent pain or loss of rotator cuff strength 3 weeks after a glenohumeral dislocation.[1–3] Toolanen found sonographic evidence of rotator cuff lesions in 24 of 63 patients older than 40 years of age at the time of anterior glenohumeral dislocation.[639]

Prompt operative repair of these acute cuff tears is usually indicated. Itoi and Tabata[285] reported 16 rotator

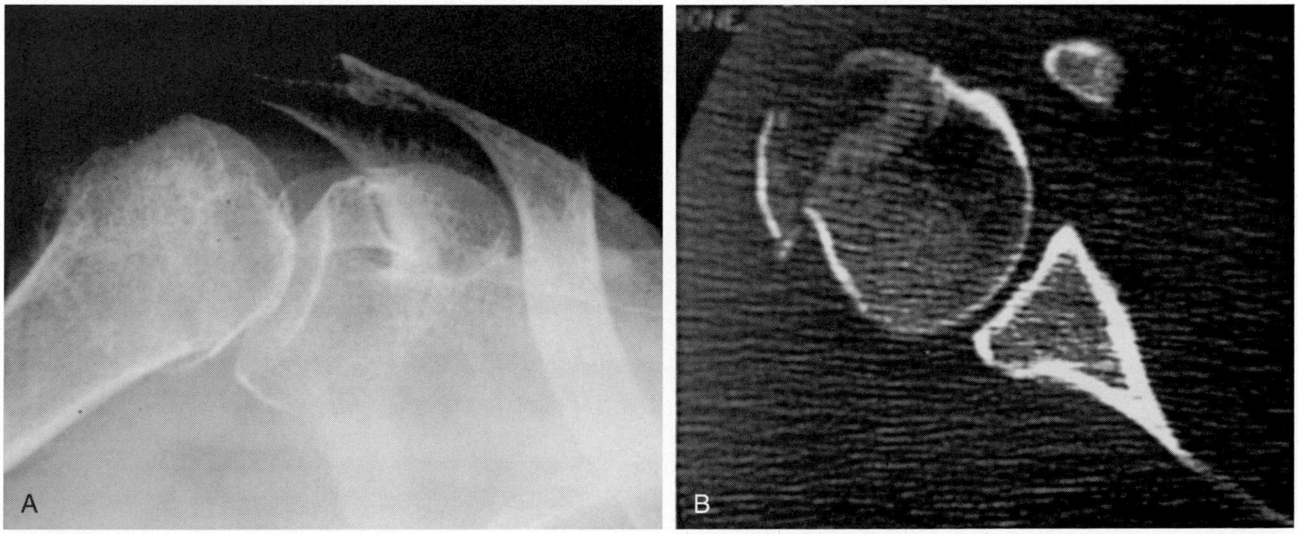

Figure 14–108

A minimally displaced greater tuberosity fracture. *A*, An anteroposterior x-ray shows a minimally displaced greater tuberosity fracture. *B*, A computed tomography scan shows the position of the greater tuberosity.

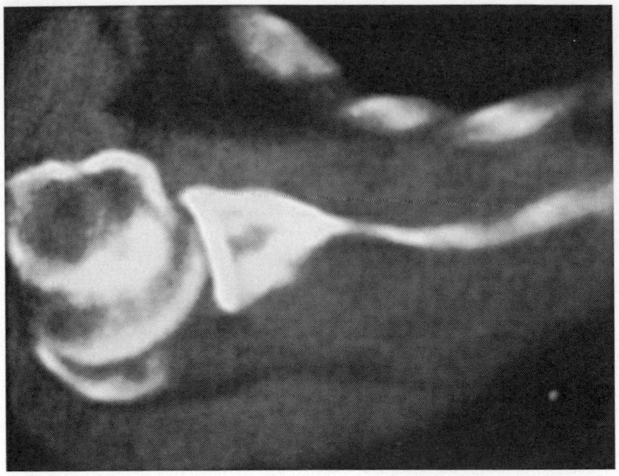

Figure 14–109

A computed tomography scan of a significantly displaced greater tuberosity fracture.

cuff tears in 109 shoulders with a traumatic anterior dislocation. The cuff was surgically repaired in 11 shoulders, and the results were graded as satisfactory in 73% of cases.

Neviaser and associates[455] reported on 37 patients older than 40 years of age in whom the diagnosis of cuff rupture was initially missed after an anterior dislocation of the shoulder. The weakness from the cuff rupture was often erroneously attributed to axillary neuropathy. Eleven of these patients developed recurrent anterior instability that was caused by rupture of the subscapularis and anterior capsule from the lesser tuberosity. None of these shoulders had a Bankart lesion. Repair of the capsule and subscapularis restored stability in all of the patients with recurrence.

Vascular Injuries

Vascular damage most frequently occurs in elderly patients with stiffer, more fragile vessels. The injury may be to the axillary artery or vein or to the branches of the axillary artery—the thoracoacromial, subscapular, circumflex, and rarely the long thoracic. These injuries can sometimes be combined, as pointed out by Kirker who described a case of rupture of the axillary artery and axillary vein along with a brachial plexus palsy.[320] Injury may occur at the time of either dislocation or reduction.[13, 110, 212, 288]

ANATOMY

The axillary artery is divided into three parts that lie medial to, behind, and lateral to the pectoralis minor muscle (Fig. 14–110). Injuries most commonly involve the second part, where the thoracoacromial trunk may be avulsed, and the third part, where the subscapular and circumflex branches may be avulsed or the axillary artery may be totally ruptured.

MECHANISM OF INJURY

Damage to the axillary artery can take the form of a complete transection, a linear tear of the artery caused by avulsion of one of its branches, or an intravascular thrombus, perhaps related to an intimal tear. The artery is relatively fixed at the lateral margin of the pectoralis minor muscle. With abduction and external rotation, the artery is taut; when the head dislocates, it forces the axillary artery forward, and the pectoralis minor acts as a fulcrum over which the artery is deformed and ruptured.[69, 288, 424]

Watson-Jones[676] reported the case of a man who had multiple anterior dislocations that he reduced himself. Finally, when the man was older, the axillary artery ruptured during one of the dislocations and he died. Vascular injuries may occur either at the time of dislocation or during attempted reduction: It is sometimes unclear which is the case.[320, 457, 615]

INJURY AT THE TIME OF DISLOCATION

Vascular injuries are commonly associated with inferior dislocation.[179, 356, 379, 416] Gardham and Scott[179] reported an axillary artery occlusion with an erect dislocation of the shoulder in a 40-year-old patient who had fallen headfirst down an escalator. Although vascular injuries are most common in older individuals, they can occur at any age.[44, 136, 167, 354, 572, 613] Baratta and co-workers[31] reported the case of a 13-year-old boy who ruptured his axillary artery with a subcoracoid dislocation sustained while wrestling.

INJURY AT THE TIME OF REDUCTION

Vascular damage at the time of reduction occurs primarily in the elderly, particularly when a chronic old anterior dislocation is mistaken for an acute injury and a closed reduction is attempted. The largest series of vascular complications associated with closed reduction of the

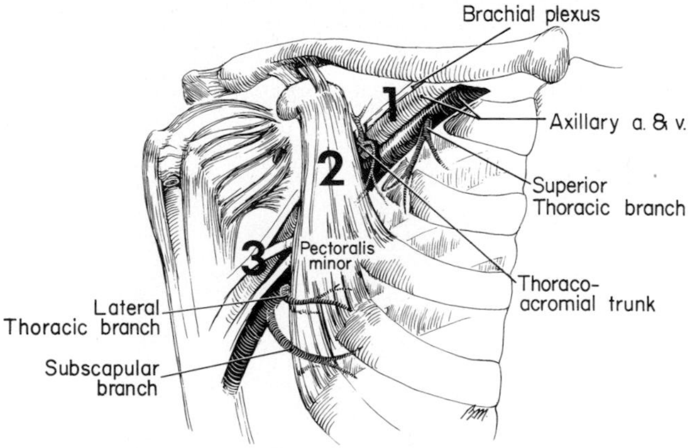

Figure 14–110

The axillary artery is divided into three parts by the pectoralis minor muscle; the second part is behind it, and the third part is lateral to it. (From Rockwood CA and Green DP [eds]: Fractures [3 vols], 2nd ed. Philadelphia: JB Lippincott, 1984.)

shoulder has been reported by Calvet and co-workers,[76] who collected 90 cases in 1941. This paper, revealing the tragic end results, must have accomplished its purpose because there have been very few reports in the literature since then dealing with the complications that occur during reduction. In their series, in which 64 of 91 reductions were performed many weeks after the initial dislocation, the mortality rate was 50%. The other patients either lost the arm or the function of the arm. Besides the long delay from dislocation to reduction, these injuries may also be caused by the use of excessive force. Delpeche observed a case in which the force of 10 men was used to accomplish the shoulder reduction, damaging the axillary vessel.[213]

SIGNS AND SYMPTOMS

Vascular damage may be obvious or subtle. Findings may include pain, expanding hematoma, pulse deficit, peripheral cyanosis, peripheral coolness and pallor, neurologic dysfunction, and shock. A Doppler or an arteriogram should confirm the diagnosis and locate the site of injury.

TREATMENT AND PROGNOSIS

Patients suspected of having major arterial injury are managed as a surgical emergency with the establishment of a major intravenous line and obtaining blood for transfusion. Jardon and co-workers[288] have pointed out that bleeding can be temporarily controlled by digital pressure on the axillary artery over the first rib. These authors also recommend that the axillary artery be explored through the subclavicular operative approach, as described by Steenburg and Ravitch.[611]

The treatment of choice for a damaged axillary artery is either by direct repair or by bypass graft after resection of the injury. Excellent results have been reported with prompt management of these vascular injuries.[69, 108, 132, 179, 192, 247, 288, 356, 403, 538, 616] The results of simple ligation of the vessels in the elderly patient have been disappointing, probably because of poor collateral circulation and the presence of arteriosclerotic vascular disease in these typically older individuals.[307, 320, 655] Even when ligation has been performed in younger patients with good collateral circulation, approximately two thirds of these patients have lost function of the upper extremity, for example, by developing upper extremity claudication.

Nerve Injuries

The brachial plexus and the axillary artery lie immediately anterior, inferior, and medial to the glenohumeral joint.[203] It is not surprising, therefore, that neurovascular injuries frequently accompany traumatic anterior glenohumeral dislocations (Fig. 14–111).

ANATOMY

The axillary nerve originates off the posterior cord of the brachial plexus. It crosses the anterior surface of the subscapularis muscle and angulates sharply posteriorly to travel along the inferior shoulder joint capsule. It then leaves the axilla to exit through the quadrangular space below the lower border of the teres minor muscle, where it hooks around the posterior and lateral humerus on the deep surface of the deltoid muscle.

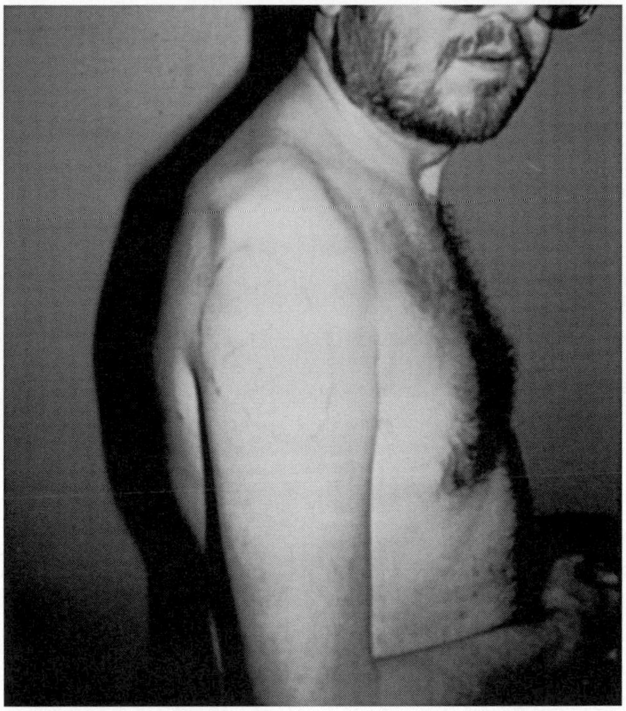

Figure 14–111

This patient sustained an axillary nerve palsy secondary to glenohumeral dislocation. Note the area of decreased sensation diagrammed on the lateral aspect of the proximal humerus. Also note the presence of significant wasting.

MECHANISM OF INJURY

The dislocated humeral head displaces the subscapularis and the overlying axillary nerve anteroinferiorly, creating traction and direct pressure on the nerve.[424, 425, 616] The injury to the nerve may be a neurapraxia (no structural damage, recovery in approximately 6 weeks), an axonotmesis (disruption of the axons, preservation of the nerve sheath, axonal regrowth at 1 inch per month), or a neurotmesis (complete nerve disruption, guarded prognosis for recovery).

INCIDENCE

The reported incidence of nerve injuries in series of acute dislocations is substantial, often as high as 33%.[70, 122, 181, 412, 444, 499, 502, 552, 646, 661, 674] If careful electrodiagnostic studies are carried out prospectively, the incidence of nerve injury may be as high as 45%.[116]

The axillary nerve is most commonly involved; up to one third of first-time anterior dislocations are associated with axillary nerve involvement.[52, 212, 351, 502, 553] The likelihood of an axillary nerve injury increases with the age of the patient, the duration of the dislocation, and the amount of trauma that initiated the dislocation.[52, 501] Other nerves injured are the radial, musculocutaneous, median, ulnar, and entire brachial plexus.

DIAGNOSIS

The diagnosis of nerve injury is considered in any patient who has neurologic symptoms or signs such as weakness or numbness after a dislocation. A nerve injury may also present as a delayed recovery of active shoulder motion after glenohumeral dislocation. Blom and Dahlback[52] demonstrated that axillary neuropathy may exist without numbness in the usual sensory distribution of the axillary nerve. Electromyography provides objective evaluation of neurologic function, provided that 3 or 4 weeks have intervened between the injury and the evaluation.[52]

TREATMENT AND PROGNOSIS

Most axillary nerve injuries resulting from anterior dislocation are traction neurapraxias, and the patients will recover completely. However, if there has been no recovery in 3 months, the prognosis is not as good.[20, 52, 70, 116]

Recurrence of Instability After Anterior Dislocations

EFFECT OF AGE

The age of the patient at the time of the initial dislocation has a major influence on the incidence of redislocation.[552, 557] Several authors have reported that individuals younger than 20 years of age at the time of the initial dislocation have up to a 90% chance of having recurrent instability.[17, 246, 262, 266, 321, 411, 412, 438, 552, 595, 684] In persons older than 40 years of age, the incidence drops sharply to 10 to 15%.[412, 557] Hovelius and associates[264] reported a careful prospective study with somewhat lower incidences of recurrences in each age group: 33% under 20 years of age, 25% between 20 and 30 years of age, and 10% between 30 and 40 years of age. The majority of all recurrences occur within the first 2 years after the first traumatic dislocation.[3, 30, 122, 154, 411, 437, 439, 552, 553, 641]

EFFECT OF TRAUMA, SPORTS, GENDER, AND DOMINANCE

Rowe[552, 557] has pointed out that the recurrence rate varies inversely with the severity of the original trauma; in other words, the more easily the dislocation occurred initially, the more easily it recurs. The recurrence rate among athletes may be higher than nonathletes[595] and higher among men than women.[438] Dominance of the affected shoulder does not seem to have a major effect on the recurrence rate.[557]

EFFECT OF POST-DISLOCATION TREATMENT

In many reports, the incidence of recurrence appears to be relatively insensitive to the type (sling versus plaster Velpeau) and duration of immobilization (0 versus 4 weeks) of the shoulder after initial dislocation.[141, 263, 411, 557] By contrast, others have reported that longer periods of immobilization (more than 3 weeks) are associated with a reduced incidence of recurrence.[315, 619]

In a definitive 10-year prospective study, Hovelius and associates studied the effect of immobilization on the incidence of recurrence.[264] After reduction, 247 primary anterior dislocations were partially randomized to either a 3- to 4-week period of immobilization or to a sling to be discarded after comfort was achieved. The authors concluded that the immobilization did not affect the rate of recurrence. The results provide useful "rules of thumb": overall half of these shoulders had recurrent dislocations; half of the recurrences had surgical treatment; half of the recurrences treated nonoperatively were stable without surgery at 10 years. One of six patients had dislocation of the opposite shoulder. Eleven per cent of the shoulders had at least mild evidence of secondary degenerative joint disease. Interestingly, this secondary DJD was observed in both surgical and nonsurgical cases.

Aronen and Regan[18] reported a 3-year average follow-up study on 20 primary dislocations in Navy midshipmen treated with a 3-month aggressive post-dislocation program. The program consisted of 3 weeks of sling immobilization followed by progressive strengthening. The patients were not allowed to return to activity until there was no evidence of weakness or atrophy and no apprehension on abduction and external rotation. In this series there were no recurrent dislocations and two recurrent subluxations. Similarly, Yoneda and associates[710] reported good results in 83% of patients in a program emphasizing post immobilization exercises.

EFFECT OF FRACTURES

The incidence of recurrence is lower when a first-time shoulder dislocation is associated with a greater tuberosity fracture.[119, 262, 264, 412, 551, 552, 556] Hovelius[262] reported that these fractures were four times as common in patients older than 30 years of age: 23% compared with 8% among patients younger than 30 years of age.

Other fractures, such as substantial posterior lateral humeral head lesions and fractures of the glenoid lip are likely to be associated with an increased incidence of recurrent instability.

In conclusion, it appears that the injuries sustained by young patients in association with traumatic dislocations are relatively unlikely to heal in a manner yielding a stable shoulder. Probably the most important of these unhealing injuries are: (1) the avulsion of the glenohumeral capsular ligaments from the anterior glenoid lip, and (2) the posterolateral humeral head defect. Older patients may tend to stretch the capsule or fracture the greater tuberosity, either of which is likely to heal yielding a stable shoulder. In atraumatic instability, there is no traumatic lesion and thus a high chance of recurrence. The degree of trauma and the age of the patient seem to be the most important factors in determining the recurrence rate.

INJURIES ASSOCIATED WITH POSTERIOR DISLOCATIONS

Fractures

Fractures of the posterior glenoid rim and of the proximal humerus (upper shaft, tuberosities, and head) are quite common in traumatic posterior dislocations of the shoulder.[475, 476, 628, 690] The commonly associated compression fracture of the anteromedial portion of the humeral head is produced by the posterior cortical rim of the glenoid. It is best seen on an axillary view or a CT scan (Fig. 14–112; see also Fig. 14–93).

This lesion, sometimes called a "reversed Hill-Sachs lesion," often occurs at the time of the original posterior dislocation. It becomes larger with multiple posterior dislocations of the shoulder. Large humeral head defects are also seen in old unreduced posterior dislocations.

The posterior rim of the glenoid may be fractured and displaced in posterior dislocations (see Fig. 14–99). This occurs not only with direct forces from an anterior direction that push the humeral head out posteriorly but also with indirect types of dislocations such as occur during seizures or accidental electrical shock.

Fracture of the lesser tuberosity of the humerus may accompany posterior dislocations. The subscapularis muscle comes under considerable tension in this dislocation and may avulse the lesser tuberosity onto which it inserts. Although the fracture may be seen on the anteroposterior and lateral x-rays of the glenohumeral joint, it is best seen on the axillary view and on a CT scan.

Posterior dislocations of the humerus may be overlooked in the presence of a comminuted fracture of the proximal humerus or humeral shaft fractures. In the series of 16 cases of posterior dislocation of the shoulder reported by O'Conner and Jacknow,[476] 12 had comminuted fractures of the proximal humerus. In 8 of the 12 cases of fracture, the diagnosis of posterior dislocation was initially missed.

Other Associated Injuries

Injuries to the rotator cuff and neurovascular structures are less common with posterior than anterior dislocations; however, they do occur. Moeller[429] reported on a patient who had an open acute posterior dislocation of the left shoulder. The shoulder was totally unstable after reduction with tears of the rotator cuff, biceps tendon, and subscapularis tendons. The patient had associated injury to the axillary and suprascapular nerves.

TREATMENT

Acute Traumatic Anterior Dislocations

TIMING OF REDUCTION AND ANALGESIA

Acute dislocations of the glenohumeral joint should be reduced as gently and expeditiously as possible, ideally after a complete set of radiographs is obtained to rule out associated bony injuries. Early relocation promptly eliminates the stretch and compression of neurovascular structures, minimizes the amount of muscle spasm that must be overcome to effect reduction, and prevents progressive enlargement of the humeral head defect in locked dislocations. The extent of anesthesia required to accomplish a gentle reduction depends on many factors, including the amount of trauma that produced the dislocation, the duration of the dislocation, the number of previous dislocations, whether the dislocation is locked, and to what extent the patient can voluntarily relax the shoulder musculature. When seen acutely, some dislocations can be reduced without the use of medication. At the other extreme, reduction of a long-standing, locked dislocation may require a brachial plexus block or general anesthetic with muscle relaxation. Many practitioners use narcotics and muscle relaxants to aid in the reduction of shoulder dislocations. A potential trap exists: The dosages required to produce muscle relaxation while the shoulder is dislocated may be sufficient to produce respiratory depression once the shoulder is reduced. Our recommendation is that if these medications are to be used, they should be administered through an established intravenous line. This produces a more rapid onset, a short duration of action, and the opportunity to adjust the required dose more appropriately. Furthermore, resusci-

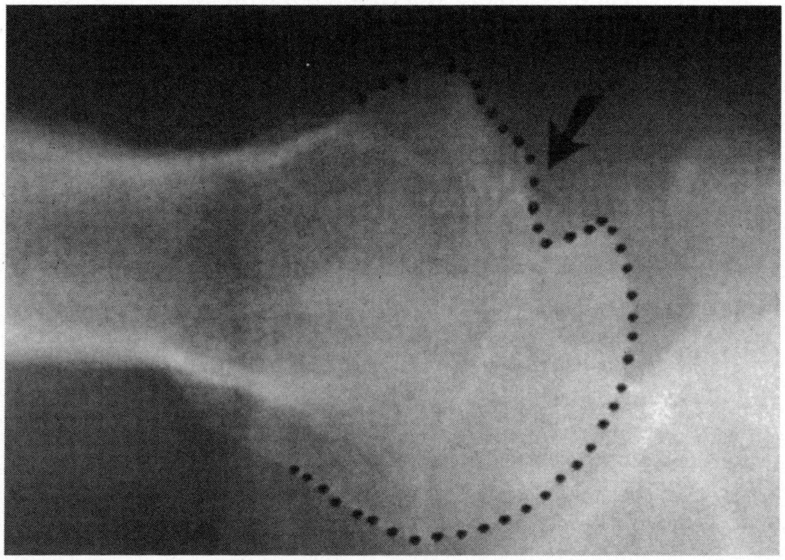

Figure 14–112

An axillary lateral x-ray film demonstrating an anteromedial compression fracture of the humeral head ("reverse Hill-Sachs lesion") after a traumatic posterior shoulder dislocation. (From Rockwood CA Jr, Green DP, and Bucholz RW [eds]: Fractures in Adults. Philadelphia: JB Lippincott, 1991.)

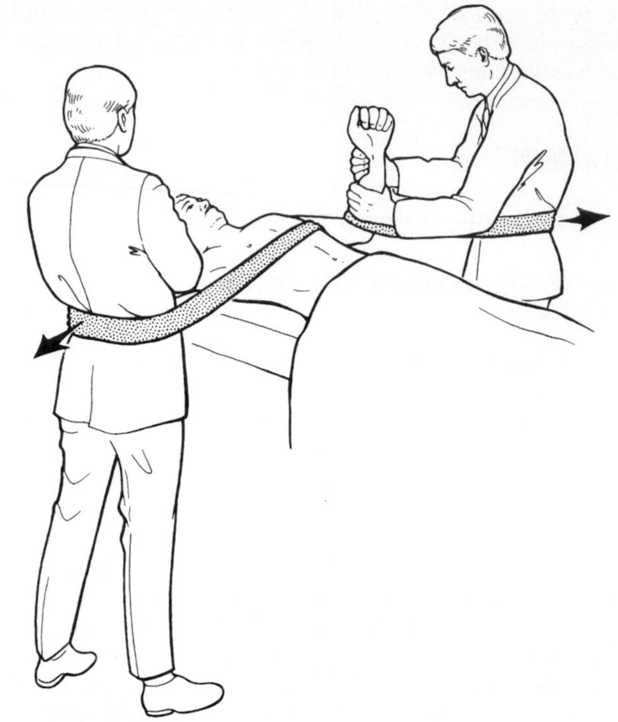

Figure 14–113

Reduction technique for an anterior glenohumeral dislocation. The patient lies supine with a sheet placed around the thorax, then around the assistant's waist; this provides countertraction. The surgeon stands on the side of the dislocated shoulder near the patient's waist with the elbow of the dislocated shoulder flexed to 90 degrees. A second sheet is tied loosely around the waist of the surgeon and looped over the patient's forearm, thus providing traction while the surgeon leans back against the sheet, grasping the forearm. Steady traction along the axis of the arm will usually cause reduction. The surgeon's hands are free to gently rock the humerus from internal to external rotation or to provide gentle outward pressure on the proximal humerus from the axilla.

tation (if necessary) is facilitated by the prospective presence of such a route of access. Airway management tools should be readily available.

Lippitt and associates[367, 368] compared two methods of analgesia for the reduction of anterior dislocations: (1) intravenous analgesia and muscle relaxation, and (2) intra-articular lidocaine. With respect to the first, they found a 75% success rate and a 37% complication rate in a retrospective series of 52 reductions in which intravenous narcotics, such as morphine (3 to 24 mg) or meperidine (12.5 to 100 mg) with or without diazepam (1.5 to 15 mg) or midazolam (1 to 10 mg), were used for analgesia. They remarked on the difficulty of determining the appropriate intravenous dose of narcotics. Level of pain, age, smoking history, alcohol consumption, cardiac disease, and regional perfusion are just a few of the factors that may influence the narcotic requirement.[24] Older patients and intoxicated patients are more sensitive to the respiratory depressant effects of narcotics. Because pain counteracts the respiratory depressant effects, patients sedated by narcotics are at increased risk of respiratory depression after removal of the painful stimulus when the shoulder is reduced. Complications from intravenous analgesia included respiratory depression, hypotension, hyperemesis, and oversedation. With respect to the second method using 20 ml of 1% plain intra-articular lidocaine, Lippitt and associates found a 100% success rate in the reduction of 40 dislocations with no complications. One patient inadvertently received 400 mg instead of 200 mg of lidocaine and developed transient tinnitus, perioral numbness, and mild dysarthria. A survey revealed that both the patients and the physicians were satisfied with this method. The authors speculated that the success of the intra-articular injection may be due to a combination of pain relief allowing reduction, relief from muscle spasm, and venting of the joint.

METHOD OF REDUCTION

Once the shoulder is relaxed, a variety of gentle methods can be used to achieve reduction. Gentle traction on the arm is common to most (Figs. 14–113 and 14–114). One such method is known as the Stimson technique. Although named for Stimson[617, 618] of New York, Stimson credited Cole, a house-staff physician of the Chambers Street Hospital. In the Stimson method, the patient is placed prone on the edge of the examining table while downward traction is gently applied.[617] The traction force may be applied by the weight of the arm, by weights taped to the wrist, or by the surgeon. It may take several minutes for the traction to produce muscle relaxation. It is important that patient is not left unattended in this position, particularly if narcotics and muscle relaxants have been administered.

AUTHORS' PREFERRED METHOD OF ANTERIOR REDUCTION

Analgesia

While analgesia may not be necessary to achieve reduction, we are impressed with the safety and effectiveness

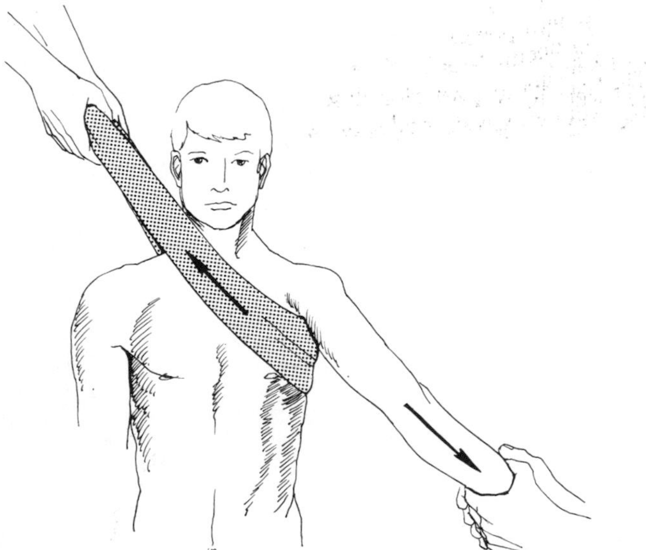

Figure 14–114

Closed reduction of the left shoulder with traction against countertraction. (From Rockwood CA and Green DP [eds]: Fractures [3 vols], 2nd ed. Philadelphia: JB Lippincott, 1984.)

of intra-articular lidocaine as described by Lippitt and associates (Fig. 14–115).[367, 368] In this method a maximum 20 ml of 1% plain lidocaine is injected using an 18-gauge needle placed 2 cm below the lateral edge of the acromion just posterior to the dislocated humeral head and directed towards the glenoid fossa. The amount of lidocaine is limited to 200 mg.[574] Placement of the needle in the joint is confirmed by a combination of: (1) feeling the needle penetrate the glenohumeral capsule, (2) aspirating joint fluid/hemarthrosis and ensuring that the injection is not intravascular, (3) gently palpating the glenoid fossa with the needle, and (4) verifying easy flow on injection and return of the injected lidocaine solution. Fifteen minutes are allowed to maximize the analgesic effect of the lidocaine prior to manipulation.

Maneuver

Reduction of either anterior or posterior glenohumeral dislocations can usually be effected by traction on the abducted and flexed arm with countertraction on the body (see Figs. 14–113 and 14–114). The patient is placed supine with a sheet around the thorax, with the loose ends on the side opposite the shoulder dislocation where they are held by an assistant. The surgeon stands on the side of the dislocated shoulder near the waist of the patient. The elbow of the dislocated shoulder is flexed to 90 degrees (to relax the neurovascular structures), and traction is applied through a sheet looped over the patient's forearm or traction can be applied directly. Steady traction along the axis of the arm will usually effect reduction. To this basic maneuver, one may add gentle rocking of the humerus from internal to external rotation or outward pressure on the proximal humerus from the axilla. These additions are particularly useful if prereduction axillary roentgenograms show that the humeral head is impaled on the glenoid rim. Postreduction roentgenograms are used to confirm reduction and to detect fractures. A postreduction neurovascular check is routine.

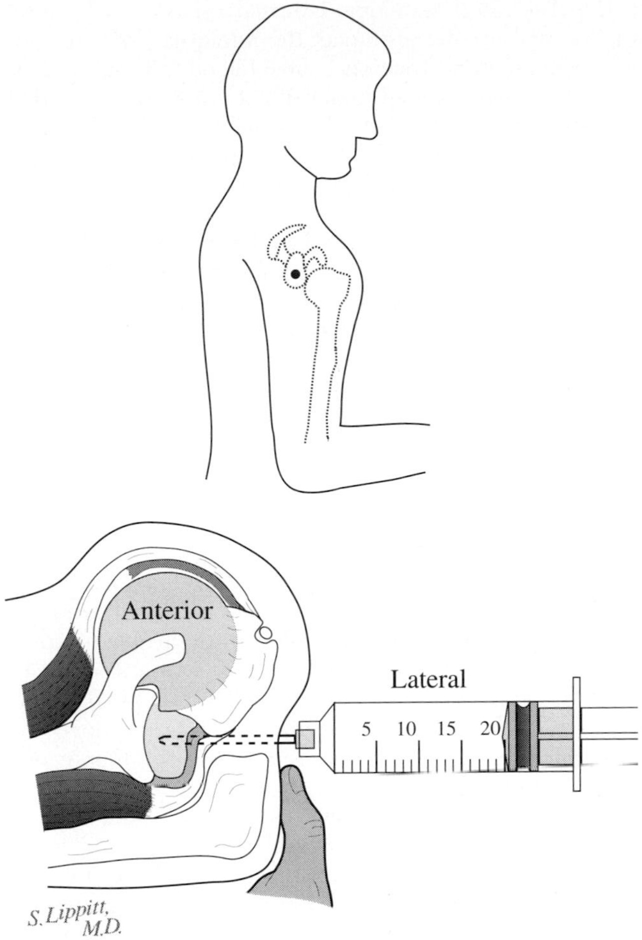

Figure 14–115

An intra-articular lidocaine injection for anesthesia during reduction of an anterior dislocation. The needle is inserted just posterior to the dislocated humeral head.

Chronic Anterior Traumatic Dislocations

REDUCTION AND ANALGESIA

A glenohumeral joint that has been dislocated for several days is a chronic dislocation. The principles and methods for reducing a chronic dislocation are similar to those relating to an acute dislocation, except for the fact that the patient and the shoulder are usually more fragile and the relocation is more difficult. As the chronicity of the dislocation increases, so do the difficulties and complications of reduction. When one encounters an elderly patient with pain in the shoulder whose x-rays reveal an anterior dislocation, a very careful history is needed to determine whether the initial injury occurred recently or quite a while earlier.

Chronic dislocations are seen most commonly in elderly people and in those whose general health or mental status may prevent them from seeking help for the injury. The event causing injury itself may be relatively trivial.[42, 427] Old age, chronicity of dislocation, and soft bone make closed reduction difficult and dangerous.[404] If a closed reduction is to be performed, it should be done with minimal traction, without leverage, and with total muscle relaxation under controlled general anesthesia. If the dislocation is more than 1 week old, the humeral head is likely to be firmly impaled on the anterior glenoid with such soft tissue contraction that gentle closed reduction is impossible.

OPEN REDUCTION

If a gentle attempt at closed reduction fails, open procedure reduction is considered. This can be a complex procedure because of the altered position of the axillary artery and branches of the brachial plexus and because the structures are tight and scarred. When the risks of attempting reduction appear to outweigh the advantages, the dislocated position may be accepted. Sometimes the symptoms of chronic dislocation are surprisingly minimal.[178]

In performing an open reduction, the subscapularis and anterior capsule are incised near their insertion to the lesser tuberosity allowing substantial external rotation of the dislocated shoulder. External rotation and lateral traction will usually disimpact the humerus from the glenoid. While lateral traction is maintained, the humerus is gently internally rotated under direct vision to ensure that the articular surface of the humerus passes safely by the anterior glenoid lip and into the glenoid fossa. Leverage is avoided because the head is usually very soft. If the posterolateral head defect is greater than 40% or if the head collapses during reduction, a humeral head prosthesis may be necessary to restore a functional joint surface. The subscapularis and capsule are then repaired. The shoulder is carefully inspected for evidence of cuff tear or vascular damage.

RESULTS OF TREATMENT OF CHRONIC DISLOCATIONS

Schulz and associates[580] reported a series of 17 posterior and 44 anterior chronic dislocations. These dislocations occurred primarily among elderly people; more than half of the dislocations were associated with fracture of the tuberosities, humeral head, humeral neck, glenoid, or coracoid process. More than one third involved neurologic deficits. Closed reduction was attempted in 40 shoulders and was successful in 20. Of the 20 shoulders successfully reduced (3 posterior and 17 anterior), the duration of dislocation exceeded 4 weeks in only one instance. Open reduction was performed in 20 and humeral head excision in 6. Eight patients were not treated, and five shoulders were irreducible.

Perniceni and co-worker[507] described the reinforcement of the anterior shoulder complex in three patients after reduction of neglected anterior dislocations of the shoulder. They used the Gosset[200] technique, which places a rib graft between the coracoid and the glenoid rim. Rowe and Zarins[560] reported on 24 patients with unreduced dislocations of the shoulder and operated on 14 of them.

Management After Reduction of an Anterior Dislocation

EVALUATION

After reducing the dislocation, anteroposterior and lateral x-ray views are obtained in the plane of the scapula to verify the adequacy of the reduction and to provide an additional opportunity to detect fractures of the glenoid and proximal humerus. The patient's neurologic status is again checked, including the sensory and motor functions of all five major nerves in the upper extremity. The strength of the pulse is verified, and evidence of bruits or an expanding hematoma is sought.[212] The integrity of the rotator cuff is initially evaluated by observing the strength of isometric external rotation and abduction.

Trimmings[644] demonstrated that aspiration of the hemarthrosis from the shoulder can be an effective means of reducing discomfort after the shoulder is reduced.

PROTECTION

Since recurrent glenohumeral instability is the most common complication of a glenohumeral dislocation, postreduction treatment focuses on optimizing shoulder stability. Thus, two potentially important elements in postreduction treatment are protection and muscle rehabilitation. Reeves demonstrated that after repair of the subscapularis in primates, 3 months were necessary before normal capsular patterns of collagen bundles were observed, 5 months before the tendon was histologically normal, and 4 to 5 months before tensile strength was regained.[527] It is unknown whether labral tears or ligamentous avulsions from the glenoid heal or how long this might take. In any event, it is apparent that the shoulder cannot be immobilized for the full length of time required for complete healing. (The reader is referred to the previous section "Recurrence of instability after anterior dislocations, effect of post dislocation treatment" for a review of some of the literature on the effectiveness of different postreduction management programs.)

The authors treat first time dislocations in a manner similar to the postoperative management for dislocation repairs. Thus, younger patients are placed on the "90-0 program" in which flexion is limited to 90 degrees and external rotation is limited to zero degrees for the first 3 weeks while strength is maintained with cuff and deltoid isometrics. The elbow is fully extended at least several times a day to prevent "sling soreness." Because persons older than 30 years of age are more likely to develop stiffness of the shoulder, elbow, and hand, the duration of immobilization is progressively reduced for individuals of increasing age.[321, 411, 412, 552, 710] Patients are checked at 3 weeks after relocation and examined for stiffness; if external rotation to zero degrees is difficult, formal stretching exercises are started. Otherwise, the patient is allowed to increase the use of the shoulder as comfort permits.

STRENGTHENING

At 3 weeks, the patient institutes more vigorous rotator cuff strengthening exercises using rubber tubing or weights. The patient is informed that strong subscapularis and infraspinatus muscles are ideally situated to increase glenohumeral stability.[569]

Burkhead and Rockwood,[71] Glousman and co-workers,[195] and Tibone and Bradley[635] have emphasized the importance of strengthening not only the rotator cuff but also the scapular stabilizing muscles because of their vital importance in providing a stable platform for shoulder function. Even in the case of recurrent instability, Rockwood and Burkhead[71] found that a complete exercise program was effective in the management of 12% of patients with traumatic subluxation, 80% with anterior atraumatic subluxation, and 90% with posterior instability.

Swimming is recommended at 6 weeks to enhance endurance and coordination. By 3 months after the dislocation, most patients should have almost full flexion and rotation of the shoulder. The patient is not allowed to use the injured arm in sports or for over-the-head labor until they have achieved: (1) normal rotator strength, (2) comfortable and nearly full forward elevation, and (3) confidence in their shoulder with it in the necessary positions. Any deviation from the expected course of recovery requires careful re-evaluation for occult fractures, loose bodies, rotator cuff tears, peripheral nerve injuries, and glenohumeral arthritis.

Indications for Early Surgery in Shoulders Dislocated Anteriorly

SOFT TISSUE INTERPOSITION

Tietjen[637] reported a case in which surgery was required to retrieve the avulsed supraspinatus, infraspinatus, and teres minor from their interposition between the humeral head and the glenoid.

Bridle and Ferris[65] reported a case of apparent successful closed reduction of an anterior shoulder dislocation that appeared to be confirmed on an anteroposterior radiograph. However, the patient continued to experience severe pain and a subsequent axillary lateral view demonstrated a persistent anterior subluxation of the glenohumeral joint. At the time of open reduction the ruptured muscle belly of the subscapularis was found interposed between the humeral head and glenoid. Inao and associates[279] reported a case of an acute anterior shoulder dislocation that was irreducible by closed treatment due to the interposition of the posteriorly displaced tendon of the long head of the biceps.

DISPLACED FRACTURE OF THE GREATER TUBEROSITY

Although fractures of the greater tuberosity are not uncommonly associated with anterior shoulder dislocation, the tuberosity usually reduces into an acceptable position when the shoulder is reduced (see Figs. 14–5 and 14–105). Occasionally, the greater tuberosity fragment displaces up under the acromion process or is pulled posteriorly by the cuff muscles. If the greater tuberosity remains displaced after reduction of the shoulder joint (see Fig. 14–109), consideration should be given to anatomic reduction and internal fixation of the fragment and repair of the attendant split in the tendons of the rotator cuff (see Fig. 14–106). It is relatively easy to determine the amount of superior displacement of the tuberosity fragment on the anteroposterior roentgenogram in the plane of the scapula. Posterior displacement can be more difficult to discern. It is important to look for the "vacant tuberosity" sign, wherein the normal contour of the greater tuberosity is lacking. If there is concern about the anteroposterior position of the tuberosity on plain films, a CT scan should be considered. If the tuberosity is allowed to heal with posterior displacement, it may produce both the functional equivalent of a rotator cuff tear and a bony block to external rotation.

GLENOID RIM FRACTURE

Aston and Gregory[21] reported three cases in which a large anterior fracture of the glenoid occurred as a result of a fall on the lateral aspect of the abducted shoulder. A fracture of the glenoid lip may require open reduction and internal fixation if it presents intra-articular incongruity or an inadequate effective glenoid arc (see Fig. 14–99).

SPECIAL PROBLEMS

Occasionally, it may be a consideration to perform an early surgical reconstruction in a patient who requires absolute and complete shoulder stability before being able to return to his or her occupation or sport. Hertz and associates[249] reported a 2.4-year follow-up on 31 patients having an initial dislocation with primary repair of an arthroscopically demonstrated Bankart lesion: none had recurrent instability. Arcierohas initiated a study at West Point in which the Bankart lesion is repaired arthroscopically after the initial dislocation.[16, 17] His initial data indicate a decrease in recurrent instability from 80% with nonoperative management to 14% with early repair.[15–17]

POSTERIOR DISLOCATIONS

Reduction

The reduction of acute, traumatic posterior dislocations may be much more difficult than the reduction of acute, traumatic anterior dislocations. Hawkins and co-workers[238] reviewed 41 cases of locked posterior shoulder dislocations. The average interval between injury and diagnosis was 1 year! In seven shoulders, the deformity was accepted. Closed reduction was successful in only 6 of the 12 cases in which it was attempted.

Intravenous narcotics combined with muscle relaxants or tranquilizers may provide insufficient analgesia and muscle relaxation; general anesthesia with muscle paralysis may be required. Atraumatic closed reduction can usually be accomplished once the muscle spasm has been eliminated. With the patient in the supine position, longitudinal and lateral traction is applied to the arm while it is gently rocked in internal and external rotation. Once the head is disimpacted, it is lifted anteriorly back into the glenoid fossa. In locked posterior dislocations, it may be necessary to gently stretch out the posterior cuff and capsule by maximally internally rotating the humerus before reduction is attempted. Care should be taken not to force the arm into external rotation before reduction is achieved; if the head is locked posteriorly on the glenoid rim, forced external rotation could produce a fracture of the head or shaft of the humerus.

If gentle closed reduction of a locked posterior glenohumeral dislocation is not possible, open reduction may be accomplished through an anterior deltopectoral approach.[131, 238, 301, 331, 337, 410, 547, 576] Because local anatomy is significantly distorted, the tendon of the long head of the biceps is used as a guide to the lesser tuberosity. The subscapularis is released either by lesser tuberosity osteotomy or by direct incision. With the glenoid thus exposed, open reduction is carried out by gently pulling the humeral head laterally and then lifting its articular surface up on the face of the glenoid.

Postreduction Care

If, after closed reduction, the shoulder is stable in the sling position, this type of postreduction management is most convenient for the patient. However, if there is concern about recurrent instability, the shoulder is immobilized in a shoulder spica or brace with the amount of external rotation necessary to provide stability.[83, 84] Scougall[583] has shown experimentally in monkeys that a surgically detached posterior glenoid labrum and capsule heal soundly without repair. He concluded that the best position of immobilization, to allow healing for all of the posterior structures, was in abduction, external rotation, and extension and that the position should be maintained for 4 weeks.

While some have recommended pin fixation for 3 weeks after reduction,[690] this method carries risk of pin breakage and infection.

Early Surgery in Acute Traumatic Posterior Dislocation

Indications for surgery include a displaced lesser tuberosity fracture, a significant posterior glenoid fracture, an irreducible dislocation, an open dislocation, or an unstable reduction.

A major cause of recurrent instability after reduction of a posterior dislocation is the presence of a large anteromedial humeral head defect. If at the time of reduction, stability cannot be obtained because of such a defect, it may be rendered extra-articular by filling it with the subscapularis tendon as described by McLaughlin[356, 405–407, 410] or the lesser tuberosity as described by Neer.[463, 541] If the humeral head defect involves more than 30% of the articular surface, prosthetic replacement may be indicated, otherwise instability may recur with internal rotation. Hawkins and associates demonstrated the use of each of these techniques in a series of locked posterior dislocations.[238]

After surgery the arm may be immobilized in a sling and swathe for 2 weeks as recommended by McLaughlin, positioning the arm at the side posterior to the coronal plane using a strip of tape or canvas restraint as recommended by Rowe and Zarins,[560] or a modified spica in neutral rotation for 6 weeks followed by an additional 3 to 6 months of rehabilitative exercises as recommended by Rockwood.[541]

Keppler and associates have suggested using rotational osteotomy of the humerus in the postreduction management of locked posterior dislocations.[317]

Chronic Posterior Dislocation

If a patient, especially an older patient, has had a chronic posterior dislocation for months or years and if there is minimal pain and a functional range of motion, then surgery may not be indicated. However, if disability exists and there is good bone stock to the glenohumeral joint, then open reduction with a subscapularis or lesser tuberosity transfer or shoulder arthroplasty can be considered.[560]

Authors' Preferred Method of Treatment

Our management of acute traumatic posterior dislocations begins with a definition of the extent and chronicity of the injury. A complete radiographic evaluation is necessary, including anteroposterior and lateral views in the plane of the scapula and an axillary view. Careful note is made of associated fractures, including the extent of the impression fracture of the anteromedial humeral head. Under anesthesia and muscle relaxation, a gentle closed reduction is attempted using axial traction on the arm. If the head is locked on the glenoid rim, gentle internal rotation may stretch out the posterior capsule to facilitate reduction. Lateral traction on the proximal humerus may unlock the humeral head. Once it is unlocked, the humerus is gently externally rotated. After reduction is achieved and confirmed by postreduction radiographs, the reduction is maintained for 3 weeks by a cummerbund "handshake" cast (Fig. 14–116) or orthotic (Fig. 14–117) in neutral rotation and slight extension. External rotation and deltoid isometrics are carried out during this period of immobilization. After removal of the cast, a vigorous internal and external rotator strengthening program is initiated. Range of motion is allowed to return with active use, beginning with elevation in the plane of the scapula. Vigorous physical activities are not resumed until the shoulder is strong and 3 months have elapsed since reduction. Swimming is encouraged to develop endurance and muscle coordination.

When there is a humeral head defect comprising 20 to 40% of the humeral head, a subscapularis transfer into the defect is considered to prevent recurrent instability. When the humeral head defect is greater than 40%, a proximal humeral prosthesis is considered to replace the lost articular surface. When the dislocation is obviously chronic, consideration can be given to accepting the dislo-

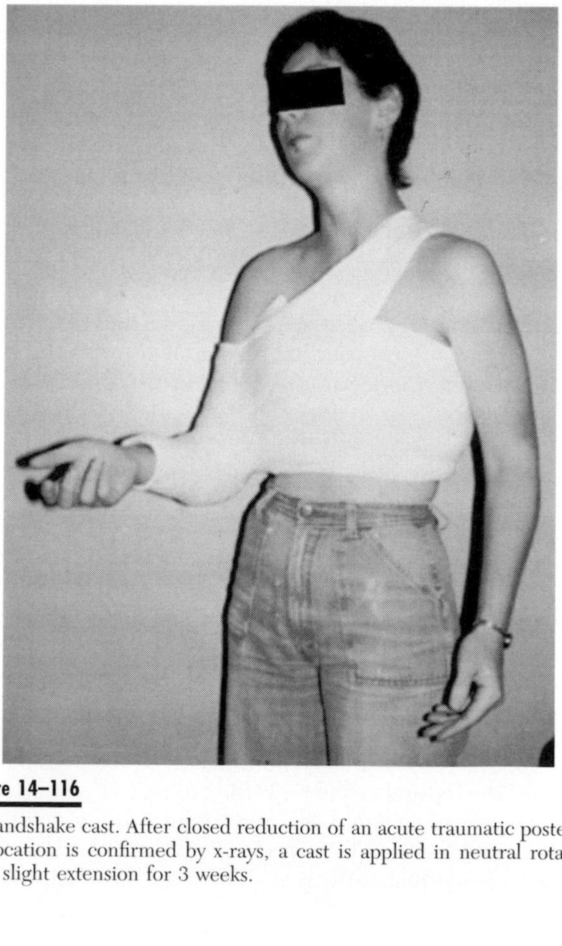

Figure 14–116

A handshake cast. After closed reduction of an acute traumatic posterior dislocation is confirmed by x-rays, a cast is applied in neutral rotation and slight extension for 3 weeks.

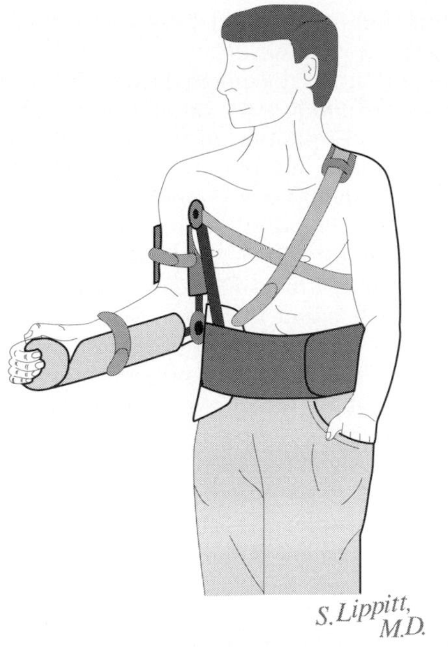

Figure 14–117

An orthosis is used to immobilize the arm after reduction of a posterior dislocation or a global capsular repair. (Modified from Matsen FA III, Lippitt SB, Sidles JA, and Harryman DT II: Practical Evaluation and Management of the Shoulder. Philadelphia: WB Saunders, 1994.)

cation and focusing on enhancing the patient's ability to carry out activities of daily living.

RECURRENT INSTABILITY: EVALUATION

After an initial dislocation, the shoulder may return to functional stability or it may fall victim to recurrent glenohumeral instability. While intermediate forms of recurrent instability do occur, the great majority of recurrently unstable shoulders may be thought of as being either atraumatic or traumatic in origin.

Recurrent Atraumatic Instability

Atraumatic instability is instability that arises without the type of trauma necessary to tear the stabilizing soft tissues or to create a humeral head defect, tuberosity fracture or glenoid lip fracture. Certain shoulders may be more susceptible to atraumatic instability. A small or functionally flat glenoid fossa may jeopardize the concavity compression, adhesion-cohesion, and glenoid suction cup stability mechanisms. Thin, excessively compliant capsular tissue may invaginate into the joint when traction is applied, limiting the effectiveness of stabilization from limited joint volume. A large, potentially capacious capsule may allow humeroscapular positions outside the range of balance stability. Weak rotator cuff muscles may provide insufficient compression for the concavity compression stabilizing mechanism. Poor neuromuscular control may fail to position the scapula to balance the net humeral joint reaction force. Voluntary or inadvertent malpositioning of the humerus in excessive anterior or posterior scapular planes may cause the net humeral joint reaction force to lie outside balance stability angles. Once initiated, the instability may be perpetuated by compression of the glenoid rim resulting from chronically poor humeral head centering. Excessive labral compliance may predispose to this loss of effective glenoid depth.

Any of these factors, individually or in combination, could contribute to instability of the glenohumeral joint. For example, posterior glenohumeral subluxation may result from the combination of a relatively flat posterior glenoid and the tendency to retract the scapula during anterior elevation of the arm, resulting in use of the elevated humerus in excessively anterior scapular planes. Excessively compliant capsular tissue in combination with relatively weak rotator cuff muscles could contribute to inferior subluxation on attempted lifting of objects with the arm at the side. If the lateral scapula is allowed to droop (whether voluntarily or involuntarily), the superior capsular structures are relaxed, permitting inferior translation of the humerus with respect to the glenoid (see Fig. 14–17).[284]

Because they usually result from loss of midrange stability, atraumatic instabilities are more likely to be multidirectional. Pathogenic factors such as a flat glenoid, weak muscles, and a compliant capsule may produce instability anteriorly, inferiorly, posteriorly, or a combination. Although the onset of atraumatic instability may be provoked by a period of disuse or a minor injury, many of the underlying contributing factors may be developmental. As a result, the tendency for atraumatic instability is likely to be bilateral and familial as well.

It is apparent that atraumatic instability is not a simple diagnosis, but rather a syndrome that may arise from a multiplicity of factors. To help recall the various aspects of this syndrome, we use the acronym AMBRII. The instability is **a**traumatic, usually associated with **m**ultidirectional laxity and with **b**ilateral findings. Treatment is predominantly by **r**ehabilitation, directed at restoring optimal neuromuscular control. If surgery is necessary, it needs to include reconstruction of the rotator **i**nterval capsule-coracohumeral ligament mechanism and tightening of the **i**nferior capsule. The diagnosis and management of this condition have been presented in detail.[96, 366, 394, 477]

HISTORY

Most patients who present with AMBRII are younger than 30 years of age (Fig. 14–118). Because the instability manifests itself in mid-range positions of the shoulder, atraumatic instability typically causes discomfort and dysfunction in ordinary activities of daily living. Commonly such patients have greatest difficulty sleeping, lifting overhead, and throwing (Table 14–2 and Fig. 14–119). Their general health status as revealed by the SF 36 is not as good on average as that of a comparable group of patients with traumatic instability (Fig. 14–120).

The onset is usually insidious, but it may occur after a minor injury or period of disuse. The unwanted translations may range from a sensation of a minor "slip" in the joint to a complete dislocation of the humeral head from

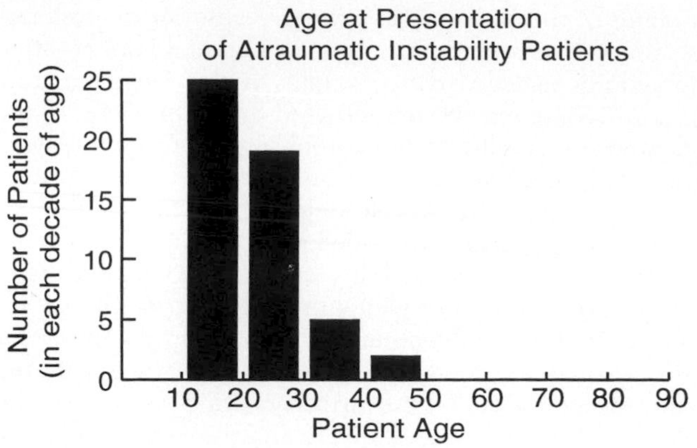

Figure 14–118

The age distribution of 51 patients with atraumatic instability. (From Matsen FA III, Lippitt SB, Sidles JA, and Harryman DT II: Practical Evaluation and Management of the Shoulder. Philadelphia: WB Saunders, 1994.)

the glenoid. The displacement characteristically reduces spontaneously after which the patient is usually able to return to his or her activities without much pain or problem. As the condition progresses, the patient notices that the shoulder has become looser and may feel it slip out and clunk back in with increasing ease and in an increasing number of activities. The shoulder may become uncomfortable, even with the arm at rest. The patient may volunteer that he or she can make the shoulder "pop out" and that at times the shoulder feels as if it "needs to be popped out" on purpose.

It is important to document from the history the circumstances surrounding the onset of the problem as well as each and every position of the shoulder in which the patient experiences instability. It is also important to note if the opposite shoulder is symptomatic as well. A family history may reveal other kindred similarly affected as well as conditions known to predispose to atraumatic instability, such as Ehlers-Danlos syndrome.

Many patients admit that they used to have a habit of dislocating the joint, but now they can no longer control the stability of the joint. The surgeon must determine if habitual dislocation remains a feature of the patient's problem. It is obvious that it is difficult for surgery to cure habitual instability.

Finally, it is important to document the patient's expectations of the shoulder to ensure that the goals are within reach before treatment is started.

PHYSICAL EXAMINATION

Demonstration of Instability

The patient is routinely asked if he or she can dislocate the shoulder at will (Fig. 14–121; see also Figs. 14–60 and 14–61). This enables the surgeon to see the different positions of concern and directions of translation. By palpating the scapula, the surgeon can estimate the relative position of the humerus and scapula when the shoul-

Table 14–2 CHARACTERISTICS OF PATIENTS WITH TRAUMATIC INSTABILITY (TUBS), ATRAUMATIC INSTABILITY (AMBRII), AND FAILED INSTABILITY REPAIRS

	TUBS	*AMBRII*	*FAILED REPAIRS*
No. of Patients	101	70	76
% Female	26%	38%	28%
% Right side	55%	68%	51%
Age	29 ± 11	27 ± 10	31 ± 8
% ABLE TO PERFORM FUNCTION	***TUBS (101)***	***AMBRII (70)***	***FAILED REPAIRS (76)***
Sleep on side	43	19	11
Comfort by side	87	71	56
Wash opposite shoulder	69	64	39
Hand behind head	77	75	48
Tuck in shirt	89	81	54
Place 8 lb on shelf	53	35	28
Place 1 lb on shelf	91	75	65
Place coin on shelf	93	77	73
Toss overhand	31	35	15
Do usual work	69	46	42
Toss underhand	83	70	44
Carry 20 lb	73	61	46
HEALTH STATUS	***TUBS (101)***	***AMBRII (70)***	***FAILED REPAIRS (76)***
Physical role	52	35	28
Comfort	60	43	43
Physical function	85	78	71
Emotional role	86	72	70
Social function	84	73	66
Vitality	67	58	55
Mental health	78	74	68
General health	81	78	68

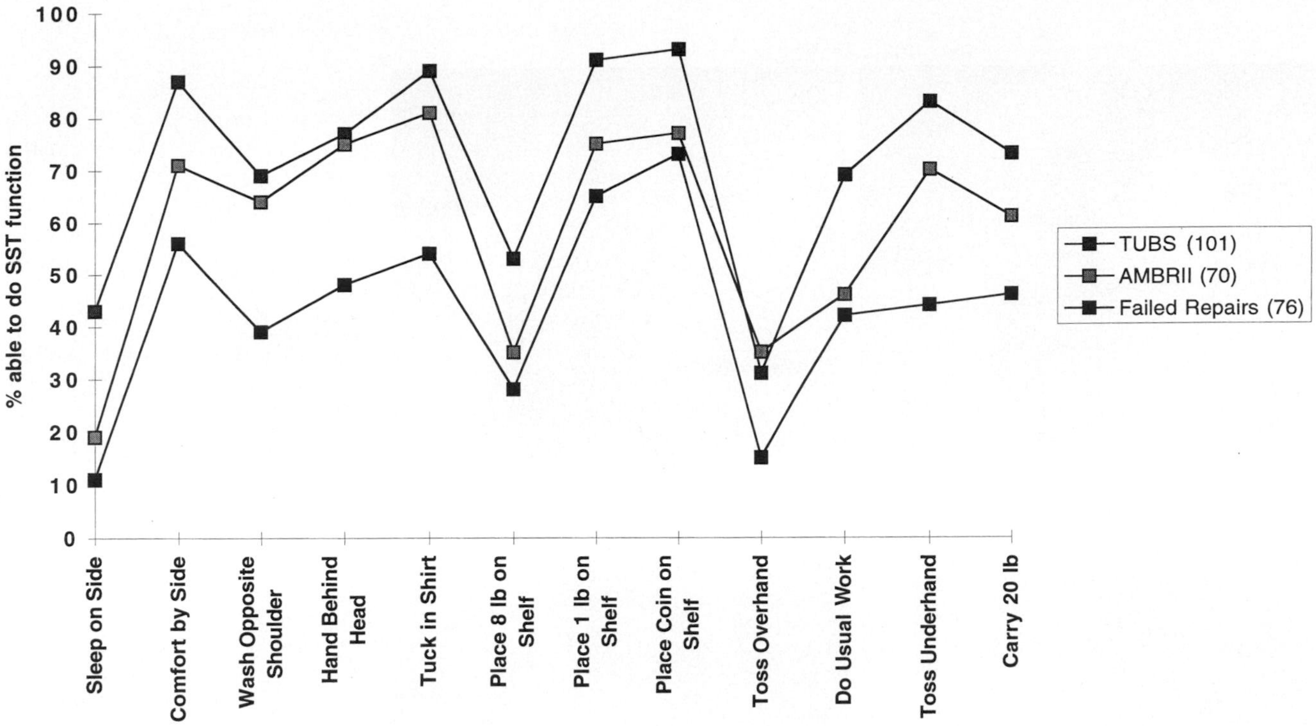

Figure 14–119

A comparison of responses to the 12 questions of the Simple Shoulder Test for groups of patients with traumatic instability (TUBS), atraumatic instability (AMBRII), and failed instability repairs.

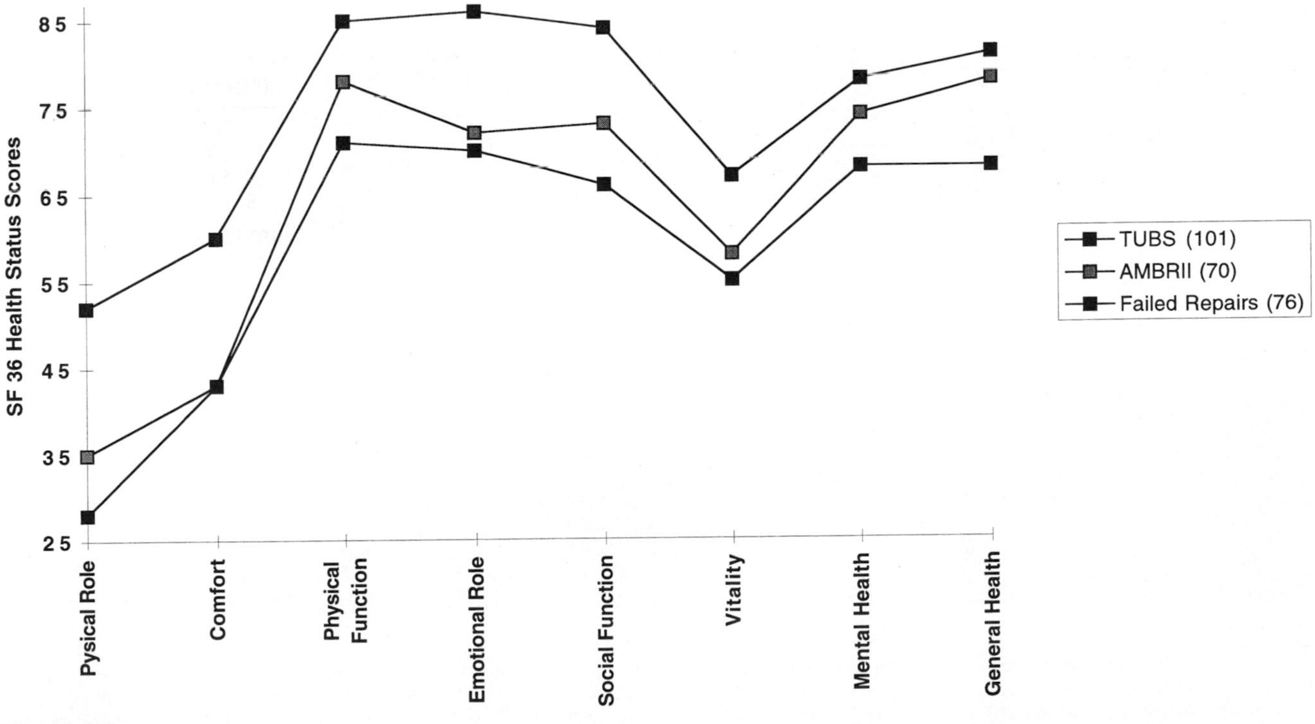

Figure 14–120

A comparison of scores on the SF 36 General Health Status Questionnaire for groups of patients with traumatic instability (TUBS), atraumatic instability (AMBRII), and failed instability repairs.

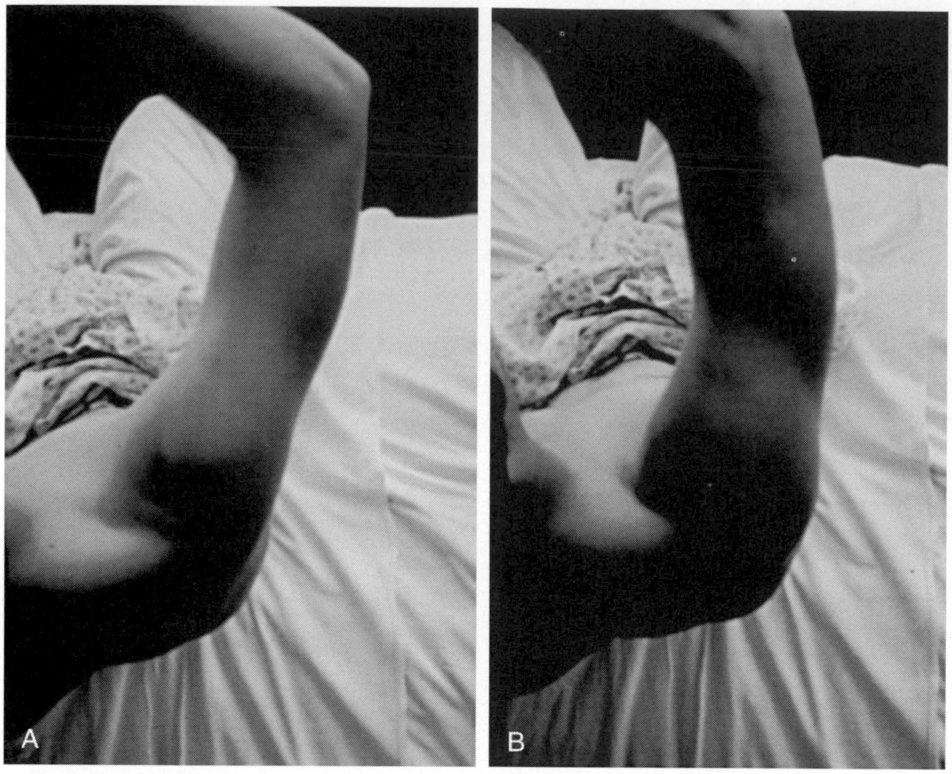

Figure 14–121

The voluntary jerk test. *A,* Normal appearance of the shoulder before the patient performs a jerk test. *B,* With movement of the arm horizontally across the body, the humeral head slides off the back of the glenoid, with a jerk of dislocation and a prominence in the posterior aspect of the patient's shoulder. When the arm is moved back to position shown in "A," a jerk of reduction occurs.

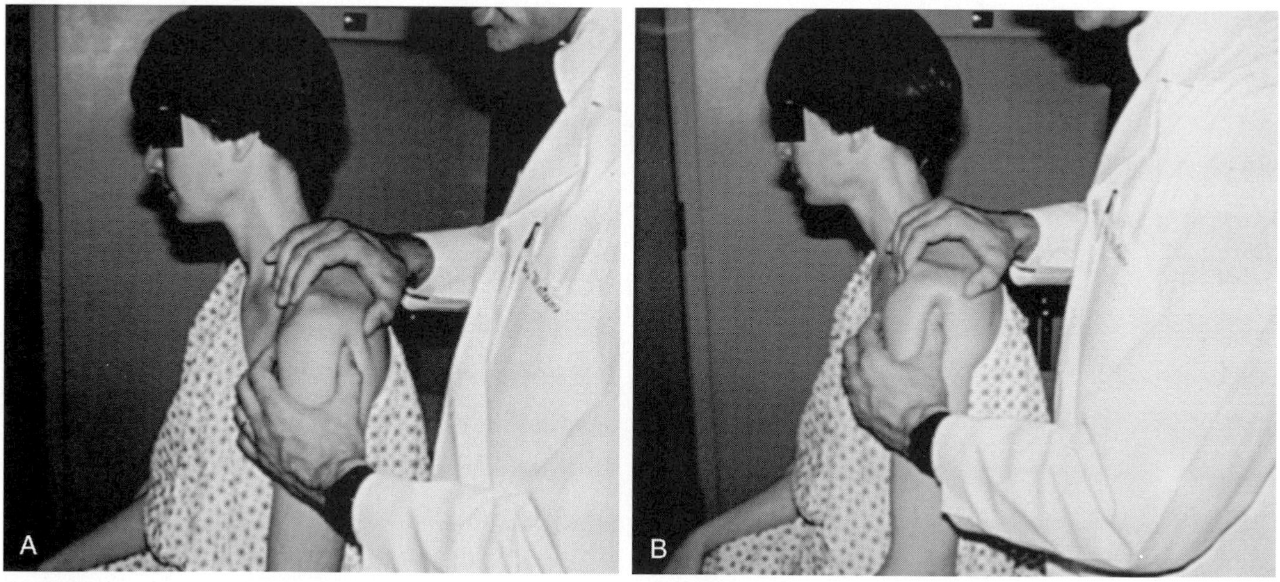

Figure 14–122

Drawer test. *A,* With the patient seated and the forearm resting in the lap, the examiner stands behind the patient and stabilizes the shoulder girdle with one hand while grasping the proximal humerus with the other, pressing the humeral head gently toward the scapula to center it in the glenoid. *B,* The head is then pushed forward to determine the amount of anterior displacement relative to the scapula. It can then be returned to the neutral position, and a posterior force is applied to determine the amount of posterior translation relative to the scapula.

der is translated and reduced. There are three common demonstrations of instability:

1. The patient may demonstrate a spontaneous "jerk" test by bringing the internally rotated arm horizontally across the chest, causing the humeral head to subluxate posteriorly; then, by returning the elevated humerus to the coronal plane, the shoulder produces a "clunk" on reduction of glenohumeral joint (much like the Ortolani and Barlow signs of the hip).
2. The patient may demonstrate that when he or she attempts to lift an object or tie a shoe, the shoulder subluxates inferiorly.
3. The patient may demonstrate that the shoulder translates when the arm is elevated in posterior humerothoracic planes with spontaneous reduction on return to the coronal plane.

Laxity Tests

These tests examine the amount of translation allowed by the shoulder starting from positions where the ligaments are normally loose. The amount of translation on laxity testing is determined by the length of the capsule and ligaments as well as by the starting position (i.e., more anterior laxity will be noted if the arm is examined in internal rotation—which relaxes the anterior structures, than if it is examined in external rotation—which tightens the anterior structures).

In interpreting the significance of the degree of translation on laxity tests, it is important to use the contralateral shoulder as an example of what is "normal" for the patient. Not infrequently, the laxity on the symptomatic side will be similar to that on the asymptomatic side. Investigations of clinical laxity tests showed that the range of translations for shoulders with atraumatic instability was similar to that of normal shoulders or shoulders with traumatic instability (see Fig. 14–46).[226] However, a distinguishing feature of many shoulders with atraumatic instability is that the resistance to translation is diminished when the humeral head is pressed into the glenoid fossa, suggesting that the effective glenoid concavity is diminished. It is helpful if the patient recognizes one or more of the directions of translation as being responsible for his or her clinical symptoms. Finally, it is important to point out that these are tests of *laxity*, not tests for *instability*: Many normally stable shoulders, such as those of gymnasts, will demonstrate substantial translation on these laxity tests even though they are asymptomatic.

Drawer Test (Fig. 14–122). The patient is seated with the forearm resting on the lap and the shoulder relaxed. The examiner stands behind the patient. One of the examiner's hands stabilizes the shoulder girdle (scapula and clavicle) while the other grasps the proximal humerus. These tests are performed with: (1) a minimal compressive load (just enough to center the head in the glenoid), and (2) with a substantial compressive load (to gain a feeling for the effectiveness of the glenoid concavity). Starting from the centered position with a minimal compressive load, the humerus is first pushed forward to determine the amount of anterior displacement relative to the scapula. The anterior translation of a normal shoulder reaches a firm end-point with no clunking, no pain, and no apprehension. A clunk or snap on anterior subluxation or reduction may suggest a labral tear or Bankart lesion. The test is then repeated with a substantial compressive load applied before translation is attempted to gain an appreciation of the competency of the anterior glenoid lip. The humerus is returned to the neutral position, and the posterior drawer test is performed, with light and again with substantial compressive loads to judge the amount of translation and the effectiveness of the posterior glenoid lip, respectively.[593]

Sulcus Test (Figs. 14–123 and 14–124). The patient sits with the arm relaxed at the side. The examiner centers the head with a mild compressive load and then pulls the arm downward. Inferior laxity is demonstrated if a sulcus or hollow appears inferior to the acromion. Competency of the inferior glenoid lip is demonstrated by pressing the humeral head into the glenoid while inferior traction is applied.

Push-Pull Test (Fig. 14–125). The patient lies supine with the shoulder off the edge of the table. The arm is in 90 degrees of abduction and 30 degrees of flexion. Standing next to the patient's hip, the examiner pulls up on the wrist with one hand while pushing down on the proximal humerus with the other. The shoulders of normal, relaxed patients often will allow 50% posterior translation on this test.

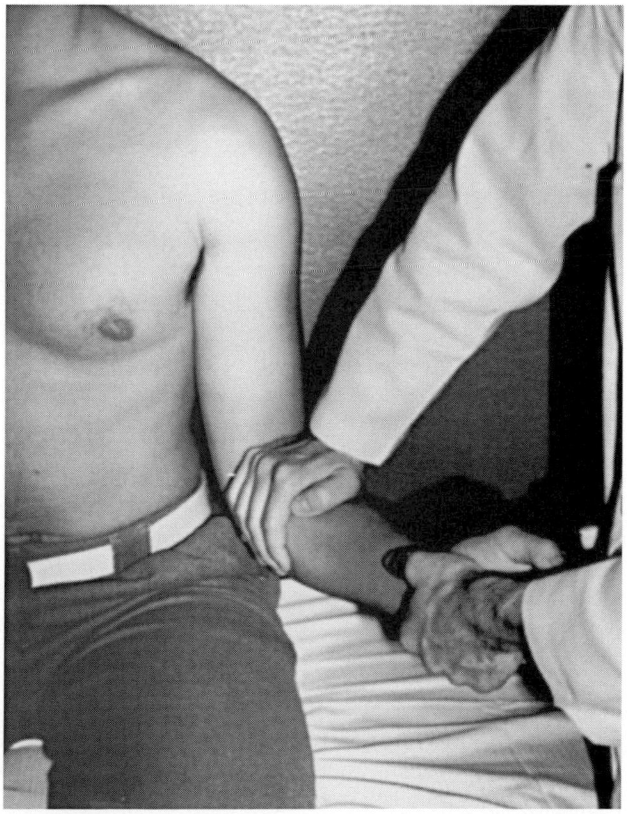

Figure 14–123

The sulcus test. The patient is seated with the arm relaxed and at the side. The examiner pulls downward on the arm. Inferior instability is demonstrated if a sulcus (or hollow) appears inferior to the acromion. The result of the sulcus test in the case of this patient is negative.

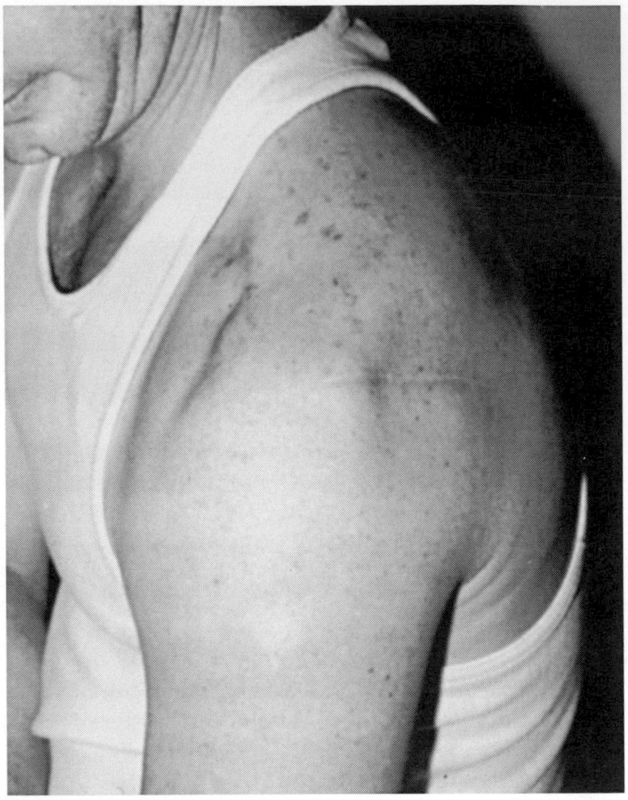

Figure 14–124

The sulcus sign. This patient had a posterior repair for glenohumeral instability. However, he continues to have inferior instability and demonstrates the sulcus (or hollow) just inferior to the anterior acromion during this sulcus test.

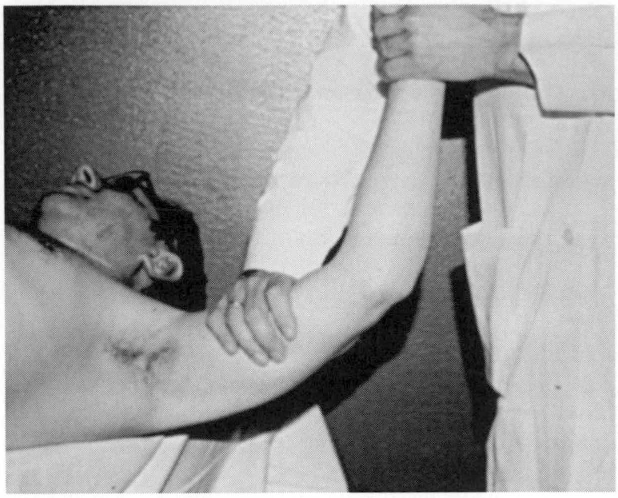

Figure 14–125

The push-pull test. The patient lies supine and relaxed with the shoulder at the edge of the examination table. The examiner pulls up on the wrist with one hand while pushing down on the proximal humerus with the other. Approximately 50% posterior translation of the humerus on the glenoid is normal in relaxed patients.

Stability Tests

These tests examine the ability of the shoulder to resist challenges to stability in positions where the ligaments are normally under tension.

Fulcrum Test (Fig. 14–126). The patient lies supine at the edge of the examination table with the arm abducted to 90 degrees. The examiner places one hand on the table under the glenohumeral joint to act as a fulcrum. The arm is gently and progressively extended and externally rotated over this fulcrum. Maintainance of gentle passive external rotation for a minute fatigues the subscapularis, challenging the capsular contribution to the anterior stability of the shoulder. The patient with anterior instability will usually become apprehensive as this maneuver is carried out (watch the eyebrows for a clue that the shoulder is getting ready to dislocate). In this test, normally no translation occurs because it is performed in a position where the anterior ligaments are placed under tension.

Crank or Apprehension Test (Fig. 14–127). The patient sits with the back toward the examiner. The arm is held in 90 degrees of abduction and external rotation. The examiner pulls back on the patient's wrist with one hand while stabilizing the back of the shoulder with the other. The patient with anterior instability will usually become apprehensive with this maneuver. As for the fulcrum test, no translation is expected in the normal shoulder because this test is performed in a position where the anterior ligaments are placed under tension.

Jerk Test (Fig. 14–128; see also Fig. 14–121). patient sits with the arm internally rotated and flexed forward to 90 degrees. The examiner grasps the elbow and axially loads the humerus in a proximal direction. While axial loading of the humerus is maintained, the arm is moved horizontally across the body. A positive result is indicated by a sudden jerk as the humeral head slides off the back of the glenoid. When the arm is returned to the original

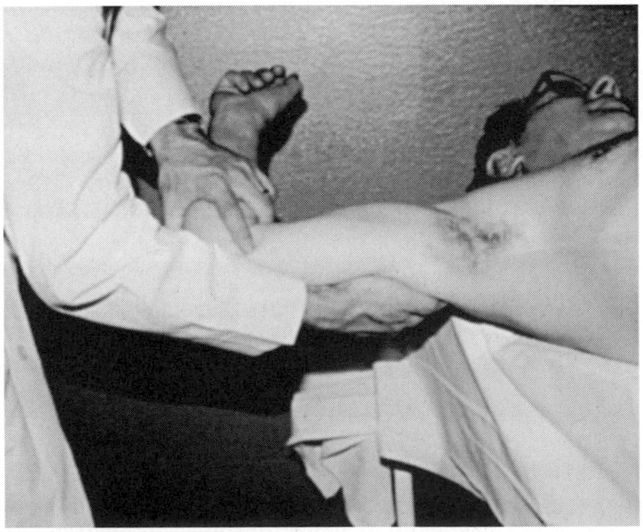

Figure 14–126

The fulcrum test. With the patient supine and the shoulder at the edge of the examination table, the arm is abducted to 90 degrees. The examiner's right hand is used as a fulcrum while the arm is gently and progressively extended and externally rotated. In the presence of anterior instability, the patient becomes apprehensive or the shoulder translates with this maneuver.

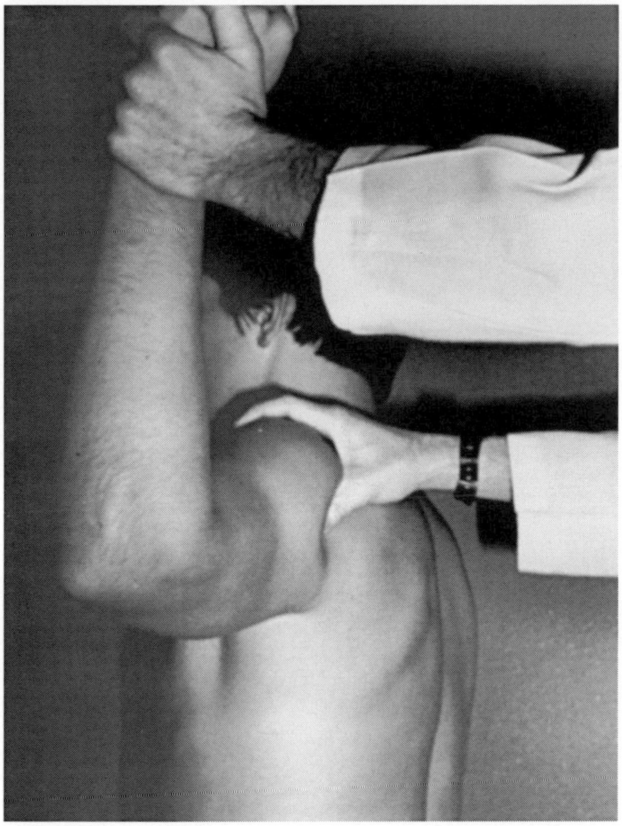

Figure 14–127

The crank test. The arm is held in 90-degree abduction and external rotation. The examiner's left hand is pulling back on the patient's wrist while his right hand stabilizes the back of the shoulder. The patient with anterior instability becomes apprehensive with this maneuver.

position of 90-degree abduction, a second jerk may be observed, that of the humeral head returning to the glenoid.

Strength Tests

The strength of abduction and rotation are tested to gauge the power of the muscles contributing to stability through concavity compression. The strength of the scapular protractors and elevators are also tested to determine their ability to position the scapula securely.

RADIOGRAPHS

In atraumatic instability shoulder radiographs characteristically show no bony pathology. Specifically, there is no posterolateral humeral head defect, no glenoid rim fracture or new bone formation, and no evidence of tuberosity fracture. Because these patients characteristically demonstrate midrange instability, radiographs may show translation of the humeral head with respect to the glenoid; for example, the axillary view may show posterior subluxation. Occasionally, radiographs may suggest factors underlying the atraumatic instability such as a relatively small or hypoplastic glenoid or a posteriorly inclined or otherwise dysplastic glenoid. The bony glenoid fossa may appear quite flat; however, it is difficult to relate the apparent depth of the bony socket to the effective depth of the fossa formed by cartilage and labrum covering the bone.

We do not use stress radiographs, arthrography, MRI, or arthroscopy in the diagnosis of atraumatic instability.

Recurrent Traumatic Instability

Traumatic instability is instability that arises from an injury of sufficient magnitude to tear the glenohumeral capsule, ligaments, labrum, or rotator cuff or to produce a fracture of the humerus or glenoid. A typical patient is a 17-year-old skier whose recurrent anterior instability began with a fall on an abducted, externally rotated arm (although the condition has been reported in individuals as young as 3 years old).[147] In order to injure these strong structures, a substantial force must be applied to them. The most common pathology associated with traumatic instability is the avulsion of the anteroinferior capsule and ligaments from the glenoid rim. Substantial force is required to produce this avulsion in a healthy shoulder. While this load may be applied directly (e.g., by having the proximal humerus hit from behind), an indirect loading mechanism is more common. Indirect loading is most easily understood in terms of a simple model of the torques involved. When the upper extremity is abducted and externally rotated by a force applied to the hand, the following equation for torque equilibrium is a useful approximation, if we attribute the major stabilizing role to the ligament (see Fig. 14–49):

$$T = B \cdot E/R$$

where "T" is the tension in the inferior glenohumeral ligament, "R" is the radius of the humeral head, "B" is the abduction external rotation load applied to the hand,

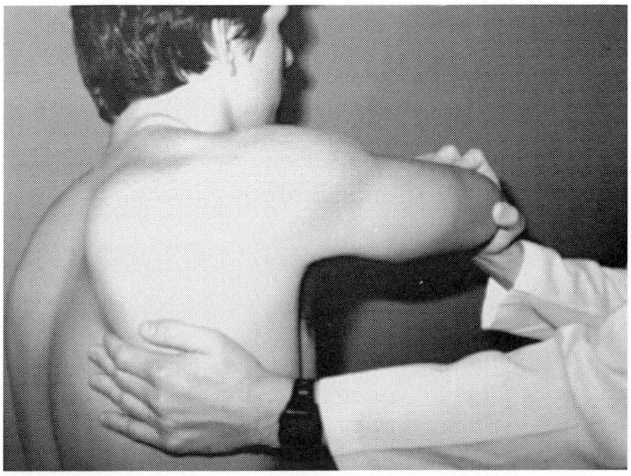

Figure 14–128

The jerk test. The patient's arm is abducted to 90 degrees and internally rotated. The examiner axially loads the humerus while the arm is moved horizontally across the body. The left hand stabilizes the scapula. A patient with a recurrent posterior instability may demonstrate a sudden jerk as the humeral head slides off the back of the glenoid or when it is reduced by moving the arm back to the starting position.

and "E" is the distance from the center of the humeral head to the hand. If the radius of the humeral head is 2.5 cm and the distance from the head center to the hand is 1 m, this formula suggests that the inferior glenohumeral ligament would experience a load 40 times greater than that applied to the hand. From this example we can see that a relatively small load is required to produce the characteristic lesion of traumatic instability if this load is applied indirectly through the lever arm of the upper extremity.

Avulsion of the anterior glenohumeral ligament mechanism (see Fig. 14–35) deprives the joint of stability in positions where this structure is a checkrein, such as in maximal external rotation and extension of the arm elevated near the coronal plane. Thus, it is evident that in recurrent traumatic instability, problems are most likely to occur when the arm is placed in a position approximating that in which the original injury occurred (see Figs. 14–126 and 14–127). Midrange instability may also result from a traumatic injury, because the glenoid concavity may be compromised by avulsion of the labrum or fracture of the bony lip of the glenoid (see Fig. 14–34). Lessening of the effective glenoid arc compromises the effectiveness of concavity compression, reduces the balance stability angles, reduces the surface available for adhesion-cohesion, and compromises the ability of the glenoid suction cup to conform to the head of the humerus.

The corner of the glenoid abuts against the insertion of the cuff to the tuberosity when the humerus is extended, abducted, and externally rotated (Fig. 14–129).[370, 394, 431, 550, 663, 664] Thus, the same forces that challenge the inferior glenohumeral ligament are also applied to the greater tuberosity-cuff insertion area. It is not surprising, therefore, that posterolateral humeral head defects, tuberosity fractures, and cuff injuries may be a part of the clinical picture of traumatic instability. The exact location and type of traumatic injury depends on the age of the patient and the magnitude, rate, and direction of force applied. Avulsions of the glenoid labrum, glenoid rim fractures, and posterolateral humeral head defects are more commonly seen in young individuals. In patients older than 35 years of age, traumatic instability tends to be associated with fractures of the greater tuberosity and rotator cuff tears. This tendency increases with increasing age at the time of the initial traumatic dislocation. Thus, as a rule, younger patients require management of anterior lesions and older patients require management of posterior lesions.

The posterior lateral humeral head defect is a common feature of traumatic instability. These lesions are often noted after the first traumatic dislocation and tend to increase in size with recurrent episodes. This impaction injury usually occurs when the anterior corner of the glenoid is driven into the posterior lateral humeral articular surface. It is evident that this injury is close to the cuff insertion. Large head defects compromise stability by diminishing the articular congruity of the humerus.

To help recall the common aspects of traumatic instability, we use the acronym TUBS. The instability arises from a significant episode of **t**rauma, characteristically from abduction and extension of the arm elevated in the coronal plane. The resultant instability is usually **u**nidirectional in the anteroinferior direction. The pathology is usually an avulsion of the labrum and capsuloligamentous complex from the anterior inferior lip of the glenoid, commonly referred to as a **B**ankart lesion. With functionally significant recurrent traumatic instability, a **s**urgical reconstruction of this labral and ligament avulsion is frequently required to restore stability.

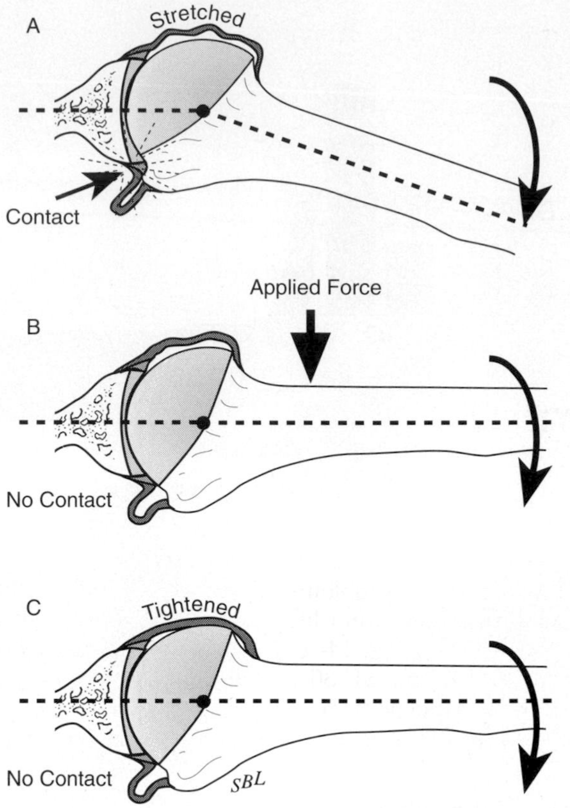

Figure 14–129

Posterior contact between the glenoid lip and the insertion of the cuff to the tuberosity occurs in the apprehension, or fulcrum, position, especially if the anteroinferior capsule has been stretched, allowing the humerus to extend to an unusually posterior scapular plane. This contact can challenge the integrity of the posterior cuff insertion and the tuberosity *(A)*. Application of a posteriorly directed force on the front of the shoulder may change the humeroscapular position enough to relieve this posterior abutment. This maneuver is similar to that described as the relocation test; however, this diagram suggests that the mechanism for relief of discomfort is the avoidance of posterior abutment rather than the elimination of subluxation *(B)*. A similar protection from posterior abutment may be achieved by tightening the anterior capsule, thus preventing the extension of the humerus to a substantially posterior scapular plane *(C)*. (From Matsen FA III, Lippitt SB, Sidles JA, and Harryman DT II: Practical Evaluation and Management of the Shoulder. Philadelphia: WB Saunders, 1994.)

The reader is referred to a review of the pathology and pathogenesis of traumatic instability by Wirth and Rockwood.[696]

HISTORY

Most patients presenting with TUBS are between the ages of 14 and 34 (Fig. 14–130). These patients characteristically have difficulty throwing overhand, but many pa-

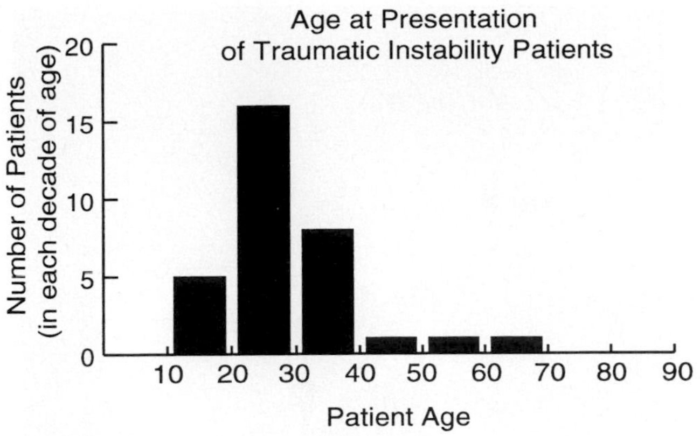

Figure 14–130

Age distribution of 32 patients with traumatic instability. (From Matsen FA III, Lippitt SB, Sidles JA, and Harryman DT II: Practical Evaluation and Management of the Shoulder. Philadelphia: WB Saunders, 1994.)

tients also have problems sleeping, putting their hand behind their head, and lifting a gallon to head level (see Table 14–2 and Fig. 14–119). Their general health status as revealed by the SF 36 self-assessment questionnaire is better on average than that of a comparable group of patients with atraumatic instability (see Fig. 14–120).

Initial Dislocation

The most important element in the history is the definition of the original injury. As is evident to anyone who has attempted to recreate these lesions in a cadaver, substantial force is required to produce a traumatic dislocation—in most cadaver specimens, it is impossible to duplicate the Bankart injury mechanism because the humerus fractures first! In characteristic anterior traumatic instability, the structure that is avulsed is the strongest part of the shoulder's capsular mechanism—the anterior inferior glenohumeral ligament. In order to tear this ligament, substantial force needs to be applied to the shoulder when the arm is in a position to tighten this ligament. Thus, the usual mechanism of injury involves the application of a large extension-external rotation force to the arm elevated near the coronal plane. Such a mechanism may occur in a fall while snow skiing, while executing a high-speed cut in water skiing, in an arm tackle during football, with a block of a volleyball or basketball shot, or in relatively violent industrial accidents in which a posteriorly directed force is applied to the hand while the arm is abducted and externally rotated. Awkward lifting on the job and rear-end automobile accidents would not be expected to provide the conditions or mechanism for this injury. Direct questioning and persistence are often necessary to elicit a full description of the mechanism of the initial injury, including the position of the shoulder and the direction and magnitude of the applied force. Yet this information is critical to establishing the diagnosis.

An initial traumatic dislocation often requires assistance in reduction, rather than reducing spontaneously as is usually the case in atraumatic instability. Radiographs from previous emergency room visits may be available to show the shoulder in its dislocated position. Axillary or other neuropathy may have accompanied the glenohumeral dislocation. Any of these findings individually or in combination support the diagnosis of traumatic as opposed to atraumatic instability.

Traumatic instability may occur without a complete dislocation. In this situation, the injury produces a traumatic lesion, but this lesion is insufficient to allow the humeral head to completely escape from the glenoid. The shoulder may be unstable because, as a result of the injury, it manifests apprehension or subluxation when the arm is placed near the position of injury. In these cases there is no history of the need for reduction nor radiographs with the shoulder in the dislocated position. Thus, the diagnosis rests to an even greater extent on a careful history that focuses on the position and forces involved in the initial episode.

Subsequent Episodes of Instability

Characteristically, the shoulder with traumatic instability is comfortable when troublesome positions are avoided. However, the apprehension or fear of instability may prevent the individual from work or sport. Recurrent subluxation or dislocation may occur when the shoulder is forced unexpectedly into the abducted externally rotated position or during sleep when the patient's active guard is less effective. There may be a history of increasing ease of dislocation as the remaining stabilizing factors are progressively compromised.

PHYSICAL EXAMINATION

The goal of the physical examination is largely to confirm the impression obtained from the history — that a certain combination of arm position and force application produces the actual or threatened glenohumeral instability that is of functional concern to the patient. If the diagnosis has been rigorously established from the history, for example by documented recurrent anterior dislocations, it is not necessary to risk redislocation on the physical examination. If such rigorous documentation is not available, however, the examiner must challenge the ligamentous stability of the shoulder in the suspected position of vulnerability being prepared to reduce the shoulder if a dislocation results.

The most common direction of recurrent traumatic instability is anteroinferior. Stability in this position is challenged by externally rotating and extending the arm elevated to various degrees in the coronal plane (see Figs. 14–126 and 14–127). It may be necessary to hold the arm in the challenging position for 1 to 2 minutes to fatigue the stabilizing musculature. When the muscle stabilizers tire, the capsuloligamentous mechanism is all that is holding the humeral head in the glenoid. At this moment the patient with traumatic anterior instability becomes apprehensive, recognizing that the shoulder is about to come out of joint. This recognition is strongly supportive of the diagnosis of traumatic anterior instability.

The magnitude of translation on the standard tests of glenohumeral laxity (see Figs. 14–122 to 14–125) does not necessarily distinguish stable from unstable shoulders (see Fig. 14–46). However, the experienced examiner may detect a diminished resistance to anterior translation on the drawer test when the humeral head is compressed into the glenoid fossa, indicating loss of the anterior glenoid lip. This maneuver may also elicit grinding as the humeral head slides over the bony edge of the glenoid from which the labrum has been avulsed or catching as the head passes over a torn glenoid labrum.

Pain on abduction, external rotation, and extension is not specific for instability. Such pain may relate to shoulder stiffness or alternatively to abutment of the glenoid against the cuff insertion to the head posteriorly.[394, 550, 663, 664] Relief of this pain by anterior pressure on the humeral head may result from diminished stretch on the anterior capsule or from relief of the abutment posteriorly (see Fig. 14–129).

In all patients with traumatic instability but particularly in those older than 35 years of age, the strength of the internal and external rotation must be examined to explore the possibility of cuff weakness or tear. Finally, a neurologic examination is performed to determine the integrity of the axillary nerve and other branches of the brachial plexus.

RADIOGRAPHS AND OTHER TESTS

Radiographs frequently help to provide confirmation of traumatic glenohumeral instability.

Humeral Head Changes

One of the commonest findings is indentation or impaction in the posterior aspect of the humeral head from contact with the anteroinferior corner of the glenoid when the joint was dislocated (Fig. 14–131; see also Figs. 14–3 and 14–92). In their classic article,[253] Hill and Sachs evaluated the relationship of humeral head defects to shoulder instability. They concluded that more than two thirds of anterior shoulder dislocations are complicated by a bony injury of the humerus or scapula. We quote:

> "Compression fractures as a result of impingement of the weakest portion of the humeral head, that is, the posterior lateral aspect of the articular surface against the anterior rim of the glenoid fossa are found so frequently in cases of habitual dislocation that they have been described as a typical defect. These defects are sustained at the time of the original dislocation. A special sign is the sharp, vertical, dense medial border of the groove known as the line of condensation, the length of which is correlated with the size of the defect."

They reported the defect in only 27% of 119 acute anterior dislocations and in 74% of 15 recurrent anterior dislocations. However, they stated that the incidence of the groove defect was low, undoubtedly because it was only in the last 6 months of their 10-year study (1930 to 1940) that they used special radiographic views. The size of the defect varied in length (cephalocaudal) from 5 mm to 3 cm, in width from 3 mm to 2 cm, and in depth from 10 mm to 22 mm.[253]

A number of special projections have been used to enhance the view of the Hill-Sachs defect.[4, 130, 219, 248, 253, 438, 484, 504, 624] Two of these views bear special mention.

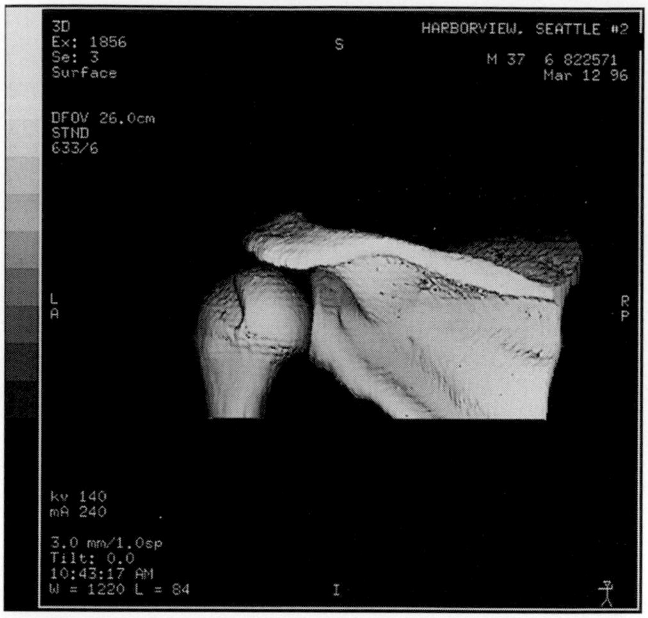

Figure 14–131

A three-dimensional computed tomography reconstruction of the left shoulder of a 37-year-old man 3 days after his first traumatic glenohumeral dislocation. The bony defect in the posterior lateral aspect of the humeral head is clearly shown. The patient went on to normal shoulder function with nonoperative management.

Stryker Notch View. The patient is supine on the table with the cassette placed under the shoulder.[219] The palm of the hand of the affected shoulder is placed on top of the head, with the fingers directed toward the back of the head. The elbow of the affected shoulder should point straight upward. The x-ray beam tilts 10 degrees toward the head, centered over the coracoid process (Fig. 14–132). This technique was developed by Stryker and

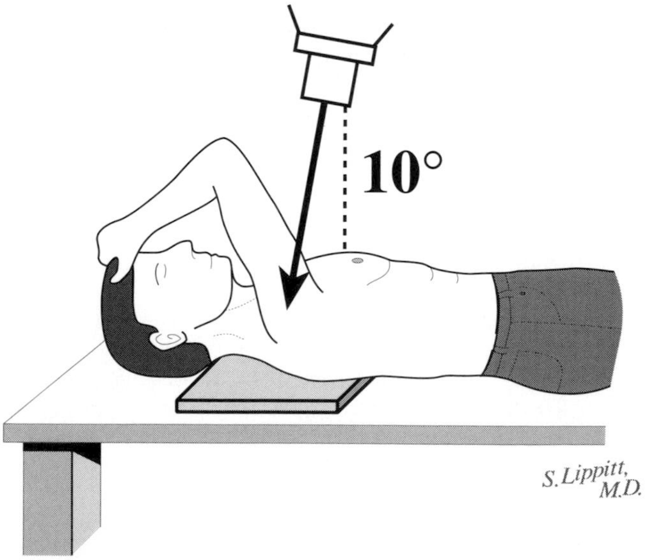

Figure 14–132

A Stryker notch view. (Modified from Hall RH, Isaac F, and Booth CR: Dislocations of the shoulder with special reference to accompanying small fractures. J Bone Joint Surg *41A*:489–494, 1959.)

reported by Hall and co-workers.[219] They stated that they could demonstrate the humeral head defect in 90% of 20 patients with a history of recurring anterior dislocation of the shoulder.

Apical Oblique View. Garth and co-workers[183, 184] described the apical oblique projection of the shoulder (Fig. 14–133). In this technique the patient sits with the scapula flat against the cassette (as for the anteroposterior view in the plane of the scapula). The arm may be in a sling. The x-ray beam is centered on the coracoid and directed perpendicular to the cassette (45 degrees to the coronal plane), except that it is angled 45 degrees caudally. The beam passes tangential to the articular surface of the glenohumeral joint and the posterolateral aspect of the humeral head. This view is likely to reveal both anterior glenoid lip defects and posterior lateral impression fractures of the humeral head.

The incidence of the Hill-Sachs defect reported depends on both the radiographic technique and the patient population. Symeonides[624] reported the humeral head defect in 23 of 45 patients who had recurrent anterior dislocations of the shoulder. However, at the time of surgery he could confirm only 18 of 45.

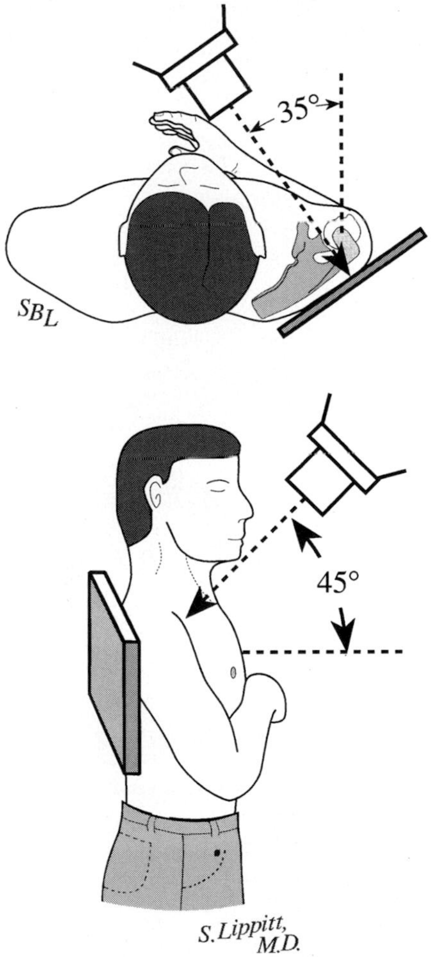

Figure 14–133

An apical-oblique x-ray: a true anteroposterior view of the glenohumeral joint with a 45-degree caudal tilt of the x-ray beam. (Modified from Garth WP Jr, Slappey CE, and Ochs CW: Roentgenographic demonstration of instability of the shoulder: The apical oblique projection. A technical note. J Bone Joint Surg 66A:1450–1453, 1984.)

Eyre-Brook[156] reported an incidence of the Hill-Sachs defect of 64% in 17 recurrent anterior dislocations, and Brav[63] recorded a rate of 67% in 69 recurrent dislocations. Rowe[554] noted the defect in 38% of 125 acute dislocations and in 57% of 63 recurrent dislocations. Adams[3] noted that the defect was found at the time of surgery in 82% of 68 patients. Palmer and Widen[493] found the defect at surgery in all of 60 patients.

Calandra and co-workers[75] prospectively studied the incidence of Hill-Sachs lesions using diagnostic arthroscopy. In a young population of 32 patients with a mean age of 28 years, the frequency of this lesion was 47% for initial anterior shoulder dislocations.

Danzig, Greenway, and Resnick[113] reported that in cadaveric and clinical studies no single view will always reveal the humeral head compression fracture. Pavlov and co-workers[504] and Rozing and associates[562] found that the Stryker notch view taken in internal rotation best revealed the posterolateral humeral head defect (see Fig. 14–132).

The demonstration of a posterior lateral humeral head defect strongly indicates that the shoulder has been subject to a traumatic anterior dislocation. When these factors are already known—for example, in a 17 year old whose recurrent anterior dislocations began with a well-documented abduction-external rotation injury in football—it is not necessary to spend a great deal of effort demonstrating the humeral head defect because: (1) it is very likely to be present even if not seen on the radiographs, and (2) the existence of such a lesion does not in itself alter our management of the patient.

Glenoid Changes

Standard radiographs may reveal a periosteal reaction to the ligamentous avulsion at the glenoid lip or a fracture (see Figs. 14–6 and 14–98), erosion (see Fig. 14–95), or new bone formation (see Figs. 14–82 and 14–94) at the glenoid rim. Modifications of the axillary view may help the identification of glenoid rim changes. Rokous[546] and colleagues described what has become known as the West Point axillary view.[541] In this technique the patient is placed prone on the x-ray table with the involved shoulder on a pad raised 7.5 cm from the top of the table. The head and neck are turned away from the involved side. With the cassette held against the superior aspect of the shoulder, the x-ray beam is centered at the axilla, 25 degrees downward from the horizontal and 25 degrees medial. The resultant x-ray is a tangential view of the anteroinferior rim of the glenoid (see Fig. 14–90). Using this view, Rokous and associates demonstrated bony abnormalities of the anterior glenoid rim in 53 of 63 patients whose histories indicated traumatic instability of the shoulder. Cyprien and co-workers[111] demonstrated lessening of the glenoid diameter and shortening of the anterior glenoid rim in shoulders with recurrent anterior dislocation. Blazina and Satzman[51] also reported anteroinferior glenoid rim fractures seen on the axillary view in nine of their patients.

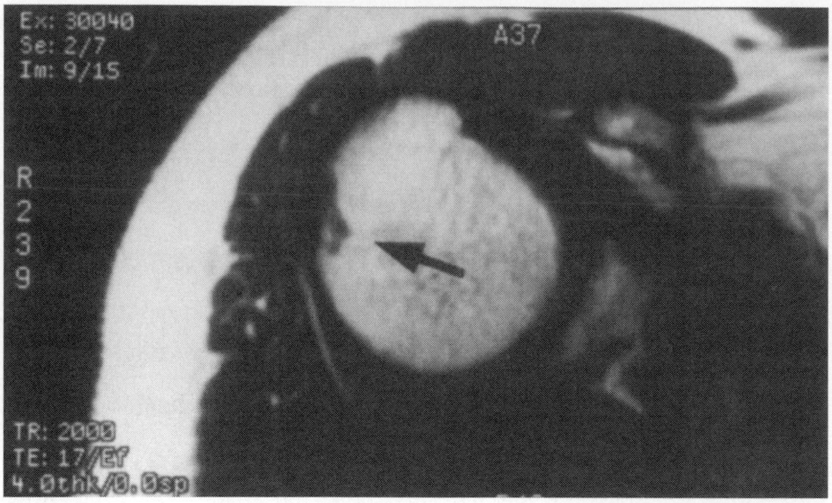

Figure 14–134

Magnetic resonance imaging demonstrating a focal abnormality in the anterolateral aspect of the humeral head that is consistent with a recent episode of anterior glenohumeral instability. The plain x-ray films were interpreted as normal. (From Rockwood CA Jr, Green DP, and Bucholz RW [eds]: Fractures in Adults. Philadelphia: JB Lippincott, 1991.)

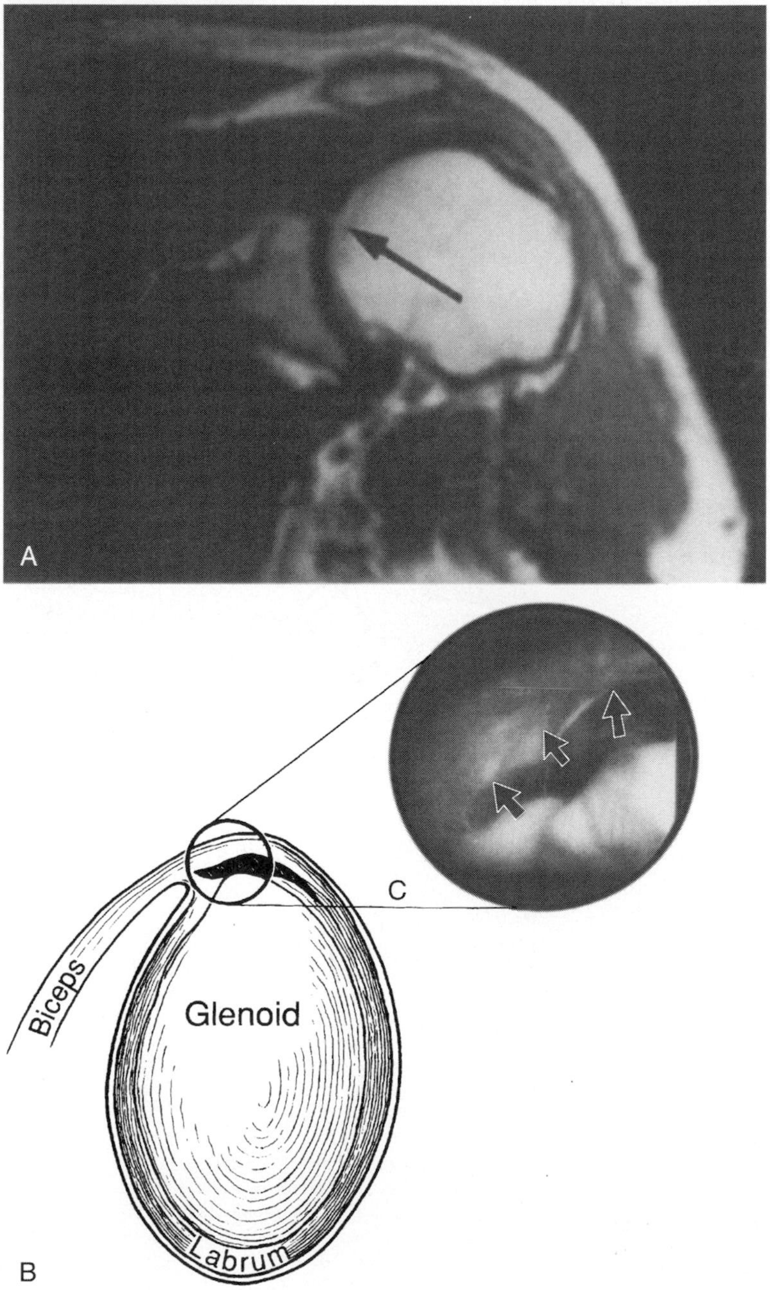

Figure 14–135

A–C, Lesion of the long head biceps tendon origin and superior glenoid labrum as seen on magnetic resonance imaging and arthroscopic examinations. (From Rockwood CA Jr, Green DP, and Bucholz RW [eds]: Fractures in Adults. Philadelphia: JB Lippincott, 1991.)

Special Radiographic Techniques

Although pathology can be seen with additional radiographic views,[207, 426, 494, 523] CT arthrography,[62, 107, 142, 316, 322, 401, 413, 521, 522, 590] fluoroscopy,[469] or MRI, these additional tests are rarely cost effective in the clinical evaluation and management of shoulders with characteristic traumatic instability.[148, 371] While CT evidence of labral or capsular pathology is unlikely to change the management of the shoulder, a contrast CT scan may help to document the flattening of the anteroinferior glenoid concavity due to loss of articular cartilage (see Fig. 14–96). CT may also be useful in defining the magnitude of bone loss when sizable humeral head or glenoid defects are suggested on plain radiographs (see Figs. 14–97 and 14–98).[201, 585] When previous glenoid bone blocks have been carried out or hardware inserted, CT is useful for examining the possibility of their encroachment on the humeral head.[106, 107, 114]

Although many articles have been written regarding the use of MRI in imaging the unstable shoulder (Fig. 14–134), the clinical usefulness of this examination awaits definition.[87, 209, 277, 318, 419, 453, 493, 534, 564, 659] Iannotti and associates[277] reported that the sensitivity and specificity of MRI in the diagnosis of lateral tears associated with glenohumeral instability were 88% and 93%, respectively (Fig. 14–135). However, in a blinded study, Garneau and associates[182] found that it was insensitive and nonspecific for labral pathology. Even if MRI reliably yielded this information, it is unclear how it would be cost effective in the management of the patient. Patients with refractory instability would be considered for surgery with or without such data.

Rotator Cuff Imaging

In a patient whose onset of traumatic instability occurred after age 35, there may be evidence on history and physical examination of rotator cuff pathology. Particular concern arises if weakness of external rotation or elevation persist longer than 1 week or so. In these situations, preoperative imaging of cuff integrity may play an important role in surgical planning: The approach for rotator cuff repair is quite different than the approach for the repair of an anterior inferior capsular lesion. Arthrography, ultrasound, or MRI may be useful in this situation.

ELECTROMYOGRAPHY

Electromyography may be helpful in the evaluation of the patient with recurrent traumatic instability if the history and physical examination suggest residual brachial plexus lesions.

ARTHROSCOPY

Diagnostic arthroscopy is not a necessary prelude to open surgical repair of documented recurrent traumatic instability. While it uncommonly changes the surgical approach, shoulder arthroscopy has helped to define some of the pathology associated with recurrent instability. Such lesions include labral tears, capsular rents, humeral head defects, and rotator cuff defects (see Fig. 14–135).[11, 77, 174, 183, 215, 256, 304, 362, 413, 428, 481, 496, 687, 688, 719]

A classification of anterior labral "Bankart" lesions was proposed by Green and Christensen.[208] In 37 cases, they described the arthroscopic appearance common to five separate groups. Type I is the normal intact labrum. Type II is a simple detachment of the labrum from the glenoid. Type III is an intrasubstance tear of the glenoid labrum. Type IV is a detachment of the labrum with significant fraying or degeneration, and Type V is a complete degeneration of absence of the glenoid labrum.

Neviaser found that occasionally the anterior labroligamentous periosteal sleeve is avulsed from the supporting anterior inferior ligamentous and labral structure.[456] Habermeyer and Gleyze found that shoulders with more than five recurrent dislocations were found to have anterior articular cartilage erosion.[194] Harryman noted labral damage in all cases treated for recurrent anterior traumatic instability (Fig. 14–136) and significant articular erosion to subchondral bone in 20% (Fig. 14–137).[223]

Other lesions may be associated with Bankart lesions. Snyder and co-workers[601] and Warner[668] found the association of superior labral detachment and Bankart lesions.

Wolf reported that 6 of 64 patients with anterior instability had avulsion of glenohumeral ligaments from the humerus, whereas 47 had true Bankart lesions (73.5%).[703]

Arthroscopy also reveals defects in the articular cartilage of the posterior lateral humeral head, which would not be detected on radiographs (Figs. 14–138 to 14–140).

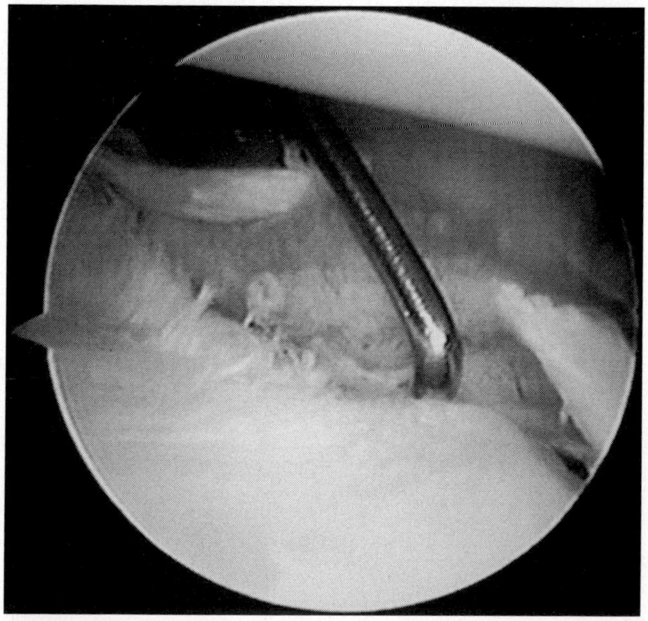

Figure 14–136

A Bankart lesion in a patient with a recurrent anteroinferior instability. Note the traumatic disruption of the glenoid labrum, articular cartilage fraying at the glenoid rim, and anterior capsular scarring with synovitis along the inferior glenohumeral ligament. (Courtesy of Douglas T. Harryman II, MD, Department of Orthopaedics, University of Washington.)

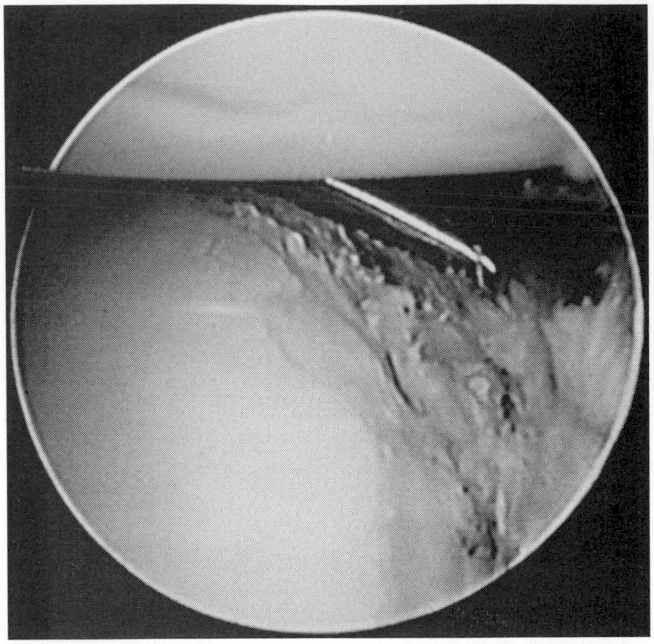

Figure 14–137

Chronic anteroinferior instability with evidence of articular cartilage erosion to the subchondral bone and degenerative erosion of the labrum. (Courtesy of Douglas T. Harryman II, MD, Department of Orthopaedics, University of Washington.)

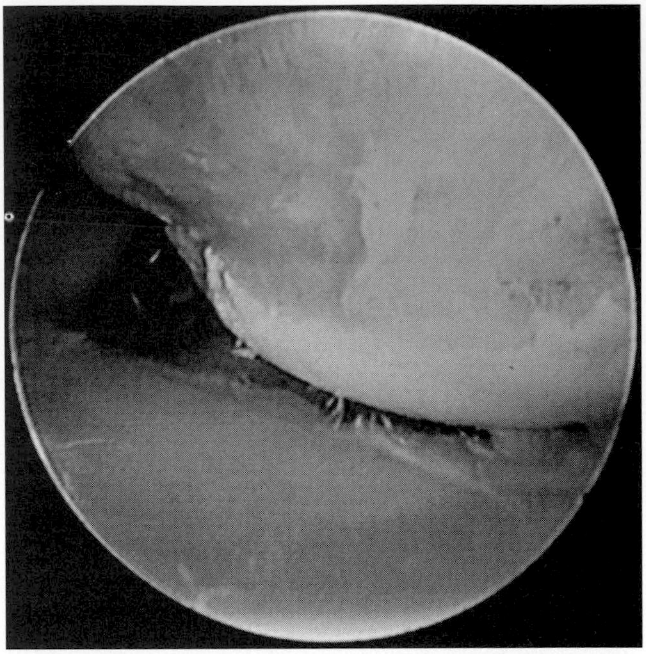

Figure 14–138

Visualizing the anterior rim of the glenoid and the posterior edge of the humeral articular surface adjacent to a large Hill-Sachs defect with the humerus in abduction-external rotation (this is the same shoulder as seen in Figure 14–136). (Courtesy of Douglas T. Harryman II, MD, Department of Orthopaedics, University of Washington.)

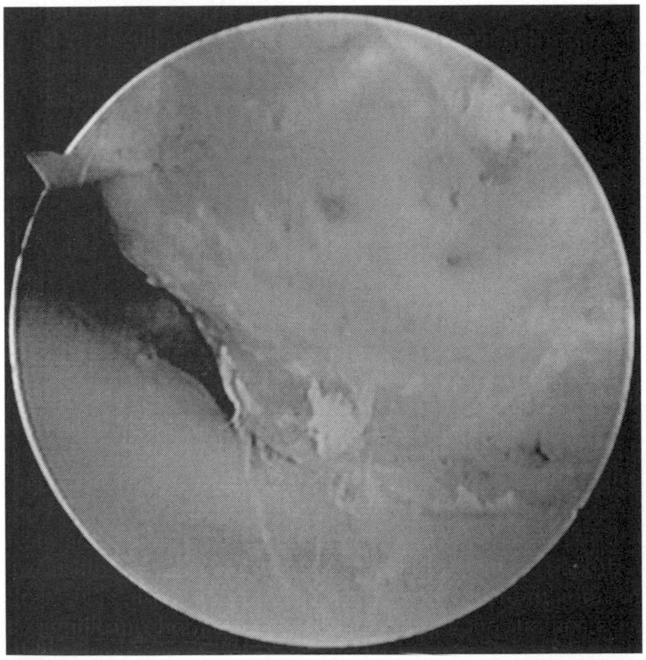

Figure 14–139

External rotation is increased until the humeral head suddenly dislocates over the edge of the anterior glenoid rim. After repair, external rotation of the glenohumeral joint must be checked adequately to maintain articular contact. (Courtesy of Douglas T. Harryman II, MD, Department of Orthopaedics, University of Washington.)

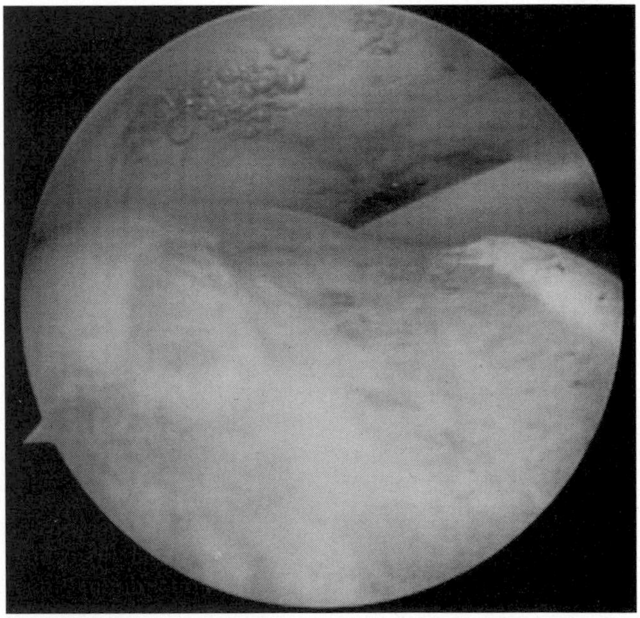

Figure 14–140

An extensive Hill-Sach's defect that crosses the superior humeral articular surface. Even with this degree of articular surface loss, an arthroscopic Bankart repair was performed using the Seattle Bankart guide and has been entirely successful. (Courtesy of Douglas T. Harryman II, MD, Department of Orthopaedics, University of Washington.)

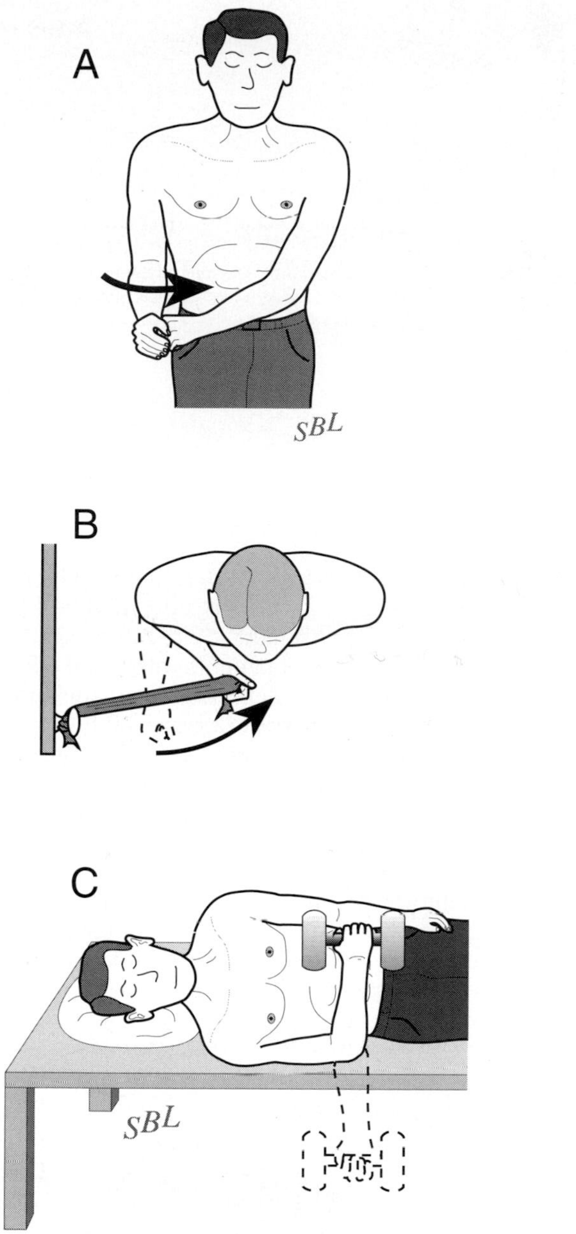

Figure 14–141

Internal rotation can be strengthened with isometrics *(A)*, rubber tubing *(B)*, or free weights *(C)*. (From Matsen FA III, Lippitt SB, Sidles JA, and Harryman DT II: Practical Evaluation and Management of the Shoulder. Philadelphia: WB Saunders, 1994.)

RECURRENT INSTABILITY: TREATMENT

Nonoperative Management

As has been emphasized in the section on "Mechanisms of Glenohumeral Stability," coordinated, strong muscle contraction is a key element of stabilization of the humeral head in the glenoid. Optimal neuromuscular control is required of the rotator cuff muscles, deltoid, pectoralis major, and scapular musculature. These dynamic stabilizing mechanisms require muscle strength, coordination, and training. Such a program is likely to be of particular benefit in patients with atraumatic (AMBRII) instability,[274, 449] because loss of neuromuscular control is one of the major features of this condition. Nonoperative management is also a particularly attractive option for children, for patients with voluntary instability,[449] for those with posterior glenohumeral instability, and for those requiring a supranormal range of motion (e.g., baseball pitchers and gymnasts) in whom surgical management often does not permit return to a competitive level of function.[235, 271, 556, 569]

Strengthening of the rotator cuff, deltoid, and scapular motors can be accomplished with a simple series of exercises (Figs. 14–141 to 14–144). During the early phases

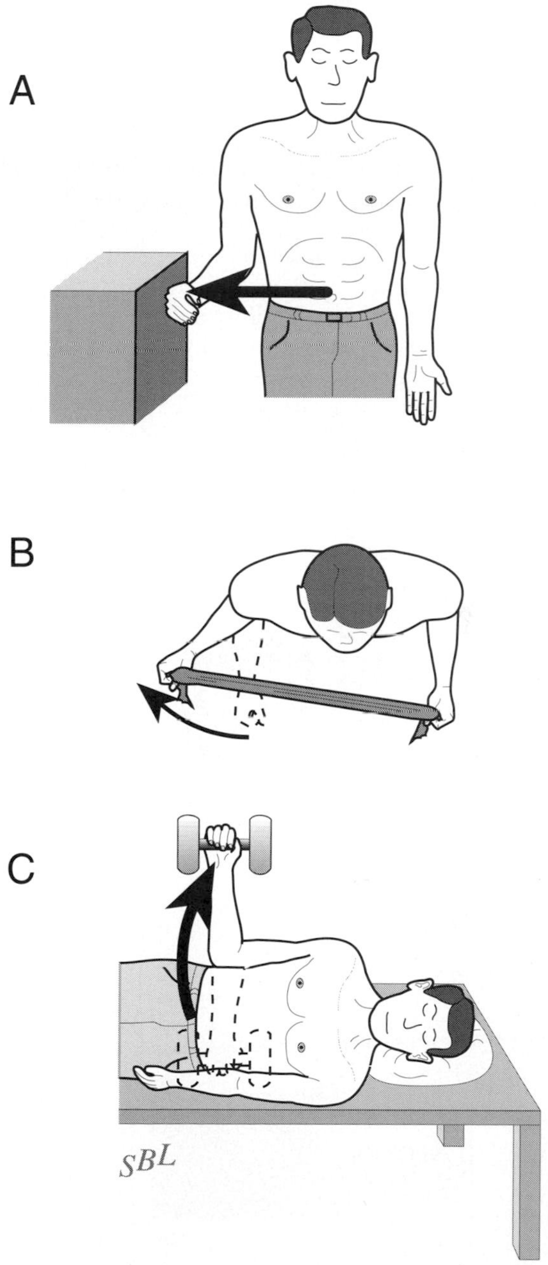

Figure 14–142

External rotation strengthening using isometrics *(A)*, rubber tubing *(B)*, or free weights *(C)*. (From Matsen FA III, Lippitt SB, Sidles JA, and Harryman DT II: Practical Evaluation and Management of the Shoulder. Philadelphia: WB Saunders, 1994.)

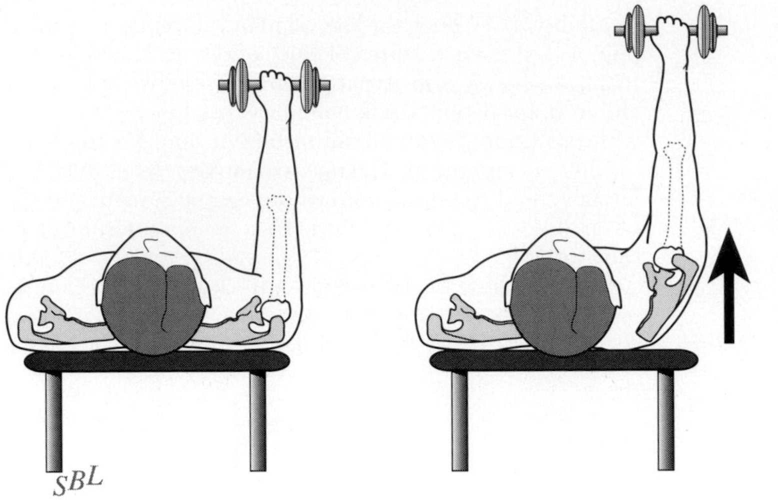

Figure 14–143

In the press plus, the arm is pushed upward until the shoulder blade is lifted off the table or bed. (From Matsen FA III, Lippitt SB, Sidles JA, and Harryman DT II: Practical Evaluation and Management of the Shoulder. Philadelphia: WB Saunders, 1994.)

of the program, the patient is taught to use the shoulder only in the most stable positions, that is those in which the humerus is elevated in the plane of the scapula (avoiding, for example, elevation in the sagittal plane with the arm in internal rotation if there is a tendency to posterior instability). As coordination and confidence improve, progressively less intrinsically stable positions are attempted. Taping may provide a useful reminder to avoid unstable positions (Fig. 14–145). The shoulder is then progressed to smooth repetitive activities, such as swimming or rowing, which can play an essential role in retraining the neuromuscular patterns required for stability.

Finally, it is important to avoid all activities and habits that promote glenohumeral subluxation or dislocation; patients are taught that each time their shoulder goes out it gets easier for it to go out the next time.

Rockwood and colleagues[543] and Burkhead and Rockwood[71] found that 16% of patients with traumatic subluxation, 80% of those with anterior atraumatic subluxation, and 90% of those with posterior instability responded to a rehabilitation program (Fig. 14–146). Brostrom and associates[68] found that exercises improved all except five of 33 unstable shoulders, including traumatic and atraumatic types. Anderson and associates have demonstrated the effectiveness of an exercise program using rubber bands in improving internal rotator strength.[10] Rockwood and associates have demonstrated that nonoperative management can be successful even when there is a congenital factor in instability. They reported 16 patients with hypoplasia of the glenoid.[695] A subset of this group consisted of five patients with bilateral glenoid hypoplasia and

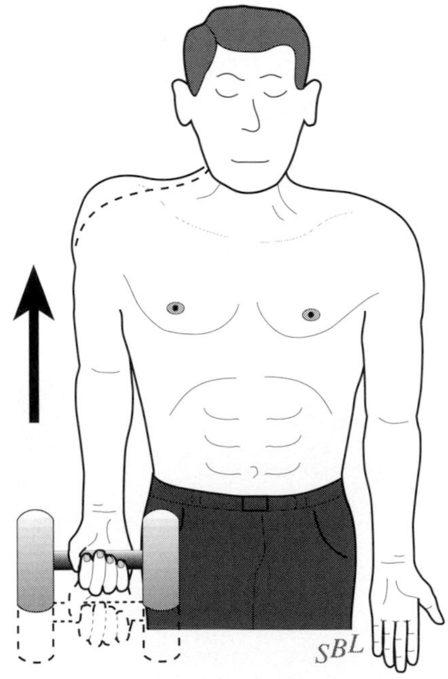

Figure 14–144

The shoulder shrug exercise—lift the tip of the shoulder toward the ear while holding the elbow straight. (From Matsen FA III, Lippitt SB, Sidles JA, and Harryman DT II: Practical Evaluation and Management of the Shoulder. Philadelphia: WB Saunders, 1994.)

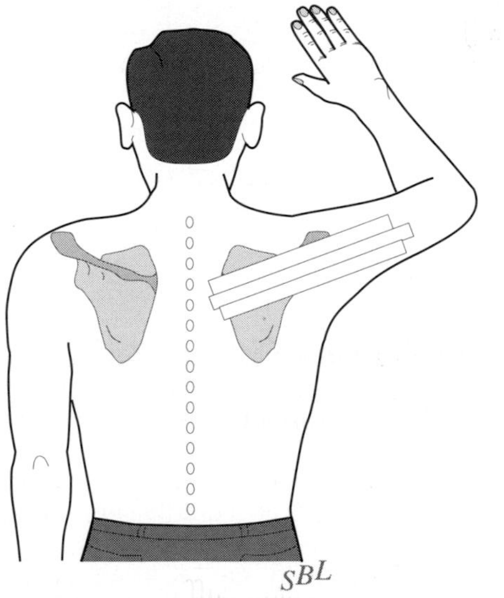

Figure 14–145

Training tape is applied across the back of the shoulder as a reminder to avoid unbalanced positions. (Modified from Matsen FA III, Lippitt SB, Sidles JA, and Harryman DT II: Practical Evaluation and Management of the Shoulder. Philadelphia: WB Saunders, 1994.)

multidirectional instability as indicated by symptomatic increased translation of the humeral head during anterior, inferior, and posterior drawer testing. In addition, generalized ligamentous laxity of the metacarpophalangeal joints, elbows, or knees was noted in all five patients. Four of the patients had been involved in occupational or recreational activities, or both, that had placed heavy demands on the shoulders. Four of these patients had considerable improvement in the ratings for pain and the ability to carry out work and sports activities at an average of 3 months after they had begun a strengthening program designed by Rockwood. None of the patients needed vocational rehabilitation, despite the heavy demands on their shoulders associated with their occupational or recreational activities.

Open Operative Management of Traumatic Anterior Instability

Surgical stabilization of the glenohumeral joint is considered in traumatic instability if the condition repeatedly compromises shoulder comfort or function in spite of a reasonable trial of internal and external rotator strengthening and coordination exercises. In contemplating a surgical approach to anterior traumatic glenohumeral instability, it is essential to identify preoperatively any factors that may compromise the surgical results, such as a tendency for voluntary dislocation, generalized ligamentous laxity, multidirectional instability, or significant bony defects of the humeral head or glenoid. When these conditions exist, it is necessary to modify the management approach. It is noteworthy that these factors can and should be identified preoperatively.

In the past, many surgical procedures have been described for the treatment of recurrent anterior glenohumeral instability. Tightening and to some degree realigning the subscapularis tendon and partially eliminating external rotation were the goals of the Magnuson-Stack and the Putti-Platt procedures. The Putti-Platt operation also tightened and reinforced the anterior capsule. Reattachment of the capsule and glenoid labrum to the glenoid lip was the goal of the DuToit staple capsulorrhaphy, and the Eyre-Brook capsulorrhaphy.[154, 155] The Bristow procedure transferred the tip of the coracoid process with its muscle attachments to create a musculotendinous sling across the anteroinferior glenohumeral joint. An anterior glenoid bone buttress was the objective of the Oudard and Trillat procedure. Augmentation of the bony anterior glenoid lip was the objective of anterior bone block procedures, such as the Eden-Hybbinette. Haaker and Eickhoff[216] used autogenous bone graft to the glenoid rim for recurrent instability. In their series recurrent instability in 24 young soldiers, they used screws to fix an anterior iliac crest graft to the anterior glenoid rim. At the conclusion of the graft placement, the glenoid labrum is replaced over the graft.

Large posterolateral humeral head defects have been approached by limiting external rotation, by filling the defect with the infraspinatus tendon, or by performing a rotational osteotomy of the humerus.[83, 84, 620, 678]

As we will see later, most of the reported series on the various types of reconstructions have yielded "excellent" results. However, it is very difficult to determine how each author graded the results. For example, if the patient has no recurrences after repair but has loss of 45 degrees of external rotation and cannot throw, is that a fair, good, or excellent result? The simple fact that the shoulder no longer dislocates cannot be equated with an excellent result. Although the older literature suggested that the goal of surgery for anterior dislocations of the shoulder was to limit external rotation, more modern literature suggests that a reconstruction can both prevent recurrent dislocation and allow a nearly normal range of motion and comfortable function.

CAPSULOLABRAL RECONSTRUCTION

The objective of anatomic repair for traumatic instability is the reconstruction of the avulsed capsule and labrum at the glenoid lip, which is often referred to as a Bankart repair. This type of repair was apparently first performed by Perthes[509] in 1906, who recommended the repair of the anterior capsule to the anterior glenoid rim. He was not in doubt about the pathology of traumatic instability: "In every case the anterior margin of the glenoid cavity will be found to be smooth, rounded, and free of any attachments, and a blunt instrument can be passed freely inwards over the bare bone on the front of the neck of the scapula." He reattached the capsule to the glenoid rim by placing drill holes through the bone. Credit for this type of repair should go to Perthes, but the popularity of the technique is due to the work of Bankart,[28, 30] who first performed the operation in 1923 on one of his former house surgeons. The procedure commonly used today is based on Bankart's 1939 article in which he discusses the repair of the capsule to the bone of the anterior glenoid through the use of drill holes and suture. The subscapularis muscle, which is carefully divided to expose the capsule, is reapproximated without any overlap or shortening. Bankart reported 27 consecutive cases with "full movements of the joint and in no case has there been any recurrence of the dislocation."[51, 546, 553, 559]

It is important to emphasize several important differences between Bankart's original method and the capsulolabral reconstruction currently recommended. Today we do not osteotomize the coracoid; we do not shave off bone from the anterior glenoid; and finally, we strive to reattach the capsule and any residual labrum up on the surface of the glenoid lip, rather than on the anterior aspect of the glenoid as shown by Bankart.

Hovelius and co-workers[267] found a 2% redislocation rate after the Bankart procedure compared with a 19% redislocation after the Putti-Platt. Over one third of patients younger than 25 years of age were dissatisfied with the results of the Putti-Platt. Rowe and Zarins[559] reported a series of 50 subluxating shoulders with good or excellent results in 94% after a Bankart repair. A Bankart lesion was found in 64% of these shoulders. Rowe and co-workers[554] reported on 51 shoulders with a fracture of the anterior rim of the glenoid. Eighteen shoulders had a fracture involving one sixth or less of the glenoid, 26 involved one fourth of the glenoid, and seven had one third of the anterior glenoid fractured off. In this group of

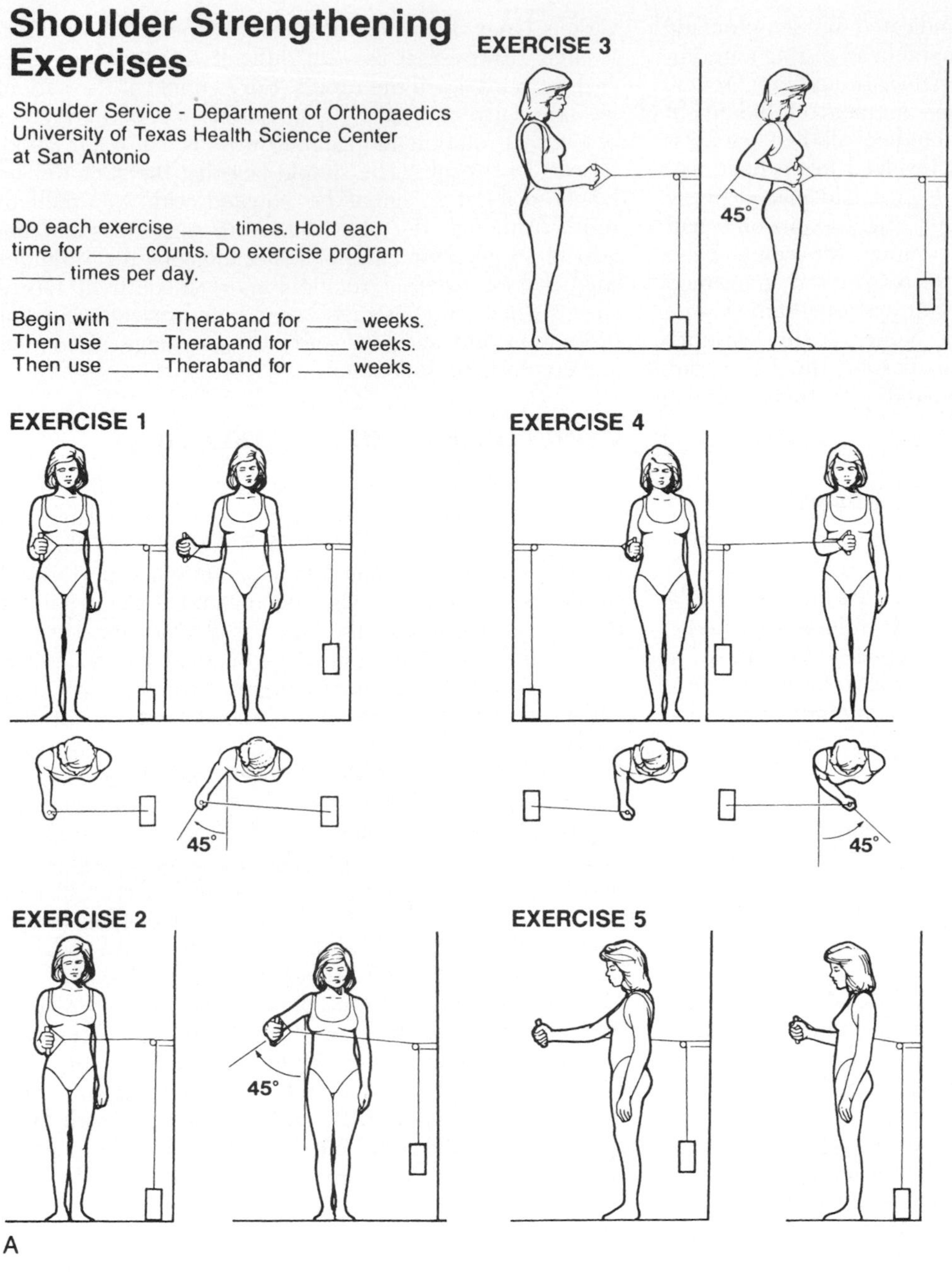
Shoulder Strengthening Exercises
Shoulder Service - Department of Orthopaedics
University of Texas Health Science Center
at San Antonio
Do each exercise ____ times. Hold each time for ____ counts. Do exercise program ____ times per day.
Begin with ____ Theraband for ____ weeks.
Then use ____ Theraband for ____ weeks.
Then use ____ Theraband for ____ weeks.
EXERCISE 1
45°
EXERCISE 2
45°
EXERCISE 3
45°
EXERCISE 4
45°
EXERCISE 5
A

Figure 14–146

A, Shoulder strengthening exercises. Initially the patient is given rubber TheraBands to strengthen the rotator cuff muscles and the three parts of the deltoid. When the patient is proficient with the rubber resistance with exercises 1 to 5, then the patient is given an exercise kit that consists of a pulley, hook, rope, and handle. The pulley is attached to the hook, which is fixed to the wall, and the five exercises are performed. Initially, the patient is instructed to use 5 or 10 lb of weight; this is gradually increased over a period of several months to as much as 25 lb. The purpose of the five exercises is to strengthen the three parts of the deltoid muscles, the internal rotators, and the external rotators.

patients who were treated with a Bankart repair without particular attention being given to the fracture, the overall incidence of failure was 2%. Prozorovskii and associates[519] reported no recurrences in the long-term follow-up of 41 Bankart repairs. Martin and Javelot[392] reported excellent results and minimal degenerative change in a 10-year follow-up of 53 patients managed with Bankart repair.

While many variations on the method of attaching the capsule to the glenoid have been described, no method has been demonstrated to be safer or more secure than suture passed through drill holes in the lip of the glenoid.[358, 399, 537] Modifications of the technique do not seem to constitute substantial improvements in the efficacy, cost, or safety of the procedure; for example, suture anchors do not have strength equal to sutures passed through holes in the glenoid lip.[196, 221, 239] Furthermore, when suture anchors are placed in the ideal location for capsulolabral reattachment, there is a substantial risk of their rubbing on the articular surface of the humerus. It is difficult to restore the effective glenoid depth using suture anchors (see Fig. 14–35*D*).

Although some have advocated the addition of a capsular shift or capsulorrhaphy to the Bankart repair,[8, 607] this does not seem necessary or advisable in the usual case of traumatic instability. In fact, one of the outstanding features of Bankart's results were that "All these cases recovered full movement of the joint, and in no case has there been any recurrence of dislocation." Excessive tightening of the anterior capsule and subscapularis can lead to limited comfort and function as well as to the form of secondary degenerative joint disease known as capsulorrhaphy arthropathy.[48, 234, 327, 378] Rosenberg and associates[549]

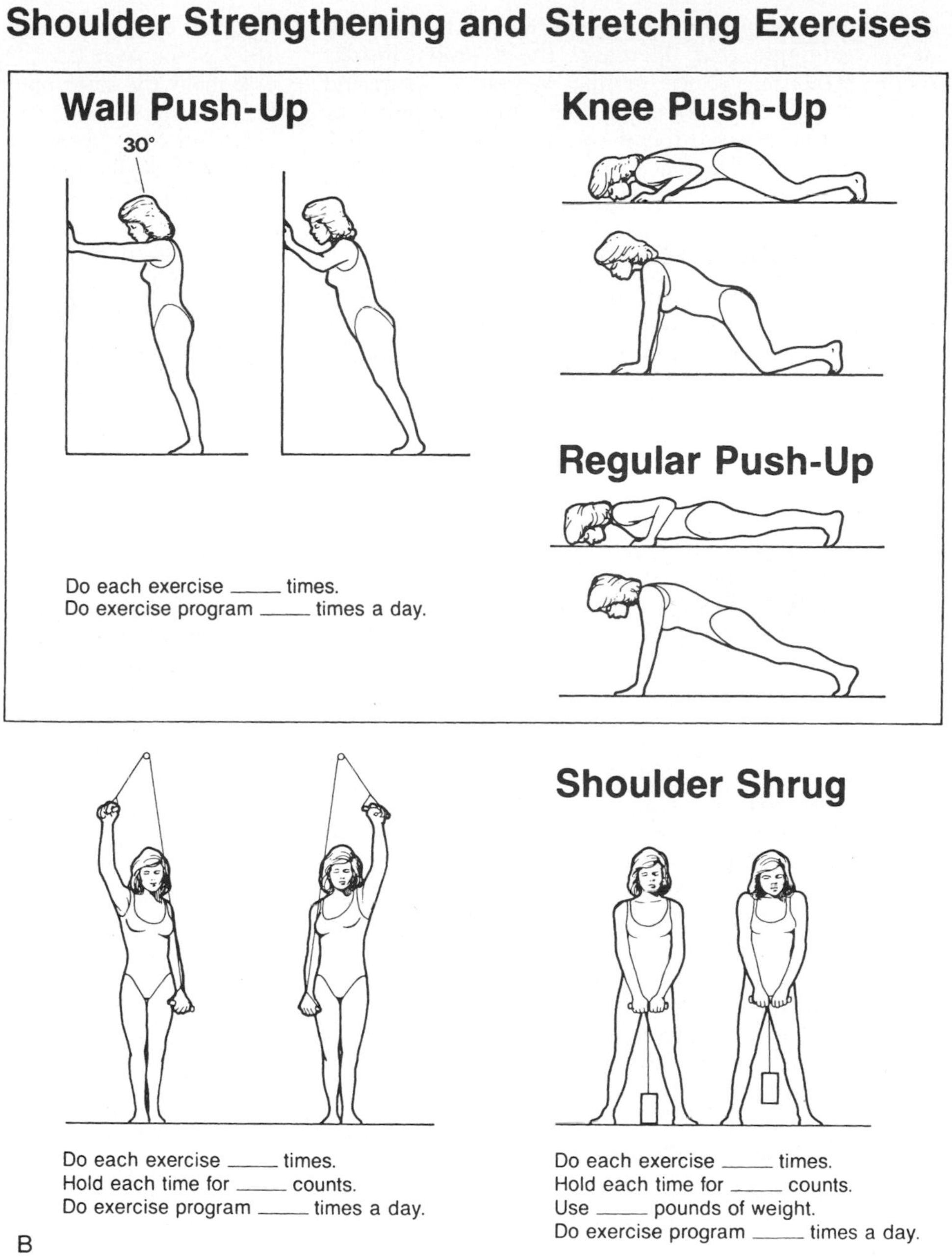

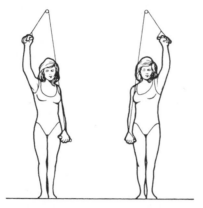

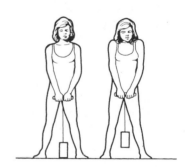

Figure 14–146

Continued B, In addition, the patient is instructed in exercises to strengthen the scapular stabilizer muscles. To strengthen the serratus anterior and rhomboids, the patient is instructed first to do wall push-ups and is then instructed to gradually do knee push-ups and then regular push-ups. The shoulder shrug exercise is used to strengthen the trapezius and the levator scapulae muscles.

found that 18 of 52 patients had at least minimal degenerative changes at an average of a 15-year follow-up; as a cautionary note against unnecessary capsular tightening, these authors found a correlation between loss of external rotation and the incidence of degenerative changes. To help guard against postoperative loss of motion, Rowe and associates[555] limit immobilization to just 2 to 3 days, after which the patient is instructed to gradually increase the motion and function of the extremity.

Thomas and Matsen described a simplified method of anatomically repairing avulsions of the glenohumeral ligaments directly to the glenoid lip without coracoid osteotomy, without splitting the capsule and the subscapularis, without metallic or other anchors, and without tightening the capsule.[43, 394, 629] This method (described in detail in the "Authors' Preferred Method" section) offers excellent range of motion and stability. Subsequently Berg and Ellison[43] have again emphasized this simplified approach to capsulolabral repair.

When pathologically increased anterior laxity is combined with a Bankart lesion, the addition of a capsular plication to the reattachment of the capsulolabral avulsion has been recommended. Jobe and colleagues[296] and Montgomery and Jobe[431] have found good or excellent results in athletes with shoulder pain secondary to anterior glenohumeral subluxation or dislocation. Two years after surgery more than 80% had returned to their preinjury sport and level of competition.

Rockwood and associates have reported their results in 108 patients (142 shoulders) with recurrent anterior shoulder instability.[691] All patients were managed by repair of capsulolabral injury, when present, and reinforcement of the anteroinferior capsular ligaments by an imbrication technique that decreases the overall capsular volume. According to the grading system of Rowe and associates, 93% of the results were rated as good or excellent at an average follow-up of 5 years (range of 2 to 12 years). The incidence of recurrent instability was approximately 1%.

OTHER ANTERIOR REPAIRS

Many other anterior repairs have been described. Most are of historical interest only. The reader is also referred to a review of the glenohumeral capsulorrhaphy by Friedman.[173]

Staple Capsulorrhaphy

In the DuToit staple capsulorrhaphy, the detached capsule is secured back to the glenoid using staples.[138, 597] Actually, the staple repair had been described 50 years earlier by Perthes. Rao and associates[525] reported follow-up on 65 patients having a DuToit staple repair of the avulsion of the capsule from the glenoid rim. Two patients showed radiographic evidence of loose staples. Ward and associates[666] reviewed 33 staple capsulorrhaphies at an average of 50 months postoperatively. Fifty per cent continued to have apprehension, and 12 had staple malposition. O'Driscoll and Evans[478, 479] reviewed 269 consecutive DuToit capsulorrhaphies in 257 patients for a median follow-up of 8.8 years. Fifty-three per cent of the patients had postoperative pain. Internal and external rotation were limited. A recurrence was reported in 28% if stapling alone was done and in 8% if a Putti-Platt procedure was added; 11% had staple loosening, migration, or penetration of cartilage. Staple complications contributed to pain, physical restrictions, and osteoarthritis. Zuckerman and Matsen have pointed out that the use of staples for surgical repairs may be associated with major complications (Figs. 14–147 and 14–148).[722]

Subscapularis Muscle Procedures

Putti-Platt Procedure. In 1948 Osmond-Clark[485] described this procedure, which was used by Platt of England and by Putti of Italy. Platt first used this technique in 1925. Some years later, Osmond-Clarke saw Putti perform essentially the same operation that had been his standard practice since 1923. Scaglietta, one of Putti's pupils, revealed that the operation may well have been performed first by Codivilla, Putti's teacher and predecessor. Neither Putti nor Platt ever described the technique in the literature.

In the Putti-Platt procedure, the subscapularis tendon is divided 2.5 cm from its insertion. The lateral stump of the tendon is attached to the "most convenient soft-tissue structure along the anterior rim of the glenoid cavity." If the capsule and labrum have been stripped from the anterior glenoid and the neck of the scapula, the tendon is sutured to the deep surface of the capsule, and "it is advisable to raw the anterior surface of the neck of the scapula, so that the sutured tendo-capsule will adhere to it." After the lateral tendon stump is secured, the medial muscle stump is lapped over the lateral stump, producing a substantial shortening of the capsule and subscapularis muscle. The exact placement of the lateral stump into the anterior soft tissues and of the medial stump into the greater tuberosity is determined so that, after conclusion of the procedure, the arm should externally rotate to the neutral position. Variations on the Putti-Platt procedure have been described by Blazina and Satzman,[51] Watson-Jones,[675] Muller,[443] and Symeonides.[624]

Quigley and Freedman[520] reported the results of 92 Putti-Platt operations; of these patients, 11 had more than a 30% loss of motion. Seven had recurrent instability after their surgery. Leach and co-workers[350] in 1981 reported a series of 78 patients who had been treated with a modified Putti-Platt procedure. Loss of external rotation averaged between 12 and 19 degrees. Collins and associates[99] reviewed a series of 58 Putti-Platt procedures and 48 Putti-Platt-Bankart procedures. The redislocation rate was 11% (some because of significant trauma), 20% had residual pain, and the average restriction of external rotation was 20 degrees. Hovelius and colleagues,[267] in a follow-up of 114 patients who underwent either a Bankart or Putti-Platt reconstruction, found a recurrence rate of 2% in 46 patients treated with the Bankart procedure and

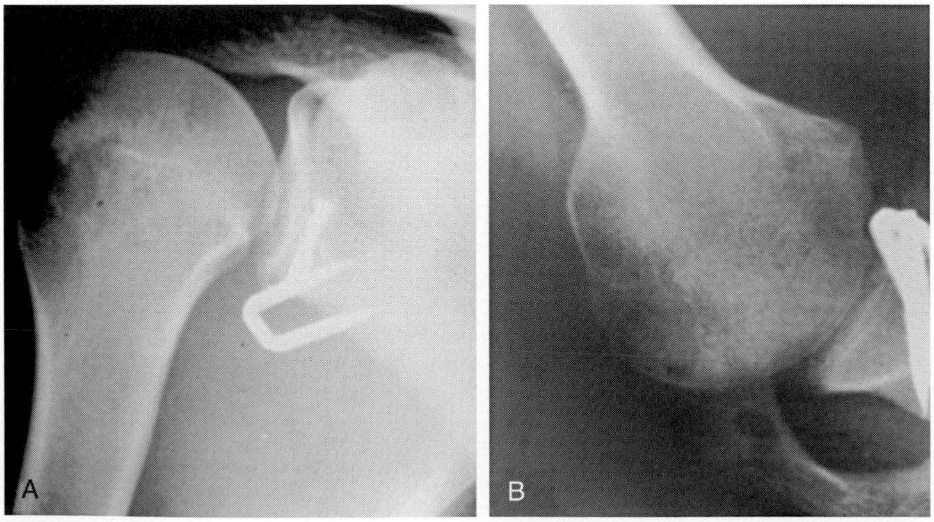

Figure 14–147

Complications of staple capsulorrhaphy. *A*, An anteroposterior x-ray showing a prominent staple on the inferior glenoid rim. *B*, An axillary view showing staple impingement on the head of the humerus.

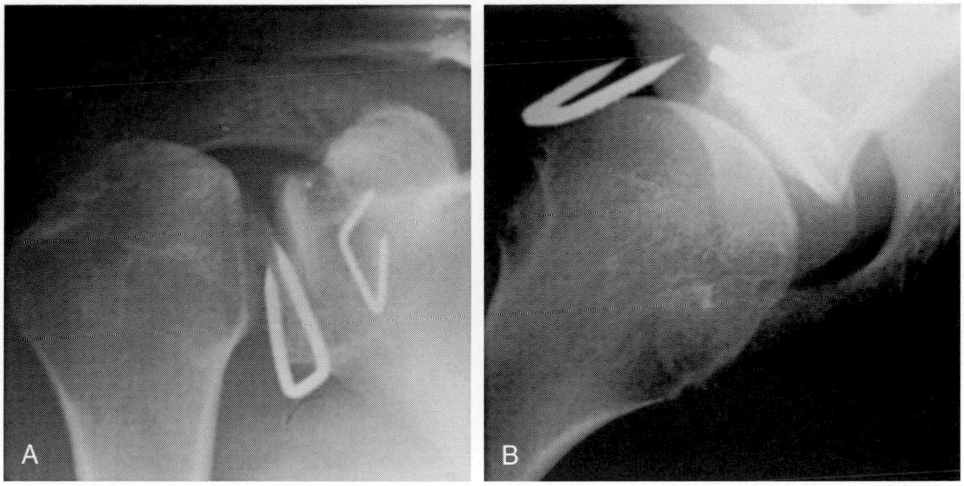

Figure 14–148

A loose staple after staple capsulorrhaphy. *A*, An anteroposterior x-ray showing a loose staple in the glenohumeral joint. *B*, Axillary view.

of 19% in 68 patients treated with a Putti-Platt procedure. The follow-up was between 1.5 and 10 years. Fredriksson and Tegner[172] reviewed 101 patients who had had a Putti-Platt procedure with a mean follow-up of approximately 8 years (range of 5 to 14 years). Recurrent instability occurred in 20% of cases, and all patients demonstrated a decrease in the range of all measured movements, especially external rotation. Additionally, a significant decrease in strength and power was noted by Cybex dynamometer assessment. The authors noted that the restricted motion after this procedure did not improve with time as previous reports had suggested and concluded that this method of reconstruction should not be recommended for young active patients.

It is important to recognize that if this operation is carried out as described, a 2.5-cm lateral stump of subscapularis tendon is attached to the anterior glenoid. Since the radius of the humerus is approximately 2.5 cm, a 2.5-cm stump of subscapularis fused to the anterior glenoid would limit the *total* humeral rotation to 1 radian, or 57 degrees. Angelo and Hawkins[12, 233] presented a series of patients who developed osteoarthritis an average of 15 years after a Putti-Platt repair. It is now recognized that limitation of external rotation in repairs for anterior instability is a predisposing factor to capsulorrhaphy arthropathy.[327, 378]

Magnuson-Stack Procedure. Transfer of the subscapularis tendon from the lesser tuberosity across the bicipital groove to the greater tuberosity was originally described by Magnuson and Stack in 1940.[312, 384–386, 422, 525] In 1955, Magnuson[525] recommended that in some cases the tendon should be transferred not only across the bicipital groove but also distally into an area between the greater tuberosity and the upper shaft. DePalma[122] recommended that the tendon be transferred to the upper shaft below the greater tuberosity. Karadimas,[312] in the largest single series of Magnuson-Stack procedures (154 patients), reported a 2% recurrence rate. Badgley and O'Connor[23] and Bailey[25] have reported on a combination of the Putti-Platt and the Magnuson-Stack operations; they used the upper half of the subscapularis muscle to perform the Putti-Platt procedure and the lower half of the muscle to perform the Magnuson-Stack procedure.

The complications of the Magnuson-Stack procedure include excessive anterior tightening with posterior subluxation or dislocation (Fig. 14–149), damage to the biceps (Fig. 14–150), and recurrent instability.

Bone Block

Eden-Hybbinette Procedure. The Eden-Hybbinette procedure was performed independently by Eden[139] in

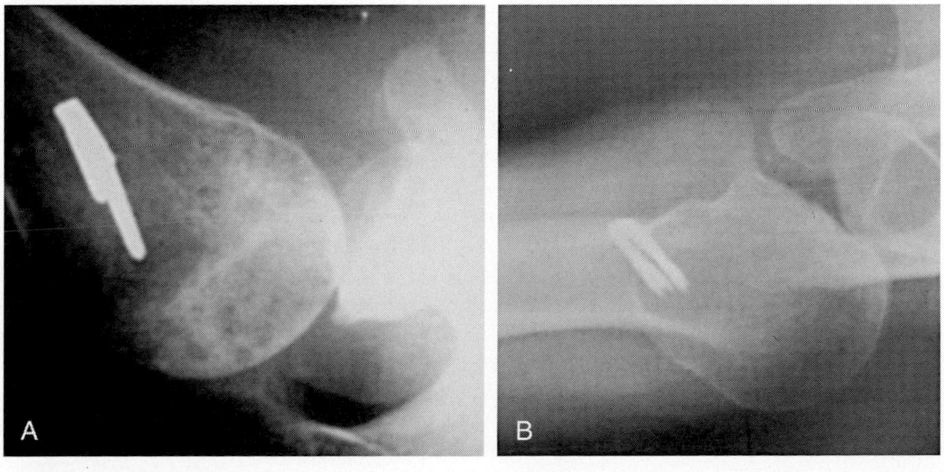

Figure 14–149

The Magnuson-Stack procedure. *A*, This axillary view shows posterior subluxation of the humeral head on the glenoid as a result of excessive anterior tightening with the Magnuson-Stack procedure. *B*, Another patient's axillary view shows excessive anterior tightening from the Magnuson-Stack procedure, resulting in posterior glenohumeral displacement of the humeral head.

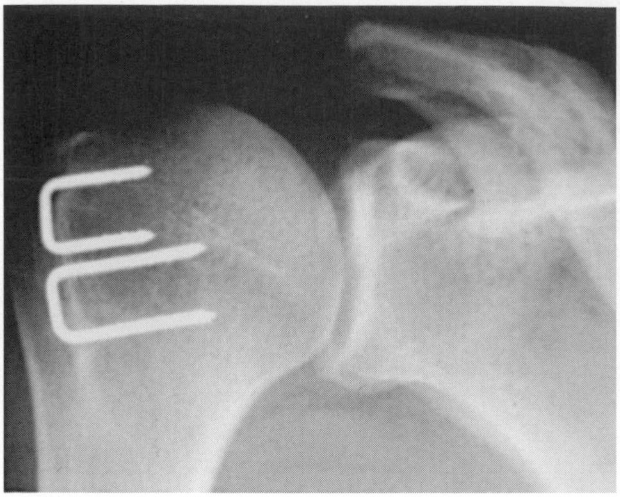

Figure 14–150

Staple impingement on the long head of the biceps tendon. This anteroposterior x-ray shows the position of the staple resulting in tendon impingement. Anterior shoulder pain resolved when the staple was removed.

1918 and by Hybbinette[276] in 1932. Eden first used tibial grafts, but both authors finally recommended the use of iliac grafts. This procedure is supposed to extend the anterior glenoid. It has been used by Palmer and Widen,[493] Lavik,[346] and Hovelius[263] in treating shoulder subluxation and dislocation. Lavik modified the procedure by inserting the graft into the substance of the anterior glenoid rim. Lange[341] inserted the bone graft into an osteotomy on the anterior glenoid. Hehne and Hubner[240] reported a comparison of the Eden-Hybbinette-Lange and the Putti-Platt procedures in 170 patients; their results seemed to favor the latter. Paavolainen and coworkers[490] reported on 41 cases of Eden-Hybbinette procedures; three had recurrent instability, and external rotation was diminished an average of 10%. They found the results similar to their series of Putti-Platt operations. Ten per cent in each group developed degenerative joint disease!

Niskanen and co-workers[465] reported a series of 52 shoulders with a mean follow-up of 6 years that had been treated with a modification of the Eden-Hybbinette procedure. The operation involved the creation of a trough through the capsule and into the anteroinferior aspects of the scapula neck. A tricortical iliac crest bone graft was then wedged into the trough without fixation. A 21% recurrence rate was attributed to one spontaneous dislocation and 10 traumatic redislocations. Postoperative arthrosis was noted in nine shoulders and early degenerative changes in an additional 18 shoulders.

Oudard Procedure. In 1924 Oudard[486] described a method in which the coracoid process was prolonged with a bone graft from the tibia. The graft (4 × 3 × 1 cm) was inserted between the sawed-off tip and the remainder of the coracoid and was directed laterally and inferiorly. The graft acted as an anterior buttress that served to prevent recurrent dislocations. Oudard also shortened the subscapular tendon. Later he published another method of obtaining the elongation of the coracoid by performing an oblique osteotomy of the coracoid and by displacing the posterolateral portion to serve as a bone block.

Bone blocks are not the procedure of choice for the routine case of recurrent anterior glenohumeral instability. One must be concerned about procedures that may bring the humeral head into contact with bone that is not covered by articular cartilage because of the high risk of degenerative joint disease. Soft tissue repairs and reconstructions are safer and more effective for dealing with the usual case of recurrent traumatic instability. However, when a major anterior glenoid deficiency reduces the anterior or anteroinferior balance stability angle to unacceptably small value, reconstruction of the anterior glenoid lip may be necessary. Matsen[395] has described a technique for using a contoured bone graft to replace the missing glenoid bone covered with joint capsule or other soft tissue in order to offer a smooth surface to articulate with the humeral head.

Coracoid Transfer

In the transfer of the coracoid process to the anterior glenoid, an attempt is made to create an anteroinferior musculotendinous sling. Some authors also refer to a bone block effect and an intentional tethering of the subscapularis in front of the glenohumeral joint. Thus it is apparent that these procedures do not address the usual pathology of traumatic instability. The redislocation rates after coracoid transfer for the usual case of traumatic instability are no lower than for soft tissue reconstructions, but the rate of serious complications is substantially higher (Figs. 14–151 to 14–156). Furthermore, in contrast to soft tissue procedures, coracoid transfer procedures are extremely difficult and hazardous to revise: The subscapularis, musculocutaneous, and axillary nerves are scarred in abnormal positions; the subscapularis muscle is scarred and tethered; and the axillary artery may be displaced in scar tissue.

Trillat Procedure. Trillat and Leclerc-Chalvet[54, 468, 642, 643] performed an osteotomy at the base of the coracoid

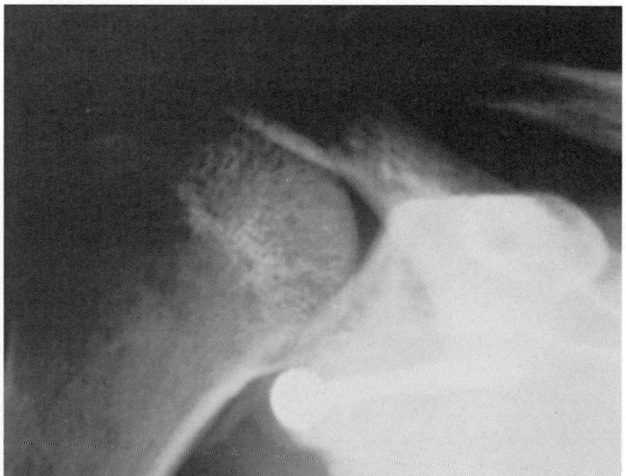

Figure 14–151

This anteroposterior x-ray shows screw impingement on the humeral head after the Bristow procedure.

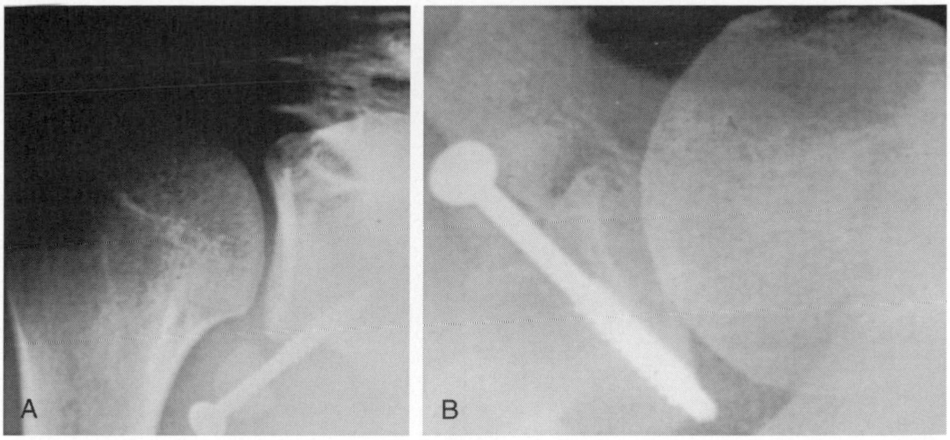

Figure 14–152

Nonunion of coracoid process after the Bristow procedure. *A,* An anteroposterior x-ray shows nonunion of the coracoid process. *B,* An axillary view of a different patient shows nonunion of the coracoid process after the Bristow procedure.

process and then displaced the coracoid downward and laterally. The displaced coracoid is held in position by a special nail-pin or screw. The pin is passed into the scapula above the inferiorly displaced subscapularis muscle, which effectively shortens the muscle.

Bristow-Helfet Procedure. This procedure was developed, used, and reported by Helfet[241] in 1958 and was named the Bristow operation after his former chief at St. Thomas Hospital, W. Rowley Bristow of South Africa. Helfet originally described detaching the tip of the coracoid process from the scapula just distal to the insertion of the pectoralis minor muscle, leaving the conjoined tendons (i.e., the short head of the biceps and the coracobrachialis) attached. Through a vertical slit in the subscapularis tendon, the joint is exposed and the anterior surface of the neck of the scapula is "rawed up." The coracoid process with its attached tendons is then passed through the slit in the subscapularis and kept in contact with the raw area on the scapula by suturing the conjoined tendon to the cut edges of the subscapularis tendon. Effectively, a subscapularis tenodesis is performed.

In 1958, T. B. McMurray (son of T. P. McMurray of hip osteotomy fame) visited Newton Mead[415] of Chicago and described modifications of the Bristow operation that were being used in Capetown, Johannesburg, and Pretoria. Mead and Sweeney[415] reported the modifications in more than 100 cases. The modifications consist of splitting the subscapularis muscle and tendon unit in line with its fibers to open the joint and firmly securing the coracoid process to the anterior glenoid rim with a screw. May[398] has modified the Bristow procedure further by vertically dividing the entire subscapularis tendon from the lesser tuberosity; after exploring the joint, he attaches the tip of

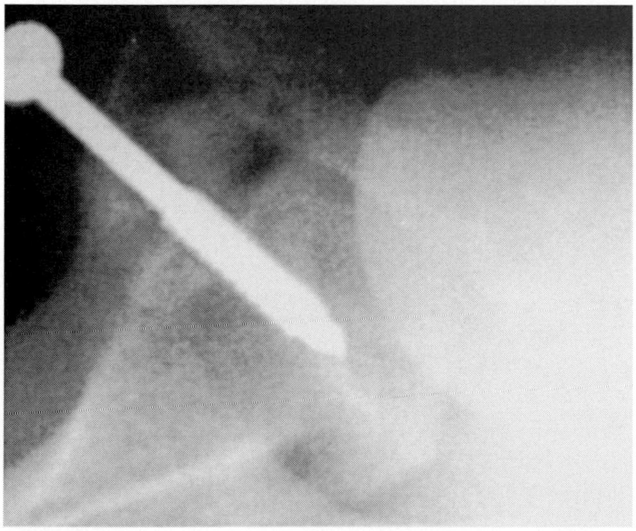

Figure 14–153

This axillary view shows the screw backing out of the glenoid after the Bristow procedure.

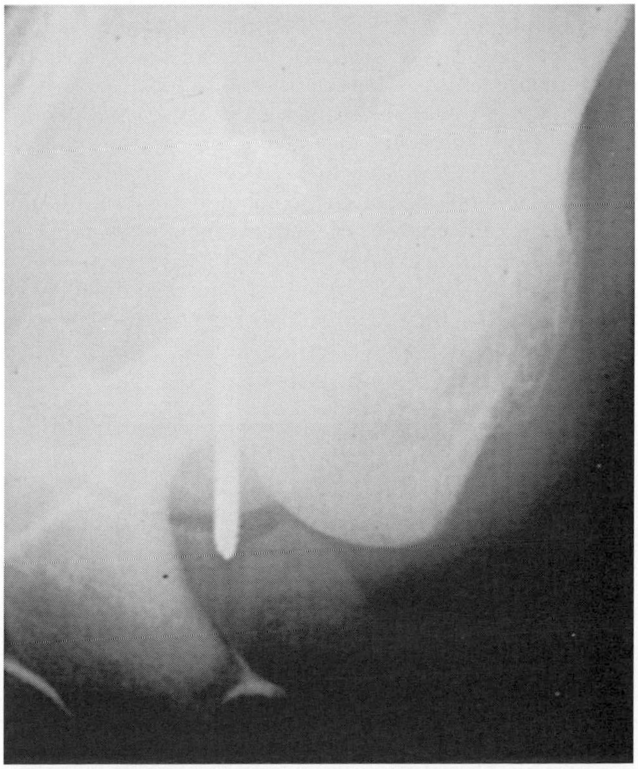

Figure 14–154

This axillary view shows an excessively long screw used during the Bristow procedure. The patient had an infraspinatus palsy as a result of injury to the nerve to this muscle.

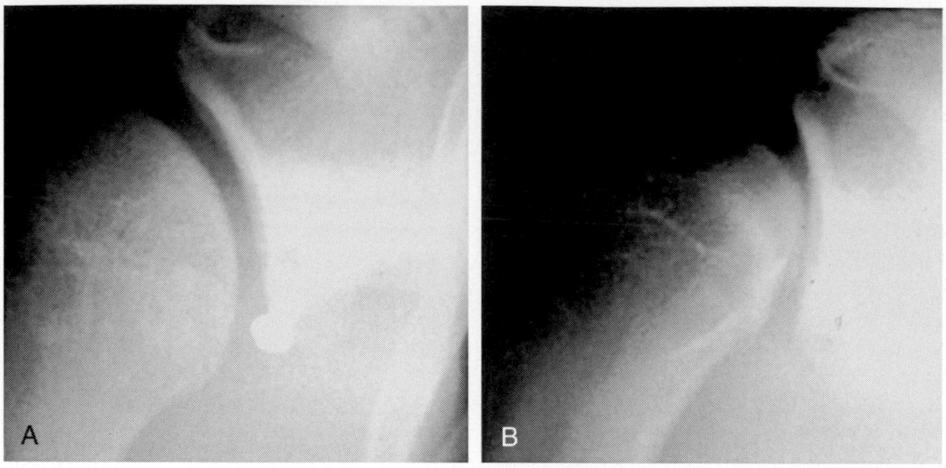

Figure 14–155

Anteroposterior x-rays showing broken screws with the humerus in external rotation *(A)* and internal rotation *(B)*.

the coracoid process with the conjoined tendon to the anterior glenoid with a screw. The subscapularis tendon is then split horizontally and reattached—half of the tendon above and half below the transferred conjoined tendon—to the site of its original insertion. Again, the net effect is a tenodesis of the subscapularis.

Helfet[241] reported that the procedure not only "reinforced" the defective part of the joint but also had a "bone block" effect. Mead,[415] however, does not regard the bone block as being a very important part of the procedure and believes that the transfer adds a muscle reinforcement at the lower anterior aspect of the shoulder joint that prevents the lower portion of the subscapularis muscle from displacing upward as the humerus is abducted. Bonnin[55, 56] has modified the Bristow procedure in the following way: he does not shorten or split the subscapularis muscle tendon unit but for exposure he divides the subscapularis muscle at its muscle-tendon junction and, following the attachment of the coracoid process to the glenoid with a screw, he reattaches the subscapularis on top of the conjoined tendon. Results with this modification in 81 patients have been reported by Hummel and associates.[272]

Torg and co-workers[640] reported their experience with 212 cases of the Bristow procedure. In their modification the coracoid was passed over the superior border rather than through the subscapularis. Their postoperative instability rate was 8.5% (3.8% redislocation and 4.7% subluxation). Ten patients required re-operation for screw-related problems; 34% had residual shoulder pain; and 8% were unable to do overhead work. Only 16% of athletes were able to return to their preinjury level of throwing. Carol and associates[78] reported on the results of the Bristow procedure performed for 32 recurrent dislocating shoulders and 15 "spontaneous" shoulder instabilities. At an average follow-up of 3.7 years, only one patient had recurrent instability, and the average limitation of external rotation was 12 degrees. Banas and associates[27] reported 4% recurrence with an 8.6-year follow-up; however, additional surgery was required in 14%. Wredmark and associates[705] found only 2 of 44 recurrent dislocations at an average follow-up of 6 years, but 28% of patients complained of pain. Hovelius and co-workers[263] reported follow-up on 111 shoulders treated with the Bristow procedure. At 2.5 years, their postoperative instability rate was 13% (6% dislocation and 7% subluxation). External rotation was limited an average of 20 degrees, and 6% required reoperation because of screw-related complications. Muscle strength was 10% less in the operated shoulder. Chen and colleagues[88] found that after the Bristow procedure, the reduced strength of the short head of the biceps was compensated for by increased activity in

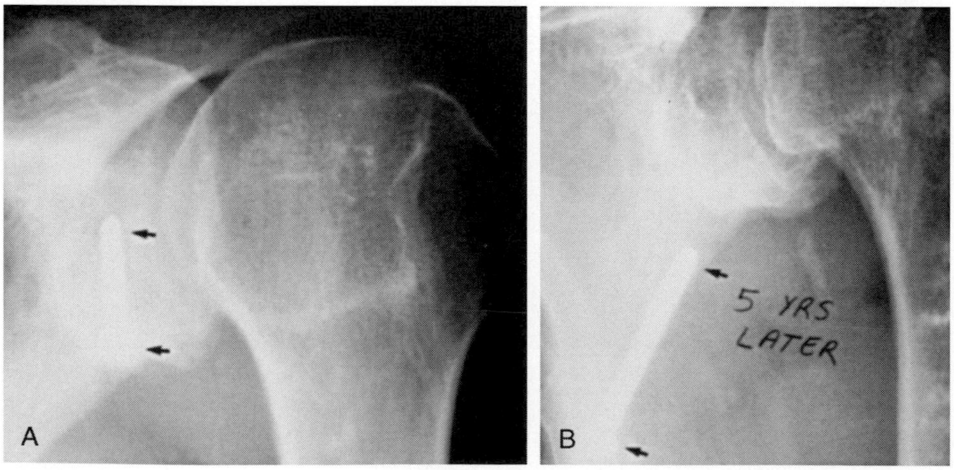

Figure 14–156

Late screw loosening after the Bristow procedure. *A,* An anteroposterior x-ray shows the position of the screw in the transferred coracoid process. *B,* An anteroposterior x-ray taken 5 years later shows the screw backed out and significant glenohumeral arthropathy.

the long head. Other series of Bristow procedures have been reported, each of which emphasizes the potential risks.[677]

Lamm and co-workers[338] and Lemmens and de Waal Malefijt[352] have described four special x-ray projections to evaluate the position of the transplanted coracoid process: anteroposterior, lateral, oblique lateral, and modified axial. Lower and co-workers[375] used CT to demonstrate the impingement of a Bristow screw on the head of the humerus. Collins and Wilde[98] and Nielsen and associates[464] reported that while they had minimal problems with recurrence of dislocation, they did encounter problems with screw breakage, migration, and nonunion of the coracoid to the scapula. Hovelius and colleagues[261, 265] reported only a 50% union rate of the coracoid to the scapula.

Norris and associates[470] evaluated 24 patients with failed Bristow repairs; only two had union of the transferred coracoid. Causes of failure included: (1) residual subluxation, and (2) osteoarthritis from screw or bone impingement or overtight repair. They pointed to the difficulty of reconstructing a shoulder after a failed Bristow procedure. Singer and associates[596] conducted a 20-year follow-up study of the Bristow-Latarjet procedure; in spite of an average Constant-Murley score of 80 points, there was radiographic evidence of degenerative joint disease in 71%.

Ferlic and DiGiovine[162] reported on 51 patients treated with the Bristow procedure. They had a 10% incidence of redislocation or subluxation and a 14% incidence of complications related to the screw. An additional surgical procedure was required in 14% of the patients. In a long-term follow-up study of 79 shoulders, Banas and colleagues[27] also reported complications necessitating reoperation in 14% of patients. Seventy-three per cent of reoperations were for hardware removal secondary to persistent shoulder pain.

There also appears to be a significant problem with recurrent subluxation after the Bristow procedure.[162, 265, 383, 400, 470] Hill and co-workers[254] and MacKenzie[382] noted failures to manage subluxation with this procedure. Schauder and Tullos[577] reported 85% good or excellent results with a modified Bristow procedure in 20 shoulders with a minimum 3-year follow-up. Interestingly, the authors attributed the success to healing of the Bankart lesion, since there were many cases in which the position of the transferred coracoid precluded it from containing the humeral head. The authors suggested that the 15% fair or poor results were secondary to persistent or recurrent subluxation.

In 1989, Rockwood and Young[544, 711] reported on 40 patients who had previously been treated with the Bristow procedure. They commented on the danger and the technical difficulty of these repairs.[19] Thirty-one underwent subsequent reconstructive procedures; 10 had a capsular shift reconstruction; four required capsular release; four had total shoulder arthroplasty; one had an arthrodesis; and six had various combined procedures. The authors concluded the Bristow procedure was nonphysiologic and was associated with too many serious complications and recommended that it not be performed for routine anterior reconstruction of the shoulder.

Latarjet Procedure. The Latarjet procedure,[344, 345, 500] described in 1954, involves the transfer of a larger portion of the coracoid process than used with the Bristow procedure with the biceps and coracobrachialis tendons to the anteroinferior aspect of the neck of the scapula. Instead of the raw cut surface of the tip of the coracoid process being attached to the scapula as is done in the Bristow-Helfet procedure, the coracoid is laid flat on the neck of the scapula and held in place with one or two screws. Tagliabue and Esposito[625] have reported on the Latarjet procedure in 94 athletes.

Wredmark and colleagues[705] analyzed 44 patients at an average follow-up of 6 years after a Bristow-Latarjet procedure for recurrent shoulder dislocation. Seventy-two per cent of patients had no discomfort, but the remaining 28% had moderate exertional pain. Vittori has modified the procedure by turning downward the subscapularis tendon and holding it displaced downward with the transferred coracoid. Pascoet and associates reported on the Vittori modification in 36 patients with one recurrence.

Other Open Repairs

Gallie Procedure. Gallie and LeMesurier[176, 177] originally described the use of autogenous fascia lata to create new ligaments between the anteroinferior aspect of the capsule and the anterior neck of the humerus in 1927. Bateman[37] of Toronto has also used this procedure. While fascia lata may not be the ideal graft material, the use of exogenous autograft or allograft to reconstruct deficient capsulolabral structures may be necessary in the management of failed previous surgical repairs.

Nicola Procedure. Nicola's name is usually associated with this operation, but the procedure was first described by Rupp[565] in 1926 and Heymanowitsch[251] in 1927. In 1929, Nicola[458] published his first article in which he described the use of the long head of the biceps tendon as a checkrein ligament. The procedure has been modified several times.[458, 460–462] Recurrence rates have been reported to be between 30% and 50%.[79, 308, 678]

Saha Procedure. Saha[567–571] has reported on the transfer of the latissimus dorsi posteriorly into the site of the infraspinatus insertion on the greater tuberosity. He reported that, during abduction, the transferred latissimus reinforces the subscapularis muscle and the short posterior steering and depressor muscles by pulling the humeral head backward. He has used the procedure for traumatic and atraumatic dislocations, and in 1969 he reported 45 cases with no recurrence.

Boytchev Procedure. Boytchev first reported this procedure in 1951 in the Italian literature,[58, 59] and later modifications were developed by Conforty.[100] The muscles that attach to the coracoid process along with the tip of the coracoid are rerouted deep to the subscapularis muscle between it and the capsule. The tip of the coracoid with its muscles is then reattached to its base in the anatomic position. Conforty[100] reported on 17 patients, none of whom had a recurrence of dislocation. Ha'eri and associates[215] reported 26 cases with a minimum of 2 years' follow-up.

Osteotomy of the Proximal Humerus. Debevoise and associates[117, 327] stated that humeral torsion is abnormal in the repeatedly dislocating shoulder. Weber[314, 422, 525, 678, 679] of Switzerland reported a rotational osteotomy whereby he increased the retroversion of the humeral head and simultaneously performed an anterior capsulorrhaphy. The indications were a moderate to severe posterior lateral humeral head defect, which he found in 65% of his patients with recurrent anterior instability. By increasing the retroversion, the posterolateral defect is delivered more posteriorly, and the anterior undisturbed portion of the articular surface of the humeral head then articulates against the glenoid. It is recognized that the effective articular surface of the humerus is reduced by the posterior lateral head defect and that the osteotomy repositions the remaining articular surface in a position more compatible with activities of daily living. Weber and colleagues[679] reported a redislocation rate of 5.7% with good to excellent results in 90%. Most patients required re-operation for plate removal.

Osteotomy of the Neck of the Glenoid. In 1933, Meyer-Burgdorff reported on decreasing the anterior tilt of the glenoid by a posterior wedge closing osteotomy.[567] Saha has written about an anterior opening wedge osteotomy with bone graft into the neck of the glenoid to decrease the tilt.[567]

COMPLICATIONS OF ANTERIOR REPAIRS

Complications of surgical repairs for anterior glenohumeral instability may be grouped into several categories.[348]

The first category includes complications that may follow any surgical procedure. Of primary importance in this category is postoperative infection. Thorough skin preparation, adhesive plastic drapes, and prophylactic antibiotics are useful in reducing contamination by axillary bacterial flora. It is also important to prevent the accumulation of a significant hematoma by achieving good hemostasis, obliterating any dead space, and using a suction drain if significant bleeding persists. Finally, it is important to keep the axilla clean and dry postoperatively by using a gauze sponge as long as the arm is held at the side.

The second category of complications consists of postoperative recurrent instability. The published incidence of recurrent dislocation after anterior repairs ranges from zero to 30%. It is noteworthy that many of the reports included in their tally only recurrent dislocation, rather than including recurrent subluxation or recurrent apprehension. A 1975 review of 1634 reconstructions compiled from the literature revealed that the incidence of redislocation averaged 3%.[541] In a 1983 review of 3076 procedures, this incidence was unchanged.[539] This review included 432 Putti-Platt operations, 571 Magnuson-Stack operations or modifications, 513 Bankart operations or modifications, 45 Saha operations, 203 Bankart-Putti-Platt combinations, 639 Bristow operations, 115 Badgley combined procedures, 254 Eden-Hybbinette operations, 277 Gallie operations or modifications, and 27 Weber operations.

The incidence of recurrence is underestimated by studies with only 2 years follow-up. Morrey and Jones,[436] in a long-term follow-up study of 176 patients that averaged 10.2 years, found a redislocation rate of 11%. The operative reconstructions were of the Bankart and Putti-Platt types. In 7 of the 20 patients, redislocation occurred 2 years or more after surgery. The need for long-term follow-up was further emphasized in a study by O'Driscoll and Evans,[478] who followed 269 consecutive staple capsulorrhaphies for a minimum of 8.8 years. Twenty-one per cent of 204 shoulders demonstrated redislocation; this incidence increased progressively with the length of follow-up.

Rowe and colleagues[561] reported on the management of 39 patients with recurrence of instability after various surgical repairs. Of 32 who were reoperated, 84% had not had effective repair of the Bankart lesion at the initial surgery. When the previously unrepaired Bankart lesion was repaired at revision surgery, almost all (22 of 24) the shoulders became stable and remained so for at least 2 years. Excessive laxity was thought to be the primary cause of instability in only four shoulders. Ungersbock and associates[649] also found that rounded or deficient glenoid rims and large unhealed Bankart lesions were associated with failure of surgical repairs for anterior instability. Zabinski and co-workers reported similar findings: more than half of their failed instability repairs were associated with unhealed Bankart lesions; most regained stability after revision repair.[714] By contrast, only nine of the 21 shoulders with recurrent multidirectional instability obtained a good/excellent result from revision surgeries.

Refractory instability can be a major problem, whether due to bone deficiency, poor quality soft tissues, musculotendinous failure, or decompensation of neuromuscular control (Fig. 14–157). Richards and associates[535] have described the challenges associated with trying to manage such cases of refractory or "terminal" instability using glenohumeral arthrodesis.

The third major category of complications arises from failure of diagnosis. It is essential to differentiate traumatic unidirectional instability (TUBS syndrome) from atraumatic multidirectional instability (AMBRII syndrome) before carrying out any surgical repair. The consequences of mistaking multidirectional instability for pure anterior instability are substantial. In this situation, if only the anterior structures are tightened, limited external rotation along with the resultant obligate posterior subluxation may lead to the rapid loss of glenohumeral articular cartilage and capsulorrhaphy arthropathy.[234, 327, 378] This complication can be prevented only by accurate preoperative diagnosis and by appropriate surgery that avoids unnecessary capsular tightening.

The importance of an accurate diagnosis and subsequent treatment cannot be overemphasized: 20 shoulders (53%) in the study of Cooper and Brems[102] and 22 shoulders (15%) in the report of Wirth and Rockwood[695] had been previously operated on for mistaken diagnosis. In the latter report, diagnostic errors included (in order of decreasing frequency) rotator cuff disease, biceps tendinitis, thoracic outlet syndrome, and cervical disk herniation.

The fourth category of operative complications consists of neurovascular injuries. The musculocutaneous nerve runs as a single or multipartite structure obliquely through the coracobrachialis, a variable distance distal to the coracoid process. In this location it may be injured by: (1) dissection to free up the coracoid process, (2)

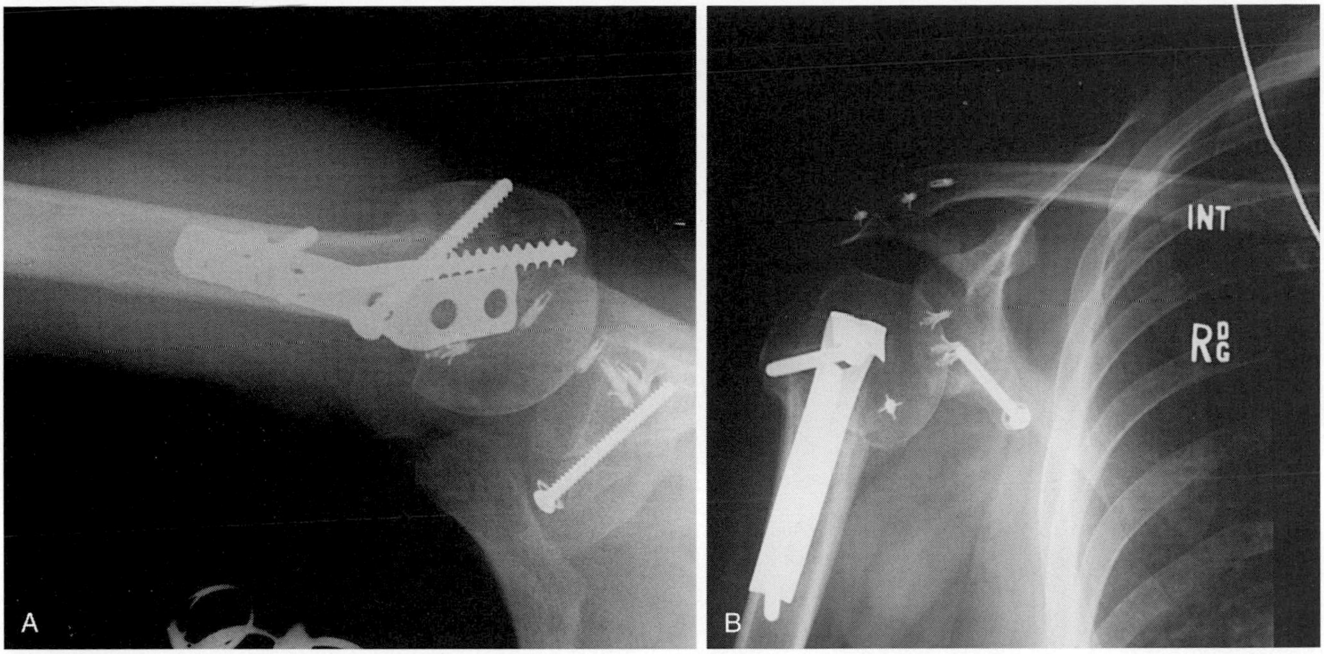

Figures 14–157

A and *B,* Anteroposterior and axillary radiographs of the shoulder of a young woman. The shoulder remained unstable after six surgeries for glenohumeral instability, including Bankart repairs, capsular shifts, a Bristow and a derotational osteotomy.

retraction, or (3) inclusion in suture.[590] Helfet[241] described one case in which the nerve had a high penetration into the coracobrachialis and became injured where the conjoined tendon entered the slit made in the subscapularis tendon for a Bristow procedure. The axillary nerve may be injured in dissection and suture of the inferior capsule and subscapularis.[373] Richards and associates[536] presented nine patients sustaining nerve injuries during anterior shoulder repair (three Bristows and six Putti-Platts). Seven involved the musculocutaneous nerve and two involved the axillary nerve. Two of the nerves were lacerated, five injured by suture, and two injured by traction. These nerve injuries are relatively more common during reoperation after a previous repair; in this situation, the nerves are tethered by scar tissue and thus are more difficult to mobilize out of harm's way. Neurovascular complications can best be avoided by good knowledge of local anatomy (including the possible normal variations), good surgical technique, and a healthy respect for the change in position and mobility of the neurovascular structures after a previous surgical procedure in the area. The authors recommend that the axillary nerve be routinely palpated and protected during all anterior reconstructions.[394, 541]

The fifth category of complications includes those related to hardware inserted about the glenohumeral joint.[86, 237] The screw used to fix the coracoid fragment in Bristow procedures has a particular potential for being problematic.[464, 520] Loosening of the screw may result from rotation of the coracoid fragment as the arm is raised and lowered; this rotation may contribute to screw loosening (Fig. 14–158). Artz and Huffer[19] and Fee and associates[160] have reported a devastating complication in which the screw became loose and caused a false aneurysm of the axillary artery with a subsequent compression of the brachial plexus and paralysis of the upper extremity. Similar complications have been reported as late as 3 years after surgery.[160] In other cases, the Bristow screw has damaged the articular surface of the glenoid and humeral head when placed too close to the glenoid lip, irritated the infraspinatus or its nerve when too long, or affected the brachial plexus when it became loose (see Figs. 14–151 to 14–156).

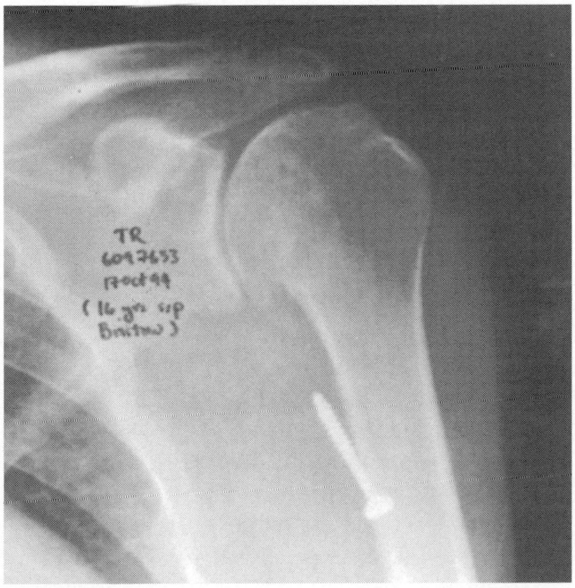

Figure 14–158

This patient experienced a pop while externally rotating the shoulder 5 months after a Bristow procedure. Shortly after this episode, he palpated a bump in his axilla while applying deodorant. (From Rockwood CA Jr, Green DP, and Bucholz RW [eds]: Fractures in Adults. Philadelphia: JB Lippincott, 1991.)

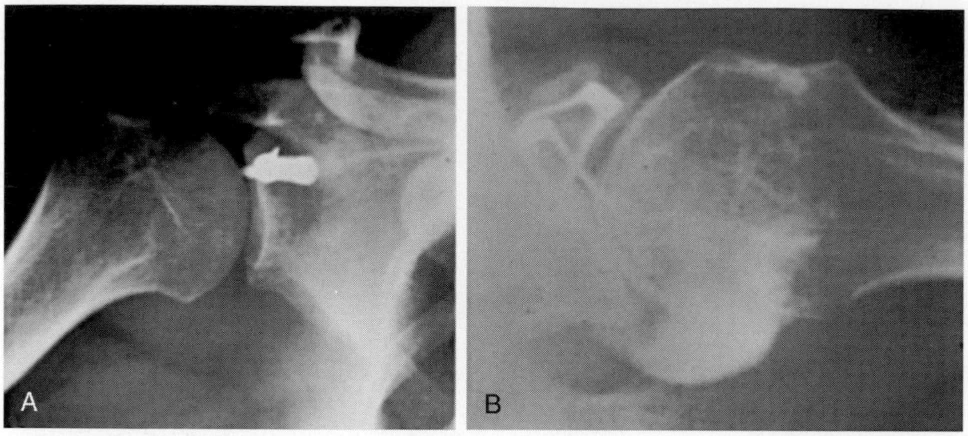

Figure 14–159

A, An anteroposterior x-ray shows the position of an arthroscopically placed staple. Impingement on the humeral head is suggested by this view. *B,* An axillary x-ray with contrast material demonstrates impingement of the staple on the humeral head.

Staples used to attach the capsule to the glenoid may miss their target, damaging the humeral or glenoid articular cartilage (Fig. 14–159; see also Figs. 14–147 to 14–149). Staples also may become loose from repeated pull of the muscles and capsule during shoulder usage, particularly if they were not well seated in the first place. O'Driscoll and Evans[478] reported an 11% incidence of staple complications after the DuToit procedure. If screws and staples migrate into the intra-articular region, significant damage to the joint surfaces may result (Fig. 14–160). Metal fixation may injure the biceps tendon in a Magnuson-Stack procedure (see Fig. 14–150).

Zuckerman and Matsen[722] reported a series of patients with problems related to the use of screws and staples about the glenohumeral joint; 21 had problems related to the Bristow procedure and 14 to the use of staples (either for capsulorrhaphy or subscapularis advancement). The time between placement and symptom onset ranged from 4 weeks to 10 years. Screws and staples had been incorrectly placed in 10 patients, had migrated or loosened in 24, and had fractured in 3. Almost all patients required reoperation, at which time 41% had a significant injury to one or both of the joint surfaces.

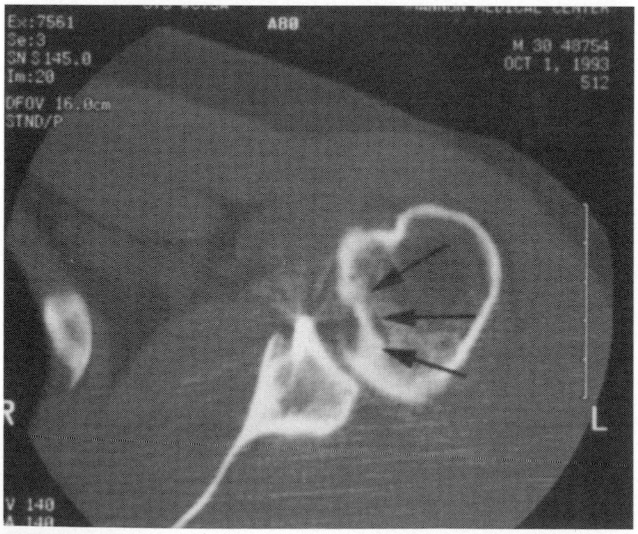

Figure 14–160

Significant humeral head erosion *(arrows)* secondary to intra-articular placement of an anterior capsular staple.

Recent attempts to "soften" the potential complications of hardware with bioabsorbable implants have been reported. However, Edwards and colleagues[140] reported the adverse effects of a polyglyconate polymer in six shoulders after repair of the glenoid labrum. All patients reported increasing pain and loss of motion requiring arthroscopic débridement. Dual-contrast arthrotomography revealed bony cystic changes around the implant, and histologic evaluation was consistent with a granulomatous reaction.

Taken together, these data suggest that primary repairs using hardware are more risky yet no more effective than are anatomic soft tissue repairs: The recurrence rates of techniques using screws and staples are no better than with hardware-free repairs. Risks are incurred with hardware that simply do not exist with other repair techniques. The depth and variable orientation of the glenoid at surgery provide substantial opportunity for hardware misplacement (into the joint, under the articular cartilage, subperiosteally, out the back, too high, too low, too medial, too prominent anteriorly, and too insecurely). The large range of motion of the shoulder with frequent vigorous challenges to its stability creates an opportunity for hardware loosening and for irreversible surface and neurovascular damage.

The sixth category of complications is limited motion. Limited range of motion, especially external rotation, has been reported after the Magnuson-Stack and the Putti-Platt procedures. It has also been noted after the Bristow procedure, which was supposed to be free of this problem.[32, 61, 255] Hovelius and colleagues[267] reported an average loss of external rotation of 21 degrees with the arm in abduction. In their series of 46 patients with continuing problems after shoulder reconstruction, Hawkins and Hawkins[232] found that 10 had stiffness related to limited external rotation.

MacDonald and colleagues[380] described release of the subscapularis muscle in 10 patients who had an internal rotation contracture after shoulder reconstruction for recurrent instability. At an average follow-up of 3 years, all patients reported less pain and demonstrated an average increase of 27 degrees of external rotation.

Lazarus and Harryman[348] pointed out that each centimeter of surgical lengthening of excessively tightened capsule regains approximately 20 degrees of rotation.

Rockwood and associates reported on 19 patients (20 shoulders) who had been treated for severe loss of external rotation of the glenohumeral joint after a previous anterior capsulorrhaphy for recurrent instability.[378] All 20 shoulders were managed by release of the anterior soft tissue. The average increase in external rotation was 45 degrees (range of 25 to 65 degrees).

The seventh complication is that of capsulorrhaphy arthropathy, or secondary degenerative joint disease resulting from surgery for recurrent instability.[12, 327, 348, 378, 394] This condition most commonly arises from excessive surgical tightening of the anterior capsule causing obligate posterior translation with secondary degenerative joint disease (see Figs. 14–48 and 14–50). This condition can be prevented by ensuring that the shoulder has a functional range of motion following repair for instability and by performing a surgical release of shoulders with major limitations of external rotation. Severe capsulorrhaphy may require shoulder arthroplasty with normalization of the posteriorly inclined glenoid version.[327, 348, 378, 394]

Angelo and Hawkins[12] reported eight patients with disabling degenerative arthritis presenting an average of 15.1 years after a Putti-Platt procedure. None of the patients had ever gained external rotation beyond zero degrees after their repair. Lusardi and associates[78] described 20 shoulders with severe loss of external rotation after anterior capsulorrhaphy and spoke to the risk of posterior subluxation and secondary degenerative joint disease under this circumstance.

Rockwood and associates[378] reported on seven shoulders in which the humeral head had been subluxated or dislocated posteriorly and 16 shoulders had been affected by mild to severe degenerative joint disease after surgical repair for recurrent anterior dislocation. Nine required shoulder arthroplasty because of severe joint surface destruction. At a mean follow-up of 48 months, all shoulders had an improvement in the ratings for pain and range of motion.

The eighth complication following surgical repair is failure of the subscapularis. As pointed out by Lazarus and Harryman[348] the clinical manifestations of subscapularis failure may include pain, weakness of abdominal press and lumbar push off, and apprehension or frank instability. A failed subscapularis can sometimes be repaired directly and on other occasions may require a hamstring autograft or allograft.

Rockwood and Wirth[699] reported a series of failed repairs in which the subscapularis was completely disrupted and contracted medially into a dense connective tissue scar that precluded mobilization. Most of the shoulders had undergone multiple previous procedures. The subscapularis deficiency was reconstructed by transfer of either the upper portion of the pectoralis major or the pectoralis minor in five shoulders.

MATSEN'S PREFERRED METHOD OF MANAGEMENT FOR RECURRENT TRAUMATIC SHOULDER INSTABILITY

The patient with traumatic anterior glenohumeral instability usually has symptoms primarily when the arm is elevated near the coronal plane, extended, and externally rotated. Characteristically the shoulder is relatively asymptomatic in other extreme positions or in midrange positions. Thus, for some patients appropriate management may consist solely of education about the nature of the lesion and identification of the positions and activities that need to be avoided.

Strengthening the shoulder musculature may help to prevent the shoulder being forced into positions of instability. The exercise program previously described for atraumatic instability may be considered as an option for traumatic instability as well.

The option of surgical repair is discussed when careful clinical evaluation has documented the diagnosis of refractory anterior instability resulting from an initial episode that was sufficiently traumatic to tear the anterior inferior glenohumeral ligament and that produces significant functional deficits (recurrent apprehension, subluxation, or dislocation) when the arm is in abduction, external rotation, and extension.

The patient desiring surgical stabilization is presented with a frank discussion of the alternatives and the risks of infection, neurovascular injury, stiffness, recurrent instability, pain, and the need for revision surgery.

Preoperative radiographs are obtained, including an anteroposterior view in the plane of the scapula, an apical oblique view (Garth view), and an axillary view. A preoperative rotator cuff ultrasound is obtained if there is suspicion of cuff disease, for example in an individual older than 40 years of age with pain between episodes of dislocation or weakness of internal rotation, external rotation, or elevation. An electromyogram is obtained if clinical evaluation suggests the possibility of nerve injury.

Surgical Technique

The goal of surgical management of traumatic anterior inferior glenohumeral instability is the safe, secure, and anatomic repair of the traumatic lesion, restoring the attachment of the glenohumeral ligaments, capsule, and labrum to the rim of the glenoid from which they were avulsed. By ensuring that reattachment occurs to the rim, the effective depth of the glenoid is restored (see Fig. 14–35). This anatomic reattachment should re-establish not only the capsuloligamentous checkrein but also the fossa-deepening effect of the glenoid labrum. Unnecessary steps are avoided, such as coracoid osteotomy and splitting the subscapularis from the capsule. No attempt is made to modify the normal laxity of the anterior capsule in the usual case of traumatic instability. The repair must be secure from the time of surgery so that it will allow the patient to resume activities of daily living while the repair is healing. Such a secure repair allows controlled mobilization, thus minimizing the possibility of unwanted stiffness. The tools needed for this repair are simple and commonly available (Fig. 14–161).

The procedure is performed under a brachial plexus block or a general anesthetic. The glenohumeral joint is examined under anesthesia. Although this examination rarely changes the procedure performed, it provides helpful confirmation of the diagnosis. **(V14-1)**

The patient is positioned in a slight head-up position

V14-2

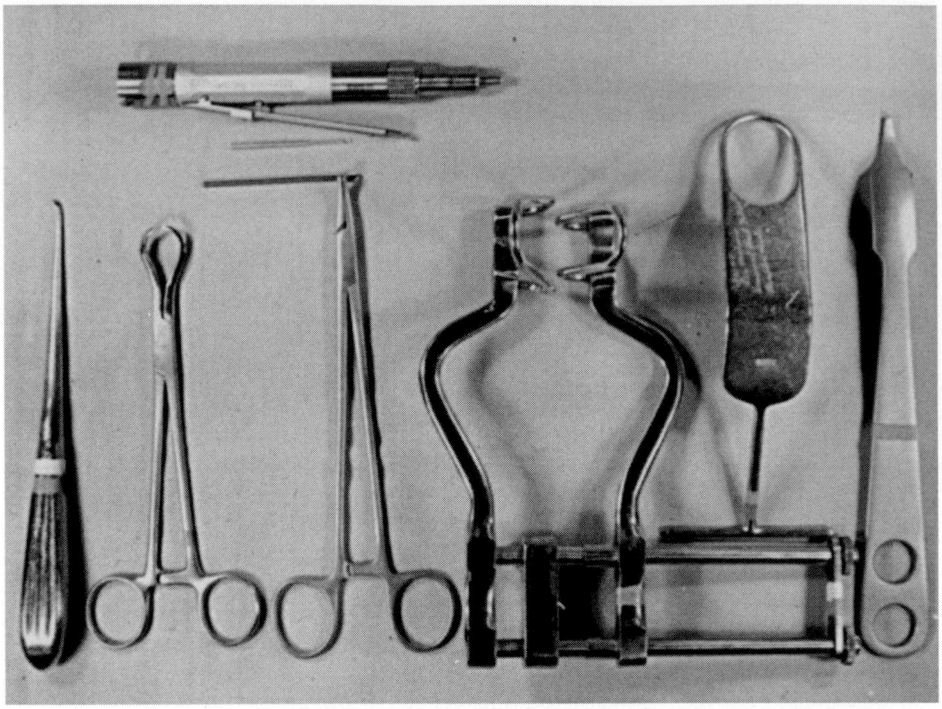

Figure 14–161

Instruments for surgical repairs of recurrent glenohumeral instability. *Top,* A high-speed drill is used for drilling holes in the glenoid rim. Left to right, A 000-angled curette and reaming tenaculum are used to connect the holes drilled in the glenoid rim; a curved-nosed needle holder for passing a No. 5 Mayo needle through these holes; self-retaining retractor; humeral head retractor; and sharp-tipped levering retractor.

(approximately 20 degrees) with the shoulder off the edge of the operating table. This position provides a full range of humeral and scapular mobility, and, if necessary, access to the posterior aspect of the shoulder. The neck, chest, axilla, and entire arm are prepared with iodine solution.

The shoulder is approached through the dominant anterior axillary crease (Fig. 14–162), which is marked prior to the application of an adherent, transparent plastic drape to facilitate a cosmetically acceptable scar.[222]

The skin is incised and the subcutaneous tissue is undermined up to the level of the coracoid process, which is then used as a guide to the cephalic vein and the deltopectoral groove (Fig. 14–163). **(V14-2)** The groove is opened by spreading with the two index fingers medial to the cephalic vein. A neurovascular bundle (a branch of the thoracoacromial artery and the lateral pectoral nerve) is commonly identified in the upper third of the groove;[203] this bundle is cauterized and transected. It is not neces-

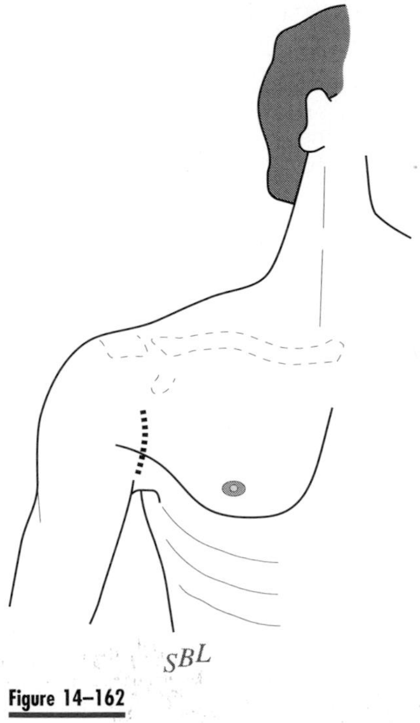

Figure 14–162

An incision in the major axillary crease.

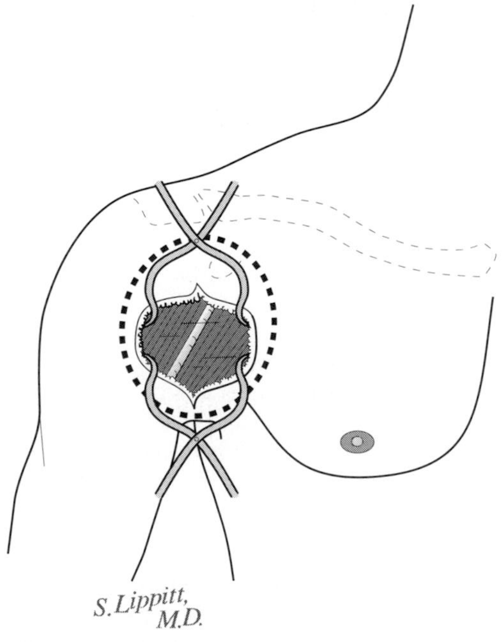

Figure 14–163

Subcutaneous tissue is undermined to the level of the coracoid. The cephalic vein is identified.

sary to release the upper pectoralis major, unless a prominent falciform border extends up to the superior extent of the bicipital groove.

The clavipectoral fascia is incised just lateral to the short head of the biceps, up to but not through the coracoacromial ligament (Fig. 14–164), entering the humeroscapular motion interface and exposing the subjacent subscapularis tendon and lesser tuberosity. The axillary nerve is routinely palpated as it crosses the anteroinferior border of the subscapularis. At this point it is useful to insert a self-retaining retractor, with one blade on the deltoid muscle and the other on the coracoid muscles. Care must be taken to ensure that the medial limb of this retractor does not compress the brachial plexus. Rotation of the arm from internal to external rotation reveals, in succession, the greater tuberosity, the bicipital groove, the lesser tuberosity, and the subscapularis. The anterior humeral circumflex vessels can usually be protected by bluntly dissecting them off of the subscapularis muscle at its inferior border. The interval between the supraspinatus and subscapularis tendons is identified by palpation, and a blunt elevator is inserted through this interval into the joint. This elevator brings the upper subscapularis into the incision (Fig. 14–165). With care to protect the tendon of the biceps, the subscapularis tendon and subjacent capsule are then incised together approximately 1 cm medial to the lesser tuberosity (Fig. 14–166), beginning at the superior rounded edge of the tendon. **(V14-3)** A tag suture is placed in the upper rolled border of the subscapularis to mark it for subsequent repair. The incision is then extended inferiorly to the level of the anterior circumflex humeral vessels. It is important that the incision through the subscapularis tendon leaves strong tendinous material on both sides of the incision to facilitate a secure repair at the conclusion of the procedure.

Without separating them, the subscapularis tendon and anterior shoulder capsule are retracted medially, providing an excellent view of the joint. If necessary for greater exposure, the joint capsule may be further divided parallel to the upper rolled border of the subscapularis. The biceps tendon is inspected and note is taken of the integrity of the transverse humeral ligament. Particularly in patients older than 40 years of age, the shoulder is inspected for evidence of rotator cuff tears. In traumatic anterior instability, a posterolateral humeral head defect is usually palpable by passing an index finger over the top of the humeral head (see Fig. 14–3). If the humeral head defect is so large that it contributes to instability in functional positions, anterior capsular tightening may be

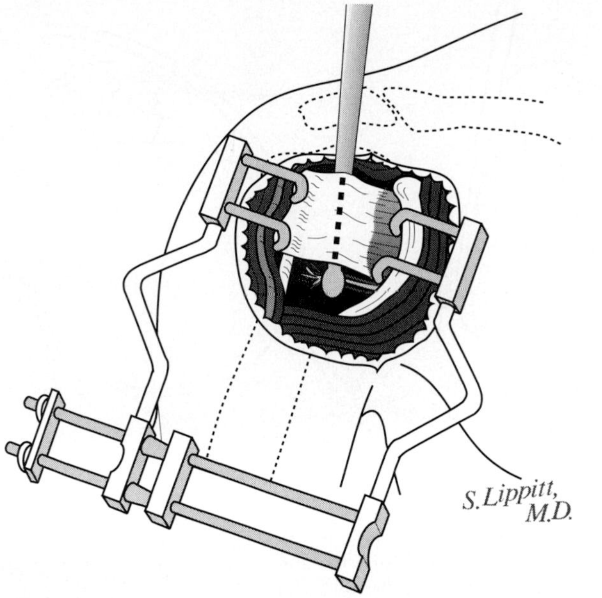

Figure 14–165

A blunt dissector is passed through the rotator interval and deep to subscapularis tendon. The tendon is divided so that strong tissue remains on either side for later repair.

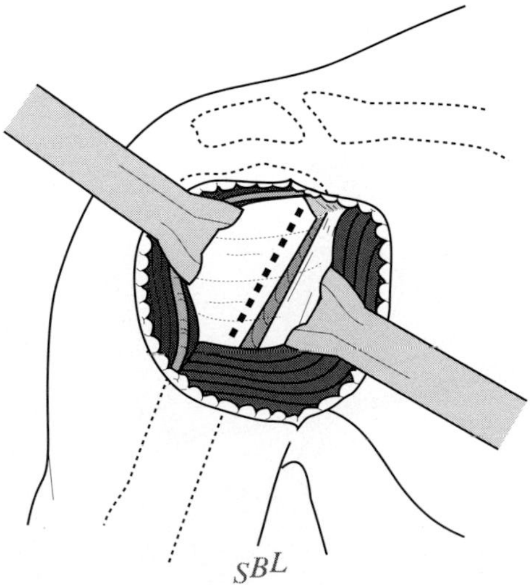

Figure 14–164

The deltopectoral groove is entered medial to the cephalic vein. An incision is made in the clavipectoral fascia just lateral to the coracoid muscles and up to the level of the coracoacromial ligament.

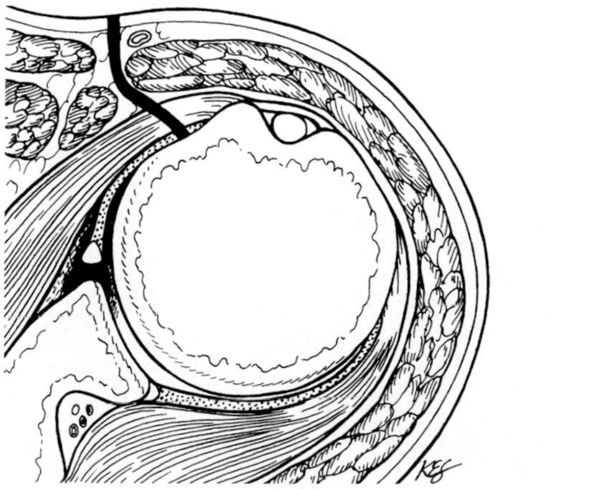

Figure 14–166

Transverse plane section from a superior view showing the incision and the plane for exposure. Note that the deltopectoral interval is utilized. The subscapularis tendon and the underlying joint capsule are incised as a unit 1 cm medial to the insertion. (From Matsen FA and Thomas SC: Glenohumeral instability. *In* Evarts CM [ed]: Surgery of the Musculoskeletal System, 2nd ed. New York: Churchill Livingstone, 1989.)

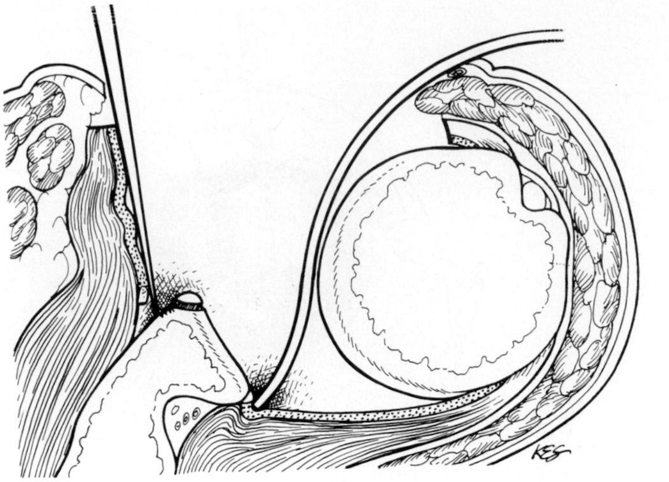

Figure 14–167

A transverse plane section showing placement of retractors and the location of drill holes. Note the area roughened by a curette along the anterior glenoid neck; also note the position of the drill hole relative to the anterior glenoid rim. (From Matsen FA and Thomas SC: Glenohumeral instability. *In* Evarts CM [ed]: Surgery of the Musculoskeletal System, 2nd ed. New York: Churchill Livingstone, 1989.)

necessary to keep the defect from entering the joint on external rotation.

The capsule and subscapularis are retracted together medially, and a humeral head retractor is placed so that it leans on the posterior glenoid lip and pushes the humeral head posterolaterally. This reveals the anterior inferior glenoid lip from which the labrum and capsule are avulsed in most patients with anterior traumatic instability (see Figs. 14–3, 14–35*B*, and 14–102). The labrum usually remains attached to the capsular ligaments but may remain on the glenoid side of the rupture, may be a separate ("bucket handle") fragment, or may be absent. Occasionally, flimsy attempts to heal the lesion will temporarily obliterate the defect. However, in these cases a blunt elevator will easily separate the capsule from the glenoid lip, revealing the typical lesion in the anterior-inferior quadrant of the glenoid. A spiked retractor is then placed through the capsular avulsion to expose the glenoid lip. The glenohumeral joint is inspected thoroughly for loose bodies, defects of the bony glenoid, and loss of cartilage from the remaining anterior glenoid.

The reconstruction of the capsulolabral detachment from the glenoid is necessary and sufficient for the surgical management of most cases of traumatic instability. This repair is carried out from inside the joint, without needing to separate the capsule from the subscapularis muscle and tendon. The glenoid is well exposed by a humeral head retractor laterally and a sharp-tipped levering retractor inserted through the capsular defect onto the neck of the glenoid (Fig. 14–167). **(V14-4)** Bucket handle or flap tears of the glenoid labrum are preserved for incorporation into the reconstruction of the glenoid lip.[1, 33]

The anterior, nonarticular aspect of the glenoid lip is roughened with a curette or a motorized burr, and care is taken not to compromise the bony strength of the

V14-4

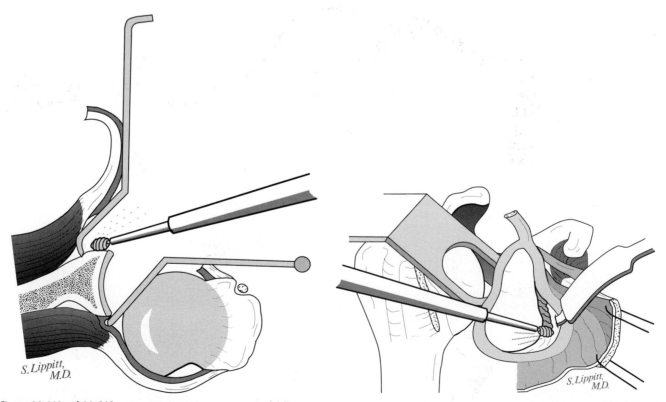

Figures 14–168 and 14–169

Roughening of the anterior, nonarticular surface of the glenoid using a pine cone burr. The capsule and subscapularis are retracted medially with a sharp-tipped retractor. The humeral head is retracted laterally with a humeral head retractor. (Modified from Matsen FA III, Lippitt SB, Sidles JA, and Harryman DT II: Practical Evaluation and Management of the Shoulder. Philadelphia: WB Saunders, 1994.)

V14-5 to V14-7

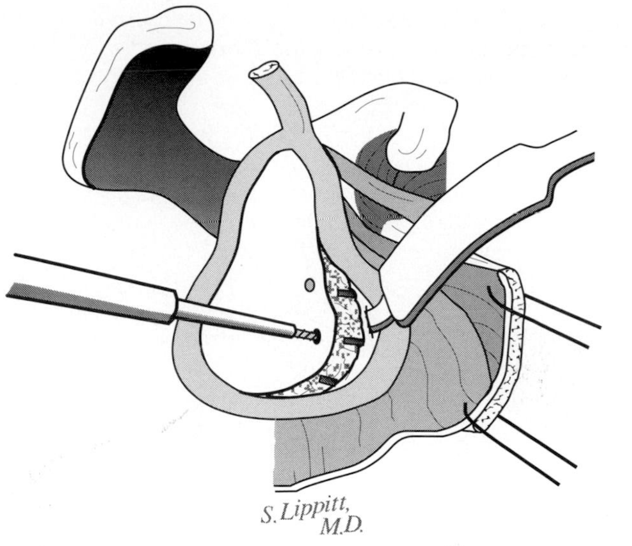

Figure 14–170

Drill holes are made in the lip of the articular glenoid 4 mm from the edge and 6 mm apart. (Modified from Matsen FA III, Lippitt SB, Sidles JA, and Harryman DT II: Practical Evaluation and Management of the Shoulder. Philadelphia: WB Saunders, 1994.)

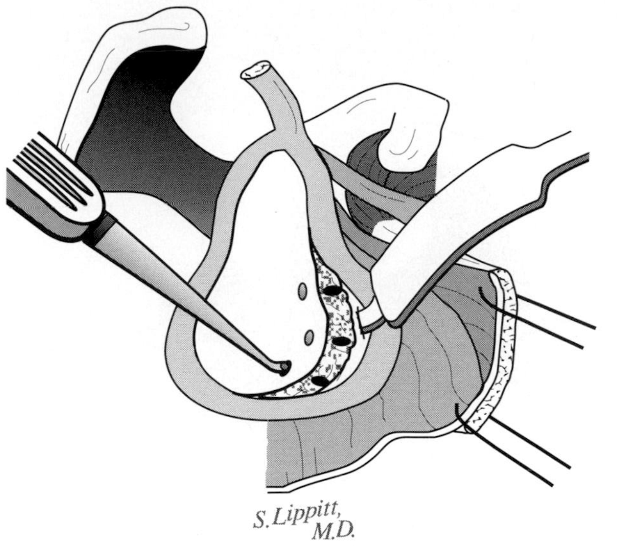

Figure 14–172

These drill holes are completed to the bony groove using a 000-angled curette. (Modified from Matsen FA III, Lippitt SB, Sidles JA, and Harryman DT II: Practical Evaluation and Management of the Shoulder. Philadelphia: WB Saunders, 1994.)

glenoid lip (Figs. 14–168 and 14–169). **(V14-5)** A 1.8-mm drill is used to make holes on the articular aspect of the glenoid 3 to 4 mm back from the edge of the lip to ensure a sufficiently strong bony bridge (Fig. 14–170). **(V14-6)** We place these holes 5 to 6 mm apart; thus, the size of the defect dictates the number of holes used for the reconstruction (Fig. 14–171). Corresponding slots are placed on the anterior nonarticular aspect of the glenoid (see Fig. 14–170). Using a 000-angled curette, continuity is established between the corresponding slots and holes (Fig. 14–172).

A strong No. 2 nonabsorbable braided suture is passed through the holes in the glenoid lip using a trocar needle and an angled needle holder (Fig. 14–173). **(V14-7)** After each suture is placed through the glenoid lip, the integrity of the bony bridge is checked by a firm pull on the suture.

When sufficient sutures have been placed to span the capsular defect, the sharp-tipped levering retractor is removed and replaced by a right-angled retractor positioned

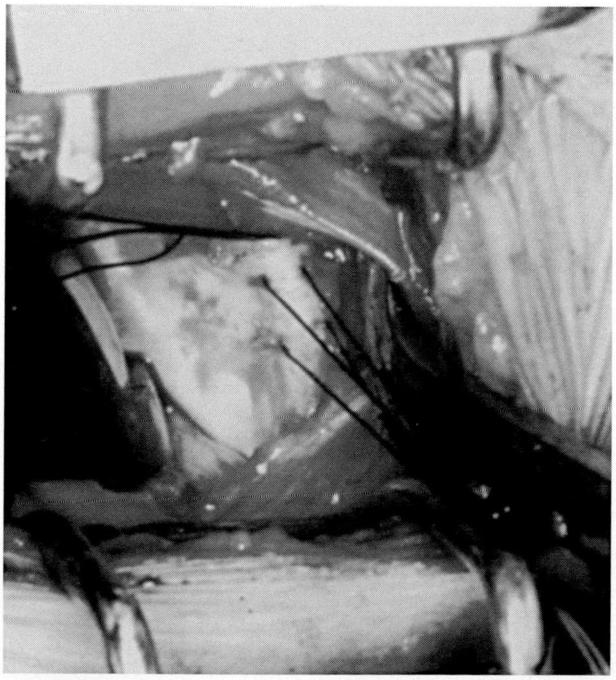

Figure 14–171

An intraoperative photograph of the Bankart procedure showing the placement of sutures through holes in the glenoid rim.

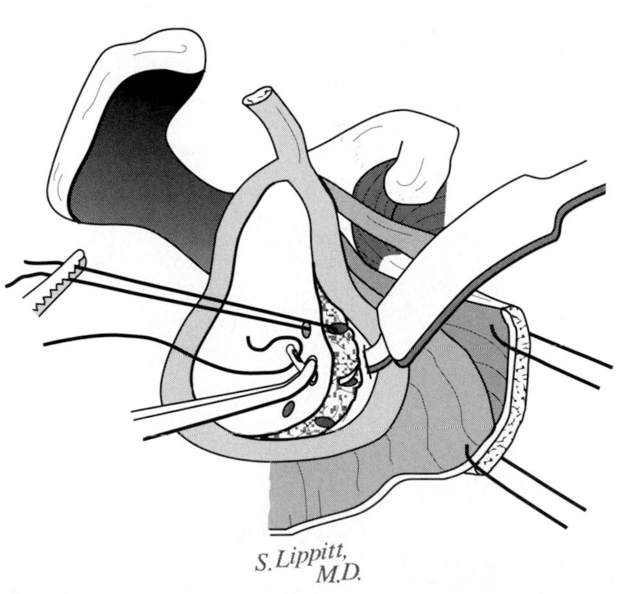

Figure 14–173

A nonabsorbable suture is passed through the drill holes. (Modified from Matsen FA III, Lippitt SB, Sidles JA, and Harryman DT II: Practical Evaluation and Management of the Shoulder. Philadelphia: WB Saunders, 1994.)

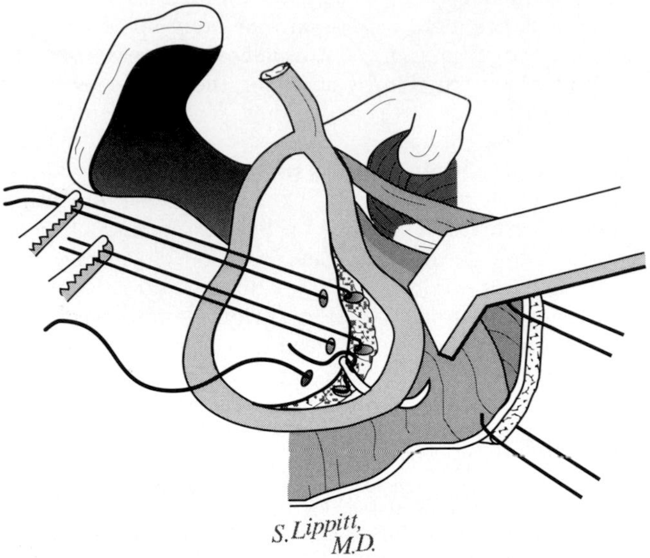

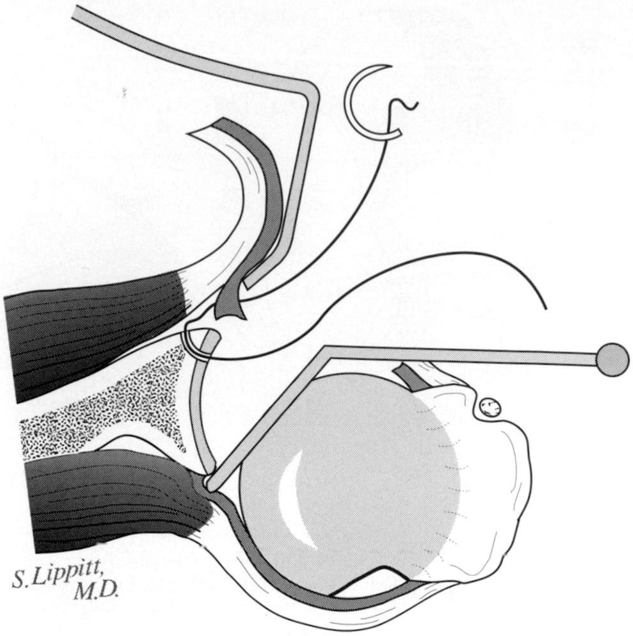

Figures 14–174 and 14–175

The sutures are then passed through the trailing medial edge of the capsule and the labrum. (Modified from Matsen FA III, Lippitt SB, Sidles JA, and Harryman DT II: Practical Evaluation and Management of the Shoulder. Philadelphia: WB Saunders, 1994.)

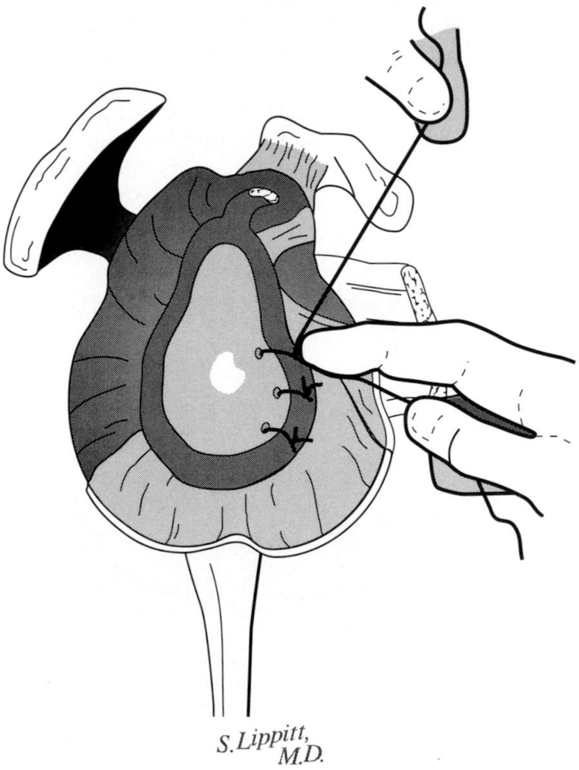

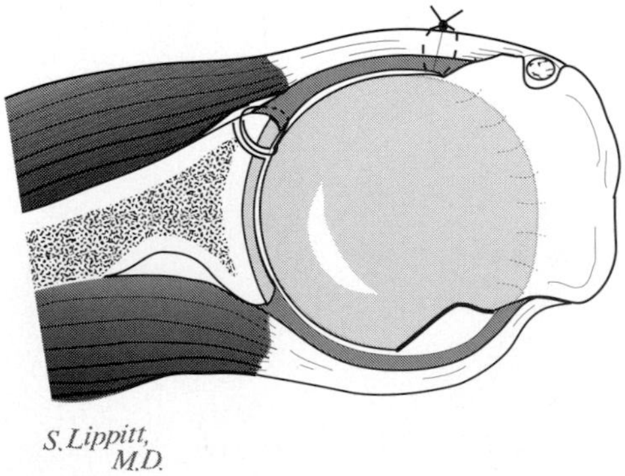

Figures 14–176 and 14–177

The suture is tied over the capsule, which securely reapproximates the detached tissues to the roughened glenoid edge and restores the fossa deepening effect of the capsule and labrum. The subscapularis and subjacent capsule are then repaired anatomically to their mates at the lesser tuberosity. (Modified from Matsen FA III, Lippitt SB, Sidles JA, and Harryman DT II: Practical Evaluation and Management of the Shoulder. Philadelphia: WB Saunders, 1994.)

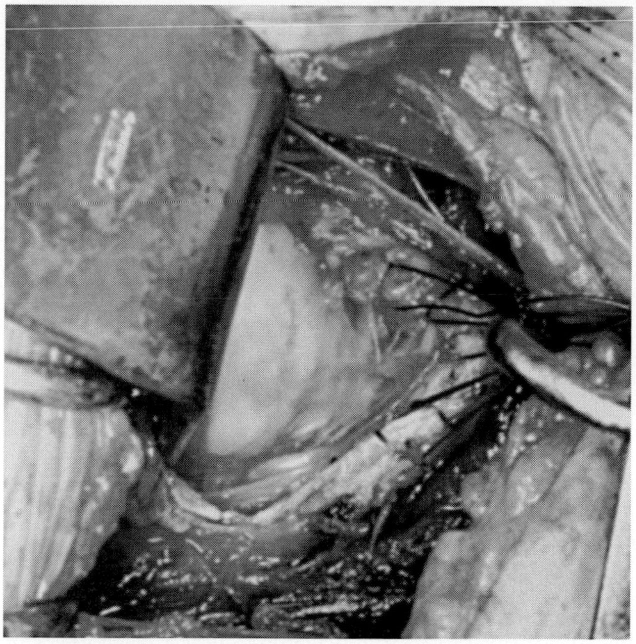

Figure 14–178

An intraoperative photograph during re-exploration of a Bankart repair. This patient ruptured the subscapularis tendon repair in a fall 2 months after a Bankart procedure. At the time of reoperation for repair of the subscapularis tendon, the anterior glenoid rim was explored and the Bankart repair was intact. The repair sutures were covered by synovium. The reconstructed labrum is strong.

to reveal the trailing medial edge of the avulsed capsule. This edge is most easily identified by tracing the intact labrum around the glenoid to its point of detachment at the Bankart defect. Next, using the trocar needle, the anterior end of the suture (the limb exiting the anterior nonarticular aspect of the glenoid lip) is passed through the trailing medial edge of the capsule, taking care to incorporate the glenoid labrum, if present, and the strong medial edge of the capsule (Figs. 14–174 and 14–175). **(V14-8)** No more capsule is taken than necessary to obtain a firm purchase. This prevents unwanted tightening of the anteroinferior capsule. In larger glenohumeral ligament avulsions, the detached medial edge of the capsule tends to sag inferiorly; in this situation, an effort is made to pass each suture through the capsule slightly inferior to the corresponding bony hole in the glenoid lip. Thus, when the sutures are tied, the inferiorly sagging medial capsule is repositioned anatomically (Fig. 14–176).

Once the sutures have been passed through the capsule, they are tied so that the labrum and medial edge of the capsule are brought up on the glenoid lip to restore the fossa-deepening effect of the labrum (Fig. 14–177).[349] **(V14-9)** The knots are tied so that they come to rest over the capsule, rather than on the articular surface of the glenoid (see Fig. 14–176). Because they lie over soft tissue, these sutures do not present a mechanical problem, even though they lie within the joint (Fig. 14–178).

Once these sutures are tied, the smooth continuity between the articular surface of the glenoid fossa and the capsule should be re-established along with a reconstructed labrum-like structure (see Figs. 14–35*C* and 14–178). No step-off or discontinuity in the capsule should be present. If a substantial anterior capsular defect exists anywhere but at the normal subcoracoid recess, it is closed.

Approximately 10% of patients with TUBS have fractures or deficiencies of the anterior bony lip of the glenoid. At the initial surgery, it usually seems reasonable to attempt reconstruction by attaching the avulsed anterior capsule to the lip of the remaining glenoid articular surface. Anterior glenoid deficiencies greater than 33% or those associated with previous surgical failure may require that the repair of the capsule to the edge of the remaining articular cartilage be backed up by the reconstruction of the lip of the glenoid using an iliac bone block. The iliac bone block is contoured flush with the normal glenoid curvature and held to the anterior glenoid with two screws placed securely and well away from the humeral joint surface. By placing the graft outside the repaired capsule, it becomes covered with periosteum or joint capsule, thus preventing direct contact with the humeral head (Figs. 14–179 to 14–181).

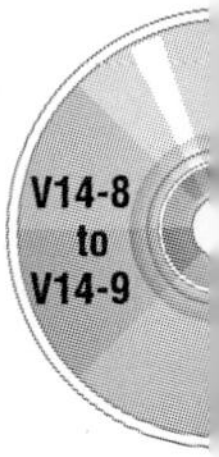

At the conclusion of the surgical repair the capsule and

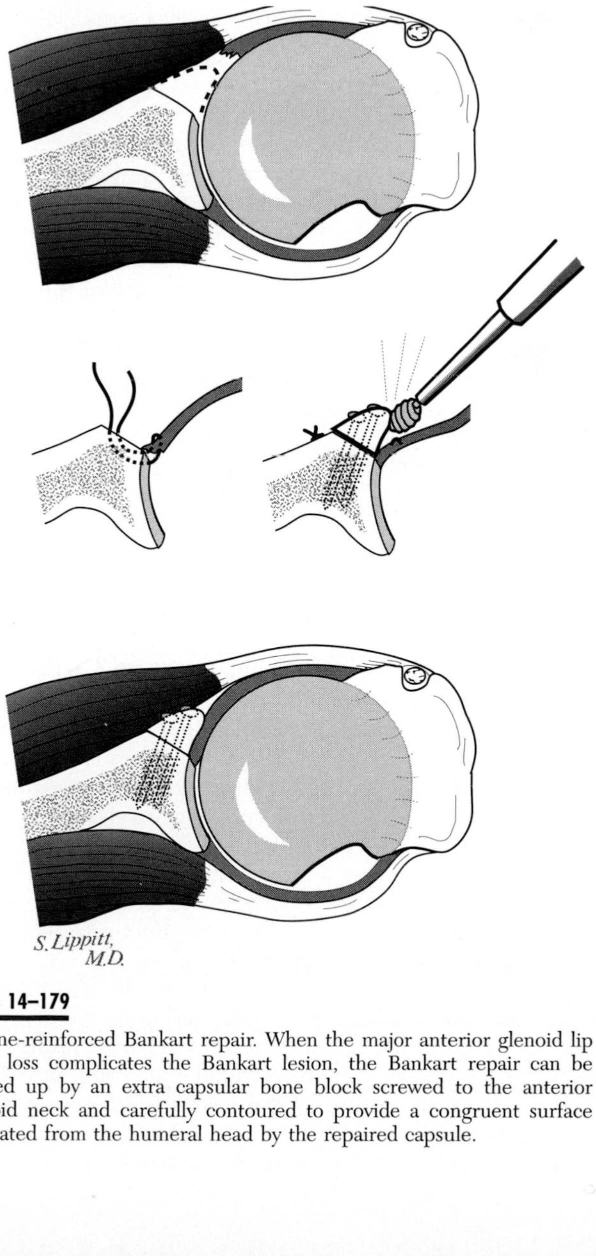

Figure 14–179

A bone-reinforced Bankart repair. When the major anterior glenoid lip bone loss complicates the Bankart lesion, the Bankart repair can be backed up by an extra capsular bone block screwed to the anterior glenoid neck and carefully contoured to provide a congruent surface separated from the humeral head by the repaired capsule.

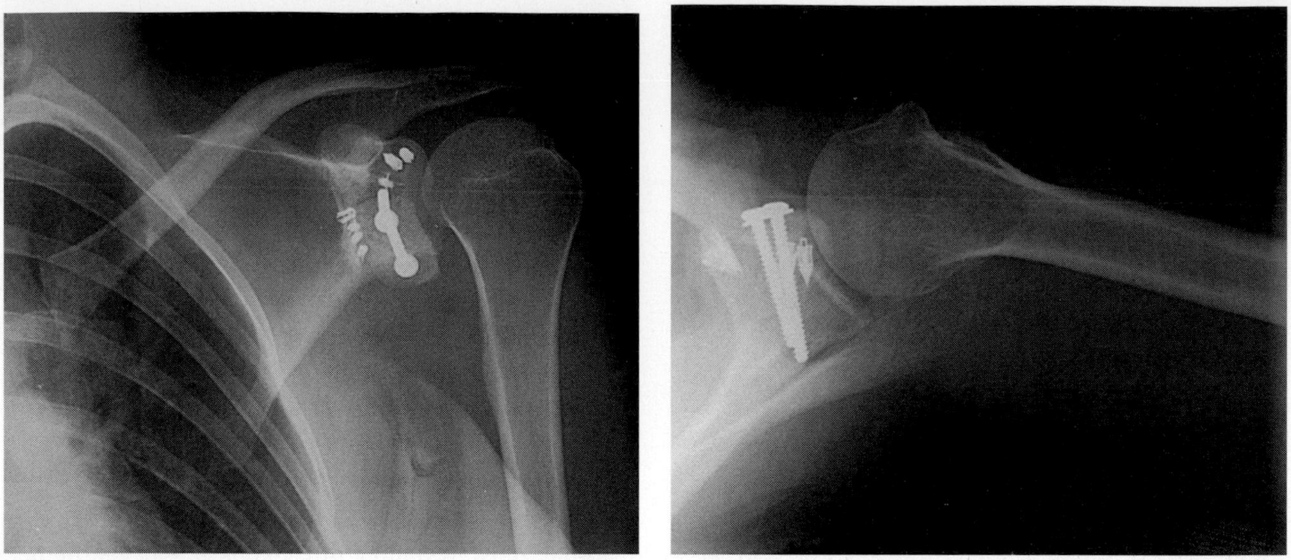

V14-10 to V14-12

Figures 14–180 and 14–181

Anteroposterior and axillary radiographs show a bone-reinforced Bankart repair (BRBR) performed for recurrent instability and anterior glenoid lip deficiency after multiple previous anterior repairs that used the suture anchors seen. In this procedure, the capsule is repaired to the lip of the remaining glenoid articular cartilage. The contoured iliac crest graft is then secured to the anterior glenoid outside the capsule, which provides a smooth covering for articulation with the humeral head. Final smoothing of the graft is carried out after it is in position to ensure that it presents the optimal congruent extension of the bony glenoid.

subscapularis tendon are repaired anatomically to their mates at the lesser tuberosity (see Fig. 14–177), using the upper rolled border of the subscapularis as a reference. **(V14-10)** At least six sutures of number two braided nonabsorbable suture are used in this repair, ensuring good bites in both the medial and lateral aspects of the repair. If the tissue on the lateral side is insufficient, the tendon and capsule are repaired to drill holes at the base of the lesser tuberosity. A strong subscapularis and capsular repair is essential to early rehabilitation. The shoulder should have at least 30 degrees of external rotation at the side after the subscapularis/capsular repair. **(V14-11)** Once this repair has been completed, the shoulder stability is examined. **(V14-12)** If excessive anterior laxity remains; for example external rotation in excess of 45 degrees (which is rarely the case), the lateral capsular and subscapularis reattachment may be advanced laterally or superolaterally as desired.

In the highly unusual situation in which a shoulder with the TUBS syndrome is found not to have capsular detachment, the shoulder should be inspected carefully for midsubstance capsular defects. If none is found, the anterior instability may be treated by reefing the anterior capsule and the subscapularis tendon (Fig. 14–182). Shortening these structures by 1 cm limits external rotation of the humerus by approximately 20 degrees. Generally, restriction of external rotation to 30 degrees at the operating table will permit a very functional shoulder after rehabilitation is complete. If the patient has marked anterior ligamentous laxity, proportionately greater anterior tightening may be necessary, although the surgeon must be certain that the patient does not have multidirectional laxity before a unidirectional tightening is carried out. A standard wound closure is carried out, using a subcuticular suture, which is removed at 3 days.

After surgery, most patients are started on a self-conducted "90-0" rehabilitation program with instructions from a physical therapist or a physician. We move the shoulder soon after surgical repair because: (1) it has proved to be safe for the reliable patient, and (2) there is evidence that early motion can increase the ultimate strength of a ligament repair.[170] On the day after surgery, five times daily exercises are started, including assisted flexion to 90 degrees and external rotation to 0 degrees. The contralateral arm is used as the "assistant" until the operated arm can conduct the exercises alone. The patient is allowed to perform many activities of daily living as comfort permits within the 90-0–degree range without lifting anything heavier than a glass of water. Allowed activities include eating and personal hygiene, as well as

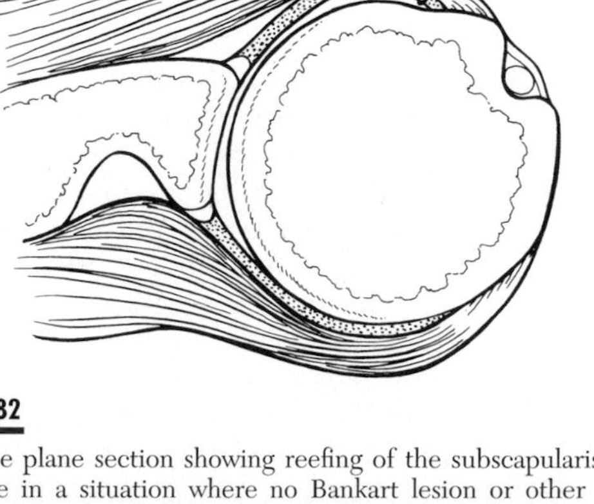

Figure 14–182

A transverse plane section showing reefing of the subscapularis tendon and capsule in a situation where no Bankart lesion or other capsular defect is found with isolated anterior instability. Note the intact anterior glenoid rim and the strong repair of the subscapularis tendon. (From Matsen FA and Thomas SC: Glenohumeral instability. *In* Evarts CM [ed]: Surgery of the Musculoskeletal System, 2nd ed. New York: Churchill Livingstone, 1989.)

certain vocational activities, such as writing and keyboarding. Gripping, isometric external rotation, and isometric abduction exercises are started immediately after surgery to minimize effects of disuse. If a patient does not appear able to comply with this restricted use program, the arm is kept in a sling for 3 weeks, otherwise a sling is used only for comfort between exercise sessions and to protect the arm when the patient is out in public and at night while sleeping. Driving is allowed as early as 2 weeks after surgery, if the arm can be used actively and comfortably, particularly if the patient's car has automatic transmission and if the operated arm is not used to set the emergency brake. This rapid return to functional activities is made possible because of the strength of the repair and helps to maintain the shoulder's strength and neuromuscular control. It minimizes the immediate postoperative disability and discomfort without jeopardizing the healing process.

At 3 weeks the patient should return for an examination and should have at least 90 degrees of elevation and external rotation to 0 degrees. From 3 to 6 weeks postoperatively, the patient is instructed to increase the range of motion to 140 degrees of elevation and 40 degrees of external rotation. Six weeks after surgery, if there is good evidence of active control of the shoulder, controlled repetitive activities such as swimming and use of a rowing machine are instituted to help rebuild coordination, strength, and endurance of the shoulder. More vigorous activities such as basketball, volleyball, throwing, and serving in tennis should not be started until 3 months and only then if there is excellent strength, endurance, range of motion, and coordination of the shoulder.

Vigilance must be exercised for patients older than 35 years of age to be sure that they do not develop unwanted postoperative stiffness. Thus, particularly for these patients, the 3-week and 6-week checks are very important to ensure that the ranges of elevation and external rotation are respectively 90 degrees and 0 degrees at 3 weeks, and 140 degrees and 40 degrees at 6 weeks.

In a 5.5-year follow-up of the first group of these repairs, we found 97% good to excellent results based on Rowe's grading system.[553] One of 39 shoulders had a single redislocation 4 years after repair while the patient was practicing karate. He became asymptomatic after completing a strengthening program and is back to full activities including karate. The average range of motion at follow-up was 171 degrees of elevation, 68 degrees of external rotation with the arm at the side, and 85 degrees of external rotation at 90 degrees of abduction. Ninety-five per cent of these patients reported that the shoulder felt stable with all activities; 80% had no shoulder pain while 20% had occasional pain with activity. None had complications of posterior subluxation due to excessive anterior tightness. None had complications related to hardware!

ROCKWOOD AND WIRTH'S PREFERRED METHOD FOR MANAGEMENT OF TRAUMATIC SHOULDER INSTABILITY

Before surgery, all our patients are instructed in a series of exercises designed to strengthen the rotator cuff, deltoid, and the scapular stabilizers (see Fig. 14–146). For the past 15 years, our preferred method of surgical repair has been an anatomic reconstruction; that is, repair of the Perthes-Bankart lesion or a double-breasting of the capsule. We rarely have to overlap, and thus shorten, the subscapularis tendon.

Surgical Incision

V14-13 to V14-15

(V14-13) The standard anterior axillary incision begins in the anterior axillary crease, extending up toward and usually stopping at the coracoid process (Fig. 14–183*A*). In large muscular men, the incision may extend proximally as far as the clavicle. In women, we use the modified axillary incision described by Leslie and Ryan.[355] The skin is undermined subcutaneously in the proximal medial corner and the distal lateral corner to expose the deltopectoral interval (see Fig. 14–183*B*). Usually, this interval is identified by the presence of the cephalic vein (see Fig. 14–183*C*), which may either be absent or lying deep in the interval out of sight. When the vein is not present we can define the deltopectoral interval proximally, because in this area, it is easier to see the difference in angles of the muscle fibers between the pectoralis major and the deltoid. **(V14-14)** The interval should be opened very carefully, taking the vein laterally with the deltoid muscle. To routinely ligate the vein produces venous congestion in the area and in the upper extremity and increases the postoperative discomfort. Preservation of the vein contributes to an easier postoperative course (i.e., less pain and swelling). We use an 8–0 nylon suture to repair any inadvertent nicks in the vein. The deltopectoral interval is developed all the way up to the clavicle, and there is no need to detach any of the deltoid from the clavicle. We usually detach the upper 2 cm of the pectoralis major tendon. This allows for better visualization of the inferior capsule and makes it easier to locate and protect the axillary nerve, which passes just inferior to the capsule. We do not find it necessary to detach the coracoid process or the conjoined tendons (see Fig. 14–183*D*). With the deltopectoral muscles retracted out of the way, the clavipectoral fascia is seen covering the conjoined tendons. This fascia is divided vertically along the lateral border of the conjoined tendons. Proximally, the clavipectoral fascia blends into the coracoacromial ligament.

Identification of the Musculocutaneous Nerve

(V14-15) Before a Richardson retractor is placed in the medial side of the incision to retract the conjoined muscles and pectoralis major muscle, we palpate for the musculocutaneous nerve as it enters the conjoined tendon. The nerve usually enters the coracobrachialis and biceps muscles from the medial aspect approximately 5 cm distal to the tip of the coracoid process. However, it must be remembered that it might penetrate immediately below the tip of the coracoid. We have even seen the nerve visible on the lateral aspect of the conjoined tendon (Fig. 14–184). Usually, by palpating just medial to the conjoined tendon and muscles, one can feel the entrance of the musculocutaneous nerve.

Text continued on page 717

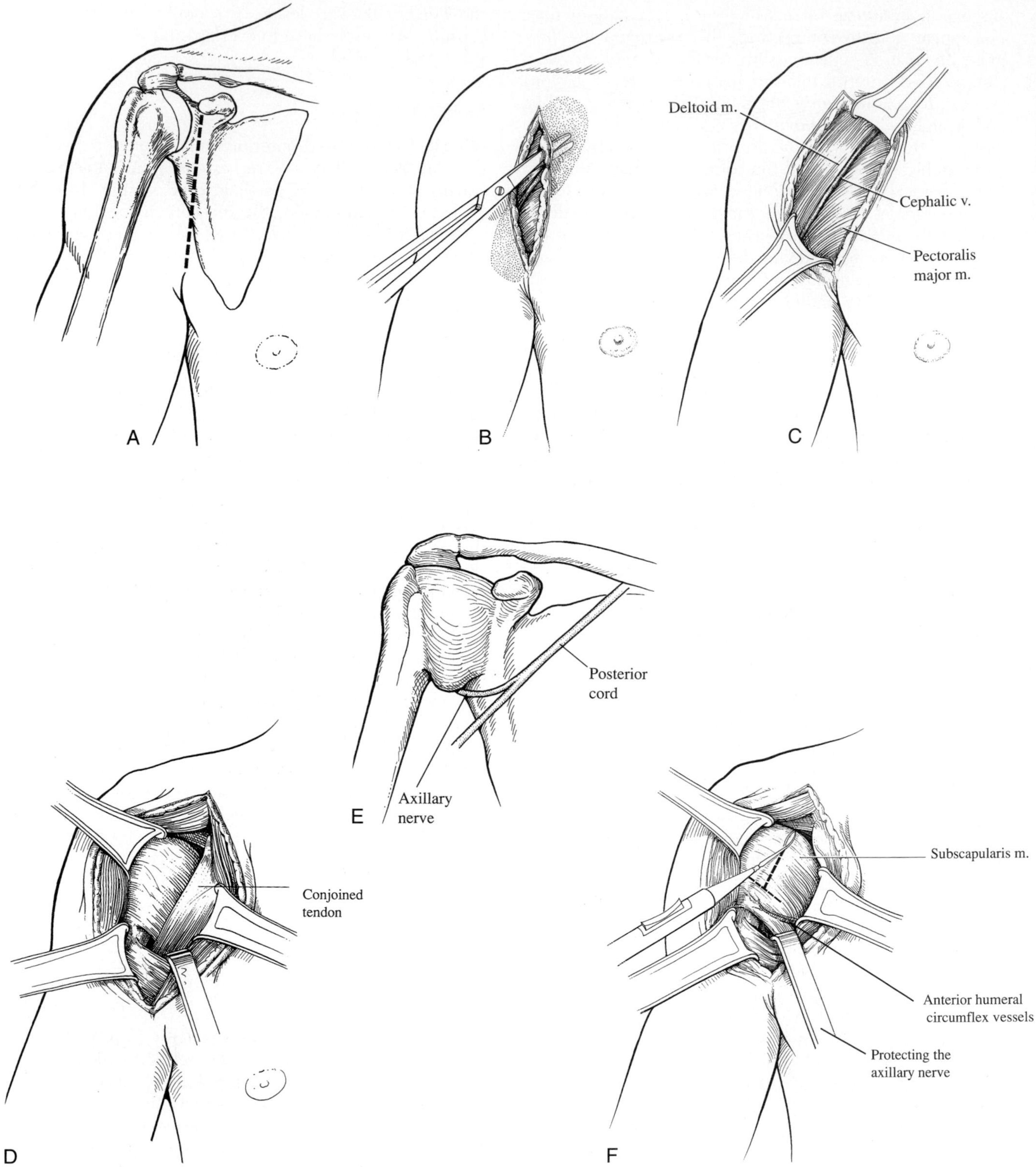

Figure 14–183

The precise details of the operative procedure can be followed in the detailed description of the author's preferred method of operative treatment in the text. *A–BB,* The procedure used if the anterior capsule is not stripped off the scapula. (From Wirth MA, Blatter G, and Rockwood CA Jr: The capsular imbrication procedure for recurrent anterior instability of the shoulder. J Bone Joint Surg 78-A:246–259, 1996.)

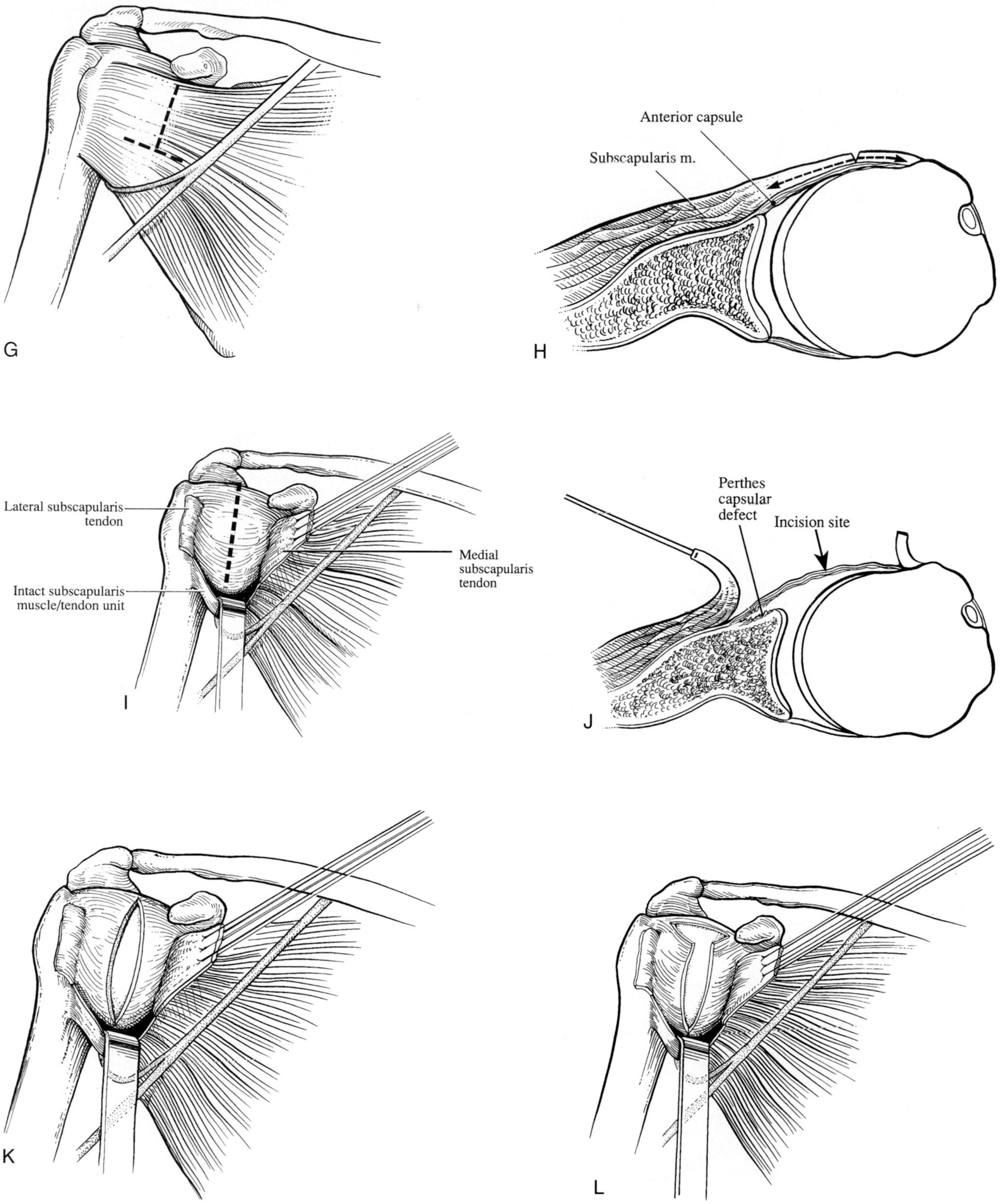

Figure 14–183

Continued

Illustration continued on following page

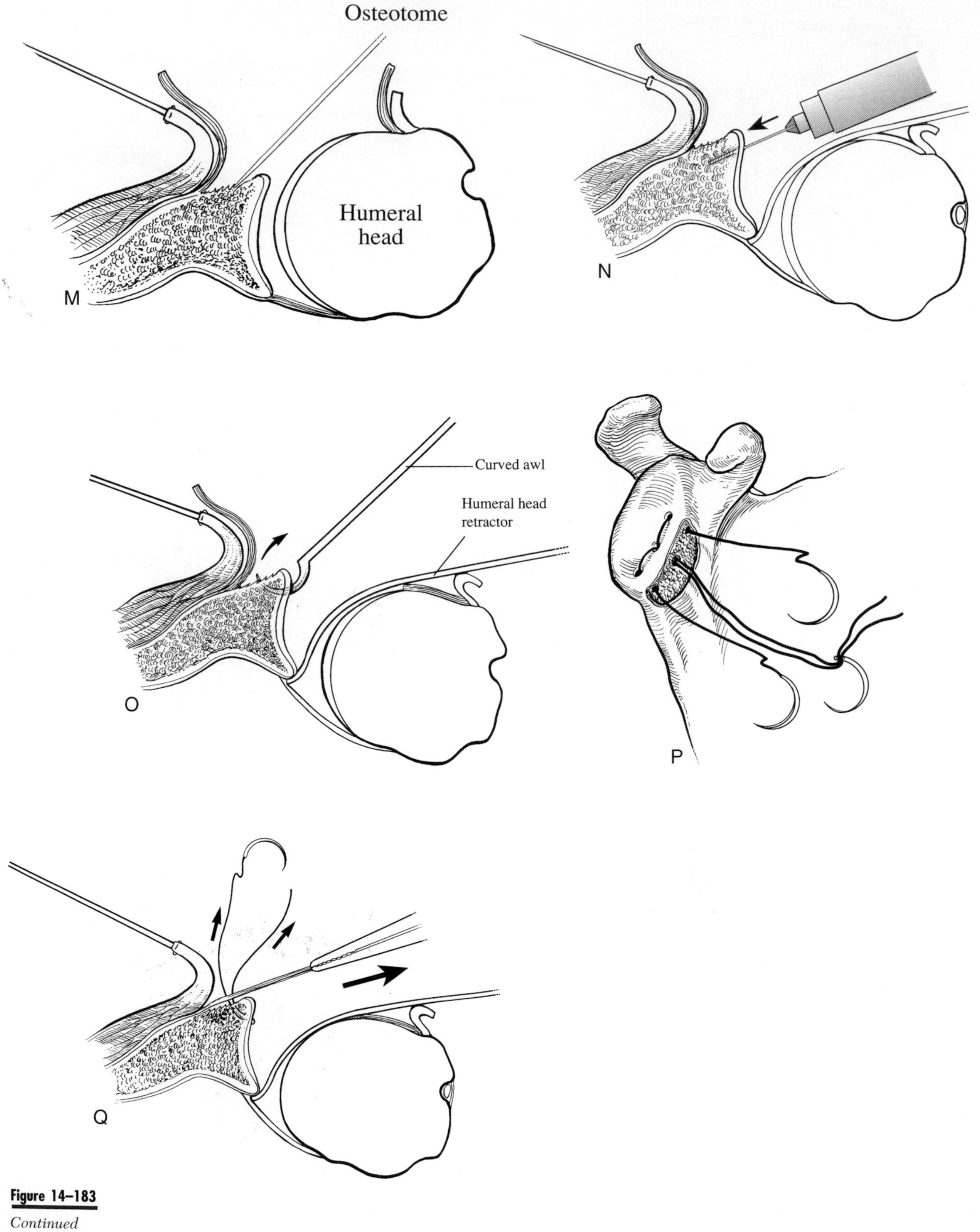

Figure 14–183

Continued

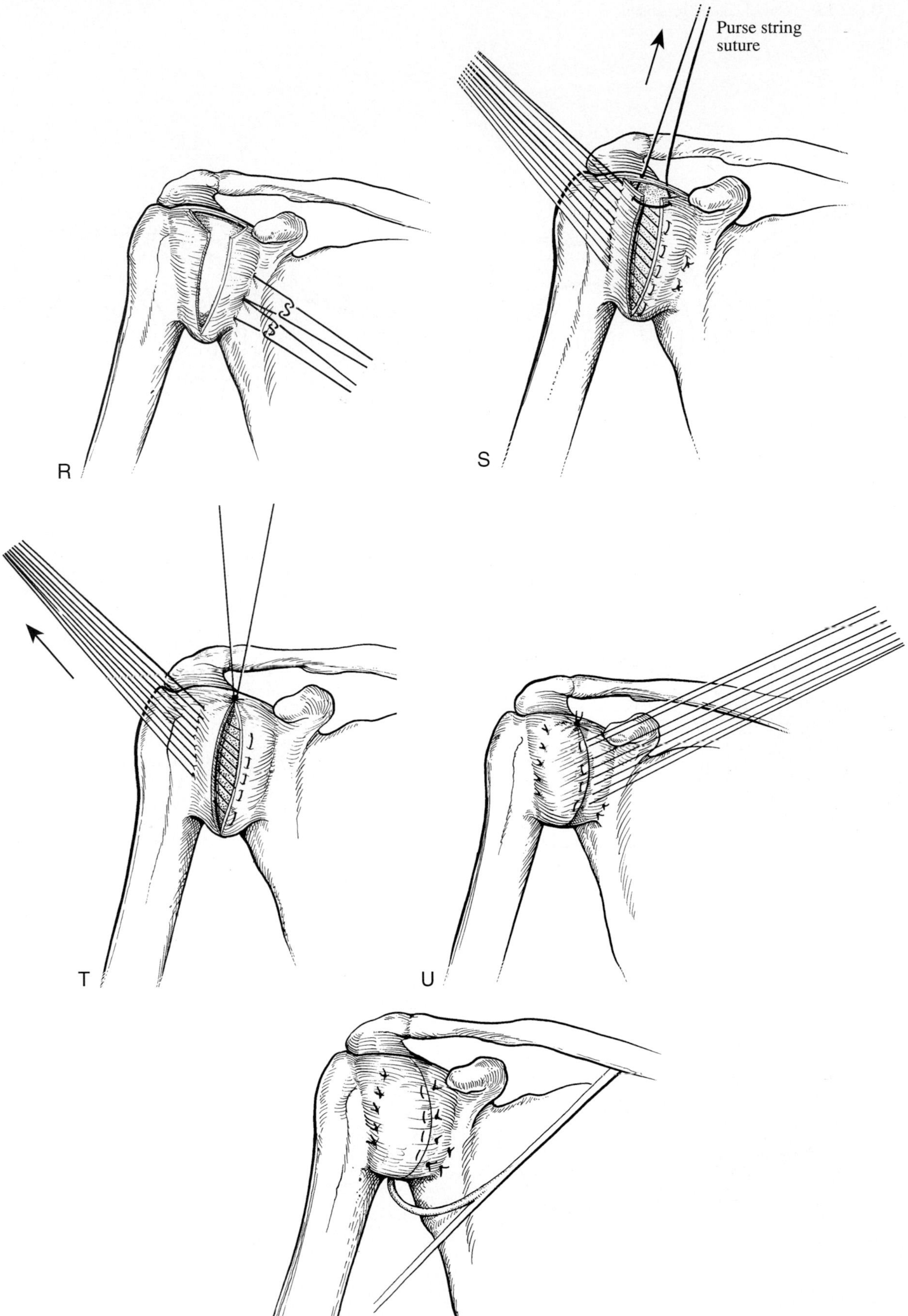

Figure 14–183

Continued

Illustration continued on following page

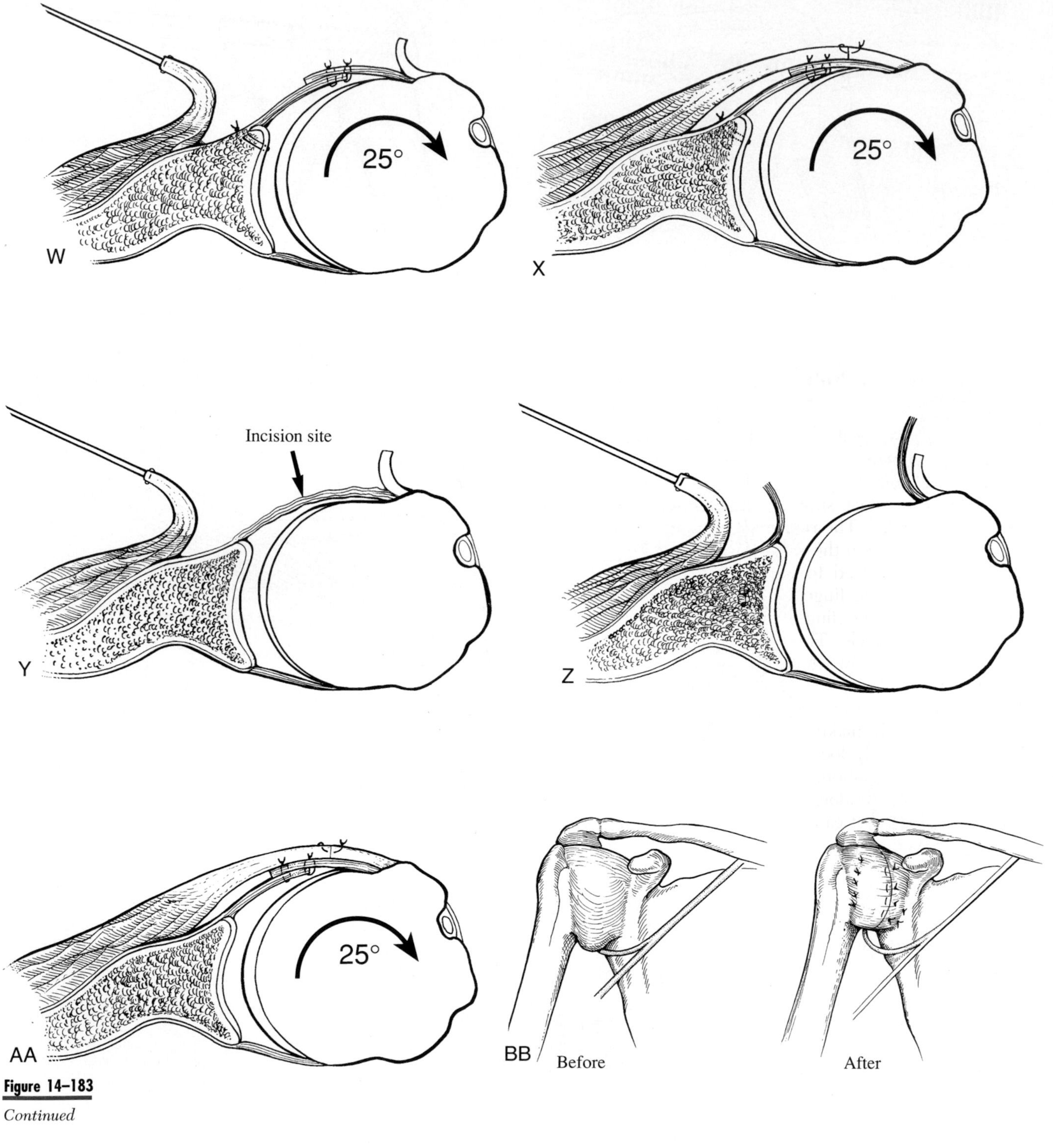

Figure 14–183

Continued

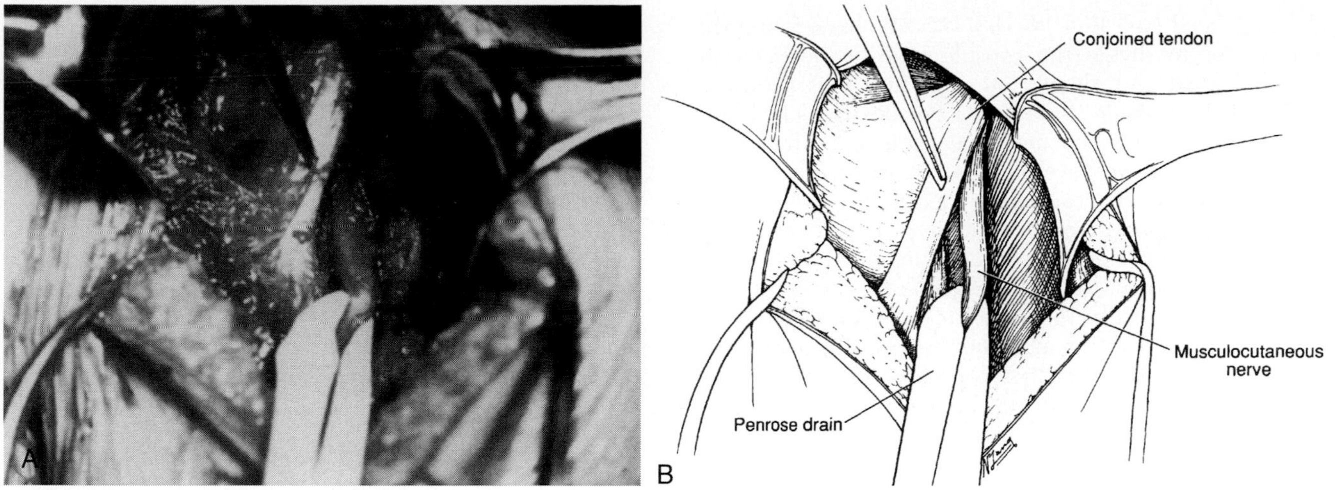

V14-16 to V14-20

Figure 14–184

A and *B*, An intraoperative photograph and a correlative diagram demonstrating the path of the musculocutaneous nerve as it courses lateral to the conjoined tendons. (From Rockwood CA Jr, Green DP, and Bucholz RW [eds]: Fractures in Adults. Philadelphia: JB Lippincott, 1991.)

Identification and Protection of the Axillary Nerve

(V14-16) Next, we locate the axillary nerve—an especially important step when performing the capsular shift procedure. This is done by passing the finger down and along the lower and intact subscapularis muscle tendon unit (see Fig. 14–183*E*). The right index finger should be used to locate the nerve in the left shoulder, and the left index finger should be used to locate the nerve in the right shoulder. When the finger is as deep as it will go, the volar surface of the finger should be on the anterior surface of the muscle. Then, the distal phalanx is flexed and rotated anteriorly, which will hook under the axillary nerve before it dives back posteriorly under the inferior capsule. With the arm in external rotation, the nerve is displaced medially, making it difficult to locate. This large nerve can be easily located with the arm in adduction and in neutral rotation. With the upper 2 cm of the pectoralis major tendon taken down, not only can the nerve be palpated, it can also be visualized. The nerve is at least 5⁄32 inch in size.

Division of the Subscapular Tendon and Preservation of the Anterior Humeral Circumflex Vessels

With the arm in external rotation, the upper and lower borders of the subscapularis tendon can be visualized and palpated. The "soft spot" at the superior border of subscapularis tendon is the interval between the subscapularis and supraspinatus tendons. The lower border of the tendon is identified by the presence of the anterior humeral circumflex artery and veins (see Fig. 14–183*F*). The upper three fourths of the subscapularis tendon will be vertically transected usually ¾ to 1 inch medial to its insertion into the lesser tuberosity. We cut only the upper two thirds of the subscapularis tendon and prefer to do this with the electric cautery (see Fig. 14–183*F* and *G*). We are very careful to divide only the tendon and usually try to leave a little of the subscapularis tendon on the capsule to add to its strength (see Fig. 14–183*H*). **(V14-17)** We avoid transecting the lower third of the subscapularis tendon, leaving it in place to prevent injury to the anterior humeral circumflex artery and veins, to preserve a portion of the tendon's proprioceptive capability, and to protect the axillary nerve. The anterior humeral circumflex artery is the primary blood supply to the head of the humerus, and we believe it should be preserved. **(V14-18)** Once the vertical cut in the tendon has been completed, we very carefully reflect the medial part of the tendon off the capsule using curved Mayo scissors, until there are no further connections between the tendon and the capsule. When applying lateral traction on the tendon, it should have a rubbery bounce to it. Three or four stay sutures of No. 2 cottony Dacron are placed in the medial edge of the tendon; these are used initially for retraction and later at the time of tendon repair. The lateral stump of the subscapularis tendon is reflected off the capsule with a small sharp knife. This is easy with the capsule intact when the arm is in external rotation and difficult when the capsule has been divided. Failure to perform this step will make the two-layer closure of the capsule and the subscapularis tendon more difficult.

(V14-19) With the divided portions of the subscapularis tendon reflected medially and laterally, and with the arm in mild external rotation, we use an elevator to gently strip the intact lower fourth of the subscapularis muscle tendon unit off the anteroinferior capsule. A narrow deep retractor (e.g., Scofield) should be used to retract the lower part of the subscapularis muscle anteriorly and distally, which allows for easy visualization of the inferior capsule. The retractor holds not only the lower part of the subscapularis muscle but also the axillary nerve anteriorly and distally out of the way, preventing injury when the inferior capsule is opened and divided and repaired (see Fig. 14–183*L*).

Division of the Capsule

(V14-20) Next, the capsule is divided vertically midway between its usual attachment on the glenoid rim and the humeral head (see Fig. 14–183*I–K*). We have found that it is easier to divide the capsule midway between the humeral head and glenoid attachments. This allows for repair of the capsule if there is a Perthes-Bankart lesion. Furthermore, after the medial capsule is reattached to the glenoid rim, we have plenty of room to add strength to the anteroinferior capsule by double-breasting it with the planned capsular reconstruction. This vertical incision begins at the superior glenohumeral ligament and extends all the way down to the most inferior aspect of the capsule. Occasionally, the superior capsular region is deficient, but this does not alter the vertical capsular incision (see Fig. 14–183*L*). **(V14-21)** We prefer to insert the horizontal mattress sutures in the medial capsule just as we complete the division of the most inferior portion of the capsule. We explore the joint carefully, removing loose bodies and glenoid labrum tears. **(V14-22)** Close attention should be paid to stripping of the labrum, capsule, and periosteum from their normal attachments on the glenoid rim and neck of the scapula (i.e., the Perthes-Bankart lesion).

V14-21 to V14-25

Capsular Shift and Reconstruction

If the capsule has a secure fixation on the glenoid rim, the capsular reconstruction can then be performed. However, if stripping of the capsule and periosteum from the glenoid rim and neck of the scapula has occurred, then the capsule must first be reattached before proceeding to the capsular reconstruction. Formerly, the senior author believed that if there was a stripping of the capsule from the neck of the scapula, all that was needed was to roughen this up with a curette or osteotome to create bleeding and then the capsule would spontaneously reattach or heal itself back to the glenoid rim. However, because of failures that required reoperation, it was obvious that this area had not healed and the capsule was still stripped off the glenoid neck. Most likely, synovial fluid within this area inhibits the usual healing process and prevents a consistent firm reattachment of the capsule and periosteum to the bony glenoid rim.

In some situations, it may be necessary to horizontally split the medial part of the capsule in its midportion to better visualize and decorticate the anterior rim and neck of the scapula with an osteotome or an air bur. There is a special retractor, developed by Rowe, which we call the "dinner fork" because of its shape and its three sharp teeth. It is used to retract the capsule and muscles out of the way while the anterior glenoid rim and neck of the scapula are decorticated, and while the drill holes are being placed in the glenoid rim. We have tried several devices, including angled dental drills and Hall drills, curved cutting gouges, clamps, and the Ellison glenoid rim punch; no matter what instrument is used, it always seems to be difficult to place these holes in the dense glenoid rim. With the Bowen, Rowe, or Fukuda retractor holding the humeral head out of the way and the "dinner fork" holding the medial capsule and muscles out of the way, an osteotome is used to decorticate the anterior surface of the neck of the scapula down to raw cancellous bone (see Fig. 14–183*M*). Usually, three holes are then made between 3 o'clock and 6 o'clock on the anterior articular surface of the glenoid. These holes are made with a small drill bit approximately 1/8 inch in from the rim of the glenoid on the articular surface (see Fig. 14–183*N*). Next, a curved Carter-Rowe awl and tenaculum are used to connect the drill holes with the decorticated neck of the anterior glenoid (see Fig. 14–183*O*). We pass the No. 2 nonabsorbable cottony Dacron sutures through these holes so that there are two loops of intra-articular sutures through the three holes (the center hole has two sutures through it) (see Fig. 14–183*P*).

The medial capsule is then pulled laterally and the needles on the intra-articular loops of sutures are passed up and through the medial capsule, so that when they are tied the capsule is reapproximated to the raw bone of the glenoid rim (see Fig. 14–183*Q* and *R*). We believe that this step is absolutely critical to eliminate the abnormal pouch in the capsule.

With the medial capsule secured back to the glenoid rim, we proceed with the capsular reconstruction. Before closure of the capsule, the joint is thoroughly irrigated with saline. **(V14-23)** The medial capsule will be double-breasted laterally and superiorly under the lateral capsule after closing the superior capsular defect, when present, with a "purse-string" ligature (see Fig. 14–183*S* and *T*). **(V14-24)** All sutures should be placed and tied, being sure that the arm is held in 25 to 30 degrees of external rotation. To carry out this step, the lateral stump of the subscapularis tendon must have been separated from the lateral portion of the capsule. It is critical that the capsular reconstruction sutures be placed under the proper tension so that the arm may easily rotate to the desired position. Next, the lateral capsule is double-breasted by taking it medially and superiorly and suturing it down to the anterior surface of the medial capsule (see Fig. 14–183*U* and *V*). These sutures are also placed with the arm in the desired rotation. This type of capsular reconstruction not only eliminates all laxity in the anterior and inferior capsular ligaments, but, because of the double-breasting, the capsule is much stronger. The wound is again carefully irrigated with several liters of saline.

(V14-25) With the arm held in 25 degrees of external rotation, the medial subscapularis tendon is brought into view by pulling on the previously placed sutures (see Fig. 14–183*W*). The two borders of the tendon are easily approximated with gentle traction, and the tendon is repaired without any overlapping (see Fig. 14–183*X*). If the tendon is loose with the arm in 25 degrees of external rotation then a double-breasting or overlapping of the tendon can be performed by using a two-layer closure with No. 2 Dacron horizontal mattress sutures. If the capsule has a secure foundation on the glenoid rim, then it will only be necessary to perform the capsular shift (see Fig. 14–183*A–BB*).

Wound Closure

Before closure of the wound, we carefully irrigate with antibiotic solution and then infiltrate the joint, muscles, and subcutaneous tissue with 25 to 30 ml of 0.5% bupivacaine (Marcaine). This aids in decreasing the immediate postoperative pain. We are convinced that the use of bupivacaine before wound closure gives the patient an easier postoperative recovery period. The effect of the bupivacaine will last for 6 to 8 hours, which allows the patient, as he or she is waking up, to have relatively little pain; later in the day, as the anesthesia begins to wear off, the patient can request pain medications. Care should be taken not to overuse the bupivacaine or to inject it directly into vessels. It is usually unnecessary to put any sutures in the deltopectoral interval. The deep subcutaneous layer is closed with 2–0 nonabsorbable sutures, which help to prevent widening of the scar. The subcutaneous fat is closed with absorbable sutures, and a running subcuticular nylon suture is used in the skin.

Surgical Technique Summary

In contrast to a number of previously reported reconstructions for anterior shoulder instability, the procedure that we advocate is an anatomic method of reconstruction that affords great latitude in correcting the pathology encountered at the time of surgery. The anatomic capsular shift procedure is a physiologic repair that includes repair of capsulolabral injury, when present, and reinforcement of the anteroinferior capsular ligaments by a double-breasting technique that decreases the overall capsule volume. This reconstruction is a modification of the published reports of Putti-Platt, Bankart, and the Neer capsular shift, and several points deserve emphasis. First, only the upper two thirds of the subscapularis tendon are detached while maintaining the inferior one third of the tendon intact. This has the theoretical advantage of preserving a portion of the tendon's proprioceptive capability and protects the anterior humeral circumflex vessels, which are the primary blood supply to the humeral head. The intact portion of the tendon is also gently stripped and retracted from the underlying capsule, which allows visualization of the inferior most capsule while protecting the axillary nerve and vessels. Second, the deltopectoral interval should be carefully developed and the cephalic vein taken laterally with the deltoid since the majority of tributaries in this region arise from this muscle. In our experience, preservation of the vein contributes to an easier postoperative course, whereas routine ligation produces venous congestion in the upper extremity and increases the postoperative discomfort. Third, it is unnecessary to detach the coracoid or conjoined tendons to gain adequate exposure. Occasionally, we will release the upper 1 cm of the pectoralis major tendon to allow better visualization of the inferior capsule. This also facilitates identification of the axillary nerve, which passes just inferior to the capsule as it exits the quadrilateral space. Fourth, proper identification of the musculocutaneous and axillary nerves cannot be overemphasized. Identification of the axillary nerve is especially critical so that it can be protected when opening and repairing the inferior capsule. Fifth, the capsule is divided in a vertical fashion midway between its glenoid and humeral site of attachment. This provides excellent intra-articular exposure to repair a Perthes-Bankart lesion, is easy to perform, and facilitates subsequent imbrication, which reinforces the capsular reconstruction. Sixth, the upper two thirds of the subscapularis tendon is repaired anatomically to itself, which helps to minimize the development of undesirable internal rotation contractures of the glenohumeral joint.

Postoperative Management

Postoperatively we prefer to use a commercial shoulder immobilizer because it is comfortable, quick, and simple to apply and prevents abduction, flexion, and external rotation. Regardless of the type of immobilization, it is very important to temporarily remove the device when the patient is seen on the afternoon or evening of the day of surgery. For some reason, a patient who awakens from surgery with the arm in the "device" does not want to wiggle any part of the arm—almost as if it were frozen in the sling-and-swathe position. The commercial immobilizer can be easily removed; this allows the patient to move the hand and wrist and then gradually extend the elbow down to the side and lay it on the bed. This almost always relieves the aching pain in the arm and the muscle tension pain. We then tell the patient to flex and extend the elbow several times, which also relieves the generalized arm and shoulder discomfort. In many instances, a patient has related that the vague ache in the shoulder and elbow is more of a problem than pain at the operative site and that this simple release of the immobilizer, allowing movement of the elbow and wrist, eliminates the discomfort. We allow the patient to remove the immobilizer three to four times a day to exercise the elbow, but otherwise we instruct him or her to always keep the immobilizer in place. Specific instructions are given to the patient to avoid abduction, flexion, and external rotation when the device is removed.

Patients are usually dismissed on the second or third postoperative day, and we allow them to remove the immobilizer two or three times a day while at home when sitting, reading, or watching television. The patient can return to school or work any time after discharge from the hospital. At 5 days after surgery the patient can remove the small dressing, take a shower, and reapply the new bandage. We usually delay removing the running subcuticular nylon stitch for 2 weeks since this seems to help to prevent a wide scar.

As a general rule, the older the patient, the shorter will be the postoperative immobilization; the younger the patient, the longer will be the immobilization. In patients younger than 20 years of age or in the competitive, aggressive athlete, we immobilize the shoulder for 3 to 4 weeks; in young, semiathletic people younger than 30 years of age, shoulders are immobilized for 3 weeks; shoulders of patients younger than 50 years of age are immobilized for 2 weeks; shoulders of patients older than 50 years of age are immobilized for 1 to 2 weeks. Following removal of the shoulder immobilizer, we allow the patient to gently use the arm for everyday living activities but do not allow any rough use (e.g., lifting, moving furniture, pushing, pulling). At the end of the immobilization period, we start the patient on a stretching exercise program using an overhead pulley and rope set. After the return of motion, we institute a resisted weight exercise and shoulder-strengthening program to strengthen the deltoid, internal rotators, external rotators and the scapular stabilizers (see Fig. 14–146). Athletes are not permitted to return to competitive sports until they have reached a full and functional range of motion and have regained normal muscle strength; this usually requires 4 to 6 months.

Results

In our series,[691] 93% of the results were rated as good or excellent at an average follow-up of 5 years with a high degree of patient satisfaction and marked improvement in ratings for pain, strength, stability, and function. The average loss of external rotation was 7 degrees, and the average loss of elevation was 6 degrees, which represents a physiologic preservation of motion and compares favorably with other reports. Results after revision surgery were encouraging, with 45 (87%) good to excellent results and 7 (13%) fair to poor results. Despite this success, revision anterior shoulder surgery is a formidable challenge with less predictable outcome since seven of ten patients graded as fair or poor had failed previous reconstructive efforts. Although progressive symptoms of discomfort were noted in the subset of patients with prior surgery and degenerative changes of the glenohumeral joint, there was no relationship between symptomatic instability after the index procedure and the length of follow-up.

Arthroscopic Repair for Traumatic Anterior Instability

Arthroscopic surgery for Bankart lesions was pioneered by Johnson as early as 1982.[303] In his initial procedure, a metal staple was used to reattach the torn labrum or capsule to the roughened edge of the glenoid. Among 106 patients thus treated there was a recurrence of instability in 21%.[542] Lane and associates[340] reported a 33% recurrence rate in 3 years after 54 arthroscopic staple capsulorrhaphies; 15% of asymptomatic patients were found to have loose staples. Detrisac and Johnson[127] found a 12% incidence of recurrence after staple capsulorrhaphy along with complications related to erosion of the humeral head and subscapularis tendon. Warner and associates[671] reviewed a series of instability repairs with arthroscopically inserted suture anchors and concluded that the failure rate remains "unacceptably high." In a companion paper, they pointed to the technical difficulty of the procedure.[670] Concern about the safety of using staples and the high redislocation rate gave rise to other arthroscopic techniques (see Fig. 14–159).

Wolf[700] reported the use of a screw to reattach the labrum. Biodegradable fixation was introduced by Warren[672] and Johnson.[305] Speer, Pagnani, and Warren[608] reported 52 patients who had had an arthroscopic shoulder surgery using a bioabsorbable tack. Eleven of the patients exhibited some degree of anterior instability at an average follow-up of 42 months.

Caspari and associates[80–82] reported 100 consecutive arthroscopic suture repairs for recurrent anterior instability with good results in 86%. Other reports of suture methods have been provided by Landsiedl,[339] Goldberg,[198] and Morgan and Bodenstab.[434] Grana and associates[202] reviewed 27 patients after an arthroscopic suturing for anterior shoulder instability; of these surgeries, 12 failed because of pain and recurrent instability.

Andrews,[11] Ellman,[143–145] Hawkins,[232, 235] Esch,[151, 152] Jobe,[294–299] and Gartsman[185–187] have provided additional reports of arthroscopic surgery for instability. Suggested advantages of arthroscopic repairs include a shorter hospitalization, lower morbidity, less postoperative pain, early recovery of strength, and minimal to no loss of motion.[236, 397, 433]

Green and Christensen reported a 1.8-fold decrease in operative time, a 10-fold decrease in blood loss, and a 2.5-fold decrease in postoperative narcotic use compared with the open procedure ($P < .001$).[206] The average hospital stay was 3.1 days with the open procedure compared with 1.1 days with the arthroscopic method ($P < .001$). Time lost from work was 25.5 days and 15.3 days for the open and arthroscopic procedures, respectively ($P < .001$).

Others have reported low rates of complications after arthroscopic Bankart repair.[41, 208, 433, 531, 623, 651] Arthroscopic repair avoids incision of the tendon. Ziegler and associates reported on the diagnostic and functional deficits in 30 patients with postoperative subscapularis failure, 26 of which followed repairs for anterior instability.[717]

The potential complications after arthroscopic repairs are similar in type to those of open repair. Of particular concern are hardware loosening and migration, staple or suture anchor abrasion of the cartilage of the humeral head, and recurrent instability.[82, 126, 175, 306, 598, 697]

The published reports of arthroscopic methods for management of glenohumeral instability indicate that: (1) many different approaches are being explored with as yet no clear consensus on the best method, (2) the learning curve is long for these procedures, (3) the return to physical activity is no more rapid than with open repairs and (4) the rates of recurrent instability after repair are inconsistent and substantially higher than with open repairs.[8, 14, 26, 105, 109, 188, 206, 210, 231, 236, 245, 305, 339, 377, 397, 402, 430, 432–434, 529, 542, 548, 575, 588, 599, 600, 602, 606, 608, 634, 647, 651, 662, 680, 681, 684, 701, 702, 709, 712]

At open revision of arthroscopic failures most have been found to have a detached inferior glenohumeral ligament at the anteroinferior labrum.[397] The open Bankart approach affords direct fixation of the detached structures to bone, whereas the majority of arthroscopic approaches do not. Resch and associates have described an anteroinferior approach to the glenoid to deal with this deficiency.[530] The authors dissected 87 cadavers to confirm the safety of their direct approach to repair through substance of the subscapularis. In 264 clinical cases, they report a 5.7% recurrence rate after excluding the first 30 cases.

A consistent challenge for arthroscopic repairs is the security of the repair to the bone. In an attempt to characterize the initial failure strength of Bankart repairs, McEleney used a canine model to compare eight common fixation repair techniques in current use for both open and arthroscopic repair.[399] The open and arthroscopic two-suture repairs were statistically equivalent in holding strength and two-suture repairs were significantly stronger than the one-suture or absorbable rivet repairs

($P < .01$). In a similar study, Shea and associates demonstrated significantly better strength of suture repair above staple fixation.[589]

Green[208] found that in 13 of 15 failed cases, significant or complete degeneration of the glenoid labrum-inferior glenohumeral ligament complex (types IV or V labra) was present. These findings indicate that redislocation after an arthroscopic Bankart procedure may be influenced by the degree of damage to the glenoid labrum-inferior glenohumeral ligament complex and by the presence of articular surface defect.

Warner and associates recommended that the success rate of an arthroscopic procedure might be improved by selecting only patients with unidirectional, post-traumatic, anterior instability who are found to have a discrete Bankart lesion and well-developed ligamentous tissue.[671] Grana[202] concluded that contact sports appeared to predispose his patients to a high risk of recurrence and recommended caution in the use of arthroscopic procedures for the competitive athlete.

In an attempt to permit a secure restoration of the labrum and capsular ligaments to the low anteroinferior rim of the glenoid, Harryman developed a posterior approach using a direct arthroscopic glenoid suture guide.[227] This technique does not rely on risky approaches, transosseous sutures adjacent to neurovascular structures or implanted devices (Fig. 14–185). Although still in the development stages, the early results are encouraging with a redislocation rate of 6% and elimination of symptoms in all but 11%.[223]

While all surgical repairs are dependent on excellent knot technique, optimizing knots is particularly challenging in arthroscopic surgery. It is possible that the relatively high rate of recurrent instability after arthroscopic repair is in part due to the difficulty in tying secure knots arthroscopically. In a most important study, Loutzenheiser and associates[374] pointed to the arthroscopic challenge of avoiding tying knots that will slip. Using rigorous criteria and mechanical testing, these authors determined that the most secure knot configurations were achieved by reversing the half-hitch throws and by alternating the strands about which the throws were made.

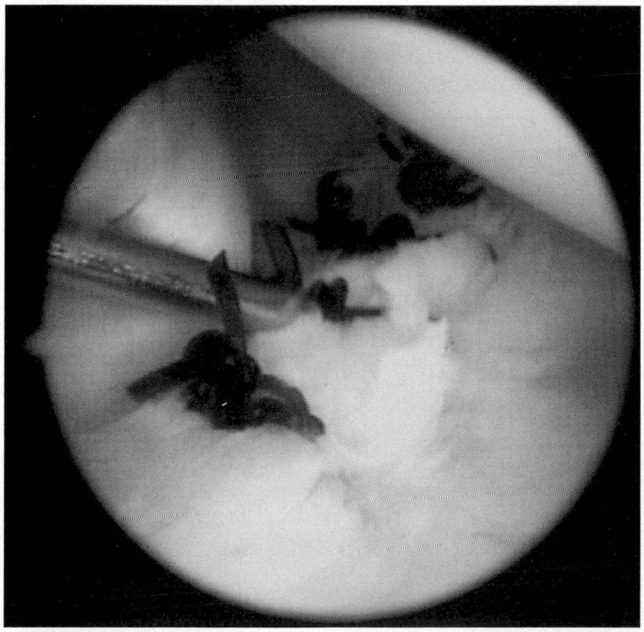

Figure 14–185

Arthroscopic intra-articular suture repair of a large Bankart lesion to the glenoid rim performed without suture anchors using the Seattle Bankart guide. Note the attachment of the labrum to reconstitute the glenoid depth. (Courtesy of Douglas T. Harryman II, MD, Department of Orthopaedics, University of Washington.)

Operative Management of Posterior Instability

CONSIDERATIONS IN THE DECISION FOR SURGERY

The choice of management for recurrent posterior instability is complicated by the facts that: (1) most often recurrent posterior instability is atraumatic: in contrast with the situation with anterior instability, only a small percentage of cases are obviously traumatic in etiology, (2) the pathogenesis of recurrent posterior instability is multifactorial, complex, and less well understood than for anterior instability, and (3) the results of the methods for posterior repair are at least 10 times worse than the average for anterior repair. As an example, Hawkins and co-workers[232, 235, 324] presented 50 shoulders in 35 patients treated for recurrent posterior instability. Only 11 of the 50 followed a traumatic event; 41 demonstrated voluntary and involuntary instability. Of those operated on, 17 patients had glenoid osteotomy, six had a reverse Putti-Platt procedure, and three had biceps tendon transfers. The dislocation rate after surgery was 50%; complications occurred in 20% of the operated cases. Two patients developed substantial degenerative osteoarthritis after glenoid osteotomy.

Many shoulders with posterior instability can be well managed by education, muscle strengthening, and neuromuscular retraining. Surgical stabilization of posterior glenohumeral instability may be considered when recurrent involuntary posterior subluxations or dislocations occur despite a concerted effort at a well-structured rehabilitation program.[512] Prior to surgery it is essential to identify all directions of instability and any anatomic factors that may predispose the joint to recurrent instability, such as humeral head or glenoid defects, abnormal glenoid version, rotator cuff tears, neurologic injuries, or generalized ligamentous laxity.[696, 697] It is important for the patient to understand the high recurrence and complication rates associated with attempted surgical correction of posterior instability. Since, the functional limitations and pain with recurrent posterior instability can be minimal, they suggested that some of these patients may do better without reconstructive procedures. Tibone and co-workers[636] stated that recurrent posterior dislocation of the shoulder is not a definite indication for surgery and emphasized the need for careful patient selection prior to surgical reconstruction.

POSTERIOR SURGICAL APPROACHES

Several surgical approaches have been described for treatment of recurrent posterior glenohumeral instability, including the posterior deltoid splitting approach (see Fig. 14–9).[692] Shaffer and associates[587] described a surgical approach to the posterior glenohumeral joint through an infraspinatus splitting incision that they found to offer safe and excellent exposure of the posterior capsule, labrum, and glenoid without requiring tendon detachment or causing neurologic compromise. Most surgeons prefer to split the deltoid at the posterior corner of the acromion and to incise the infraspinatus tendon near its attachment to the greater tuberosity.

Posterior Soft Tissue Repairs

The goal of these procedures is to tighten the posterior capsule (the infraspinatus and posterior capsule), restricting the range of positions attainable by the humerus in relation to the scapula.[197, 268, 359, 451, 561, 652] In some cases, the infraspinatus and teres minor tendon may be used together in the plication. Boyd and Sisk[57] described transplanting the long head biceps tendon posteriorly around the humerus to the posterior glenoid rim.

One of the difficulties with these procedures is that the repair tends to stretch out as the shoulder resumes normal usage. Hurley and associates[274] retrospectively reviewed 50 patients with recurrent posterior shoulder instability. Of the 25 patients treated surgically, 72% experienced recurrent instability. Tibone and co-workers[635] reported a failure rate of 30% following posterior staple capsulorrhaphy. Bayley and Kessel[38] stated that the failure to distinguish between traumatic and habitual (atraumatic) types of instability led to inappropriate surgery and was a major cause of recurrence after the operative repairs. Bigliani and associates[46] reported a 20% failure rate for the management of recurrent posterior inferior instability with a posterior capsular shift; most of the failures were in patients with previous attempts at surgical stabilization.

Tibone and Bradley[635] reviewed their experience with the management of posterior subluxation in athletes. They pointed to the difficulty in diagnosis, the unclear pathology, the importance of nonoperative management with exercises, and a 40% failure rate of surgical management with a posterior capsular shift. Eleven of the failures were secondary to instability, eight having a recurrence of their posterior instability and three demonstrating anterior subluxation. These cases of conversion of posterior instability to anterior instability emphasize the importance of recognition and the challenge of management of multidirectional instability.

Rotation Osteotomy of the Humerus[515, 621, 678]

Sunn and colleagues[622] evaluated 12 shoulders that had recurrent posterior shoulder instability and were treated with external rotation osteotomy of the humerus. Recurrent instability occurred in one shoulder with multidirectional instability.

Glenoid Osteotomy and Bone Blocks[447]

Kretzler and co-workers,[325, 326] Scott,[582] English and Macnab,[150] Bestard,[45] Vegter,[658] and Ahlgren and associates[6] and others[157, 190, 197, 214, 447] have reported using an opening, posterior wedge, glenoid osteotomy in recurrent posterior dislocations of the shoulder. In 1966, Kretzler and Blue[326] reported the use of this procedure in six patients with cerebral palsy. They used the acromion as the source of the graft to hold the wedge open. Kretzler[325] reported on 31 cases of the posterior glenoid osteotomy in voluntary (15 cases) and involuntary (16 cases) posterior dislocations with recurrences in four patients, two from each category.

Extreme care must be taken during this procedure to prevent the osteotome from entering into the glenoid, although cracks of the subchondral bone may be experienced as the osteotomy is displaced (Fig. 14–186). The suprascapular nerve above and the axillary nerve below are also at risk. English and Macnab[150] have pointed out that there may be a tendency for the humeral head to subluxate anteriorly after the osteotomy of the glenoid. Gerber and associates[189] demonstrated that with major angular changes posterior glenoid osteotomy can thrust the humeral head forward and potentially cause impingement of the humeral head on the coracoid, producing pain and dysfunction. Their cadaver studies demonstrated that glenoplasty "consistently produced impingement of the subscapularis between the coracoid tip and the humeral head."

The posterior bone block or the glenoid osteotomy has been combined with the various soft tissue reconstructions.[129] Mowery and associates[442] reported a series of five patients having a bone block for recurrent posterior dislocation. One patient had a subsequent anterior dislocation. Wirth and associates[698] reported the use of glenoid osteotomy to manage recurrent posterior glenohumeral instability (Fig. 14–187).

COMPLICATIONS OF POSTERIOR REPAIRS

The principal cause of failure after a posterior soft tissue repair is recurrent instability.[235, 451] Unless excellent dy-

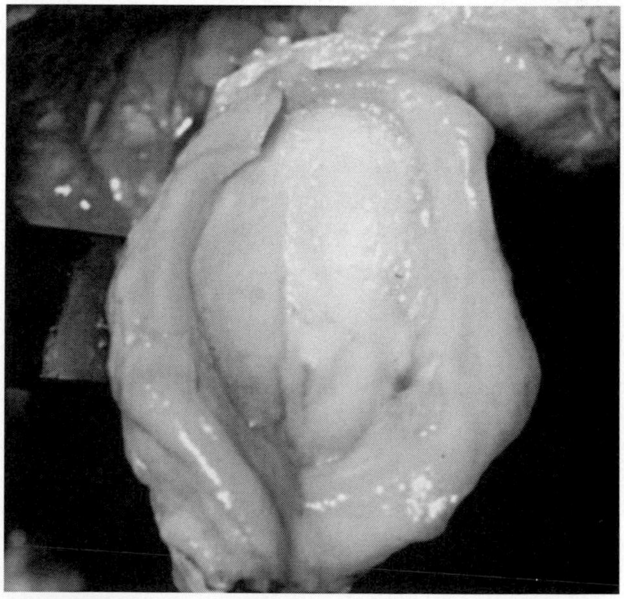

Figure 14–186

The articular surface of the glenoid after a posterior opening wedge osteotomy in a cadaver specimen.

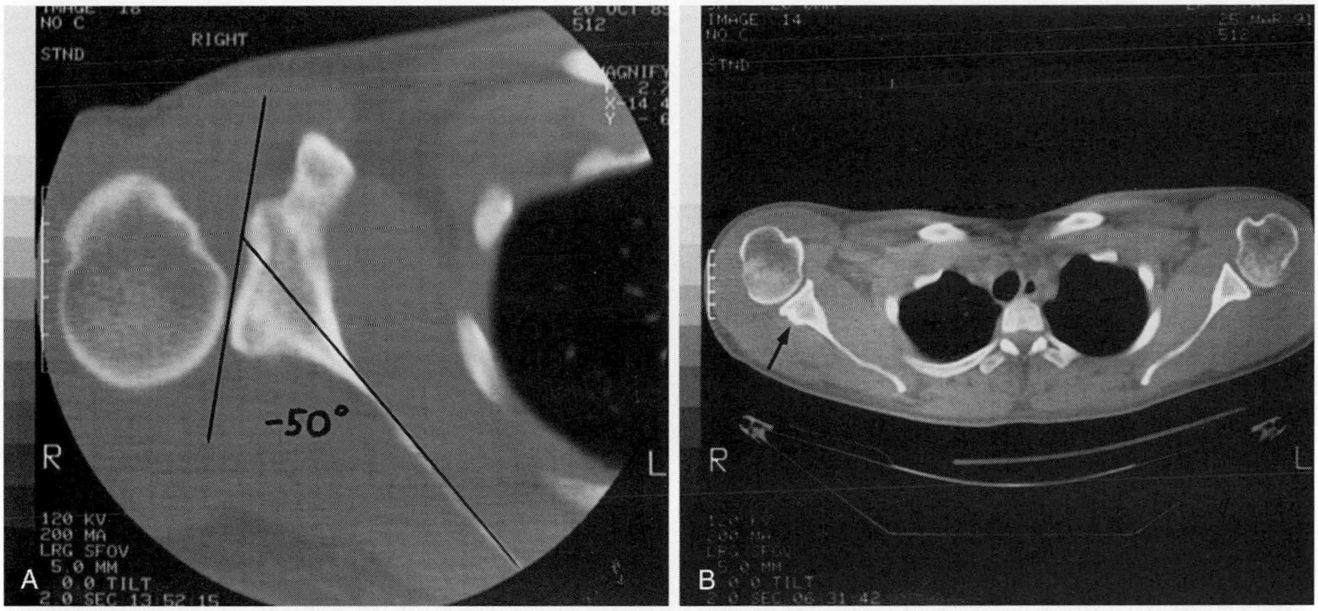

Figure 14–187

A, A preoperative computed tomography (CT) scan demonstrating a moderate glenoid retrotilt. *B*, A postoperative CT scan revealing a significant degree of correction in the glenoid version and incorporation of the tricortical bone graft after a posterior opening wedge osteotomy of the glenoid.
Illustration continued on following page

namic stabilization is regained, so that concavity compression, rather than capsular restraint, is the dominant mechanism of stability, the tightened posterior soft tissues are likely to stretch out as motion is regained. Even in its normal state, the posterior capsule is thin, often translucent. Its stretching out after surgical tightening is hastened if the posterior soft tissues are of poor quality, if the patient voluntarily or habitually tries to translate the shoulder posteriorly, or if large bony defects cause unphysiologic dependency on soft tissues for stability.

Occasionally the opposite outcome can occur: posterior repair may produce a shoulder that is too tight, which may push the shoulder out anteriorly. Insufficient posterior laxity can limit flexion, cross-body adduction, and internal rotation.

Complications may also result from bony procedures for posterior instability. Attempted posterior opening wedge osteotomy of the glenoid may result in an intra-articular fracture, in avascular necrosis of the osteotomized fragment, or in excessive anterior inclination and anterior instability. Posterior bone blocks placed in an excessively prominent position may cause severe degenerative joint disease.

Neurovascular injuries may also complicate posterior instability surgery. The axillary nerve may be injured as it exits the quadrangular space, or the nerve to the infraspinatus may be injured in the spinoglenoid notch.[280, 451]

MATSEN'S PREFERRED METHOD OF TREATMENT FOR RECURRENT POSTERIOR GLENOHUMERAL INSTABILITY

Care is taken to identify the circumstances and directions of instability, the presence of generalized ligamentous laxity, and any anatomic factors that might potentially compromise the surgical result. We evaluate the possibilities of multidirectional and voluntary instability in each patient with posterior instability. All patients with posterior instability are placed on the rehabilitation program described previously for atraumatic instability. A substantial number of patients with recurrent posterior instability respond to this program, particularly those with relatively atraumatic initiation of their condition. Straightforward patients who continue to have major symptomatic posterior instability after a reasonable rehabilitation effort may be considered for surgery. The type of posterior repair is influenced by the pathophysiology:

- Those with traumatic posterior instability may in fact have pathology very similar to that of traumatic anterior instability (avulsion of the capsule and labrum from the glenoid rim), which is amenable to primary repair. This condition must be diagnosed primarily from a history of an initial forcible posterior displacement of the humeral head on the glenoid but may be corroborated by a painful snap on posterior drawer.
- Those with lax posterior capsules may be managed with posterior capsulorrhaphy, but this capsular tightening is subject to stretching out again postoperatively with resultant recurrent instability. This condition is suggested if the shoulder has an excessive range of cross-body adduction or internal rotation in abduction. If atraumatic multidirectional laxity is present, the surgery is better performed from the front so that the rotator interval can be closed.
- Those shoulders without an effective posterior glenoid lip may require augmentation of the posterior lip with a labral reconstruction or posterior glenoid osteotomy. This situation is suggested if there is little

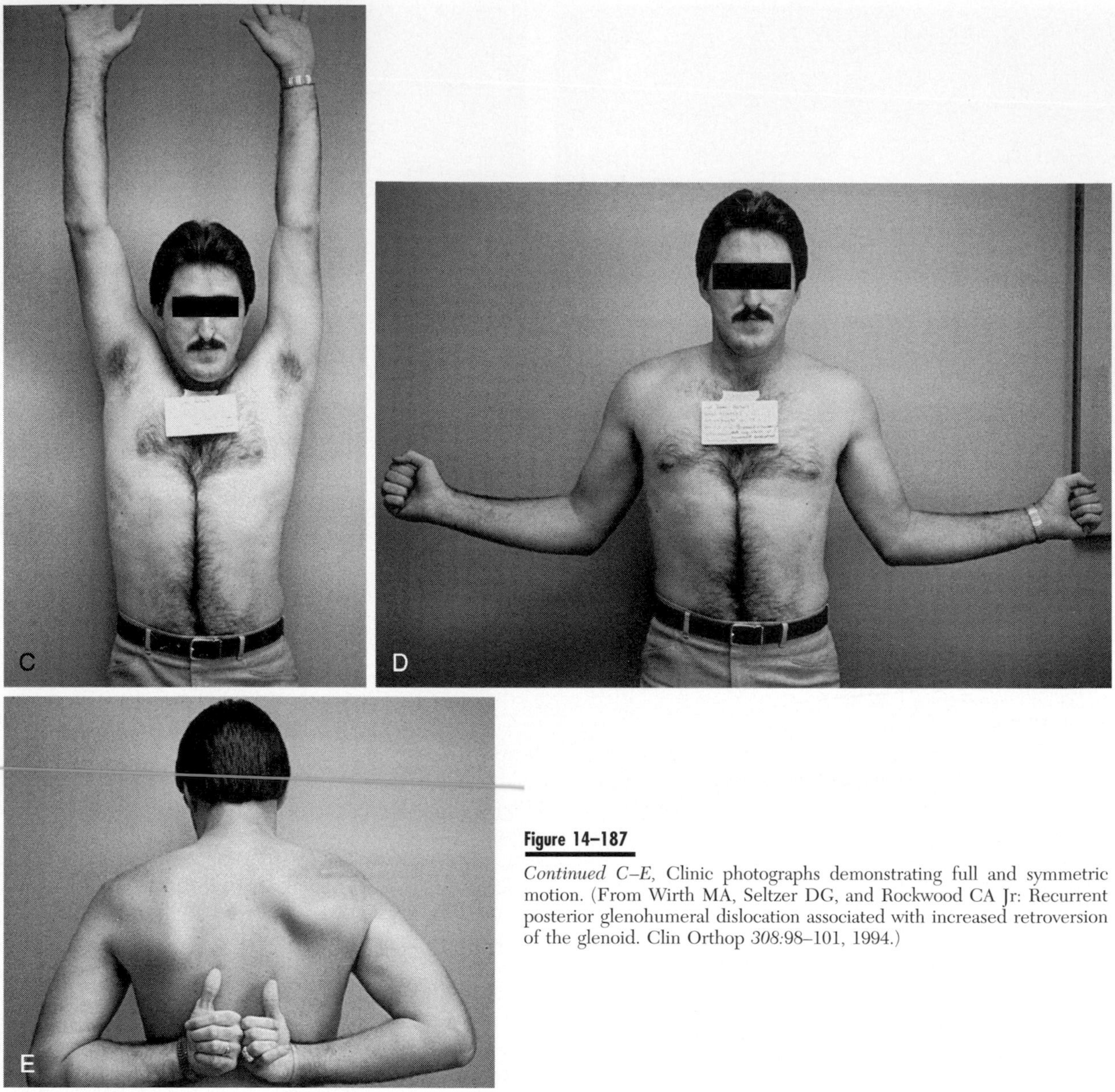

Figure 14–187

Continued C–E, Clinic photographs demonstrating full and symmetric motion. (From Wirth MA, Seltzer DG, and Rockwood CA Jr: Recurrent posterior glenohumeral dislocation associated with increased retroversion of the glenoid. Clin Orthop *308:*98–101, 1994.)

resistance to posterior translation when the humeral head is pressed into the glenoid.

- Those with major anterior medial humeral head defects (e.g., over one third of the humeral articular surface) may require the insertion of a proximal humeral prosthesis. This situation needs to be identified preoperatively because the preferred surgical approach for this procedure is anterior.

Preoperatively patients are informed of the alternatives and the risks of recurrent instability, excessive tightness with limited flexion and internal rotation, pain, neurovascular injury, infection, and the need for revision surgery.

Before the patient is placed prone, the shoulder is examined under anesthesia, with particular attention to the resistance to posterior translation with the humeral head pressed into the glenoid—this indicates the competence of the posterior glenoid lip. The patient is then placed prone with the shoulder off the operating table to allow a full range of humeral and scapular motion. After routine preparation of the arm, shoulder, neck, and back, a 10-cm incision is made in the extended line of the posterior axillary crease (see Fig. 14–9). The deltoid muscle is split for a distance of 4 cm between its middle and posterior thirds. If necessary, additional exposure may be obtained by carefully dissecting the muscle for a short distance from the scapular spine and posterior acromion (Fig. 14–188). Retraction of the deltoid muscle inferiorly and laterally reveals the infraspinatus muscle, the teres minor muscle, and the axillary nerve emerging from the quadrangular space. The spinoglenoid notch is palpated to determine the location of the important nerve to the infraspinatus.

The infraspinatus, the teres minor, and the attached capsule are incised 1 cm from the greater tuberosity to expose the posterior glenohumeral joint (see Fig. 14–

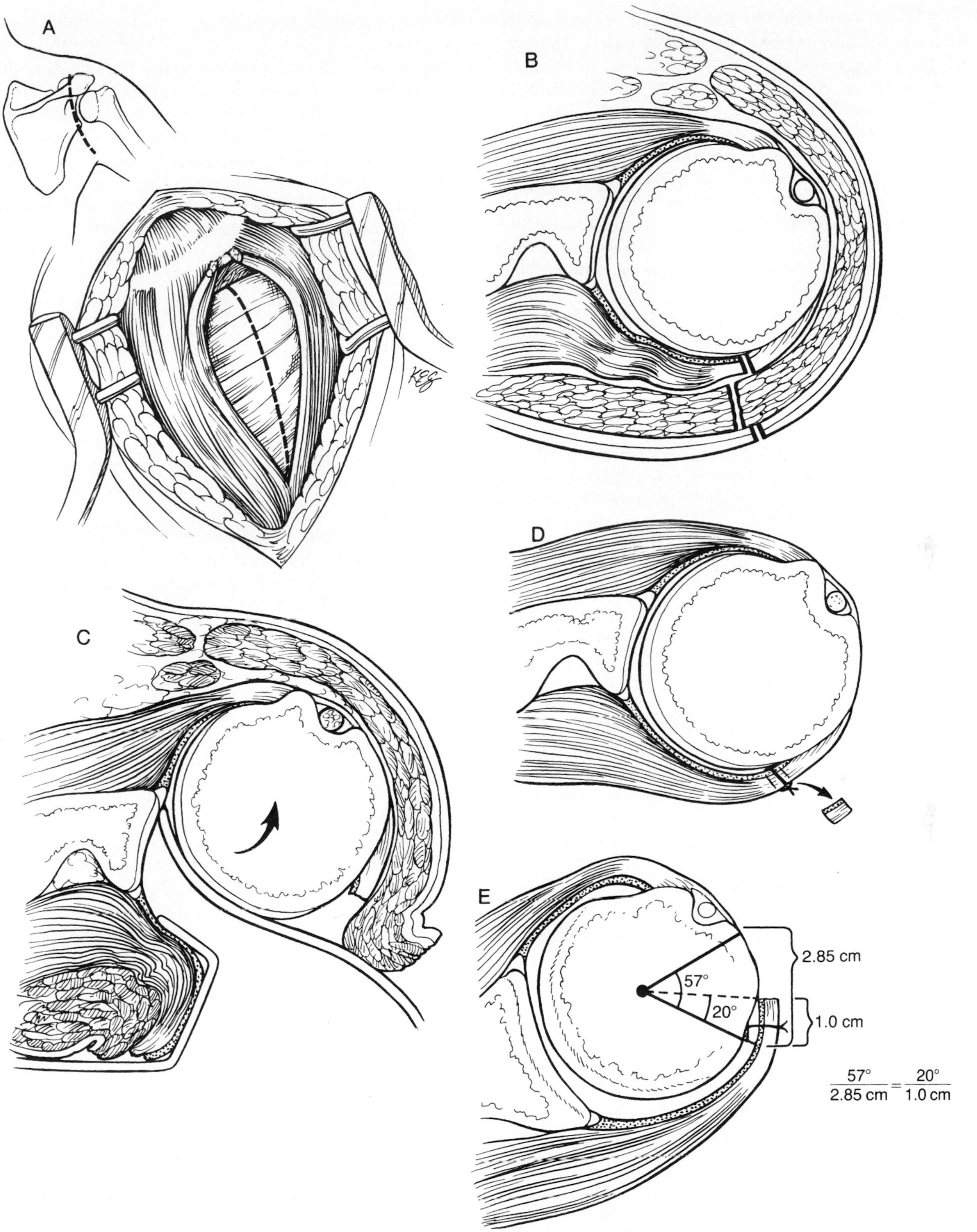

Figure 14–188

Operative repair for recurrent posterior glenohumeral instability. *A,* A 10-cm skin incision is made in the extended line of the posterior axillary crease *(inset).* The deltoid muscle is split between its middle and posterior thirds. *B,* A transverse plane section shows the interval through the deltoid muscle and the infraspinatus tendon. *C,* A transverse plane section shows placement of the retractors exposing the glenoid. *D,* A transverse plane section shows repair of the infraspinatus tendon after resecting the desired amount for capsular and tendon advancement. Shortening the posterior capsule and tendon by 1 cm will limit internal rotation by approximately 20 degrees. *E,* The effect of shortening capsular structures on limitation to rotation. The average radius of the humerus is 2.85 cm; this is the length of an arc equal to 1 radian, or approximately 57 degrees. If the capsule was shortened by 2.85 cm, rotation would be restricted by 57 degrees. Proportionally, a 1-cm shortening of the capsule would restrict rotation by 20 degrees. A posterior reefing of approximately 1 cm, decreasing internal rotation by approximately 20 degrees, is shown here.

188). Excessive traction on the axillary nerve and the nerve to the infraspinatus is carefully avoided. The joint is inspected for humeral head defects, wear of the anterior or posterior glenoid, tears in the glenoid labrum, loose bodies, and tears of the rotator cuff. Traumatic posterior capsular avulsions are repaired to the lip of the glenoid by a technique similar to that described for anterior repair. Excessive capsular laxity may be managed by reefing the capsule along with the attached infraspinatus and teres minor tendons. This is accomplished by overlapping the medial and lateral flaps by the desired amount or by advancing the capsule and tendon into a bony groove at the desired length. We usually try to limit internal rotation of the adducted humerus to 45 degrees. Internal rotation is limited by approximately 20 degrees for each centimeter of shortening of the posterior capsule and tendon. Greater tightening may be used in patients with generalized ligamentous instability.

If the patient demonstrates excessive posterior inferior capsular laxity, the capsule is released from the inferior neck of the humerus under direct visualization as the humerus is progressively internally rotated. The capsule and muscle tendons are then advanced superiorly as well as laterally, tightening the axillary recess. If significant multidirectional instability is present, a formal inferior capsular shift may be performed; however, this situation should be recognized preoperatively in that a capsular shift is preferably performed from the front so that the rotator interval can be closed and so that the posterior inferior capsule becomes tightened with flexion (Figs. 14–189 and 14–190).[1, 2, 449]

Anteromedial humeral head defects of moderate size are managed by tightening the posterior capsule so that internal rotation is limited to 30 degrees. A shoulder with an anterior humeral head defect constituting more than a third of the articular surface often cannot be stabilized by soft tissue surgery. In these instances insertion of a prosthetic head through the anterior approach will be required to restore stability and function to the glenohumeral joint. Because it changes the surgical approach, a lesion of this size needs to be identified preoperatively.

When there is deficiency of the posterior glenoid lip, increased glenoid retroversion, or undependable posterior soft tissues, a posterior inferior glenoid osteotomy can be considered. This osteotomy increases the effective glenoid arc posterior inferiorly. It is most safely performed by exposing the posterior inferior glenoid neck and joint surface simultaneously and inserting an osteotome parallel to the joint surface and about 6 mm medial to it. The depth of the osteotomy needs to be judged carefully to avoid excessive anterior penetration of the osteotome. The osteotome is advanced slowly, and the posterior-inferior glenoid lip is pried laterally with each advancement. This technique optimizes the reconstruction of the posterior inferior glenoid lip. The opening wedge osteotomy is held open by a wedge-shaped bone graft from the posterior acromion inserted so that its cortex is tucked just anterior to that of the posterior glenoid. Posterior humeral head displacement is attempted while the head is pressed into the glenoid to ensure that the correction is sufficient and that the bone graft is secure. If the amount of correction needs to be modified, this can easily be accomplished at this time. After the osteotomy, routine soft tissue repair is carried out.

When the indicated procedure is complete with maximal strength of the soft tissue reattachments, the deltoid is carefully repaired to the scapular spine and acromion, using drill holes as necessary. After surgery, the patient is immobilized in a "handshake" cummerbund cast (see Fig. 14–116) or orthotic (see Fig. 14–117) with the shoulder in adduction, neutral rotation, and slight extension for 3 weeks, during which time internal rotation isometric exercises are instituted. After the cast is removed, the patient is allowed to perform more vigorous rotator-strengthening exercises and to use the shoulder below the horizontal. The patient is encouraged to regain motion in abduction where stability against posterior displacement is optimal, avoiding early on forward flexion and internal rotation. As strength of external rotation and confidence are developed, more anterior planes of elevation are used. Vigorous shoulder activity is prohibited until normal rotator strength, coordination, and confidence in anterior planes is developed. The patient is advised to continue

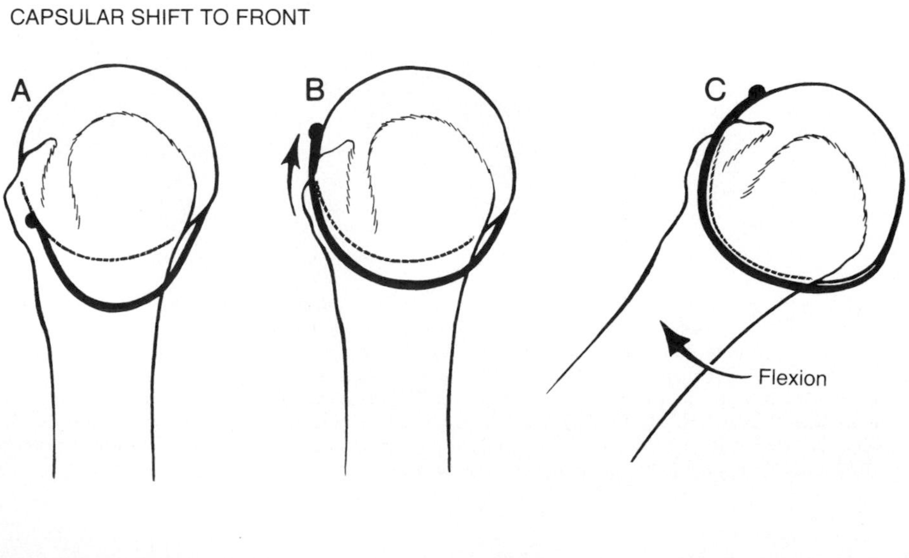

Figure 14–189

An inferior capsular shift, when performed from the anterior approach, advances the capsule anteriorly on the humerus. This produces additional posterior capsular tightening with shoulder flexion. *A,* Lax inferior capsule. *B,* Inferior capsule brought anteriorly on the humerus on an anterior approach. *C,* With humeral flexion, the posterior and inferior capsule is further tightened.

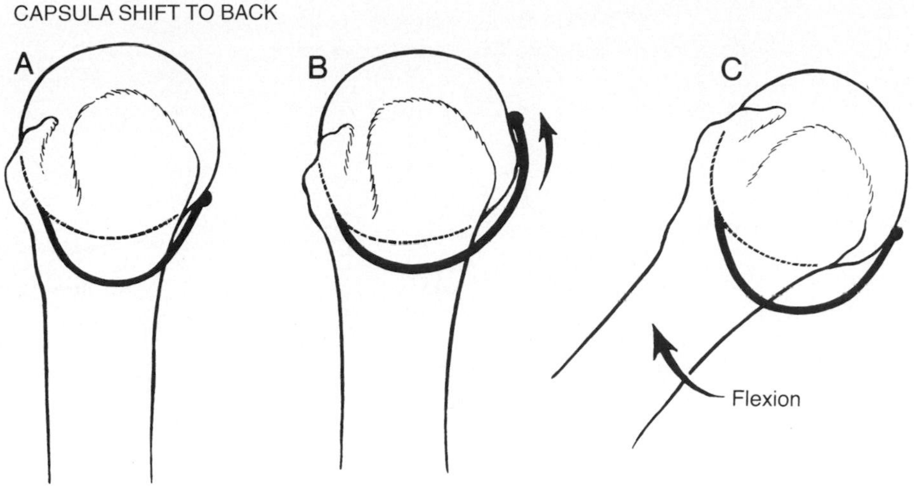

Figure 14–190

When the inferior capsular shift is performed from the posterior approach and the capsule is advanced posteriorly on the humerus, the tightened capsule loosens with shoulder flexion. *A*, Lax inferior capsule. *B*, From the posterior approach the lax inferior capsule is advanced posteriorly on the humerus. *C*, Humeral flexion loosens the posterior and inferior capsule.

rotator strengthening exercises on a daily basis to optimize dynamic shoulder stability.

ROCKWOOD AND WIRTH'S TECHNIQUE OF POSTERIOR RECONSTRUCTION FOR TRAUMATIC INSTABILITY[692]

Standard Posterior Repair

The patient is placed in the lateral decubitus position with the operative shoulder upward. The best way to support the patient in this position is to use the kidney supports and the "bean bag."

The incision begins 1 inch medial to the posterolateral corner of the acromion and extends downward 3 inches toward the posterior axillary creases (Fig. 14–191).[72] If a bone graft is to be taken from the acromion, the incision extends a little farther superiorly so that the acromion can be exposed. Next, the subcutaneous tissues are dissected medially and laterally so that the skin can be retracted to visualize the fibers of the deltoid.

A point 1 inch medial to the posterior corner of the acromion is selected, and the deltoid is then split distally for 4 inches in the line of its fibers. The deltoid can be easily retracted medially and laterally to expose the underlying infraspinatus and teres minor muscles. This deltoid split can be made down to the midportion of the teres minor muscle. Remember that the axillary nerve exits the quadrangular space at the lower border of the teres minor muscle.

In performing a posterior reconstruction, the teres minor tendon should be reflected inferiorly down to the level of the inferior joint capsule. If the infraspinatus tendon is divided and reflected medially and laterally, care should be taken not to injure the suprascapular nerve. When the infraspinatus tendon is very lax, it can be reflected off the capsule and retracted superiorly without having to divide the tendon.

With the infraspinatus and teres minor muscles retracted out of the way, a vertical incision can be made in the posterior capsule to expose and explore the joint. We prefer to make the incision midway between the humeral and glenoid attachment so that at closure we can double-breast it and make it stronger. In doing the posterior capsular shift procedure, it is essential to have the teres minor muscle reflected sufficiently inferior so that the vertical cut in the capsule will go all the way down to the most inferior recess of the capsule. If the capsule is thin and friable, and it appears that a capsular shift alone will be insufficient, then the infraspinatus tendon can be divided so that it can be double-breasted to shorten it.

With the capsule divided all the way down inferiorly, horizontal mattress sutures of No. 2 cottony Dacron are inserted in the edge of the medial capsule. The arm should be held in neutral rotation, and the medial capsule is sutured laterally and superiorly under the lateral capsule. Next, the lateral capsule is reflected and sutured medially and superiorly over the medial capsule and again held in place with horizontal mattress sutures. This capsular shift procedure has effectively eliminated any of the posterior and inferior capsular redundancy.

The infraspinatus tendon is next repaired; this should also be performed with the arm in neutral rotation. If laxity exists, the tendon can be double-breasted. The wound is thoroughly irrigated, and the muscle and subcutaneous tissues are infiltrated with 25 to 30 ml of 0.25% bupivacaine (Marcaine). Care must be taken not to overuse the bupivacaine or inject it directly into vascular channels.

When the retractors are withdrawn, the deltoid falls nicely together and a subcutaneous closure is performed. Care must be taken throughout the closure of the capsule, infraspinatus tendon, and skin to maintain the arm in neutral rotation. The patient is then gently rolled into the supine position, making sure that the arm is in neutral rotation. When the anesthetic is completed, the patient is transferred to his or her bed, where the arm is maintained in the neutral position and supported by skin traction. Usually within 24 hours after surgery the patient can stand, and a modified shoulder immobilizer cast is applied.

Posterior Glenoid Osteotomy

We do not use this as a routine part of the posterior reconstruction. Occasionally when there is a posterior

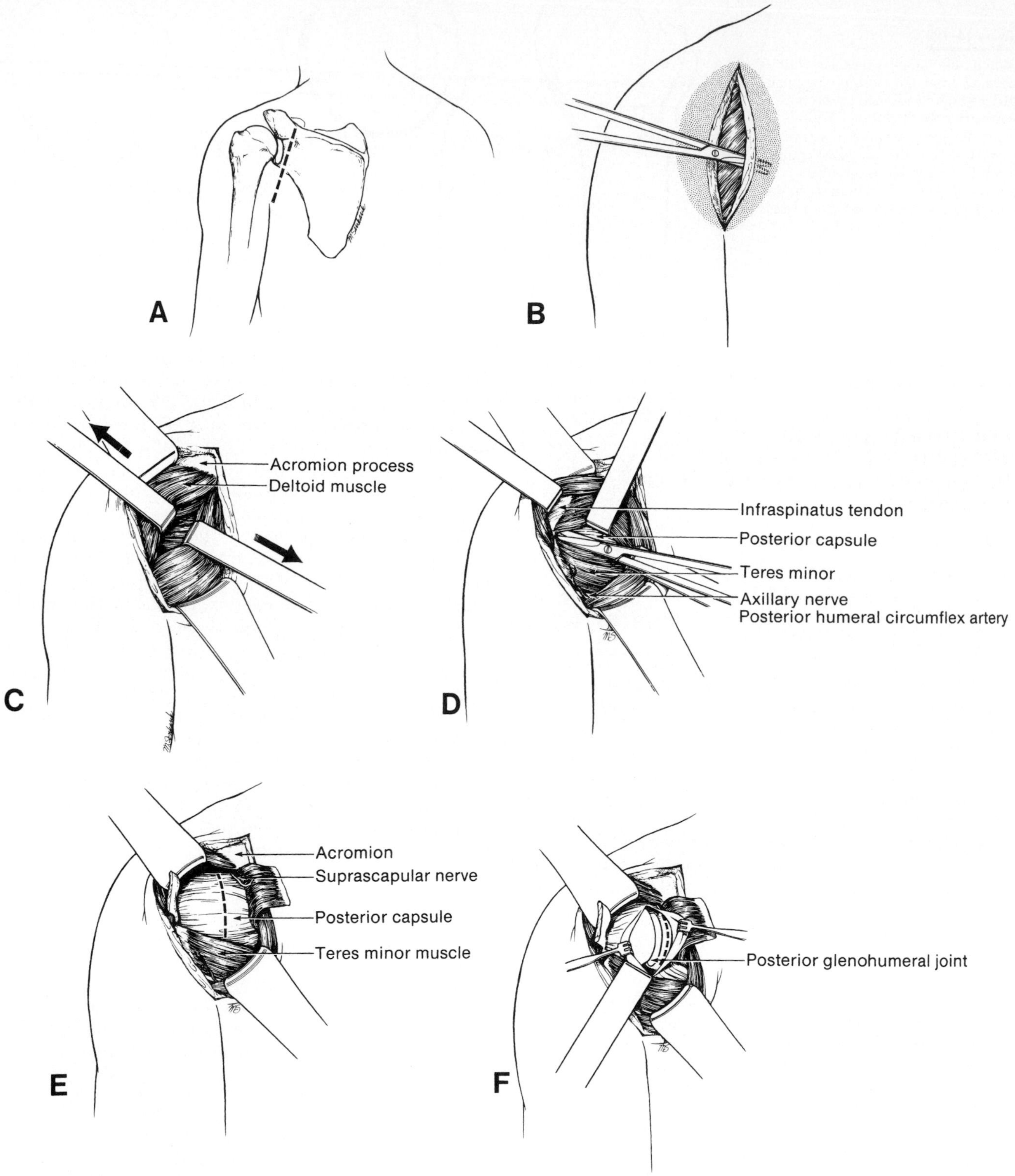

Figures 14–191

A–R, Rockwood's preferred posterior shoulder reconstruction. (See the text for a detailed description of each step of the procedure.) (From Rockwood CA and Green DP [eds]: Fractures [3 vols], 2nd ed. Philadelphia: JB Lippincott, 1984.)

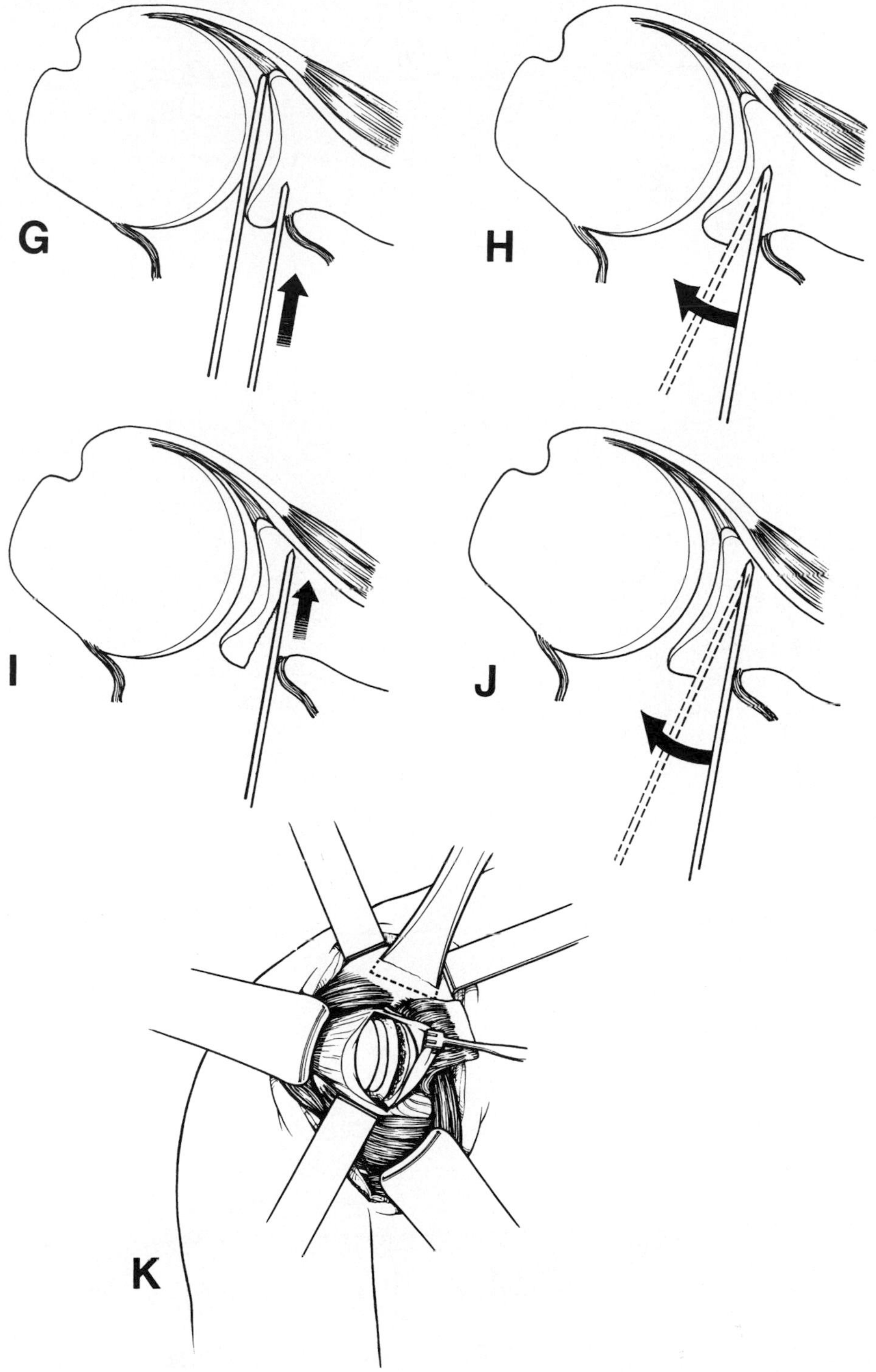

Figure 14–191
Continued

Illustration continued on following page

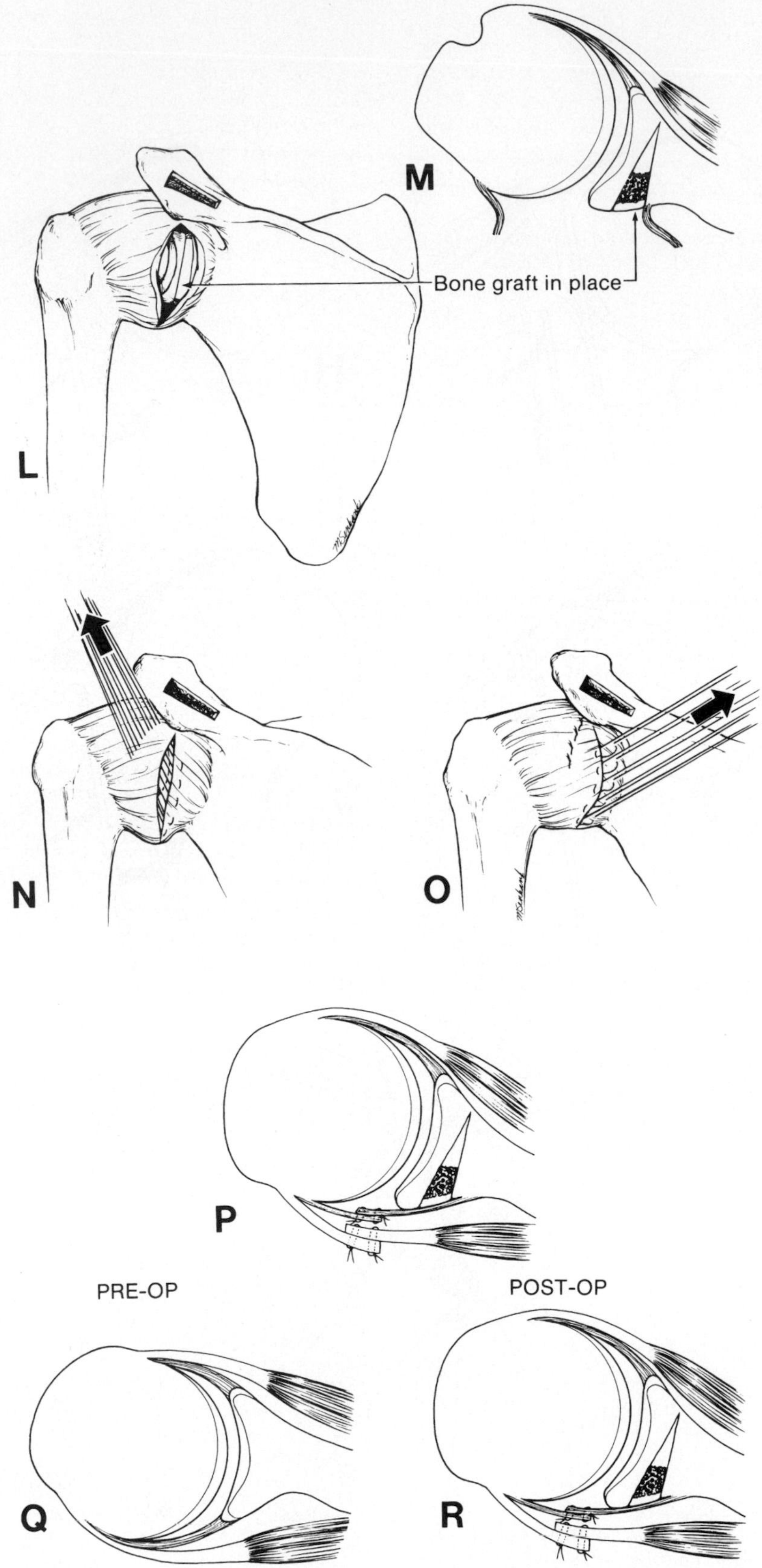

Figure 14–191

Continued

glenoid deficiency, or in cases where there is a congenital retrotilt of the glenoid (i.e., greater than 30 degrees), a posterior osteotomy should be considered. We have reported a patient who had failed two previous attempts at posterior capsulorrhaphy for recurrent posterior shoulder instability.[698] The patient demonstrated a previously unrecognized unilateral increase in glenoid fossa retrotilt and was treated successfully with a posterior opening wedge osteotomy of the scapular neck (see Fig. 14–187).

When performing a posterior glenoid osteotomy, care must be taken not to overcorrect the retroversion, because it may force the head out anteriorly. If a posterior osteotomy is to be performed, it is absolutely essential to know the anatomy and angle of the slope of the glenoid. This can best be determined by placing a straight, blunt instrument into the joint so that it lies on the anterior and posterior glenoid rim (see Fig. 14–191). Next, the osteotome is placed intracapsularly and directed parallel to the blunt instrument. If one is unsure of the angle and does not have a guide instrument in place, there is the possibility of the osteotomy entering the joint (see Fig. 14–186). The osteotomy site is not more than ¼ inch medial to the articular surface of the glenoid. If the osteotomy is more medial than this, the possibility exists of injuring the suprascapular nerve as it passes around the base of the spine of the scapula to supply the infraspinatus muscle. Each time that the osteotome is advanced, the osteotomy site is pried open (see Fig. 14–191); this helps to create a lateral plastic deformation of the posterior glenoid. The osteotomy should not exit anteriorly but should stop just at the anterior cortex of the scapula (see Fig. 14–191). The intact anterior cortex periosteum and soft tissue will act as a hinge, which allows the graft to be secure in the osteotomy without the need for internal fixation. We usually use an osteotome that is 1 inch wide to make the original cut, and then we use smaller ½-inch osteotomes superiorly and inferiorly to complete the posterior division of bone. Osteotomes are used to open up the osteotomy site, and the bone graft is placed into position (see Fig. 14–191). If the anterior cortex is partially intact, there is no need for any internal fixation of the graft because it is held securely in place by the osteotomy. We prefer to take the bone graft from the acromion (see Fig. 14–191). Either a small piece (8 × 30 mm) for the osteotomy or a large piece (15 × 30 mm) for a posteroinferior bone block can be taken from the top or the posterior edge of the acromion. If a larger piece of graft is required, it should be taken from the ilium. Following completion of the osteotomy, the capsular shift, as described earlier, is performed.

After surgery the patient lies supine with the forearm supported by the overhead bed frame, holding the arm in neutral rotation. We usually let the patient sit up on the bed the evening of surgery while maintaining the arm in neutral rotation. We let him or her sit up in a chair the next day, again holding the arm in neutral rotation. Either 24 or 48 hours after surgery, when the patient can stand comfortably, we apply a lightweight long arm cast. Next, a well-padded iliac crest band that sits around the abdomen and iliac crest is applied. The arm is then connected to the iliac crest band with a broom handle support to maintain the arm in 10 to 15 degrees of abduction and in neutral rotation. The cast is left in place for 6 to 8 weeks. Following removal of the plaster, the patient is allowed to use the arm for 4 to 6 weeks for everyday living activities. A rehabilitation program is begun that includes pendulum exercises, isometric exercises, and stretching of the shoulder with the use of an overhead pulley, after which resistive exercises are gradually increased.

Anterior Capsular Shift Reconstruction

We have used a capsular shift reconstruction in patients whose primary pathology is posterior shoulder instability if there is a recognizable component of multidirectional shoulder laxity (Fig. 14–192).[693] This procedure is indicated when instability or apprehension repeatedly compromises shoulder comfort or function in spite of an adequate trial of rotator cuff strengthening and coordination exercises. The mainstay of the capsular shift procedure is reduction of the excessive joint volume through a symmetric and anatomic plication of the redundant capsule. We have found it unnecessary to perform a combined anterior and posterior approach but rather reserve posterior capsular reconstruction for patients with recurrent traumatic posterior shoulder instability who do not demonstrate concomitant generalized ligamentous laxity and multidirectional laxity of the shoulder.

One explanation for the difficulties encountered with traditional posterior reconstructions has been the poor quality and unsubstantial nature of the posterior capsule that precludes a strong surgical reconstruction. Additionally, surgically addressable lesions known to contribute to recurrent instability such as associated fractures involving the posterior glenoid rim or anteromedial humeral head are less frequent. In contrast to the capsulolabral injuries seen with traumatic anterior shoulder instability, posterior glenoid lateral pathology is often limited to degenerative

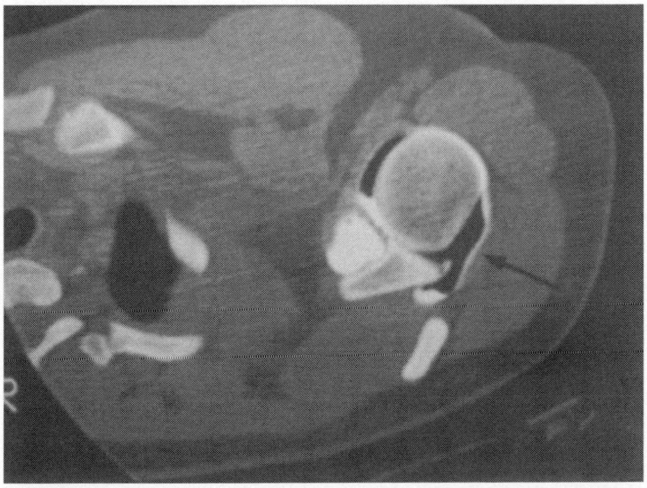

Figure 14–192

A computed tomography arthrogram in a patient with symptomatic posterior shoulder instability and multidirectional glenohumeral laxity. Note the overall capsular volume and the posterior capsular redundancy *(arrow)*. (From Rockwood CA Jr, Green DP, and Bucholz RW [eds]: Fractures in Adults. Philadelphia: JB Lippincott, 1991.)

changes rather than capsulolabral avulsions, which lend themselves to stable surgical repair. Finally, and perhaps the most subtle reason for poor surgical results, is failure to recognize that some shoulders demonstrate multidirectional laxity though the patient may present with a history, physical examination, and radiographs consistent with symptomatic posterior shoulder instability.

The basis for this seemingly unorthodox approach is supported by several reports in the literature. In 1988, Schwartz and colleagues[581] performed arthroscopically assisted selective sectioning of the shoulder capsule to quantitate the relative contribution of specific structures to glenohumeral stability. The superior glenohumeral ligament was found to provide secondary restraint to posterior shoulder instability. In addition, posterior glenohumeral dislocation did not occur after incision of the posterior capsule until the anterosuperior capsular structures were also sectioned. More recently, Harryman and associates[225] investigated the role of selective capsular sectioning and imbrication of the interval capsule. Surgical modifications were found to alter several different parameters of shoulder motion, including rotation and translation, which ultimately affected the stability of the shoulder joint. Specifically, the intrarotator interval was found to be a major component of stability against posterior and inferior glenohumeral displacement. Posterior and inferior glenohumeral dislocations usually occurred after sectioning of the rotator interval capsule, while imbrication of this structure increased the resistance to translation in these directions. These authors concluded that patients with inferior or posterior shoulder instability may benefit from an anterior reconstruction of the interval capsule.

Nonoperative Treatment of the AMBRII Syndrome: Recurrent Multidirectional Instability

The goal of treatment for patients with atraumatic instability is the restoration of shoulder function. Many patients with AMBRII syndrome have simply become deconditioned from their normal state of dynamic glenohumeral stability. They have lost the proper neuromuscular control of humeroscapular positioning; concavity compression has become dysfunctional. Neuromuscular control cannot be restored surgically; rather, it requires prolonged adherence to a well-constructed reconditioning program. The patient may need to be convinced that training and exercises constitute a reasonable therapeutic approach. Many would prefer a surgical "cure." It is often useful to demonstrate that the contralateral shoulder has substantial laxity on examination yet is clinically stable. In this way the patient and family can appreciate that a loose shoulder is not necessarily unstable; for example, gymnasts usually have very lax, yet very stable shoulders.

The nonoperative management of glenohumeral instability has been discussed earlier in this chapter. In general, but particularly in atraumatic instability, glenohumeral stability is dependent on dynamic compression of the humeral head into the glenoid concavity (concavity compression) and excellence in neuromuscular control. Thus the nonoperative and postoperative programs for an AMBRII shoulder need to optimize both.

Operative Treatment of Atraumatic Instability

PRESURGICAL CONSIDERATIONS

The ability of surgery alone to *cure* atraumatic instability is limited. Usually there is no single lesion that can be repaired. Most of the factors providing midrange stability cannot be enhanced by surgical reconstruction. Problems of neuromuscular control or relative glenoid flatness do not have easy surgical solutions. Even after a snug capsulorrhaphy, the midrange stabilizing mechanisms of balance and concavity compression must be optimized through muscle strengthening and kinematic training. Otherwise, excessive loads will be applied to the surgically tightened glenohumeral capsule, leading to stretching and failure of the surgical reconstruction.

In this light, the indications for surgical treatment of atraumatic instability need to be carefully considered. First, the patient must have major functional problems that are clearly related to atraumatic glenohumeral instability. Second, the patient must clearly understand that good strength and kinematic technique are the primary stabilizing factors for the shoulder rather than capsular tightness. Third, the patient must have conscientiously participated in a strengthening and training program and recognize that strength and proper technique will continue to be major stabilizing factors for the shoulder even after reconstructive surgery is performed. The patient must also recognize that capsulorrhaphy is designed to stiffen the shoulder: the surgery will compromise the range of motion in the hope of gaining stability. If attempts to regain totally normal range are made in the first postoperative year, instability is likely to recur. Thus, the limitations imposed by surgical capsulorrhaphy may be incompatible with the goals of normal or supernormal range of motion. Therefore, gymnasts, dancers, and baseball pitchers may not be good candidates for this surgical procedure. Similarly, this procedure has a limited ability to hold up under the demands of heavy physical labor unless it is accompanied by a superb strength and kinematic rehabilitation program. Finally, the patient must understand that rehabilitation after a capsular shift procedure is protracted. It is important that the shoulder be immobilized in a brace for 1 month, during which time muscles get weak and normal kinematics are lost. After this month of immobilization many months are required for the re-establishment of good strength and shoulder kinematics. In spite of the best operative and postoperative management, the success of this procedure in reestablishing normal shoulder function is substantially less than procedures for traumatic instability.

The foregoing is a large amount of very important information that must be understood by the patient considering the surgical procedure. The situation is further complicated by the fact that many patients who present with atraumatic midrange instability are young and may have difficulty understanding and accepting the ramifications of this information. Thus, during the preoperative discussions with young patients it may be important that parents participate actively. We find that many families who present requesting that "the shoulder be fixed" are prepared to work more diligently on the nonoperative program after this discussion.

When the history and physical examination indicate that the shoulder is loose in all directions and when the patient has failed to respond to vigorous internal and external rotator-strengthening, endurance, and coordination exercises, an inferior capsular shift procedure may be considered as originally described by Neer and Foster.[449] The principle of the procedure is to symmetrically tighten the anterior, inferior, and posterior aspects of the capsule by advancing its humeral attachment.

RESULTS OF RECONSTRUCTIONS FOR ATRAUMATIC INSTABILITY

A capsular shift procedure is often considered in the surgical management of atraumatic instability. However, most of the existing reports of inferior capsular shift surgery include patients with both traumatic and atraumatic forms of instability.[8, 102, 450] Therefore, the results are substantially better than would be expected in the treatment of atraumatic instability. Cooper and Brems[102] reported a 2-year follow-up of inferior capsular-shift procedure finding that 9% continued to have significant instability. Altchek and colleagues[8] utilized a T-plasty modification of the Bankart procedure for multidirectional instability on 42 shoulders injured during athletics. Four patients experienced episodes of instability after the procedure and the throwing athletes suffered from decreased throwing velocity. Despite these shortcomings, patient satisfaction was noted to be excellent in 95% of shoulders. Bigliani and associates[46] managed 68 shoulders in 63 athletes with anterior and inferior instability with an inferior capsular shift procedure. Fifty-eight patients returned to their major sports, 75% at the same competitive level, but only 50% of elite throwing athletes returned to their prior level of competition.

In general, better results are obtained with surgery whenever trauma is a contributing factor. In an attempt to evaluate the effectiveness of a homogenous series of primary capsular shift surgeries for purely atraumatic instability, Obremskey[480] reviewed 26 patients with no history, radiographic or surgical evidence of a traumatic etiology. The patients in this series had failed an average of 17 months of vigorous physical rehabilitation prior to proceeding with surgery. Fifty-seven per cent of the patients had bilateral symptoms. The average age was 22 ± 6 years (range of 13 to 34). Twenty-nine per cent had generalized ligamentous laxity; 15% had an industrial claim. At an average of 27 months after a standard capsular shift was performed,[450] Seventy-four per cent of the patients were satisfied with the condition of their shoulder; 46% were able to return to recreation and 69% to their previous job. Thirty-nine per cent had persistent pain, and 57% had night pain that interfered with sleeping. Sixty-eight per cent had at least occasional symptoms of instability, and 10% required further surgery. Using regression analysis, the most important correlates with patient dissatisfaction was not recurrent instability but rather persistent pain and stiffness. These results suggest that a key in management of patients with atraumatic multidirectional instability is not the degree of surgical tightness achieved but rather the restoration of comfort and motion.

MATSEN'S APPROACH TO OPERATIVE TREATMENT OF RECURRENT ATRAUMATIC MULTIDIRECTIONAL GLENOHUMERAL INSTABILITY

The goals of the surgery are to tighten the capsule symmetrically around the joint and to close the rotator interval, creating a new, stronger rotator interval capsule and coracohumeral ligament (Fig. 14–193). These goals can only be accomplished through an anterior surgical ap-

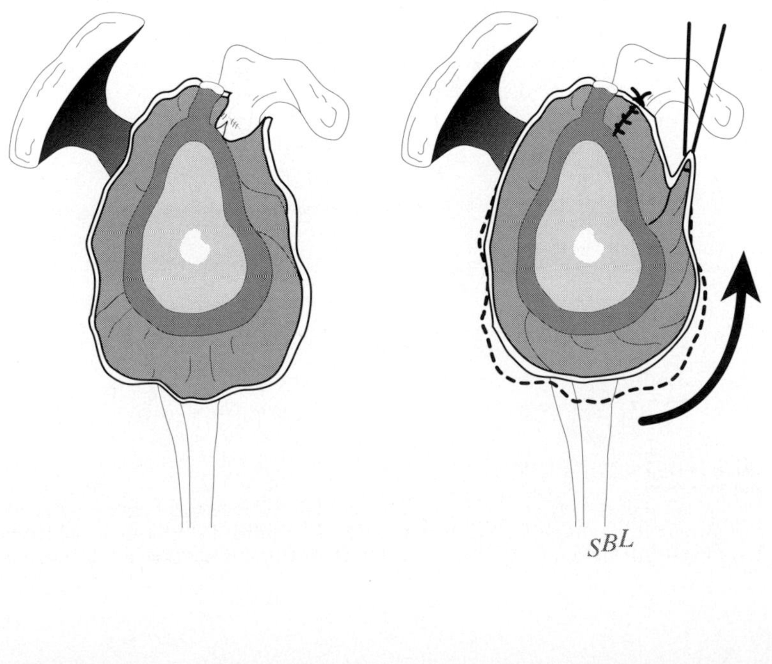

Figure 14–193

The essence of the reconstruction of atraumatic instability is the reduction of the posteroinferior recess by anterosuperior advancement of the capsule combined with closure of the rotator interval capsule. This reconstruction has the advantage of becoming additionally tight as the arm is elevated in anterior planes (see Fig. 14–189). (From Matsen FA III, Lippitt SB, Sidles JA, and Harryman DT II: Practical Evaluation and Management of the Shoulder. Philadelphia: WB Saunders, 1994.)

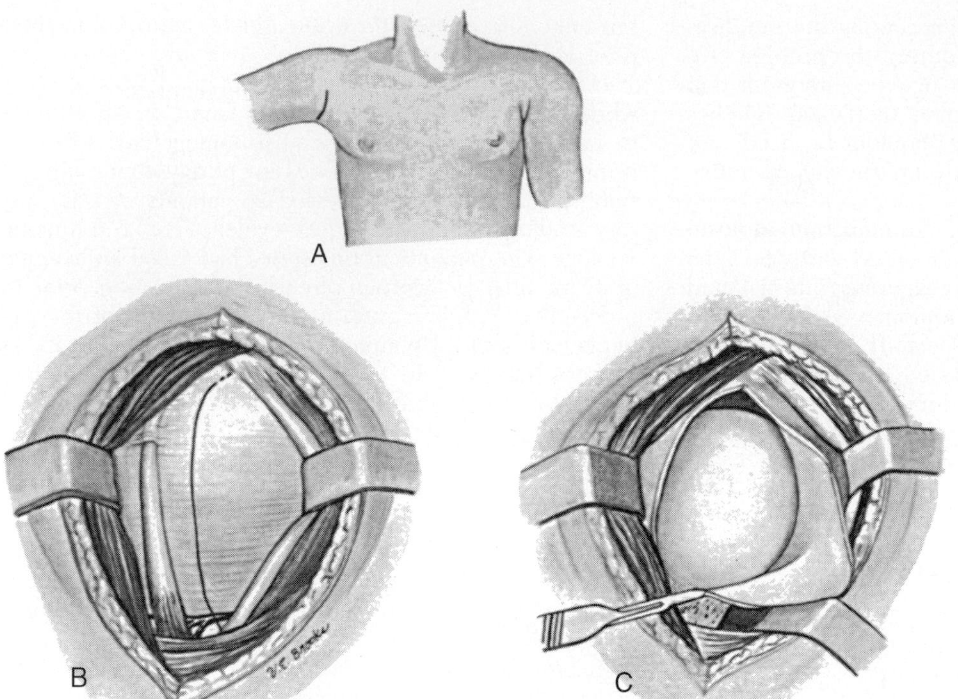

Figure 14–194

A, Axillary incision. *B,* Incision through the subscapularis. *C,* Release of the anterior and inferior capsule from the neck of the humerus.

proach. Thus, we routinely approach a repair for atraumatic instability from the front, even if the predominant direction of instability appears to be posterior. In addition, the anterior approach is cosmetically superior to the posterior approach. Furthermore, it can be accomplished without incising the critical external rotator cuff musculature. Finally, when the capsule is advanced anterosuperiorly on the humeral side, elevation of the arm anteriorly results in desirable additional tightening of the inferior and posterior capsule (see Fig. 14–189). In contrast, when the procedure is performed from a posterior approach, the capsule is advanced posterior superiorly on the humerus so that it loosens as the humerus is flexed (see Fig. 14–190).

The shoulder is approached through a low anterior axillary incision, entering the deltopectoral groove medial to the cephalic vein (Fig. 14–194). The clavipectoral fascia is divided up to the level of the coracoacromial ligament

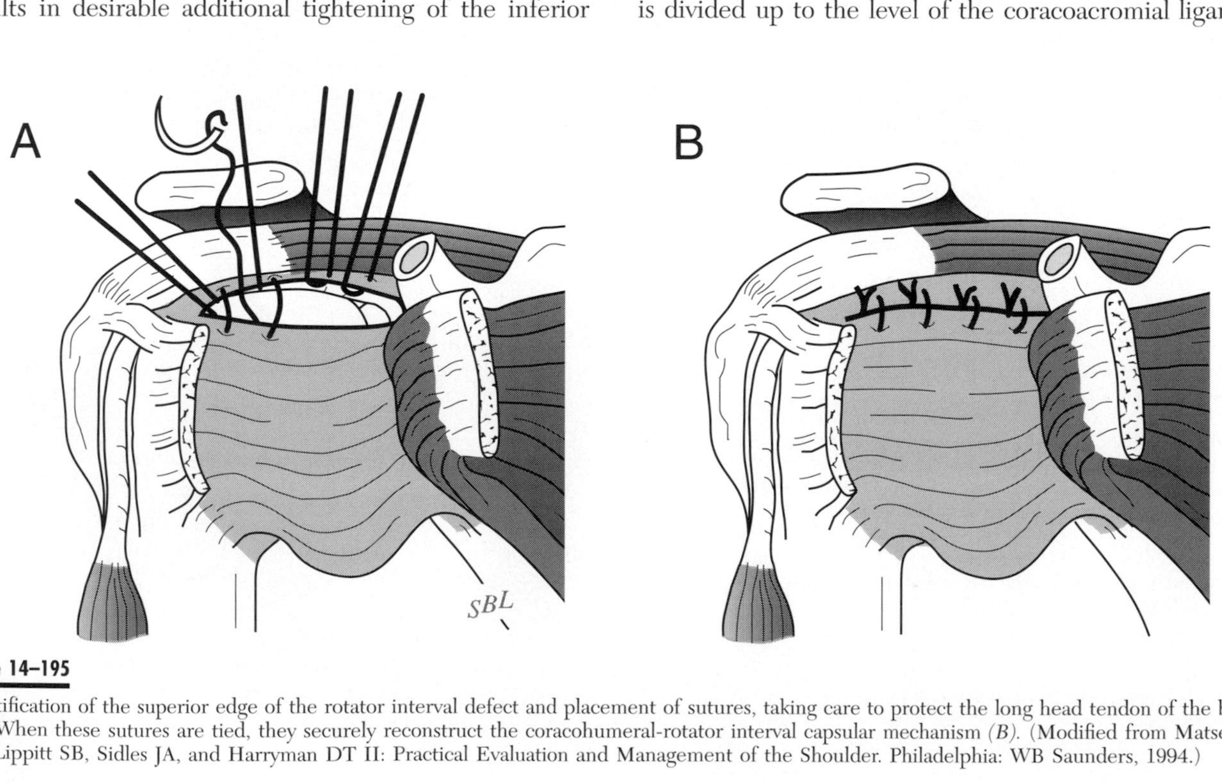

Figure 14–195

Identification of the superior edge of the rotator interval defect and placement of sutures, taking care to protect the long head tendon of the biceps *(A).* When these sutures are tied, they securely reconstruct the coracohumeral-rotator interval capsular mechanism *(B).* (Modified from Matsen FA III, Lippitt SB, Sidles JA, and Harryman DT II: Practical Evaluation and Management of the Shoulder. Philadelphia: WB Saunders, 1994.)

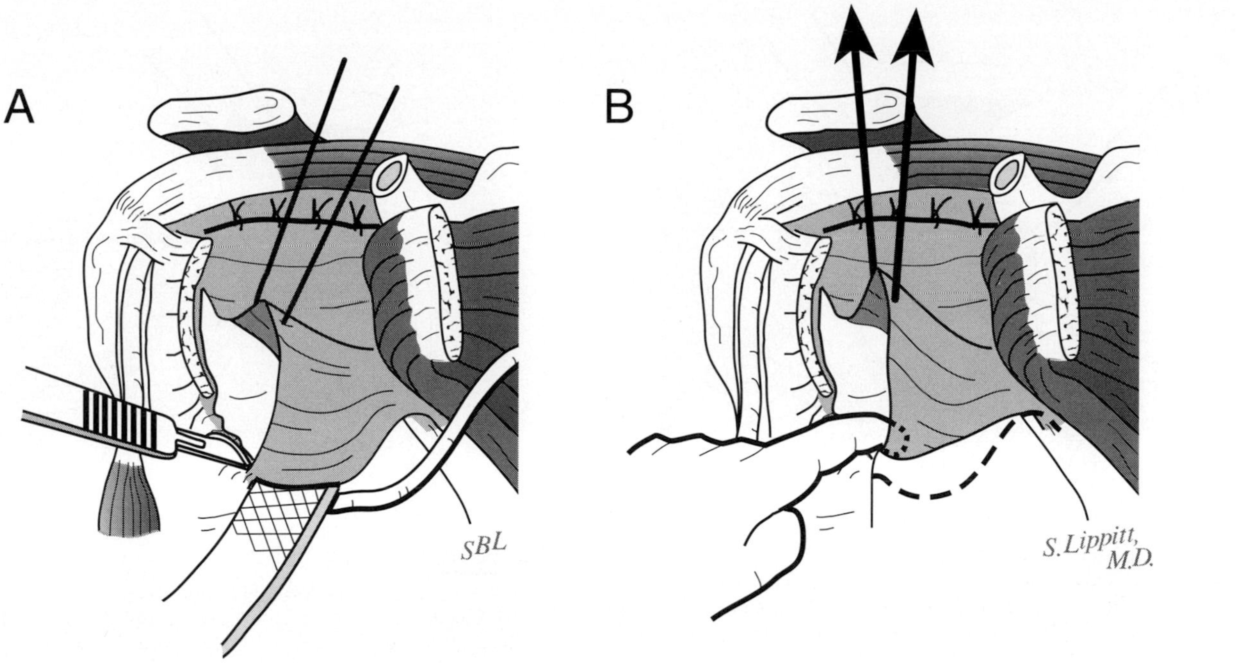

Figure 14–196

Release of the capsule from the humeral neck laterally. This dissection is carried beyond the inferior (6 o'clock) position *(A)* until traction on the anterior capsular flap reduces the posteroinferior recess *(B)*. (From Matsen FA III, Lippitt SB, Sidles JA, and Harryman DT II: Practical Evaluation and Management of the Shoulder. Philadelphia: WB Saunders, 1994.)

providing access to the humeroscapular motion interface. The axillary nerve is palpated medially as it courses across the subscapularis and passes inferiorly toward the quadrangular space. The superior edge of the subscapularis is then identified by palpating the rotator interval lateral to the coracoid process and medial to the bicipital groove. The triad of anterior humeral circumflex vessels mark the inferior border of the subscapularis where they can be prospectively cauterized. The subscapularis tendon is sharply and carefully dissected from the capsule, ensuring that the thickness of the capsule is not compromised.

A substantial defect in the rotator interval is seen consistently in AMBRII syndrome. This defect is bordered by the capsule adjacent to the supraspinatus overlying the biceps tendon superiorly, the anterior capsule and subscapularis anteroinferiorly, the coracoid process medially, and the transverse humeral ligament laterally. This defect is accentuated by pushing the humeral head posteriorly. Sutures of No. 2 nonabsorbable material are securely placed in the superior edge of the defect and then passed across to the inferior edge of the defect (Fig. 14–195; see also Fig. 14–194). When these sutures are tied, a strong rotator interval capsule is reconstructed.

The anterior capsule is incised from the humeral neck, and traction sutures are placed in the incised margin as the anterior capsule is released. The axillary nerve is identified and protected during this dissection. The dissection is continued until superiorly directed traction on the capsular flap causes the capsule to tighten on a finger placed in the posteroinferior capsular recess (Fig. 14–196). Usually this point is reached when the capsule is released just past the inferior (6 o'clock position) on the humeral neck, sectioning the posterior band of the inferior glenohumeral ligament.

After the capsular release, a bony trough is created in the anteroinferior humeral neck adjacent to the articular surface using a power burr (Fig. 14–197). Holes are made in the humeral neck lateral to the groove, and sutures are passed through these holes into the groove for reattachment of the capsule securely to bone. With the arm at the side and in neutral rotation and with strong anterior superior traction on the sutures to obliterate the posterior inferior recess, the sutures from the groove are passed through the lateral edge of the capsule (Fig. 14–198). Tying these sutures securely fixes the capsule in its advanced position (Fig. 14–199). This step needs to be accomplished with excellent direct vision to be sure that the bites in the capsule are sufficiently inferior to tighten it to the groove and to ensure the safety of the axillary nerve. The surgeon must ensure that pulling up on these sutures obliterates the posterior inferior recess. If this is not the case, either the inferior capsular release was insufficient or the sutures were not placed sufficiently inferior. This repair to the groove is continued anteriorly up the humeral neck. Redundant anterior superior capsule is folded down over the previous repair to reinforce it (Fig. 14–200).

At this point the shoulder is checked to ensure that internal rotation of the abducted arm is limited to 45 degrees below the horizontal, that the posterior drawer is less than 50% of the humeral head diameter, and that external rotation of the arm at the side is 30 degrees. Excessive internal rotation of the abducted arm indicates the inferior capsule was not advanced sufficiently anterior.

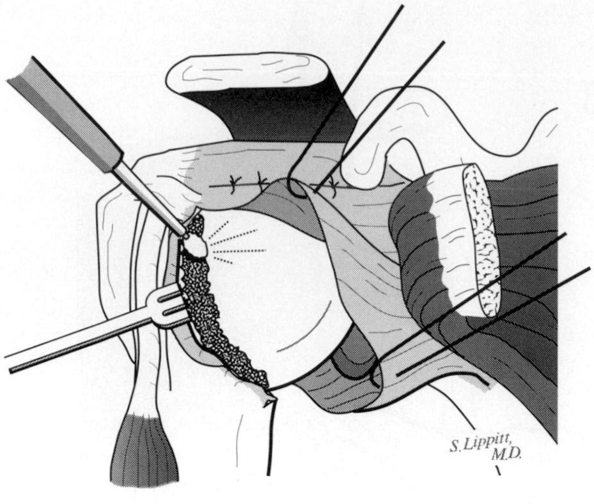

Figure 14–197

Preparation of the humeral neck with a groove at the margin of the articular surface. (Modified from Matsen FA III, Lippitt SB, Sidles JA, and Harryman DT II: Practical Evaluation and Management of the Shoulder. Philadelphia: WB Saunders, 1994.)

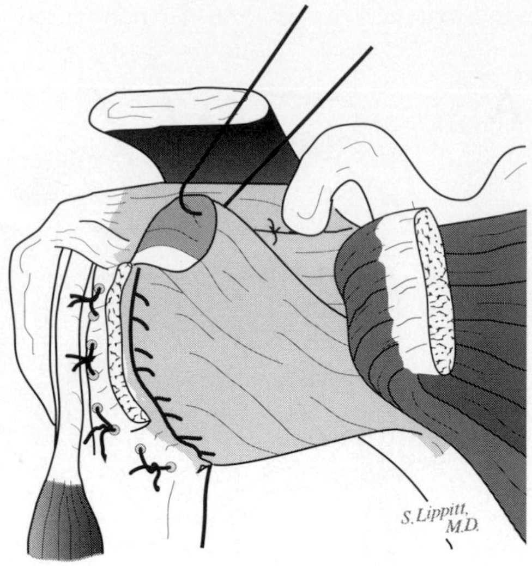

Figure 14–199

Tying the sutures fixes the advanced capsule to the groove. (From Matsen FA III, Lippitt SB, Sidles JA, and Harryman DT II: Practical Evaluation and Management of the Shoulder. Philadelphia: WB Saunders, 1994.)

Excessive translation on the sulcus test indicates that the rotator interval capsule was insufficiently tightened. Excessive limitation of external rotation indicates that the anterior capsule was tightened too much.

The subscapularis is then repaired to its normal anatomic insertion. After a standard wound closure, the arm is placed in a prefitted "handshake" orthosis (see Fig. 14–117) or cast (see Fig. 14–116) with the arm in neutral rotation and slight abduction.

With the arm in the orthosis or cast, the patient is started on grip strengthening, elbow range of motion, isometric external rotation, and isometric abduction shoulder exercises. Immobilization is usually continued for 1 month, although longer periods may be used for individuals who are extremely lax, and shorter periods may be used for individuals older than 25 years of age who may be prone to excessive stiffness.

The patient is then weaned from immobilization over a period of 1 week. During this time the patient is taught to elevate the arm in the plane of the scapula (the plane of maximal stability), to continue the cuff and deltoid strengthening, and to avoid any activities that may challenge the repair. From this point, range of motion is gained only with active exercises; no passive stretching is used. Lifting of more than 10 lb is delayed for 6 months. Sports are delayed for at least 1 year after surgery and are permitted only if the patient has excellent strength and dynamic control of the shoulder. The patient is asked

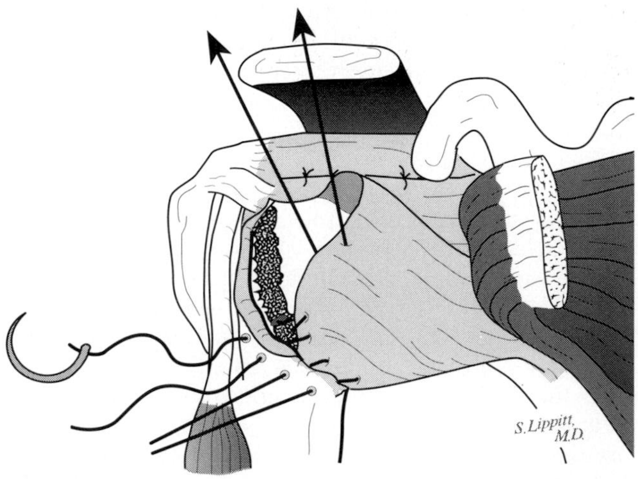

Figure 14–198

Sutures are placed through drill holes so that they exit the groove and pass through the advanced capsule and then back out through adjacent drill holes. (Modified from Matsen FA III, Lippitt SB, Sidles JA, and Harryman DT II: Practical Evaluation and Management of the Shoulder. Philadelphia: WB Saunders, 1994.)

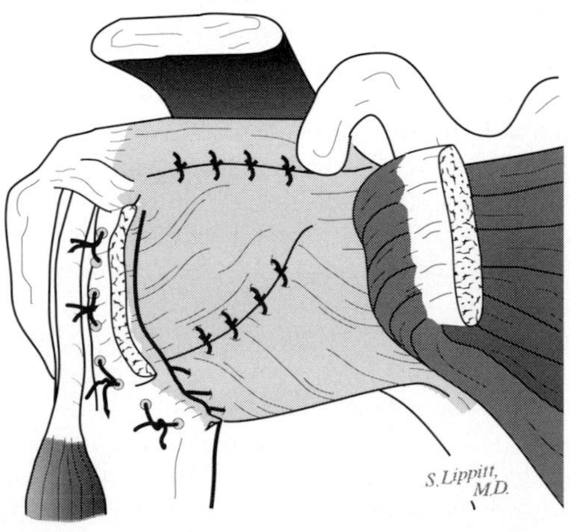

Figure 14–200

Any redundant anterosuperior capsule is folded down to reinforce the previous repair. (From Matsen FA III, Lippitt SB, Sidles JA, and Harryman DT II: Practical Evaluation and Management of the Shoulder. Philadelphia: WB Saunders, 1994.)

to learn and maintain the program for nonoperative management of glenohumeral instability.

ROCKWOOD'S APPROACH TO TREATMENT OF ATRAUMATIC AND MULTIDIRECTIONAL GLENOHUMERAL INSTABILITY

The treatment of patients with atraumatic instability requires that the physician differentiate between the voluntary and the involuntary types. Certainly, the patient with voluntary instability who has psychiatric problems should never be treated with surgery. Rowe and Yee[558] reported on disasters in patients with psychiatric problems who had been treated with surgical reconstructions. Patients with emotional disturbances and psychiatric problems should be referred for psychiatric help. Rowe and Yee also pointed out that there are patients with voluntary instability who do not have psychiatric problems who can be significantly helped with a rehabilitation program.

Consistent with this recommendation, we place all patients with atraumatic instability problems on a very specific rehabilitation program used to strengthen the three parts of the deltoid, the rotator cuff, and the scapular stabilizers. If the patient has an obvious psychiatric or emotional problem, we do our best to explain the problem to the patient and the family and help them to seek psychiatric help. Under no circumstances do we ever tell the patient or family that surgery is a possibility for the emotionally disturbed patient. When we have ruled out congenital or developmental causes for the instability problem, we personally teach the patient how to perform the shoulder-strengthening exercises and give him or her a copy of the exercise diagrams (see Fig. 14–146). We give the patient a set of TheraBands, which includes yellow, red, green, blue, and black bands, and the diagrams of the exercises to be performed. Each TheraBand is a strip 3 inches wide and 5 ft long that is tied into a loop. The loop can be fastened over a door knob or any fixed object to offer resistance to the pull. The patient does five basic exercises to strengthen the deltoid and the rotator cuff. The yellow TheraBand is the weakest and offers 1 lb of resistance; the red, 2 lb; the green, 3 lb; the blue, 4 lb; and, finally, the black offers 5 lb of resistance to the pull. The patient is instructed to do the five exercises two to three times a day. Each exercise should be performed five to ten times and each held for a count of five to ten. The patient is instructed to gradually increase the resistance (i.e., yellow to red and green, and so on) every 2 to 4 weeks. After the black TheraBand becomes easy to use, the patient is given a pulley kit and is instructed to do the same five basic exercises, but now lifting weights, as shown in Figure 14–146. The pulley kit consists of a pulley, an open eye screw hook, a handle, and a piece of rope, all in a plastic bag. The patient begins by attaching 7 to 10 lb of weight to the end of the rope and proceeds on to the five basic exercises. Gradually over several months, the patient increases the weights of resistance, up to 15 lb for women and 20 to 25 lb for men. When we start the basic strengthening of the rotator cuff and the deltoid, we also instruct the patient how to do the exercises to strengthen the scapular stabilizer muscles. The push-ups (i.e., wall push-ups, knee push-ups, and regular push-ups) are used to strengthen the serratus anterior, rhomboids, etc., and the shoulder-shrugging exercises are done to strengthen the trapezius muscles. We have learned that the rehabilitation program is 80% successful in managing anterior instability problems and 90% successful in managing the atraumatic posterior instability problems.[543] Regardless of any prior "rehabilitation program" that the patient has participated in, we always start the patient on our strengthening routine.

If the patient still has the signs and symptoms of instability after 6 months of doing the exercises, a very specific capsular shift procedure is performed. One must always remember that it is possible for a patient with laxity of the major joints to have a superimposed traumatic episode, which ordinarily does not respond to a rehabilitation program. A patient with atraumatic instability who has a history of significant trauma, pain, swelling, and so forth, probably will require a surgical reconstruction, but only after a trial with the rehabilitation program.

The details of the incision, surgical approach, protection of the axillary nerve, and preservation of the anterior humeral circumflex vessels are essentially the same as we use for the management of a recurrent traumatic anterior instability problem (Fig. 14–201). The main difference is noted after the capsule is opened and the surgeon notices that there is no Perthes-Bankart lesion. The deficiency is simply a very redundant capsule anteriorly, inferiorly, or posteroinferiorly. The principle of the capsular shift is to divide the capsule all the way down inferiorly, midway between its attachment on the humerus and on the glenoid rim. The joint is carefully inspected and then the shift is performed. As is demonstrated in Figure 14–183*P* and *Q*, we prefer to take the medial capsule superiorly and laterally under the lateral capsule, and then take the lateral capsule superiorly and medially over the medial capsule. We are careful that the placement and tying of the sutures are done with the arm in approximately 15 to 20 degrees of external rotation for an anterior reconstruction and in neutral rotation for a posterior reconstruction. Ordinarily, the subscapularis is simply repaired to itself, but if there is laxity of the subscapularis with the arm in 15 to 20 degrees of external rotation, then the subscapularis can be double-breasted. Ordinarily, in doing the posterior capsular shift, the infraspinatus tendon can be reflected superiorly and the teres minor reflected inferiorly off the posterior capsule. As with the anterior shift, the posterior capsule is divided midway between its attachments, thus allowing a double-breasting or strengthening of the midportion of the capsule. The reader must remember, however, that posterior shifts are rarely required because most patients do so well with the rehabilitation program.

The surgical management of patients with atraumatic instability demands that the shoulder not be put up too tight, as can be done with the Magnuson-Stack, Putti-Platt, or Bristow procedure. If the surgeon fails to recognize that the patient has an atraumatic instability problem, and if a routine muscle-tightening procedure is performed, the result may be that the humeral head will be pushed out in the opposite direction. The surgeon must also be careful, even in patients with atraumatic instabil-

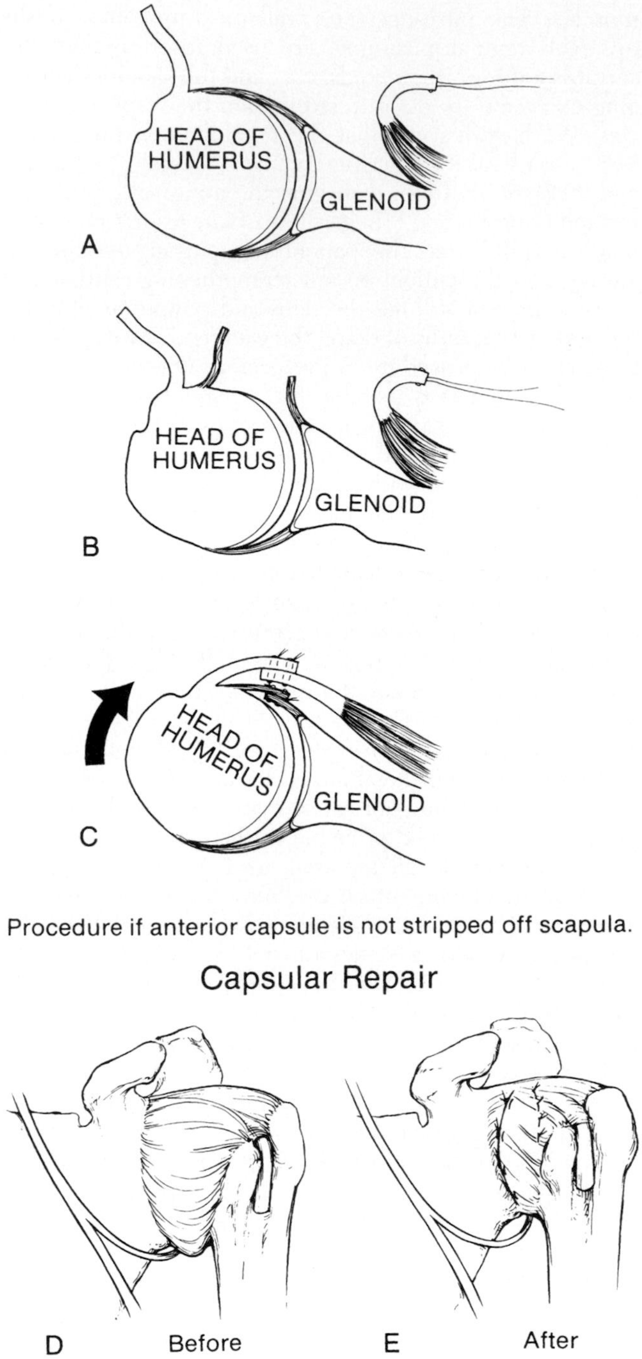

Figure 14–201

Capsular shift reconstruction for atraumatic anterior subluxation or dislocation. The Bankart-Perthes lesion is not present, and the capsule is shifted to eliminate the anterior inferior laxity.

ity, not to perform a capsular shift that is so tight as to force the head out in the opposite direction. As mentioned, we prefer to place and tie the sutures in the anterior capsular shift procedure with the arm in 15 to 20 degrees of external rotation and held in neutral rotation during the posterior capsular shift reconstruction. The reader must also be warned that it is essential to isolate and protect the axillary nerve when doing the anterior or posterior capsular shift.

Arthroscopic Repair of Atraumatic Instability

Arthroscopists have described redundancy in shoulders with atraumatic instability.[127, 137, 626, 634, 635] Methods for intra-articular plication, shifting, and suturing the capsule or actually shrinking the redundant tissue using thermal energy have been reported.[137, 159, 220, 223, 390]

In the laboratory, Lippitt and associates and Lazarus and co-workers have documented the essential stabilizing effect of the glenoid labrum with increased stability rations.[349, 369] Arthroscopic examination of shoulders with atraumatic instability frequently reveal insufficient posterior and inferior labral tissue. Snyder, Wolf, and Harryman have relied on this principle clinically and coupled capsular reduction in volume to augment the depth of the glenoid and reduce laxity simultaneously.[223] This procedure has been called arthroscopic capsular plication and capsulolabral augmentation.

Harryman, Pond, Metcalf, Smith, and Sidles have quantitated the effect of arthroscopic posterior-inferior capsulolabral reconstruction in six cadavers. Although the shoulders were elderly, these investigators were able to demonstrate substantial increases in the glenoid depth (Fig. 14–202) and in the stability ratios (Fig. 14–203).

Reports in the literature of arthroscopic management for atraumatic instability have been few and preliminary. Tauro and Carter described a modification of the arthroscopic Bankart repair that includes an inferior capsular split and shift to remove capsular redundancy for patients with anterior instability associated inferior laxity.[626] Duncan and Savoie reported on 10 consecutive patients with involuntary multidirectional instability who were managed by an arthroscopic modification of the inferior capsular shift procedure using the Caspari suture punch.[137] All of their patients had a satisfactory result according to Neer's outcome scoring.

Early studies, which mixed atraumatic and traumatized shoulders, attempted to address posterior and multidirectional instability arthroscopically using a staple to shift and repair the capsule.[127, 634, 635] Detrisac and Johnson reported a 12% failure rate attributing problems to inadequate immobilization, a lack of sufficient posterior capsule, and the presence of a metal staple. Tibone and associates also used a metal staple in 40 athletes with posterior instability.[634, 635] They reported a 40% failure rate and a high number of complications that were attributed to ligamentous laxity and unrecognized and untreated multidirectional instability. They found that the higher the competitive level of athlete, the worse was the overall result. They concluded that staple capsulorrhaphy was not acceptable treatment for posterior instability of the shoulder.

At the University of Washington, Harryman has enrolled patients in a prospective study after having failed a thorough nonoperative treatment course for functionally incapacitating atraumatic instability. All patients were treated with: (1) education regarding activities to be avoided, and (2) a conditioning exercise program of rotator cuff and periscapular muscle strengthening.[394] Patients met specific diagnostic criteria. The operative goals were to stabilize the glenohumeral joint by removing capsular redundancy, effectively deepened the glenoid concavity

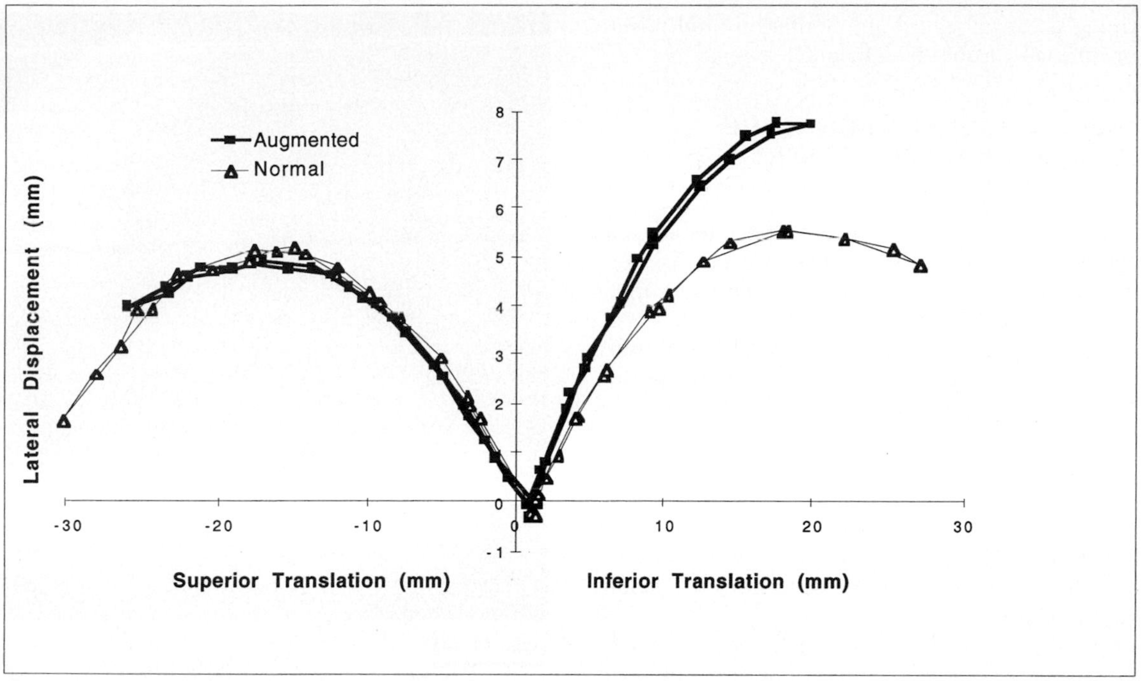

Figure 14–202

Glenoidograms indicate the path of the center of the humeral head as it is translated across the face of the glenoid in superiorly (left abscissa) and inferiorly (right abscissa). The height of the curves indicates the effective depth of the glenoid in the respective directions. Results are shown before (normal) and after (augmented) arthroscopic capsulolabral reconstruction, a procedure that increases the effective glenoid depth inferiorly.

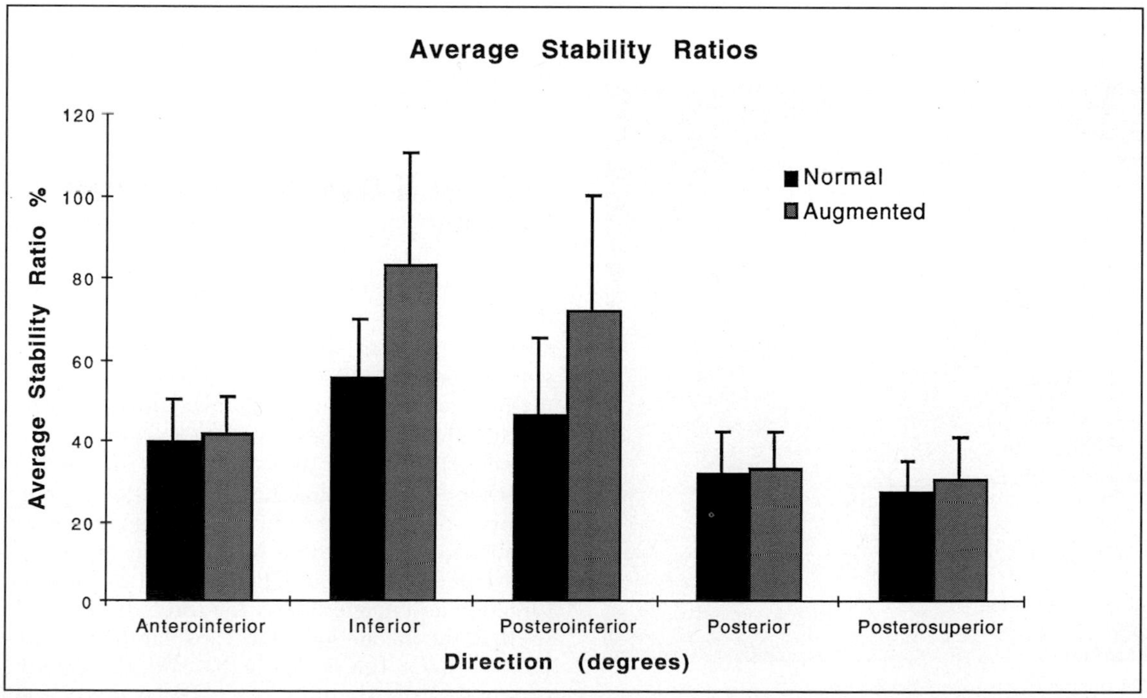

Figure 14–203

Stability ratios are the ratios of the force necessary to displace the head from the glenoid divided by the compressive load pressing the humeral head into the glenoid. These ratios are different for different directions of displacement due to differences in effective glenoid depth. This graph shows the variations in stability ratio for different directions of displacement in the intact cadaver shoulder (normal) as well as in the increment in inferior and posteroinferior stability ratios seen after arthroscopic posteroinferior capsulolabral reconstruction *(cross-hatched)*.

by performing a capsulolabral augmentation, and plicate the rotator interval capsule if deficient.

HARRYMAN'S SURGICAL TECHNIQUE FOR ARTHROSCOPIC ATRAUMATIC INSTABILITY REPAIR

Each shoulder was compared with the opposite side under anesthesia. All patients demonstrated a positive jerk test[396] with displacement either over the glenoid rim or frank dislocation posteroinferiorly.

Only a single anterior and posterior portal is necessary for scope and instrument access. Arthroscopic inspection revealed posterior and inferior labral flattening or rounding or a partial or complete detachment from the articular cartilage, but no anteroinferior labral detachments were found (Fig. 14–204). The synovium and capsule were typically redundant and partially stripped away from the labrum, resulting in a large posterior and inferior recess. Only three patients were found to have a deficient rotator interval capsule.

The peripheral rim of the glenoid labrum was roughened with a motorized shaver. Next, a suture hook was used to bring up approximately 1 cm of the inferior capsule in a posterosuperior direction to buttress the glenoid labrum. Additionally, the posterior and anterior capsule was shifted in a similar manner about the labrum. Five to nine sutures were placed through the capsule and between the deepest annular fibers of the glenoid labrum adjacent to the articular cartilage (Fig. 14–205). When necessary, rotator interval capsule plication was performed with a 30-degree straight suture hook by working within the subacromial space. Postoperative management must avoid capsular stretching and emphasize an early active rotator cuff, deltoid, and scapular strengthening program.

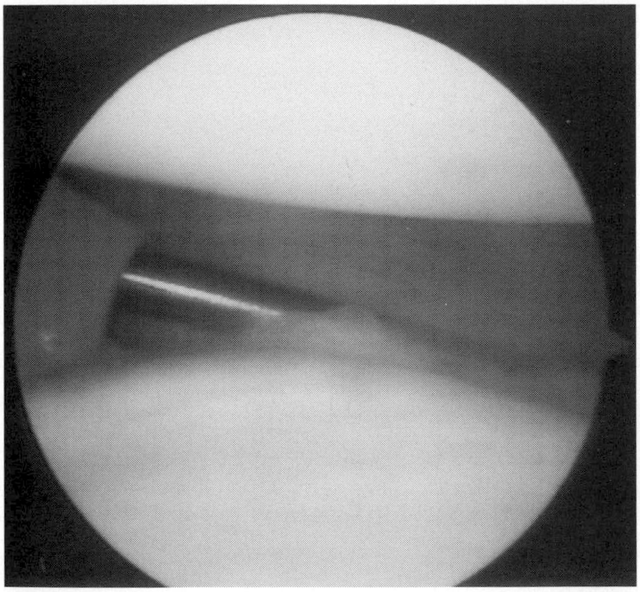

Figure 14–204

A shoulder with chronic posteroinferior atraumatic instability. Notice the synovial stripping adjacent to the labrum (glenoid on the bottom with flaps of synovium in the center) and the appearance of labral flattening to the right of center. The posteroinferior capsular recess is enlarged. (Courtesy of Douglas T. Harryman II, MD, Department of Orthopaedics, University of Washington.)

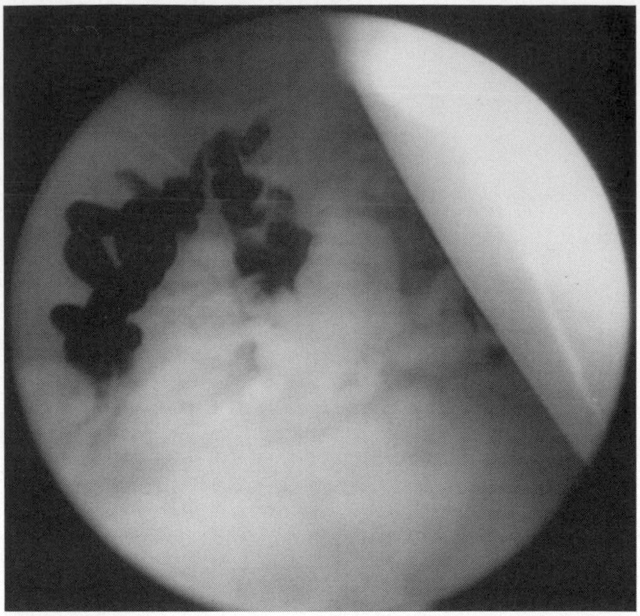

Figure 14–205

Posteroinferior capsulolabral augmentation. Notice how the capsule is bunched up and attached to the peripheral annual fibers of the labrum to increase the glenoid depth and reduce the capsular redundancy. (Courtesy of Douglas T. Harryman II, MD, Department of Orthopaedics, University of Washington.)

Twenty patients with a mean follow-up of 21 months (range of 12 to 52) are included in this review. At present, two patients (who had failed a previous open instability repair) developed recurrent instability (10%); no primary repairs have failed to date.

Treatment of Other Types of Recurrent Instability

The AMBRII and TUBS syndromes represent clearly defined clinical pathologic entities, each of which has specific diagnostic features and treatment strategies. Together, they comprise the great majority of patients who present with glenohumeral instability. Patients who do not fit into one of these two categories have highly individualized problems and cannot be grouped effectively together. When evaluating these patients, a meticulous history and physical examination take on even greater importance. When there has been an initiating injury, it is essential to determine the position of the arm and the direction and magnitude of the force producing the injury so that the likelihood of a capsular tear can be determined. Unless this is clearly the case, the default assumption is that the shoulder has become dysfunctional without a substantial anatomic lesion and therefore needs to be managed with a rehabilitative approach emphasizing strength, balance, endurance, and good technique. Unless a functionally significant instability can be determined on history and physical examination, the emphasis on

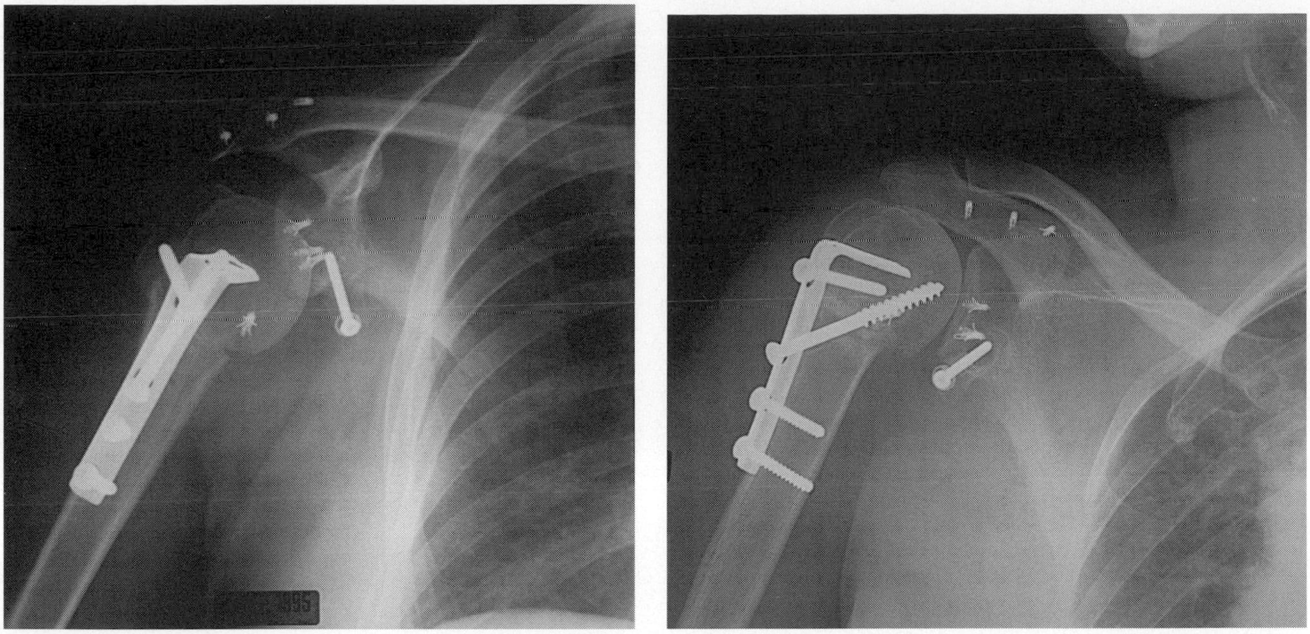

Figures 14–206 and 14–207

Radiographs of a shoulder with continued instability after five operations, including a capsular shift, a Bristow procedure, and a rotational osteotomy.

rehabilitation must continue. When the history and physical examination do not indicate the nature of the functional instability "studies" (e.g., contrast CT, MRI), examination under anesthesia and arthroscopy are unlikely to be helpful in determining the treatment. "Findings" on these tests, such as "increased translation," "increased laxity," "a large axillary pouch," or "labral fraying" may be identified even in functionally normal shoulders and as such may have no relation to the patient's functional problem. The risk, therefore, is that findings on these tests may distract the clinician from findings on history and physical examination. Unless the functional instability can be rigorously characterized by the history and physical examination, it is unlikely that surgical treatment will be curative.

In summary, the history and physical examination constitute the most efficient and cost-effective mechanisms for identifying treatable problems of glenohumeral instability. When these clinical tools do not clearly define the nature of the patient's functional problem, management by techniques other than physical rehabilitation and activity modification are unlikely to be effective. Using this approach, use of expensive diagnostic approaches is reduced to a minimum and surgery is reserved for those who can most benefit from it. This highly selective approach improves the overall results of surgical treatment of instability by helping to minimize the situations where an operation fails to restore the patient's function (Figs. 14–206 and 14–207).

References and Bibliography

1. Adams F: The Genuine Works of Hippocrates, Vol. 2. New York: William Woods, 1891.
2. Adams FL: The Genuine Works of Hippocrates, Vols. 1 and 2. New York: William Wood, 1886.
3. Adams JC: Recurrent dislocation of the shoulder. J Bone Joint Surg *30B*:26, 1948.
4. Adams JC: The humeral head defect in recurrent anterior dislocations of the shoulder. Br J Radiol 23:151–156, 1950.
5. Ahlgren O, Lorentzon R, and Larsson SE: Posterior dislocation of the shoulder associated with general seizures. Acta Orthop Scand 52:694–695, 1981.
6. Ahlgren SA, Hedlund T, and Nistor L: Idiopathic posterior instability of the shoulder joint. Acta Orthop Scand *49*:600–603, 1978.
7. Albert E: Arthodese bei einer Habituellen Luxation der Schultergelenkes. Klin Rundschau 2:281–283, 1898.
8. Altchek DW, Warren RF, Skyhar MJ, and Ortiz G: T-plasty modification of the Bankart procedure for multidirectional instability of the anterior and inferior types. J Bone Joint Surg Am *73*:105–112, 1991.
9. Anderson D, Zvirbulis R, and Ciullo J: Scapular manipulation for reduction of anterior shoulder dislocations. Clin Orthop *164*:181–183, 1982.
10. Anderson L, Rush R, Sherer L, and Highes CJ: The effects of a TheraBand exercise program on shoulder internal rotation strength. Phys Ther (Suppl)72:S40, 1992.
11. Andrews J, Carson WCM, and Hughston JC: Operative Shoulder Arthroscopy. Homestead, VA: American Orthopaedics Association, 1983.
12. Angelo RN and Hawkins RJ: Osteoarthritis Following an Excessively Tight Putti-Platt Repair. American Shoulder and Elbow Surgeons 4th Open Meeting, Atlanta, GA, 1988.
13. Antal CS, Conforty B, and Engelberg M: Injuries to the axillary due to anterior dislocation of the shoulder. J Trauma *13*:564, 1973.
14. Arciero RA: Arthroscopic Stabilization of Initial Anterior Shoulder Dislocations. Presented at the American Academy of Orthopaedic Surgeons Specialty Day, Arthroscopy Association of North America, New Orleans, LA, 1994.
15. Arciero RA: Arthroscopic Stabilization of Acute, Initial Anterior Shoulder Dislocation in Current Techniques in Arthroscopy, 2nd ed. New York: Churchill Livingstone, 1996, pp 117–124.
16. Arciero RA, Taylor DC, Snyder RJ, and Uhorchak JM: Arthroscopic bioabsorbable tack stabilization of initial anterior shoulder dislocations: A preliminary report. Arthroscopy *11*:410–417, 1995.
17. Arciero RA, Wheeler JH, Ryan JB, and McBride JT: Arthroscopic Bankart repair vs. nonoperative treatment for acute, initial, anterior shoulder dislocations. Am J Sports Med *22*:589–594, 1994.
18. Aronen JG and Regan K: Decreasing the incidence of recurrence of first time anterior shoulder dislocations with rehabilitation. Am J Sports Med *12*:283–291, 1984.

19. Artz T and Huffer JM: A major complication of the modified Bristow procedure for recurrent dislocation of the shoulder: A case report. J Bone Joint Surg *54A*:1293–1296, 1972.
20. Assmus H and Meinel A: Schulterverletzung und Axillarparese. Hefte Unfallheilkd *79*:183–187, 1976.
21. Aston JW and Gregory CF: Dislocation of the shoulder with significant fracture of the glenoid. J Bone Joint Surg *55A*:1531–1533, 1973.
22. Atwater AE: Biomechanics of overarm throwing movements and of throwing injuries. Exerc Sports Sci Rev *71*:43–85, 1980.
23. Badgley CE and O'Connor GA: Combined procedure for the repair of recurrent anterior dislocation of the shoulder. J Bone Joint Surg *47A*:1283, 1965.
24. Bailey PL and Stanley TH: Pharmacology of the intravenous narcotic anesthetics. *In* Miller R (ed): Anesthesia. New York: Churchill Livingstone, pp 745–797, 1986.
25. Bailey RW: Acute and recurrent dislocation of the shoulder. Instr Course Lect *18*:70–74, 1962–1969.
26. Baker CL, Uribe JW, and Whitman C: Arthroscopic evaluation of acute initial anterior shoulder dislocations. Am J Sports Med *18*:25–28, 1990.
27. Banas MP, Dalldorf PG, Sebastianelli WJ, and DeHaven KE: Long-term followup of the modified Bristow procedure (see comments). Am J Sports Med *21*:666–671, 1993.
28. Bankart ASB: Recurrent or habitual dislocation of the shoulder joint. BMJ *2*:1132–1133, 1923.
29. Bankart ASB: The pathology and treatment of recurrent dislocation of the shoulder joint. Br J Surg *26*:23–29, 1938.
30. Bankart ASB: The pathology and treatment of recurrent dislocation of the shoulder joint. Br J Surg *26*:23–29, 1939.
31. Baratta JB, Lim V, Mastromonaco E, and Edillon E: Axillary artery disruption secondary to anterior dislocation of the shoulder. J Trauma *23*:1009–1011, 1983.
32. Bardenheuer BA: Die Verletzungen Der Oberen Extremitaten. Dtsch Chir *63*:268–418, 1886.
33. Barrett J: The clavicular joints. Physiotherapy *57*:268–269, 1971.
34. Basmajian JV and Bazant FJ: Factors preventing downward dislocation of the adducted shoulder joint. J Bone Joint Surg Am *41*:1182–1186, 1959.
35. Basmajian JV and DeLuca CJ: Muscles Alive, 5th ed. Baltimore: Williams & Wilkins, 1985, pp 270–271.
36. Bassett RW, Browne AO, Morrey BF, and An KN: Glenohumeral muscle force and moment mechanics in a position of shoulder instability. J Biomech *23*:405–415, 1990.
37. Bateman JE: Gallie technique for repair of recurrent dislocation of the shoulder. Surg Clin North Am *43*:1655–1662, 1963.
38. Bayley JIL and Kessel L: Posterior dislocation of the shoulder: The clinical spectrum. J Bone Joint Surg *60B*:440, 1978.
39. Beattie TF, Steedman DJ, McGowan A, and Robertson CE: A comparison of the Milch and Kochner techniques for acute anterior dislocation of the shoulder. Injury *17*:349–352, 1986.
40. Benechetrit E and Friedman B: Fracture of the coracoid process associated with subglenoid dislocation of the shoulder. J Bone Joint Surg *61A*:295–296, 1979.
41. Benedetto KP and Glotzer W: Arthroscopic Bankart procedure by suture technique: Indications, technique, and results. Arthroscopy *8*:111–5, 1992.
42. Bennett GE: Old dislocations of the shoulder. J Bone Joint Surg *18*:594–606, 1936.
43. Berg EE and Ellison AE: The inside-out Bankart procedure. Am J Sports Med *18*:129–133, 1990.
44. Bertrand JC, Maestro M, Pequignot JP, and Moviel J: Les complications vasculaires des luxations artérieures fermes de l'épaule. Ann Chir *36*:329–333, 1981.
45. Bestard EA: Glenoplasty: A simple reliable method of correcting recurrent posterior dislocation of the shoulder. Orthop Rev *5*:29–34, 1976.
46. Bigliani LU, Pollock RG, McIlveen SJ, et al: Shift of the posteroinferior aspect of the capsule for recurrent posterior glenohumeral instability. J Bone Joint Surg *77*:1011–1020, 1995.
47. Bigliani LU, Pollock RG, Soslowsky LJ, et al: Tensile properties of the inferior glenohumeral ligament. J Orthop Res *10*:187–197, 1992.
48. Bigliani LU, Weinstein DM, Glasgow MT, et al: Glenohumeral arthroplasty for arthritis after instability surgery. J Shoulder Elbow Surg *4*:87–94, 1995.
49. Blasier RB, Carpenter JE, and Huston LJ: Shoulder proprioception: Effect of joint laxity, joint position, and direction of motion. Orthop Rev *23*:45–50, 1994.
50. Blasier RB, Guldberg RE, and Rothman ED: Anterior shoulder stability: Contributions of rotator cuff forces and the capsular ligaments in a cadaver model. J Shoulder Elbow Surg *1*:140–150, 1992.
51. Blazina ME and Satzman JS: Recurrent anterior subluxation of the shoulder in athletes—a distinct entity. J Bone Joint Surg *51A*:1037–1038, 1969.
52. Blom S and Dahlback LO: Nerve injuries in dislocations of the shoulder joint and fractures of the neck of the humerus. Acta Chir Scand *136*:461–466, 1970.
53. Bloom MH and Obata WG: Diagnosis of posterior dislocation of the shoulder with use of Velpeau axillary and angle-up roentgenographic views. J Bone Joint Surg *49A*:943–949, 1967.
54. Bodey WN and Denham RA: A free bone block operation for recurrent anterior dislocation of the shoulder joint. Injury *15*:184, 1983.
55. Bonnin JG: Transplantation of the tip of the coracoid process for recurrent anterior dislocation of the shoulder. J Bone Joint Surg *51B*:579, 1969.
56. Bonnin JG: Transplantation of the coracoid tip: A definitive operation for recurrent anterior dislocation of the shoulder. R Soc Med *66*:755–758, 1973.
57. Boyd HB and Sisk TD: Recurrent posterior dislocation of the shoulder. J Bone Joint Surg *54A*:779, 1972.
58. Boytchev B: Treatment of recurrent shoulder instability. Minerva Orthop *2*:377–379, 1951.
59. Boytchev B, Conforty B, and Tchokanov K: Operatiunaya Ortopediya y Travatologiya. Meditsina y Fizkultura, 2nd ed. Sofia, 1962.
60. Bradley JP and Tibone JE: Electromyographic analysis of muscle action about the shoulder. Clin Sports Med *10*:789–805, 1991.
61. Braly WG and Tullos HS: A modification of the Bristow procedure for recurrent anterior shoulder dislocation and subluxation. Am J Sports Med *13*:81, 1985.
62. Braunstein EM and O'Conner G: Double-contrast arthrotomography and the shoulder. J Bone Joint Surg *64A*:192–195, 1982.
63. Brav EA: Ten years' experience with Putti-Platt reconstruction procedure. Am J Surg *100*:423–430, 1960.
64. Brewer BJ, Wubben RC, and Carrera GF: Excessive retroversion of the glenoid cavity: A cause of non-traumatic posterior instability of the shoulder. J Bone Joint Surg *68*:724–731, 1986.
65. Bridle SH and Ferris BD: Irreducible acute anterior dislocations of the shoulder: Interposed scapularis. J Bone Joint Surg *72B*:1078–1079, 1990.
66. Broca A and Hartmann H: Contribution a l'étude des luxations de l'épaule. Bull Soc Anat Paris *4*:312–336, 1890.
67. Brockbank W and Griffiths DL: Orthopaedic surgery in the 16th and 17th centuries. J Bone Joint Surg *30B*:365–375, 1948.
68. Brostrom LA, Kronberg M, Nemeth G, and Oxelback U: The effect of shoulder muscle training in patients with recurrent shoulder dislocations. Scand J Rehab Med *24*:11–15, 1992.
69. Brown FW and Navigato WJ: Rupture of the axillary artery and brachial plexus palsy associated with anterior dislocation of the shoulder—report of a case with successful vascular repair. Clin Orthop *60*:195–199, 1968.
70. Brown JT: Nerve injuries complicating dislocation of the shoulder. J Bone Joint Surg *34B*:526, 1952.
71. Burkhead WZ and Rockwood CA Jr: Treatment of instability of the shoulder with an exercise program. J Bone Joint Surg Am *74*:890–896, 1992.
72. Butters KP, Curtis RJ, and Rockwood CA Jr: Posterior deltoid splitting shoulder approach. J Bone Joint Trans *11*:233, 1987.
73. Cain PR, Mitschler T, Fu FH, and Lee SK: Anterior stability of the glenohumeral joint: A dynamic model. Am J Sports Med *15*:144–148, 1987.
74. Caird FM: The shoulder joint in relation to certain dislocations and fractures. Edinb Med J *32*:708–714, 1887.
75. Calandra JJ, Baker CL, and Uribe J: The incidence of Hill-Sachs lesions in initial anterior shoulder dislocations. Arthroscopy *5*:254–257, 1989.
76. Calvet J, Leroy M, and Lacroix L: Luxations de l'épaule et lesions vasculaires. J Chir *58*:337–346, 1942.
77. Carew-McColl M: Bilateral shoulder dislocations caused by electrical shock. Br J Clin Prac *34*:251–254, 1980.

78. Carol EJ, Falke LM, Kortmann JH, et al: Bristow-Laterjet repair for recurrent anterior shoulder instability; an 8 year study. Neth J Surg *37*:109–113, 1985.
79. Carpenter GI and Millard PH: Shoulder subluxation in elderly inpatients. J Am Geriatr Soc *30*:441–446, 1982.
80. Caspari RB: Shoulder arthroscopy: A review of the present state of the art. Contemp Orthop *4*:523–531, 1982.
81. Caspari RB: Arthroscopic reconstruction for anterior shoulder instability. Tech Orthop *3*:59–66, 1988.
82. Caspari RB: Arthroscopic reconstruction of anterior shoulder instability. Fourth International Conference on Surgery of the Shoulder, New York, NY, 1989.
83. Cautilli RA, Joyce MF, and Mackell JV Jr: Posterior dislocation of the glenohumeral joint. Jefferson Orthop J *7*:15–20, 1978.
84. Cautilli RA, Joyce MF, and Mackell JV Jr: Posterior dislocations of the shoulder: A method of postreduction management. Am J Sports Med *6*:397–399, 1978.
85. Cave EF, Burke JF, and Boyd RJ: Trauma Management. Chicago: Year Book Medical Publishers, 1974, p 437.
86. Cayford EH and Tees FJ: Traumatic aneurysm of the subclavicular artery as a late complication of fractured clavicle. Can Med Assoc J *25*:450–452, 1931.
87. Chandnani VP, Yeager TD, DeBerardino T, et al: Glenoid labral tears: Prospective evaluation with MRI imaging, MR arthrography, and CT arthrography. Am J Roentgenol *161*:1229–1235, 1993 Dec.
88. Chen SK, Perry J, Jobe FW, et al: Elbow flexion analysis in Bristow patients: A preliminary report. Am J Sports Med *12*:347–350, 1984.
89. Clairmont P and Ehrlich H: Ein Neues Operations-Verfahren zur Behandlung der Habituellen Schulterluxation Mittels Muskelplastik. Verh Dtsch Ges Chir *38*:79–103, 1909.
90. Clark JM and Harryman DT II: Tendons, ligaments, and capsule of the rotator cuff. Gross and microscopic anatomy. J Bone Joint Surg Am *74*:713–725, 1992.
91. Clark JM, Sidles JA, and Matsen FA III: The relationship of the glenohumeral joint capsule to the rotator cuff. Clin Orthop *254*:29–34, 1990.
92. Clark KC: Positioning in Radiography, 2nd ed. London: William Heinemann, 1941.
93. Cleaves EN: A new film holder for roentgen examination of the shoulder. Am J Roentgenol Rad Ther Nucl Med *45*:288–290, 1941.
94. Clotteau JE, Premont M, and Mercier V: A simple procedure for reducing dislocations of the shoulder without anesthesia. Nouv Presse Med *11*:127–128, 1982.
95. Codman EA: Rupture of the Supraspinatus Tendon and Other Lesions In or About the Subacromial Bursa. Boston: Thomas Todd & Co, 1934.
96. Cofield RH: Physical examination of the shoulder: Effectiveness in assessing shoulder stability. *In* Matsen FA III, Fu F, and Hawkins R (eds): The Shoulder: A Balance of Mobility and Stability. Rosemont, IL: American Academy of Orthopaedic Surgeons, 1993, pp 331–344.
97. Cofield RH, Nessler JP, and Weinstabl R: Diagnosis of shoulder instability by examination under anesthesia. Clin Orthop *291*:45–53, 1993.
98. Collins HR and Wilde AH: Shoulder instability in athletes. Orthop Clin North Am *4*:759–773, 1973.
99. Collins KA, Capito C, and Cross M: The use of the Putti-Platt procedure in the treatment of recurrent anterior dislocation, with special reference to the young athlete. Am J Sport Med *14*:380–382, 1986.
100. Conforty B: The results of the Boytchev procedure for treatment of recurrent dislocation of the shoulder. Int Orthop *4*:127–132, 1980.
101. Cooper A: On the dislocation of the os humeri upon the dorsum scapula, and upon fractures near the shoulder joint. Guy's Hosp Rep *4*:265–284, 1839.
102. Cooper RA and Brems JJ: The inferior capsular-shift procedure for multidirectional instability of the shoulder. J Bone Joint Surg Am *74*:1516–1521, 1992.
103. Costigan PS, Binns MS, and Wallace WA: Undiagnosed bilateral anterior dislocation of the shoulder. Injury *21*:409, 1990.
104. Cotton FJ: Subluxation of the shoulder downward. Boston Med Surg J *185*:405–407, 1921.
105. Coughlin L, Rubinovich M, Johansson J, et al: Arthroscopic staple capsulorrhaphy for anterior shoulder instability. Am J Sports Med *20*:253–256, 1992.
106. Cramer F: Resection des Oberamkopfes wegen Habitueller Luxation (Nach einem im Arzlichen Verein zu Wiesbaden Gehaltenen Vortrage). Berl Klin Wochenschr *19*:21–25, 1882.
107. Cramer F, Von BM, and Kramps HA: CT diagnosis of recurrent subluxation of the shoulder. Fortschr Rontgenstr *136*:440–443, 1982.
108. Cranley JJ and Krause RF: Injury to the axillary artery following anterior dislocation of the shoulder. Am J Surg *95*:524–526, 1958.
109. Cuckler JM, Bearcroft J, and Asgian CM: Femoral head technologies to reduce polyethylene wear in total hip arthroplasty. Clin Orthop *317*:57–63, 1995.
110. Curr JF: Rupture of the axillary artery complicating dislocation of the shoulder. Report of a case. J Bone Joint Surg *52B*:313–317, 1970.
111. Cyprien JM, Vasey HM, and Burdet A: Humeral retrotorsion and glenohumeral relationship in the normal shoulder and in recurrent anterior dislocation. Clin Orthop *175*:8–17, 1983.
112. D'Angelo D: Luxacaorecidivante Anterior de Ombro. Rio de Janeiro: Brazil University of Rio de Janeiro, 1970.
113. Danzig LA, Greenway G, and Resnick D: The Hill-Sachs lesion: An experimental study. Am J Sports Med *8*:328–332, 1980.
114. Danzig LA, Resnick D, and Greenway G: Evaluation of unstable shoulders by computed tomography. Am J Sports Med *10*:138–141, 1982.
115. Das SP, Roy GS, and Saha AK: Observations on the tilt of the glenoid cavity of scapula. J Anat Soc India *15*:114, 1966.
116. de Laat EA, Visser CP, Coene LN, et al: Nerve lesions in primary shoulder dislocations and humeral neck fractures: A prospective clinical and EMG study. J Bone Joint Surg Br *76*:381–383, 1994.
117. Debevoise NT, Hyatt GW, and Townsend GB: Humeral torsion in recurrent shoulder dislocation. Clin Orthop *76*:87–93, 1971.
118. Delorme D: Die Hemmungsbander des Schultergelenks und ihre Bedeutung fur die Schulterluxationen. Arch Klin Chir *92*:79–101, 1910.
119. DePalma AF: Recurrent dislocation of the shoulder joint. Ann Surg *132*:1052–1065, 1950.
120. DePalma AF: Surgery of the Shoulder. Philadelphia: JB Lippincott, 1950.
121. DePalma AF: The Management of Fractures and Dislocations: An Atlas, Vol. 1, 2nd ed. Philadelphia: WB Saunders, 1970.
122. DePalma AF: Surgery of the Shoulder, 2nd ed. Philadelphia: JB Lippincott, 1973.
123. DePalma AF: Surgery of the Shoulder, 3rd ed. Philadelphia: JB Lippincott, 1983.
124. DePalma AF, Callery G, and Bennett GA: Variational anatomy and degenerative lesions of the shoulder joint, Vol 6. Ann Arbor: 1949, pp 255–281.
125. DePalma AF, Cooke AJ, and Prabhakar M: The role of the subscapularis in recurrent anterior dislocations of the shoulder. Clin Orthop *54*:35–49, 1967.
126. Detrisac DA: Arthroscopic Shoulder Staple Capsulorrhaphy for Traumatic Anterior Instability. New York: Raven Press, 1991.
127. Detrisac DA and Johnson LL: Arthroscopic shoulder capsulorrhaphy using metal staples. Orthop Clin North Am *24*:71–88, 1993.
128. Dias JJ, Mody BS, Finlay DB, and Richardson RA: Recurrent anterior glenohumeral joint dislocation and torsion of the humerus. J Orthop Sports Phys Ther *18*:379–385, 1993 July.
129. Dick W and Baumgartner R: Hypermobilitat und Wilkurliche Hintere Schulterluxation. Orthop Prax *16*:328–330, 1980.
130. Didiee J: Le radiodiagnostic dans la luxation récidivante de l'épaule. J Radiol Electrol *14*:209–218, 1930.
131. Doege KW: Irreducible shoulder joint dislocations. Lancet *49*:191–195, 1929.
132. Dolk T and Stenberg B: Arterial injury in fracture dislocation of the shoulder. Acta Orthop Scand *62*(Suppl 246):17, 1991.
133. Dorgan JA: Posterior dislocation of the shoulder. Am J Surg *89*:890–900, 1955.
134. Dowdy PA and O'Driscoll SW: Shoulder instability: An analysis of family history. J Bone Joint Surg Br *75*:782–784, 1993 Sept.
135. Dowdy PA and O'Driscoll SW: Recurrent anterior shoulder instability. Am J Sports Med *22*:489–492, 1994.
136. Drury JK and Scullion JE: Vascular complications of anterior dislocation of the shoulder. Br J Surg *67*:579–581, 1980.
137. Duncan R and Savoie FHD: Arthroscopic inferior capsular shift for multidirectional instability of the shoulder: A preliminary report. Arthroscopy *9*:24–7, 1993.

138. DuToit GT and Roux D: Recurrent dislocation of the shoulder: A 24 year study of the Johannesburg stapling operation. J Bone Joint Surg *38A*:1–12, 1956.
139. Eden R: Zur Operation der Habituellen Schulterluxation unter Mitteilung Eines Neuen Verfahrens bei Abriss am Inneren Pfannenrande. Dstch Ztschr Chir *144*:269, 1918.
140. Edwards DJ, Hoy G, Saies AD, and Hayes MG: Adverse reactions to an absorbable shoulder fixation device. J Shoulder Elbow Surg *3*:230–233, 1994.
141. Ehgartner K: Has the duration of cast fixation after shoulder dislocations had an influence on the frequency of recurrent dislocation? Arch Orthop Unfallchir *89*:187–190, 1977.
142. El-Khoury GY, Kathol MH, Chandler JB, and Albright JP: Shoulder instability: impact of glenohumeral arthrotomography on treatment. Radiology *160*:669–673, 1986.
143. Ellman H: Arthroscopic subacromial decompression: Analysis of one to three year results. Arthroscopy *3*:173–181, 1987.
144. Ellman H: Arthroscopic Subacromial Decompression: New Techniques and Result. Arthroscopy Association of North America, Instructional Course, 8th Annual Meeting, Seattle, WA, 1989.
145. Ellman H and Kay SP: Arthroscopic treatment of calcific tendinitis (Abstract). Orthop Trans *13*:240, 1989.
146. Emery RJ and Mullaji AB: Glenohumeral joint instability in normal adolescents. Incidence and significance. J Bone Joint Surg Br *73*:406–408, 1991.
147. Endo S, Kasai T, Fujii N, et al: Traumatic anterior dislocation of the shoulder in a child. Arch Orthop Trauma Surg *112*:201–202, 1993.
148. Engebretsen L and Craig EV: Radiologic features of shoulder instability. Clin Orthop *291*:29–44, 1993.
149. Engelhardt MB: Posterior dislocation of the shoulder: Report of six cases. South Med J *71*:425–427, 1978.
150. English E and Macnab I: Recurrent posterior dislocation of the shoulder. Can J Surg *17*:147–151, 1974.
151. Esch JC: Shoulder Arthroscopy: Treatment of Rotator Cuff Pathology. Arthroscopy Association of North American, Instructional Course, 8th Annual Meeting, Seattle, WA, 1989.
152. Esch JC, Ozerkis LR, Helgager JA, et al: Arthroscopic subacromial decompression: Results according to the degree of rotator cuff tear. Arthroscopy *4*:241–249, 1988.
153. Eve FS: A case of subcoracoid dislocation of the humerus with the formation of an indentation on the posterior surface of the head. Medico-Chirurg Trans Soc Lond *63*:317–321, 1880.
154. Eyre-Brook AL: The morbid anatomy of a case of recurrent dislocation of the shoulder. Br J Surg *29*:32–37, 1943.
155. Eyre-Brook AL: Recurrent dislocation of the shoulder: Lesions discovered in seventeen cases. Surgery employed, and intermediate report on results. J Bone Joint Surg *30B*:39, 1948.
156. Eyre-Brook AL: Recurrent dislocation of the shoulder. Physiotherapy *57*:7–13, 1971.
157. Fairbank HAT: Birth palsy: Subluxation of the shoulder joint in infants and young children. Lancet *1*:1217–1223, 1913.
158. Fairbank TJ: Fracture-subluxations of the shoulder. J Bone Joint Surg *30B*:454–460, 1948.
159. Fanton GS: Shoulder arthroscopy using the holmium-YAG laser method. State of the art 1994. Orthopade *25*:79–83, 1996.
160. Fee HJ, McAvoy JM, and Dainko EA: Pseudoaneurysm of the axillary artery following a modified Bristow operation: Report of a case and review. Cardiovasc Surg *19*:65, 1978.
161. Ferkel RD, Hedley AK, and Eckardt JJ: Anterior fracture-dislocations of the shoulder: Pitfalls in treatment. J Trauma *24*:363–367, 1984.
162. Ferlic DC and DeGiovine NM: A long-term retrospective study of the modified Bristow procedure. Am J Sports Med *16*:469–474, 1988.
163. Ferrari DA: Capsular ligaments of the shoulder: Anatomical and functional study of the anterior superior capsule. Am J Sports Med *18*:20–24, 1990.
164. Fick R: Handbuch der Anatomie und Mechanik der Gelenke unter Berucksichtigung der Bewegenden Muskeln. Jena: Fischer, 1904.
165. Finsterer H: Die operative behandlung der habituellen schulterluxation. Dtsch Ztschr Chir *141*:354–497, 1917.
166. Fipp GJ: Simultaneous posterior dislocation of both shoulders. Clin Orthop *44*:191–195, 1966.
167. Fitzgerald JF and Keates J: False aneurysm as a late complication of anterior dislocation of the shoulder. Ann Surg *181*:785–786, 1975.
168. Flatow EL, Raimondo RA, Kelkar R, et al: Active and Passive Restraints Against Superior Humeral Translation: The Contributions of the Rotator Cuff, the Biceps Tendon, and the Coracoacromial Arch. Presented at the Annual American Academy of Orthopaedic Surgeons meeting, Atlanta, GA, 1996.
169. Flower WH: On pathologic changes produced in the shoulder joint by traumatic dislocation. Trans Path Soc Lond *12*:179–200, 1861.
170. Frank CB: Ligament healing: Current knowledge and clinical applications. J Am Acad Orthop Surg *4*:74–83, 1996.
171. Franke GH: Dislocations of shoulder. Dtsch Ztschr Chir *48*:399, 1898.
172. Fredriksson AS and Tegner Y: Results of the Putti-Platt operation for recurrent anterior dislocation of the shoulder. Int Orthop (SICOT) *15*:185–188, 1991.
173. Friedman RJ: Glenohumeral capsulorrhaphy. *In* Matsen III FA, Fu FH, and Hawkins RJ (eds): The Shoulder: A Balance of Mobility and Stability. Rosemont, IL: American Academy of Orthopaedic Surgeons, 1993, pp 445–458.
174. Frizziero L, Zizzi F, and Facchini A: Arthroscopy of the shoulder joint: A review of 23 cases. Rheumatologie *11*:267–276, 1981.
175. Fu FH and Klein BS: Shoulder Arthroscopy: Complications and Pitfalls. Gaithersburg, MD: Aspen Publishers, 1991.
176. Gallie WE and LeMesurier AB: An operation for the relief of recurring dislocations of the shoulder. Trans Am Surg Assoc *45*:392–398, 1927.
177. Gallie WE and LeMesurier AB: Recurring dislocation of the shoulder. J Bone Joint Surg Br *30B*:9–18, 1948.
178. Ganel A, Horoszowski H, and Heim M: Persistent dislocation of the shoulder in elderly patients. J Am Geriatr Soc *28*:282–284, 1980.
179. Gardham JRC and Scott JE: Axillary artery occlusion with erect dislocation of the shoulder. Injury *11*:155–158, 1980.
180. Gardner E: The prenatal development of the human shoulder joint. Surg Clin North Am *43*:1465–1470, 1963.
181. Gariepy R, Derome A, and Laurin CA: Brachial plexus paralysis following shoulder dislocation. Can J Surg *5*:418–421, 1962.
182. Garneau RA, Renfrew DL, Moore TE, et al: Glenoid labrum: Evaluation with MR imaging. Radiology *179*:519–522, 1991.
183. Garth WP Jr, Allman FL, and Armstrong WS: Occult anterior subluxations of the shoulder in noncontact sports. Am J Sports Med *15*:579–585, 1987.
184. Garth WP Jr, Slappey CE, and Ochs CW: Roentgenographic demonstration of instability of the shoulder: The apical oblique projection. A technical note. J Bone Joint Surg *661*:1450–1453, 1984.
185. Gartsman GM: Arthroscopic acromioplasty for rotator cuff lesions. Unpublished paper, 1989.
186. Gartsman GM: Arthroscopic subacromialdecompression for advanced rotator cuff disease (Abstract). Orthop Trans *13*:240, 1989.
187. Gartsman GM, Blair M, Bennett JB, et al: Arthroscopic subacromial decompression: An anatomical study. Am J Sports Med *16*:48–50, 1988.
188. Geiger DF, Hurley JA, Tovey JA, and Rao JP: Results of Arthroscopic Versus Open Bankart Suture Repair. Presented at the American Academy of Orthopaedic Surgeons Specialty Day, San Francisco, CA, 1993.
189. Gerber C, Ganz R, and Vinh TS: Glenoplasty for recurrent posterior shoulder instability. Clin Orthop Rel Res *216*:70–79, 1987.
190. Ghormley RK, Black JR, and Cherry JH: Ununited fractures of the clavicle. Am J Surg *51*:343–349, 1941.
191. Gibb TD, Harryman DT II, Sidles JA, et al: The effect of capsular venting on glenohumeral laxity. Clin Orthop *268*:120–127, 1991.
192. Gibson JMC: Rupture of the axillary artery following anterior dislocation of the shoulder. J Bone Joint Surg *44B*:114–115, 1962.
193. Glessner JR: Intrathoracic dislocation of the humeral head. J Bone Joint Surg *42A*:428–430, 1961.
194. Gleyze P and Habermeyer P: Aspects arthroscopiques et évolution chronologique des lesions du complexe labro-ligamentaire dans l'instabilite antero-inférieure post-traumatique de l'épaule. Rev Chir Orthop *82*:288–298, 1996.
195. Glousman R, Jobe F, and Tibone J: Dynamic electromyographic analysis of the throwing shoulder with glenohumeral instability. J Bone Joint Surg *70A*:220–226, 1988.

196. Gohlke F, Schneider P, Siegel K, and Balzer C: Tensile strength of various anchor systems in surgical correction of instability of the shoulder joint. Unfallchirurg *96*:546–550, 1993.
197. Gold AM: Fractured neck of the humerus with separation and dislocation of the humeral head (fracture-dislocation of the shoulder, severe type). Bull Hosp Joint Dis *32*:87–99, 1971.
198. Goldberg BJ, Nirschl RP, McConnell JP, and Pettrone FA: Arthroscopic transglenoid suture capsulolabral repairs: preliminary results. Am J Sports Med *21*:656–664, 1993.
199. Gonzalez D and Lopez R: Concurrent rotator-cuff tear and brachial plexus palsy associated with anterior dislocation of the shoulder: A report of two cases. J Bone Joint Surg Am *73*:620–621, 1991.
200. Gosset J: Une technique de greffe coraco-glenordienne dans le traitement des luxations récidivantes de l'époule. Mem Acad Chir *86*:445–447, 1960.
201. Gould R, Rosenfield AT, and Friedlaender GE: Loose body within the glenohumeral joint in recurrent anterior dislocation: CT demonstration. J Comput Assist Tomogr *9*:404–405, 1985.
202. Grana WA, Buckley PD, and Yates CK: Arthroscopic Bankart suture repair. Am J Sports Med *21*:348–353, 1993.
203. Grant JCB: Grant's Atlas of Anatomy, 6th ed. Baltimore: Williams & Wilkins, 1972.
204. Grashey R: Atlas Typischer Rontgenfilder. 1923.
205. Grasshoff H, Buhtz C, Gellerich I, and von Knorre C: CT diagnosis in instability of the shoulder joint. Rofo Fortschr Geb Rontgenstr Neuen Bildgeb Verfahr *155*:523–526, 1991.
206. Green MR and Christensen KP: Arthroscopic versus open Bankart procedures: a comparison of early morbidity and complications. Arthroplasty 9:371–374, 1993.
207. Green MR and Christensen KP: Magnetic resonance imaging of the glenoid labrum in anterior shoulder instability. Am J Sports Med *22*:493–498, 1994.
208. Green MR and Christensen KP: Arthroscopic Bankart procedure: Two- to five-year followup with clinical correlation to severity of glenoid labral lesion. Am J Sports Med *23*:276–81, 1995.
209. Gross ML, Seeger LL, Smith JB, et al: Magnetic resonance imaging of the glenoid labrum. Am J Sports Med *18*:229–234, 1990.
210. Gross RM: Arthroscopic shoulder capsulorrhaphy: Does it work? Am J Sports Med *17*:495–500, 1989.
211. Guanche C, Knatt T, Solomonow M, et al: The synergistic action of the capsule and the shoulder muscles. Am J Sports Med *23*:301–306, 1995.
212. Gugenheim S and Sanders RJ: Axillary artery rupture caused by shoulder dislocation. Surgery *95*:55, 1984.
213. Guibe M: Des lesions des vaisseaux de l'aiselle qui compliquent les luxations de l'épaule. Rev Chir *4*:580–583, 1911.
214. Guilfoil PH and Christiansen T: An unusual vascular complication of fractured clavicle. JAMA *200*:72–73, 1967.
215. Ha'eri GB and Maitland A: Arthroscopy findings in the frozen shoulder. J Rheumatol *8*:149–152, 1981.
216. Haaker RG, Eickhoff U, and Klammer HL: Intraarticular autogenous bone grafting in recurrent shoulder dislocations. Mil Med *158*:164–169, 1993.
217. Habermeyer P and Schuller U: Significance of the glenoid labrum for stability of the glenohumeral joint: An experimental study. Unfallchirurg *93*:19–26, 1990.
218. Habermeyer P, Schuller U, and Wiedemann E: The intra-articular pressure of the shoulder: An experimental study on the role of the glenoid labrum in stabilizing the joint. J Arthroscopy *8*:166–172, 1992.
219. Hall RH, Isaac F, and Booth CR: Dislocations of the shoulder with special reference to accompanying small fractures. J Bone Joint Surg *41A*:489–494, 1959.
220. Hardy P, Thabit Gr, Fanton GS, et al: Arthroscopic management of recurrent anterior shoulder dislocation by combining a labrum suture with antero-inferior holmium: YAG laser capsular shrinkage. Orthopade *25*:91–3, 1996.
221. Harner CD and Fu FH: The Bankart lesion of the shoulder: A biochemical analysis following repair. Knee Surg Sports Traumatol Arthrosc *3*:117–120, 1995.
222. Harryman DT II: Common surgical approaches to the shoulder. *In* Eilert RE (ed): Instructional Course Lectures. Park Ridge, IL: American Academy of Orthopaedic Surgeons, 1992, pp 3–11.
223. Harryman DT II: Arthroscopic management of shoulder instability. Univ Washington Res Rep *1*:24–26, 1996.
224. Harryman DT II, Sidles JA, Clark JM, et al: Translation of the humeral head on the glenoid with passive glenohumeral motion. J Bone Joint Surg Am *72A*:1334–1343, 1990.
225. Harryman DT II, Sidles JA, Harris S, and Matsen FA III: The role of the rotator interval capsule in passive motion and stability of the shoulder. J Bone Joint Surg Am *74*:53–66, 1992.
226. Harryman DT II, Sidles JA, and Matsen FA III: Laxity of the normal glenohumeral joint: A quantitative in vivo assessment. J Shoulder Elbow Surg *1*:66–76, 1992.
227. Harryman DT II, Ballmer FP, Harris SL, and Sidles JA: Arthroscopic labral repair to the glenoid rim. J Arthroscopy *10*:20–30, 1994.
228. Harryman DT II, Lazarus MD, Sidles JA, and Matsen FA III: Pathophysiology of Shoulder Instability, Vol 2. McGinty JB (ed), 1996, pp 677–693.
229. Hashimoto T, Hamada T, Sasaguri Y, and Suzuki K: Immunohistochemical approach for the investigation of nerve distribution in the shoulder joint capsule. Clin Orthop *305*:273–282, 1994.
230. Hauser EDW: Avulsion of the tendon of the subscapularis muscle. J Bone Joint Surg *36A*:139–141, 1954.
231. Hawkins RB: Arthroscopic stapling repair for shoulder instability: A retrospective study of 50 cases. Arthroscopy *5*:122–128, 1989.
232. Hawkins RH and Hawkins RJ: Failed anterior reconstruction for shoulder instability. J Bone Joint Surg *67*:709–714, 1985.
233. Hawkins RJ and Angelo RL: Glenohumeral osteoarthritis: A late complication of the Putti-Platt repair. J Bone Joint Surg *72A*:1193–1197, 1990.
234. Hawkins RJ and Angelo RL: Glenohumeral osteoarthrosis: A late complication of the Putti-Platt repair. J Bone Joint Surg Am *72A*:1193–1197, 1990.
235. Hawkins RJ, Koppert G, and Johnston G: Recurrent posterior instability (subluxation) of the shoulder. J Bone Joint Surg *66A*:169, 1984.
236. Hawkins RJ and Mohtadi NGH: Controversy in anterior shoulder instability. Clin Orthop *272*:152–161, 1991.
237. Hawkins RJ, Neer CS II, Pianta R, and Mendoza FX: Missed posterior dislocations of the shoulder. Presented at the American Academy of Orthopaedic Surgery Annual Meeting, New Orleans, LA, 1982.
238. Hawkins RJ, Neer CS II, Pianta RM, and Mendoza FX: Locked posterior dislocation of the shoulder. J Bone Joint Surg *69A*:9, 1987.
239. Hecker AT, Shea M, Hayhurst JO, et al: Pull-out strength of suture anchors for rotator cuff and Barkart lesion repairs. Am J Sports Med *21*:874–879, 1993.
240. Hehne HJ and Hubner H: Die Behandlung der Rezidivieremden Schulterluxation nach Putti-Platt-Bankart und Eden-Hybinette-Lange. Orthop Prax *16*:331–335, 1980.
241. Helfet AJ: Coracoid transplantation for recurring dislocation of the shoulder. J Bone Joint Surg *40B*:198–202, 1958.
242. Heller KD, Forst J, Forst R, and Cohen B: Posterior dislocation of the shoulder. Arch Orthop Trauma Surg *113*:228–231, 1994.
243. Henderson MS: Habitual or recurrent dislocation of the shoulder. Surg Gynecol Obstet *33*:1–7, 1921.
244. Henderson MS: Tenosuspension operation for recurrent or habitual dislocation of the shoulder. Surg Clin North Am *5*:997–1007, 1949.
245. Henderson WD: Arthroscopic stabilization of the anterior shoulder. Clin Sports Med *6*:581–586, 1987.
246. Henry JH and Genung JA: Natural history of glenohumeral dislocation—revisited. Am J Sports Med *10*:135–137, 1982.
247. Henson GF: Vascular complications of shoulder injuries: A report of two cases. J Bone Joint Surg *38B*:528–531, 1956.
248. Hermodsson I: Rontgenologische Studein uber die Traumatischen und Habituellen Schultergelenk-Verrenkungen Nach Vorn und Nach Unten. Acta Radiol (Suppl) *20*:1–173, 1934.
249. Hertz H, Kwasny O, and Wohry G: Therapeutic procedure in initial traumatic shoulder dislocation (arthroscopy–limbus refixation). Unfallchirurgie *17*:76–79, 1991.
250. Hertz H, Weinstabl R, Grundschober F, and Orthner E: Macroscopic and microscopic anatomy of the shoulder joint and the limbus glenoidalis. Acta Anat (Basel) *125*:96–100, 1986.
251. Heymanowitsch Z: Ein beitrag zur operativen behandlung der habituellen schulterluxationen. Zentralbl Chir *54*:648–651, 1927.
252. Hildebrand: Zur operativen behandlung der habituellen schuterluxation. Arch Klin Chir *66*:360–364, 1902.

253. Hill HA and Sachs MD: The grooved defect of the humeral head. A frequently unrecognized complication of dislocations of the shoulder joint. Radiology *35*:690–700, 1940.
254. Hill JA, Lombardo SJ, Kerlan RK, et al: The modified Bristow-Helfet procedure for recurrent anterior shoulder subluxations and dislocations. Am J Sports Med *9*:283–287, 1981.
255. Hill NA and McLaughlin HL: Locked posterior dislocation simulating a "frozen shoulder." J Trauma *3*:225–234, 1963.
256. Hintermann B and Gachter A: Theo van Rens Prize. Arthroscopic assessment of the unstable shoulder. Knee Surg Sports Traumatol Arthrosc *2*:64–69, 1994.
257. Hippocrates: Works of Hippocrates with an English Translation. London: William Heinemann, 1927.
258. Hirakawa M: On the etiology of the loose shoulder-biochemical studies on collagen from joint capsules. Nippon Seikeigeka Gakkai Zasshi *65*:550–60, 1991.
259. Hirschfelder H and Kirsten U: Biometric analysis of the unstable shoulder. Z Orthop Ihre Grenzgeb *129*:516–520, 1991.
260. Honner R: Bilateral posterior dislocation of the shoulder. Aust N Z J Surg *38*:269–272, 1969.
261. Hovelius L: Incidence of shoulder dislocation in Sweden. Clin Orthop *166*:127–131, 1982.
262. Hovelius L: Anterior dislocation of the shoulder in teenagers and young adults. Five-year prognosis. J Bone Joint Surg *69A*:393, 1987.
263. Hovelius L, Akermark C, and Albrektsson B: Bristow-Latarjet procedure for recurrent anterior dislocation of the shoulder. Acta Orthop Scand *54*:284–290, 1983.
264. Hovelius L, Augustini BG, Fredin H, et al: Primary anterior dislocation of the shoulder in young patients. J Bone Joint Surg *78A*:1677–1684, 1996.
265. Hovelius L, Eriksson K, Fredin H, et al: Recurrences after initial dislocation of the shoulder. Results of a prospective study of treatment. J Bone Joint Surg *65A*:343–349, 1983.
266. Hovelius L, Malmqvist B, and Augustaini BG: Ten Year Prognosis of Primary Anterior Dislocation of the Shoulder in Young (Abstract 7). Presented at the 10th Open Meeting of the American Shoulder and Elbow Surgeons, New Orleans, 1994.
267. Hovelius L, Thorling J, and Fredin H: Recurrent anterior dislocation of the shoulder: Results after the Bankart and Putti-Platt operations. J Bone Joint Surg *61A*:566–569, 1979.
268. Howard FM and Shafer SJ: Injuries to the clavicle with neurovascular complications. J Bone Joint Surg *47A*:1335–1346, 1965.
269. Howell SM and Galinat BJ: The glenoid-labral socket: A constrained articular surface. Clin Orthop *43*:122–125, 1989.
270. Howell SM, Galinat BJ, Renzi AJ, and Marone PJ: Normal and abnormal mechanics of the glenohumeral joint in the horizontal plane. J Bone Joint Surg *70A*:227–232, 1988.
271. Huber H and Gerber C: Voluntary subluxation of the shoulder in children. J Bone Joint Surg *76B*:118–1220, 1994.
272. Hummel A, Bethke RO, and Kempf L: Die behandlung der habituellen schulterluxation nach dem Bristow-Verfahren. Unfallheikunde *85*:482–484, 1982.
273. Humphry GM: A Treatise on the Human Skeleton (Including the Joints), Vol 410. London: Macmillan, 1858, pp 73–74.
274. Hurley JA, Anderson TE, Dear WA, et al: Posterior shoulder instability. Surgical versus conservative results with evaluation of glenoid version. Am J Sports Med *20*:396–400, 1992.
275. Hussein MK: Kocher's method is 3,000 years old. J Bone Joint Surg *50B*:669–671, 1968.
276. Hybbinette S: De la transplantation d'un fragment osseux pour remedier aux luxations récidivantes de l'épaule; constations et résultats operatoires. Acta Chir Scand *71*:411–445, 1932.
277. Iannotti JP, Zlatkin MB, Esterhai JL, et al: Magnetic resonance imaging of the shoulder. Sensitivity, specificity, and predictive value. J Bone Joint Surg Am *73*:17–29, 1991.
278. Imazato Y: Etiological considerations of the loose shoulder from a biochemical point of view—biochemical studies on collagen from deltoid and pectoral muscles and skin. Nippon Seikeigeka Gakkai Zasshi *66*:1006–1015, 1992.
279. Inao S, Hirayama T, and Takemitsu Y: Irreducible acute anterior dislocation of the shoulder: Interposed bicipital tendon. J Bone Joint Surg *72B*:1079–1080, 1990.
280. Inman VT, Saunders JB, and Abbott LC: Observations on the function of the shoulder joint. J Bone Joint Surg *26*:1–30, 1994.
281. Itoi E, Motzkin NE, Morrey BP, and An KN: Scapular inclination and inferior stability of the shoulder. J Shoulder Elbow Surg *1*:131–139, 1992.
282. Itoi E, Newman SR, Kuechle DK, et al: Dynamic anterior stabilizers of the shoulder with the arm in abduction. J Bone Joint Surg *76B*:834–836, 1994.
283. Itoi E, Kuechle DK, Newman SR, et al: Stabilizing function of the biceps in stable and unstable shoulders. J Bone Joint Surg Br *75*:546–550, 1993.
284. Itoi E, Motzkin NE, Morrey BF, and An K: Bulk effect of rotator cuff on inferior glenohumeral stability as function of scapular inclination angle: A cadaver study. Tohoku J Exp Med *171*:267–276, 1993.
285. Itoi E and Tabata S: Rotator cuff tears in anterior dislocation of the shoulder. Int Orthop (SICOT) *16*:240–244, 1992.
286. Itoi EA, Motzkin NE, Browne AO, et al: Intraarticular pressure of the shoulder. Arthroscopy *9*:406–413, 1993.
287. Janecki CJ and Shahcheragh GH: The forward elevation maneuver for reduction of anterior dislocations of the shoulder. Clin Orthop *164*:177–180, 1982.
288. Jardon OM, Hood LT, and Lynch RD: Complete avulsion of the axillary artery as a complication of shoulder dislocation. J Bone Joint Surg *55*:189, 1973.
289. Jens J: The role of the subscapularis muscle in recurring dislocation of the shoulder (Abstract). J Bone Joint Surg *34B*:780, 1964.
290. Jerosch J, Castro WH, Grosse-Hackman A, and Clahsen H: Function of the glenohumeral ligaments in active protection of shoulder stability. Z Orthop Ihre Grenzgeb *133*:67–71, 1995.
291. Jerosch J, Goertzen M, and Marquardt M: Possibilities of diagnostic sonography in assessment of instability of the shoulder joint. Unfallchirurg *94*:88–94, 1991.
292. Jerosch J, Marquardt M, and Winklemann W: Ultrasound documentation of translational movement of the shoulder joint: Normal values and pathologic findings. Ultraschall Med *12*:31–35, 1991.
293. Jerosch J, Moersler M, and Castro WH: The function of passive stabilizers of the glenohumeral joint—a biomechanical study. Z Orthop Ihre Grenzgeb *128*:206–212, 1990.
294. Jobe FW: Unstable shoulders in the athletes. Instr Course Lect *XXXIV*:228–231, 1985.
295. Jobe FW, Giangarra CE, Glousman RE, and Kvitne RS: Anterior capsulolabral reconstruction in throwing athletes (Abstracts). Orthop Trans *13*:230, 1989.
296. Jobe FW, Giangarra CE, Kvitne RS, and Glousman RE: Anterior capsulolabral reconstruction of the shoulder in athletes in overhand sports. Am J Sports Med *19*:428–434, 1991.
297. Jobe FW, Moynes DR, and Brewster CE: Rehabilitation of shoulder joint instabilities. Orthop Clin North Am *18*:473–482, 1987.
298. Jobe FW, Tibone JE, Perry J, and Moynes D: An EMG analysis of the shoulder in throwing and pitching. Am J Sports Med *11*:3–5, 1983.
299. Jobe FW and Zeman B: How to detect and manage an unstable shoulder. J Musculoskel Med *2*:60–68, 1985.
300. Joessel D: Ueber die recidine der humerus-luxationen. Dtsch Ztschr Chir *13*:167–184, 1880.
301. Johnson HF: Unreduced dislocation of the shoulder. Nebr State Med J *16*:220–224, 1931.
302. Johnson JR and Bayley JIL: Loss of shoulder function following acute anterior dislocation. J Bone Joint Surg *63B*:633, 1981.
303. Johnson JR and Bayley JIL: Early complications of acute anterior dislocation of the shoulder in the middle-aged and elderly patient. Injury *13*:431–434, 1982.
304. Johnson LL: Arthroscopy of the shoulder. Orthop Clin North Am *11*:197–204, 1980.
305. Johnson LL: Symposium: The Controversy of Arthroscopic Versus Open Approaches to Shoulder Instability and Rotator Cuff Disease: A New Perspective, a New Opportunity, a New Challenge. American Shoulder and Elbow Surgeons 4th Open Meeting, Atlanta, GA, 1988.
306. Johnson LL, Schneider DA, Austin MD, et al: Two percent glutaraldehyde: A disinfectant in arthroscopy and arthroscopic surgery. J Bone Joint Surg *64A*:237, 1982.
307. Johnston GW and Lowry JH: Rupture of the axillary artery complicating anterior dislocation of the shoulder. J Bone Joint Surg *44B*:116–118, 1962.
308. Jones FW: Attainment of upright position of man. Nature *146*:26–27, 1940.

309. Jordan H: New technique for the roentgen examination of the shoulder joint. Radiology *25*:480–484, 1935.
310. Jorgensen U and Bak K: Shoulder instability: Assessment of anterior-posterior translation with a knee laxity tester. Acta Orthop Scand *66*:398–400, 1995.
311. Kaltsas DS: Comparative study of the properties of the shoulder joint capsule with those of other joint capsules. Clin Orthop *173*:20–26, 1983.
312. Karadimas J, Rentis G, and Varouchas G: Repair of recurrent anterior dislocation of the shoulder using transfer of the subscapularis tendon. J Bone Joint Surg *62A*:1147–1149, 1980.
313. Karlsson D and Peterson B: Towards a model for force predictions in the human shoulder. J Biomech *25*:189–199, 1992.
314. Kavanaugh JH: Posterior shoulder dislocation with ipsilateral humeral shaft fracture. Clin Orthop *131*, 1978.
315. Kazar B and Relovszky E: Prognosis of primary dislocation of the shoulder. Acta Orthop Scand *40*:216, 1969.
316. Kelley JP: Fractures complicating electroconvulsive therapy and chronic epilepsy. J Bone Joint Surg *36B*:70–79, 1954.
317. Keppler P, Holz U, Thieleman FW, and Meinig R: Locked posterior dislocation of the shoulder. J Orthop Trauma *8*:286–292, 1994.
318. Kiett GJ, Bloem JL, Rozing PM, et al: MR Imaging of recurrent anterior dislocation of the shoulder: Comparison with CT arthrography. AJR Am J Roentgenol *150*:1083–1087, 1988.
319. Kinnard P, Gordon D, Levesque RY, and Bergeron D: Computerized arthrotomography in recurring shoulder dislocations and subluxations. Can J Surg *27*:487–488, 1984.
320. Kirker JR: Dislocation of the shoulder complicated by rupture of the axillary vessels. J Bone Joint Surg *34B*:72–73, 1952.
321. Kiviluoto O, Pasila M, Jaroma H, and Sundholm A: Immobilization after primary dislocation of the shoulder. Acta Orthop Scand *51*:915–919, 1980.
322. Kleinman PD, Kanzaria PK, Goss TP, and Pappas AM: Axillary arthrotomography of the glenoid labrum. AJR Am J Roentgenol *142*:993–999, 1984.
323. Kocher T: Eine neue reductions methode fur schulterverrenkung. Berl Klin *7*:101–105, 1870.
324. Koppert G and Hawkins RJ: Recurrent posterior dislocating shoulder. J Bone Joint Surg *62B*:127–128, 1980.
325. Kretzler HH: Posterior Glenoid Osteotomy. Dallas. TX: American Academy of Orthopaedic Surgeons Meeting, 1944.
326. Kretzler HH and Blue AR: Recurrent posterior dislocation of the shoulder in cerebral palsy. J Bone Joint Surg *48A*:1221, 1966.
327. Kronberg M and Brostrom LA: Humeral head retroversion in patients with unstable humeroscapular joints. Clin Orthop *260*:207–211, 1990.
328. Kronberg M, Brostrom LA, and Nemeth G: Differences in shoulder muscle activity between patients with generalized joint laxity and normal controls. Clin Orthop *269*:181–192, 1991.
329. Kubin Z: Luxatio humeri erecta: kasuisticke sdeleni. Acta Chir Orthop Traumatol Cech *31*:565, 1964.
330. Kuboyama M: The role of soft tissues in downward stability of the glenohumeral joint—an experimental study with fresh cadavers. Igaku Kenkyu *61*:20–33, 1991.
331. Kuhnen W and Groves RJ: Irreducible acute anterior dislocation of the shoulder: Case report. Clin Orthop *139*:167–168, 1979.
332. Kumar VP and Balasubramaniam P: The role of atmospheric pressure in stabilizing the shoulder. J Bone Joint Surg Br *67*:719–721, 1985.
333. Kumar VP and Balasubramaniam P: The role of atmospheric pressure in stabilizing the shoulder. An experimental study. J Bone Joint Surg Br *67*:719–721, 1985.
334. Kuster E: Ueber Habituelle Schulter Luxation. Verh Dtsch Ges Chir *11*:112–114, 1882.
335. L'Episcopo JB: Restoration of muscle balance in the treatment of obstetrical paralysis. N Y J Med *39*:357–363, 1939.
336. Lacey T II: Reduction of anterior dislocation of the shoulder by means of the Milch abduction technique. J Bone Joint Surg *34A*:108–109, 1952.
337. Lam SAS: Irreducible anterior dislocation of the shoulder. J Bone Joint Surg *48B*:132, 1966.
338. Lamm CR, Zaehrisson BE, and Korner L: Radiography of the shoulder after Bristow repair. Acta Radiol Diagn *23*:523–528, 1982.
339. Landsiedl F: Arthroscopic therapy of recurrent anterior luxation of the shoulder by capsular repair. Arthroscopy *8*:296–304, 1992.
340. Lane JG, Sachs RA, and Riehl B: Arthroscopic staple capsulorrhaphy: A long-term follow-up. Arthroscopy *9*:190–194, 1993.
341. Lange M: Die Operative Behandlung der Gewohnheitsmabigen Verrenkung an Schulter. Knie und Fub Z Orthop *75*:162, 1944.
342. Langfritz HV: Die Doppelseitige Traumatische Luxatio Humeri Erecta eine Seltene Verletzungsform. Monatschr Unfallheilkunde *59*, 1956.
343. Laskin RS and Sedlin ED: Luxatio erecta in infancy. Clin Orthop *80*:126–129, 1971.
344. Latarjet M: Technique de la butée coracoidienne preplenoidienne dans le traitement des luxations récidivantes de l'épaule. Lyon Chir *54*:604–607, 1958.
345. Latarjet M: Résultat du traitement des luxations récidivantes de l'épaule par le procède de Latarjet, à propos de 42 cas. Lyon Chir *(64)*, 1968.
346. Lavik K: Habitual shoulder luxation. Acta Orthop Scand *30*:251–264, 1961.
347. Lawrence WS: New position in radiographing the shoulder joint. Am J Roentgenol *2*:728–730, 1915.
348. Lazarus MD and Harryman DT II: Complications of open anterior repairs for instability and their solutions. *In* Warner J, Iannotti J, and Gerber R (eds): Complex and Revision Problems in Shoulder Surgery. Philadelphia: Lippincott-Raven, 1996.
349. Lazarus MD, Sidles JA, Harryman DT II, and Matsen FA III: Effect of a chondral-labral defect on glenoid concavity and glenohumeral stability: A cadaveric model. J Bone Joint Surg *78A*:94–102, 1996.
350. Leach RE, Corbett M, Schepsis A, and Stockel J: Results of a modified Putti-Platt operation for recurrent shoulder dislocation and subluxation. Clin Orthop *164*:20–25, 1982.
351. Leffert RD and Seddon H: Infraclavicular brachial plexus injuries. J Bone Joint Surg *47B*:9–22, 1965.
352. Lemmens JA and de Waal Malefitj J: Radiographic evaluation of the modified Bristow procedure for recurrent anterior dislocation of the shoulder. Diagn Imaging Clin Med *53*:221–225, 1984.
353. Lerat JL, Chotel F, Besse JL, et al: Dynamic anterior jerk of the shoulder. A new clinical test for shoulder instability: Preliminary study. Rev Chir Orthop Reparatrice Appar Mot *80*:461–467, 1994.
354. Lescher TJ and Andersen OS: Occlusion of the axillary artery complicating shoulder dislocation: Case report. Milit Med *144*:621–622, 1979.
355. Leslie JT and Ryan TJ: The anterior axillary incision to approach the shoulder joint. J Bone Joint Surg *44A*:1193–1196, 1962.
356. Lev-El A and Rubinstein Z: Axillary artery injury in erect dislocation of the shoulder. J Trauma *21*:323–325, 1981.
357. Levick JR: Joint pressure-volume studies: Their importance, design and interpretation. J Rheumatol *10*:353–357, 1983.
358. Levine WN, Richmond JC, and Donaldson WR: Use of the suture anchor in open Bankart reconstruction: A follow-up report. Am J Sports Med *22*:723–726, 1994.
359. Leyder P, Augereau B, and Apoil A: Traitement des luxations postérieures inveterées de l'épaule par double abord et butée osseuse retro-glenoidienne. Ann Chir *34*:806–809, 1980.
360. Lieber R: Skeletal Muscle Structure and Function. Baltimore: Williams & Wilkins, 1992, p 314.
361. Liedelmeyer R: External rotation method of shoulder dislocation reduction (Letter to the editor). Ann Emerg Med *10*:228, 1981.
362. Lilleby H: Arthroscopy of the shoulder joint. Acta Orthop Scand *53*:708–709, 1982.
363. Lindholm TS and Elmstedt E: Bilateral posterior dislocation of the shoulder combined with fracture of the proximal humerus. Acta Orthop Scand *51*:485–488, 1980.
364. Lippert FG: A modification of the gravity method of reducing anterior shoulder dislocations. Clin Orthop *165*:259–260, 1982.
365. Lippitt SB, Harris SL, Harryman DT II, Sidles JA, et al: In vivo quantification of the laxity of normal and unstable glenohumeral joints. J Shoulder Elbow Surg *3*:215–223, 1994.
366. Lippitt SB, Harryman DT II, Sidles JA, and Matsen FA III: Diagnosis and management of AMBRI syndrome techniques. Techniques Orthop *6*:61–73, 1991.
367. Lippitt SB, Kennedy JP, and Thompson TR: Intraarticular lidocaine versus intravenous analgesia in the reduction of dislocated shoulders. Orthop Trans *15*:804, 1991.
368. Lippitt SB, Kennedy JP, and Thompson TR: Intraarticular lidocaine versus intravenous analgesia in the reduction of dislocated shoulders. Orthop Trans *16*:230, 1992.

369. Lippitt SB, Vanderhooft JE, Harris SL, et al: Glenohumeral stability from concavity—compression: A quantitative analysis. J Shoulder Elbow Surg *2*:27–35, 1993.
370. Liu SH and Boynton E: Posterior superior impingement of the rotator cuff on the glenoid rim as a cause of shoulder pain in the overhead athlete. Arthroscopy *9*:697–699, 1993.
371. Liu SH and Henry MH: Anterior shoulder instability. CORR *323*:327–337, 1996.
372. Löbker K: Einige Práparate von habitueller Schulterluxation. Arch Klin Chir *34*:658–667, 1887.
373. Loomer R and Graham B: Anatomy of the axillary nerve and its relation to inferior capsular shift. Clin Orthop *243*:100–105, 1989.
374. Loutzenheiser TD, Harryman DT II, Yung SW, et al: Optimizing arthroscopic knots. Arthroscopy *11*:199–206, 1995.
375. Lower RF, McNiesh LM, and Callaghan JJ: Computed tomographic documentation of intra-articular penetration of a screw after operations on the shoulder: A report of two cases. J Bone Joint Surg *67*:1120–1122, 1985.
376. Lucas GL and Peterson MD: Open anterior dislocation of the shoulder. J Trauma *17*:883–884, 1977.
377. Luetzow WF, Atkin DM, and Sachs RA: Arthroscopic versus open Bankart repair of the shoulder for recurrent anterior dislocations. Presented at the American Academy of Orthopaedic Surgeons Specialty Day, ASES annual open meeting, 1995.
378. Lusardi DA, Wirth MA, Wurtz D, and Rockwood CA Jr: Loss of external rotation following anterior capsulorrhaphy of the shoulder. J Bone Joint Shoulder *75*:1185–1192, 1993.
379. Lynn FS: Erect dislocation of the shoulder. Surg Gynecol Obstet *39*:51–55, 1921.
380. MacDonald PB, Hawkins RJ, Fowler PJ, and Miniaci A: Release of the subscapularis for internal rotation contracture and pain after anterior repair for recurrent dislocation of the shoulder. J Bone Joint Surg *74*:734–737, 1992.
381. Mack LA, Matsen FA III, and Kilcoyne RF: Ultrasound: US evaluation of the rotator cuff. Radiology *157*:205, 1985.
382. Mackenzie DB: The Bristow-Helfet operation for recurrent anterior dislocation of the shoulder. J Bone Joint Surg *62B*:273–274, 1980.
383. Mackenzie DB: The treatment of recurrent anterior shoulder dislocation by the modified Bristow-Helfet procedure. S Afr Med J *65*:325, 1984.
384. Magnuson PB: Treatment of recurrent dislocation of the shoulder. Surg Clin North Am *25*:14–20, 1945.
385. Magnuson PB and Stack JK: Bilateral habitual dislocation of the shoulder in twins, a familial tendency. JAMA *144*:2103, 1940.
386. Magnuson PB and Stack JK: Recurrent dislocation of the shoulder. JAMA *123*:889–892, 1943.
387. Maki S and Gruen T: Anthropomorphic studies of the glenohumeral joint. Trans Orthop Res Soc *1*:173, 1976.
388. Malgaigne JF: Traite des Fractures et des Luxations. Paris: JB Bailliere, 1855.
389. Manes HR: A new method of shoulder reduction in the elderly. Clin Orthop *147*:200–202, 1980.
390. Markel MD, Hayashi K, Thabit GR, and Thielke RJ: Changes in articular capsular tissue using holmium:YAG laser at non-ablative energy densities. Potential application in non-ablative stabilization procedures. Orthopade *25*:37–41, 1996.
391. Marquardt M and Jerosch J: Ultrasound evaluation of multidirectional instability of the shoulder. Unfallchirurg *94*:295–301, 1991.
392. Martin B, Javelot T, and Vidal J: Long-term results obtained with the Bankart method for the treatment of recurring anterior instability of the shoulder. Chir Organi Mov *76*:199–207, 1991.
393. Matsen FA III, Fu FH, and Hawkins RJ (eds): The Shoulder: A Balance of Mobility and Stability. Rosemont, IL: American Academy of Orthopaedic Surgeons, 1993.
394. Matsen FA III, Lippitt SB, Sidles JA, and Harryman DT II: Practical Evaluation and Management of the Shoulder. Philadelphia: WB Saunders, 1994.
395. Matsen FA III and Thomas SC: Glenohumeral instability. *In* Evarts CMC (ed): Surgery of the Musculoskeletal System, Vol 3. New York: Churchill Livingstone, 1990, pp 1439–1469.
396. Matsen FA III, Thomas SC, and Rockwood CA Jr: Glenohumeral instability. *In* Rockwood CA Jr and Matsen FA III (eds): The Shoulder, Vol 1. Philadelphia: WB Saunders, 1990, pp 547–551.
397. Matthews L, Vetter W, Oweida S, et al: Arthroscopic staple capsulorrhaphy for recurrent anterior shoulder instability. Arthroscopy *4*:106–111, 1988.
398. May VR: A modified Bristow operation for anterior recurrent dislocation of the shoulder. J Bone Joint Surg *52A*:1010–1016, 1970.
399. McEleney ET, Donovan MJ, Shea KP, and Nowak MD: Initial failure strength of open and arthroscopic Barkart repairs. Arthroscopy *11*:426–431, 1995.
400. McFie J: Bilateral anterior dislocation of the shoulders: A case report. Injury *8*:67–69, 1976.
401. McGlynn FJ, El-Khoury G, and Albright JP: Arthrotomography of the glenoid labrum in shoulder instability. J Bone Joint Surg *64A*:506–518, 1982.
402. McIntyre LF and Caspari RB: The rationale and technique for arthroscopic reconstruction of anterior shoulder instability using multiple sutures. Orthop Clin North Am 1993.
403. McKenzie AD and Sinclair AM: Axillary artery occlusion complicating shoulder dislocation. Am Surg *148*:139–141, 1958.
404. McLaughlin HL: Discussion of acute anterior dislocation of the shoulder by Toufick Nicola. J Bone Joint Surg *31A*:172, 1949.
405. McLaughlin HL: On the "frozen" shoulder. Bull Hosp Joint Dis *12*:383–393, 1951.
406. McLaughlin HL: Posterior dislocation of the shoulder. J Bone Joint Surg *34A*:584, 1952.
407. McLaughlin HL: Trauma. Philadelphia: WB Saunders, 1959.
408. McLaughlin HL: Recurrent anterior dislocation of the shoulder. I. Morbid anatomy. Am J Surg *99*:628–632, 1960.
409. McLaughlin HL: Dislocation of the shoulder with tuberosity fractures. Surg Clin North Am *43*:1615–1620, 1963.
410. McLaughlin HL: Locked posterior subluxation of the shoulder—diagnosis and treatment. Surg Clin North Am *43*:1621, 1963.
411. McLaughlin HL and Cavallaro WU: Primary anterior dislocation of the shoulder. Am J Surg *80*:615–621, 1950.
412. McLaughlin HL and MacLellan DI: Recurrent anterior dislocation of the shoulder. II. A comparative study. J Trauma *7*:191–201, 1967.
413. McMaster WC: Anterior glenoid labrum damage: A painful lesion in swimmers. Am J Sports Med *14*:383–387, 1986.
414. McMurray TB: Recurrent dislocation of the shoulder (Proceedings). J Bone Joint Surg *43B*:402, 1961.
415. Mead NC and Sweeney HJ: Bristow procedure. Spectator Letter 1964.
416. Meadowcroft JA and Kain TM: Luxatio erecta shoulder dislocation: report of two cases. Jefferson Orthop J *6*:20–24, 1977.
417. Merrill V: Atlas of Roentgenographic Positions and Standard Radiologic Procedures, Vol 1, 4th ed. St. Louis: CV Mosby, 1975.
418. Mestdagh H, Maynou C, Delobelle JM, et al: Traumatic posterior dislocation of the shoulder in adults. A propos of 25 cases. Ann Chir *48*:355–363, 1994.
419. Meyer SJ and Dalinka MK: Magnetic resonance imaging of the shoulder. Orthop Clin North Am *21*:497–513, 1990.
420. Middeldorpf M and Scharm B: De Nova Humeri Luxationis Specie. Clinique Europenne, Inaugural Dissertation, Vol 2, Breslau, 1859.
421. Milch H: Treatment of dislocation of the shoulder. Surgery *3*:732–740, 1938.
422. Miller LS, Donahue JR, Good RP, and Staerk AJ: The Magnuson-Stack procedure for treatment of recurrent glenohumeral dislocation. Am J Sports Med *12*:133, 1984.
423. Mills KLG: Simultaneous bilateral posterior fracture dislocation of the shoulder. Injury *6*:39–41, 1974–1975.
424. Milton GW: The mechanism of circumflex and other nerve injuries in dislocation of the shoulder and the possible mechanism of nerve injuries during reduction of dislocation. Aust N Z J Surg *23*:24–30, 1953–1955.
425. Milton GW: The circumflex nerve and dislocation of the shoulder. Br J Phys Med *17*:136–138, 1954.
426. Minkoff J and Cavaliere G: Glenohumeral instabilities and the role of magnetic resonance imaging techniques. The orthopedic surgeon's perspective. Magn Reson Imaging Clin N Am *1*:105–123, 1993.
427. Mirick MJ, Clinton JE, and Ruiz E: External rotation method of shoulder dislocation reduction. J Am Coll Emerg Physicians *8*:528–531, 1979.
428. Mital MA and Karlin LI: Diagnostic arthroscopy in sports injuries. Orthop Clin North Am *11*:771–785, 1980.

429. Moeller JC: Compound posterior dislocation of the shoulder. J Bone Joint Surg *57A*:1006–1007, 1975.
430. Mologne TS, Lapoint JM, Morin WD, and Zilberfarb J: Arthroscopic Anterior Labral Reconstruction Using a Transglenoid Suture Technique: Results in the Active Duty Military Patient. Presented at the American Academy of Orthopaedics Surgeons Specialty Day, ASES, Orlando, FL, 1995.
431. Montgomery WH and Jobe FW: Functional outcomes in athletes after modified anterior capsulolabral reconstruction. Am J Sports Med *22*:352–357, 1994.
432. Moran MC and Warren RF: Development of a synovial cyst after arthroscopy of the shoulder. J Bone Joint Surg *71*:127–129, 1989.
433. Morgan CD: Arthroscopic transglenoid Bankart suture repair. Oper Tech Orthop *1*:171–179, 1991.
434. Morgan CD and Bordenstab AB: Arthroscopic Barkart suture repair: Technique and early results. Arthroscopy 3:111–122, 1987.
435. Morgan CD, Rames RD, and Snyder SJ: Arthroscopic assessment of anatomic variants of the glenohumeral ligaments associated with recurrent anterior shoulder instability. Orthop Trans *15*:727, 1992.
436. Morrey BF and Janes JM: Recurrent Anterior Dislocation of the Shoulder: Long-Term Follow-Up of the Putti-Platt and Bankart Procedures. J Bone Joint Surg *58A*:252–256, 1976.
437. Moseley HF: Shoulder Lesions. Springfield IL: Charles C. Thomas, 1945.
438. Moseley HF: Recurrent Dislocations of the Shoulder. Montreal: McGill University Press, 1961.
439. Moseley HF: The basic lesions of recurrent anterior dislocation. Surg Clin North Am *43*:1631–1634, 1963.
440. Moseley HF: Shoulder Lesions. Edinburgh: Churchill Livingstone, 1972.
441. Moseley HF and Overgaard B: The anterior capsular mechanism in recurrent anterior dislocation of the shoulder: Morphological and clinical studies with special reference to the glenoid labrum and glenohumeral ligaments. J Bone Joint Surg Br *44*:913–927, 1962.
442. Mowery CA, Garfin SR, Booth RE, and Rothman RH: Recurrent posterior dislocation of the shoulder: treatment using a bone block. J Bone Joint Surg *67*:777–781, 1985.
443. Müller W: Über den negativen Luftdruck im Gelenkraum. Dtsch A Chir *217*:395–401, 1929.
444. Mumenthaler M and Schliack H: Lasionen Peripherer Nerven. Stuttgart: Georg Thieme Verlag, 1965.
445. Murrard J: Un cas de luxatio erecta de l'épaule double et symmétrique. Rev Orthop *7*:423, 1920.
446. Mynter H: Subacromial dislocation from muscular spasm. Ann Surg *36*:117–119, 1902.
447. Neer CS II: Degenerative lesions of the proximal humeral articular surface. Clin Orthop *20*:116–124, 1961.
448. Neer CS II: Fractures of the distal third of the clavicle. Clin Orthop *58*:43–50, 1968.
449. Neer CS II: Displaced proximal humeral fractures. I. Classification and evaluation. J Bone Joint Surg *52A*:1077–1089, 1970.
450. Neer CS II and Foster CR: Inferior capsular shift for involuntary inferior and multidirectional instability of the shoulder: A preliminary report. J Bone Joint Surg *62A*:897–908, 1980.
451. Neer CS II and Horwitz BS: Fracture of the proximal humeral epiphyseal plate. Clin Orthop *41*:24–31, 1965.
452. Neer CS II, Satterlee CC, Dalsey RM, and Flatow EL: On the value of the coracohumeral ligament release. Ortho Trans *13*:235–236, 1989.
453. Neumann CH, Petersen SA, and Jahnke AH: MR imaging of the labral capsular complex: Normal variation. AJR Am J Roentgenol *157*:1015–1021, 1991.
454. Neviaser RJ, Neviaser TJ, and Neviaser JS: Concurrent rupture of the rotator cuff and anterior dislocation of the shoulder in the older patient. J Bone Joint Surg *70(A)*:1308–1311, 1988.
455. Neviaser RJ, Neviaser TJ, and Neviaser JS: Anterior dislocation of the shoulder and rotator cuff rupture. Clin Orthop *291*:103–6, 1993.
456. Neviaser TJ: The anterior labroligamentous periosteal sleeve avulsion lesion: A cause of anterior instability of the shoulder. Arthroscopy 9:17–21, 1993.
457. Ng KC, Singh S, and Low YP: Axillary artery damage from shoulder trauma—a report of 2 cases. Chirurgie *116*:190–193, 1990.
458. Nicola FG, Ellman H, Eckardt J, and Finerman G: Bilateral posterior fracture-dislocation of the shoulder treated with a modification of the McLaughlin procedure. J Bone Joint Surg *63A*:1175–1177, 1981.
459. Nicola T: Recurrent anterior dislocation of the shoulder. J Bone Joint Surg *11*:128–132, 1929.
460. Nicola T: Recurrent dislocation of the shoulder—its treatment by transplantation of the long head of the biceps. Am J Surg *6*:815, 1929.
461. Nicola T: Anterior dislocation of the shoulder: The role of the articular capsule. J Bone Joint Surg *24*:614–616, 1942.
462. Nicola T: Acute anterior dislocation of the shoulder. J Bone Joint Surg *31A*:153–159, 1949.
463. Nicola T: Recurrent dislocation of the shoulder. Am J Surg *86*:85–91, 1953.
464. Nielsen AB and Nielsen K: The modified Bristow procedure for recurrent anterior dislocation of the shoulder. Acta Orthop Scand *53*:229–232, 1982.
465. Niskanen RO, Lehtonen JY, and Kaukonen JP: Alvik's glenoplasty for humeroscapular dislocation. Acta Orthop Scand *62*:279–283, 1991.
466. Nobel W: Posterior traumatic dislocation of the shoulder. J Bone Joint Surg *44A*:523–538, 1962.
467. Nobuhara K and Ikeda H: Rotator interval lesion. Clin Orthop *223*:44–50, 1987.
468. Noesberger B and Mader G: Die Modifizierte Operation nach Trillat bei Habitueller Schulterluxation. Zschr Unf Med Berufskr *69*:34–36, 1976.
469. Norris TR: C-arm Fluoroscopic Evaluation Under Anesthesia for Glenohumeral Subluxations. Philadelphia: BC Decker, 1984, pp 22–25.
470. Norris TR, Bigliani LU, and Harris E: Complications following the modified Bristow repair for shoulder instability. Presented at the American Shoulder and Elbow Surgeons 3rd Open Meeting, San Francisco, 1987.
471. O'Brien SJ, Neves MC, Arnoczky SP, et al: The anatomy and histology of the inferior glenohumeral ligament complex of the shoulder. Am J Sports Med *18*:449–456, 1990.
472. O'Brien SJ, Neves MC, Arnoczky SP, et al: The anatomy and histology of the inferior glenohumeral ligament complex of the shoulder. Am J Sports Med *18*:449–456, 1990.
473. O'Connell PW, Nuber GW, Mileski RA, and Lautenschlager E: The contribution of the glenohumeral ligaments to anterior stability of the shoulder joint. Am J Sports Med *18*:579–584, 1990.
475. O'Conner SJ: Posterior dislocation of the shoulder. Arch Surg *72*:479–491, 1956.
476. O'Conner SJ and Jacknow AS: Posterior dislocation of the shoulder. J Bone Joint Surg *37A*:1122, 1955.
477. O'Driscoll SW: Atraumatic instability: pathology and pathogenesis. *In* Matsen III FA, Fu FH, and Hawkins RJ (eds): The Shoulder: A Balance of Mobility and Stability. Rosemont, IL: American Academy of Orthopaedic Surgeons, 1993, pp 305–318.
478. O'Driscoll SW and Evans DC: The DuToit Staple Capsulorrhaphy for Recurrent Anterior Dislocation of the Shoulder: Twenty Years of Experience in Six Toronto Hospitals. Presented at the American Shoulder and Elbow Surgeons 4th Open Meeting, Atlanta, 1988.
479. O'Driscoll SW and Evans DC: Long-term results of staple capsulorrhaphy for anterior instability of the shoulder. J Bone Joint Surg *75*:249–258, 1993.
480. Obremskey WT, Lippitt SB, Harryman DT II, and Matsen FA III: Follow-up of the inferior capsular shift procedure for atraumatic multidirectional instability. Submitted to Clin Orthop 1995.
481. Older MWJ: Arthroscopy of the shoulder joint. J Bone Joint Surg *58B*:253, 1976.
482. Olsson O: Degenerative changes of the shoulder joint and their connection with shoulder pain. Acta Chir Scand [Suppl] *181*:1–130, 1953.
483. Onabowale BO and Jaja MOA: Unreduced bilateral synchronous shoulder dislocations. Niger Med J *9*:267–271, 1979.
484. Oppenheim WL, Dawson EG, Quinlan C, and Graham SA: The cephaloscapular projection: A special diagnostic aid. Clin Orthop *195*:191–193, 1985.
485. Osmond-Clarke H: Habitual dislocation of the shoulder. The Putti-Platt operation. J Bone Joint Surg Br *30*:19–25, 1948.

486. Oudard P: La luxation récidivante de l'épaule (variete anterointerne) procède opératoire. J Chir *23*:13, 1924.
487. Ovesen J and Nielsen S: Experimental distal subluxation in the glenohumeral joint. Arch Orthop Trauma Surg *104*:82–84, 1985.
488. Ovesen J and Nielsen S: Stability of the shoulder joint: Cadaver study of stabilizing structures. Acta Orthop Scand *56*:149–151, 1985.
489. Ozaki J: Glenohumeral movement of the involuntary inferior and multidirectional instability. Clin Orthop *238*:107–111, 1989.
490. Paavolainen P, Bjorkenheim JM, Ahovuo J, and Slatis P: Recurrent anterior dislocation of the shoulder. Results of Eden-Hybinette and Putti-Platt operations. Acta Orthop Scand *55*:556–560, 1984.
491. Pagden D, Halaburt AS, Wiroszo R, and Karyn A: Posterior dislocation of the shoulder complicating regional anesthesia. Anesth Analg *65*:1063–1065, 1986.
492. Pagnani MJ, Deng XH, Warren RF, et al: Effect of lesions of the superior portion of the glenoid labrum on glenohumeral translation. J Bone Joint Surg Am *77*:1003–1010, 1995.
493. Palmer I and Widen A: The bone block method for recurrent dislocation of the shoulder joint. J Bone Joint Surg *30B*:53, 1948.
494. Palmer WE and Caslowitz PL: Anterior shoulder instability: Diagnostic criteria determined from prospective analysis of 121 MR arthrograms. Radiology *197*:819–825, 1995 Dec.
495. Pappas AM, Goss TP, and Kleinman PK: Symptomatic shoulder instability due to lesions of the glenoid labrum. Am J Sports Med *11*:279–288, 1983.
496. Parisien JS: Shoulder arthroscopy technique and indications. Bull Hosp Joint Dis *43*:56–69, 1983.
497. Parisien VM: Shoulder dislocation: An easier method of reduction. J Maine Med Assoc *70*:102, 1979.
498. Parrish GA and Skiendzielewski JJ: Bilateral posterior fracture-dislocations of the shoulder after convulsive status epilepticus. Ann Emerg Med *14*:264–266, 1985.
499. Parsons SW and Rowley DI: Brachial plexus lesions in dislocations and fracture dislocation of the shoulder. J R Coll Surg Edinb *31*:85–87, 1986.
500. Pascoet G, Jung F, Foucher G, and Kehr P: Treatment of recurrent dislocation of the shoulder by preglenoid artificial ridge using the Latarjet-Vittori technique. J Med Strasbourg *6*:501–504, 1975.
501. Pasila M, Jaroma H, and Kiviluoto O: Early complications of primary shoulder dislocations. Acta Orthop Scand *49*:260–263, 1978.
502. Pasila M, Kiviluoto O, Jaroma H, and Sundholm A: Recovery from primary shoulder dislocation and its complications. Acta Orthop Scand *51*:257–262, 1980.
503. Patel MR, Pardee ML, and Singerman RC: Intrathoracic dislocation of the head of the humerus. J Bone Joint Surg *45A*:1712–1714, 1963.
504. Pavlov H, Warren RF, Weiss CBJ, and Dines DM: The roentgenographic evaluation of anterior shoulder instability. Clin Orthop *194*:153–158, 1985.
505. Peiro A, Ferrandis R, and Correa F: Bilateral erect dislocation of the shoulders. Injury *6*:294, 1975.
506. Percy LR: Recurrent posterior dislocation of the shoulder. J Bone Joint Surg *42B*:863, 1960.
507. Perniceni B and Augereau A: Treatment of old unreduced anterior dislocations of the shoulder by open reduction and reinforced rib graft: Discussion of three cases. Ann Chir *36*:235–239, 1983.
508. Perry J and Glousman RE: Biomechanics of Throwing. St. Louis: CV Mosby, 1989, pp 727–751.
509. Perthes G: Uber operationen bei habitueller schulterluxation. Dtsch Ztschr Chir *85*:199–222, 1906.
510. Pettersson G: Rupture of the tendon aponeurosis of the shoulder joint in anterior inferior dislocation. Acta Chir Scand (Suppl) *77*:1–187, 1942.
511. Pilz W: Zur Rontgenuntersschung der Habituellen Schulterverrenkung. Arch Klin Chir *135*:1–22, 1925.
512. Pollock RG and Bigliani LU: Recurrent posterior shoulder instability: Diagnosis and treatment. Clin Orthop *291*:85–96, 1993.
513. Poppen NK and Walker PS: Normal and abnormal motion of the shoulder. J Bone Joint Surg *58A*:195, 1976.
514. Poppen NK and Walker PS: Forces at the glenohumeral joint in abduction. Clin Orthop *135*:165–170, 1978.
515. Porteous MJL and Miller AJ: Humeral rotation osteotomy for chronic posterior dislocation of the shoulder. J Bone Joint Surg 72:181–186, 1990.
516. Post M: The Shoulder. Surgical and Non-surgical Management. Phildelphia: Lea & Febiger, 1978.
517. Prodromos CC, Ferry JA, Schiller AL, and Zarins B: Histological studies of the glenoid labrum from fetal life to old age. J Bone Joint Surg Am *72*:1344–1348, 1990.
518. Protzman RR: Anterior instability of the shoulder. J Bone Joint Surg *62A*:909–918, 1980.
519. Prozorovskii VF, Khvisiuk NI, and Gevorkian AD: Surgical treatment of anterior instability of the shoulder joint. Ortop Traumatol Protez *4*:14–18, 1991.
520. Quigley TB and Freedman PA: Recurrent dislocation of the shoulder. Am J Surg *128*:595–599, 1974.
521. Rafii M, Firooznia H, and Bonamo JJ: CT arthrography of capsular structures of the shoulder. AJR Am J Roentgenol *146*:361–367, 1986.
522. Rafii M, Firooznia H, and Bonamo JJ: Athlete shoulder injuries: CT arthrographic findings. Radiology *162*:559–564, 1987.
523. Rafii M, Firooznia H, Golimbu C, and Weinreb J: Magnetic resonance imaging of glenohumeral instability. Magn Reson Imaging Clin N Am *1*:87–104, 1993.
524. Randelli M and Gambrioli PL: Glenohumeral osteometry by computed tomography in normal and unstable shoulders. Clin Orthop *208*:151, 1986.
525. Rao JP, Francis AM, Hurley J, and Daczkewycz R: Treatment of recurrent anterior dislocation of the shoulder by duToit staple capsulorrhaphy: Results of long-term follow-up study. Clin Orthop *204*:169, 1986.
526. Reeves B: Arthrography in acute dislocation of the shoulder. J Bone Joint Surg *48B*:182, 1968.
527. Reeves B: Experiments on the tensile strength of the anterior capsular structures of the shoulder in man. J Bone Joint Surg Br *50*:858–865, 1968.
528. Reeves B: Acute anterior dislocation of the shoulder. Ann R Coll Surg Engl *43*:255, 1969.
529. Resch H: Current aspects in the arthroscopic treatment of shoulder instability. Orthopade *20*:273–281, 1991.
530. Resch H, Wykypiel HF, Maurer H, and Wambacher M: The antero-inferior (transmuscular) approach for arthroscopic repair of the Bankart lesion: An anatomic and clinical study. J Arthroscopy *12*:309–319, 1996.
531. Rhee KJ, Ahn SR, and Lee JK: Arthroscopic capsular suture for anterior instability of the shoulder. Orthopedics *15*:217–24, 1992.
532. Rhee YG, Harryman II DT, Romeo AA, et al: Translational laxity of the glenohumeral joint. Submitted to Am J Sports Med, 1994.
533. Ribbans WJ, Mitchell R, and Taylor GJ: Computerized arthrotomography of primary anterior dislocation of the shoulder. J Bone Joint Surg *72B*:181–185, 1990.
534. Richards RD, Sartoris DJ, Pathria MN, and Resnick D: Hill-Sachs lesion and normal humeral groove: MR imaging features allowing their differentiation. Radiology *190*:665–668, 1994.
535. Richards RR, Beaton D, and Hudson AR: Shoulder arthrodesis with plate fixation: Functional outcome analysis. J Shoulder Elbow Surg *2*:225–239, 1993.
536. Richards RR, Waddell JP, and Hudson MB: Shoulder Arthrodesis for the Treatment of Brachial Plexus Palsy: A review of Twenty-two Patients. Presented at the American Shoulder and Elbow Surgeons 3rd Open Meeting, San Francisco, 1987.
537. Richmond JC, Donaldson WR, Fu F, and Harner CD: Modification of the Barkart reconstruction with a suture anchor: Report of a new technique. Am J Sports Med *19*:343–346, 1991.
538. Rob CG and Standeven A: Closed traumatic lesions of the axillary and brachial arteries. Lancet *1*:597–599, 1956.
539. Roca LA and Ramos-Vertiz JR: Luxacion erecta de hombro. Rev San Mil Arg *61*:135, 1962.
540. Rockwood CA Jr: Subluxation of the shoulder–the classification, diagnosis and treatment. Orthop Trans *4*:306, 1979.
541. Rockwood CA Jr: Part 2: Dislocations about the shoulder, Vol 1, 2nd ed. Rockwood CA and Green DP (eds): Fractures. Philadelphia: JB Lippincott, 1984.
542. Rockwood CA Jr: Shoulder arthroscopy. J Bone Joint Surg *70A*:639–640, 1988.
543. Rockwood CA Jr, Burkhead WZ Jr, and Brna J: Subluxation for the Glenohumeral Joint; Response to Rehabilitative Exercise in Traumatic vs. Atraumatic Instability. Presented at the American Shoulder and Elbow Surgeons 2nd Open Meeting, New Orleans, 1986.

544. Rockwood CA Jr and Young DC: Complications and management of the failed Bristow shoulder reconstructions. Orthop Trans *13*:232, 1989.
545. Rodosky MW, Harner CD, and Fu FH: The role of the long head of the biceps muscle and superior glenoid labrum in anterior stability of the shoulder. Am J Sports Med *22*:121–130, 1994.
546. Rokous JR, Feagin JA, and Abbott HG: Modified axillary roentgenogram. A useful adjunct in the diagnosis of recurrent instability of the shoulder. Clin Orthop *82*:84–86, 1972.
547. Romanes GJ(ed): Cunningham's Textbook of Anatomy, 11th ed. London: Oxford University Press, 1972.
548. Rose DJ: Arthroscopic Suture Capsulorrhaphy for Recurrent Anterior and Anteroinferior Shoulder Instability: 2–6 Year Followup. Presented at the American Academy of Orthopaedic Surgeons Specialty Day, Arthroscopy Association of North America, 1994.
549. Rosenberg BN, Richmond JC, and Levine WN: Long-term follow up of Barkart Reconstruction. Am J Sports Med *23*:538–544, 1995.
550. Rossi F, Ternamian PJ, Cerciello G, and Walch G: Posterosuperior glenoid rim impingement in athletes: The diagnostic value of traditional radiology and magnetic resonance. Radiol Med (Torino) *87*:22–27, 1994.
551. Roston JB and Haines RW: Cracking in the metacarpo-phalangeal joint. J Anat *81*:165–173, 1947.
552. Rowe CR: Prognosis in dislocations of the shoulder. J Bone Joint Surg *38A*:957–977, 1956.
553. Rowe CR: Instabilities of the glenohumeral joint. Bull Hosp Joint Dis *39*:180–186, 1978.
554. Rowe CR, Patel D, and Southmayd WW: The Bankart procedure—a study of late results (Proceedings). J Bone Joint Surg *59B*:122, 1977.
555. Rowe CR, Patel D, and Southmayd WW: The Bankart procedure: Long-term end-result study. J Bone Joint Surg Am *60*, 1978.
556. Rowe CR, Pierce DS, and Clark JC: Voluntary dislocation of the shoulder: A preliminary report on a clinical, electromyographic, and psychiatric study of 26 patients. J Bone Joint Surg *55A*:445–460, 1973.
557. Rowe CR and Sakellarides HT: Factors related to recurrences of anterior dislocations of the shoulder. Clin Orthop *20*:40, 1961.
558. Rowe CR and Yee LBK: A posterior approach to the shoulder joint. J Bone Joint Surg *26A*:580, 1944.
559. Rowe CR and Zarins B: Recurrent transient subluxation of the shoulder. J Bone Joint Surg *63A*:863–872, 1981.
560. Rowe CR and Zarins B: Chronic unreduced dislocations of the shoulder. J Bone Joint Surg *64A*:494–505, 1982.
561. Rowe CR, Zarins B, and Ciullo JV: Recurrent anterior dislocation of the shoulder after surgical repair: Apparent causes of failure and treatment. J Bone Joint Surg *66A*:159, 1984.
562. Rozing PM, De Bakker HM, and Obermann WR: Radiographic views in recurrent anterior shoulder dislocation: Comparison of six methods for identification of typical lesions. Acta Orthop Scand *57*:328–330, 1986.
563. Rubin SA, Gray RL, and Green WR: Scapular Y—a diagnostic aid in shoulder trauma. Radiology *110*:725–726, 1974.
564. Runkel M, Kreitner KF, Wenda K, et al: Nuclear magnetic tomography in shoulder dislocation. Unfallchirurg *96*:124–128, 1993.
565. Rupp F: Ueber ein Vereinfachtes Operationverfahren bei Habitueller Schulterluxatuion. Dtsch Z Chir *198*:70–75, 1926.
566. Russell JA, Holmes EMI, and Keller DJ: Reduction of acute anterior shoulder dislocations using the Milch technique: A study of ski injuries. J Trauma *21*:802–804, 1981.
567. Saha AK: Theory of Shoulder Mechanism. Springfield, IL: Charles C. Thomas, 1961.
568. Saha AK: Anterior recurrent dislocation of the shoulder. Acta Orthop Scand *39*:479–493, 1967.
569. Saha AK: Dynamic instability of the glenohumeral joint. Acta Orthop Scanda *42*:491–505, 1971.
570. Saha AK: Mechanics of elevation of glenohumeral joint: Its application in rehabilitation of flail shoulder in upper brachial plexus injuries and poliomyelitis and in replacement of the upper humerus by prosthesis. Acta Orthop Scand *44*:668, 1973.
571. Saha AK, Das NN, and Chakravarty BF: Treatment of recurrent dislocation of shoulder: past, present, and future: Studies on electromyographic changes of muscles acting on the shoulder joint complex. Calcutta Med J *53*:409–413, 1956.
572. Sarma A, Savanchak H, Levinson ED, and Sigman R: Thrombosis of the axillary artery and brachial plexus injury secondary to shoulder dislocation. Conn Med *45*:513–514, 1981.
573. Sarrafian AK: Gross and functional anatomy of the shoulder. CORR *173*:11–19, 1983.
574. Savarsee JJ and Covino BG: Basic and clinical pharmacology of local anesthetic drugs. *In* Miller RD (ed): Anesthesia. New York: Churchill Livingstone, 1986.
575. Savoie III FH: Arthroscopic Reconstruction of Recurrent Traumatic Anterior Instability. Presented at the American Academy of Orthopaedic Surgeons Specialty Day, ASES, 1995.
576. Saxena K and Stavas J: Inferior glenohumeral dislocation. Ann Emerg Med *12*:718–720, 1983.
577. Schauder KS and Tullow HS: Role of the coracoid bone block in the modified Bristow procedure. Am J Sports Med *20*:31–34, 1992.
578. Schlemm F: Ueber die Verstarkungsbander am Schultergelenk. Arch Anat Physiol Wissenschaft Med *22*:45, 1853.
579. Schüller M: Berl Klin Wochenschr *33*:760, 1896.
580. Schulz TJ, Jacobs B, and Patterson RL: Unrecognized dislocations of the shoulder. J Trauma *9*:1009–1023, 1969.
581. Schwartz RE, O'Brien SJ, Warren RF, and Torzilli PA: Capsular restraints to anterior-posterior motion in the shoulder. Orthop Trans *12*:727, 1988.
582. Scott DJJ: Treatment of recurrent posterior dislocations of the shoulder by glenoplasty. J Bone Joint Surg *49A*:471, 1967.
583. Scougall S: Posterior dislocation of the shoulder. J Bone Joint Surg *39B*:726–732, 1957.
584. Segal D, Yablon IG, Lynch JJ, and Jones RP: Acute bilateral anterior dislocation of the shoulders. Clin Orthop *140*:21–22, 1979.
585. Seltzer SE and Weissman BN: CT findings in normal and dislocating shoulders. J Can Assoc Radiol *36*:41–46, 1985.
586. Sever JW: Obstetrical paralysis. Surg Gynecol Obstet *44*:547–549, 1927.
587. Shaffer BS, Conway J, Jobe FW, et al: Infraspinatus muscle-splitting incision in posterior shoulder surgery: An anatomic and electromyographic study. Am J Sports Med *22*:113–120, 1994.
588. Shea KP and Lovallo JL: Scapulothoracic penetration of a beath pin: an unusual complication of arthroscopic Bankart suture repair. Arthroscopy 7:115–117, 1991.
589. Shea KP, O'Keefe RM Jr, and Fulkerson JP: Comparison of initial pull-out strength of arthroscopic suture and staple Bankart repair techniques. Arthroscopy 8:179–82, 1992.
590. Shively J and Johnson J: Results of modified Bristow procedure. Clin Orthop *187*:150, 1984.
591. Shuman WP, Kilcoyne RF, Matsen FA III, et al: Double-contrast computed tomography of the glenoid labrum. AJR Am J Roentgenol *141*:581–584, 1983.
592. Sidles JA, Harryman DT, and Simkin PA: Passive and active stabilization of the glenohumeral joint. Submitted to J Bone Joint Surg, 1989.
593. Silliman JF and Hawkins RJ: Classification and physical diagnosis of instability of the shoulder. CORR *291*:7–19, 1993.
594. Simkin PA: Structure and function of joints. *In* Schumacher HR (ed): Primer on the Rheumatic Diseases, 9th ed. Atlanta: Arthritis Foundation, 1988.
595. Simonet WT and Cofield RH: Prognosis in Anterior Shoulder Dislocation. Homestead, VA: American Orthopaedic Society for Sports Medicine, 1983.
596. Singer GC, Kirkland PM, and Emery RJH: Coracoid transposition for recurrent anterior instability of the shoulder. J Bone Joint Surg *77B*:73–76, 1995.
597. Sisk TD and Boyd HB: Management of recurrent anterior dislocation of the shoulder. DuToit-type or staple capsulorrhaphy. Clin Orthop *103*:150, 1974.
598. Small NC: Complications in arthroscopy: The knee and other joints. Arthroscopy 2:253, 1986.
599. Small NC: Complications in arthroscopic surgery performed by experienced arthroscopists. Arthroscopy *4*:215–221, 1988.
600. Small NC: Complications in arthroscopic surgery of the knee and shoulder. Orthopedics *16*:985–988, 1993.
601. Snyder SJ, Banas MP, and Karzel RP: An analysis of 140 injuries to the superior glenoid labrum. J Shoulder Elbow Surg *4*:243–8, 1995.
602. Snyder SJ and Strafford BB: Arthroscopic management of instability of the shoulder. Orthopedics *16*:993–1002, 1993.
603. Sonnabend DH: Treatment of primary anterior shoulder disloca-

tion in patients older than 40 years of age. Clin Orthop *304*:74–77, 1994.
604. Soslowsky LJ, Bigliani LU, Flatow EL, and Mow VC: Articular geometry of the glenohumeral joint. Clin Orthop *285*:181–190, 1992.
605. Speed K: Fractures and Dislocation, 4th ed. Philadelphia: Lea & Febiger, 1942.
606. Speer KP, Deng X, Borrero S, et al: A Biomechanical Evaluation of the Bankart Lesion. Presented at the American Academy of Orthopaedic Surgeons Specialty Day, ASES, 1995.
607. Speer KP, Deng X, Torzilli PA, et al: Strategies for an anterior capsular shift of the shoulder: A biomechanical comparison. Rev Chir Orthop Reparatice Appar Mot *80*:602–609, 1994.
608. Speer KP, Pagnani M, and Warren RF: Arthroscopic Anterior Shoulder Stabilization: 2–5 Year Follow-up Using a Bioabsorbable Tac. American Shoulder and Elbow Surgeons 10th Open Meeting, New Orleans, 1994.
609. Sperber A and Wredmark T: Capsular elasticity and joint volume in recurrent anterior shoulder instability. Arthroscopy *10*:598–601, 1994.
610. Staffel F: Verh Dtsch Ges Chir *24*:651–656, 1895.
611. Steenburg RW and Ravitch MM: Cervicothoracic approach for subclavian vessel injury from compound fracture of the clavicle: Considerations of subclavian axillary exposures. Ann Surg *157*:839–846, 1963.
612. Stefko JM, Tibone JE, McMahon PJ, et al: Strain of the Anterior Band of the Glenohumeral Ligament at the Time of Capsular Failure. Presented at the American Shoulder and Elbow Surgeons Closed Meeting, LaQuinta, CA, 1995.
613. Stein E: Case report 374: Posttraumatic pseudoaneurysm of axillary artery. Skeletal Radiol *15*:391–393, 1986.
614. Steiner D and Hermann B: Collagen fiber arrangement of the human shoulder joint capsule—an anatomical study. Acta Anat (Basel) *136*:300–302, 1989.
615. Stener B: Dislocation of the shoulder complicated by complete rupture of the axillary artery. J Bone Joint Surg *39B*:714–717, 1957.
616. Stevens JH: Brachial Plexus Paralysis. New York: G. Miller, 1934.
617. Stimson LA: Fractures and Dislocations, 3rd ed. Philadelphia: Lea Brothers, 1900.
618. Stimson LA: A Practical Treatise on Fractures and Dislocations, 7th ed. Philadelphia: Lea & Febiger, 1912.
619. Stromsoe K, Senn E, Simmen B, and Matter P: Rezidivhaufigkeit nach Erstmaliger Traumatischer Schulter-luxation. Helv Chir Acta *47*:85–88, 1980.
620. Stufflesser H and Dexel M: The treatment of recurrent dislocation of the shoulder by rotation osteotomy with internal fixation. Ital J Orthop Traumatol *39*:191, 1977.
621. Sudarov Z: The results of the modified Nosske-Oudard-Bazy-savic operation for recurrent dislocation of the shoulder (Abstract). J Bone Joint Surg *48B*:855, 1966.
622. Surin V, Blader S, Markhede G, and Sundholm K: Rotational osteotomy of the humerus for posterior instability of the shoulder. J Bone Joint Surg *72*:181–186, 1990.
623. Swenson TM and Warner JJ: Arthroscopic shoulder stabilization: Overview of indications, technique, and efficacy. Clin Sports Med *14*:841–62, 1995.
624. Symeonides PP: The significance of the subscapularis muscle in the pathogenesis of recurrent anterior dislocation of the shoulder. J Bone Joint Surg Br *54*:476–483, 1972.
625. Tagliabue D and Esposito A: L'intervento di Latarjet nella lussazione recidivante di spalla-dello sportivo. Ital J orthop Traumatol 2:91–100, 1980.
626. Tauro JC and Carter FMN: Arthroscopic capsular advancement for anterior and anterior-inferior shoulder instability: A preliminary report. Arthroscopy *10*:513–7, 1994.
627. Terry GC, Hammon D, and France P: The stabilizing function of passive shoulder restraints. Am J Sports Med *19*:26–34, 1991.
628. Thomas MA: Posterior subacromial dislocation of the head of the humerus. AJR Am J Roentgenol *37*:767–773, 1937.
629. Thomas SC and Matsen III FA: An approach to the repair of glenohumeral ligament avulsion in the management of traumatic anterior glenohumeral instability. J Bone Joint Surg Am *71A*:506–513, 1989.
630. Thomas TT: Habitual or recurrent anterior dislocation of the shoulder. Am J Med Sci *137*:229–246, 1909.
631. Thomas TT: Habitual or recurrent dislocation of the shoulder: Forty-four shoulder operations in 42 patients. Surg Gynecol Obstet *32*:291–299, 1921.
632. Thompson FR and Winant WM: Unusual fracture-subluxations of the shoulder joint. J Bone Joint Surg Am *32*:575–582, 1950.
633. Thompson FR and Winant WM: Comminuted fractures of the humeral head with subluxation. Clin Orthop *20*:94–96, 1961.
634. Tibone J and Ting A: Capsulorrhaphy with a staple for recurrent posterior subluxation of the shoulder. J Bone Joint Surg *72*:999–1002, 1990.
635. Tibone JE and Bradley JP: The treatment of posterior subluxation in athletes. Clin Orthop *291*:124–137, 1993.
636. Tibone JE, Prietto C, Jobe FW, et al: Staple capsulorrhaphy for recurrent posterior shoulder dislocation. Am J Sports Med *9*:135–139, 1981.
637. Tietjen R: Occult glenohumeral interposition of a torn rotator cuff. J Bone Joint Surg *64A*:458–459, 1982.
638. Tijmes J, Loyd HM, and Tullos HS: Arthrography in acute shoulder dislocations. South Med J *72*:564–567, 1979.
639. Toolanen G, Hildingsson C, Hedlund T, et al: Early complications after anterior dislocation of the shoulder in patients over 40 years: An ultrasonographic and electromyographic study. Acta Orthop Scand *64*:549–552, 1993.
640. Torg JS, Balduini FC, Bonci C, et al: A modified Bristow-Helfet-May procedure for recurrent dislocations and subluxation of the shoulder: Report of 212 cases. J Bone Joint Surg *69*:904–913, 1987.
641. Townley CO: The capsular mechanism in recurrent dislocation of the shoulder. J Bone Joint Surg Am *32*:370–380, 1950.
642. Trillat A: Traitement de la luxation récidivante de l'épaule: Considerations, techniques. Lyon Chir *49*:986, 1954.
643. Trillat A and Leclerc-Chalvet F: Luxation Récidivante de L'Épaule. Paris: Masson, 1973.
644. Trimmings NP: Hemarthrosis aspiration in treatment of anterior dislocation of the shoulder. J R Soc Med *78(12)*, 1985.
645. Turkel SJ, Panio MW, Marshall JL, and Girgis FG: Stabilizing mechanisms preventing anterior dislocation of the glenohumeral joint. J Bone Joint Surg Am *63*:1208–1217, 1981.
646. Tuszynski W: Anterior dislocation of the shoulder complicated by temporary brachial paresis. Chir Narzadow Ruchu Orthop Pol *46*, 1981.
647. Uhorchak JM, Arciero RA, and Taylor DC: Recurrent Instability After Open Shoulder Stabilization in Athletes. Presented at the American Academy of Orthopaedic Surgeons Specialty Day, ASES, 1995.
648. Uhthoff HK and Piscopo M: Anterior capsular redundancy of the shoulder: Congenital or traumatic? An embryological study. J Bone Joint Surg *67*:363–366, 1985.
649. Ungersbock A, Michel M, and Hertel R: Factors influencing the results of a modified Barkart procedure. J Shoulder Elbow Surg *4*:365–369, 1995.
650. Unsworth A, Dowson D, and Wright V: "Cracking joints": A bioengineering study of cavitation in the metacarpophalangeal joint. Ann Rheum Dis *30*:348, 1971.
651. Uribe JW and Hechtman KS: Arthroscopically assisted repair of acute Bankart lesion. Orthopedics *16*:1019–1023, 1993.
652. Valls J: Acrylic prosthesis in a case with fracture of the head of the humerus. Bal Soc Orthop Trauma *17*:61, 1952.
653. Van der Helm FC: A finite element musculoskeletal model of the shoulder mechanics. J Biomech *27*:551–569, 1994.
654. Van der Helm FC, Veeger HE, Pronk GM, Van der Woude LH, et al: Geometry parameters for musculoskeletal modeling of the shoulder system. J Biomech *25*:129–144, 1992.
655. Van der Spek K: Rupture of the axillary artery as a complication of dislocation of the shoulder. Arch Chir Neerl *16*:113–118, 1964.
656. Vangsness CTJ, Ennis M, Taylor JG, and Atkinson R: Neural anatomy of the glenohumeral ligaments, labrum, and subacromial bursa. Arthroscopy *11*:180–184, 1995.
657. Veeger HE, Van der Helm FC, Van der Woude LH, et al: Inertia and muscle contraction parameters for musculoskeletal modeling of the shoulder mechanism. J Biomech *24*:615–629, 1991.
658. Vegter J and Marti RK: Treatment of posterior dislocation of the shoulder by osteotomy of the neck of the scapula. J Bone Joint Surg *63*:288, 1981.
659. Vellet AD, Munk PL, and Marks P: Imaging techniques of the shoulder: Present perspectives. Clin Sports Med *10*:721–756, 1991.

660. Verrina F: Para-articular ossification following simple dislocation of the shoulder. Minerva Orthop *210*:480–486, 1975.
661. Volpin G, Langer R, and Stein H: Complete infraclavicular brachial plexus palsy with occlusion of axillary vessels following anterior dislocation of the shoulder joint. J Orthop Trauma *4*:121–123, 1990.
662. Walch G, Boileau P, Levigne C, et al: Arthroscopic stabilization for recurrent anterior shoulder dislocation. J Arthrosc Related Surg *11*:173–179, 1995.
663. Walch G, Liotard JP, Boileau P, and Noel E: Postero-superior glenoid impingement: Another shoulder impingement. Rev Chir Orthop Reparatrice Appar Mot 77:571–574, 1991.
664. Walch G, Liotard JP, Boileau P, and Noel E: Postero-superior glenoid impingement: Another impingement of the shoulder. J Radiol *74*:47–50, 1993.
665. Waldron VD: Dislocated shoulder reduction—a simple method that is done without assistants. Orthop Rev *11*:105–106, 1982.
666. Ward WG, Bassett FHI, and Garrett WEJ: Anterior staple capsulorrhaphy for recurrent dislocation of the shoulder: a clinical and biomechanical study. South Med J *83*:510–518, 1990.
667. Warner JJ, Deng XH, Warren RF, and Torzilli PA: Static capsuloligamentous restraints to superior-inferior translation of the glenohumeral joint. Am J Sports Med *20*:675–685, 1992.
668. Warner JJ, Kann S, and Marks P: Arthroscopic repair of combined Bankart and superior labral detachment anterior and posterior lesions: Technique and preliminary results. Arthroscopy *10*:383–91, 1994.
669. Warner JJ, Micheli LJ, Arslanian LE, et al: Scapulothoracic motion in normal shoulders and shoulders with glenohumeral instability and impingement syndrome: A study using Moir'e topographic analysis. Clin Orthop *285*:191–199, 1992.
670. Warner JJ, Miller MD, and Marks P: Arthroscopic Barkart repair with the Suretac device. Part II. Experimental Observations. Arthroscopy *11*:14–20, 1995.
671. Warner JJ, Miller MD, Marks P, and Fu FH: Arthroscopic Barkart repair with the Suretac device. Part I. Clinical Observations. Arthroscopy *11*:2–13, 1995.
672. Warren RF: The Role of Shoulder Arthroscopy. American Academy of Orthopaedic Surgeons Instructional Course, Minneapolis, 1989.
673. Warren RF, Kornblatt IB, and Marchand R: Static factors affecting posterior shoulder stability. Orthop Trans *8*:89, 1984.
674. Watson-Jones R: Dislocation of the shoulder joint. Proc R Soc Med *29*:1060–1062, 1936.
675. Watson-Jones R: Recurrent dislocation of the shoulder. J Bone Joint Surg *30B*:6–8, 1948.
676. Watson-Jones R: Fractures and Joint Injuries, 4th ed. Baltimore: Williams & Wilkins, 1957.
677. Weaver JK and Derkash RS: Don't forget the Bristow Latarjet procedure. Clin Orthop *308*:102–110, 1994.
678. Weber BG: Operative treatment for recurrent dislocation of the shoulder. Injury *1*:107–109, 1969.
679. Weber BG, Simpson LA, and Hardegger F: Rotational humeral osteotomy for recurrent anterior dislocation of the shoulder associated with a large Hill-Sachs lesion. J Bone Joint Surg *66A*:1443, 1984.
680. Weber S: The gold standard revisited: Recent Experience with the Open Bankart Repair for Recurrent Anterior Glenohumeral Dislocation. Presented at the American Academy of Orthopaedic Surgeons Specialty Day, ASES, 1995.
681. Weber SC: Open Versus Arthroscopic Repair of Traumatic Anterior Glenohumeral Instability. Presented at the American Academy Meeting of Orthopaedic Surgeons Specialty Day, Arthroscopy Association of North America, 1995.
682. Weitbrecht J: Syndesmology; or, a Description of the Ligaments of the Human Body (trans E. B. Kaplan). Philadelphia: WB Saunders, 1969.
683. West EF: Intrathoracic dislocation of the humerus. J Bone Joint Surg *31B*:61–62, 1949.
684. Wheeler JH, Ryan JB, Arciero RA, and Molinari RN: Arthroscopic versus nonoperative treatment of acute shoulder dislocations in young athletes. Arthroscopy *5*:213–217, 1989.
685. White ADN: Dislocated shoulder—a simple method of reduction. Med J Aust *2*:726–727, 1976.
686. Wickstrom J: Birth injuries of the brachial plexus: Treatment of defects in the shoulder. Clin Orthop *23*:187–196, 1962.
687. Wiley AM and Austwick DH: Shoulder Surgery Through the Arthroscope. Toronto: Department of Surgery, University of Toronto and Toronto Wester Hospital, 1982.
688. Wiley AM and Older MWJ: Shoulder arthroscopy. J Sports Med *8*:31–38, 1980.
689. Williams MM, Snyder SJ, and Buford DJ: The Buford complex—the cord-like middle glenohumeral ligament and absent anterosuperior labrum complex: In a normal anatomic capsulolabral variant. Arthroscopy *10*:241–247, 1994.
690. Wilson JC and McKeever FM: Traumatic posterior (retroglenoid) dislocation of the humerus. J Bone Joint Surg *31A*:160–172, 1949.
691. Wirth MA, Blatter G, and Rockwood CA Jr: The capsular imbrication procedure for recurrent anterior instability of the shoulder. J Bone Joint Surg *78A*:246–259, 1996.
692. Wirth MA, Butters KP, and Rockwood CA Jr: The posterior deltoid-splitting approach to the shoulder. Clin Orthop *296*:92–98, 1993.
693. Wirth MA, Groh GI, and Rockwood CA Jr: The Treatment of Symptomatic Posterior Glenohumeral Instability With an Anterior Capsular Shift. Presented at the Western Orthopaedic Association 58th Annual Meeting, 1994.
694. Wirth MA, Jensen KL, Agarwal A, et al: Fracture-dislocation of the proximal humerus with retroperitoneal humeral head displacement. J Bone Joint Surg (In press).
695. Wirth MA, Lyons FR, and Rockwood CA Jr: Hypoplasia of the glenoid: A review of sixteen patients. J Bone Joint Surg Am *75*:1175–1184, 1993.
696. Wirth MA and Rockwood CA Jr: Traumatic glenohumeral instability. *In* Matsen FA III, Fu FH, and Hawkins RJ (eds): The Shoulder: A Balance of Mobility and Stability. Rosemont: American Academy of Orthopaedic Surgeons, 1993, pp 279–304.
697. Wirth MA and Rockwood CA Jr: Complications of treatment of injuries of the shoulder. *In* Epps CH (ed): Complications in Orthopaedic Surgery. Philadelphia: JB Lippincott, 1994, pp 229–255.
698. Wirth MA, Seltzer DG, and Rockwood CA Jr: Recurrent posterior glenohumeral dislocation associated with increased retroversion of the glenoid. Clin Orthop *308*:98–101, 1994.
699. Wirth MA, Seltzer DG, and Rockwood CA Jr: Replacement of the Subscapularis with Pectoralis Muscle in Anterior Shoulder Instability. Presented at the 62nd Annual Meeting of the American Academy of Orthopaedics Surgeons, Orlando, FL, 1995.
700. Wolf EM: Arthroscopic anterior shoulder capsulorrhaphy. Tech Orthop *3*:67–73, 1988.
701. Wolf EM: Arthroscopic capsulolabral repair using suture anchors. Orthop Clin North Am *24*:59–69, 1993.
702. Wolf EM: Arthroscopic Capsulolabral Reconstruction Using Suture Anchors. Presented at the American Academy of Orthopaedic Surgeons Specialty Day, ASES Annual Meeting, 1994.
703. Wolf EM, Cheng JC, and Dickson K: Humeral avulsion of glenohumeral ligaments as a cause of anterior shoulder instability. Arthroscopy *11*:600–7, 1995.
704. Wong-Pack WK, Bobechko PE, and Becker EJ: Fractured coracoid with anterior shoulder dislocation. J Can Assoc Radiol *31*:278–279, 1980.
705. Wredmark T, Tornkvist H, Johansson C, and Brobert B: Long-term functional results of the modified Bristow procedure for recurrent dislocations of the shoulder. Am J Sports Med *20*:157–161, 1992.
706. Wulker N, Rossig S, Korell M, and Thren K: Dynamic stability of the glenohumeral joint: A biomechanical study. Sportverletz Sportschaden *9*:1–8, 1995.
707. Wulker N, Sperveslage C, and Brewe F: Passive stabilizers of the glenohumeral joint: A biomechanical study. Unfallchirurg *96*:129–133, 1993.
708. Yadav SS: Bilateral simultaneous fracture-dislocation of the shoulder due to muscular violence. J Postgrad Med *23*:137–139, 1977.
709. Yahiro MA and Matthews LS: Arthroscopic stabilization procedures for recurrent anterior shoulder instability. Orthop Rev *18*:1161–1168, 1989.
710. Yoneda B, Welsh RP, and MacIntosh DL: Conservative treatment of shoulder dislocation in young males (Proceedings). J Bone Joint Surg *64B*:254–255, 1982.
711. Young DC and Rockwood CA Jr: Complications of a failed Bristow procedure and their management. J Bone Joint Surg *73A*:969–981, 1991.

712. Youssef JA, Carr CF, Walther CE, and Murphy JM: Arthroscopic Bankart suture repair for recurrent traumatic unidirectional anterior shoulder dislocations. Arthroscopy *11*:561–3, 1995.
713. Yung SW and Harryman DT II: The Surgical Anatomy of the Subscapular Nerves. Presented at the 62nd Annual Meeting of the American Academy of Orthopaedic Surgeons, Orlando, FL, 1995.
714. Zabinski SJ, Callaway GH, Cohen S, and Warren RF: Long Term Results of Revision Shoulder Stabilization. Presented at the American Shoulder and Elbow Surgeons Closed Meeting, La Quinta, CA, 1995.
715. Zachary RB: Transplantation of teres major and latissimus dorsi for loss of external rotation at the shoulder. Lancet *2*:757–761, 1947.
716. Ziegler DW, Harrington RM, and Matsen FA III: The superior rotator cuff tendon and acromion provide passive superior stability to the shoulder. Submitted to J Bone Joint Surg, 1996.
717. Ziegler DW, Harryman DT II, and Matsen FA III: Subscapularis Insufficiency in the Previously Operated Shoulder. Presented at the American Shoulder and Elbow Surgeons Twelfth Open Meeting, Atlanta, GA, 1996.
718. Zimmerman LM and Veith I: Great Ideas in the History of Surgery: Clavicle, Shoulder, Shoulder Amputations. Baltimore: Williams & Wilkins, 1961.
719. Zizzi F, Frizziero L, Facchini A, and Zini GL: Artroscopia della spalla: indicazioni e limiti. Reumatismo *33*:429–432, 1981.
720. Zorowitz RD, Idank D, Ikai T, et al: Shoulder subluxation after stroke: A comparison of four supports. Arch Phys Med Rehabil *76*:763–771, 1995.
721. Zuckerman JD, Gallagher MA, Cuomo F, and Rokito AS: Effect of Instability and Subsequent Anterior Shoulder Repair on Proprioceptive Ability. Presented at the American Shoulder and Elbow Surgeons 12th Open Meeting, Atlanta, GA, 1996.
722. Zuckerman JD and Matsen FAI: Complications about the glenohumeral joint related to the use of screws and staples. J Bone Joint Surg *66A*:175, 1984.

CHAPTER

15

FREDERICK A. MATSEN III, M.D.
CRAIG T. ARNTZ, M.D.
STEVEN B. LIPPITT, M.D.

Rotator Cuff

Ay, there's the rub.

HAMLET, III. i. 47, SHAKESPEARE

The coracoacromial ligament has an important duty and should not be thoughtlessly divided at any operation.

EA CODMAN, 1934

The wise surgeon, realizing that he may find little but rotten cloth to sew, will operate only by necessity and make a carefully guarded prognosis.

HL MCLAUGHLIN, 1962

HISTORICAL REVIEW

Rotator Cuff Tears

It is often difficult to tell where concepts actually begin. It is certainly not obvious who first used the term rotator or musculotendinous cuff. Credit for first describing ruptures of this structure is often given to Smith, who in 1834 described the occurrence of tendon ruptures after shoulder injury in the *London Medical Gazette*.[378] In 1924, Meyer published his attrition theory of cuff ruptures.[255] In his 1934 classic monograph, Codman summarized his 25 years of observations on the musculotendinous cuff and its components and discussed ruptures of the supraspinatus tendon.[62] Beginning 10 years after the publication of Codman's book and for the next 20 years, McLaughlin wrote on the etiology of cuff tears and their management.[247, 251] Arthrography was first carried out by Oberholtzer in 1933 using air as the contrast medium.[295] Lindblom and Palmer[230] used radio-opaque contrast and described partial-thickness, full-thickness, and massive tears of the cuff.

Codman recommended early operative repair for complete cuff tears. He carried out what may have been the first cuff repair in 1909.[62] Current views of cuff tear pathogenesis, diagnosis, and treatment are quite similar to those that he proposed over 50 years ago.

Pettersson has provided an excellent summary of the early history of published observations on subacromial pathology. Because of its completeness, his account is quoted here.[323]

As already mentioned, the tendon aponeurosis of the shoulder joint and the subacromial bursa are intimately connected with each other. An investigation on the pathological changes in one of these formations will necessarily concern the other one also. A historical review shows that there has been a good deal of confusion regarding the pathological and clinical observations on the two.

The first to observe morbid processes in the subacromial bursa was Jarjavay,[185] who on the basis of a few cases gave a general description of subacromial bursitis. His views were modified and elaborated by Heineke[170] and Vogt.[421] Duplay introduced the term "periarthritis humeroscapularis" to designate a disease picture characterized by stiffness and pain in the shoulder joint following a trauma.[100] Duplay based his observations on cases of trauma to the shoulder joint and on other cases of stiffness in the shoulder following dislocation, which he had studied at autopsy. The pathological foundation for the disease was believed by Duplay to lie in the subacromial and subdeltoid bursa. He thought that the cause was probably destruction or fusion of the bursa.

Duplay's views, which were supported by his followers, Tillaux[402] and Desché,[93] were hotly disputed. His opponents, Gosselin and his pupil Duronea[101] and Desplats,[94] Pingaud and Charvot,[326] tried to prove that the periarthritis should be regarded as a rheumatic affection, neuritis, etc.

In Germany, Colley[72] and Küster[211] were of practically the same opinion regarding periarthritis humeroscapularis as Duplay. Roentgenography soon began to contribute to the problem of humeroscapular periarthritis. It was not long before calcium shadows began to be observed in the soft parts between the acromion and the greater tuberosity.[310] The same finding was made by Stieda,[385] who assumed that these calcium masses were situated in the wall and in the lumen of the subacromial bursa. These new findings were indiscriminately termed "bursitis calcarea subacromialis" or "subdeltoidea." The term "bursoliths" was even used by Haudek[160] and Holzknecht.[174] Later, however, as the condition showed a strong resemblance to humeroscapular periarthritis, it became entirely identified with the latter.

In America, Codman[64] made a very important contribution to the question when he drew attention to the important role played by changes in the supraspinatus in the clinical picture of subacromial bursitis. Codman was the first to point out that many cases of inability to abduct the arm are due to incomplete or complete ruptures of the supraspinatus tendon.

With Codman's findings it was proved that humeroscapular periarthritis was not only a disease condition localized in the subacromial bursa, but that pathologic changes also occurred in the tendon aponeurosis of the shoulder joint. This theory was further supported by Wrede,[445] who, on the basis of one surgical case and several cases in which roentgenograms had revealed calcium shadows in the region of the greater tuberosity, was able to show that the calcium deposits were localized in the supraspinatus tendon.

More and more disease conditions in the region of the shoulder joint have gradually been distinguished and separated from the general concept, periarthritis humeroscapularis. For example, Sievers[373] drew attention to the fact that arthritis deformans in the acromioclavicular joint may give a clinical picture reminiscent of periarthritis humeroscapularis. Bettman[26] and Meyer and Kessler[254] pointed to the occurrence of deforming changes in the intertubercular sulcus, the canal in which the biceps tendon glides. Payr[318] attempted to isolate the clinical picture that appears when the shoulder joint without any previous trauma is immobilized too long in an unsuitable position. Julliard[192] demonstrated apophysitis in the coracoid process (coracoiditis) as forming a special subdivision of periarthritis. Wellisch[437] described apophysitis at the insertion of the deltoid muscle on the humerus, giving it the name of "deltoidalgia." Schár and Zweifel[365] described deforming changes in connection with certain cases of os acromiale.

In addition to this excellent review, Pettersson himself made several important contributions to the study of the rotator cuff, as will be seen subsequently in this chapter.

The cuff story continues with the recognition of subacromial abrasion as an element in rotator cuff disease by a number of well-known surgeons including Codman,[64] Armstrong,[6] Hammond,[155, 156] McLaughlin,[247] Moseley,[270] Smith-Petersen and colleagues,[379] and Watson-Jones.[431] Some of these surgeons proposed a complete acromionectomy, whereas others advocated a lateral acromionectomy for relief of these symptoms.[6, 95, 155, 156, 247, 379, 431] The term "impingement syndrome" was popularized by Neer in 1972.[275] In 100 dissected scapulas, Neer found 11 with a "characteristic ridge of proliferative spurs and excrescences on the undersurface of the anterior process (of the acromion), apparently caused by repeated impingement of the rotator cuff and the humeral head, with traction of the coracoacromial ligament. . . . Without exception it was the anterior lip and undersurface of the anterior third that was involved." Neer emphasized that the supraspinatus insertion to the greater tuberosity and the bicipital groove lie anterior to the coracoacromial arch with the shoulder in the neutral position and that with forward flexion of the shoulder these structures must pass beneath the arch, providing the opportunity for abrasion. He suggested a continuum from chronic bursitis and partial tears to complete tears of the supraspinatus tendon, which may extend to involve rupture of other parts of the cuff. He pointed out that the physical examination and plain radiographic findings were not reliable in differentiating chronic bursitis and partial tears from complete tears. Importantly, he emphasized that patients with partial tears seemed more susceptible to increased shoulder stiffness and that surgery in this situation was inadvisable until the stiffness had resolved. He described the use of a subacromial lidocaine injection to help localize the clinical problem and before acromioplasty as a "useful guide of what the procedure would accomplish."

Neer described three different stages of the "impingement syndrome." In stage 1, reversible edema and hemorrhage are present in a patient younger than 25 years of age. In stage 2, fibrosis and tendinitis affect the rotator cuff of a patient typically in the 25- to 40-year age group. Pain often recurs with activity. In stage 3, bone spurs and tendon ruptures are present in the individual older than 40 years of age. He emphasized the importance of nonoperative management of cuff tendinitis. If surgery was performed, Neer pointed out the importance of preserving a secure acromial origin of the deltoid, a smooth resection of the undersurface of the anteroinferior acromion, the careful inspection for other sources of abrasion (e.g., the undersurface of the acromioclavicular joint), and careful postoperative rehabilitation.[275, 277, 280]

In 1972, Neer[275] described the indications for acromioplasty as: (1) long-term disability from chronic bursitis and partial tears of the supraspinatus tendon, or (2) complete tears of the supraspinatus. He pointed out that the physical and roentgenographic findings in these two categories were indistinguishable, including crepitus and tenderness over the supraspinatus with a painful arc of active elevation from 70 to 120 degrees and pain at the anterior edge of the acromion on forced elevation. Neer's report[277] in 1983 described candidates for acromioplasty as: (1) patients with an arthrographically demonstrated cuff tear, (2) patients older than 40 years of age with negative arthrograms but persistent disability for 1 year despite adequate conservative treatment (including efforts to eliminate stiffness), provided that the pain can be temporarily eliminated by the subacromial injection of lidocaine, (3) certain patients younger than 40 years of age with refractory stage II impingement lesions, and (4) patients undergoing other procedures for conditions in which impingement is likely (e.g., total shoulder replacement in patients with rheumatoid arthritis or old fracture). The proposed goal of acromioplasty was to relieve mechanical wear at the critical area of the rotator cuff. Surgery was not considered until any stiffness had resolved and until the disability had persisted for at least 9 months. Even in patients who had had a previous lateral acromionectomy with continuing symptoms, Neer considered anterior acromioplasty, having found that many still had problems related to subacromial impingement. Neer also reported that the rare patient with an irreparable tear in the rotator cuff could be made more comfortable and could gain surprising function if impingement were relieved, as long as the deltoid origin was preserved.[277]

Neer recommended resection of small unfused acromial growth centers and internal fixation of larger unfused segments in a manner that tilted the acromion upwards to avoid impingement.[277] His indications for resections of the lateral clavicle included: (1) arthritis of the acromioclavicular joint, (2) a need for greater exposure of the supraspinatus in a cuff repair, and (3) nonarthritic enlargement of the acromioclavicular joint resulting in impingement on the supraspinatus (in this situation only the undersurface of the joint was resected).[277]

Additional approaches to subacromial abrasion have been proposed including coracoacromial ligament section,[164, 184, 200, 320] resection arthroplasty of the acromioclavicular joint,[200] extensive acromionectomy,[6, 95, 155, 156, 247, 257, 270, 379, 431] and combined procedures such as acromioplasty, incision of the coracoacromial ligament, acromioclavicular resection arthroplasty, and excision of the intra-articular portion of the biceps tendon with tenodesis of the distal portion of the bicipital groove.[151, 290, 333]

Comparison of the results of these procedures is difficult owing to the heterogeneous patient groups and varying methods of evaluation. In 16 patients with chronic bursitis with fraying or partial tear of the supraspinatus, Neer[275] found that 15 attained satisfactory results (no significant pain, less than 20 degrees of limitation of overhead extension, and at least 75% of normal strength). Thorling and co-workers[399] found good to excellent results in 33 of 51 patients after acromioplasty (in 11 resection of the acromioclavicular joint was performed as well).

Recently, arthroscopic acromioplasty has been introduced. The frequency with which this procedure is performed has increased dramatically as the strictness of Neer's original indications for acromioplasty have been allowed to relax. Ellman[104] presented the initial results on 50 consecutive cases of arthroscopic acromioplasty for stage II impingement without a cuff tear (40 cases) and for a full-thickness cuff tear (20 cases). Eighty-eight per cent of the patients had excellent or good results, and the rest were unsatisfactory at a 1- to 3-year follow-up. He pointed out that the technique was technically demanding. Difficulties with arthroscopic acromioplasty range from inadequate subacromial smoothing on one hand to transection of the acromion or virtually total acromionectomy on the other. In his early series of 100 arthroscopic acromioplasties, Gartsman[130] found that at an average of 18.5 months' follow-up, 85 shoulders were improved and 15 were failures, of which nine required subsequent open acromioplasty. The procedure took longer than open acromioplasty and did not hasten the patient's return to work or sport. Morrison[267] reported a series of arthroscopic acromioplasties in which the quality of the result was closely correlated with the conversion of a curved or hooked acromion to a flat undersurface.

Even though the indications for its performance are still being defined, arthroscopic acromioplasty is currently one of the commonest of all orthopedic procedures, being applied to shoulder pain, bursal hypertrophy, partial-thickness cuff tears, calcific tendinitis, as well as reparable and irreparable rotator cuff tears.

RELEVANT ANATOMY AND MECHANICS

Skin

Rotator cuff surgery can usually be accomplished through cosmetically acceptable incisions in the lines of the skin (Fig. 15–1). These skin lines run obliquely from superior lateral to inferomedial. The usual "superior" approach to the cuff is made through such an oblique incision that runs over the anterior corner of the acromion.

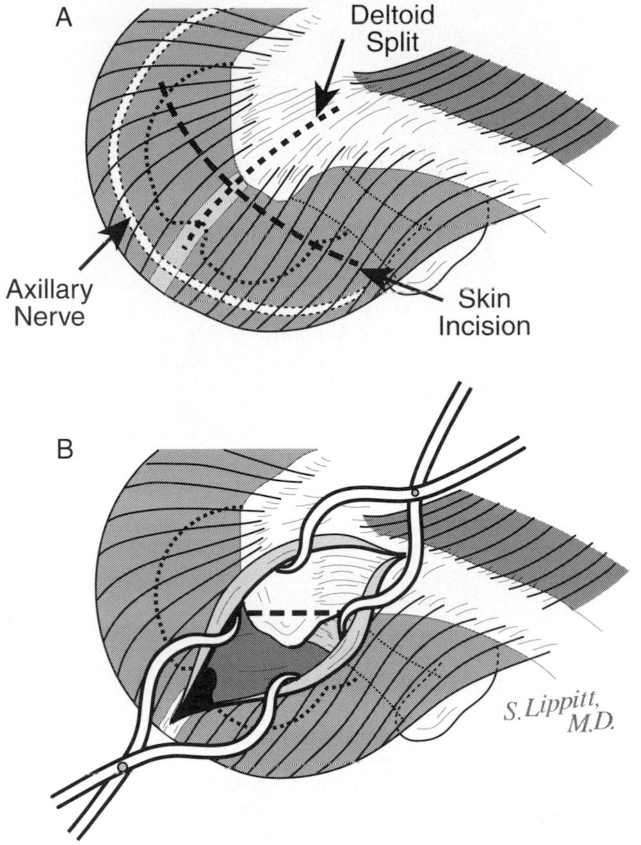

Figure 15–1

The deltoid on approach. *A*, Skin incision in Langer's lines across the front of the acromion. The deltoid is split along the tendon at the junction of the anterior and middle thirds. *B*, The deltoid origin can be sharply dissected from the acromion for greater exposure. It is desirable to preserve Sharpey's fibers of origin on the muscle and continuity of the medial and lateral flaps with trapezius insertion. (Modified from Matsen FA III, Lippitt SB, Sidles JA, and Harryman DT II: Practical Evaluation and Management of the Shoulder. Philadelphia: WB Saunders, 1994.)

Deltoid Muscle

The deltoid arises from the lateral half of the clavicle and the acromion and posteriorly from the scapular spine. The origin of the deltoid is over the entire anterior height of the acromion; thus, in the performance of an acromioplasty, a substantial amount of the deltoid origin must be detached, whether the procedure is performed open or arthroscopically.[407] The deltoid has an important and constant tendon of origin separating its anterior and lateral thirds. This tendon attaches to the anterior lateral corner of the acromion in which location it provides the key to the anterior deltoid-splitting approach to the cuff. By making the deltoid split down the center of the tendon, the surgeon can be assured of having strong tendinous "handles" on the muscle for use in deltoid closure (see Fig. 15–1). While it is often said that the location of the axillary nerve is on the average 5 cm distal to the acromion, its anterior branches swoop upwards so that it is desirable to limit the inferior extent of the deltoid split to minimize the risk of injury to the axillary nerve branches (see Fig. 15–1).

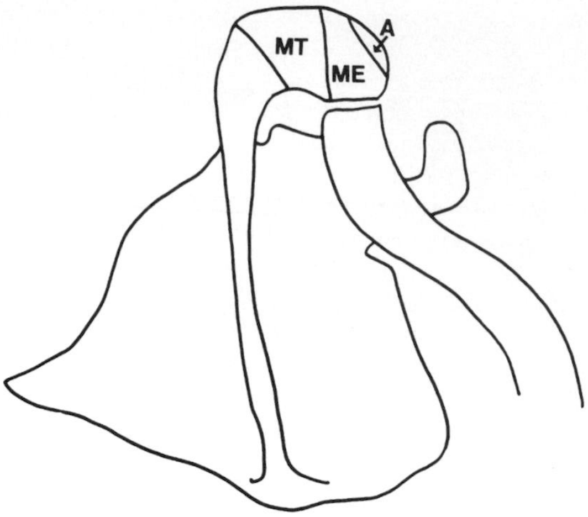

Figure 15–2

A superior view of the scapula and clavicle. A, Acro-os acromiale; meso-os acromiale; MT, meta-os acromiale. (From Iannotti JP: Rotator Cuff Disorders: Evaluation and Treatment. Rosemont, IL: American Academy of Orthopaedic Surgeons, 1991.)

Acromion, Coracoid, and Coracoacromial Ligament

The *acromion* is a scapular process arising from three separate centers of ossification—a preacromion, a mesoacromion, and a meta-acromion.[55, 272, 362] These centers of ossification are usually united by 22 years of age. When these centers fail to unite, the un-united portion is referred to as an os acromiale (Fig. 15–2). This condition may have been first recognized by Schár and Zweifel[365] in 1936, as was mentioned by Pettersson.[323] Grant[148] found that 16 of 194 cadavers older than 30 years of age demonstrated incomplete fusion of the acromion; the condition was bilateral in five subjects and unilateral in 11 subjects. In a large review of 1000 radiographs, Liberson found unfused acromia in 2.7%; of these, 62% were bilateral.[223] Most commonly the lesion is a failure of fusion of the mesoacromion to the meta-acromion. He found the axillary view to be most helpful in revealing the condition. The size of the unfused fragment may be substantial, up to 5 × 2 cm.[275] Resection of a fragment this large creates a serious challenge for deltoid reattachment.

Norris and co-workers[294] and Bigliani and associates[29] have pointed to an association between cuff degeneration and unfused acromial epiphysis. Mudge and co-workers[272] found that 6% of 145 shoulders with cuff tears had an os acromiale, whereas Liberson found a 2.7% incidence of this finding in unselected scapulas.[223] The statistical and clinical significance of this association remains unclear.

An additional anatomic feature of importance is the acromial branch of the thoracoacromial artery. This artery runs in close relation to the coracoacromial ligament and is often transected in the course of an acromioplasty and coracoacromial ligament section.

The *coracoid* arises from two or three ossification centers.[362] It provides the medial attachment site for both the coracohumeral ligament and the coracoacromial ligament. In that their muscle bellies lie medial to it, the neighboring supraspinatus and subscapularis tendons must be able to glide by the coracoid with their full excursion during shoulder movement. Scarring of one or both these tendons to the coracoid can inhibit passive and active shoulder motion. While the coracoid does not normally make contact with the anterior subscapularis tendon, forced internal rotation, particularly in the presence of a tight posterior capsule, can produce such contact due to obligate translation.[139, 159]

The *coracoacromial ligament* spans from the undersurface of the acromion to the lateral aspect of the coracoid and is continuous with the less dense clavipectoral fascia. It forms a substantial part of the superficial aspect of the humeroscapular motion interface (Figs. 15–3 and 15–4).

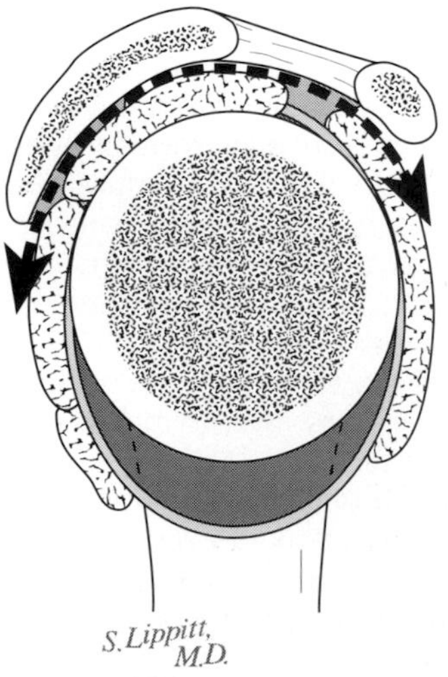

Figure 15–3

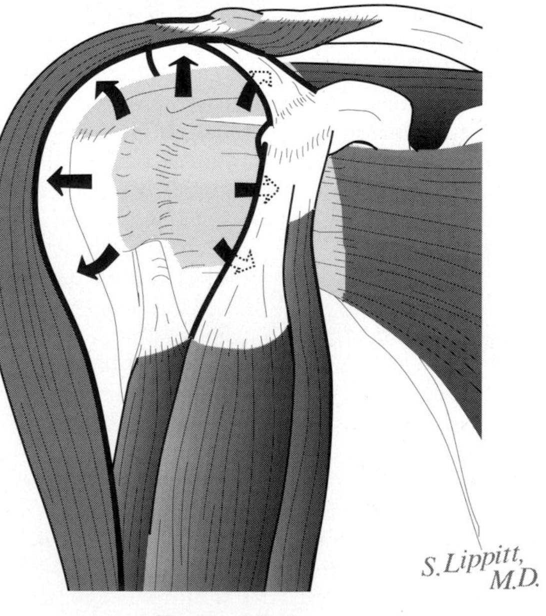

Figure 15–4

Figures 15–3 and 15–4

The humeroscapular motion interface is an important location of motion between the humerus and the scapula. The deltoid, acromion, coracoacromial ligament, coracoid process, and tendons attaching to the coracoid lie on the superficial side of this interface, whereas the proximal humerus, rotator cuff, and biceps tendon sheath lie on its deep side. These two groups of structures are essentially in contact, separated only by lubricating bursal surfaces.

This ligament may be thought of as the "spring" ligament of the shoulder, maintaining the normal relationships between the coracoid and the acromion. Separation of these two scapular processes has been observed on sectioning this ligament in cadavers.[117]

The *coracoacromial arch* is the inferiorly concave smooth surface consisting of the anterior undersurface of the acromion and the coracoacromial ligament. It provides a strong ceiling for the shoulder joint along which the cuff tendons must glide during all shoulder movements (see Figs. 15–3 and 15–4). Passage of the cuff tendons and proximal humerus under this arch is facilitated by the subacromial-subdeltoid bursa, which normally is not a space, as is often shown in diagrams, but rather two serosal surfaces in contact with each other, one on the undersurface of the coracoacromial arch and deltoid and the other on the cuff. These sliding surfaces are lubricated by bursal surfaces and synovial fluid.

The recognition of the gliding articulation between the arch and the cuff is not new. Renoux and associates credited Ludkewitch, who in 1900 recognized that the proper functioning of the "scapulohumeral articulation" requires the presence of a "secondary socket," which extends the glenoid fossa of the scapula above, in front, and behind, and of which the coracoacromial arch forms the ceiling.[342] In 1934 Codman stated that the coracoacromial arch was an auxiliary joint of the shoulder and that its roughly hemispheric shape was "almost a counterpart in the size and curvature of the articular surface of the true joint." He referred to the "gleno-coraco-acromial socket."[62] His belief in the importance of the coracoacromial arch was great enough to state that "the coracoacromial ligament has an important duty and should not be thoughtlessly divided at any operation." Wiley has pointed to the severe superior instability when the ceiling of the shoulder is lost in association with cuff deficiency.[440] In 1961, Kernwein and associates stressed the importance of the "suprahumeral gliding mechanism," consisting of the coracoacromial arch on one side and the rotator cuff and biceps tendon on the other separated by the subacromial bursa.[198] They believed that these two opposing, gliding surfaces and interposed bursa constituted a fifth joint that contributed to shoulder motion. DePalma, in 1967, also recognized the intimate relationship between the arch and the structures below it.[88] He referred to the arch, together with the head of the humerus, the rotator cuff, and the subacromial bursa, as the "superior humeral articulation."

Matsen and Romeo described the humeroscapular motion interface as an articulation (see Figs. 15–3 and 15–4) between the cuff, humeral head, and biceps on the inside and the coracoacromial arch, deltoid, and coracoid muscles on the outside and measured up to 4 cm of gliding at this articulation in normal shoulders in vivo.[244]

Recent investigations have pointed to the importance of contact and load transfer between the rotator cuff and the coracoacromial arch in the function of normal shoulders, including the provision of superior stability.[48, 117, 118, 340, 446, 457] Because there is normally no gap between the superior cuff and the coracoacromial arch, the slightest amount of superior translation compresses the cuff tendon between the humeral head and the arch. Superior displacement is opposed by a downward force exerted by the coracoacromial arch through the cuff tendon to the humeral head. Ziegler and associates[457] demonstrated this passive resistance effect in cadavers by showing that the acromion bent upwards when a superiorly directed force was applied to the humerus in the neutral position. The amount of *acromial deformation* was related directly to the amount of superior force applied to the humerus; the load being transmitted through the intact superior cuff tendon. Furthermore, these authors found that the amount of *superior humeral displacement* resulting from a superiorly directed humeral load of 80 N was increased from 1.7 to 5.4 mm when the cuff tendon was excised ($P < .0001$) (Figs. 15–5 and 15–6). These results indicate that: (1) the intact superior cuff tendon is subject to compressive loading between the humeral head and the coracoacromial arch, and (2) the presence of this tendon provides passive resistance against superior displacement of the humeral head when superiorly directed loads are applied.

Flatow and associates also noted that, in a dynamic cadaver model, the presence of the supraspinatus tendon limited superior translation of the humeral head, even when there was no tension in the tendon from simulated muscle action.

The spacer effect of the superior cuff tendon is evident when comparing shoulders with intact cuffs with those in which the superior tendon is deficient (Figs. 15–7 and 15–8).

Both Ziegler and co-workers and Flatow and associates cautioned that the superior stability of the shoulder is dependent on an intact coracoacromial arch. Surgical sacrifice of the arch can lead to severe superior stability (Fig. 15–9).

Changes in the coracoacromial arch have been described in association with cuff disease along with variations of acromial shape.[29, 275, 382] Bigliani and colleagues studied 140 shoulders in 71 cadavers.[28] The average age was 74.4 years. They identified three acromial shapes: type I (flat) in 17%, type II (curved) in 43%, and type III (hooked) in 40%. Fifty-eight per cent of the cadavers had the same type of acromion on each side. Thirty-three per cent of the shoulders had full-thickness tears, of which 73% were seen in the presence of type III acromia, 24% in type II, and 3% in type I. The anterior slope of the acromion in shoulders with cuff tears averaged 29 degrees, slightly more than the slope of those without cuff tears that averaged 23 degrees. The clinical significance of this relatively small difference is not known. Several other authors have reported that patients with cuff defects are more likely to have hooked or angled acromia.[268, 405, 408] Nicholson and associates[291] demonstrated on a review of 420 scapulas that spur formation of the anterior acromion was an age-related process such that individuals younger than 50 years of age had less one quarter the prevalence of those older than 50 years of age. The status of the cuffs of these shoulders is unknown.

Although these data indicate a strong association between aging, the presence of cuff tears, and alterations of acromial contour, it has been unclear whether the change in acromial shape was caused by or resulted from the cuff defect or whether both were consequences of aging. As

Text continued on page 763

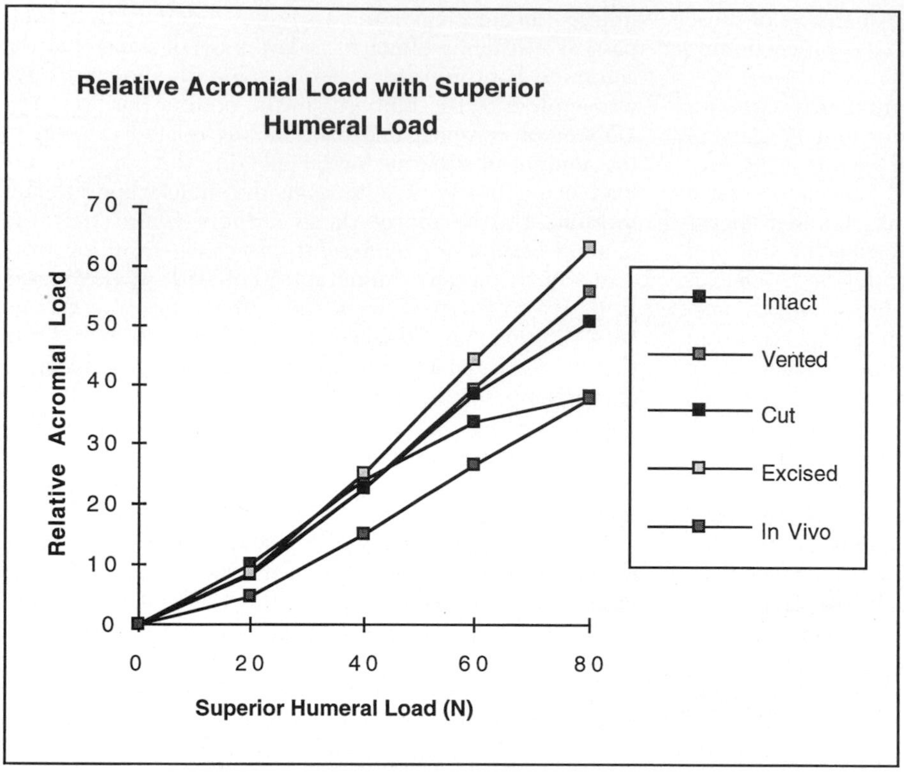

Figure 15–5

Superiorly directed humeral loads are transmitted to the acromion. If the superior cuff is intact, the load is transferred through the cuff tendon. If the cuff tendon is not interposed, the humeral head loads the acromion directly. The chart compares the relative acromial load as a function of superiorly directed humeral load for: (1) intact specimens; (2) after venting of the joint to air; (3) after cutting (but not excising the cuff tendon); and (4) after excising the superior cuff tendon; also included are the data from (5) a single in vivo experiment done with the identical instrumentation. Note that there is minimal difference in these acromial load—humeral load relationships, even when the cuff tendon has been excised.

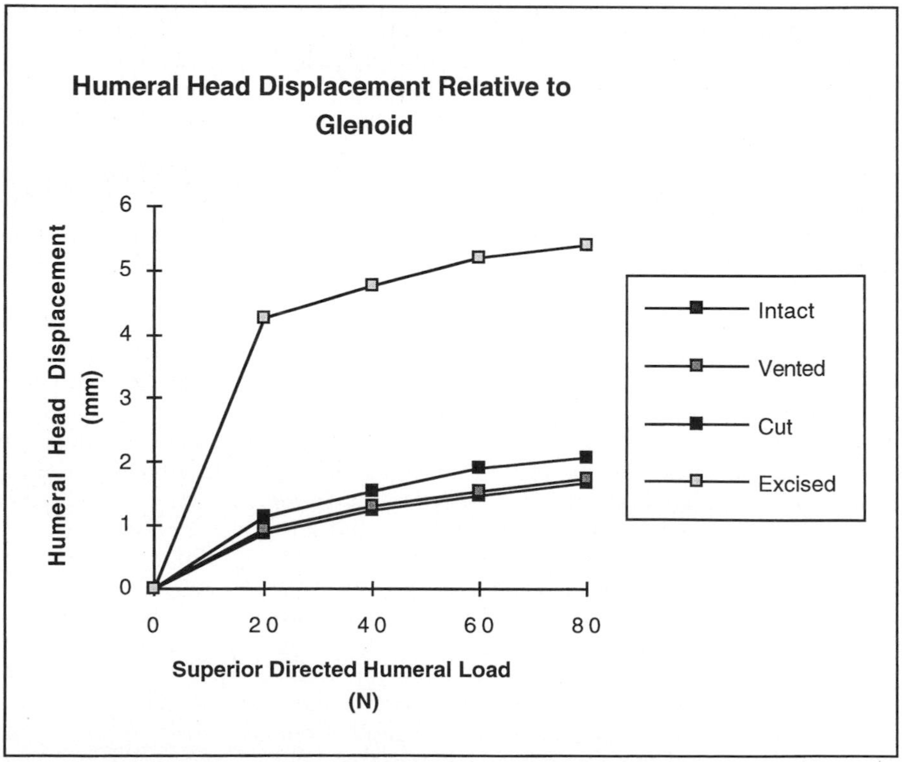

Figure 15–6

The intact superior cuff tendon stabilizes the humeral head against upward-directed humeral loads. When the tendon is removed, this "passive resistance" effect is lost. The chart compares mean superior humeral displacement (relative to the scapula) as a function of superior humerus load for: (1) intact specimens, (2) after venting of the joint to air; (3) after cutting (but not excising the cuff tendon); and (4) after excising the superior cuff tendon.

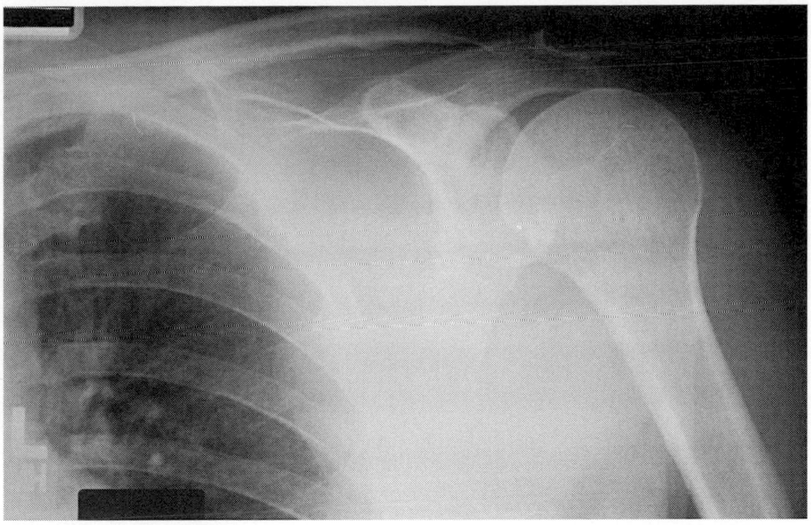

Figure 15–7

The passive resistance effect of the intact cuff tendon. The acromiohumeral interval of the left shoulder preserved by the interposed superior cuff tendon in a 58-year-old man.

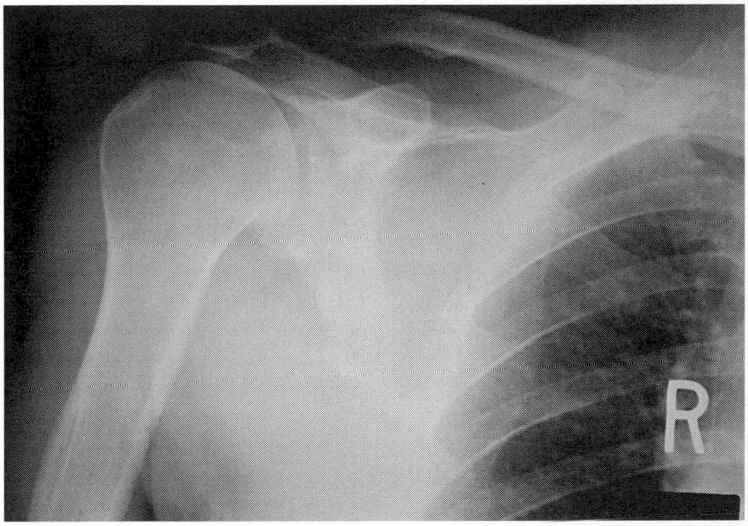

Figure 15–8

Loss of the passive resistance effect. The acromiohumeral interval of the right shoulder is narrowed because of the loss of the interposed superior cuff tendon in the same individual as in Figure 15–7.

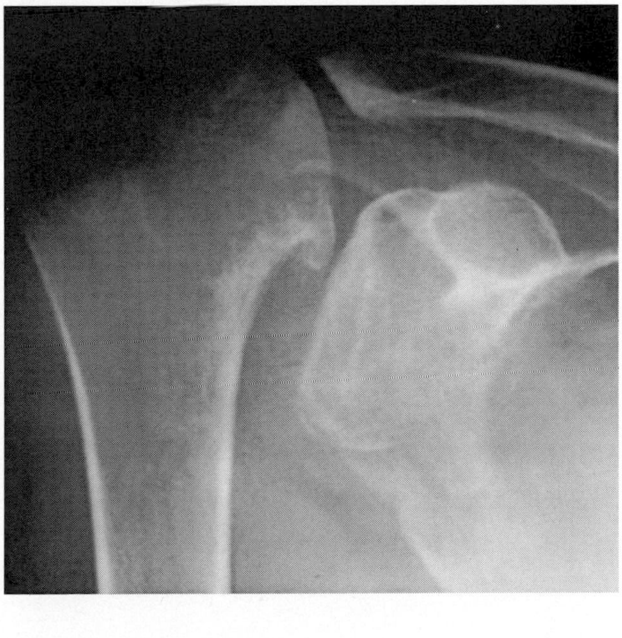

Figure 15–9

An anteroposterior roentgenogram after radical acromionectomy. This procedure removes the origin of the deltoid muscles and may fail to provide complete subacromial smoothing. This patient's symptoms were much more severe after surgery than before.

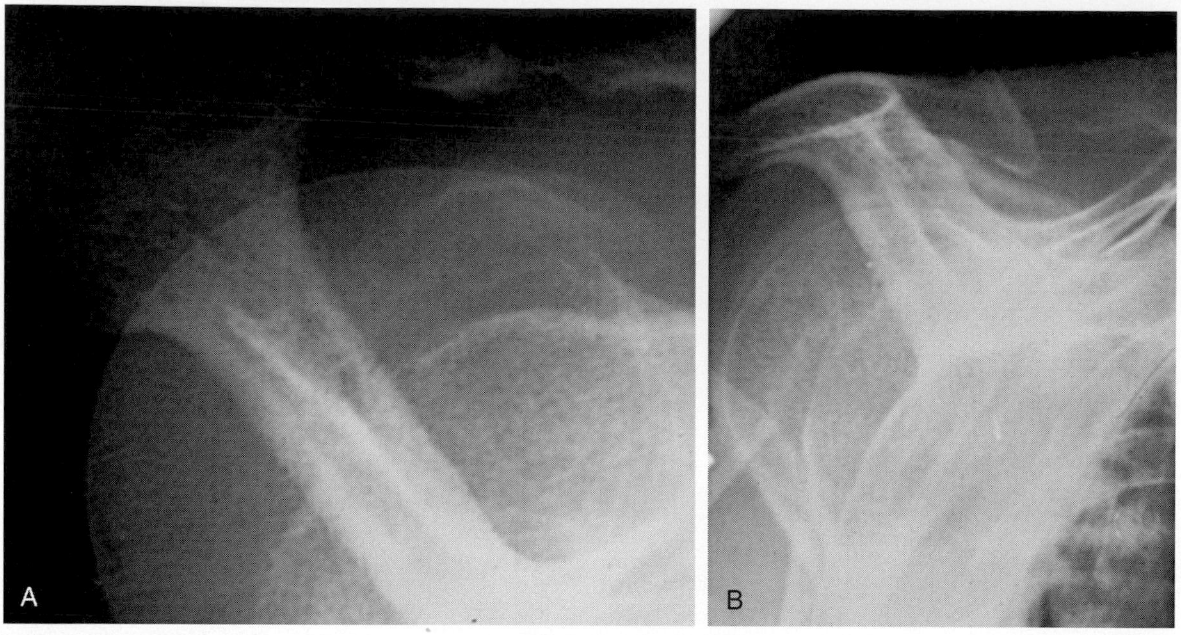

Figure 15–10

A, Variations of the acromial shape are commonly observed in patients with cuff disease. The supraspinatus outlet view is helpful in defining this anatomy. *B*, In this arthrogram (lateral view), one can see indentation of the supraspinatus by the anteroinferior acromion.

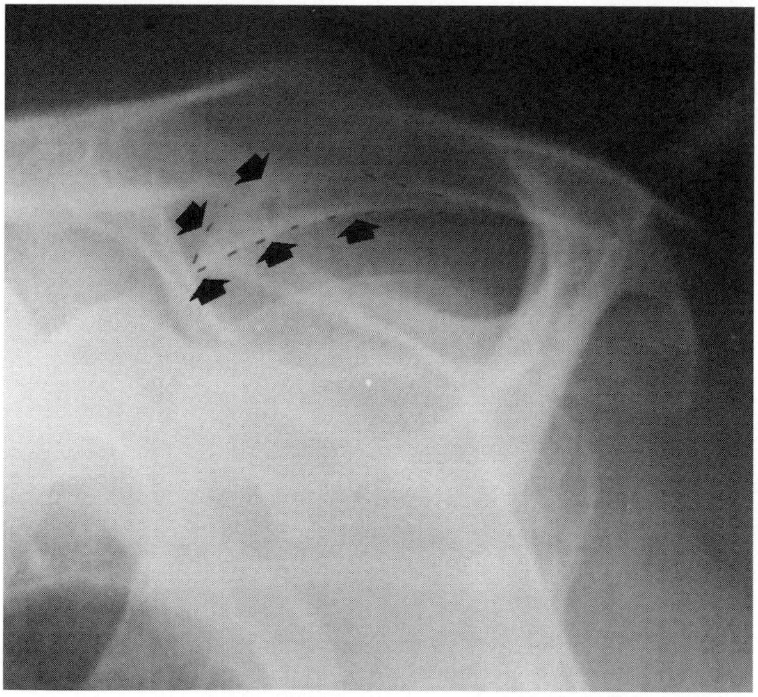

Figure 15–11

A supraspinatus outlet radiograph demonstrating a large anterior inferior osteophyte *(arrows)*. (From Iannotti JP: Rotator Cuff Disorders: Evaluation and Treatment. Rosemont, IL: American Academy of Orthopaedic Surgeons, 1991.)

pointed out by Neer,[275] disease of the rotator cuff causes characteristic changes on the undersurface of the coracoacromial arch. In a remarkable study, Ozaki and associates[306] correlated the histology of the acromial undersurface with the status of the rotator cuff in 200 cadaver shoulders. Cuff tears that did not extend to the bursal surface were associated with normal acromial histology, whereas those that extended to the bursal surface were associated with changes in pathologic changes in the acromial undersurface. They concluded that most cuff tears are related to tendon degeneration and that acromial changes are secondary to pathology of the bursal side of the cuff. These results are similar to those reported by Fukuda and associates.[127]

Studies suggest that type II and type III acromia are acquired, rather than being developmental.[455] In that most acromial "hooks" lie within the coracoacromial ligament (Figs. 15–10 and 15–11), it seems likely that they are actually traction spurs in this ligament (analogous to the traction spur seen in the plantar ligament at its attachment to the calcaneus) (Fig. 15–12). The traction loads producing this "hook" may result from loading of the arch by the cuff and may be increased with growing dependency on the coracoacromial arch for superior stability in the presence of cuff degeneration.[117, 118, 457] The concept of the "hook" as a traction phenomenon was first forwarded by Neer more than 25 years ago.[275] More recently, Putz and Reichelt[334] reported that three quarters of 133 operative specimens of the coracoacromial ligament showed chondroid metaplasia near the acromial insertion, suggesting that this metaplastic area becomes the acromial "hook" by enchondral bone formation.[296] Because this "hook" lies within the ligament and points toward the coracoid (see Fig. 15–11), it seems unlikely that it would jeopardize the passage of the cuff beneath the coracoacromial arch (see Fig. 15–12). Even in the severest cases of cuff tear arthropathy, the undersurface of the coracoacromial arch commonly presents a smooth articulating concavity (Fig. 15–13; see also Fig. 15–12).

In view of the forgoing, it is instructive to consider the humeroscapular articulation as consisting of *two concentric spheres*, the humeral head sphere and the sphere represented by the inferior surface of the coracoacromial arch. Together these two spheres enhance both shoulder stability and the surface available for scapulohumeral load transfer (Fig. 15–14).[62] Normally, the spheres of the humeral head and coracoacromial arch share the same center. The difference in radius of the two spheres is provided by the thickness of the rotator cuff, which serves as a spacer (see Fig. 15–14). In the presence of posterior

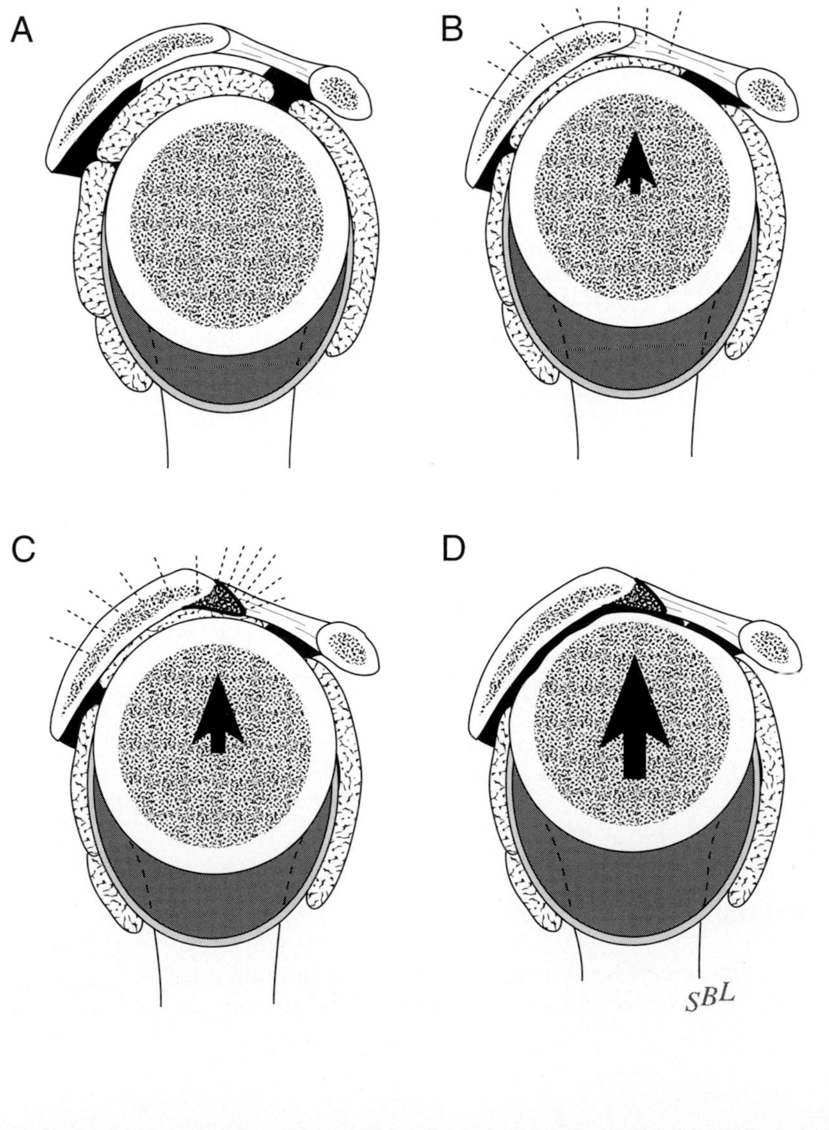

Figure 15–12

The progression of cuff fiber failure. *A*, Normal relationships of the cuff and the coracoacromial arch. *B*, Upward displacement of the head, squeezing the cuff against the acromion and the coracoacromial ligament. *C*, Greater contact and abrasion, giving rise to a traction spur in the coracoacromial ligament. *D*, Still greater upward displacement, resulting in abrasion of the humeral articular cartilage and cuff tear arthropathy. (Modified from Matsen FA III, Lippitt SB, Sidles JA, and Harryman DT II: Practical Evaluation and Management of the Shoulder. Philadelphia: WB Saunders, 1994.)

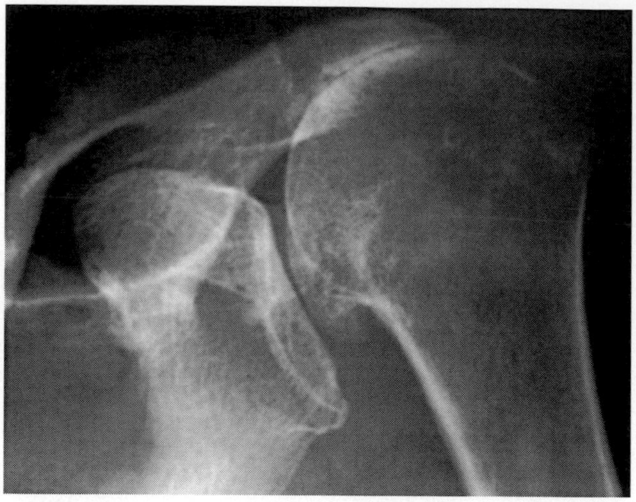

Figure 15–13

Chronic massive tears result in upward displacement of the humeral head until it articulates with the acromion. Humeral osteophytes result from abnormal glenohumeral articulation. Note the smooth undersurface of the coracoacromial arch.

capsular tightness, shoulder flexion or internal rotation causes obligate anterosuperior translation of the humeral head and loss of the concentricity of the two spheres (Fig. 15–15).[69, 159] As a result, the convex cuff-covered head is forced against the anterior undersurface of the concave coracoacromial arch, rather than rotating concentrically beneath it (see Fig. 15–14). In the presence of degeneration of the cuff tendon, the shoulder may lose the concentricity of the humeral head and coracoacromial arch spheres (Figs. 15–16 and 15–17). Taken together, these observations reinforce the shoulder's need for: (1) normal posterior capsular laxity, (2) a smooth, concentric and congruent coracoacromial undersurface, and (3) a normally thick and uniform cuff interposed between the humeral head and coracoacromial arch.

Acromioclavicular Joint. Osteophytes from the acromioclavicular joint may encroach on the space normally occupied by the cuff tendons (Fig. 15–18). In a series of 47 patients with arthrographically confirmed supraspinatus tendon ruptures, Peterson and Gentz[322] found that 51% had distally pointing acromioclavicular joint osteophytes. A similar incidence was found in their series of 170 autopsy specimens with cuff defects. The incidence of distally pointing acromioclavicular osteophytes in normal shoulders was 14% and 10% in the clinical and cadaver studies, respectively. It is recognized, however, that degenerative changes in the cuff and degenerative changes in the acromioclavicular joint may coexist in the aging population without the former being causally related to the latter. It is furthermore recognized that acromioclavicular osteophytes may be sufficiently medial that they do not jeopardize the cuff.

Rotator Cuff

The rotator cuff is the complex of four muscles that arise from the scapula and whose tendons blend in with the subjacent capsule as they attach to the tuberosities of the humerus. The *subscapularis* arises from the anterior aspect of the scapula and attaches over much of the lesser tuberosity. It is innervated by the upper and lower subscapular nerves.[456] The *supraspinatus* muscle arises from the supraspinatus fossa of the posterior scapula, passes beneath the acromion and the acromioclavicular joint, and attaches to the superior aspect of the greater tuberos-

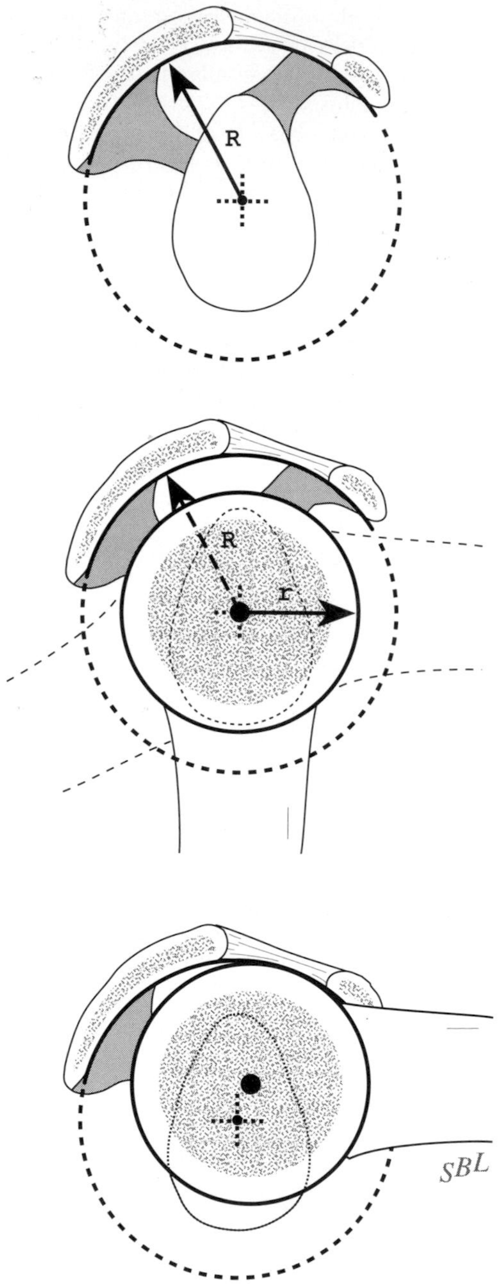

Figure 15–14

The two concentric spheres of the humeroscapular articulation. The coracoacromial arch sphere has a somewhat larger radius (R) than the humeral head sphere (r). In normal shoulder movement, these two spheres share the same center. When the posterior capsule is tight, obligate translation of the humeral head occurs in the anterior superior direction as the shoulder is flexed. In this situation the centers no longer coincide and the cuff (not shown) is squeezed between the humeral head and the anterior undersurface of the coracoacromial arch.

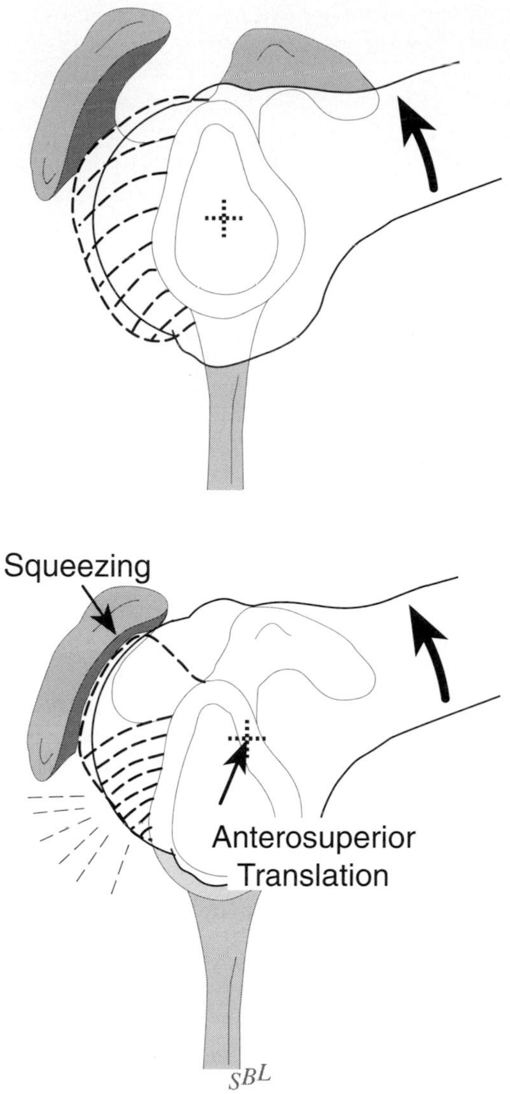

Figure 15–15

Normal capsular laxity allows the humeral head to remain centered during elevation. Tightness of the posterior capsule can create obligate anterosuperior translation with shoulder flexion. This may cause squeezing of the cuff (not shown) between the humerus and the undersurface of the coracoacromial arch. (Modified from Matsen FA III, Lippitt SB, Sidles JA, and Harryman DT II: Practical Evaluation and Management of the Shoulder. Philadelphia: WB Saunders, 1994.)

ity. It is innervated by the suprascapular nerve after it passes through the suprascapular notch. The *infraspinatus* muscle arises from the infraspinous fossa of the posterior scapula and attaches to the posterolateral aspect of the greater tuberosity. It is innervated by the suprascapular nerve after it passes through the spinoglenoid notch. The *teres minor* arises from the lower lateral aspect of the scapula and attaches to the lower aspect of the greater tuberosity. It is innervated by a branch of the axillary nerve.

The insertion of these tendons as a continuous cuff around the humeral head (see Fig. 15–3) permits the cuff muscles to provide an infinite variety of moments to rotate the humerus and to oppose unwanted components of the deltoid and pectoralis muscle forces. For an excel-

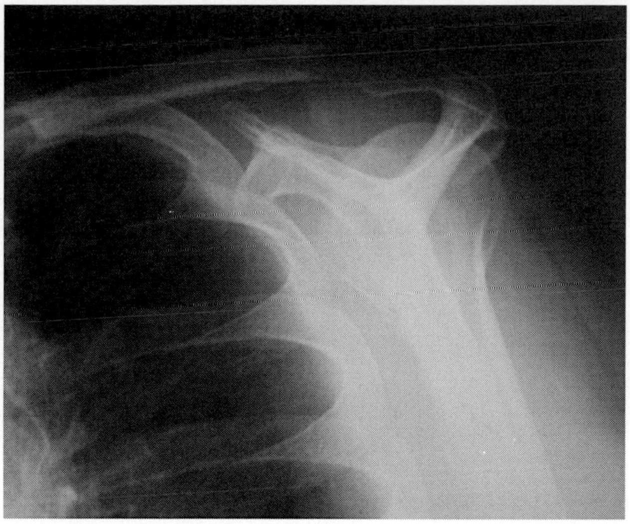

Figure 15–16

Concentricity of the humeral head and coracoacromial arch spheres. The scapular lateral radiograph of the normal left shoulder of a 58-year-old man.

lent review of the anatomy and histology of the rotator cuff, the reader is referred to the works of Clark and Harryman[56–58] and Warner's chapter on shoulder anatomy in *The Shoulder: A Balance of Mobility and Stability*.[426]

The *long head of the biceps* tendon may be considered a functional part of the rotator cuff. It attaches to the supraglenoid tubercle of the scapula, runs between the subscapularis and the supraspinatus, and exits the shoulder through the bicipital groove under the transverse humeral ligament, attaching to its muscle in the proximal arm. Slátis and Aalto point out that the coracohumeral ligament and the transverse humeral ligament keep the biceps tendon aligned in the groove.[376] Tension in the

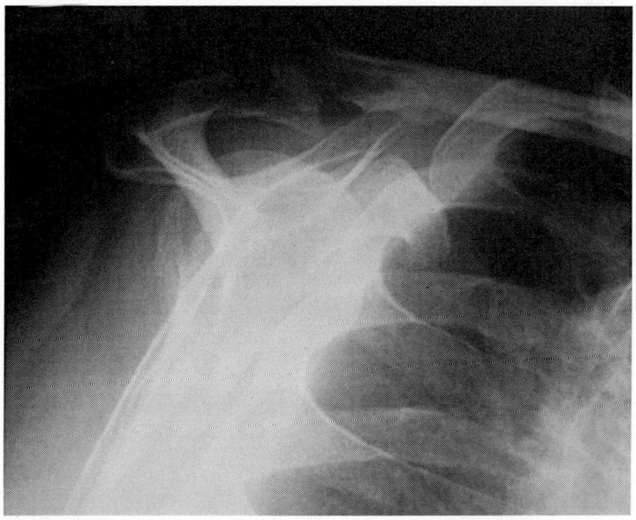

Figure 15–17

The scapular lateral radiograph of a right shoulder (same patient as in Figure 15–16) that has a full-thickness tear of the supraspinatus tendon. Note the loss of concentricity of the humeral head and the arc of the coracoacromial undersurface.

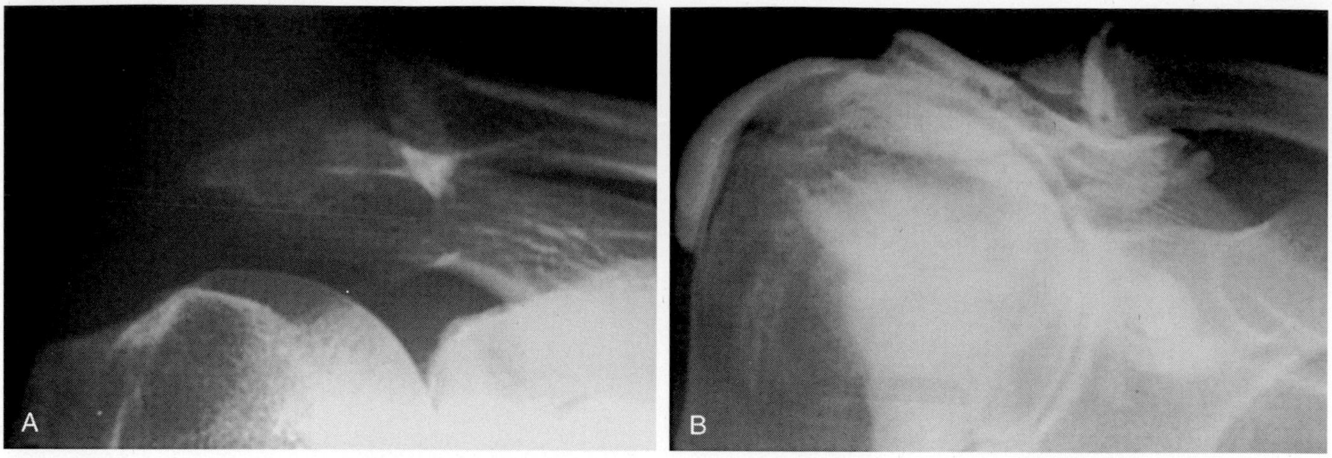

Figure 15–18

A, This anteroposterior roentgenogram shows acromioclavicular joint arthritis. *B*, An arthrogram in the same patient reveals dye leakage into the acromioclavicular joint ("geyser sign"), confirming the clinical suspicion of a rotator cuff tear. Note the indentation of the cuff caused by the acromioclavicular joint osteophytes.

long head of the biceps can help to compress the humeral head into the glenoid. Furthermore, this tendon has the potential for guiding the head of the humerus as it is elevated, the bicipital groove traveling on the biceps tendon like a monorail on its track. This mechanism helps to explain why the humerus is capable of substantial rotation when it is adducted and allows very little rotation when it is maximally abducted (in which position the tuberosities are constrained as they straddle the biceps tendon near its attachment to the supraglenoid tubercle).

The *mechanics of cuff action* are complex. The humeral torque resulting from a cuff muscle's contraction is determined by the moment arm (the distance between the effective point of application of this force and the center of the humeral head) and the component of the muscle force that is perpendicular to it (Fig. 15–19).[448]

The magnitude of force deliverable by a cuff muscle is determined by its size, health, and condition as well as by the position of the joint. The cuff muscles' contribution to shoulder strength has been evaluated by Colachis and associates,[70, 71] who used selective nerve blocks and found that the supraspinatus and infraspinatus provide 45% of abduction and 90% of external rotation strength. Howell and co-workers[175] measured the torque produced by the supraspinatus and deltoid muscles in forward flexion and elevation. They found that the supraspinatus and deltoid muscles are equally responsible for producing torque about the shoulder joint in the functional planes of motion. Other estimates of the relative contributions of the rotator cuff to shoulder strength have been published.[28, 67, 418]

There are at least three factors that complicate the analysis of the contribution of a given muscle to shoulder strength:

1. The force and torque that a muscle can generate vary with the position of the joint: muscles are usually stronger near the middle of their excursion and weaker at the extremes (Fig. 15–20).[225]

2. The direction of a given muscle force is determined by the position of the joint; for example, the supraspinatus can contribute to abduction or external rotation, depending on the initial position of the arm.[303]

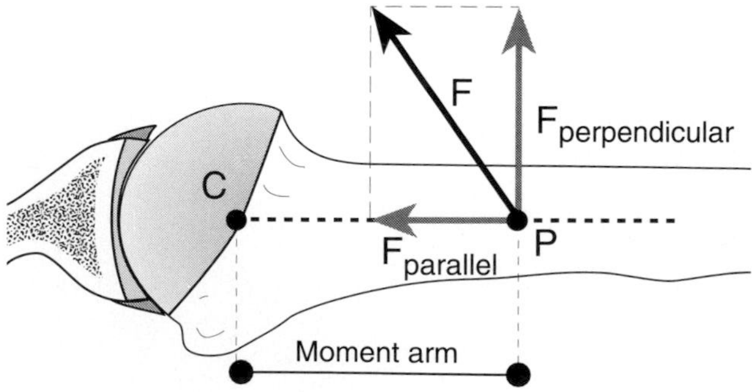

Figure 15–19

The moment arm is the distance between the point of application of a force (P) and the center of movement (C). Torque is the product of the moment arm and the component of the muscle force perpendicular to it (F perpendicular). The component of the muscle force that is parallel to the moment arm (F parallel) can contribute to joint stability through concavity compression. (Modified from Matsen FA III, Lippitt SB, Sidles JA, and Harryman DT II: Practical Evaluation and Management of the Shoulder. Philadelphia: WB Saunders, 1994.)

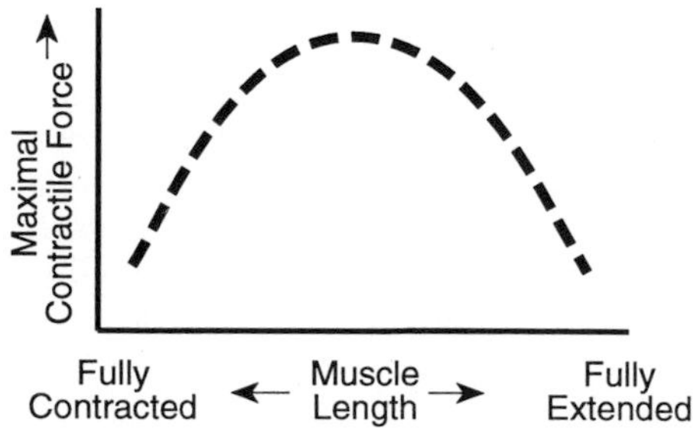

Figure 15–20

A typical relationship between a muscle's length and the maximal force that it can produce. The muscle's length is determined by its origin, insertion, and the position of the joint(s) it spans. (From Matsen FA III, Lippitt SB, Sidles JA, and Harryman DT II: Practical Evaluation and Management of the Shoulder. Philadelphia: WB Saunders, 1994.)

3. The *effective* humeral point of application for a cuff tendon wrapping around the humeral head is not its anatomic insertion, but rather is the point where the tendon first contacts the head, a point that usually lies on the articular surface (Fig. 15–21).

The cuff muscles may be thought of as having three functions:

1. They *rotate the humerus* with respect to the scapula.
2. They *compress the head into the glenoid fossa*, providing a critical stabilizing mechanism to the shoulder, known as concavity compression. While in the past the cuff muscles were referred to as head depressors, it is evident that the inferiorly directed component of the cuff muscle force is small; instead, the primary stabilizing function of the cuff muscles is through head compression into the glenoid (Fig. 15–22).[371, 447]
3. They *provide muscular balance*, a critical function that is discussed in some detail here. In the knee, the muscles generate torques primarily about a single axis: that of flexion-extension. If the quadriceps pull is slightly off-center, the knee still extends. By contrast, in the

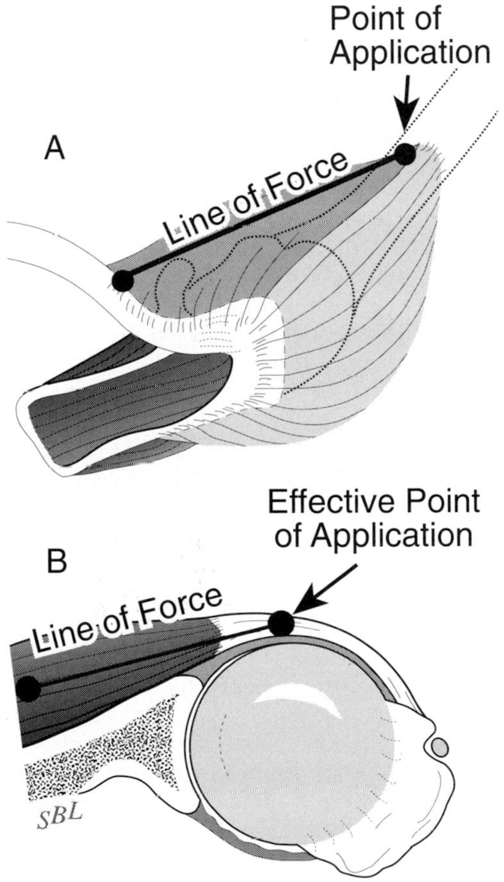

Figure 15–21

Point of application of muscle force. *A*, Determination of the point of force application is simple when the line of force is collinear with its origin and insertion. *B*, However, the rotator cuff tendons wrap around the head of the humerus so that their effective point of attachment usually lies on the humeral articular surface. (Modified from Matsen FA III, Lippitt SB, Sidles JA, and Harryman DT II: Practical Evaluation and Management of the Shoulder. Philadelphia: WB Saunders, 1994.)

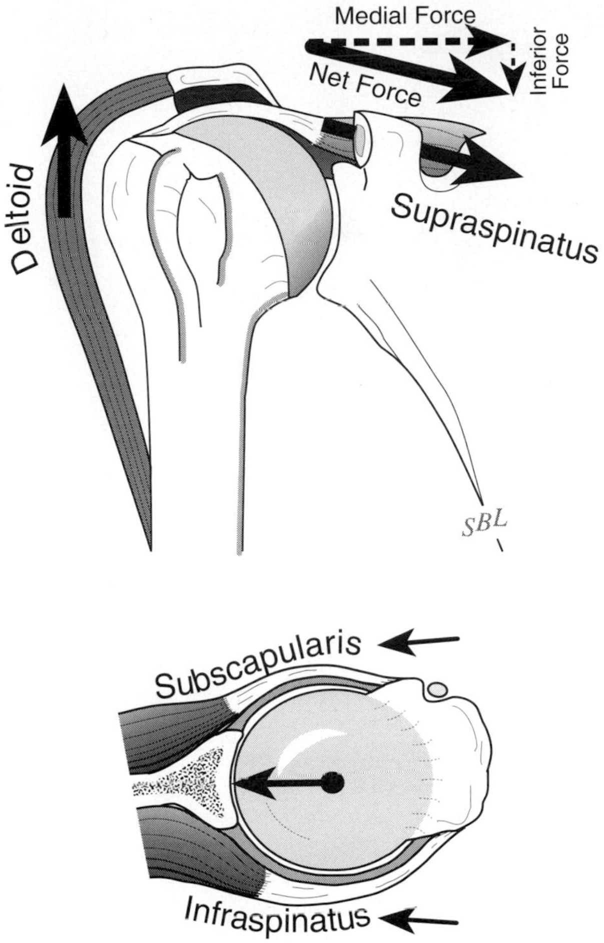

Figure 15–22

Concavity compression. The supraspinatus muscle is not optimally oriented to depress the head of the humerus against the upward pull of the deltoid, because the inferiorly directed component of the supraspinatus force is small. Instead, the humeral head is stabilized in the concave glenoid fossa by the compressive action of the cuff muscles. (Modified from Matsen FA III, Lippitt SB, Sidles JA, and Harryman DT II: Practical Evaluation and Management of the Shoulder. Philadelphia: WB Saunders, 1994.)

shoulder, no fixed axis exists. In a specified position, activation of a muscle creates a unique set of rotational moments. For example, the anterior deltoid can exert moments in forward elevation, internal rotation, and cross-body movement (Fig. 15–23). If forward elevation is to occur without rotation, the cross-body and internal rotation moments of this muscle must be neutralized by other muscles, such as the posterior deltoid and the infraspinatus (Fig. 15–24).[371] As another example, use of the latissimus dorsi in a movement of pure internal rotation requires that its adduction moment be neutralized by the superior cuff and the deltoid. Conversely, use of the latissimus in a movement of pure adduction requires that its internal rotation moment be neutralized by the posterior cuff and posterior deltoid muscles.

The timing and magnitude of these balancing muscle effects must be precisely coordinated to avoid unwanted directions of humeral motion. For a gymnast to hold her arm motionless above her head, all the forces and torques

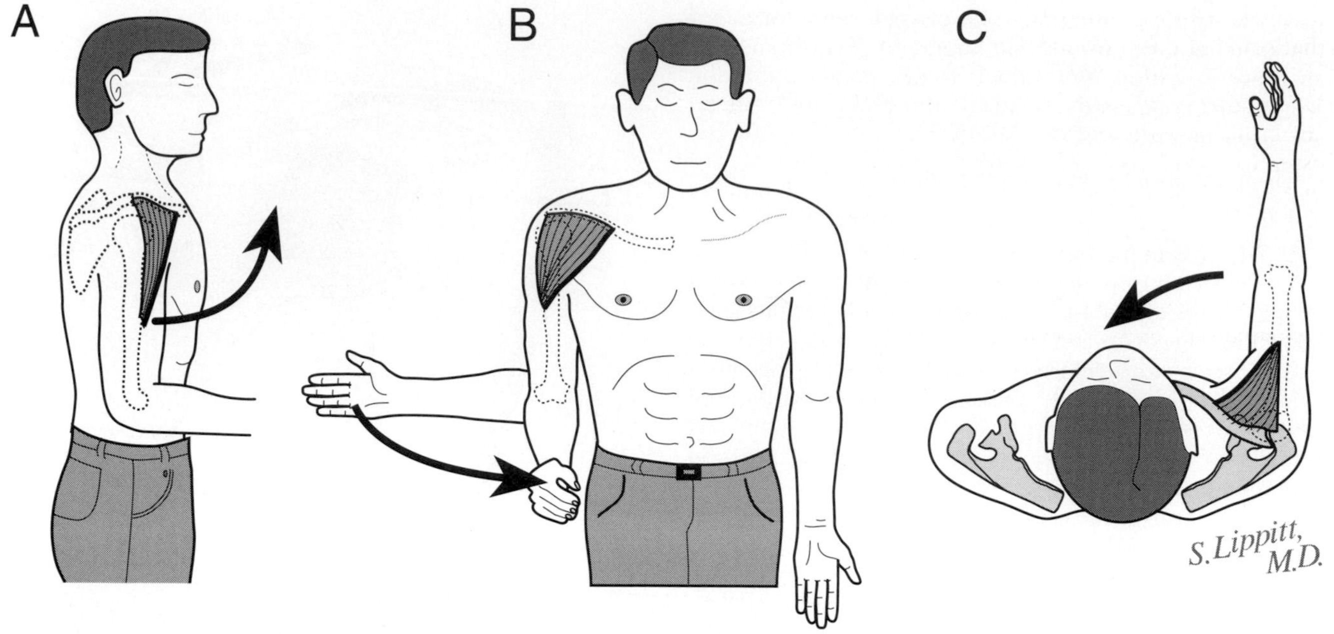

Figure 15–23

The anterior deltoid generates moments in forward elevation *(A)*, internal rotation *(B)*, and cross-body movement *(C)*. (Modified from Matsen FA III, Lippitt SB, Sidles JA, and Harryman DT II: Practical Evaluation and Management of the Shoulder. Philadelphia: WB Saunders, 1994.)

exerted by each of her shoulder muscles must add up to zero. Thus the simplified view of muscles as isolated motors or as members of "force couples" must give way to an understanding that all shoulder muscles function together in a precisely coordinated way: opposing muscles canceling out undesired elements leaving only the net torque necessary to produce the desired action.[356]

This degree of coordination requires a preprogrammed

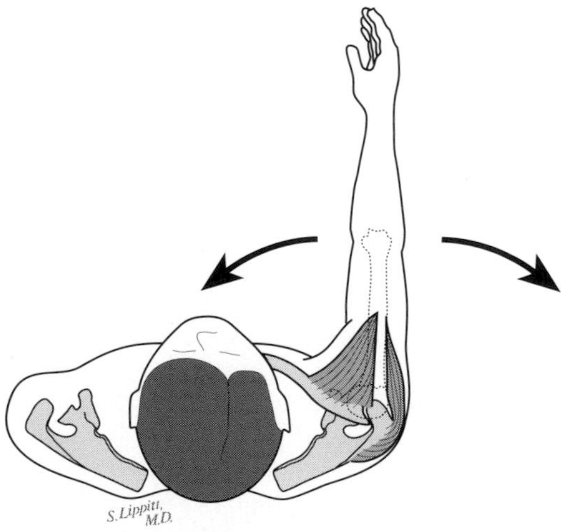

Figure 15–24

Pure elevation requires that the internal rotation and cross-body moments of the anterior deltoid be opposed by other muscle action. For example, even though it is an antagonist to the anterior deltoid, the posterior deltoid must contract during elevation in a plus 90-degree thoracic plane to resist the cross-body moment of the anterior deltoid. (From Matsen FA III, Lippitt SB, Sidles JA, and Harryman DT II: Practical Evaluation and Management of the Shoulder. Philadelphia: WB Saunders, 1994.)

strategy of muscle activation or engram that must be established before the motion is carried out. The rotator cuff muscles are critical elements of this shoulder muscle balance equation.[14, 88, 116, 150, 178, 186, 190, 226, 360, 383, 392, 423]

The *vascular anatomy* of the cuff tendons has been described by a number of investigators.[40, 233, 271, 338, 355] Lindblom described an area of relative avascularity in the supraspinatus tendon near its insertion.[228, 229] Rothman and Parke[355] found contributions to the cuff vessels from the suprascapular, anterior circumflex, and posterior circumflex arteries in all cases. The thoracoacromial contributed in 76% to the cuff's blood supply, the suprahumeral in 59%, and the subscapular in 38%. These authors found that the area of the supraspinatus just proximal to its insertion was markedly undervascularized in relation to the remainder of the cuff. Uhthoff and co-workers[411] observed relative hypovascularity of the deep surface of the supraspinatus insertion compared with its superficial aspect.

By contrast, Moseley and Goldie studied the vascular pattern in the cuff tendons, including the "critical zone" of the supraspinatus (i.e., the anterior corner of the tendon near its insertion that is prone to ruptures and calcium deposits). They found a vascular network that received contributions from the anterior humeral circumflex, subscapular, and suprascapular arteries.[271] They concluded that the critical zone was not much less vascularized than were other parts of the cuff; rather, it was rich in anastomoses between the osseous and tendinous vessels. Rathbun and Macnab[338] found that the filling of cadaveric cuff vessels was dependent on the position of the arm at the time of injection. They noted a consistent zone of poor filling near the tuberosity attachment of the supraspinatus when the arm was adducted; with the arm in abduction, however, there was almost full filling of vessels to the point of insertion. They suggested that some of the previous data suggesting hypovascularity was, in fact, due to this artifact of positioning. Nixon and DiStefano[292] suggested that the "critical zone" of Codman corresponds with the area of anastomoses between the osseous vessels (the anterolateral branch of the anterior humeral circumflex and the posterior humeral circumflex) and the muscular vessels (the suprascapular and the subscapular vessels).

Recently, the vascularity of the supraspinatus tendon has been reconfirmed by the laser Doppler studies of Swiontkowski and associates.[391] The laser Doppler assesses red blood cell motion at a depth of 1 to 2 mm. These investigators found substantial flow in the "critical zone" of the normal tendon and increased flow at the margins of cuff tears. Furthermore, Clark and associates found no avascular areas on extensive histologic studies of the supraspinatus tendon.[56–58]

Uhthoff and Sarkar[413] examined biopsy specimens obtained during surgery on 115 patients with complete rotator cuff rupture. They found vascularized connective tissue covering the area of rupture and proliferating cells in the fragmented tendons. They concluded that the main source of fibrovascular tissue for tendon healing was the wall of the subacromial bursa.

The *histology* of the supraspinatus insertion has been studied in some detail. Codman[61] observed that there were "transverse fibers in the upper portion of the tendon." He stated that "the insertion of the infraspinatus overlaps that of the supraspinatus to some extent. Each of the other tendons also interlaces its fibers to some extent with its neighbor's tendons." In detailed anatomic studies, Clark and Harryman[57] and Clark and associates[56, 58] studied the tendons and capsule of the rotator cuffs from shoulders aged 17 to 72 years. They found that the tendons splayed out and interdigitated to form a common continuous insertion on the humerus. The biceps tendon was ensheathed by interwoven fibers derived from the subscapularis and the supraspinatus. Blood vessels were noted throughout the tendons with no avascular zones. When dissecting what initially appeared to be an intact cuff, the authors frequently encountered a deep-substance tear in which fibers were avulsed from the humerus.

Benjamin and co-workers[23] have analyzed four zones of the supraspinatus attachment to the greater tuberosity: (1) the tendon itself, (2) uncalcified fibrocartilage, (3) calcified fibrocartilage, and (4) bone. Whereas there were blood vessels in the other three zones, the zone of uncalcified fibrocartilage appeared avascular. A tidemark existed between the uncalcified and calcified fibrocartilage that was continuous with the tidemark between the uncalcified and calcified portions of articular cartilage. The collagen fibers often meet this tidemark approximately at right angles. In the tendon of the supraspinatus, there was an abrupt change in fiber angle just before the tendon becomes fibrocartilaginous and only a slight change in angle within fibrocartilage. When interpreting the significance of these findings, these authors point out that the angle between the humerus and the tendon of the supraspinatus changes constantly in shoulder movement (Fig. 15–25). While the belly of the muscle remains parallel to the spine of the scapula, the tendon must bend to reach its insertion. This bending appears to take place above the level of the fibrocartilage so that the collagen fibers meet the tidemark at right angles. The fibrocartilage provides a transitional zone between hard and soft tissues, protecting the fibers from sharp angulation at the interface between bone and tendon. The fibrocartilage pad keeps the tendon of the supraspinatus from rubbing on the head of the humerus during rotation as well as keeping it from bending, splaying out, or becoming compressed at the interface with hard tissue.

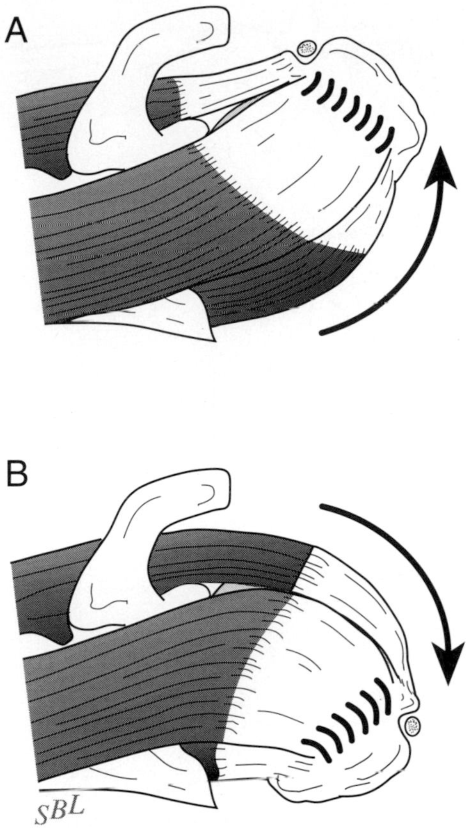

Figure 15–25

The cuff fibers bend at their insertion as the humerus rotates from internal rotation *(A)* to external rotation *(B)*. (Modified from Matsen FA III, Lippitt SB, Sidles JA, and Harryman DT II: Practical Evaluation and Management of the Shoulder. Philadelphia: WB Saunders, 1994.)

The *loading environment* of the cuff tendon fibers is complex, even in the normal shoulder. These fibers sustain *concentric tension loads* when the humerus is moved actively in the direction of action of the cuff muscle (Fig. 15–26). They sustain *eccentric tension loads* as they resist humeral motion or displacement in directions opposite the direction of action of the cuff muscles (Fig. 15–27). The tendon fibers are subjected to *bending loads* when the humeral head rotates with respect to the scapula (see Fig. 15–25). As observed by Sidles[244] in magnetic resonance imaging (MRI) scans positioned with the arm positioned at the limits of motion, the glenoid rim can apply a *shearing load* to the deep surface of the tendon insertion (Fig. 15–28). This abutment of the labrum of the cuff against the cuff insertion may be a better ex-

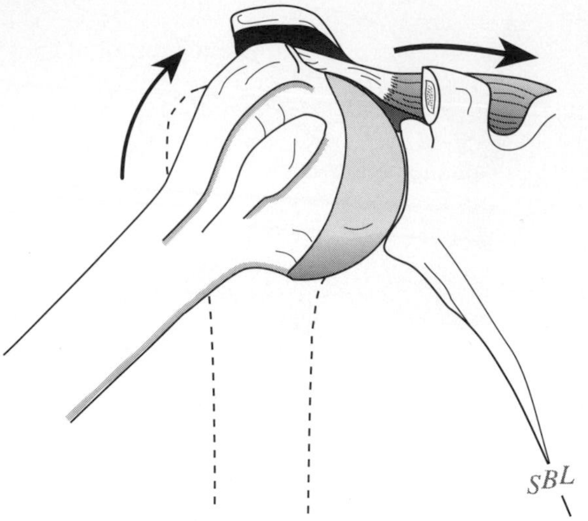

Figure 15–26

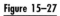

Concentric action of the cuff muscles: the muscle shortens under active tension. (Modified from Matsen FA III, Lippitt SB, Sidles JA, and Harryman DT II: Practical Evaluation and Management of the Shoulder. Philadelphia: WB Saunders, 1994.)

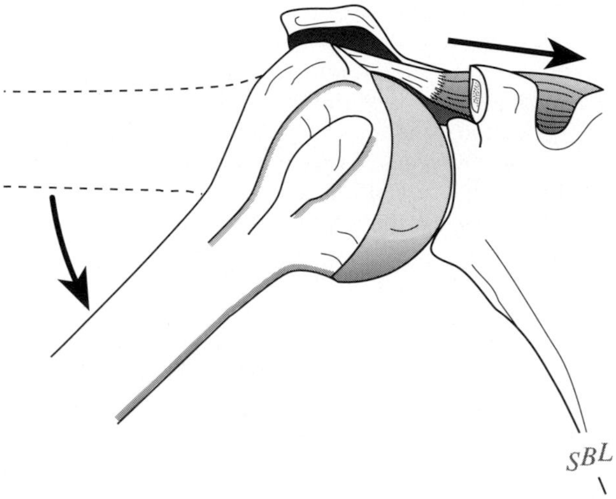

Figure 15–27

Eccentric action of the cuff muscles: the muscle lengthens under active tension. (Modified from Matsen FA III, Lippitt SB, Sidles JA, and Harryman DT II: Practical Evaluation and Management of the Shoulder. Philadelphia: WB Saunders, 1994.)

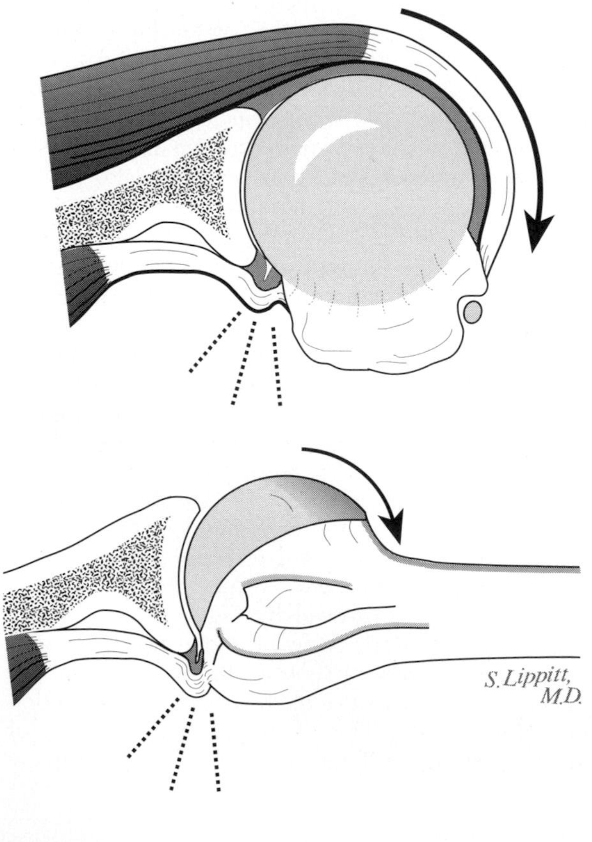

Figure 15–28

Abutment of the deep surface of cuff insertion against the glenoid rim at the extremes of motion. (Modified from Matsen FA III, Lippitt SB, Sidles JA, and Harryman DT II: Practical Evaluation and Management of the Shoulder. Philadelphia: WB Saunders, 1994.)

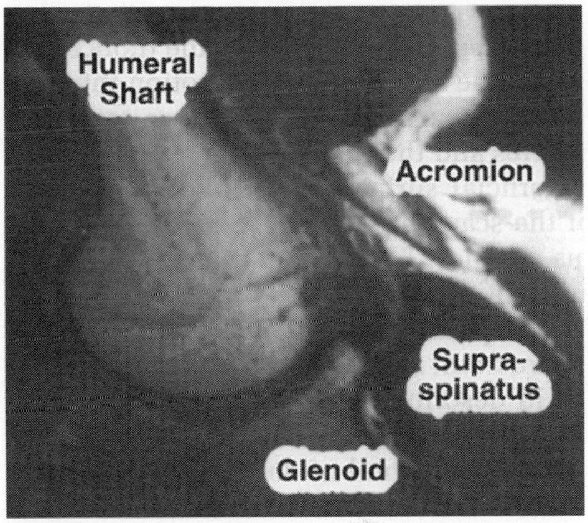

Figure 15–29

This magnetic resonance imaging view of the glenohumeral joint at maximal elevation shows abutment of the acromion against the humerus, which limits elevation. Note, however, that the supraspinatus tendon has cleared the acromion, so that the acromion contacts the humerus distal to the cuff insertion, rather than impinging on the tendon. (From Matsen FA III, Lippitt SB, Sidles JA, and Harryman DT II: Practical Evaluation and Management of the Shoulder. Philadelphia: WB Saunders, 1994.)

planation than acromial impingement for the deep surface cuff defects seen in throwers (Figs. 15–29 and 15–30).[115, 187, 232, 353, 404, 422]

Ziegler and associates have suggested that the superior cuff tendon also experiences *compressive loads* as it is squeezed between the humeral head and the coracoacromial arch when superiorly directed loads are applied to the humerus.[457] In a cadaver model, they found that the preponderance of an upward directed humeral load was transmitted through the cuff tendon to the overlying acromion. When the cuff tendon was excised, the humeral head moved cephalad 6 mm until the superior humeral

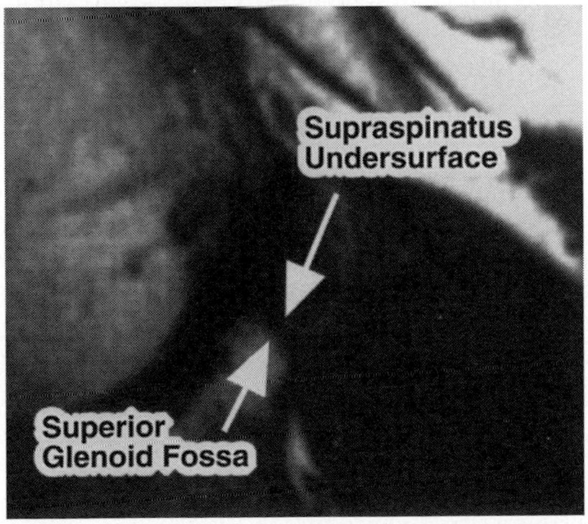

Figure 15–30

In the same shoulder as shown in Figure 15–29, abutment of the undersurface of the supraspinatus tendon against the superior glenoid fossa occurs at the extremes of motion. (From Matsen FA III, Lippitt SB, Sidles JA, and Harryman DT II: Practical Evaluation and Management of the Shoulder. Philadelphia: WB Saunders, 1994.)

load was applied directly to the acromion (see Figs. 15–5 and 15–6). Using completely different methodologies Lazarus and co-workers[214] and Poppen and Walker[327] also found that the humeral head translated 6 mm superiorly when the cuff tendon was absent. Flatow and associates[118] referred to this phenomenon as the "spacer" effect of the cuff tendon. Kaneko and co-workers[193] found that superior displacement of the humeral head was one of the most significant plain radiographic signs of massive cuff deficiency (see Figs. 15–7 and 15–8). Sigholm and colleagues found evidence of this normal tendon compression in vivo.[374] Using a micropipette infusion technique, they found that the normal subacromial resting pressure of 8 mm Hg was elevated to 39 mm Hg by active shoulder flexion to 45 degrees and to 56 mm Hg by the addition of a 1-kg weight to the hand in the elevated position. Recently, morphologic evidence has emerged that supports the concept of compressive loading of the supraspinatus tendon. Okuda[300] described fibrocartilaginous areas in areas of tendons subjected to compression. Riley and co-workers[346] found such areas in the supraspinatus tendon and noted that they had the proteoglycan/glycosaminoglycan of tendon fibrocartilage. They indicated that these morphologic features were an adaptation to mechanical forces, including compression. It has been questioned whether or not compression of the cuff by the acromion could produce the type of cuff defects commonly seen in clinical practice. Recent investigations with a rat model demonstrated that increasing the loading and abrasion of the cuff tendon by the addition of bone plates between the acromion and the tendon produced only bursal side lesions and never the intratendinous or articular side cuff tendon defects that are most frequently seen clinically.[1]

Although young healthy tendons seem to tolerate their complex loading situation without difficulty, structurally inferior tissue,[210, 346] tissue with compromised repair potential,[84, 154] or tendons frequently subjected to unusually large loads (e.g., in an individual with paraplegia)[18] may degenerate in their hostile mechanical environment.[141, 306, 345]

Tendon Degeneration. A normal tendon is exceedingly strong. The work of McMaster is often quoted in this regard.[252] He conducted experiments showing that loads applied to the Achilles tendons of normal rabbits produced failure at the musculotendinous junction, at the insertion into bone, at the muscle origin, or at the bone itself, but not at the tendon midsubstance. In his preparation, one half of the tendon's fibers had to be severed before the tendon failed in tension. If the tendon was crushed with a Kocher clamp, pounded, and then doubly ligated above and below the injury, rupture could be produced in one half of the specimens when tested over 4 weeks later. A normal tendon is obviously tough stuff!

It is estimated that in normal activities, the force transmitted through the cuff tendon is in the range 140 to 200 N.[213, 223, 233, 362] The ultimate tensile load of the supraspinatus tendon in specimens from the sixth or seventh decade of life has been measured between 600 and 800 N.[180]

Although cuff strength may be compromised by inflammatory arthritis[68, 246] and steroids,[106, 196] the primary cause of tendon degeneration is aging. Like the rest of the body's connective tissues, rotator cuff tendon fibers become weaker with disuse and age; as they become weaker, less force is required to disrupt them (Fig. 15–31).[55, 276, 338, 391] Hollis and associates[172] showed that the anterior cruciate ligament of a 70 year old is only 20 to 25% as strong as that of a 20 year old. Others have shown similar loss of tendon strength with age.[62, 89, 228–230, 241, 275, 277, 292, 323, 432] Uhthoff and Sarkar concluded that "Aging is the single most important contributing factor in the pathogenesis of tears of the cuff tendons."[414]

Pettersson[323] provided an excellent summary of the early work on the pathology of degenerative changes in the cuff tendons. Citing the research of Loschke, Wrede, Codman, Schaer, Glatthaar, Wells, and others, he built a convincing case for primary, age-related degeneration of the tendon manifested by changes in cell arrangement, calcium deposition, fibrinoid thickening, fatty degeneration, necrosis, and rents. He stated that "the degenerative changes in the tendon aponeurosis of the shoulder joint, except for calcification and rupture, give no symptoms, as far as is known at present. On the other hand the tensile strength and elasticity of a tendon aponeurosis that exhibits such degenerative lesions are unquestionably less than in a normal tendon aponeurosis."

The major role of tendon degeneration in the production of cuff defects was promoted as a concept by Meyer[255, 256] and corroborated by the studies of DePalma and others.[76, 90–92, 149, 278, 306, 412, 458] Nixon and DiStefano, reviewing the literature on the microscopic anatomy of cuff deterioration,[292] found loss of the normal organizational and staining characteristics of bone, fibrocartilage, and tendon without evidence of repair. They summarized these degenerative changes as follows:

> Early changes are characterized by granularity and a loss of the normal clear wavy outline of the collagen fibers and bundles of fibers. The structures take on a rather homogenous appearance; the connective tissue cells become distorted and the parallelism of the fibers is lost. The cell nuclei become distorted in appearance—some rounded, others pyknotic or fasciculated. Some areas of the tendon have a gelatinous or edematous appearance with loosening of fibers that contain broken, frayed elements separated by a pale staining homogeneous material.

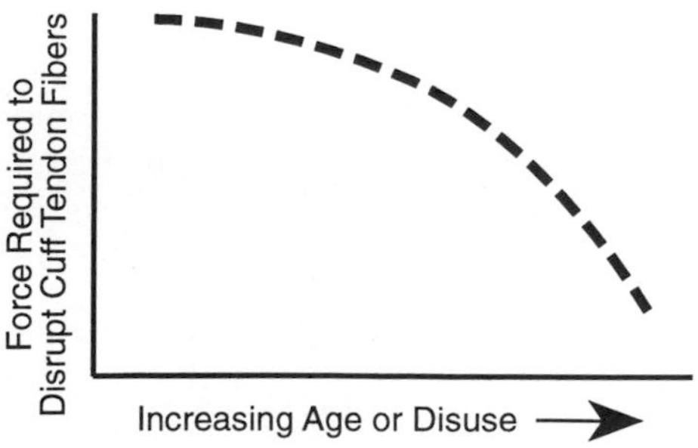

Figure 15–31

The force necessary to disrupt the rotator cuff tendon fibers diminishes with age, disuse, or both. (From Matsen FA III, Lippitt SB, Sidles JA, and Harryman DT II: Practical Evaluation and Management of the Shoulder. Philadelphia: WB Saunders, 1994.)

This histologic picture is reminiscent of that described for tennis elbow, Achilles tendinitis, and patellar tendinitis.

Brewer[38] has demonstrated age-related changes in the rotator cuff. These changes include diminution of fibrocartilage at the cuff insertion, diminution of vascularity, fragmentation of the tendon with loss of cellularity and staining quality, and disruption of the attachment to bone via Sharpey's fibers. The bone at the insertion becomes osteoporotic and susceptible to fracture.[194]

Kumagai and colleagues[210] studied the attachment zone of the rotator cuff tendons to determine how degenerative changes affected the pattern of collagen fiber distribution. Degenerative changes were found in all tendons in the elderly but not in tendons from younger subjects. Changes in insertional fibrocartilage included calcification, fibrovascular proliferation, and microtears. In degenerative tendons, the normal distribution of collagen fiber types was greatly altered with fibrovascular tissue containing type III collagen instead of the usually predominant type II collagen. The authors concluded that severe degenerative changes in the cuff tendons of elderly individuals alter the collagen characteristic of the rotator cuff and that the changes could be associated with impairment of biomechanical properties of the attachment zone. Virtually identical findings were reported by Riley.[345]

In all clinical reports, the incidence of cuff defects is relatively rare before the age of 40 and begins to rise in the 50- to 60-year age group and continues to increase in the 70-year and older age group. Of 55 patients with arthrographically verified cuff tears, Bakalim and Pasila[11] found only three patients who were younger than 40 years of age. Yamada and Evans found no cuff tears in 42 shoulders of patients younger than 40 years of age.[450] In Hawkins and co-workers' series of 100 cuff repairs, only two patients were in their third or fourth decade.[165] In their series of shoulder dislocations, Reeves[339] and Moseley[270] found the incidence of cuff tears among patients younger than 30 years of age to be very low. These authors found that the incidence of cuff failure in dislocated shoulders rose dramatically with the age of the patient. As noted by DePalma, even massive injuries to young healthy shoulders "seem more likely to produce glenohumeral ligament tears and fractures than ruptures of the rotator cuff." Pettersson[323] stated that "even in cases of traumatic rupture . . . the age distribution indicates that changes in the elasticity and tensile strength are prerequisites for the appearance of the rupture." Pettersson reported further that in patients with anteroinferior dislocations, the incidence of arthrographically proven partial- or full-thickness cuff tears was 30% in the fourth decade and 60% in the sixth decade.[323]

Many cuff defects occur in 50- to 60-year-old individuals who have led quite sedentary lives without a history of injury or heavy use. In one of his clinical series, Neer provided substantial evidence for a degenerative etiology of cuff defects[277]: (1) 40% of those with cuff defects have "never done strenuous physical work," (2) cuff defects are frequently bilateral, (3) many heavy laborers never develop cuff defects, and (4) 50% of patients with cuff defects had no recollection of shoulder trauma. In their 1988 report to the American Shoulder and Elbow Surgeons (ASES), Neer and co-workers[280] found that of 233 patients with cuff defects, all except eight patients were older than 40 years of age; 70% of the defects occurred in sedentary individuals doing light work, 27% in females, and 28% in the nondominant arm.

As expected, the deterioration in cuff quality is usually bilateral. Harryman found that 55% of patients presenting with cuff tears on one side had ultrasonographic evidence of cuff defects on the contralateral side.[244] Age-related degeneration can also be observed by MRI.[410]

The pattern of degenerative cuff failure is distinctive. Codman described the "rim rent" in which the deep surface of the cuff is torn at its attachment to the tuberosity.[62] Codman's wonderful book contains many photomicrographs of these rim rents, providing a convincing argument that cuff tears most frequently begin on the deep surface and extend outward until they become full-thickness defects (Fig. 15–32). Codman pointed out that: "It would be hard to explain this . . . by erosion from contact with the acromion process." Similarly, McLaughlin[247] observed that partial tears of the cuff "commonly involve only the deep surface of the cuff. . . ." Wilson and Duff[442] also described partial tears near the insertion of the cuff. These occurred on the articular surface, on the bursal surface, and in the substance of the tendon. Cotton and Rideout[76] also described "slight" tears on the deep surface of the supraspinatus adjacent to the biceps tendon in their necropsy studies. Pettersson and DePalma noted that the innermost fibers of the cuff begin to tear away from their bony insertion to the humeral head in the fifth decade and that these partial-thickness tears increase in size over the next several decades.[89, 323] The partial-thickness tears observed by Uhthoff and co-workers[411] were always on the articular side; none occurred on the bursal side despite the occasional presence of spurs or osteophytes on the acromion. Other authors have also described partial-thickness tears.[34, 35, 62, 125, 129, 212, 262, 307, 387, 393, 394, 397, 451–453] These observations suggest that the deep fibers of the cuff near its insertion to the tuberosity are most vulnerable to failure, either because of the loads to which they are exposed or because of their relative lack of strength or because of their limited capacity for repair.

An important study by Fukuda and associates documented the patterns of intratendinous tears and observed that these lesions tend not to heal.[126] Further evidence of the nonhealing of cuff lesions was provided by Yamanaka and Matsumoto[454] who demonstrated progression of partial-thickness tears. After initial arthrography, they followed 40 tears (average patient aged 61 years) managed without surgery. Repeat arthrograms an average of 1 year later showed apparent healing in only 10%, reduction of apparent tear size in 10%, and enlargement of the tear size in more than 50% with over 25% progressing to full-thickness tears. Interestingly, the clinical pain and function scores of these patients were *improved* at follow-up. These observations lend "proof" to Codman's statement 60 years earlier, "It is my unproved opinion that many of these lesions never heal, although the symptoms caused by them usually disappear after a few months. Otherwise, how could we account for their frequent presence at autopsy?"[62] These studies also demonstrate the critical point that scores based on clinical symptoms are an unreliable way of determining the integrity of the cuff tendon.

The traumatic and the degenerative theories of cuff tendon failure can be synthesized into a unified view of pathogenesis. Through its life the cuff is subjected to various adverse factors such as traction, compression, contusion, subacromial abrasion, inflammation, injections, and, perhaps most importantly, age-related degeneration. Lesions of the cuff typically start where the loads are presumably the greatest: at the deep surface of the anterior insertion of the supraspinatus near the long head of the biceps (Figs. 15–33 and 15–34). Tendon fibers fail when the applied load exceeds their strength. Fibers may fail a few at a time or en masse (Fig 15–35). Because these fibers are under load even with the arm at rest, they retract after their rupture. Each instance of fiber failure has at least four adverse effects: (1) it increases the load on the neighboring as yet unruptured fibers, giving rise to the "zipper" phenomenon, (2) it detaches muscle fibers from bone (diminishing the force that the cuff muscles can deliver), (3) it compromises the tendon

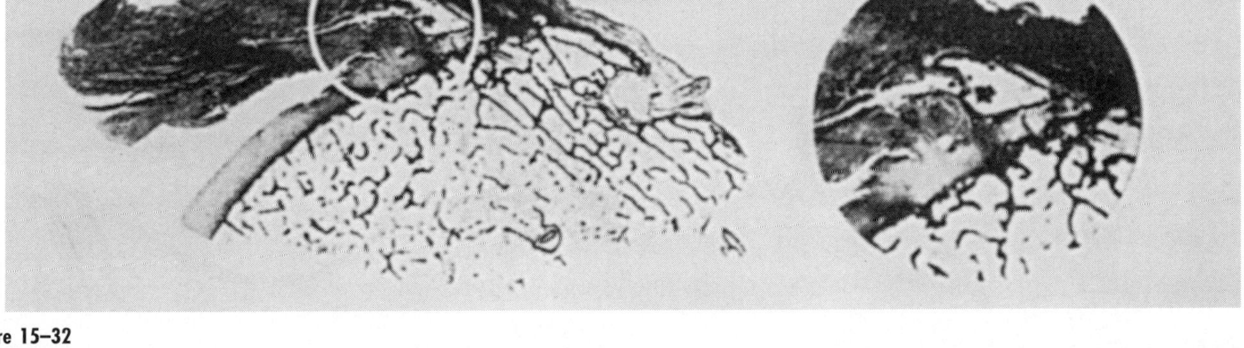

Figure 15–32

Codman's illustration of "A rim rent where all the tendon is torn away from the sulcus except the superficial portion which extends into the periosteum." These photomicrographs provide a convincing argument that cuff tears frequently begin on the deep surface and extend outward until they become full-thickness defects. (From Codman EA: The Shoulder: Rupture of the Supraspinatus Tendon and Other Lesions In or About the Subacromial Bursa. Malabar, FL: Robert E Krieger, 1984.)

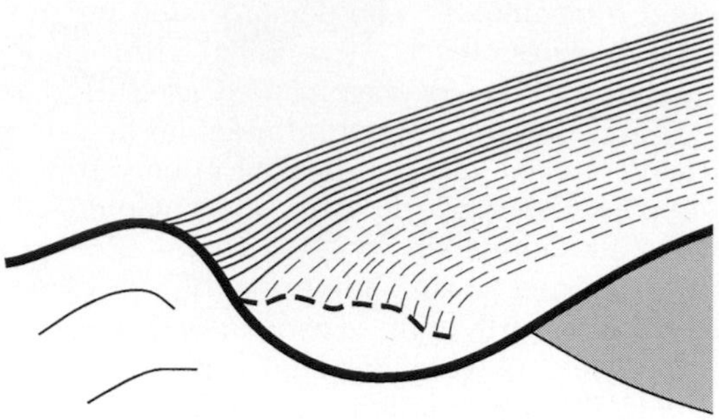

Figure 15–33

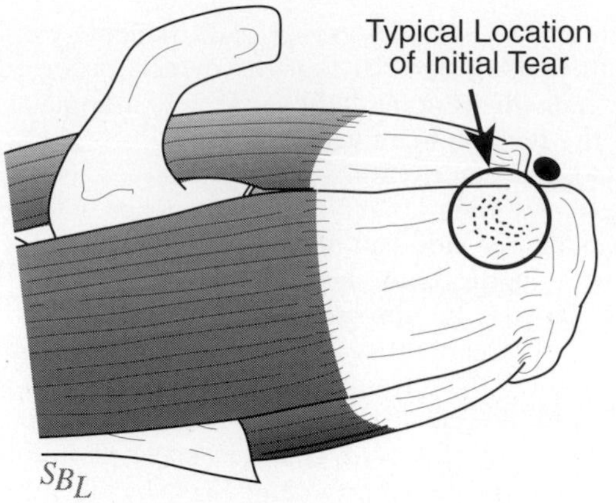

Figure 15–34

Figures 15–33 and 15–34

In degenerative cuff disease, the tendon fibers fail a few at a time, usually starting at the deep surface of the supraspinatus near its insertion near the long head of the biceps. (Modified with permission from Matsen FA III, Lippitt SB, Sidles JA, and Harryman DT II: Practical Evaluation and Management of the Shoulder. Philadelphia: WB Saunders, 1994.)

fibers' blood supply by distorting the anatomy contributing to progressive local ischemia (Fig. 15–36), and (4) it exposes increasing amounts of the tendon to joint fluid containing lytic enzymes, which remove any hematoma that could contribute to tendon healing (Fig. 15–37). Even when the tendon heals, its scar tissue lacks the normal resilience of tendon and is, therefore, under increased risk for failure with subsequent loading. These events weaken the substance of the cuff, impair its function, and diminish its ability to effectively repair itself. In the absence of repair, the degenerative process tends to continue through the substance of the supraspinatus tendon to produce a full-thickness defect in the anterior supraspinatus tendon (Fig. 15–38). This full-thickness defect tends to concentrate loads at its margin, facilitating additional fiber failure with smaller loads than those that produced the initial defect (Fig. 15–39). With subsequent episodes of loading, this pattern repeats itself, rendering the cuff weaker, more susceptible to additional failure with less load, and less able to heal. Once a supraspinatus defect is established, it typically propagates posteriorly through the remainder of the supraspinatus, then into the infraspinatus (Fig. 15–40).

With progressive dissolution of the cuff tendon, the spacer effect of the cuff tendon is lost, allowing the humeral head to displace superiorly (see Figs. 15–8 and 15–12), placing increased load on the biceps tendon. As a result, the breadth of the long head tendon of the biceps is often greater in patients with cuff tears in com-

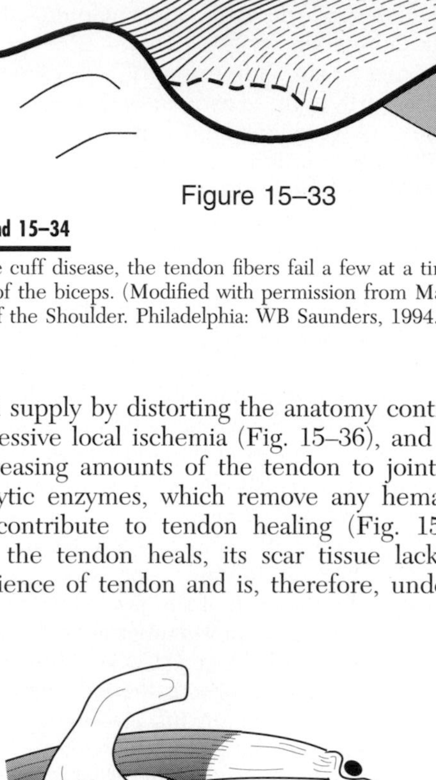

Figure 15–35

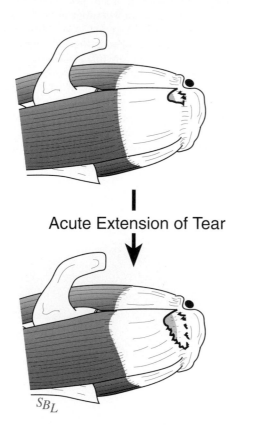

Acute extension of a defect in the rotator cuff. (Modified from Matsen FA III, Lippitt SB, Sidles JA, and Harryman DT II: Practical Evaluation and Management of the Shoulder. Philadelphia: WB Saunders, 1994.)

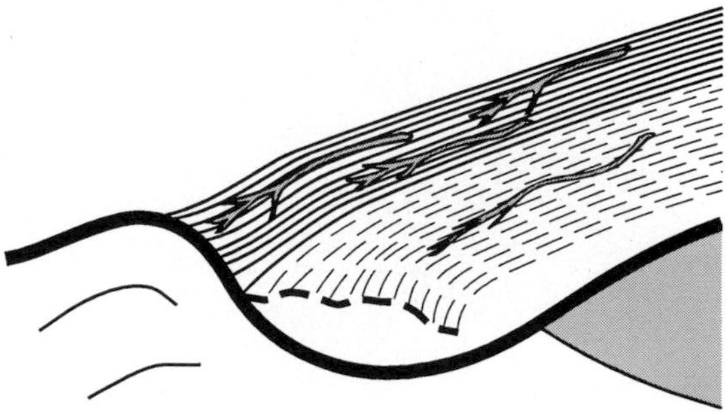

Figure 15–36

Excessive tension at the margin of the tear can compromise the local tendon circulation. (From Matsen FA III, Lippitt SB, Sidles JA, and Harryman DT II: Practical Evaluation and Management of the Shoulder. Philadelphia: WB Saunders, 1994.)

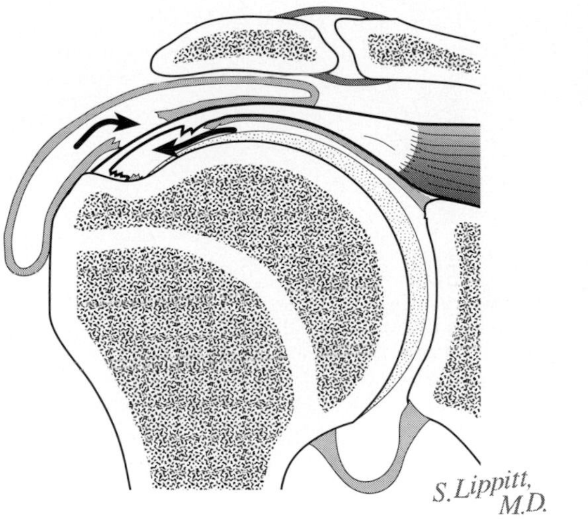

Figure 15–37

The tendon defect is bathed in joint fluid, preventing the formation of a fibrin clot and further compromising the tear's healing potential. (Modified from Matsen FA III, Lippitt SB, Sidles JA, and Harryman DT II: Practical Evaluation and Management of the Shoulder. Philadelphia: WB Saunders, 1994.)

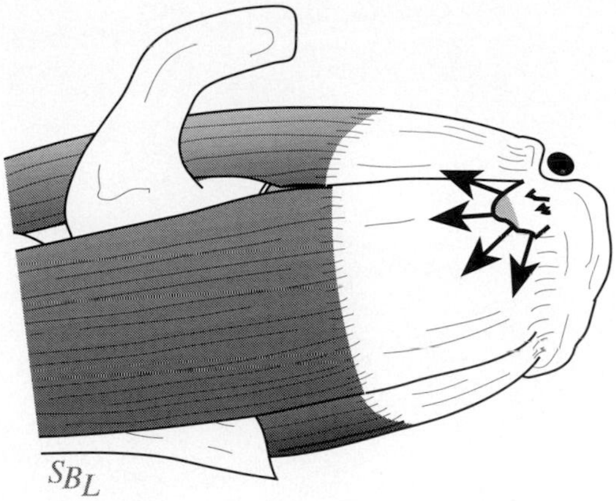

Figure 15–39

The notch phenomenon: the stress on the tendon is channeled toward the edges of the defect, leading to further fiber failure. (From Matsen FA III, Lippitt SB, Sidles JA, and Harryman DT II: Practical Evaluation and Management of the Shoulder. Philadelphia: WB Saunders, 1994.)

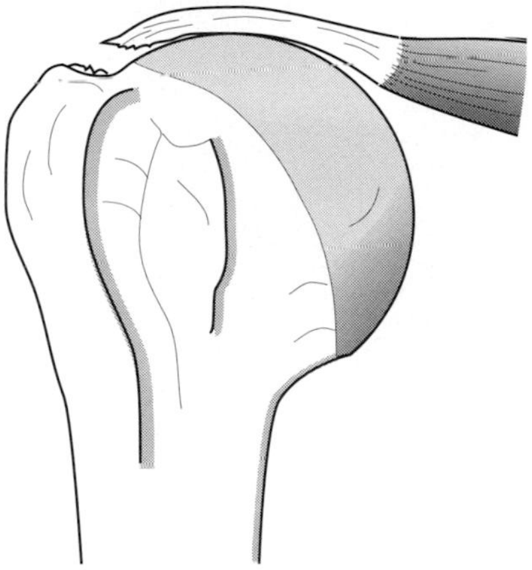

parison with uninjured shoulders (Fig. 15–41).[403] In chronic cuff deficiency, the long head tendon of the biceps is frequently ruptured.

Further propagation of the cuff defect crosses the bicipital groove to involve the subscapularis, starting at the top of the lesser tuberosity and extending inferiorly. As the defect extends across the bicipital groove, it may be associated with rupture of the transverse humeral ligament and destabilization of the long head tendon of the biceps allowing its medial displacement (Fig. 15–42).[376]

The concavity compression mechanism of glenohumeral stability is compromised by cuff disease (see Fig. 15–22). Beginning with the early stages of cuff fiber failure, the compression of the humeral head becomes less effective in resisting the upward pull of the deltoid. Partial-thickness cuff tears cause pain on muscle contraction similar to that seen with other partial tendon injuries

Figure 15–38

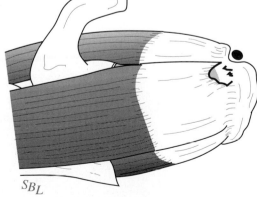

A full-thickness defect in the supraspinatus tendon. (Modified from Matsen FA III, Lippitt SB, Sidles JA, and Harryman DT II: Practical Evaluation and Management of the Shoulder. Philadelphia: WB Saunders, 1994.)

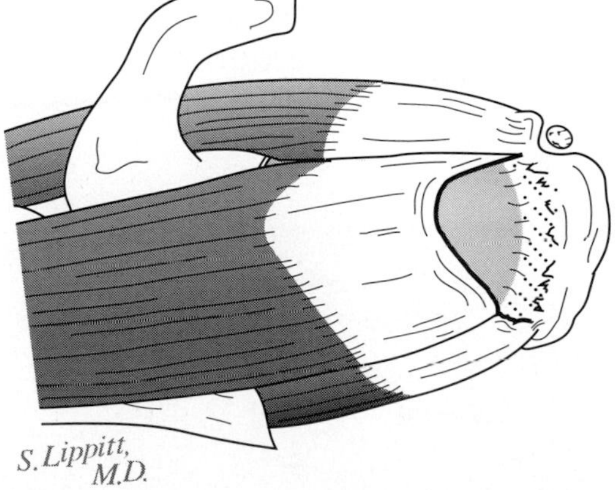

Figure 15–40

The defect propagates through the remainder of the supraspinatus and into the infraspinatus tendon. (Modified from Matsen FA III, Lippitt SB, Sidles JA, and Harryman DT II: Practical Evaluation and Management of the Shoulder. Philadelphia: WB Saunders, 1994.)

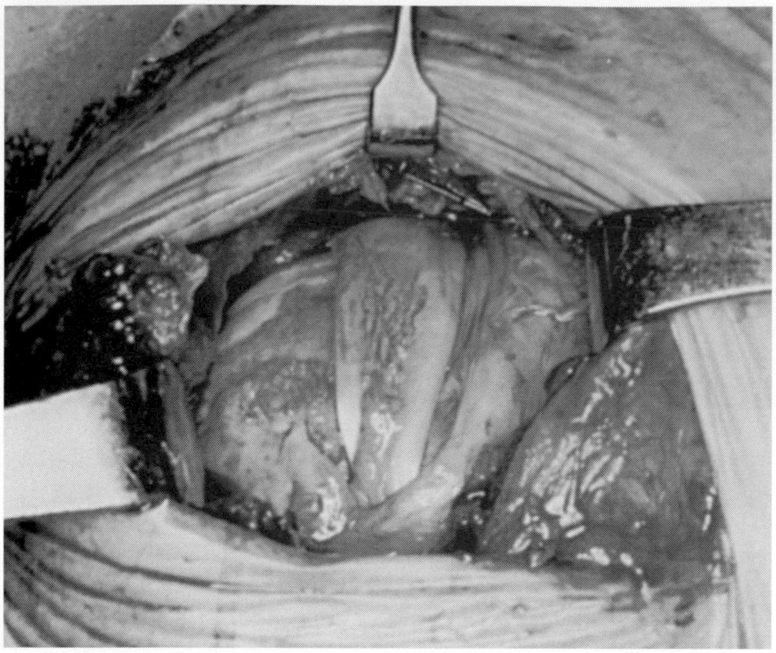

Figure 15–41

Rotator cuff tears are frequently accompanied by changes in the long head tendon of the biceps as it exits the bicipital groove. In many cases, the biceps is seen to be hypertrophied and flattened to the contour of the humeral head—almost as if it were trying to become a substitute cuff.

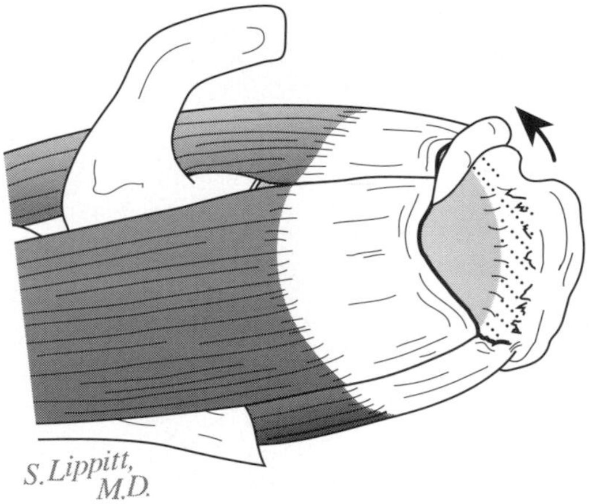

Figure 15–42

The defect further propagates across the bicipital groove to the subscapularis, destabilizing the tendon of the long head of the biceps. (Modified from Matsen FA III, Lippitt SB, Sidles JA, and Harryman DT II: Practical Evaluation and Management of the Shoulder. Philadelphia: WB Saunders, 1994.)

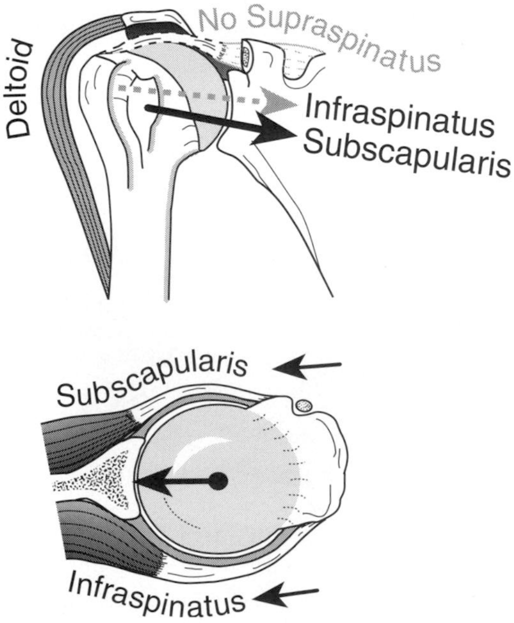

Figure 15–43

Compression by the infraspinatus and the subscapularis can help to stabilize the humeral head in the absence of a supraspinatus, provided that the glenoid concavity is intact. (From Matsen FA III, Lippitt SB, Sidles JA, and Harryman DT II: Practical Evaluation and Management of the Shoulder. Philadelphia: WB Saunders, 1994.)

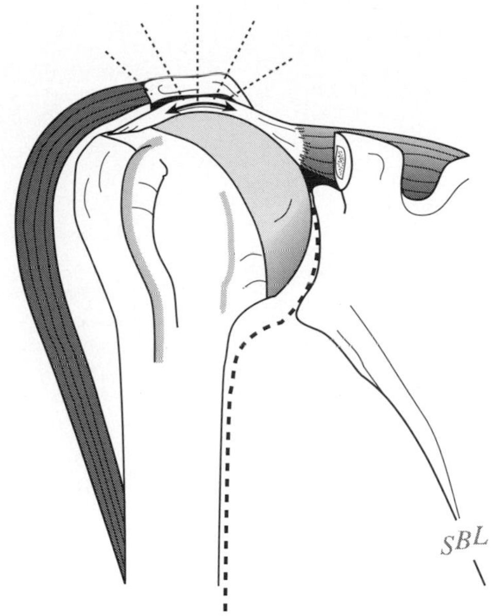

Figure 15–44

Abrasion of the superficial surface of the cuff by the coracoacromial arch associated with superior displacement of head relative to glenoid. (Modified from Matsen FA III, Lippitt SB, Sidles JA, and Harryman DT II: Practical Evaluation and Management of the Shoulder. Philadelphia: WB Saunders, 1994.)

(e.g., those of the Achilles tendon or extensor carpi radialis brevis). This pain produces reflex inhibition of the muscle action. In turn, this reflex inhibition along with the absolute loss of strength from fiber detachment makes the muscle less effective in balance and stability. However, as long as the glenoid concavity is intact, the compressive action of the residual cuff muscles may stabilize the humeral head (Fig. 15–43). When the weakened cuff cannot prevent the humeral head from rising under the pull of the deltoid, the residual cuff becomes squeezed between the head and the coracoacromial arch. Under these circumstances, abrasion occurs with humeroscapular motion, further contributing to cuff degeneration (Fig. 15–44). Degenerative traction spurs develop in the coracoacromial ligament, which is loaded by pressure from the humeral head (analogous to the calcaneal traction spur that occurs with chronic strains of the plantar fascia) (see Fig. 15–12). Upward displacement of the head also wears on the upper glenoid lip and labrum (Fig. 15–45), reducing the effectiveness of the upper glenoid concavity. Further deterioration of the cuff allows the tendons to slide down below the center of the humeral head, producing a boutonnière deformity (Fig. 15–46).[294] The cuff tendons become head elevators rather than head compressors. Just as in the boutonnière of the finger, the shoulder with a buttonholed cuff is victimized by the conversion of balancing forces into unbalancing forces. Erosion of the superior glenoid lip may thwart attempts to keep the humeral head centered after cuff repair (Fig. 15–47). Once the full thickness of the cuff has failed, abrasion of the humeral articular cartilage against the coracoacromial arch may lead to a secondary degenerative joint disease known as cuff tear arthropathy (Fig. 15–48; see also Fig. 15–12).[279]

The cuff muscle deterioration that inevitably accompanies chronic cuff tears is one of the most important limiting factors in cuff repair surgery. Atrophy, fatty degeneration, retraction, loss of excursion are all commonly associated with chronic cuff tendon defects.[218, 274] To a large extent, these factors are irreversible.[145] These changes increase with the duration of the tear and do not rapidly reverse after cuff repair.[146]

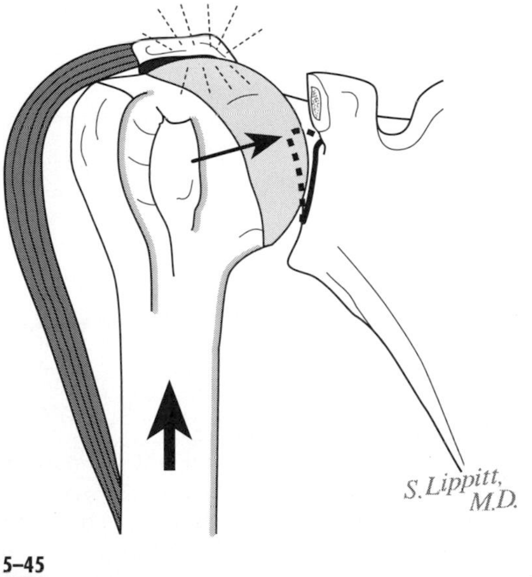

Figure 15–45

Erosion of the superior glenoid concavity compromises the concavity compression stability mechanism, allowing upward translation. The destabilizing effect of this permanent loss of the effective glenoid concavity cannot be offset by rotator cuff repair (see also Fig. 15–47). (Modified from Matsen FA III, Lippitt SB, Sidles JA, and Harryman DT II: Practical Evaluation and Management of the Shoulder. Philadelphia: WB Saunders, 1994.)

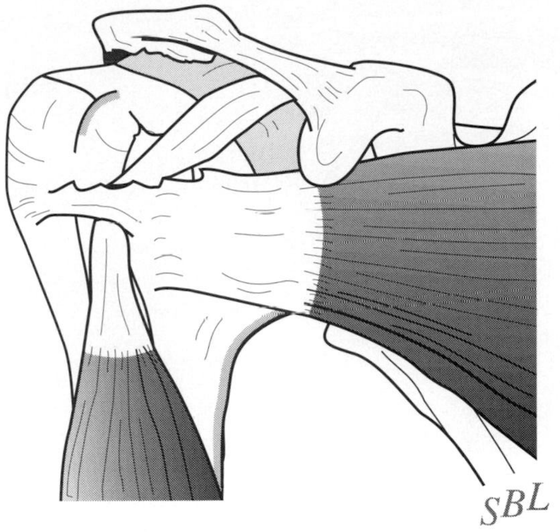

Figure 15–46

The boutonnière deformity, in which the subscapularis and infraspinatus tendons slide below the center of the humeral head. (Modified from Matsen FA III, Lippitt SB, Sidles JA, and Harryman DT II: Practical Evaluation and Management of the Shoulder. Philadelphia: WB Saunders, 1994.)

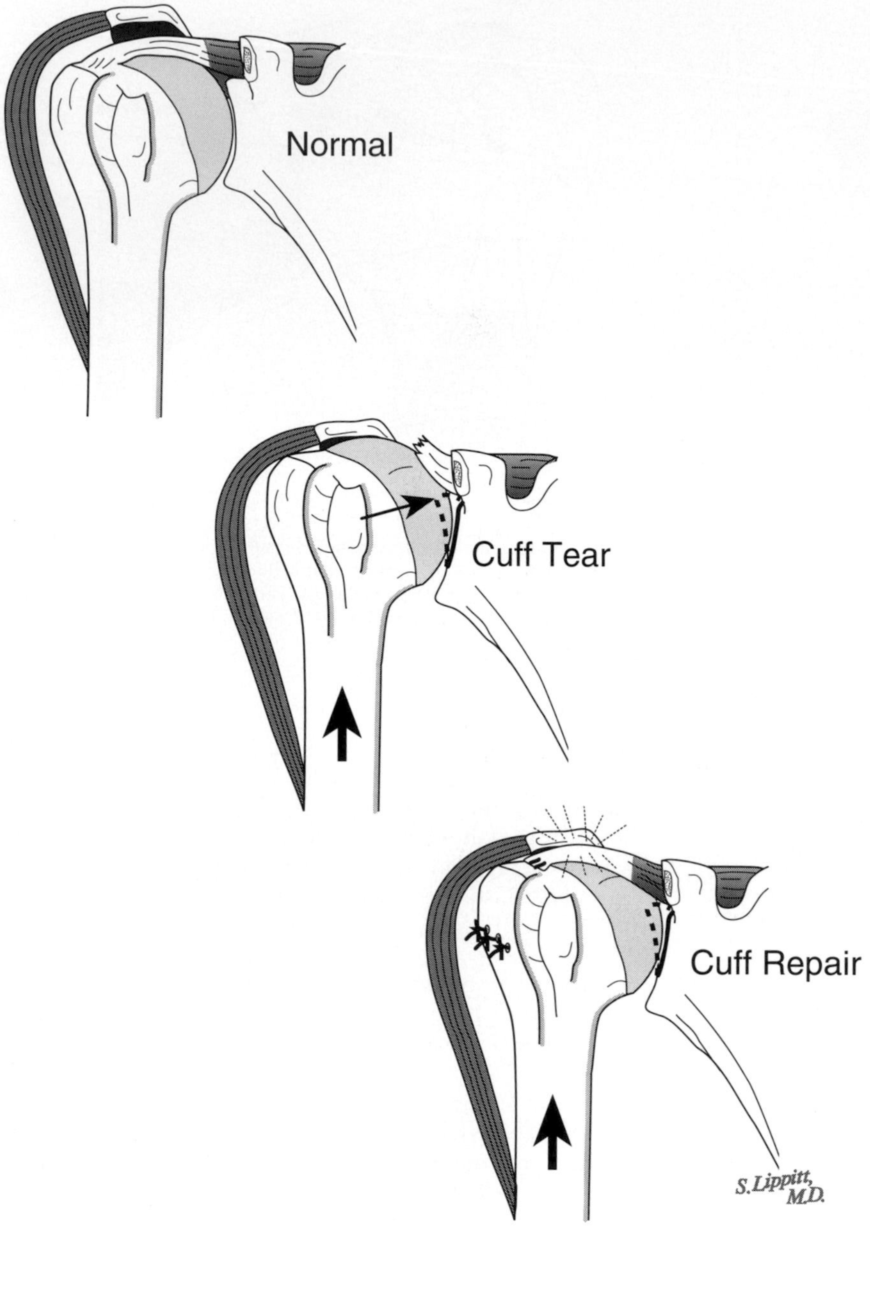

Figure 15–47

In chronic cuff deficiency, erosion of the upper glenoid may leave the shoulder with a permanent tendency to superior subluxation that cannot be reversed by cuff repair surgery.

CLINICAL CONDITIONS INVOLVING THE CUFF

The requisites for normal cuff function are stringent, including healthy, strong cuff muscles, normal capsular laxity, intact cuff tendons, a smooth contour of the undersurface of the coracoacromial arch, a thin, lubricating bursa, a smooth upper surface of the cuff and tuberosities, and concentricity of the glenohumeral and cuff-coracoacromial spheres of rotation (see Figs. 15–3, 15–4, 15–14, 15–15, and 15–22). Disorders of this complex mechanism constitute the most common source of shoulder problems.[52, 176]

Cuff disruption may be partial or full thickness, acute or chronic, and traumatic or degenerative.[67, 244] The magnitude of cuff disruption ranges from the mildest strain to total absence of the cuff tendons. In younger patients, partial-thickness cuff lesions may include the avulsion of a small chip of bone from the tuberosity, the radiographic appearance of which should not be confused with that of calcific tendinitis (Fig. 15–49). Contributing factors may include trauma,[60, 63] attrition,[91, 202, 255, 269] ischemia,[228, 230, 271, 338, 355] and subacromial abrasion.[77, 275, 277, 287, 322, 429]

Degenerative cuff failure almost always starts with a partial-thickness defect on the deep surface near the attachment of the supraspinatus to the greater tuberosity. Codman's view of the frequency of this lesion and the potential range of pathology is indicated by the following passage.[62] In Figure 15–50 there is:

> an extensive tear so that the rent has come through to the most superficial fibers of the tendon. The reader should visualize this vertical section so as to understand that the rent also extends along the curve of the edge of the joint cartilage

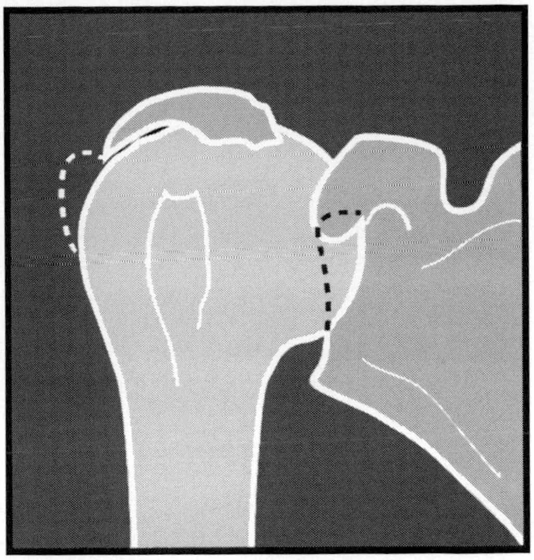

Figure 15–48

Radiographic appearance of cuff tear arthropathy with acetabularization of the upper glenoid and the coracoacromial arch and femuralization of the proximal humerus. (Modified from Matsen FA III, Lippitt SB, Sidles JA, and Harryman DT II: Practical Evaluation and Management of the Shoulder. Philadelphia: WB Saunders, 1994.)

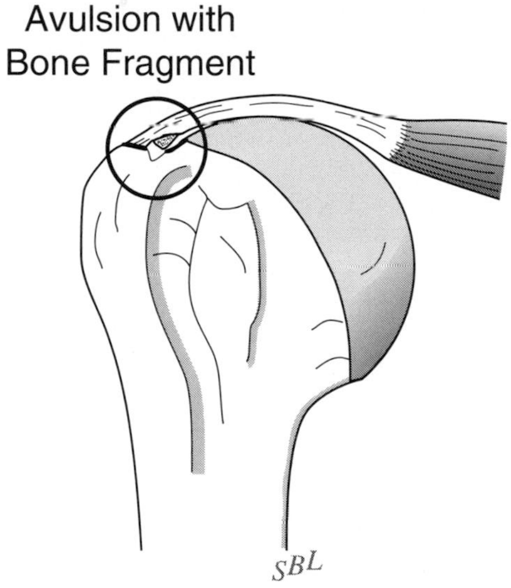

Figure 15–49

A partial-thickness cuff tear with avulsion of bony fragment from the tuberosity. (Modified from Matsen FA III, Lippitt SB, Sidles JA, and Harryman DT II: Practical Evaluation and Management of the Shoulder. Philadelphia: WB Saunders, 1994.)

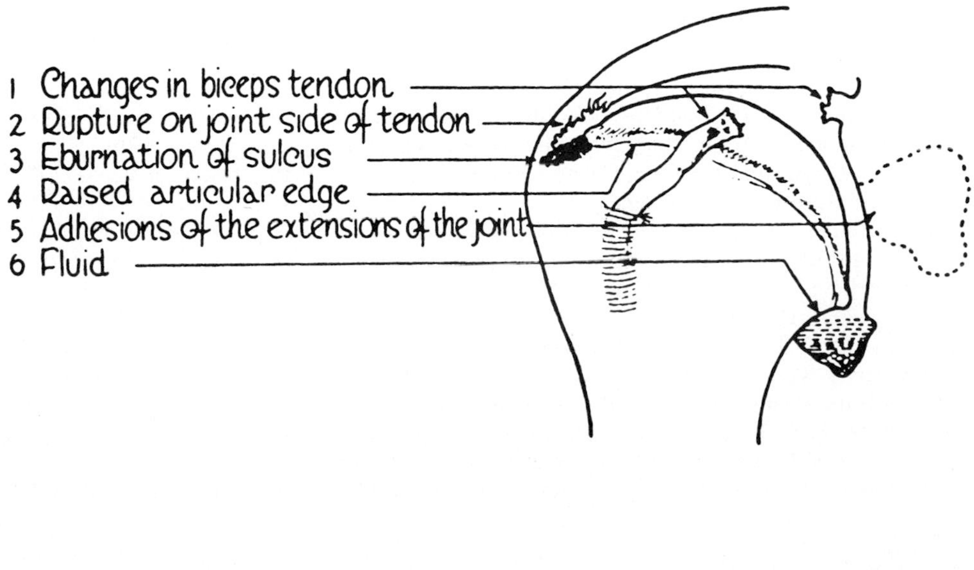

Figure 15–50

In 1934, Codman described the "rim rent" wherein the deep surface of the cuff is torn at its attachment to the tuberosity. (From Codman EA: The Shoulder: Rupture of the Supraspinatus Tendon and Other Lesions In or About the Subacromial Bursa. Malabar, FL: Robert E Krieger, 1984.)

> to a considerable extent, leaving the sulcus bare, perhaps for an inch or more. This condition I like to call a "rim rent," and I am confident that these rim rents account for the great majority of sore shoulders. It is my unproved opinion that many of these lesions never heal, although the symptoms caused by them usually disappear after a few months. Otherwise, how could we account for their frequent presence at autopsy?

The anatomically observed prevalence of partial-thickness cuff lesions leads one to Codman's suggestion that commonly diagnosed diagnoses of shoulder pain, referred to as "cuff tendinitis," "bursitis," or "impingement syndrome," may actually represent failure of the deep surface fibers of the rotator cuff.[126] The degree to which the fibers that remain intact may hypertrophy, strengthen, or adapt to stabilize the tear and take up the function of the damaged fibers is unknown.[45] It appears likely that repeated failure of small groups of fibers leads not only to self-limited, acute symptoms (perhaps interpreted as "tendinitis" or "bursitis"[165]) but also to progressive weakness of the rotator cuff, making it increasingly susceptible to damage from lesser loads. This gives rise to the "creeping tendon ruptures" described by Pettersson.[323] The observation by Pettersson[323] and others that major cuff defects may occur without symptoms or recognized injury suggests that previous minor, often subclinical, fiber failure leaves the shoulder weaker and the cuff tendons progressively less able to withstand the loads encountered in daily living.

Incidence of Rotator Cuff Defects

The incidence of rotator cuff tendon defects has been described in various reports of cadaver dissections: Smith[378] found an incidence of 18%; Keyes,[201] 19%; Wilson,[441, 442] 20% in a series of autopsy dissections and 26.5% in a series of cadaver dissections; Cotton and Rideout,[76] 8%; Yamanaka and co-workers,[453] 7%; Fukuda and associates,[129] 7%; and Uhthoff and colleagues,[411] 20%. Neer found that the incidence of complete cuff tears in more than 500 cadaver shoulders was less than 5%.[277] Lehman and associates[217] found that the incidence of full-thickness rotator cuff tears in 235 male and female cadavers ranging in age from 27 to 102 years (average of 64.7 years) was 17% (53 female, 26 male). The average age of those cadavers with tears was 77.8 years compared with 64.7 years in the intact group. Recognizing the importance of age in the prevalence of cuff lesions, these authors noted that in cadavers younger than 60 years of age the incidence of rotator cuff tears was 6% as opposed to 30% in those older than 60 years of age.

Partial-thickness tears appear to be about twice as common as full-thickness defects. Yamanaka and co-workers[453] and Fukuda[125, 128, 129] reported on 249 cadaver left shoulders in which they found a 13% incidence of partial-thickness tears. Thirty per cent of shoulders in patients older than 40 years of age had cuff tears, whereas there were no tears seen in those younger than 40 years of age. Three per cent had tears on the bursal side; 3% had tears on the joint side; and 7% had intratendinous tears. In another clinical series of partial-thickness cuff tears, Fukuda and associates[128] found nine tears on the bursal side, 11 tears on the joint side, and one intratendinous tear. The bursal side tears had the most severe symptoms. All of these tears were localized in the critical area of the supraspinatus tendon. In studies of 96 shoulders in patients ranging in age from 18 to 74 years, DePalma found a 37% incidence of partial-thickness tears of the supraspinatus and infraspinatus, a 21% incidence of partial-thickness tears in the subscapularis, and a 9% incidence of full-thickness tears. Uhthoff and associates[411] found a 32% incidence of partial-thickness tears in 306 autopsy cases with a mean age of 59 years. Other studies have reported partial-thickness tears in approximately 20 to 30% of cadaver shoulders.[63, 67, 76, 128, 149, 165, 201, 228–230, 411] The data from studies in which the cuff was sectioned to demonstrate the prevalence of intrasubstance lesions indicate that cadaver or clinical examinations confined to the bursal and articular sides of the tendon will overlook the common intratendinous form of cuff defect.

The incidence of cuff defects in *living* subjects is more difficult to study. In a community survey of 644 individuals older than 70 years of age, Chard and associates[53] found 21% had shoulder symptoms (25% in women, 17% in women), the majority of which were attributed to the rotator cuff. However, fewer than 40% of these subjects sought medical attention for these symptoms.

Distorted views of the incidence of cuff disease and of the relationship of cuff tears to clinical symptoms are obtained if only *symptomatic* patients are studied. Thus, some of the most important studies have concerned the prevalence of cuff lesions in *asymptomatic* patients. Pettersson[323] performed arthrography on 71 apparently healthy, asymptomatic shoulders ranging in age from 15 to 85 years. He found that of 27 asymptomatic, untraumatized shoulders in patients aged 55 to 85 years, 13 had arthrographically proven partial- or full-thickness rotator cuff defects and that most were observed between the ages of 70 and 75 years. All these shoulders were symptom free and had no history of trauma. Repeated episodes of fiber failure lead to progressive cuff weakness but not necessarily to pain, unless the extension of the defect is acute and substantial. Milgrom and colleagues[263] found that the prevalence of partial- or full-thickness tears increased greatly after 50 years of age: more than 50% of subjects in their seventh decade and more than 80% in subjects older than 80 years of age. They concluded that "rotator-cuff lesions are a natural correlate of aging, and are often present with no clinical symptoms." Sher and associates[372] used MRI to evaluate asymptomatic shoulders over a wide age range and found that 15% had full-thickness tears and 20% had partial-thickness tears. The frequency of full-thickness tears and partial-thickness tears increased significantly with age ($P < 0.001$ and 0.05, respectively). Twenty-five (54%) of the 46 individuals who were more than 60 years old had a tear of the rotator cuff: 13 (28%) had a full-thickness tear and 12 (26%) had a partial-thickness tear. Of the 25 individuals who were 40 to 60 years old, one (4%) had a full-thickness tear and six (24%) had a partial-thickness tear. Of the 25 individuals who were 19 to 39 years old, none had a full-thickness tear and one (4%) had a partial-thickness tear. They concluded that: (1) MRI identified a high prevalence of tears of the rotator cuff in asymptomatic individuals, (2) these tears were increasingly frequent with advancing age, and (3) these defects were compatible with normal, painless, functional activity.

In another most important study, Yamanaka and Matsumoto[454] demonstrated the progression of partial-thickness tears. After initial arthrography, they followed 40 tears (average patient with an age of 61 years) managed without surgery repeating the arthrogram at an average of more than 1 year later. Although the patients had improved average shoulder scores at follow-up, follow up arthrographies revealed apparent resolution of the tear in only four patients, reduction of the tear size in only four patients, enlargement of the tear size in 21 patients, and progress to full-thickness cuff tear in 11 patients. The authors concluded that tears were likely to progress with increasing age in the absence of a history of trauma.

Thus, it must be concluded that cuff defects become increasingly common after the age of 40 and that many of these occur without substantial clinical manifestations.

Certain occupations seem to be particularly problematic for the rotator cuff, including tree pruning, fruit picking, nursing, grocery clerking, longshoring, warehousing, carpentry, and painting.[236] Some patients relate the onset to some type of athletic activity, such as throwing, tennis, skiing, and swimming. Richardson and associates[344] reviewed 137 of the best swimmers in the United States. The incidence of shoulder problems was 42%. These authors calculated that the average national-level swimmer puts his or her shoulder through about 500,000 cycles per season. Although subluxation is a recognized problem in this group, many were found to have symptoms and signs suggesting cuff involvement. The technique that an athlete uses has a major relationship to the development of or freedom from symptoms, as discussed by Richardson and co-workers,[344] Albright and colleagues,[3] Cofield and Simonet,[69] Penny and Welsh,[320] Neer and Welsh,[282] and Penny and Smith.[319]

CLINICAL PRESENTATION

The clinical manifestations of the various clinical forms of cuff disease include difficulties with shoulder stiffness, weakness, instability, and roughness.[244, 363]

Stiffness

Stiffness limits passive range of motion and frequently causes pain at the end point of motion as well as difficulty sleeping. Stiffness is most common in partial-thickness cuff lesions but may also be associated with full-thickness cuff defects.[184] Stiffness may be demonstrable as limitations of: (1) internal rotation with the arm in abduction (degrees from the neutral position) (Fig. 15–51), (2) reach up the back (posterior segment reached with the thumb) (Fig. 15–52), (3) cross-body adduction (centimeters from the ipsilateral antecubital fossa to the contralateral acromion or coracoid)(Fig. 15–53), (4) flexion (degrees from the neutral position) (Fig. 15–54), or (5) external rotation (degrees from the neutral position) (Fig. 15–55).

Weakness or Pain

Weakness or pain on muscle contraction limits the function of the shoulder with cuff disease. Tendon fibers weakened by degeneration may fail without clinical manifestations or may produce only transient symptoms interpreted as "bursitis" or "tendinitis." A greater injury is required to tear the cuff of individuals at the younger

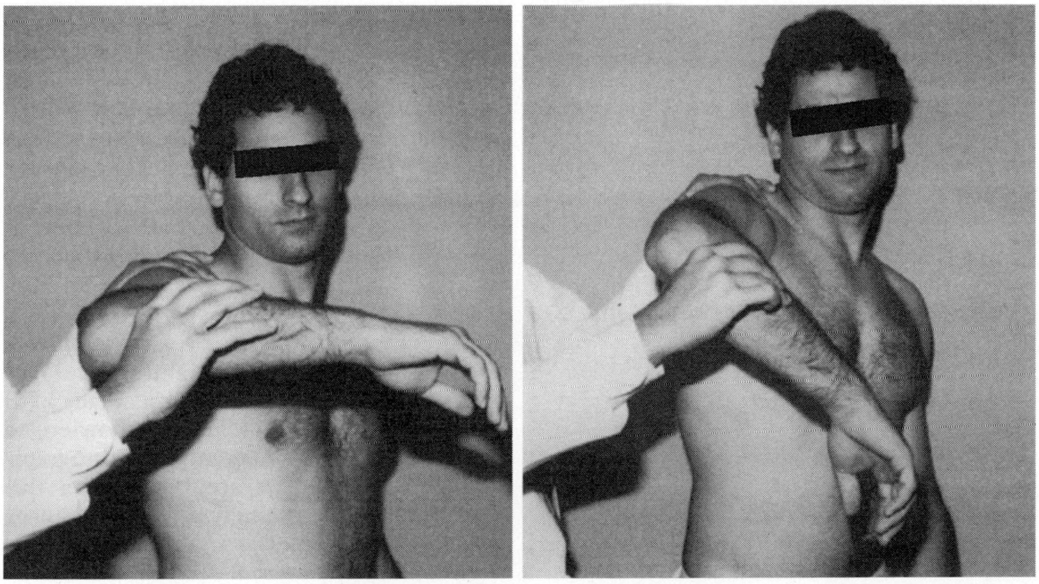

Figure 15–51

Internal rotation in abduction is limited when the posterior capsule is tight. (From Iannotti JP: Rotator Cuff Disorders: Evaluation and Treatment. Rosemont, IL: American Academy of Orthopaedic Surgeons, 1991.)

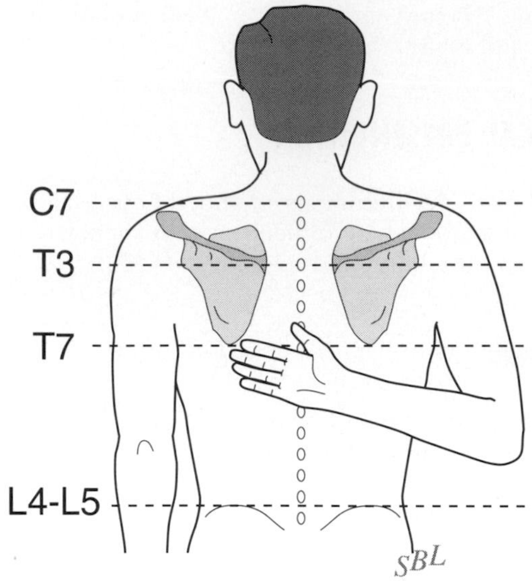

Figure 15–52

Maximal internal rotation is measured by the highest segment of posterior anatomy reached with the thumb, for example, L4-L5, T3, T7, or C7. (From Matsen FA III, Lippitt SB, Sidles JA, and Harryman DT II: Practical Evaluation and Management of the Shoulder. Philadelphia: WB Saunders, 1994.)

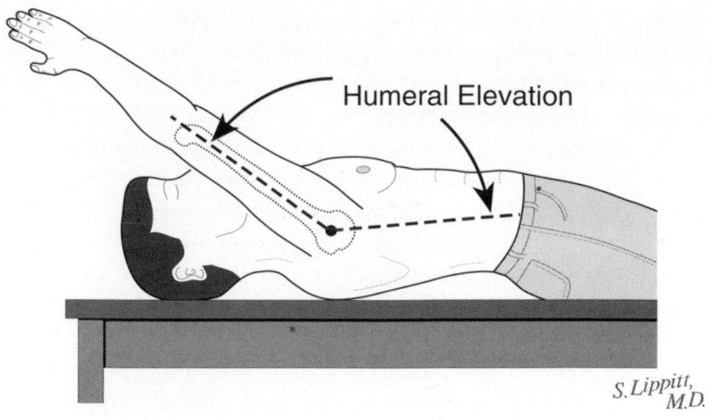

Figure 15–54

Maximum elevation (flexion) is measured with the patient supine and with the opposite arm assisting in elevation, if necessary, to gain maximal range. (From Matsen FA III, Lippitt SB, Sidles JA, and Harryman DT II: Practical Evaluation and Management of the Shoulder. Philadelphia: WB Saunders, 1994.)

end of the age distribution. Traumatic glenohumeral dislocations in individuals older than 40 years of age have a strong association with rotator cuff tears. These traumatic cuff tears commonly involve the subscapularis, producing weakness in internal rotation. Neviaser and associates[288] reported on 37 patients older than 40 years of age in whom the diagnosis of cuff rupture was initially missed after an anterior dislocation of the shoulder. The weakness from the cuff rupture was often erroneously attributed to axillary neuropathy. Eleven of these patients developed recurrent anterior instability that was due to rupture of the subscapularis and anterior capsule from the lesser tuberosity. None of these shoulders had a Bankart lesion. Repair of the capsule and subscapularis restored stability in all of the patients with a recurrence.

Sonnabend reported a series of primary shoulder dislocations in patients older than 40 years of age.[381] Of the 13 patients who had complaints of weakness or pain after 3 weeks, 11 had rotator cuff tears. Toolanen found sonographic evidence of rotator cuff lesions in 24 of 63 patients older than 40 years of age at the time of anterior glenohumeral dislocation.[406]

Even though patients with full-thickness cuff defects may still retain the ability to actively abduct the arm,[284] significant tendon fiber failure is usually manifest by weakness on manual muscle testing.[36, 165, 219, 220] *Isometric* testing of muscle strength prevents confusion with symptoms that may arise from shoulder movement (e.g., those associated with subacromial abrasion). While the individual cuff muscles cannot be specifically isolated, the following isometric tests are reasonably selective (Fig. 15–56):

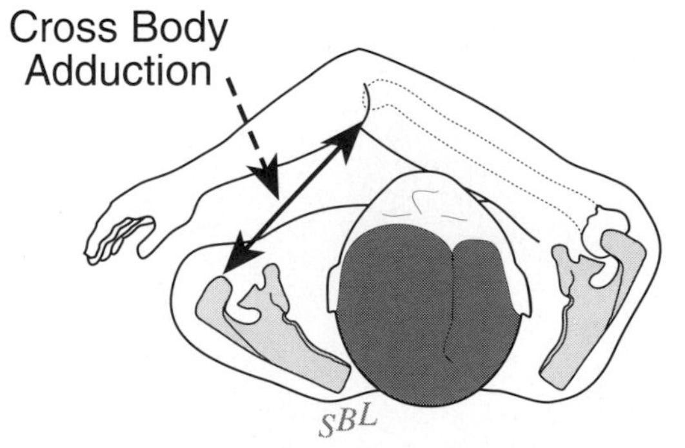

Figure 15–53

Maximal cross-body adduction is measured as the minimal distance from the antecubital fossa to the contralateral acromion when the arm is adducted horizontally across the body. (From Matsen FA III, Lippitt SB, Sidles JA, and Harryman DT II: Practical Evaluation and Management of the Shoulder. Philadelphia: WB Saunders, 1994.)

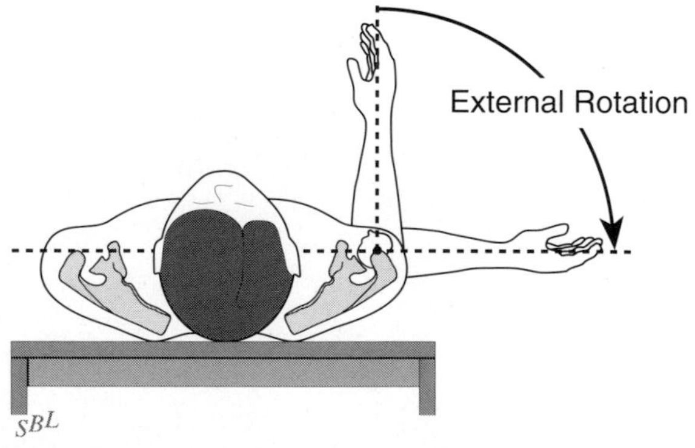

Figure 15–55

Maximal external rotation is measured with the arm at the side (zero degrees being the position in which the forearm of the flexed elbow points straight ahead). We prefer to make this measurement with the patient supine to help fix the thorax. (From Matsen FA III, Lippitt SB, Sidles JA, and Harryman DT II: Practical Evaluation and Management of the Shoulder. Philadelphia: WB Saunders, 1994.)

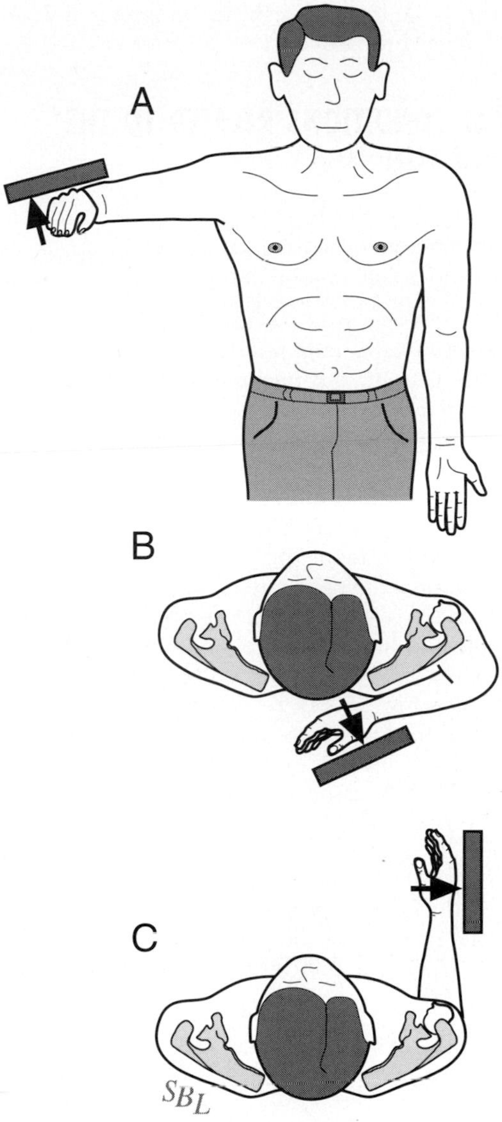

Figure 15–56

Tendon signs: *A*, Supraspinatus tendon sign: pain and weakness on isometric elevation of the arm that is internally rotated and elevated to the horizontal position in the plane of the scapula. *B*, Subscapularis tendon sign: pain and weakness on isometric internal rotation of the arm with the hand held away from the body at the posterior waist. *C*, Infraspinatus tendon sign: pain and weakness on the isometric external rotation with the arm at the side and the forearm pointing ahead. (Modified from Matsen FA III, Lippitt SB, Sidles JA, and Harryman DT II: Practical Evaluation and Management of the Shoulder. Philadelphia: WB Saunders, 1994.)

- *Supraspinatus*—isometric elevation of the arm held in 90 degrees of elevation in the plane of the scapula and in mild internal rotation
- *Subscapularis*—isometric internal rotation of the arm with the elbow flexed to 90 degrees and the hand held posteriorly just off the waist
- *Infraspinatus*—isometric external rotation of the arm held at the side in neutral rotation with the elbow flexed to 90 degrees

These simple manual tests are helpful in characterizing the size of the tendon defects, from single tendon tears involving only the supraspinatus to two tendon tears involving the supraspinatus and infraspinatus to three tendon tears involving the subscapularis as well.

Individuals with partial-thickness cuff lesions have substantially more pain on resisted muscle action than do those with full-thickness lesions. This phenomenon is analogous to the observation that partial tears of the Achilles tendon, partial tears of the patellar tendon, and partial tears of the origin of the extensor carpi radialis brevis are more painful on muscle contraction than when the complete structure is ruptured or surgically released. Fukuda and co-workers[129] characterized patients with partial-thickness cuff tears as having pain on motion, crepitus, and stiffness. They observed that patients with bursal side tears seemed to be more symptomatic than were those with deeper tears, owing to the resultant problems with roughness of the articulation between the upper surface cuff and the undersurface of the coracoacromial arch.

Some have suggested that weakness from pain inhibition can be distinguished from weakness from tendon defect by a subacromial injection of local anesthetic.[22, 230] If cuff dysfunction has been present for more than 1 month or so, it may be accompanied by supraspinatus and infraspinatus muscle atrophy. Subtle atrophy can be seen most easily by casting a shadow from a light over the head of the patient.

As pointed out by Codman,[62] defects in the cuff can often be palpated by rotating the proximal humerus under the examiner's finger placed at the anterior corner of the acromion. The perimeters of the "divot" left by a defect in the supraspinatus are particularly easy to palpate. The defect is usually just posterior to the bicipital groove and medial to the greater tuberosity (Fig. 15–57).

Instability

The inability to keep the head centered in the glenoid may result from cuff disease. Acute tears of the subscapularis may contribute to recurrent anterior instability.[288, 381, 406]

Chronic loss of the normal compressive effect of the cuff mechanism and of the stabilizing effect of the superior cuff tendon interposed between the humeral head and the coracoacromial arch may contribute to superior glenohumeral instability.[117, 118, 214, 327, 457] Superior instability is magnified in the presence of wear of the upper glenoid rim (see Figs. 15–12, 15–13, and 15–45)[279] and when the normal supportive function of the coracoacromial arch is lost from erosion or surgical removal.[440]

Roughness

Roughness associated with cuff disease manifests itself as symptomatic crepitus on passive glenohumeral motion. Bursal hypertrophy, secondary changes in the undersurface of the coracoacromial arch, loss of the integrity of the upper aspect of the cuff tendons, and degenerative changes of the tuberosities may all contribute to *subacromial abrasion*. Crepitus from subacromial abrasion is easily detected by placing the examiner's thumb and fingers on the anterior and posterior aspects of the acromion

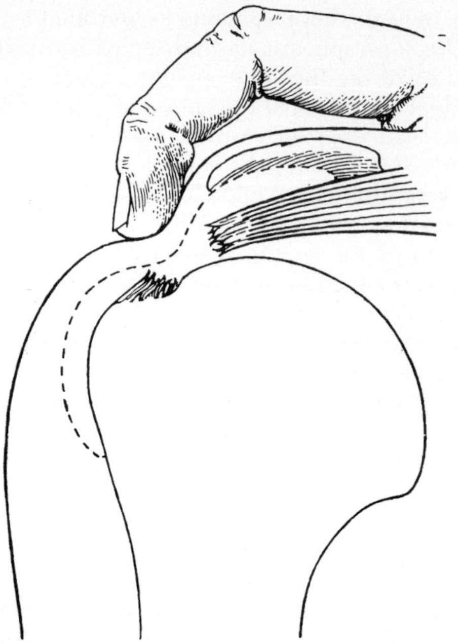

Figure 15–57

Tip of the finger pressing on the eminence and on the sulcus. The plane of this diagram is halfway between the coronal and sagittal. The *dotted line* represents the contour of the bursa. (From Codman EA: Rupture of the Supraspinatus Tendon and Other Lesions In or About the Subacromial Bursa. Malabar, FL: Robert E Krieger, 1984.)

while the humerus is moved relative to the scapula (Figs. 15–58 and 15–59). Since many shoulders demonstrate asymptomatic subacromial crepitus, it is important during the examination to ask whether the crepitus noted by the examiner is directly related to the patient's complaints.

Rotator cuff tear arthropathy is another cause of roughness associated with cuff disease. This term, coined by Neer and co-workers,[279] denotes the loss of the glenohumeral articular surface in association with a massive rotator cuff deficiency (Fig. 15–60). These authors described 26 shoulders of which more than 75% were in female patients. The average age was 69 years; 20% had evidence of contralateral cuff arthropathy, and 75% had no history of trauma. Typically the shoulders were swollen; the muscles were atrophic; and the long head biceps were ruptured. Passive elevation was limited to an average of 90 degrees of elevation and 20 degrees of external rotation (a degree of limitation atypical of uncomplicated cuff tears). The shoulder often demonstrated anteroposterior instability. Collapse of the proximal humeral subchondral bone was a common observation. Glenoid, greater tuberosity, acromial, and lateral clavicular erosion were also commonly observed. The authors hypothesized that the arthropathy resulted from both mechanical factors (e.g., anteroposterior instability and superior migration of the humeral head) (see Figs. 15–12, 15–13, 15–45, 15–46, 15–48) and nutritional factors (e.g., loss of a closed joint space, lack of normal diffusion of nutrients to the joint surface, and disuse). To this list could be added the disruption of the tendinous-osseous circulation entering through the subscapular, anterior humeral circumflex, and suprascapular vessels. This condition is distinct from osteoarthritis, rheumatoid arthritis, avascular necrosis, and neurogenic arthropathy.[277]

CLINICAL CONDITIONS RELATED TO THE ROTATOR CUFF

When discussing the broad spectrum of clinical involvement of the rotator cuff, it is useful to speak of eight clinical entities that can be easily identified by simple criteria:

1. *Asymptomatic cuff failure*—the shoulder does not bother the patient, but imaging studies document a full-thickness defect in the cuff tendon.
2. *Posterior capsular tightness*—the shoulder is limited in its range of internal rotation in abduction (see Fig. 15–51), cross-body adduction (see Fig. 15–53), internal rotation up the back (see Fig. 15–52), and flexion (see Fig. 15–54) (in approximate order of decreasing frequency).
3. *Subacromial abrasion (without a significant defect in the cuff tendon)*—the shoulder demonstrates symptomatic crepitus as the humerus is rotated beneath the acromion (see Figs. 15–58 and 15–59); isometric testing of the cuff muscles (see Fig. 15–56) reveals no pain or weakness.
4. *Partial-thickness cuff lesion*—resisted isometric contraction of the involved cuff muscles is painful or weak (see Fig. 15–56); associated posterior capsular tightness is common (see Figs. 15–51 to 15–53); imaging studies may indicate cuff tendon thinning, but the lesion does not extend through the full thickness of the tendon.
5. *Full-thickness cuff tear*—resisted isometric contraction of one or more of the cuff muscles is painful or weak (see Fig. 15–56); a full-thickness defect of one or more

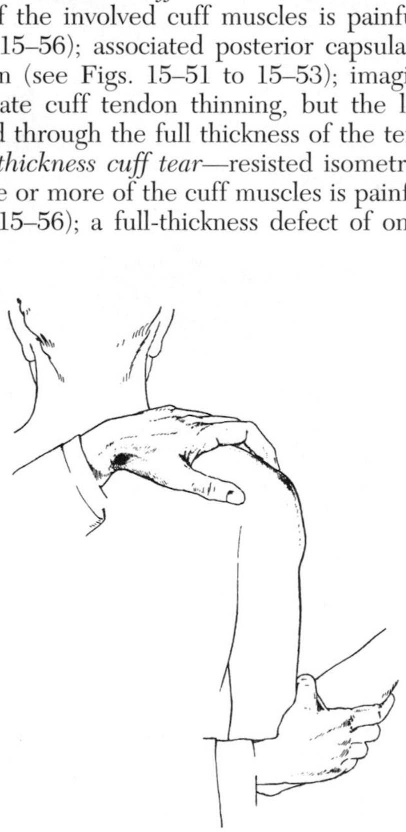

Figure 15–58

Position of the hands for examination of the shoulder. The left thumb lies along the depression below the spine of the scapula, and the tip of the forefinger is just anterior to the acromion. The other three fingers cross and hold the clavicle. Thus, the shoulder girdle is firmly held and any motion of the scapulohumeral joint is at once detected. (From Codman EA: Rupture of the Supraspinatus Tendon and Other Lesions In or About the Subacromial Bursa. Malabar, FL: Robert E Krieger, 1984.)

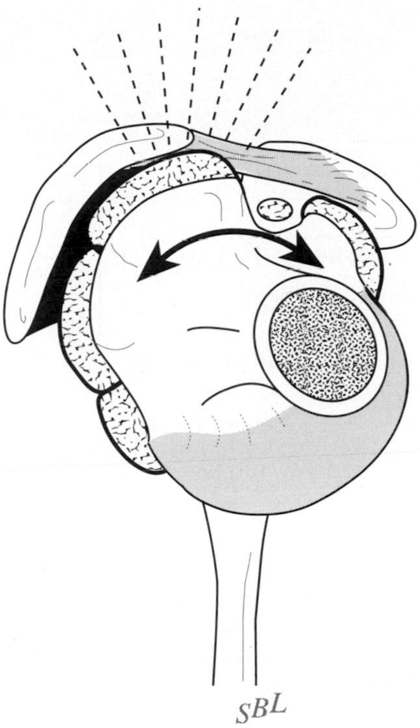

Figure 15–59

Abrasion sign: symptomatic subacromial crepitance on rotation of the arm elevated to 90 degrees with respect to the thorax, a position in which the capsule and ligaments are normally not under tension. (Modified from Matsen FA III, Lippitt SB, Sidles JA, and Harryman DT II: Practical Evaluation and Management of the Shoulder. Philadelphia: WB Saunders, 1994.)

of the cuff tendons is demonstrated on ultrasonography, arthrography, MRI, arthroscopy, or open surgery.

6. *Cuff tear arthropathy*—resisted isometric contraction of the cuff muscles is weak (see Fig. 15–56); acromiohumeral (see Figs. 15–58 and 15–59) and often glenohumeral movements produce crepitance; radiographs demonstrate superior translation of the head of the humerus with respect to the acromion, loss of the articular cartilage of the superior humeral head, direct articulation of the head with the coracoacromial arch, "femoralization" of the proximal humerus and "acetabularization" of the upper glenoid and coracoacromial arch (see Figs. 15–12, 15–13, 15–45, 15–46, and 15–48).

7. *Failed acromioplasty*—the patient is dissatisfied with the result from a previous arthroscopic or open acromioplasty and presents for consideration of additional surgery.

8. *Failed cuff surgery*—the patient is dissatisfied with the result from a previous arthroscopic or open operation on the rotator cuff and presents for consideration of additional surgery.

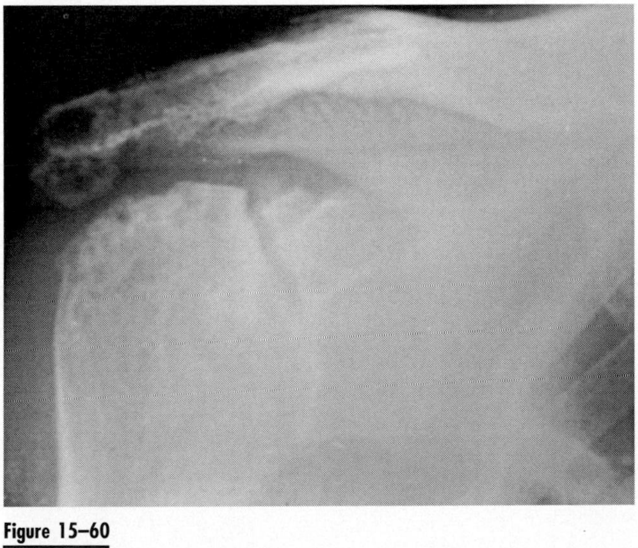

Figure 15–60

Collapse of the humeral head in combination with a massive cuff deficiency—cuff tear arthropathy.

SHOULDER FUNCTION AND HEALTH STATUS IN CLINICAL CONDITIONS OF THE ROTATOR CUFF

To better understand the function and health status of patients with various conditions involving the rotator cuff, Simple Shoulder Test (SST)[244] and short form (SF) 36[425] self-assessments were obtained on 355 consecutive patients presenting to one of us (FAM) with subacromial abrasion, partial-thickness cuff lesions, full-thickness cuff tears, failed acromioplasties, failed cuff repairs, and cuff tear arthropathy. The numbers and average ages of patients with each diagnosis are shown in Table 15–1.

The SST data and SF 36 data for these patients are shown in Figures 15–61 and 15–62, respectively. The SST data indicate that individuals presenting with rotator cuff problems have difficulty with most of the standardized shoulder functions questioned by the SST, especially sleeping comfortably, lifting 8 lb to a shelf, and throwing. More than one half of patients presenting with full-thickness tears are unable to lift 1 lb to a shelf, toss underhand, wash the back of the opposite shoulder, or do their usual work. The severity of functional loss is least for subacromial abrasion followed by partial-thickness cuff lesions, full-thickness cuff tears, failed acromioplasties, failed cuff repairs, and finally, the most severely limiting of this family of conditions, cuff tear arthropathy.

The SF 36 data indicate that patients presenting with cuff disease are most severely compromised with respect to their physical role function and their comfort. Even though the differences among diagnoses are not large,

Table 15–1 PREVALENCE AND AVERAGE AGE OF PATIENTS WITH SIX TYPES OF CUFF LESIONS

	NO. OF PATIENTS	AGE AT PRESENTATION
Subacromial abrasion	18	43
Partial-thickness cuff lesion	104	48
Rotator cuff tear	133	62
Failed acromioplasty	29	49
Failed cuff repair	47	60
Cuff tear arthropathy	24	74

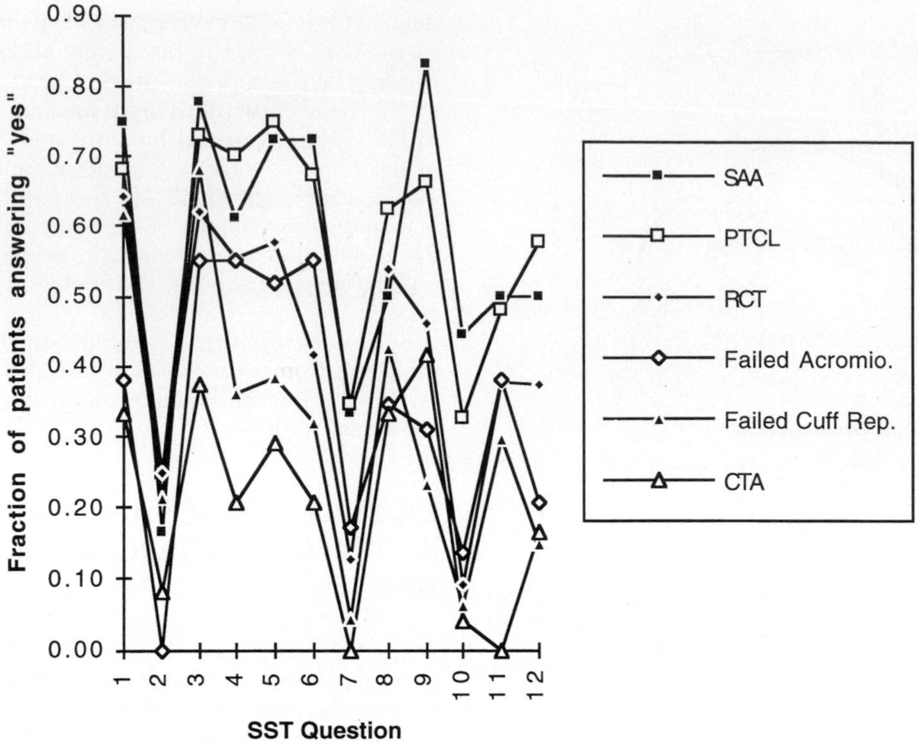

Figure 15–61

Self-assessed shoulder function of 355 patients with six different rotator cuff diagnoses: (1) subacromial abrasion (SAA); (2) partial-thickness cuff lesion (PTCL); (3) complete-thickness cuff tear (RCT); (4) failed acromioplasty; (5) failed cuff repair; and (6) cuff tear arthropathy (CTA).

SST questions: (1) Is your shoulder comfortable with your arm at rest by your side?; (2) Does your shoulder allow you to sleep comfortably?; (3) Can you reach the small of your back to tuck in your shirt with your hand?; (4) Can you place your hand behind your head with the elbow straight out to the side?; (5) Can you place a coin on a shelf at the level of your shoulder without bending your elbow?; (6) Can you lift 1 lb (a full pint container) to the level of your shoulder without bending your elbow?; (7) Can you lift 8 lb (a full gallon container) to the level of the top of your head without bending your elbow?; (8) Can you carry 20 lb (a bag of potatoes) at your side with the affected extremity?; (9) Do you think you can toss a softball underhand 10 yards with the affected extremity?; (10) Do you think you can throw a softball overhand 20 yards with the affected extremity?; (11) Can you wash the back of your opposite shoulder with the affected extremity?; and (12) Would your shoulder allow you to work full-time at your regular job?

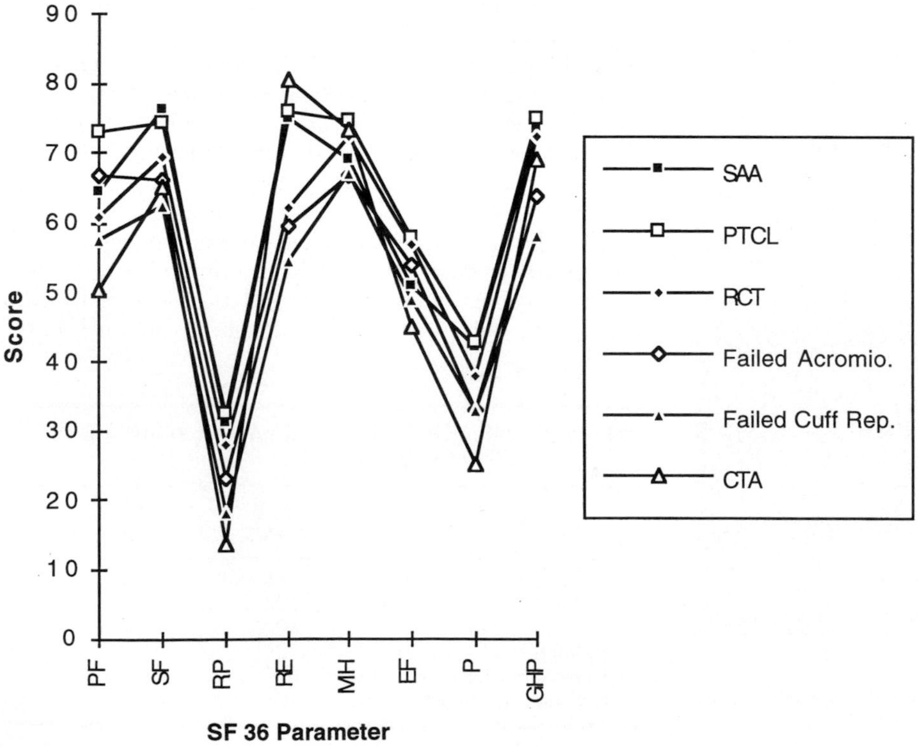

Figure 15–62

The patient population is the same as for Figure 15–61. The SF 36 parameters on this graph include: physical function (PF), social function (SF), physical role function (RP), emotional role function (RE), mental health (MH), energy/fatigue (EF), pain (P), and general health perception (GHP).

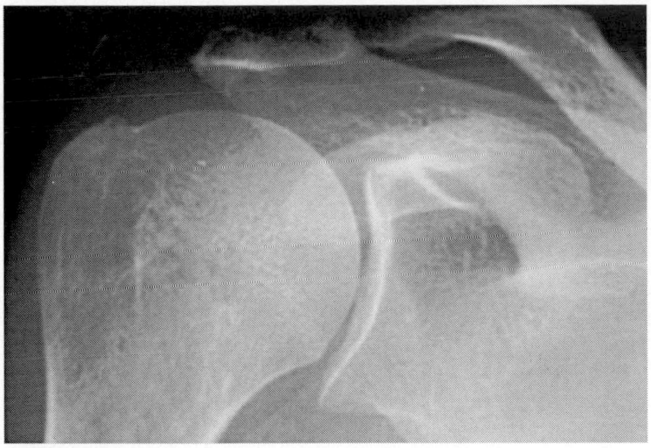

Figure 15–63

A roentgenogram demonstrating subacromial sclerosis, the so-called "sourcil" or "eyebrow" sign, from chronic loading of the undersurface of the acromion by the rotator cuff. Corresponding sclerosis or cystic changes involving the greater tuberosity may also occur.

those with cuff tear arthropathy and failed surgery have worse scores than do those with unoperated cuff lesions and subacromial abrasion.

IMAGING TECHNIQUES

Plain Radiographs

Standard radiographs can provide limited assistance when evaluating shoulder weakness. Small avulsed fragments of the tuberosity may be seen in younger patients with cuff lesions (see Fig. 15–49) (not to be confused with calcific deposits). Chronic cuff disease may be accompanied by sclerosis of the undersurface of the acromion (the "sourcil" or eyebrow sign) (Fig. 15–63), traction spurs in the coracoacromial ligament from forced contact with the cuff and the humeral head, and changes at the cuff insertion to the humerus (Fig. 15–64; see also Figs. 15–10 to 15–12).[95, 178, 191, 256, 435] Radiographs may also reveal evidence of some of the conditions possibly associated with cuff disease, such as acromioclavicular arthritis, chronic calcific tendinitis, tuberosity displacement, and the like (Figs. 15–65 to 15–67; see also 15–18). With larger tears, radiographs reveal upward displacement of the head of the humerus with respect to the glenoid and the acromion (Fig. 15–68; see also Figs. 15–7, 15–8, and 15–13).[70, 95, 179, 192, 227, 435] Kaneko and associates[193] found that superior migration of the humerus and deformity of the greater tuberosity were the most sensitive and specific manifestations of massive cuff deficiency. In cuff tear arthropathy, the humeral head may have lost the prominence of the tuberosities (become "femoralized"), and the coracoid, acromion, and glenoid may have formed a deep spherical socket (become "acetabularized") (Figs. 15–69 and 15–70; see also Figs. 15–12 and 15–48).

Cuff Tendon Imaging

A number of different studies are available for imaging the rotator cuff. Each of these tests adds both information

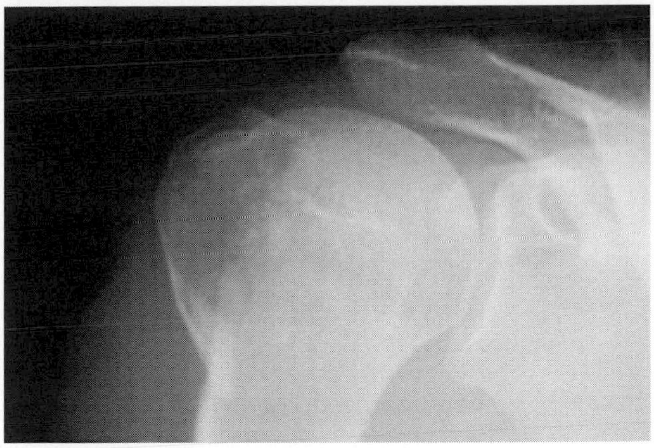

Figure 15–65

An anteroposterior roentgenogram shows malunion of a fractured greater tuberosity and malunion associated with abrasion, loss of motion, and weakness.

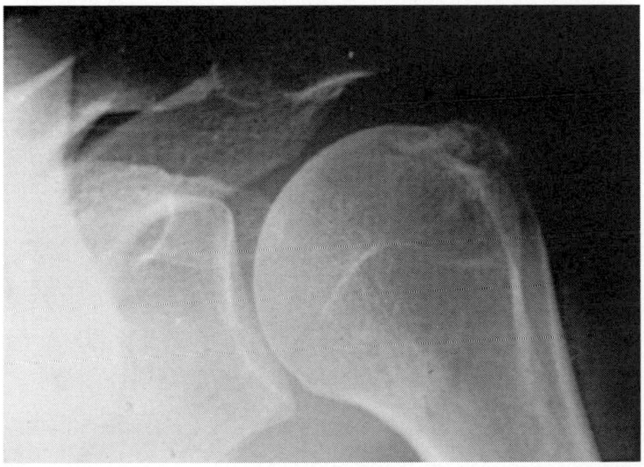

Figure 15–64

Even with small rotator cuff tears, radiographs may reveal bony cysts at the normal cuff insertion, subacromial sclerosis, and acromial spurs.

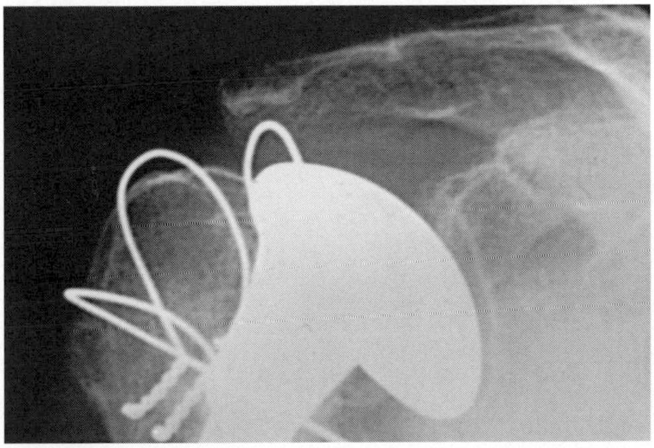

Figure 15–66

This patient developed refractory subacromial abrasion and stiffness due to the relative prominence of fracture fixation wires. The symptoms resolved after the subacromial wires were removed.

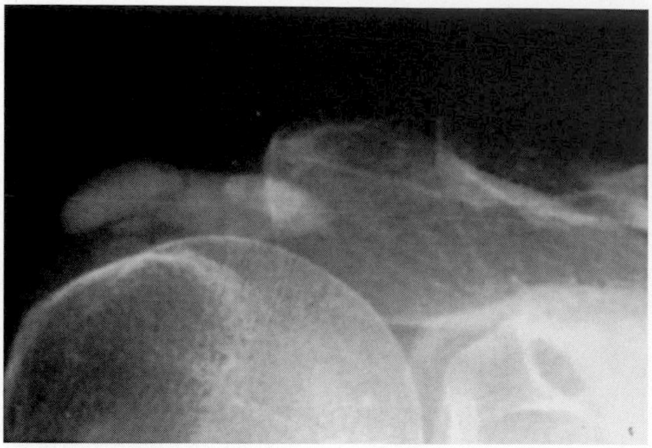

Figure 15–67

This anteroposterior roentgenogram shows chronic calcific deposits in the supraspinatus tendon. These deposits may increase the thickness of the tendon and thus contribute to subacromial abrasion and loss of motion.

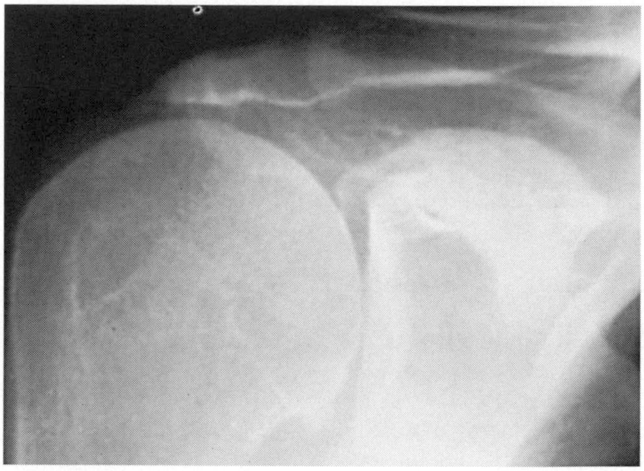

Figure 15–68

With larger cuff tears, radiographs reveal upward displacement of the humeral head with marked narrowing of the interval between the humeral head and the acromion. Note the marked cystic changes and sclerosis involving the undersurface of the acromion.

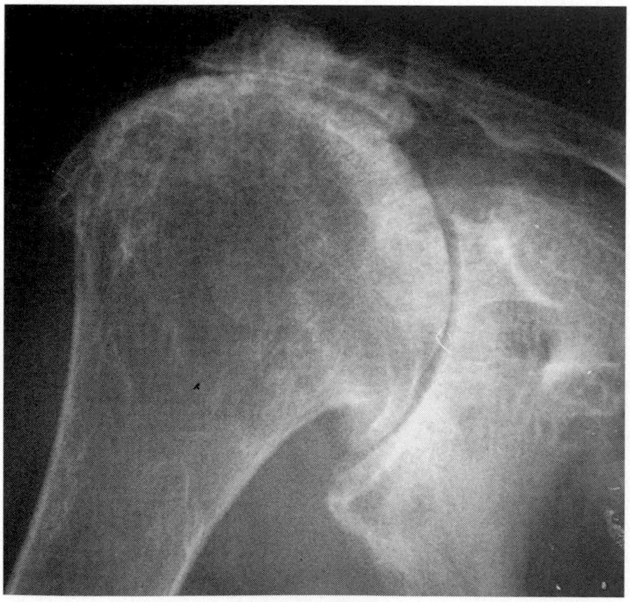

Figure 15–69

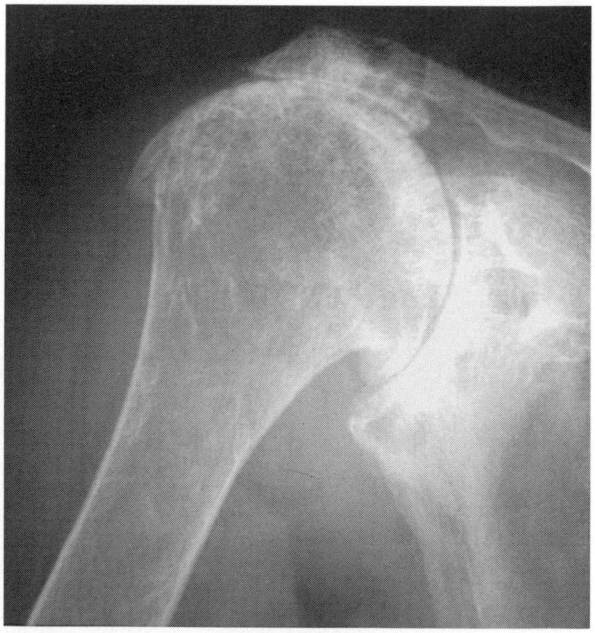

Figure 15–70

Figures 15–69 and 15–70

Cuff tear arthropathy showing "femoralization" of the proximal humerus and "acetabularization" of the coracoacromial arch and glenoid.

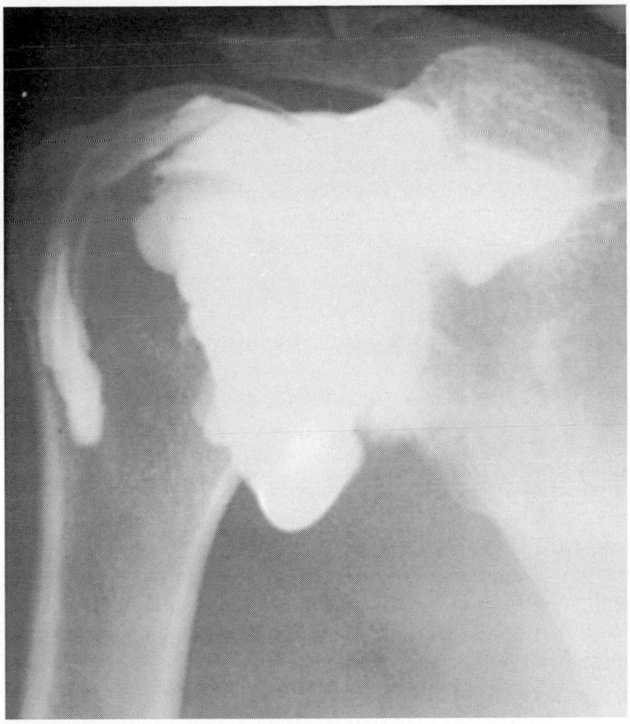

Figure 15–71

An arthrogram of a normal shoulder in neutral position. Note the normal extension of dye beneath the coracoid into the subscapularis bursa. Also note the normal extension of dye beneath the transverse humeral ligament and into the biceps sheath. The superolateral extension of dye is limited by the normal cuff attachment.

and expense to the evaluation of the patient; health care resources can be conserved by only ordering imaging tests if the results are likely to change the management of the patient. Patients younger than 40 years of age without a major injury or weakness are unlikely to have significant cuff defects; thus, cuff imaging is less likely to be helpful in their evaluation. At the other extreme, patients with weak external rotation and atrophy of the spinatus muscles whose plain radiographs show the head of the humerus in contact with the acromion (see Figs. 15–69 and 15–70) do not need cuff imaging to establish the diagnosis of a rotator cuff defect. Finally, the initial management of patients with nonspecific shoulder symptoms and an unremarkable physical examination is unlikely to be changed by the results of a cuff imaging test. Cuff imaging is strongly indicated when it would affect treatment, such as in the case of a 47 year old with immediate weakness of flexion and external rotation after a major fall on the outstretched arm or shoulder dislocation. Imaging the cuff is also important when symptoms and signs of cuff involvement do not respond as expected; for example, symptoms of "tendinitis" or "bursitis" that do not respond to 3 months of rehabilitation.

A review of the literature suggests that, in experienced hands, arthrography, MRI, ultrasound, and arthroscopy each yield sufficient accuracy for making the diagnosis of a full-thickness cuff tear.[54, 81, 83, 147, 240, 304, 308, 312, 335, 347, 409, 420, 424]

ARTHROGRAPHY

For many years the single contrast shoulder *arthrogram* has been the standard technique for diagnosing rotator cuff tears. In this test, contrast material is injected into the glenohumeral joint (Fig. 15–71); after brief exercise, radiographs are taken to reveal intravasation of the dye into the tendon (Figs. 15–72 and 15–73) or extravasation of the contrast agent through the cuff into the subacromial subdeltoid bursa (Fig. 15–74). In 1933, Oberholtzer[295] used air as a contrast agent, injecting it into the glenohumeral joint prior to radiographic evaluation. Air contrast is still useful in patients who are allergic to iodine. In 1939, Lindblom used an opaque contrast opaque medium.[228–230] Since then, iodinated contrast media have

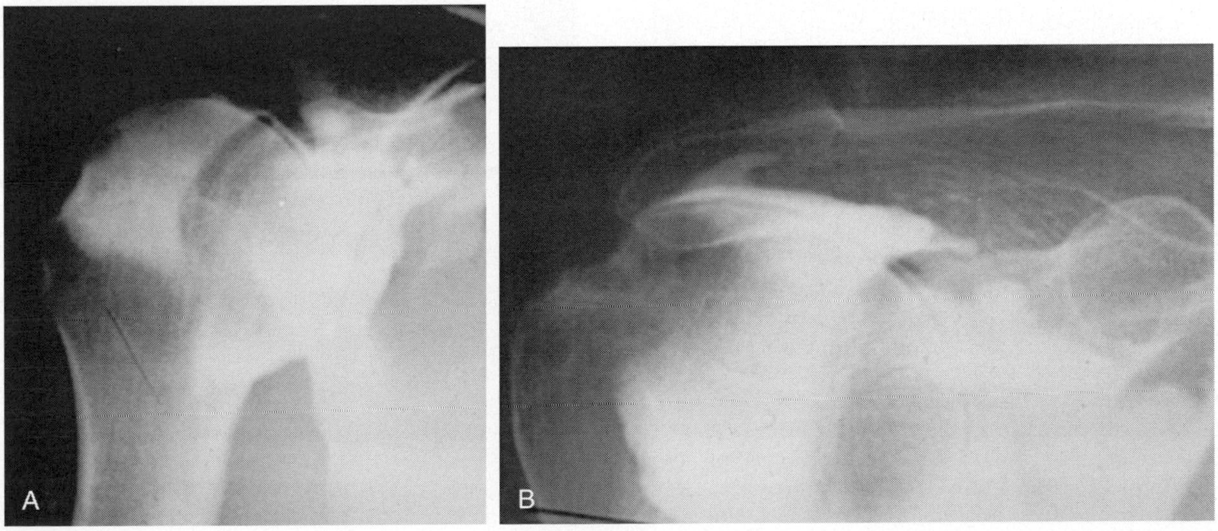

Figure 15–72

Arthrograms of two different shoulders showing partial-thickness, deep surface tears of the cuff. *A*, Note the "feathered" edge of the contrast material laterally, indicating the loss of the normal insertion at the base of the tuberosity. The absence of filling of the bursa suggests that the tendon defect is not full thickness. These findings were confirmed at surgery. *B*, Another patient had a falciform-shaped deep surface tear.

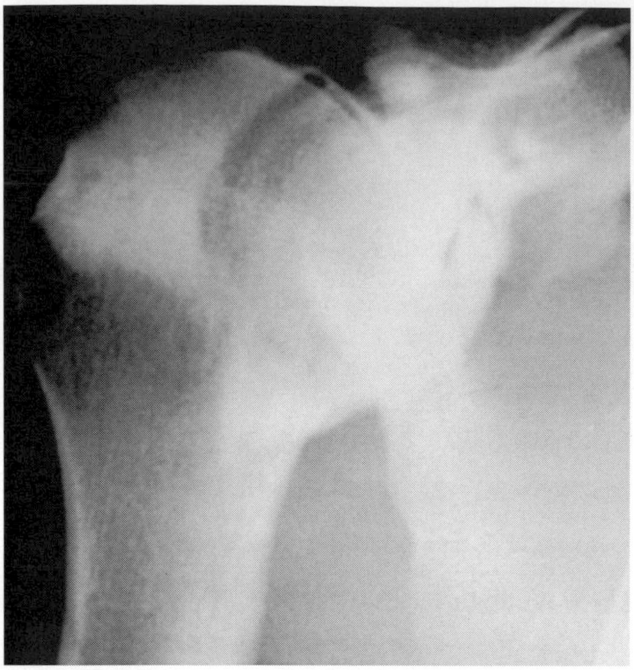

Figure 15–73

This arthrogram shows evidence of a partial-thickness rotator cuff tear originating at the articular surface of the cuff. Leakage of dye is seen to extend beyond the normal deep surface cuff attachment and is restrained by the more superficial cuff fibers that insert further laterally (see Fig. 15–50). These findings were confirmed at surgery.

been the standard for single-contrast arthrography. Several extensions of the basic technique have been published.[2, 199, 205, 277, 286, 343, 364]

Pettersson[323] and Neviaser and colleagues[289] demonstrated the effectiveness of arthrography in revealing deep surface partial-thickness cuff tears (see Figs. 15–72 and 15–73); however, arthrography cannot reveal isolated midsubstance tears or superior surface tears. Craig[77] described the "geyser sign" in which dye leaks from the shoulder joint through the cuff into the acromioclavicular joint. The presence of this sign suggests a large tear with erosion of the undersurface of the acromioclavicular joint (Fig. 15–75; see also Fig. 15–18). Double-contrast arthrography using both air and iodinated material may enhance the resolution of arthrography.[2, 106, 140, 199] Berquist and associates[24] reported on the use of single- and double-contrast arthrograms to evaluate the size of the cuff tears seen at surgery. Their ability to accurately predict one of four cuff tear sizes (small, medium, large, and massive) was just over 50%. The reported incidence of false-negative arthrograms in the presence of surgically proven cuff tears ranges from 0 to 8%.[165, 167, 264, 284, 331, 363, 444] The anatomic resolution of shoulder arthrography can be enhanced to a certain degree by obtaining tomograms with the contrast material in place to give information about the size and location of the tear and the quality of the remaining tissue. Further resolution can be obtained by performing double-contrast arthrotomography.[124, 142, 143, 204] Kilcoyne and Matsen[204] used arthropneumotomography to evaluate the size of the cuff tear and the quality of the residual tissue. They found a good correlation with the surgical appearance. The accuracy of arthrography does not seem to be enhanced by digital subtraction.[113]

The subacromial injection of contrast material (bursography) has been used to evaluate the subacromial zone and the upper surface of the rotator cuff.[125, 129, 224, 228–230, 262, 283, 387] Fukuda reported six patients who had normal arthrograms and positive bursograms, which he defined as pooling of the subacromially injected contrast in the cuff tissue. He reported an overall accuracy for bursography of 67% when compared with operative findings. Although lesions can be identified on this type of examination, criteria for making diagnoses have not been rigorously defined.

MAGNETIC RESONANCE IMAGING

MRI can reveal information about the tendon and muscle. Seeger and co-workers[369] and Kneeland and associates[207] provided initial information on the use of MRI to image the cuff; however, they did not document the sensitivity and selectivity of this method. Crass and Craig[78] concluded that the accuracy of MRI in diagnosing cuff pathology is unknown. Kieft and associates[203] reported on 10 patients with shoulder symptoms evaluated with MRI and arthrography. Arthrography showed a tear in three patients, whereas MRI detected none of them.

In a retrospective study by Robertson and associates,[347] the authors found that full-thickness tears of the rotator cuff can be accurately identified at MRI with little ob-

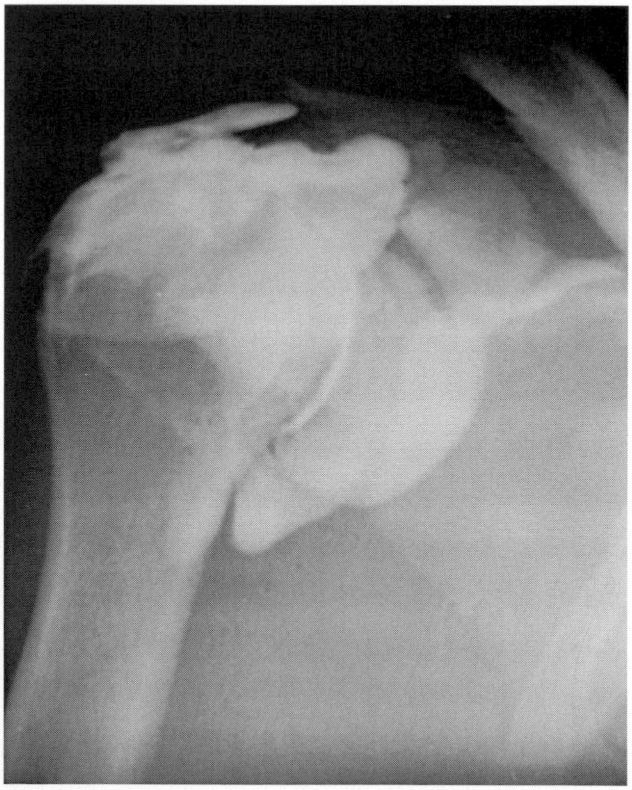

Figure 15–74

This arthrogram shows dye leakage into the subacromial space and beyond the normal cuff attachment at the greater tuberosity. This finding indicates a full-thickness cuff defect.

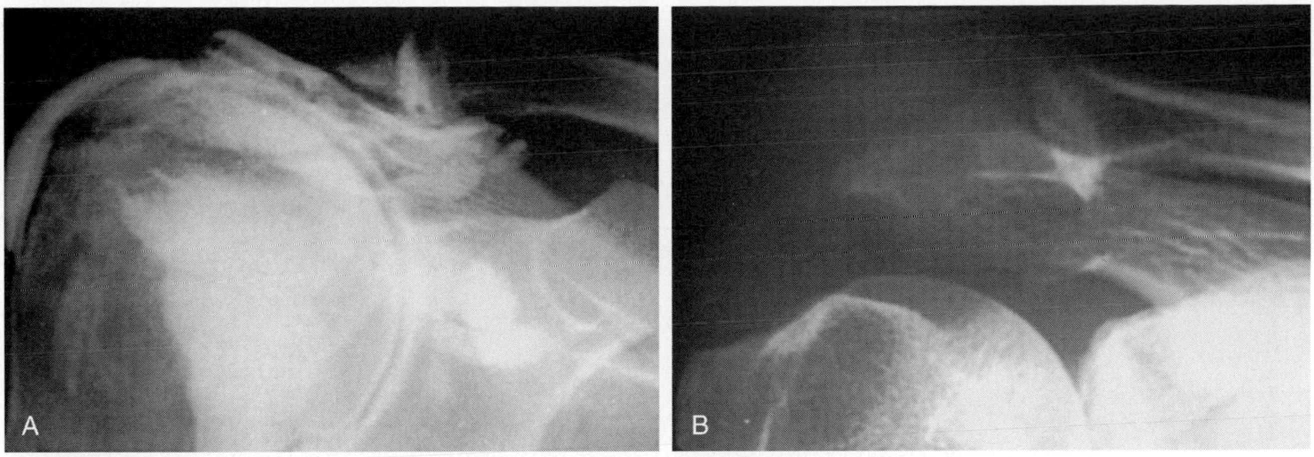

Figure 15–75

A, This arthrogram shows leakage of dye into the subacromial space and beyond the normal cuff attachment at the greater tuberosity. Note the dye leakage into the acromioclavicular joint, the "geyser" sign. Also note the marked inferior displacement of the cuff outline caused by this arthritic acromioclavicular joint. *B*, A plain radiograph of the same joint.

server variation; however, consistent differentiation of normal rotator cuff, tendinitis, and partial-thickness tears is difficult. Iannotti and associates described the sensitivity, specificity, and predictive value of MRI for different clinical conditions.[177]

ULTRASONOGRAPHY

In experienced hands, *ultrasonography* can noninvasively and nonradiographically reveal not only the integrity of the rotator cuff but also the thickness of its various component tendons. In 1982, one of us (FAM) observed during prenatal ultrasonography that movement dramatically enhanced the resolution during real-time imaging of a fetal hand. Similarly, adding a dynamic element to the sonographic evaluation of the rotator cuff significantly improves its resolution: moving the shoulder through even a small arc helps to distinguish the cuff tendons from the humeral head, deltoid, and acromion. The importance of movement during the ultrasound examination was re-emphasized by Drakeford and colleagues.[98] Our initial series of ultrasound examinations of the shoulder was presented in 1983.[114] Since then, the criteria for diagnosing cuff lesions have evolved, as have the quality of the equipment and the technique. Much of this work was carried out by and as a result of the stimulation of the late Lawrence Mack.[237, 238, 240] He demonstrated that by careful positioning and by knowledge of the dynamic anatomy of the cuff, the experienced ultrasonographer can image selectively the upper and lower subscapularis, the biceps tendon, the anterior and posterior supraspinatus, the infraspinatus, and the teres minor. Defects are revealed as absence of the normal tissue echoes and failure of the tissue to move appropriately with defined humeral movements (Figs. 15–76 to 15–78). In his series of 141 patients from the University of Washington Shoulder Clinic,[238] Mack demonstrated a specificity of 98% and a sensitivity of 91% in comparison with surgical findings. Most of the false-negative results occurred in patients who were found to have tears less than 1 cm in size.[238]

Ultrasonography has the advantages of speed and safety. In addition, it provides the important benefit of practical bilateral examinations (which, although theoretically possible with arthrography, MRI, and arthroscopy, are usually not done for reasons of cost, risk, and time). Ultrasonography also allows the shoulder to be examined dynamically and provides the opportunity to show the results to the patient in real time. Yet another advantage is its low cost: a bilateral shoulder ultrasound is usually half of the cost of a unilateral arthrogram and one eighth of the cost of an MRI of the unilateral shoulder. While some series have reported less accuracy with ultrasonography than arthrography, others have pointed to its high degree of accuracy, noninvasiveness, and effectiveness in experienced hands.[37, 73, 78, 81, 259–261, 301, 308, 395, 438] Ultrasonography has been applied to the evaluation of recurrent tears as well as incomplete tears.[79, 80] Seitz and co-workers[370] compared arthrography, ultrasonography, and MRI for the detection of cuff tears in 25 patients. They found that ultrasonography was the most helpful study in accurately documenting the size and location of the tear when it existed. MRI suffered from problems of image resolution. Arthrography was reliable in determining full-thickness tears, but correlation with size and location of the tear was difficult. Middleton[258] concluded that:

> Shoulder sonography is a valuable means of evaluating the rotator cuff and biceps tendon. In experienced hands, it is as sensitive as arthrography and magnetic resonance imaging for detecting rotator cuff tears and abnormalities of the biceps tendon. Because sonography is rapid, noninvasive, relatively inexpensive, and capable of performing bilateral examinations in one sitting, it should be used as the initial imaging test when the primary question is one of rotator cuff or biceps tendon abnormalities.

In a review of the literature, Stiles and Otte concluded that the accuracy of ultrasound in experienced hands was at least as good as that of MRI.[386]

Recent investigations have again confirmed the value of sonography. In a study of 4588 shoulders, Hedtmann and Fett[168] found that the overall sensitivity in diagnosing

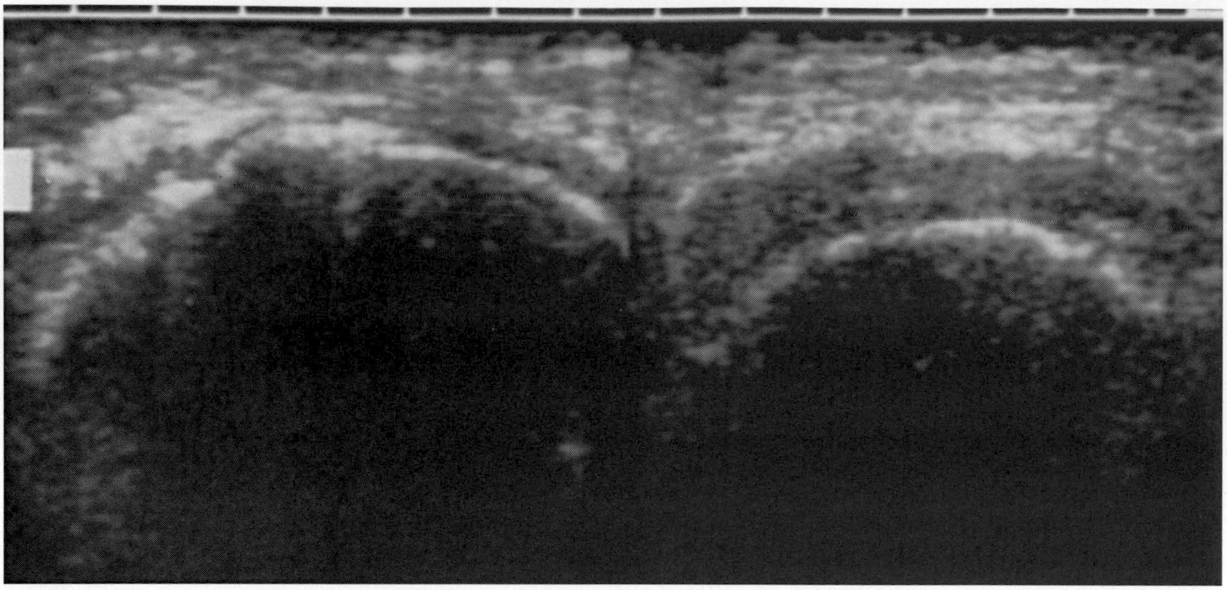

Figure 15–76

A sonogram with the transducer perpendicular to the long axis of the supraspinatus demonstrates the tendon as an arc of soft tissue overlying the humeral head on the normal side *(right)* and absent on the side with a large cuff tear *(left)*.

cuff tears was 97% in full-thickness tears and 91% in partial-thickness tears. The false-negative rate was less than 2% for an overall accuracy of 95%. The supraspinatus was involved in 96%; the infraspinatus in 39%; the subscapularis in 10%; and the long head of the biceps in 34%. The authors also developed an approach for measuring the degree of retraction of the torn tendon. Farin and Jaroma[112] examined 184 patients for possible acute traumatic tears. Ultrasonography demonstrated 42 (91%) of 46 full-thickness tears and seven (78%) of nine partial-thickness tears. Ultrasonography showed more extensive tears than were found at surgery in four (4%) of 98 patients and less extensive tears in seven (7%) of 98 patients. Sonographic patterns consisted of a defect in 31 (63%), focal thinning in 10 (21%), and nonvisualization in 8 (16%).

Van Holsbeeck and associates[419] found that a 7.5-MHz commercially available linear-array transducer and a standardized study protocol yielded a sensitivity for partial-thickness tears of 93% and a specificity of 94%. The positive predictive value was 82%, and the negative predictive value was 98%. Similar results are reported by others.[420] Hollister and associates[173] studied the association between sonographically detected joint fluid and rotator cuff disease. In 163 shoulders they found that the sonographic finding of intraarticular fluid alone (without

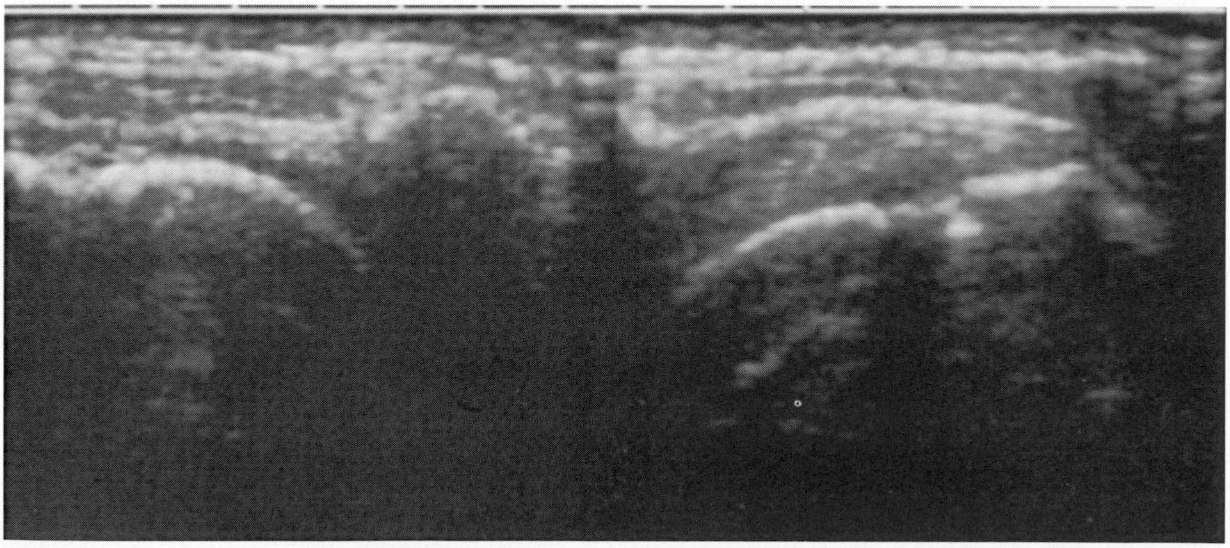

Figure 15–77

A sonogram in the plane of the supraspinatus. The normal attachment to the greater tuberosity is shown on the right. An absent supraspinatus insertion is shown in the shoulder with a large cuff tear *(left)*.

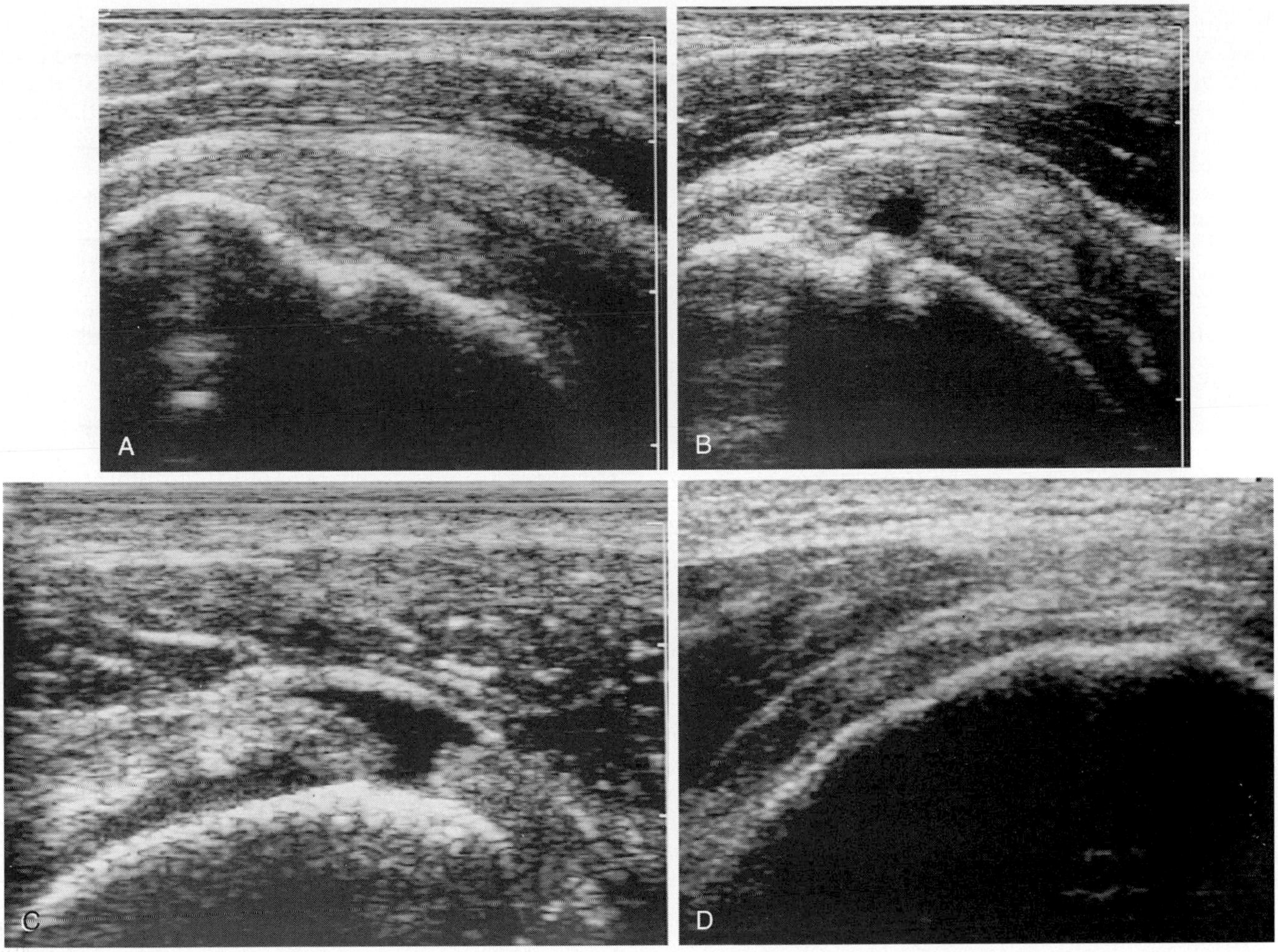

Figure 15–78

The spectrum of rotator cuff appearances in four different patients. All images are of the right supraspinatus tendon and were obtained with linear, high-frequency (10MHz), broad bandwidth transducers. *A*, A normal tendon. The hyperechoic line at the deep portion of the image represents the humeral cortex, while the nearly parallel hyperechoic curve approximately 1 cm superficial to that represents the subdeltoid bursa. Intermediate density echoes between these two lines represent the normal supraspinatus tendon. *B*, A small (5 mm) tear is seen best along the inferior surface of the supraspinatus tendon. The tear is well delineated because it is filled with anechoic (black) fluid. *C*, An approximately 1-cm full-thickness tear. Note the tendon remnants at either side of the tear, which are again well outlined by fluid. *D*, A massive rotator cuff tear. No normal supraspinatus tendon is seen. Instead, the thickened subdeltoid bursa is directly opposed to the humeral cortex. (Ultrasound images courtesy of Dr. Tom Winter, Department of Radiology, University of Washington.)

bursal fluid) has both a low sensitivity and a low specificity for the diagnosis of rotator cuff tears. However, the finding of fluid in the subacromial/subdeltoid bursa, especially when combined with a joint effusion, is highly specific and has a high positive predictive value for associated rotator cuff tears.

We find that expert ultrasonography provides the most efficient and cost-effective approach to imaging of the cuff tendons. The real-time, dynamic, and interactive examination of the rotator cuff provides the physician and the patient with the information needed to make the necessary management decisions in both primary and postsurgical cuff conditions.

DIFFERENTIAL DIAGNOSIS

Traditionally, it is stated that rotator cuff tears must be differentiated from cuff *tendinitis* and *bursitis* and that tests such as arthrography or ultrasonography are necessary to make this distinction. Perhaps a more realistic view is that many of the symptoms often attributed to tendinitis and bursitis are, in actuality, episodes of acute fiber failure that are not clinically detected.

Patients with a *frozen shoulder* demonstrate, by definition, a restricted range of passive motion with normal glenohumeral radiographs. Patients with partial-thickness cuff defects may similarly demonstrate motion restriction, whereas patients with major full-thickness defects usually have a good range of passive shoulder motion but may be limited in strength or range of active motion. An arthrogram in the case of frozen shoulder shows a diminished volume and obliteration of the normal recesses of the joint.

A snapping scapula may produce shoulder pain on elevation and a catching sensation somewhat reminiscent of the subacromial snap of a cuff tear. However, the latter can usually be elicited with the scapula stabilized while the arm is rotated in the flexed and somewhat abducted position. Scapular snapping usually arises from the superomedial corner of the scapula, producing local discomfort, and is elicited on scapular movement without glenohumeral motion.

Glenohumeral arthritis may also produce shoulder pain, weakness, and catching. This diagnosis can be reliably differentiated from rotator cuff disease by a careful history, physical examination, and roentgenographic analysis (Fig. 15–79).

Acromioclavicular arthritis may imitate cuff disease. Characteristically, however, the shoulder is most painful with cross-body movements and with activities requiring strong contraction of the pectoralis major. Tenderness is commonly limited to the acromioclavicular joint. Relief of pain on selective lidocaine injection and coned-down radiographs may help to establish the diagnosis of acromioclavicular arthritis.

Suprascapular neuropathy and cervical radiculopathy are common imitators of cuff disease. The suprascapular nerve and the fifth and sixth cervical nerve roots supply two of the most important cuff muscles: the supraspinatus and the infraspinatus. Thus, patients with involvement of these structures may have lateral shoulder pain and lack strength of elevation and external rotation.

In the presence of weakness, the neurologic examination should test the cutaneous distribution of the nerve roots from C5 to T1. The biceps reflex and the triceps reflex help to screen C5-C6 and C7-C8, respectively. The next component of the neurologic examination requires recognition of the segmental innervation of joint motion: abduction at C5; adduction at C6, C7, and C8; external rotation at C5; internal rotation at C6, C7, and C8; elbow flexion at C5 and C6; elbow extension at C7 and C8; wrist extension and flexion at C6 and C7; finger flexion and extension at C7 and C8; and finger adduction and abduction at T1.

A set of screening tests checks the motor and sensory components of the major peripheral nerves: (1) the axillary nerve (the anterior, middle, and posterior parts of the deltoid and the skin just above the deltoid insertion); (2) the radial nerve (the extensor pollicis longus and the skin over the first dorsal web space); (3) the median nerve (the opponens pollicis and the skin over the pulp of the index finger); (4) the ulnar nerve (the first dorsal interosseous and the skin over the pulp of the little finger); and (5) the musculocutaneous nerve (the biceps muscle and the skin over the lateral forearm). The long thoracic nerve is checked by having the patient elevate the arm 60 degrees in the anterior sagittal plane while the examiner pushes down on the arm seeking winging of the scapula posteriorly. The nerve of the trapezius is checked by observing the strength of the shoulder shrug. Lesions of the suprascapular nerve produce weakness of elevation and external rotation without sensory loss.

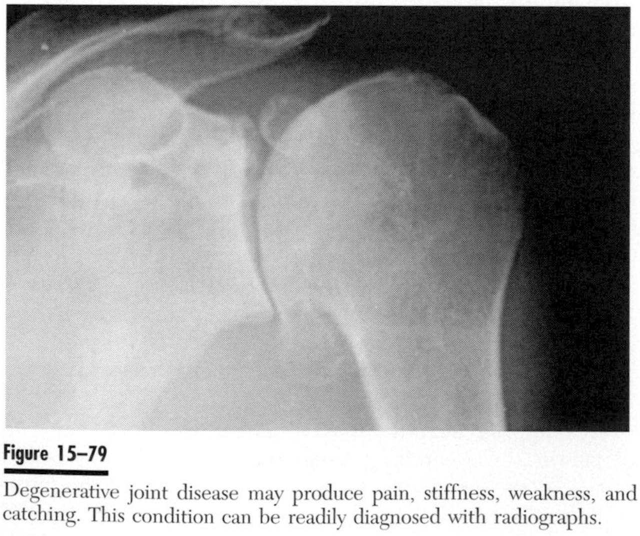

Figure 15–79

Degenerative joint disease may produce pain, stiffness, weakness, and catching. This condition can be readily diagnosed with radiographs.

Clinical conditions affecting these structures include: (1) cervical spondylosis involving C5 and C6, (2) brachial plexopathy involving the suprascapular nerve, (3) traction injuries (e.g., in the mechanism of Erb's palsy), (4) suprascapular nerve entrapment at the suprascapular notch, (5) pressure on the inferior branch of the suprascapular nerve from a ganglion cyst at the spinoglenoid notch, (6) traumatic severance in fractures, or (7) iatrogenic injury[10, 17, 39, 59, 97, 99, 103, 111, 136, 183, 208, 209, 241, 242, 273, 325, 337, 341, 367, 368, 380, 388, 433]

Cervical spondylosis involving the fifth and sixth cervical nerve route may imitate or mask rotator cuff involvement by producing pain in the lateral shoulder as well as weakness of shoulder flexion, abduction, and external rotation. Cervical radiculopathy is suggested if the patient has pain on neck extension or on turning the chin to the affected side. Pain of cervical origin more commonly includes the area of the trapezius muscle along with the area of the deltoid and may radiate down the arm to the hand. Sensory, motor, or reflex abnormalities in the distribution of the fifth or sixth cervical nerve root provide additional diagnostic support for the diagnosis of cervical radiculopathy. Inasmuch as many asymptomatic patients have degenerative changes at the C5 to C6 area, cervical spine radiographs are not a specific diagnostic tool. When mild cervical spondylosis is suspected, it is practical to implement a rehabilitation program, without an extensive diagnostic work-up. This program includes gentle neck mobility exercises, isometric neck-strengthening exercises, home traction, and protection of the neck from aggravation positions during sleep. If the condition is unresponsive or severe, additional evaluation by electromyography or MRI may be indicated.

Suprascapular neuropathy is characterized by dull pain over the shoulder exacerbated by movement of the shoulder, weakness in overhead activities, wasting of the supraspinatus and infraspinatus muscles, weakness of external rotation, and normal radiographic evaluation. This condition may arise from suprascapular nerve traction injuries, suprascapular nerve entrapment, brachial neuritis affecting the suprascapular nerve, or a spinoglenoid notch ganglion cyst. The first three should involve the nerve supply to both the supraspinatus and infraspinatus and are most easily differentiated by the history. Traction injuries to the suprascapular nerve are usually associated with a history of a violent downward pull on the shoulder and may be a part of a larger Erb palsy–type injury to the brachial plexus. Suprascapular nerve entrapment may produce chronic recurrent pain and weakness aggravated by shoulder use. Finally, brachial neuritis often produces

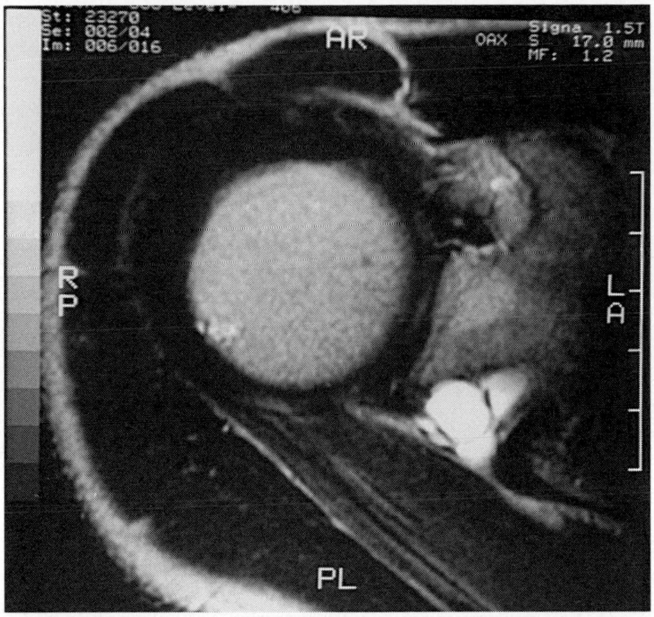

Figure 15–80

Magnetic resonance imaging showing a ganglion cyst in the spinoglenoid notch. Cysts in this location can press on the nerve to the infraspinatus that runs through this notch. Symptoms can include pain and weakness of external rotation that are somewhat similar to the symptoms of cuff disease.

a rather intense pain that lasts for several weeks, with the onset of weakness being noted as the pain subsides. A spinoglenoid notch ganglion usually arises from a defect in the posterior shoulder joint capsule and may press on the nerve to the infraspinatus as it passes through the notch. These cysts are well seen on an MRI scan (Fig. 15–80). Depending on the site of the suprascapular nerve lesion, electromyography may indicate involvement of the infraspinatus alone or involvement of this muscle along with the supraspinatus. None of these conditions should produce cuff defects on shoulder ultrasonography or arthrography.

TREATMENT

The discussion of treatment is divided in terms of the eight clinical entities previously identified: asymptomatic cuff failure, posterior capsular tightness, subacromial abrasion, failed acromioplasty, partial-thickness cuff lesions, full- thickness cuff tears, failed cuff repair, and cuff tear arthropathy.

Asymptomatic Cuff Failure

In this condition, the shoulder does not bother the patient, but imaging studies document a full-thickness defect in the cuff tendon.[157, 244, 263, 323, 372]

The realization that full-thickness cuff tears may be asymptomatic poses substantial questions regarding the prevalence of cuff tears in the general population and the indications for rotator cuff surgery. It is difficult to improve patients who have minimal symptoms. The case for surgery to prevent future problems in such patients has not been convincingly made.

Posterior Capsular Tightness

In this condition the shoulder is limited in its range of internal rotation in abduction, cross-body adduction, internal rotation up the back, and flexion (in approximate order of decreasing frequency). The symptoms and physical examination of this "slightly frozen shoulder" may be similar to those described for the "impingement syndrome,"[69] including difficulties sleeping and reaching across the body and up the back.

The patient with posterior capsular tightness is informed that this condition is a common result of a mild injury to the rotator cuff, but that, in the absence of weakness or pain on isometric muscle testing, nonoperative management is usually successful. The most effective program is one that is taught by the surgeon or therapist but is carried out by the patient. The recommended treatment consists of gentle stretches performed five times a day by the patient (Figs. 15–81 to 15–86). Each stretch is performed to the point where the patient feels a pull against the shoulder tightness, but not to the point of pain. Each stretch is performed for 1 minute, so that the patient invests about 30 min/day working on the shoulder. Obvious improvement commonly occurs within the first month, but 3 months may be required to com-

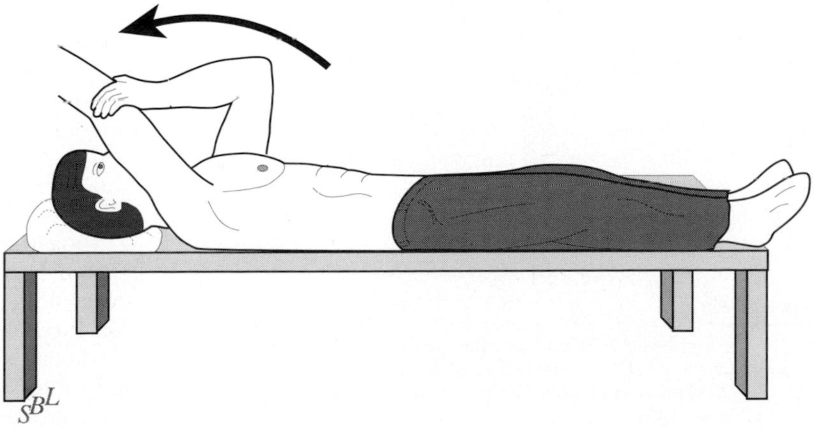

Figure 15–81

Stretching in overhead reach using the opposite arm as the therapist. (From Matsen FA III, Lippitt SB, Sidles JA, and Harryman DT II: Practical Evaluation and Management of the Shoulder. Philadelphia: WB Saunders, 1994.)

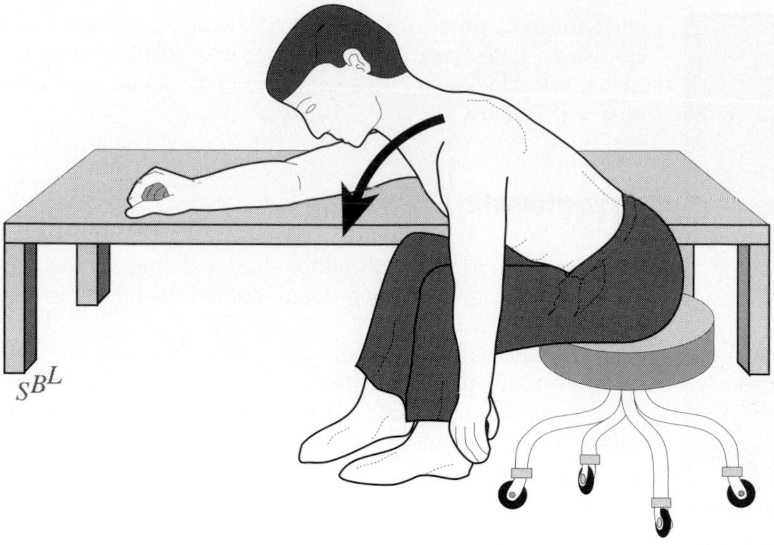

Figure 15–82

Stretching in overhead reach using the progressive forward lean to apply a gentle elevating force to the arm. (From Matsen FA III, Lippitt SB, Sidles JA, and Harryman DT II: Practical Evaluation and Management of the Shoulder. Philadelphia: WB Saunders, 1994.)

pletely eliminate the condition. The rare refractory case may be considered for an arthroscopic capsular release as described by Harryman.[158]

Subacromial Abrasion (Without a Significant Defect in the Cuff Tendon)

In this condition, the shoulder demonstrates symptomatic crepitus as the humerus is rotated beneath the acromion; isometric testing of the cuff muscles reveals no pain or weakness.

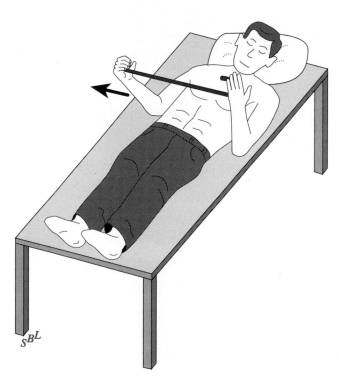

Figure 15–83

Stretching in external rotation using the opposite hand as the therapist. (From Matsen FA III, Lippitt SB, Sidles JA, and Harryman DT II: Practical Evaluation and Management of the Shoulder. Philadelphia: WB Saunders, 1994.)

NONOPERATIVE TREATMENT

Patients in whom the primary complaint is symptomatic subacromial crepitance (see Fig. 15–59) will usually benefit from reassurance and a home program of gentle stretching and strengthening exercises. Various nonoperative rotator cuff programs have been described for the general population and for athletes, including throwers.[3, 9, 25, 30, 67, 69, 121, 164, 189, 197, 277, 290, 313, 314, 344, 348, 366] Exercises must address specifically any shoulder stiffness that may cause obligate translation and loss of concentricity on shoulder movement (see Figs. 15–14 and 15–60). The effectiveness of nonoperative treatment was recognized many years ago by Neer who, in his initial article on anterior acromioplasty, pointed out that "Many patients . . . were suspected of having impingement, but responded well to conservative treatment."[275] Furthermore, he stated that patients were advised not to have an acromioplasty until the stiffness of the shoulder had disappeared and the disability had persisted for at least 9 months. As a result of these conservative surgical indications, during the period covered by his report, this most active shoulder surgeon operated on an average of only 10 shoulders a year with this diagnosis: the effectiveness of nonoperative management is worthy of emphasis!

The low success rate in returning athletes to competition after acromioplasty reinforces the importance of nonoperative management in this population.[401] Similar principles apply to workers who are required to use their shoulders in positions that aggravate subacromial abrasion.

Subacromial injections of corticosteroids have been reported by some to produce symptomatic relief.[171] However, Withrington and co-workers[443] reported a double-blind trial of steroid injections and found no evidence of the efficacy of such treatment. Valtonen[416] found no difference between subacromial and gluteal injections of steroids. Berry and colleagues compared acupuncture,

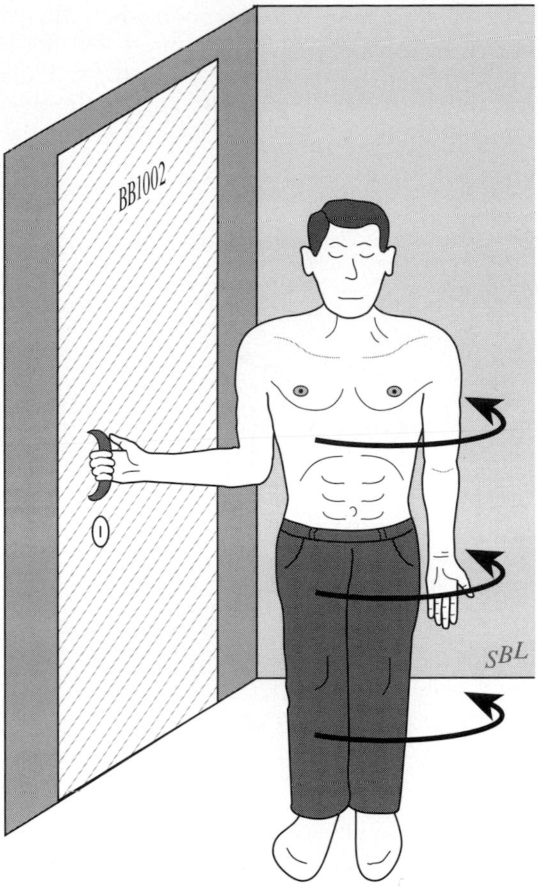

Figure 15–84

Stretching in external rotation by turning the body away from a fixed object to apply a gentle stretching force. (From Matsen FA III, Lippitt SB, Sidles JA, and Harryman DT II: Practical Evaluation and Management of the Shoulder. Philadelphia: WB Saunders, 1994.)

physiotherapy, steroid injections, and anti-inflammatory medications and found no difference among these treatments.[25]

Steroid injections in or near the cuff and biceps tendons may produce tendon atrophy or may reduce the ability of damaged tendon to repair itself. Such changes have been well documented in other tissues.[234, 354, 415] Uitto and colleagues demonstrated corticosteroid-induced inhibition of the biosynthesis of collagen in human skin.[415] The harmful effects of repetitive intra-articular injection of steroids have been noted.[20, 82, 243, 361, 390]

Ford and DeBender[120] reported 13 patients who developed 15 ruptured tendons subsequent to nearby injection of steroids. Other authors have reported spontaneous ruptures of the Achilles tendon and patellar tendon after injections of steroids.[19, 179, 215, 253, 377] Although Matthews and colleagues[245] failed to find a deleterious effect of corticosteroid injections on rabbit patellar tendons, Kennedy and Willis[196] found a substantial effect in the Achilles tendon of the rabbit. They concluded that physiologic doses of local steroid placed directly in a normal tendon weaken it significantly for up to 14 days after the injection.

Watson[430] reviewed the surgical findings in 89 patients with major ruptures of the cuff. He found that all seven

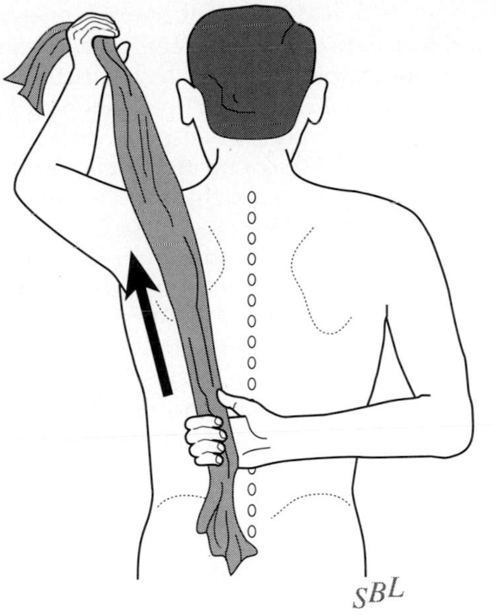

Figure 15–85

Stretching in internal rotation using a towel to apply a gentle stretching force. (From Matsen FA III, Lippitt SB, Sidles JA, and Harryman DT II: Practical Evaluation and Management of the Shoulder. Philadelphia: WB Saunders, 1994.)

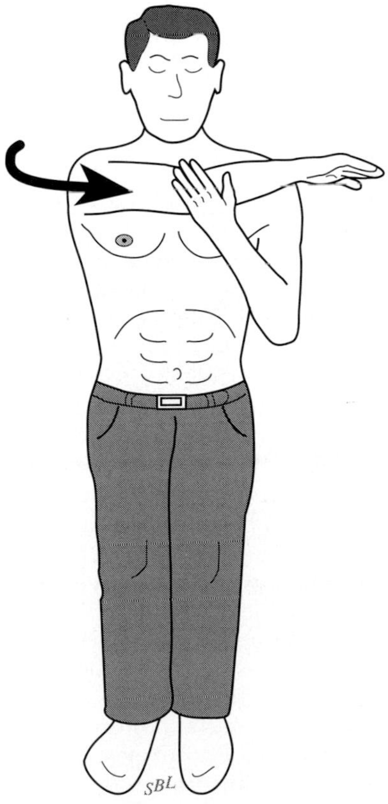

Figure 15–86

Stretching in cross-body reach using the opposite arm as the therapist. (From Matsen FA III, Lippitt SB, Sidles JA, and Harryman DT II: Practical Evaluation and Management of the Shoulder. Philadelphia: WB Saunders, 1994.)

patients who had had no local steroid injections had strong residual cuff tissue. Thirteen of 62 patients who had one to four steroid injections had soft cuff tissue that held suture poorly; 17 of the 20 patients who had more than four steroid injections had very weak cuff tissue; these shoulders with weak cuff tissue had poorer results after surgical repair. In this light, one can appreciate the potential hazard of making a diagnosis of "bursitis" or "bicipital tendinitis" and treating the situation with repeated steroid injections until the reality of a major cuff tendon deterioration becomes inescapable.[85, 196]

The patient with subacromial abrasion is informed that this condition can usually be resolved with nonoperative management directed toward the restoration of normal mobility, strength, coordination, and fitness.

AUTHORS' PREFERRED METHOD OF NONOPERATIVE MANAGEMENT OF SUBACROMIAL ABRASION

In our approach to subacromial abrasion, we recognize the important interplay between cuff weakness, stiffness of the posterior capsule, and subacromial roughness. We use a program designed by Jackins, a physical therapist who has worked with the University of Washington Shoulder and Elbow Service since its inception in 1975. This treatment regimen is analogous to one that would be used for managing a tennis elbow or Achilles tendinitis and includes: (1) avoidance of repeated injury, (2) restoration of normal flexibility, (3) restoration of normal strength, (4) aerobic exercise, and (5) modification of work or sport. The emphasis is on simple, low-technology exercises that the patient can perform unassisted.

Jackins Program

Step 1: Avoidance of Repeated Injury

Although it seems obvious that an affected shoulder must be rested, we see patients each week who are trying to continue vigorous overhead work or swimming hundreds of miles per week in the presence of cuff symptoms. It is difficult to treat these symptoms when the affected area is repeatedly irritated; activities may need to be temporarily modified—light duty, reducing mileage, less throwing, using the kickboard for a major part of the workout rather than continuing to try to "swim through" the problem, or working on the forehand and footwork rather than beating away at the serve. Once symptoms have subsided, the activity is progressively resumed with an emphasis on proper technique and a paced resumption of normal levels of performance.

Step 2: Restoration of Normal Flexibility

The goal of step 2 is to stretch out all directions of tightness. Shoulders with subacromial abrasion are frequently stiff, especially in the posterior capsule (see Fig. 15–60). As described earlier for posterior capsular tightness, the most effective program is one that taught by the surgeon or therapist but is carried out by the patient. The goal of the flexibility program is to restore the range of motion to that of the unaffected shoulder. The recommended treatment consists of gentle stretches performed five times a day by the patient (see Figs. 15–81 to 15–86). Each stretch is performed to the point where the patient feels a pull against the shoulder tightness, but not to the point of pain. Each stretch is performed for 1 minute, thus the patient invests about 30 min/day in the shoulder. Obvious improvement commonly occurs within the first

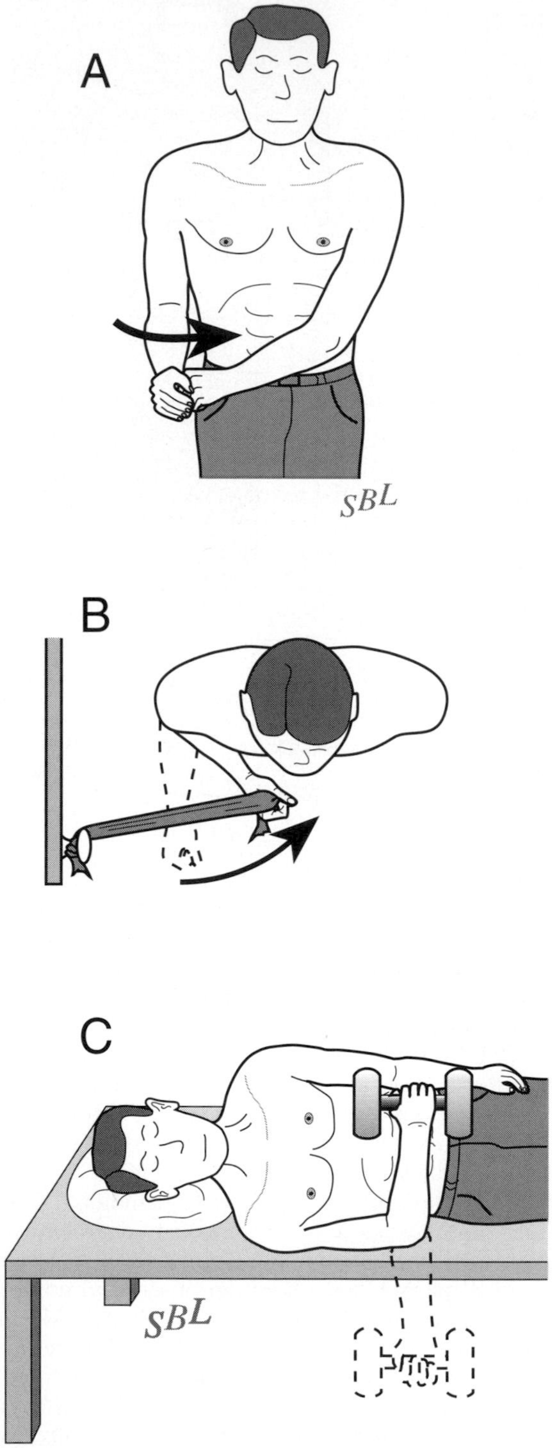

Figure 15–87

Internal rotation can be strengthened with isometrics *(A)*, rubber tubing *(B)*, or free weights *(C)*. (From Matsen FA III, Lippitt SB, Sidles JA, and Harryman DT II: Practical Evaluation and Management of the Shoulder. Philadelphia: WB Saunders, 1994.)

month, but 3 months may be required to completely eliminate the condition.

Step 3: Restoration of Normal Strength

When near-normal passive flexibility of the shoulder is restored, the patient's attention is directed toward regaining muscle strength. As is the case in managing tennis elbow, it is most effective to delay strengthening exercises until normal range of motion is achieved. As with the flexibility exercises, the patient is given the responsibility for strengthening the shoulder. Internal and external rotator-strengthening exercises are carried out with the arm at the side to strengthen the anterior and posterior cuff muscles without the potential for subacromial grinding that exists with exercises in abduction and flexion (Figs. 15–87 and 15–88). These exercises are most conveniently performed against the resistance of rubber tubing, sheet rubber, bicycle inner tubes, springs, or weights. It is convenient if the resistance device can be carried in a pocket or purse for frequent use through the day. As strength increases, the patient is advanced to more resistance: thicker tubing, tougher rubber sheets, or more springs. Deltoid strengthening is added when it can be performed comfortably (Fig. 15–89) as are exercises to strengthen the scapular motors (Figs. 15–90 and 15–91). Athletes are not returned to full activity until the shoulder has full mobility and strength.

Step 4: Aerobic Exercise

If a patient has got out of shape as a result of the shoulder problem, it is important to emphasize the need to regain normal fitness. To get back in shape and to improve the sense of well-being, 30 minutes of "sweaty" exercise 5 days a week is recommended. Brisk walking may be the safest and most effective type of aerobic exercise, but other suitable forms include jogging, biking, and stationary biking. Aerobic calisthenics as usually defined must be carefully reviewed to ensure that the patient does not require arm positions that aggravate his or her symptoms.

Step 5: Modification of Work or Sport

Obviously, the purpose of the program is to return the patient to the comfortable pursuit of normal activities. Not infrequently, this requires some analysis of working and recreational techniques. Occasionally, this is as simple as having the short grocery clerk stand on a platform at work. The technique of swimmers is reviewed to ensure, for example, adequate roll on the freestyle stroke. Throwers are taught the importance of body position and rotator cuff strength. Adequate knee bend and lumbar extension are reinforced in the execution of the tennis serve. If the patient has an occupation that requires vigorous or repeated use of the shoulder in painful positions, vocational rehabilitation to a different job may be required.

Subsequent Steps

It may take 6 weeks before substantial benefit is realized. As long as the patient is making progress, we continue this program. If improvement is not forthcoming, the program is reviewed to ensure that it is being conducted in an ideal way. The shoulder and the patient are also re-evaluated to make sure that no other factors may be interfering with recovery. If a repeat clinical evaluation indicates positive tendon signs (see Fig. 15–56) or other evidence of cuff fiber failure, tendon imaging studies may be considered if the results would change the patient's management. If a well-motivated patient continues to have symptomatic subacromial abrasion after 6 months of a well-conducted program, subacromial smoothing may

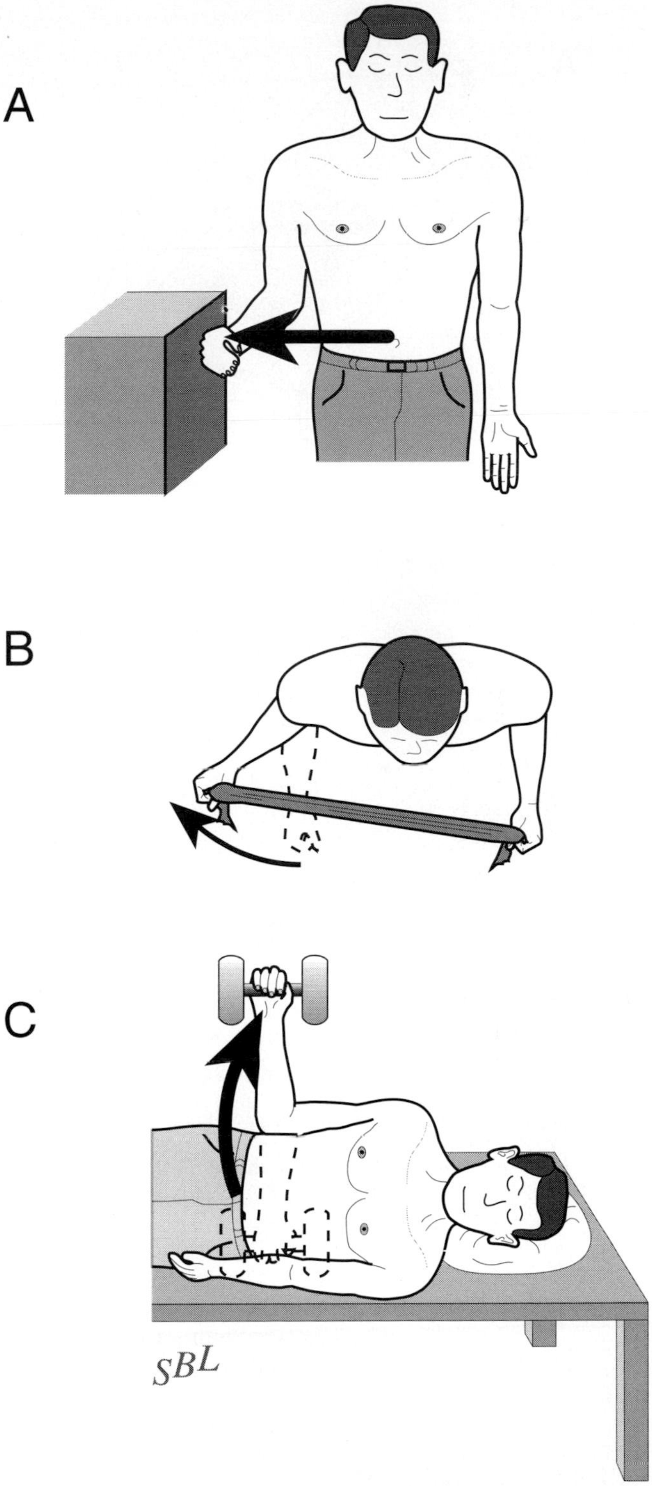

Figure 15–88

External rotation strengthening using isometrics (*A*), rubber tubing (*B*), or free weights (*C*). (From Matsen FA III, Lippitt SB, Sidles JA, and Harryman DT II: Practical Evaluation and Management of the Shoulder. Philadelphia: WB Saunders, 1994.)

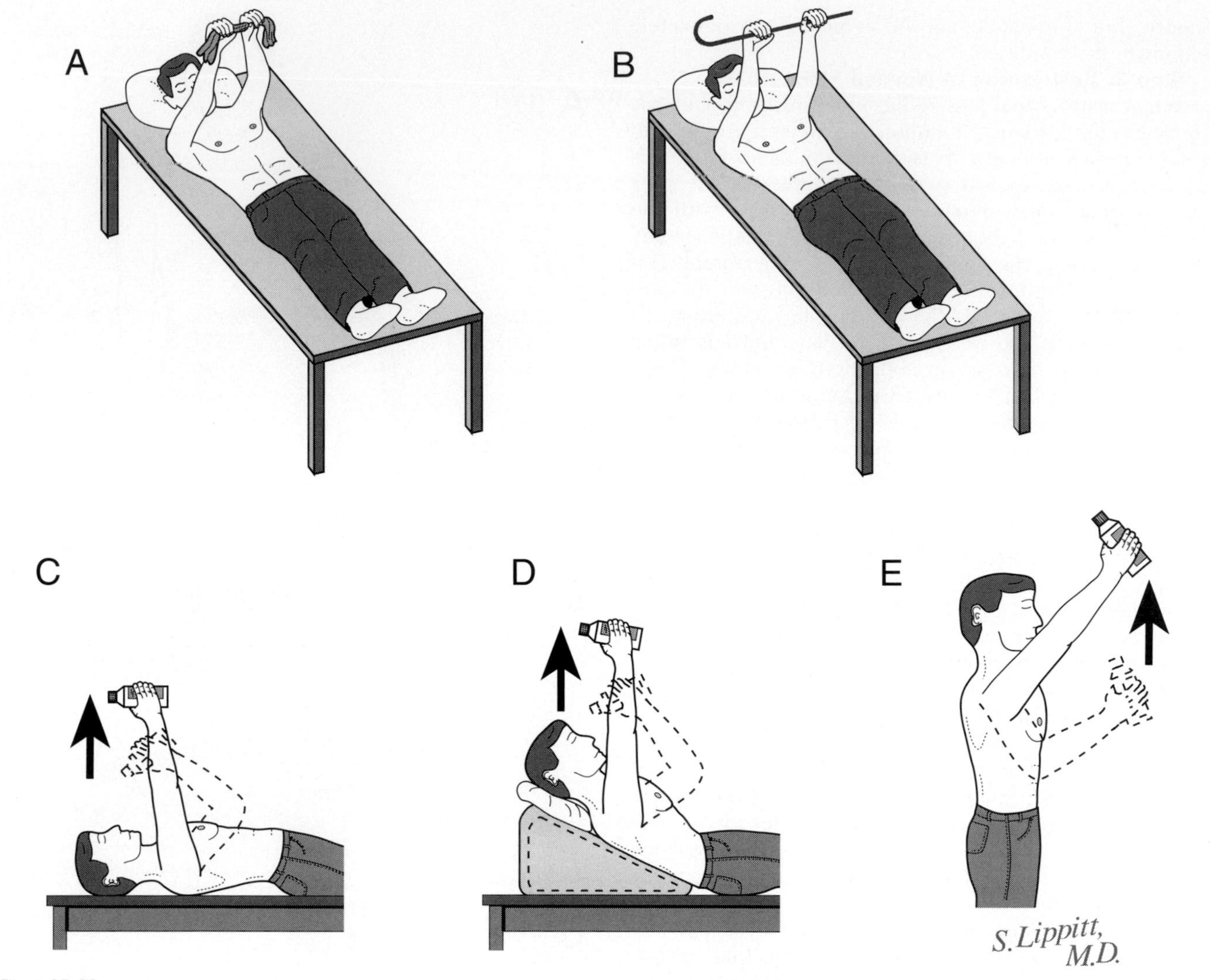

Figure 15–89

Progressive supine press exercises to strengthen flexion. The motion is always pushing up toward the ceiling, ending with a lift of the shoulder blade off the bed. *A*, Start with two hands together holding a wash cloth; *B*, then two hands apart; *C*, then one hand with a 1-pint (i.e., 1 lb) weight; *D*, then one hand with a 1-pint weight with greater degrees of sitting up; and finally, *E*, one hand with a 1-pint weight while standing. (Modified from Matsen FA III, Lippitt SB, Sidles JA, and Harryman DT II: Practical Evaluation and Management of the Shoulder. Philadelphia: WB Saunders, 1994.)

be discussed as an alternative to continued nonoperative management. Poor compliance with an exercise program may foretell an equally poor result from surgical treatment.

OPERATIVE TREATMENT

Open Acromioplasty

In his classic description of acromioplasty, Neer[275] described approaching the shoulder through a 9-cm incision made in Langer's lines from the anterior edge of the acromion to a point just lateral to the coracoid. The deltoid is split for 5 cm distal to the acromioclavicular joint in the direction of its fibers. It is then dissected from the front of the acromion and the acromioclavicular joint capsule. The stump of the deltoid's tendinous origin is elevated upward and preserved for the deltoid repair. Using an osteotome, a wedge-shaped piece of bone 0.09 × 2 cm is resected from the anterior undersurface of the acromion, along with the entire attachment of the coracoacromial ligament. If acromioclavicular osteophytes are present, the distal 2.5 cm of the clavicle are also excised along with the prominences on the acromial side of the joint. After the procedure, the deltoid is carefully repaired to the acromioclavicular joint capsule, the trapezius, and its tendon of origin.

Many reports regarding the results of open acromioplasty have been published.[6, 95, 151, 155, 156, 164, 184, 200, 247, 257, 270, 275, 277, 290, 320, 333, 375, 379, 399, 431] However, the interpretation of these reports is made difficult by the admixture of patients with intact cuffs, partial-thickness cuff lesions, and full-thickness cuff tears as well as by the inclusion of a wide range of additional elements to the surgery. Stuart and associates[389] reported a series that included acromioplasty with or without cuff repair, distal clavicle exci-

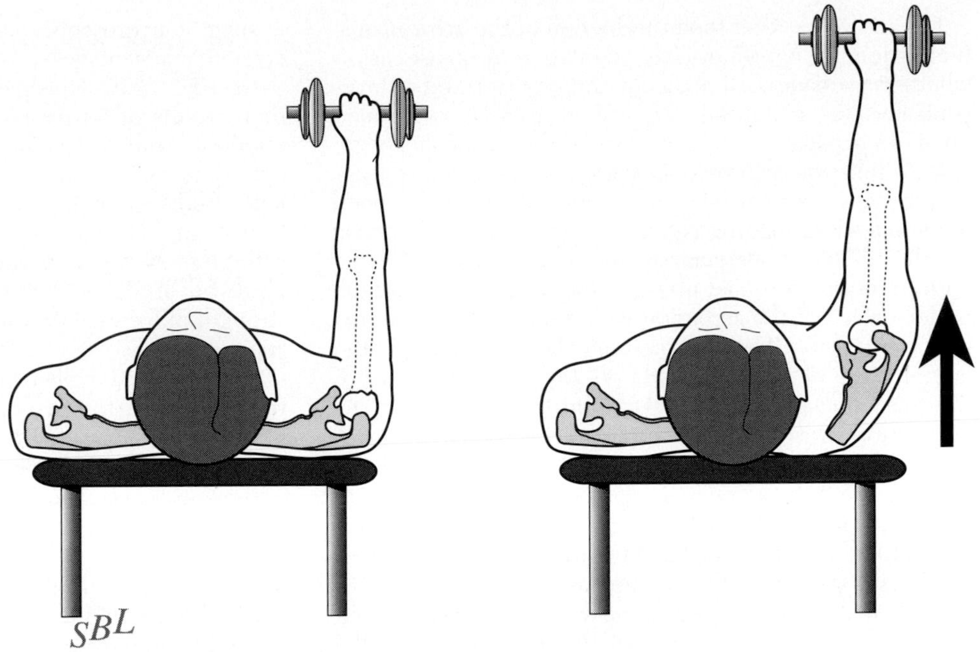

Figure 15–90

In the press plus, the arm is pushed upward until the shoulder blade is lifted off the table or bed. (From Matsen FA III, Lippitt SB, Sidles JA, and Harryman DT II: Practical Evaluation and Management of the Shoulder. Philadelphia: WB Saunders, 1994.)

sion, and biceps tenodesis; 23% were still painful. Rockwood and Lyons[350] reported on a series of 71 patients who had a modified acromioplasty with or without cuff repair and concluded that cuff repair did not influence the percentage of excellent results. Bosley[33] reported on 35 patients with total acromionectomy, including patients with and without long-standing massive cuff tears; most failures were attributed to either the underlying pathology or to failure of deltoid reattachment. Bjorkenheim and associates[31] reported a failure rate of more than 25%, attributing the failures to "associated bony as well as soft-tissue subacromial lesions." Ogilvie-Harris and associates[298] evaluated 67 shoulders in 65 patients who had pain and dysfunction for more than 2 years after an initial acromioplasty for impingement syndrome without a rotator cuff tear. In almost half of the cases, there were "diagnostic errors" and even in those where there was a correct diagnosis and no operative errors, the failure rate was almost 20%.

Arthroscopic Acromioplasty

Ellman,[104] in 1987, published the first large series of 50 patients (average age of 50 years) with mixed shoulder pathology who underwent arthroscopic acromioplasty; 10 had full-thickness tears. At an average follow-up of 17 months, 88% had good or excellent results. These results persisted at 2.5-year follow-up of the same treatment group.[107]

Since then others have reported results of arthroscopic acromioplasty.[104, 110] Gartsman,[131] Speer and associates,[384] Altchek and colleagues,[4] and Roye and co-workers[357] reported series of arthroscopic acromioplasties on shoulders without cuff tears; each finding that 83 to 94% of the results were satisfactory. Approximately 75% of the patients were able to return to sports activity. Recovery times in these series ranged from 2 to 4 months. Most authors describe the procedure as technically demanding. The control of bleeding and the determination of the amount of bone to resect are two commonly technical difficultics in performing arthroscopic subacromial decompression. Many describe a learning curve associated with this technique and have recommended that this procedure be performed on cadaver shoulders before it is used clinically.

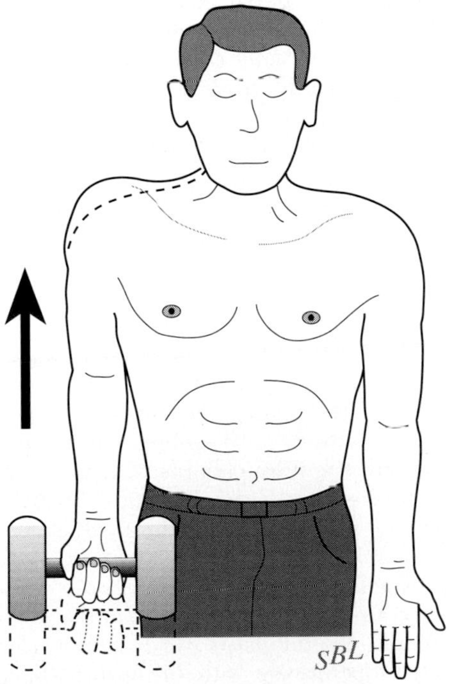

Figure 15–91

The shoulder shrug exercise: lift the tip of the shoulder toward the ear while holding the elbow straight. (From Matsen FA III, Lippitt SB, Sidles JA, and Harryman DT II: Practical Evaluation and Management of the Shoulder. Philadelphia: WB Saunders, 1994.)

In early years, after the introduction of the arthroscopic technique of acromioplasty, controversy arose as to whether a subacromial decompression performed arthroscopically was technically equivalent to that performed open. In a cadaver study, Gartsman and associates were able to perform arthroscopic bony resection with release of the coracoacromial ligament equivalent to the open technique described by Neer.[131, 132] He suggested criteria for the technical adequacy of the acromioplasty: (1) the entire anterior acromial protuberance is resected, (2) the undersurface of the acromion is flattened, (3) the deltoid fibers are visible from the acromioclavicular joint to the lateral edge of the acromion, (4) the inferior aspect of the acromioclavicular joint is débrided to remove any downward protrusion, (5) the coracoacromial ligament is completely released from the anterior portion of the acromion and the acromioclavicular joint, (6) a portion of the ligament is resected, (7) an adequate subacromial bursectomy is performed to allow complete inspection of the bursal surface of the rotator cuff, and (8) finally, no subacromial abrasion is observed when the arm is taken through a range of motion at the completion of the procedure.

Most authors state that the *indications* for arthroscopic acromioplasty should be identical to those for the open procedure described by Neer in 1972. However, compared with the rate with which Neer used open acromioplasty in his practice, it is apparent that arthroscopic acromioplasty is performed much more commonly with broader indications. Although overall satisfactory results were obtained in most reports, some authors were uncertain whether relief was obtained from the modifications of the acromial shape or from other aspects of the treatment.

To keep things in perspective, Brox and associates[43] compared the effectiveness of arthroscopic acromioplasty, an exercise program, and a placebo in a randomized clinical trial. The study group consisted of 125 patients aged 18 to 66 who had had rotator cuff disease for at least 3 months and whose condition was resistant to treatment. The authors concluded that surgery or a supervised exercise regimen significantly, and equally, improved rotator cuff disease compared with a placebo; however, the surgical treatment was substantially more costly.

Comparison of Open and Arthroscopic Acromioplasty

In 1994, Sachs and associates[359] reported on a series of 44 patients with stage II impingement prospectively randomized into open (22 patients with an average age of 49) and arthroscopic treatment groups (19 patients with an average age of 51). In both groups, full recovery took at least 1 year for most patients. In both groups more than 90% of patients achieved a satisfactory result (good or excellent). Final analysis showed that the main benefits of arthroscopic acromioplasty were evident in the first 3 months postoperatively with the arthroscopic patients regaining flexion and strength more rapidly than did patients treated with open decompression. Furthermore, the arthroscopic treatment group had shorter hospitalizations, used fewer narcotics, and returned more quickly to both work and activities of daily living, leading the authors to suggest arthroscopic acromioplasty may have significant economic advantages.

In 1992, Van Holsbeeck and associates[417] compared their results of 53 patients treated by arthroscopic acromioplasty and 53 patients treated by an open acromioplasty. Based on the UCLA rating scale, good or excellent results were identical for both groups at a 2-year follow-up. The authors suggested that arthroscopic acromioplasty was associated with a shorter recovery time; however, in the long term, there was no difference in strength of forward flexion between the open and arthroscopic groups.

Hawkins and colleagues[166] reported 40% satisfactory results with arthroscopic subacromial decompression, while they reported 87% satisfactory results with a concurrent series of open acromioplasty.

Roye and associates[357] reported a series of 90 arthroscopic acromioplasties and found that the most of the patients who were not throwing athletes obtained satisfactory results and that the presence or absence of a cuff tear did not affect the result.

Lindh and co-workers, in 1993, reported on a series of 20 patients who were randomly selected for either open or arthroscopic acromioplasty (10 patients in each group). The average duration of symptoms before surgery was over 5 years. Functional results in both the arthroscopic and open surgery groups were good and similar. Patients in the arthroscopic group were observed to demonstrate earlier restoration of full range of motion and reduction in time away from work.

Proponents of arthroscopic acromioplasty have argued this procedure requires less surgical dissection and produces less scarring and less postoperative morbidity. In most cases, the procedure can be performed on an outpatient basis. Postoperative discomfort is moderate and can usually be controlled by oral analgesics. Additionally, cosmesis is good, and patient acceptance is high.

A countervailing advantage of open acromioplasty is the advantage of being able to observe directly the subacromial space during motions that preoperatively caused the patient's symptomatic subacromial crepitance and the ability to ensure that the crepitance is resolved before the procedure is concluded.

Deltoid retraction can be a significant problem after open procedures that require detachment and subsequent reattachment of the deltoid to the anterior acromion.[27] Arthroscopic acromioplasty has the theoretical advantage of leaving the deltoid origin almost totally undisturbed. However, in a report by Torpey and associates,[407] it was pointed out that much of the deltoid arose from the anterior acromion. Their analysis indicated that a 4-mm anterior acromioplasty would detach approximately half of the deltoid fibers, whereas a 6-mm anterior acromioplasty would detach approximately 75% of the fibers. They concluded that neither an open nor an arthroscopic acromioplasty can be performed without substantial compromise of the anterior deltoid origin.

Arthroscopy offers the ability to directly inspect the glenohumeral joint as well as the subacromial space. During an open acromioplasty, the deep surface of the cuff (where most cuff lesions begin) is not visible. By contrast at arthroscopy, partial- or complete-thickness tears of either surface of the rotator cuff as well as other findings can be identified by the experienced observer. However, even with arthroscopy, the common intratendinous lesions remain inaccessible. Paulos and Franklin[315] in their series of 80 arthroscopic acromioplasties reported a high number of unsuspected diagnoses that were made during arthroscopy. These included 26 partial rotator cuff tears; 12 labral tears; 8 cases of humeral chondrosis; 4 cases of biceps tendon fraying; and 2 loose bodies in the glenohumeral joint. They reported that for most of these shoulders these findings would have been missed with the open technique.

Altchek and associates[4] in their series of 44 patients treated by arthroscopic acromioplasty; 11 patients had lesions of the glenoid labrum. Preoperatively, these patients had no evidence of instability, either by history or physical examination in action. Five of these patients had a tear involving the inferior part of the labrum and failed to recover completely after the acromioplasty and were unable to return to full participation in sports. The authors felt that undetected slight instability may have played a role in the production of these patients' symptoms. The authors argued that arthroscopic inspection of the glenohumeral joint makes it possible to detect such problems, thus providing information that is important for prognosis. Others have reported a higher than anticipated percentage of unsuspected associated lesions in those shoulders being treated arthroscopically for impingement symptoms.[188] Burns and Turba[47] reported on their findings in 29 patients treated with arthroscopic acromioplasty, which included the anterior glenoid labrum tear (15), undersurface rotator cuff tear (8), chondromalacia of the humerus (3), biceps rupture (1), posterior glenoid labrum tear (1), and acromioclavicular arthritis (1).

These results indicate that the preoperative diagnosis of "impingement syndrome" has been associated with a wide range of shoulder pathologies. They leave unanswered the question of the prevalence of these same findings in asymptomatic shoulders and the role played by each of the findings in producing clinical symptoms. Hopefully in the future, methodical clinicopathologic correlation will lead to improved accuracy in preoperative diagnosis and greater specificity in treatment.

The primary difficulty in interpreting these studies on open and arthroscopic acromioplasty is that, although the *outcome* of the procedure is characterized in terms such as of good or excellent, the *effectiveness* of the procedure is often undetermined because the preoperative status (or *ingo)* was not characterized in the same way. Ideally, a good result from surgery would indicate the *change* in the patient's condition as a result of the procedure, rather than the status of the shoulder postoperatively.

The definition of the indications for and the effectiveness of acromioplasty must await multipractice studies that define accurately the pretreatment clinical findings and shoulder functional status, the nature of and compliance with a nonoperative program, the nature of the surgery, and the *change* in the shoulder function realized after the procedure using the same parameters of comfort and function before and after surgery. The *effectiveness* of a treatment is the difference between the *outcome* and the *ingo*.

AUTHORS' PREFERRED METHOD FOR SUBACROMIAL SMOOTHING

In our experience, the results of subacromial smoothing are likely to be best in the following circumstances: (1) a well-motivated patient older than 40 years of age, (2) absence of posterior capsular stiffness, (3) presence of symptomatic subacromial crepitus (see Fig. 15–59) that the patient agrees is the dominant clinical problem, (4) absence of tendon signs (see Fig. 15–56) and other shoulder pathology, and (5) symptoms that are not associated with a work-related injury. Poor prognostic signs include: (1) age younger than 40, (2) stiffness, (3) absence of subacromial crepitus, (4) presence of tendon signs or evidence of other shoulder pathology, (5) attribution of the problem by the patient to his or her occupation, (6) concomitant evidence of glenohumeral instability, and (7) neurogenic cuff muscle weakness.

We use an open approach to subacromial smoothing. The patient is positioned with the head up at 30 degrees and the arm draped free. Before making the incision, we note the positions and motions in which subacromial crepitus can be palpated through the acromion. The shoulder is approached through an incision in the skin lines over the anterolateral corner of the acromion (see Fig. 15–1). The acromion is exposed in an attempt to maintain the continuity of the deltoid fascia, the acromial periosteum, and the trapezius fascia. The deltoid tendon is split in line with its fibers along the strong tendon of origin that divides the anterior and middle deltoid. This allows two strong "handles" on the deltoid for repair. This split is deepened under direct vision until the bursa is entered. Rotating the humerus provides easy differentiation between the deltoid (which does not move with humeral rotation) and the superficial surface of the cuff (which does).

On entering the subacromial aspect of the humeroscapular motion interface (see Figs. 15–3 and 15–4), the subacromial space is observed while the preoperatively identified crepitus-producing movements are carried out. This step reveals the cause of the crepitance, which is usually some combination of roughness on the undersurface of the acromion, hypertrophic bursa, adhesions between the cuff and the acromion, roughness of the superior surface of the rotator cuff, or a prominent tuberosity. By gently rotating the arm, most of the cuff can be brought to the incision as pointed out by Codman (Figs. 15–92 and 15–93). The rotator cuff is thoroughly explored and palpated for evidence of superior surface blisters, partial tears, thinning, or full-thickness defects. Although deep surface cuff fiber failure cannot be seen through this approach, it is also true that such fiber disruption cannot cause the subacromial crepitance. Fukuda's methylene blue "dye test" or more recently the "Fukudalite" test with saline is used to evaluate shoulders with suspicious cuff integrity.[128] In this test, fluid is injected to distend the glenohumeral joint to further explore suspected thinning or small cuff defects.

A hypertrophic bursa is resected. Superior surface cuff defects are smoothed by either resection of their protruding aspects or occasionally by reattaching a superior surface cuff flap. Prominences of the tuberosity are

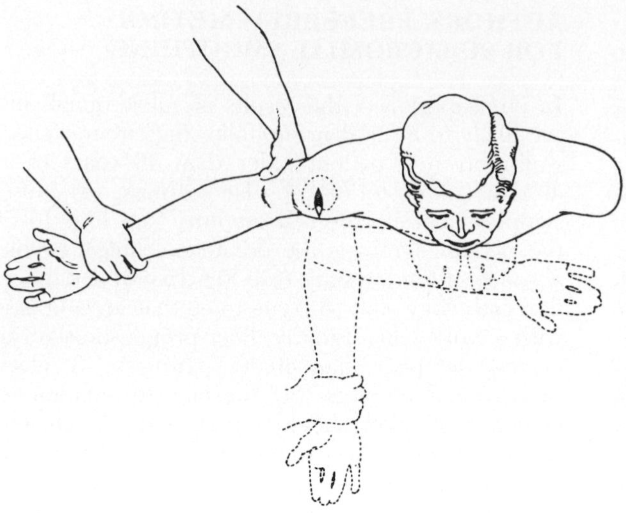

Figure 15–92

A, Operative position, superior view. *B*, Rotation of the humerus beneath the incision. (From Codman EA: Rupture of the Supraspinatus Tendon and Other Lesions In or About the Subacromial Bursa. Malabar, FL: Robert E Krieger, 1984.)

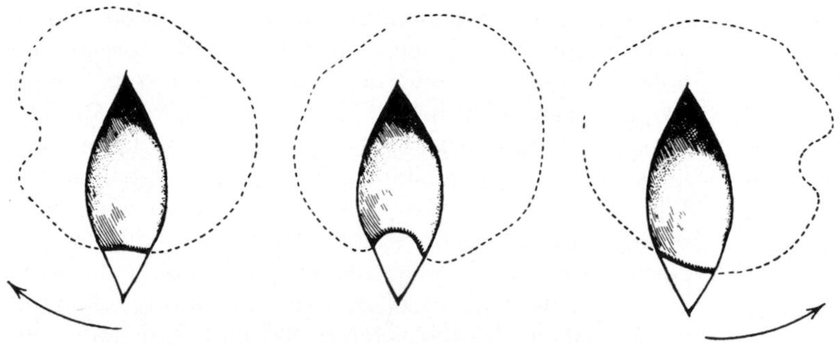

smoothed so that the tuberosity passes easily beneath the coracoacromial arch. The undersurface of the coracoacromial arch is palpated to identify areas of roughness or prominence. These are smoothed with a "pine cone" burr, although an osteotome or rongeur may be useful for larger lesions. No attempt is made to resect the coracoacromial ligament unless it can be demonstrated to be the cause of the subacromial roughness.

If a substantial amount of bone needs to be removed, a thin-bladed osteotome is used (Fig. 15–94). The osteotomy is oriented in line with the extrapolated undersurface of the posterior acromion (identified by palpation and direct vision). Care is taken that the osteotomy does not continue into the posterior acromion or scapular spine. The undersurface of the acromion is then smoothed using a "pine cone" power burr, taking care that no spurs are left laterally in the deltoid origin or medially at the acromioclavicular joint. The shoulder is thoroughly irrigated to remove all bone fragments.

Additional surgery is avoided unless clearly indicated. Inferiorly directed acromioclavicular osteophytes are resected if they scrape on the cuff. The biceps is left undisturbed unless it appears to be seriously inflamed, obviously unstable, or doomed to imminent rupture, in which case we perform a tenodesis to the proximal humerus.

The shoulder is gently manipulated through a complete range of motion to ensure the absence of stiffness or additional adhesions. The entire humeroscapular motion interface (see Figs. 15–3 and 15–4) is inspected to ensure

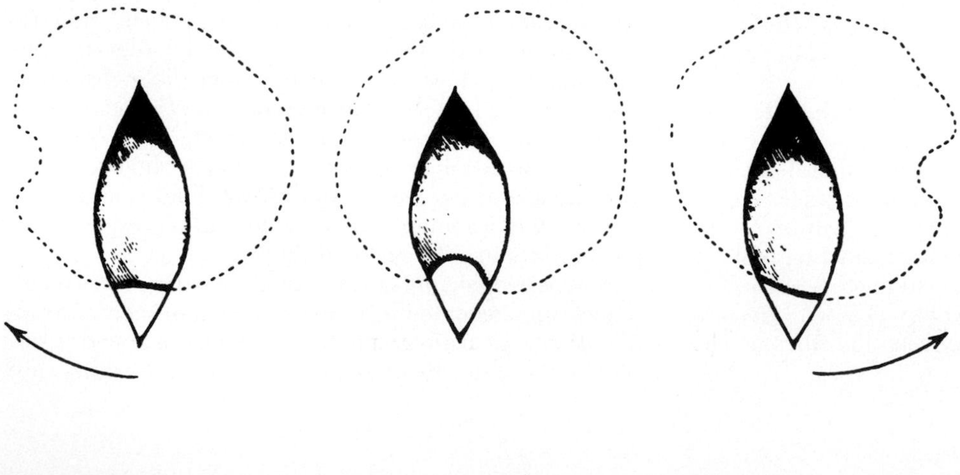

Figure 15–93

The underlying cuff is systematically explored and palpated. This is accomplished by rotating the arm to bring the different parts of the cuff into view (rather than by extending the incision). (From Codman EA: Rupture of the Supraspinatus Tendon and Other Lesions In or About the Subacromial Bursa. Malabar, FL: Robert E Krieger, 1984.)

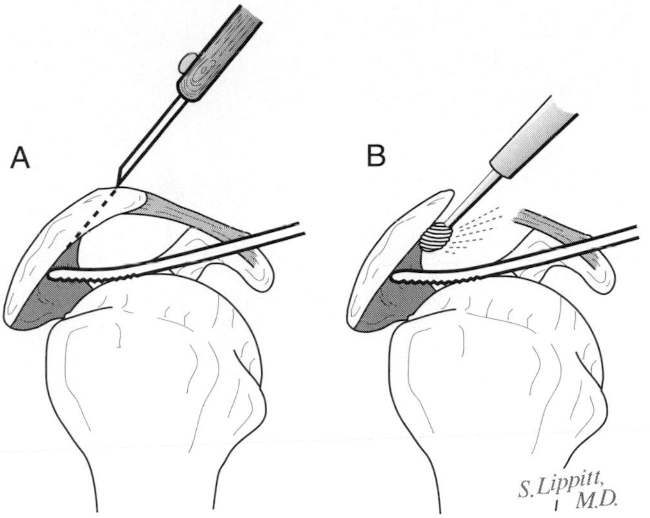

Figure 15–94

A thin-bladed osteotome is used to resect the anteroinferior surface of the acromion. The coracoacromial ligament is resected along with the acromial fragment. The osteotomy is oriented in line with the extrapolated undersurface of the posterior acromion. Exposure and access are facilitated by employing a Darrach retractor to gently depress the humeral head. (Modified from Matsen FA III, Lippitt SB, Sidles JA, and Harryman DT II: Practical Evaluation and Management of the Shoulder. Philadelphia: WB Saunders, 1994.)

the absence of adhesions and for other pathology. Before the procedure is concluded, the upper surface of the cuff and tuberosities and the undersurface of the coracoacromial arch are carefully palpated to ensure the absence of residual roughness. The entire range of passive shoulder motion must be free of subacromial crepitance.

On closure, a secure deltoid reconstitution is top priority so that early postoperative motion may be instituted. The deltoid is repaired by side-to-side closure of the medial and lateral aspects of the tendon split using a No. 2 nonabsorbable suture (Fig. 15–95). The tendon is secured to the acromion, using suture to bone as necessary. Suture from the medial hole is passed through the lateral part of the deltoid tendon, and suture from the lateral hole is passed through the medial part of the deltoid tendon to effect a criss-cross closure. This avoids the tell-tale "V" defect that reveals a poor deltoid closure. All knots are placed on the superficial aspect to avoid recreating subacromial roughness.

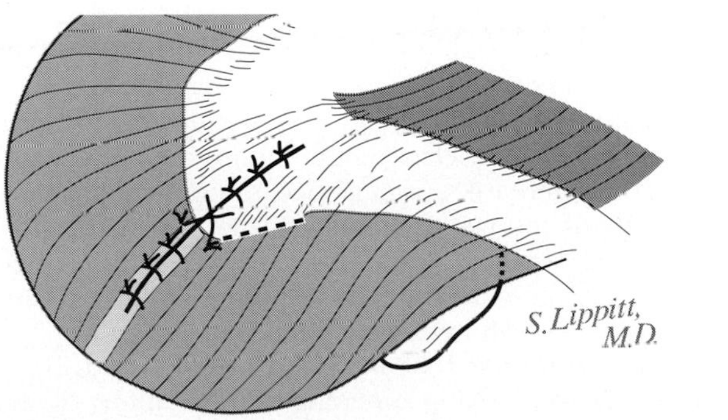

Figure 15–95

A secure deltoid reconstruction is essential so that immediate postoperative motion can be instituted. (Modified from Matsen FA III, Lippitt SB, Sidles JA, and Harryman DT II: Practical Evaluation and Management of the Shoulder. Philadelphia: WB Saunders, 1994.)

Postoperative Program

After any type of subacromial surgery, there is a great potential for adhesions between the cuff and the arch. In cases of failed acromioplasty, such scarring seems to be a dominant feature and appears to be often related to delay in the institution of motion after the surgery. To avoid such problems, we begin motion as soon as possible, preferably with continuous passive motion (CPM) in the recovery room (Fig. 15–96). CPM is set to move the arm slowly through an arc of 0 to 90 degrees of elevation and from 50 to 0 degrees of internal rotation. CPM is applied whenever the patient is in bed during hospitalization but is not continued after the patient is discharged. On the day of surgery, the patient is instructed in the "140/40 passive program" in which the opposite hand is used to assist the operated shoulder in achieving 140 degrees of elevation and 40 degrees of external rotation (see Figs. 15–81 and 15–83). Emphasis is also placed on posterior capsular stretching, including cross-body adduction (see Fig. 15–86), reaching up the back (see Fig. 15–85), and internal rotation of the abducted arm.

The early implementation of passive motion is facilitated if the procedure is performed under brachial plexus block,[398] which lasts from 12 to 18 hours. The postoperative exercises are already familiar to the patient, having been performed as part of the preoperative trial of the Jackins program. The patient is allowed active use of the shoulder within the realm of comfort, unless there is concern for the strength of the deltoid reattachment. Internal and external rotation strengthening exercises are also begun immediately (see Figs. 15–87 and 15-88). Deltoid strengthening is initiated at 6 weeks after the repair is secure (see Fig. 15–89). As soon as they can be performed comfortably, exercises to strengthen the scapular motors are added (see Figs. 15–90 and 15–91). Athletics are not allowed for 3 months after surgery and not until normal motion and strength are regained.

Failed Acromioplasty

In this condition, the patient is dissatisfied with the result from a previous arthroscopic or open acromioplasty and presents for consideration of additional surgery. Such results occur in every series of acromioplasty, even if the technique of the procedure seems appropriate. The incidence of these failures ranges from 3 to 11%.[275, 329, 336, 399] In Post and Cohen's series, 11% continued to have significant pain after surgery.[329, 330] Fifty-six per cent of those with weakness before surgery still had weakness postoperatively; 29% of those with preoperative limitations of motion still had limitation of motion after surgery. The rate of return to high-level athletics or challenging occupations is lower. Tibone and colleagues[401] found that of 35 athletes having impingement syndrome treated by anterior acromioplasty, 20% still had moderate to severe

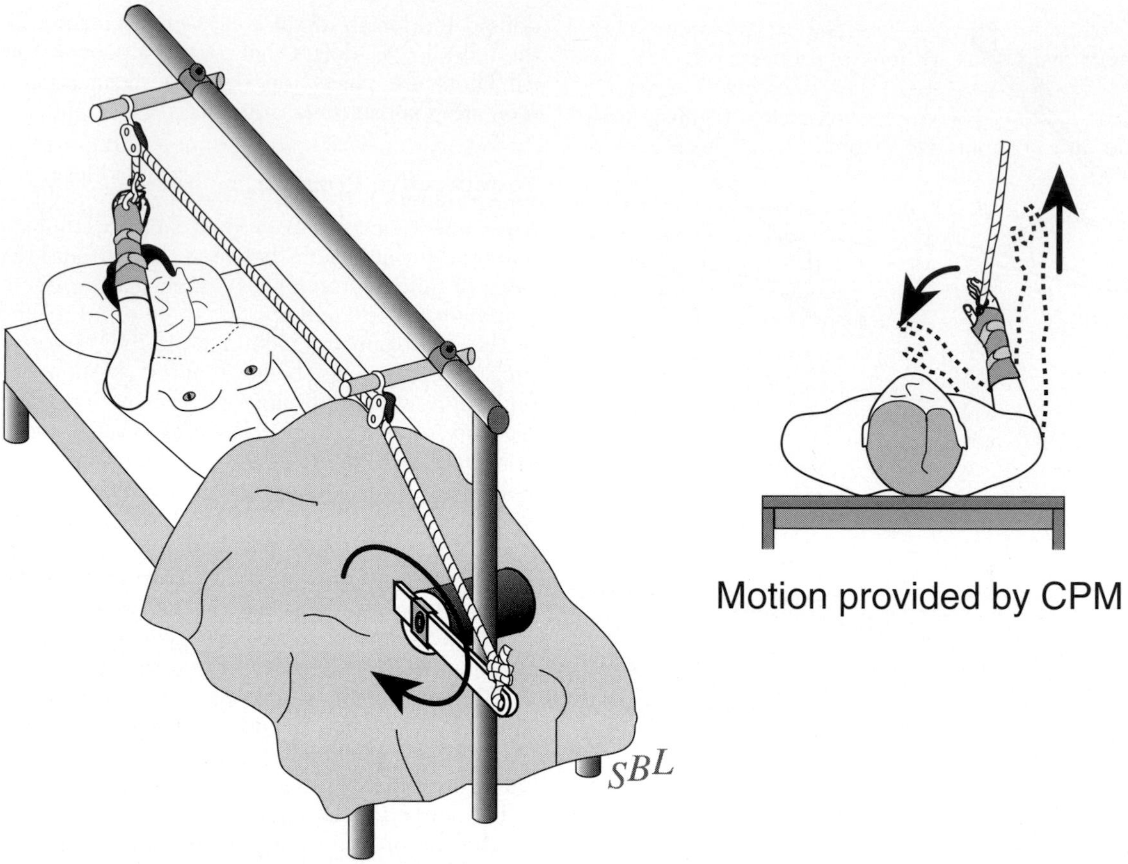

Figure 15–96

Continuous passive motion (CPM) is helpful for the first 24 to 48 hours after a procedure to mobilize the shoulder. Elevation to 90 degrees is easily achieved using a simple pulley system with a motor-driven eccentric cam. (Modified from Matsen FA III, Lippitt SB, Sidles JA, and Harryman DT II: Practical Evaluation and Management of the Shoulder. Philadelphia: WB Saunders, 1994.)

pain, and 9% had pain at rest and with activities of daily living. Only 43% returned to their preinjury level of competitive athletics, and only 4 of 18 returned to competitive throwing. Hawkins and co-workers[163] have shown that it is difficult for patients injured on the job to return to their original occupations after an acromioplasty.

Why is this? Failure to achieve complete relief of symptoms through acromioplasty may indicate: (1) pathology other than subacromial roughness, (2) failure to achieve subacromial smoothness, (3) failure of deltoid reattachment, (4) excessive acromial resection, (5) postoperative complications such as dense scarring between the cuff and the acromion, or (6) failure of rehabilitation. Many of these problems can leave the patient more symptomatic than before the surgery (see Fig. 15–9).

Acromioclavicular joint problems were thought to be responsible for five failures in Post's series, a "frequent cause of failure of surgical treatment" in the series of Penny and Welsh,[320] and the cause of the only unsatisfactory result in Neer's series. In their series of patients who had persistent problems after acromioplasty, Hawkins and colleagues[163] reported that 45% of the patients had a diagnosis other than continuing impingement, including acromioclavicular joint problems, cervical spondylosis, reflex sympathetic dystrophy, rotator cuff tear, thoracic outlet syndrome, glenohumeral osteoarthritis, and glenohumeral instability. Thirty-three per cent were thought to have continuing subacromial abrasion. The striking finding in this series was the relative lack of improvement in patients on workmen's compensation after revision acromioplasty. Even in these authors' series of primary acromioplasties, 22% of the workmen's compensation cases had an unsatisfactory result, compared with 8% failure rate with nonworkmen's compensation cases.[162] Post and Cohen[330] also observed that worse results were obtained from surgery performed for work-related impingement syndrome. This inability to return to work may be due to partial-thickness cuff tears, residual tendon scarring, and residual weakness. Post and Cohen emphasized the need for recovery of muscle strength before the laborer returns to work; otherwise, a recurrence can be anticipated. The difficulty of returning workers to their jobs after acromioplasty is reminiscent of the problems described by Tibone and co-workers[401] in returning athletes to a competitive level of function.

Bosley reported that most failures were attributed to either the underlying pathology or to failure of deltoid reattachment.[33] Bjorkenheim and associates[31] reported a failure rate of more than 25%, attributing the failures to "associated bony as well as soft-tissue subacromial lesions." Ogilvie-Harris and colleagues[298] evaluated 67 shoulders in 65 patients who had pain and dysfunction for more than 2 years after an initial acromioplasty for impingement syndrome without a rotator cuff tear. In almost half of the cases, there were "diagnostic errors," and even in patients for whom a correct diagnosis had been made and no operative errors, the failure rate was almost 20%.

Radical acromionectomy may worsen a patient's comfort and function (see Fig. 15–9). This procedure removes the origin of the deltoid muscle and facilitates scar formation between the deltoid muscle and the rotator cuff. Neer and Marberry have pointed out that a radical acromionectomy may seriously compromise shoulder function without achieving subacromial smoothness.[281] In their series of 30 patients, all had marked shoulder weakness and almost all had persistent pain. In the 20 shoulders reoperated upon, all had a retracted and scarred middle deltoid that was adherent to the cuff and the humerus. Fifteen of the patients had residual cuff tears. Attempts to reconstruct these severely damaged shoulders were disappointing. The effects of loss of the deltoid attachment and the permanent contracture could not be reversed. In addition, these authors observed a high incidence of wound problems and infections after the radical acromionectomy, which further complicated their attempts at revision.

To help understand some of the other causes of unsuccessful acromioplasty, Flugstad and co-workers[119] reviewed 19 patients referred to the University of Washington Shoulder and Elbow Service because of persistent pain and stiffness after open acromioplasty performed elsewhere. The average age was 42; 16 patients were male. Eleven patients had a traumatic onset of their shoulder problem; eight of these were work related. The average time of postoperative immobilization was 4 weeks. At the time of presentation, the patients complained of pain and stiffness. Physical examination revealed an average of 126 degrees of forward flexion and 36 degrees of external rotation and internal rotation so that the thumb could touch T12. In 13 of these patients, revision surgery was performed after an exercise program failed to improve their symptoms. The average interval between the initial surgery and revision surgery was 15 months. At the revision surgery, 10 patients had roughness of the undersurface of the acromion. Five patients had distinct spurs protruding from the lateral or medial acromion; eight patients had large amounts of subacromial scarring in which heavy bands of cicatrix connected the undersurface of the acromion to the rotator cuff. Three patients had acromioclavicular joint spurs; one patient had a large un-united acromial fragment; and another patient had an os acromial. Although no patients had a full-thickness cuff tear, the incidence of partial-thickness deep surface or midsubstance cuff tears is unknown. The revision surgical procedure included excision of scar tissue, revision of the acromioplasty to ensure adequate resection of the anterior and inferior acromion, resection of acromioclavicular spurs, inspection of the rotator cuff, and careful deltoid repair. Immediately after surgery, gentle range-of-motion exercises were initiated to minimize restriction from postoperative scar. A follow-up at an average of 10 months' postoperatively revealed substantial although incomplete improvement in comfort, range of motion, and ability to work.

This report emphasizes the importance of accurate diagnosis and effective subacromial smoothing. However, the key lesson was the importance of rapid restoration of full joint motion before restricting adhesions have the opportunity to form: the average patient in this series had a 1-month delay between surgery and the implementation of motion.

AUTHORS' PREFERRED METHOD FOR THE MANAGEMENT OF FAILED ACROMIOPLASTY

Patients who have had previous acromioplasty with unsatisfactory results need to be carefully re-evaluated to determine presence of stiffness, weakness, instability, or persistent roughness. The social and vocational context of the shoulder problem must also be re-evaluated.

The Jackins nonoperative program is instituted, even if the patient already has "had therapy"; because surgery has failed once already, there is plenty of time for conservatism and a period of observation.

Patients with positive tendon signs may be considered for cuff imaging studies if these signs are refractory to rehabilitation (see Fig. 15–56). Vocational rehabilitation may be essential; if one procedure has not helped the patient to get back to his or her job, the odds would seem not much better during the second attempt.

Reoperation is considered in well-motivated patients with evidence of residual subacromial roughness or stiffness that is attributable to postoperative scarring in the humeroscapular motion interface (see Figs. 15–3 and 15–4). In contrast to primary acromioplasty, we are willing to operate again on patients with refractory shoulder stiffness, because this stiffness may be caused by dense scarring between the cuff and the acromion, which cannot be managed nonoperatively. Our revision procedure is identical with the primary subacromial smoothing described earlier.

Partial-Thickness Cuff Lesions

In this condition, partial-thickness disruption of the cuff is manifest by pain or weakness on resisted isometric contraction of the involved cuff muscles. The shoulder commonly demonstrates associated posterior capsular tightness. Imaging studies may indicate cuff tendon thinning or partial-thickness defects, but the lesion does not extend through the full thickness of the tendon.

Judging from the cadaver studies reviewed earlier in this chapter, intrasubstance and articular surface partial-thickness cuff tears represent the commonest forms of cuff involvement. These lesions usually involve the supraspinatus tendon near its anterior insertion but may also involve the infraspinatus and subscapularis. Clinical observation of patients with documented partial-thickness cuff lesions suggests that they produce symptoms analogous to other partial-thickness tendon lesions, such as a partial Achilles tear, a partial tear of the patellar tendon, or a partial tear of the tendon of origin of the extensor carpi radialis brevis (tennis elbow). These partial tendon lesion symptoms include *stiffness* of the joint on passive motion in a direction that stretches the tendon and *tendon signs* (i.e., pain or weakness on isometric contraction of the tendon's muscle) (see Fig. 15–56). These partial tendon lesions are often much more painful than are full-thickness tears. This is because, in contrast with full-thickness tears, partial-thickness defects of the cuff give rise to stiffness and unphysiologic tension on the remaining fibers.

In its less common form involving the bursal aspect of the cuff tendon, partial-thickness cuff lesions may be associated with *subacromial abrasion*, yielding subacromial crepitance on passive joint motion.

There is not a lot of published information regarding the results of operative treatment for partial-thickness cuff lesions. Fukuda and colleagues[128, 129] described the management of six patients with partial-thickness bursal-side tears by acromioplasty or wedge resection with tendon repair to bone. They used an intraoperative "color test" in which dye was injected into the shoulder joint to indicate the extent of joint side tears. The results were satisfactory in 90% of cases. Itoi and Tabata[182] reported their results in managing 38 shoulders with partial-thickness cuff lesions. The average follow-up period was 4.9 years, and the average age at operation was 52.2 years. Three types of lesions were identified: superficial (12 shoulders), intratendinous (three), and deep surface tears (23). The authors performed full-thickness resection of the cuff including the lesion and repaired the defect with side-to-side suture (13 shoulders), side-to-bone suture (eight), fascial patch grafting (16), or side-to-bone suture with fascial patch grafting (one). The overall results were satisfactory in 31 shoulders (82%). The results were not affected by the tear types, operative methods, or follow-up period.

ARTHROSCOPIC TREATMENT

Andrews and associates[5] presented 36 patients with partial-thickness tears of the supraspinatus portion of the cuff treated with arthroscopic débridement of the rotator cuff defect. No acromioplasty was performed. The average age was 22.5 years, and 64% of the patients were baseball pitchers. Of the 34 patients available for follow-up, 85% had an excellent (26 patients) or good (three patients) result and were able to return to sports. The authors suggested that the débridement may initiate a healing response. Arthroscopy revealed a tear of some part of the glenoid labrum in all patients. Six had partial tears of the long head of the biceps tendon. These observations point to the difficult of deciding which surgical findings are responsible for the patient's symptoms.

Ogilvie-Harris and Wiley[297] reported on arthroscopic treatment of 57 incomplete tears of the rotator cuff with symptoms of impingement. These tears were débrided, and no acromioplasty was performed. One half of the patients improved.

Wiley[439] reported on 33 patients treated arthroscopically for partial tears of the rotator cuff. Only three patients achieved a satisfactory result.

Ellman reported good results from arthroscopic acromioplasty performed in conjunction with arthroscopic débridement of partial-thickness tears of the rotator cuff.[108]

In 1988, Esch and colleagues reported on 34 patients with stage II rotator cuff disease and partial-thickness rotator cuff tears treated with arthroscopic acromioplasty and tear débridement.[110] Twenty-eight patients were satisfied with their results; 16 patients were rated excellent; 10 were good; six were fair; and two were rated as poor.

Gartsman[131] presented 40 patients with partial-thickness rotator cuff tears in a group of 125 patients treated with arthroscopic acromioplasty. Of these partial-thickness tears, 32 involved the articular surface of the supraspinatus tendon and four tears involved the bursal side. Four infraspinatus tears were identified, three of which involved the articular surface. Notably, in these 40 patients, there were 27 cases of labral fraying with six cases of biceps/labral complex detachment, again indicating the difficulty of relating symptoms to surgical findings. Of the 40 patients, 33 (83% satisfactory results) had major improvement in their ratings for pain, activities of daily living, work, and sports, at an average of 28.9 months of postarthroscopic débridement. Two patients, who had an unsatisfactory result, had a second operation: one had an open acromioplasty, and the other had a repair of the rotator cuff with satisfactory results. Of the 30 patients in this group engaged in sports preoperatively, 10 patients returned to those sports at the same level of performance as before the symptoms had started.

Altchek and associates[4] reported four of six good or excellent results in patients with partial-thickness rotator cuff tears treated with arthroscopic acromioplasty and débridement of the rotator cuff defect.

Roye and co-workers[357] presented 38 patients with partial-thickness rotator cuff tears (32 involving the supraspinatus) treated with arthroscopic acromioplasty. A satisfactory result was achieved in 95%.

As part of a larger series, Ryu,[358] reported on 35 patients with partial-thickness rotator cuff tears treated with arthroscopic acromioplasty. Thirty of 35 patients (86%) were rated with excellent or good results (five fair, no poor) at a minimum follow-up of 12 months. Of the group with partial tears, four were found to involve only the articular surface. Three of these four were considered failures.

In 1994, Olsewski and Depew[302] reported on their experience with 61 consecutive patients treated with arthroscopic acromioplasty and débridement of the rotator cuff defect (17 of 21 patients (81%) with a partial-thickness rotator tear rated a satisfactory result (UCLA rating scale). This was identical to the result achieved in 27 patients treated with arthroscopic acromioplasty for rotator cuff "tendinitis" with an intact rotator cuff. As was the case with the series of Roye and associates,[357] the extent of the tear did not statistically affect the result.

From this group of reports it is difficult to define: (1) the indications for surgery, (2) which aspects of the patients' pathologies were responsible for their symptoms, (3) why from 15 to 50% of patients failed to achieve a satisfactory result, and (4) which aspect of the surgery (acromioplasty or débridement) was responsible for improvement after surgery. It seems likely that the patients who benefited from this procedure were able to heal their tendon débridement in a way that stabilized the insertional mechanism, distributing the loads from muscle to bone in a way that prevented disproportionately large loads from being concentrated on the neighboring intact tendon fibers.

AUTHORS' PREFERRED METHOD OF TREATING PARTIAL-THICKNESS CUFF LESIONS

Nonoperative Treatment

The nonoperative management of partial-thickness cuff tears is similar to that for subacromial abrasion described earlier in this chapter. Just as with partial lesions of the Achilles, patellar, or extensor radialis brevis tendons, the program must emphasize stretching against all directions of tightness, including internal rotation (see Fig. 15–85), cross-body adduction (see Fig. 15–86), elevation (see Figs. 15–81 and 15–82), and occasionally external rotation (see Fig. 15–83). As in a tennis elbow rehabilitation program, when a comfortable normal range of passive motion is re-established, gentle progressive muscle strengthening is instituted (see Figs. 15–87 and 15–88). An emphasis is always placed on gentle and comfortable progress of this rehabilitation program. The goal of this program is to ensure that the scar collagen that forms in the defect will become as supple as a normal tendon; otherwise, scar contracture will tend to concentrate the loads of the cuff on the lesion leading to a recurrence and propagation of injury.

Operative Treatment

Open Surgery

Just as is the case for partial Achilles, patellar and extensor carpi radialis brevis tendon lesions, there is no surgical treatment that reliably restores the tendon to its normal condition. Preoperatively, it is important to determine whether the patient's primary problem is due to stiffness or to difficulties upon active muscle contraction so that the procedure can be biased accordingly. On the one hand, sectioning of the fibers that remain intact (e.g., in a tennis elbow release) may worsen the problem of weakness; however, this may be the basis of the arthroscopic débridement advocated by some surgeons for this lesion. On the other hand, excision of the defect and repair would worsen the problem of stiffness.[459] Furthermore, such surgical tightening of involved part of the cuff would cause the area of damage and repair to bear the majority of the load when the cuff muscles contract (reminiscent of the "quadregia" phenomenon in hand surgery). Thus, excision and repair of partial-thickness cuff lesions should include efforts to ensure that the tendon load is distributed evenly at the insertion, by carrying out a repair that is isometric, allowing uniform load distribution, and carrying out a release of the capsule tightened in the repair.[158]

The surgical exposure to the partial-thickness cuff lesion is identical to that described for the management of subacromial roughness (see Fig. 15–1). If symptoms are related to subacromial abrasion (i.e., symptomatic subacromial crepitance), subacromial smoothing is performed as described previously in this chapter.

The decision to convert a partial-thickness cuff defect to a full-thickness defect and then to repair it is based on the patient's preoperative evaluation and surgical findings (Fig. 15–97). The thickness of the cuff can be determined at surgery by inspection, palpation, and the Fukuda test described earlier. A depth gauge or calibrated nerve hook inserted in the area of the lesion may help to determine the percentage of the tendon that remains intact. If the decision is made to perform an open repair, a tenotomy is performed in the most suspicious area along the line of the tendon fibers to explore the full-thickness of the tissue. If, as is usually the case, the defect is within the substance of the tendon or on its deep surface near the anterior insertion of the supraspinatus, a longitudinal tenotomy and capsulotomy are performed along the anterior aspect of the supraspinatus near the rotator interval. This cut is then extended at right angles posteriorly through the partially detached cuff at its insertion to the greater tuberosity, turning back the flap of cuff until normal tendon of full thickness is encountered. Next an attempt is made to retrieve and consolidate any split laminations of cuff that may have retracted medially (see Fig. 15–97). These are usually on the deep articular

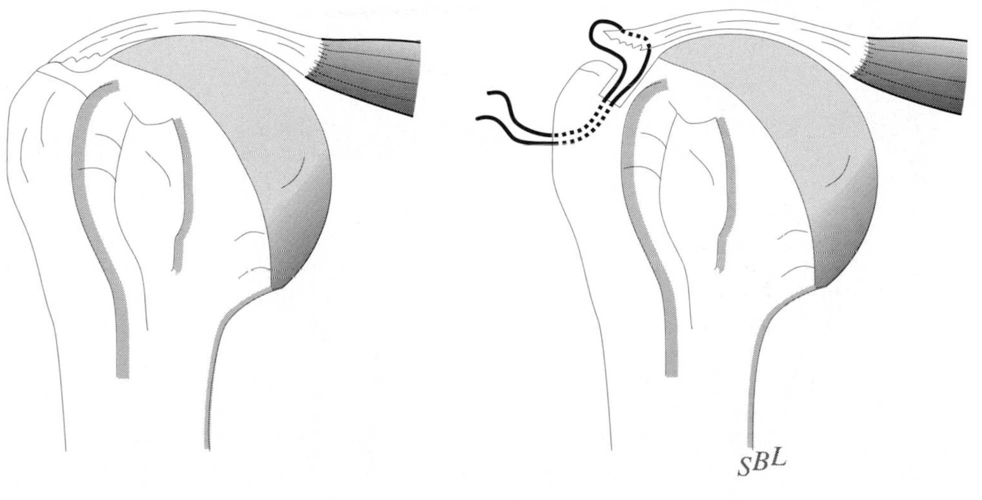

Figure 15–97

Repair of a partial-thickness defect by converting it to a full-thickness defect and gathering the medially retracted deep fibers with suture. (Modified from Matsen FA III, Lippitt SB, Sidles JA, and Harryman DT II: Practical Evaluation and Management of the Shoulder. Philadelphia: WB Saunders, 1994.)

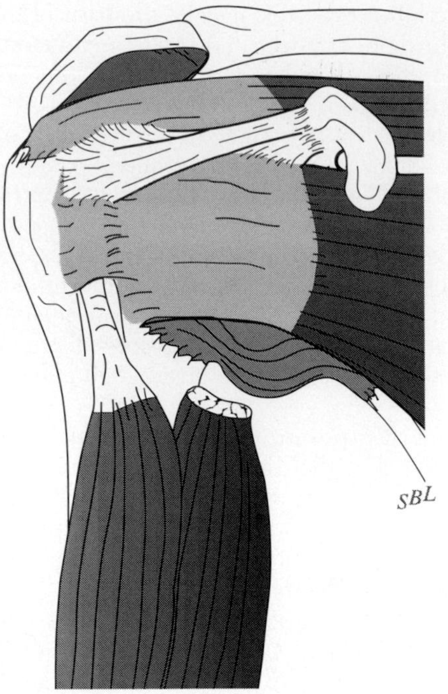

Figure 15–98

The rotator interval capsule–coracohumeral ligament complex lies between the coracoid process, the bicipital groove, the subscapularis tendon, and the supraspinatus tendon. This is not a separate structure but rather a particular area of the glenohumeral capsule. Tightness of this structure can limit external rotation of the adducted arm, adduction, and humeral elevation in anterior and posterior scapular planes. (From Matsen FA III, Lippitt SB, Sidles JA, and Harryman DT II: Practical Evaluation and Management of the Shoulder. Philadelphia: WB Saunders, 1994.)

surface where the cuff lesion begins and may have retracted up to 1 cm. Release of the coracohumeral ligament and the rotator interval capsule from the base of the coracoid (Figs. 15–98 and 15–99) as well as release of the capsule from the glenoid lip (Fig. 15–100) will minimize tension on the repair. The full-thickness defect is then repaired with care to render the cuff insertion isometric with respect to all its fibers and smooth on its superior surface (Figs. 15–101 and 15–102). Finally, with the anterior undersurface of the acromion in full view, the shoulder is put through a full range of motion to verify the elimination of any subacromial abrasion and to ensure that the repair has not restricted shoulder motion (see Fig. 15–59).

Postoperative management is the same as for the repair of full-thickness defects with a particular emphasis on continuous passive motion (see Fig. 15–96) and on the early restitution of a full range of motion to prevent stiffness and adhesions (see Figs. 15–81 to 15–86).

Full-Thickness Cuff Tear

Characteristically, full-thickness cuff tears present as pain or weakness on resisted isometric contraction of one or more of the cuff muscles. A full-thickness defect of one or more of the cuff tendons can be demonstrated on ultrasonography, arthrography, MRI, arthroscopy, or open surgery.

While the diagnosis is not difficult, several key factors must be considered when selecting the appropriate treatment for cuff defects. Some defects cannot be repaired, because as McLaughlin pointed out they offer only "rotten cloth to sew."[247–249, 251] The recognition that full-thickness cuff tears may exist without clinical symptoms cautions that cuff defects need not be repaired just because they are there.[157, 244, 263, 323, 372]

NONOPERATIVE TREATMENT

Substantial data are available on the results of nonoperative treatment for full-thickness cuff defects. The programs generally include some combination of "compound tincture of time" along with physical therapy, administration of nonsteroidal anti-inflammatory medications, rest,

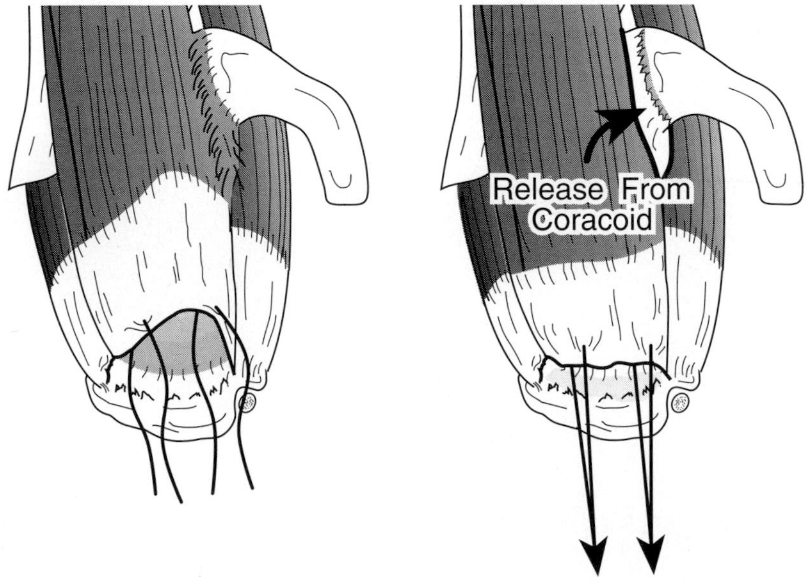

Figure 15–99

Release of the cuff tendons from the coracoid allows their lateral advancement. (Modified from Matsen FA III, Lippitt SB, Sidles JA, and Harryman DT II: Practical Evaluation and Management of the Shoulder. Philadelphia: WB Saunders, 1994.)

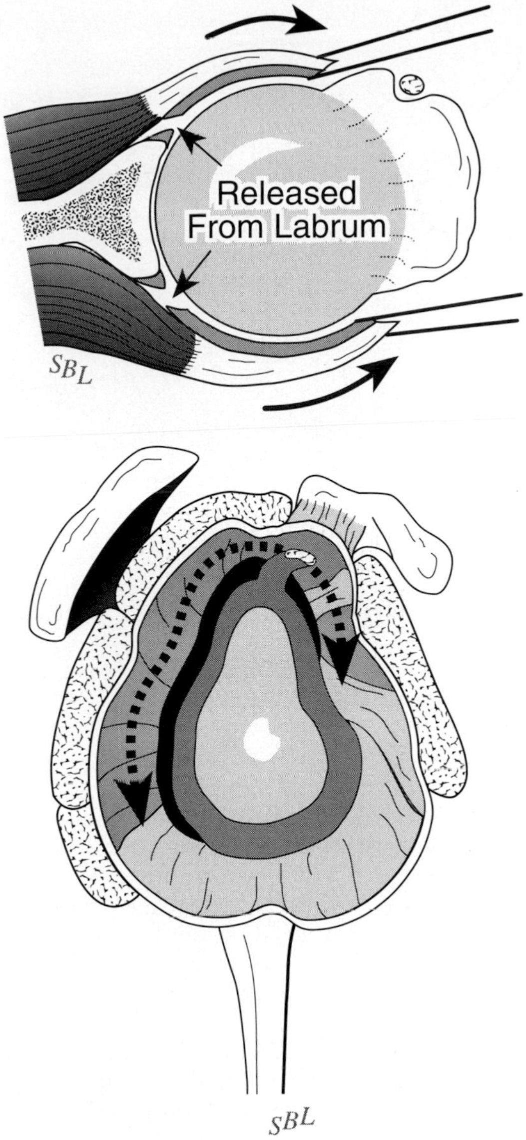

Figure 15–100

Release of the capsule from the labrum allows further lateral advancement. (Modified from Matsen FA III, Lippitt SB, Sidles JA, and Harryman DT II: Practical Evaluation and Management of the Shoulder. Philadelphia: WB Saunders, 1994.)

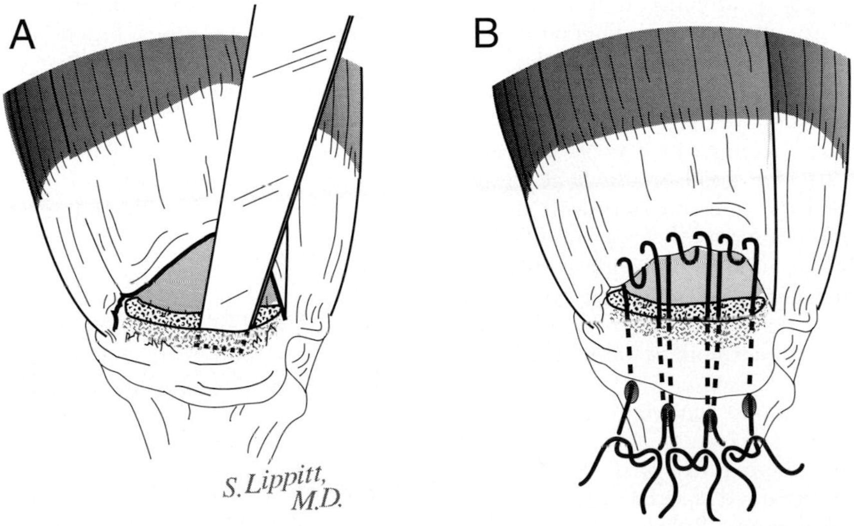

Figure 15–101

A, A groove is created in the sulcus just lateral to the articular surface. *B*, Sutures draw the tendon edge into this groove. (Modified from Matsen FA III, Lippitt SB, Sidles JA, and Harryman DT II: Practical Evaluation and Management of the Shoulder. Philadelphia: WB Saunders, 1994.)

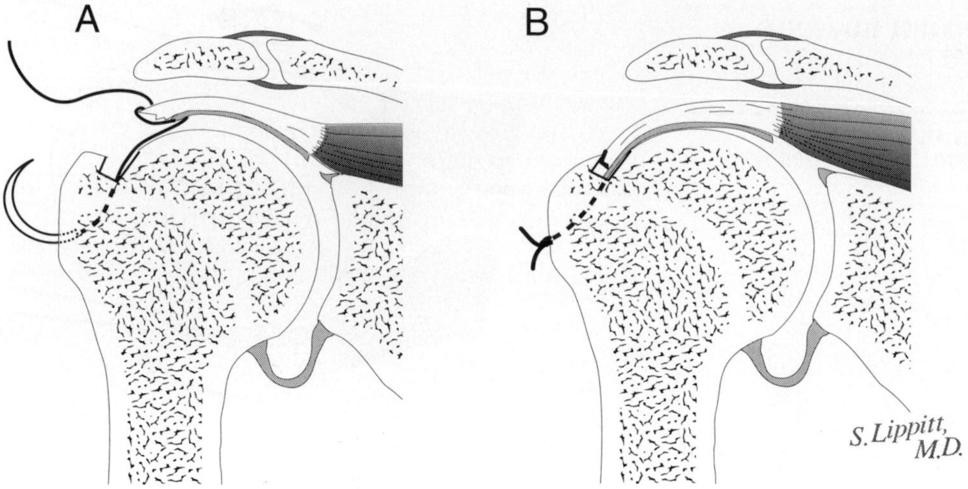

Figure 15–102

The sutures are placed low on the tuberosity *(A)* and tied laterally *(B)* to leave a smooth upper surface for the cuff insertion. The bony eminence above the groove is smoothed as necessary. (Modified from Matsen FA III, Lippitt SB, Sidles JA, and Harryman DT II: Practical Evaluation and Management of the Shoulder. Philadelphia: WB Saunders, 1994.)

avoidance of precipitating activities, and steroid injections.

Improvement with nonoperative management was noted to be 33% in Wolfgang's series,[444] 44% in Takagishi's series,[396] 59% in Samilson and Binder's series,[363] and 90% in Brown's series.[41]

Steroid injections do not seem to be a major enhancement to the nonoperative management program. Although Weiss[436] presented some evidence that patients with arthrographically proven cuff tears are symptomatically improved by intra-articular injections, there is little evidence for a protracted benefit from this method. Other observers found that steroid injections offered no benefit to patients with cuff tears. Coomes and Darlington,[75, 85] Lee and colleagues,[216] and Connolly[74] compared steroid and local anesthetic injections in patients with tendinitis and tendon tears. They found a small subjective benefit in relief of pain but no effect on function in the steroid-treated group.

There has been a recent resurgence of reports confirming the value of nonoperative management for chronic cuff tears. Bartolozzi and associates[13] studied the factors predictive of outcome in 136 patients with cuff disease who were treated nonoperatively. The mean follow-up time was 20 months (range of 6 to 41 months). The authors found 66 to 75% good or excellent results with indication that the clinical result improved significantly as follow-up duration increased. Prognostic factors that were associated with an unfavorable clinical outcome included a rotator cuff tear over 1 cm^2, a history of pretreatment clinical symptoms for longer than 1 year, and significant functional impairment at initial presentation.

Hawkins and Dunlop[161] found that more than half of the patients with full-thickness cuff tears who were treated with a supervised nonoperative program of rotator strengthening exercises obtained satisfactory results at an average of 4 years' follow-up. Bokor and associates[32] managed 53 patients (average age of 62 years) with full-thickness cuff tears documented arthroscopically using a program of nonsteroidal medications, stretching, strengthening, and occasional steroid injections. At an average of 7.6 years later, 39 of the 53 patients (74%) had only slight or no shoulder discomfort. Of the 28 shoulders presenting within 3 months of injury, 24 (86%) were rated as satisfactory at the time of latest evaluation. Of the 16 patients who initially had had shoulder pain for more than 6 months, only nine (56%) were rated as satisfactory. Most patients showed improvement with regard to their ability to perform activities of daily living. Average active total elevation was 149 degrees compared with 121 degrees at initial presentation. Thirty-two of the 34 patients examined (94%) had evidence of weakness on muscle testing, and 19 (56%) had demonstrable muscle atrophy.

Itoi and Tabata[181] followed 62 shoulders with complete rotator cuff tears that were treated conservatively from 1980 until 1989. The average follow-up period was 3.4 years. Fifty-one shoulders (82%) rated satisfactory. The overall scores of pain, motion, and function improved significantly. The authors concluded that conservative treatment affords satisfactory results when it is given to the patients with well-preserved motion and strength, although in some cases function may deteriorate with time.

In our own practice we have follow-up data on 56 patients (23 female, 33 male) with full-thickness cuff tears managed nonoperatively. The average age was 61 ± 10 years (range of 45 to 84 years), and the mean follow-up time was 25 months. The initial and final responses to the questions of the SST are shown in Table 15–2 and Figure 15–103.

Taken together, these results clearly offer encouragement for a trial of nonoperative management for chronic full-thickness cuff tears, particularly in cases where the prospect of achieving a durable cuff repair appears doubtful.

OPERATIVE TREATMENT

Cuff Repair

Patient Selection

Substantial information bearing on the potential reparability of a rotator cuff defect can be obtained from the

Table 15–2 EFFECTIVENESS OF NONOPERATIVE MANAGEMENT OF FULL-THICKNESS CUFF TEARS (56 PATIENTS WITH AN AVERAGE FOLLOW-UP OF 25 MONTHS)

FUNCTION	*% ABLE INITIALLY*	*% ABLE AT FOLLOW-UP*
Sleep on side	27	48
Arm comfortable at side	57	80
Wash back of opposite shoulder	36	41
Place hand behind head	52	65
Tuck in shirt	57	70
Place 8 lb on shelf	7	22
Place 1 lb on shelf	45	56
Place coin on shelf	63	69
Toss overhand	9	19
Do usual work	38	50
Toss underhand	46	57
Carry 20 lb	45	54

history along with the physical examination and plain radiographs (Table 15–3). Acute tears in younger, healthy individuals without prior shoulder disease are more likely to be repairable. Long-standing tears associated with major weakness in older patients carry a poorer prognosis. The prognosis for a durable repair is even worse if the history reveals the administration of local or systemic steroids, smoking, or difficulties in healing previous injuries or surgeries.

These guidelines are derived from our experience but are also supported by the literature. Postacchini and associates[332] found in a study of 73 cuff repairs, that whereas 73% of the cases had satisfactory results, rotator cuff repair is almost always successful in patients with more than 60 degrees of active arm flexion and either small- or medium-sized tears. Less than two thirds of the patients with major tears and less than 60 degrees of motion achieved satisfactory results, particularly if there was cuff muscle atrophy.

Watson[430] reviewed the surgical findings in 89 patients with major ruptures of the cuff. He found that all seven patients who had had no local steroid injections had strong residual cuff tissue. Thirteen of 62 patients who had one to four steroid injections had soft cuff tissue that held suture poorly; 17 of the 20 patients who had more than four steroid injections had very weak cuff tissue; these shoulders with weak cuff tissue had poorer results after surgical repair.

Misamore and colleagues[265] evaluated 107 consecutive cuff repairs, including 24 patients on workers' compensation and 79 who were not. Although other factors such as the age and sex of the patients, the size of the tear of the rotator cuff, and the preoperative strength, pain, and active range of motion of the shoulder were comparable, only 54% of the shoulders covered by workers' compensation were rated good or excellent, compared with 92% who were not. Forty-two per cent of the patients on workers' compensation returned to full activity, compared with 94% who were not.

Samilson and Binder listed the following most reasonable indications for operative repair of nonacute cuff tears[363]: (1) a patient "physiologically" younger than 60 years, (2) clinically or arthrographically demonstrable full-thickness cuff tear, (3) failure of patient to improve under nonoperative management for a period not less than 6 weeks, (4) patient's need to use the involved shoulder in overhead elevation in his or her vocation or avocation, (5) full passive range of shoulder motion, (6) patient's willingness to exchange decreased pain and increased external rotator strength for some loss of active abduction, and (7) ability and willingness of the patient to cooperate.

Grana and associates[147] reviewed their experience with

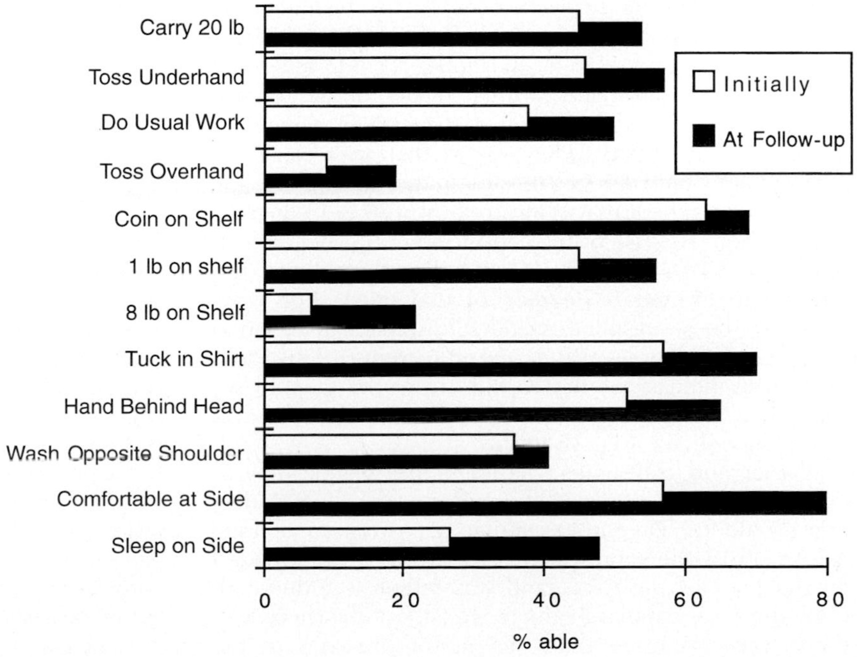

Figure 15–103

Effectiveness of nonoperative management of full-thickness cuff tears (56 patients with an average follow-up time of 25 months).

Table 15–3 PROGNOSTIC FACTORS RELATED TO THE DURABILITY OF ROTATOR CUFF REPAIR

ENCOURAGING	DISCOURAGING
History	
Age less than 55	Age over 65
Acute traumatic onset	Insidious atraumatic onset
No relation to work	Attribution of tear to work
Short duration of weakness	Weakness over 6 months
No history of smoking	Many smoking pack-years
No steroid injections	Repeated steroid injections
No major medications	Systemic steroids or antimetabolites
No concurrent disease	Inflammatory joint disease; other chronic illnesses
No infections	History of previous shoulder infection
No previous shoulder surgery	Previous cuff repair attempts
Benign surgical history	History of failed soft tissue repairs (e.g., dehiscence, infections complicating herniorrhaphy)
Physical Examination	
Good nutrition	Poor nutrition
Mild to moderate weakness	Severe weakness
No spinatus atrophy	Severe spinatus atrophy
Stable shoulder	Anterior superior instability
Intact acromion	Previous acromial resection
No stiffness	Stiffness
X-Rays	
Normal radiographs	Upwards displacement of head against the coracoacromial arch; cuff tear arthropathy

54 patients having open repair of chronic cuff tears. They concluded that pre-repair arthroscopic evaluation did not affect the functional outcome but did increase the cost by about $2000 per patient.

Laboratory Studies on Repair Techniques

Gerber and associates[138] studied the mechanical properties of several techniques of tendon-to-bone suture employed in rotator cuff repair in cadavers. Two simple stitches failed at 184 N; four simple stitches failed at 208 N. Two Mason-Allen stitches failed at 359 N. These results indicate that in addition to the quality of the bone and the quality of the cuff tissue, the number of sutures, and the suture technique affect the load to failure.

A most important study bearing on the technique of cuff repair was published by Zuckerman and associates.[459] These authors used a cadaver model to determine the effect of arm position and capsular release on the tension in the repaired tendon as reflected by strain gauges on the greater tuberosity. They found that with repair of supraspinatus-only defects, tension in the repair increased significantly as the arm was lowered from 30 to 15 degrees of abduction. Release of the capsule from the glenoid rim (see Figs. 15–99 and 15–100) significantly reduced the tension at 15 and 0 degrees of abduction. For tears involving the supraspinatus and infraspinatus, abduction of at least 30 degrees was required to reduce tension in the repair. Release of the capsule from the glenoid resulted in a 30% reduction in repair tension when the arm was adducted (see Fig. 15–100).

Warner and colleagues[427] studied the relationships of the suprascapular nerve to the cuff muscles in 31 cadaveric shoulders. The suprascapular nerve ran an oblique course across the supraspinatus fossa, was relatively fixed on the floor of the fossa, and was tethered underneath the transverse scapular ligament. In 84% of the shoulders, there were no more than two motor branches to the supraspinatus muscle, and the first was always the larger of the two. In 84, the first motor branch originated underneath the transverse scapular ligament or very near it. In one shoulder (3%), the first motor branch passed over the ligament. The average distance from the origin of the long tendon of the biceps to the motor branches of the supraspinatus was 3 cm. In 48%, the infraspinatus muscle had three or four motor branches of the same size. The average distance from the posterior rim of the glenoid to the motor branches of the infraspinatus muscle was 2 cm. The motor branches to the supraspinatus muscle were fewer, usually smaller, and significantly shorter than those to the infraspinatus muscle. The standard anterosuperior approach allowed only 1 cm of lateral advancement of either tendon and limited the ability of the surgeon to dissect safely beyond the neurovascular pedicle. The advancement technique of Debeyre and associates, or a modification of that technique, permitted lateral advancement of each muscle of as much as 3 cm and was limited by tension in the motor branches of the suprascapular nerve. In some situations, the safe limit of advancement may be even less. The authors concluded that lateral advancement of the rotator cuff is limited anatomically and may place the neurovascular structures at risk.

Surgical Approaches

The surgical approaches to the complete cuff tear vary substantially. These include a saber cut,[60] an anterior approach through the acromioclavicular joint,[16] a posterior approach,[86] and an "extensile" approach.[152] Many authors prefer the anterior acromioplasty approach, taking care to preserve the deltoid attachment and acromial lever arm.[65, 67, 275, 281] This technique provides excellent exposure of the common sites of lesions—the anterior cuff, biceps groove, undersurface of the acromion, and acromioclavicular joint.

Packer and co-workers,[309] reporting on 63 cuff repairs

followed for an average of 32.7 months, found that those performed with acromioplasty yielded more pain relief than did cuff repair without acromioplasty. If greater access to the supraspinatus is needed, the acromioclavicular joint can be excised.[277] Debeyre and associates[86] described a posterior approach with acromial osteotomy. Ha'eri and Wiley described an approach that is extensile through the acromioclavicular joint to the supraspinous fossa.[152]

Repair Methods

Operative techniques for repairing full-thickness cuff defects include tendon-to-tendon repair and tendon advancement to bone. McLaughlin[247–251] described his approaches to transverse ruptures (reinsertion into bone), longitudinal rents (side-to-side repair), and tears with retraction (side-to-side repair followed by reinsertion of the retracted portion of cuff into the head wherever it will reach with ease with the arm at the side). Although many of his principles are still applied today, most authors would not concur with his use of the transacromial approach or his belief that "distinct benefits are gained by excising and discarding the outer fragment of the divided acromion."[247, 249] Hawkins and colleagues used side-to-side repair for small tears and tendon-to-bone repair for larger defects.[165] Cofield has emphasized the identification of the tear pattern and the use of direct repair and flaps as indicated by the tear pattern.[66, 67] Nobuhara and associates[293] reviewed, at an average of 7 years, 187 patients (189 shoulders) treated surgically for massive rotator cuff tears using either a tendon-to-tendon repair or the McLaughlin procedure. Ninety-five per cent of the patients were 45 years or older. Excellent or good functional results were attained in 93% of patients. Thirty-three per cent of those who underwent tendon to tendon repair had pain after overuse compared with only 18% who had the McLaughlin procedure.

Several authors have described extensive tendon mobilization or advancement of major tendon flaps to repair large defects. Cofield recommended the transposition of the subscapularis for repair of large cuff defects.[66] In this technique the subscapularis and the anterosuperior capsule are freed from the anteroinferior capsule, leaving the middle and inferior glenohumeral ligaments intact. The tendon is then transferred superiorly to the anterior aspect of the greater tuberosity. Most patients required postoperative protection in an abduction splint or cast for 4 to 5 weeks. These patients, who had severe symptoms of pain and limitation of function preoperatively, had less pain and slight improvement in active motion; 12 of 26 patients gained more than 30 degrees of active abduction, and four lost this amount of motion. Two patients disrupted their repair during the acute postoperative period. Of the 26, 25 were satisfied with the procedure.

Karas and Giachello[195] reported their results with 20 patients treated with acromioplasty and subscapularis transfer for massive (>5 cm) tears of the cuff in which direct tendon to bone reconstruction could not be achieved. At a mean of 30 months after surgery, 17 patients were satisfied. Nine had weakness and discomfort with overhead activities, and two had lost active elevation despite relief of pain. The authors found that this procedure was useful when "traditional" methods of repair were insufficient, but cautioned against its use when patients had full functional elevation preoperatively.

In fewer than 5% of his cuff repairs, Neer[277] shifted the infraspinatus and upper half of the subscapularis superiorly to close a defect in the supraspinatus, leaving the lower half of the subscapularis, the teres minor, and the intervening capsule intact. He described the use of a second incision posteriorly for better mobilization of the infraspinatus toward the top of the greater tuberosity. Neviaser and Neviaser[287] described the transposition of both the subscapularis and the teres minor to close the defect. Debeyre and colleagues and others described the use of a supraspinatus muscle slide to help close major cuff defects.[86, 152, 153] Ha'eri and Wiley[153] used the supraspinatus advancement technique of Debeyre; most of their 18 patients achieved satisfactory results.

Latissimus transfers as described for Erb's palsy[324] have been used to manage large cuff defects. Gerber[137] reported on 16 irreparable, massive rotator cuff tears treated with latissimus dorsi transfer and reviewed after an average of 33 months. Pain relief was satisfactory in 94% of the shoulders at rest and in 81% on exertion. Flexion was 83 degrees preoperatively and 135 degrees postoperatively. If the subscapularis was torn and could not be adequately repaired, a latissimus dorsi transfer was of no value. In cases with good subscapularis function but irreparable defects in the external rotator tendons, restoration of approximately 80% of normal shoulder function was obtained.

A flap of deltoid has been used to cover cuff defects. Thur and Julke[400] analyzed the results of shoulder reconstruction using an anterolateral deltoid muscle flap plasty in 100 patients with rotator cuff lesions that were at least 5 × 5 cm. Ninety per cent of patients were satisfied. Shoulder function improved significantly, and 72% recovered their strength completely. Most of the patients were able to work after 6 months. The overall result was good to very good in 83%.

Dierickx and Vanhoof[96] reviewed 20 patients with a painful massive, irreparable rotator cuff tear treated with an open partial acromionectomy and an anterior deltoid muscle inlay flap. After follow-up averaging 12 months, 17 of 20 patients were satisfied, and the UCLA score improved from an average of 9.35 to an average of 25.7 Active forward flexion improved in 17, and strength of forward flexion improved in 15 patients.

As an alternative approach to surgery for massive tears, Burkhart and associates[46] repaired the margins of the tear to restore force transmission, believing that complete coverage of the defect was not essential. In 14 patients, this procedure led to improvement in active elevation from 59.6 to 150.4 degrees. Strength improved an average of 2.3 grades on a 0- to 5-point scale. The average score on the UCLA Shoulder Rating Scale improved from a preoperative value of 9.8 to a postoperative value of 27.6. All except one patient was very satisfied with the result.

Some authors have used biologic and prosthetic grafts to repair large cuff defects. Neviaser,[284] Bush,[49] and McLaughlin and Asherman[251] employed grafts from the long head tendon of the biceps to patch cuff defects. Ting and co-workers[403] found that the electromyographic activity and size of the long head tendon of the biceps is significantly greater in patients with cuff tears compared with the uninjured shoulder. Their study suggests that the long head of the biceps may be a greater contributor to abduction and flexion in the shoulder with cuff tear than in the normal shoulder and that sacrificing the intracapsular portion of the tendon for grafting material may not be advisable. Heikel[169] used fascia lata to close cuff defects, and both Heikel and Bateman described the use of the coracoacromial ligament. A freeze-dried rotator cuff has been used by Neviaser and co-workers.[285] In this report, 16 patients with massive tears had cadaver grafts, producing decrease in nocturnal pain in all 16. The change in shoulder function and strength was not reported. Post reported on preliminary results in five patients in whom a carbon fiber prosthesis was used to manage massive cuff deficiencies.[328] Three had excellent to good results and two failed, one because of possible infection. The author stated that these results are no better than with conventional repairs. Finally, synthetic cuff prostheses have been used by Ozaki and colleagues[305] and by Post.[328] The former found that of 168 shoulders with cuff tears (almost all of which were "chronic" and "massive"), 25 could not be repaired by standard surgical techniques. Their defects were typically 6 × 5 cm. These patients had cuff reconstruction with Teflon fabric, Teflon felt, or Marlex mesh. This procedure was followed by a structured postoperative program, including the use of an abduction orthosis to keep the arm elevated in the plane of the scapula for 2 to 3 months and continued rehabilitation for 3 to 6 months. At an average of 2.1 years' follow-up, 23 of 25 patients gained 120 to 160 degrees of abduction (the other two having had axillary nerve injury). Whereas 20 had reported continual or intolerable pain preoperatively, pain was absent in 23 patients at follow-up. The authors found that results were better with the thicker felt and now recommend the use of 3- to 5-mm–thick Teflon felt in patients with massive defects.

Some authors recommend postoperative immobilization in an abduction splint,[11, 16, 86, 169] whereas others advise against this.[249, 292]

Results of Treatment

Neer and co-workers[280] reported the results of 233 primary cuff repairs with an average follow-up of 4.6 years. Results were excellent (essentially normal) in 77%, satisfactory in 14%, and unsatisfactory in 9%. The unsatisfactory ratings were usually due to lack of strength rather than pain and usually occurred in patients with longstanding, neglected tears. Hawkins and co-workers found that 86% of their patients had relief of pain after repair.[165] Recovery of strength was more common in patients with smaller tears.[165] In other series, pain relief was reported in 58%,[321] 60%,[169] 66%,[86] 74%,[141] and 85%.[363]

Gore and associates[144] reviewed the results from 63 primary cuff repairs with an average of 5.5 years' follow-up. The shoulders without a traumatic onset were repaired an average of 32 months after the onset of symptoms, whereas those with a traumatic onset were repaired an average of 6 months after the traumatic episode. The surgical approach and technique varied somewhat but usually consisted of acromioplasty and tendon repair to bone or to adjacent tendon. Six shoulders had biceps tendon grafts. Most shoulders were immobilized at the side for 4 to 6 weeks, but 12 had immobilization in abduction. Subjective improvement was seen in 95% of shoulders with repaired cuffs. Flexion averaged 126 degrees actively and 147 degrees passively. Most patients had marked relief of pain and minimal or no problems with activities of daily living. Patients with tears less than 2.5 cm long had better results than did those with larger tears. The superior result with repair of smaller tears is consistent with the observations of Godsil and Linscheid[141] and Post and co-workers.[331] Watson[430] found that results were worse in patients with larger cuff defects, with multiple preoperative steroid injections, and with preoperative weakness of the deltoid. Ellman and colleagues[106] reported a 3.5-year follow-up of 50 patients who had rotator cuff repair. Techniques of repair included tendon-to-tendon suture, reimplantation into bone, grafts, and tendon flaps. Comfort and function were usually improved by these procedures. Their report provided additional support for timely repair: patients with symptoms of longer standing had larger tears and more difficult repairs. Shoulders with grade 3 or less strength of abduction before surgery had poorer results; those with an acromiohumeral interval of 7 mm or less also had poorer results. Arthrography was not consistently accurate in estimating the size of the tear.

Hawkins found that acromioplasty and cuff repair relieved pain and restored the ability to sleep on the affected side in most patients. Seventy-eight per cent were able to use the arm above shoulder level after surgery, whereas only 16% were able to do so before surgery. Hawkins and co-workers[165] found that the results of cuff repair were worse in patients on Workmen's Compensation. Only two of 14 patients unable to work because of cuff tears could return to work after surgery, whereas eight of nine patients not on Workmen's Compensation did return to work after operation. Other series of cuff repairs include those of Codman,[62] Moseley,[269] Neviaser,[284] Wolfgang,[444] Bakalim and Pasila,[11] Bassett and Cofield,[15] Earnshaw and co-workers,[102] Packer and associates,[309] Post and colleagues,[331] Samilson and Binder,[363] and Weiner and Macnab.[434] Cofield[67] averaged the results of many reports in the literature and found that pain relief occurred in 87% (range of 71 to 100%), and patient satisfaction averaged 77% (range of 72 to 82%). The reader is encouraged to compare and contrast these results with those following nonoperative treatment that was described earlier.

Some reports have focused on the results of acute repairs. Bakalim and Pasila reviewed their series of 55 patients with arthrographically verified rupture of the cuff tendons treated surgically.[11] Whereas only half of the workers were able to return to their previous work, all workers operated upon within 1 month of a traumatic rupture of the cuff were able to return to their jobs. Bassett and Cofield[15] presented a series of 37 patients having surgical repair within 3 months of cuff rupture. At an average follow-up of 7 years, active abduction averaged 168 degrees for those who had repair within 3 weeks and 129 degrees for those who had repair within 6 to 12 weeks after injury. Patients with small tears averaged 148 degrees, and those with large tears averaged 133 degrees of elevation. The authors concluded that surgical repair

Table 15–4 RECOVERY OF TORQUE AFTER CUFF REPAIR*

	FLEXION	ABDUCTION	EXTERNAL ROTATION
Preoperative	54	45	64
6 Months	78	80	79
12 Months	84	90	91

*From Rokito AS, Zuckerman JD, Gallagher MA, and Cuomo F: Strength after surgical repair of the rotator cuff. J Shoulder Elbow Surg *5*:12–17, 1996.

must be considered within 3 weeks of injury to obtain maximal return of shoulder function.

The importance of continued postoperative exercises is emphasized by the data of Walker and associates,[423] who measured the isokinetic strength of the shoulder after cuff repair. They found a significant increase in strength between 6 and 12 months after surgery. One year after operation, abduction was 80% of normal and external rotation was 90% of normal. Brems[36] found that the strength of external rotation after cuff repair averaged 20% at 3 months, 38% at 6 months, 57% at 9 months, and 71% at 1 year.

Rokito and co-workers[352] followed at 3-month intervals the isokinetic strength of 42 patients who had repair of full-thickness defects. The torques for the operated shoulder (as a percentage of the opposite uninvolved shoulder) are shown in Table 15–4). Recovery of strength correlated primarily with the size of the tear: for small- and medium-sized tears, the recovery of strength was almost complete during the first year. For large and massive tears, recovery was slower and less consistent. The authors concluded that at least 1 year is required to regain strength after a cuff repair.

Kirschenbaum and associates[206] came up with very similar results in their evaluation of 25 shoulders tested isokinetically with a pain-relieving subacromial lidocaine injection before and after cuff repair (Table 15–5).

The analysis of the results of cuff repair is hampered by lack of a uniform approach to the description of: (1) the shoulder's preoperative functional status, (2) the magnitude and location of the cuff defect, (3) the quality of the tissue available for repair, (4) the anatomic integrity at follow-up, and (5) the postoperative functional status. The need for correlation of anatomic and functional outcomes is demonstrated by the surprisingly good results obtained with débridement for irreparable cuff tears. Neer,[275] Rockwood,[349] and others have reported that in

Table 15–5 RECOVERY OF TORQUE AFTER CUFF REPAIR*

	FLEXION	ABDUCTION	EXTERNAL ROTATION
Preoperative	33	37	36
6 Months	66	68	76
12 Months	97	104	142

*From Kirschenbaum D, Coyle MPJ, Leddy JP, et al: Shoulder strength with rotator cuff tears. Pre- and postoperative analysis. Clin Orthop *288*:174–178, 1993.

certain cases when the cuff cannot be repaired, comfort and function may be improved by débridement of the shreds of residual cuff and subacromial smoothing followed by muscle strengthening and range-of-motion exercises. The realization that patients may have good function and comfort in the presence of major cuff defects makes the definition of "success" after a cuff repair challenging.

Interestingly, there have been few follow-up studies of the relationship of cuff integrity to the quality of the result after cuff surgery. Lundberg[235] followed 21 cuff repairs with arthrography and found leakage in seven cases. The results in the leaking cuffs were not as good as in those with sealed cuffs. Calvert and associates[50] performed double-contrast arthrograms in 20 patients at an average of 30 months after operative repair of a torn cuff. In 17 of 20 shoulders the contrast leaked into the bursa, indicating a cuff defect. These defects were estimated to be small in eight cases, medium in eight cases, and large in two cases. However, 17 patients had complete relief of pain, 15 had a full range of shoulder elevation, and 10 felt that they had regained full function. The authors suggest that a complete closure of the cuff is not essential for a good functional result and that arthrography may not be helpful in the investigation of failure of repair.

Ultrasonography appears to offer a greater potential for evaluating postoperative cuff integrity. Mack and co-workers[239] investigated the accuracy of ultrasonography in this regard. In a group of symptomatic postoperative shoulders that were subsequently reoperated, ultrasonography accurately diagnosed recurrent cuff tears in 25 of 25 cases and correctly confirmed cuff integrity in 10 of 11. Using expert ultrasonography, Harryman[157] correlated the integrity of the cuff with functional status after 105 surgical repairs of chronic rotator cuff tears in 89 patients at an average of 5 years postoperatively. The patients' ages at the time of repair averaged 60 years (range of 32 to 80). The numbers of patients in each age decade were as follows: 30 to 39:1, 40 to 49:16, 50 to 59:31, 60 to 69:42, 70 to 79:14, and 80 to 89:1. Eighty-six (82%) of the shoulders had no prior attempt at repair of the cuff.

In all of the surgeries, an anteroinferior acromioplasty was carried out. The involved tendon or tendons were mobilized as necessary. A bony trough was created in the humerus to reattach the mobilized tendons. The site of reattachment was usually in the sulcus adjacent to the humeral articular surface. In some cases the trough was placed somewhat more medially, if after mobilization the tendons did not reach their original anatomic attachment without undue tension when the arm was at the side. The cuff was protected from active use for 3 months postoperatively.

The status of the cuff at surgery and at follow-up was characterized in terms of the integrity of the different tendons: Type O was a cuff of normally full thickness; type 1A was thinning or a partial-thickness defect of the supraspinatus tendon, type 1B was a full-thickness defect of the supraspinatus; type 2 was a full-thickness two-tendon defect involving the supraspinatus and the infraspinatus; and type 3 was a full-thickness defect involving

Table 15–6 INTEGRITY OF CUFF REPAIRS AT FOLLOW-UP*

				SIZE OF CUFF DEFECT AT FOLLOW-UP EXAMINATION						
SIZE OF DEFECT REPAIRED AT SURGERY (ALL CASES)	*PRIMARY REPAIRS (86)*	*REPEAT REPAIRS (19)*	*TOTAL NO. OF REPAIRS (105)*	*None (0)* 40	*Partial (1A)* 28	*Supraspinatus Tear (1B)* 12	*Supraspinatus and Infraspinatus Tear (2)* 14	*Supraspinatus, Infraspinatus, and Subscapularis Tear (3)* 11	*% INTACT (0 OR 1A) (65)*	*YEARS OF FOLLOW-UP AVERAGE AND RANGE 5 (2–11)*
Partial tears (1A)	5	1	6	4	2	0	0	0	100	2.7 (2–6)
Supraspinatus tears (1B)	39	10	49	23	16	3	5	2	80	5.1 (2–10.5)
Supraspinatus and infraspinatus (2)	25	3	28	7	9	6	5	1	57	5.9 (2–6)
Supraspinatus, infraspinatus, and subscapularis (3)	17	5	22	6	1	3	4	8	32	4.1 (2–11)
Intact at follow-up	60	8	68							

*From Matsen FA III, et al: Practical Evaluation and Management of the Shoulder. Philadelphia: WB Saunders, 1994.

Table 15–7 INFLUENCE OF SIZE OF CUFF DEFECT AT FOLLOW-UP ON ACTIVE RANGE, COMFORT, AND SATISFACTION AT FOLLOW-UP*

		ACTIVE RANGE OF MOTION AT FOLLOW-UP					
SIZE OF CUFF DEFECT AT FOLLOW-UP	NUMBER	Flexion	External Rotation at Side	External Rotation at 90° Abduction	Internal Rotation	TOTAL PAINLESS	TOTAL SATISFIED
None (0)	40	132°	41°	71°	T7	37	39
Partial (1A)	28	124°	38°	68°	T7	21	23
Supraspinatus (1B)	12	107°	34°	63°	T8	8	12
Supraspinatus and infraspinatus (2)	14	109°	25°	48°	T9	10	10
Supraspinatus, infraspinatus, and subscapularis (3)	11	71°	27°	61°	T10	8	10
Total	105					84	94

*From Matsen FA III, et al: Practical Evaluation and Management of the Shoulder. Philadelphia: WB Saunders, 1994.

three tendons: the supraspinatus, the infraspinatus, and the subscapularis.

The results are summarized in Table 15–6. No patient who had a partial-thickness tear repaired had a full-thickness retear. In 80% of shoulders with repaired full-thickness supraspinatus tears, the cuff was found to be intact (no full-thickness defect) at follow-up. Only 57% of cuffs that had tears involving both the supraspinatus and infraspinatus were intact at an average follow-up of 6 years. Less than one third of the cuffs that had tears involving all three major tendons were intact after repair at an average of 4 years of follow-up.

Patients were generally satisfied with the results of surgery, even when expert sonography showed that the cuff was no longer intact (Table 15–7). Shoulders with intact repairs (no full-thickness defect) at follow-up had the greatest range of active flexion (129 ± 20 degrees) compared with those with large recurrent defects (71 ± 41 degrees) (Fig. 15–104). Shoulders with intact repairs also demonstrated the best function in activities of daily living. Where the cuff was not intact, the degree of functional loss was related to the size of the recurrent defect (Fig. 15–105).

Although the chances of having an intact repair at follow-up was less for those with large tears, patients with intact repairs of large tears had just as good function as did those with intact repairs of small tears. Similarly, there was an overall greater incidence of recurrent defects in shoulders with repeat repairs, yet shoulders with intact cuffs after repeat repairs functioned as well as did those with intact primary repairs (Fig. 15–106).

From this study it can be concluded that: (1) the integrity of the rotator cuff at follow-up (and not the size of the tear at the time of repair) is a major determinant of the functional outcome of surgical repair, (2) the chances of the repair of a large tear remaining intact, however, are not as good as those for a small tear, and (3) older patients tended to have larger tears and to have a higher incidence of recurrent defects (Table 15–8).

In very comparable study, Gazielly and associates[133–135] examined the anatomic condition by ultrasonography and the function of the rotator cuff at 4 years after surgical repair in a series of 100 full-thickness rotator cuff tears. The series comprised 98 patients, (62 men and 36 women) whose average age was 56 years. Sixty-nine tears were less than 2 cm in size (39 cases) or between 2 and 4 cm (3 cases) of the supraspinatus, 22 tears of the supraspinatus and infraspinatus measuring between 2 and 4 cm, and nine massive tears. All 98 patients were operated on by the same surgeon using the same repair technique. Ultrasonography revealed intact cuffs in 65%, thinned cuffs in 11%, and recurrent full-thickness tears in 24% of cases. The risk of a recurrent tear increased with the extent of the tear to be repaired (57%), in older patients (25%) and with a higher level of postsurgical occupational use (18%). At follow-up, they noted a close

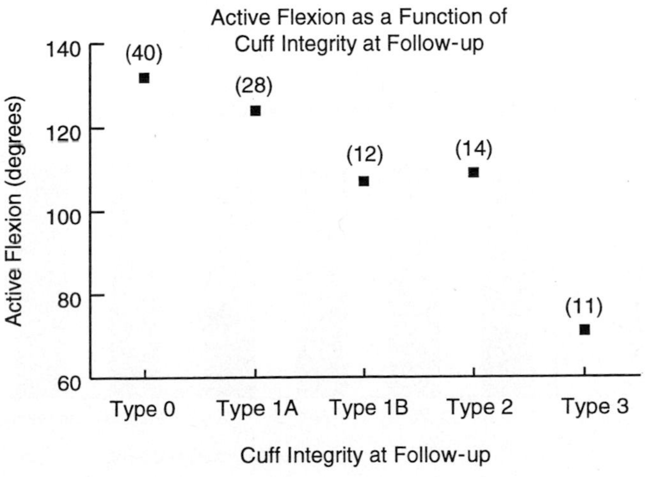

Figure 15–104

Active flexion after cuff repair as a function of cuff integrity at follow-up. The numbers of shoulders are in parentheses. Type O represents a cuff of normally full thickness; type 1A is thinning or partial-thickness lesions of the cuff; type 1B is a full-thickness cuff defect of the supraspinatus. Type 2 is a full-thickness defect of the supra- and infraspinatus. Type 3 is a full-thickness defect of the subscapularis, supraspinatus, and infraspinatus. (From Matsen FA III, Lippitt SB, Sidles JA, and Harryman DT II: Practical Evaluation and Management of the Shoulder. Philadelphia: WB Saunders, 1994.)

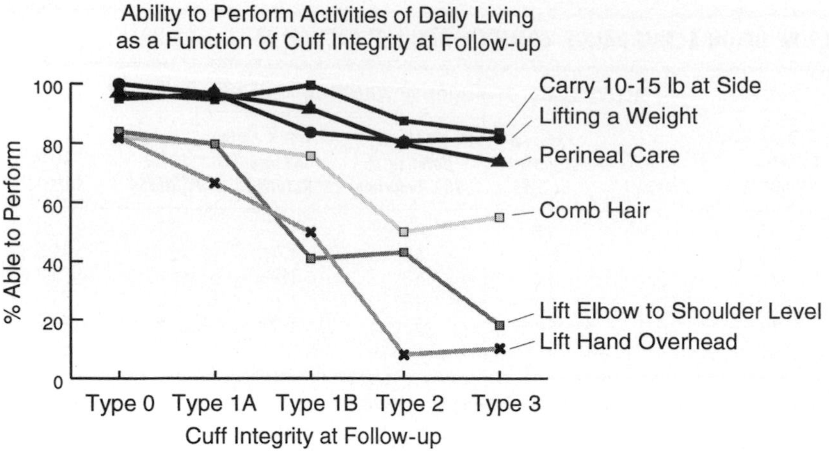

Figure 15–105

The ability to perform activities of daily living as a function of cuff integrity at follow-up. The ordinate indicates the percentage of shoulders that were functional enough for the patient to perform the activity. (From Matsen FA III, Lippitt SB, Sidles JA, and Harryman DT II: Practical Evaluation and Management of the Shoulder. Philadelphia: WB Saunders, 1994.)

correlation between the anatomic condition of the cuff by ultrasound and Constant's functional score.

Similar results have been reported by Cammerer and associates[51] and Bellumore and co-workers.[21]

Wulker and associates[449] followed 97 of 116 shoulders operated on for rotator cuff lesions after an average follow-up time of 37 months. Seventy per cent had a good or excellent clinical result; however, an ultrasonographic examination revealed that only 37 had a normal rotator cuff, 31 had thinning or hyperdensity, and 29 had a complete rupture of the cuff. The authors concluded that rotator cuff tears should be closed only if this can be achieved without undue tension and without extensive tissue mobilization or coverage, otherwise they recommended that the lesion should be débrided and left open, and only an anterior acromioplasty should be performed.

Taken together these studies provide strong evidence that after cuff repair surgery, a high percentage of patients have a satisfactory clinical result despite a recurrence of the cuff defect. Several conclusions are evident: (1) one cannot infer integrity of the repaired cuff from a "good" or "excellent" clinical result, (2) factors other than cuff integrity must contribute to the quality of the clinical result from rotator cuff surgery, and (3) if we are to learn more about the value of cuff repair, analysis of cuff integrity and change in functional status must become essential elements in outcome studies of cuff repair surgery.

Arthroscopically Assisted Repair

Some authors have reported short term follow-up of arthroscopic-assisted rotator cuff repair.[222, 311] These authors have suggested that required components of the repair include an adequate smoothing of the undersurface of the acromion and the acromioclavicular joint; arthroscopic (or open) resection of the distal clavicle in the presence of significant acromioclavicular joint arthrosis; mobilization of the entire rotator cuff with release of adhesions and scar tissue; and repair of strong tendon to a properly placed, well-prepared, bleeding bone trough.

The rotator cuff repair is often performed through a lateral deltoid muscle–splitting incision. The deltoid is not detached from the acromion. The deltoid muscle is split with blunt dissection with careful attention to the axillary nerve, which crosses on the deep surface of the deltoid as close as 5 cm to the lateral edge of the acromion. A bony trough is developed in the greater tuberosity. Reapposition of the torn cuff edge to the greater tuberosity is accomplished with nonabsorbable sutures passed through drill holes and tied over bone.

Alternative methods for arthroscopically assisted cuff repair include the percutaneous insertion of absorbable tacks and metallic staples. Use of fixation implants of this type carries the potential for loss of fixation, particularly in patients with soft cancellous bone. Loss of fixation can result in failure of tendon repair as well as mechanical

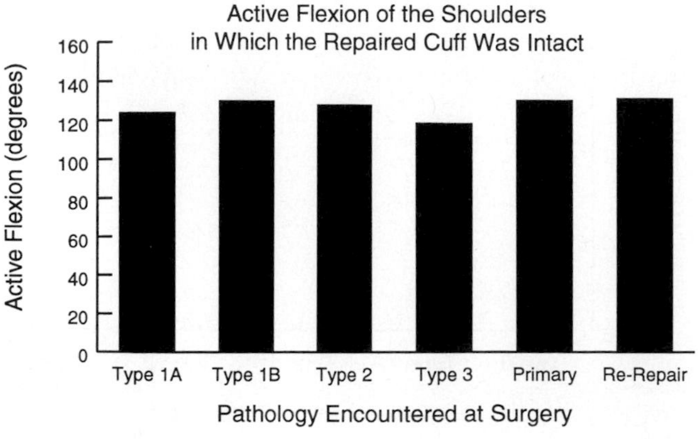

Figure 15–106

Active flexion of the shoulders in which the repaired cuff remained intact (no full-thickness recurrent defect) was independent of the pathologic conditions encountered at surgery. (From Matsen FA III, Lippitt SB, Sidles JA, and Harryman DT II: Practical Evaluation and Management of the Shoulder. Philadelphia: WB Saunders, 1994.)

Table 15–8 INFLUENCE OF SIZE OF CUFF TEAR REPAIRED AT SURGERY ON ACTIVE RANGE OF MOTION AT FOLLOW-UP*

			ACTIVE RANGE OF MOTION AT FOLLOW-UP			
SIZE OF DEFECT REPAIRED AT SURGERY	NUMBER	AGE AT REPAIR (MEANS ± SD)	Flexion	External Rotation at Side	External Rotation at 90° Abduction	Internal Rotation
Partial (1A)	6	49 ± 13	126°	38°	68°	T8
Supraspinatus (1B)	49	57 ± 8	129°	40°	70°	T7
Supraspinatus and infraspinatus (2)	28	64 ± 8	119°	28°	60°	T8
Supraspinatus, infraspinatus, and subscapularis (3)	22	64 ± 8	92°	33°	60°	T10°

*From Matsen FA III, et al: Practical Evaluation and Management of the Shoulder. Philadelphia: WB Saunders, 1994.
SD, standard deviation.

irritation caused by displacement of these devices in the subacromial space.

Palette and associates reported success in the arthroscopic management of small tears.[311] Levy and colleagues[222] in 1990 reported on 25 patients with full-thickness rotator cuff tears treated with an arthroscopically assisted rotator cuff repair. After performing an arthroscopic acromioplasty, the rotator cuff was identified, débrided, mobilized with arthroscopically placed sutures, and then repaired to a bony trough through a limited deltoid splitting approach. The patients, with an average age of 57.7 years (range of 21 to 74 years), were evaluated at an average of 18 months (range of 12 to 27 months). Based on the UCLA shoulder rating scale, 80% of the patients were rated as excellent or good, with reported significant improvements in pain, function, motion, and strength. Ninety-six per cent of the patients were satisfied with their result. Of the 15 large tears (3 to 5 cm), four were excellent, six were good (67% satisfactory), four were fair, and one was poor (33% unsatisfactory). Of the patients with small- (<1 cm) or moderate- (1 to 3 cm) sized tears, 100% received a satisfactory rating.

Warren and associates[428] reported good or excellent results in 13 of 17 patients who underwent arthroscopic acromioplasty and arthroscopic-assisted rotator cuff repair who were followed for a minimum of 2 years with an average follow-up of 25 months. Tear size was small in four, moderate in five, large in six, and massive in two. The rotator cuff was repaired into a prepared bony trough using arthroscopically placed sutures through a limited deltoid muscle–splitting incision and in some cases, using percutaneous fixation with a cannulated tack. Eight of nine tennis players and all the golfers returned to their previous sports.

Paulos and Kody,[317] in 1994, reported their results of 18 consecutive patients who underwent arthroscopic acromioplasty and rotator cuff repair through a 4-cm deltoid muscle–splitting approach with an average follow-up of 46 months (range of 36 to 72 months) and a mean age of 47.2 years (range of 26 to 74 years). Sixteen repairs were tendon-to-bone; two repairs were tendon-to-tendon. Sixteen patients (88%) scored good to excellent on the UCLA shoulder rating scale with significant improvement in pain and function scores. Two patients had poor results; both had workers' compensation cases pending. One patient with a poor result had two complications: superficial infection and failure of repair that required reoperation. Seventeen of the 18 patients (94%) were satisfied with the result.

In 1994, Liu,[231] reported on 44 patients (average age of 58 years, range of 35 to 76) with full-thickness rotator cuff tears at an average of 4.2 years (range of 2.5 to 6.1 years) after arthroscopic-assisted rotator cuff repair. Eighty-five per cent of the patients were discharged from the hospital immediately after the operation. The results were rated as good or satisfactory in 84% (37 of 44) (eight of eight in those with small tears (<1 cm), 15 of 17 with moderate tears (1 to 3 cm), 12 of 15 with large tears (3 to 5 cm), and two of five with massive tears (>5 cm). Eighty-eight per cent of the patients were satisfied with the result, and 64% of the athletes returned to their previous sport. The size of the tear seemed to be a determining factor in the functional outcome: the small and moderate tears did better than did the large and massive tears. The patients' satisfaction, however, did not seem to relate to the size of the tear repair; those with small, moderate, and large tears were equally satisfied.

In 1995, Baker and Liu[12] compared the results of open and arthroscopically assisted rotator cuff repair in 36 patients with a minimum follow-up of 2 years. The open repair group (average age of 60 years) comprised 20 shoulders with an average follow-up of 3.3 years; the arthroscopic-assisted repair group (average age of 59 years) comprised 17 shoulders with an average follow-up of 3.2 years. Overall the open repair group had 88% good-to-excellent results and 88% patient satisfaction; the arthroscopically assisted repair group had 85% good-to-excellent and 92% patient satisfaction (based on the UCLA rating scale). The functional outcome with regard to shoulder flexion, strength of abduction, and size of the rotator cuff tear repaired did not differ significantly between the two treatment groups. In general, however, small- and moderate-sized tears (<3 cm) demonstrated earlier return to full function after arthroscopically assisted rotator cuff repair; this group was hospitalized 1.2 days less and returned to previous activities an average of 1 month earlier. In the patients with large tears, two of four patients (50%) in the arthroscopically assisted repair group and four of five (80%) in the open repair group had good-to-excellent results. In general, the authors found arthroscopically assisted rotator cuff repair to be as effective as open repair in the treatment of small and moderated-sized tears (<3 cm), whereas large tears did better after open repair.

These studies suggest that arthroscopic acromioplasty combined with arthroscopically assisted rotator cuff repair can provide acceptable clinical results in the management of small full-thickness rotator cuff tears in the presence of excellent quality tissue with minimal tissue retraction and scarring. These results, however, are not directly comparable with the results of traditional open surgery, because studies involving open techniques include larger numbers of older patients, many of whom have large chronic tears requiring extensive soft tissue mobilization. The long-term clinical results and the integrity of the cuff after these arthroscopically assisted repairs have yet to be determined.

Open Operative Treatment When Repair Is Not Possible

While it used to be said by some that the term "irreparable cuff" reflects more on the surgeon than on the patient, the fact is that some rotator cuff tears may be impossible to repair. Rockwood and associates[349, 351] reported on their experience using a modified Neer acromioplasty and débridement of massive irreparable lesions involving the supraspinatus and infraspinatus tendons in 53 shoulders (average age of 60). At an average of 6.5 years of follow-up the comfort, function, and satisfaction were satisfactory in 83%. Good prognostic findings were an intact biceps, an intact anterior deltoid, and no previous shoulder surgery. Active forward flexion improved from 105 to 140 degrees. These results indicate that subacromial smoothness and vigorous postsurgical rehabilitation can substantially improve comfort and function, even when large cuff defects are irreparable.

In a small series Hawkins and associates[165] reported only 50% satisfactory results with open subacromial decompression alone in patients with massive full-thickness rotator cuff tears. Bakalim and Pasila found that acromial excision alone gave relief of night pain in certain cases.[11]

Arthroscopic Operative Treatment When Repair Is Not Possible

Several authors have reported acceptable clinical results with full-thickness cuff defects when arthroscopic acromioplasty and débridement were performed without rotator cuff repair, especially for the sedentary, low-demand patients whose main complaint is pain.[105, 110, 131, 166, 384, 417]

In one of the earliest studies, Wiley,[439] in 1985, reported on 20 patients with full-thickness rotator cuff tears who underwent arthroscopic, rotator cuff débridement and shoulder manipulation without acromioplasty. Within 24 months, 16 patients had pain relief (five complete, 11 partial), 12 had increased range of motion, and 11 were able to return to work. He concluded that arthroscopic treatment was useful in treating older patients with chronic shoulder pain associated with full-thickness rotator cuff tears.

Ellman,[104] in 1987, presented 10 patients with full-thickness tears of the rotator cuff treated with arthroscopic acromioplasty and rotator cuff débridement. Based on the UCLA shoulder rating scale, 80% were rated satisfactory (eight good) and 20% unsatisfactory (two poor). It was noted that none of the eight satisfactory results achieved an excellent objective rating.

Esch and associates,[110] in 1988, presented their results according to the degree of rotator cuff tendon failure. Their patients with complete tears were divided into groups of tears less than 1 cm, tears greater than 1 cm, and massive tears. The patients were treated with an arthroscopic acromioplasty, coracoacromial ligament resection, and débridement of acromioclavicular spurs. All patients were followed for a minimum of 1 year. Four patients with tears less than 1 cm had a satisfactory result and an excellent rating. Of the 16 patients with tears greater than 1 cm, 14 were satisfied and objectively 13 had a good or excellent result (based on the UCLA shoulder rating scale). There were three fair objective ratings and no poor ratings. Of the six patients with massive tears, five were satisfied but only three had a satisfactory score. Thus, patients with complete rotator cuff tears had an overall patient satisfaction rate of 88% and an objective satisfactory rating of 77%. Esch subsequently concluded that results are related to tear size. Patients with small full-thickness tears may achieve excellent results with arthroscopic acromioplasty and cuff débridement. Of the patients with large tears, only four of the 13 obtained an excellent objective result.

Gartsman,[131] as part of a larger series, reported on 25 patients with full-thickness rotator cuff tears treated with arthroscopic acromioplasty, resection of the coracoacromial ligament and subacromial bursa, removal of osteophytes, and a minimal débridement of the rotator cuff defect. The tears were divided into four groups based on size of the tear: (1) small tears of less than 1 cm (three total); (2) tears between 1 and 3 cm (13 total); (3) tears between 3 and 5 cm (six total); and three massive tears that were larger than 5 cm. At an average of 31 months, there were 14 satisfactory and 11 unsatisfactory results. Seven of these patients were subsequently treated with open rotator cuff repair, six of which had a satisfactory result. Notably, there was no correlation between the final result and the patient's age, sex, hand dominance, or the location of the tear. Only rotator cuff tear size correlated with outcome—13 of 16 patients with a tear less than 3 cm had a satisfactory result while only one of nine patients with a larger tear (>3 cm) did well.

Montgomery and associates[266] reported on 87 patients with 89 full-thickness rotator cuff tears who failed to respond to conservative treatment. Fifty patients (group I) were treated with open rotator cuff repair and Neer acromioplasty. Thirty-eight patients (group II) were managed by arthroscopic débridement, acromioplasty, and abrasion of the greater tuberosity. With similar size rotator cuff tears represented in each group at 1 year follow-up, the authors found no statistically significant difference between the two groups. However, on re-evaluation 2 years after surgery, the open surgical repair group (I) was statistically much better than the arthroscopic débridement group (II) with regard to pain and function. Four of the 38 patients in the arthroscopic débridement group developed rotator cuff tear arthropathy, which was thought to occur secondary to the instability and abnormal movement of the humeral head on the glenoid.

In 1991, Levy and co-workers[221] reported on 25 patients with full-thickness tears of the rotator cuff treated with arthroscopic acromioplasty and rotator cuff tendon débridement alone. There was significant improvement in pain, function, motion, and strength. Eighty-four per cent of the cases were rated as excellent or good (and 88% of the patients were satisfied with the procedure). Although all tear sizes were improved significantly, small tears fared better than did larger tears.

In a follow-up series,[460] Zvijac, Levy, and Lemak reevaluated all 25 patients from the original study group with full-thickness rotator cuff tears who underwent arthroscopic acromioplasty. At mean follow-up of 45.8 months, 68% of the patients were rated as excellent or good, representing a significant decrease from the initial report of 84% satisfactory result at a mean follow-up of 24.6 months. The authors found a significant decrease in rating with regard to pain and function. Ratings for motion and strength did not change significantly with time. Large and massive rotator cuff tears fared worse over time when compared with small and moderate-sized tears. These findings led the authors to abandon support for the use of arthroscopic acromioplasty and rotator cuff débridement alone in the treatment of repairable full-thickness rotator cuff tears.

In 1993, Ellman and associates[109] reported their follow-up results of 40 full-thickness rotator cuff tears treated by arthroscopic acromioplasty and débridement in a selected group of patients. The patients were divided into three groups based on the size of their tear. Ten small (0 to 2 cm) tears in older patients that were not involved in strenuous activities were rated satisfactory in 90% of cases. Patients with eight larger (2 to 4 cm) reparable tears did poorly (50% satisfactory results). Arthroscopic treatment in 22 patients with massive irreparable tears did not improve range of motion or restore strength but did result in significant pain relief, and 86% were satisfied with the results on a "limited goals basis." Ellman and co-workers concluded that for patients with medium-sized tears, pain relief from arthroscopic acromioplasty alone is inadequate, and the "procedure probably should not be offered." In carefully selected patients described as "relatively older and very sedentary," however, with small rotator cuff tears (0 to 2 cm), arthroscopic acromioplasty can have a useful role. Ellman emphasized that even for these patients, and certainly for most patients, repairable rotator cuff tears are best treated with open surgical repair.

In a series of 80 consecutive arthroscopic acromioplasties in 76 patients with stage II and III impingement syndrome, Paulos and associates[315] identified seven patients with full-thickness rotator cuff tears. Three of these patients, all with small (1 cm) tears, remained symptomatic and required reoperation for open repair of the rotator cuff tear.

In 1993, Ogilvie-Harris and associates,[299] in a prospective cohort study, compared the results of arthroscopic acromioplasty and rotator cuff débridement (22 patients) and open repair and acromioplasty (23 patients) as treatment for tears of the rotator cuff 1 to 4 cm in size. Follow-up varied from 2 to 5 years. The two treatment groups showed no significant differences in age, size of tear, preoperative pain, function, range of active forward flexion, and strength of forward flexion. At follow-up, both groups had similar pain relief and range of active forward flexion. The open repair group scored significantly better for function, strength, and overall score; however, patient satisfaction was similar in both groups. These authors found no significant difference in the final result in relation to the age of the patient or the size of the rotator cuff tears. On the basis of their results, the authors consider use of arthroscopic acromioplasty and débridement for patients with demands whose main complaints are pain and loss of range of movement. For patients, however, who need good function and strength, arthroscopic débridement and acromioplasty are not sufficient, and open repair and acromioplasty are advised.

In 1994, Olsewski and Depew[302] reported on their results of arthroscopic acromioplasty and rotator cuff débridement performed on 61 consecutive patients with a minimum of 2-year follow-up (mean of 27.7 months). In this study, 13 full-thickness rotator cuff tears were identified. Of the 13 full-thickness tears treated, 10 were rated satisfactory (77%) and three were rated unsatisfactory (33%). Of the 10 satisfactory results, eight were in patients who were either retired or worked at sedentary jobs that did not demand above-shoulder activities and strength and whose main preoperative complaint was pain. All 10 of these patients had relief of their pain. The three unsatisfactory results were all in active patients with demands on strength and overhead activity.

Burkhart[44] described 10 patients with massive (irreparable or >5 cm) complete rotator cuff tears involving primarily the supraspinatus treated with arthroscopic acromioplasty with débridement of redundant nonfunctional rotator cuff tissue. All patients except one had normal active motion and strength preoperatively, and all had a roentgenographically normal acromiohumeral distance and an anteroinferior acromial osteophyte. The procedure was offered to a subset of older patients, with activity limiting pain, who were preoperatively found to have a full range of active shoulder motion and normal strength of external rotation. Arthroscopic débridement and decompression were accompanied by pain relief without loss of motion or strength in all 10 patients. The follow-up period ranged from 8 to 33 months (mean of 17.6 months). Patients ranged from 53 to 77 years of age (average of 65 years). There were seven excellent results and three good results. All patients were satisfied with their results.

COST-EFFECTIVENESS OF TREATMENT OF FULL-THICKNESS CUFF TEARS

Rotator cuff disease is one of the commonest afflictions of the shoulder. Many health care dollars are spent on its evaluation and management. It is apparent that a large number of variables affect the effectiveness of treatment of cuff lesions. The cost of various treatment methods varies substantially as well. To initiate a practical investigative method by which the cost-effectiveness might be

Table 15–9 DATA ON 67 PATIENTS TREATED FOR DOCUMENTED FULL-THICKNESS TEARS OF THE ROTATOR CUFF

	NO. OF PATIENTS	AVERAGE AGE	% FEMALE	AVERAGE FOLLOW-UP (YR)
Nonoperative	36	62.4	36	1.7
Subacromial smoothing	11	67.8	45	1.7
Cuff repair	20	60.3	10	2.0

compared among treatment methods, we conducted a preliminary study of 67 unmatched patients presenting for treatment of documented, symptomatic full-thickness tears. Based on our clinical assessment and the desires of the patient, one of three treatment methods was selected for each patient: nonoperative management, subacromial smoothing without repair, and surgical repair. The number of patients, average age, gender, and length of follow-up for the patients in each of the three groups is given in Table 15–9.

All patients completed SSTs and SF 36 questionnaires preoperatively and at follow-up. The effectiveness of treatment was measured in terms of the postoperative-preoperative change in the number of affirmative responses on the SST and the postoperative-preoperative change in the SF 36 comfort score. This analysis indicated that the greatest improvement was found in the group that had surgical repair (see solid bars in Figs. 15–107 and 15–108). The change in SST and SF 36 comfort score results for each patient were then divided by the total hospital, office, and physician charges for the treatment to yield the average change/$1000 charge. In this analysis, nonoperative treatment was associated with the greatest change per unit charge (see hollow bars in Figs. 15–107 and 15–108).

While no conclusions should be drawn from these preliminary results, it is hoped that further studies of this type will help to determine the cost-effectiveness of different treatment methods.

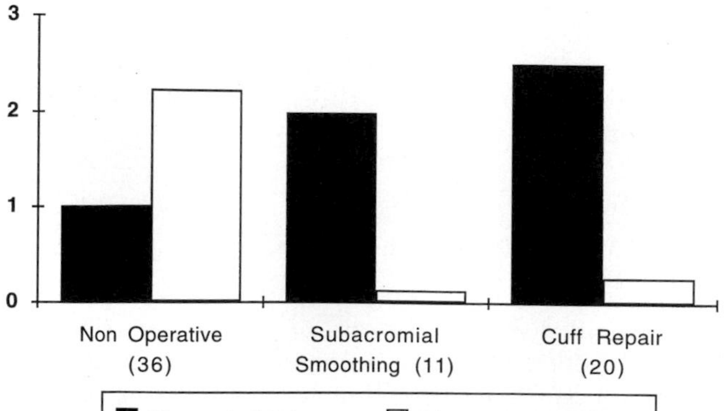

Figure 15–107

Median change in the number of positive SST responses.

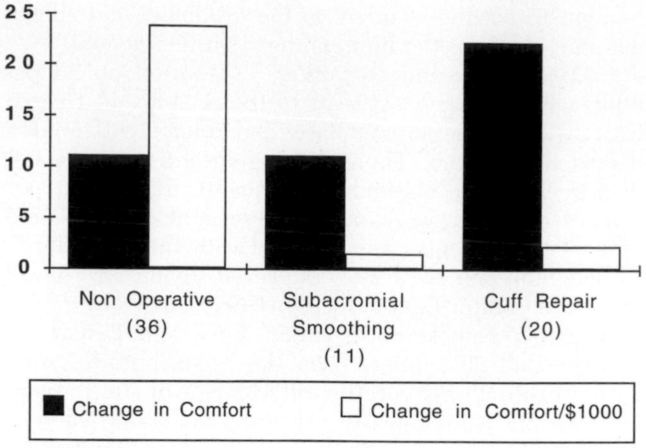

Figure 15–108

Median change in the SF 36 comfort score.

AUTHORS' PREFERRED METHOD OF TREATMENT FOR SURGICAL MANAGEMENT OF FULL-THICKNESS ROTATOR CUFF TEARS

The goal of rotator cuff surgery is to improve comfort and function of the shoulder. Surgery is considered: (1) in the patient with a significant acute cuff tear, and (2) in the patient with a chronic cuff defect associated with significant symptoms that have been refractory to a 3-month course of nonoperative management. In the situation of an acute cuff tear in a previously normal shoulder, the quality and quantity of tendon for repair should be excellent. Repair should be carried out promptly before tissue loss, retraction, and atrophy occur.

For tears older than 6 months, surgical repair is not an emergency: there is time to explore nonoperative management, including a general shoulder stretching and strengthening program. This nonoperative program may be the treatment of choice in patients with chronic weakness who are not candidates for surgery or for those in whom achieving a durable repair seems unlikely (see Table 15–3). This regime has been described earlier in this chapter as the Jackins program; it emphasizes stretching and strengthening the muscle groups that provide elevation and rotation of the shoulder. Surgical exploration is considered for patients with functionally significant symptoms from longer-standing tears refractory to nonoperative management, provided that their expectations are realistic. While a successful cuff repair may increase the strength of the shoulder, patients with repairs of chronic tears are advised against returning to heavy lifting, pushing, pulling, or overhead work after surgery for fear of re-rupturing the abnormal tendon tissue. Thus, we initiate vocational rehabilitation as soon as the diagnosis is made, indicating that, despite optimal treatment, there is a substantial risk of re-tearing if the cuff is again subjected to major loads. It is important to remind both the patient and the employer that a cuff tear usually occurs through abnormal cuff tendon. Repair of the tear does not restore the quality of the tendon tissue; thus, the repaired cuff remains permanently vulnerable to sudden or large loads.

Critical determinants of a durable repair are the quality of the tendon and muscle and the amount of cuff tendon tissue that has been lost. The strength of the cuff tendon diminishes with age and disuse; as a result, the chances of a durable cuff repair also decrease in older and less active shoulders. This is particularly the case if the cuff defect has been long-standing.

Table 15–3 lists some of the factors that contribute to a durable repair, as well as those that predispose to failure. None of the factors in this table requires special imaging of the rotator cuff; all are discernible from the history, physical examination, and plain radiographs. Although none of these factors is a contraindication to surgery, each works to some degree against the chances of a durable repair. The choice of treatment of shoulder weakness caused by cuff failure is determined by the functional needs of the patient and the likeliness of a durable surgical repair. Patients with low functional requirements and a substantial number of the "discouraging" factors from Table 15–3 are given a nonoperative program to help optimize the strength and coordination of the muscles about the shoulder that remain intact. At the opposite extreme, patients with major functional demands and mostly "encouraging" factors are presented with the option of an attempt at surgical repair and informed that the success of this repair will be determined primarily by the quality of the tendon and muscle and by the amount of tissue lost.

We recall that cuff repair is a shoulder tightening operation—in a sense it is a capsulorrhaphy. Thus it is not a treatment for the shoulder whose primary functional limitation is caused by tightness, even if a cuff defect is also present. If the shoulder demonstrates stiffness, a shoulder mobilization program is instituted before consideration of surgery.

For surgery, the patient is positioned in a semisitting (beach chair) position. Both the anterior and posterior aspects of the chest and the arm are prepared to allow access to the back of the shoulder and full motion of the arm. Surgery begins with an inspection of the cuff through a "deltoid on" acromioplasty approach (see Fig. 15–1). This incision offers excellent exposure and the opportunity for a cosmetic closure. Great care is taken to preserve the tendon fibers of the deltoid origin to permit a strong repair. The deltoid has an important tendon of origin between its anterior and middle thirds. Arising from the anterior lateral corner of the acromion, this tendon is not only the guide to exposure of the cuff but is also the key to reattachment of the deltoid origin at the conclusion of the surgery. This tendon is split longitudinally for 2 cm distal to the acromion in line with its fibers, taking care to leave some of the tendon on each side of the split. The split is continued up over the acromion and into the trapezius insertion. Although it is usually unnecessary for inspection of the cuff, additional exposure can be achieved by sharply dissecting the deltoid origin off the acromion for 1 cm on either side of this split so that the strong bony attachment fibers remain with the muscle. These fibers provide a strong "handle" on the muscle, thus a solid repair can be achieved at the conclusion of the procedure. Splitting the parietal layer of the bursa on the deep aspect of the deltoid provides a view of the rotator cuff. Later closure of the split is facilitated if at this point in the procedure a suture is placed on each side of the split fixing the incised bursal layer to the deltoid.

Before a "reflex" acromioplasty is performed, this window is used to inspect the cuff and determine its reparability without further compromising the deltoid or the coracoacromial arch. Hypertrophic bursa and scar tissue are resected to allow a good view of the cuff tendon involvement, tendon quality, and tendon tissue loss. Cuff tendon involvement is conveniently characterized using the system introduced by Harryman and associates,[157] which is based on the number of tendons torn. In type 1, only one tendon (almost always the supraspinatus) is torn. In type 2, two tendons (usually the supraspinatus and infraspinatus) are torn. In type 3, the supraspinatus, infraspinatus and subscapularis are torn. Type 1 is broken down into type 1A (a partial thickness) and type 1B (the full-thickness tear confined to a single tendon). The quality of the cuff tissue is judged in terms of its ability to hold a strong pull applied to a suture passed through its edge. Finally, it is critical to note the amount of tissue that has been lost. The extent of tissue loss and the ability of the remaining tissue to hold suture are the major determinants of cuff reparability.

If inspection of the cuff at surgery reveals good quality tissue in sufficient quantity and quality for a robust repair, a standard anteroinferior acromioplasty may be performed if necessary to improve exposure and to protect the repair from abrasion. A flexible osteotome is directed so that the anterior undersurface of the acromion is resected in the same plane as the posterior acromion (see Fig. 15–94). Rough spots are smoothed with a motorized burr.

The goal of repair is a strong fixation of the tendon to the humerus under normal tension with the arm at the side. The desired attachment site is at the sulcus near the base of the tuberosity. This goal is facilitated by using three stages of sequential release. These releases are required because the cuff is usually retracted and because tissue is lost in chronic cuff disease. Unless these releases are carried out, increased tension in the repaired tendon will predispose to tightness of the glenohumeral joint and will additionally challenge the repair site.[459] The humeral head is rotated to present successively the margins of the cuff defect through the incision (see Fig. 15–93), rather than enlarging the exposure to show the entire lesion at one time. The deep surface of the cuff is searched for retracted laminations. All layers of the cuff are assembled and tagged with sutures. By applying traction to these sutures, the cuff is mobilized sequentially as necessary to allow the torn tendon edge to reach the desired insertion at the base of the tuberosity. First, the humeroscapular motion interface is freed between the cuff and the deltoid, acromion, coracoacromial ligaments, coracoid, and coracoid muscles (see Figs. 15–3 and 15–4). Next, the coracohumeral ligament/rotator interval capsule (see Fig. 15–98) is sectioned around the coracoid process to eliminate any restriction to the excursion of the cuff tendons and to minimize tension on the repair during passive movement (see Fig. 15–99). This release of the coracohumeral ligament and rotator interval capsule also contributes to the comfort and ease of motion after the surgical repair by minimizing the capsular tightening effect of cuff repair.[459] At this point the ease with which the cuff margins can be approximated to their anatomic insertion at the base of the tuberosity is evaluated. If good tissue cannot reach the sulcus, the third release is carried out. This release divides the capsule from the glenoid just outside the glenoid labrum (see Fig. 15–100), which allows the capsule and tendon of the cuff to be drawn further laterally toward the desired tuberosity insertion without restricting range of motion.

After the necessary releases have been completed, a judgment is made concerning the site at which the cuff can be implanted into the bone without undue tension while the arm is at the side. Ideally, the site of implantation will be in the sulcus at the base of the tuberosity. In large cuff defects, a somewhat more medial insertion site may be necessary. Often, when a medial insertion site is required for a large cuff defect, the new insertion lies in an area where the articular cartilage has been damaged by abrasion against the undersurface of the acromion.

The repair is accomplished as a tongue in groove, with the cuff tendon drawn into a trough near the tuberosity, providing a smooth upper surface to glide beneath the acromion (see Fig. 15–101). This groove provides the additional advantage that if some slippage occurs in the suture fixation of the cuff to bone, contact between these two structures is not lost. Nonabsorbable sutures woven through the tendon margin are passed through drill holes in the distal tuberosity so that the knots will not catch beneath the acromion (see Fig. 15–102). The knots are tied over the tuberosities so that they will lie out of the subacromial space. If the bone of the tuberosities is osteopenic, the sutures can be passed through bone more distally, even down to the junction of the metaphysis and diaphysis. If there is a longitudinal component to the tear, it is repaired side-to-side with the knots buried out of the humeroscapular motion interface. The repair is checked throughout a range of motion to 140 degrees of elevation and 40 degrees of external rotation to ensure that it is strong, that it is not under excessive tension, and that it will permit smooth subacromial motion. If additional subacromial smoothing is required to allow smooth passage of the repaired tendon, it is performed at this time.

After a careful and robust deltoid repair using nonabsorbable sutures (see Fig. 15–95) and cosmetic skin closure, the patient is returned to the recovery room with the affected arm in continuous passive motion (see Fig. 15–96). Immediate postoperative motion is valuable because there is a tendency for scarring between the raw undersurface of the acromion and the upper aspect of the rotator cuff or proximal humerus. Immediate postoperative continuous passive motion is facilitated if the surgery is performed under a brachial plexus block, which lasts up to 18 hours after surgery. CPM is continued for up to 48 hours after surgery but does not appear to be necessary after that. The patient is expected to perform passive exercises in flexion and external rotation. Before discharge from the medical center, the patient should be able to attain comfortably 140 degrees of passive flexion and 40 degrees of passive external rotation. A progress chart mounted on the patient's wall helps to document progress toward these discharge goals (Fig. 15–109).

Postdischarge management must consider the magnitude of the tear and the strength of the repair. It is unlikely that the repair will have substantial strength until at least 3 months after surgery.[122] As is the case with repairs of the anterior cruciate ligament, major cuff repairs may require 6 to 12 months to regain useful strength. Thus, in the first several postoperative months, the emphasis is placed on maintaining passive motion and avoiding loading of the repair. Posterior capsular stretching is not started until 3 months after surgery. Gentle progressive strengthening of the repaired cuff muscles is also started at 3 months. Work and sports are not resumed until the shoulder is comfortable, flexible, and strong.

WHEN CUFF REPAIR CANNOT BE ACHIEVED

If the initial inspection of the cuff reveals major tissue loss and residual tendon of poor quality and if it becomes evident that a robust repair cannot be performed, the coracoacromial arch is preserved. When primary stability from an intact cuff cannot be restored, it is important to avoid a "reflex" acromioplasty. Sacrifice of the coracoacromial arch jeopardizes the secondary stabilization required in cuff deficiency. Without this secondary restraint, the shoulder is susceptible to anterosuperior "escape" of the humeral head when superiorly directed loads are applied to the humerus (see Fig. 15–9). Therefore, when a strong rotator cuff repair cannot be performed because of limited quantity and quality of the residual cuff tissue, we preserve the coracoacromial arch and ensure the smoothness of its undersurface to allow unimpeded passage of the humeral head and residual cuff beneath. Any debris, scar, useless fronds of cuff, or thickened bursa in the subacromial area is excised. It is important to also ensure smoothness of the upper surface of the uncovered proximal humerus, particularly if the tuberosities are prominent or irregular.

A strong repair of the deltoid is accomplished using a side-to-side repair of the surgical split in the deltoid tendon and a secure reattachment to the acromion using drill holes in the bone as necessary (see Fig. 15–95). The full thickness of the deltoid, including the deltoid side of the bursa, is incorporated in the sutures to be certain that it does not impede smooth motion in the humeroscapular motion interface.

A subcuticular skin closure reinforced with paper tapes provides optimal cosmesis. The patient is returned to the recovery room with the arm in CPM to minimize the tendency to form adhesions in the humeroscapular motion interface (see Fig. 15–96).

The patient is taught passive mobilization of the shoulder to 140 degrees of elevation (see Figs. 15–81 and 15–82) and 40 degrees of external rotation (see Fig. 15–83) as well as stretching of the posterior capsule (see Figs. 15–85 and 15–86) and is discharged from the medical center when these goals are achieved. Active use of the shoulder with the arm at the side is instituted immediately. Sling immobilization is unnecessary.

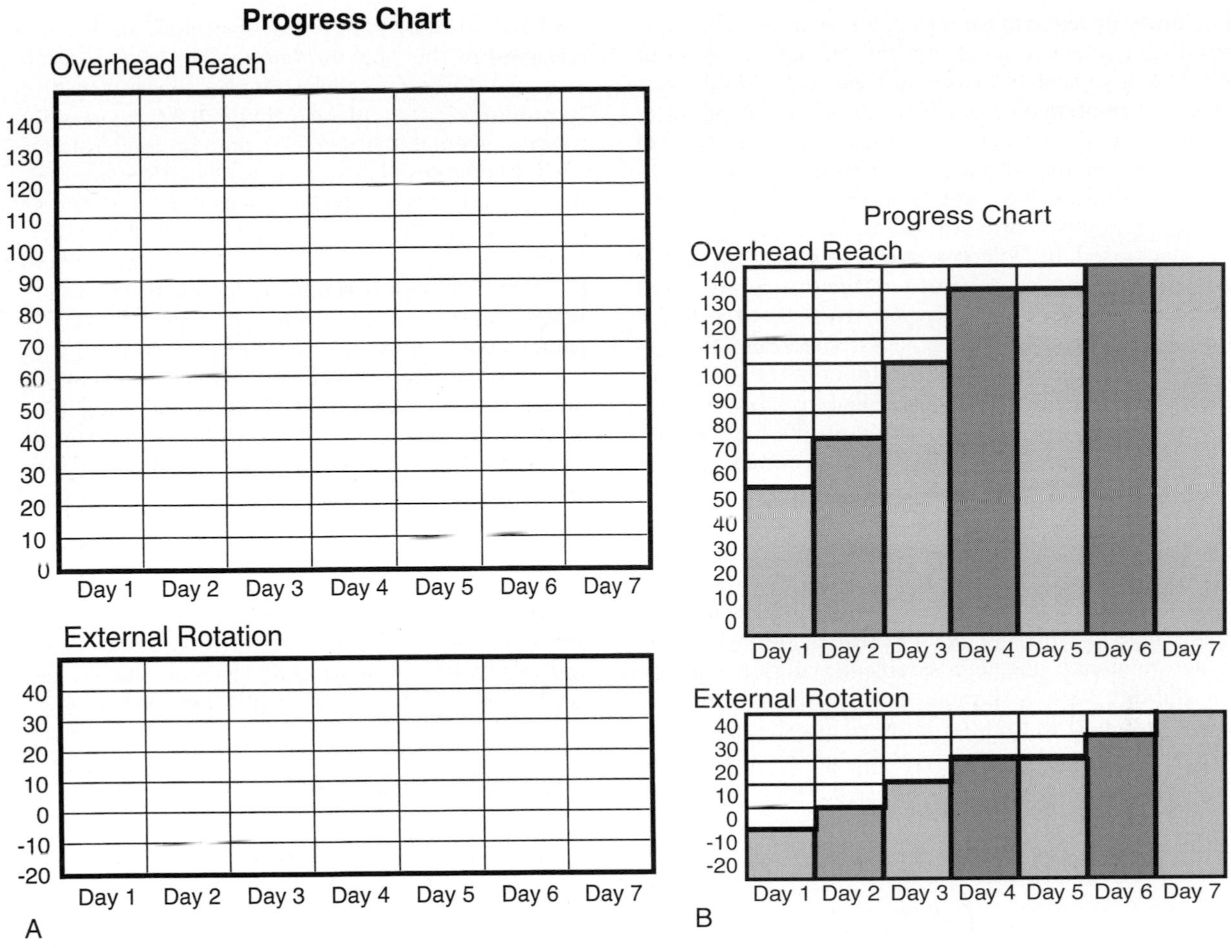

Figure 15–109

A, Wall charts are used to display the patient's overhead reach *(top)* and external rotation *(bottom)*. These charts are posted in the patient's room to provide positive feedback to the patient. Using a colored marker, the physical therapist, nurse, or physician charts the range of motion achieved each day. *B*, Typical wall charts showing the improvement in overhead reach and external rotation after an open release. (From Matsen FA III, Lippitt SB, Sidles JA, and Harryman DT II: Practical Evaluation and Management of the Shoulder. Philadelphia: WB Saunders, 1994.)

Strengthening of the deltoid and residual cuff muscles is started 6 weeks after surgery. An ideal exercise for optimizing the strength of active elevation is the progressive supine press (see Fig. 15–89). In this exercise, small increments are used to train the remaining muscles to optimal advantage. Note that the scapular muscles are also put to work in these exercises (see Figs. 15–90 and 15–91). This program is easy for the patient to learn and to carry out alone.

Failed Cuff Surgery

In this condition, the patient is dissatisfied with the result from a previous arthroscopic or open operation on the rotator cuff and presents for consideration of additional surgery.

CAUSES OF FAILURE

Rotator cuff repair may fail to yield a satisfactory result for many reasons including failure to obtain preoperative expectations of strength and comfort, infection, deltoid denervation, deltoid detachment, loss of the acromial lever arm, adhesions in the humeroscapular motion interface, persistent subacromial roughness, denervation of the cuff, failure of the cuff repair, retear of abnormal tendon, failure of grafts to "take," failure of rehabilitation, and loss of superior stability. Effective treatment of these failures depends on the establishment of the proper diagnosis. *Infection* requires culture-specific antibiotics and irrigation and drainage if purulence is present. A prompt definitive approach may prevent joint surface destruction. Acute *failure of the deltoid reattachment* requires prompt repair before muscle retraction becomes fixed. Chronically painful and functionally limiting *postoperative scarring* often responds to gentle, frequent stretching at home. Shoulder manipulation in this situation is inadvisable because of the risk of cuff damage. However, in certain shoulders that are refractory to rehabilitation, substantial improvement in comfort and function can be achieved by an open lysis of adhesions and subacromial smoothing, followed by early assisted motion. *Weakness* of shoulder elevation often responds to gentle, progressive strengthening of the anterior deltoid and external rotators. Persistent weakness requires evaluation for possible neurologic injury or cuff failure. *Denervation of the deltoid* is diagnosed by selective electromyography of the anterior muscle fibers. In selected cases, anterior deltoid denervation may be treated by anterior transfer of the origin of the middle deltoid with closure to the clavicular head of the pectoralis major, although consistently good results from this procedure have not been documented. *Denervation* of the supraspinatus and infraspinatus or subscapularis is diagnosed by selective electromyography and is difficult to manage. Postoperative *cuff failure* is suggested by failure of the patient to regain strength of external rotation or elevation of the shoulder, subacromial snapping, and upward instability of the humeral head. In this situation arthrography may not be reliable; false-negative results from scarring or false-positive results from inconsequential leaks reduce the diagnostic accuracy. In our experience, expert dynamic cuff ultrasonography provides the most specific data on cuff thickness and integrity. Repeat cuff exploration with smoothing or repair may be considered, although the patient is warned that the tissue may be of insufficient quantity and quality for a durable re-repair. Loss of superior stability can result when the coracoacromial arch has been sacrificed without re-establishing stability with a durable cuff repair. The deltoid becomes stretched so that the humeral head seems to be just below the skin. Patients who lose stability and deltoid function are some of the most unhappy patients that we encounter after previous repair attempts.

The results of surgery for failure of previous cuff repairs are inferior to those of primary repair. DeOrio and Cofield[87] reviewed their experience with re-repairs. At a minimum of 2 years' follow-up (average of 4 years), 76% of patients had substantial diminution of pain; however, 63% still had moderate or severe pain. Only seven patients gained more than 30 degrees of abduction, and only four patients were considered to have a good result. The authors suggested that the main benefit of repeat cuff surgery is likely to be a reduction in discomfort.

Harryman and associates,[157] however, showed that if cuff integrity is durably established at revision surgery, the results are comparable with those of primary repairs (see Fig. 15–106).

ARTHRODESIS

When a shoulder has been devastated by infection, deltoid detachment or denervation, intractable cuff failure or denervation, or acromionectomy, consideration is given to shoulder arthrodesis. Under these circumstances, a glenohumeral arthrodesis provides a salvage option: by securing the humeral head to the scapula, the scapular motors can be used to power the humerus through a very limited range of humerothoracic motion.

The best candidates for this procedure are patients with: (1) permanent and severe weakness due to loss of cuff and deltoid function, (2) good bone stock, (3) a good understanding of the limitations and potential complications of a shoulder fusion, (4) intact scapular motors, (5) good motivation, (6) minimal complaints of pain, and (7) a functional contralateral shoulder.

To establish the limitations of shoulder fusions, we studied 12 patients who had glenohumeral arthrodeses at least 2 years prior to the time of study.[244] In these patients, elevation in the plus 90 degrees (anterior sagittal) plane averaged 47 degrees. Elevation in the minus 90 degrees (posterior sagittal) plane averaged 22 degrees. External rotation averaged 9 degrees, and internal rotation averaged 46 degrees. These ranges of motion were similar to the scapulothoracic motion measured in normal subjects. Only one of the patients could reach his hair without bending his neck forward; only five patients could reach the perineum; six patients could reach the back pocket; seven patients could reach the opposite axilla; and 10 patients could reach the side pocket.

We also studied normal in vivo shoulder kinematics to predict the functions that would be allowed by various positions of glenohumeral arthrodesis, assuming that the scapulothoracic motion would remain unchanged. Using the normal scapulothoracic motions, we were able to model the functional effects of fusion positions. We found that activities of daily living could be best performed if the joint was fused in 15 degrees of flexion, 15 degrees of abduction, and 45 degrees plane and 45 degrees of internal rotation (Fig. 15–110). This low angle of elevation and relatively high degree of internal rotation facilitated reaching the face, opposite axilla, and perineum.

Cuff Tear Arthropathy

In this condition resisted isometric contraction of the cuff muscles is weak; acromiohumeral and often glenohumeral movements produce crepitance; radiographs demonstrate superior translation of the head of the humerus with respect to the acromion, loss of the articular cartilage of the superior humeral head, direct articulation of the head with the coracoacromial arch, "femoralization" of the proximal humerus, and "acetabularization" of the upper glenoid and coracoacromial arch (Fig. 15–111; see also Figs. 15–12, 15–13, 15–48, 15–60, 15–69, and 15–70).

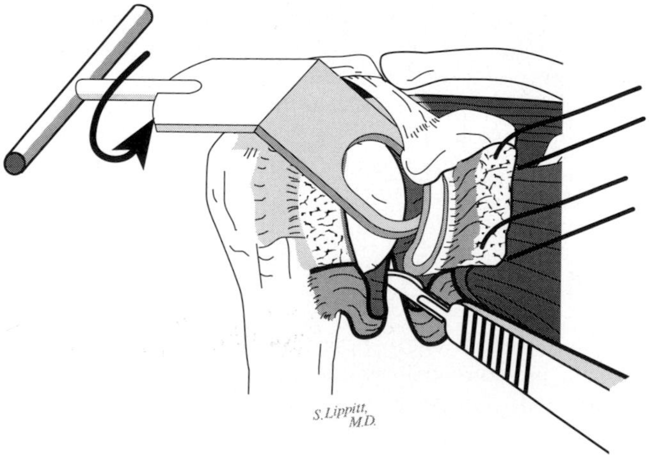

Figure 15–110

Recommended arthrodesis position: 15 degrees of humerothoracic flexion *(left)*, 15 degrees of humerothoracic abduction *(middle)*, and 45 degrees of internal rotation *(right)*. (From Matsen FA III, Lippitt SB, Sidles JA, and Harryman DT II: Practical Evaluation and Management of the Shoulder. Philadelphia: WB Saunders, 1994.)

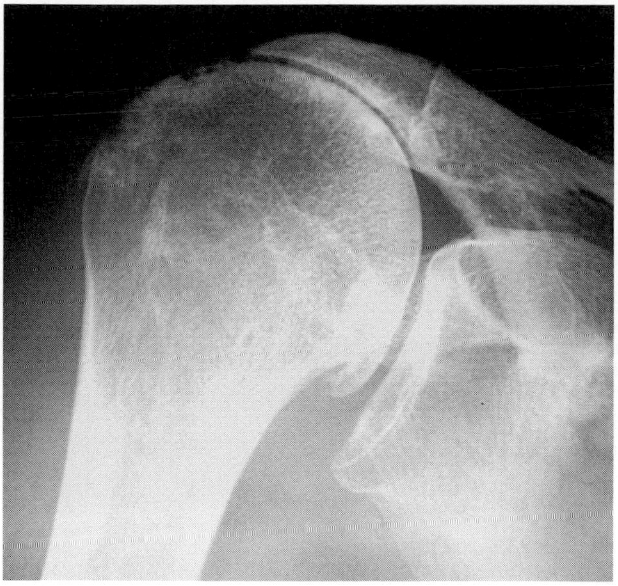

Figure 15–111

Cuff tear arthropathy.

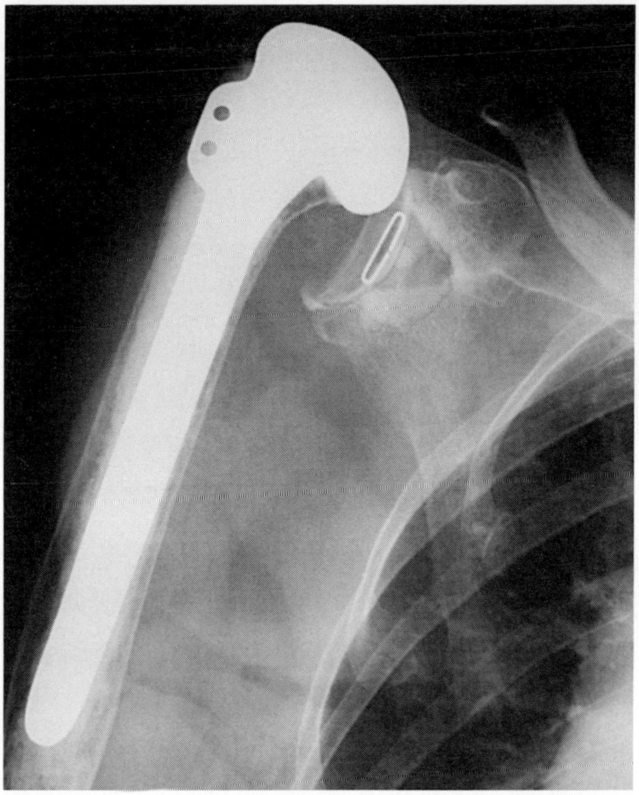

Figure 15–112

Glenoid component loosening via a "rocking horse" mechanism after shoulder replacement performed in the presence of a massive cuff deficiency (see Chapter 16).

The combination of glenohumeral joint surface destruction and massive cuff deficiency can be devastating.[279] Yet, each patient has an individual combination of pain and functional losses. Patients with mild pain are managed with mild analgesics and gentle, function-maintaining exercises.

When chronic cuff deficiency with upward displacement of the humeral head leads to repeated abrasive contact between the upper humerus and the coracoacromial arch and symptomatic destruction of the humeral articular cartilage, reconstructive options are seriously limited. Shoulder arthrodesis is unattractive because these patients are often older and the condition may be bilateral.[277] Constrained total shoulder arthroplasty is an option, but the failure rate is very high. Secure cuff reconstruction with unconstrained total shoulder arthroplasty is usually impossible owing to massive cuff tissue deficiency.[123] Unconstrained arthroplasty without a secure cuff repair carries a high incidence of eccentric loading and "rocking horse" loosening of the component (Fig. 15–112).[123, 244]

In a 1986 report to the ASES, Brownlee and Cofield reported on 20 surgical procedures for cuff tear arthropathy.[42] These included Neer-type total shoulder arthroplasty, total shoulder arthroplasty using a hooded glenoid, and proximal humeral replacement without a glenoid. Extensive mobilization of tendons was attempted for repair. Pain relief was substantial in each group. Active abduction was best in the group with proximal humeral replacement. Three of the glenoid components loosened.

Arntz and associates reported our results in 19 patients, 54 to 84 years of age who had disabling pain attributable to a massive tear of the rotator cuff, accompanied by loss of the surface of the glenohumeral joint.[7] These patients were not considered candidates for total shoulder replacement because of the massive deficiency in the cuff and the fixed upward displacement of the humeral head (Fig. 15–113; see also Figs. 15–12, 15–13, 15–48, 15–60, 15–69, 15–70, and 15–111). A prerequisite for hemiarthroplasty was a functionally intact coracoacromial arch to provide superior secondary stability for the prosthesis. One im-

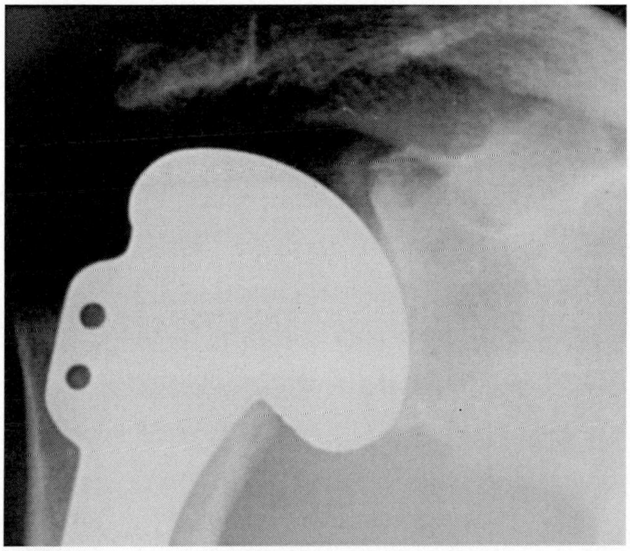

Figure 15–113

Resurfacing of the humeral head improved the comfort and function of the shoulder shown in Figure 15–60.

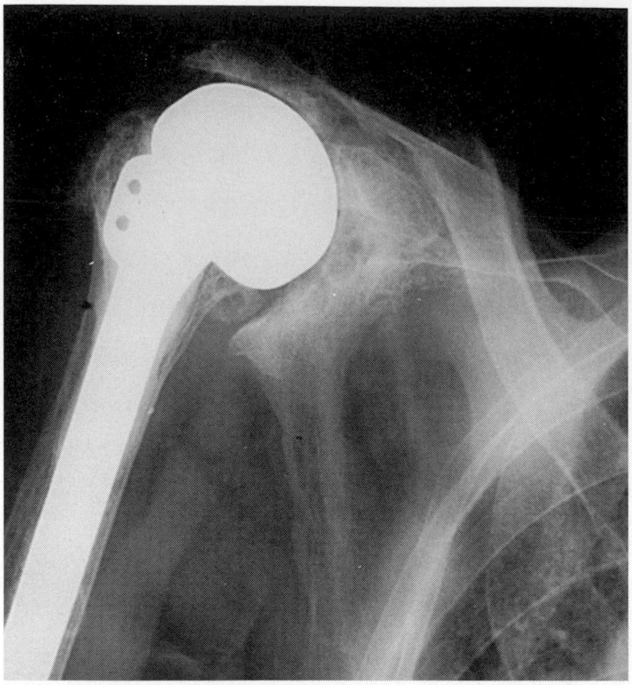

Figure 15–114

Resurfacing hemiarthroplasty for cuff tear arthropathy (same patient as in Fig. 15–69).

portant aspect of the operative technique was the selection of a sufficiently small prosthetic head volume so that excessive tightness of the posterior aspect of the capsule could be avoided (see Chapter 16 for discussion of "overstuffing"). Eighteen shoulders in 16 patients were available for follow-up, which ranged from 25 to 122 months. Pain decreased from marked or disabling in 14 shoulders preoperatively to none or slight in 10 and to pain only after unusual activity in four. Active forward elevation improved from an average of 66 degrees preoperatively to an average of 109 degrees postoperatively. One patient, who had had an excellent result, fell and sustained an acromial fracture, thus the functional result changed to poor. Three patients had persistent, substantial pain in the shoulder that led to a revision. Neither infection nor prosthetic loosening developed in any shoulder.

In a separate report, Arntz and colleagues[8] reviewed 23 shoulders in 23 patients with disabling pain associated with irreparable tears of the musculotendinous cuff. Twelve shoulders with preserved passive motion, normal deltoid function, loss of glenohumeral joint surfaces, and sculpturing of the coracoacromial arch received a reconstruction with a humeral hemiarthroplasty. In another 11 shoulders that failed to meet these prerequisites or that demanded heavy use after operation, glenohumeral arthrodesis was selected. Comfort level and overall function were improved in both groups. Active forward eleva-

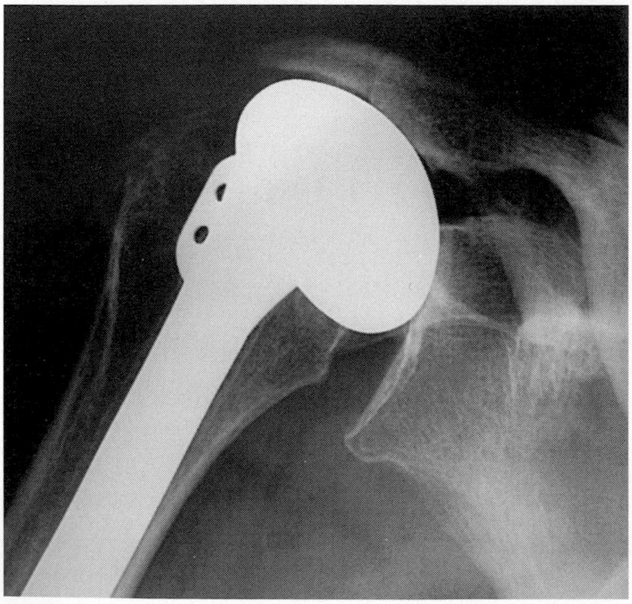

Figure 15–115

Resurfacing hemiarthroplasty for cuff tear arthropathy (same patient as in Fig. 15–111).

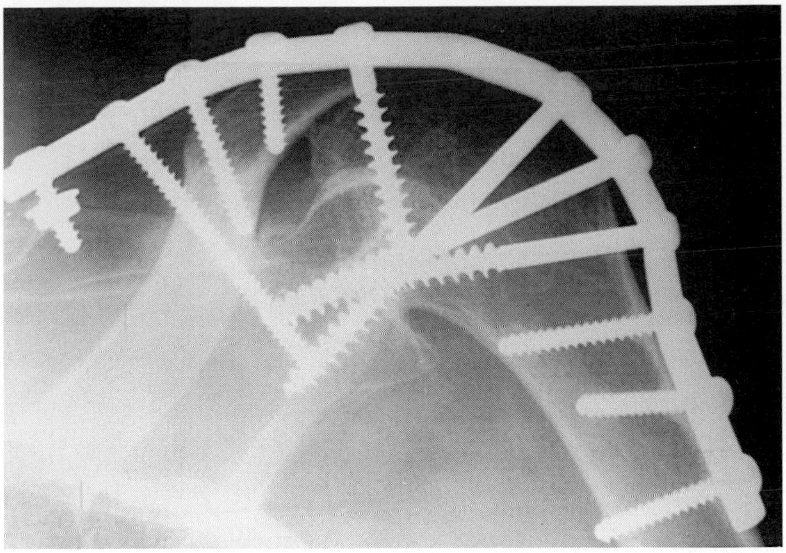

Figure 15–116

Shoulder arthrodesis for a young patient with a combined deficiency of the cuff and the deltoid.

tion improved an average of 44 degrees in the hemiarthroplasty group and an average of 15 degrees in the arthrodesis group. These results combined with the problems of glenoid loosening reported when total shoulder arthroplasty (see Fig. 15–112) is performed in the presence of cuff deficiency with upward head displacement suggest that humeral hemiarthroplasty is the preferred method for managing complex irreparable tears of the rotator cuff in which the articular surface is destroyed, yet the deltoid muscle is functional (Figs. 15–114 and 15–115; see also Figs. 15–69 and 15–111). Shoulder arthrodesis is reserved for patients who have both irreparable tears of the rotator cuff and irreparable deficiencies of the deltoid muscle or for the younger patient with demands for substantial strength at low angles of flexion (Fig. 15–116).

AUTHORS' PREFERRED METHOD FOR CUFF TEAR ARTHROPATHY

In the reconstruction for cuff tear arthropathy we attempt to make use of the "femoralization" of the proximal humerus (i.e., rounding so that the prominence of the tuberosities is lost) and the "acetabularization" of the glenocoracoacromial socket (i.e., erosion of the upper aspect of the glenoid and congruent concavity of the coracoacromial arch) (see Figs. 15–48, 15–69, 15–70, and 15–111). We have found that this adaptive ball-and-socket joint can be effectively and safely resurfaced using a humeral hemiarthroplasty (see Figs. 15–114 and 15–115). The goals of surgery are: (1) ensuring a smooth coracoacromial arch (usually already created by the process itself), avoiding acromioplasty and coracoacromial ligament section, which would destroy the superior constraint of the humeral head; (2) débriding useless fragments of cuff and bursa; and (3) anatomically resurfacing the destroyed humeral articular surface with a humeral endoprosthesis that will articulate with the coracoacromial arch and that will at all costs preserve the deltoid. We do not advocate cuff repair in this context, nor the use of double cups, nor oversized humeral head prostheses. Instead, the goal is to maintain the normal capsular laxity allowing internal rotation of the abducted arm to approximately 60 degrees.

Postoperatively, the patient is started on continuous passive motion (see Fig. 15–96) and allowed activities as comfort permits.

References and Bibliography

1. Structural changes of the rotator cuff caused by experimental subacromial impingement in the rat. Clin Orthop (in press).
2. Ahovou J, Paavolainen P, and Slätis P: The diagnostic value of arthrography and plain radiography in rotator cuff tears. Acta Orthop Scand 55:220–223, 1984.
3. Albright JA, Jokl P, Shaw R, and Albright JP: Clinical study of baseball pitchers: Correlation of injury to the throwing arm with method of delivery. Am J Sports Med 6:15–21, 1978.
4. Altchek DW, Warren RF, Wickiewicz TL, et al: Arthroscopic acromioplasty. J Bone Joint Surg Am *72(A)*:1198–1207, 1990.
5. Andrews JR, Broussard TS, and Carson WG: Arthroscopy of the shoulder in the management of partial tears of the rotator cuff: A preliminary report. Arthroscopy *1*:117–122, 1985.
6. Armstrong JR: Excision of the acromion in treatment of the supraspinatus syndrome: Report of ninety-five excisions. J Bone Joint Surg *31B*:436–442, 1949.
7. Arntz CT, Jackins S, and Matsen III FA: Prosthetic replacement of the shoulder for the treatment of defects in the rotator cuff and the surface of the glenohumeral joint. J Bone Joint Surg 75:485–491, 1993.
8. Arntz CT, Matsen III FA, and Jackins S: Surgical management of complex irreparable cuff deficiency. J Arthroplasty *6*:363–370, 1991.
9. Atwater AE: Biomechanics of overarm throwing movements and of throwing injuries. Exerc Sport Sci Rev *7*:43–85, 1979.
10. Bacevich BB: Paralytic brachial neuritis. J Bone Joint Surg Am *58A*:262, 1976.
11. Bakalim G and Pasila M: Surgical treatment of rupture of the rotator cuff tendon. Acta Orthop Scand *46*:751–757, 1975.
12. Baker CL and Liu SH: Comparison of open and arthroscopic assisted rotator cuff repairs. Am J Sports Med 23:99–104, 1995.
13. Bartolozzi A, Andreychik D, and Ahmad S: Determinants of outcome in the treatment of rotator cuff disease. Clin Orthop *308*:90–97, 1994.
14. Basmajian JV and Bazant FJ: Factors preventing downward dislocation of the adducted shoulder joint: An electromyographic and morphological study. J Bone Joint Surg *41A*:1182–1186, 1959.
15. Bassett RW and Cofield RH: Acute tears of the rotator cuff: The timing of surgical repair. Clin Orthop *175*:18–24, 1983.

16. Bateman JE: The diagnosis and treatment of ruptures of the rotator cuff. Surg Clin North Am *43*:1523–1530, 1963.
17. Bauer B and Vogelsang H: Die Lahmung des N. Suprascapularis als Taumafloge. Unfallheilkunde *65*:461–465, 1962.
18. Bayley JC, Cochran TP, and Seldge CB: The weight-bearing shoulder: The impingement syndrome in paraplegics. J Bone Joint Surg *69A*:676–678, 1987.
19. Bedi SS and Ellis W: Spontaneous rupture of calcaneal tendon in rheumatoid arthritis after local steroid injection. Ann Rheum Dis *29*:494, 1970.
20. Behrens F, Shepherd N, and Mitchell N: Alteration of rabbit articular cartilage by intra-articular injections of glucocorticoids. J Bone Joint Surg *57A1*:70, 1975.
21. Bellumore Y, Mansat M, and Assoun J: Results of the surgical repair of the rotator cuff. Radio-clinical correlation. Rev Chir Orthop Reparatrice Appar Mot *80*:582–594, 1994.
22. Ben-Yishay A, Zuckerman JD, Gallagher M, and Cuomo F: Pain inhibition of shoulder strength in patients with impingement syndrome. Orthopaedics *17*:685–688, 1994.
23. Benjamin M, Evans EJ, and Copp L: The histology of tendon attachments to bone in man. J Anat *149*:89–100, 1986.
24. Berquist TH, McCough PF, Hattrup SH, and Cofield RH: Arthrographic Analysis of Rotator Cuff Tear Size. American Shoulder and Elbow Surgeons 4th meeting, Atlanta, 1988.
25. Berry H, Fernandes L, and Bloom B: Clinical study comparing acupuncture, physiotherapy, injection and oral anti-inflammatory therapy in shoulder-cuff lesions. Curr Med Res Opin *7*:121–126, 1980.
26. Bettman: Monatsschr Unfallheilk. 14, 1926.
27. Bigliani LU, Cordasco FA, McIlveen SJ, et al: Operative management of failed rotator cuff repairs. Orthop Trans *12*:1974, 1988.
28. Bigliani LU, Morrison D, and April EW: The morphology of the acromion and its relationship to rotator cuff tears. Orthop Trans *10*:228, 1986.
29. Bigliani LU, Norris TR, and Fischer J: The relationship between the unfused acromial epiphysis and subacromial impingement lesions. Orthop Trans 7:138, 1983.
30. Binder A, Parr G, Hazleman B, and Fitton-Jackson S: Pulsed electromagnetic field therapy of persistent rotator cuff tendinitis. Lancet *1*:695–698, 1984.
31. Bjorkenheim JM, Paavolainen P, Ahovuo J, and Slatis P: Subacromial impingement decompressed with anterior acromioplasty. Clin Orthop *252*:150–155, 1990.
32. Bokor DJ, Hawkins RJ, Huckell GH, et al: Results of nonoperative management of full-thickness tears of the rotator cuff. Clin Orthop *294*:103–110, 1993.
33. Bosley RC: Total acromionectomy: A twenty-year review. J Bone Joint Surg *73*:961–968, 1991.
34. Bosworth DM: An analysis of twenty-eight consecutive cases of incapacitating shoulder lesions, radically explored and repaired. J Bone Joint Surg *22*:369–392, 1940.
35. Bosworth DM: The supraspinatus syndrome—symptomatology, pathology, and repair. JAMA *117*:422, 1941.
36. Brems JJ: Digital Muscle Strength Measurement in Rotator Cuff Tears. Paper presented at the ASES 3rd Open Meeting, San Francisco, 1987.
37. Brenneke SL and Morgan CJ: Evaluation of ultrasonography as a diagnostic technique in the assessment of rotator cuff tendon tears. Am J Sports Med *20*:287–289, 1992.
38. Brewer BJ: Aging of the rotator cuff. Am J Sports Med *7*:102–110, 1979.
39. Brogi M, Laterza A, and Neri C: Entrapment neuropathy of the suprascapular nerve. Riv Neurobiol *25*:318, 1979.
40. Brooks CH, Revell WJ, and Heatley FW: A quantitative histological study of the vascularity of the rotator cuff tendon. J Bone Joint Surg Br *74*:151–153, 1992.
41. Brown JT: Early assessment of supraspinatus tears: Procaine infiltration as a guide to treatment. J Bone Joint Surg *31B*:423, 1949.
42. Brownlee C and Cofield MD: Shoulder Replacement in Cuff Tear Arthropathy. Paper presented at ASES meeting, New Orleans, 1986.
43. Brox JI, Staff PH, Ljunggren AE, and Brevik JI: Arthroscopic surgery compared with supervised exercises in patients with rotator cuff disease (stage II impingement syndrome). BMJ *307*(6909):899–903, 1993.
44. Burkhart SS: Arthroscopic treatment of massive rotator cuff tears. Clin Orthop *267*:45–46, 1991.
45. Burkhart SS, Fischer SP, Nottage WM, et al: Tissue fixation security in transosseous rotator cuff repairs: A mechanical comparison of simple versus mattress sutures. Arthroscopy (in press).
46. Burkhart SS, Nottage WM, Ogilvie-Harris DJ, et al: Partial repair of irreparable rotator cuff tears. Arthroscopy *10*:363–370, 1994.
47. Burns TP and Turba JE: Arthroscopic treatment of the shoulder impingement in athletes. Am J Sports Med *20*:13–16, 1992.
48. Burns WC and Whipple TL: Anatomic relationships in the shoulder impingement syndrome. Clin Orthop *294*:96–102, 1993.
49. Bush LF: The torn shoulder capsule. J Bone Joint Surg Am *57A*:256–259, 1975.
50. Calvert PT, Packer NP, Stoker DJ, et al: Arthrography of the shoulder after operative repair of the torn rotator cuff. J Bone Joint Surg Br *68B*:147–150, 1986.
51. Cammerer U, Habermeyer P, Plenk A, and Huber R: Ultrasound assessment of recontructed rotator cuffs. Unfallchirurg *95*:608–12, 1992.
52. Chakravarty K and Webley M: Shoulder joint movement and its relationship to disability in the elderly. J Rheum *20*:1359–1361, 1993.
53. Chard MD, Hazleman R, Hazleman BL, et al: Shoulder disorders in the elderly: A community survey. Arthritis Rheum *34*:766–769, 1991.
54. Chiodi E and Morini G: Lesions of the rotator cuff: Diagnostic validity of echography. Surgical findings. Radiol Med *88*:733–735, 1994.
55. Chung SMK and Nissenbaum MM: Congenital and developmental defects of the shoulder. Orthop Clin North Am *6*:382, 1975.
56. Clark JC: Fibrous Anatomy of the Rotator Cuff. Abstract presented to the American Academy of Orthopaedic Surgeons, 1988.
57. Clark JM and Harryman II DT: Tendons, ligaments, and capsule of the rotator cuff. Gross and microscopic anatomy. J Bone Joint Surg *74-A*:713–725, 1992.
58. Clark JM, Sidles JA, and Matsen III FA: The relationship of the glenohumeral joint capsule to the rotator cuff. Clin Orthop *254*:29–34, 1990.
59. Clein LJ: Suprascapular entrapment neuropathy. J Neurosurg *43*:337–342, 1975.
60. Codman EA: Complete rupture of the supraspinatus tendon: Operative treatment with report of two successful cases. Boston Med Surg J *164*:708–710, 1911.
61. Codman EA: The Shoulder, Rupture of the Supraspinatus Tendon and Other Lesions In or About the Subacromial Bursa. Boston: Thomas Todd, 1934.
62. Codman EA: The Shoulder, Rupture of the Supraspinatus Tendon and Other Lesions In or About the Subacromial Bursa. Boston: Thomas Todd, 1934.
63. Codman EA: Rupture of the supraspinatus—1834–1934. J Bone Joint Surg *19*:643–652, 1937.
64. Codman EA: Rupture of the supraspinatus tendon. *In* The Shoulder: Rupture of the Supraspinatus Tendon and Other Lesions In or About the Subacromial Bursa. Malabar, FL: Robert E Krieger, supplement edition, 1984, pp 123–177.
65. Cofield RH: Tears of rotator cuff. Instr Course Lect *30*:258–273, 1981.
66. Cofield RH: Subscapular muscle transposition for repair of chronic rotator cuff tears. Surg Gynecol Obstet *154*:667–672, 1982.
67. Cofield RH: Current concepts review: Rotator cuff disease of the shoulder. J Bone Joint Surg *67A*:974–979, 1985.
68. Cofield RH: Glenohumeral Arthroplasty for Rheumatoid Arthritis: Incidence of Rotator Cuff Tears. 54th Annual Meeting of the American Academy of Orthopaedic Surgeons, San Francisco, 1987.
69. Cofield RH and Simonet WT: Symposium on sports medicine. Part 2. The Shoulder in Sports. Mayo Clin Proc *59*:157–164, 1984.
70. Colachis SCJ and Strohm BR: Effect of suprascapular and axillary nerve blocks and muscle force in upper extremity. Arch Phys Med Rehabil *52*:22, 1971.
71. Colachis SCJ, Strohm BR, and Brechner VL: Effects of axillary nerve block on muscle force in the upper extremity. Arch Phys Med Rehabil *50*:647, 1969.
72. Colley F: Die Periarthritis humeroscapularis. Rose E and Helferich von FCW. Leipzig, 1899.
73. Collins RA, Gristina AG, Carter RE, et al: Ultrasonography of the shoulder. Orthop Clin North Am *18*:351, 1987.

74. Connolly JF: Humeral head defects associated with shoulder dislocations—their diagnostic and surgical significance. Instr Course Lect *21*:42, 1972.
75. Coomcs EN and Darlington LG: Effects of local steroid injection for supraspinatus tears: Controlled study. Ann Rheum Dis *35*: 943, 1976.
76. Cotton RE and Rideout D: Tears of the humeral rotator cuff: A radiological and pathological necropsy survey. J Bone Joint Surg *46(B)*:314–328, 1964.
77. Craig EV: The geyser sign and torn rotator cuff: Clinical significance and pathomechanics. Clin Orthop *191*:213–215, 1984.
78. Crass JR and Craig EV: Noninvasive imaging of the rotator cuff. Orthopaedics *11*:57–64, 1988.
79. Crass JR, Craig EV, Bretzke C, et al: Ultrasonography of the rotator cuff. Radiographics *5*:941–953, 1985.
80. Crass JR, Craig EV, and Feinberg SB: Sonography of the postoperative rotator cuff. AJR *146*:561–564, 1986.
81. Crass JR, Craig EV, Thompason RC, et al: Ultrasonography of the rotator cuff: Surgical correlation. J Clin Ultrasound *12*:497–491, 1984.
82. Cruess RL, Blennerhassett J, and MacDonald FR: Aseptic necrosis following renal transplantation J Bone Joint Surg 50A:1577, 1968.
83. D'Erme M, DeCupis V, DeMaria M, et al: Echography, magnetic resonance and double-contrast arthrography of the rotator cuff. A prospective study in 30 patients. Radiol Med *86*:72–80, 1993.
84. Dalton S, Cawston TE, Riley GP, et al: Human shoulder tendon biopsy samples in organ culture produce procollagenase and tissue inhibitor of metalloproteinases. Ann Rheum Dis *54*:571–577, 1995.
85. Darlington LG and Coomes EN: The effects of local steroid injection for supraspinatus tears. Rheumatol Rehabil *16*:172–179, 1977.
86. Debeyre J, Patte D, and Emelik E: Repair of ruptures of the rotator cuff with a note on advancement of the supraspinatus muscle. J Bone Joint Surg *47B*:36–42, 1965.
87. DeOrio JK and Cofield RH: Results of a second attempt at surgical repair of a failed initial rotator cuff repair. J Bone Joint Surg *66A*:563–567, 1984.
88. DePalma AF: Surgical anatomy of the rotator cuff and the natural history of degenerative periarthritis. Surg Clin North Am *43*:1507–1520, 1967.
89. DePalma AF: Surgery of the Shoulder, 2nd ed. Philadelphia: JB Lippincott, pp 206–210, 229, 234–235, 1973.
90. DePalma AF: Surgery of the Shoulder, 3rd ed. Philadelphia: JB Lippincott, 1983.
91. DePalma AF, Gallery G, and Bennett CA: Variational anatomy and degenerative lesions of the shoulder joint. AAOS Instr Course Lect *6*:255–281, 1949.
92. DePalma AF, White JB, and Callery G: Degenerative lesions of the shoulder joint at various age groups which are compatible with good function. AAOS Instr Course Lect, 1950.
93. Desché: Contribution à l'étude au traitement de la periarthrite scapulohumerale. Paris, p 1892.
94. Desplats H: De L'atrophie musculaire dans la péri-arthrite scapulo humérale. Gazette Hebdomadaire de Médicine et de Chir *24*:371, 1878.
95. Diamond B: The Obstructing Acromion. Springfield, IL: Charles C Thomas, 1964.
96. Dierickx C and Vanhoof H: Massive rotator cuff tears treated by a deltoid muscular inlay flap. Acta Orthop Belg *60*:94–100, 1994.
97. Donovan WH and Kraft GH: Rotator cuff tear vs. suprascapular nerve injury. Arch Phys Med Rehabil 55:424, 1974.
98. Drakeford MK, Quinn MJ, Simpson SL, and Pettine KA: A comparative study of ultrasonography in evaluation of the rotator cuff. Clin Orthop *253*:118–122, 1990.
99. Drez D: Suprascapular neuropathy in the differential diagnosis of rotator cuff injury. Am J Sports Med *4*:43, 1976.
100. Duplay: Arch Gén Méd 2:513, 1872.
101. Duronea: Essai sur la scapulalgie. 1873.
102. Earnshaw P, Desjardins D, Sarkar K, and Uhthoff HK: Rotator cuff tears: The role of surgery. Can J Surg *25*:60–63, 1982.
103. Edeland HG and Zachrisson BE: Fracture of the scapular notch associated with lesion of the suprascapular nerve. Acta Orthop Scand *46*:758–763, 1975.
104. Ellman H: Arthroscopic subacromial decompression: Analysis of one- to three-year results. J Arthrosc Rel Surg 3:173–181, 1987.
105. Ellman H: Arthroscopic subacromial decompression: Analysis of one- to three-year results. Arthroscopy 3:173–181, 1988.
106. Ellman H, Hanker G, and Bayer M: Repair of the rotator cuff: End-result study of factors influencing reconstruction. J Bone Joint Surg *68(A)*:1136–1144, 1986.
107. Ellman H and Kay SP: Arthroscopic subacromial decompression 2–5 year results. Orthop Trans *13*:239, 1989.
108. Ellman H and Kay SP: Arthroscopic subacromial decompression for chronic impingement: Two to five year results. J Bone Joint Surg *73(B)*:395–398, 1991.
109. Ellman H, Kay SP, and Wirth M: Arthroscopic treatment of full thickness rotator cuff tears: Two to seven year follow-up study. Arthroscopy 9:195–200, 1993.
110. Esch JC, Ozerkis LR, Helgager JA, et al: Arthroscopic subacromial decompression: Results according to degree of rotator cuff. Arthroscopy *4*:241–249, 1988.
111. Esslen E, Flachsmann H, Bischoff A, et al: Die Einklemmungsneuropathie des N. Suprascapularis: Eine Klinisch-Therapeutische Studie. Nervenarzt *38*:311–314, 1967.
112. Farin PU and Jaroma H: Acute traumatic tears of the rotator cuff: Value of sonography. Radiology *197*:269–273, 1995.
113. Farin PU and Jaroma H: Digital subtraction shoulder arthrography in determining site and size of rotator cuff tear. Invest Radiol *30*:544–547, 1995.
114. Farrer IL, Matsen FAI, Rogers JV, et al: Dynamic Sonographic Study of Lesion of the Rotator Cuff (Abstract). Paper presented at the American Academy of Orthopedic Surgeons 50th Annual Meeting, Anaheim, CA, 1983.
115. Ferrari JD, Ferrari JA, Coumas J, and Pappas AM: Posterior ossification of the shoulder: The Bennett lesion. Etiology, diagnosis, and treatment. Am J Sports Med *22*:171–175, 1994.
116. Flanders M: Shoulder muscle activity during natural arm movements: What is optimized? *In* Matsen FA III, Fu FH, and Hawkins RJ (eds): The Shoulder: A Balance of Mobility and Stability. Rosemont, IL: American Academy of Orthopaedic Surgeons, 1993, pp 635–646.
117. Flatow EL, Raimondo RA, Kelkar R, et al: Active and Passive Restraints Against Superior Humeral Translation: The Contributions of the Rotator Cuff, the Biceps Tendon, and the Coracoacromial Arch. 12th Open Meeting, American Shoulder and Elbow Surgeons, Atlanta, GA, 1996.
118. Flatow EL, Soslowsky LJ, Ticker JB, et al: Excursion of the rotator cuff under the acromion. Patterns of subacromial contact. Am J Sports Med 22:779–788, 1994.
119. Flugstad D, Matsen III FA, Larry I, and Jackins SE: Failed Acromioplasty and the Treatment of the Impingement Syndrome. Paper presented at ASES, 2nd Open Meeting, New Orleans, 1986.
120. Ford LT and DeBender J: Tendon rupture after local steroid injection. South Med J 72:827–830, 1979.
121. Fowler P: Swimmer problems. Am J Sports Med 7:141–142, 1979.
122. Frank CB: Ligament healing: Current knowledge and clinical applications. J Am Acad Orthop Surg *4*:74–83, 1996.
123. Franklin JL, Barrett WP, Jackins SE, and Matsen FA, III: Glenoid loosening in total shoulder arthroplasty; association with rotator cuff deficiency. J Arthroplasty *3*:39–46, 1988.
124. Freiberger RH, Kaye JJ, and Spiller J: Arthrography. New York: Appleton-Century-Crofts, 1979.
125. Fukuda H: Rotator cuff tears. Geka Chiryo (Osaka) *43*:28, 1980.
126. Fukuda H, Hamada K, Nakajima T, and Tomonaga A: Pathology and pathogenesis of the intratendinous tearing of the rotator cuff viewed from en bloc histologic sections. Clin Orthop *304*:60–67, 1994.
127. Fukuda H, Hamada K, and Yamanada K: Pathology and pathogenesis of bursal side rotator cuff tears viewed from en bloc histologic sections. Clin Orthop *254*:75–80, 1990.
128. Fukuda H, Mikasa M, Ogawa K, et al: The partial thickness tear of rotator cuff. Orthop Trans *7*:137, 1983.
129. Fukuda H, Mikasa M, and Yamanaka K: Incomplete thickness rotator cuff tears diagnosed by subacromial bursography. Clin Orthop *223*:51–58, 1987.
130. Gartsman GM: Arthroscopic Treatment of Stage II Subacromial Impingement. Paper presented at ASES, 4th meeting, Atlanta, 1988.
131. Gartsman GM: Arthroscopic acromioplasty for lesion of the rotator cuff. J Bone Joint Surg *72(A)*:169–180, 1990.

132. Gartsman GM, Blair ME, Noble PC, et al: Arthroscopic subacromial decompression: An anatomical study. Am J Sports Med *16*:48–50, 1988.
133. Gazielly DF, Gleyze P, and Montagnon C: Functional and anatomical results after rotator cuff repair. Clin Orthop *304*:43–53, 1994.
134. Gazielly DF, Gleyze P, Montagnon C, et al: Functional and anatomical results after surgical treatment of ruptures of the rotator cuff. 1. Preoperative functional and anatomical evaluation of ruptures of the rotator cuff. Rev Chir Orthop Reparatrice Appar Mot *81*:8–16, 1995.
135. Gazielly DF, Gleyze P, Montagnon C, et al: Functional and anatomical results after surgical treatment of ruptures of the rotator cuff. 2. Postoperative functional and anatomical evaluation of ruptures of the rotator cuff. Rev Chir Orthop Reparatrice Appar Mot *81*:17–26, 1995.
136. Gelmers HJ and Buys DA: Suprascapular entrapment neuropathy. Acta Neurochir (Wien) *38*:121–124, 1977.
137. Gerber C: Latissimus dorsi transfer for the treatment of irreparable tears of the rotator cuff. Clin Orthop *275*:152–160, 1992.
138. Gerber C, Schneeberger AG, Beck M, and Schlegel U: Mechanical strength of repairs of the rotator cuff. J Bone Joint Surg *76*:371–380, 1994.
139. Gerber C, Terrier F, and Ganz R: The role of the coracoid process in the chronic impingement syndrome. J Bone Joint Surg *67B*:703–708, 1985.
140. Ghelman B and Goldman AB: The double contrast shoulder arthrogram: Evaluation of rotary cuff tears. Radiology *124*:251–254, 1977.
141. Godsil RD and Linscheid RL: Intratendinous defects of the rotator cuff. Clin Orthop *69*:181–188, 1970.
142. Goldman AB, Dines DM, and Warren RF: Shoulder Arthrography. *In* Technique, Diagnosis and Clinical Correlation. Boston: Little, Brown, 1982, pp 1–3.
143. Goldman AB and Gehlman B: The double-contrast shoulder arthrogram. Radiology *127*:655–663, 1978.
144. Gore DR, Murray MP, Sepic SB, et al: Shoulder-muscle strength and range of motion following surgical repair of full-thickness rotator cuff tears. J Bone Joint Surg *68*:266–272, 1986.
145. Goutallier D, Postel JM, Bernageau J, et al: Fatty muscle degeneration in cuff ruptures. Pre- and postoperative evaluation by CT scan. Clin Orthop *304*:78–83, 1994.
146. Goutallier D, Postel JM, Bernageau J, et al: Fatty infiltration of disrupted rotator cuff muscles. Rev Rhum Engl Ed *62*:415–422, 1995.
147. Grana WA, Teague B, King M, and Reeves RB: An analysis of rotator cuff repair. Am J Sports Med *22*:585–588, 1994.
148. Grant JCB: Grant's Atlas of Anatomy, 6th ed. Baltimore: Williams & Wilkins, 1972.
149. Grant JCB and Smith CG: Age incidence of rupture of the supraspinatus tendon (Abstract). Anat Rec *100*:666, 1948.
150. Grigg P: The role of capsular feedback and pattern generators in shoulder kinematics. *In* Matsen FA III, Fu FH, and Hawkins RJ (eds): The Shoulder: A Balance of Mobility and Stability. Rosemont, IL: American Academy of Orthopaedic Surgeons, 1993, pp 173–184.
151. Ha'eri GB, Orth MC, and Wiley AM: Shoulder impingement syndrome. Clin Orthop *168*:128–132, 1982.
152. Ha'eri GB and Wiley AM: An extensile exposure for subacromial derangements. Can J Surg *23*:458–461, 1980.
153. Ha'eri GB and Wiley AM: Advancement of the supraspinatus muscle in the repair of ruptures of the rotator cuff. J Bone Joint Surg *63A*:232–238, 1981.
154. Hamada K, Okawara Y, Fryer JN, et al: Localization of mRNA of procollagen alpha 1 type I in torn supraspinatus tendons. In situ hybridization using digoxigenin labeled oligonucleotide probe. Clin Orthop *304*:18–21, 1994.
155. Hammond G: Complete acromionectomy in the treatment of chronic tendinitis of the shoulder. J Bone Joint Surg *44A*:494–504, 1962.
156. Hammond G: Complete acromionectomy in the treatment of chronic tendinitis of the shoulder. A follow-up of ninety operations of eighty-seven patients. J Bone Joint Surg *53A*:173–180, 1971.
157. Harryman DT II, Mack LA, Wang KY, et al: Repairs of the rotator cuff. J Bone Joint Surg *73-A*:982–989, 1991.
158. Harryman DT II, Matsen FA III, and Sidles JA: Arthroscopic management of refractory shoulder stiffness. J Arthrosc (in press).
159. Harryman DT II, Sidles JA, Clark JM, et al: Translation of the humeral head on the glenoid with passive glenohumeral motion. J Bone Joint Surg *72A*:1334–1342, 1990.
160. Haudek: Wien klin Wochenschr 43, 1911.
161. Hawkins RH and Dunlop R: Nonoperative treatment of rotator cuff tears. Clin Orthop *321*:178–188, 1995.
162. Hawkins RJ and Brock RM: Anterior acromioplasty: early results for impingement with intact rotator cuff. Orthop Trans *3*:274, 1979.
163. Hawkins RJ, Chris AD, and Kiefer G: Failed Anterior Acromioplasty. Paper presented at ASES, 3rd meeting, San Francisco, 1987.
164. Hawkins RJ and Kennedy JC: Impingement syndrome in athletes. Am J Sports Med *8*:151–158, 1980.
165. Hawkins RJ, Misamore GW, and Hobeika PE: Surgery of full thickness rotator cuff tears. J Bone Joint Surg *67A*:1349–1355, 1985.
166. Hawkins RJ, Saddamis S, Moor J, et al: Arthroscopic Subacromial Decompression: A Two-to-Four-Year Follow-up. Presented at the Annual Meeting of Arthroscopy Association of North America, 1992.
167. Hazlett JW: Tears of the rotator cuff. *In* Proceedings of the Dewar Orthopaedic Club. J Bone Joint Surg *53B*:772, 1971.
168. Hedtmann A and Fett H: Ultrasonography of the shoulder in subacromial syndromes with disorders and injuries of the rotator cuff. Orthopade *24*:498–508, 1995.
169. Heikel HVA: Rupture of the rotator cuff of the shoulder: Experiences of surgical treatment. Acta Orthop Scand *39*:477–492, 1968.
170. Heineke: Die Anatomie und Pathologie der Schleimbeutel und Sehnenscheiden. Erlangen, 1868.
171. Hollingworth GR, Ellis RM, and Hattersley TS: Comparison of injection techniques for shoulder pain: results of a double blind, randomized study. BMJ *287*:1339–1341, 1983.
172. Hollis JM, Lyon RM, Marcin JP, et al: Effect of age and loading axis on the failure properties of the human ACL. *In* Transactions of 34th Annual Meeting, Orthopedic Research Society, Atlanta, Georgia, 1988.
173. Hollister MS, Mack LA, Patten RM, et al: Association of sonographically detected subacromial/subdeltoid bursal effusion and intraarticular fluid with rotator cuff tear. Am J Roentgenol *165*:605–608, 1995.
174. Holzknecht G: Uber Bursitis mit Konkrementbildung. Wien Med Wochenschr *43*:2757, 1911.
175. Howell SM, Imobersteg AM, Segar DH, and Marone PJ: Clarification of the role of the supraspinatus muscle in shoulder function. J Bone Joint Surg *68*:398–404, 1986.
176. Iannotti J: Full-thickness rotator cuff tears: Factors affecting surgical outcome. J Am Acad Orthop Surg *2*:87–95, 1994.
177. Iannotti JP, Zlatkin MB, Esterhai JL, et al: Magnetic resonance imaging of the shoulder. Sensitivity, specificity, and predictive value. J Bone Joint Surg *73*:17–29, 1991.
178. Inman VT, Saunders JBDCM, and Abbott LC: Observations on the function of the shoulder joint. J Bone Joint Surg *26A*:1–30, 1944.
179. Ismail AM, Balakishnan R, and Rajakumar MK: Rupture of patellar ligament after steroid infiltration. J Bone Joint Surg *51B*:503, 1969.
180. Itoi E, Berglund LJ, Grabowski JJ, et al: Tensile properties of the supraspinatus tendon. J Orthop Res *13*:578–584, 1995.
181. Itoi E and Tabata S: Conservative treatment of rotator cuff tears. Clin Orthop *275*:165–173, 1992.
182. Itoi E and Tabata S: Incomplete rotator cuff tears. Results of operative treatment. Clin Orthop *284*:128–135, 1992.
183. Jackson DL, Farrage J, Hynninen BC, and Caborn DN: Suprascapular neuropathy in athletes: Case reports. Clin J Sports Med *5*:134–136, 1995.
184. Jackson DW: Chronic rotator cuff impingement in the throwing athlete. Am J Sports Med *4*:231–240, 1976.
185. Jarjavay JF: Sur la luxation du tendon de la longue portion du muscle biceps humeral; sur la luxation des tendons des muscles peroniers latéraux. Gazette Hebdomadaire de Médecine et de Chir *21*:325, 1867.
186. Jens J: The role of the subscapularis muscle in recurring dislocation of the shoulder (Abstract). J Bone Joint Surg *34B*:780, 1964.
187. Jobe CM: Posterior superior glenoid impingement: Expanded spectrum. Arthroscopy *11*:530–536, 1995.

188. Jobe FW and Kvitne RS: Shoulder pain in the overhand or throwing athlete. Orthop Rev *18*:963–975, 1989.
189. Jobe FW and Moynes DR: Delineation of diagnostic criteria and a rehabilitation program for rotator cuff injuries. Am J Sports Med *10*:336–339, 1982.
190. Joessel D: Uber die Recidine der Humerus-Luxationen. Dtsch Ztschr Chir *13*:167–184, 1880.
191. Johansson JE and Barrington TW: Coracoacromial ligament division. Am J Sports Med *12*:138–141, 1984.
192. Julliard: La coracoidite. Rev Med Suisse Romande *12*:47, 1933.
193. Kaneko K, DeMouy EH, and Brunet ME: Massive rotator cuff tears. Screening by routine radiographs. Clin Imaging *19*:8–11, 1995.
194. Kannus P, Leppala J, Lehto M, et al: A rotator cuff rupture produces permanent osteoporosis in the affected extremity, but not in the those with whom shoulder function has returned to normal. J Bone Miner Res *10*:1263–1271, 1995.
195. Karas SE and Giachello TA: Subscapularis transfer for reconstruction of massive tears of the rotator cuff. J Bone Joint Surg *78-A*:239–245, 1996.
196. Kennedy JC and Willis RB: The effects of local steroid injections on tendons: A biomechanical and microscopic correlative study. Am J Sports Med *4*:11–21, 1976.
197. Kerlan RK, Jobe FW, and Blazina ME: Throwing injuries of the shoulder and elbow in adults, Vol 6. St. Louis: CV Mosby, 1975.
198. Kernwein GA, Roseberg B, and Sneed WR: Aids in the differential diagnosis of the painful shoulder syndrome. Clin Orthop *20*:11–20, 1961.
199. Kerwein GH, Rosenburg B, and Sneed WR: Arthrographic studies of the shoulder joint. J Bone Joint Surg *39A*:1267–1279, 1957.
200. Kessel L and Watson M: The painful arc syndrome. Clinical classification as a guide to management. J Bone Joint Surg *59B*:166–172, 1977.
201. Keyes EL: Observations on rupture of supraspinatus tendon. Based upon a study of 73 cadavers. Ann Surg *97*:849–856, 1933.
202. Keyes EL: Anatomical observations on senile changes in the shoulder. J Bone Joint Surg Am *17*:953, 1935.
203. Kieft GJ, Bloem JL, Rozing PM, and Oberman WR: Rotator cuff impingement syndrome: MR imaging. Radiology *166*:211–214, 1988.
204. Kilcoyne RF and Matsen FA III: Rotator cuff tear measurement by arthropneumotomography. AJR Am J Roentgenol *140*:315–318, 1983.
205. Killoran PJ, Marcove RC, and Freiberger RH: Shoulder arthroscopy. Am J Roentgenol *103*:658–668, 1968.
206. Kirschenbaum D, Coyle MPJ, Leddy JP, et al: Shoulder strength with rotator cuff tears. Pre- and postoperative analysis. Clin Orthop *288*:174–178, 1993.
207. Kneeland JB, Middleton WD, and Carnera GF: MR imaging of the shoulder: Diagnosis of rotator cuff tears. AJR Am J Roentgenol *149*:333–337, 1987.
208. Komar J: Eine Wichtige Urasache des Schulterschmerzes: Incisurascapulae-Syndrom. Fortschr Neurol Psychiatr *44*:644–648, 1976.
209. Kopell HP and Thompson WAL: Suprascapular nerve. *In* Peripheral Entrapment Neuropathies. Baltimore: Williams & Wilkins, 1963, pp 130–142.
210. Kumagai J, Sarkar K, and Uhthoff HK: The collagen types in the attachment zone of rotator cuff tendons in the elderly: An immunohistochemical study. J Rheumatol *21*:2096–2100, 1994.
211. Kuster E: Ueber habituelle Schutter Luxation. Verh Dtsch Ges Chir *11*:112–114, 1882.
212. Kutsuma T, Akaoka K, Kinoshita H, et al: The results of surgical management of rotator cuff tear. The Shoulder Joint *6*:136, 1982.
213. Laing PG: The arterial supply of the adult humerus. J Bone Joint Surg *38(A)*:1105–1116, 1956.
214. Lazarus MD, Harryman II DT, Yung SW, et al: Anterosuperior Humeral Displacement: Limitation by the Coracoacromial Arch. AAOS Annual Meeting, Orlando, FL, 1995.
215. Lee HB: Avulsion and rupture of the tendo calcaneus after injection of hydrocortisone. BMJ *2*:395, 1957.
216. Lee PN, Lee M, Haq AMMM, et al: Periarthritis of the shoulder. Ann Rheum Dis *33*:116–119, 1974.
217. Lehman C, Cuomo F, Kummer FJ, and Zuckerman JD: The incidence of full thickness rotator cuff tears in a large cadaveric population. Bull Hosp Jt Dis *54*:30–31, 1995.
218. Leivseth G and Reikeras O: Changes in muscle fiber cross-sectional area and concentrations of Na, K-ATPase in deltoid muscle in patients with impingement syndrome of the shoulder. J Orthop Sports Phys Ther *19*:146–149, 1994.
219. Leroux JL, Codine P, Thomas E, et al: Isokinetic evaluation of rotational strength in normal shoulders and shoulders with impingement syndrome. Clin Orthop *304*:108–115, 1994.
220. Leroux JL, Thomas E, Bonnel F, and Blotman F: Diagnostic value of clinical tests for shoulder impingement syndrome. Rev Rhum Engl Ed *62*:423–428, 1995.
221. Levy HJ, Gardner RD, and Lemak LJ: Arthroscopic subacromial decompression in the treatment of full thickness rotator tears. Arthroscopy *7*:8–13, 1991.
222. Levy HJ, Urie JW, and Delaney LG: Arthroscopic-assisted rotator cuff repair: Preliminary results. Arthroscopy *6*:55–60, 1990.
223. Liberson F: Os acromiale—a contested anomaly. J Bone Joint Surg *19*:683–689, 1937.
224. Lie S and Mast WA: Subacromial bursography: Technique and clinical application. Tech Dev Instrum *144*:626–630, 1982.
225. Lieber RL: Skeletal Muscle Structure and Function. Baltimore: Williams & Wilkins, 1992, p 314.
226. Lieber RL and Friden J: Neuromuscular stablization of the shoulder girdle. *In* Matsen FA III, Fu FH, and Hawkins RJ (eds): The Shoulder: A Balance of Mobility and Stability. Rosemont, IL: American Academy of Orthopaedic Surgeons, 1993, pp 91–106.
227. Lilleby H: Shoulder arthroscopy. Acta Orthop Scand *55*:561–566, 1984.
228. Lindblom K: Arthrography and roentgenography in ruptures of the tendon of the shoulder joint. Acta Radiol *20*:548, 1939.
229. Lindblom K: On pathogenesis of ruptures of the tendon aponeurosis of the shoulder joint. Acta Radiol *20*:563, 1939.
230. Lindblom K and Palmer I: Ruptures of the tendon aponeurosis of the shoulder joint—the so-called supraspinatus ruptures. Acta Chir Scand *82*:133–142, 1939.
231. Liu SH: Arthroscopically assisted rotator cuff repair. J Bone Joint Surg *76(B)*:592–595, 1994.
232. Liu SH and Boynton E: Posterior superior impingement of the rotator cuff on the glenoid rim as a cause of shoulder pain in the overhead athlete. Arthroscopy *9*:697–699, 1993.
233. Lohr JF and Uhthoff HK: The microvascular pattern of the supraspinatus tendon. Clin Orthop *254*:35–38, 1990.
234. Lund IM, Donde R, and Knudsen EA: Persistent local cutaneous atrophy following corticosteroid injection for tendinitis. Rheumatol Rehab *18*:91–93, 1979.
235. Lundberg BJ: The correlation of clinical evaluation with operative findings and prognosis in rotator cuff rupture. *In* Bayley I and Kessel L (eds): Shoulder Surgery. Berlin: Springer-Verlag, 1982, pp 35–38.
236. Luopajarvi T, Kuorinka I, Virolainen M, and Holmberg M: Prevalence of tenosynovitis and other injuries of the upper extremities in repetitive work. Scand J Work Environ Health *5*:48–55, 1979.
237. Mack LA and Matsen III FA: Rotator cuff. Clin Diagn Ultrasound *30*:113–133, 1995.
238. Mack LA, Matsen III FA, and Kilcoyne RF: Ultrasound: US evaluation of the rotator cuff. Radiology *157*:205–209, 1985.
239. Mack LA, Nuberg DS, Matsen FA III, et al: Sonography of the Postoperative Shoulder (Abstract). Paper presented at American Roentgen Ray Society Annual Meeting, Miami Beach, Florida, 1987.
240. Mack LA, Nyberg DA, and Matsen III FA: Sonography of the postoperative shoulder. AJR Am J Roentgenol *150*:1089–1093, 1988.
241. Macnab I: Rotator cuff tendinitis. Ann R Coll Surg Engl 53:271–287, 1973.
242. Macnab I and Hastings D: Rotator cuff tendinitis. Can Med Assoc J 99:91–98, 1968.
243. Mankin HJ and Conger KA: The acute effects of intra-articular hydrocortisone on articular cartilage in rabbits. J Bone Joint Surg 48A:1383, 1966.
244. Matsen FA, III, Lippitt SB, Sidles JA, and Harryman DT, II: Practical Evaluation and Management of the Shoulder. Philadelphia: WB Saunders, 1994, pp 1–242.
245. Matthews LS, Sonstegard DA, and Phelps DB: A biomechanical study of rabbit patellar tendon: effects of steroid injection. J Sports Med 2:9, 1974.

246. McCarty DJ, Haverson PB, Carrera GF, et al: "Milwaukee Shoulder": Association of microspheroids containing hydroxyapatite crystals, active collagenase, and neutral protease with rotator cuff defects. I. Clinical aspects. Arthritis Rheum *24*:353–354, 1981.
247. McLaughlin HL: Lesions of the musculotendinous cuff of the shoulder. I. The exposure and treatment of tears with retraction. J Bone Joint Surg *26*:31–51, 1944.
248. McLaughlin HL: Rupture of the rotator cuff. J Bone Joint Surg *44A*:979–983, 1962.
249. McLaughlin HL: Repair of major cuff ruptures. Surg Clin North Am *43*:1535–1540, 1963.
250. McLaughlin HL: Lesions of the musculotendinous cuff of the shoulder. The exposure and treatment of tears with retraction. Clin Orthop *304*:3–9, 1994.
251. McLaughlin HL and Asherman EG: Lesions of the musculotendinous cuff of the shoulder. IV. Some observations based upon the results of surgical repair. J Bone Joint Surg *33A*:76–86, 1951.
252. McMaster PE: Tendon and muscle ruptures: Clinical and experimental studies on the causes and location of subcutaneous ruptures. J Bone Joint Surg *15A*:705–722, 1933.
253. Melmed EP: Spontaneous bilateral rupture of the calcaneal tendon during steroid therapy. J Bone Joint Surg *47B*:104, 1965.
254. Meyer and Kessler: Strassbourg Méd *2*:205, 1926.
255. Meyer AW: Further evidence of attrition in the human body. Am J Anat *34*:241–267, 1924.
256. Meyer AW: The minute anatomy of attrition lesions. J Bone Joint Surg *13A*:341, 1931.
257. Michelsson JE and Bakalim G: Resection of the acromion in the treatment of persistent rotator cuff syndrome of the shoulder. Acta Orthop Scand *48*:607–611, 1977.
258. Middleton WD: Ultrasonography of rotator cuff pathology. Top Magn Reson Imaging *6*:133–138, 1994.
259. Middleton WD, Edelstein G, Reinus WR, et al: Sonographic detection of rotator cuff tears. AJR Am J Roentgenol *144*:349–353, 1985.
260. Middleton WD, Reinus WR, Melson GL, et al: Pitfalls of rotator cuff sonography. AJR Am J Roentgenol *146*:555–560, 1986.
261. Middleton WD, Reinus WR, Totty WG, et al: Ultrasonographic evaluation of the rotator cuff and biceps tendon. J Bone Joint Surg *68A*:440–450, 1986.
262. Mikasa M: Subacromial bursography. J Jpn Orthop Assoc *53*:225, 1979.
263. Milgrom C, Schaffler M, Gilbert S, and van Holsbeeck M: Rotator cuff changes in asymptomatic adults. The effect of age, hand dominance and gender. J Bone Joint Surg Br *77*:296–298, 1995.
264. Mink JH, Harris E, and Rappaport M: Rotator cuff tears: Evaluation using double-contrast shoulder arthrography. Radiology *153*:621–623, 1985.
265. Misamore GW, Ziegler DW, and Rushton II JL: Repair of the rotator cuff. A comparison of results in two populations of patients. J Bone Joint Surg *77*:1335–1339, 1995.
266. Montgomery TJ, Yerger B, and Savoie FH: Management of Full Thickness Tears of the Rotator Cuff: A Comparison of Arthroscopic Debridement with Open Repair. Presented at the 8th Annual Open Meeting of the American Shoulder and Elbow Surgeons, Washington, DC, 1992.
267. Morrison DS: The Use of Magnetic Resonance Imaging in the Diagnosis of Rotator Cuff Tears. Paper presented at ASES, 4th Meeting, Atlanta, 1988.
268. Morrison DS and Bigliani LU: The Clinical Significance of Variations in Acromial Morphology. Paper presented at ASES, 3rd Open Meeting, San Francisco, 1987.
269. Moseley HF: Ruptures to the Rotator Cuff. Springfield, IL: Charles C Thomas, 1952.
270. Moseley HF: Shoulder Lesions, 3rd ed. Edinburgh and London: Livingstone, 1969.
271. Moseley HF and Goldie I: The arterial pattern of the rotator cuff of the shoulder. J Bone Joint Surg *45B*:780, 1963.
272. Mudge MK, Wood VE, and Frykman GK: Rotator cuff tears associated with os acromiale. J Bone Joint Surg *66A*:427–429, 1984.
273. Murray JWG: A surgical approach for entrapment neuropathy of the suprascapular nerve. Orthop Rev *3*:33–35, 1974.
274. Nakagaki K, Tomita Y, Sakurai G, et al: Anatomical study on the atrophy of supraspinatus muscle belly with cuff tear. Nippon Seikeigeka Gakkai Zasshi *68*:516–521, 1994.
275. Neer CS II: Anterior acromioplasty for the chronic impingement syndrome in the shoulder: A preliminary report. J Bone Joint Surg *54A*:41–50, 1972.
276. Neer CS II: Unfused Acromial Epiphysis in Impingement and Cuff Tears. 45th Annual Meeting of the American Academy of Orthopaedic Surgeons, Dallas, 1978.
277. Neer CS II: Impingement lesions. Clin Orthop *173*:70–77, 1983.
278. Neer CS II: Shoulder Reconstruction. Philadelphia: WB Saunders, 1990, pp 73–77.
279. Neer CS II, Craig EV, and Fukuda H: Cuff-tear arthropathy. J Bone Joint Surg *65A*:1232–1244, 1983.
280. Neer CS II, Flatow EL, and Lech O: Tears of the Rotator Cuff. Long-Term Results of Anterior Acromioplasty and Repair. Paper presented at ASES 4th Meeting, Atlanta, GA, 1988.
281. Neer CS II and Marberry TA: On the disadvantages of radical acromionectomy. J Bone Joint Surg *63A*:416–419, 1981.
282. Neer CS II and Welsh RP: The shoulder in sports. Orthop Clin North Am *8*:583–591, 1977.
283. Nelson DH: Arthography of the shoulder. Br J Radiol *25*:134, 1952.
284. Neviaser JS: Ruptures of the rotator cuff of the shoulder. New concepts in the diagnosis and operative treatment of chronic ruptures. Arch Surg *102*:483–485, 1971.
285. Neviaser JS, Neviaser RJ, and Neviaser TJ: The repair of chronic massive ruptures of the rotator cuff of the shoulder by use of a freeze-dried rotator cuff. J Bone Joint Surg *60A*:681–684, 1978.
286. Neviaser RJ: Tears of the rotator cuff. Orthop Clin North Am *11*:295–306, 1980.
287. Neviaser RJ and Neviaser TJ: Transfer of subscapularis and teres minor for massive defects of rotator cuff. *In* Bayley I and Kessel L (eds): Shoulder Surgery. Berlin: Springer-Verlag, 1982, pp 60–63.
288. Neviaser RJ, Neviaser TJ, and Neviaser JS: Anterior dislocation of the shoulder and rotator cuff rupture. Clin Orthop *291*:103–106, 1993.
289. Neviaser TJ, Neviaser RJ, and Neviaser JS: Incomplete rotator cuff tears. A technique for diagnosis and treatment. Clin Orthop *306*:12–16, 1994.
290. Neviaser TJ, Neviaser RJ, and Neviaser JS: The four-in-one arthroplasty for the painful arc syndrome. Clin Orthop *163*:107–112, 1982.
291. Nicholson GP, Goodman DA, Flatow EA, and Bigliani LU: The acromion: Morphologic condition and age-related changes: A study of 420 scapulas. J Shoulder Elbow Surg 5:1–11, 1996.
292. Nixon JE and DiStefano V: Ruptures of the rotator cuff. Orthop Clin North Am *6*:423–447, 1975.
293. Nobuhara K, Hata Y, and Komai M: Surgical procedure and results of repair of massive tears of the rotator cuff. Clin Orthop *304*:54–59, 1994.
294. Norris TR, Fischer J, and Bigliani LU: The unfused acromial epiphysis and its relationship to impingement syndromes. Orthop Trans *7*:505, 1983.
295. Oberholtzer J: Die Arthropneumoradiographe bei habitueller Schulterluxatio. Röntgenpraxis *5*:589–590, 1933.
296. Ogata S and Uhthoff HK: Acromial enthesopathy and rotator cuff tear. A radiologic and histologic postmortem investigation of the coracoacromial arch. Clin Orthop *254*:39–48, 1990.
297. Ogilvie-Harris DJ and Wiley AM: Arthroscopic surgery of the shoulder: A general appraisal. J Bone Joint Surg *68(B)*:201–207, 1986.
298. Ogilvie-Harris DJ, Wiley AM, and Sattarian J: Failed acromioplasty for impingement syndrome. J Bone Joint Surg *72*:1070–1072, 1990.
299. Ogilvie-Harris DL and Demaziere A: Arthroscopic debridement versus open repair for rotator cuff tears. J Bone Joint Surg *75(B)*:416–420, 1993.
300. Okuda Y, Gorski JP, An KN, and Amadio PC: Biochemical histological and biochemical analysis of canine tendon. J Orthop Res *5*:60–68, 1987.
301. Olive RJJ and Marsh HO: Ultrasonography of rotator cuff tears. Clin Orthop 282:110–3, 1992.
302. Olsewski JM and Depew AD: Arthroscopic subacromial decompression and rotator cuff debridement for stage II and stage III impingement. Arthroscopy *10*:61–68, 1994.
303. Otis JC, Jiang CC, Wickiewicz TL, et al: Changes in the moment arms of the rotator cuff and deltoid muscles with abduction and rotation. J Bone Joint Surg *76*:667–676, 1994.
304. Owen RS, Iannotti JP, Kneeland JB, et al: Shoulder after surgery: MR imaging with surgical validation. Radiology *186*:443–447, 1993.

305. Ozaki J, Fujimoto S, and Masuhara K: Repair of chronic massive rotator cuff tears with synthetic fabrics. *In* Bateman JE and Welsh RP (eds): Surgery of the Shoulder. Philadelphia: BC Decker, 1984, pp 185–191.
306. Ozaki J, Fujimoto S, Nakagawa Y, et al: Tears of the rotator cuff of the shoulder associated with pathological changes in the acromion. J Bone Joint Surg *70*:1224–1230, 1988.
307. Ozaki J, Fujimoto S, Tomita K, and al: Non-perforated superficial surface cuff tears associated with hydrops of the subacromial bursa. Katakansetsu (Fukuoka) *9*:52, 1985.
308. Paavolainen P and Ahovuo J: Ultrasonography and arthrography in the diagnosis of tears of the rotator cuff. J Bone Joint Surg *76*:335–340, 1994.
309. Packer NP, Calvert PT, Bayley JIL, and Kessel L: Operative treatment of chronic ruptures of the rotator cuff of the shoulder. J Bone Joint Surg Br *65B*:171–175, 1983.
310. Painter: Boston Med Surg J *156*:345, 1907.
311. Palette GA Jr, Warner JP, Altchek DW, et al: Arthroscopic Rotator Cuff Repair: Evaluation of Results and Comparison of Techniques. Presented at the 60th Annual Meeting of the American Academy of Orthopaedic Surgeons, San Francisco, 1993.
312. Palmer WE, Brown JH, and Rosenthal DI: Rotator cuff: Evaluation with fat-suppressed arthrography. Radiology *188*:683–687, 1993.
313. Pappas AM, Zawacki RM, and McCarthy CF: Rehabilitation of the pitching shoulder. Am J Sports Med *13*:223–235, 1985.
314. Pappas AM, Zawacki RM, and Sullivan TJ: Biomechanics of baseball pitching. A preliminary report. Am J Sports Med *13*:216–222, 1985.
315. Paulos LE and Franklin JL: Arthroscopic shoulder decompression development and application. Am J Sports Med *18*:235–244, 1990.
316. Paulos LE, Harner CD, and Parker RD: Arthroscopic subacromial decompression for impingement syndrome of the shoulder. Tech Orthop *3*:33–39, 1988.
317. Paulos LE and Kody MH: Arthroscopically enhanced "miniapproach" to rotator cuff repair. Am J Sports Med *22*:19–25, 1994.
318. Payr E: Gelenk "Sperren" und "Ankylosen" Uber die "Schultersteifen verschiedener Ursache und die sogenannte "Periarthrities humero-scapularis," Ihre Behandlung. Zentralbl Chir *58*:2993–3003, 1931.
319. Penny JN and Smith C: The prevention and treatment of swimmer's shoulder. Can J Appl Sport Sci 5:195–202, 1980.
320. Penny JN and Welsh RP: Shoulder impingement syndromes in athletes and their surgical management. Am J Sports Med *9*:11–15, 1981.
321. Peterson C: Long-term results of rotator cuff repair. *In* Bayley I and Kessel L (eds): Shoulder Surgery. Berlin: Springer-Verlag, 1982, pp 64–69.
322. Peterson CJ and Gentz CF: Ruptures of the supraspinatous tendon—the significance of distally pointing acromioclavicular osteophytes. Clin Orthop *174*:143, 1983.
323. Pettersson G: Rupture of the tendon aponeurosis of the shoulder joint in antero-inferior dislocation. Acta Chir Scand (Suppl) *77*:1–187, 1942.
324. Phipps GJ and Hoffer MM: Latissimus dorsi and teres major transfer to rotator cuff for Erb's palsy. J Shoulder Elbow Surg *4*:124–129, 1995.
325. Picot C: Neuropathie canalaire du nerf sus-scapulaire. Rhumatologie *21*:73–75, 1969.
326. Pingaud and Charvot: Scapulalgie. *In* Dechambre: Dictionaire Encyclopédique des Sciences Médicales, Vol. 11. Paris, 1879, p 232.
327. Poppen NK and Walker PS: Normal and abnormal motion of the shoulder. J Bone Joint Surg *58A*:195, 1976.
328. Post M: Rotator cuff repair with carbon filament: A preliminary report of five cases. Clin Orthop *196*:154–158, 1985.
329. Post M and Cohen J: Impingement Syndrome—A Review of Late Stage II and Early Stage III Lesions, ASES, First Open Meeting, 1985.
330. Post M and Cohen J: Impingement syndrome. Clin Orthop *207*:126–132, 1986.
331. Post M, Silver R, and Singh M: Rotator cuff tear: Diagnosis and treatment. Clin Orthop *173*:78, 1983.
332. Postacchini F, Perugia D, and Rampoldi M: Rotator cuff tears: Results of surgical repairs. Ital J Orthop Traumatol *18*:173–188, 1992.
333. Pujadas GM: Coraco-acromial ligament syndrome. J Bone Joint Surg *52A*:1261–1262, 1970.
334. Putz R and Reichelt A: Structural findings of the coracoacromial ligament in rotator cuff rupture, tendinosis calcarea and supraspinatus syndrome. Z Orthop Ihre Grenzgeb *128*:46–50, 1990.
335. Quinn SF, Sheley RC, Demlow TA, and Szumowski J: Rotator cuff tendon tears: Evaluation with fat-suppressed MR imaging with arthroscopic correlation in 100 patients. Radiology *195*:497–500, 1995.
336. Raggio CL, Warren RF, and Sculco T: Surgical Treatment of Impingement Syndrome: a Four Year Follow-up. ASES, First Open Meeting, 1985.
337. Rask MR: Suprascapular nerve entrapment: A report of two cases treated with suprascapular notch resection. Clin Orthop *123*:73–75, 1977.
338. Rathbun JB and Macnab I: The microvascular pattern of the rotator cuff. J Bone Joint Surg *52-B*:540–553, 1970.
339. Reeves B: Arthrography of the shoulder. J Bone Joint Surg *48B*:424–435, 1966.
340. Regan WD and Richards RR: Subacromial pressure pre and post acromioplasty: A cadaveric study. Orthop Trans *13*:671, 1989.
341. Rengachary SS, Neff JP, Singer PA, and Brackett CE: Suprascapular entrapment neuropathy: A clinical, anatomical, and comparative study. Neurosurgery *5*:441–446, 1979.
342. Renoux S, Monet J, Pupin P, et al: Preliminary note on the biometric data relating to the human coracoacromial arch. Surg Radiol Anat *8*:189–195, 1986.
343. Resnick D: Shoulder arthrography. Radiol Clin North Am 19:243–252, 1981.
344. Richardson AB, Jobe FW, and Collins HR: The shoulder in competitive swimming. Am J Sports Med 8:159–163, 1980.
345. Riley GP, Harrall RL, Constant CR, et al: Tendon degeneration and chronic shoulder pain: Changes in the collagen composition of the human rotator cuff tendons in rotator cuff tendinitis. Ann Rheum Dis 53:359–66, 1994.
346. Riley GP, Harrall RL, Constant CR, et al: Glycosaminoglycans of human rotator cuff tendons: changes with age and in chronic rotator cuff tendinitis. Ann Rheum Dis *53*:367–376, 1994.
347. Robertson PL, Schweitzer ME, Mitchell DG, et al: Rotator cuff disorders: Interobserver and intraobserver variation in diagnosis with MR imaging. Radiology *194*:831–835, 1995.
348. Rocks JA: Intrinsic shoulder pain syndrome. Phys Ther *59*:153–159, 1979.
349. Rockwood CA Jr: Personal communication. 1983 and 1987.
350. Rockwood CA Jr and Lyons FR: Shoulder impingement syndrome: Diagnosis, radiographic evaluation, and treatment with a modified Neer acromioplasty. J Bone Joint Surg 75:473–474, 1993.
351. Rockwood CA Jr, Williams GR Jr, and Burkhead WZ Jr: Debridement of degenerative, irreparable lesions of the rotator cuff. J Bone Joint Surg *77-A*:857–866, 1995.
352. Rokito AS, Zuckerman JD, Gallagher MA, and Cuomo F: Strength after surgical repair of the rotator cuff. J Shoulder Elbow Surg 5:12–17, 1996.
353. Rossi F, Ternamian PJ, Cerciello G, and Walch G: Posterosuperior glenoid rim impingement in athletes: The diagnostic value of traditional radiology and magnetic resonance. Radiol Med (Torino) *87*:22–27, 1994.
354. Rostron PK, Orth MCH, Wigan FRCS, and Calver RF: Subcutaneous atrophy following methylprednisolone injection in Osgood-Schlatter epiphysitis. J Bone Joint Surg *61A*:627–628, 1979.
355. Rothman RH and Parke WW: The vascular anatomy of the rotator cuff. Clin Orthop *41*:176–186, 1965.
356. Rowlands LK, Wertsch JJ, Primack SJ, et al: Kinesiology of the empty can test. Am J Phys Med Rehabil *74*:302–304, 1995.
357. Roye RP, Grana WA, and Yates C: Arthroscopic subacromial decompression: Two-to-seven-year follow-up. Arthroscopy *11*:301–306, 1995.
358. Ryu RK: Arthroscopic subacromial decompression: A clinical review. Arthroscopy *8*:141–147, 1992.
359. Sachs RA, Stone ML, and Devine S: Open vs. arthroscopic acromioplasty: A prospective, randomized study. Arthroscopy *10*:248–254, 1994.
360. Saha AK: Dynamic stability of the glenohumeral joint. Acta Orthop Scand *42*:491–505, 1971.

361. Salter RB, Gross A, and Hall JH: Hydrocortisone arthropathy: An experimental investigation. Can Med Assoc J 97:374, 1967.
362. Samilson RL: Congenital and developmental anomalies of the shoulder girdle. Orthop Clin North Am *11*:219–231, 1980.
363. Samilson RL and Binder WF: Symptomatic full thickness tears of the rotator cuff: An analysis of 292 shoulders in 276 patients. Orthop Clin North Am 6:449–466, 1975.
364. Samilson RL, Raphael RL, Post L, et al: Arthrography of the shoulder. Clin Orthop *20*:21–31, 1961.
365. Schär W and Zweifel C: Das os acromiale und seine klinische Bedeutung. *In* Breitner B and Nordmann O (eds): Bruns Beiträse zur Klinischen Chir. Berlin: Urban & Schwarzenberg, 1936, p 101.
366. Scheib JS: Diagnosis and rehabilitation of the shoulder impingement syndrome in the overhand and throwing athletes. Rheum Dis Clin North Am *16*:971–988, 1990.
367. Schilf E: Über eine Einseitige Lähmung des Nervus Suprascapularis. Nervenarzt 23:306–307, 1952.
368. Schneider JE, Adams OR, and Easley KJ: Scapular notch resection for suprascapular nerve decompression in 12 horses. JAMA *187*:1019–1020, 1985.
369. Seeger LL, Gold RH, Bassett LW, and Ellman H: Shoulder impingement syndrome: MR findings in 53 shoulders. AJR Am J Roentgenol *150*:343–347, 1988.
370. Seitz WHJ, Abram LJ, Froimson AI, et al: Rotator Cuff Imaging Techniques: A Comparison of Arthrography, Ultrasonography and Magnetic Resonance Imaging. Paper presented at ASES, 3rd Open Meeting, San Francisco, CA, 1987.
371. Sharkey NA, Marder RA, and Hanson PB: The entire rotator cuff contributes to elevation of the arm. J Orthop Res *12*:699–708, 1994.
372. Sher JS, Uribe JW, Posada A, et al: Abnormal findings on magnetic resonance images of asymptomatic shoulders. J Bone Joint Surg Am *77*:10–15, 1995.
373. Sievers: Verh dtsch Ges Chir 43. Kongr :243, 1914.
374. Sigholm G, Styf J, Korner L, and Herberts P: Pressure recording in the subacromial bursa. J Orthop Res *6*:123–128, 1988.
375. Skoff HD: Conservative open acromioplasty. J Bone Joint Surg *77*:933–936, 1995.
376. Slatis P and Aalto K: Medial dislocation of the tendon of the long head of the biceps brachii. Acta Orthop Scand *50*:73–77, 1979.
377. Smaill GB: Bilateral rupture of Achilles tendon. BMJ *1*:1657, 1961.
378. Smith JG: Pathological appearances of seven cases of injury of the shoulder joint with remarks. London Med Gazette *14*:280, 1834.
379. Smith-Petersen MN, Aufranc OE, and Larson CB: Useful surgical procedures for rheumatoid arthritis involving joints of the upper extremity. Arch Surg *46*:764–770, 1943.
380. Solheim LF and Roaas A: Compression of the suprascapular nerve after fracture of the scapular notch. Acta Orthop Scand *49*:338–340, 1978.
381. Sonnabend DH: Treatment of primary anterior shoulder dislocation in patients older than 40 years of age. Conservative versus operative. Clin Orthop *304*:74–77, 1994.
382. Soslowsky LJ, An CH, Johnston SP, and Carpenter JE: Geometric and mechanical properties of the coracoacromial ligament and their relationship to rotator cuff disease. Clin Orthop *304*:10–17, 1994.
383. Speer KP and Garrett WE Jr: Muscular control of motion and stability about the pectoral girdle. *In* Matsen FA, III, Fu FH, and Hawkins RJ (eds): The Shoulder: A Balance of Mobility and Stability. Rosemont, IL: American Academy of Orthopaedic Surgeons, 1993, pp 159–172.
384. Speer KP, Lohnes J, and Garrett WE: Arthroscopic subacromial decompression: Results in advanced impingement syndrome. Arthroscopy *7*:291–296, 1991.
385. Stieda A: Zur Pathologie der Schulter gelenkschlembeutel. *In* Langebeck B (ed): Archiv für Klinische Chirurgie. Berlin: Verlag von August Hirschwald, 1908, p 910.
386. Stiles RG and Otte MT: Imaging of the shoulder. Radiology 188:603–613, 1993.
387. Strizak AM, Danzig L, and Jackson DW: Subacromial bur-sography: An anatomic and clinical study. J Bone Joint Surg *64A*:196, 1982.
388. Strohm BR and Colachis SCJ: Shoulder joint dysfunction following injury to the suprascapular nerve. Phys Ther *45*:106–111, 1965.
389. Stuart MJ, Azevedo AJ, and Cofield RH: Anterior acromioplasty for treatment of the shoulder impingement syndrome. Clin Orthop *260*:195–200, 1990.
390. Sweetnam R: Corticosteroid arthropathy and tendon rupture. J Bone Joint Surg *51B*:397, 1969.
391. Swiontkowski M, Iannotti JP, Boulas JH, et al: Intraoperative Assessment of Rotator Cuff Vascularity Using Laser Doppler Flowmetry. St Louis: Mosby–Year Book, 1990, pp 208–212.
392. Symeonides PP: The significance of the subscapularis muscle in the pathogenesis of recurrent anterior dislocation of the shoulder. J Bone Joint Surg *54B*:476–483, 1972.
393. Tabata S and Kida H: Diagnosis and treatment of partial thickness tears of rotator cuff. Orthop Traumatol Surg (Tokyo) *26*:1199, 1983.
394. Tabata S, Kida H, Sasaki J, et al: Operative treatment for the incomplete thickness tears of the rotator cuff. Katakansetsu (Fukuoka) *5*:29, 1981.
395. Taboury J: Ultrasonography of the shoulder: Diagnosis of rupture of tendons of the rotator muscles. Ann Radiol (Paris) *35*:133–140, 1992.
396. Takagishi N: Conservative treatment of the ruptures of the rotator cuff. J Jpn Orthop Assoc *52*:781–787, 1978.
397. Tamai K and Ogawa K: Intratendinous tear of the supraspinatus tendon exhibiting winging of the scapula. Clin Orthop *194*:159–163, 1985.
398. Tetzlaff JE, Yoon HJ, and Brems J: Interscalene brachial plexus block for shoulder surgery. Reg Anesth *19*:339–343, 1994.
399. Thorling J, Bjerneld H, and Hallin G: Acromioplasty for impingement syndrome. Orthop Scand *56*:147–148, 1985.
400. Thur C and Julke M: The anterolateral deltoid muscle flap-plasty: The procedure of choice in large rotator cuff defects. Unfallchirurg *98*:415–421, 1995.
401. Tibone JE, Jobe FW, and Kerlan RK: Shoulder impingement syndrome in athletes treated by an anterior acromioplasty. Clin Orthop *198*:134–140, 1985.
402. Tillaux: Traite de la chirurgie clinique. Paris, 1888.
403. Ting A, Jobe FW, Barto P, et al: An EMPG Analysis of the Lateral Biceps in Shoulders with Rotator Cuff Tears. Paper presented at ASES, 3rd Open Meeting, San Francisco, 1987.
404. Tirman PF, Bost FW, Garvin GJ, et al: Posterosuperior glenoid impingement of the shoulder: Findings at MR imaging and MR arthrography with arthroscopic correlation. Radiology *193*:431–436, 1994.
405. Toivonen DA, Tuite MJ, and Orwin JF: Acromial structure and tears of the rotator cuff. J Shoulder Elbow Surg *4*:376–383, 1995.
406. Toolanen G, Hildingsson C, Hedlund T, et al: Early complications after anterior dislocation of the shoulder in patients over 40 years. An ultrasonographic and electromyographic study. Acta Orthop Scand *64*:549–552, 1993.
407. Torpey BM, McFarland EG, Ikeda K, et al: Deltoid Muscle Origin: Histology and Subacromial Decompression. ASES, 12th Open meeting, Atlanta, GA, 1996.
408. Tuite MJ, Toivonen DA, Orwin JF, and Wright DH: Acromial angle on radiographs of the shoulder: Correlation with the impingement syndrome and rotator cuff tears. Am J Roentgenol *165*:609–613, 1995.
409. Tuite MJ, Yandow DR, DeSmet AA, et al: Diagnosis of partial and complete rotator cuff using combined gradient echo and spin echo. Skeletal Radiol *23*:541–545, 1994.
410. Tyson LL and Crues III JV: Pathogenesis of rotator cuff disorders. Magnetic resonance imaging characteristics. Magn Reson Imaging Clin N Am *1*:37–46, 1993.
411. Uhthoff HK, Loehr J, and Sarkar K: The Pathogenesis of Rotator Cuff Tears. *In* Proceedings of the Third International Conference on Surgery of the Shoulder, Fukuora, Japan, 1986.
412. Uhthoff HK and Sarkar K: Pathology of rotator cuff tendons. *In* Watson MS (ed): Surgical Disorders of the Shoulder. Edinburgh: Churchill Livingstone, 1991, pp 259–270.
413. Uhthoff HK and Sarkar K: Surgical repair of rotator cuff ruptures. The importance of the subacromial bursa. J Bone Joint Surg Br *73*:399–401, 1991.
414. Uhthoff HK and Sarkar K: The effect of aging on the soft tissues of the shoulder. *In* Matsen FA III, Fu FH, Hawkins RJ (eds): The Shoulder: A Balance of Mobility and Stability. Rosemont, IL: American Academy of Orthopaedic Surgeons, 1993, pp 269–278.
415. Uitto J, Teir H, and Mustakallio KK: Corticosteroid induced inhibi-

tion of the biosynthesis of human skin collagen. Biochem Pharmacol *21*:2161, 1972.
416. Valtonen EJ: Double acting betamethasone (Celestone Chronodose) in the treatment of supraspinatus tendinitis: A comparison of subacromial and gluteal single injections with placebo. J Int Med Res *6*:463–467, 1978.
417. van Holsbeeck E, DeRycke J, Declercy G, et al: Subacromial impingement: Open versus arthroscopic decompression. Arthroscopy *8*:173–178, 1992.
418. Van Linge B and Mulder JD: Function of the supraspinatus muscle and its relation to the supraspinatus syndrome: An experimental study in man. J Bone Joint Surg *45(B)*:750–754, 1963.
419. Van-Holsbeeck MT, Kolowich PA, Eyler WR, et al: US Depiction of partial thickness tear of the rotator cuff. Radiology *197*:443–436, 1995.
420. van-Moppes FL, Veldkamp O, and Roorda J: Role of shoulder ultrasonography in the evaluation of the painful shoulder. Eur J Radiol *19*:142–146, 1995.
421. Vogt: Deutsche Chirurgie Lief 64, 1881.
422. Walch G, Liotard JP, Boileau P, and Noel E: Postero-superior glenoid impingement: Another shoulder impingement. Rev Chir Orthop Reparatrice Appar Mot *77*:571–574, 1991.
423. Walker SW, Couch WH, Boester GA, and Sprowl DW: Isokinetic strength of the shoulder after repair of a torn rotator cuff. J Bone Joint Surg *69*:1041–1044, 1987.
424. Wang YM, Shih TT, Jiang CC, et al: Magnetic resonance imaging of rotator cuff lesions. J Formos Med Assoc *93*:234–239, 1994.
425. Ware JE, Snow KK, Kosinski M, and Gandek B: *In* Institute TH (ed): SF 36 Health Survey Manual and Interpretation Guide. Boston: New England Medical Center, 1993.
426. Warner JP: The gross anatomy of the joint surfaces, ligaments, labrum, and capsule. *In* Matsen FA III, Fu FH, and Hawkins RJ (eds): The Shoulder: A Balance of Mobility and Stability. Rosemont, IL: American Academy of Orthopaedic Surgeons, 1993, pp 7–28.
427. Warner JP, Krushell RJ, Masquelet A, and Gerber C: Anatomy and relationships of the suprascapular nerve: Anatomical constraints to mobilization of the supraspinatus and infraspinatus muscles in the management of massive rotator cuff tears. J Bone Joint Surg *74*:36–45, 1992.
428. Warren JP, Altchek DW, and Warren RF: Arthroscopic management of rotator cuff tears with emphasis on the throwing athlete. Oper Tech Orthop *1*:235–239, 1991.
429. Watson M: The refractory painful arc syndrome. J Bone Joint Surg *60B*:544–546, 1978.
430. Watson M: Major ruptures of the rotator cuff: The results of surgical repair in 89 patients. J Bone Joint Surg *67B*:618–624, 1985.
431. Watson-Jones R: Fractures and Joint Injuries, 4th ed. Baltimore: Williams & Wilkins, 1960, pp 449–451.
432. Watson-Jones R: Injuries in the region of the shoulder joint: Capsule and tendon injuries. BMJ *2*:29–31, 1961.
433. Weaver HL: Isolated suprascapular nerve lesions: Injury. Br J Accident Surg *15*:117–126, 1983.
434. Weiner DS and Macnab I: Ruptures of the rotator cuff: Follow-up evaluation of operative repairs. Can J Surg *13*:219–227, 1970.
435. Weiner DS and Macnab I: Superior migration of the humeral head: A radiological aid in the diagnosis of tears of the rotator cuff. J Bone Joint Surg *52B*:524–527, 1970.
436. Weiss JJ: Intra-articular steroids in the treatment of rotator cuff tear: reappraisal by arthrography. Arch Phys Med Rehabil *62*:555–557, 1981.
437. Wellisch: Wien Med Wochenschr 974, 1934.
438. Wiener SN and Seitz WH Jr: Sonography of the shoulder in patients with tears of the rotator cuff: Accuracy and value for selecting surgical options. Am J Roentgenol *160*:103–107, 1993.
439. Wiley AM: Arthroscopic evaluation and surgery for rotator cuff disease. *In* Shoulder Surgery in the Athlete. Aspen Press, 1985, pp 83–91.
440. Wiley AM: Superior humeral dislocation. A complication following decompression and debridement for rotator cuff tears. Clin Orthop *263*:135–141, 1991.
441. Wilson CL: Lesions of the supraspinatus tendon: Degeneration, rupture and calcification. Arch Surg *46*:307, 1943.
442. Wilson CL and Duff GL: Pathologic study of degeneration and rupture of the supraspinatus tendon. Arch Surg *47*:121–135, 1943.
443. Withrington RH, Girgis FL, and Seifert MH: A placebo-controlled trial of steroid injections in the treatment of supraspinatus tendinitis. Scand J Rheumatol *14*:76–78, 1985.
444. Wolfgang GL: Rupture of the musculotendinous cuff of the shoulder. Clin Orthop *134*:230–243, 1978.
445. Wrede L: Ueber Kalkablagerungen in der Umgebung des Schultergelenks und ihre Beziehungen zur Periarthritis. Berlin: Verlag von August Hirschwald, 1912, p 259.
446. Wuelker N, Plitz W, and Roetman B: Biomechanical data concerning the shoulder impingement syndrome. Clin Orthop *303*:242–249, 1994.
447. Wuelker N, Roetman B, Plitz W, and Knop C: Function of the supraspinatus muscle in a dynamic. Unfallchirurgie *97*:308–313, 1994.
448. Wuelker N, Wirth CJ, Plitz W, and Roetman B: A dynamic shoulder model: Reliability testing and muscle force study. J Biomech *28*:489–499, 1995.
449. Wulker N, Melzer C, and Wirth CJ: Shoulder surgery for rotator cuff tears. Ultrasonographic 3 year follow-up of 97 cases. Acta Orthop Scand *62*:142–147, 1991.
450. Yamada H and Evans F: Strength of Biological Materials. Baltimore: Williams & Wilkins, 1972, pp 67–70.
451. Yamamoto R: Rotator cuff rupture. J Joint Surg *1*:93, 1982.
452. Yamanaka K and Fukuda H: Histological study of the supraspinatus tendon. The Shoulder Joint 5:9, 1981.
453. Yamanaka K, Fukuda H, Hamada K, and Mikasa M: Incomplete thickness tears of the rotator cuff. Orthop Traumatol Surg (Tokyo) *26*:713, 1983.
454. Yamanaka K and Matsumoto T: The joint side tear of the rotator cuff: A followup study by arthrography. Clin Orthop *304*:68–73, 1994.
455. Yazici M, Kapuz C, and Gulman B: Morphologic variants of acromion in neonatal cadavers. J Pediatr Orthop *15*:644–647, 1995.
456. Yung SW and Harryman DT II: The Surgical Anatomy of Subscapular Nerves. Presented at the 62nd Annual meeting of the American Academy of Orthopaedic Surgeons, Orlando, FL, 1995.
457. Ziegler DW, Matsen III FA, and Harrington RM: The superior rotator cuff tendon and acromion provide passive superior stability to the shoulder. Submitted to J Bone Joint Surg, 1996.
458. Zuckerman JD, Kummer FJ, Cuomo F, et al: The influence of coracoacromial arch anatomy on rotator cuff tears. J Shoulder Elbow Surg *1*:4–14, 1992.
459. Zuckerman JD, Leblanc JM, Choueka J, and Kummer F: The effect of arm position and capsular release on rotator cuff repair. J Bone Joint Surg *73(B)*:402–405, 1991.
460. Zvijac JE, Levy HJ, and Lemak LJ: Arthroscopic subacromial decompression in the treatment of full thickness rotator cuff tears: A 3- to 6-year follow-up Arthroscopy *10*:518–523, 1994.

C H A P T E R

16

FREDERICK A. MATSEN III, M.D.
CHARLES A. ROCKWOOD, Jr., M.D.
MICHAEL A. WIRTH, M.D.
STEVEN B. LIPPITT, M.D.

Glenohumeral Arthritis and Its Management

The humeral head and the glenoid normally articulate through smooth, congruent, and well-lubricated joint surfaces. Glenohumeral arthritis results when these joint surfaces are damaged by congenital, metabolic, traumatic, degenerative, vascular, septic, or nonseptic inflammatory factors. These conditions are common, especially in older populations in which the prevalence is approximately 20%.[60, 172, 347] In *degenerative joint disease*, the glenoid cartilage and subchondral bone are typically worn posteriorly, sometimes leaving intact articular cartilage anteriorly. The cartilage of the humeral head is eroded in a pattern of central baldness, which is often surrounded by a rim of remaining cartilage and osteophytes. In *inflammatory arthritis*, the cartilage is usually destroyed evenly across the humeral and glenoid joint surfaces. *Cuff tear arthropathy* occurs when a chronic large rotator cuff defect subjects the uncovered humeral articular cartilage to abrasion by the undersurface of the coracoacromial arch. The erosion of the humeral articular cartilage begins superiorly rather than centrally. *Neurotrophic arthropathy* arises in association with syringomyelia, diabetes, or other causes of joint denervation. The joint and subchondral bone are destroyed because of the loss of the trophic and protective effects of its nerve supply. In *capsulorrhaphy arthropathy*, prior surgery for glenohumeral instability leads to joint surface destruction. In this situation excessive anterior or posterior capsular tightening forces the head of the humerus out of its normal concentric relationship with the glenoid fossa. The eccentric glenohumeral contact increases contact pressure and joint surface wear. Most commonly, overtightening of the anterior capsule produces obligate posterior translation, posterior glenoid wear, and central wear of the humeral articular cartilage.

MECHANICS OF ARTHRITIS AND ARTHROPLASTY

Four basic mechanical characteristics are essential to the function of the normal shoulder: motion, stability, strength, and smoothness. Each of these is commonly compromised in the arthritic shoulder and can potentially be restored by shoulder arthroplasty. The approach to glenohumeral arthritis is guided by an understanding of the necessary elements for optimal shoulder mechanics.

Motion

The requisites of a normal range of glenohumeral motion include the following.

Normal Capsular Laxity. Normal capsular laxity allows a full range of rotation. The glenohumeral capsule is normally lax through most of the functional range of shoulder motion.[155, 208] As the joint approaches the limit of its range, the tension in the capsule and its ligaments increases sharply, serving to check the range of rotation (Fig. 16–1). In many conditions that require shoulder arthroplasty, the capsule and ligaments are contracted, thus limiting the range of rotation. Shoulder arthroplasty tends to further tighten the capsule, because a degenerated and collapsed humeral head is replaced by a relatively larger prosthesis and because a glenoid component is added to the surface of the glenoid bone, which may consume more space than the degenerated cartilage that it replaces (Fig. 16–2) and "stuff" the joint. Unless sufficient capsular releases (Figs. 16–3 and 16–4) have been performed to accommodate this stuffing, the joint is "overstuffed." If the joint is overstuffed, joint motion is limited (Fig. 16–5) and more torque (muscle force) is required to move the arm (Fig. 16–6).

Harryman and associates determined that all motions, including flexion, external and internal rotation, and maximal elevation, are diminished when an oversized humeral head prosthesis is implanted.[54] Furthermore, this overstuffing causes obligate translation of the humeral head to occur on the glenoid; for example, forced posterior translation occurs when external rotation is attempted against a tight anterior capsule (Figs. 16–7 and 16–8). Thus, if normal capsular laxity is lacking, unwanted translation and eccentric glenoid loading may result.

In arthroplasty surgery, the amount of stuffing can be estimated by adding the thickness of the glenoid component to the difference between the amount of intra-articular humerus replaced and the amount of humerus resected. To be comparable, the measurement of the

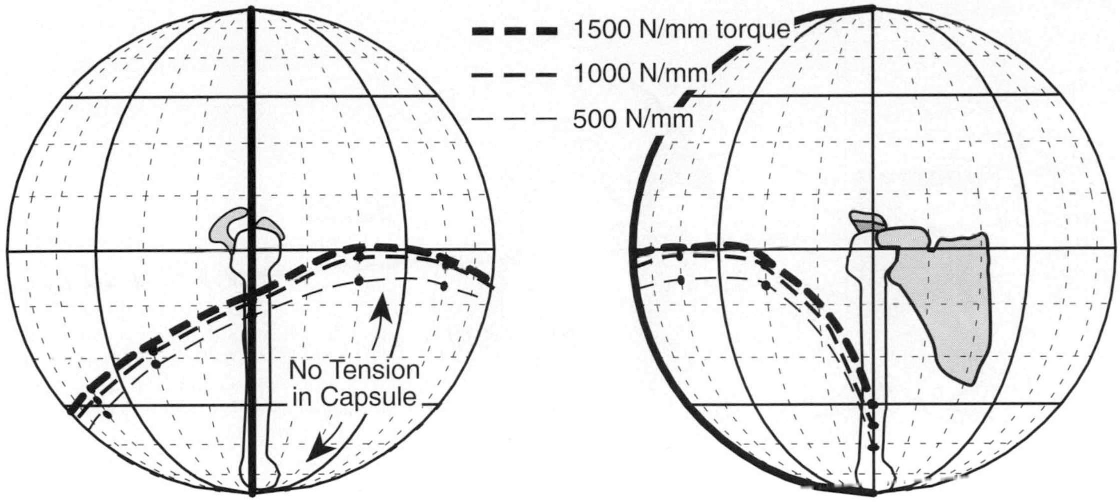

Figure 16–1

Range of humeroscapular elevation with no capsular tension. This global diagram represents data from a cadaver experiment in which the humerus was elevated in a variety of scapular planes, allowing free axial rotation. Elevation was performed until the torque reached 500, 1000, and 1500 N/mm. The positions associated with these torque levels are indicated by the isobars. The area within the inner isobar indicates the range of positions in which there was effectively no tension in the capsuloligamentous structures. For further details, please see Matsen FA III, Lippitt SB, Sidles JA, and Harryman DT II: Practical Evaluation and Management of the Shoulder. Philadelphia: WB Saunders, 1994.

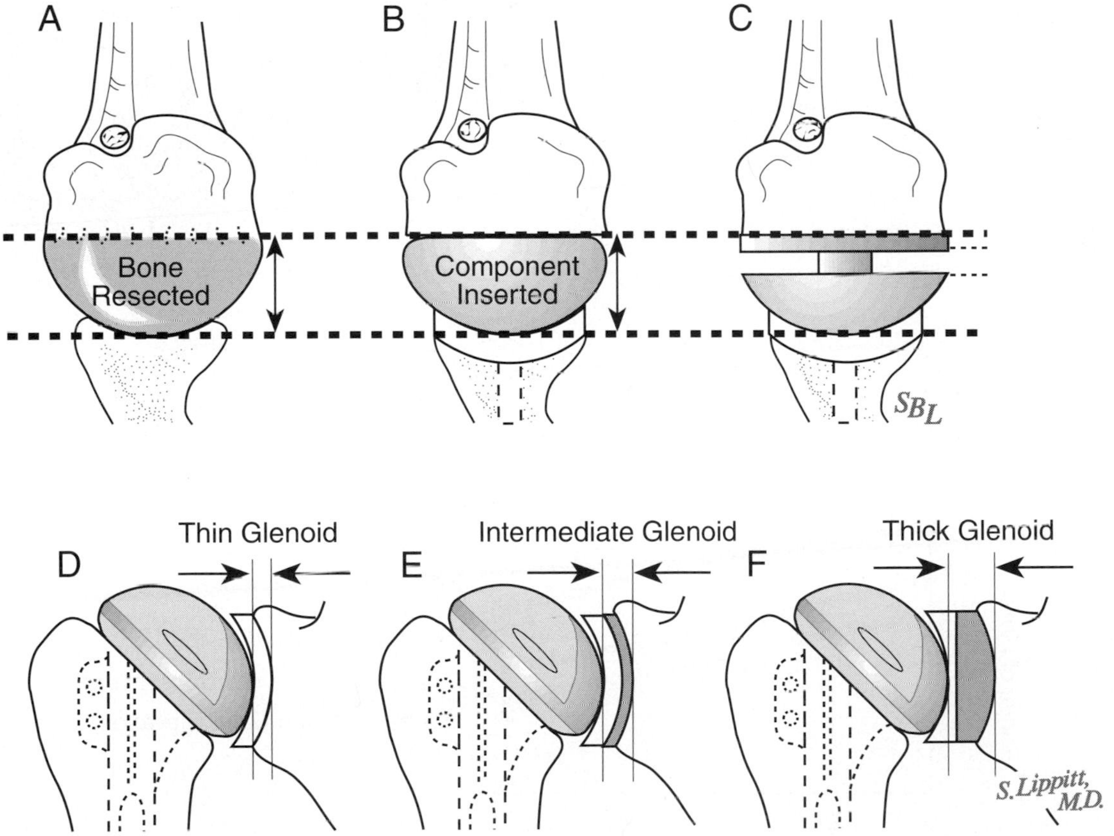

Figure 16–2

The amount of humeral stuffing is measured by comparing the amount of humerus resected (*A*) to the amount of intra-articular humeral prosthesis added (*B*). In modular systems, the amount of prosthesis added must include the collar and the exposed part of the Morse taper as well as the prosthetic head (*C*). The amount of glenoid stuffing is determined by the distance between the bone surface and the prosthetic articular surface. This distance is greater in proportion to the thickness of the glenoid components (*D–F*). (From Matsen FA III, Lippitt SB, Sidles JA, and Harryman DT II: Practical Evaluation and Management of the Shoulder. Philadelphia: WB Saunders, 1994.)

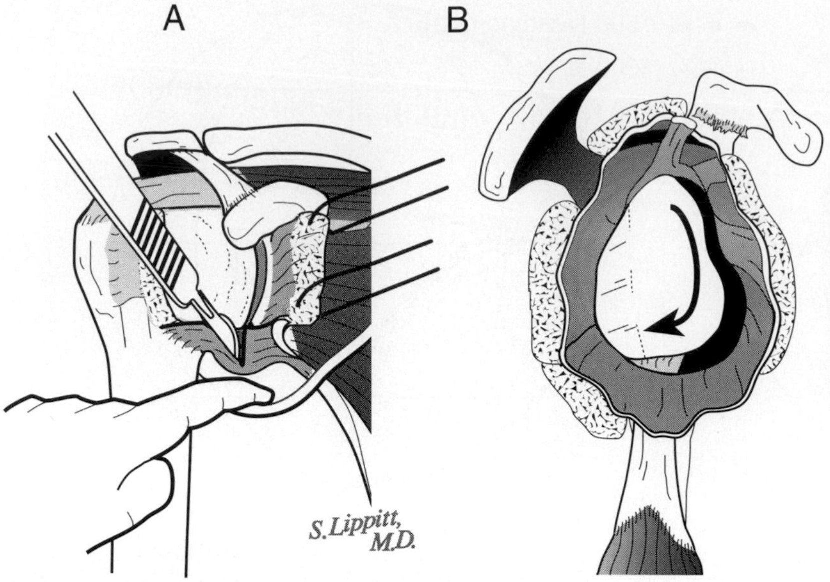

Figure 16–3

A, Division of the anteroinferior capsular attachments to the glenoid under direct vision while the axillary nerve is protected and retracted. *B*, Capsular release to the 7 o'clock position on the glenoid exposes the origin of the long head of the triceps. (Modified from Matsen FA III, Lippitt SB, Sidles JA, and Harryman DT II: Practical Evaluation and Management of the Shoulder. Philadelphia: WB Saunders, 1994.)

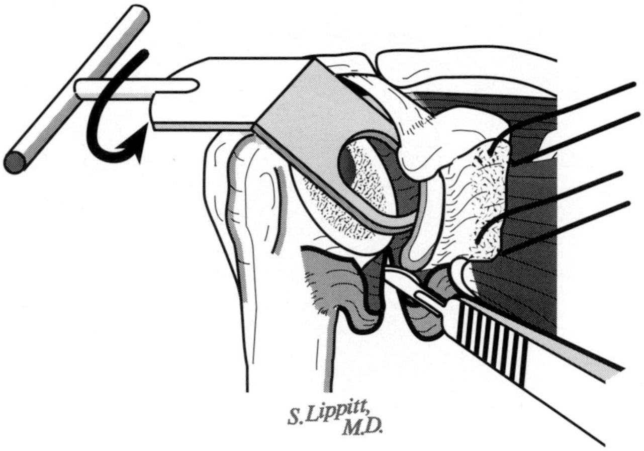

Figure 16–4

If necessary, the sequential posterior release is accomplished at the glenoid rim (release at the humerus would jeopardize the cuff insertion). During this release, the capsule is tensed by twisting the humeral retractor. Care is taken to protect the axillary nerve below and the cuff behind. (Modified from Matsen FA III, Lippitt SB, Sidles JA, and Harryman DT II: Practical Evaluation and Management of the Shoulder. Philadelphia: WB Saunders, 1994.)

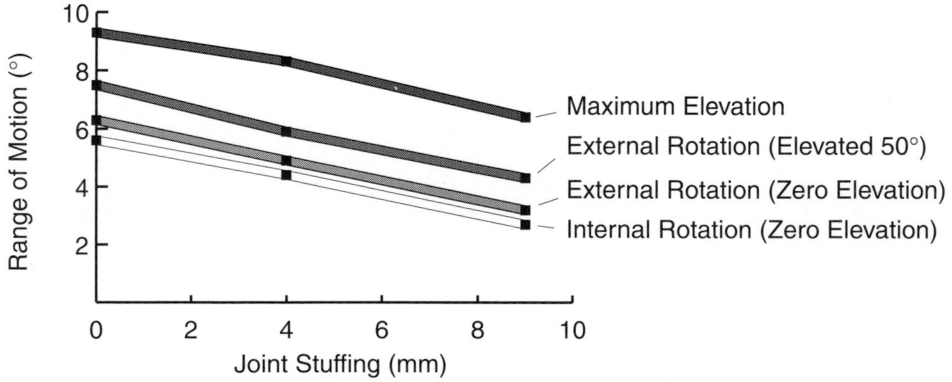

Figure 16–5

The effect of joint stuffing on the range of motion. This graph compares the ranges of four humeroscapular motions that could be achieved with an applied torque of 1500 N/mm for: (1) an anatomic joint (0 mm of joint stuffing), (2) an anatomic humeral arthroplasty with a 4-mm-thick glenoid component (4 mm of overstuffing), and (3) an arthroplasty with a 4-mm-thick glenoid and a 5-mm oversized humeral neck (total overstuffing is 9 mm). Note the sequential loss of each of the motions with increasing degrees of stuffing. (From Matsen FA III, Lippitt SB, Sidles JA, and Harryman DT II: Practical Evaluation and Management of the Shoulder. Philadelphia: WB Saunders, 1994.)

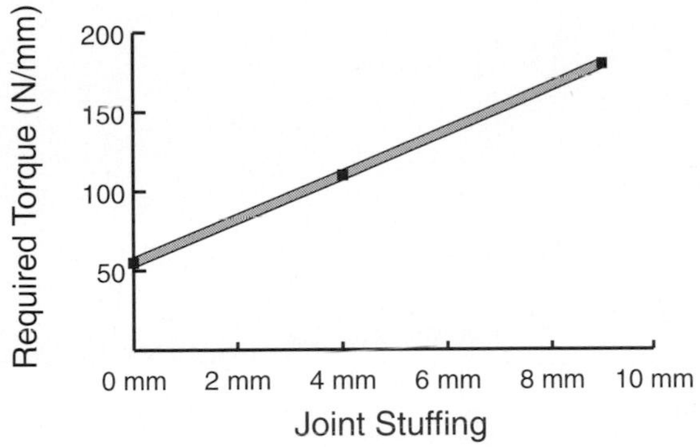

Figure 16–6

Comparison of the average torque necessary to achieve 60 degrees of elevation in the +90-degree scapular plane for the anatomic shoulder (0 mm of stuffing), an anatomic shoulder arthroplasty with 4 mm of glenoid stuffing, and an arthroplasty with 4 mm of glenoid and 5 mm of humeral overstuffing (total overstuffing is 9 mm). The required torque is almost three times higher for the joint overstuffed with 9 mm of component than for the anatomic joint. (From Matsen FA III, Lippitt SB, Sidles JA, and Harryman DT II: Practical Evaluation and Management of the Shoulder. Philadelphia: WB Saunders, 1994.)

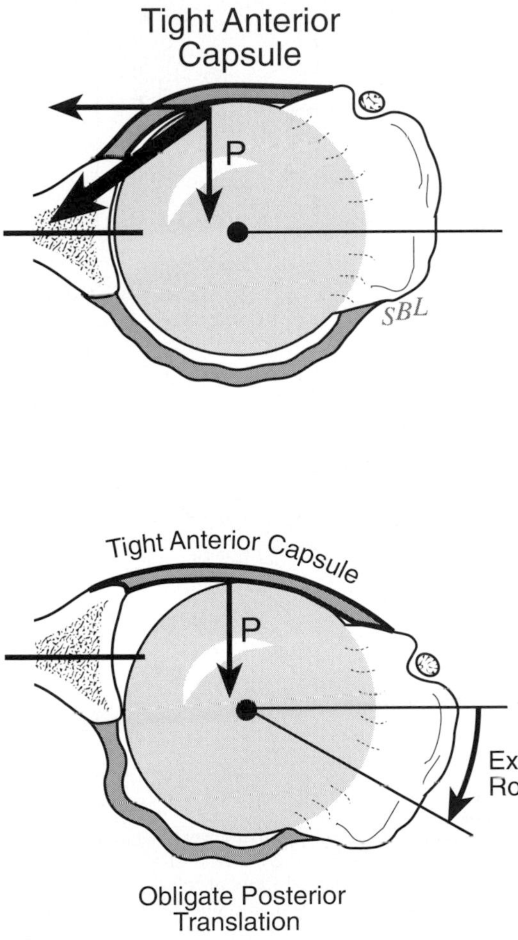

Figure 16–7

If the humerus is rotated beyond the point where the ligaments become tight, the displacing force (P) can push the humeral head out of the glenoid center — a phenomenon known as obligate translation. (Modified from Matsen FA III, Lippitt SB, Sidles JA, and Harryman DT II: Practical Evaluation and Management of the Shoulder. Philadelphia: WB Saunders, 1994.)

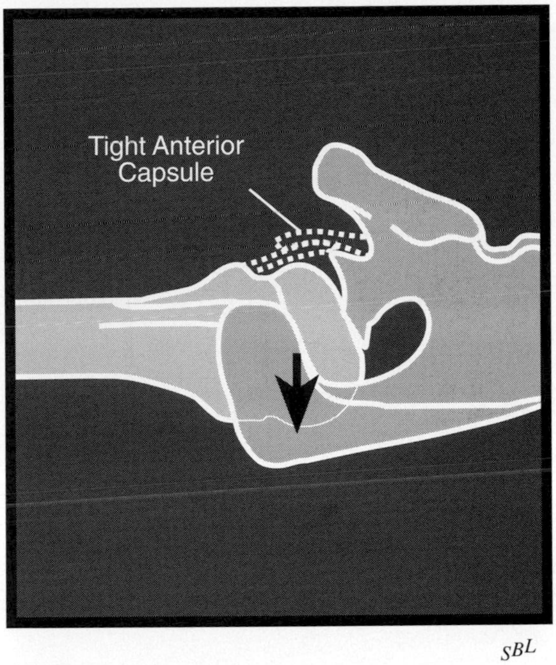

Figure 16–8

Axillary view of capsulorrhaphy arthropathy, in which an excessively tight anterior capsular repair forces the head of the humerus posteriorly. This effect is accentuated by forced external rotation. Note also the typical posterior glenoid erosion. (From Matsen FA III, Lippitt SB, Sidles JA, and Harryman DT II: Practical Evaluation and Management of the Shoulder. Philadelphia: WB Saunders, 1994.)

amount of humeral head resected and the measurement of the amount of intra-articular humeral prosthesis added must both be made from the cut surface of the humeral neck to the articular surface. In modular humeral heads, the amount of bone replaced must include the thickness of the collar and the exposed part of the Morse taper stem as well as the head itself (see Fig. 16–2).

The amount of stuffing from the glenoid component is related primarily to its thickness as well as to the amount of reaming, the presence or absence of cement between the component and the bone, and the use of bone grafts. The thickness of currently available glenoid components varies from 3 mm to more than 15 mm. Thicker glenoid polyethylene may help to manage contact stresses and may have superior wear properties.[129] Metal-backed glenoid components affect load transfer and offer opportunities for screw fixation and tissue ingrowth.[81] However, both thicker polyethylene and metal backing contribute to joint stuffing, which becomes particularly problematic in shoulders that remain tight even after soft tissue releases. Overstuffing may also predispose the reconstructed shoulder to instability.[81]

The amount of stuffing from the humeral component is determined both by the geometry of the component and by the position in which it is placed. The size of the intra-articular aspect of the humeral component is related to its design, including its radius of curvature, the percentage of the sphere represented by its articular surface, and the distance between the base of its collar and the articular surface of the prosthesis (Fig. 16–9; see also Fig. 16–2). The position of the component also has a major

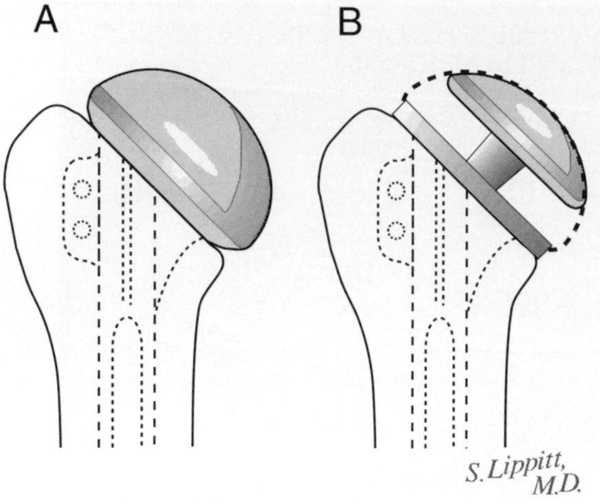

Figure 16–9

A, Ideally, the humeral component provides a maximal articular surface area. *B*, Significant portions of the intra-articular space can be consumed by nonarticular aspects of the prosthesis. (From Matsen FA III, Lippitt SB, Sidles JA, and Harryman DT II: Practical Evaluation and Management of the Shoulder. Philadelphia: WB Saunders, 1994.)

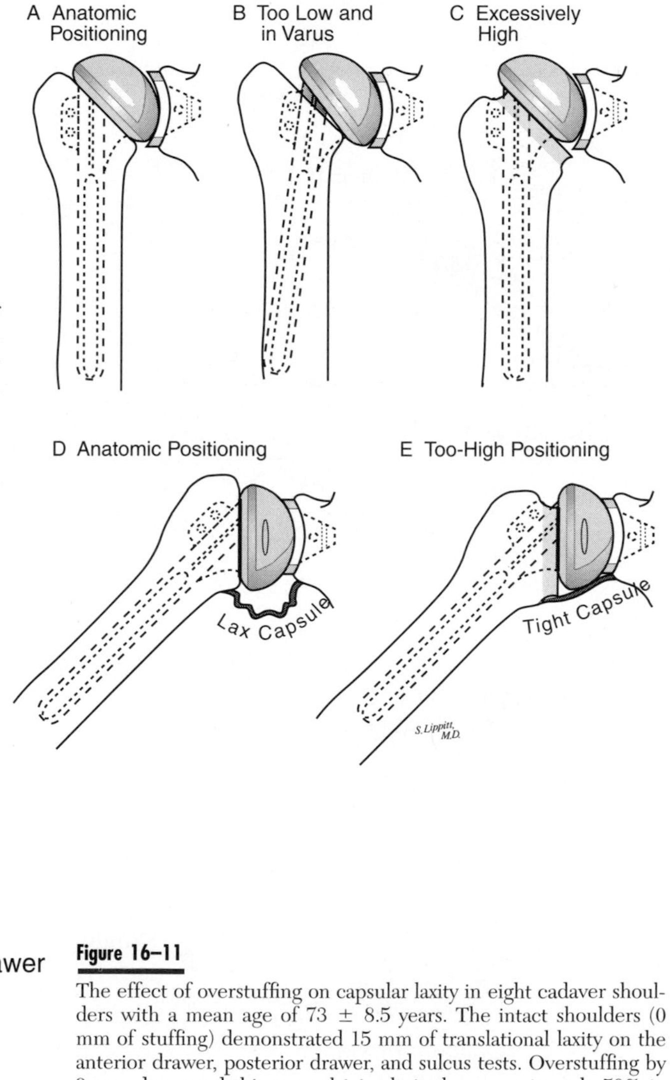

Figure 16–10

The position of the humeral component is an important determinant of the amount of stuffing. *A*, Anatomic positioning of the humeral component. *B*, A component placed low and in varus will disproportionately stuff the shoulder while the arm is at the side. *C*, A component placed excessively high. *D*, Normal anatomic relationships in humeral elevation. *E*, A humeral component that is too high causes tightening of the capsule as the humerus is elevated. (From Matsen FA III, Lippitt SB, Sidles JA, and Harryman DT II: Practical Evaluation and Management of the Shoulder. Philadelphia: WB Saunders, 1994.)

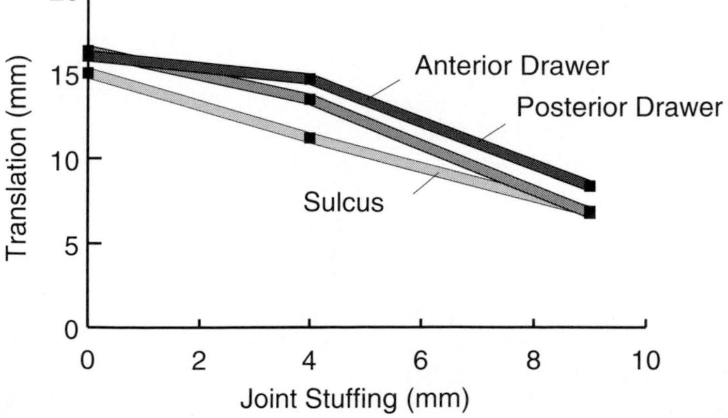

Figure 16–11

The effect of overstuffing on capsular laxity in eight cadaver shoulders with a mean age of 73 ± 8.5 years. The intact shoulders (0 mm of stuffing) demonstrated 15 mm of translational laxity on the anterior drawer, posterior drawer, and sulcus tests. Overstuffing by 9 mm decreased this normal joint laxity by approximately 50% in all directions. (From Matsen FA III, Lippitt SB, Sidles JA, and Harryman DT II: Practical Evaluation and Management of the Shoulder. Philadelphia: WB Saunders, 1994.)

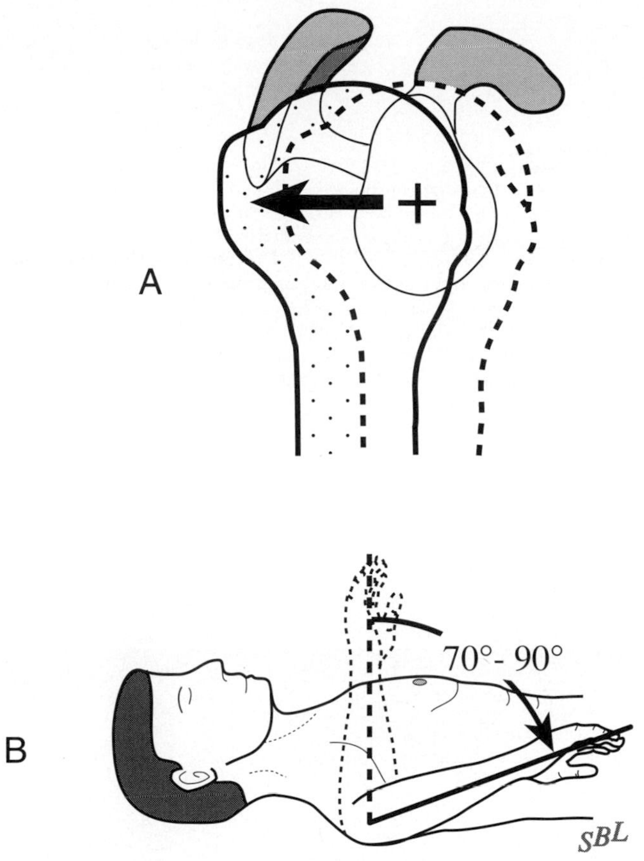

Figure 16–12

A, Proper soft tissue tension allows 50% posterior translation of the humeral head component on the glenoid and a spontaneous return to the centered position (the "springbok" test). *B*, The patient should have sufficient laxity in the posterior capsule after arthroplasty to allow internal rotation in the abducted position in the range of 70 to 90 degrees (the "scarecrow" test). (From Pearl ML and Lippitt SB: Shoulder arthroplasty with a modular prosthesis. Tech Orthop 8[3]:151–162, 1994. Original illustrator—SB Lippitt.)

Table 16–1 RANGE OF ANGULAR MOTION BEFORE ONSET OF OBLIGATE TRANSLATION*

	ANATOMIC SHOULDER (DEGREES)	*JOINT OVERSTUFFED 9 mm (DEGREES)*
Elevation in the plus 90 degree scapular plane	60	30
External rotation of the arm elevated 50 degrees	60	32

*Values represent the maximal elevation achieved with no more than 2 mm of obligate translation.

effect on the degree to which it stuffs the joint. A component inserted into varus will disproportionately stuff the joint when the arm is at the side; this outcome is more likely when the stem of the prosthesis does not fit the humeral canal snugly. A component inserted excessively high will tighten the capsule as the arm is elevated (similar to a mechanical cam) and limit the range of elevation (Fig. 16–10).

Cadaver studies[221] indicate that less than 10 mm of overstuffing can reduce normal capsular laxity by as much as 50% (Fig. 16–11). The overstuffed shoulder is predisposed to obligate translation (Table 16–1).

The variables of component size and capsular release are under the control of the surgeon. As a rule of thumb for judging capsular laxity at the time of surgery: (1) the humeral head should translate approximately 15 mm on the posterior drawer, (2) the abducted arm should allow 70 degrees of internal rotation, and (3) the arm should allow 40 degrees of external rotation at the side after the anterior structures have been repaired (Fig. 16–12).

Humeral Articular Surface. A substantial and properly located humeral articular surface area allows a large unimpeded rotational range. Humeral articular surfaces that comprise only a small portion of the sphere (Fig. 16–13) predispose to abutment of the rim of the glenoid against the tuberosities or anatomic neck of the humerus (Figs. 16–14 and 16–15).[12] The normal extent of the humeral joint surface can be restored with appropriate positioning of the appropriate prosthesis at the time of joint replacement (see Fig. 16–9).

Glenoid Articular Surface. A glenoid articular surface comprises a relatively small portion of the sphere in comparison with that of the humerus. If the prosthetic glenoid joint surface area is large compared with that of the humerus, abutment of the prosthesis against the humeral neck or tuberosities can restrict joint motion (Fig. 16–16; see also Fig. 16–14).

Absence of Blocking Osteophytes. Osteophytes predispose to contact with the glenoid and can impair motion (Fig. 16–17). Blocking osteophytes must be completely resected at the time of joint reconstruction (Fig. 16–18).

Unrestricted Humeroscapular Motion Interface. Normally, 3 to 4 cm of excursion takes place at the upper aspect of this interface between the coracoid muscles and the subscapularis (Fig. 16–19). Adhesions or "spot welds" between the proximal humerus and cuff on one hand and

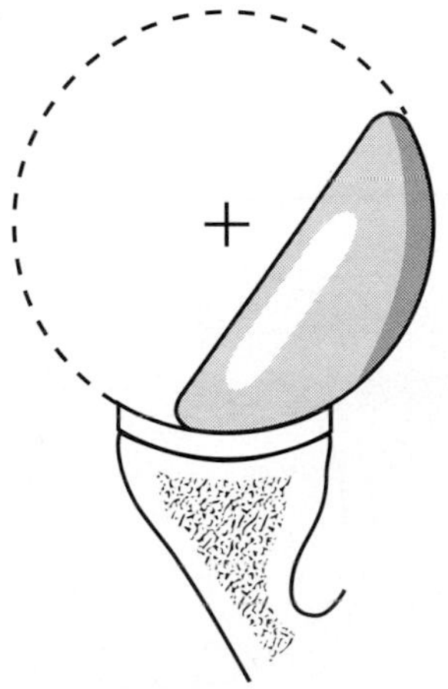

Figure 16–13

Each prosthetic head represents a portion of a sphere. Different prostheses comprise different percentages of the surface of the sphere. (Modified from Ballmer FT, Lippitt SB, Romeo AA, and Matsen FA III: Total shoulder arthroplasty: Some considerations related to glenoid surface contact. J Shoulder Elbow Surg 3:299–306, 1994.)

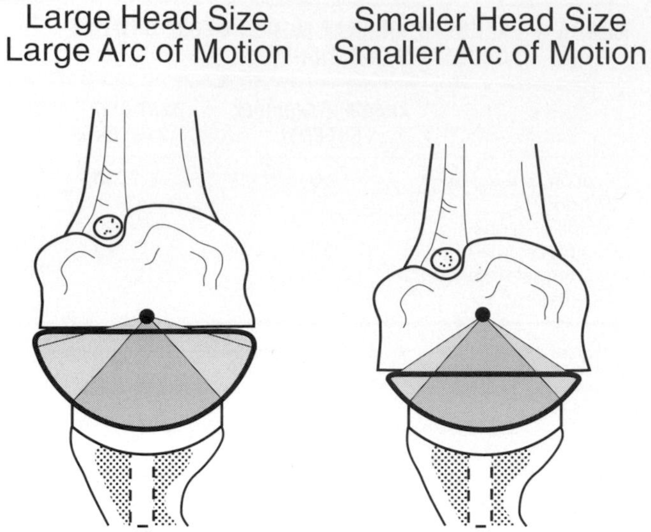

Figure 16–14

The arc of motion that can be accomplished at the glenohumeral joint before running out of humeral articular surface is determined by the difference between the angles subtended by the humeral and the glenoid articular surfaces in the direction of motion. Thus, although a smaller humeral head component may increase capsular laxity, its smaller surface arc may actually diminish the glenohumeral motion allowed before the bone of the humerus makes contact with the glenoid. (From Matsen FA III, Lippitt SB, Sidles JA, and Harryman DT II: Practical Evaluation and Management of the Shoulder. Philadelphia: WB Saunders, 1994.)

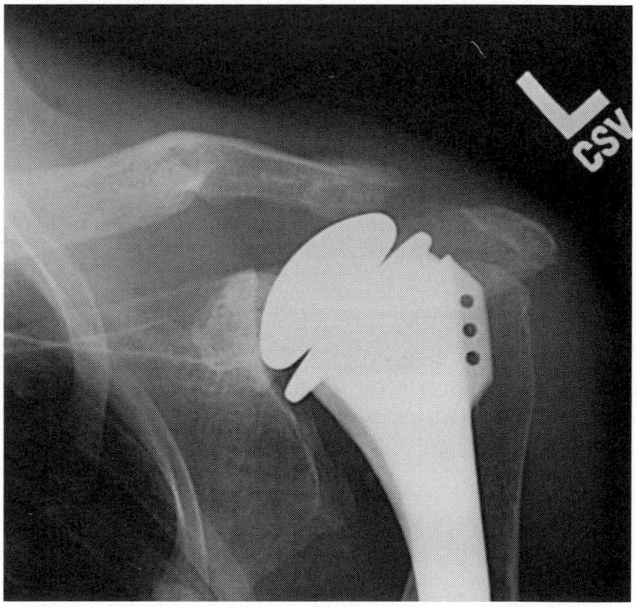

Figure 16–15

A humeral component with an articular surface comprising only a small portion of the potential spherical articular surface may predispose the prosthesis to unwanted translation as well as contact between the prosthetic collar and the glenoid.

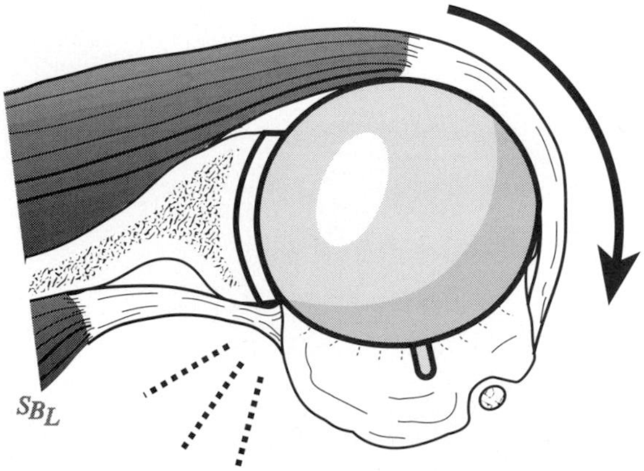

Figure 16–16

Motion-limiting abutment between the glenoid component and soft tissue or bone. (Modified from Ballmer FT, Lippitt SB, Romeo AA, and Matsen FA III: Total shoulder arthroplasty: Some considerations related to glenoid surface contact. J Shoulder Elbow Surg 3:299–306, 1994.)

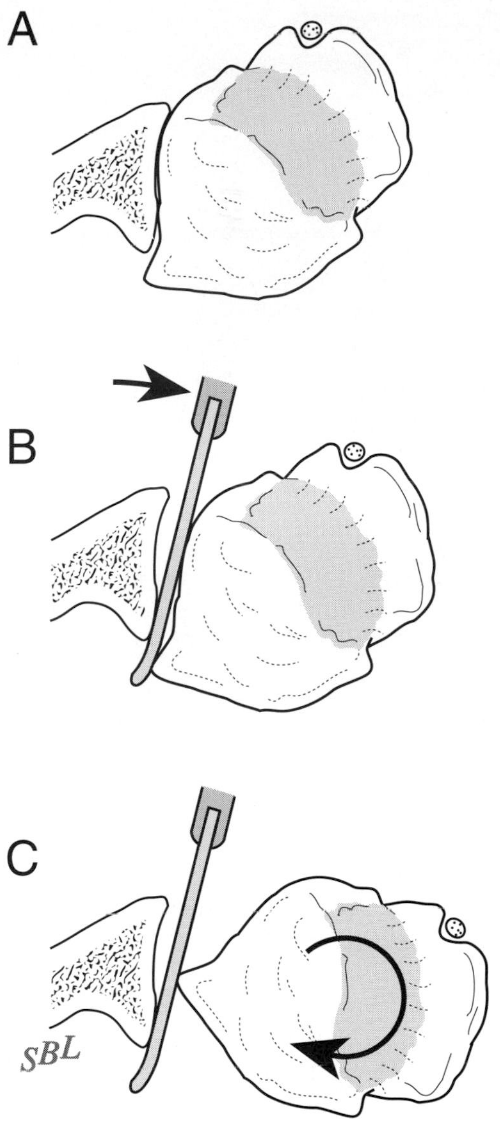

Figure 16–17

Osteophyte blocking range of motion. A "shoe horn" elevator may be required to ease them into the joint at the time of surgical arthroplasty. (Modified from Matsen FA III, Lippitt SB, Sidles JA, and Harryman DT II: Practical Evaluation and Management of the Shoulder. Philadelphia: WB Saunders, 1994.)

the deltoid and coracoacromial arch on the other can limit motion, even if the intra-articular aspect of the arthroplasty is perfectly balanced. Lysis of humeroscapular spot welds is an important early step in arthroplasty of the shoulder.

Stability

The requisites of glenohumeral stability follow.

Anatomically Oriented and Sufficiently Extensive Humeral Articular Surface Area. The orientation of the humeral articular surface can be described in terms of the humeral head center line; a line passing through the center of the humeral articular cartilage and through the center of the anatomic neck. This line usually makes a valgus angle of about 130 degrees with the humeral shaft. The humeral head center line usually makes a retroversion angle of about 30 degrees with the axis of elbow flexion.[72, 86, 119, 130, 159, 253, 256, 270, 309, 355] Studies point out that mean humeral retroversion varies widely from 7 to 50 degrees.[197, 272, 300] Hernigou and associates pointed out the importance of clearly defining the reference system when measuring humeral version.[162]

The extent of the humeral articular surface area is another critical determinant of stability. In the arthritic glenohumeral joint, stability can be compromised by a reduced amount of available humeral articular surface. Similarly, a prosthetic surface area that comprises only a small part of the total sphere (see Figs. 16–9, 16–13, and 16–15) can predispose to instability in the same way that a Hill-Sachs defect does in traumatic instability by offering less contact area for joint surface contact (Fig. 16–20).

Anatomically Oriented Glenoid. The glenoid center line, the line perpendicular to the center of the glenoid fossa, is usually relatively closely aligned with the plane of the scapula (Figs. 16–21 and 16–22). In the arthritic glenohumeral joint, stability may be compromised by abnormal glenoid version (Figs. 16–23 and 16–24; see also Fig. 16–8). Friedman and colleagues[128] and Mullaji and associates[242] have used computed tomography (CT) to document that arthritic involvement may alter the glenoid version. The orientation of the glenoid prosthesis should be normalized as a part of the arthroplasty procedure (Figs. 16–25 to 16–27).

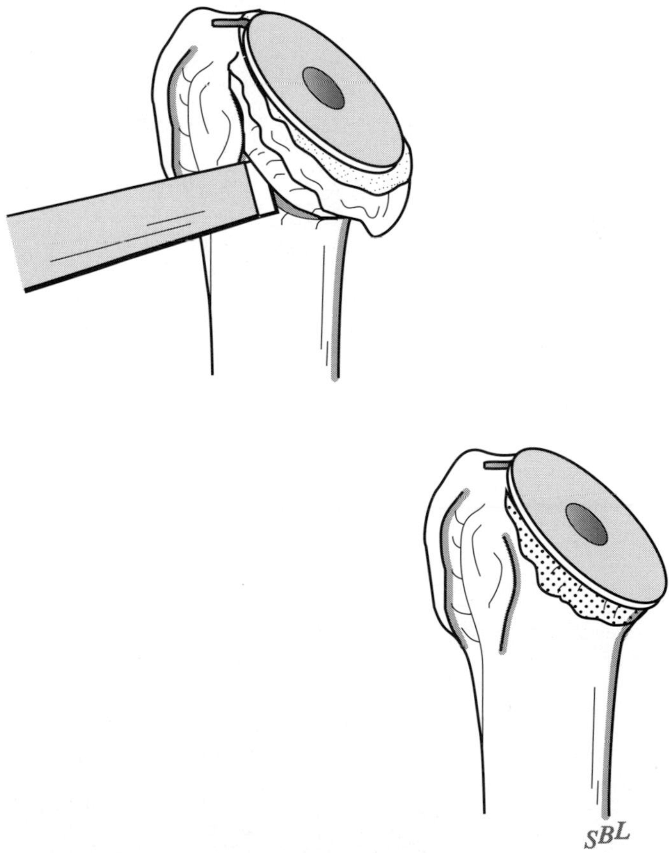

Figure 16–18

Resection of osteophytes using the rim of the prosthetic collar as a girdle. (From Pearl ML and Lippitt SB: Shoulder arthroplasty with a modular prosthesis. Tech Orthop 8[3]:151–162, 1994. Original illustrator—SB Lippitt.)

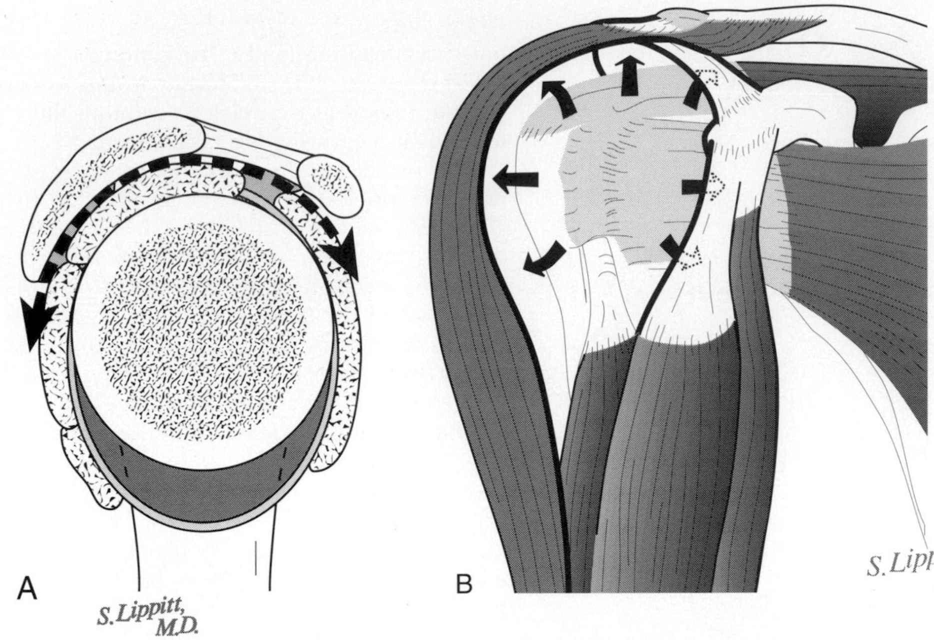

Figure 16–19

A and *B*, The humeroscapular motion interface is an important location of motion between the humerus and the scapula. The deltoid, acromion, coracoacromial ligament, coracoid process, and tendons attaching to the coracoid lie on the superficial side of this interface, whereas the proximal humerus, rotator cuff, and biceps tendon sheath lie on its deep side.

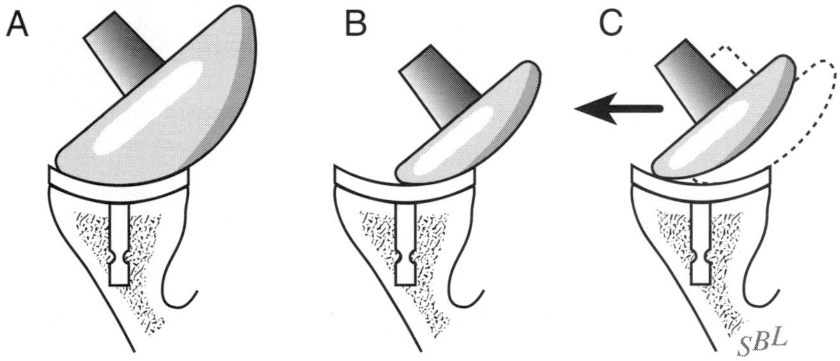

Figure 16–20

The effect of humeral contact area on translational stability. Full surface contact provides maximal joint stability (*A*). When full surface contact is lacking because of a small humeral joint surface angle (*B*), the humeral component can be translated in the direction of the empty part of the glenoid (*C*). (Modified from Matsen FA III, Lippitt SB, Sidles JA, and Harryman DT II: Practical Evaluation and Management of the Shoulder. Philadelphia: WB Saunders, 1994.)

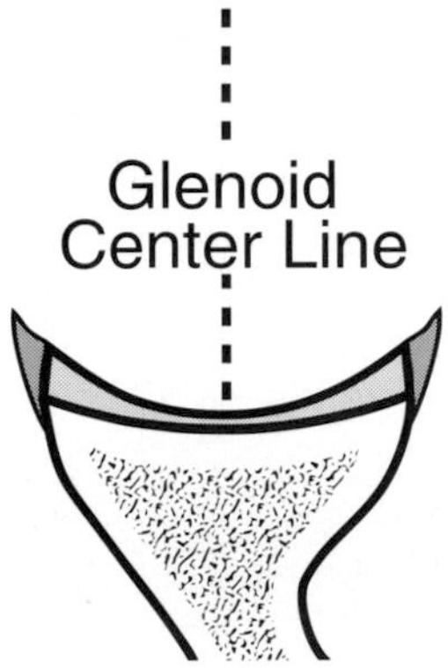

Figure 16–21

The *glenoid center line* is a line perpendicular to the surface of the glenoid fossa at its midpoint. (Modified from Matsen FA III, Lippitt SB, Sidles JA, and Harryman DT II: Practical Evaluation and Management of the Shoulder. Philadelphia: WB Saunders, 1994.)

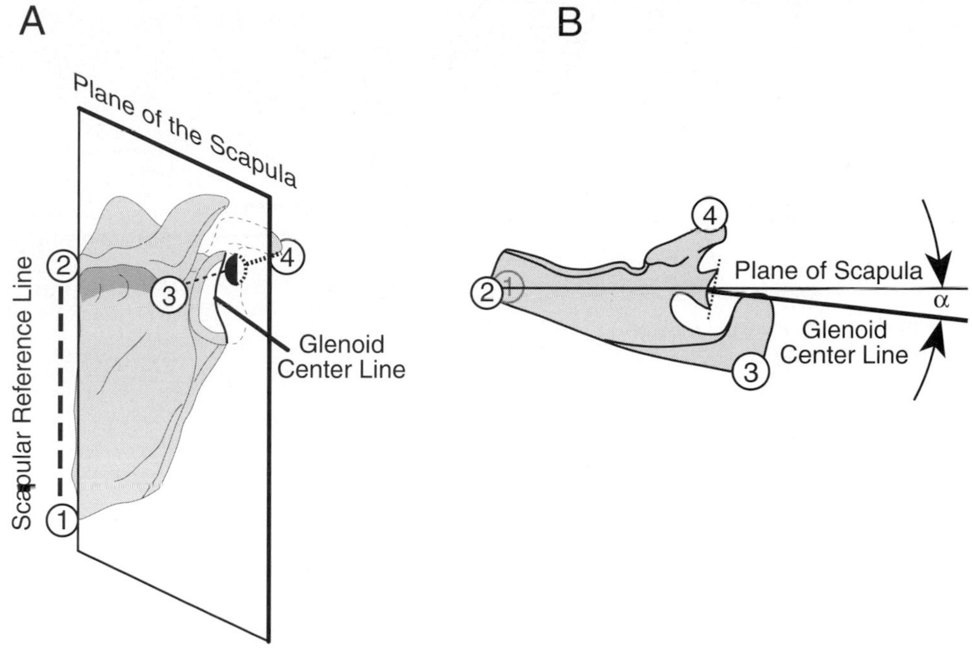

Figure 16–22

The glenoid center line can be related to scapular coordinates and to the plane of the scapula. These reference points are all easily palpated: *A*, (1) the inferior pole of the scapula, (2) the medial end of the spine of the scapula, (3) the posterior angle of the acromion, and (4) the coracoid tip. *B*, The scapular reference line connects reference points 1 and 2. The plane of the scapula passes through points 1 and 2 and halfway between points 3 and 4. The glenoid center line usually makes a slightly posterior angle (α) with the plane of the scapula. (Modified from Matsen FA III, Lippitt SB, Sidles JA, and Harryman DT II: Practical Evaluation and Management of the Shoulder. Philadelphia: WB Saunders, 1994.)

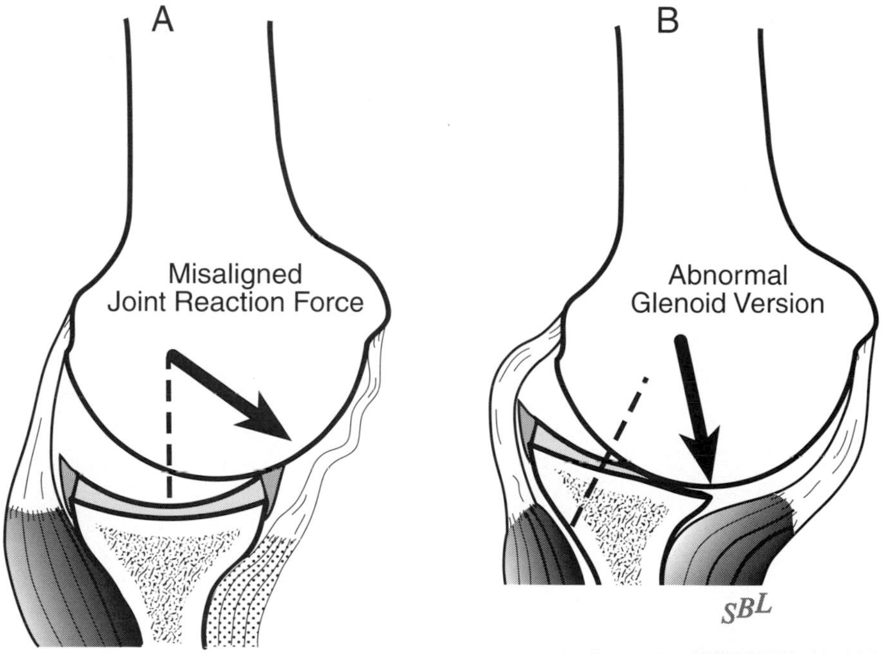

Figure 16–23

A, Stability is compromised by muscle imbalance. In this example, the humerus is aligned with the glenoid center line, but the net humeral joint reaction force is misaligned owing to weakness of the posterior cuff musculature. *B*, Balance stability is also compromised by the abnormal glenoid version. In this example, the humerus is aligned with the plane of the scapula, but severe glenoid retroversion results in a posteriorly directed glenoid center line that is divergent from the net humeral joint reaction force. (Modified from Matsen FA III, Lippitt SB, Sidles JA, and Harryman DT II: Practical Evaluation and Management of the Shoulder. Philadelphia: WB Saunders, 1994.)

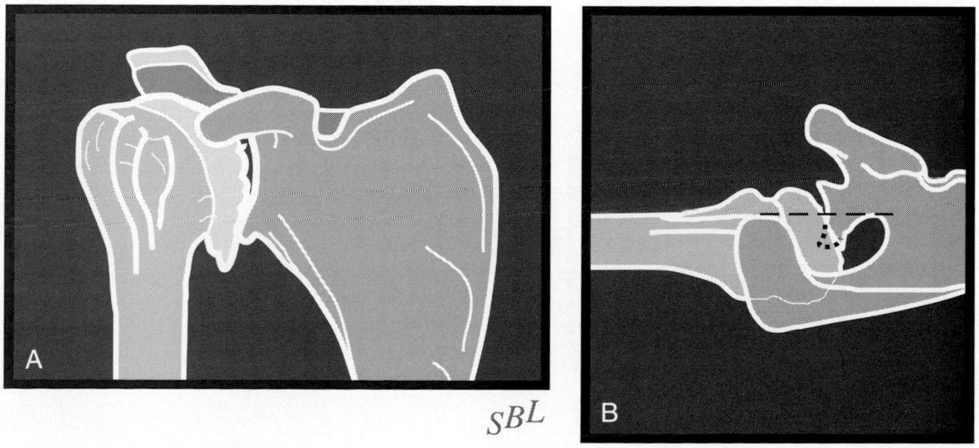

Figure 16–24

Glenohumeral degenerative joint disease. *A*, An anteroposterior view showing the typical "goat's beard" osteophyte enlarging the apparent superoinferior dimension of the head. *B*, Axillary view showing posterior subluxation and posterior rim wear. (Modified from Matsen FA III, Lippitt SB, Sidles JA, and Harryman DT II: Practical Evaluation and Management of the Shoulder. Philadelphia: WB Saunders, 1994.)

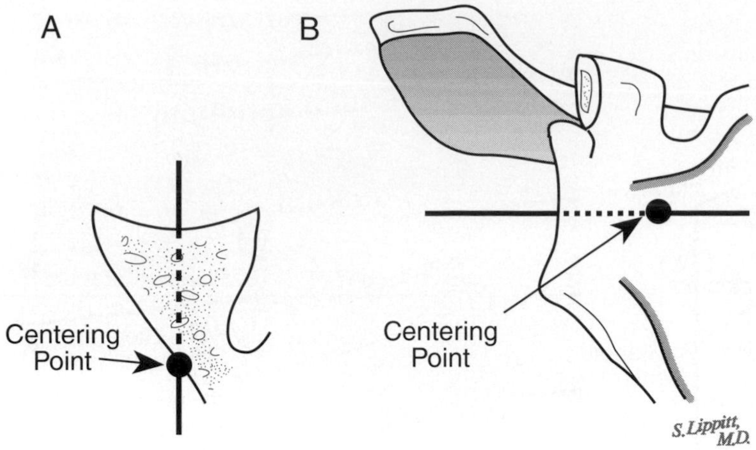

Figure 16–25

The normal glenoid center line passes perpendicular to the center of the glenoid articular surface and exits the glenoid neck at the "centering point" between the upper and lower crura of the scapula in the lateral aspect of the subscapularis fossa. (From Matsen FA III, Lippitt SB, Sidles JA, and Harryman DT II: Practical Evaluation and Management of the Shoulder. Philadelphia: WB Saunders, 1994.)

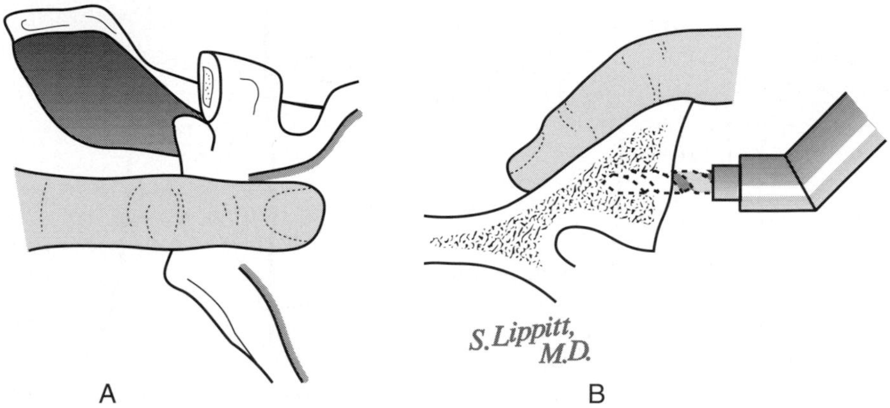

Figure 16–26

Use of the glenoid centering point to help orient the central hole for glenoid component fixation. *A*, The index finger is inserted anterior to the glenoid so that its tip palpates the centering point in the sulcus bounded by the thick upper and lower crura of the scapula and the flare of the glenoid vault. *B*, This centering point serves as a useful guide for drilling the normal glenoid center line, particularly when the anatomic structure is distorted by eccentric glenoid wear. The normal glenoid center line connects the center of the glenoid face with the centering point. (Modified from Matsen FA III, Lippitt SB, Sidles JA, and Harryman DT II: Practical Evaluation and Management of the Shoulder. Philadelphia: WB Saunders, 1994.)

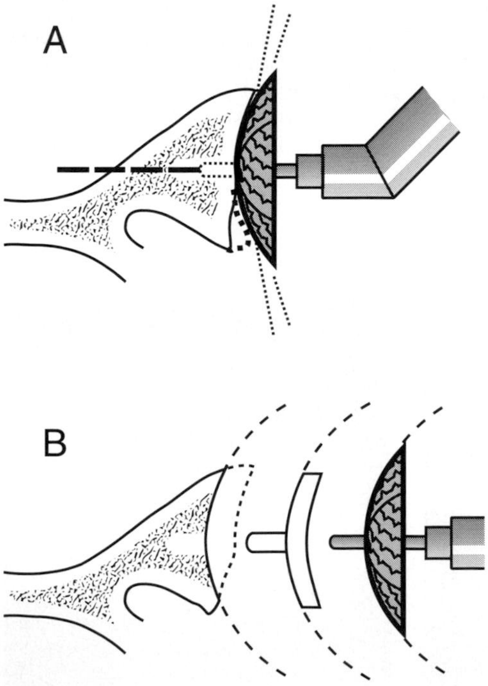

Figure 16–27

A, Reaming along the normalized glenoid center line. The objective is to normalize the glenoid orientation and to contour the glenoid face to match the back of glenoid component. *B*, Accurate contouring of the glenoid face improves the quality of bone support for the glenoid component. (Modified from Matsen FA III, Lippitt SB, Sidles JA, and Harryman DT II: Practical Evaluation and Management of the Shoulder. Philadelphia: WB Saunders, 1994.)

Glenoid Concavity with Sufficiently Large Effective Arcs. The arc of the glenoid determines the maximal angles that the net humeral joint reaction force can make with the glenoid center line before dislocation occurs (Fig. 16–28).

In the arthritic joint, the effective glenoid arc can be diminished by wear or inflammation; for example, posterior wear is typical of glenohumeral osteoarthritis (see Figs. 16–23*B* and 16–24) and capsulorrhaphy arthropathy (see Fig. 16–8), whereas central erosion of the glenoid is typical of rheumatoid arthritis (Fig. 16–29). At arthroplasty, the effective glenoid arcs need to be restored (see Fig. 16–27).

Control of the Net Humeral Joint Reaction Force. The direction of the net humeral joint reaction force is controlled actively by the elements of the rotator cuff and other shoulder muscles (Fig. 16–30). Neural control of the magnitude of the different muscle forces provides the mechanism by which the direction of the net humeral joint reaction force is modulated. For example, by increasing the force of contraction of a muscle whose force direction is parallel to the glenoid center line, the body can change the direction of the net humeral joint reaction force to an orientation of closer alignment with the glenoid fossa (Fig. 16–31).

In glenohumeral arthritis, control of the net humeral joint reaction force may be compromised by tendon ruptures, tuberosity detachment, and deconditioning (see Fig. 16–23). The most striking example is in cuff tear arthropathy where the normally stabilizing cuff muscle forces are compromised (Figs. 16–32 to 16–34).

If, following glenohumeral arthroplasty, the net humeral joint reaction force is not centered in the glenoid fossa, eccentric loading may produce "rocking horse" loosening of the glenoid component (Fig. 16–35). A slight degree of mismatch of the glenoid and humeral diameters

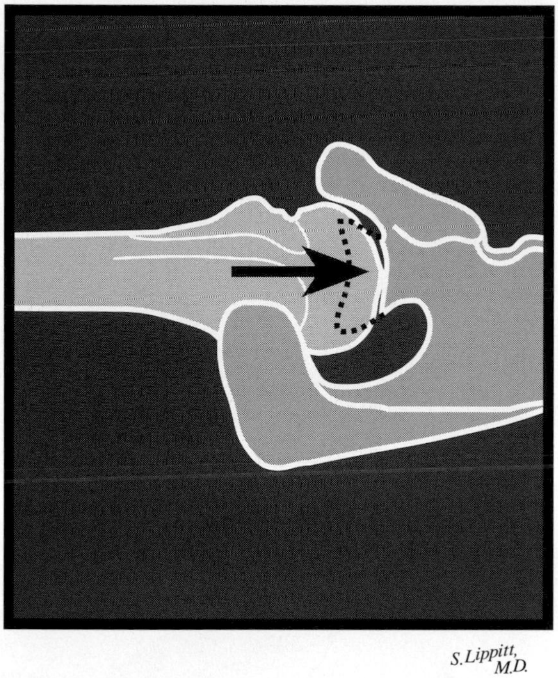

Figure 16–29

Axillary view of glenohumeral rheumatoid arthritis showing medial erosion of the glenoid. (From Matsen FA III, Lippitt SB, Sidles JA, and Harryman DT II: Practical Evaluation and Management of the Shoulder. Philadelphia: WB Saunders, 1994.)

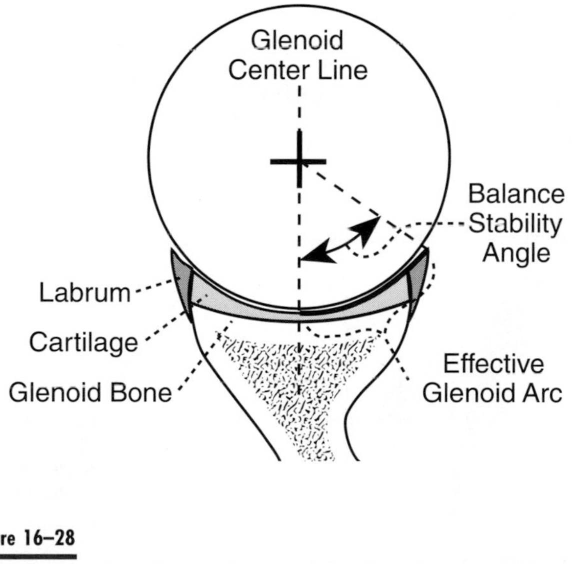

Figure 16–28

The effective glenoid arc is the arc of the glenoid able to support the net humeral joint reaction force. The balance stability angle is the maximal angle that the net humeral joint reaction force can make with the glenoid center line before dislocation occurs. (Modified from Matsen FA III, Lippitt SB, Sidles JA, and Harryman DT II: Practical Evaluation and Management of the Shoulder. Philadelphia: WB Saunders, 1994.)

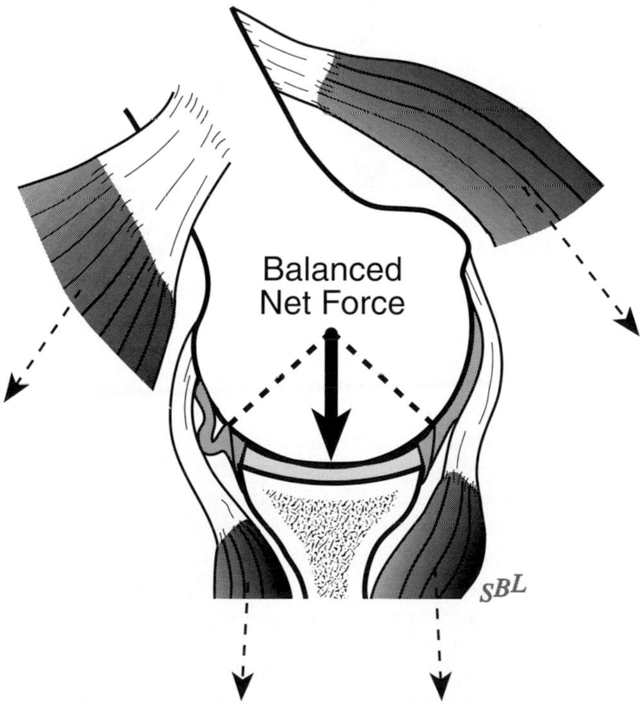

Figure 16–30

The vector sum of the deltoid and the cuff muscle forces lies close to the axis of the humerus in many functional positions of the shoulder. (Modified from Matsen FA III, Lippitt SB, Sidles JA, and Harryman DT II: Practical Evaluation and Management of the Shoulder. Philadelphia: WB Saunders, 1994.)

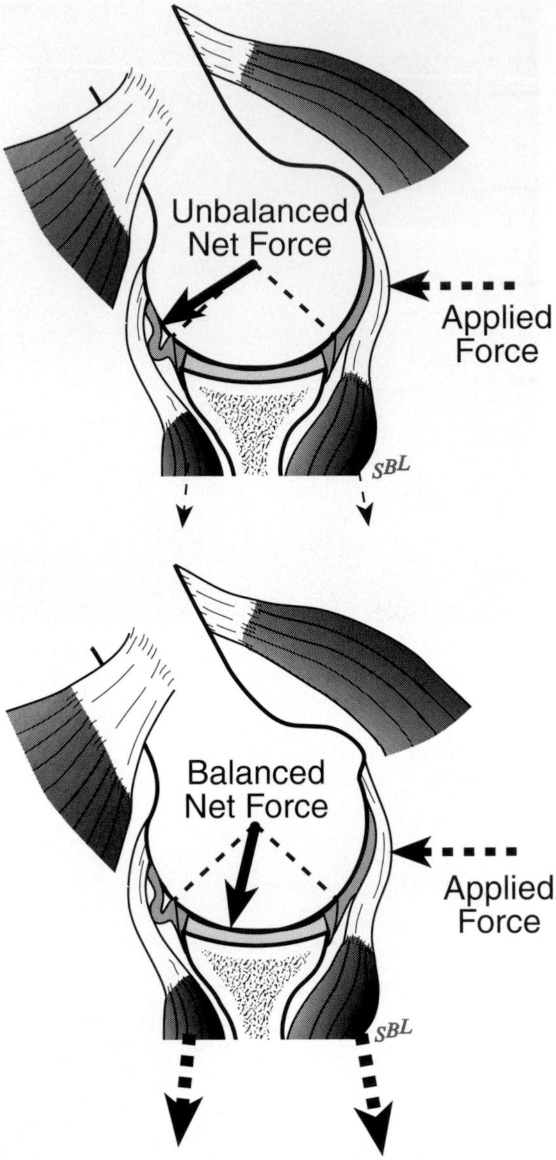

Figure 16–31

Stabilizing the glenohumeral joint against an applied translational force. Strong contraction of the cuff muscles provides an increased compression force into the glenoid concavity. As a result, the net humeral force is balanced within the glenoid concavity.

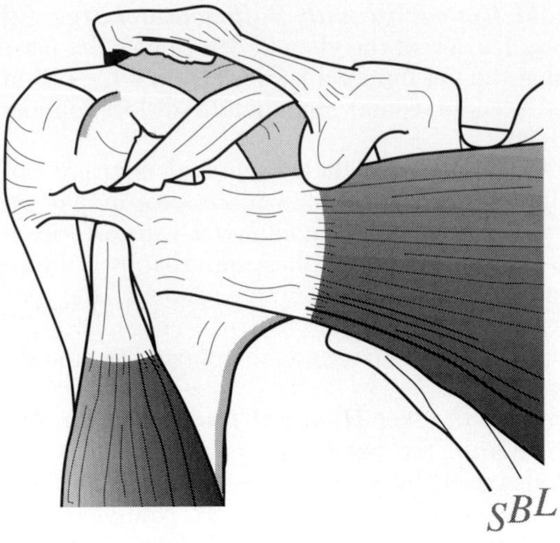

Figure 16–32

The boutonnière deformity, in which the subscapularis and infraspinatus tendons slide below the center of the humeral head. (Modified from Matsen FA III, Lippitt SB, Sidles JA, and Harryman DT II: Practical Evaluation and Management of the Shoulder. Philadelphia: WB Saunders, 1994.)

of curvature allows for minor amounts of force malalignment before rim contact occurs (Figs. 16–36 and 16–37). Severt and associates[323] pointed out that high degrees of conformity between the glenoid and humeral joint surfaces increases the translational forces and frictional torque applied to the glenoid component and on this basis advocated the use of less conforming and less constrained designs.

Severe degrees of mismatch may have adverse effects on the glenohumeral contact area (Fig. 16–38) and on peak stresses in the polyethylene (Fig. 16–39).

Strength

The requisites of strength include:

1. A functional deltoid
2. A functional rotator cuff
3. Normal length relationships of muscle origin and insertions

In the arthritic shoulder, strength can be compromised by cuff deterioration, disuse, previous injury, and previous surgery. The surgeon may be able to enhance the strength of the shoulder through muscle balancing, tendon repairs, tuberosity reattachment, and effective rehabilitation.[42] It

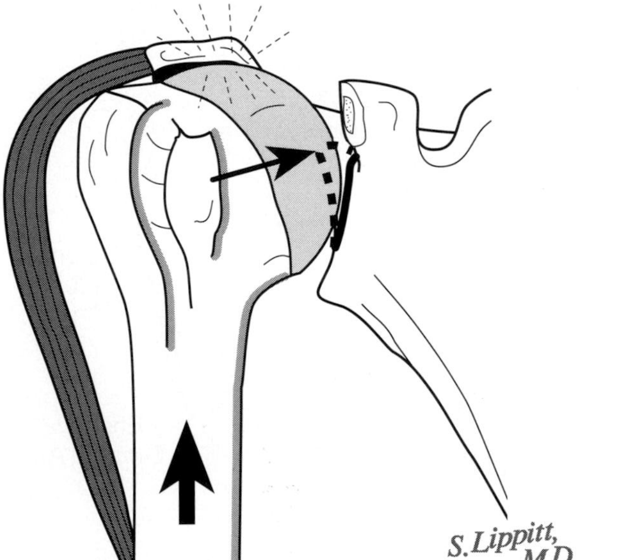

Figure 16–33

Erosion of the superior glenoid concavity compromises the concavity compression stability mechanism, allowing upward translation when the deltoid contracts. (Modified from Matsen FA III, Lippitt SB, Sidles JA, and Harryman DT II: Practical Evaluation and Management of the Shoulder. Philadelphia: WB Saunders, 1994.)

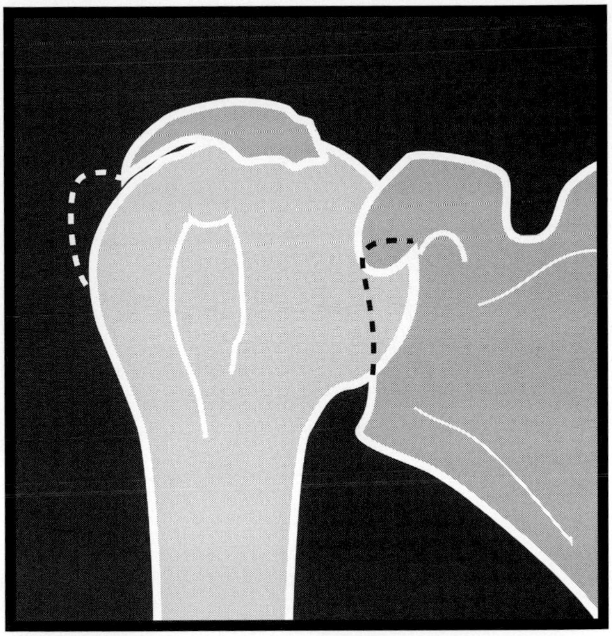

Figure 16–34

Radiographic appearance of cuff tear arthropathy with "acetabularization" of the upper glenoid and the coracoacromial arch and "femoralization" of the proximal humerus. (Modified from Matsen FA III, Lippitt SB, Sidles JA, and Harryman DT II: Practical Evaluation and Management of the Shoulder. Philadelphia: WB Saunders, 1994.)

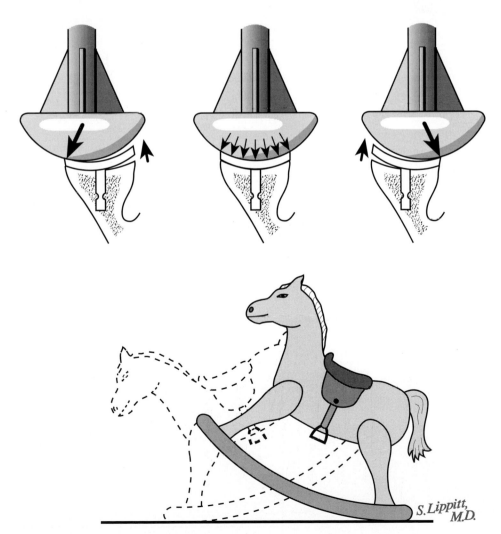

Figure 16–35

"Rocking horse" loosening of the glenoid component results when translation of the head on the glenoid produces eccentric forces on the glenoid component. (From Matsen FA III, Lippitt SB, Sidles JA, and Harryman DT II: Practical Evaluation and Management of the Shoulder. Philadelphia: WB Saunders, 1994.)

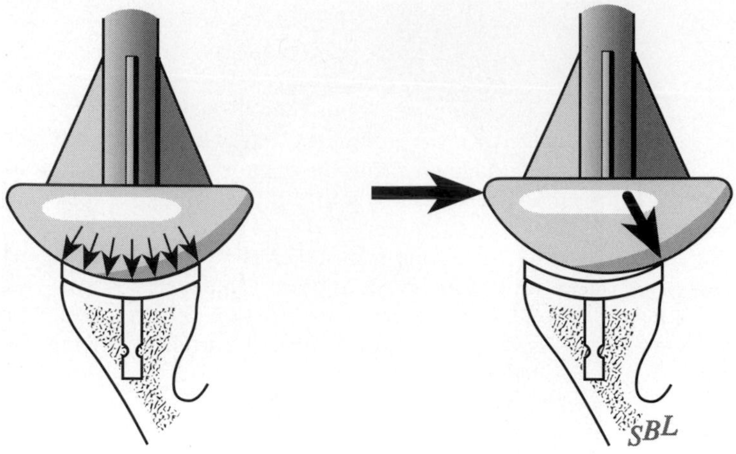

Figure 16–36

When the radii of curvature of the glenoid component and the humeral head conform, any translation results in glenoid component rim loading.

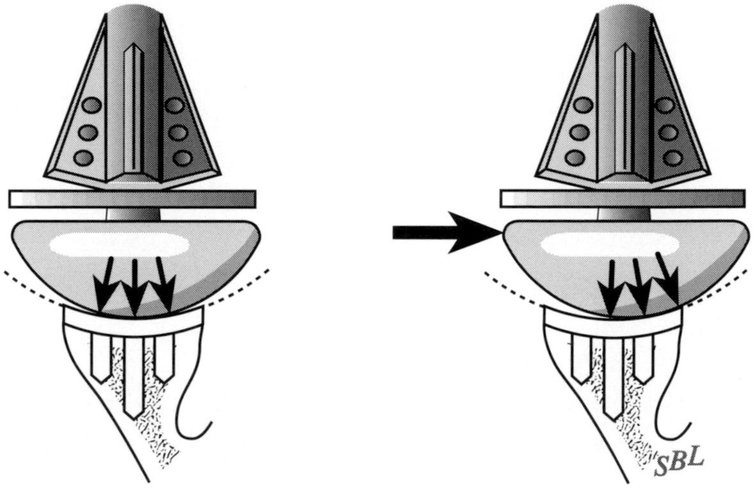

Figure 16–37

A slight increase in the diameter of curvature of the glenoid component over that of the humeral head allows some translation before rim loading occurs.

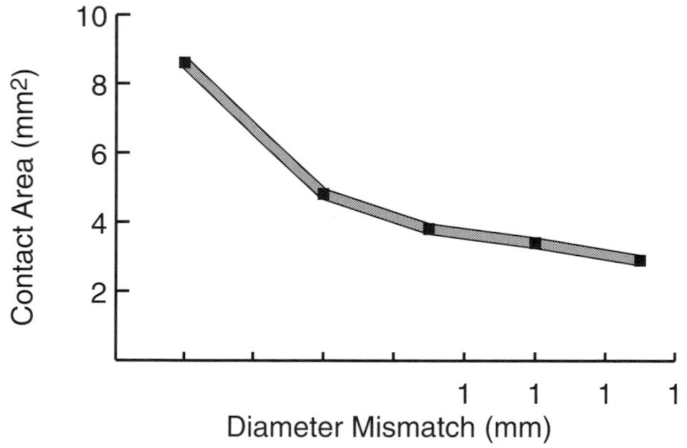

Figure 16–38

Results of a finite element model analysis of a polyethylene glenoid showing the effect of diameter mismatch on the contact area. Even a slight increase in the glenoid diameter relative to that of the humerus dramatically reduces the contact area. Any further increase in the mismatch further reduces the contact area. (From Matsen FA III, Lippitt SB, Sidles JA, and Harryman DT II: Practical Evaluation and Management of the Shoulder. Philadelphia: WB Saunders, 1994.)

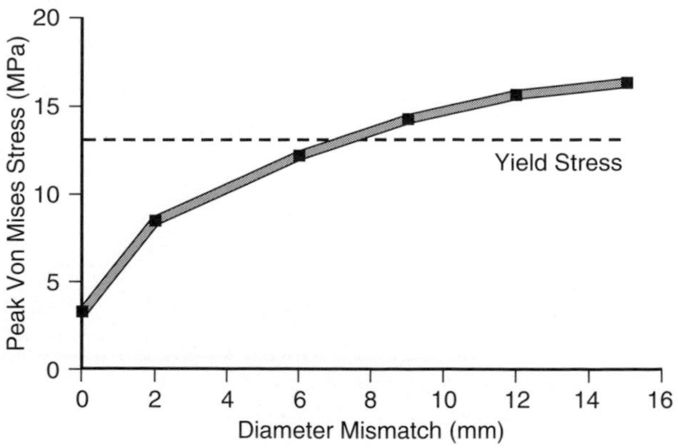

Figure 16–39

Results of a finite element model analysis of the effect of diameter mismatch on the peak contact stresses (pressure-modified Von Mises stress) in a polyethylene glenoid component. The applied compressive load is 625 N (approximately one body weight). The predicted yield stress for the component is shown. A load of one body weight with diametral mismatch in excess of 6 mm is predicted to exceed the yield stress of ordinary polyethylene. (From Matsen FA III, Lippitt SB, Sidles JA, and Harryman DT II: Practical Evaluation and Management of the Shoulder. Philadelphia: WB Saunders, 1994.)

is critical that the procedure not impair the function of the muscle-tendon units (Fig. 16–40).

The amount of stuffing of the joint sets the resting length of the cuff muscles and to a lesser extent that of the deltoid. If the components are too small, the cuff will be slack at rest and thus place the muscles at the low end of the ideal length-tension relationship. If the joint is overstuffed, the cuff muscles may be at the high end of their length-tension curve. The distance between the effective cuff insertion and the humeral head center establishes the moment arm for the cuff.

Jacobson and Mallon have provided a method for measuring the glenohumeral offset ratio,[171] while Hsu and associates have reviewed the influence of abductor lever arm changes after shoulder arthroplasty.[165]

Smoothness

The anatomic requisites of smooth motion follow.

Smooth Joint Surfaces. In the normal shoulder, intact articular cartilage covering the humeral head and glenoid lubricated with normal joint fluid provide the lowest possible resistance to motion at the joint surface. In arthritis, these factors are compromised. Although prosthetic joint surfaces offer much less friction than bone rubbing on bone, they have a coefficient of friction approximately ten times greater than that of normal cartilage moving on normal cartilage.

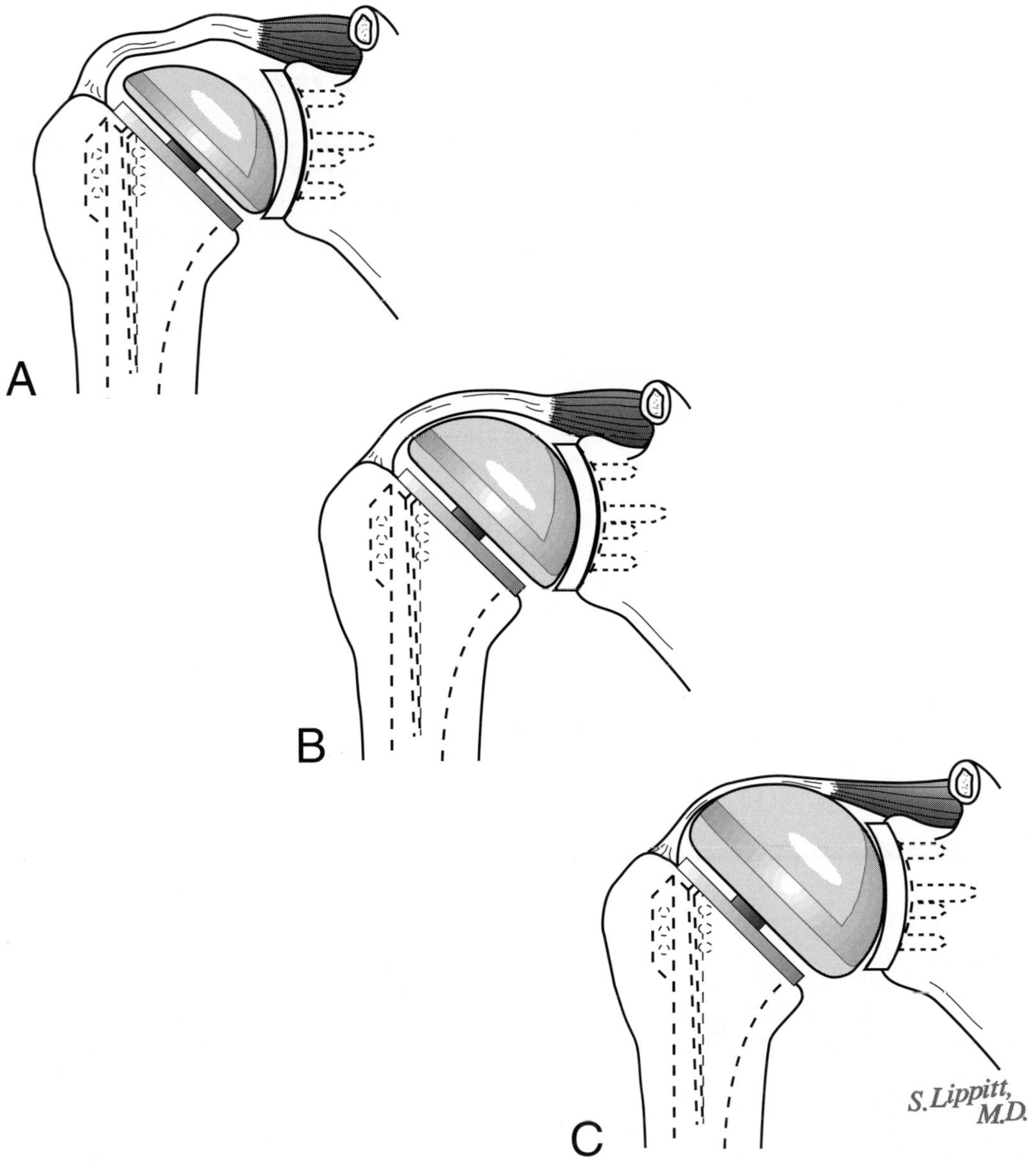

Figure 16–40

A, A humeral head that is too small leaves the joint with excessive laxity and reduced resting muscle tension. *B*, The correct size of head balances the soft tissues. *C*, Overstuffing the joint places excessive tension on the soft tissues, limiting their excursion, decreasing range of motion, and predisposing them to rupture. (Modified from Matsen FA III, Lippitt SB, Sidles JA, and Harryman DT II: Practical Evaluation and Management of the Shoulder. Philadelphia: WB Saunders, 1994.)

Smooth and Unimpaired Humeroscapular Motion Interface. The proximal humerus and rotator cuff must slide smoothly beneath the deltoid, acromion, coracoacromial ligament, coracoid, and coracoid muscles (see Fig. 16–19). Smoothness of the humeroscapular motion interface is often compromised in postsurgical and posttraumatic arthritis. The surfaces of this important interface must glide smoothly on each other at the conclusion of the arthroplasty procedure.

CLINICAL PRESENTATION AND EVALUATION

History

The patient with significant glenohumeral arthritis usually presents with pain and loss of function, which are refractory to rest, anti-inflammatory medications, and exercise. The history should include a description of the onset of the problem, the mechanism of any injuries, and the nature and progression of functional difficulties. Systemic or polyarticular manifestations of sepsis, degenerative joint disease, or rheumatoid arthritis may provide helpful clues. A past history of steroid medication, fracture, or working at depths may suggest the diagnosis of avascular necrosis. Past injury or surgery suggest the possibility of secondary arthritis or capsulorrhaphy arthropathy.

Standardized methods have been developed by which patients can assess their health status and shoulder function. Bostrom and associates[35] found that standardized assessments of shoulder function are more reliable and reproducible than are conventional range-of-motion measurements. Matsen and colleagues reported the self-assessment of 103 patients with primary glenohumeral degenerative joint disease.[221, 224] More than half reported that their SF-36 pain and physical role function scores were more than one standard deviation below those of age- and sex-matched controls. These patients consistently reported the inability to perform standard shoulder functions, such as sleeping comfortably, lifting 8 lb to shoulder height, washing the back of the opposite shoulder, throwing overhand, and tucking in a shirt behind. Matsen and associates used self-assessment of shoulder function and health status to compare patients with rheumatoid arthritis and degenerative joint disease of the shoulder.[222]

Physical Examination

The physical examination often reveals mild or moderate muscle wasting about the shoulder, crepitus on joint motion, and limited range of motion. The limitation of glenohumeral motion is most easily identified if one of the examiner's hands is used to stabilize the scapula while the flexion/extension and internal/external rotation of the humerus relative to the scapula are documented with the other.

Isometric strength is documented in flexion, extension, abduction, and rotation. Individuals being considered for prosthetic arthroplasty should have good anterior deltoid and rotator cuff strength. Strong internal and external rotators are particularly important if a glenoid prosthesis is being considered.

It is important to emphasize that shoulder arthritis may coexist with other medical conditions, many of which will substantially alter the patient's disability and their potential to respond positively to treatment. Thus, a thorough evaluation of each individual is essential. As will be seen later, the SF-36 provides a standardized documentation of the patient's self-assessed health status. The importance of factors, such as the SF-36 scales of emotional role function, mental health, and social function, is well demonstrated in the work of Summers and associates,[333] who found that the objective severity of the disease showed little relationship to patients' reports of pain, whereas psychological variables were much more closely correlated with measures of pain and functional impairment.

Radiographic Evaluation

In the evaluation of glenohumeral arthritis, standardized radiographic views are necessary to understand the disease process and its severity. Standard views include an anteroposterior view in the plane of the scapula and a true axillary view (Fig. 16–41). These views indicate the thickness of the cartilage space between the humerus and the glenoid; the relative positions of the humeral head and the glenoid; the presence of osteophytes; the degree of osteopenia; and the extent of bony deformity and erosion. Superior displacement of the humeral head relative to the scapula suggests major cuff deficiency and argues against the use of a glenoid prosthesis (see Fig. 16–34). If a humeral arthroplasty is being considered, a templating anteroposterior view of the humerus in 35 degrees of external rotation relative to the x-ray beam with a magnification marker is obtained (Fig. 16–42). This view places the humeral neck in maximal profile, allowing a comparison of the proximal humeral anatomy to that of various humeral prostheses. If this view is taken with the arm in 45 degrees of abduction, placing the middle of the humeral articular surface in the middle of the glenoid fossa, it can reveal thinning of the central aspect of the humeral articular cartilage typical of degenerative joint disease (the "Friar Tuck" pattern), whereas radiographs with the arm in other positions may suggest the presence of a thicker layer of cartilage at the periphery of the head.

CT scans are obtained if there is a question about the amount or quality of bone available for reconstruction. These questions can usually be answered from plain radiographs alone. Friedman and associates[128] and Mullaji and colleagues[242] have used CT to characterize the changes in version in a group of patients with degenerative and inflammatory arthritis. The most important conclusion from these two studies is that glenoid version varies through a range of 30 degrees in these populations! Mallon and associates[215] have also conducted detailed studies of the articular surface of the glenoid and related this shape to the anatomy of the scapula.

Galinat reported variation in the glenoid version depending on the angle of the x-ray beam during positioning of the machine for the axillary x-ray.[132] Glenoid version can be measured by connecting a line drawn down the

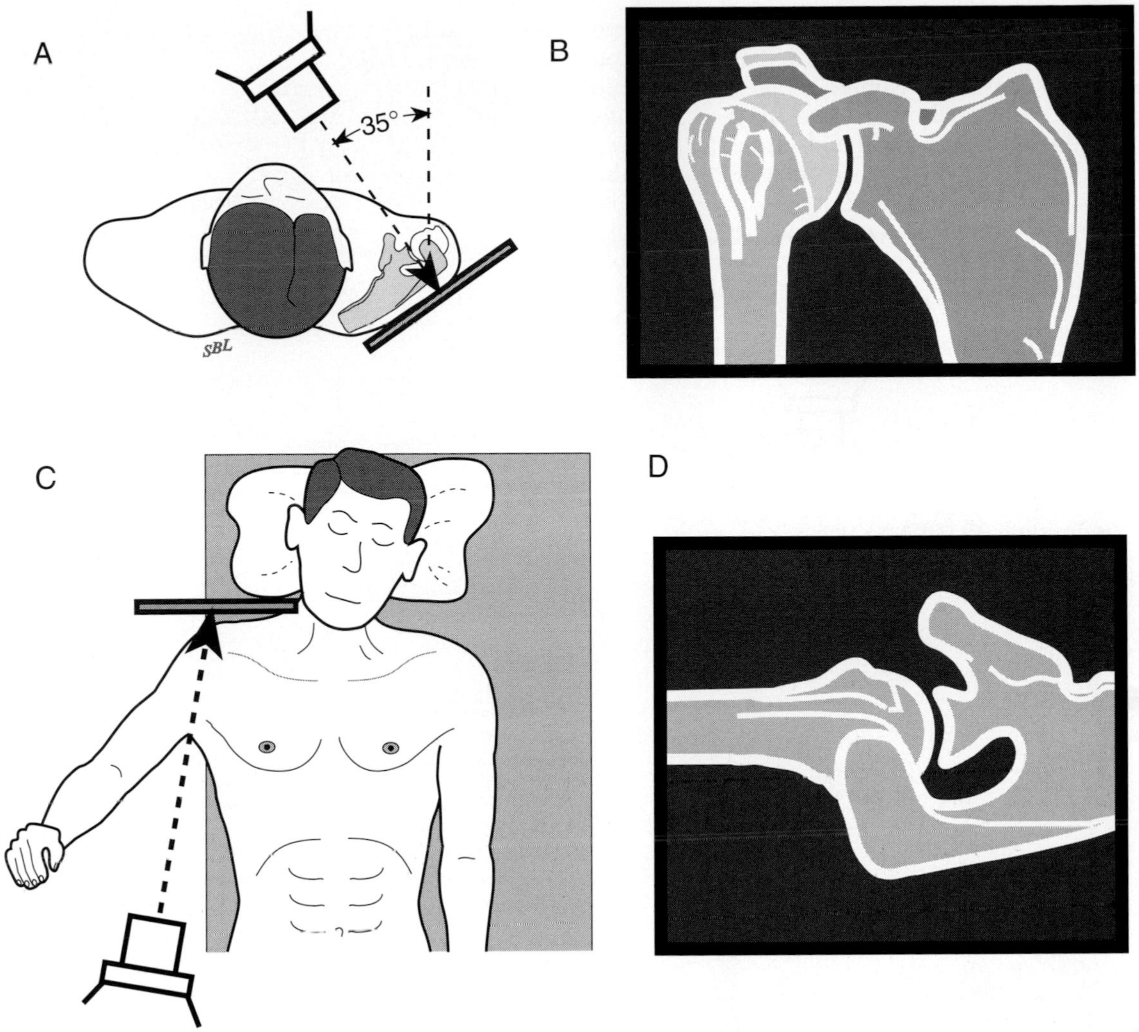

Figure 16–41

Radiographic series for a stiff shoulder. *A*, The anteroposterior view in the plane of the scapula is obtained by orienting the beam perpendicular to the plane of the scapula and centering it on the coracoid tip while the film is parallel to the plane of the scapula. *B*, The resultant radiograph should clearly reveal the radiographic joint space between the humeral head and the glenoid. *C*, The axillary view is obtained by centering the beam between the coracoid tip and the posterior angle of the acromion. *D*, The resultant radiograph should project the glenoid midway between the coracoid and the acromion, providing a clear view of the joint space. (From Matsen FA III, Lippitt SB, Sidles JA, and Harryman DT II: Practical Evaluation and Management of the Shoulder. Philadelphia: WB Saunders, 1994.)

line of the body of the scapula with a line between the anterior and posterior glenoid rim. Normal version at the level just below the coracoid process varies from 0 degrees to −7 degrees (Fig. 16–43). In a series of 200 patients undergoing shoulder arthroplasty, Jensen and Rockwood obtained a CT scan in 78 patients to define glenoid version.[173] These 78 patients also had severe loss of external rotation and posterior subluxation of the head of the humerus. Sixty-three per cent, or 49 shoulders, required specific alterations during their arthroplasty (i.e., decreasing the amount of humeral retroversion or changing the version of the glenoid with special reamers).

Imaging of the rotator cuff by arthrography, magnetic resonance imaging (MRI), or ultrasound is carried out if it will affect management of the patient. The status of the rotator cuff can usually be understood from an evaluation of the history, the physical examination, and the plain radiographs.

Green and Norris[139] and Slawson and associates[325] have provided a review of imaging techniques for glenohumeral arthritis and for glenohumeral arthroplasty.

Disease Characteristics

A number of different processes can destroy the glenohumeral joint surface. Clinical evaluation, management, and effectiveness measurement is facilitated by establishing necessary and sufficient criteria that enable us to standardize the assignment of each diagnosis. Table 16–2 lists the necessary and sufficient criteria for six of the more common types of glenohumeral joint destruction: primary degenerative joint disease, secondary degenerative joint disease, rheumatoid arthritis, cuff tear arthropathy, capsulorrhaphy arthropathy, and avascular necrosis.

In an extension of a study on self-assessment of patients

with glenohumeral osteoarthritis,[224] patients presenting with these conditions assessed their shoulder function using the 12 questions of the Simple Shoulder Test (Table 16–3).[221] These individuals with glenohumeral arthritis had greatest difficulty with overhand throwing, sleeping comfortably on the affected side, washing the back of the opposite shoulder, and placing 8 lb on a shelf (Table 16–4). Interestingly, the degree of functional compromise at the time of presentation for evaluation was comparable for the different diagnoses. Apparently, it is this level of functional impairment, irrespective of the diagnosis, that brings the patient in for evaluation.

These individuals also assessed their health status using the SF-36.*

The self-assessed overall health status of individuals with glenohumeral arthritis is most compromised in the domains of physical role function and overall comfort (Table 16–5). For patients with primary and secondary degenerative joint disease and cuff tear arthropathy, the other SF-36 parameters (e.g., vitality and overall health) were relatively close to population-based age and sex-matched controls. The health status of patients with rheumatoid arthritis, capsulorrhaphy arthropathy, and avascular necrosis was poorer than that of controls of the same age and sex.[222]

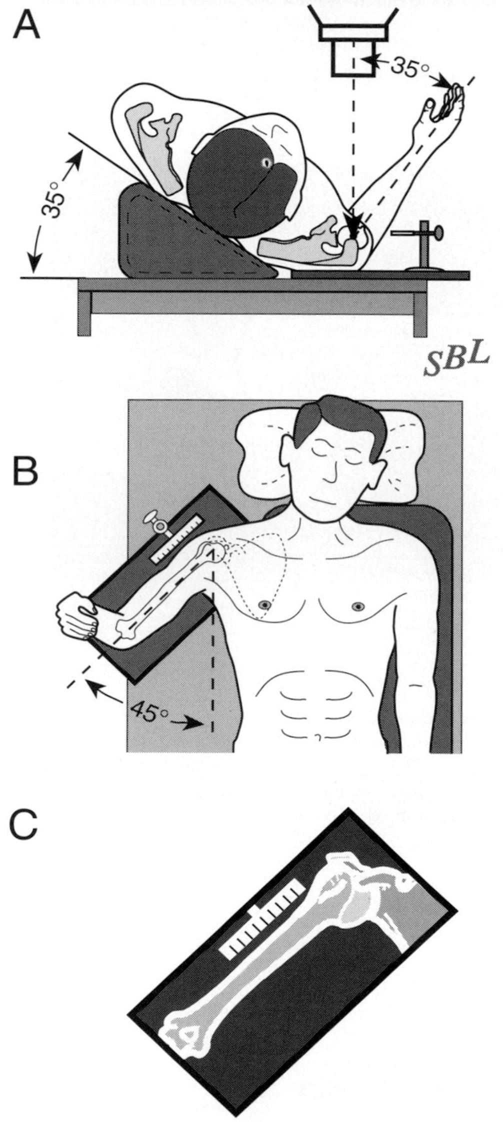

Figure 16–42

Templating view, the anteroposterior radiograph in the "centered position." The humerus is positioned in neutral rotation with respect to the thorax and is abducted 45 degrees. The anteroposterior radiograph in the plane of the scapula is obtained by positioning the scapula flat on the cassette and by aiming the beam at the joint. The beam makes a 35-degree angle with the forearm, and the thorax makes a 35-degree angle with the cassette. A centimeter marker held adjacent to the lateral humerus indicates the radiographic magnification when templates for various components are compared. The final radiographic appearance is as shown in *C*. (From Matsen FA III, Lippitt SB, Sidles JA, and Harryman DT II: Practical Evaluation and Management of the Shoulder. Philadelphia: WB Saunders, 1994.)

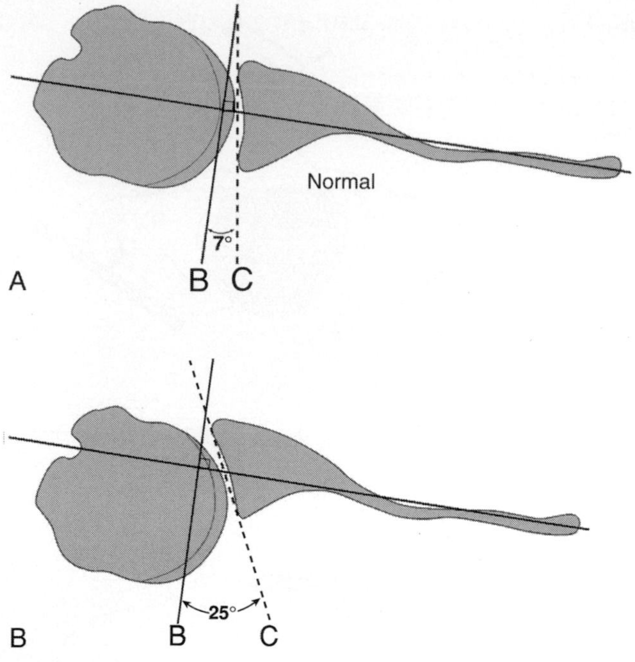

Figure 16–43

A, Normal glenoid version varies from 0 to -7 degrees of retroversion. Using a computed tomography scan, the measurement of version is accomplished by drawing a line along the axis of the scapular body and then drawing a line perpendicular to it (B). A third line is drawn along the anterior and posterior rims of the glenoid (C). The angle between B and C is the glenoid version. *B*, An increase in retroversion to 25 degrees is usually accompanied by posterior subluxation of the head of the humerus.

DEGENERATIVE JOINT DISEASE

In degenerative joint disease, the glenoid cartilage and subchondral bone are typically worn posteriorly, often leaving intact articular cartilage anteriorly (see Fig. 16–24). The cartilage of the humeral head is eroded in a

*The SF-36 is a general health status self-assessment used in many fields of medicine.[289, 350] It is very useful in orthopedics for documenting the general health deficits of patients before and after reconstructive surgery. The overall comfort and physical role function scales are most commonly affected by arthritic conditions of the shoulder. Other SF-36 scores are useful in documenting the patient's vitality, mental health, general health, and social, emotional, and physical function.

Table 16–2 NECESSARY AND SUFFICIENT DIAGNOSTIC CRITERIA FOR CLINICALLY SIGNIFICANT INVOLVEMENT FROM SIX MAJOR TYPES OF GLENOHUMERAL ARTHRITIS

DEGENERATIVE JOINT DISEASE (PRIMARY)

History

1. Absence of major joint trauma, previous surgery, or other known causes of secondary degenerative joint disease
2. Limited motion and function

Physical Examination

1. Limited glenohumeral motion
2. (Diagnosis is supported by bone-on-bone crepitance)

Radiographs (see Figs. 16–24, 16–44, 16–45)

1. Joint space narrowing
2. Periarticular sclerosis
3. Periarticular osteophytes
4. Absence of other pathology
5. (Diagnosis is supported by posterior glenoid erosion with posterior subluxation of the humeral head)

SECONDARY DEGENERATIVE JOINT DISEASE

History

1. Evidence of major joint trauma or other known causes of secondary degenerative joint disease
2. Limited motion and function

Physical Examination

1. Limited glenohumeral motion
2. (Diagnosis is supported by bone-on-bone crepitance)

Radiographs (see Figs. 16–46 to 16–50)

1. Joint space narrowing
2. Periarticular sclerosis
3. Periarticular osteophytes
4. (Diagnosis is supported by radiographic evidence of previous trauma or other known causes of secondary degenerative joint disease)

RHEUMATOID ARTHRITIS

History

1. Established diagnosis rheumatoid arthritis
2. Limited motion and function

Physical Examination (see Fig. 16–62)

1. Limited glenohumeral motion
2. (Diagnosis is supported by findings of muscle atrophy and weakness or bone-on-bone crepitance)

Radiographs (see Figs. 16–29, 16–51 to 16–62)

1. Joint space narrowing
2. Periarticular osteopenia
3. (Diagnosis is supported by the absence of osteophytes and sclerosis)
4. (Diagnosis is supported by the presence of periarticular erosions and medial erosion of the glenoid)

CUFF TEAR ARTHROPATHY

History

1. Limited motion and function
2. Weakness in elevation and rotation
3. Diagnosis is supported by previously confirmed cuff tear

Physical Examination

1. Limited glenohumeral motion
2. Evidence of large cuff defect, such as:
   - Supraspinatus and infraspinatus atrophy
   - Weakness of external rotation and elevation
   - Superior position of humeral head relative to scapula
   - Palpable rotator cuff defect
3. Bone-on-bone crepitance

Radiographs (see Figs. 16–33, 16–34, 16–46, 16–64, 16–65)

1. Superior displacement of humeral head relative to the glenoid leading to contact with coracoacromial arch
2. Secondary degenerative changes of the glenohumeral joint
3. (Diagnosis is supported by erosion of the greater tuberosity ("femoralization" of proximal humerus)
4. (Diagnosis is supported by a contoured coracoacromial arch and upper glenoid to produce a socket for the proximal humerus ["acetabularization"])
5. (Diagnosis is supported by the collapse of the superior subchondral bone of the humeral head)

CAPSULORRHAPHY ARTHROPATHY

History

1. Functionally significant restricted glenohumeral motion
2. History of previous repair for glenohumeral instability

Physical Examination

1. Limited motion and function (especially external rotation)
2. (Diagnosis is supported by bone-on-bone crepitance)

Radiographs (see Figs. 16–7, 16–8, 16–46, 16–47)

1. Joint space narrowing
2. Periarticular sclerosis
3. Periarticular osteophytes
4. (Diagnosis is supported by posterior glenoid erosion with posterior subluxation of the humeral head)

AVASCULAR NECROSIS (ATRAUMATIC)

History

1. Limited shoulder function
2. (Diagnosis is supported by the presence of risk factors, such as steroid use)

Physical Examination

1. (Diagnosis is supported by glenohumeral crepitance)

Radiographs (see Figs. 16–68 to 16–71)

1. Sclerosis within head of humerus
2. Collapse of subchondral bone of humeral head
3. Absence of other pathology (e.g., tumor, cuff tear arthropathy)

"Friar Tuck" pattern of central baldness, often surrounded by a rim of remaining cartilage and osteophytes. Degenerative cysts may occur in the humeral head or glenoid. Osteophytes typically surround the anterior, inferior, and posterior aspects of the humeral head and the inferior and posterior glenoid. As a result the humeral and glenoid articular surfaces have a flattened configuration that blocks rotation (Figs. 16–44 and 16–45). Loose bodies are often found in the axillary or subscapularis recesses. The triad of anterior capsular contracture, posterior glenoid wear, and posterior humeral subluxation is common in primary degenerative joint disease. Rotator cuff defects are uncommon in primary degenerative joint disease. Cofield summarized the pathoanatomy of degenerative joint disease in Table 16–6.[77]

SECONDARY DEGENERATIVE JOINT DISEASE

In contrast with primary degenerative joint disease, secondary degenerative joint disease arises when previous injury, surgery, or another condition affects the joint sur-

Table 16–3 SIMPLE SHOULDER TEST

1. Is your shoulder comfortable with your arm at rest by your side?
2. Does your shoulder allow you to sleep comfortably?
3. Can you reach the small of your back to tuck in your shirt with your hand?
4. Can you place your hand behind your head with the elbow straight out to the side?
5. Can you place a coin on a shelf at the level of your shoulder without bending your elbow?
6. Can you lift 1 lb (a full pint container) to the level of your shoulder without bending your elbow?
7. Can you lift 8 lb (a full gallon container) to the level of the top of your head without bending your elbow?
8. Can you carry 20 lb (a bag of potatoes) at your side with the affected extremity?
9. Do you think you can toss a softball underhand 10 yards with the affected extremity?
10. Do you think you can throw a softball overhand 20 yards with the affected extremity?
11. Can you wash the back of your opposite shoulder with the affected extremity?
12. Would your shoulder allow you to work full time at your regular job?

face and precipitates its degeneration. In chronic, unreduced dislocations,[161, 287, 313] the humeral head may be indented and worn (Fig. 16–46). The cartilage of the joint surfaces may be replaced with scar tissue, or the subchondral bone may be so weakened by bone atrophy that it will collapse after reduction, leading to an incongruous joint surface (Fig. 16–47). Samilson and Prieto[319] identified 74 shoulders with a history of single or multiple dislocations that exhibited radiographic evidence of glenohumeral arthritis (Fig. 16–48). The dislocations had been anterior in 62 shoulders and posterior in 11 cases, and one had multidirectional instability. The number of dislocations was not related to the severity of the arthrosis. Shoulders with posterior instability had a higher incidence of moderate or severe arthritis, as did shoulders with previous surgery in which internal fixation devices intruded on the joint surface. Hawkins and co-workers[161] have suggested hemiarthroplasty if the dislocation is more than 6 months old or if the humeral head defect involves more than 45% of the articular surface. If the glenoid is destroyed, a total shoulder arthroplasty may be indicated.

Tanner and Cofield reviewed 28 shoulders with chronic fracture problems that required prosthetic arthroplasty.[339] Sixteen had malunions with a joint incongruity (Fig. 16–49); eight had post-traumatic osteonecrosis (Fig. 16–50); and four had nonunion of a surgical neck fracture with a small, osteopenic head fragment. Cofield summarized some features of post-traumatic arthritis in Table 16–7.[77]

Shoulders with secondary degenerative joint disease

Table 16–4 PERCENTAGE OF PATIENTS WITH SIX DIFFERENT TYPES OF GLENOHUMERAL ARTHRITIS WHO WERE ABLE TO PERFORM FUNCTIONS OF THE SIMPLE SHOULDER TEST AT THE TIME OF PRESENTATION

FUNCTION	DJD	SDJD	RA	CTA	CA	AVN
Sleep comfortably	12	13	18	8	0	29
Arm comfortable at side	67	36	61	33	65	79
Wash back of shoulder	13	20	13	0	18	7
Hand behind head	35	38	26	21	35	50
Tuck in shirt	32	33	39	38	29	50
8 lb on shelf	19	16	3	0	18	7
1 lb on shelf	54	36	26	21	53	50
Coin on shelf	59	44	29	29	53	64
Throw overhand	7	9	3	4	0	0
Do usual work	39	44	21	17	41	21
Throw underhand	53	44	13	42	29	21
Carry 20 lb	62	62	21	33	41	29

AVN, avascular necrosis; CA, capsulorrhaphy arthropathy; CTA, cuff tear arthropathy; DJD, degenerative joint disease; RA, rheumatoid arthritis; SDJD, secondary degenerative joint disease.

Table 16–5 SELF-ASSESSED HEALTH STATUS OF PATIENTS WITH SIX DIFFERENT TYPES OF GLENOHUMERAL ARTHRITIS REVEALED BY THE SF-36. DATA ARE PRESENTED AS THE AVERAGE PERCENT OF AGE- AND SEX-MATCHED POPULATION CONTROLS [289]

SF-36 PARAMETER	DJD	SDJD	RA	CTA	CA	AVN
Physical role function	44	33	23	30	39	28
Comfort	54	47	34	39	40	47
Physical function	78	73	38	81	62	50
Emotional role function	83	76	58	100	64	40
Social function	84	73	63	81	71	62
Vitality	86	83	44	81	65	60
Mental health	92	90	87	97	76	84
General health	100	93	65	100	71	63

AVN, avascular necrosis; CA, capsulorrhaphy arthropathy; CTA, cuff tear arthropathy; DJD, degenerative joint disease; RA, rheumatoid arthritis; SDJD, secondary degenerative joint disease.

Table 16–6 PATHOANATOMY OF GLENOHUMERAL OSTEOARTHRITIS

- Humeral head
  - Cartilage loss—central, superior, or complete
  - Sclerosis—central, superior
  - Peripheral osteophytes—most prominent inferiorly
  - Increased size
  - Erosion with central flattening
  - Subchondral cysts
- Glenoid
  - Cartilage loss—central, posterior, or complete
  - Sclerosis—central or posterior
  - Peripheral osteophytes—lower two thirds
  - Erosion—central or posterior with flattening
  - Subchondral cysts
- Joint position
  - Central or posterior subluxation
- Capsule
  - Enlarged, especially inferiorly
  - Anterior contracture
- Rotator cuff and biceps tendon
  - Complete-thickness tearing unusual (approximately 5%)
  - Degeneration or fibrosis (especially subscapularis) may be present
- Loose bodies within joint or subscapularis bursa

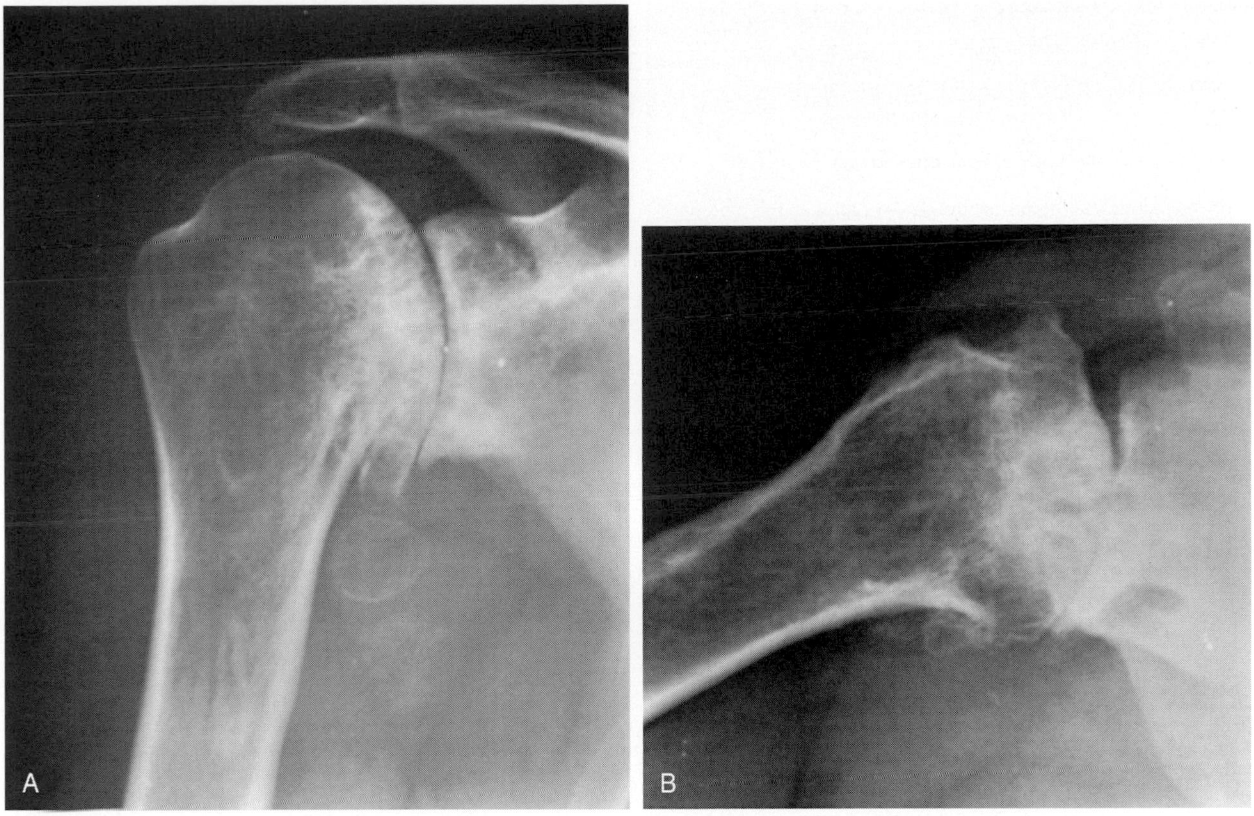

Figure 16–44

Osteoarthritis of the shoulder. *A*, A stereotypical radiographic, pathoanatomic appearance. The humeral head is somewhat enlarged and flattened. Peripheral osteophytes are particularly prominent inferiorly. There is flattening of the humeral head with subchondral sclerosis, particularly rest centrally and central-superiorly. There may be intraosseous cysts. These cysts are best seen on the axillary projection. *B*, In the axillary view, one also sees asymmetric glenoid wear with slightly greater wear of the posterior aspect of the glenoid. In addition, the glenoid is also flattened. There is a suggestion of posterior humeral subluxation, but this is not a striking feature in these radiographs.

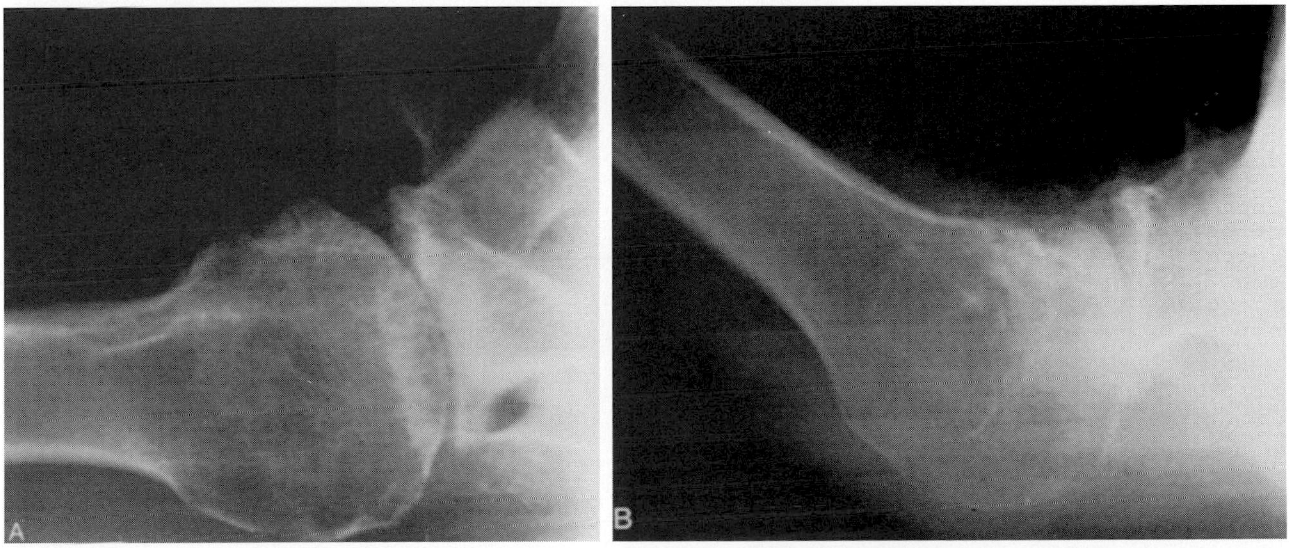

Figure 16–45

In osteoarthritis of the shoulder, there may be varying amounts of asymmetric posterior glenoid erosion and posterior humeral instability. In *A*, there has been a moderate amount of asymmetric posterior glenoid erosion and subluxation of the humeral head into the area of wear. In *B*, there is a lesser amount of glenoid erosion but a much larger amount of posterior humeral subluxation, suggesting significant elongation of the posterior shoulder capsule and the overlying rotator cuff. Reconstructive steps should take these changes—the glenoid erosion and the instability—into consideration.

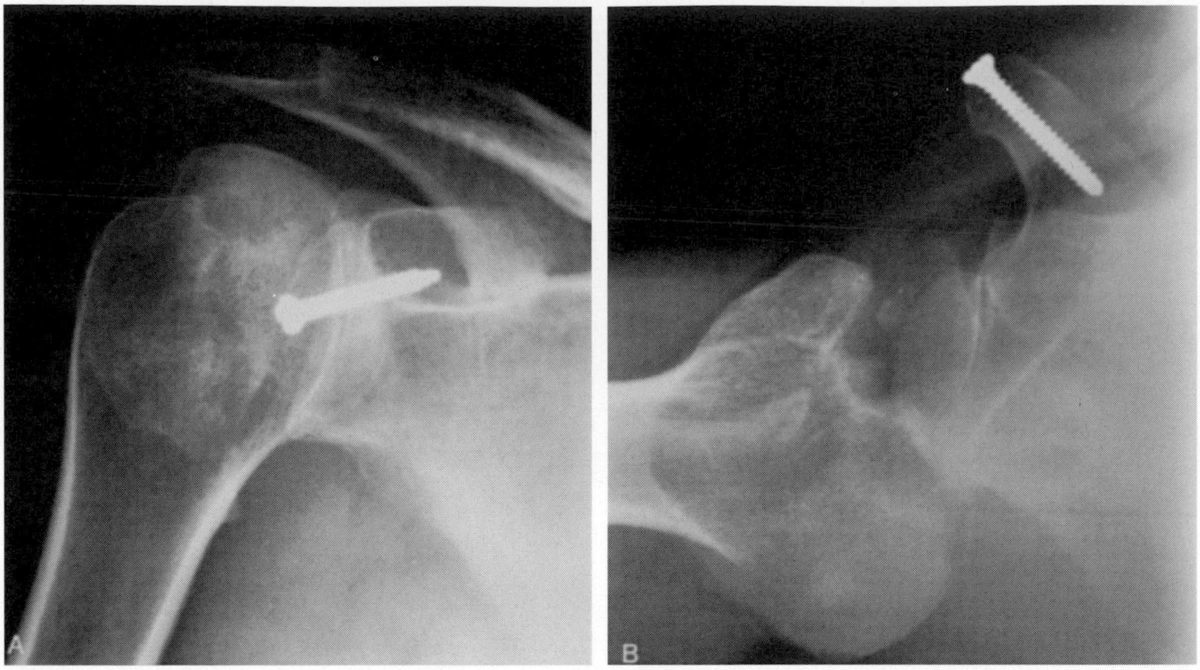

Figure 16–46

A chronic posterior shoulder dislocation in a 26-year-old man. The injury occurred approximately 1 year earlier. A recent previous anterior approach to the shoulder was ineffective in reducing the dislocation. At the time of the second surgical procedure, the shoulder was reduced, but the cartilage of the humeral head had been replaced with fibrous tissue. A proximal humeral prosthesis was placed as a part of the reconstructive procedure. *A*, A 40-degree posterior oblique x-ray illustrating the overlap between the humeral head and the glenoid. *B*, Clearly illustrates the posterior dislocation, the slight malunion between the head and shaft fragments, and the evidence of fracturing of the lesser tuberosity with healing of this tuberosity to the shaft but somewhat displaced from the humeral head segment.

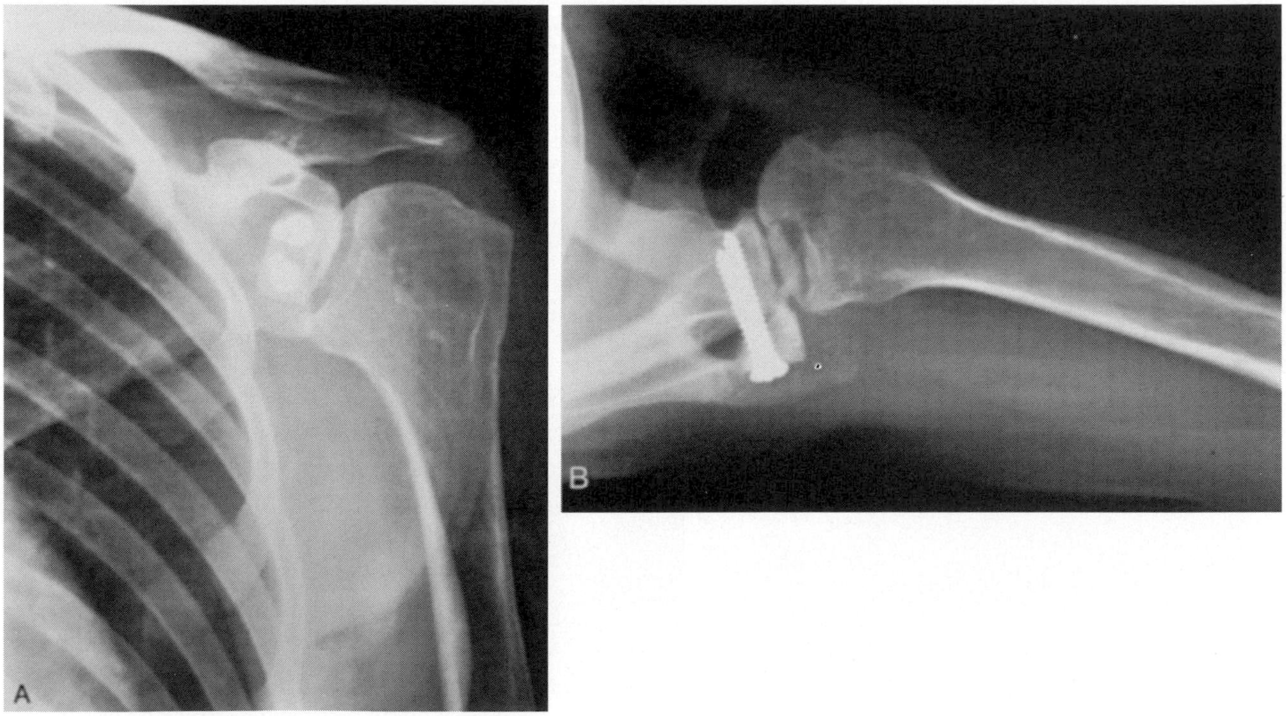

Figure 16–47

This young woman underwent open reduction of a posterior shoulder dislocation that had been unreduced for approximately 2 months. At the time of the reduction, the cartilage surfaces were intact; the humeral head was noted to be somewhat softened. A bone graft was added to the posterior aspect of the shoulder to substitute for an area of glenoid wear. Within the first month after open reduction, it was apparent on the anteroposterior view, *A*, and the axillary view, *B*, that the humeral head, because of its softness, had collapsed, and traumatic arthritis was developing. Subsequently, a proximal humeral prosthesis was placed.

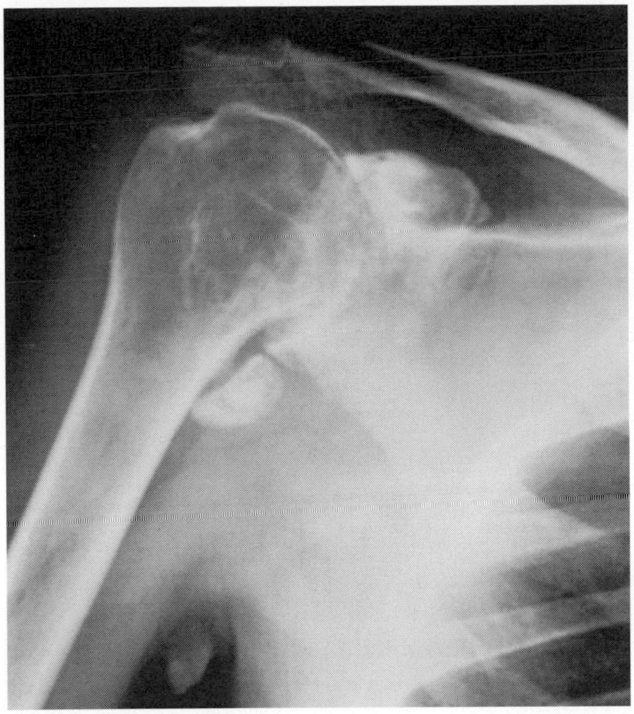

Figure 16–48

This elderly man had a 5- to 10-year history of progressively severe shoulder pain and limitation of motion. As an adolescent, he had had recurrent dislocations of this shoulder, and presumably his current arthritis has developed subsequent to his recurrent instability. This sequence of events certainly can occur but is surprisingly uncommon.

often present complex pathology and difficult surgical management.[168, 256] Difficulties may be related to a number of factors: muscle contracture, scarring, malunion requiring osteotomy, nonunion, or bone loss, especially humeral shortening. Dines and associates[102] reported

Table 16–7 GLENOHUMERAL ARTHRITIS FOLLOWING TRAUMA

POTENTIAL ETIOLOGIES
Recurrent subluxations or dislocations
Chronic dislocations
Fracture malunion with joint incongruity
Osteonecrosis of the humeral head
Proximal humeral nonunion with fibrous ankylosis

their results with shoulder arthroplasty in 20 patients with post-traumatic changes. They emphasize the difficulty of these cases and the advisability of avoiding tuberosity osteotomy. Other series of arthroplasty for late sequelae of trauma include that of Norris and co-workers,[263] Habermeyer and Schweiberer,[148] and Frich and associates.[126]

RHEUMATOID AND OTHER TYPES OF INFLAMMATORY ARTHRITIS

Rheumatoid arthritis is a systemic disease with highly variable clinical manifestations. It may be isolated to the glenohumeral joint or may affect most of the tissues in the body. In rheumatoid arthritis and many other types of inflammatory arthritis, the cartilage is characteristically destroyed evenly across all joint surfaces. The glenoid is eroded medially (see Fig. 16–29) rather than posteriorly, such as in degenerative joint disease (see Fig. 16–24). The condition is often bilaterally symmetric. The arthritic process erodes not only the cartilage but also the subchondral bone and renders it osteopenic (Figs. 16–51 to 16–61). The glenohumeral, acromioclavicular, sternoclavicular, elbow, wrist, and hand articulations may all be affected, greatly amplifying the resultant functional losses. Soft tissues, including the rotator cuff, may likewise be swollen, contracted, weakened, or torn (Fig. 16–62; see

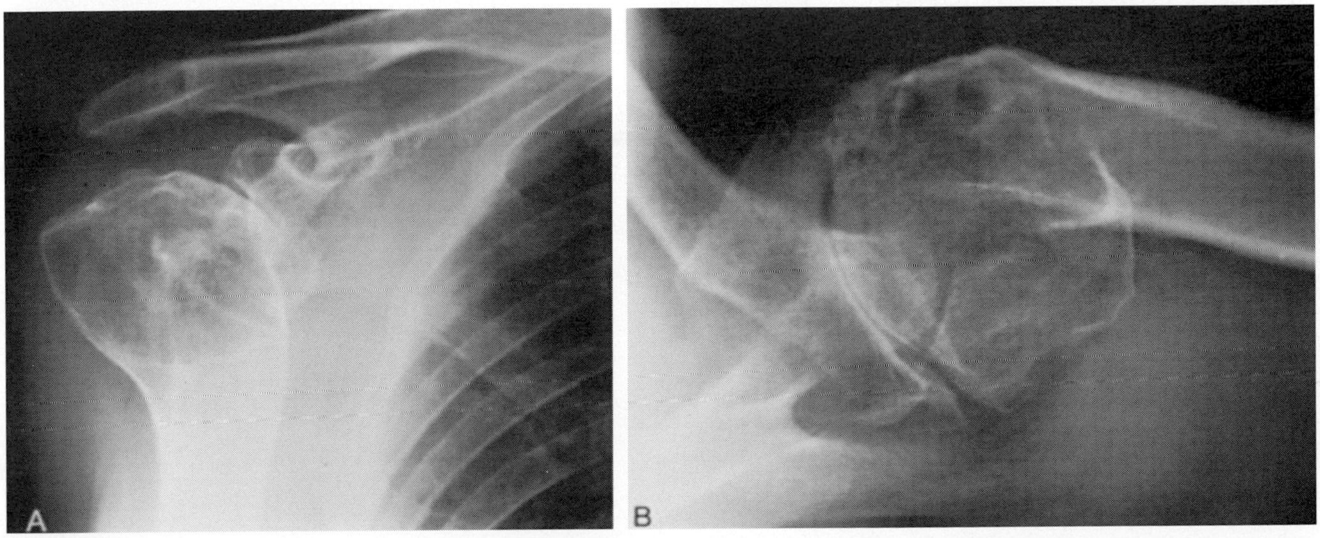

Figure 16–49

A and *B*, Traumatic arthritis with loss of glenohumeral cartilage has developed after malunion of a comminuted proximal humeral fracture.

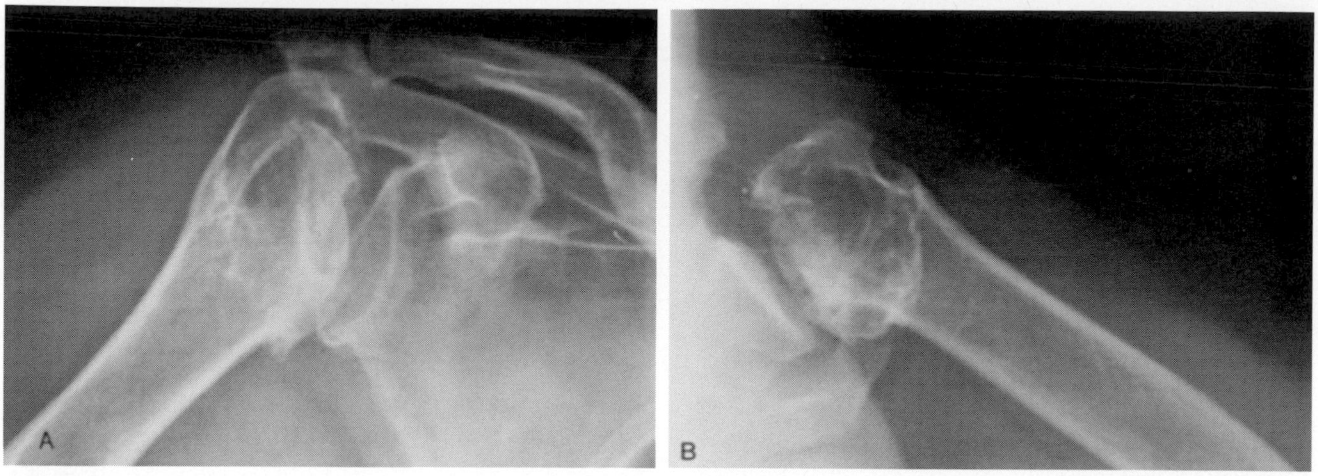

Figure 16–50

Traumatic arthritis with malunion and osteonecrosis of the head segment. Radiograph *A* shows the collapse of the head segment and the slight malunion of the greater tuberosity relative to the shaft. Radiograph *B* again shows collapse of the humeral head segment but reasonable positions of the tuberosities on this view. Damage to the glenoid articular surface is underestimated on these radiographic projections. At reconstructive surgery for situations such as this, either proximal humeral prosthetic replacement or total shoulder arthroplasty might be needed, depending on the extent of glenoid surface involvement.

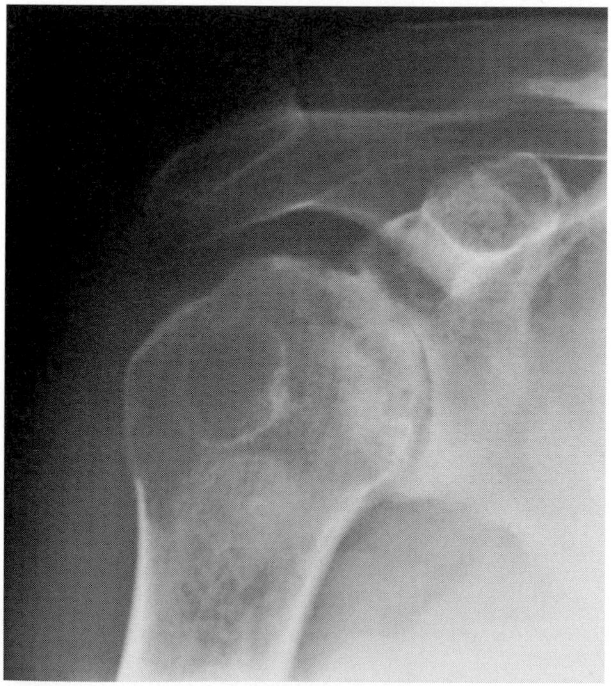

Figure 16–51

Rheumatoid arthritis of the shoulder with glenohumeral cartilage loss and joint stiffness, the so-called dry form of the disease.

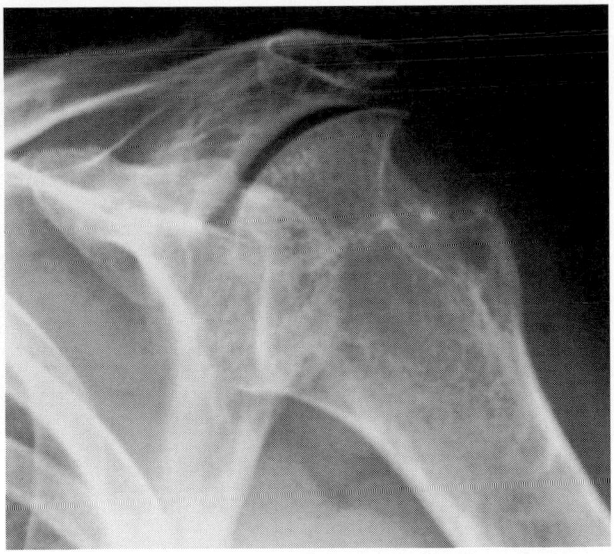

Figure 16–52

Rheumatoid arthritis in the shoulder with cartilage loss, extensive periarticular erosions, and an extremely hypertrophic synovitis, the so-called wet form of joint involvement.

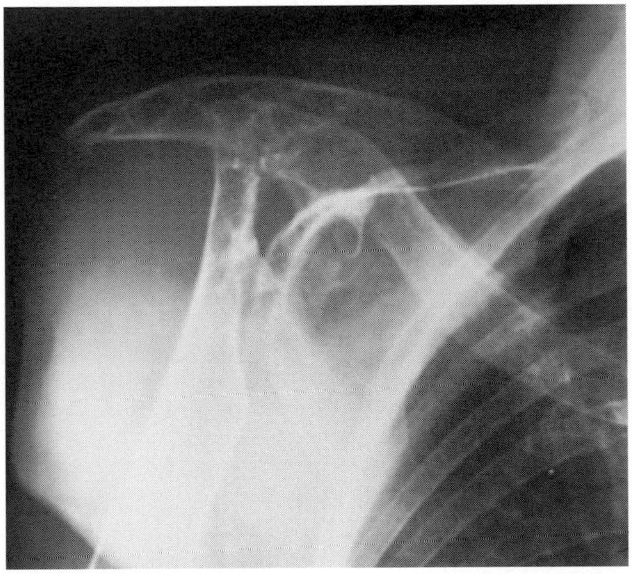

Figure 16–53

This radiograph of the shoulder of an elderly woman with long-standing rheumatoid arthritis shows extreme resorption involving the humeral head, a portion of the proximal humerus, and the lateral aspect of the scapula, including the entire glenoid.

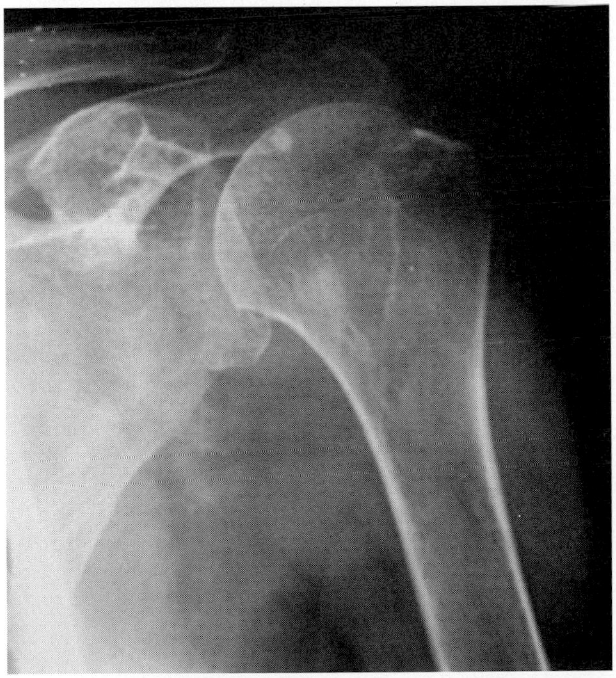

Figure 16–54

A middle-aged woman with long-standing rheumatoid arthritis and multiple joint involvement. When these radiographs were taken, the woman presented with severe shoulder pain and mild restriction of movement. The radiographs essentially show only osteopenia. There is maintenance of the joint space and only the slightest suggestion of marginal joint erosion. The extent of pathologic changes seen here is rather mild. Unfortunately, the patient's symptoms did not respond to conservative management. Significant synovitis was demonstrated on the arthrogram, and a shoulder synovectomy was undertaken.

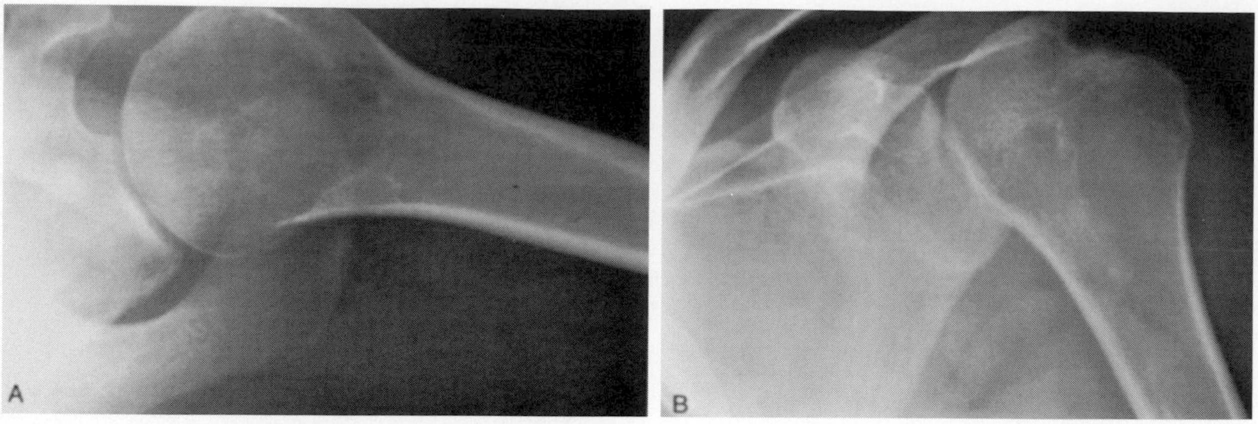

Figure 16–55

Rheumatoid arthritis involving the shoulder of a 26-year-old man with oligoarticular disease. His symptoms were moderate. The radiographs show slight cartilage loss, particularly on the axillary projection (*A*), and erosion of the humeral head near the articular surface margin on the anteroposterior radiograph (*B*). Extensive synovitis was present (see Fig. 16–59).

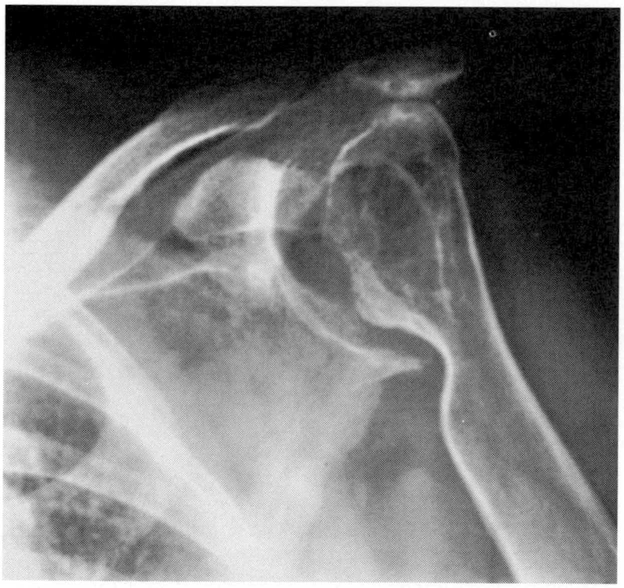

Figure 16–56

Long-standing rheumatoid arthritis of the shoulder with erosion of subchondral and adjacent bone structures. This is notable on the humeral head but is most pronounced in the scapula with extreme central resorption. In patients such as this, there may not be enough remaining bone to allow placement of a glenoid component at the time of reconstructive surgery.

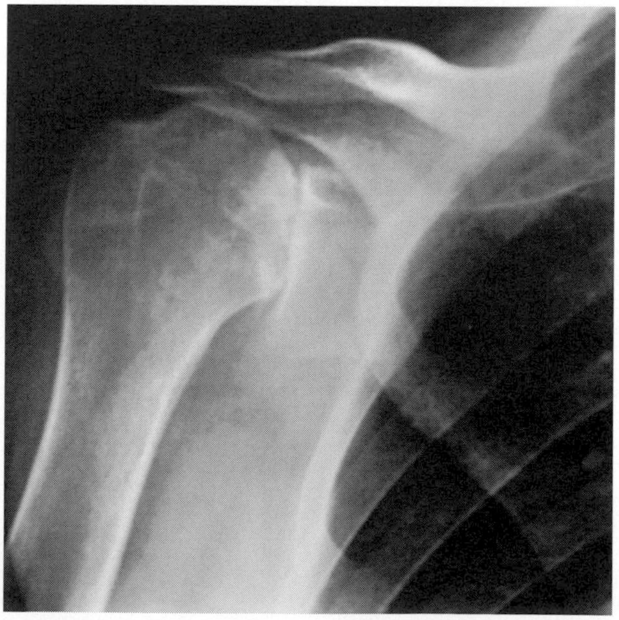

Figure 16–57

Rheumatoid arthritis of the shoulder. The radiograph shows a slight amount of osteopenia, cartilage loss, mild subchondral bone loss, and upward subluxation of the humeral head. In this patient, as in many with rheumatoid arthritis of the shoulder, the rotator cuff has become thin, with attrition, stretching, and fibrosis, but without full-thickness rotator cuff tearing.

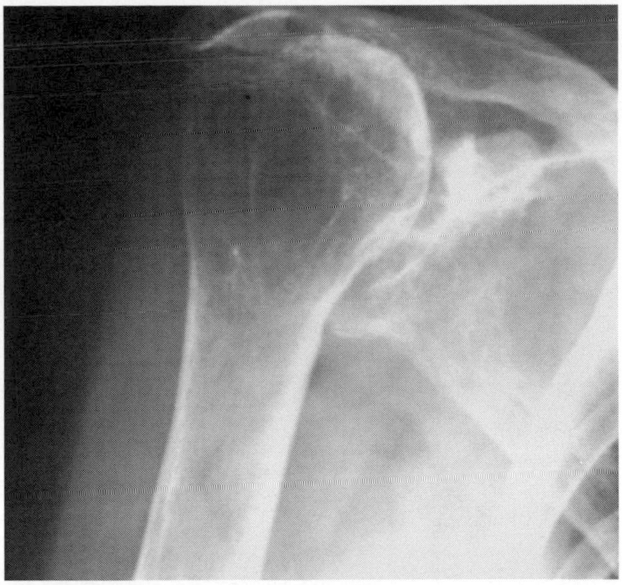

Figure 16–58

Rheumatoid arthritis of the shoulder in association with rotator cuff tearing. The radiogram shows cartilage loss, central-superior erosion of the glenoid, upward subluxation of the humeral head, and some erosion of the overlying acromion and distal clavicle. At surgery, a large rotator cuff tear was found involving the infraspinatus, supraspinatus, and subscapularis.

also Fig. 16–60). In a clinical and arthrographic study of 200 painful shoulders in patients with rheumatoid arthritis, Ennevarra found that only 26% of patients had full-thickness rotator cuff defects.[112] In two series of patients with rheumatoid arthritis that required total shoulder arthroplasty, the rotator cuff had full-thickness tearing in 29 of 69 shoulders (42%) and in 18 of 66 shoulders (27%).[71, 259] Even the skin may be fragile and subject to compromise in wound healing. The fragility of the patient with rheumatoid arthritis is frequently compounded by long-term use of steroids and other antimetabolic medication. Because the condition itself involves the immune system, the patient is often on immunosuppressive medication, and the clinical manifestations of rheumatoid arthritis are similar to those of infectious arthritis, the physician must be aware of the possible coexistence of joint infection. Cofield summarized the characteristics of rheumatoid arthritis of the shoulder in Table 16–8.[77] Petersson[274] pointed to the prevalence and progression of rheumatoid involvement of the shoulder. Winalski and Shapiro[361] and Mulliaji and associates[242] used CT to characterize the rheumatoid involvement of the sternoclavicular and glenohumeral joints. Alasaarela and Alasaarela[2] have used ultrasound to define the soft tissue changes associated with rheumatoid arthritis of the shoulder.

Other conditions may produce shoulder findings quite

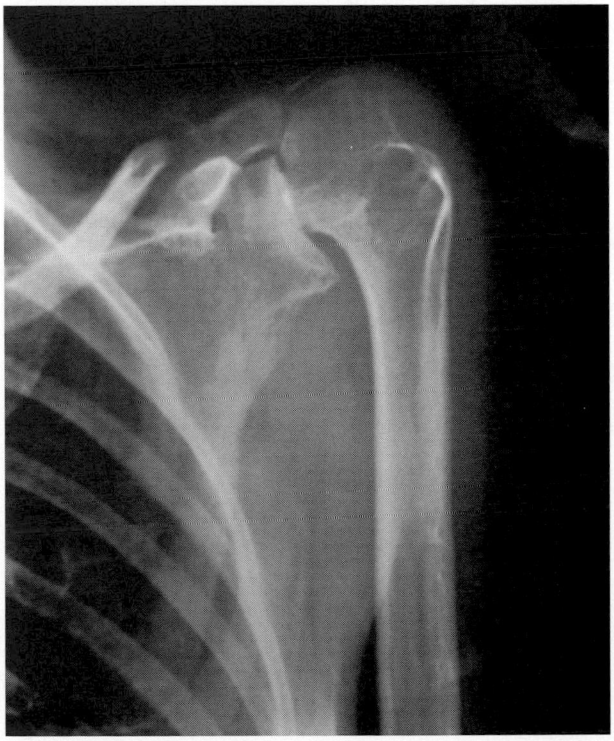

Figure 16–59

Juvenile rheumatoid arthritis with extreme rotator cuff and capsular involvement, even to the extent of acromial erosion. The humeral head is now beneath the skin across the superior aspect of the shoulder.

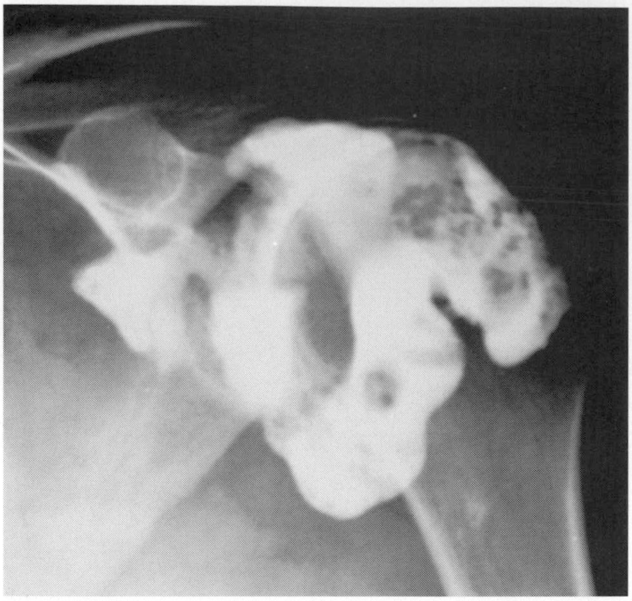

Figure 16–60

Shoulder arthrogram showing active synovitis in a patient with rheumatoid arthritis. The plain x-rays (see Fig. 16–54) showed only minor joint changes.

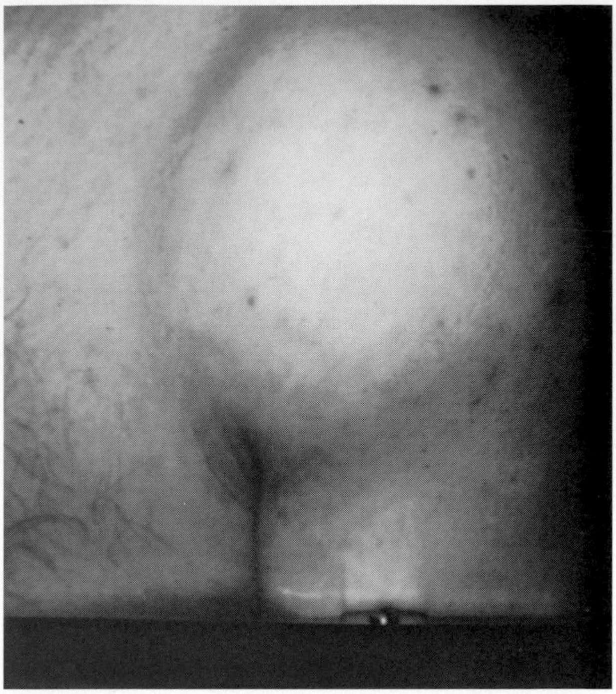

Figure 16–62

A clinical photograph of the shoulder of a young man with rheumatoid arthritis and primary rheumatoid involvement of the subacromial-subdeltoid bursa. The rotator cuff was intact, and the glenohumeral joint had minimal involvement with rheumatoid synovitis. There was a full, minimally painful range of motion in the shoulder, with excellent shoulder strength. The hypertrophic bursitis did not respond to medical management, and surgical excision of the bursa was done.

similar to those of rheumatoid arthritis (Fig. 16–63). Included in the list are localized processes, such as pigmented villonodular synovitis,[105, 106] synovial chondrometaplasia,[164] and pseudogout.[167] The shoulder may be a site of manifestation of systemic disorders such as hemophilia and hemachromatosis,[113, 290] primary hyperparathyroidism,[264] acromegaly,[276] amyloid arthropathy,[98] gout,[108] chondrocalcinosis,[91] ankylosing spondylitis,[122, 216] psoriasis,[122] and Lyme arthritis.[98] Sethi and associates[322] have reported a "dialysis arthropathy" that affects multiple joints, including the shoulder, in individuals on long-term dialysis.

Because of the fragility of the skin and other soft tissues, osteopenia, and severe bone erosion common with this condition, the patient with substantial involve-

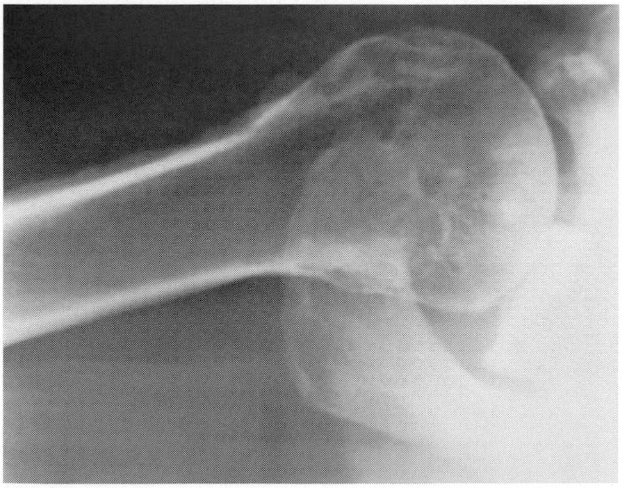

Figure 16–61

Axillary x-ray projection of the shoulder of a young woman with rheumatoid arthritis. Rheumatoid destruction of the anterior shoulder capsule and the anterior aspect of the rotator cuff has occurred such that anterior instability now exists. Enough cartilage loss had occurred that treatment included proximal humeral prosthetic replacement, glenohumeral joint synovectomy, and anterior capsule and rotator cuff repair.

Table 16–8 RHEUMATOID ARTHRITIS OF THE SHOULDER

TISSUE	*TYPE OF PATHOLOGIC CHANGE*
Subdeltoid bursa	Inflammation
	Fibrosis
	Synovial hypertrophy
Bone	Osteopenia
	Erosions
	Resorption
	Sclerosis
	Cysts
	Fracture
Cartilage	Loss, partial or complete
Rotator cuff	Inflammation
	Fibrosis
	Thinning, stretching
	Tearing
Synovial lining	Inflammation
	Fibrosis
	Synovial hypertrophy
Shoulder capsule	Inflammation
	Fibrosis
	Thinning, stretching
	Instability

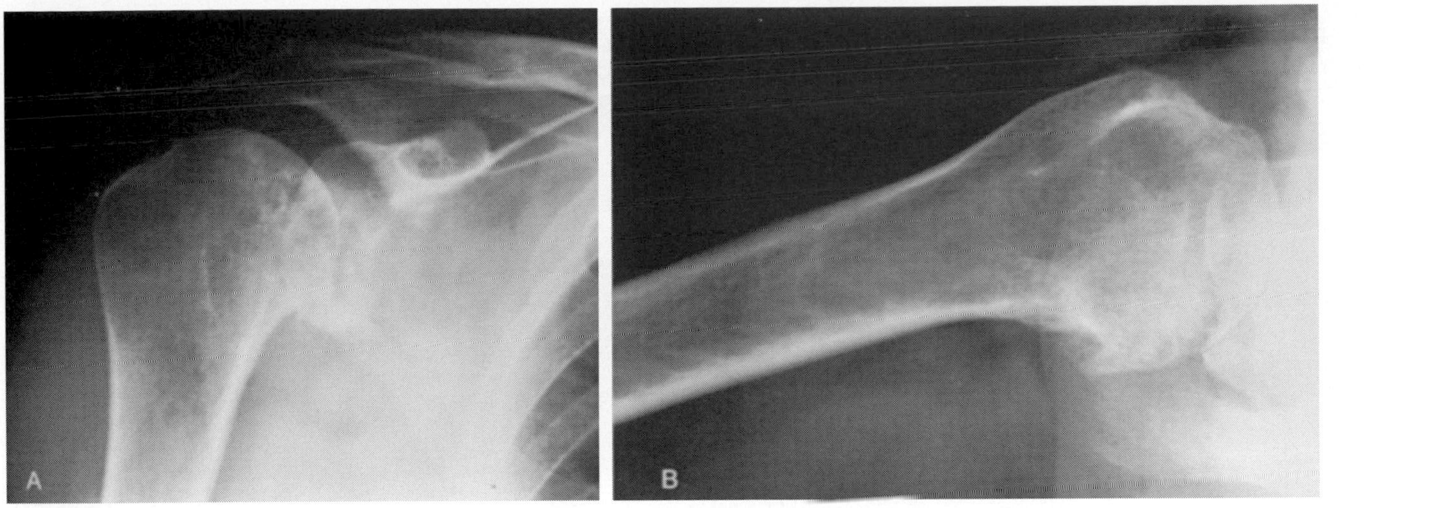

Figure 16–63

An upper-middle-aged woman with 4 years of progressively severe shoulder pain. She now has pain with any arm activity and at rest. There is no history of a previous injury or any history of multiple joint arthritic involvement. The sedimentation rate is slightly elevated; the rheumatoid factor is negative. At surgery, the synovium exhibited histologic changes of a mild chronic synovitis but was not diagnostic for a specific type of arthritic disease. As seen on the anteroposterior view, *A*, and the axillary view, *B*, this patient's disease has many of the characteristics of a nonspecific inflammatory arthritis with osteopenia, cartilage loss, granulation tissue within a cyst in the humeral head and glenoid, and minimal hypertrophic or sclerotic changes. A presentation such as this is somewhat uncommon but is not rare.

ment from rheumatoid arthritis or similar types of arthritis must be treated with extreme gentleness, thoroughness, and care. These admonitions are referred to as "rheumatoid rules."

In a review, Sneppen and associates[327] pointed to the challenges of arthroplasty in rheumatoid disease. In their series of Neer arthroplasties, at 92-month follow-up, 55% showed proximal migration of the humerus relative to the glenoid; 40% showed progressive loosening of the glenoid component; and 5 of 12 press-fit humeral components showed progressive loosening (but none in 50 cemented humeral components). Despite these problems, 89% of the patients demonstrated good pain relief. Boyd and associates[36] found that of 111 Neer total shoulders with an average follow-up of 55 months, progressive proximal migration occurred in 22% of patients (29 shoulders).

As shown in Table 16–5, individuals with rheumatoid arthritis characteristically have substantially lower self-assessed vitality and overall physical function than the other causes of glenohumeral arthritis. The compromised general health and strength of individuals with rheumatoid arthritis must be considered in their management as has been emphasized by a comparison study of rheumatoid arthritis and degenerative joint disease conducted by Smith and associates.[222]

CUFF TEAR ARTHROPATHY

Cuff tear arthropathy occurs when a chronic, massive rotator cuff defect subjects the uncovered humeral articular cartilage to abrasion by the undersurface of the coracoacromial arch (Figs. 16–64 and 16–65). The humeral head becomes "femoralized" and the coracoacromial arch "acetabularized" (see Fig. 16–34). The erosion of the humeral articular cartilage begins superiorly rather than centrally, such as is the case in degenerative joint disease and capsulorrhaphy arthropathy.

In 1981, McCarty and co-workers described a shoulder condition: the "Milwaukee shoulder." This condition included significant rotator cuff disease and shoulder arthritis in older patients and often in women.[133, 150, 231] The synovial fluid contained aggregates of hydroxyapatite crystals, active collagenase, and neutral protease. At that time, these authors hypothesized that the crystals within the synovial fluid were phagocytized by the macrophage-like synovial cells, and the cells in turn released enzymes, resulting in damage of the joint and joint-related structures. The inciting process could not be identified.

In 1983, the hypothesis was further refined. The crystals were identified as basic calcium phosphate (BCP).[230] It was thought these crystals would form in the synovial fluid by unknown mechanisms. They would then be phagocytosed by the synovial lining cells. These cells would then secrete the collagenase and neutral protease. This would damage the tissues and, in addition, cause the release of additional crystals. The importance of this concept may be a more universal understanding of crystal-related arthropathies and a better understanding of how multiple joint structures can be affected by an underlying problem.[149, 151, 152, 192]

Nguyen and Nguyen[261] and Campion and colleagues[58] have described an "idiopathic destructive arthritis" of the shoulder, which may be another form of the same condition.

In 1983, Neer and co-workers published an article on cuff tear arthropathy describing pathologic changes in 26 patients.[255] These changes included massive rotator cuff tearing, glenohumeral instability, loss of articular cartilage of the glenohumeral joint, humeral head collapse, and related bone loss. This entity was distinctly different from osteoarthritis, which he had defined earlier. Neer believed that mechanical factors associated with extensive rotator cuff tearing played a prominent role in the creation of

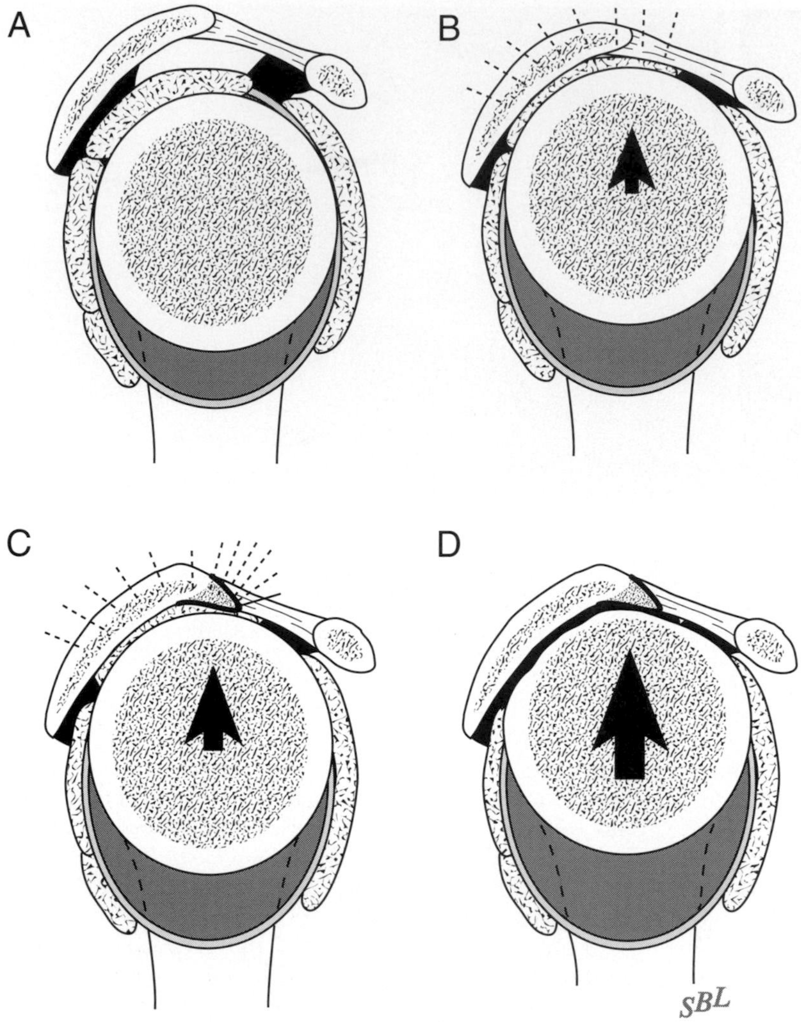

Figure 16–64

With progressive cuff fiber failure, the head moves upward against the coracoacromial arch. *A*, Normal relationships of the cuff and the coracoacromial arch. *B*, Upward displacement of the head, squeezing the cuff against the acromion and the coracoacromial ligament. *C*, Greater contact and abrasion, giving rise to a traction spur in the coracoacromial ligament. *D*, Still greater upward displacement, resulting in abrasion of the humeral articular cartilage and cuff tear arthropathy. (Modified from Matsen FA III, Lippitt SB, Sidles JA, and Harryman DT II: Practical Evaluation and Management of the Shoulder. Philadelphia: WB Saunders, 1994.)

this problem and that secondary nutritional changes may augment the pathologic changes that occur.

The relationship between "Milwaukee shoulder" syndrome, crystal deposition arthritis, and cuff tear arthropathy is unclear. They may be the same process or a different process with similar end stages. For the surgeon, however, the challenge is an eroded joint lacking normal bone stock and reconstructable rotator cuff tissue. In this condition, the glenohumeral joint is deprived of several of its major stabilizing factors: (1) the normal cuff muscle force vector compressing the humeral head into the glenoid (Fig. 16–66), (2) the superior lip of the glenoid concavity, which is typically worn away by chronic superior subluxation (see Fig. 16–33), and (3) the cuff tendon interposed between the humeral head and the coracoacromial arch (Fig. 16–67). As a result of these deficits, the superior instability is of sufficient severity that it cannot be reversed in a dependable way at the time of reconstructive surgery.

Arntz and associates[8] reported their results from 21 shoulders with cuff tear arthropathy. These shoulders were not candidates for glenoid replacement because of the massive deficiency in the cuff and the fixed upward displacement of the humeral head; thus, they were treated with a special hemiarthroplasty, allowing the prosthesis to articulate with the coracoacromial arch. The prerequisites for successful hemiarthroplasty were an intact deltoid and a functionally intact coracoacromial arch to provide superior secondary stability for the prosthesis. One important aspect of the operative technique was the selection of a sufficiently small prosthesis so that excessive tightness of the posterior aspect of the capsule could be avoided. Eighteen shoulders in 16 patients were available for follow-up, which ranged from 25 to 122 months. Pain decreased from marked or disabling in 14 shoulders preoperatively to none or slight in 10 and to pain only after unusual activity in four. Active forward elevation improved from an average of 66 degrees preoperatively to an average of 109 degrees postoperatively. One patient, who had an excellent result, fell and sustained an acromial fracture, thus the functional result changed to poor. Three patients had persistent, substantial pain in the shoulder that led to a revision. Neither infection nor prosthetic loosening developed in any shoulder.

CAPSULORRHAPHY ARTHROPATHY

Capsulorrhaphy arthropathy is recognized as a special subset of secondary degenerative joint disease in which deterioration of the joint surface is related to a previous

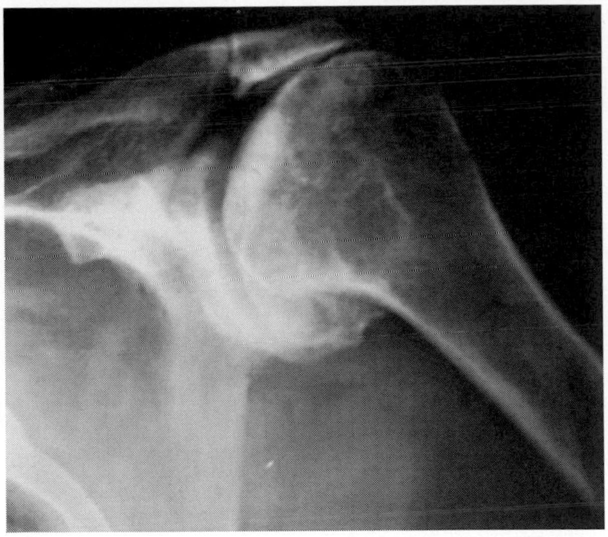

Figure 16–65

Rotator cuff tear arthropathy. The radiograph depicts the cartilage loss, mild but definite bone loss of the humeral head and glenoid, severe upward subluxation of the humeral head against the acromion with rotator cuff tearing, and some erosion of the abutting acromion. This patient has significant multitissue involvement of the cartilage, bone, capsule, and rotator cuff. Reconstructive surgery should address all these deficiencies.

repair for recurrent dislocations. This is one of the commonest causes of severe arthritis in the individual younger than 55 years of age (Table 16–9). Capsulorrhaphy arthropathy may be caused by overtightening the anterior capsule; for example, in a Putti-Platt repair, limiting external rotation and causing obligate posterior translation that forces the humeral head out of its normal concentric relationship with the glenoid fossa (see Figs. 16–7, 16–8, and 16–46). The posterior glenoid is typically eroded from this chronic posterior humeral subluxation; occasionally, major posterior bone deficiencies result (see Fig. 16–8). The converse situation may arise when obligate anterior translation results from excessive posterior capsular tightening. Lusardi and associates[212] reported a retrospective study of 20 shoulders in 19 patients who had been managed for severe loss of external rotation of the glenohumeral joint after a previous anterior capsulorrhaphy for recurrent instability. All patients had noted a restricted range of motion, and 17 shoulders had been painful. In seven shoulders, the humeral head had been subluxated or dislocated posteriorly, and 16 shoulders had been affected by mild to severe glenohumeral osteoarthrosis. All 20 shoulders were treated with a reoperation, which consisted of a release of the anterior soft tissue. In addition, eight shoulders had a total arthroplasty, and one had a hemiarthroplasty. At an average duration of follow-up of 48 months, all shoulders showed an improvement in the ratings for pain and range of motion. The average increase in external rotation was 45 degrees.

Capsulorrhaphy arthropathy may also be related to intra-articular positioning of metallic internal fixation devices (screws or staples) or bone graft used in repairs of recurrent instability (see Fig. 16–47).[375]

Bigliani and associates,[30] Hawkins and Angelo,[158] and

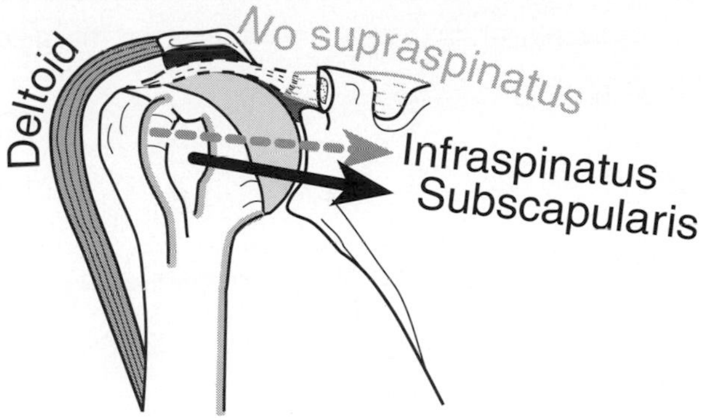

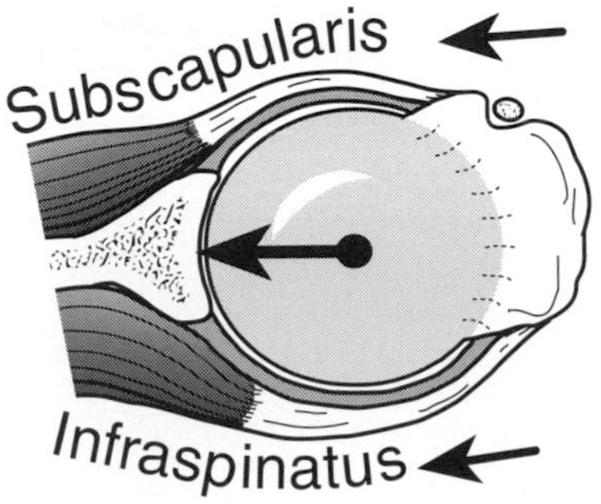

Figure 16–66

Compressive forces from the infraspinatus and subscapularis can stabilize the humeral head in the absence of a supraspinatus, provided that the glenoid concavity is intact. (Modified from Matsen FA III, Lippitt SB, Sidles JA, and Harryman DT II: Practical Evaluation and Management of the Shoulder. Philadelphia: WB Saunders, 1994.)

Rockwood and Lusardi and colleagues[212] reported their results from reconstruction of shoulders damaged by capsulorrhaphy arthropathy.

AVASCULAR NECROSIS

Nontraumatic avascular necrosis of the humeral head may be idiopathic or may be associated with the systemic use of steroids, dysbaric conditions, transplantation, or systemic illnesses with vasculitis. Other implicated conditions include alcoholism, sickle cell disease, hyperuricemia, Gaucher's disease, pancreatitis, familial hyperlipid-

Table 16–9 SIX DIAGNOSES WITH THE RELATIVE PREVALENCE, AGE, AND GENDER FOR 306 PATIENTS PRESENTING TO ONE OF US (FAM) FOR EVALUATION AND MANAGEMENT OF SHOULDER ARTHRITIS

		NO. OF PATIENTS	
DIAGNOSIS	***AGE***	***Male***	***Female***
Degenerative joint disease	63 ± 12	125	42
Secondary degenerative joint disease	54 ± 15	36	9
Rheumatoid arthritis	59 ± 12	7	32
Cuff tear arthropathy	75 ± 9	9	13
Capsulorrhaphy arthropathy	46 ± 9	13	4
Avascular necrosis	51 ± 15	6	8

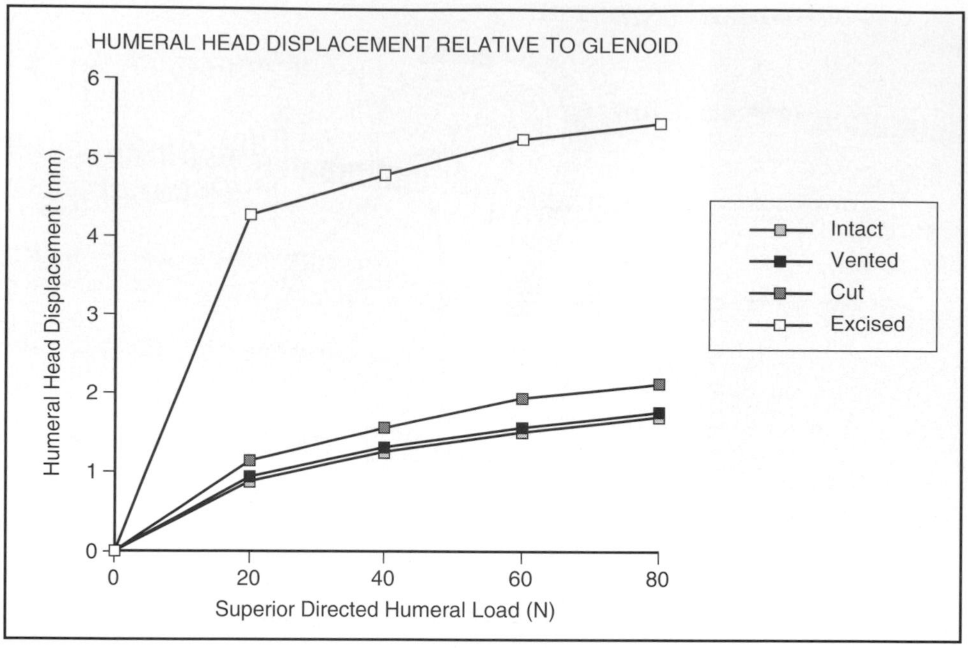

Figure 16–67

The cuff tendon interposed between the humeral head and the coracoacromial arch stabilizes the head against superiorly directed loads. This graph shows the mean superior humeral displacement (relative to the scapula) as a function of superior humerus load. The chart compares displacements for: (1) intact specimens, (2) after venting of the joint to air, (3) after cutting (but not excising the cuff tendon), and (4) after excising the superior cuff tendon. Note the marked superior displacement after excision of the cuff tendon.

emia, renal or other organ transplantation, and lymphoma.[40, 95, 97, 310]

The pathology may first be detected by MRI before collapse is seen radiographically. Later, osteoporosis or osteosclerosis may be seen on plain radiographs. Next, there is evidence of a fracture through the abnormal subchondral bone superocentrally (Fig. 16–68). Later, collapse of the subchondral bone occurs, often with a separated osteocartilaginous flap (Fig. 16–69). In end-stage avascular necrosis, the irregular humeral head destroys glenoid articular cartilage and results in secondary degenerative joint disease (Figs. 16–70 and 16–71).[95, 316]

OTHER TYPES OF ARTHRITIS

Neurotrophic arthropathy arises in association with syringomyelia, diabetes, or other causes of joint denervation. The joint and subchondral bone are destroyed because of the loss of the trophic and protective effects of its nerve supply. It has been suggested that the injection of corticosteroids may contribute to the development of this condition.[268] The Charcot joint presents with functional limitation and pain (despite the denervation). Cervical spine trauma may have occurred in the past,[293] or unrecognized syringomyelia may exist.[226, 343] There is usually significant bone destruction and osseous debris about the joint area

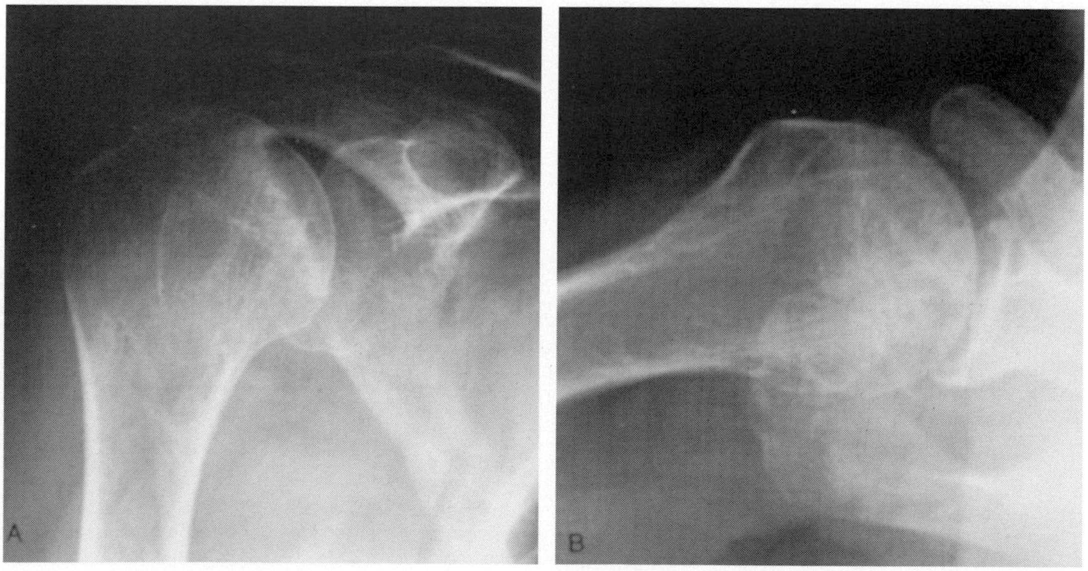

Figure 16–68

Osteonecrosis of the proximal humerus. There is an osteochondral fracture with minimal distortion of the articular surface of the humerus. This is best seen in *A*, the anteroposterior view. In *B*, the axillary view, there is a crescent sign in the anterocentral part of the humeral head.

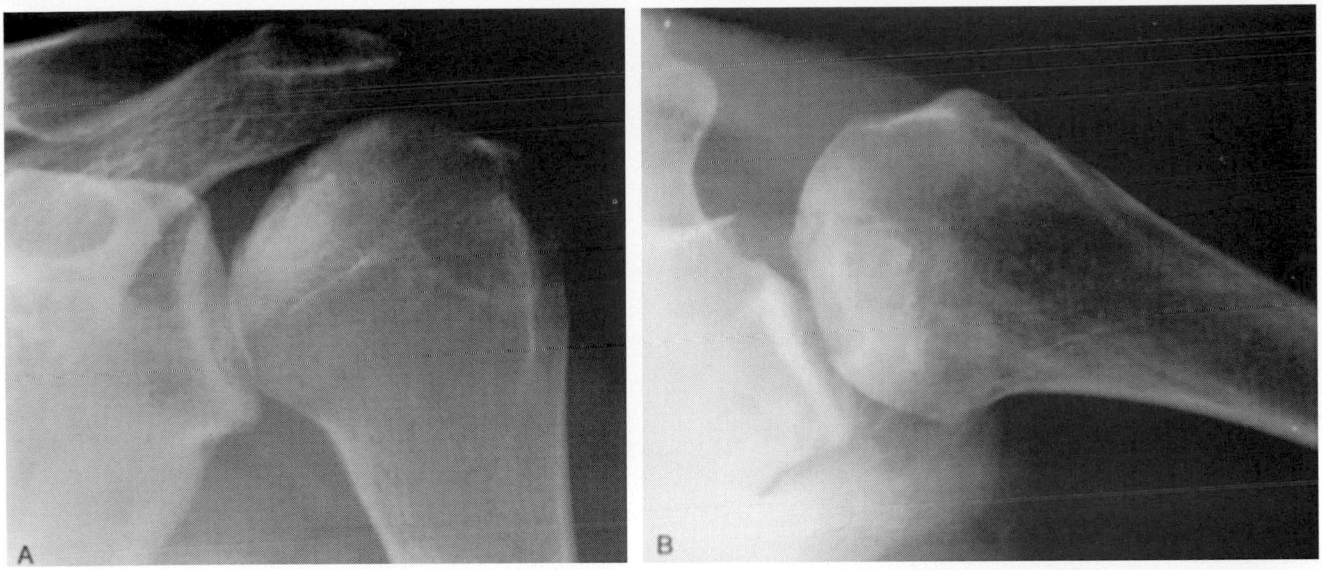

Figure 16–69

Osteonecrosis of the humeral head associated with chronic steroid use. A subchondral fracture has occurred in the past. There is distortion of the humeral articular surface shape and early glenohumeral arthritis. Symptoms were significant in this young man, and treatment with a proximal humeral prosthesis was quite effective. *A*, Anteroposterior view; *B*, axillary view.

(Fig. 16–72). This condition may resemble infectious arthritis.[210]

Radiation therapy, especially for the treatment of breast cancer, may cause a number of shoulder problems: brachial plexopathies, osteonecrosis, malignant bone tumors, and fibrous replacement of many tissues. Glenohumeral cartilage and subchondral bone are occasionally affected by these changes and may require treatment by prosthetic arthroplasty or other alternative methods (Fig. 16–73).

Septic arthritis of the shoulder is uncommon; however, when it occurs, it is often in a person debilitated from a generalized disease,[11, 52] in a person on immunosuppressive medications, or in a person who has an underlying shoulder disease process such as rotator cuff tearing or rheumatoid arthritis.[6, 196] In this latter setting, there appears to be an exacerbation of the underlying shoulder disease; and in the absence of fever or an elevated white blood count (WBC), the diagnosis will depend on a high level of suspicion, joint aspiration, and bacteriologic testing. Leslie and associates[202] reviewed 18 cases of shoulder sepsis, of which 11 had *S. aureus*. Some cases were initially confused with nonseptic arthritis and were treated with anti-inflammatory agents. The results of treatment

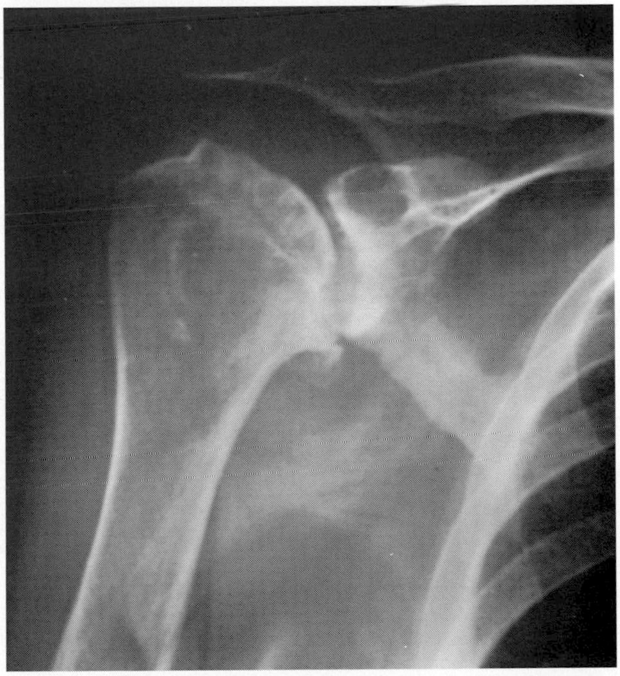

Figure 16–70

Long-standing osteonecrosis of the proximal humerus with only slight distortion of the articular surface but, unfortunately, progression to significant arthritis involving both the humeral and glenoid articular surfaces.

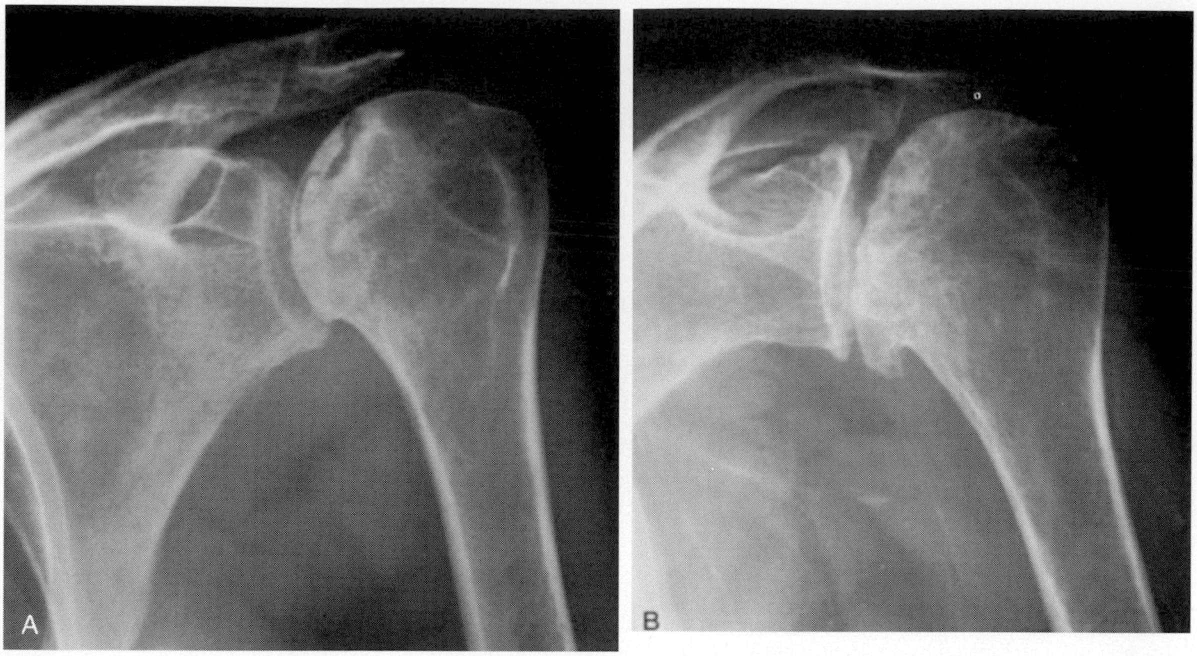

Figure 16–71

Steroids were used as a part of the treatment for this middle-aged woman with multiple sclerosis. She presented (*A*) with mild shoulder symptoms associated with osteonecrosis of the proximal humerus. There is minimal distortion of the articular surface shape. *B*, The same shoulder is shown about 8 years later. There has been greater distortion of the articular surface shape and the development of some glenohumeral arthritis. However, the symptoms are still mild, and nonoperative treatment continues to be appropriate for this patient.

were poor, but somewhat better with arthrotomy than repeated aspiration.

Neoplasia presents insidiously and is often characterized by nonmechanical pain. The tumor may incite a synovial response, mimicking an arthritic condition.[26, 236] The pain may be more intense than the usual arthritic pain and decidedly unresponsive to rest. The diagnosis will depend on access to the patient's general health, high-quality plain x-rays, and additional imaging modes including tomography, CT scanning, bone scanning, or MRI. Identification of the primary lesion in metastatic disease is desirable, but sometimes a biopsy of the shoul-

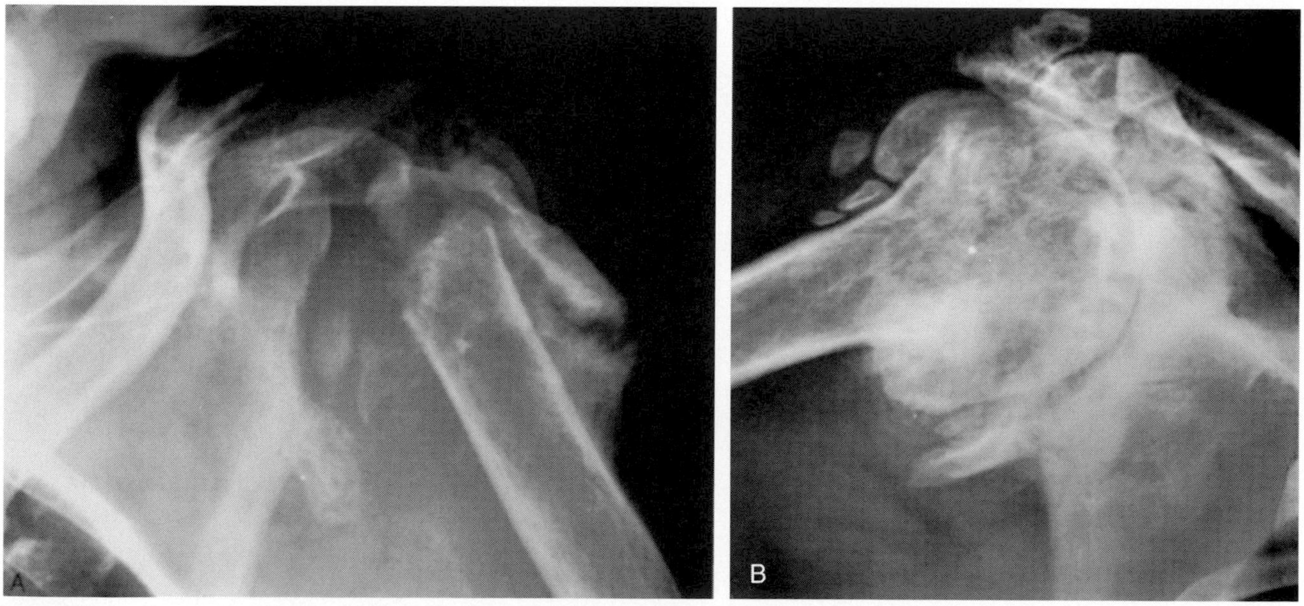

Figure 16–72

Occasionally, neuropathic arthritis can be confused with the more common forms of glenohumeral arthritis. *A*, Fragmentation of the proximal humerus with bone debris scattered throughout the joint region. *B*, Bone fragmentation is shown but also a predominantly sclerotic response is associated with neuropathic arthritis. The underlying condition in both of these patients was syringomyelia of the cervical portion of the spinal cord.

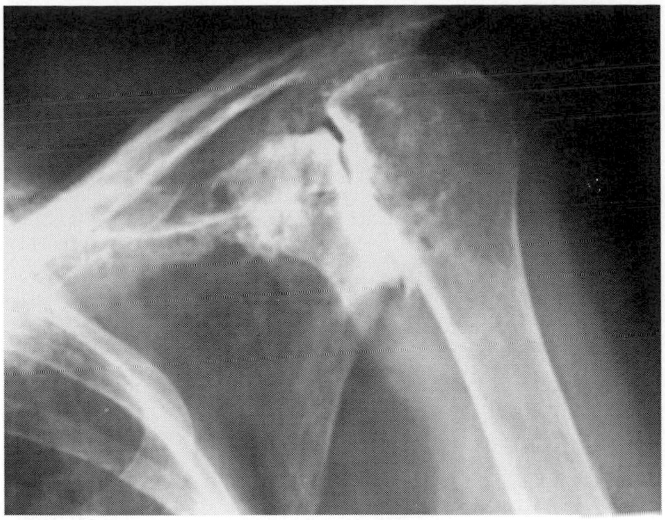

Figure 16–73

Cartilage loss, alteration of subchondral bone shape with segmental collapse, and alteration in bone texture secondary to irradiation that was done as a part of the treatment for breast cancer. Symptoms were quite significant in this elderly woman and were relieved effectively with total shoulder arthroplasty.

der lesion is the most direct route when making a diagnosis (Fig. 16–74).

MANAGEMENT

Nonoperative Treatment

Glenohumeral joint arthritis is commonly accompanied by stiffness related to contracture and adhesions involving the glenohumeral capsule, the cuff muscles, and the nonarticular humeroscapular motion interface. Weakness of the cuff muscles results from disuse or fiber failure. Instability patterns may also complicate glenohumeral roughness, such as the posterior subluxation characteristic of degenerative joint disease and capsulorrhaphy arthropathy or the superior subluxation characteristic of cuff tear arthropathy. There is a lot about these conditions that needs management!

Because glenohumeral roughness is usually of insidious onset and chronic duration, there is ample opportunity to try nonoperative management. In many cases of glenohumeral arthritis, the mechanics of the shoulder can be improved by a program of patient-conducted gentle range-of-motion and strengthening exercises (Figs. 16–75 to 16–84). It is important that vigorous torques and forces not be applied in an attempt to regain motion because of the concern for causing obligate translation and accelerated wear. Nonsteroidal anti-inflammatory medication and mild analgesics may be useful adjuncts.

Surgical Treatment

Surgery is considered for well-informed, well-motivated, cooperative, sufficiently healthy, and socially supported patients with refractory and functionally significant glenohumeral roughness. Surgical reconstruction offers the potential to optimize capsular laxity and muscle mechanics, as well as the smoothness, size, shape, and orientation of the joint surface. Although prosthetic arthroplasty is the primary surgical option to be considered when major pain and functional loss result from glenohumeral arthritis, other surgical alternatives have been described in the management of arthritis. Kelly,[186, 187] Bennett and Gerber,[28] and Thomas and associates[340] have reviewed some of the surgical options for surgical management of the rheumatoid shoulder.

SYNOVECTOMY

Rheumatoid arthritis and other inflammatory arthropathies produce synovial tissue hyperplasia and its attendant symptoms. A benchmark article on care for rheumatoid joint problems was published in 1943.[326] This article offered great insight into the surgical care of patients with rheumatoid arthritis during the preprosthetic era. The

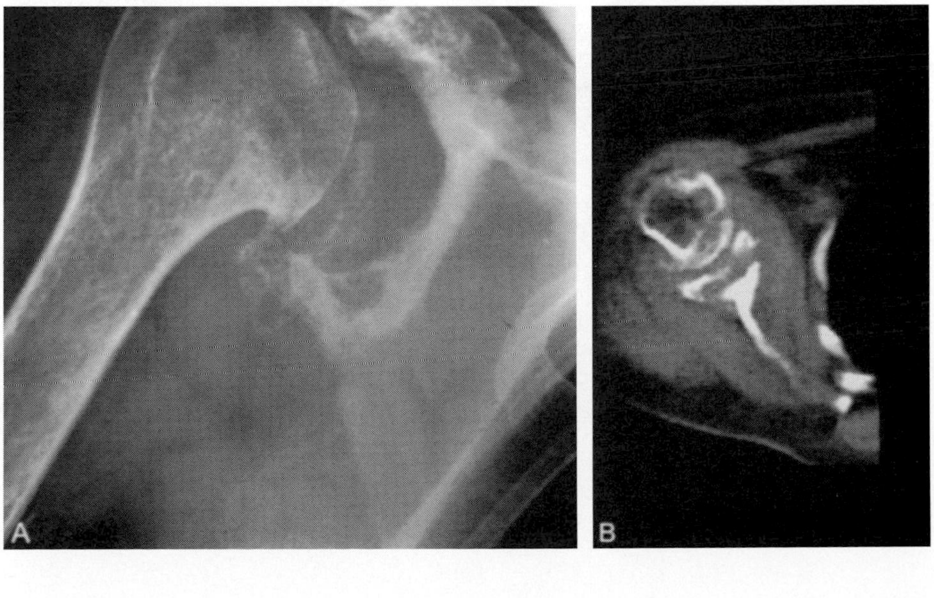

Figure 16–74

This upper-middle-aged woman presented with the gradual onset of shoulder pain and reduction of movement. The shoulder was more painful with use and was also painful at rest (often typical of shoulder arthritis). She had no known systemic illness. *A*, Arthritic involvement of the glenohumeral joint is shown with some collapse of the humeral head articular surface; however, what is more important is that it shows destruction of the bone of the glenoid. *B*, A computed tomography image shows this bone destruction quite well. Biopsy revealed metastatic thyroid carcinoma. A neoplastic process must always be considered in the evaluation of a patient with supposed glenohumeral arthritis.

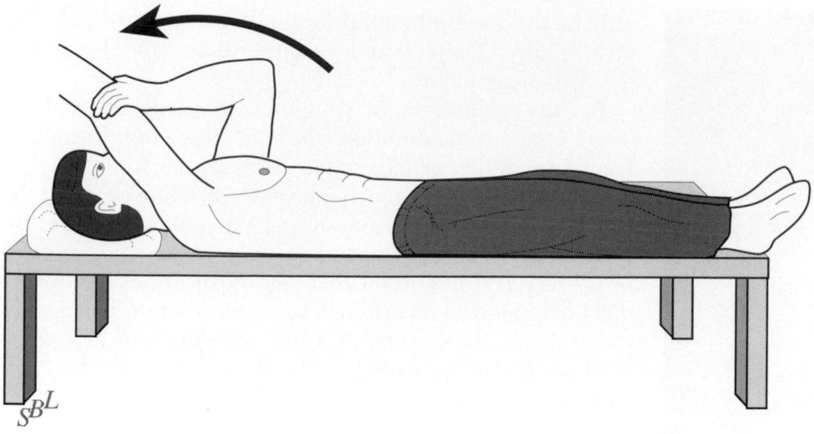

Figure 16–75

Stretching in overhead reach using the opposite arm as the "therapist." (From Matsen FA III, Lippitt SB, Sidles JA, and Harryman DT II: Practical Evaluation and Management of the Shoulder. Philadelphia: WB Saunders, 1994.)

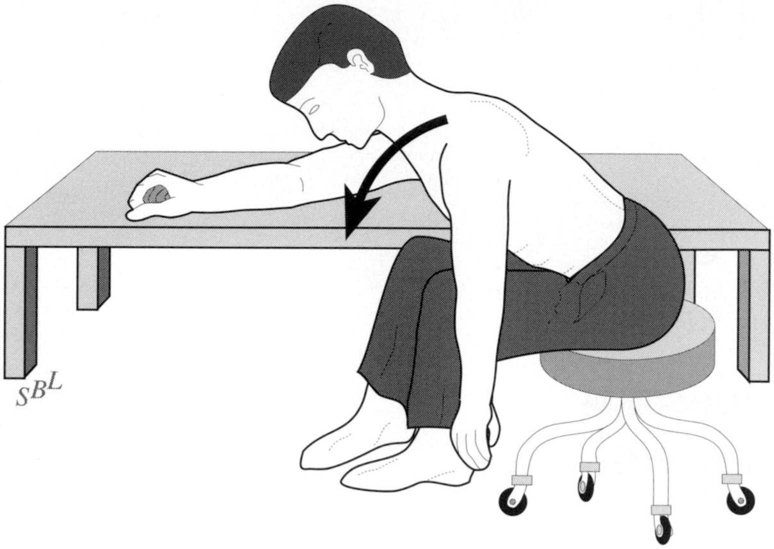

Figure 16–76

Stretching in overhead reach using the progressive forward lean to apply a gentle force to the arm. (From Matsen FA III, Lippitt SB, Sidles JA, and Harryman DT II: Practical Evaluation and Management of the Shoulder. Philadelphia: WB Saunders, 1994.)

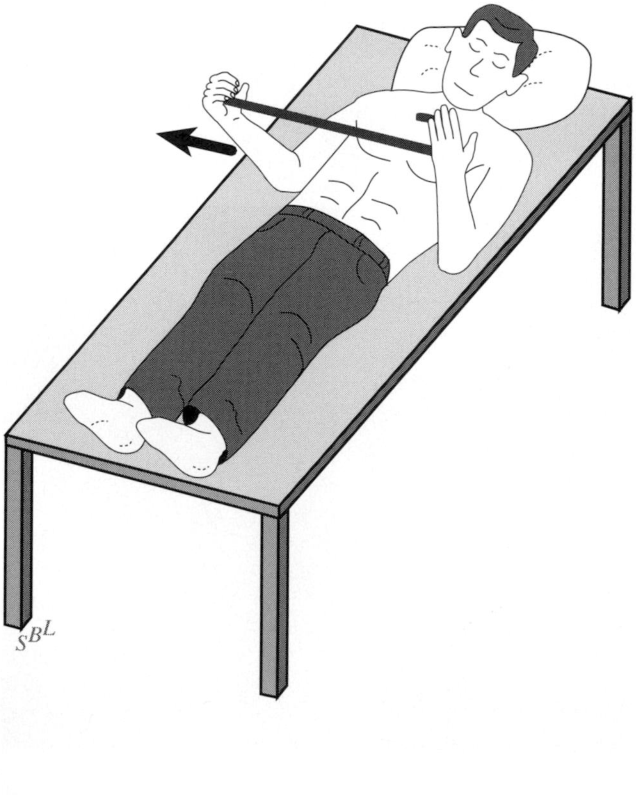

Figure 16–77

Stretching in external rotation using the opposite hand as the "therapist." (From Matsen FA III, Lippitt SB, Sidles JA, and Harryman DT II: Practical Evaluation and Management of the Shoulder. Philadelphia: WB Saunders, 1994.)

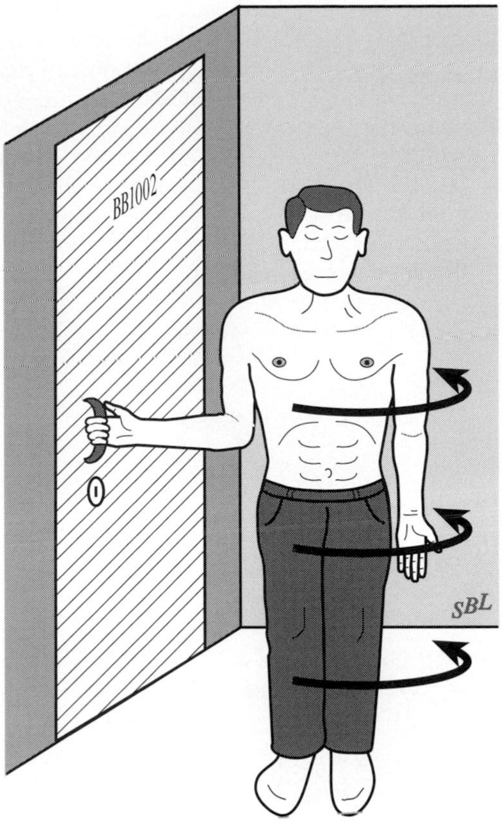

Figure 16–78

Stretching in external rotation by turning the body away from a fixed object to apply a gentle stretching force. (From Matsen FA III, Lippitt SB, Sidles JA, and Harryman DT II: Practical Evaluation and Management of the Shoulder. Philadelphia: WB Saunders, 1994.)

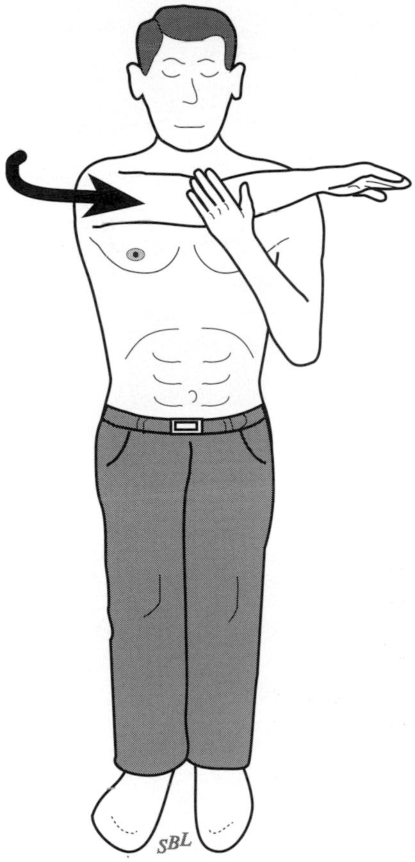

Figure 16–80

Stretching in cross-body reach using the opposite arm as the "therapist." (From Matsen FA III, Lippitt SB, Sidles JA, and Harryman DT II: Practical Evaluation and Management of the Shoulder. Philadelphia: WB Saunders, 1994.)

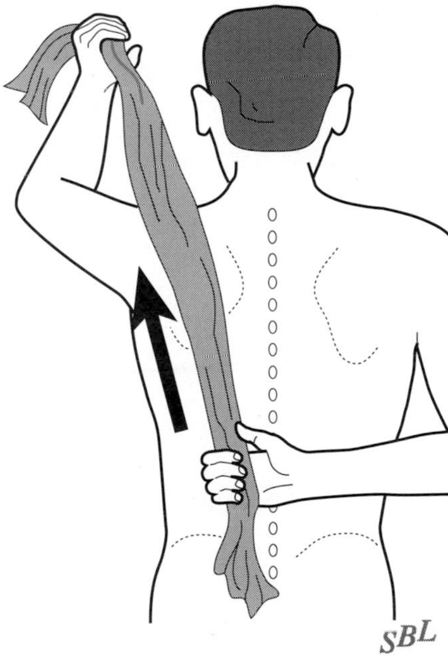

Figure 16–79

Stretching in internal rotation using a towel to apply a gentle stretching force. (From Matsen FA III, Lippitt SB, Sidles JA, and Harryman DT II: Practical Evaluation and Management of the Shoulder. Philadelphia: WB Saunders, 1994.)

authors observed that surgery was not always necessary or desirable, and surgery of the joint in and of itself would be unlikely to change the long-term course of the disease for the patient. When shoulder symptoms were severe and persistent, shoulder synovectomy, bursectomy, and acromioplasty seemed to alleviate pain and allow the patient improved use of the involved limb.

Patients may be considered for synovectomy if they have chronic refractory synovitis. Clinically, this is evident as an enlarged, boggy-feeling shoulder, indicating either primary bursal hypertrophy or rotator cuff tearing with extension of synovial tissue and fluid into the subdeltoid bursa (see Fig. 16–62). A shoulder arthrogram (see Fig. 16–60) may help to define the severity and extent of the synovitis as well as information about the presence or absence of rotator cuff tearing.

Pahle and Kvarnes[267] reported on the application and relative effectiveness of shoulder synovectomy. Their method included a subdeltoid and subacromial bursectomy, arthrotomy through the subscapularis, and synovectomy of all joint areas. In addition, any osteophytes or other joint irregularities are removed or smoothed. If there is tenosynovial hypertrophy surrounding the long head of the biceps brachii, this tissue is also removed. Postoperatively, a light abduction pillow is placed, and exercises are commenced 2 to 3 days after surgery. Pain

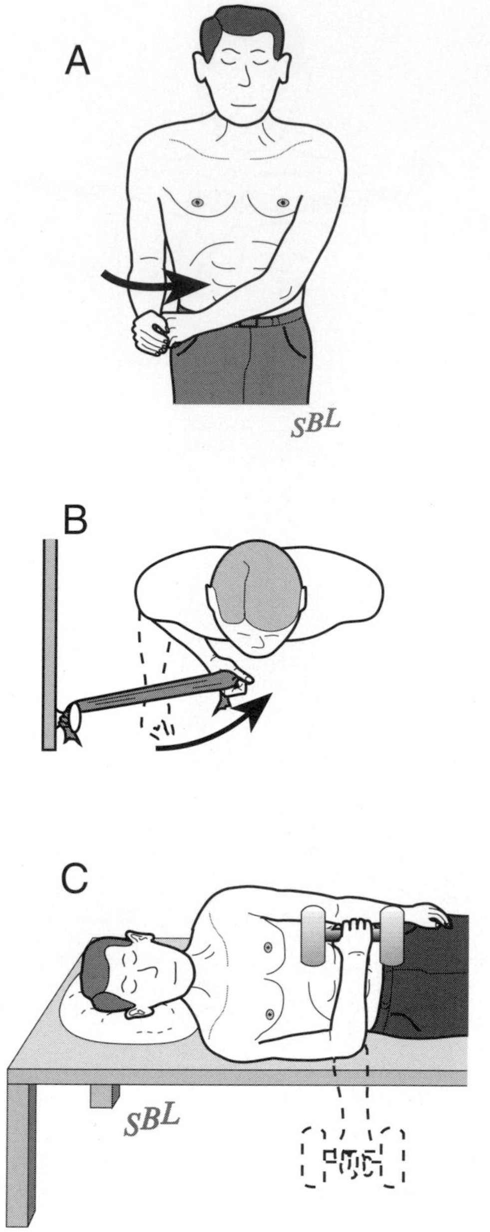

Figure 16–81

Internal rotation can be strengthened with isometrics (*A*), rubber tubing (*B*), or free weights (*C*). (From Matsen FA III, Lippitt SB, Sidles JA, and Harryman DT II: Practical Evaluation and Management of the Shoulder. Philadelphia: WB Saunders, 1994.)

relief in their patients was often quite good, with significant residual pain in only 10 of 54 shoulders (approximately one half had significant joint surface irregularity). Motion in these patients was slightly improved but not dramatically so. A lessening of the pain did improve limb function.

Currently, synovectomy is reserved for patients with intact articular cartilage or cartilage that is at least one half of its normal thickness. Synovectomy may be accomplished arthroscopically, although great care is necessary to avoid nerve damage. Open synovectomy is approached through the deltopectoral interval. The subdeltoid bursal tissue is excised carefully, protecting the axillary nerve on the undersurface of the deltoid muscle. Rotator cuff defects are identified. Usually, the arthrotomy will include division of the subscapularis near its insertion and division of the anterior shoulder capsule at its humeral attachments. The capsular incision will extend up to the intra-articular portion of the long head of the biceps tendon and along this tendon to its glenoid origin. The incision will also extend inferiorly to the 6 o'clock position on the humeral head. Synovium is removed from the anterior portion of the shoulder and the subscapularis recess and then from the inferior aspect of the joint. By preserving the fibrous layer beneath the synovial tissue, the axillary

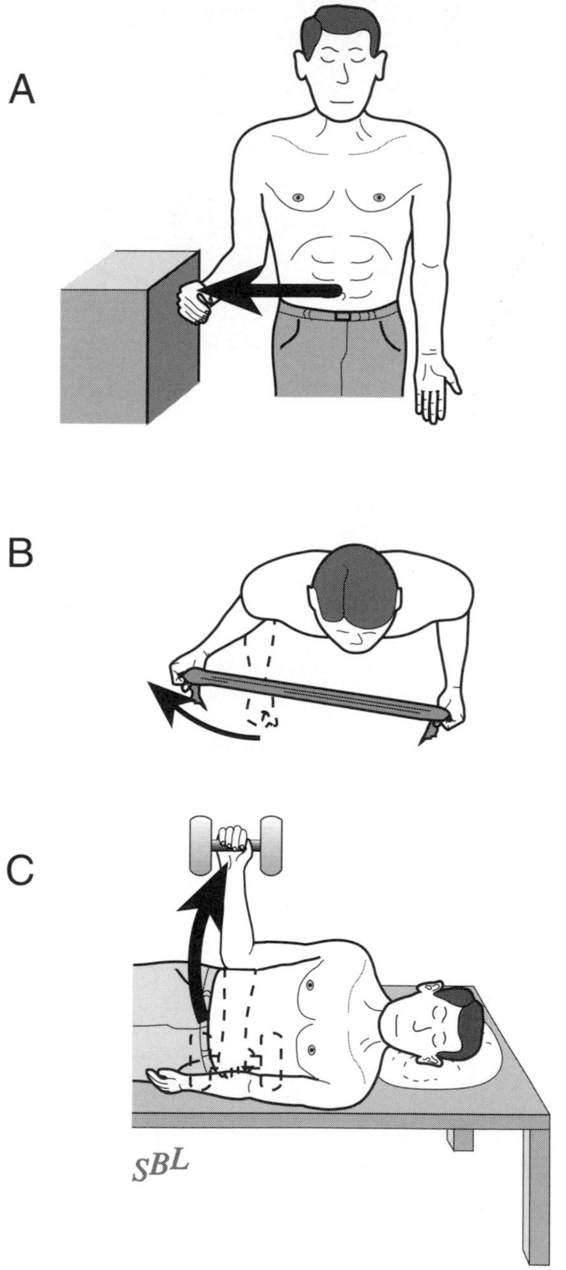

Figure 16–82

External rotation strengthening using isometrics (*A*), rubber tubing (*B*), or free weights (*C*). (Reproduced with permission from Matsen FA III, Lippitt SB, Sidles JA, and Harryman DT II: Practical Evaluation and Management of the Shoulder. Philadelphia: WB Saunders, 1994.)

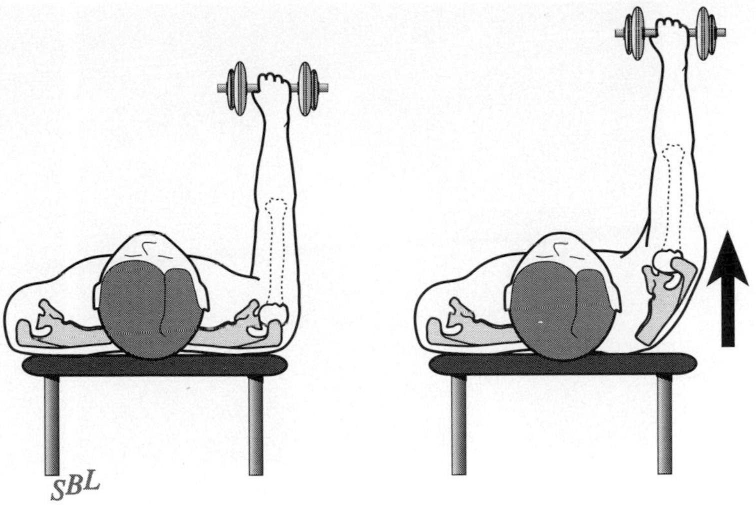

Figure 16–83

In the press plus, the arm is pushed upward until the shoulder blade is lifted off the table or bed. (From Matsen FA III, Lippitt SB, Sidles JA, and Harryman DT II: Practical Evaluation and Management of the Shoulder. Philadelphia: WB Saunders, 1994.)

nerve is protected. By working around the humeral head, the posterior synovial hypertrophy is removed. Exposure may be facilitated by partially dislocating the joint. Reparable cuff defects may be addressed by direct suturing or subscapularis transposition upward.[76] Drains are kept in place as long as fluid is being retrieved. Sutures are left in place for 10 days. Postoperative care includes early passive range of motion. Active exercises are delayed until healing of tendon repairs is complete.

RESECTION ARTHROPLASTY

Before prostheses were available, resection of the humeral head was used to manage severe fractures and uncontrollable infection.[94, 219, 330] Several authors have reported on excision of the glenoid in conjunction with a synovectomy.[134, 349] Milbrink and Wigren[237] reported reasonable short-term results from 13 resection arthroplasties for advanced rheumatoid arthritis. Pain relief was reported to be good.

Resection arthroplasty of the shoulder is useful as an adjunct to the care for septic arthritis of the shoulder with extensive humeral head and glenoid osteomyelitis. A joint resection also results after the removal of infected or mechanically compromised implants (Fig. 16–85).[70, 94, 203] The initial problem after resection is joint instability. Later, stiffness usually develops, and a few shoulders actually go on to bony arthrodesis.[249] Pain relief is variable.[203] Maximum active abduction is typically 60 to 80 degrees.[70, 94, 203, 238, 334] However, moderate weakness persists. Suturing the rotator cuff to the remaining portion of the upper humerus may increase strength, but the results have been variable.[177, 178, 193, 254]

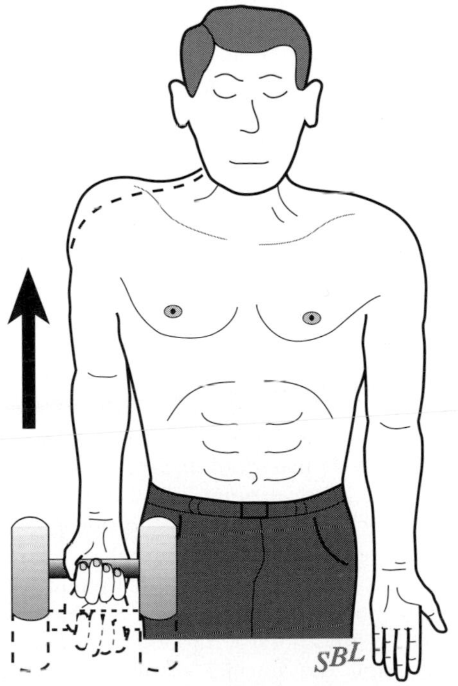

Figure 16–84

In the shoulder shrug exercise, the tip of the shoulder is lifted toward the ear while holding the elbow straight. (From Matsen FA III, Lippitt SB, Sidles JA, and Harryman DT II: Practical Evaluation and Management of the Shoulder. Philadelphia: WB Saunders, 1994.)

GLENOHUMERAL ARTHRODESIS

Glenohumeral arthrodesis is usually reserved for attempts at salvaging septic arthritis or complex deficiencies of the joint surface associated with permanent loss of the cuff and deltoid. Early in this decade, there were many indications for arthrodesis of the shoulder, but now there are only a few.[73, 80] Cofield demonstrated this trend in Table 16–10.[77] Most shoulder fusions today are done for one of four reasons: (1) paralysis of the deltoid and rotator cuff, (2) infection with loss of glenohumeral cartilage, (3) refractory instability, or (4) failed reconstructive procedures.[303] Seldom, if ever, is shoulder fusion undertaken for treatment of the more usual causes of shoulder arthritis, even in younger individuals who wish to be active. An exception to this is expressed in the article by Rybka and co-workers from Finland.[317] These authors defined the results of arthrodesis in a group of patients with rheumatoid arthritis. Thirty-seven of 41 shoulders fused. Complications were few. A brace was used for postoperative support in an attempt to avoid potential elbow stiffness. This investigation suggested that arthrodesis was easily achieved, inexpensive, and a reliable method for the treatment of severely involved rheumatoid shoulders.

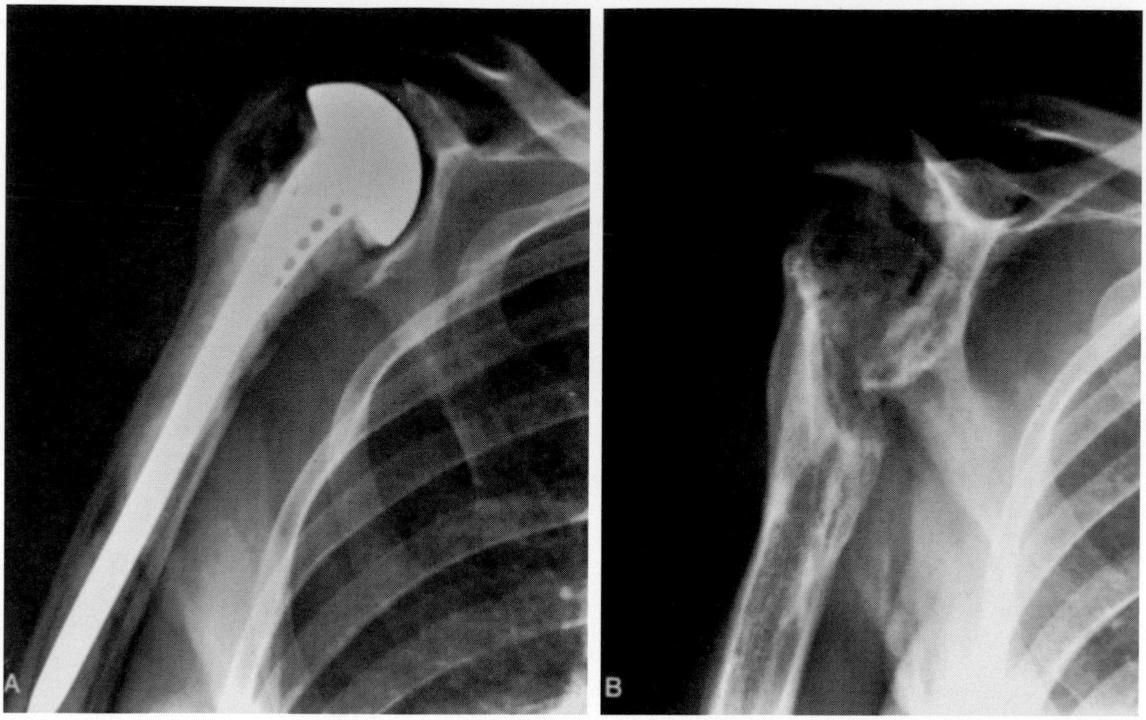

Figure 16–85

A previous proximal humeral prosthetic replacement was done in an elderly woman with multiple joint osteoarthritis. Her total knee arthroplasty became infected, and the infection spread to the proximal humeral prosthetic replacement (*A*). The shoulder region was brawny and erythematous, and there was a draining sinus on the anterolateral aspect of the arm. The region was débrided; the prosthesis and cement were removed; and, after delayed primary closure, the radiographic appearance of the joint was as seen in *B*. Fortunately, the patient had only mild pain, and the shoulder was stable because of fibrosis. There was active abduction of 65 degrees and external rotation of 10 degrees.

Some consensus has been reached about the desirable position of shoulder fusion. Rowe was the first to firmly state the advantages of less abduction and flexion for the surgically arthrodesed shoulder: 20 degrees of abduction, 30 degrees of flexion, and internal rotation of 40 degrees (Fig. 16–86).[312] Hawkins and Neer[160] recommended 25 to 40 degrees of abduction for the arm, 20 to 30 degrees of flexion, and 25 to 30 degrees of internal rotation. When determining arm position, the trunk is commonly used as the source of reference, with the scapula being held in the anatomic position. Jonsson and associates[181] described a method for documenting the position of fusion using Moire photography.

The best candidates for this procedure are patients with: (1) permanent and severe weakness due to loss of cuff and deltoid function; (2) good scapular motors (e.g., trapezius, pectoralis, serratus, rhomboids); (3) a good understanding of the limitations and potential complications of a shoulder fusion; (4) good motivation; and (5) minimal complaints of pain.

Table 16–10 INDICATIONS FOR SHOULDER ARTHRODESIS (AT THE MAYO CLINIC, ROCHESTER, MINNESOTA)

DIAGNOSIS	*1950–1974**	*1975–1983†*
Paralysis	21	20
Infection	8	15
Severe rotator cuff tearing	12	9
Traumatic or osteoarthritis	18	5
Neoplasia	0	3
Recurrent dislocations	7	0
Rheumatoid arthritis	5	0
	71	52

*Cofield RH and Briggs BT: J Bone Joint Surg *61A*:668–677, 1979.
†From Cofield RH: AAOS Instruct Course Lect *34*:268–277, 1985.

To establish the limitations of shoulder fusions, Haryman and associates[156, 221] studied 12 shoulders that had glenohumeral arthrodeses at least 2 years before the time of study. Elevation in the plus 90-degree (anterior sagittal) plane averaged 47 degrees. Elevation in the minus 90-degree (posterior sagittal) plane averaged 22 degrees. The average external rotation was 9 degrees, and the average internal rotation was 46 degrees. These ranges of motion were similar to the scapulothoracic motion measured in normal subjects.[156] Only one of the patients could reach his hair without bending his neck forward; only five patients could reach their perineum; six patients could reach the back pocket; seven patients could reach the opposite axilla; and 10 patients could reach the side pocket.

These same authors studied normal in vivo shoulder kinematics to predict the functions that would be allowed by various positions of glenohumeral arthrodesis, assuming that the scapulothoracic motion would remain unchanged.[221] Using the normal scapulothoracic motions, they were able to model the functional effects of different fusion positions. They found that activities of daily living could be best performed if the joint was fused in 15 degrees of flexion, 15 degrees of abduction, and 45 degrees of internal rotation (Fig. 16–87). This low angle of

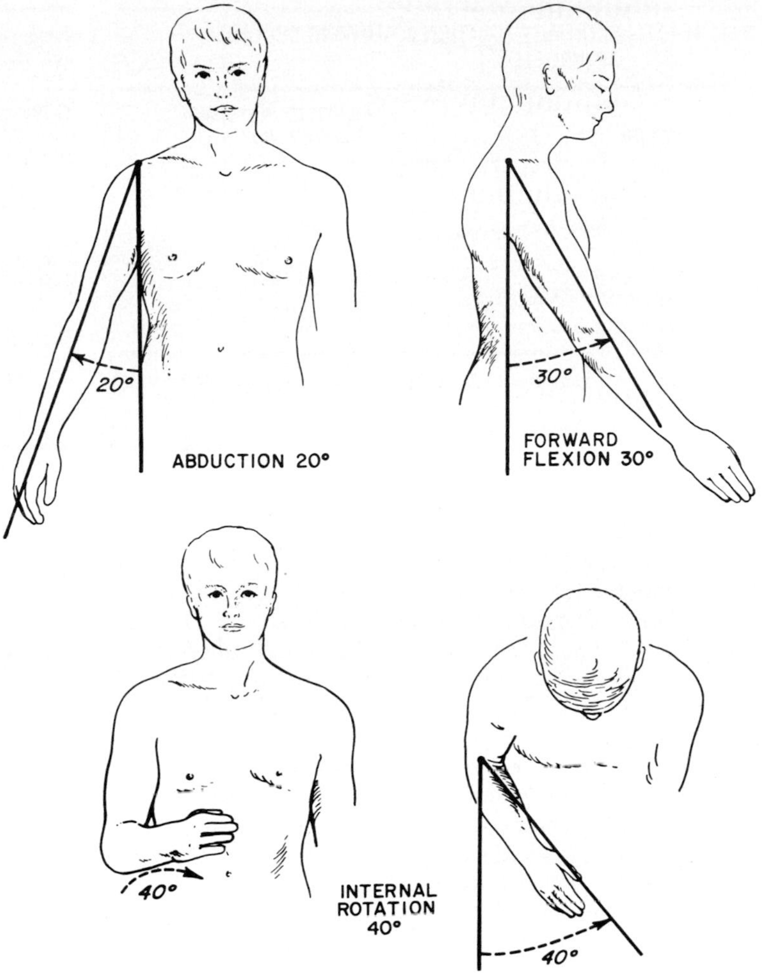

Figure 16–86

Rowe re-evaluated the position of the arm in arthrodesis of the shoulder in the adult. From his experience, he recommended that less abduction and forward flexion be incorporated into the fusion position and that internal rotation (not external rotation) was necessary. (From Rowe CR: Re-evaluation of the position of the arm in arthrodesis of the shoulder in the adult. J Bone Joint Surg *56A*:913–922, 1974.)

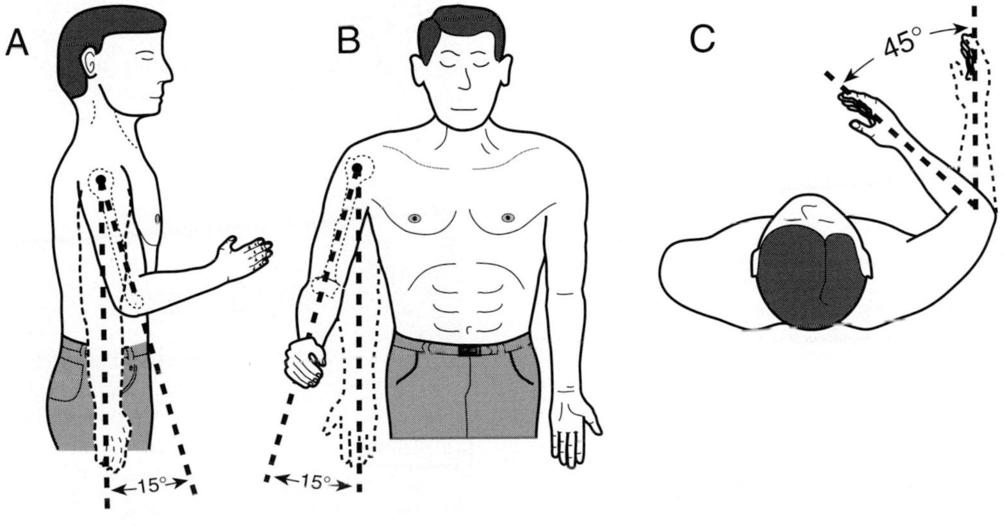

Figure 16–87

The recommended arthrodesis position: 15 degrees of humerothoracic flexion (*A*), 15 degrees of humerothoracic abduction (*B*), and 45 degrees of internal rotation (*C*). (From Matsen FA III, Lippitt SB, Sidles JA, and Harryman DT II: Practical Evaluation and Management of the Shoulder. Philadelphia: WB Saunders, 1994.)

Table 16–11 EXTREMITY FUNCTION FOLLOWING SHOULDER ARTHRODESIS*†

FUNCTION	ABILITY TO PERFORM FUNCTION NO. (%)
Sleep on limb	46 (73)
Dress	45 (71)
Eat using limb	45 (71)
Toilet care	44 (70)
Lift 5 to 7.5 kg	43 (68)
Comb hair	28 (44)
Use hand at shoulder level	13 (21)

*Adapted from Cofield RH and Briggs BT: J Bone Joint Surg *61A*:668, 1979.
†No. of shoulders = 63.

elevation and relatively high degree of internal rotation facilitated sitting comfortably in a chair, lying flat in bed, as well as reaching the face, the opposite axilla, and the perineum. However, all positions represented major compromises of normal function (Table 16–11). This is the primary reason for avoiding fusion in individuals with conditions such as osteoarthritis, rheumatoid arthritis, or traumatic arthritis when adequate bone stock and muscle function are present. Function after total shoulder arthroplasty is much better (Table 16–12).

There are many techniques for shoulder arthrodesis (Table 16–13). These techniques are best classified as extra-articular, intra-articular, or a combination of the two. Extra-articular arthrodesis techniques, such as that of Putti,[288] Watson-Jones,[353] or Brittain,[46] had greatest usefulness as adjunctive care for infection, especially tuberculosis. With an extra-articular arthrodesis, the surgeon hoped to avoid the infectious focus and to accomplish a fusion about the affected joint. Now, effective antimicrobial medications essentially obviate the need for this approach.

Intra-articular fusion offers the simplest and most direct method. The joint is débrided and remaining cartilage, scar, and dense subchondral bone are removed. Cancellous bone of the humeral head and glenoid are placed against each other, and with the arm in the desired position, fixation is placed. Different forms of fixation have been used, including screws,[21, 157, 225] wires,[59] bone grafts,[166, 311] and pins.[100] Currently, the use of screws seems to be favored. A cast is usually used after this technique and is continued for 3 to 6 months. This technique still seems reasonable for the individual with an excellent rotator cuff and capsule who might later be a candidate for prosthetic replacement (Fig. 16–88).

Intra-articular fusion can be combined with extra-articular fusion. Extra-articular bone contact is achieved by bringing the humeral head against the acromion (Fig. 16–89) or by adding bone grafts between the humeral head and the acromion or between the humeral neck and the medial scapula adjacent to the glenoid. Fixation is obtained by screws,[19, 80, 182, 227, 317, 345] staples, bone grafts,[25, 44] external fixation,[61, 64, 176] or bone plates.[101, 199, 297–299, 315, 354] Tension band wiring has been suggested if the bone is osteoporotic (Fig. 16–90).[31] External fixation may be preferred if the shoulder is infected or in the presence of

Table 16–12 EXTREMITY FUNCTION FOLLOWING TOTAL SHOULDER ARTHROPLASTY*†

FUNCTION	ABILITY TO PERFORM FUNCTION NO. (%)
Sleep on limb	64 (90)
Dress	69 (97)
Eat using limb	70 (99)
Toilet care	68 (96)
Lift 5 to 7.5 kg	60 (85)
Comb hair	56 (79)
Use hand at shoulder level	53 (75)

*Adapted from Cofield RH: J Bone Joint Surg *66A*:899–906, 1984.
†No. of shoulders = 71.

Table 16–13 TECHNIQUES FOR SHOULDER FUSION

EXTRA-ARTICULAR	INTRA-ARTICULAR	COMBINED EXTRA- AND INTRA-ARTICULAR
Acromion-humeral[175]	Suture[203]	Suture[89]
Spine of scapula-humeral[217]	Screws[14, 100, 136]	Screws[10, 39, 57, 138, 190, 213]
Axillary border of scapula or humeral plus tibial graft[27]	Pin[81]	Staples
	Tibial graft[185]	Wire[32]
	Bone bank graft[105]	Pins and tension band[22]
		Bone graft[18, 26]
		External fixator[34, 35, 110]
		Plate or plates[58, 73, 181, 182, 130, 183, 188, 218]

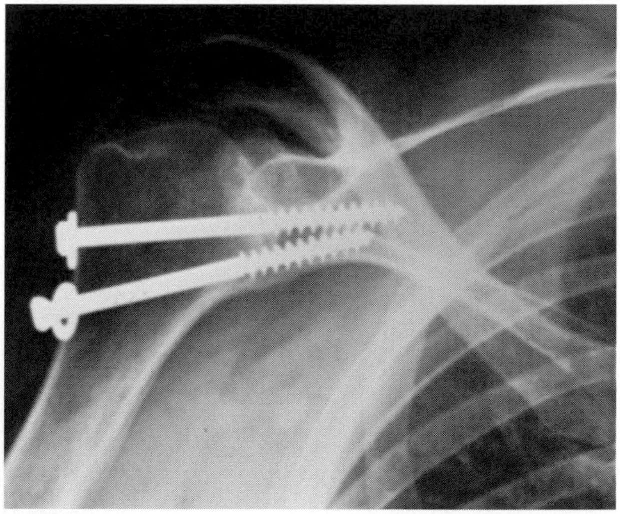

Figure 16–88

Intra-articular shoulder arthrodesis using screws for internal fixation. This young man had recurrent shoulder instability and, after anterior capsule repair, developed an infection that eventuated in cartilage loss at the glenohumeral joint. This simple form of fusion was undertaken to preserve the largely intact surrounding joint capsule and rotator cuff. His neuromuscular function is, of course, normal, and there may be a possibility in the future of reconstruction with prosthetic joint replacement.

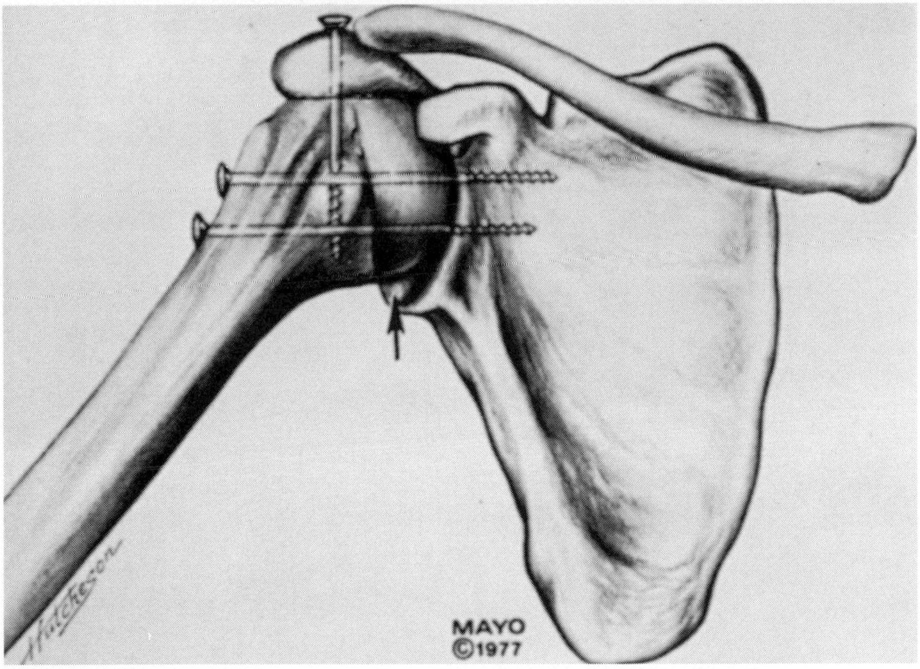

Figure 16–89

A technique of combined intra-articular and extra-articular shoulder arthrodesis using screws for internal fixation. (From Cofield RH and Briggs BT: Glenohumeral arthrodesis: Operative and long term functional results. J Bone Joint Surg *61A*:668–677, 1979. By permission of the Mayo Foundation.)

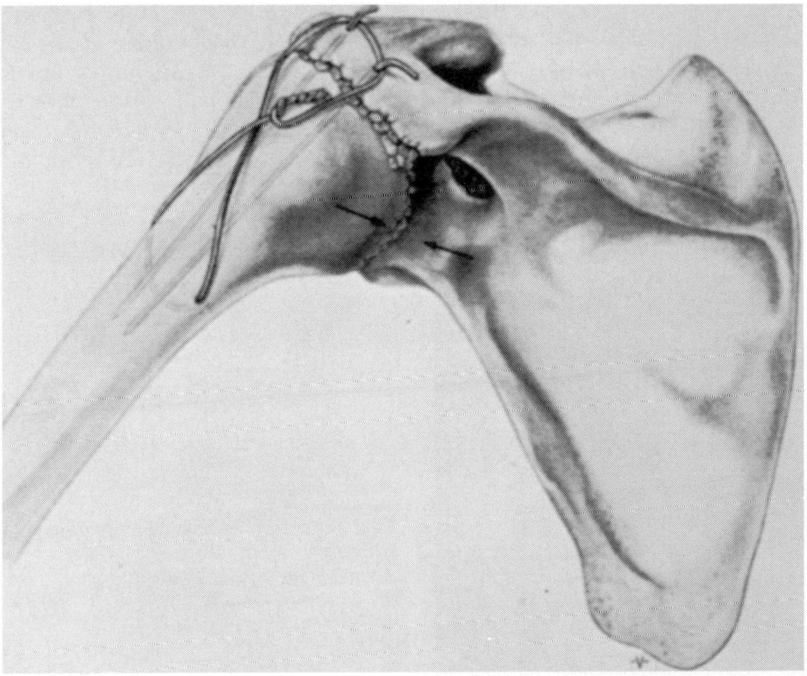

Figure 16–90

When the bones of the shoulder are extremely osteoporotic and one is attempting a shoulder arthrodesis, it has been suggested that pins and tension band wiring may be a satisfactory solution to obtain continued coaptation of the joint surfaces. Supplemental fixation with a cast will be necessary. (From Blauth W and Hepp WR: Arthrodesis of the shoulder joint by traction absorbing wire. *In* Chapchal G [ed]: The Arthrodesis in the Restoration of Working Ability. Stuttgart: Georg Thieme, 1975, p 30.)

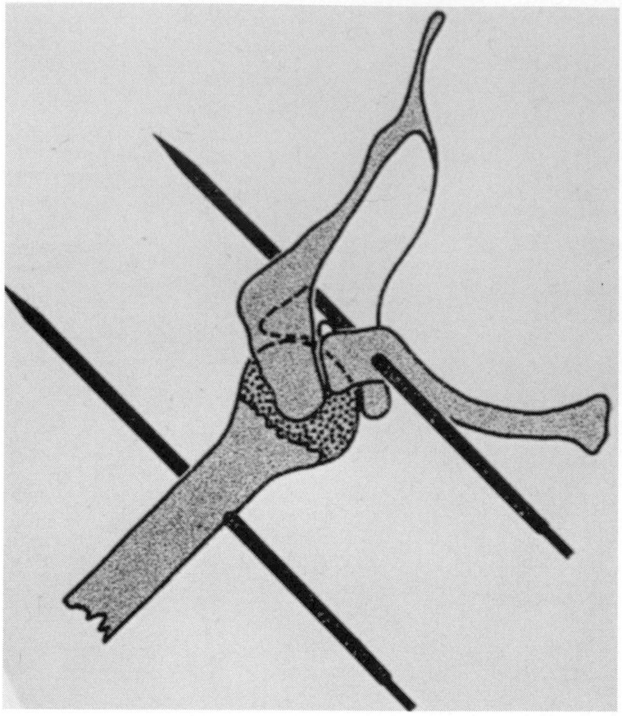

Figure 16–91

The first method of placing pins for compression arthrodesis of the shoulder as suggested by Charnley. A simple external fixator was then applied. (From Charnley J: Compression arthrodesis of the ankle and shoulder. J Bone Joint Surg *33B*:180–191, 1951.)

wound problems (Figs. 16–91 to 16–94). External rotation carries the risk of radial nerve injury.[61]

Internal fixation with one or more plates has the potential to obviate the need for a long-term external cast or brace support during the postoperative period.[358] The arm position can be fixed securely in the position that the surgeon wishes without worry that the position of the arm will change during healing. Narrow dynamic compression plates are often used (Fig. 16–95). It has been suggested that pelvic reconstruction plates are easier to apply and may be equally effective (Fig. 16–96).[297]

The rate of bone fusion after many of these methods of shoulder arthrodesis is 80 to 90% (Table 16–14). Shoulder fusion carries the risks of infection, reflex dystrophy, acromioclavicular arthritis, and symptomatic internal fixation that must be removed later. Fracture of the operated extremity below the fusion has been reported.[73]

Patient satisfaction can never be perfect after a procedure such as this, but it does approach 80%.[73] Some patients have shoulder girdle pain despite a successful bone fusion.[19, 73] Richards and associates[296] reviewed 57 patients who had fusion with a single plate to achieve glenohumeral and acromiohumeral arthrodesis. They used a 30,30,30 position (abduction, internal rotation, and

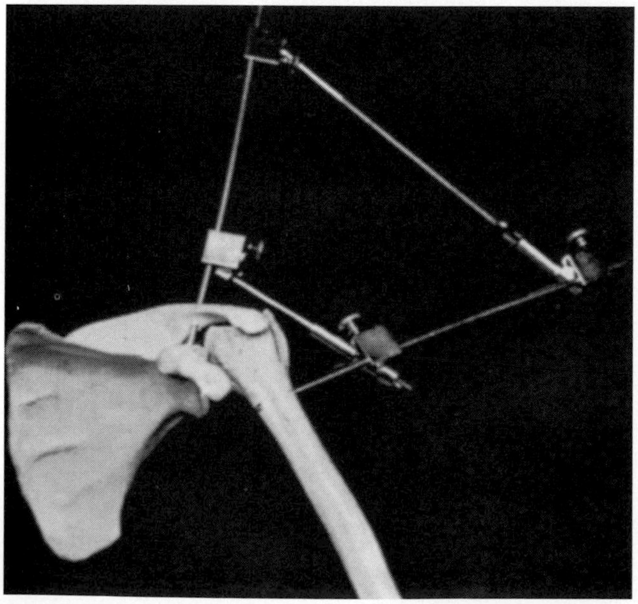

Figure 16–92

Charnley's second technique to apply pins as a part of a shoulder arthrodesis procedure so that an external fixator might be used to apply compression across the arthrodesis site. (From Charnley J and Houston JK: Compression arthrodesis of the shoulder. J Bone Joint Surg *46B*:614–620, 1964.)

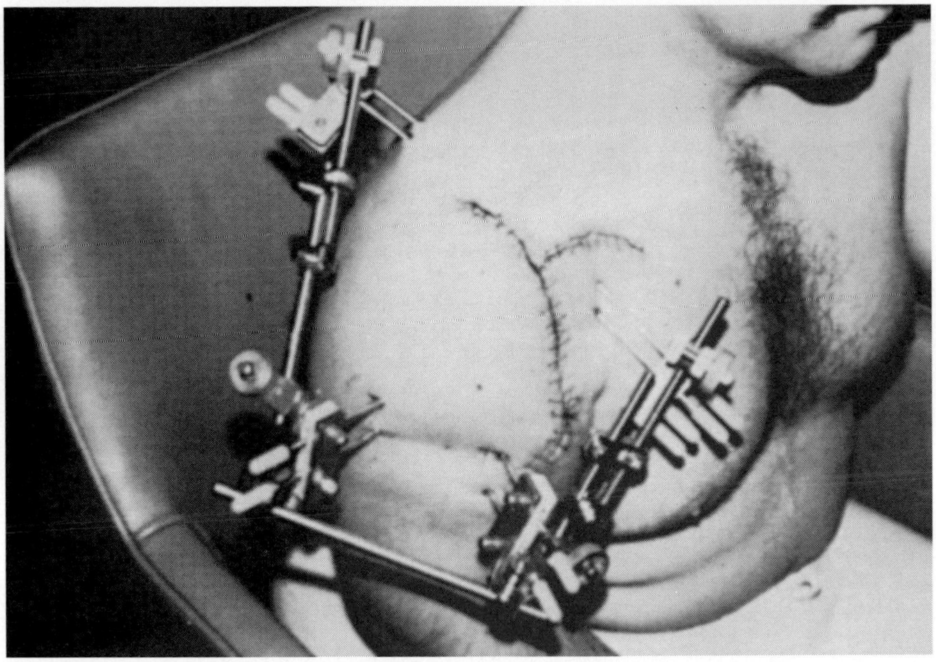

Figure 16–93

An external fixation device used for shoulder arthrodesis. Half pins are placed in the proximal humerus, then more proximal pins are inserted into the acromion and exit through the spine of the scapula. (From Johnson CA, Healy WL, Brooker AF Jr, and Krackow KA: External fixation shoulder arthrodesis. Clin Orthop *211*:219–223, 1986.)

flexion). Only two of these fusions were for arthritis, and two for failed shoulder arthroplasty (the rest were for brachial plexus palsy, refractory instability, or sepsis). There were 14% complications, and three required regrafting. Most patients, except those in the instability group, were satisfied. Persistent pain after a fusion is often difficult to explain. It used to be thought that resection of the distal clavicle would improve motion after shoulder fusion; however, our experience indicates that gains are minimal.

Matsen's Technique for Shoulder Arthrodesis

The patient is positioned in a beach-chair position with the scapula in the field and the arm draped free. The operative approach is through an anterior deltopectoral incision with superior extension of the incision if plate fixation is used (Fig. 16–97). Any residual articular cartilage on the humerus or glenoid is resected down to raw subchondral bone (removing the subchondral bone

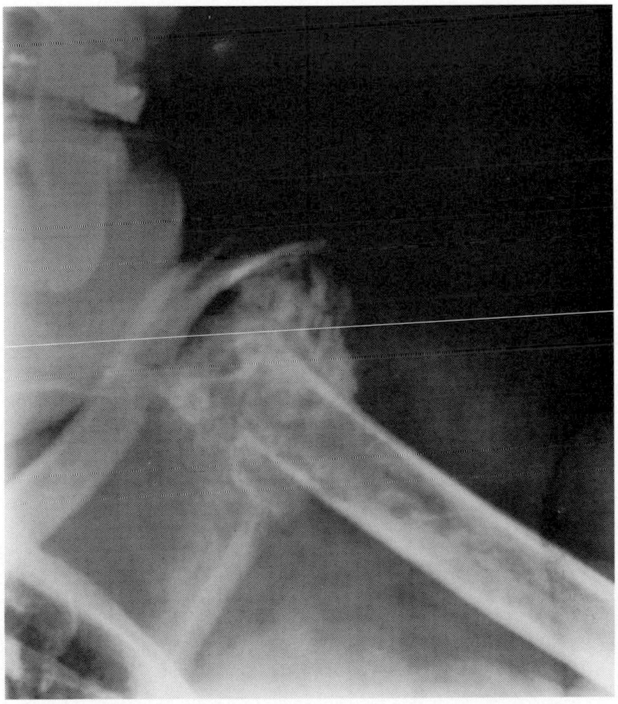

Figure 16–94

External fixation may prove to be a useful adjunct to obtain shoulder fusion in certain patients. Certainly, patients with open wounds who need sequential débridements might be considered for this form of support for shoulder arthrodesis. This patient had previous trauma and previous surgery, with a significant amount of bone loss. She had also lost function of her deltoid and rotator cuff. At the time of shoulder arthrodesis, pins were placed as suggested by Charnley (his revised technique). Also, an iliac crest graft was placed around the junction of the remaining humerus and scapula. The patient went on to develop a solid bone fusion.

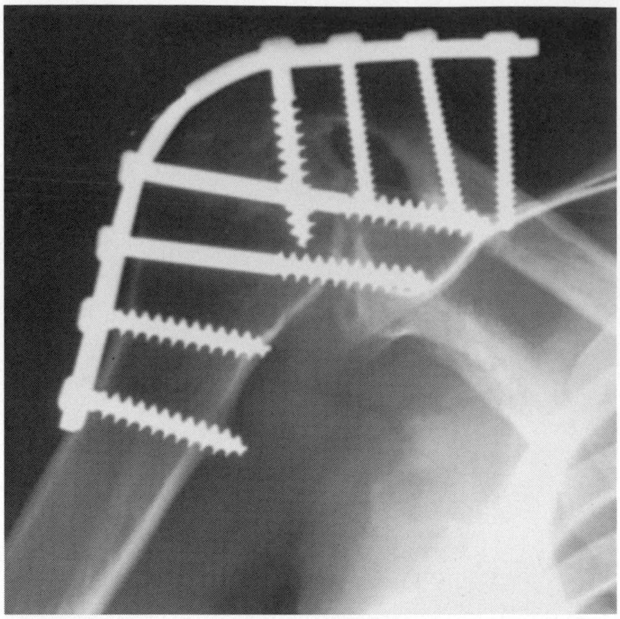

Figure 16–95

A radiographic illustration of a shoulder fusion incorporating both intra- and extra-articular bone contact. Fixation with a plate has provided immediate stability. This could preclude the use of cast support; however, a number of surgeons consider a 1- to 2-month period of spica cast immobilization as an adjunct to this fixation.

weakens the construct and makes solid glenohumeral compression more difficult to achieve). The supraspinatus tendon is resected from between the humeral head and the acromion. The undersurface of the acromion is stripped down to raw bone. The soft tissues are lifted from the anterior glenoid neck so that the subscapularis fossa can be palpated. The humeral head is positioned in

Table 16–14 PSEUDOARTHROSIS FOLLOWING SHOULDER ARTHRODESIS

SERIES	NO. OF SHOULDERS	NO. OF PSEUDOARTHROSES
Ten series*	87	0
Hauge (1961)[157]	34	1
Cofield and Briggs (1979)[80]	71	3
Charnley and Houston (1964)[64]	19	1
Steindler (1944)[330]	82	5
Becker (1975)[21]	47	3
Rybka and co-workers (1979)[317]	41	4
De Velasco Polo and Cardoso Monterrubio (1973)[100]	31	6
Barton[16a]	10	2
AOA report	102	23
Totals	524	48

*Johnson and co-workers (1986),[176] Hucherson (1959),[166] Kalamchi (1978),[182] Matsunaga (1972),[225] May (1962),[227] Richards and associates (1985),[298] Richards and associates (1988),[297] Riggins (1976),[299] Uematsu (1979),[345] Weigert and Gronert (1974)[354].

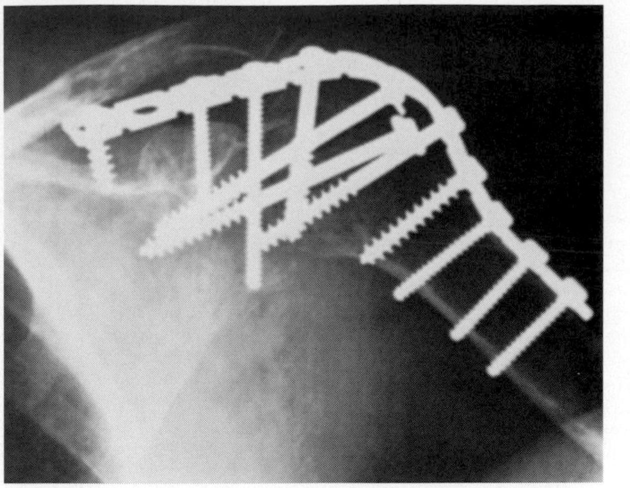

Figure 16–96

A radiograph of a shoulder arthrodesis using a pelvic reconstruction plate for internal fixation. This plate is more easily contoured than the standard DCP plate yet seems to offer enough rigidity for arthrodesis of the shoulder.

the glenoid in 15 degrees of abduction, 15 degrees of flexion, and 45 degrees of internal rotation position (see Fig. 16–87) and is temporarily fixed with three long 3.2-mm drills that intentionally exit the neck of the scapula

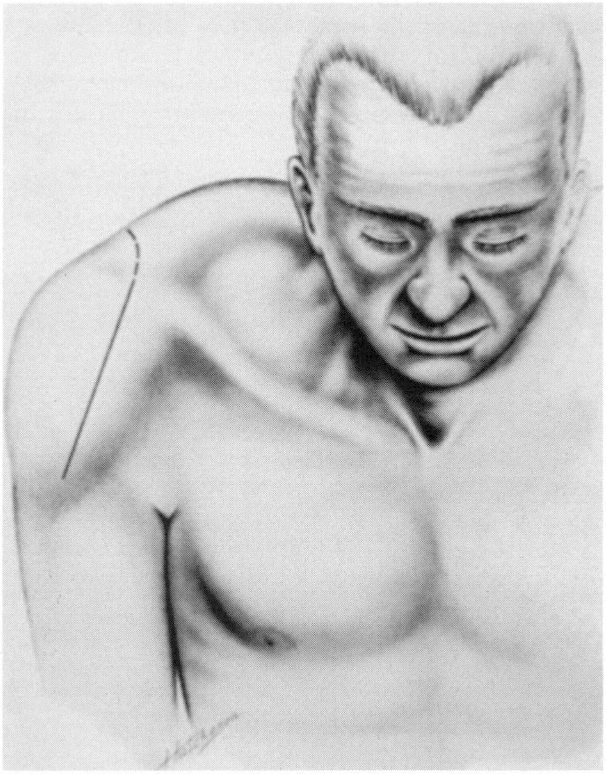

Figure 16–97

An anterior incision for shoulder arthrodesis. The incision can be extended over the superior aspect of the shoulder to expose the scapular spine if a plate is to be used for internal fixation. (From Cofield RH: Shoulder arthrodesis and resection arthroplasty. Instr Course Lect *34*:268–277, 1985.)

anteriorly approximately 2 cm medial to the glenoid lip where their tips can be palpated and controlled. When used in this manner, the known length of the drills can serve as depth gauges to determine the length of screws needed. The position of the arm is checked by making sure that the hand can reach the mouth, the anterior perineum, and the contralateral axilla. The 3.2-mm drills are sequentially replaced by fully threaded 6.5-mm cancellous screws with washers. Because the humeral head is softer than the glenoid, compression can usually be achieved without formally "lagging" the screw and without needing to use a smooth shank. An iliac crest bone graft is fashioned to fit between the humeral head and the acromion, resting in the position normally occupied by the supraspinatus tendon. The interposition of the iliac crest graft maximizes humeroscapular contact by preserving the normal concave-convex glenohumeral relationships while allowing for stabilizing contact between the head, the graft, and the acromion (if the humeral head is moved upward to make contact with the acromion without a graft, the glenohumeral contact area is diminished). The graft is held in position with another screw placed from the acromion, through the graft, and out the anteromedial humeral neck. Depending on the circumstances, a neutralization plate (usually an 8- to 12-hole dynamic compression plate or pelvic reconstruction plate may be used (Fig. 16–98). If so, there are a few key points that are helpful. The plate needs about a 90-degree bend at the acromion and often about a 45-degree internal rotation twist to fit on the anterior humerus. The strongest fixation for the plate on the scapula is obtained by a screw down the base of the spine of the scapula just medial to the spinoglenoid notch. Postoperatively, if there is concern about the fixation or the patient, a spica cast is applied and continued for 6 to 12 weeks or until fusion has occurred. When the fusion is solid, function and comfort can be enhanced by strengthening all muscle groups surrounding the fused glenohumeral joint.

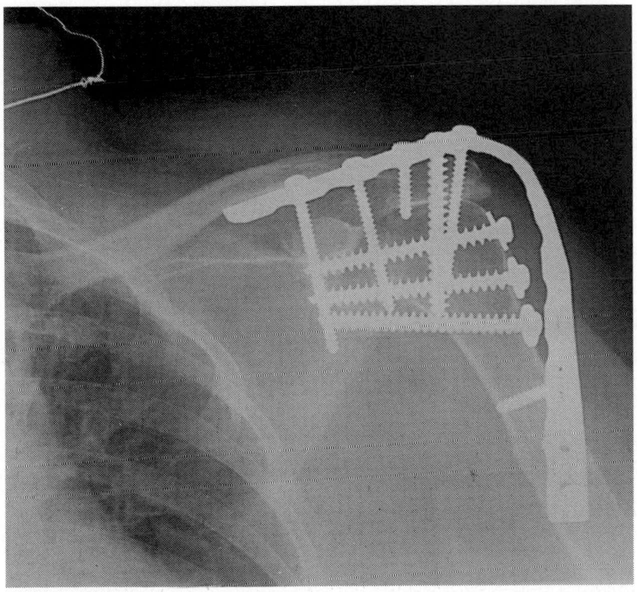

Figure 16–98

A glenohumeral and acromiohumeral arthrodesis using a contoured iliac crest bone graft inserted between the acromion and the humeral head. The arthrodesis is stabilized securely with three washered fully threaded cancellous humeroglenoid screws; one fully threaded cancellous screw through the acromion, graft, and humeral head; and a contoured reconstruction plate.

Rockwood's Technique for Shoulder Arthrodesis

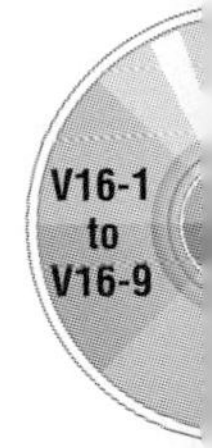

Rockwood prefers the anterior or oblique technique for shoulder fusions.[243] **(V16-1)** A straight skin incision is made along the spine of the scapular across the acromion and down the lateral shaft of the humerus to the insertion of the deltoid. **(V16-2)** The deltoid is elevated from the scapular spine and the acromion in a subparietal fashion, and a wide capsulotomy is performed. **(V16-3)** The shaft of the humerus is exposed and, if possible, the axillary nerve should be preserved. **(V16-4)** The residual portion of the rotator cuff, lying between the humeral head and the glenoid, and the inferior acromion must be resected. **(V16-5)** The bursal surface of the acromion is decorticated, and all articular cartilage is resected from the humeral head and the glenoid. **(V16-6)** The arm is placed in 15 to 20 degrees of flexion and 15 to 20 degrees of abduction. The amount of internal rotation should be such that the hand can easily be brought up to the level of the mouth. This is usually at approximately 40 to 45 degrees of internal rotation. Once sufficient decortication has taken place, the head is jammed up under the acromion adjacent to the upper portion of the glenoid and is fixed provisionally with one or two threaded Steinmann pins.

(V16-7) A malleable template is then used to match the contour of the temporarily stabilized scapula and humerus. A 4.5 pelvic reconstruction plate is then contoured to match the curve of the malleable template. The plate should be long enough to allow purchase of three or four screws in the scapula, two screws from the plate through the humeral head and into the glenoid fossa, and at least four screws into the humeral shaft. **(V16-8)** With the pelvic reconstruction plate temporarily in place, a hole is selected in the plate that will allow a drill to be passed down through the acromion, down into the neck of the scapular approximately 1 to 2 cm medial to the surface of the glenoid. This is a critical anchor hole for the plate medially, and it must be accurately placed to ensure a stable, surgical construct. The plate is then laid back on the scapula and humerus, and a screw of approxiate length is placed down through the plate acromion and then to the scapula. **(V16-9)** Two or three additional screws should be used to stabilize the plate through the scapula and, if possible, down into the glenoid. Three or four cortical screws are used to secure the plate to the shaft of the humerus, and then one or two cancellous screws are used through the plate across the head of the humerus and into the glenoid.

PERIARTICULAR OSTEOTOMY

Benjamin and associates have described the use of osteotomies adjacent to the glenohumeral joint for relief of pain in shoulder arthritis.[26, 27] In the 16 shoulders that they

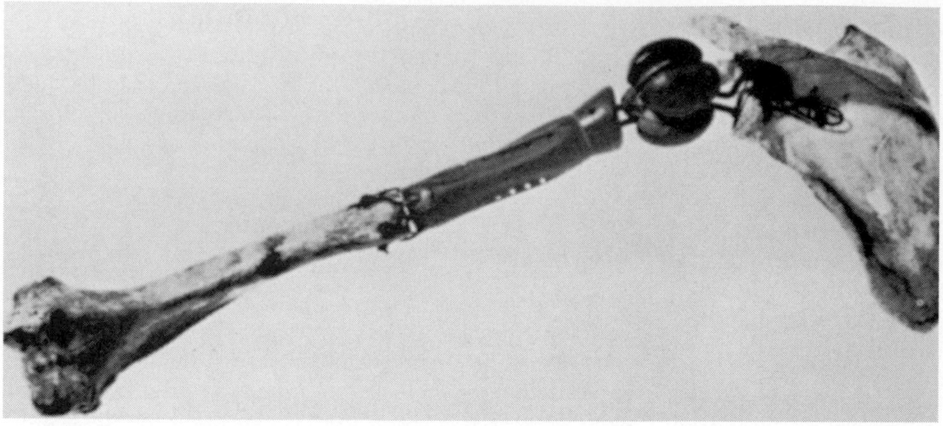

Figure 16–99

The first total shoulder arthroplasty, an artificial joint composed of platinum and rubber inserted by the French surgeon Péan in the late 1800s. (From Lugli T: Artificial shoulder joint by Péan [1893]. The facts of an exceptional intervention and the prosthetic method. Clin Orthop *133*:215–218, 1978.)

treated with this method, all had advanced arthritic destruction (rheumatoid arthritis in 12 and osteoarthritis in four). The average age of patients was 51 years; the average time for evaluation was 2 years and 11 months. Thirteen patients showed an improvement in range and comfort.

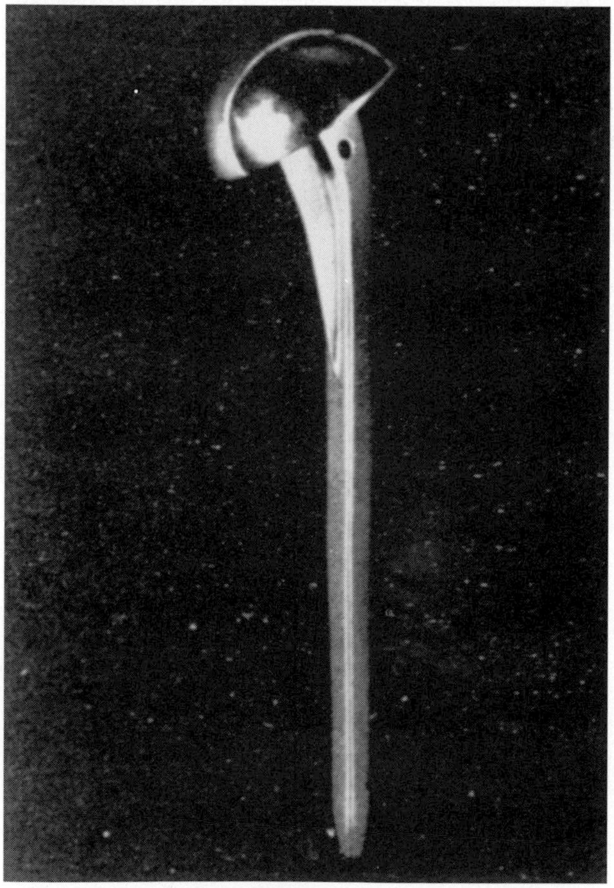

Figure 16–100

The early design of the Neer articular surface replacement for the proximal humerus. This implant was used initially in the care of patients with severely comminuted fractures of the humeral head. (From Neer CS, Brown TH Jr, and McLaughlin HL: Fracture of the neck of the humerus with dislocation of the head fragment. Am J Surg 85:252–258, 1953.)

ARTHROPLASTY

Historical Review

In 1893, one of the first prosthetic shoulder replacements was performed by the French surgeon Péan.[211] Péan was the subject of a painting called "Une Opération de Tracheotomie" by Henri de Toulouse-Lautrec.[14] A platinum and rubber total joint and proximal humeral implant was fashioned for him by J. Porter Micheals, a dentist from Paris, and inserted by Pean in a 37-year-old baker after his tuberculous arthritis had been débrided (Fig. 16–99). The patient gained increased strength and range of the arm. However, the infection recurred. After one of the first x-ray machines documented an overwhelming reactive process, the prosthesis was removed 2 years after implantation.

In 1953, Neer presented the option of replacement of a fractured humeral head with a Vitallium prosthesis.[254] Use of this prosthesis (Fig. 16–100) was next applied to patients with irregular articular surfaces as a result of fractures and osteonecrosis.[249] In 1971 and 1974, Neer described the results of the use of this proximal humeral implant for patients with rheumatoid arthritis and osteoarthritis of the glenohumeral joint (Table 16–15).[250, 251] In

Table 16–15 INDICATIONS FOR HUMERAL REPLACEMENT ARTHROPLASTY (1953–1963)*

DIAGNOSIS	***NO. OF SHOULDERS***
Arthritides	
Osteoarthritis	9
Traumatic arthritis	9
Rheumatoid arthritis	2
Radiation necrosis	1
Sickle cell infarction	1
Ochronosis	1
Trauma	
Fracture-dislocation	26
"Head-splitting" fracture	4
Displaced "shell fragment" with retracted tuberosities	2
Previous humeral head resection	1

*Adapted from Neer CS II: Articular replacement of the humeral head. J Bone Joint Surg *46A*:1607–1610, 1964.

these articles, Neer also described the use of a high-density polyethylene glenoid in the management of osteoarthritis of the glenohumeral joint (Fig. 16–101). Also in 1974, Kenmore and associates published a brief article reporting on the development of a polyethylene glenoid liner for use with a Neer humeral replacement in the treatment of degenerative joint disease of the shoulder.[189, 190, 259] Other early descriptions of shoulder arthroplasty components include prostheses of Vitallium as reported by Krueger[198] and acrylic as reported by Richard and Judet (Fig. 16–102).[294]

The initial Neer prosthesis had three sizes (Fig. 16–103), and two more were added. In the early 1970s, the implant was redesigned to better use the alternative of cement fixation, and the articular portion was made spherical.[251] This implant proved its versatility over time. It was used initially for acute fractures but subsequently has been shown to be effective for the care of patients with chronic fracture problems,[161, 287, 313, 339] osteoarthritis,[251, 373] rheumatoid arthritis,[250, 373] osteonecrosis,[95, 97, 316] and a variety of the more rare forms of disease affecting the shoulder joint. A number of other shoulder implant systems include a metallic humeral component that can be used without a glenoid replacement.[3–5, 18, 74, 75, 141, 143] Bipolar implants have also been described (Fig. 16–104).[201, 336–338]

Some authors suggested that a cup arthroplasty might be a satisfactory alternative for prosthetic shoulder surgery.[179, 180] Initially, hip cups were used,[329] and then cups were manufactured specifically for the shoulder (Fig. 16–105).[329] Rydholm and Sjogren [318] described a surface replacement for the humeral head. At an average of 4.2 years after surgery, 72 rheumatoid shoulders demonstrated substantial improvement. Twenty-five per cent of the cups were loose at follow-up. However, neither cup loosening, nor proximal migration of the humerus, nor central glenoid wear apparently affected the clinical result.

Several plastics and other softer materials have been used as implants. Swanson designed an all-silicon rubber humeral head implant in extension of the concept of flexible implants as an adjunct to resection arthroplasty.[335] Apparently, this design was used only rarely, and no results are available for a series of patients. Varian reported on a clinical trial of the use of a Silastic cup in patients with rheumatoid arthritis of the shoulder.[348] Early results were promising, but another series by Spencer and Skirving described a number of complications, and the authors recommended restricted use of the device.[328]

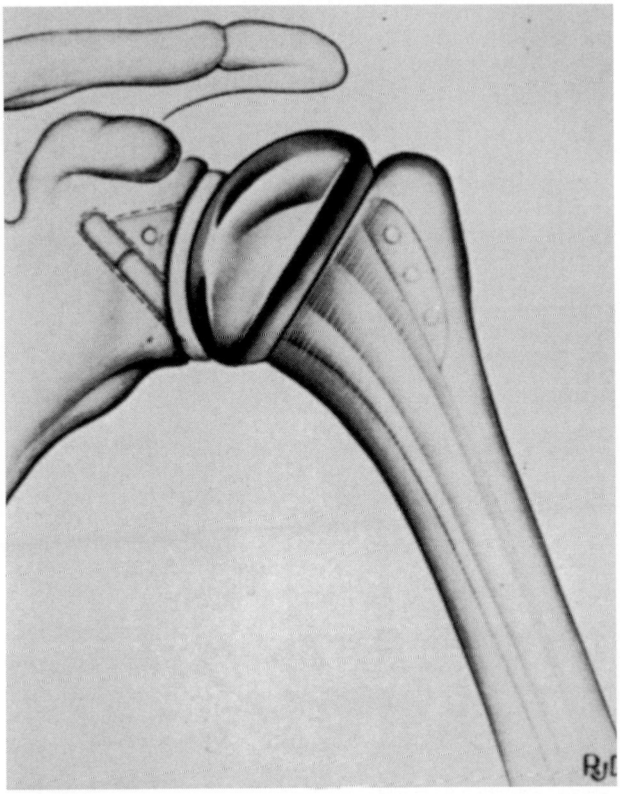

Figure 16–101

The first illustration depicting the use of a high-density polyethylene glenoid component in conjunction with a proximal humeral prosthesis—a total shoulder arthroplasty. (From Neer CS II: Replacement arthroplasty for glenohumeral osteoarthritis. J Bone Joint Surg 56A:1–13, 1974.)

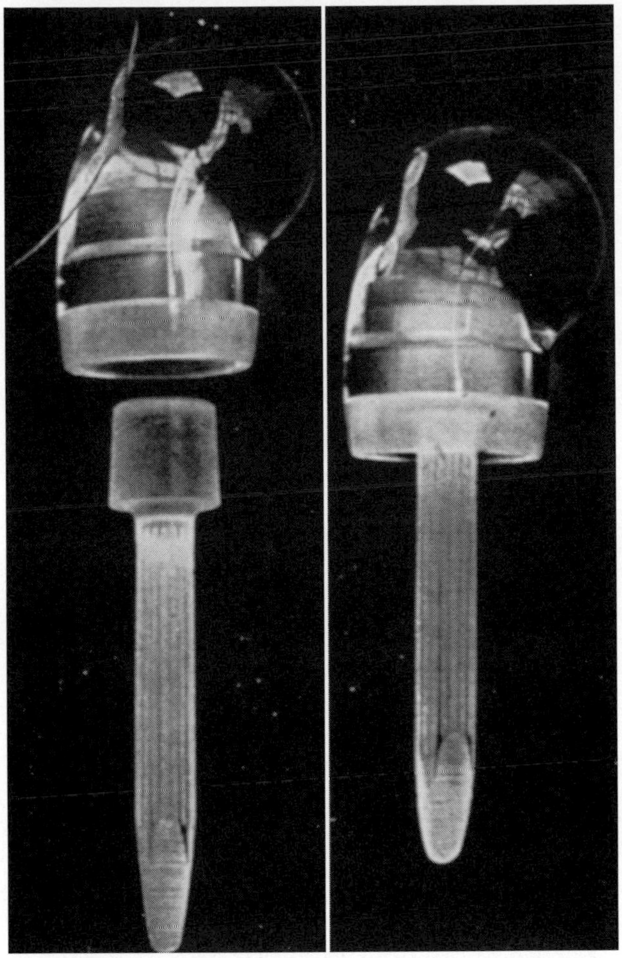

Figure 16–102

An acrylic prosthesis developed for the treatment of severe fracture-dislocations of the proximal humerus. (From Richard A, Judet R, and René L: Acrylic prosthetic reconstruction of the upper end of the humerus for fracture-luxations. J Chir 68:537–547, 1952.)

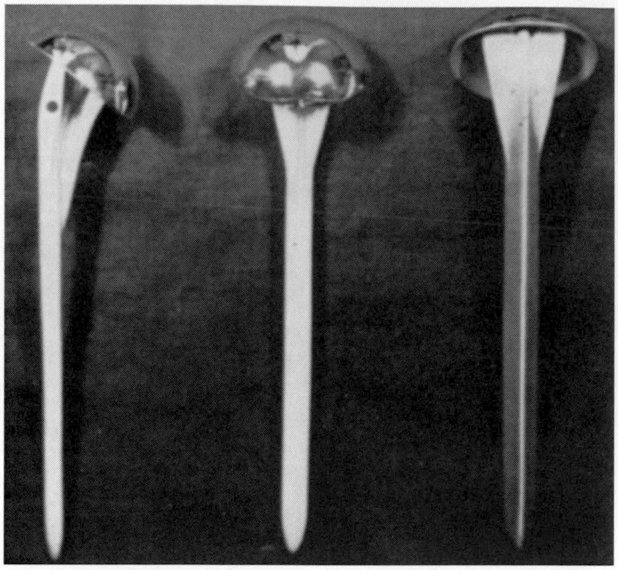

Figure 16–103

Neer replacement prosthesis for the articular surface of the humeral head. Small, medium, and large models are shown in the 1955 article. (From Neer CS II: Articular replacement for the humeral head. J Bone Joint Surg 37A:215–228, 1955.)

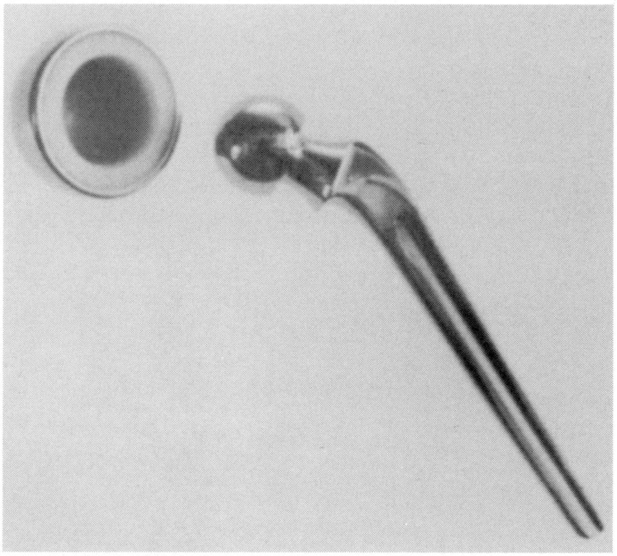

Figure 16–104

The bipolar shoulder implant system developed by Swanson. Proposed advantages include smooth concentric contact for the entire shoulder joint cavity including the coracoacromial arch as well as the glenoid, a decrease in force concentration over any one contact area, a lengthening of the glenoid joint moment arm, and avoidance of abutment of the greater tuberosity against the acromion. (From Swanson AB: Bipolar implant shoulder arthroplasty. *In* Bateman JE and Welsh RP [eds]: Surgery of the Shoulder. St. Louis: CV Mosby, 1984, pp 211–223.)

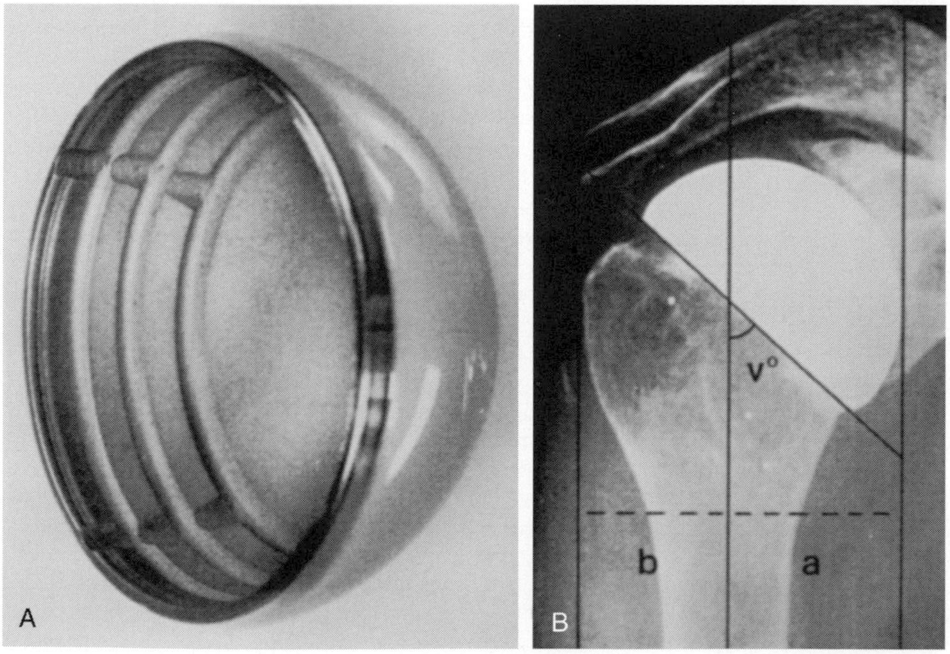

Figure 16–105

A cup arthroplasty of the shoulder. Illustrated are the cup (*A*) and a radiograph after implantation of a cup in a patient with rheumatoid arthritis (*B*). (From Jónsson E: Surgery of the Rheumatoid Shoulder with Special Reference to Cup Hemiarthroplasty and Arthrodesis. The University Department of Orthopaedics, Lund, Sweden, 1988.)

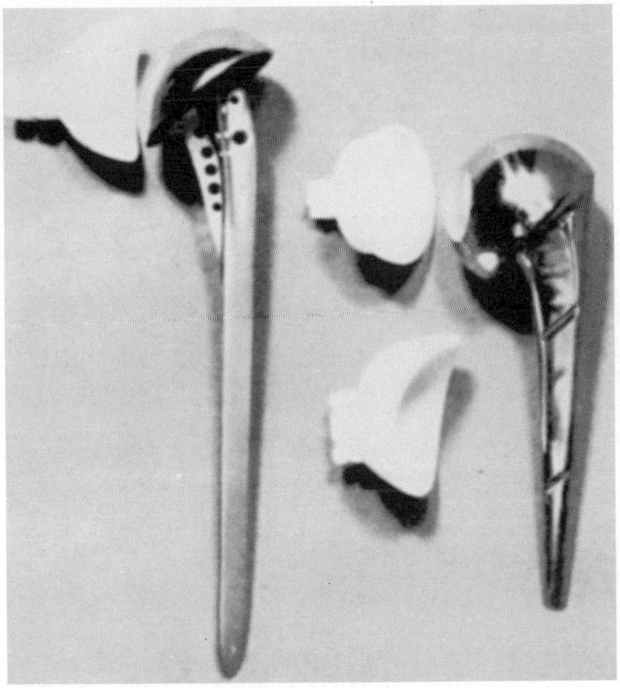

Figure 16–106

The St. Georg total shoulder prosthesis from Hamburg, Germany. Polyethylene sockets were constructed to mate with the Neer prosthesis (*left*) or the St. Georg model (*right*). (From Engelbrecht E and Stellbrink G: Totale Schulterendoprosthese Modell [St. Georg.] Chirurg *47*:525–530, 1976.)

After these pioneering efforts, many additional shoulder prostheses were constructed. Some mirrored the implants used by Neer, including the St. Georg[111] (Fig. 16–106), the Bechtol[20] prosthesis, the DANA,[340] the Cofield[74, 75] (Fig. 16–107), and the Monospherical.[141, 143] Isoelastic shoulder implants have been used in Europe.[56, 66, 341] Other designs included a captive ball-in-socket unit to replace the stabilizing functions of the rotator cuff and shoulder capsule (Figs. 16–108 to 16–112).[22, 23, 51, 84, 92, 109, 115, 136, 142, 191, 194, 195, 203, 281–284, 286, 292, 356, 371] Of these, many included complex and extensive attachments to the scapula by cementing within the glenoid (Fig. 16–113) and by stems (Fig. 16–114), wedges (Fig. 16–115), a screw (Fig. 16–116), and bolted flanges (Fig. 16–117). Some designs reversed the ball-and-socket configuration and have attached the ball part of the implant to the glenoid (see Figs. 16–114 to 16–117).[292] Others incorporated two ball-in-socket units (Fig. 16–118; see also Fig. 16–109).[51, 142] Engelbrecht and associates suggested a hemiarthroplasty with modification of the glenoid by osteotomy and bone graft to buttress the humeral prosthesis (Fig. 16–119).[109] Burkhead and Hutton[54] performed biologic resurfacing of the glenoid in association with humeral hemiarthroplasty.

Some designs had a hood on the glenoid component in an attempt to prevent upward humeral subluxation associated with rotator cuff weakness or absence (Figs. 16–120 and 16–121).[3–5, 111, 229, 233, 259] Implants could be classified as anatomic, semiconstrained (hooded glenoid), or constrained (ball and socket) (Fig. 16–122). Some of the early investigators of these designs are listed in Table 16–16.

The nonretentive prosthesis of Mazas and Caffiniére also included a superiorly placed hood on the glenoid component. Of 38 shoulders operated, nine developed instability, and 14 shoulders remained stiff after surgery.[229] A third early system including a hooded component was the English-Macnab. This system also has a nonhooded glenoid implant and incorporates porous ingrowth surfaces on the glenoid component and the humeral stem (Fig. 16–123).[114, 233]

The Neer system originally included 200% and 600% enlarged glenoids. These components were used in only 12 of 273 shoulders reported,[259] suggesting that the need for them was quite uncommon. The DANA total shoulder arthroplasty (Fig. 16–124) includes a semiconstrained, hooded component designed to enhance stability in shoulders with irreparable rotator cuff tears.[3] The Monospherical total shoulder also incorporated a slight hood on the glenoid component (Fig. 16–125), imparting somewhat greater stability to the articulation.[131, 141] Laurence[200] has described a "snap" fit prosthesis for arthroplasty in the cuff deficient shoulder; the cup is secured to the glenoid and the acromion.

Text continued on page 900

Table 16–16 VARIATIONS IN TOTAL SHOULDER ARTHROPLASTY DESIGN

UNCONSTRAINED (ANATOMIC)	***SEMICONSTRAINED (HOODED OR CUP-SHAPED GLENOID)***	***CONSTRAINED (BALL-IN-SOCKET)***
Bechtol[20]	DANA[3–5]	Bickel[84]
Bipolar[18]	English-Macnab[114, 233]	Fenlin[115]
Cofield[74, 75]	Mazas[229]	Floating-socket[51]
DANA[3–5]	Neer[259]	Gerard[136]
Kenmore[190]	St. Georg[109–111]	Kessel[191]
Monospherical[141]		Kölbel[194, 195]
Neer[259]		Liverpool[22, 23]
Saha[318a]		Michael Reese[281–285]
St. Georg[109–111]		Reeves[292]
		Stanmore[84, 92, 203]
		Trispherical[142]
		Wheble-Skorecki[356]
		Zippel[371]
		Zimmer

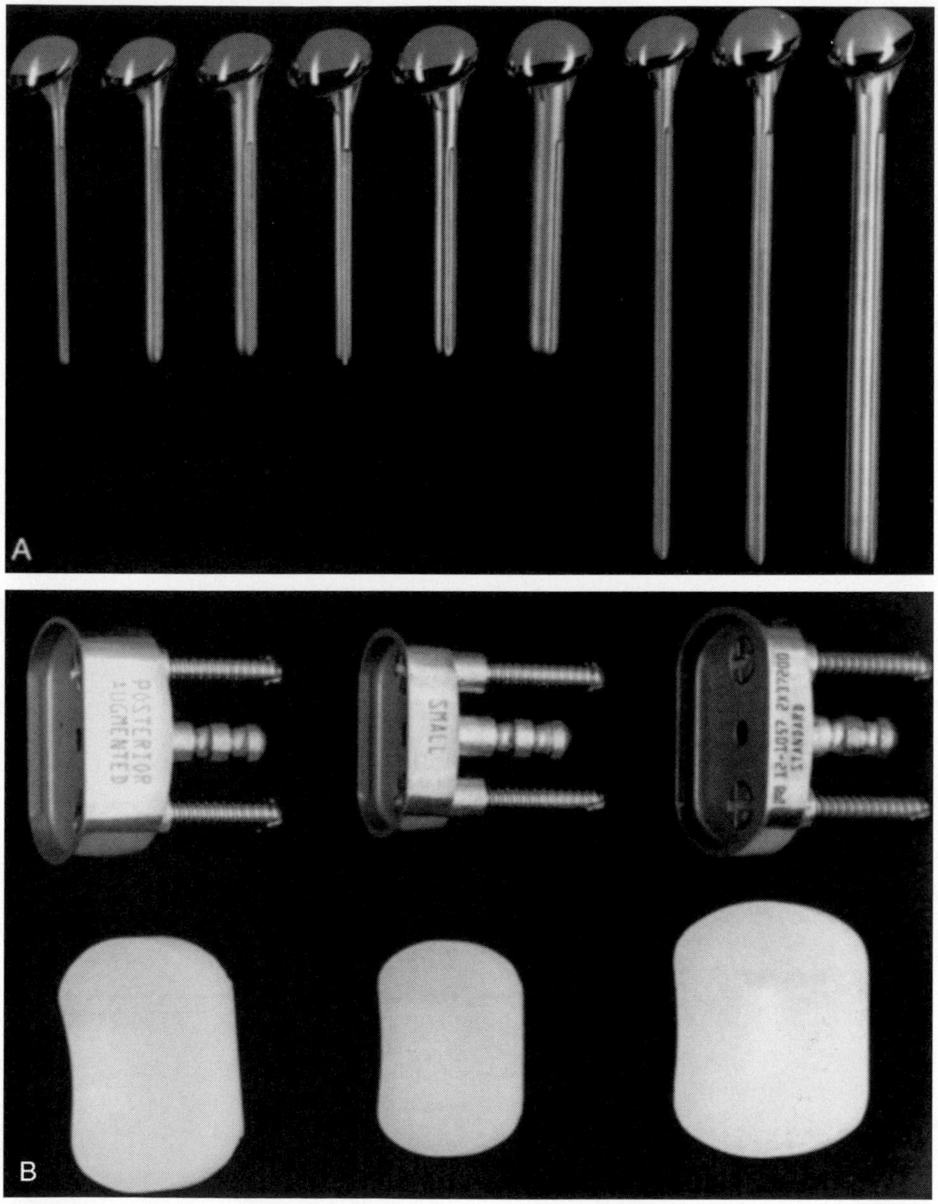

Figure 16–107

The Cofield total shoulder arthroplasty system. In this system, there are two humeral neck lengths, four humeral stem widths, and two humeral stem lengths (*A*). There are two glenoid component sizes and one glenoid component with an asymmetric construction to compensate for uneven glenoid wear (*B*). The ingrowth material in the humeral head is only on the undersurface of the head and does not extend down onto the shaft. The ingrowth material on the glenoid component only abuts against the prepared face of the glenoid and does not extend into the scapular neck.

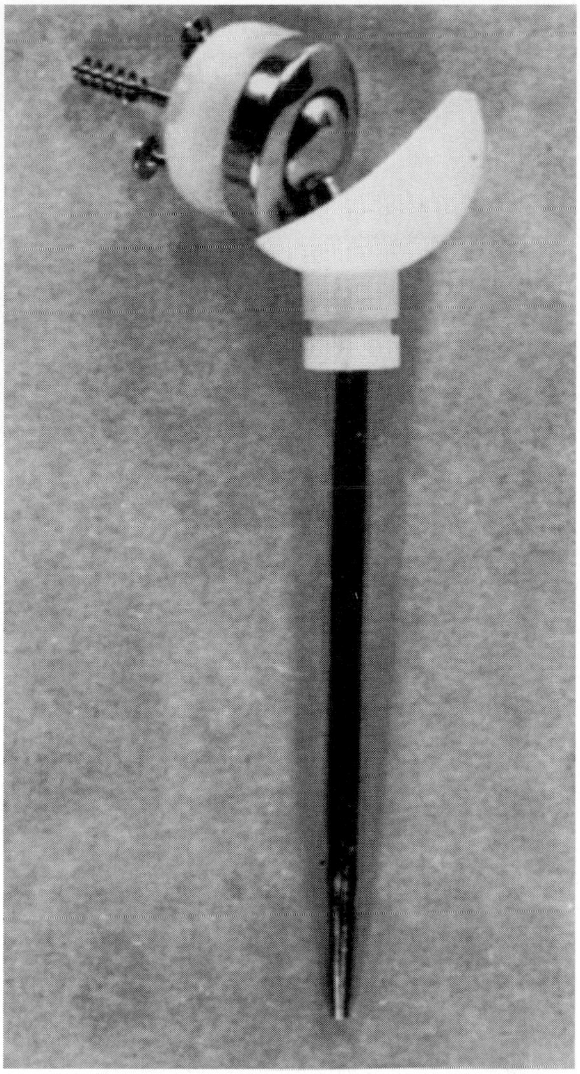

Figure 16–108

Model BME total shoulder arthroplasty designed by Zippel of Hamburg, Germany. This is an early captive ball-in-socket type of total shoulder arthroplasty. (From Zippel J: Luxationssichere Schulterendoprosthese Modell BME. Z Orthop *113*:454–457, 1975.)

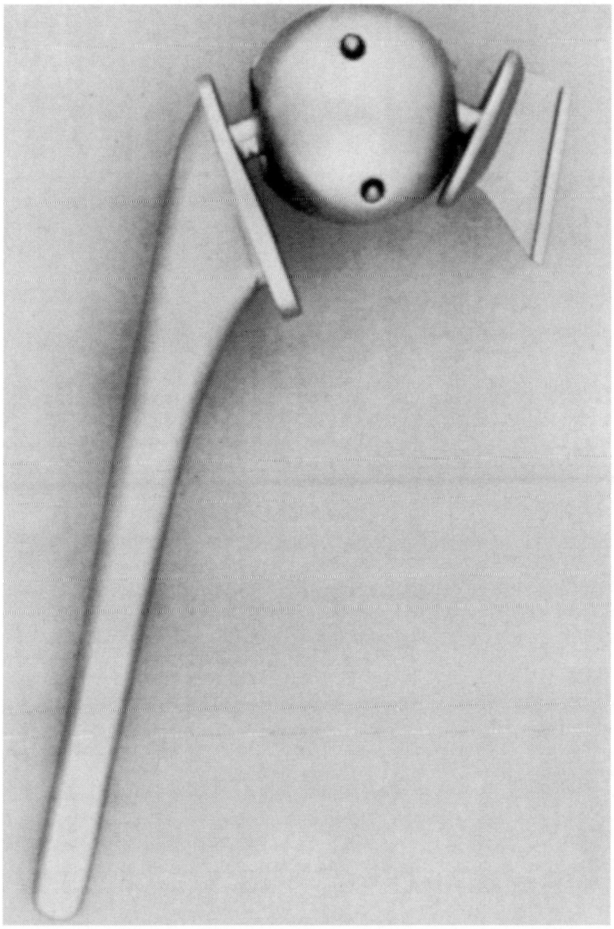

Figure 16–109

This trispherical total shoulder prosthesis was designed by Gristina and coworkers. Two spheres are held captive within a third larger sphere. The design thus allows an extremely large range of motion in a captive ball-in-socket constrained implant system. (From Gristina AG and Webb LX: The trispherical total shoulder replacement. *In* Bayley I and Kessel L [eds]: Shoulder Surgery. New York: Springer-Verlag, 1982, pp 153–157.)

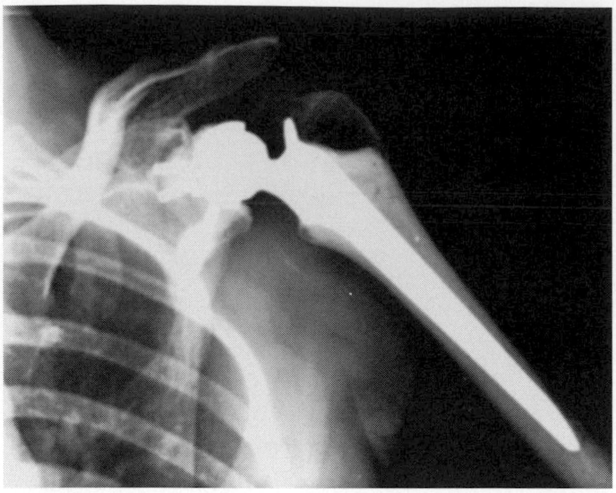

Figure 16–110

The Stanmore total shoulder replacement. The glenoid component was cemented and relied on a large amount of methyl methacrylate for support. The two components snapped together after being implanted. (From Cofield RH: Status of total shoulder arthroplasty. Arch Surg *112*:1088–1091, 1977.)

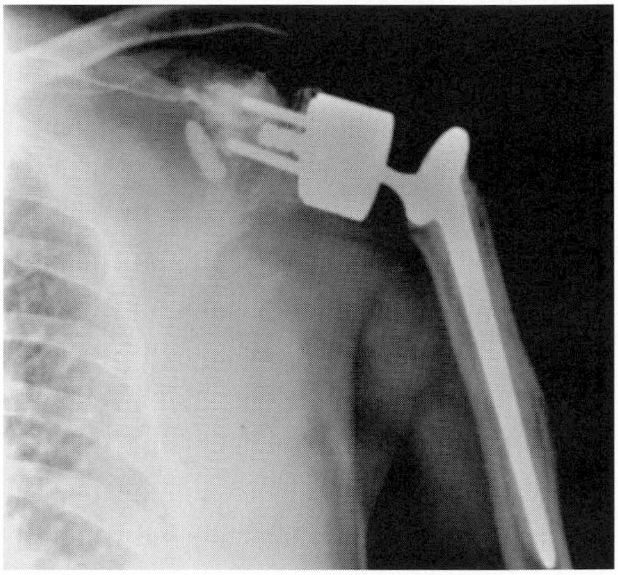

Figure 16–111

Michael Reese total shoulder replacement, perhaps the most widely used constrained total shoulder system in North America. Its placement requires resection of more proximal humerus than with many alternative prosthetic designs. (From Cofield RH: Status of total shoulder arthroplasty. Arch Surg *112*:1088–1091, 1977.)

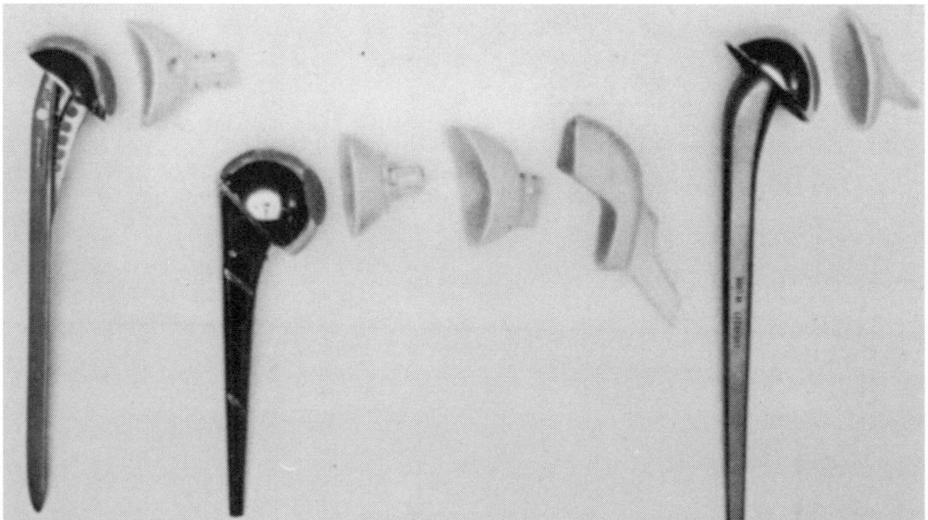

Figure 16–112

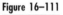

With more than 10 years' experience using unconstrained shoulder replacement, Engelbrecht and co-workers have continued to use unconstrained systems. Initially, the Neer prosthesis was used in conjunction with a high-density polyethylene component of these workers' design (*left*). This evolved to the St. Georg implant with various glenoid components including those with rather deep hoods (*center*). Currently, these workers have returned to a proximal humeral prosthetic replacement (*right*) with a rather simple and unconstrained polyethylene glenoid component. (From Engelbrecht E and Heinert TK: More than ten years' experience with unconstrained shoulder replacement. *In* Kölbel R, Helbig B, and Blauth W [eds]: Shoulder Replacement. New York: Springer-Verlag, 1987, pp 85–91.)

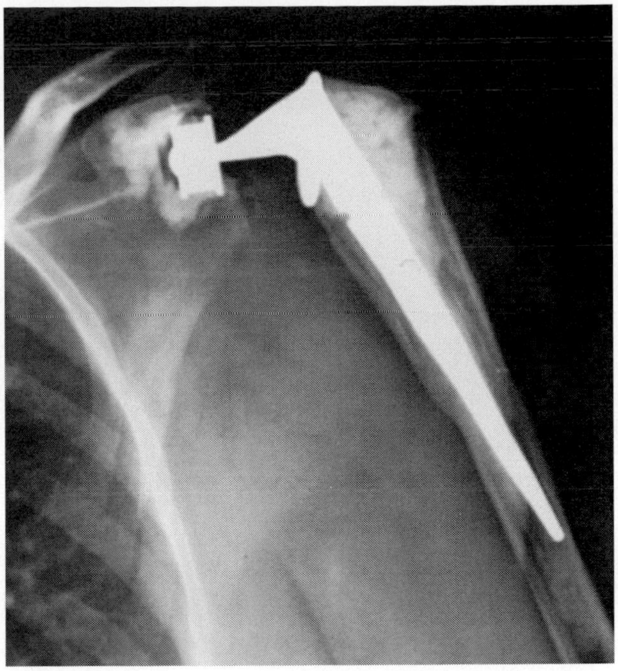

Figure 16–113

The Bickel glenohumeral prosthesis. The design included a very small ball to decrease friction between components, and the glenoid component was designed to be incorporated entirely within the glenoid cavity and, ideally, to maximize prosthesis-bone contact area. (From Cofield RH: Status of total shoulder arthroplasty. Arch Surg *112*:1088–1091, 1977.)

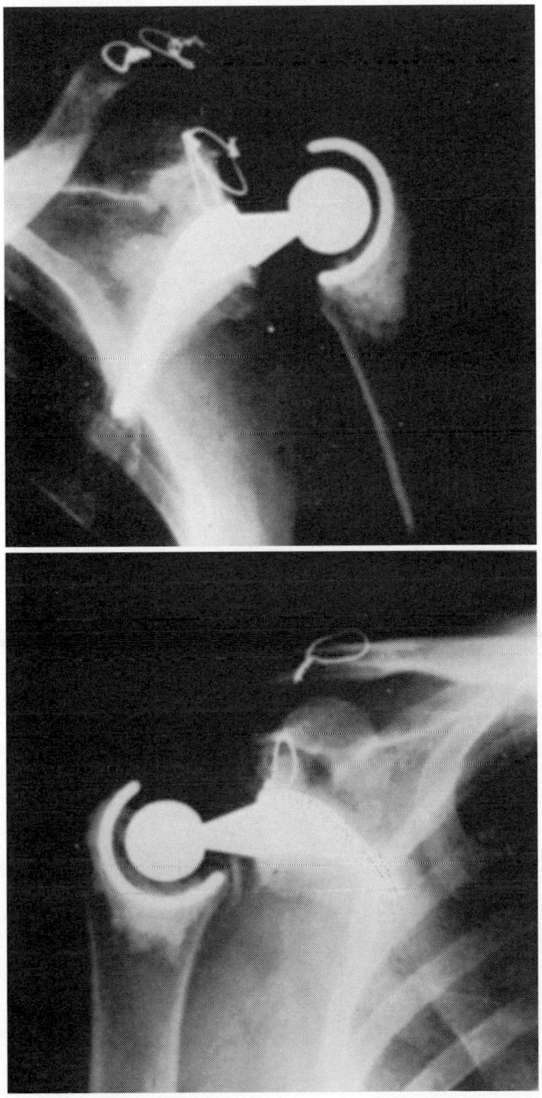

Figure 16–114

The Liverpool shoulder replacement. A reverse ball-in-socket design. The glenoid component has a stem that is inserted into the medullary cavity of the axillary border of the scapula to a depth of approximately 50 mm. (From Beddow FH and Elloy MA: Clinical experience with the Liverpool shoulder replacement. *In* Bayley I and Kessel L [eds]: Shoulder Surgery. New York: Springer-Verlag, 1982, pp 164–167.)

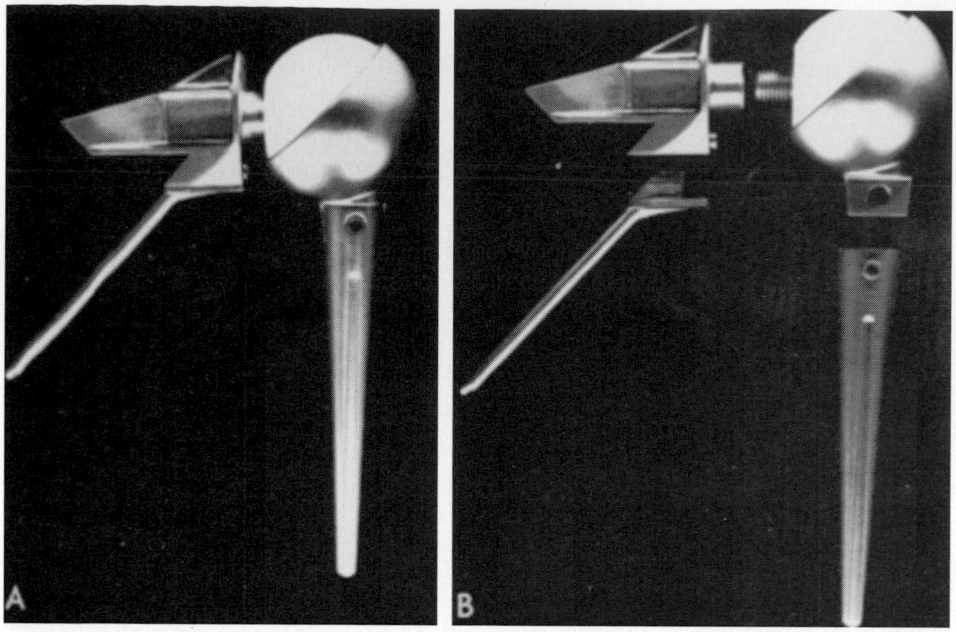

Figure 16–115

Reverse ball-in-socket total shoulder arthroplasty designed by Fenlin. *A*, The prosthesis has been assembled. *B*, The prosthesis has been disassembled. A wedge is driven into the bone of the scapula for fixation, and a column is placed down the axillary border of the scapula. (From Fenlin JM Jr: Total glenohumeral joint replacement. Orthop Clin North Am *67*:565–583, 1975.)

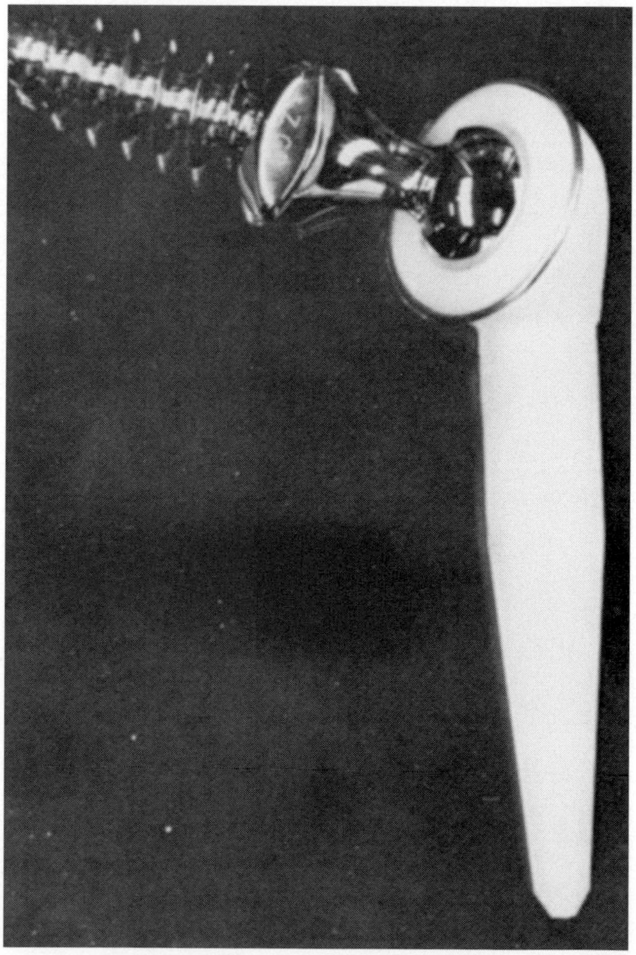

Figure 16–116

The Kessel total shoulder replacement. A reversed ball-in-socket design. The glenoid component is screwed into the glenoid, and the humeral stem is cemented in place. The components then snap together. (From Bayley JIL and Kessel L: The Kessel total shoulder replacement. *In* Bayley I and Kessel L [eds]: Shoulder Surgery. New York: Springer-Verlag, 1982, pp 160–164.)

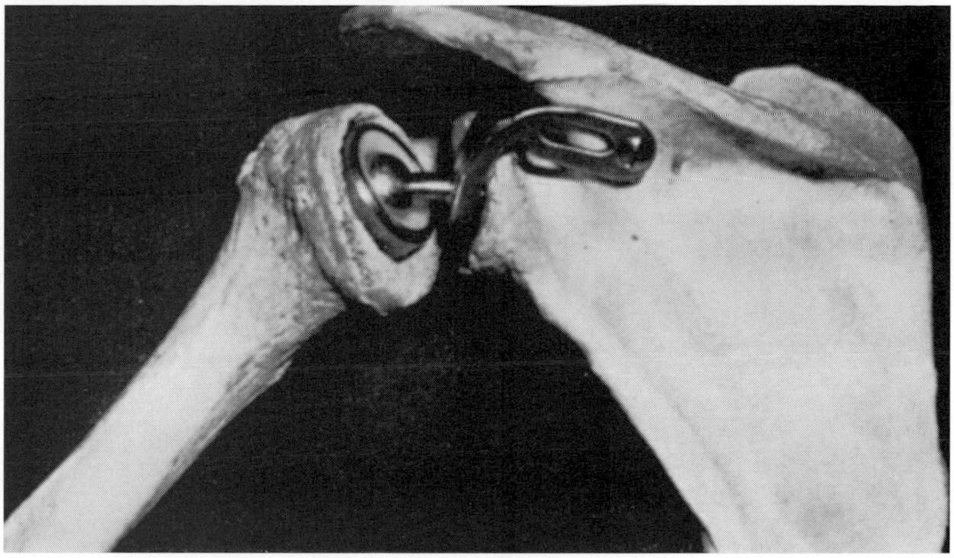

Figure 16–117

The total shoulder arthroplasty designed by Kölbel. This is a reversed ball-in-socket unit. Scapular component fixation includes a flange bolted to the base of the spine of the scapula. (From Wolff R and Kölbel R: The history of shoulder joint replacement. *In* Kölbel R, Helbig B, and Blauth W [eds]: Shoulder Replacement. New York: Springer-Verlag, 1987, pp 2–13.)

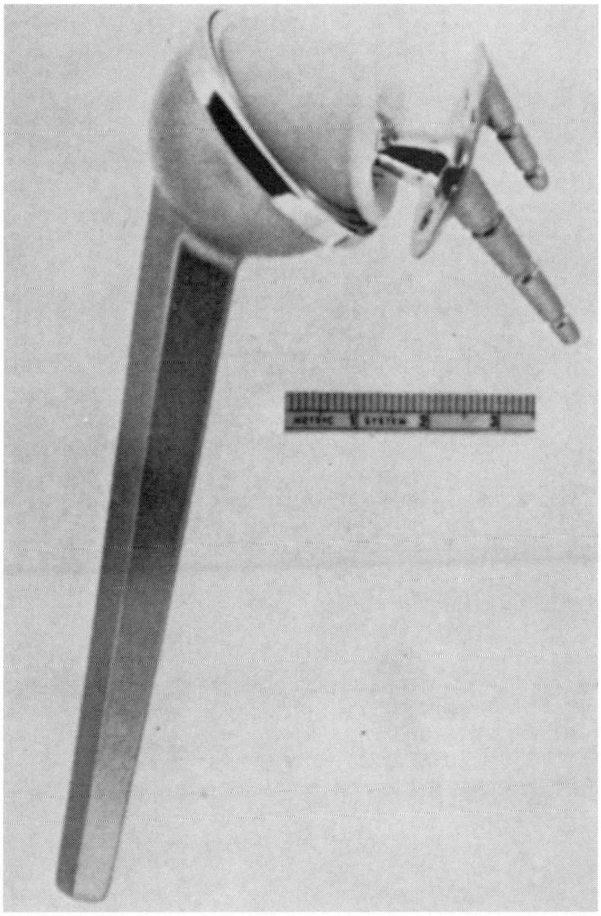

Figure 16–118

The floating socket total shoulder replacement. This implant contains a dual spherical bearing system to provide a "floating fulcrum." This configuration allows the prosthesis to have motion in excess of normal anatomic limits. (From Buechel FF, Pappas MJ, and DePalma AF: "Floating socket" total shoulder replacement: Anatomical, biomechanical, and surgical rationale. J Biomed Mater Res *12*:89–114, 1978.)

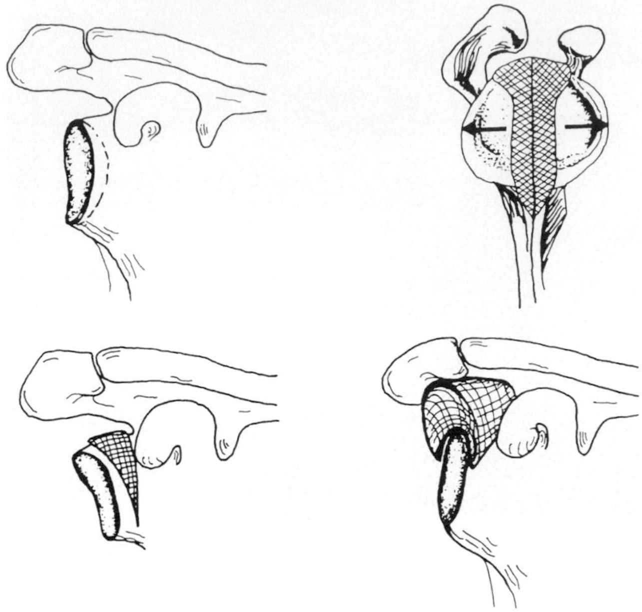

Figure 16–119

In the face of unusually frequent glenoid loosening, Engelbrecht and coworkers have tended to treat patients with shoulder arthritis with glenoid reshaping (*upper left*), glenoid osteotomies (*upper right* and *lower left*), or glenoid bone grafting (*upper right* and *lower left* and *right*) as an adjunct to proximal humeral prosthetic replacement rather than using a cemented glenoid component. (From Engelbrecht E and Heinert TK: More than ten years' experience with unconstrained shoulder replacement. *In* Kölbel R, Helbig B, and Blauth W [eds]: Shoulder Replacement. New York: Springer-Verlag, 1987, pp 85–91.)

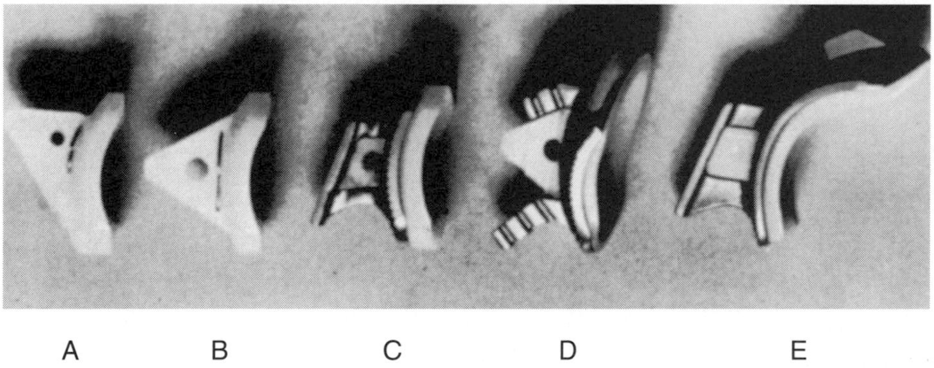

Figure 16–120

The Neer design of total shoulder arthroplasty includes a number of types of glenoid components. Five glenoid components were used in the series of patients reported in 1982. These included (A) the original 1973 polyethylene component; (B) the standard polyethylene component; (C) the metal-backed standard-sized glenoid component; (D) the metal-backed 200% larger glenoid component; and (E) the metal-backed 600% larger glenoid component. These latter two hooded components were designed for additional joint constraint against superior humeral subluxation. (From Neer CS II, Watson KC, and Stanton FJ: Recent experience in total shoulder replacement. J Bone Joint Surg *64A*:319–337, 1982.)

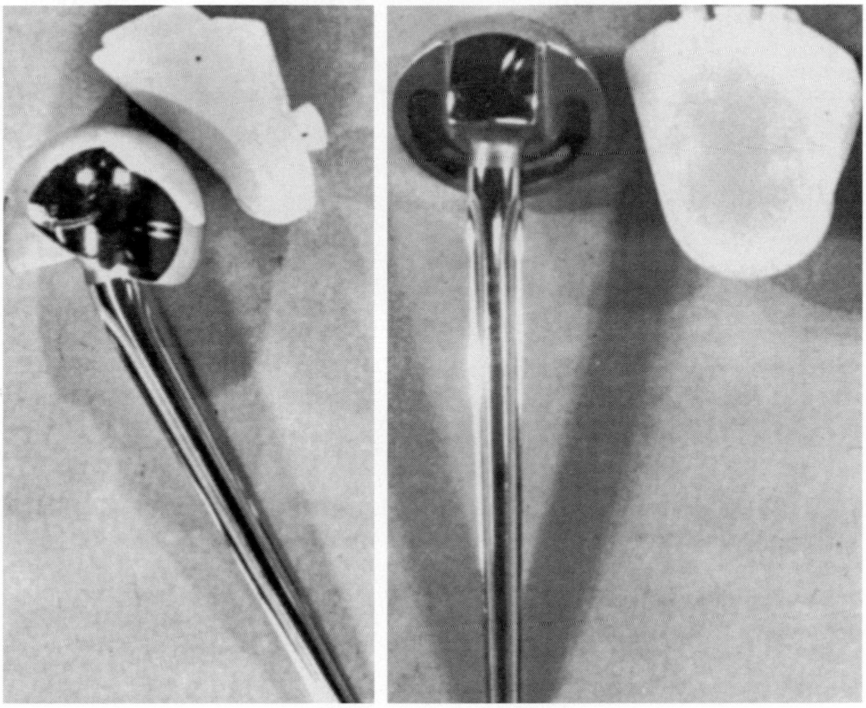

Figure 16–121

The nonretentive total shoulder arthroplasty designed by Mazas. (From Mazas F and de la Caffiniére JY: Un prothèse totale d'épaule non rétentive: À propos de 38 cas. Rev Chir Orthop 68:161–170, 1982.)

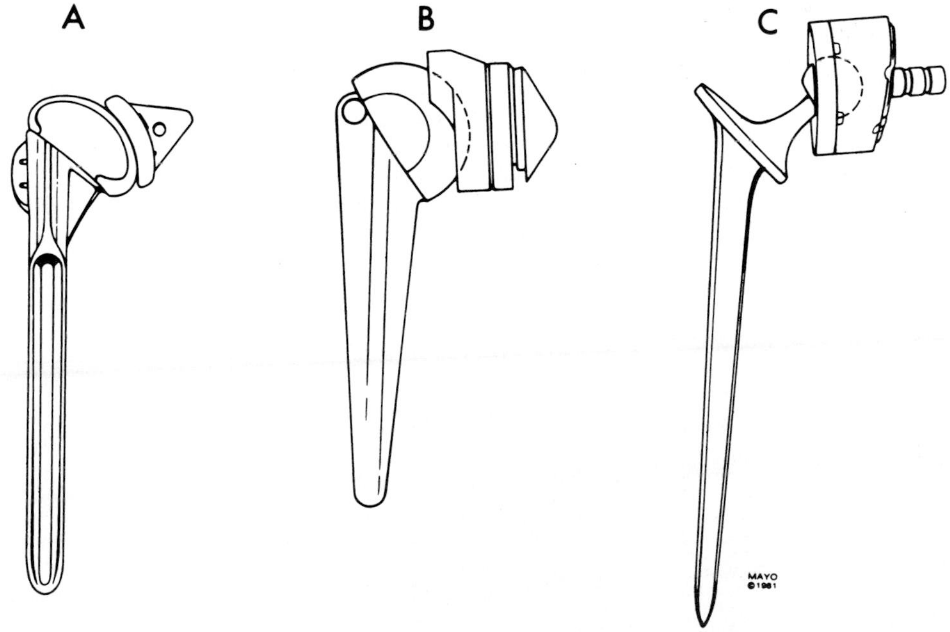

Figure 16–122

A variable amount of constraint is incorporated in the various designs of total shoulder replacement. Many implants have their articular surfaces shaped much like a normal joint surface (*A*). The system may be partially constrained by virtue of a hooded or more cup-shaped socket (*B*), or the components may be secured to one another as in the ball-in-socket prosthesis (*C*). (From Cofield RH: The shoulder and prosthetic arthroplasty. *In* Evarts CM [ed]: Surgery of the Musculoskeletal System. New York: Churchill Livingstone, 1983, pp 125–143.)

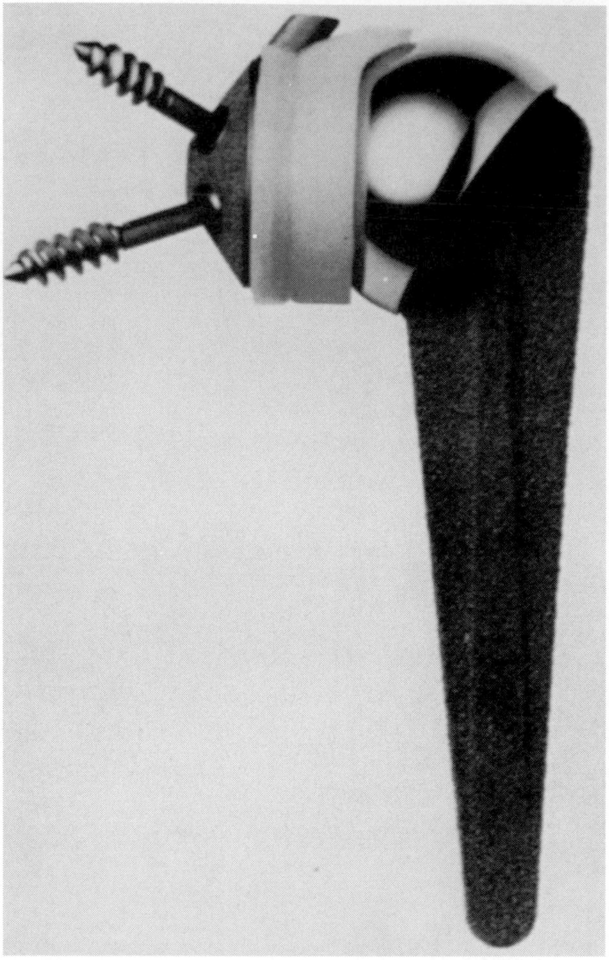

Figure 16–123

English-Macnab cementless total shoulder arthroplasty. (From Faludi DD and Weiland AJ: Cementless total shoulder arthroplasty: Preliminary experience with 13 cases. Orthopedics 6:431–437, 1983.)

Neer defined many of the challenges of shoulder reconstruction, including the management of malversion of the glenoid (Fig. 16–126), cementing the glenoid (Fig. 16–127), and proximal humeral deficiency (Fig. 16–128).[259] He expanded the diagnoses that could be managed by prosthetic shoulder reconstruction (Table 16–17).

Table 16–17 DIAGNOSTIC INDICATIONS FOR TOTAL SHOULDER REPLACEMENT (1973–1981)*

	NO. OF SHOULDERS
Rheumatoid arthritis	69
Osteoarthritis (primary and secondary)	62
Old trauma	60
Prosthetic revision	32
Arthritis of recurrent dislocation	26
Cuff-tear arthropathy	16
Neoplasm	4
Congenital dysplasia	2
Glenohumeral fusion	2
Total	273

*Adapted from Neer CS II et al: Recent experience in total shoulder replacement. J Bone Joint Surg *64A*:319–337, 1982.

Cofield also pioneered the extended application of shoulder arthroplasty with an expanded implant system (Table 16–18).[77] Pearl and Lippitt[271] and Collins and colleagues[86] have outlined many of the elements of modern arthroplasty technique.

The 1980s saw the advent of a number of modular humeral component designs, which tried to accommodate the variations in humeral anatomy and space available for the joint and humeral medullary canal diameters. On the glenoid side, some designs offered cementless fixation using screws and porous coatings on metal backing to the polyethylene (see Fig. 16–107). In the 1990s, increased emphasis is being placed on restoring normal kinematics with anatomic location and orientation of the humeral and glenoid joint surfaces, advanced soft tissue balancing methods, and physiologic stabilization of the joint. Zuckerman and Cuomo have provided a review of the indications and preoperative planning for glenohumeral arthroplasty.[374] Brems has conducted a review of the evolution of the glenoid component.[41] Rodosky and Bigliani have reviewed the indications for glenoid resurfacing.[307]

Unfortunately, the results of most of the tens of thousands of surgeries performed for glenohumeral arthritis are not available. This is due in large part to the fact that most "outcome" systems are too burdensome for most of the surgeons carrying out shoulder reconstructions. During the 20 years since the advent of shoulder arthroplasty,

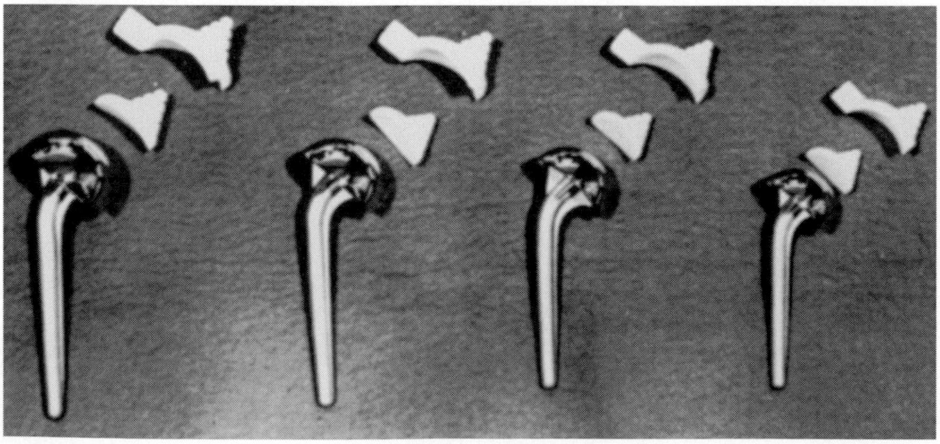

Figure 16–124

The DANA total shoulder arthroplasty. Illustrated are the four available sizes with the standard and the "hooded" glenoid components. (From Amstutz HC, Thomas BJ, Kabo JM, et al: The DANA total shoulder arthroplasty. J Bone Joint Surg *70A*:1174–1182, 1988.)

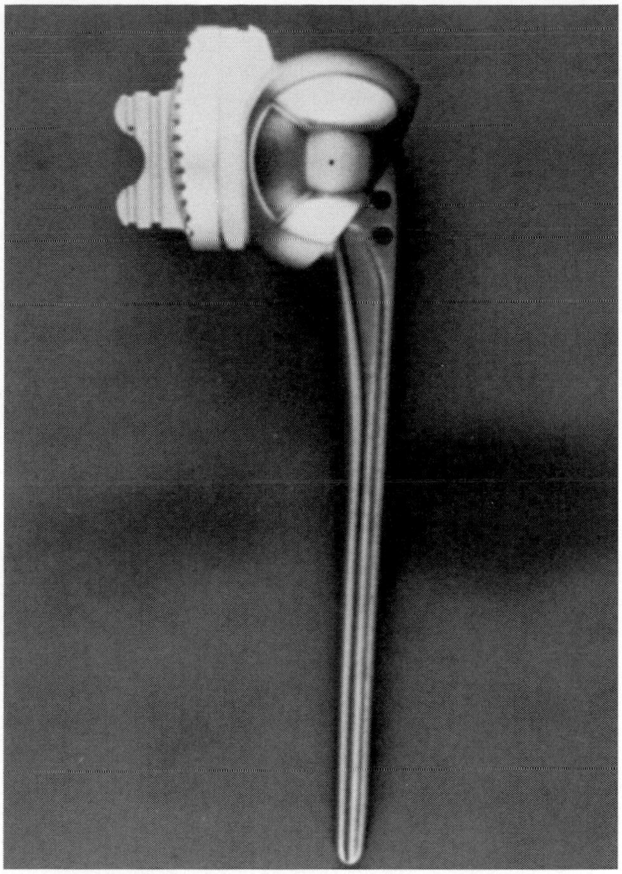

Figure 16–125

The monospherical total shoulder replacement. A slight amount of hooding has been incorporated into the design of the glenoid component. (From Gristina AG, Romano RL, Kammire GC, and Webb LX: Total shoulder replacement. Orthop Clin North Am *18*:445–453, 1987.)

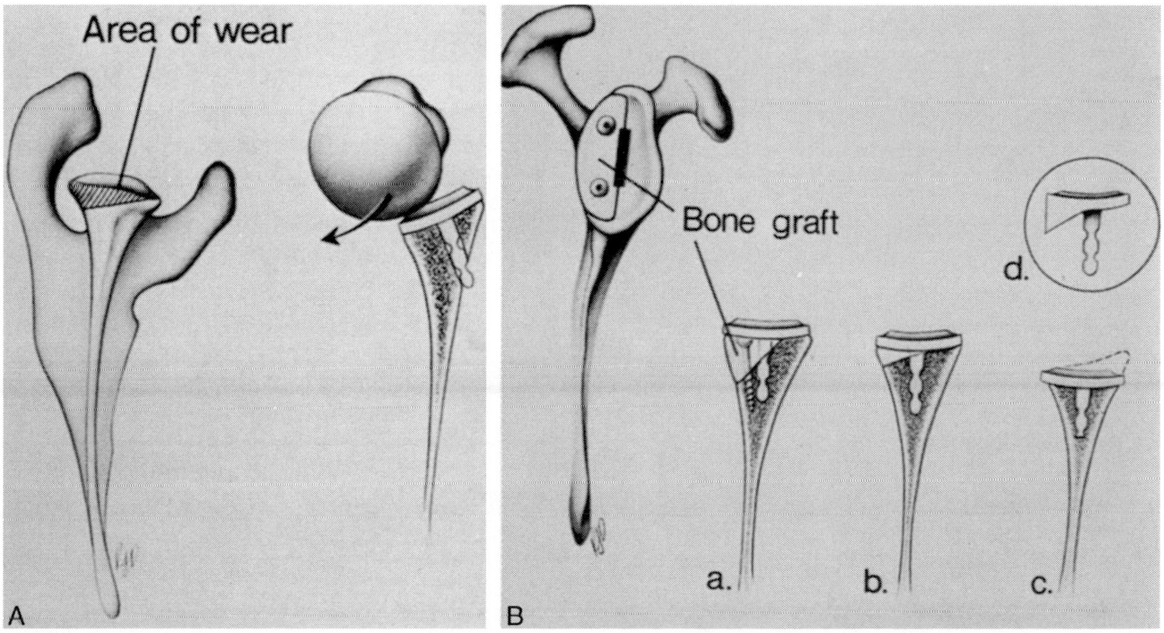

Figure 16–126

In arthritis of the shoulder, the glenoid may show uneven wear. If the glenoid component is cemented upon the remaining subchondral bone surface, as illustrated in *A*, the prosthesis may subluxate in the direction of glenoid wear and the stem of the glenoid prosthetic component may perforate the scapular neck in the opposite direction. Neer and associates pointed out that, as illustrated in *B*, this may be corrected by applying a bone graft to the area of wear, by building up the worn area with methyl methacrylate as illustrated in *B*, grinding away the prominent remaining bone in the area that has not been subject to wear as in *C*, or by using a custom-designed glenoid component as illustrated in *D*. (From Neer CS II, Watson KC, and Stanton FJ: Recent experience in total shoulder replacement. J Bone Joint Surg *64A*:319–337, 1982.)

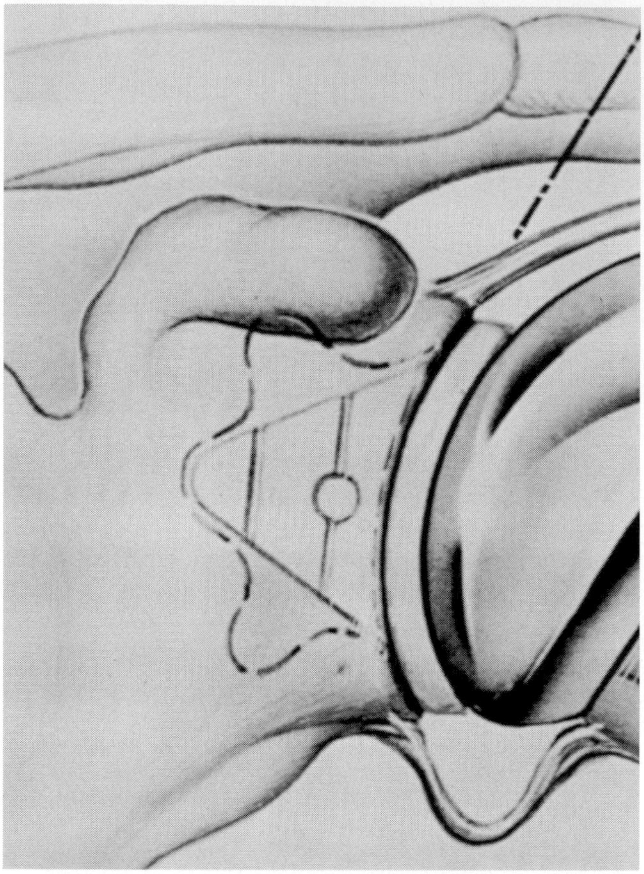

Figure 16–127

A demonstration of the cementing technique as used by Neer and associates. Subchondral bone is preserved, except for the slot for the keel portion of the component. Soft cancellous bone is removed from beneath a portion of the subchondral plate, from the base of the coracoid process, and, to some degree, from the axillary border of the scapula. The remaining cancellous bony bed is carefully dried, and blood is removed. In this illustration, the *broken line* within the neck of the scapula shows the area of cancellous bone removal, which will be occupied by a prosthesis and polymethyl methacrylate. (From Neer CS II, Watson KC, and Stanton FJ: Recent experience in total shoulder replacement. J Bone Joint Surg *64A*:319–337, 1982.)

the results of the procedure have been published for less than 2000 cases performed in the United States, an estimated 5% of the total. In that most of the published reports come from centers where relatively large numbers of these procedures are performed, it would be of immense interest to know to what degree the results of the other 95% were similar.

An important advance is that simple and practical systems are now available by which surgeons can easily document the status of their patients before and sequentially after shoulder arthroplasty.[209, 220, 222, 224, 295] This documentation of treatment effectiveness will permit the comparison of different management approaches for defined groups of patients. If data on more than 6000 shoulder arthroplasties being performed each year can be gathered, analyzed, and compared, shoulder surgeons will be in a powerful position to understand and to progressively improve the effectiveness of the care that they offer their patients.

Milne and Gartsman[239] reviewed the costs of arthroplasty in 1992 and 1993 in a private practice in Houston, Texas. They found that the average cost for hemiarthroplasty was $15,656 and that for total shoulder arthroplasty was $16,606. Of this cost, 20% was for the surgeon, 75% for the hospital, 3% for the anesthesia, and 2% for consultations. Four per cent of the patients were on workers' compensation; 43% were on private pay; and 53% were on Medicare. The average length of stay was 5 days with a range from 3 to 14 days.

Indications for Surgery

Glenohumeral arthroplasty is a technically demanding and powerful tool for the reconstruction of the arthritic shoulder. Shoulder arthroplasty is indicated when the following conditions are met:

1. *Substantial disability of the shoulder exists and is clearly related to loss of the normal glenohumeral articulation.* It is useful to document both the disability and the glenohumeral destruction using standardized tools, such as the Simple Shoulder Test (see Table 16–4), the SF-36 (see Table 16–5), and defined radiographic views (see Figs. 16–41 and 16–42).
2. *The anatomy of the shoulder is amenable to reconstruction using shoulder arthroplasty* (i.e., there is sufficient bone stock, muscle strength, and tendon integrity to provide for a functional and robust reconstruction). In certain situations the presence of anatomic deficiencies may favor a hemiarthroplasty as opposed to a total shoulder; for example, when there is insufficient glenoid bone to support a glenoid component; when the humeral head is fixed in a superiorly displaced position relative to the glenoid (e.g., in cuff tear arthropathy), in patients with degenerative arthritis and an irreparable cuff,[360] in patients with rheumatoid arthritis and an irreparable cuff that is still concentric in shape,[17, 327] and in patients with degenerative arthritis and a glenoid that has not eroded.[138, 173]
3. *The patient is committed to the success of the procedure, has no contraindications, understands the limitations of a shoulder prosthesis, and has sufficient social*

Table 16–18 DIAGNOSES IN PATIENTS REQUIRING TOTAL SHOULDER ARTHROPLASTY*

	NO. OF SHOULDERS
Osteoarthritis	173
Rheumatoid arthritis	165
Traumatic arthritis	46
Cuff-tear arthropathy	42
Failed surgery	
Total	34
Proximal humeral	21
Resection	3
Fusion	4
Osteonecrosis	15
Old sepsis	5
Other	8
Total	516

*December 1965–June 1988.

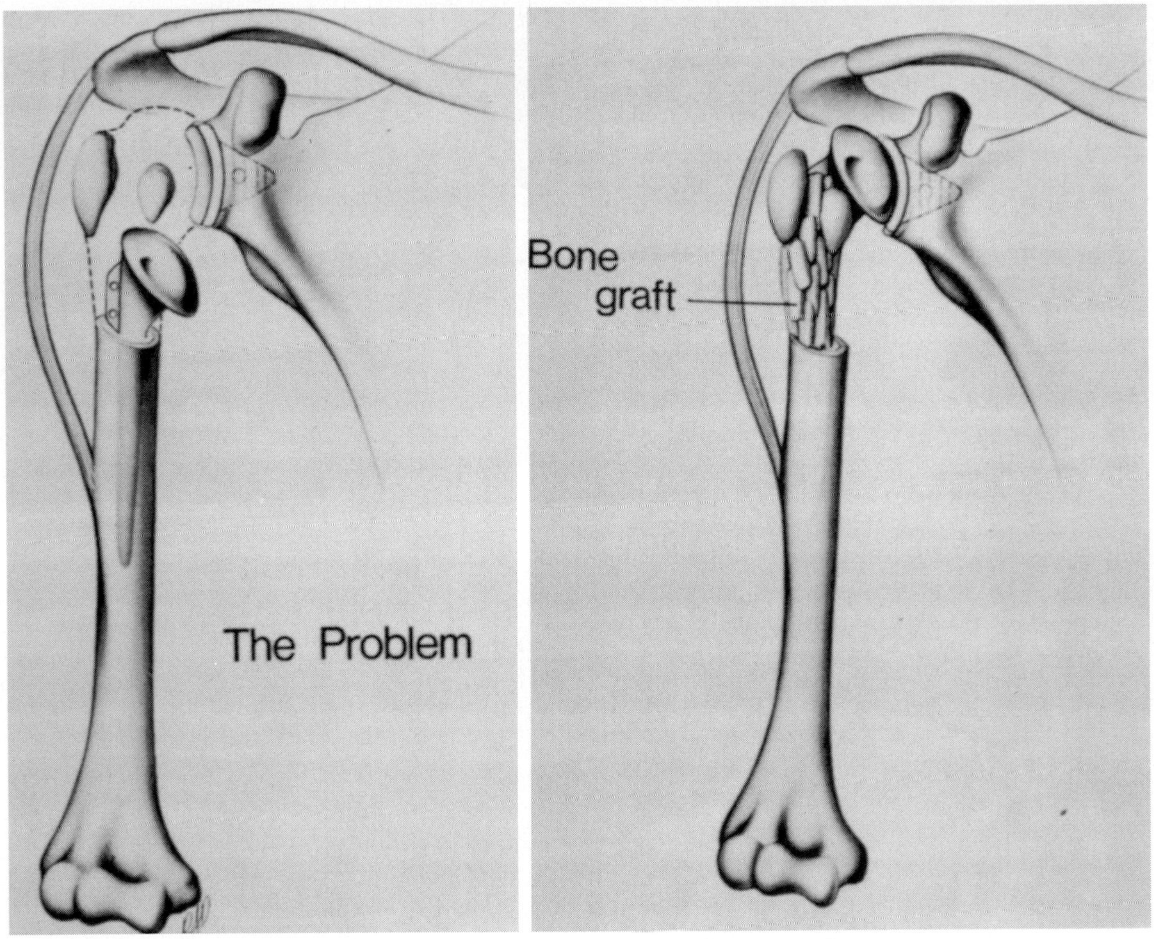

Figure 16–128

In certain shoulder arthritis problems, especially those associated with trauma, there may be loss of proximal humeral bone. If the prosthesis is set low to match the remaining bone, the prosthesis will subluxate inferiorly and the deltoid will be too long to develop any force. As illustrated on the right, Neer and associates proposed restoring humeral length, setting the prosthesis opposite the glenoid, and replacing deficient proximal humerus with bone graft. (From Neer CS II, Watson KC, and Stanton FJ: Recent experience in total shoulder replacement. J Bone Joint Surg *64A*:319–337, 1982.)

support for the postoperative period. The ideal patient for a prosthetic arthroplasty has a positive attitude combined with the understanding that a shoulder arthroplasty is not meant to be used for heavy or jerky pushing, pulling, lifting, or overhead work. Active or recent infection, absent deltoid function and poor general health are considered contraindications. Patients with rheumatoid arthritis and other systemic diseases can be expected to have poorer general health and vitality those with uncomplicated degenerative joint disease. Poor general health may lessen the desirability of shoulder reconstruction even if the joint involvement is severe. Poor tissue quality, cuff deficiency, tuberosity nonunion or malunion, remote infection, previous shoulder surgery, previous trauma, alcoholism, smoking, narcotic use, significant parkinsonism, neuropathic arthropathy, obesity, crutch dependency, and unrealistic expectations all lessen the chances of a good result. Poor mental or emotional health may need management before shoulder reconstruction is undertaken; again, the routine preoperative use of the SF-36 may provide the surgeon with a "heads up" that these conditions exist (see Table 16–5).

4. *The surgeon is experienced and prepared to provide a technically excellent arthroplasty.* In that reconstruction of the shoulder is greater in complexity than that of the hip or knee, a similar type of learning and number of cases are necessary before mastery is achieved. According to the October 1993 to September 1994 National Inpatient Profile (HCIA INC 1995), the number of total knees performed in 12 months in the United States was 211,872, whereas the number of total shoulders was only 5895.* These data indicate that surgeons have only 3% of the opportunity to master the total shoulder as they have to master the total knee. Expressed in another way, if the cases were distributed evenly, each of the 16,731 members of the AAOS would perform, on the average, just over one total knee per month and one total shoulder every 3 years.

The shoulder arthroplasty surgeon must have a command of the anatomy as well as the techniques to safely manage the exposure, capsular contractures, abnormalities of glenoid version, cuff pathology, humeral deformi-

*Similar data are presented by Madhok and associates,[214] who reviewed the trends in utilization in upper limb replacements at the Mayo Clinic from 1972 to 1990.

ties, and intraoperative problems. Although the approximate number of cases to achieve mastery has not been determined, it is recognized that for shoulder as well as for hip and knee reconstruction, "the surgeon is the method."

Goals of Surgery

Shoulder arthroplasty provides the surgeon with the opportunity to restore the mechanics of glenohumeral motion, strength, stability, and smoothness.

Motion is re-established and obligate translation prevented by:

1. Releasing all adhesions and contractures at the humeroscapular motion interface (see Fig. 16–19).
2. Inserting a smooth humeral prosthesis whose articular surface area comprises a substantial portion of the sphere (see Figs. 16–13 and 16–14).
3. Inserting a smooth glenoid prosthesis whose articular surface comprises a relatively small portion of the sphere (see Fig. 16–14).
4. Removal of blocking osteophytes (see Fig. 16–18).
5. Avoiding overstuffing of the joint (see Fig. 16–2).

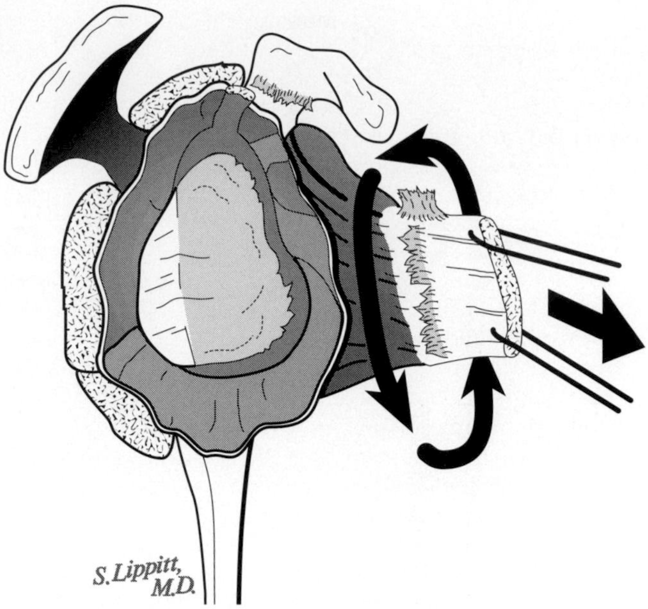

Figure 16–130

360-Degree subscapularis tendon release. (Modified from Matsen FA III, Lippitt SB, Sidles JA, and Harryman DT II: Practical Evaluation and Management of the Shoulder. Philadelphia: WB Saunders, 1994.)

Stability and **strength** are achieved by:

1. Normalizing glenoid and humeral joint surface location and orientation so that full surface contact occurs throughout the useful range of joint motion (see Fig. 16–20). Ballmer and associates[12] have studied in detail the effect of component articular surface geometry on the extent of glenohumeral joint surface contact. They found that for some commercially available prosthetic combinations, there was no position in which full surface contact existed, whereas others offer a 117-degree range of positions of full surface contact. They pointed out that in the range of positions in which full surface contact exists, there is no possibility for abutment of humeral bone or surrounding soft tissues against the glenoid edge. Furthermore, within this range, joint contact area is maximal; joint pressures are minimal; and the joint offers maximal stability. Conversely, outside the range of full surface contact, the edge of the glenoid may abut against humeral bone or soft tissue; there is increased joint contact pressure; and instability may result.
2. Selecting and positioning the new glenoid joint surface (see Figs. 16–26 and 16–27) so that effective arcs are available to balance the range of net humeral joint reaction forces usually encountered.
3. Re-establishing normal compressive muscle force (see Fig. 16–30) by releasing, repairing, balancing, and rehabilitating the cuff muscles (Figs. 16–129 and 16–130).

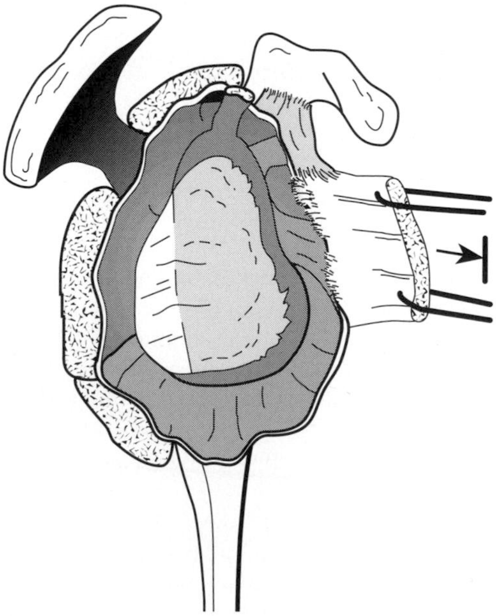

Figure 16–129

Contracted subscapularis tendon. (Modified from Matsen FA III, Lippitt SB, Sidles JA, and Harryman DT II: Practical Evaluation and Management of the Shoulder. Philadelphia: WB Saunders, 1994.)

The deltoid is the most important motor of the shoulder arthroplasty. The integrity of its origin, insertion, and nerve supply must be maintained. This is most easily accomplished by gently approaching the joint through the deltopectoral interval and by identifying and protecting the axillary nerve both anteromedially as it crosses the subscapularis and the inferior capsule and laterally as it exits the quadrangular space and winds around the tuberosities on the deep surface of the deltoid. Rehabilitation of the deltoid is critical to the active motion after arthroplasty.

The rotator cuff mechanism is in jeopardy in shoulder arthroplasty for several reasons. The suprascapular nerve, which supplies the supraspinatus and infraspinatus, is at risk during surgical releases as it courses medial to the coracoid and then down the back of the glenoid 1 cm medial to the glenoid lip. The cuff tendons are at risk during surgery because the humeral cut must come close to their insertion to the tuberosities superiorly and posteriorly. A humeral cut made in excessive retroversion is likely to detach the cuff posteriorly, and a cut made too low on the humerus is likely to detach the cuff superiorly (Fig. 16–131). Overstuffing the joint places the cuff under tension when the arm is adducted or rotated (see Fig. 16–40). Most shoulder arthroplasties are performed for older individuals in whom the quality of the cuff tissue may be compromised not only from age-related changes but also from disuse enforced by chronic glenohumeral roughness. Shoulder arthroplasty may quickly restore motion and smoothness to the joint, placing new and substantial demands on the disused cuff tissue. Thus, the rehabilitation program and the patient's activities after arthroplasty must *gradually* increase the loads on the cuff, allowing the tissue the opportunity to toughen over time.

If a cuff defect exists at the time of the arthroplasty, a cuff repair to bone should be carried out, provided the quantity and quality of the cuff tissue are sufficient to allow a secure repair under physiologic tension with the arm at the side. If these conditions are not met, an attempted cuff repair may not be worthwhile. If a cuff repair is carried out or if fixation of the tuberosities is performed, the rehabilitation after arthroplasty must be changed dramatically to allow for secure reattachment of the cuff mechanism to the humerus before active use is allowed. For these reasons, if the rotator cuff is deficient, repair is not usually attempted. In these circumstances, a hemiarthroplasty is often considered instead of a total shoulder arthroplasty.

4. Ensuring that capsular ligaments that are neither too short (in which case obligate translation may occur at the limits of motion) (see Fig. 16–7) nor too loose (in which case the joint may over-rotate beyond the positions in which the muscles can stabilize the head in the socket).

These considerations are critical. Reports suggest that almost one third of glenoid failures are associated with chronic glenohumeral instability after shoulder arthroplasty.[306–308]

Smoothness is provided by

1. Inserting smooth prosthetic joint surfaces
2. Managing all humeroscapular motion interface roughness
3. Implementing immediate postoperative motion to prevent unwanted scar formation (Fig. 16–132). Early postoperative motion not only reduces the likelihood of adhesion formation but may also increase the strength of soft tissue repairs.[123]

Types of Arthroplasty

Three levels of glenohumeral arthroplasty are commonly used. The basic surgical approach, capsular balancing, and osteophyte removal are similar for all three:

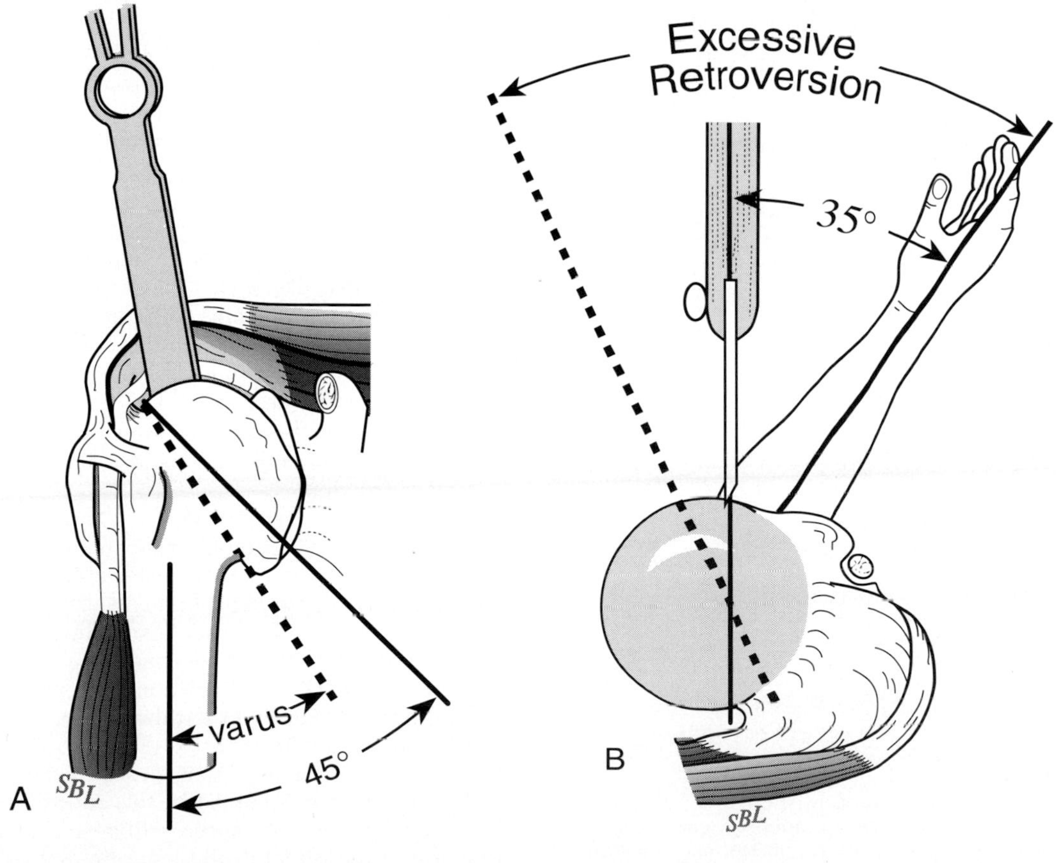

Figure 16–131

A, A cut that is too lateral risks detaching the cuff insertion superiorly. *B*, A humeral cut made in excessive retroversion risks detaching the cuff posteriorly. (From Matsen FA III, Lippitt SB, Sidles JA, and Harryman DT II: Practical Evaluation and Management of the Shoulder. Philadelphia: WB Saunders, 1994.)

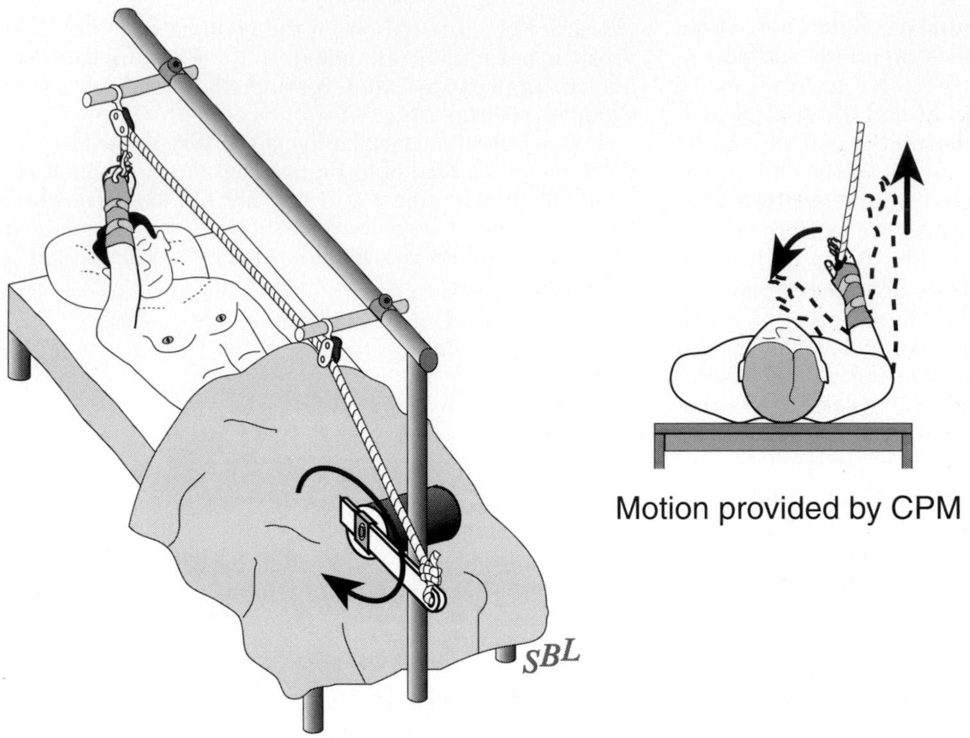

Figure 16–132

Continuous passive motion (CPM) is helpful for the first 24 to 48 hours after a procedure to mobilize the shoulder. Elevation to 90 degrees is easily achieved using a simple pulley system with a motor-driven eccentric cam. (From Matsen FA III, Lippitt SB, Sidles JA, and Harryman DT II: Practical Evaluation and Management of the Shoulder. Philadelphia: WB Saunders, 1994.)

Nonprosthetic arthroplasty is considered when osteophytes and capsular contractures block motion and function in the presence of congruent glenohumeral contact and reasonable cartilaginous space on radiographs. This option is particularly desirable in a young individual who plans to place heavy demands on the shoulder.

Prosthetic humeral hemiarthroplasty is considered when:

1. The humeral joint surface is rough, but the cartilaginous surface of the glenoid is intact* and there is sufficient glenoid arc to stabilize the humeral head.† In this situation, there is an even greater need to match the normal anatomy than that which exists with total glenohumeral replacement.‡
2. There is insufficient bone to support a glenoid component (e.g., after severe medial erosion of the glenoid in rheumatoid arthritis) (see Figs. 16–29 and 16–53).
3. There is fixed upward displacement of the humeral head relative to the glenoid as in cuff tear arthropathy (see Fig. 16–34) or severe rheumatoid arthritis (see Fig. 16–58).
4. There is a history of remote joint infection.
5. Heavy demands will be placed on the joint (e.g., in motion disorders or anticipated heavy loading from occupation, sport, or lower extremity paresis).

Humeral hemiarthroplasty may be stabilized in cuff tear arthropathy, even though the superior lip of the glenoid is eroded away by superior humeral subluxation. In this situation, the prosthetic humeral head is captured by an acetabular-like socket consisting of the eroded upper glenoid, the coracoid, the coracoacromial ligament, and the acromion, provided these structures have not been sacrificed by acromioplasty. It is vital that the surgeon not compromise this "socket" by sacrificing the anterior acromion or the coracoacromial ligament; otherwise, the humeral head is likely to be destabilized in an anterosuperior direction.

In hemiarthroplasty for cuff tear arthropathy, the undersurface of the "acetabularized" coracoacromial arch is found to be polished smooth with a consistent radius of curvature. The prosthetic humeral articular surface and the tuberosities must provide a smooth congruent surface to mate with this arch. Achieving this goal requires attention to the selection and positioning of the humeral component and to sculpting the tuberosities. The best choice is a humeral prosthesis that duplicates the size and position of the humeral head that is excised. The large smooth joint contact area achieved in this procedure appears to be responsible for its success in restoring comfort and function in the difficult problem of cuff tear arthropathy. Care should be taken to avoid replacement of the head of the humerus with a "big head" that can overstuff the joint!

*The articular cartilage is assessed by preoperative radiographs, including CT scans, and at surgery by observation, palpation, and by listening to the sound when it is struck with a small blunt elevator: Thin cartilage or bare bone will cause the elevator to ring, whereas normal cartilage will yield only a dull "thunk."

†Frequently in degenerative joint disease and in capsulorrhaphy arthropathy the posterior half of the glenoid concavity is eroded away, depriving the shoulder of the effective glenoid arc (see Figs. 16–24 and 16–44). Thus, even if excellent articular cartilage exists on the anterior half of the glenoid, a humeral hemiarthroplasty cannot be stable without this posterior glenoid lip.

‡When performing a hemiarthroplasty, the goal is to restore the humeral articular surface to its normal location and configuration. Because the glenoid is not replaced, the size, radius, and orientation of the prosthetic humeral joint surface must duplicate that of the original biologic humeral head. Information regarding the patient's normal humeral head anatomy may be obtained from radiographs of the opposite shoulder.

Total glenohumeral arthroplasty is desirable when both joint surfaces are damaged and when both are reconstructable.

Some studies have attempted to compare hemiarthroplasty and total shoulder arthroplasty. Boyd and associates[37] found in a "similar" but unmatched series comparison that at 44-month follow-up, hemiarthroplasty and total shoulder arthroplasty produced similar results in terms of functional improvement. Pain relief, range of motion, and patient satisfaction were better with total shoulder arthroplasty than with hemiarthroplasty in the rheumatoid population. Progressive glenoid loosening was found in 12% of total shoulder arthroplasties, but no correlation with pain relief or range of motion was noted.

In an article, Rodosky and Bigliani[307] reviewed the indications for glenoid resurfacing. They pointed out that early on in the history of shoulder arthroplasty it was recognized that when the glenoid was significantly diseased, problems with excessive excursion of the prosthetic head were noted. The goal of inserting a glenoid prosthesis was to provide a better fulcrum and therefore better strength and greater stability[252] along with decreased friction and elimination of "glenoid socket pain."[307] Other potential benefits of the glenoid component include avoiding the progressive glenoid erosion seen when arthritis or fractures are treated with proximal humeral replacement alone.[29, 87, 241]

Comparison of Hemiarthroplasty and Total Shoulder Arthroplasty

At this point the literature comparing hemiarthroplasty and total shoulder arthroplasty seems to favor the former when arthritis and cuff deficiency are coexistent[7, 8, 48, 67, 79, 116, 118, 183, 184, 217, 277, 327, 360] and the latter in osteoarthritis and rheumatoid arthritis when the cuff is intact.[24, 37, 65, 83, 147, 252, 253, 259, 275, 278] It is recognized that badly eroded glenoid bone cannot support a glenoid prosthesis.[252, 253, 259]

PROSTHESIS SELECTION

Many of the concepts guiding prosthesis selection have been presented in the section of this chapter on Mechanics. A few additional comments are offered here regarding the selection of the prosthesis.

Desirable Characteristics of the Glenoid Prosthesis

- As thin as structural properties will allow to minimize joint stuffing (see Fig. 16–2). For this reason, all polyethylene components have an advantage, because metal backing takes up needed room in the joint.
- Supported directly and intimately by bone (Fig. 16–133; see also Fig. 16–27) to avoid cracking away of a thin cement mantle. The high incidence of failure of metal-backed glenoid components has been recognized.[306–308] Preservation of the subchondral bone and use of all polyethylene components results in loading patterns most similar to those found in a normal glenoid, whereas metal-backed components lead to high nonphysiologic stresses.[129] Bone-prosthesis contact must be optimized by appropriate design, sizing, and bone preparation. Free-hand bone preparation is too uncertain to routinely provide optimal stability without resorting to the interposition of cement (see Fig. 16–133). Drill guides can ensure that the fixation system achieves the desired relationship to the prepared glenoid face and minimizes the amount of bone removed.
- Fixation that preserves bone stock and minimizes the need for cement
- Appropriate articular surface area[12] and diameter of curvature relative to the humeral prosthesis (Figs. 16–134 and 16–135; see also Figs. 16–14, 16–36, and 16–37)

In order for the glenoid to stabilize the humeral head against transverse loads, it must be well supported by the bone beneath it. Clinical observations suggest that a primary mechanism of glenoid loosening is via the rocking horse mechanism when eccentric loads are applied. In a series of 10 cadaver glenoids, the authors studied the effect of glenoid bone preparation on the stability of a 3-mm-thick, nonclinical, glenoid component with a diameter of curvature of 60 mm on the surface apposed to bone.[221] To emphasize the effect of glenoid surface preparation, the component was secured to the bony glenoid with only a single, flexible, uncemented central peg. The component was loaded with an eccentric force of 200 N applied at an angle of 14 degrees with the glenoid center line. While the component was loaded, the wobble of the component with respect to the bone and the warp or deformation of the component were measured using displacement transducers. The stability of the component was measured sequentially after three different glenoid preparations: (1) curettage of the articular cartilage, (2) meticulous burring of the bone by hand to fit the back of the component, and (3) preparation using a reamer with a diameter of curvature of 60 mm centered in a hole along the glenoid center line. Spherical reaming dramatically diminished both the wobble and the warp of the glenoid component with eccentric loading, in comparison with the other two methods of bone preparation (see Fig. 16–133). It is likely that an even greater increment in stability would accrue with concentric reaming in a deformed bony glenoid, such as that found in degenerative joint disease. This study demonstrates that precise contouring of the bone to fit the back of the glenoid component provides excellent support of the prosthesis, even without the potential benefits of fixation using multiple pegs, keels, cement, screws, or tissue ingrowth. Spherical reaming along the anatomic glenoid center line has two important advantages: (1) it normalizes glenoid version, and (2) it provides "bone back" support of the glenoid component with the opportunity for optimal stability and load transfer without the use of metal backing.

Fixation anterior and posterior to the meridian is used to prevent anterior and posterior rocking or "lift off" during eccentric loading (see Fig. 16–35).

Glenohumeral arthroplasty provides the surgeon the opportunity to control the shape of the prosthetic glenoid

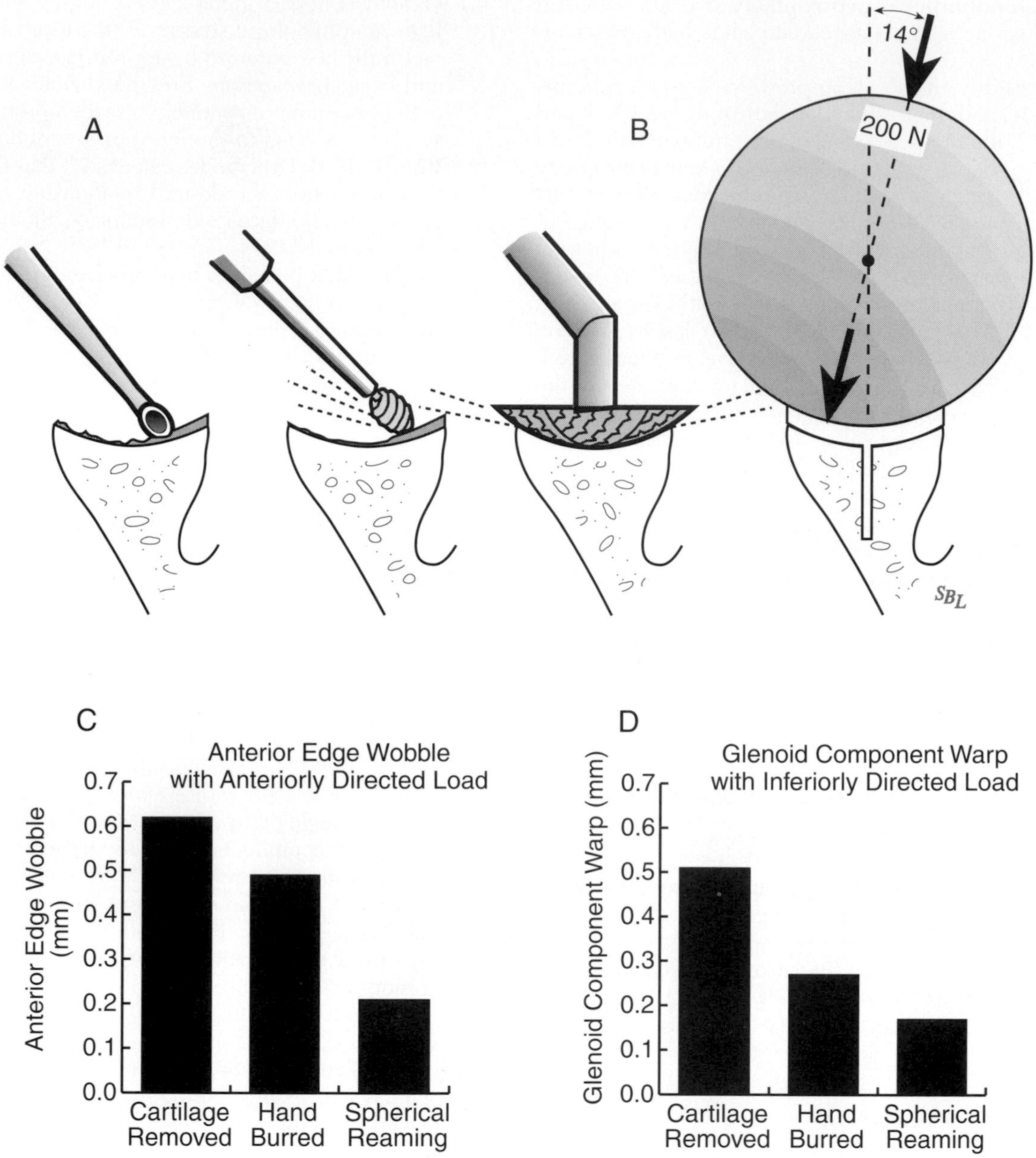

Figure 16–133

The effect of glenoid-bone preparation on component stability. *A*, Three methods of bone preparation were compared: curettage, hand burring, and spherical reaming. *B*, Loads of 200 N were applied through a metal ball at an angle of 14 degrees with respect to the glenoid center line. The glenoid was fixed only with a single uncemented flexible central peg. Displacement transducers measured the change in position of the edges of the glenoid component. *C* and *D*, Data on the stability of a glenoid component with three different types of glenoid surface preparation. Spherical reaming of the glenoid along the glenoid center line significantly reduced the wobble (*C*) and warp (*D*) of the glenoid component and thus provided more glenoid component stability than did curettage or hand burring. (From Matsen FA III, Lippitt SB, Sidles JA, and Harryman DT II: Practical Evaluation and Management of the Shoulder. Philadelphia: WB Saunders, 1994.)

concavity. The depth of the glenoid concavity is related to dimensions of the face of the glenoid (superoinferior and anteroposterior breadth) and to the radius of curvature (Fig. 16–136). For a given radius of joint surface curvature, larger components are deeper than smaller ones. For a given glenoid size, components with a smaller radius of curvature are deeper than those with larger radii of joint surface curvature.

If the glenoid and humeral radii of curvature are equal, the head will be held precisely in the center by concavity compression; no translation can occur unless the humeral head is allowed to lift out of the fossa (Fig. 16–137). Although this tight conformity provides excellent stability, it has the potential disadvantage that displacing loads applied to the humerus will be transmitted fully to the glenoid and thence to the glenoid-bone interface. In the biologic glenoid, the compliance of the articular cartilage and glenoid labrum provide shock absorption for these

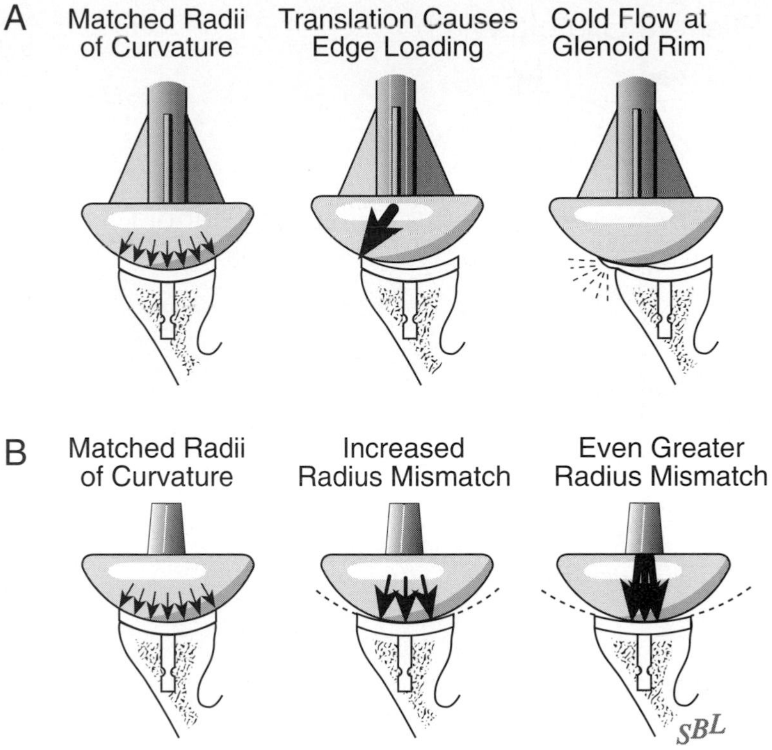

Figure 16–134

A, When the joint surfaces of the glenoid and humeral components have identical radii of curvature, any amount of translation (however small) causes rim loading. Rim loading in turn results in high contact pressures, rim wear, and cold flow. *B*, When the radius of curvature of the glenoid component surface is larger than that of the humerus, there is an increase in joint pressure (load per unit area) related to the degree of mismatch (see Figs. 16–38 and 16–39). (Modified from Matsen FA III, Lippitt SB, Sidles JA, and Harryman DT II: Practical Evaluation and Management of the Shoulder. Philadelphia: WB Saunders, 1994.)

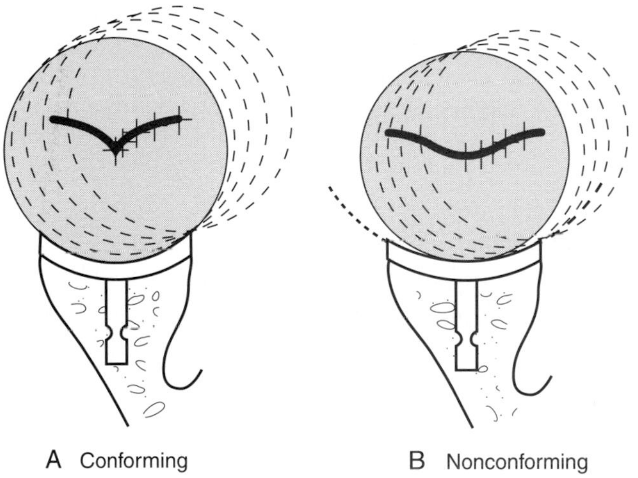

Figure 16–135

The path that the center of the humeral head takes during translation relative to the glenoid (the "glenoidogram" path). *A*, Conforming surfaces yield a tight V on the glenoidogram. *B*, When the glenoid diameter of curvature is slightly larger than that of the humerus, the glenoidogram yields a U shape. (From Matsen FA III, Lippitt SB, Sidles JA, and Harryman DT II: Practical Evaluation and Management of the Shoulder. Philadelphia: WB Saunders, 1994.)

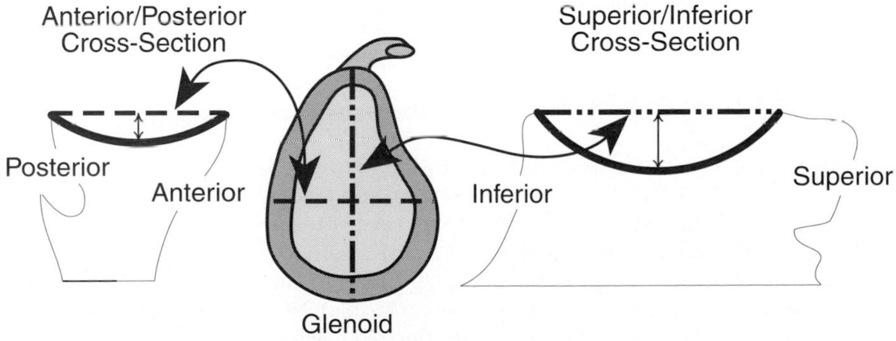

Figure 16–136

The width of the glenoid in the superoinferior direction is greater than the width of the glenoid in the anteroposterior direction. For a given radius of curvature, an increase in width results in an increase in depth. Thus, the depth of the glenoid as measured along the superoinferior direction is greater than the depth measured along the anteroposterior direction. (From Matsen FA III, Lippitt SB, Sidles JA, and Harryman DT II: Practical Evaluation and Management of the Shoulder. Philadelphia: WB Saunders, 1994.)

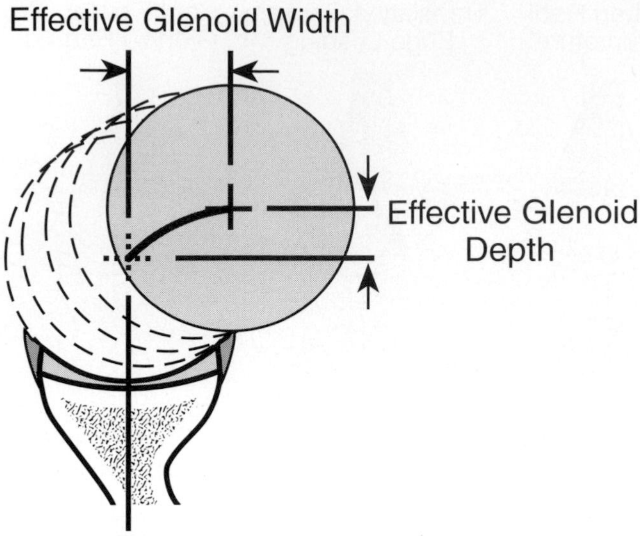

Figure 16–137

The glenoidogram is the path of the humeral head as it translates in a specified direction across the face of the glenoid away from the glenoid center line under defined loads. The glenoidogram shows the effective glenoid depth and width for the specified direction of translation and loading conditions. (Modified from Matsen FA III, Lippitt SB, Sidles JA, and Harryman DT II: Practical Evaluation and Management of the Shoulder. Philadelphia: WB Saunders, 1994.)

transverse displacing loads. Because polyethylene is much stiffer than cartilage and labrum, this shock absorption is not present in a prosthetic glenoid arthroplasty. Thus glenoid fixation is at risk for substantial peak loads when the glenoid and humeral joint surfaces are totally conforming.

Some degree of shock absorption can be provided by a slight mismatch between the humeral and glenoid radii of curvature, that of the glenoid being slightly larger. This allows some translation before the humeral head must lift out of the fossa (the glenoidogram becomes more a "U" than a tight "V"; see Fig. 16–135). This too is a compromise, however, in that the degree of mismatch decreases the contact area and increases the contact pressures with potential risk of polyethylene failure. In a finite element model using conventional polyethylene, the surface area of contact with a load of typical body weight 625 N (140 lb) was predicted to decrease dramatically with increasing degrees of radial mismatch (see Fig. 16–38). This drop in contact area gives rise to a corresponding increase in the contact stresses (see Fig. 16–39). For loads of 625 N, the contact stress exceeds the predicted yield stress for conventional polyethylene when the radial mismatch is greater than 3 mm.

- Optimal articular surface diameter of curvature relative to that of the humerus. Harryman and associates[153, 221] demonstrated glenohumeral translation in normal shoulders with passive motion. Friedman[127] have used a radiographic technique to measure anteroposterior translation in 13 patients who had Neer or Cofield total shoulder arthroplasties (in each of which the diameters of curvature of the glenoid and humeral surfaces were equal). They measured an average of 4 mm (range of 0 to 12 mm) of posterior translation between horizontal elevation in the −30 degree (posterior) plane and horizontal elevation in the 60-degree (anterior) plane. Along with Matsen and associates[221] they pointed out that this translation could contribute to loosening or to asymmetric wear (see Figs. 16–36, 16–37, and 16–134) as demonstrated by Collins and associates.[85] Such a tendency for rim loading may be lessened if there is a slight diametric mismatch between the humerus and the glenoid (see Figs. 16–36, 16–37, and 16–135).
- Sufficient yield stress for the anticipated loading conditions (see Figs. 16–38 and 16–39)
- Normal orientation with respect to the scapula

A simple cadaver study demonstrated a practical method for normalizing the glenoid orientation. The center of the face of the glenoid was located in each of 10 normal cadaveric scapulas. A drill was then inserted perpendicular to the face, starting at the glenoid center. In each case, the drill emerged from the anterior glenoid neck at the lateral aspect of the subscapularis fossa at a point midway between the upper and lower crus of the scapula (see Fig. 16–25). This spot is known as the "centering point." This point is easily palpated at arthroplasty surgery after an anterior capsular release has been performed (see Fig. 16–26). The line connecting it to the center of the glenoid face is the normalized glenoid center line. Orienting the prosthetic glenoid to this normalized glenoid center line enables the surgeon to correct pathologic glenoid version, which is frequently encountered in degenerative joint disease and other conditions that require shoulder arthroplasty (see Fig. 16–27).

Desirable Characteristics of the Humeral Prosthesis

- Maximizes the percentage of the sphere represented by the humeral articular surface area (see Figs. 16–9 and 16–13)[12]
- Positions the humeral articular surface in the anatomic location and orientation (see Figs. 16–2 and 16–10)
- Provides secure humeral fixation in a way that preserves humeral bone stock
- If the component is press-fit in the medullary canal, the surgeon must recognize the restrictions that this poses on the positioning of the prosthesis. Ballmer and colleagues[13, 221] pointed out that in a press-fit situation, the canal rather than the neck cut becomes the primary determinant of the mediolateral, anteroposterior, flexion-extension, and varus-valgus position of the component. In fact, with a snug canal fit, only 2 of the 6 potential degrees of freedom remain: component height and component version. Canal-fitting components are usually inserted after reaming the canal to the necessary depth and to a diameter judged to be safe and snug by the surgeon. The axis of this reamed proximal humeral canal is the "orthopedic axis" of the humerus (Fig. 16–138).

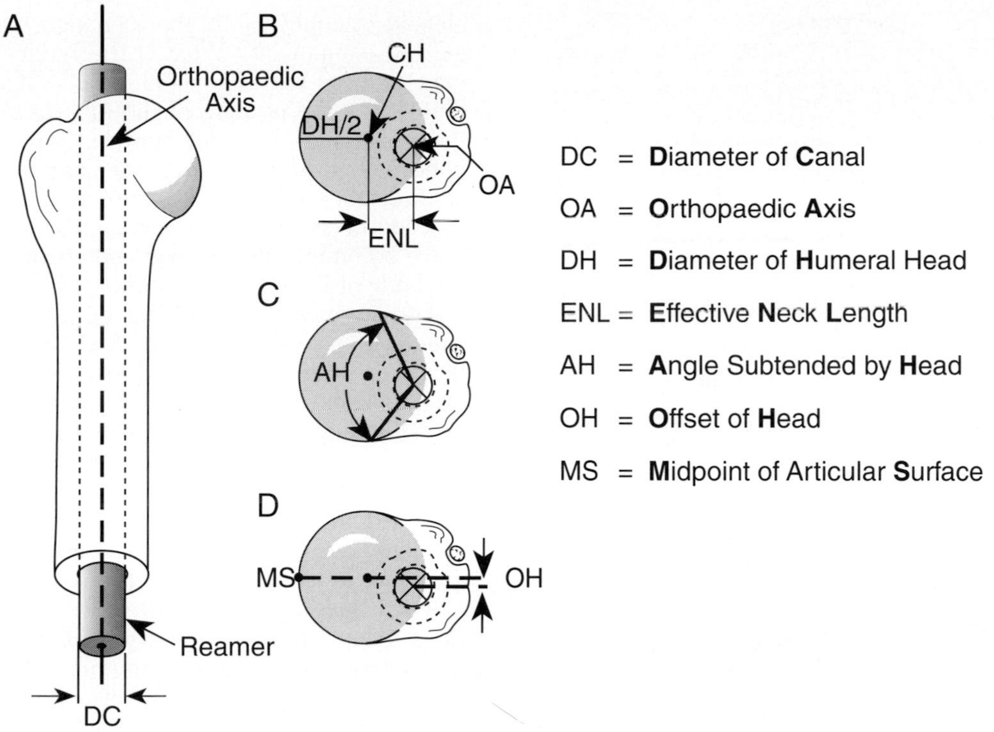

Figure 16–138

A, The humeral medullary canal is reamed to a diameter (DC) defining the orthopedic axis (OA). *B,* The diameter of curvature of the humeral articular surface is DH (radius is DH/2). The effective neck length (ENL) is the distance between the center of the humeral head (CH) and the orthopedic axis (OA). *C,* The angle based at the orthopedic axis and subtended by the humeral articular surface is AH. *D,* The offset of the center of the humeral head (OH) is defined as the perpendicular distance between the orthopedic axis (OA) and a line connecting the midpoint of the articular surface (MS) and the center of the humeral head (CH). (From Matsen FA III, Lippitt SB, Sidles JA, and Harryman DT II: Practical Evaluation and Management of the Shoulder. Philadelphia: WB Saunders, 1994.)

Again, the significance of this axis is that it defines much of the positional geometry of a humeral component press-fit into it.

Good fit and fill of the humerus can often provide secure fixation without cement, but press fitting does increase the risk of humeral fracture. Whether the medullary canal needs to be sealed to prevent entry of polyethylene debris remains a theoretical consideration. Using this axis as a reference, several geometric parameters were measured in 10 cadaveric humeri ranging in age from 37 to 78 years (mean of 60 years). The results are shown in Table 16–19.

For components that fit snugly within the medullary canal, changes in humeral version must take place about the orthopedic axis. This does not allow much latitude in the version if the humeral articular surface is to be optimized (Fig. 16–139). For this reason and because the center of rotation of the head lies close to the orthopedic axis, the soft tissue tension is not substantially changed by alterations in humeral version (a very different situation from that encountered in the hip where the center of rotation of the head is distant from the medullary axis of the shaft). Ballmer and colleagues[13] found that only a 2-mm change in combined head/neck length could be achieved by a change in the version of a prosthesis press-fit in the canal.

Zuckerman[372] compared hospital reimbursement by Medicare for diagnostic-related group (DRG) 491 (shoulder arthroplasty) and found an overall range from $4699 to $9856 with a mean of $6906 for urban locations and a mean of $5198 for rural locations. He found that the cost of humeral components ranged from $950 to $2250, whereas the glenoid components ranged from $520 to $1250. Total shoulder systems ranged from $1470 to $2900. Thus, if the least costly implant system was used in a location with the greatest DRG reimbursement, it would account for $1470/$9856 or 15% of the hospital reimbursement. At the opposite extreme, if the most costly implant was used where DRG reimbursement was the least, it would account for $2900/$4699 or 62% of the total hospital reimbursement.

Table 16–19 RESULTS OF SEVERAL GEOMETRIC PARAMETERS MEASURED IN 10 CADAVERIC HUMERI RANGING IN AGE FROM 37 TO 78 YEARS (MEAN OF 60 YEARS), USING THE "ORTHOPEDIC AXIS" OF THE HUMERUS AS A REFERENCE

	RANGE	*MEAN*	*STANDARD DEVIATION*
Canal diameter (DC) (mm)	8–14	11	2
Head diameter (DH) (mm)	39–41	44	4
Neck length (ENL) (mm)	7–14	11	2
Joint surface angle (AH) (°)	104–120	113	5
Posterior head offset (OH) (mm)	(−3)−4	2	2

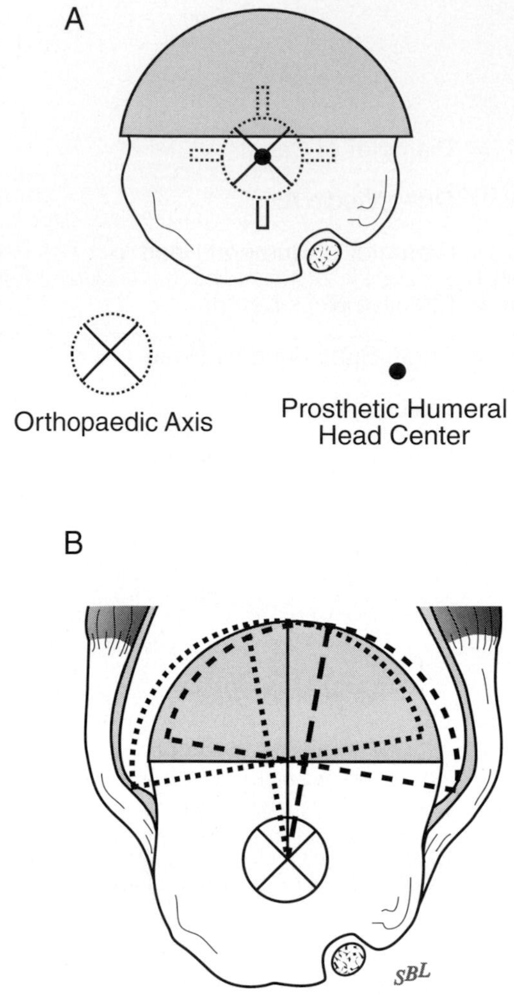

Figure 16–139

The effect of changing the humeral version in a canal-fitting prosthesis is determined by the effective neck length of the prosthesis (the distance between the orthopedic axis and the center of curvature of the head) and the amount of change in the version. *A*, If the effective neck length is zero, no amount of change in version will affect the distance between the tuberosities and the glenoid that the soft tissues must span. *B*, For anatomic humeri, the effective neck length is small (average 11 mm). If the humeral neck cut is made just inside the cuff insertion to the tuberosities, little angular change of the humeral component can be accomplished without jeopardizing the integrity of the cuff insertion. Thus, in a canal-fitting humeral component, changes in version do not have a major effect on soft tissue balance. (From Matsen FA III, Lippitt SB, Sidles JA, and Harryman DT II: Practical Evaluation and Management of the Shoulder. Philadelphia: WB Saunders, 1994.)

MATSEN'S SURGICAL TECHNIQUE

Standardized preoperative radiographs are obtained to reveal the amount, quality, and orientation of the glenoid bone as well as the size and configuration of the humerus down to where the tip of the humeral prosthesis will rest (see Figs. 16–41 and 16–42). Drawing the cuts and the implants on the preoperative radiographs using the manufacturer's templates helps the surgeon to determine where the humeral and glenoid components should be positioned and whether any particular problems in their placement can be anticipated. Is there significant glenoid erosion or altered version? Are there potentially confusing glenoid osteophytes? Is there enough bone to support a glenoid component? What is the radius of the humeral joint surface? Is the humeral canal straight? What size is it? What is the position of the tuberosities in relation to the canal and the joint surface? How much humeral bone will need to be excised? Are there other major abnormalities of bone structure that could change the procedure? In press-fit components, will the medullary space accommodate the size and shape of the stem and the body of the prosthesis without risk of fracture?

After a brachial plexus block or general anesthetic, the patient is placed in the beach-chair position with the thorax up at an angle of 30 degrees. The shoulder is just off the edge of the operating table so that it can be moved freely through an entire range of motion. The anesthesiologist is positioned at the side of the neck on the opposite side from the shoulder being operated. A careful double-skin preparation includes the entire arm and forequarter, anteriorly and posteriorly. Draping allows access to the entire scapula, clavicle, and humerus.

A *skin incision* is made over the deltopectoral groove along a line connecting the midpoint of the clavicle to the midpoint of the lateral humerus and crossing over the coracoid process (Fig. 16–140). The deltopectoral interval is developed medial to the cephalic vein, preserving its major tributaries from the deltoid muscle (Fig. 16–141). No deltoid detachment is needed proximally or distally.

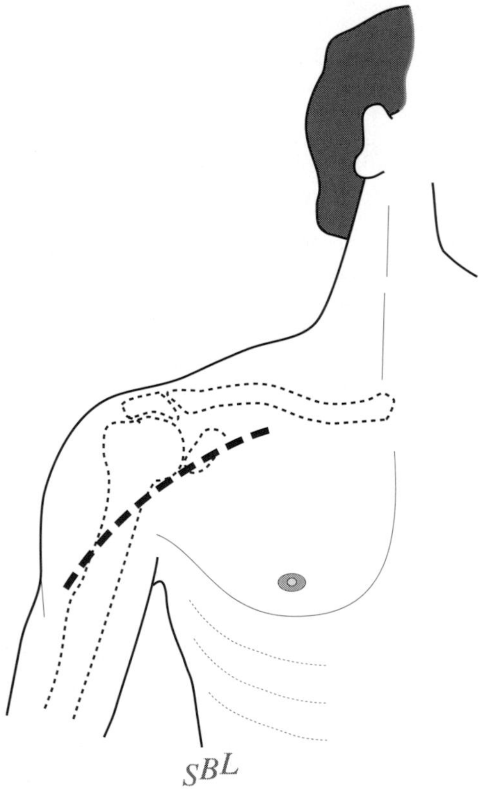

Figure 16–140

The skin incision for the extended deltopectoral approach utilizes the midclavicle, the tip of the coracoid process, and the deltoid tuberosity of the midhumerus as landmarks. (Modified from Matsen FA III, Lippitt SB, Sidles JA, and Harryman DT II: Practical Evaluation and Management of the Shoulder. Philadelphia: WB Saunders, 1994.)

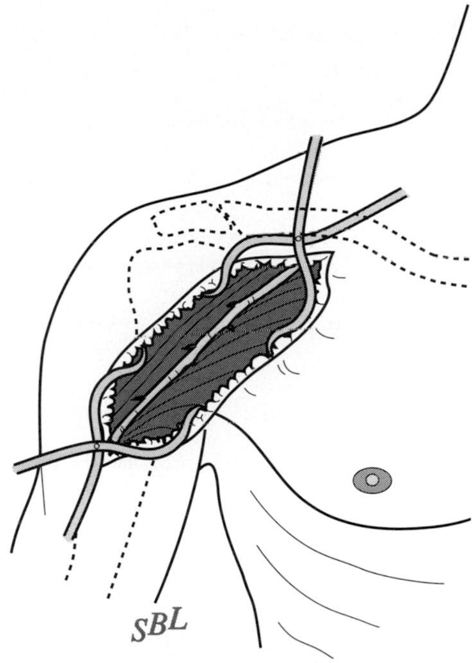

Figure 16–141

The cephalic vein identified in the deltopectoral groove. (Modified from Pearl ML and Lippitt SB: Shoulder arthroplasty with a modular prosthesis. Tech Orthop 8[3]:151–162, 1994. Original illustrator SB Lippitt.)

Incising the clavipectoral fascia at the lateral edge of the conjoined tendon up to, but not through, the coracoacromial ligament provides entry to the nonarticular humeroscapular motion interface (Fig. 16–142; see also Fig. 16–19). All adhesions in this interface are lysed from the axillary nerve medially to the axillary nerve as it exits the quadrilateral space posterior laterally. Burkhead and associates[55] have provided an excellent review of the surgical anatomy of this nerve.

The subscapularis is incised at its insertion to the lesser tuberosity along with the subjacent capsule (Fig. 16–143). **(V16-10)** This method of detachment maximizes the potential for a strong repair, in that as Hinton and associates[163] point out, the inferior 40% of the belly of the subscapularis extends all the way to the bone, rather than inserting as a tendon. A 360-degree release of the subscapularis tendon is then performed, ensuring that it moves freely with respect to the glenoid, the coracoid, the coracoid muscles, the axillary nerve, and the inferior capsule (see Figs. 16–129 and 16–130).

Humeral preparation is the next step in the arthroplasty. The humeral head is exposed anteriorly by *gentle* external rotation and slight extension. Special care is exercised in old patients and in those with rheumatoid arthritis or other causes of fragile bone. Barriers to gentle external rotation may be an unreleased anterior capsule or posterior osteophytes (see Fig. 16–17).

The humeral osteotomy requires attention to detail. Although the degree of retroversion is often approximately 35 degrees, it may vary from 10 to 50 degrees. **(V16-11)** The ideal humeral cut is that which will allow positioning of the humeral prosthetic articular surface in the anatomic position. The cut plane must pass just inside the rotator cuff insertion to the tuberosity, resecting the humeral articular surface without damaging the cuff insertion (Figs. 16–144 and 16–145). **(V16-12)** In degenerative joint disease, the apparent articular surface may not provide an accurate indication of the plane of humeral head resection. The angle of the cut with the humeral shaft must match that of the prosthesis being used—often about 45 degrees. The amount of humeral bone to be resected is compared for the different prosthetic options (see Fig. 16–2). **(V16-13)**

V16-10 to V16-13

After the humeral osteotomy, the surgeon can get an idea of the joint volume remaining for the glenoid and humeral head components by pushing the humeral neck laterally with a finger. This step is helpful in determining the need for further soft tissue releases. If the capsule is so tight that even the smallest head will not fit, more release is required (see Figs. 16–3 and 16–4). Cutting away more humerus is not an option, because the humeral head has already been resected at the cuff insertion and further resection will jeopardize this essential attachment.

With the proximal humerus displaced medially into the joint, the rotator cuff is palpated to establish its integrity. If a repairable defect through quality cuff tissue is identified, the retracted tendon is mobilized so that it will reach the tuberosity without undue tension with the arthroplasty components in place and with the arm at the side (Fig. 16–146). However, the two potential downsides of cuff repair in this circumstance are recognized: (1) in the presence of deficient tendon, cuff repair tightens the glenohumeral joint, and (2) cuff repair changes the

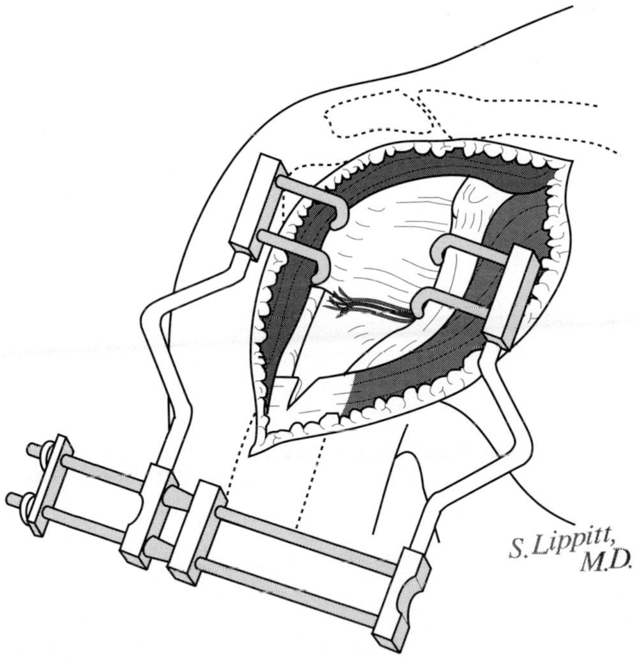

Figure 16–142

Self-retaining retractor below the conjoined tendon medially and the deltoid muscle laterally. (From Pearl ML and Lippitt SB: Shoulder arthroplasty with a modular prosthesis. Tech Orthop 8[3]:151–162, 1994. Original illustrator—SB Lippitt.)

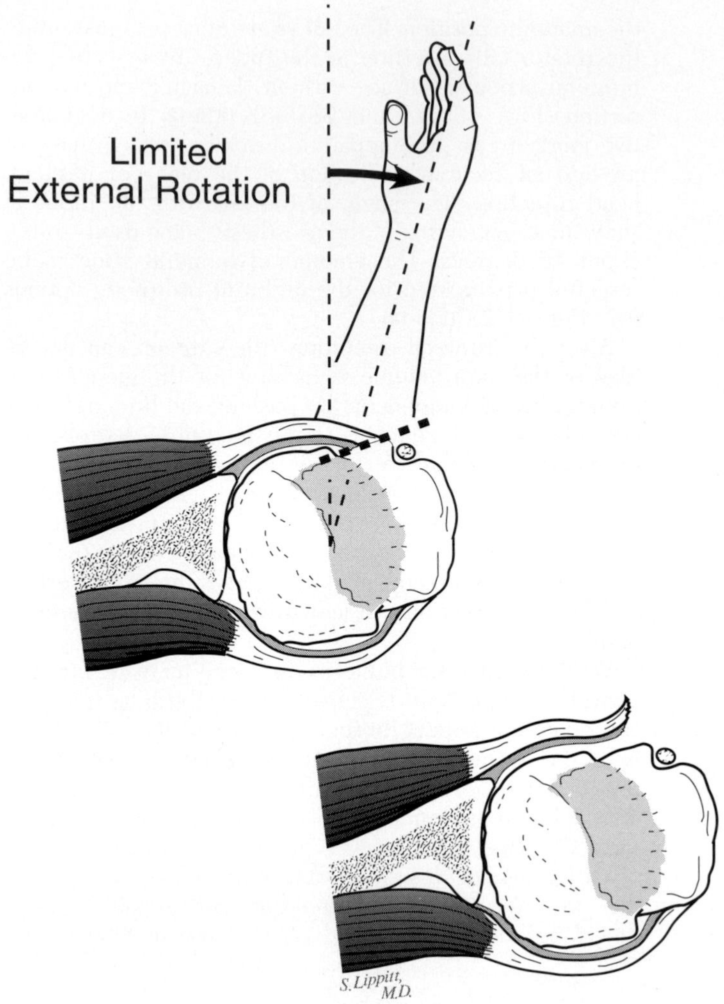

Figure 16–143

The subscapularis incision. The subscapularis and the subjacent capsule are incised directly from the lesser tuberosity, striving for maximal length of the tendon. (Modified from Matsen FA III, Lippitt SB, Sidles JA, and Harryman DT II: Practical Evaluation and Management of the Shoulder. Philadelphia: WB Saunders, 1994.)

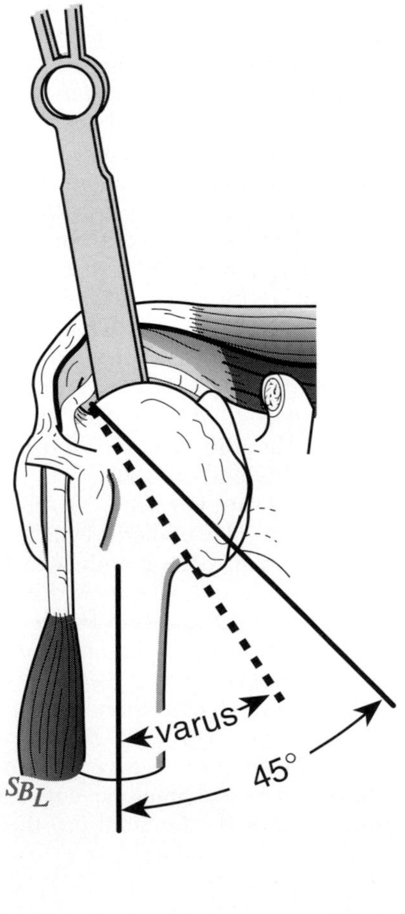

Figure 16–144

Humeral osteotomy planes. (*A*) The preferred osteotomy plane starts just inside the insertion of the cuff to the greater tuberosity and proceeds medially at a 45-degree angle with respect to the long axis of the humeral shaft. If the osteotomy is incorrectly oriented such that it emerges at the margin of the osteophytes instead of the articular cartilage (*dotted line*), the resulting cut will be in excessive varus. (Modified from Matsen FA III, Lippitt SB, Sidles JA, and Harryman DT II: Practical Evaluation and Management of the Shoulder. Philadelphia: WB Saunders, 1994.)

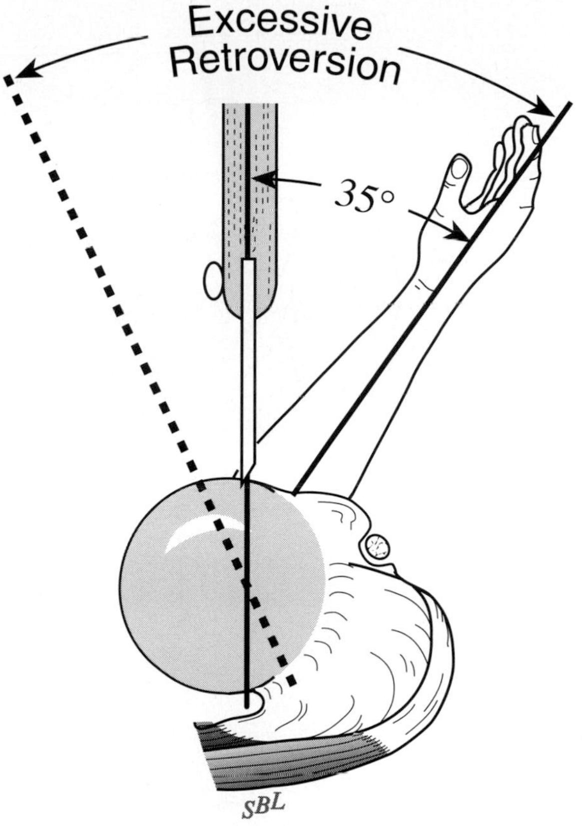

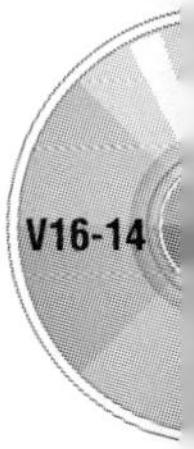

Figure 16–145

Humeral osteotomy planes. Humeral osteotomy also requires careful attention to version. An excessively retroverted cut (*dotted line*) will compromise the cuff insertion. (Modified from Matsen FA III, Lippitt SB, Sidles JA, and Harryman DT II: Practical Evaluation and Management of the Shoulder. Philadelphia: WB Saunders, 1994.)

postoperative rehabilitation from active to passive motion until the tendon has healed.

The medullary canal of the humerus is reamed, starting at a point lateral on the cut surface just behind the bicipital groove (Fig. 16-147). **(V16-14)** Starting with a small-diameter reamer, reaming is continued up to the diameter appropriate to the component, using a slight valgus bias and while protecting the biceps and cuff (Fig. 16–148). For prostheses that have press-fit stems, medullary reaming continues until a snug fit is achieved.

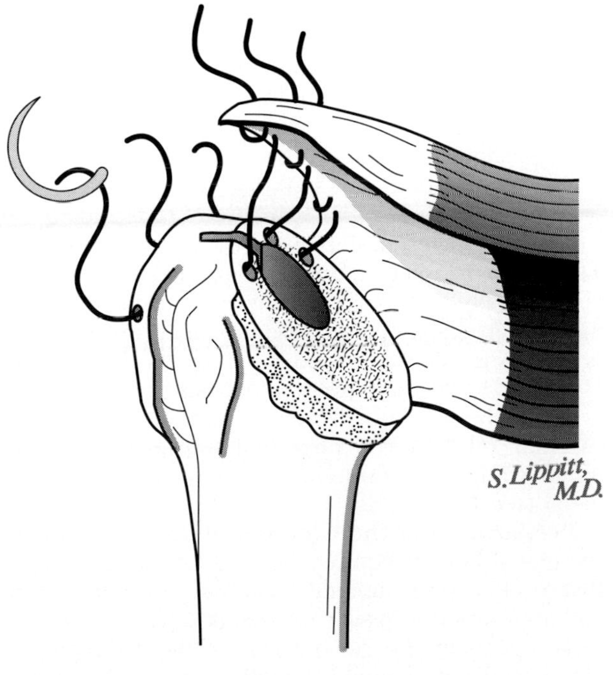

Figure 16–146

Repair of a rotator cuff tear. If tissue is of sufficient quantity and quality for a durable repair, drill holes are placed in the tuberosities for cuff attachment before the insertion of the humeral component. (Modified from Matsen FA III, Lippitt SB, Sidles JA, and Harryman DT II: Practical Evaluation and Management of the Shoulder. Philadelphia: WB Saunders, 1994.)

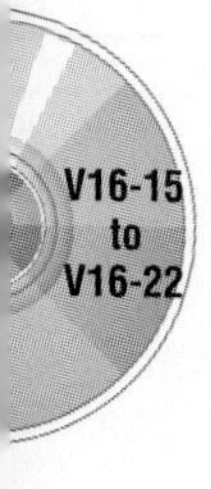

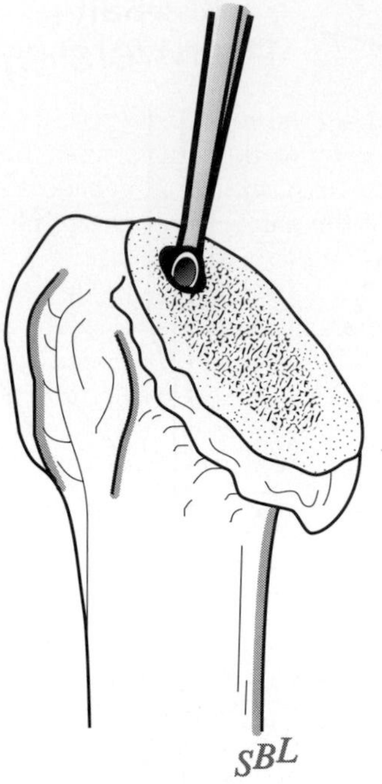

Figure 16–147

Making the pilot hole into the superior lateral cancellous surface just posterior to the bicipital groove to gain entrance into the humeral medullary canal. (From Pearl ML and Lippitt SB: Shoulder arthroplasty with a modular prosthesis. Tech Orthop 8[3]:151–162, 1994. Original illustrator—SB Lippitt.)

This press-fit limits the degrees of freedom for placing the humeral component (see Fig. 16–139). If necessary, slots are made in the tuberosity to accommodate the fins and throat of the component (Fig. 16–149). **(V16-15)** The slot for the lateral fin should be just posterior to the bicipital groove. A trial component body is inserted so that the prosthetic neck is centered on the neck of the bony humerus. **(V16-16)** The trial component is used as a guide to the excision of the osteophytes all around the humeral neck (see Fig. 16–18). **(V16-17)** Ideally, the horizontal and vertical distances between the tuberosity and the joint surface should be normalized (Fig. 16–150).

By placing various trial humeral heads, the surgeon can select the size that allows 70 degrees of internal rotation of the abducted arm (the "scarecrow" test) and 15 mm of translation on the posterior drawer test (see Fig. 16–12). These two parameters are guides to the posterior capsular laxity usually necessary to achieve a satisfactory range of motion. A global periglenoid capsular release may be necessary to achieve this laxity (see Figs. 16–3 and 16–4). However, in degenerative joint disease, preoperative posterior subluxation usually obviates the need for posterior capsular release. The important interplay between humeral component position and capsular laxity is recognized (see Fig. 16–10).

Preparation of the Glenoid. Accurate preparation of the glenoid bone requires the excellent surgical exposure that results from humeral head and osteophyte excision and appropriate capsular release. **(V16-18)**

The goals of the glenoid part of the arthroplasty are: (1) normalized glenoid orientation, (2) direct support of the component by precisely contoured bone, (3) secure fixation, and (4) avoidance of overstuffing (see Fig. 16–2).

Glenoid orientation is defined in terms of the glenoid center line: the line perpendicular to the center of the normally oriented glenoid face. The shoulder arthroplasty surgeon should practice verifying the landmarks for a normal glenoid center line by drilling holes perpendicular to the glenoid face of normal cadaveric scapulas and observing their exit in a consistent spot just medial to the anterior scapular neck: the "centering point" (see Fig. 16–25). This spot lies between the upper and lower crus of the body of the scapula as they approach the neck. After the capsular releases have been performed at surgery, this centering point can be palpated at the lateral extent of the subscapularis fossa. Because the location of this centering point is unaffected by arthritis, it is of great value in normalizing the orientation of a distorted glenoid face. It is particularly useful in correcting the posterior facing of the glenoid face that commonly results from posterior erosion in degenerative joint disease.

An index finger identifies the centering point on the anterior scapular neck while a hole is drilled from the center of the glenoid face toward it (see Fig. 16–26). **(V16-19** to **V16-22)** The orientation of the glenoid face is normalized using a spherical reamer with a guiding peg inserted along the glenoid center line drill hole (see Fig.

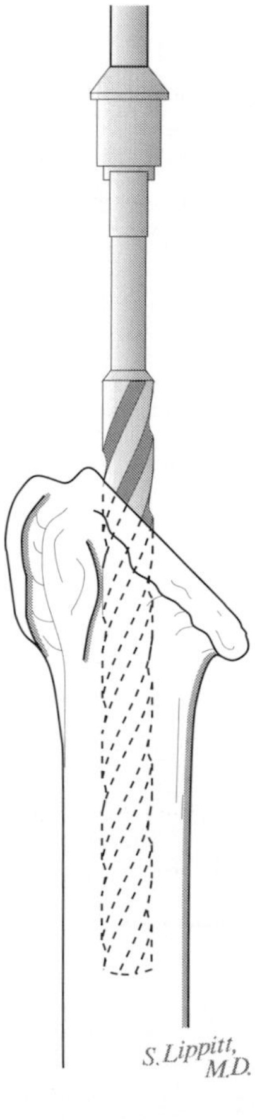

Figure 16–148

Reaming the humeral medullary canal. (From Pearl ML and Lippitt SB: Shoulder arthroplasty with a modular prosthesis. Tech Orthop 8[3]:151–162, 1994. Original illustrator—SB Lippitt.)

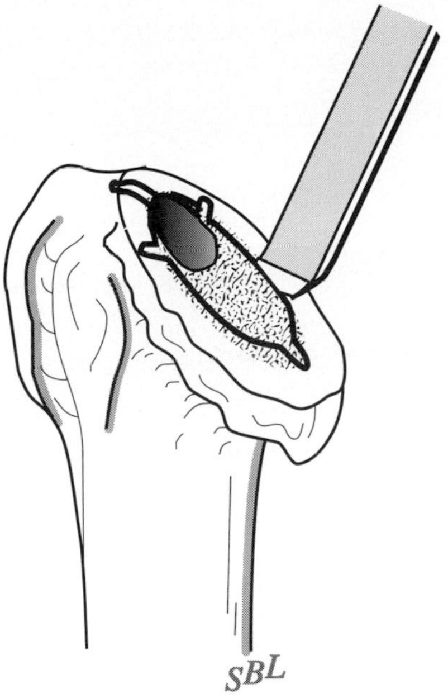

Figure 16–149

A small curved osteotome is used to remove the cancellous bone outlined by the body sizing osteotome. (From Pearl ML and Lippitt SB: Shoulder arthroplasty with a modular prosthesis. Tech Orthop 8[3]:151–162, 1994. Original illustrator—SB Lippitt.)

16–27). Appropriate positioning of retractors facilitates this reaming (Fig. 16–151). This technique is usually sufficient to manage posterior erosion; posterior glenoid bone grafting (Fig. 16–152) is rarely necessary. If there are reasons not to insert a glenoid component, this normalizing reaming provides an excellent nonprosthetic glenoidplasty.

Once the reaming is completed, the glenoid center line hole and the reamed glenoid surface can be used to orient precisely a drill guide for making additional fixation holes as required by the particular glenoid component design. **(V16-23)** Each hole is checked to determine whether it penetrates the scapula at its depth. Penetrating holes are cemented, but the cement is not pressurized.

A glenoid component is selected that covers the maximal amount of the prepared glenoid face with minimal overhang. The quality of the glenoid bone preparation is checked by inserting the glenoid trial and ensuring that it does not rock even when the surgeon's finger applies an eccentric load to the rim.

After water spray irrigation, the holes are cleaned and dried with a spray of sterile CO_2 gas (Innovative Surgical Devices, Stillwater, MN 55082). **(V16-24)** A small amount of cement is injected into each of the holes with a large-tipped syringe. Holes that do not penetrate the scapula can be pressurized by the syringe. No cement is placed on the bony face of the glenoid; if the back of the glenoid component matches the prepared bony face, there is no advantage of an interposed layer of cement, which could fail and displace, leaving the glenoid component relatively unsupported. Contact between precisely contoured bone and polyethylene ("bone backing" as opposed to metal backing) provides an optimal load transfer mechanism (see Fig. 16–133). After the glenoid component is pressed into position, the absence of residual cement bits in the posterior shoulder is verified.

Insertion of the humeral body is the next step in the arthroplasty. Prior to the insertion of the body, the surgeon places at least six No. 2 nonabsorbable sutures in secure bone at the anterior humeral neck for later attachment of the subscapularis tendon (Fig. 16–153). Final balancing of the soft tissues must be verified before the definitive humeral component is inserted. **(V16-25, V16-26)** A shoulder arthroplasty with balanced soft tissues should allow: (1) 70 degrees of internal rotation of the arm elevated in the coronal plane ("scarecrow" test), **(V16-27)** (2) 15 mm of posterior subluxation of the humeral head on the posterior drawer test, **(V16-28)** (3) 140 degrees of elevation, and (4) 40 degrees of external rotation of the unelevated arm with the subscapularis approximated (see Fig. 16–12). A tighter shoulder will not only have limited range of motion but may also challenge the rotator cuff (see Fig. 16–40) and foster obligate translation at the extremes of motion with resultant rim loading, risking glenoid loosening and component deformation (see Fig. 16–35). Some component systems are designed to allow a small amount of translation before rim loading occurs (see Figs. 16–36, 16–37, and 16–134). **V16-23 to V16-28**

The humeral component is then inserted into the prepared proximal humerus. The height, version, and fixation are carefully checked. If sufficient stability of the prosthesis in the bone is not achieved with a press-fit, bone graft or cement may be used.

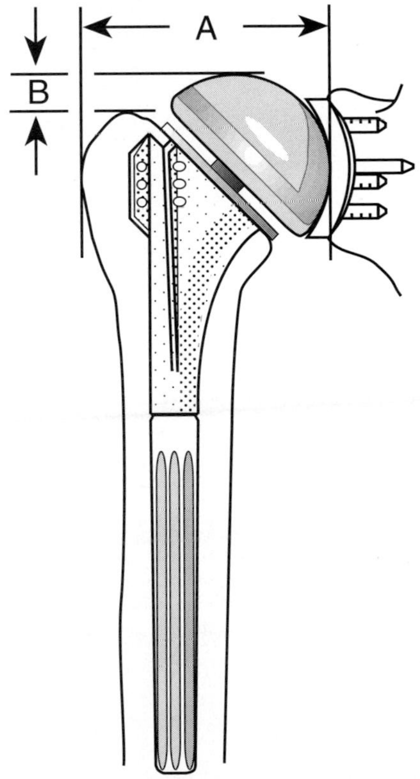

Figure 16–150

The prosthesis in position, reproducing normal tuberosity offset *(A)* and head height *(B)*.

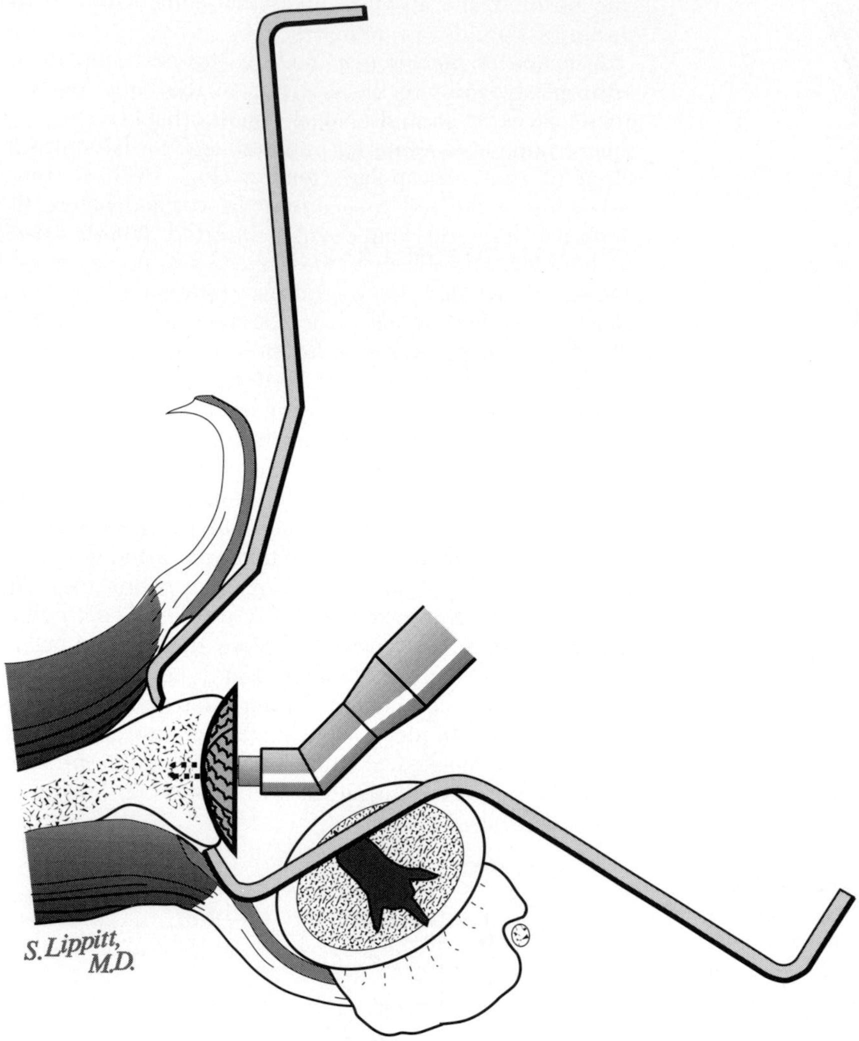

Figure 16–151

Anterior glenoid neck retractor and the posterior glenoid retractor allowing exposure of the glenoid fossa in reaming.

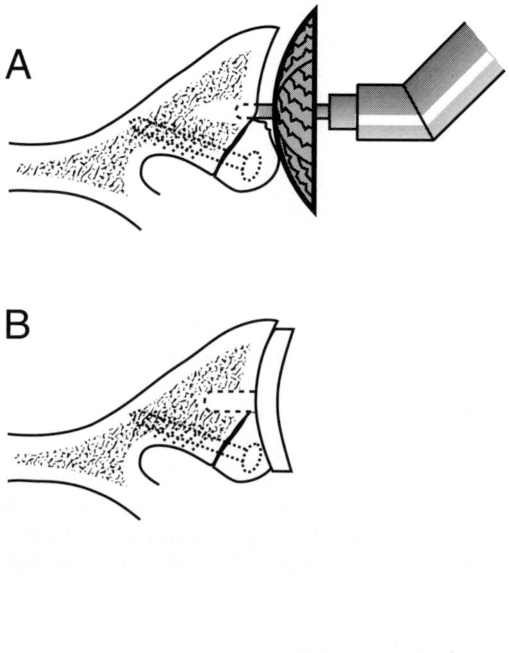

Figure 16–152

Posterior glenoid bone grafting. When there is a major defect of the posterior glenoid, a humeral head or iliac bone graft can be used to replace a deficient glenoid lip. If the fixation screw is recessed, the bone graft can be contoured and reamed for balanced support of glenoid component. (Modified from Matsen FA III, Lippitt SB, Sidles JA, and Harryman DT II: Practical Evaluation and Management of the Shoulder. Philadelphia: WB Saunders, 1994.)

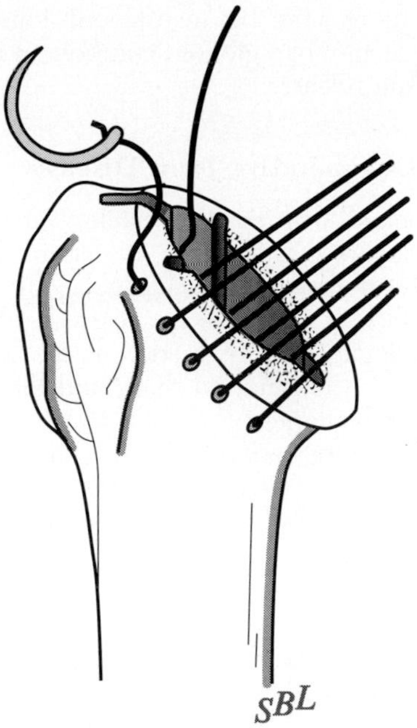

Figure 16–153

Placing sutures in the humeral neck through drill holes before insertion of the final humeral component.

Prior to *closure*, the wound is thoroughly inspected for debris. The joint is put through a full range of motion to verify smoothness and lack of unwanted contact (e.g., between the medial humerus and inferior glenoid or "Pooh Corner"). The wound is drained. The subscapularis is repaired securely to the humeral neck so that the unelevated arm can be externally rotated by 40 degrees (Fig. 16–154). **(V16-29)** If additional subscapularis length is required, a "Z-plasty" can be performed (Fig. 16–155), although this compromises the strength of the tendon. The wound is closed in layers. Simple interrupted skin sutures are preferred when substantial drainage is anticipated or when wound healing may be impaired (e.g., in an individual on corticosteroids or with thin rheumatoid skin).

V16-29

SPECIAL CONSIDERATIONS

Degenerative Joint Disease

In this condition, the glenoid face is typically flattened and often eroded posteriorly from chronic posterior subluxation (see Fig. 16–24). The glenoid may be distorted by peripheral osteophytes masking the location of the anatomic fossa. The humeral head may be flattened in a corresponding manner and effectively enlarged by the proliferation of "goat's beard" osteophytes from the anterior, inferior, and posterior articular rim. Intra-articular loose bodies may lie hidden in the subcoracoid or axillary recesses. Anterior capsular and subscapularis contractures are common in degenerative joint disease and require release; however, posterior capsular release is not performed if there is posterior humeral subluxation preoperatively.

Rheumatoid Arthritis

The basic principles of shoulder arthroplasty in rheumatoid arthritis are similar to those in degenerative arthritis, but some important differences exist. Rheumatoid tissues are much more fragile. The bone is more likely to frac-

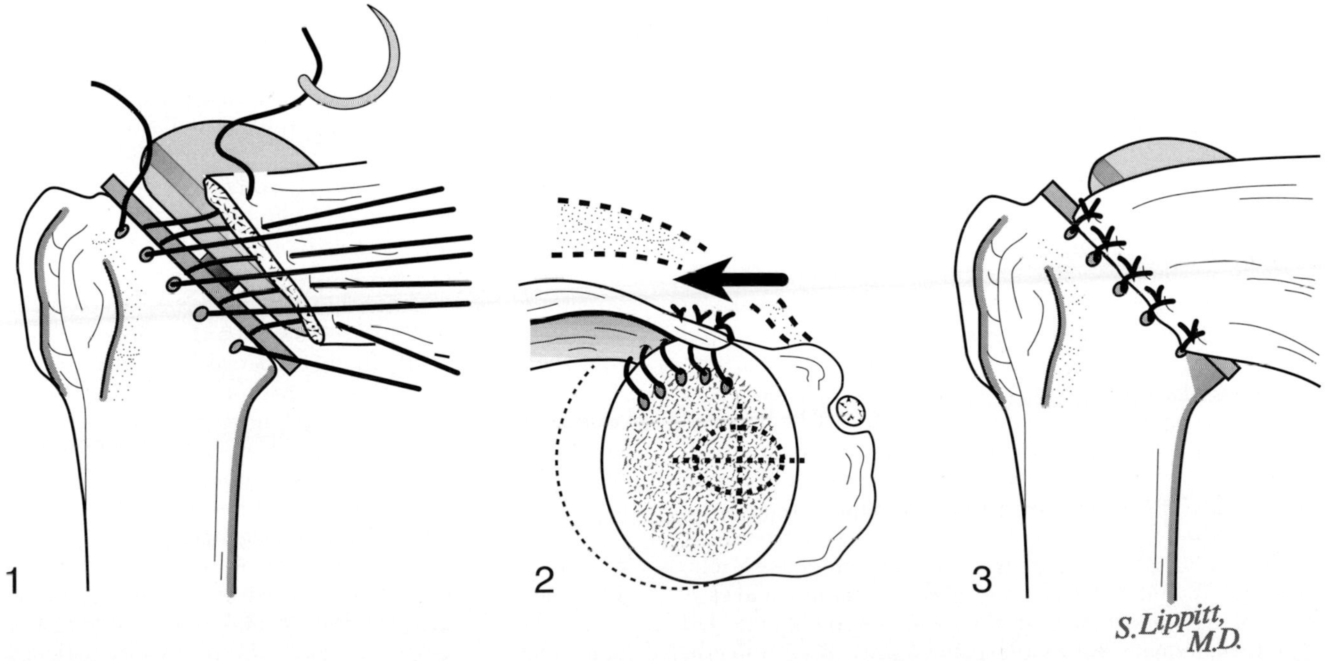

Figure 16–154

Subscapularis tendon repair to drill holes in the anterior humeral neck medial to the lesser tuberosity. (Modified from Matsen FA III, Lippitt SB, Sidles JA, and Harryman DT II: Practical Evaluation and Management of the Shoulder. Philadelphia: WB Saunders, 1994.)

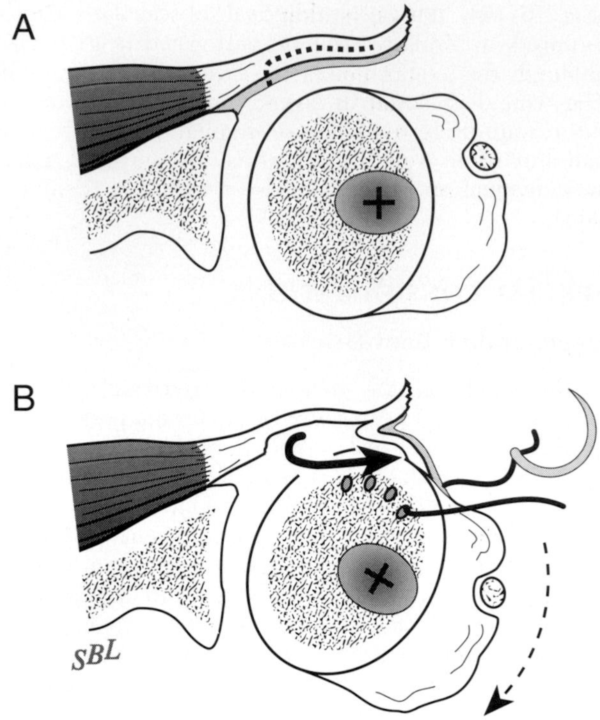

Figure 16–155

The inside-out Z-plasty. *A*, Additional length of the subscapularis tendon can be gained by splitting the capsule from the tendon medially, leaving their connection laterally. *B*, The medial end of the split capsule is reflected and attached to the humeral neck. (Modified from Matsen FA III, Lippitt SB, Sidles JA, and Harryman DT II: Practical Evaluation and Management of the Shoulder. Philadelphia: WB Saunders, 1994.)

ture, and the muscle and tendons are more susceptible to tear. Thus, from the outset, extreme care must be taken to preserve bone and soft tissue integrity. We refer to these requirements for extraordinary gentleness as "rheumatoid rules."

Because rheumatoid arthritis is an erosive and destructive disease, tissue deficiencies of the bone and rotator cuff are more likely to occur than in degenerative joint disease. Thus, the soft tissues anteriorly may be insufficient to allow for a subscapularis lengthening. The glenoid bone may be so eroded that there is insufficient stock to support a glenoid component. The rotator cuff may be partially or totally deficient. Thus, in the preoperative evaluation and in discussion with the patient concerning the possible outcomes of surgery, all of these factors need to be considered.

The standard preoperative scapular anteroposterior and axillary radiographs are required to evaluate the humeral and glenoid bone stock. In rheumatoid arthritis, the glenoid erosion is usually medial (rather than posterior as in degenerative joint disease). For this reason, only minimal glenoid reaming may be necessary to achieve an excellent quality fit to the back of the glenoid component. The potential fragility of the bone and soft tissues makes it particularly important that the joint not be overstuffed and that adequate soft tissue laxity be present for immediate postoperative motion. This is particularly a challenge in diminutive patients with juvenile rheumatoid arthritis who may also have a tiny humeral medullary canal. In some cases there may be insufficient joint volume to permit the insertion of a glenoid component despite complete soft tissue releases.

Secondary Degenerative Joint Disease

In post-traumatic arthritis, the challenges may be even greater. The anatomy is likely to be distorted by previous fracture and surgery. The nonarticular humeroscapular motion interface is likely to be scarred, obscuring important neurologic structures, such as the axillary nerve. The tuberosities, the humeral shaft, and the glenoid may be ununited or malunited.

As a first step, the motion interface must be carefully freed, and the axillary nerve is identified both as it crosses the subscapularis and as it courses laterally on the deep surface of the deltoid. Case by case judgments must be made concerning the need for osteotomy to try to restore more normal anatomic relationships, recognizing that additional healing and postoperative protection may be required. Again, the goal is restoration of anatomic relationships, firm fixation of components, soft tissue balance, stability, and smooth gliding in the humeroscapular motion interface.

Capsulorrhaphy Arthropathy

Shoulders affected by capsulorrhaphy arthropathy present additional challenges, such as neurovascular scarring from previous surgery, soft tissue contractures, bone deficiencies, implants from previous surgery, changes of glenoid version, and an increased potential for glenohumeral instability after the arthroplasty (see Fig. 16–8).

Cuff Tear Arthropathy

In this condition there are several unique challenges for regaining glenohumeral smoothness. The humeral head is subluxated in a superior position so that it is articulating with the coracoacromial arch. The rotator cuff is almost never amenable to a strong repair, and the glenoid is eroded superiorly, so that an acetabular-like structure is formed in continuity with the coracoacromial arch. Under these circumstances, normal glenohumeral relationships are very difficult to normalize and maintain by a durable cuff reconstruction. More often it is preferable to accept the altered joint relationship that uses the "acetabulum" for secondary stability in the absence of primary stability from the rotator cuff. In this "special hemiarthroplasty," the articular surface of the proximal humerus is resurfaced with a component matching the preoperative humeral joint surface size and position. The tuberosities are smoothed so that they are congruous with the humeral articular surface. This allows for the proximal humerus to match the "acetabulum" and to articulate smoothly within it. It is very important to avoid using "oversized" humeral components, because they overstuff the joint, do not match the concavity of the "acetabulum," and restrict joint motion. In a special hemiarthroplasty, the patient is spared the necessity of protecting a rotator cuff repair, so that immediate passive and active exercises can be instituted after surgery. The patient is also spared the risk of

Table 16–20 INCREMENT IN FUNCTION AFTER SPECIAL HEMIARTHROPLASTY FOR CUFF TEAR ARTHROPATHY

	PREOPERATIVE	*POSTOPERATIVE*
Active elevation	71° (Range of 50–100)	115° (Range of 50–160)
External rotation	30°	41°
Internal rotation	L-5	L-1
Perineal care	2/10 Patients	9/10 Patients
Reach opposite axilla	3/10 Patients	10/10 Patients
Comb hair	2/10 Patients	8/10 Patients
Sleep on side	2/10 Patients	9/10 Patients
Use above shoulder level	0/10 Patients	6/10 Patients

glenoid loosening from the rocking horse mechanism (see Fig. 16–35).

The ideal patient for this procedure has a normal deltoid muscle, a concentric coracoacromial "acetabulum" stabilizing the proximal humerus, which is superiorly displaced with respect to the glenoid, concentric erosion of the upper glenoid fossa, a "femoralized" upper humerus with rounding off of the greater tuberosity, an irreparable rotator cuff defect, no previous surgical compromise of the acromion or coracoacromial ligament, good patient motivation, and realistic expectations.

In a series of 10 patients with special hemiarthroplasty for rotator cuff tear arthropathy, the range of active motion and function were substantially improved by this procedure (Table 16–20). These results are not as good as those for total glenohumeral arthroplasty, because the patient lacks the benefit of both prosthetic glenoid smoothness as well as the function of the rotator cuff.

POSTOPERATIVE REHABILITATION

Rehabilitation is started immediately after surgery in the recovery room with the initiation of slow and gentle continuous passive motion (see Fig. 16–132).

For patients who have had an interscalene block before surgery, this early motion is pain free. Continuous passive motion should be stopped and the wrist brace removed every 2 to 3 hours for approximately 15 to 20 minutes to relieve any skin and nerve compression. A sling is worn between exercise sessions until active muscle control is regained.

The patient-conducted rehabilitation program is started on the day of surgery under instructions given by the surgeon or therapist. Although the program may vary with the details of the surgery performed, the following is a description of the basic program for shoulder arthroplasty. The stretching exercises include: (1) elevation, (2) external rotation limited to 40 degrees, (3) internal rotation, (4) cross-body adduction, (5) grip strengthening, (6) elbow range of motion, (7) external rotator isometrics, and (8) anterior, middle, and posterior deltoid isometrics. The patient is instructed to perform a total of five exercise sessions spread evenly throughout the day both while in the hospital as well as at home after discharge.*

Charts are placed on the wall in full view from the patient's bed to graph the progress of external rotation and elevation (Fig. 16–156) as measured by the surgeon or therapist. This provides positive feedback for rehabilitative progress.

For the routine arthroplasty, the range-of-motion goals to be achieved before discharge are 140 degrees of elevation, 40 degrees of external rotation, and functional internal rotation and cross-body adduction. These goals may be modified according to the specific surgical procedure. Because the desired range has been achieved on the operating table, the patient's task is simplified, he or she has only to maintain this range during the postoperative period.

Elevation (overhead reach) is performed in the supine position (lying flat on the back), grasping the wrist or elbow of the operative shoulder with the hand of the unoperated arm, pulling up toward the ceiling, and reaching overhead as high as possible to the goal of 140 degrees with the arm relaxed (see Fig. 16–75). A pulley or the forward lean (see Fig. 16–76) may also be useful in achieving elevation, especially if the opposite shoulder is involved.

External rotation (rotation away from the body) is performed in the supine position (see Fig. 16–77) with the

*For example, if tuberosity or cuff fixation has been part of the procedure, external rotation isometrics and active elevation may be delayed.

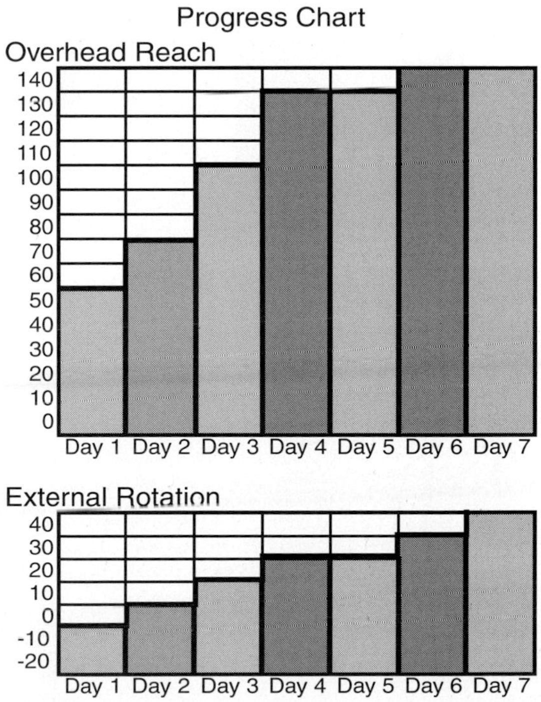

Figure 16–156

Typical wall charts showing the improvement in overhead reach and external rotation after surgery. (From Matsen FA III, Lippitt SB, Sidles JA, and Harryman DT II: Practical Evaluation and Management of the Shoulder. Philadelphia: WB Saunders, 1994.)

operative side elbow held against or close to the side and flexed to 90 degrees. A stick is held in both hands so that the unaffected extremity pushes on the operative arm to externally rotate it to the goal of 40 degrees. Holding on to a door and turning away is another useful way to stretch external rotation (see Fig. 16–78).

Internal rotation is performed by grasping the wrist of the relaxed involved arm with the nonoperative side hand; the hands are lifted up the back as high as possible. A towel can also be used to assist with pulling the involved arm into internal rotation behind the back (see Fig. 16–79).

Cross-body adduction is performed sitting or standing, grasping the elbow of the involved arm with the other hand. The involved arm is relaxed and the elbow is extended and pulled across the body until a stretch is felt (Fig. 16–80).

Active elbow motion is performed standing in order to allow unimpeded or unrestricted flexion/extension and supination/pronation. Grip strengthening is performed to maintain forearm tone and can be accomplished using a foam pad or tennis ball.

External rotator isometrics are performed with the forearm at neutral rotation. An attempt is made to move the wrist out to the side against the resistance of the other hand or a fixed object (see Fig. 16–82). Deltoid isometrics are also performed standing or sitting. The arm is held in a neutral position and pushed forward, to the side, and to the back to exercise the anterior, middle, and posterior deltoid respectively.

Supine presses are performed initially holding a cloth or stick between both hands with the hands held close together (Fig. 16–157). From a starting position with the elbows bent and the hands lying across the chest, the stick is pushed straight to the ceiling with both hands in a slow and controlled manner and then slowly lowered back to the resting position at the chest. The space between the two hands is progressively increased. As the

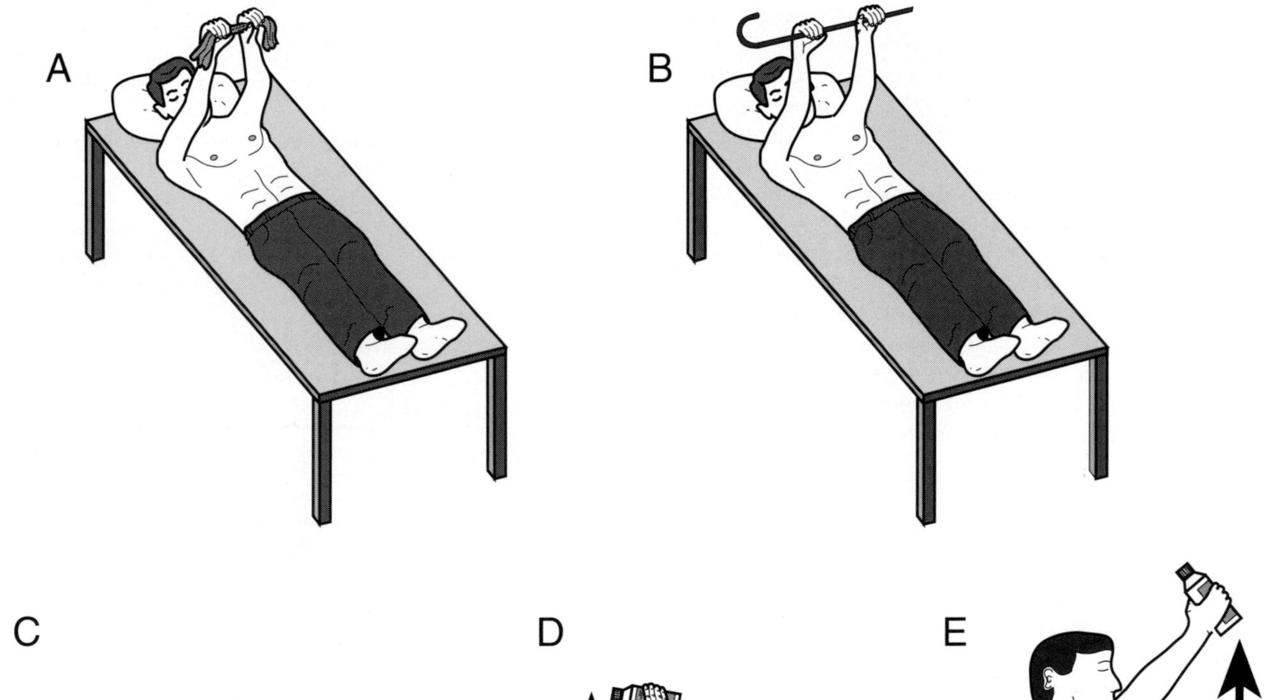

Figure 16–157

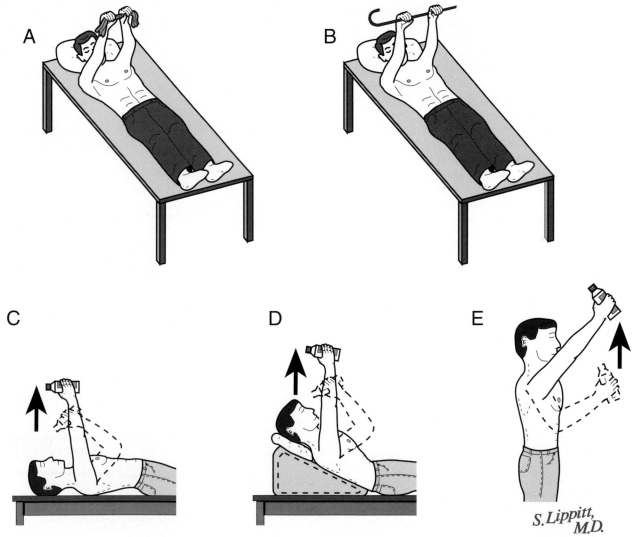

Progressive supine press exercises to strengthen flexion. The motion is always pushing up toward the ceiling, ending with a lift of the shoulder blade off the bed. *A*, Start with two hands together holding a wash cloth; *B*, then two hands apart; *C*, then one hand with a 1-pint (i.e., 1 lb) weight; *D*, then one hand with a 1-pint weight with greater degrees of sitting up; and finally, *E*, one hand with a 1-pint weight while standing. (Modified from Matsen FA III, Lippitt SB, Sidles JA, and Harryman DT II: Practical Evaluation and Management of the Shoulder. Philadelphia: WB Saunders, 1994.)

shoulder becomes stronger, the hands are pushed to the ceiling in a slow and controlled manner independent of each other. With increasing strength, the exercise is conducted with a 1-lb weight that is held in the involved hand as it is pressed to the ceiling. When the patient is comfortable, the incline is gradually increased to eventually reach the upright position. All presses should be performed in a slow and controlled manner; they are progressed to the next level only when 20 repetitions can be performed comfortably.

The patient is instructed in all these exercises on three occasions: (1) before surgery, (2) immediately after surgery, and (3) before leaving the hospital. Before discharge, the goals of assisted external rotation to 40 degrees and assisted elevation to 140 degrees must be accomplished.

The patient is placed in charge of his or her own rehabilitation and taught to progressively return to normal use of the shoulder. Typically, keyboarding and driving are achieved at 2 weeks; swimming is started at 6 weeks; golf or tennis are started at 3 to 6 months; and chopping wood is precluded.

ROCKWOOD'S PREFERRED TECHNIQUE FOR SHOULDER ARTHROPLASTY

Although a number of surgical approaches for performing arthroplasty of the shoulder have been described, most procedures are performed through an anterior approach to the joint. The anterior, long deltopectoral approach without detaching the origin of the deltoid as described by Neer[258, 259, 305] is currently our preferred approach for shoulder arthroplasty. Two important principles of this approach are preservation of the anterior attachment of the deltoid to the clavicle and the acromion and protection of the axillary and musculocutaneous nerves.

The anterior portion of the deltoid must be preserved, because there is no muscle to effectively compensate for the loss of this powerful shoulder flexor.[55] Weakness of the posterior portion of the deltoid is less disabling, because the latissimus dorsi is a strong synergistic muscle. Detachment of the anterior deltoid is problematic, because secure reattachment of this muscle after shoulder arthroplasty is difficult and impairs postoperative rehabilitation for the patient.[82] Patients with a detached or denervated anterior deltoid after shoulder arthroplasty have a poor outcome in that they have limited motion and decreased strength, and they are extremely dissatisfied with the procedure.[145, 363]

The relationship of the axillary and musculocutaneous nerves must always be of concern to the surgeon. Although positioning the arm in adduction and external rotation may make anterior approaches to the glenohumeral joint safer,[50, 253, 258, 363] it is much better to identify the nerves and protect them during the entire surgical procedure. Burkhead and associates[53, 55] have described in detail the tremendous variation, from one specimen to another, in the course and position of these nerves. Laceration of the axillary nerve denervates the entire deltoid muscle. Because all important shoulder function requires elevation in the scapular plane, injury to the axillary nerve is the most catastrophic neurogenic injury that can occur during shoulder arthroplasty. Disastrous consequences await those surgeons who embark on a shoulder arthroplasty without exact knowledge of the location of the axillary nerve and fail to protect it.[145]

Anatomic Landmarks

Three anterior prominences—the clavicle, acromion, and coracoid—are excellent guides to the placement of the incision and are intimately related to important structures in developing the exposure. The clavicle is just superior to the upper portion of the deltopectoral groove. Its position is readily palpable and marks the most superior aspect of the incision.

The acromion serves as a large surface area for attachment of the deltoid, increasing the muscle's efficiency. If wide reflection of the deltoid becomes necessary, the deltoid should never be released from the acromion during arthroplasty; rather, the partial deltoid insertion can be released.[77, 253, 258] The interval between the acromion and the coracoid process is spanned by the tough, wide coracoacromial ligament. It is rarely necessary to divide or resect this ligament, because it serves as a buttress to anterior displacement of the humeral head.

The coracoid serves as a "lighthouse" to the deltopectoral interval.[258] It lies within the deltopectoral groove, and its palpation is a landmark for the position of the cephalic vein and the brachial plexus. The cephalic vein is intimately attached to the deltoid and directly overlies the coracoid. The brachial plexus and its terminal divisions lie medial to the base of the coracoid.

Nerves

The axillary nerve is one of the two terminal branches of the posterior cord of the brachial plexus. It arises posterior to the coracoid process and crosses the anteroinferior border and then the lateral border of the subscapularis muscle. At this point, the nerve joins the posterior humeral circumflex artery, and together they exit posteriorly through the quadrangular space where the axillary nerve sends two branches to supply the capsule. The axillary nerve then splits into two major trunks. The posterior trunk gives off branches to the teres minor and posterior deltoid, terminating as the superior lateral cutaneous nerve. The anterior trunk passes forward around the humerus and supplies first the middle deltoid and then the anterior deltoid.[53, 55, 206]

The musculocutaneous nerve originates from the lateral cord of the brachial plexus and innervates the coracobrachialis muscle as well as the biceps brachii and brachialis muscles. The coracobrachialis muscle is occasionally innervated directly from the lateral cord of the brachial plexus. Flatow and associates[121] noted that the lateral portion of the musculocutaneous nerve penetrates into the coracobrachialis muscle at a distance of 3.1 to 8.2 cm from the tip of the coracoid. However, we have seen cases in which the nerve comes from under the coracoid to then penetrate the conjoined tendon from the lateral side. The most common cause of damage to this nerve during shoulder arthroplasty is overzealous retraction. We

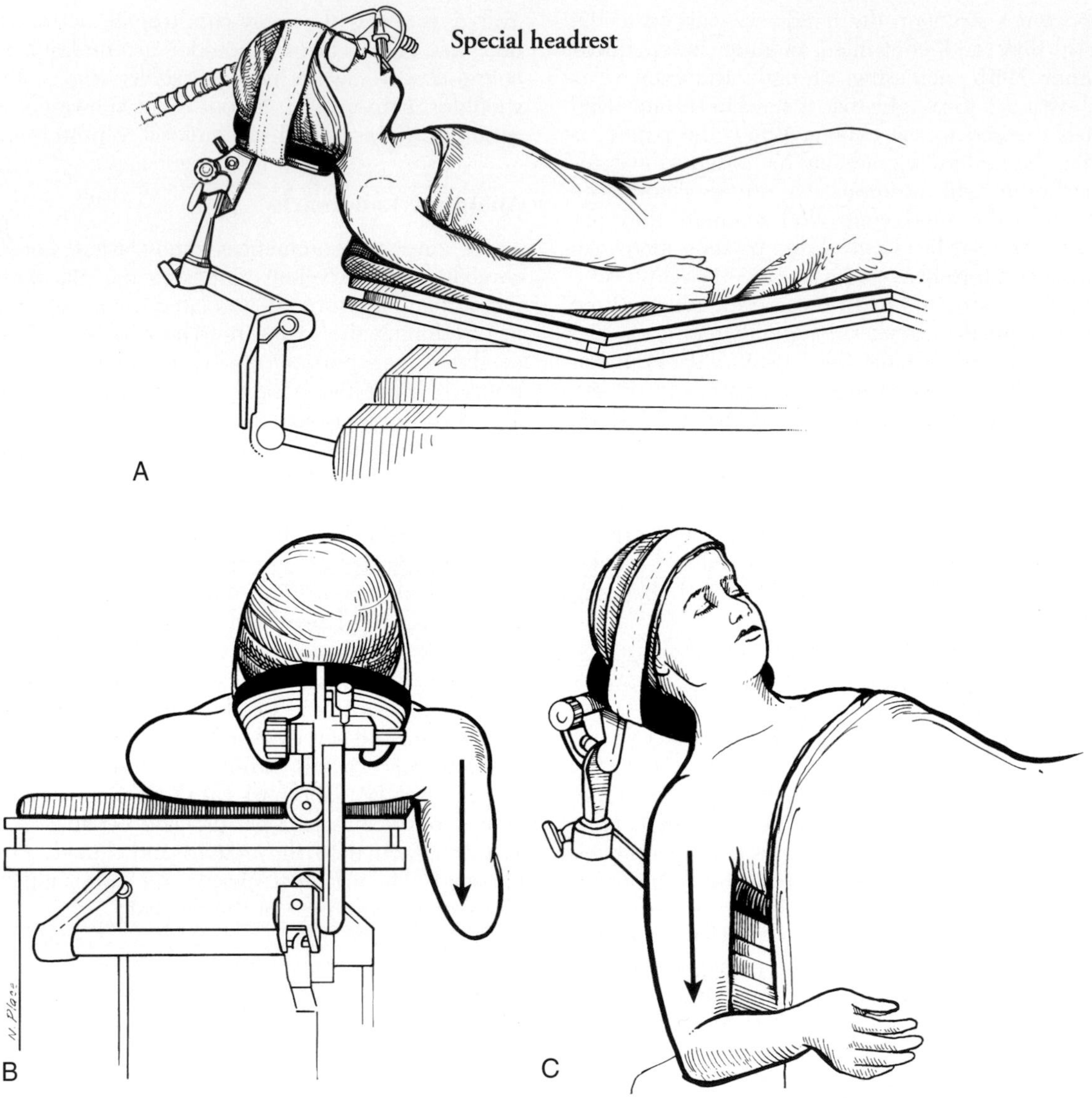

Figure 16–158

A, Proper positioning of the patient on the operating room table with the head supported by a McConnell headrest (*B*). *C*, The patient is on the top outer corner of the table so that the arm can be extended off the table down towards the floor.

prefer not to detach the conjoined tendons because they protect the neurovascular bundle during medial retraction of the pectoralis major muscle. Powerful retraction on the conjoined tendons, which are made up by the short head of the biceps and the coracobrachialis, may produce a traction injury to the musculocutaneous nerve. Careful attention to retraction should minimize this possibility.

Surgical Approach

Neer and associates[258, 259, 305] described the development of the currently preferred anterior deltopectoral surgical approach. Initially, a short deltopectoral approach with detachment of the anterior portion of the deltoid from the clavicle was used; however, this weakened the muscle and delayed the postoperative rehabilitation. In 1976 and 1977, Neer utilized a superior approach with detachment of the middle section of the deltoid; however, this approach was found to weaken the middle part of the deltoid. In September 1977, Neer began to exclusively utilize the long deltopectoral approach, which has become the standard for shoulder arthroplasty because of the greater ease of rehabilitation after surgery and is the technique described here.[253]

In 1977, the author (CAR) recalls chatting with Neer about his approach, and it seemed incredible because I had trouble doing the arthroplasty procedure after detaching the majority of the anterior deltoid. I had to visit him and observe his technique before I could use it on my patients.

Surgical Technique

The patient is positioned on the operating room table in the semi-Fowler position with the knees flexed to avoid dependency (Fig. 16–158*A*). The standard headrest from the operating table is removed and replaced with the McConnell headrest (McConnell Orthopaedic Equipment Co., Greenville, TX). This allows the patient to be positioned at the top and edge of the table (see Fig. 16–158*B*, *C*), which is necessary in order to be able to extend the externally rotated arm off the side of the table down toward the floor, enabling the surgeon to ream the intramedullary canal and insert the prosthesis. The patient's head should be secured to the headrest with tape, and tape can be used to secure the anesthesia tube to the headrest. Care should be taken to rest the head in a position that avoids hyperextension or tilting of the neck, which may cause compression of the cervical roots. We have found it best to position the table in the proper semi-Fowler position before securing the head to the headrest.

Plastic towel drapes are used to block out the area being prepared and to isolate the hair and the anesthesia equipment from the operative field. The entire upper extremity is prepared, and the arm is draped free. The axilla is separated as much as possible from the sterile surgical field. After the skin incision is marked, the surgical site is covered with sterile adherent plastic drapes. A special shoulder drape pack is available and includes towel drapes, body drapes, gowns, gloves, and a marking pen (Shoulder Drape Pack, DePuy Co., Warsaw, IN).

(V16-30) The skin incision is made in a straight line with the arm held in 30 degrees of abduction (Fig. 16–159*A*). The incision should begin from the superior aspect of the clavicle, then over the top of the coracoid; the incision should extend down the anterior aspect of the arm. Once the incision has been made, the cephalic vein near the deltopectoral interval should be identified (see Fig. 16–159*B*) and protected, because postoperative extremity swelling and pain will be decreased by its preservation. The vein is usually intimately associated with the deltoid, because of the many feeding vessels from the deltoid into the cephalic vein. It is for this reason that we recommend the cephalic vein be taken laterally with the deltoid muscle. The feeding vessels coming into the vein from the region of the pectoralis major muscle should be damped and tied, allowing lateral retraction of the deltoid muscle with the vein. The deep surface of the deltoid is then freed from the underlying tissues using a combination of blunt and sharp dissection all the way from its origin on the clavicle down to its insertion onto the humeral shaft. On occasion, as recommended by Neer, it may be necessary to partially free the insertion of the deltoid from the humeral shaft.

V16-30 to V16-31

When the deep surface of the deltoid has been completely freed, abduct and externally rotate the arm. Protect the exposed surface of the deltoid with a moist laparotomy sponge, and retract the deltoid laterally with two Richardson retractors. We routinely use moist lap sponges during the procedure because they seem to be easier on the soft tissue. Then, retract the conjoined tendon medially with a Richardson retractor. It is rarely necessary to release a portion of the conjoined tendon or divide the coracoid process for additional exposure.

(V16-31) The tendon of the upper portion of the pecto-

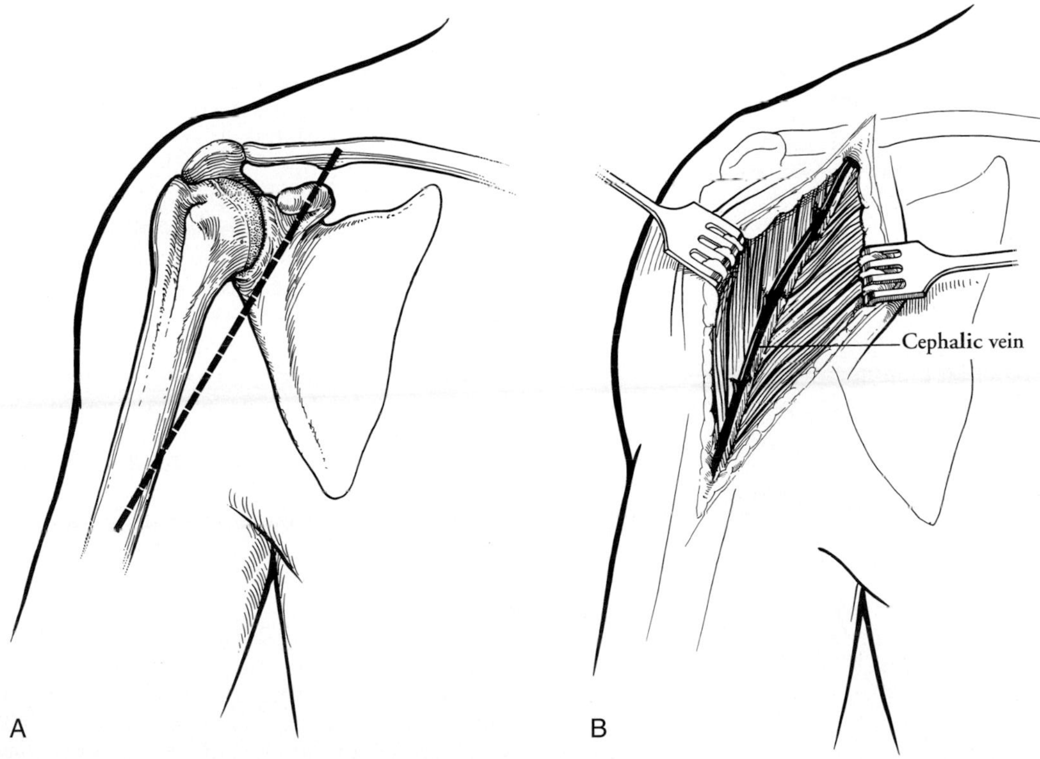

Figure 16–159

A, Placement of the surgical incision from the clavicle across the top of the coracoid down to the anterior aspect of the arm. *B*, The cephalic vein should be preserved and placed laterally with the deltoid muscle.

ralis major is identified, and the upper portion of the tendon is released with an electrocautery cutting blade to aid in the exposure of the inferior aspect of the joint (Fig. 16–160). Care must be taken to avoid injury to the long head of the biceps tendon during this maneuver. If the patient has a marked internal rotation contracture (i.e., −30 degrees or more), then the entire pectoralis major tendon can be released from its insertion. This tendon release should not be repaired at the completion of the operation.

V16-32 to V16-34

(V16-32) The anterior humeral circumflex vessels are then identified on the lower third of the subscapularis tendon. The vessels are isolated, clamped, and ligated (Fig. 16–161). Due to the extensive anastomoses of blood supply in this area, other sources of bleeding should be expected and controlled with electrocautery during release of the subscapularis tendon.

It is now important to identify the musculocutaneous and axillary nerves. Palpate the musculocutaneous nerve as it comes from the brachial plexus into the medial aspect of the conjoined tendon (Fig. 16–162*A*). The nerve usually penetrates the muscle about 4 to 5 cm inferior to the tip of the coracoid; however, as previously mentioned, the nerve may have a higher penetration into the conjoined muscle-tendon unit. The proximity of this nerve must be kept in mind during retraction of the conjoined tendon.

(V16-33) The axillary nerve is then located by passing the volar surface of the index finger down along the anterior surface of the subscapularis muscle (see Fig. 16–162*B*). As the hand and wrist are supinated, the finger is rotated and hooked anteriorly to identify the axillary nerve (see Fig. 16–162*A*). Scarring and adhesions may result in the nerve being plastered onto the anterior surface of the subscapularis so that identification of the nerve is difficult. When this occurs, an elevator should be passed along the anterior surface of the subscapularis muscle to create an interval between the muscle and the nerve. Always identify the axillary nerve and carefully retract and hold it out of the way, especially during the critical steps of releasing and resecting the anteroinferior capsule. We have found that a Scoffield type of retractor works well to protect the axillary nerve.

The amount of passive external rotation present at this point in the procedure determines the specific technique for subscapularis tendon release. **(V16-34)** We currently release the tendon from its insertion into the lesser tuberosity, just medial to the long head of the biceps tendon (Fig. 16–163*A*). When a good stump of the subscapularis tendon has been freed up, heavy nonabsorbable 1-mm Dacron tape should be secured to the tendon with two or three "W" stitches or modified Kessler stitches. These sutures can then be used as traction sutures when freeing up the rest of the tendon from the underlying capsule and scar tissue. At the time of closure, the tendon is repaired back to the cut surface of the humerus with these sutures (see Fig. 16–163*B*). The release of the tendon from the lesser tuberosity and its repair back to the cut surface of the neck of the humerus allows greater excursion of external rotation. If the patient's shoulder has marked limitation of external rotation, then lengthen the tendon using a coronal Z-plasty technique (see Fig.

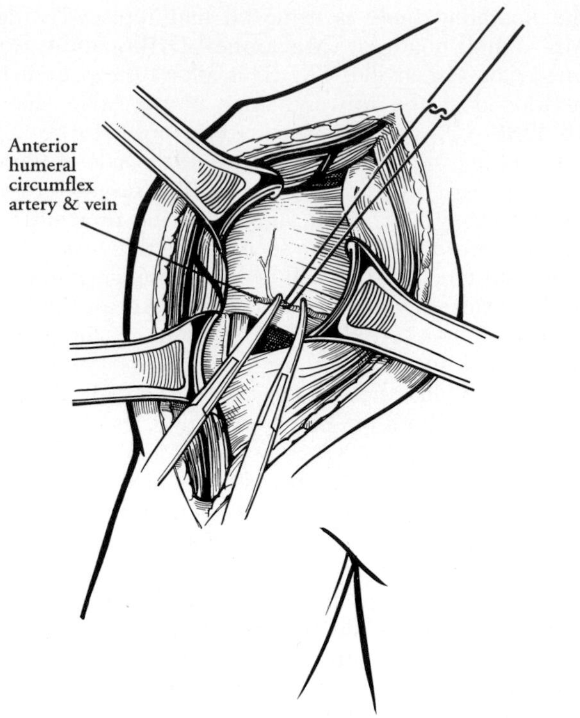

Figure 16–161

The anterior humeral circumflex vessels, lying on the inferior portion of the subscapularis tendon, should be isolated and coagulated or ligated.

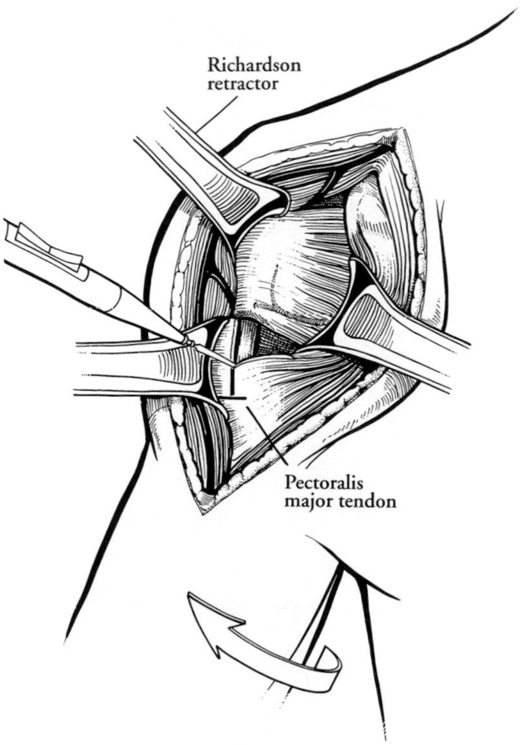

Figure 16–160

The deltoid and pectoralis major tendons are retracted and the upper portion of the pectoralis major tendon should be released. Care should be taken not to injure the underlying long head of the biceps tendon.

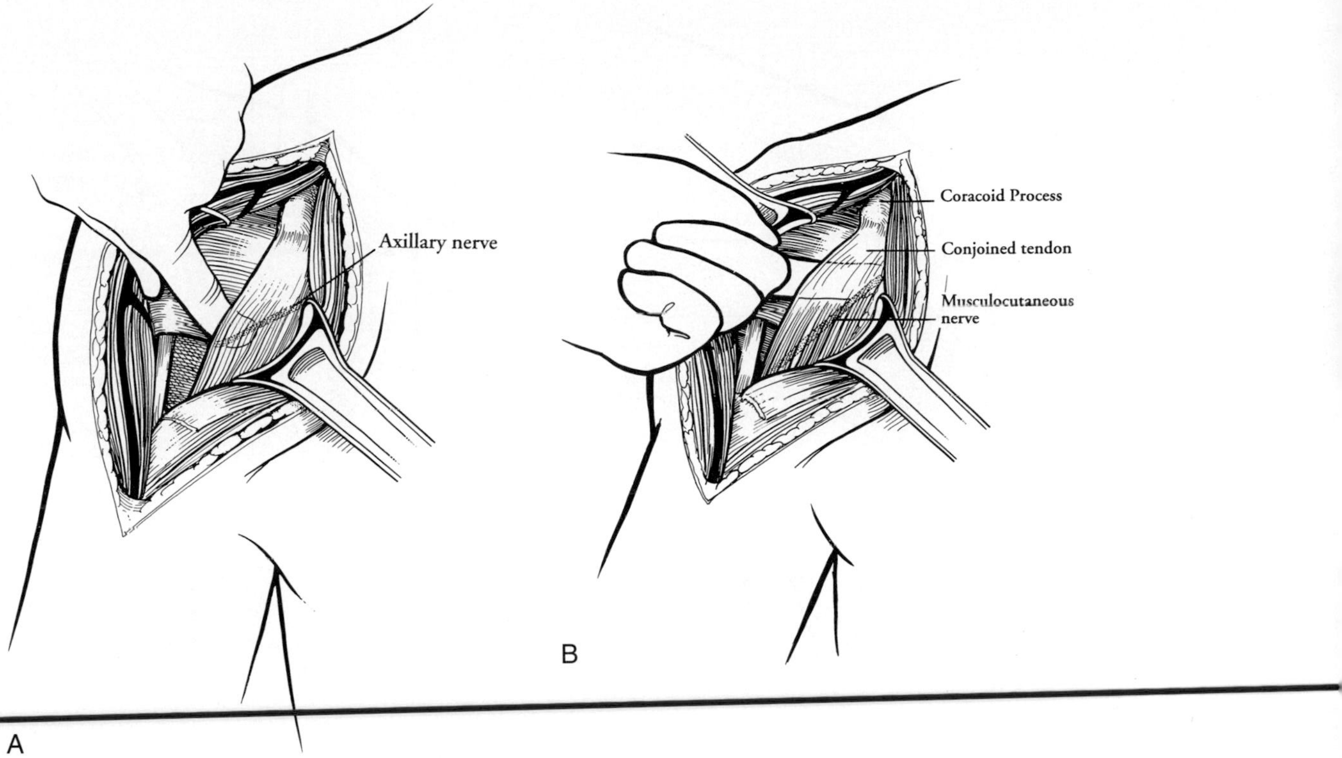

Figure 16–162

A and *B*, The identification of the musculocutaneous and axillary nerves.

16–163*C, D*). Each centimeter of tendon lengthened will equal approximately 20 degrees of additional external rotation. When the coronal Z-plasty procedure is performed, include the capsule on the lateral stump of the tendon for additional strength. At the time of closure, the subscapularis tendon should be repaired with heavy nonabsorbable 1-mm surgical tape.

After the subscapularis tendon has been released, it

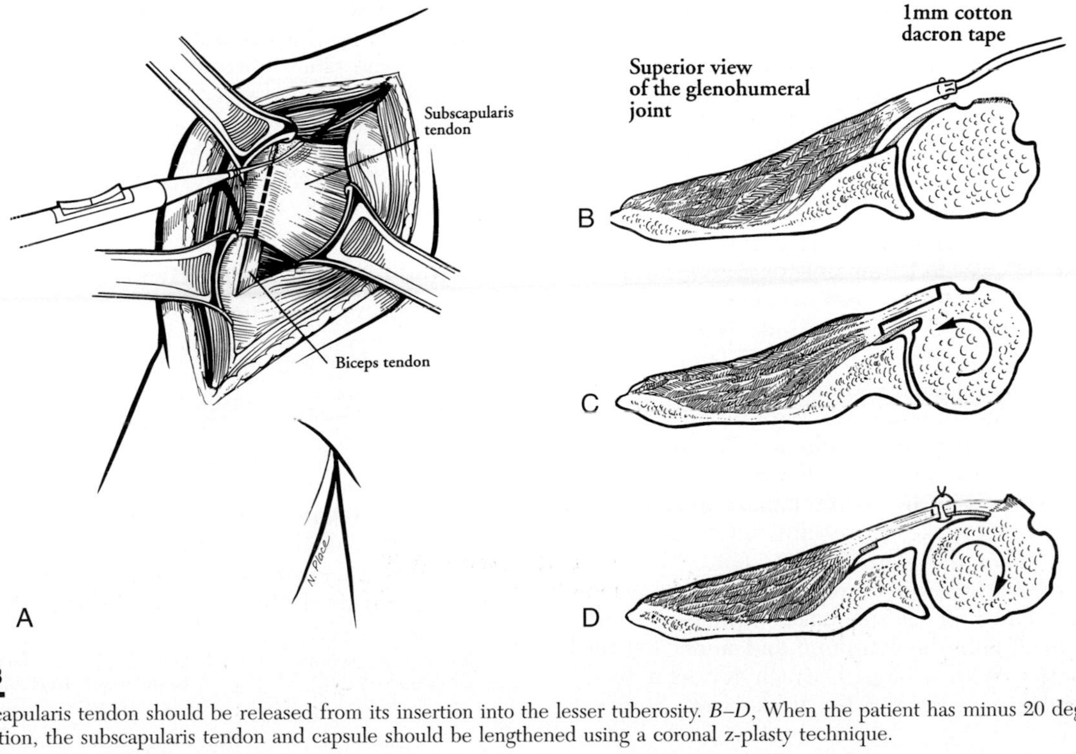

Figure 16–163

A, The subscapularis tendon should be released from its insertion into the lesser tuberosity. *B–D*, When the patient has minus 20 degrees or less of external rotation, the subscapularis tendon and capsule should be lengthened using a coronal z-plasty technique.

V16-35 to V16-36

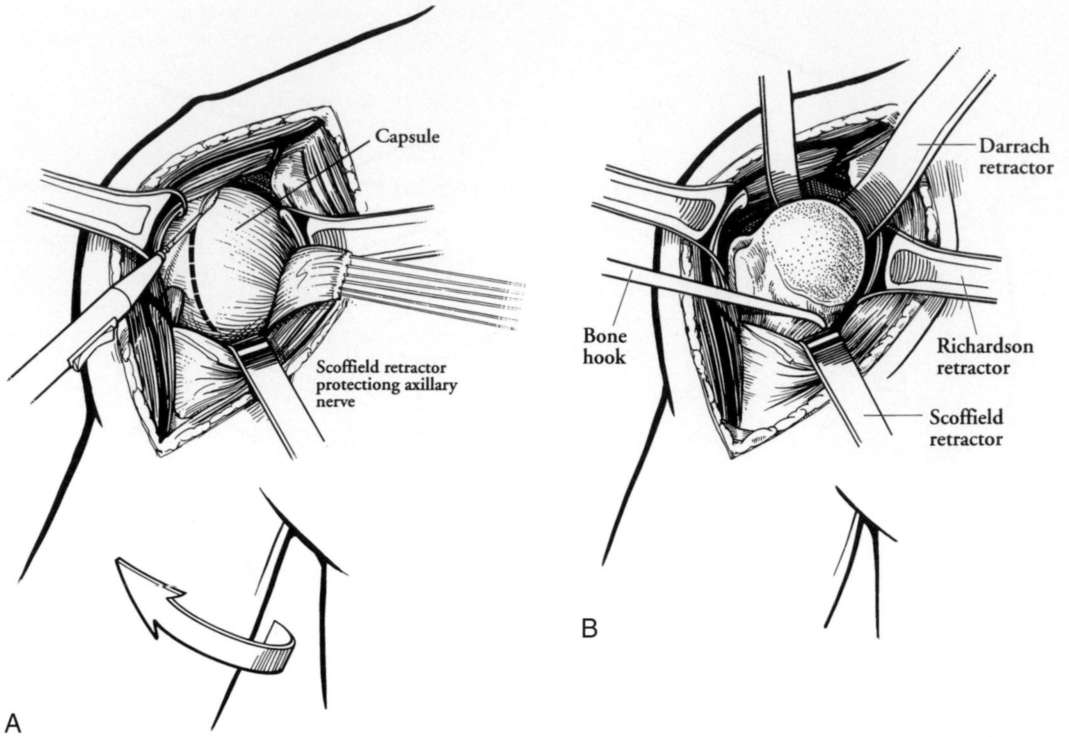

Figure 16–164

A, The capsule should be released from the neck of the humerus from the top to the bottom. Failure to release the capsule all the way inferiorly will lead to difficulty in displacing the head of the humerus up and out of the glenoid fossa. *B*, With Darrach retractors in the shoulder as a skid, a bone hook can be used to lift the head of the humerus out of the glenoid fossa while the arm is externally rotated and extended off the edge of the table.

must be completely freed up from the capsule and the anterior glenoid rim, so that it once again becomes a dynamic muscle-tendon unit. This process requires that the subscapularis muscle-tendon unit be released 360 degrees around its circumference. This usually requires a fair amount of soft tissue dissection along the anterior aspect of the neck of the scapula. During this dissection, it is imperative to identify, protect, and retract the axillary nerve with a Scoffield-type retractor. It is important to have a free, dynamic, and functioning subscapularis muscle-tendon unit at the time of its repair.

On occasion, the capsule will be released at the time of the subscapularis release. If that occurs, the anterior capsule must be resected from the posterior surface of the subscapularis so that a free, dynamic subscapularis tendon can be obtained. If the capsule is just released from the glenoid and left in place, it will later scar back to the humerus and glenoid and once again limit external rotation. **(V16-35)** The anteroinferior capsule must then be released from the humerus all the way inferiorly to at least the 6 o'clock position, even in the presence of a large inferior osteophyte (Fig. 16–164*A*). Failure to release the inferior capsule will make it very difficult to deliver the head up and out of the glenoid fossa. Later, the entire anterior inferior capsule will be released from the glenoid and discarded. Once the capsule has been released inferiorly, pass a small bone hook around and under the neck of the humerus. With a large Darrach retractor in the joint and a bone hook around the neck of the humerus, the arm is externally rotated, adducted, and extended off the edge of the table to deliver the head up and out of the glenoid fossa (see Fig. 16–164*B*). If the humeral head cannot be delivered in this fashion, the inferior capsule is likely still intact and must be further released. It is important to obtain this exposure with the arm extended off the side of the table in external rotation before proceeding with humeral head resection.

TECHNIQUE FOR NONCONSTRAINED SHOULDER ARTHROPLASTY*

Resection of the Humeral Head

Resection of the humeral head is a critical part of the procedure. When there is no posterior glenoid erosion, as determined by the CT scan, the humeral head should be removed with the arm in 20 to 25 degrees of external rotation. This can be accomplished by flexing the elbow 90 degrees and then externally rotating the arm 20 to 25 degrees (Fig. 16–165). The varus-valgus angle of the head to be removed is determined using a humeral osteotomy template (Fig. 16–166*A*). **(V16-36)** Place the template along the anterior aspect of the arm parallel to the shaft of the humerus, and mark the angle at which the head will be

*The surgical technique used in this chapter is adapted from the manual entitled *Global Shoulder Arthroplasty System* of DePuy, Inc., 1994.[304]

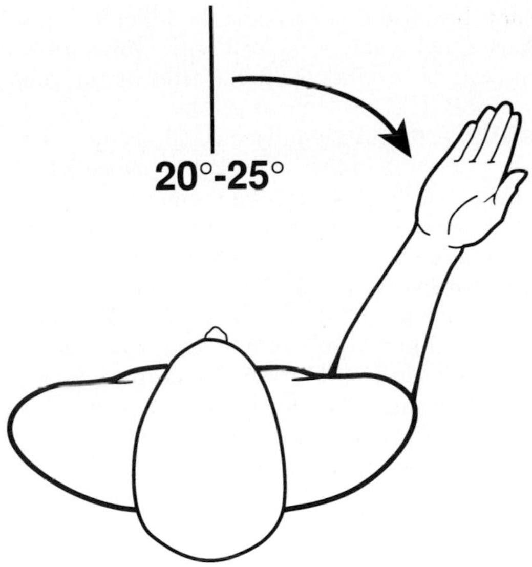

Figure 16–165

Prior to head resection, the arm should be held parallel to the floor and should be externally rotated 20 to 25 degrees.

removed with an electrocautery blade. The superolateral portion of the mark should be at the sulcus of the top of the shoulder (i.e., at the junction of the articular surface with the attachment of the rotator cuff on the greater tuberosity). In most cases, the inferior portion of the mark will be medial to the inferior osteophyte of the flattened and deformed humeral head (see Fig. 16–166*B*). Use of the osteotomy template will ensure that the prosthesis sits properly on the supporting medial neck of the humerus. If the resection is in too much of a varus position, then support for the collar of the prosthesis will be compromised (see Fig. 16–166*C*, *D*).

If a preoperative axillary CT scan has shown posterior glenoid erosion, then several options are available for the surgeon; that is, remove the anterior half of the glenoid with an air bur and glenoid reamer, bone graft to the posterior glenoid, or resect the humeral head with the arm in less than 20 to 25 degrees of external rotation. For example, if there is 10 degrees of posterior glenoid erosion, then the head should be resected with the arm externally rotated only 10 to 15 degrees. If there is more than 25 degrees of posterior glenoid erosion, then we usually use the air bur and special glenoid reamer to remove some of the anterior glenoid.

V16-37 to V16-38

Before the oscillating saw is used to remove the head, the biceps tendon and insertions of the supraspinatus, infraspinatus, and teres minor into the proximal part of the humerus must be protected. **(V16-37)** Pass the large curved modified Crego retractor under the biceps, and curl it around to protect these structures during humeral head resection (Fig. 16–167). **(V16-38)** With the Darrach retractors in the joint, a sagittal power saw is then used to remove the humeral head at the predetermined angle. During removal of the head, the arm must be parallel to the floor and the saw must be perpendicular to the floor.

Once the humeral head has been removed, and with the Darrach retractors acting as a skid, use a bone hook in combination with extension and external rotation of

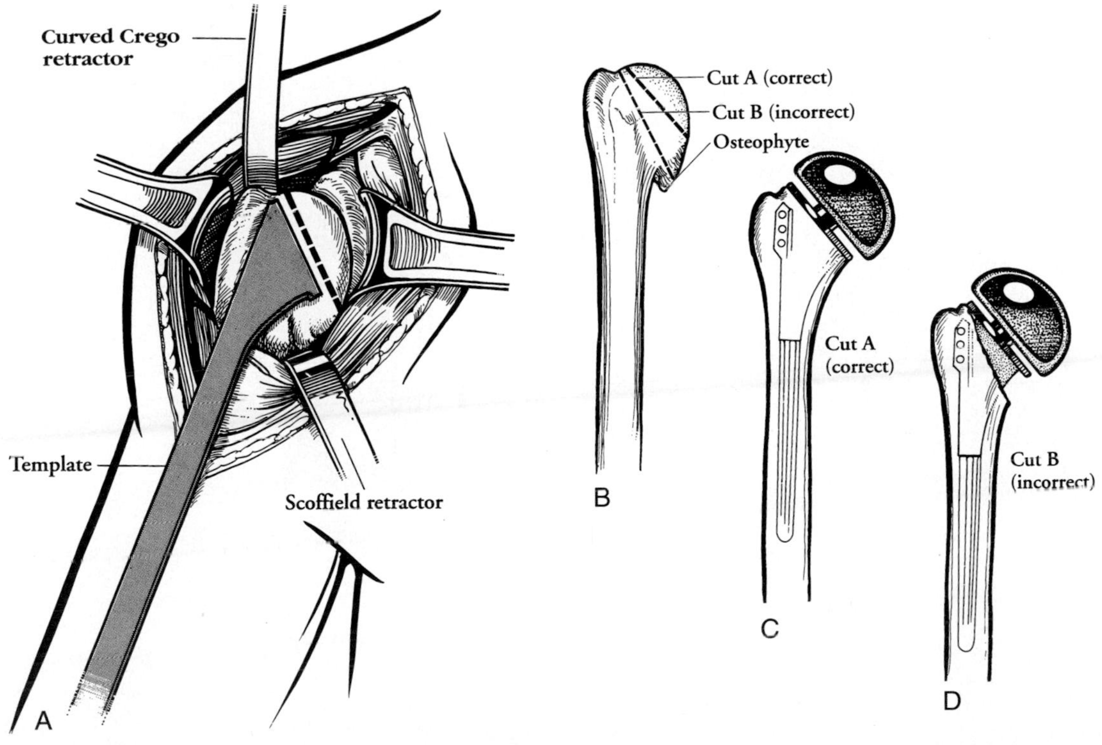

Figure 16–166

A, The template should be used to determine the proper angle of head resection. *B–D*, Failure to use the template in removing the head would lead to insufficient bone to support the neck of the prosthesis.

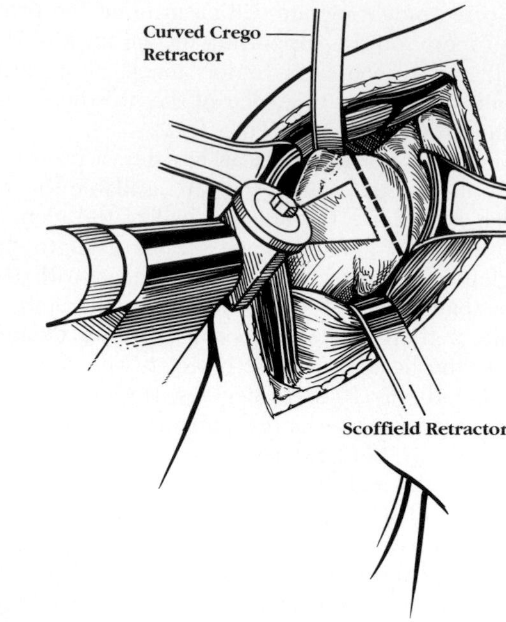

V16-39 to V16-40

Figure 16–167

A modified Crego retractor should be passed under the biceps tendon and then curl around the back of the neck of the humerus. This will protect the biceps and the rotator cuff from being divided during removal of the head with an oscillating saw.

the arm off the side of the table to deliver the cancellous bone surface of the proximal end of the humerus up and out of the incision (Fig. 16–168). Once again, positioning of the patient on the operating room table is extremely important, because it is exceedingly difficult to insert the medullary canal reamers, as well as the prosthesis, unless the arm can be extended off the side of the table (see Fig. 16–158*B, C*).

(V16-39) The 6-mm medullary canal reamer is used to make the pilot hole in the superolateral cancellous surface of the humerus. In this way, the reamer will pass directly down the intramedullary canal (Fig. 16–169*A, B*). The humeral reamer is inserted down the humerus until the top flute pattern is at the level of the cut surface of the bone. Once the initial reamer is seated, proceed with the 8-mm, 10-mm, and 12-mm reamers until one of the reamers begins to bite on the cortical bone of the intramedullary canal. The final reamer size that bites into the cortex will determine the stem size of the body sizing osteotome and the implant. The reaming is done by hand and should not be performed with motorized equipment. Caution should be used NOT to over-ream the canal. Remember that the arm is being supported in external rotation, and the reaming is in an internal rotation direction. Over-reaming puts torque on the humerus and could create a stress riser or fracture.

(V16-40) The body-sizing osteotome matching the size of the final reamer is selected; that is, if a 12-mm reamer was used, then a 12-mm body-sizing osteotome and 12-mm intramedullary rod would be selected. The rod is then threaded into the osteotome body and is then inserted down the intramedullary canal (Fig. 16–170*A*). The rod placed down into the reamed canal prevents the sizing osteotome from drifting into a varus position. The collar on the body-sizing osteotome is used to determine

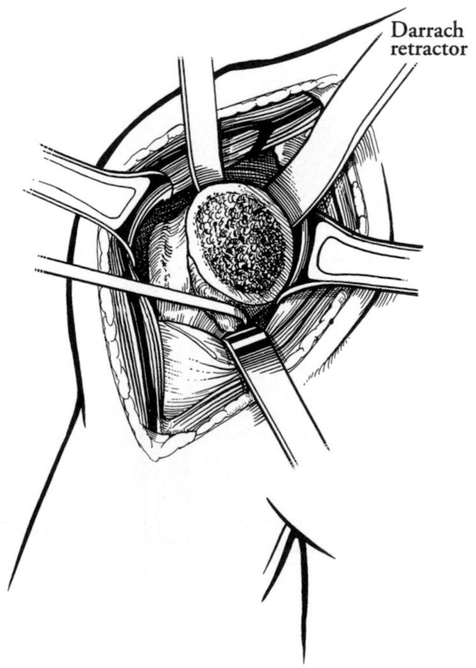

Figure 16–168

The Darrach retractor in the glenoid humeral joint will act as a skid. The bone hook can again be used to deliver the cut surface of the proximal humerus up and out of the wound.

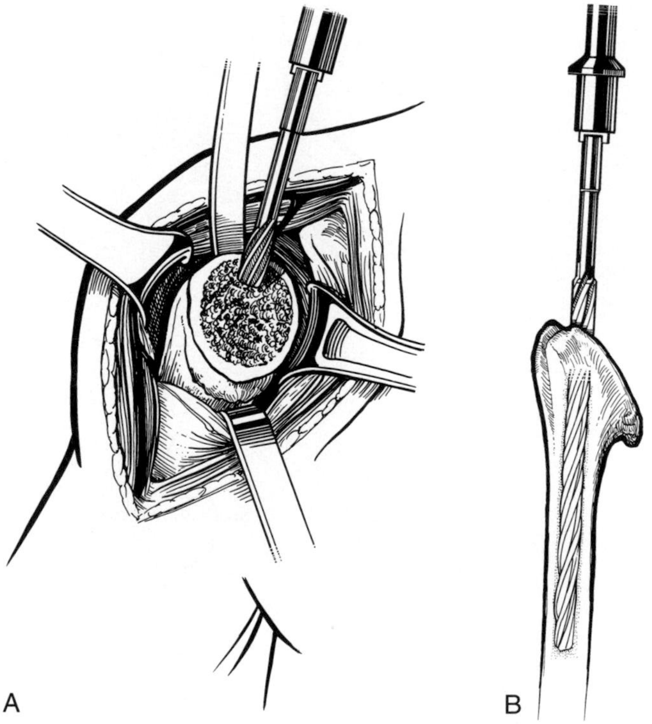

Figure 16–169

A, Initially, the 6-mm intramedullary reamer is placed eccentrically and superior as possible into the proximal humerus. *B*, Progressive reamers are used until the reamer begins to obtain purchase in the cortical bone.

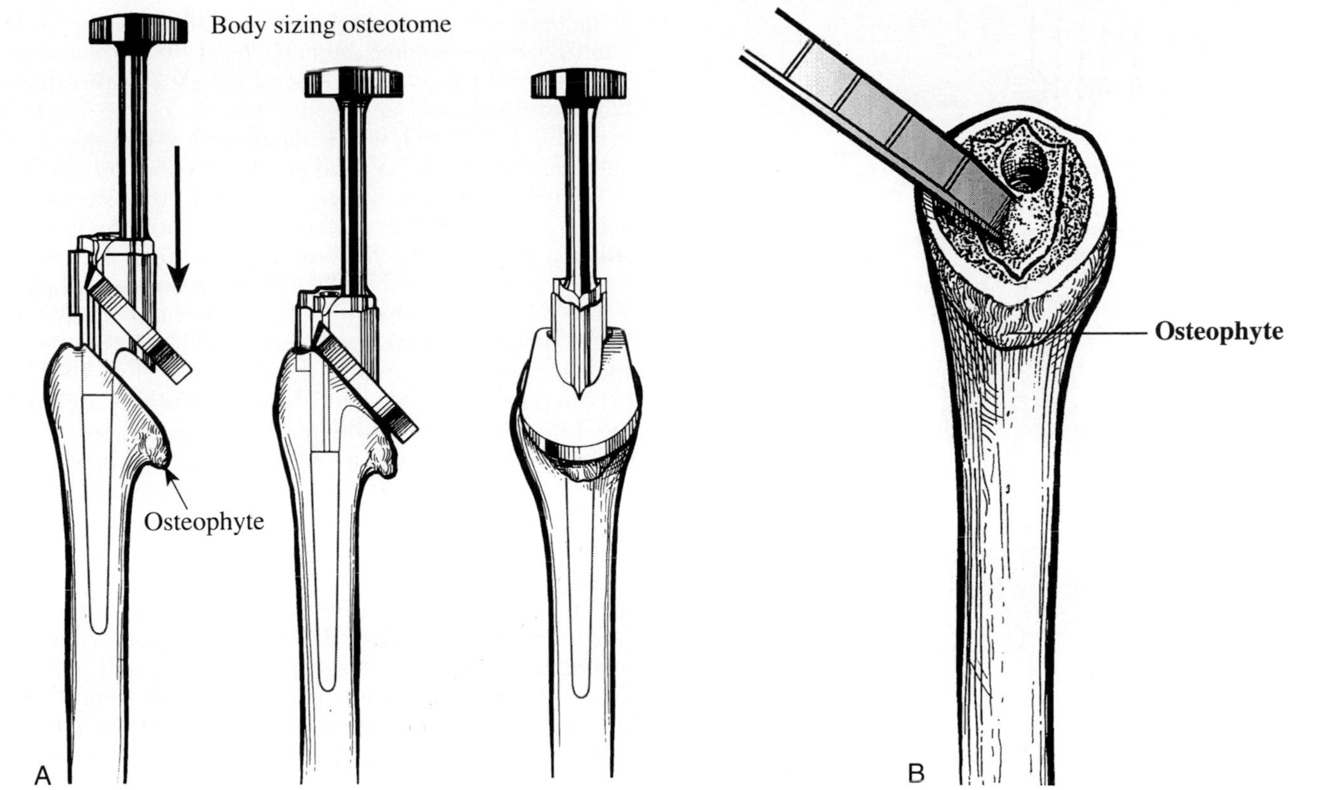

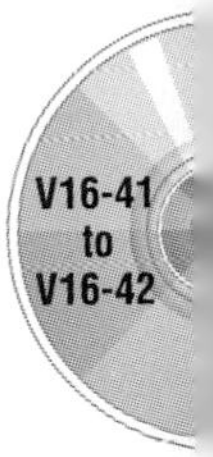

Figure 16–170

A, The stem of the body sizing osteotome, which is the same size as the appropriate intramedullary canal reamer, is inserted down into the intramedullary canal of the humerus. *B*, The osteotome should be rotated until the collar lies flat on the cut surface of the bone. This ensures that you have maintained the proper version for the prosthesis.

proper rotation before cutting the bone. When the lateral fin of the osteotome touches the greater tuberosity, slide the collar down the osteotome until it touches the cancellous bone. Then rotate the body-sizing osteotome until the collar lies flat on the cut-bone surface. The body-sizing osteotome is tapped a few times with a mallet to drive the osteotome down into the cancellous bone. Driving the body-sizing osteotome down into the cancellous bone identifies the appropriate amount of bone to be removed to receive the body broach and creates the anterior, posterior, and inferior fin tracks. Before inserting the body broach, the cancellous bone can be removed with a small osteotome (see Fig. 16–170*B*).

Broaching with the trial body is an important step in the procedure. If a 12-mm reamer and 12-mm body-sizing osteotome have been used, then a 12-mm broach should be used. With the broach locked into place (Fig. 16–171) in the driver-extractor tool, the fin tracks of the broach should carefully be lined up with the fin tracks previously established with the body-sizing osteotome.

(V16-41) The broach should be carefully driven into place, being sure to maintain proper version of the broach by following the previously cut fin tracks. If the proximal part of the humerus is large in proportion to the intramedullary canal, a mismatched humeral body-stem combination is available. If the intramedullary canal was reamed to 12 mm and the proximal part of the humerus is quite large, then a 14/12 broach and prosthesis could be used. The final humeral prosthesis is approximately 1 mm larger than the corresponding broach size; thus, if the body broach is tight, you can obtain a stable press-fit of the prosthesis. Because the medullary canal is filled with the proper-sized stem and the body of the prosthesis fills the cancellous bone proximally, a press-fit of the prosthesis can usually be obtained. However, in the case of deficient cancellous bone proximally that may be seen in patients with rheumatoid arthritis, cement may be required. If cement is required, we (CAR and MW) do not use cement restricters or cement pressurization—we just use enough cement with finger pressure to prevent proximal rotation of the prosthesis.

(V16-42) With the final broach in place, remove any osteophytes that extend inferiorly from the cut surface of the medial humeral neck using an osteotome or rongeurs (see Fig. 16–171*B*). While the glenoid fossa is being evaluated and prepared, the body broach should be left in place to protect the proximal humerus from compression fractures or deformation by the humeral head retractors.

With the broach in place, use a humeral head retractor to displace the proximal end of the humerus posteriorly to expose the glenoid fossa (i.e., Carter Rowe, Fukuda, or DePuy retractor) (Fig. 16–172). The Scoffield retractor should again be utilized to protect the axillary nerve as the labrum and thickened anteroinferior capsule are removed. If the capsule is not excised and is left in place, it can become reattached to the glenoid and the humerus

V16-43 to V16-45

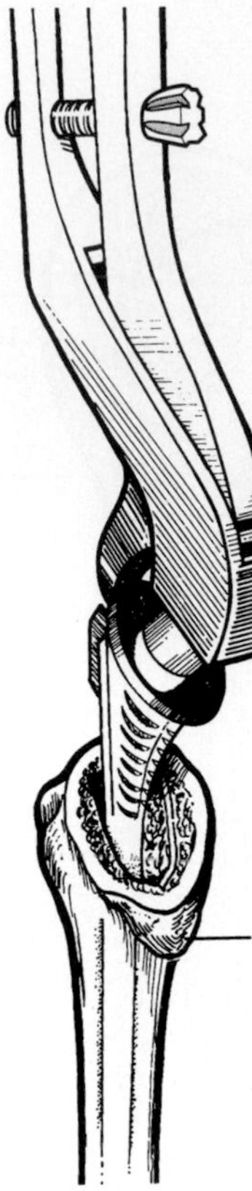

Figure 16–171

After insertion of the trial broach body with the driver extractor tool, the osteophytes should be removed using an osteotome and a rongeur.

and can once again restrict external rotation postoperatively. Resection of the anteroinferior capsule has not led to any instability of the joint.

Hemiarthroplasty Versus Total Shoulder Arthroplasty

If a hemiarthroplasty is the procedure of choice, then you are ready for the final insertion of the prosthesis and the reattachment of the subscapularis tendon. However, if a total shoulder replacement is planned, then the following describes the steps of replacement of the glenoid.

TECHNIQUE FOR USING THE FIVE-PEGGED GLENOID PROSTHESIS

(V16-43) A variety of glenoid sizer disks are utilized to determine the proper size of the glenoid. Select the one that best fits the size of the glenoid fossa. The disk that is used must be the same size or slightly smaller than the glenoid fossa. A larger disk and glenoid prosthesis could interfere with cuff function. Since the normal shoulder joint allows 6 mm of anteroposterior translation of the head in the glenoid fossa, the glenoid prostheses have been developed with a diameter of curvature 6 mm larger than the corresponding humeral head.[153] Each of the glenoid sizer disks and trial prostheses is numbered 40xs, 40, 44, 48, 52, 56, or 56EL, and each has a different color. The numbers do not mean that the size is marked in millimeters; rather, each is 6 mm in diameter larger than the corresponding humeral head, which automatically allows for head translation in the glenoid prosthesis. If a No. 52 glenoid is selected, then a 52-mm humeral head should be used, which allows for a 6-mm mismatch between the prosthetic head and the glenoid prosthesis.

With the humerus sufficiently displaced posteriorly, a hole is created in the center of the glenoid fossa using either a punch or an air bur (Fig. 16–173). Attach the gold-colored, anodized drill guide to the handle and place it into the glenoid fossa over the centering hole. **(V16-44)** Insert the gold-colored anodized drill bit into the guide, and drill until the guard hits the drill guide (Fig. 16–174). It is important that the drill bit is perfectly centered in the drill guide and that the power is engaged before the drill bit comes into contact with the bone. If the drill bit is not properly aligned, the bit will bind in the guide, which can cause damage to the drill.

If the joint is so tight that the longer gold-colored, anodized drill bit cannot be inserted, the shorter silver bit may be used to create the central drill hole. After "bottoming out" the silver drill bit, the central drill guide should be removed and the drilling resumed until the silver drill bit bottoms out. The depth of the central drill hole using the silver bit without using the central drill guide will be the same as if the longer gold anodized drill bit with the guide had been used.

(V16-45) Next, attach to the drill the glenoid reamer that best fits the size of the glenoid fossa. Insert the hub of the reamer into the central hole, and ream the glenoid until it has a smooth configuration that matches the size

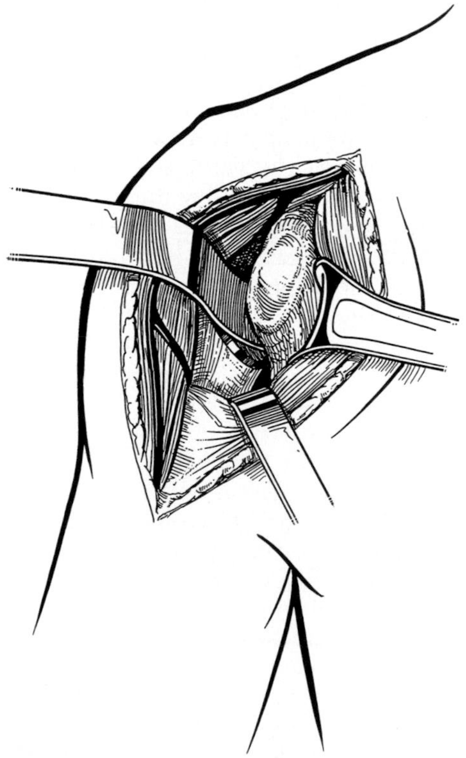

Figure 16–172

When replacing the glenoid fossa with a prosthesis, various types of humeral head retractors can be used to expose the glenoid fossa.

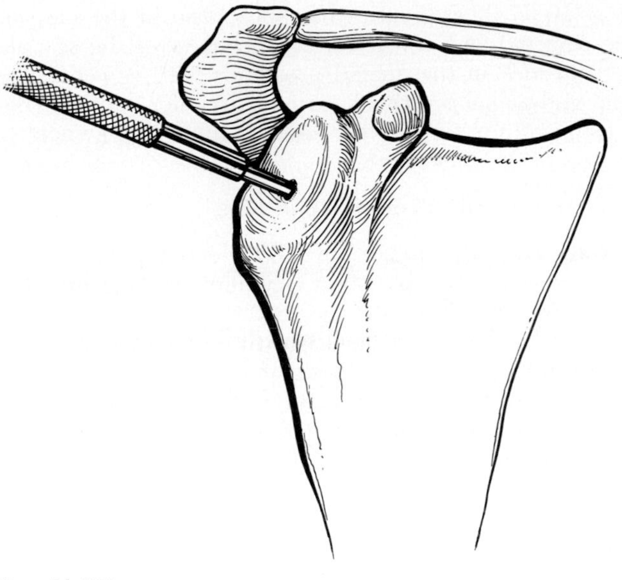

Figure 16–173

A central hole is placed in the glenoid fossa using a punch or an air burr.

of the previously selected trial glenoid prosthesis (Fig. 16–175). This ensures a perfect fit between the back of the glenoid prosthesis and the face of the glenoid. The power should be engaged to the glenoid reamer while the tip of the reamer is in the pilot hole but before it comes in contact with the bone. If the reamer is held

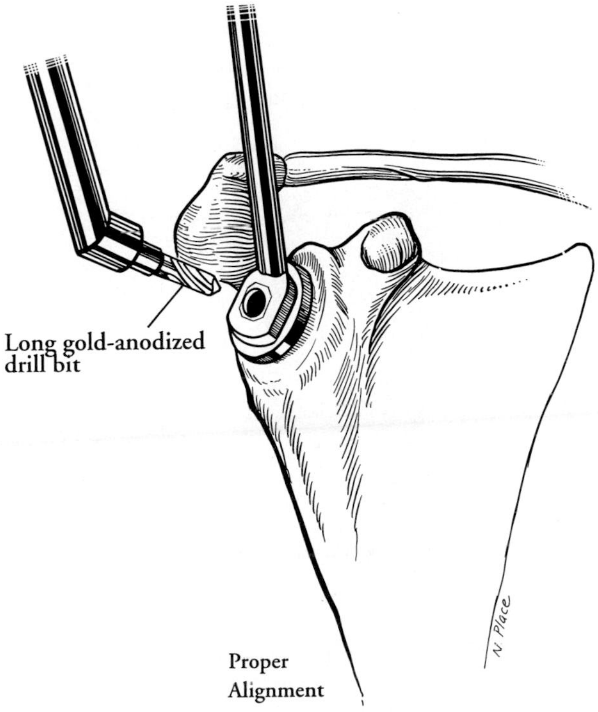

Figure 16–174

The long gold-anodized drill bit must be placed perfectly straight into the drill guide. If it is inserted at an angle, the drill bit can bind up in the drill guide and break the drill. A straight or 45-degree-angled drill is available.

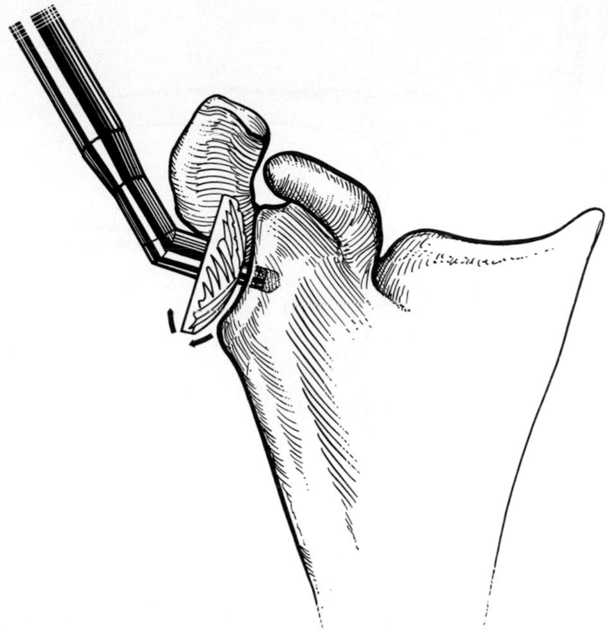

Figure 16–175

The hub of the glenoid reamer should be placed into the central hole. Reaming of the glenoid should be performed until the glenoid fossa is perfectly smooth and will match the back surface of the glenoid prosthesis.

V16-46 to V16-47

tightly against the glenoid before the power is started, then the reamer may bind and cause damage to the power drill and bone.

The silver-colored peripheral drill guide is now attached to the handle. The central peg on the drill guide slips into the hole previously drilled in the center of the glenoid fossa. **(V16-46)** Use the silver-colored drill bit, which is shorter than the gold anodized drill bit, to create four peripheral holes in the glenoid fossa (Fig. 16–176). Drill the superior hole first, and then place the antirotation peg to prevent any rotation of the guide while the other holes are being drilled.

Note that with the peripheral guide in place, it is a good idea to see if there is sufficient room to drill the posterior hole. The shoulder joint is sometimes so tight that it is very difficult to displace the proximal humerus enough posteriorly to be able to drill the posterior hole. If that is the case, you have several options; for example, release more of the posterior capsule; remove the posterior peg from the final prosthesis and utilize the remaining four pegs for fixation; or abandon the use of the pegged glenoid and plan on using the keeled glenoid prosthesis.

Insert the previously selected, trial-pegged glenoid prosthesis and keep it in place during sizing of the trial humeral head (Fig. 16–177). The final pegged glenoid prosthesis is slightly smaller than the trial prosthesis in order to allow room for cement.

TECHNIQUE FOR USING THE KEELED GLENOID PROSTHESIS

(V16-47) To utilize the keeled component, use an air bur to partially create a slot in the glenoid fossa. Then insert

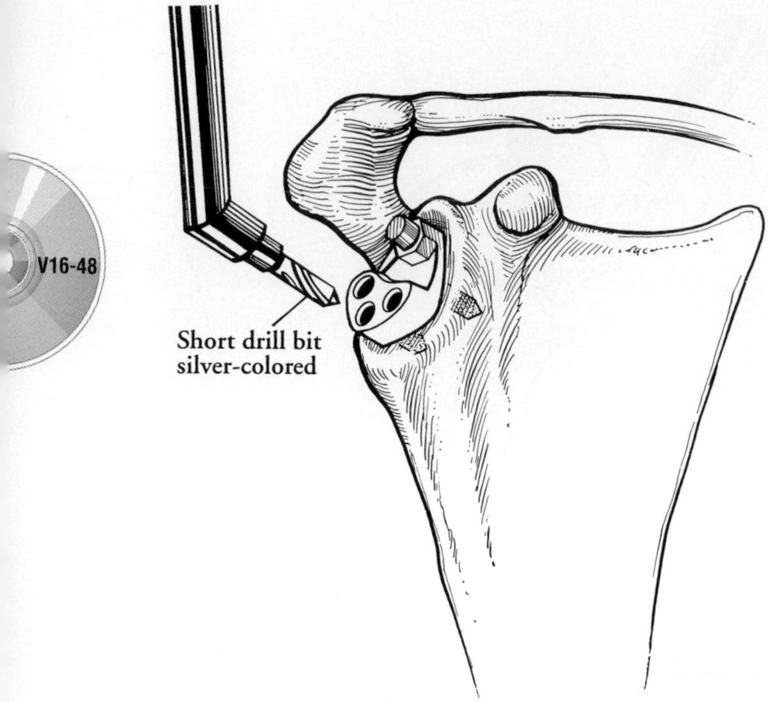

Figure 16–176

With the peripheral drill guide in place, the short silver drill bit should be used to drill the peripheral four holes into the glenoid fossa.

the hub of the appropriate size of glenoid reamer into the slot and ream the glenoid until it has a smooth configuration that matches the size of the previously selected glenoid component. Continue to use the air bur with curettes to remove enough bone to receive the keel (Fig. 16–178). Evacuate cancellous bone in the base of the coracoid and down the lateral border of the scapula to help lock in the keeled prosthesis with cement. The keel of the final prosthesis is slightly smaller than the trial prosthesis in order to accommodate the use of cement.

Selection of the Proper Head Size

(V16-48) With the trial body and glenoid prosthesis in place, select a suitable short, medium, or long humeral head (Fig. 16–179).

Note that the short head is **only** to be used with the 6- or 8-mm humeral prosthesis. If you use the short head with a size 10-mm or greater body, the collar of the humeral prosthesis is larger than the humeral head, which could damage the surface of the glenoid. If the medium and long heads are too tight, then you will have to remove more of the neck of the humerus and release more capsular tissue rather than using a short head.

The numeric size of the head is determined by the glenoid sizer disk selection. Selection of a humeral head of the appropriate length allows the soft tissues to be balanced with proper tension. With the correct head size in place, a stable configuration of the joint without gross anterior or posterior instability should be achieved. However, you should be able to displace the prosthesis posteriorly 50% out of the glenoid fossa. In addition, it should be possible to reapproximate the subscapularis tendon back to bone and have at least 30 to 50 degrees of external rotation, and you should be able to place the patient's hand on the opposite shoulder without any tension. If the fit of the humeral head is so tight that

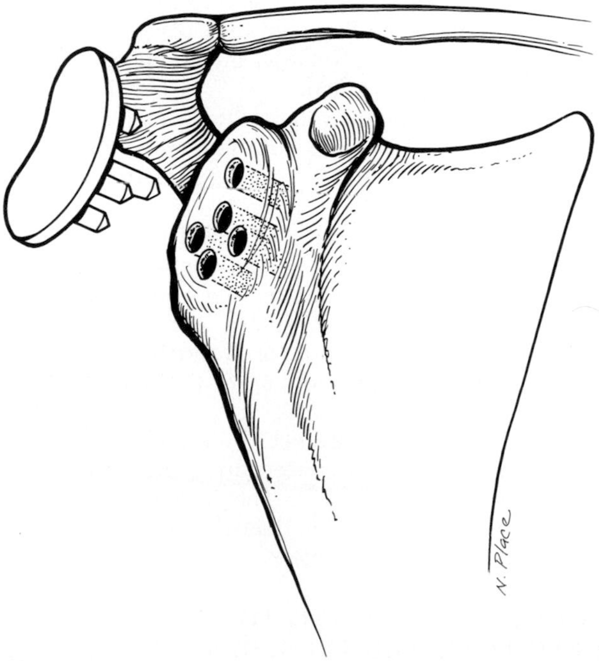

Figure 16–177

A trial pegged glenoid prosthesis is placed into position.

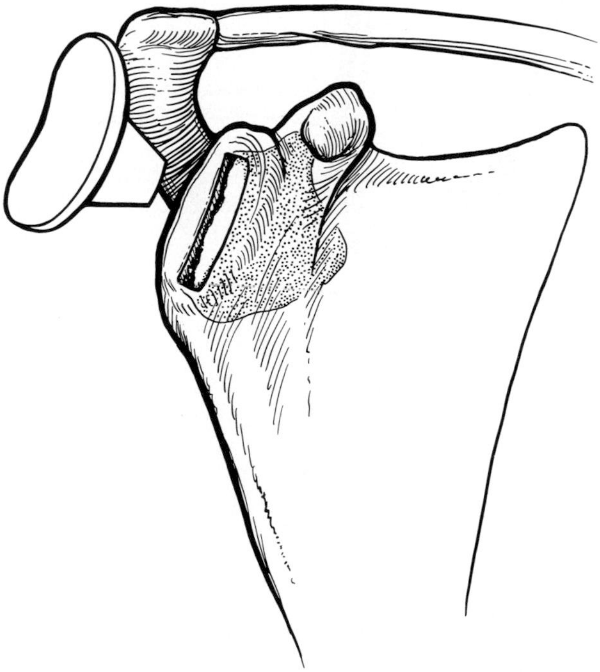

Figure 16–178

If a keeled glenoid prosthesis has been selected, then the air burr is used to create a slot in the glenoid fossa. After the glenoid fossa has been reamed, a trial keel prosthesis is placed into position.

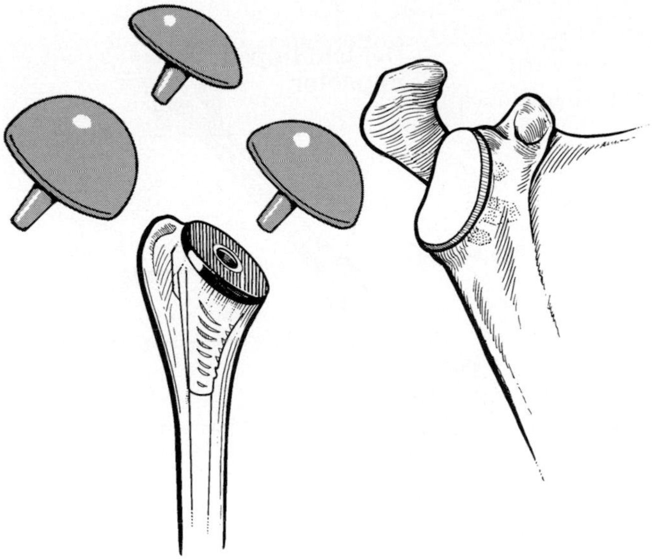

Figure 16–179

With the trial glenoid and broach body in place, the appropriate sized humeral head (i.e., short, medium, or long) is selected, which will balance the soft tissues.

functional internal or external rotation cannot be obtained, then more posterior capsule must be released or a shorter head should be used. Remember that the short head should only be used with a size 6 or 8 humeral body. If gross anterior or posterior instability exists, a longer head should be utilized.

Insertion of the Final Prosthesis

With the broach in place and the trial humeral head removed, displace the humerus posteriorly to prepare the glenoid fossa for insertion of the glenoid prosthesis. Insert a probe into each of the drilled holes to determine if the holes have exited the anterior or posterior cortex of the glenoid. If exit holes are found, it is important not to put an excessive amount of cement into the holes, where it could extrude out and possibly damage the surrounding soft tissues.

(V16-49) Carefully irrigate or use pulsatile lavage to remove any clotted blood from the holes. For hemostasis, spray thrombin and insert Surgicel gauze into each of the holes. Mix half a package of methyl methacrylate; remove the gauze from the holes; and place a small amount of methyl methacrylate into each of the holes using your fingertip (Fig. 16–180). Only a small amount of methyl methacrylate is necessary in each hole to create the proper cement mantle around each peg. Excessive cement extruding out of the holes and lying between the prosthesis and the glenoid fossa is undesirable for two reasons. First, it could create an uneven seat for the glenoid prosthesis, and second, the thin segments of cement from between the back of the glenoid prosthesis and the face of the glenoid may become fragmented and loosen in the joint, causing damage to the polyethylene. Insert the glenoid prosthesis and hold it in position with finger pressure until the cement is cured and the prosthesis is secure (see Fig. 16–180).

If the keeled glenoid prosthesis is to be used, hemostasis in the keel hole must be obtained. The slot should be irrigated to remove any clots and then sprayed with thrombin and packed with Surgicel gauze and a lap sponge. When the methyl methacrylate is ready, remove the Surgicel gauze and the sponge and impact the cement into the slot with finger pressure. Firm finger pressure and several small batches of cement will ensure a good cement mantle in the slot to receive and secure the keeled prosthesis. As mentioned, cement between the glenoid fossa and the back of the prosthesis is undesirable. Insert the keeled prosthesis, and hold it in position with finger pressure until the cement is set and the prosthesis is secure (Fig. 16–181).

V16-49 to V16-50

Repair of the Subscapularis Tendon

Before the humeral component is inserted, you must prepare for the repair of the subscapularis back to the cut surface of the proximal humerus. Since the tendon was released from its insertion onto the lesser tuberosity, we can gain length of the tendon and hence gain external rotation by reattaching it medially on the cut surface of the neck of the humerus. **(V16-50)** Three or four drill holes should be made into the anterior neck of the humerus with a small drill. Use a suture passer to pull loops of suture through these drill holes (Fig. 16–182). These loops of suture will be used later to pull the 1-mm nonabsorbable Dacron tape sutures in the subscapularis

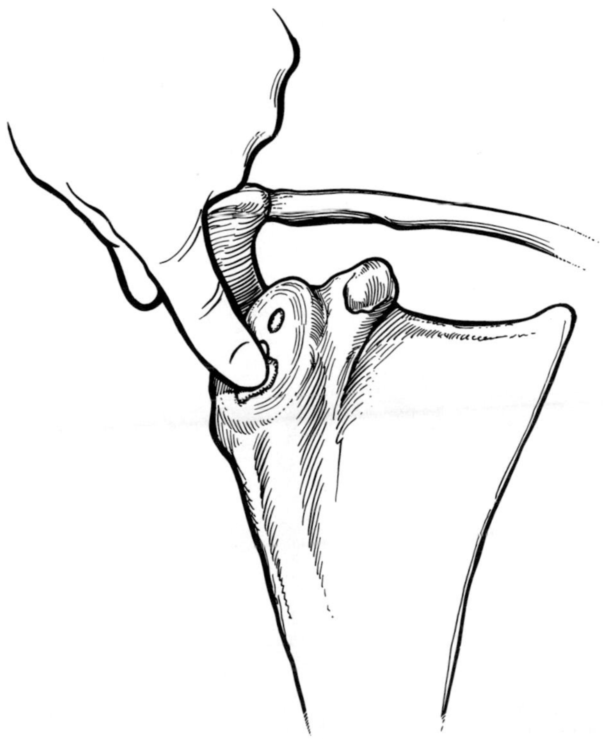

Figure 16–180

The drill holes are thoroughly irrigated, sprayed with thrombin, and packed with Surgicel gauze. This will dry up the drill holes. A small amount of bone cement is placed into each of the holes using fingertip pressure.

V16-51 to V16-53

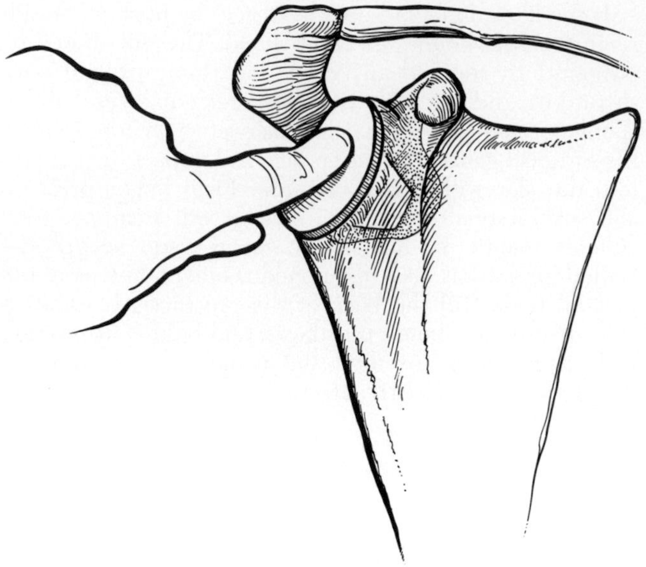

Figure 16–181

When a keeled prosthesis is used, the slot is cleaned, dried, and then packed with cement. The prosthesis is held in place with finger pressure until it has set up.

tendon out through the bone for secure fixation of the tendon back to bone.

(V16-51) Attach the humeral prosthesis that is the same size as the final broach size into the driver-extractor and insert the prosthesis down the humeral canal. The fins of the prosthesis must be aligned with the fin tracks previously created by the body broach. The final prosthesis is 1 mm larger overall than the broach so that a press-fit

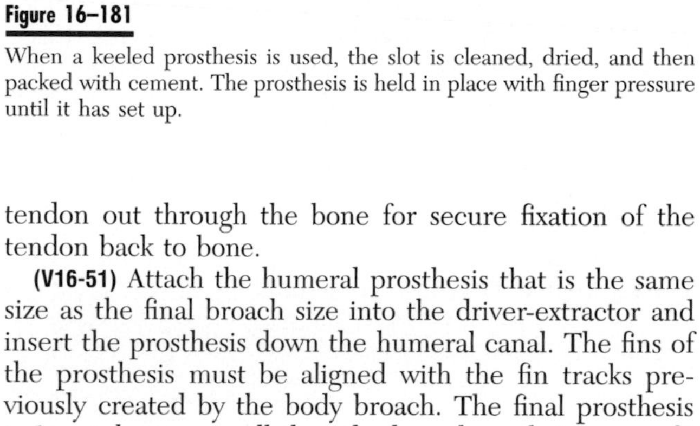

Figure 16–182

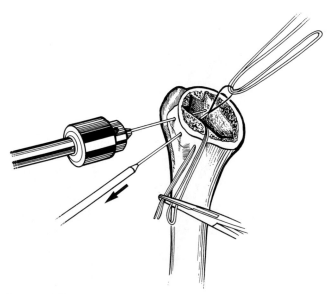

In preparation for repair of the subscapularis tendon, three or four drill holes are placed in the anterior neck of the humerus. Using a suture passer, loops of sutures are to be placed through the drill holes. These loops of suture will be used later to pull the Dacron tape sutures into the subscapularis tendon through the bone for secure fixation of the tendon to bone.

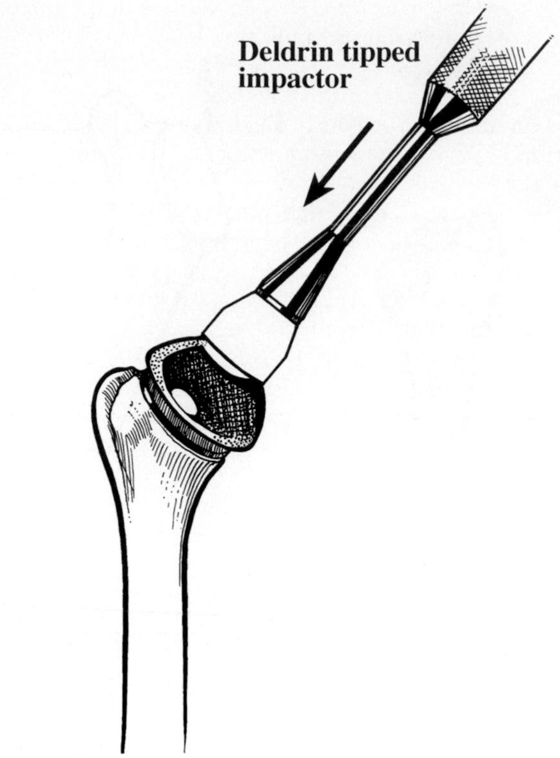

Figure 16–183

The head of the prosthesis is then impacted into the humeral body using the Deldrin tipped impactor.

without cement can be obtained. Cancellous bone from the resected humeral head can be used as graft to help fill in any defects in the proximal part of the humerus or to ensure a good tight press-fit. The decision to use cement or a press-fit technique is up to the individual surgeon. In some cases, it may be necessary to use methyl methacrylate due to a previous surgical procedure, fractures, osteoporosis, rheumatoid arthritis, or degenerative cysts in the humerus. A set of long-stem humeral prostheses is available for revision cases or in case of fractures of the shaft of the humerus.

(V16-52) Before the final humeral head is inserted, thoroughly clean the Morse taper socket in the humeral prosthesis with a dry sponge and insert the appropriate size of head. Use a plastic-tipped driver to secure the head in place by sharply striking it four to five times with a 2-lb mallet (Fig. 16–183). Make sure to impact the head down in the direction of the Morse taper. Grasp the head to ensure that it is securely attached to the humeral prosthesis. The pull-out strength of the properly attached head into the body has been tested to be approximately 1400 lb. If for some reason the head needs to be removed, a special forked sled driver should be placed between the head and the body and tapped.

With gentle traction, internal rotation, and finger pressure on the humeral prosthesis, reduce the head into the glenoid fossa. A special plastic skid is available and should be used in place of the Darrach retractor to avoid scratching the humeral head. **(V16-53)** After joint irrigation, pass the previously placed Dacron tape sutures in the subscapularis tendon into the loop of sutures in the proximal part of the humerus; pull the loops and sutures through the bone; and secure the tendon back to bone (Fig. 16–184).

If the tendon was previously divided or was lengthened with a coronal Z-plasty technique, then repair and secure it with heavy nonabsorbable sutures, such as 1-mm Dacron tape. Use of the heavy 1-mm tape sutures allows immediate passive movement beginning the day of surgery without fear of detaching the subscapularis tendon.

Before wound closure, palpate the axillary nerve a final time to be sure that it is intact. Thoroughly irrigate the wound with antibiotic solution. Infiltrate the subcutaneous and muscle tissues with 0.25% bupivacaine solution to ease immediate postoperative pain. One or two portable wound evacuation units are used to prevent the formation of a postoperative hematoma.

The wound may be dosed according to the surgeon's preference. The deltopectoral fascia can be closed with a running 0 absorbable suture, and the deep layer of fat with a 0 or 2–0 absorbable suture. The subcuticular fat is closed as a separate layer, and the skin is closed with a running subcuticular nylon suture. Careful attention to wound closure will result in a cosmetically acceptable incision.

If a humeral prosthesis needs to be removed, a special slap hammer extractor is available (Fig. 16–185). After the head has been removed, you should remove the Deldrin tip of the driver-extractor tool and replace it with a steel tip. The driver-extractor should be attached to the prosthesis. The slap hammer is screwed into the top of the driver-extractor, and then the handle is used to apply upward blows to remove the prosthesis. It may be necessary to use small osteotomes to loosen the prosthesis from bone or cement.

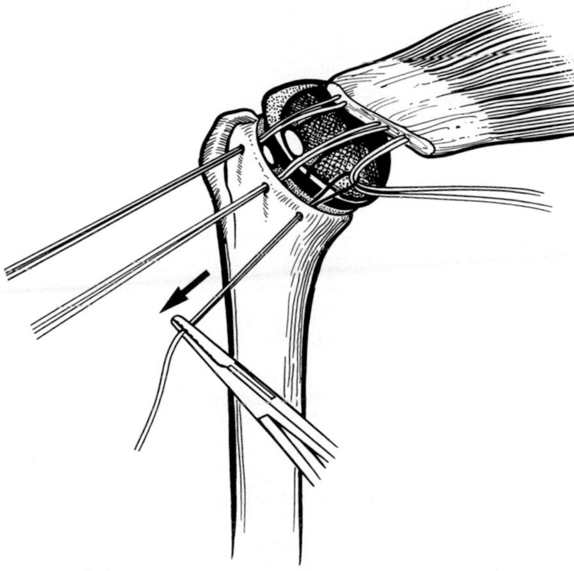

Figure 16–184

Using the loops of suture in the anterior surface of the neck of the humerus, the Dacron tape sutures previously placed in the subscapularis tendon are pulled out through the neck of the humerus and tied.

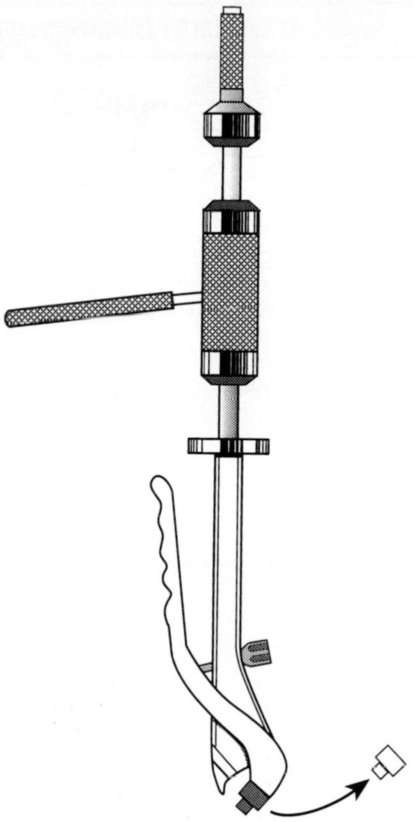

Figure 16–185

To remove a secure or cemented prosthesis, a special slap hammer is available. It requires that the driver-extractor tool be modified by tapping a hole in the top of the tool to receive the slaphammer.

RESULTS

Hemiarthroplasty Results

The results for the Neer design of hemiarthroplasty, or proximal humeral prosthetic replacement, are reported in Table 16–21. The results have been reported for osteonecrosis, osteoarthritis, rheumatoid arthritis, and the residuals of trauma. When this procedure is applied to the treatment of proximal humeral osteonecrosis, the pain relief has been quite good, ranging from 91 to 100%, and the range of motion of the shoulder approaches normal. When this operation is applied to patients with rheumatoid arthritis, osteoarthritis, or the residuals of trauma, satisfactory pain relief is less consistently achieved but, with the exception of 3 of the 11 reported series, is still quite acceptable. Range of motion in these latter patients tends to be less and varies from one series to another; average active abduction ranged from one third to three quarters normal.

In 1996, Williams and Rockwood[360] reported on treating 21 shoulders in 20 patients with glenohumeral arthritis rotator cuff–deficient shoulders with a hemiarthroplasty procedure. After an average of 4 years of follow-up, using the limited goal criteria of Neer, 86% of the patients had achieved a satisfactory result (i.e., pain was improved; deflection improved from an average of 70 degrees preoperatively to 120 degrees postoperatively).

Table 16–21 RESULTS OF SHOULDER HEMIARTHROPLASTY—NEER DESIGN

AUTHOR, YEAR	DIAGNOSIS	NO. OF SHOULDERS	NO OR SLIGHT PAIN (%)	AVERAGE ACTIVE ABDUCTION (°) OR OVERALL RATING
Neer, 1955[249]	Osteonecrosis	3	100	Excellent, good, good
Neer, 1974[251]	Osteoarthritis	47		20 excellent 20 satisfactory 6 unsatisfactory
Cruess, 1976[95]	Osteonecrosis	5	100	Approached normal
Bodey and Yeoman, 1983[23]	Osteoarthritis Rheumatoid arthritis	8	88	63°
Tanner and Cofield, 1983[339]	Old trauma	28	89	112°
Bell and Gschwend, 1986[24]	Mixed	17	59	91°
Petersson, 1986[274]	Rheumatoid arthritis	11	36	74°
Zuckerman and Cofield, 1986[373]	Osteoarthritis	39	82	134°
	Rheumatoid arthritis	44	91	112°
Hawkins et al, 1987[161]	Chronic dislocation	9	67	140°
Pritchett and Clark, 1987[287]	Chronic dislocation	7	100	5 good, 2 fair
Rutherford and Cofield, 1987[316]	Osteonecrosis	11	91	161°
Total		229	Weighted mean, 82%; median, 89%	Weighted mean of 8 series, 115°; median, 112°

External rotation improved preoperatively from an average of 27 degrees to a postoperative average of 45 degrees. None of the patients developed postoperative instability of the shoulder.

In 1996, Bigliani, Glasson, and associates[138] treated 31 shoulders with osteoarthritis and intact cuff with a hemiarthroplasty procedure. The patients were evaluated by the American Shoulder and Elbow Surgeons, Neer and Constant end result scoring methods. They reported that the outcome varied with the amount of glenoid wear. However, in the patients with a smooth concentric glenoid, they reported that 86% had excellent results and 7% had good results.

Total Shoulder Arthroplasty Results

The most commonly used total shoulder arthroplasty has been the Neer design. The results for this system are tabulated in Table 16–22. Most patient series contain a mixed diagnostic grouping, including patients with rheumatoid arthritis, osteoarthritis, old trauma, and a variety of less common diagnostic categories. As can be seen from Table 16–22, the percentage of patients who achieved satisfactory pain relief is quite high, and, quite typically, slightly more than 90% of patients reported no or only slight pain after surgery. Motion data after surgery have not been as consistently reported as one might desire, but the amount of motion regained seems variable and dependent on the diagnostic category. For example, in the series reported by Cofield, the mean active abduction after surgery for the entire group of patients reported was 120 degrees.[72] The average return of active abduction varied greatly according to the diagnosis: 141 degrees for patients with osteoarthritis, 109 degrees for those with post-traumatic arthritis, and 103 degrees for patients with rheumatoid arthritis. The return of movement in Cofield's series was not only dependent on diagnosis but was also highly dependent on the condition of the rotator cuff and shoulder capsule and on the avoidance of complications.[72]

The largest series of total shoulder arthroplasties of this category has been reported by Neer.[259] He has suggested two systems for grading results. Patients who received a full rehabilitation program were graded as excellent, satisfactory, or unsatisfactory. To achieve an excellent result, the patient was enthusiastic about the operation and had no significant pain; the patient could use the arm

Table 16–22 RESULTS OF TOTAL SHOULDER ARTHROPLASTY—NEER DESIGN

AUTHOR, YEAR	MEAN FOLLOW-UP (YR)	DIAGNOSIS	NO. OF SHOULDERS	NO OR SLIGHT PAIN (%)	AVERAGE ACTIVE ELEVATION* (°)	AVERAGE EXTERNAL ROTATION (°)
Neer et al, 1982[259]	3.1	Mixed	194			
Bade et al, 1984[10]	4.5	Mixed	38	93	118	
Cofield, 1984[72]	3.8	Mixed	73	92	120	48
Wilde et al, 1984[357]	3.0	Mixed	38	92		
Adams et al, 1986[1]	2.7	Mixed	33	91	96	
Hawkins et al, 1986[101]	3.0	Rheumatoid arthritis Osteoarthritis	70			
Barrett et al, 1987[15]	3.5	Mixed	50	88	100	54
Kelly et al, 1987[188]	3.0	Rheumatoid arthritis	40	88	75	40
Frich et al, 1988[125]	2.3	Mixed	50	92	58–78†	17–21†

*Elevation = abduction with 30 to 60 degrees of horizontal flexion.
†Range, depending on diagnosis.

Table 16–23 FOLLOW-UP ON 194 TOTAL SHOULDER ARTHROPLASTIES* (CLINICAL RATINGS)

DIAGNOSIS	NO. OF SHOULDERS	EXCELLENT	FULL EXERCISE PROGRAM		LIMITED GOALS REHABILITATION	
			Satisfactory	Unsatisfactory	Successful	Unsuccessful
Osteoarthritis (primary and secondary)	40	36	3	0	1	0
Arthritis of recurrent dislocation	18	13	3	1	1	0
Rheumatoid arthritis	50	28	12	3	7	0
Old trauma	41	16	7	12	6	0
Prosthetic revision	26	7	3	5	11	0
Cuff-tear arthropathy	11	—	—	—	10	1
Miscellaneous (tumor, glenoid dysplasia, failed arthrodesis)	8	1	—	—	6	1
Total	194	101	28	21	42	2

*Adapted from Neer CS, Watson KC, and Stanton FJ: Recent experience in total shoulder replacement. J Bone Joint Surg *64A*:319–337, 1982.

without limitations; strength approached normal; active elevation of the arm was within 35 degrees of the opposite normal side; and external rotation was 90% of the normal side. In patients with a satisfactory result, there was no more than occasional pain or aching with weather changes, good use of the shoulder for daily activities, elevation of at least 90 degrees, and rotation to 50% of the normal side. Muscle strength was at least 30% of the normal side, and the patients expressed satisfaction with the operation. In an unsatisfactory result, the aforementioned criteria were not achieved. Neer has suggested a separate evaluation category for patients who have total shoulder replacement but whose muscles could be classified as detached and not capable of recovering function after repair because of fixed contracture or denervation. Patients with substantial bone loss, particularly bone loss in the proximal humerus, might also be included within this evaluative category. In this setting, rehabilitation is aimed at achieving limited goals, the purpose being to gain a lesser range of motion but maintain stability. Neer has suggested that this limited-goals rehabilitation is successful when patients with these muscle or bone deficiencies achieve 90 degrees of elevation and 20 degrees of external rotation, maintain reasonable stability, and achieve satisfactory pain relief. The results achieved for Neer's large series of patients, including the numerous diagnostic categories, are displayed in Table 16–23. Other series of results with this type of prosthesis have been reported.[355]

Roentgenographic analyses for a number of series of total shoulder arthroplasties using the Neer design are displayed in Table 16–24. All series report lucent lines or lucent zones at the glenoid-bone cement junction. These vary considerably in frequency among the different series, ranging from 30 to 93% of shoulders reported. The keel portion of this implant serves as the significant means of attachment to the scapula, and the lucent zones seen at the cement-bone junction surrounding the keel are of great concern. The median percentage of the number of shoulders analyzed in which a lucent line was identified at the bone-cement junction of the keel part of the component is 36. The argument has been presented that when these lucent lines or zones are seen in patients, they are almost always present immediately postoperatively and clearly represent an error in surgical technique.[259] This may be the most common sequence of events associated with roentgenographic lucent zones at the glenoid bone-cement junction and speaks for the need for meticulous preparation of the bone bed and cementing at the time of surgery. However, it has also been reported that these lucent zones have not been present immediately after surgery but rather have developed over time.[72] Green and Norris[140] and Slawson and associates[325] have provided a review of imaging techniques for evaluating a glenohumeral arthroplasty.

Franklin and co-authors have suggested a classification system for describing the radiographic appearance of the glenoid component.[124] In class 0, there is no lucency. In

Table 16–24 RESULTS OF ROENTGENOGRAPHIC ANALYSIS OF NEER TOTAL SHOULDER ARTHROPLASTY

AUTHOR, YEAR	NO. OF SHOULDERS	GLENOID BONE-CEMENT JUNCTION LUCENT ZONES (%)			SHIFT IN POSITION
		None	Any Area	Keel	
Neer et al, 1982[259]	194	70	30	12	
Bade et al, 1984[10]	38	33	67		
Cofield, 1984[72]	73	29	71	33	11
Wilde et al, 1984[357]	38	7	93	68	
Adams et al, 1986[1]	33			36	
Brems, 1993[41]	69	31	69		
Barrett et al, 1987[15]	50	26	74	36	10
Kelly et al, 1987[188]	40	17	83	63	

class 1, there is lucency at the superior or inferior flange only. In class 2, there is incomplete lucency at the keel. In class 3, there is complete lucency up to 2 mm around the component. In class 4, there is complete lucency greater than 2 mm around the component. In class 5A, the component has translated, tipped, or shifted in position. And in class 5B, the component has become dislocated from the bone.

In the series by Barrett and co-workers[15] and Cofield,[72] analyses have also included a shift in glenoid component position relative to the position achieved immediately after surgery. Analysis of component movement relative to the bone requires the viewing of sequential x-rays over time, because often a lucent zone is not seen. This finding implies component loosening, but it can easily be overlooked if serial x-rays are not studied.

Comparison of Hemiarthroplasty Versus Total Shoulder Arthroplasty in Patients with Osteoarthritis

In 1996, Jensen and Rockwood[174] reported the end results of patients with osteoarthritis who were treated with hemiarthroplasty against those who were treated with total shoulder arthroplasty. This was a retrospective review of 87 consecutive patients (117 shoulders). Forty-two patients were treated with a hemiarthroplasty, and 75 patients were treated with a total shoulder arthroplasty. A Neer prosthesis was used in 72 shoulders, and a modular global prosthesis was used in 45 shoulders. The average age was 63.5 years, and the average follow-up was 58 months. In 38 shoulders (25%), an irreparable rotator cuff was noted and the majority of these patients were treated with a hemiarthroplasty. At follow-up, which included comparing range of motion before and after the operative procedure, the relief of pain, the ability to perform 15 different activities of daily living, and a review of x-rays, we found that there was no statistical difference between patients treated with a hemiarthroplasty and total shoulder arthroplasty.

Norris and Iannotti[262] reported on a prospective outcome study comparing humeral head replacement and total shoulder arthroplasty for primary osteoarthritis. This was a report to the American Shoulder and Elbow Surgeons open meeting in 1996. They evaluated the functional outcome, patient satisfaction, shoulder motion, strength, stability, and postoperative radiographs in this series of patients and compared the results of humeral head replacement and total shoulder arthroplasty. They concluded that the outcome for prosthetic replacement for primary osteoarthritis yields excellent results. Patients are greatly improved by 3 months after the procedure and continue to improve over the first 12 months and have stable functional outcome thereafter. Full-thickness rotator cuff tears are uncommon with primary osteoarthritis; however, when present, will result in less favorable results. Glenoid erosion is common in primary osteoarthritis and when moderate or severe in degree will adversely affect functional outcome in humeral head replacement and is associated with a higher degree of glenoid component lucent lines when associated with a thick cement mantle beneath the base of the glenoid component. A thick cement mantle at the base of the component should be avoided in this situation, because it adds to the increased incidence of glenoid lucent lines. The results of humeral head replacement for the osteoarthritis having an intact rotator cuff and minimal glenoid wear are essentially equivalent to total shoulder arthroplasty. Humeral lucent lines are uncommon but are more often seen with total shoulder arthroplasty. This may be associated with polyethylene wear debris.

Comparison of Hemiarthroplasty Versus Total Shoulder Arthroplasty in Patients with Rheumatoid Arthritis

Sneppen and associates[327] reported a prospective study of 62 shoulders with grade IV and V Larsen rheumatoid arthritis who were treated with a Neer total shoulder arthroplasty. At an average of 92 months, Charles Neer reported that proximal migration had occurred in 55% of the patients and 40% showed radiographic loosening, translation or displacement of the glenoid prosthesis. However, despite the glenoid loosening and displacement and loosening of the press-fit humeral components, 89% of the patients had good pain relief. The loosening did not influence range of motion or function. He concluded that a cemented hemiarthroplasty may be better treatment in end stages of rheumatoid arthritis of the shoulder.

Basamania, Rockwood, and associates[17] reported that patients with rheumatoid arthritis who were treated with hemiarthroplasty had better results compared with patients who were treated with total shoulder arthroplasty. Their data were reported to the 1994 Open Meeting of the American Shoulder and Elbow Surgeons and were based on 45 shoulders in 37 patients with rheumatoid arthritis. There were 28 women and 9 men ranging from 22 to 77 years of age with an average age of 54 years. The average follow-up was 5.5 years (range of 2 to 14 years). In an effort to avoid the loosening of the glenoid component secondary to proximal migration of the humeral prosthesis, 32 shoulders were treated with a hemiarthroplasty and 13 shoulders were treated with a total shoulder arthroplasty. Preoperatively, the average active flexion for all shoulders was 50 degrees, 21 degrees of external rotation and internal rotation to the lateral hip. Postoperatively, the average gain in motion for all shoulders was 42 degrees of active flexion, 10 degrees of external rotation, and six spinal levels for internal rotation. Twenty-four shoulders (53%) did not have the rotator cuff repaired secondary to massive irreparable effects that were associated with superior migration of the humeral head.

Patients treated with a hemiarthroplasty had greater improvement in their postoperative range of motion. For these patients, the average gain in shoulder flexion was 53 degrees compared with 38 degrees in shoulders treated with total shoulder arthroplasty. At latest follow-up, satisfaction was reported in 85% of patients treated with total shoulder arthroplasty and 94% of patients treated with hemiarthroplasty.

Methods of Assessing Functional Outcome

Codman will be remembered in the annals or orthopedic history as a pioneer in the study of shoulder disorders, but few except the most ardent of his followers are familiar with the role that he played as a visionary and champion of what is currently described as outcomes research.[69] Central to what Codman described in the early 1900s as an "end-result" system was the admonition that every patient should be followed to determine if the treatment was a success and if not to determine the reasons for failure so that such occurrences could be prevented in the future. Despite Codman's admonition almost 100 years ago, there continues to exist a lack of standardized methods for measuring results and reporting complications associated with total shoulder implants. Unfortunately, the lack of a universally accepted outcome measurement system for shoulder arthroplasty increases methodologic flaws in structured literature reviews and often precludes meaningful retrospective or prospective comparisons between various arthroplasty series. The desirability of research methodologies that will improve the quality and comparability of multicenter studies is underscored by our review of almost 50 total shoulder replacement series.[37, 43, 47, 49, 65, 81, 84, 92, 96, 110, 114, 115, 120, 125, 141, 142, 159, 188, 195, 200, 203, 207, 218, 228, 232–234, 256, 257, 266, 277, 281, 284–286, 309, 342, 352, 357] The results of this review revealed that only 33 of these reports assessed the outcome of treatment by applying a specific grading system. Moreover, there was a great lack of unanimity with regard to these evaluation schemes because 22 different grading systems were utilized. Another disconcerting factor was the variability in reported data, variations in terminology, and ill-defined standards of assessing complications that made it difficult to systematically analyze many of these studies.

The necessity for improving study design, defining the important constituents of outcome measurement, and increasing the validity of orthopedic clinical research has been emphasized by several authors.[93, 99, 135, 314] It has been suggested that the current emphasis of orthopedic clinical studies should be directed toward outcome research that documents the effect of treatment on the health of those treated and the subsequent quality of their lives.[135] The American Shoulder and Elbow Surgeons proposed a standardized form for assessment of the shoulder that is applicable to all patients regardless of their diagnosis.[295] Such standardized forms represent assessment tools that will facilitate the analysis of multicenter studies, permit validity testing of measurement tools, and provide documentation of patient outcome in terms of economics and improved quality of life.

Survivorship Analysis

The validity of survivorship analysis in the evaluation of long-term clinical studies involving total hip replacements is well established.[90, 103, 104, 175, 269] Although nonparametric estimates of survivorship based on life tables and the Kaplan-Meier curve have proved useful in predicting the longevity of hip arthroplasties, the application of these instruments to total shoulder arthroplasty studies is limited to two series.[43, 78]

In 1983, Cofield performed a nonparametric estimation of survivorship in 176 unconstrained total shoulder arthroplasties and predicted a 9.6% cumulative probability of failure at 5 years.[78] The criteria for failure were defined as the need for a major reoperation, which occurred in eight (4.5%) cases. The indication for reoperation included early dislocation in three shoulders, glenoid component loosening in three shoulders, and muscle transfer for axillary nerve paralysis and resectional arthroplasty for sepsis in one shoulder each. In a more recent article by the same author, this figure did not significantly change at an 11-year end-point.[342] In 1989, Brenner and colleagues[43] analyzed the results of 53 unconstrained total shoulder arthroplasties using the Kaplan-Meier survivorship curve. Employing a more rigid definition that considered failure as not only the need for reoperation but also patient dissatisfaction with the degree of pain relief, the authors reported an 11-year survival of only 73%.

In a large multicenter prospective study involving more than 470 unconstrained total shoulder arthroplasties, the 5-year survival was estimated at 97% (95% confidence interval).[301] A more rigid definition of failure, similar to the criteria proposed by Brenner and associates,[43] was applied to a subset of these patients whose diagnosis was restricted to osteoarthritis. For these patients, failure was defined by one of two parameters. The first parameter, as with the two previous studies, simply involved the need for reoperation after the index procedure. The second parameter was based on a patient self-assessment visual analog scale for pain. For this analysis, failure was defined as the point in time at which the patient reported shoulder pain that was equal or worse than the preoperative condition. For the osteoarthritis subgroup, the probability of 5-year survival was 92% using the more stringent criteria.

Patient Self-Assessment

As a practical approach to effectiveness measurement that can easily be applied in an active practice, one of us (FAM) has used patient self-assessment methods (see earlier sections of this chapter). Since January 1992, all new patients with shoulder problems have been asked to complete the Simple Shoulder Test (SST)[209, 221] to define their pretreatment shoulder function and the SF-36 to characterize their overall health status. The results from these pretreatment questionnaires serve as the baseline on "ingo" for evaluating treatment effectiveness from the perspective of the patient. Follow-up questionnaires reveal the "outcome" of treatment from the patient's perspective. The difference between the outcome and the ingo is the effectiveness of the treatment. Table 16–25 indicates some of these early data for the effectiveness of total or hemiarthroplasty for each of the indicated diagnoses. The preoperative scores are shown to the left of each arrow, and the follow-up score is shown to the right. The data include the SF-36 parameters for total body physical role function and comfort as well as the 12 SST parameters that are specific to the shoulder. The SF-36 scores are the average of the scores of the patients. The SST scores are the percentage of the patients answering "yes" to the indicated question.

A convenient way to display these data is in the Cod-

Table 16–25 EFFECTIVENESS OF TOTAL OR HEMIARTHROPLASTY FOR EACH OF THE INDICATED DIAGNOSES

Diagnosis	*DJD*	*2° DJD*	*RA*	*CTA*	*CA*	*AVN*
Treatment	Total	Total	Total	Hemi	TSA	Hemi
Number of patients	87	20	11	14	6	4
Average follow-up (months)	17	18	19	15	24	14
Physical role						
Preoperative average score	31	25	25	18	25	25
Postoperative average score	58	29	41	29	13	56
Comfort						
Preoperative average score	38	36	33	25	39	36
Postoperative average score	62	54	47	40	44	64
Sleep comfortably						
Preoperative average score	9	15	18	14	0	0
Postoperative average score	89	60	73	64	67	100
Comfort by side						
Preoperative average score	70	40	82	29	67	50
Postoperative average score	95	75	100	64	100	100
Wash opposite shoulder						
Preoperative average score	7	35	0	0	17	0
Postoperative average score	61	55	36	14	33	50
Hand behind head						
Preoperative average score	22	30	27	21	17	50
Postoperative average score	84	50	55	21	67	75
Tuck in shirt						
Preoperative average score	24	40	55	36	17	50
Postoperative average score	79	60	36	50	50	50
8 lb to shelf						
Preoperative average score	13	25	0	0	0	0
Postoperative average score	59	45	9	7	33	25
1 lb to shelf						
Preoperative average score	46	45	36	29	33	75
Postoperative average score	91	65	82	29	83	100
Coin to shelf						
Preoperative average score	55	50	27	36	33	75
Postoperative average score	92	70	91	29	83	75
Overhand toss						
Preoperative average score	5	15	0	7	0	0
Postoperative average score	44	25	18	14	33	0
Usual work						
Preoperative average score	36	45	36	21	67	25
Postoperative average score	71	40	64	14	67	75
Underhand toss						
Preoperative average score	52	45	27	36	33	25
Postoperative average score	72	55	55	29	50	75
Carry 20 lb						
Preoperative average score	62	60	45	43	33	50
Postoperative average score	82	60	73	36	67	75

AV, avascular necrosis; CA, capsulorrhaphy arthropathy; CTA, cuff tear arthropathy; DJD, degenerative joint disease; RA, rheumatoid arthritis; TSA, total shoulder arthroplasty.

man graph (Fig. 16–186), which shows the ingo and the outcome for each patient.

COMPLICATIONS

At the present time, complications associated with prosthetic devices or implants account for approximately 5% of the more than 3.5 million hospitalizations secondary to musculoskeletal conditions.[247] This fact is interesting in light of the increasing patient population with permanent implants and the knowledge that the average age of patients undergoing total shoulder arthroplasty is the lowest of all major joint replacement groups.[235, 248] Cofield and Edgerton have reviewed many of these complications in an instructional course lecture.[82]

Mirroring the increase in volume of total joint arthroplasties in general, the number of shoulder replacement procedures has increased substantially in recent years. However, despite this growth, there was an annual average of less than 5000 total shoulder replacements performed in the United States from 1990 to 1992, compared with 136,000 each for total hip and total knee arthroplasties over the same time period.[246] Although early and midrange follow-up studies of total shoulder arthroplasty have been encouraging with good and excellent results in more than 90% of shoulders, widespread experience and long-term evaluations approaching that of lower extremity joint replacement are not presently available in the literature.[5, 15, 16, 43, 72, 125, 159, 232, 233, 259]

A review of 43 series involving 1858 total shoulder arthroplasties, which were reported over a 20-year period from 1975 to 1995, revealed a mean follow-up of only 3.5 years.[9, 10, 15, 16, 37, 43, 47, 49, 65, 81, 84, 92, 96, 110, 114, 115, 120, 125, 141, 159, 188, 195, 200, 203, 207, 218, 228, 232–234, 256, 257, 266, 277, 281, 284–286, 309, 342, 352, 357] Additionally, less than 50% of these reports met the generally accepted minimum 2-year follow-up criteria established by the peer review process. Of the 21 reports with a minimum follow-up of 2 years, only five studies (391 shoulders) had an average follow-up of 5 years or more.[16, 43, 47, 200, 342] It has been suggested that the duration of follow-up must be sufficient to allow assessment of all clinically relevant outcomes, including those that may occur long after the therapeutic intervention.[135] The use of an inappropriately short follow-up may fail to detect a potentially important difference in prosthetic survivorship or the long-term complication rate of various methods of treatments.[291] In the context of this concern, Neer and associates[256] stated in 1982 that an average follow-up of 3 years was not sufficient to assess many of the complications associated with total shoulder arthroplasty, and it is our opinion that this statement is just as relevant today. Nonetheless, it is our purpose to review the most common problems associated with this procedure in the hope of providing a framework for understanding not only the rectifiable complications but also the failures in patients who have experienced an unfavorable outcome.

Complications of Constrained Total Shoulder Arthroplasty

Since the 1970s, several constrained total shoulder prostheses have been employed in the treatment of various shoulder disorders. These implants include the Fenlin,[115, 117] Bickel,[207] Stanmore,[84, 92, 203, 266] Michael-Reese,[281, 284–286] Kolbel,[195] Kessel,[47] Laurence,[200] Zippel,[370] Liverpool,[23] Trispherical,[142] and three different fixed-Fulcrum prostheses designed by Neer and Averill.[253]

The development of these constrained shoulder prostheses resulted from the commonly held view that glenohumeral instability would be a natural sequela of shoulders with ineffective, attenuated, or torn rotator cuffs. This incomplete understanding of shoulder kinematics led to a variety of non-anatomic shoulder arthroplasty devices which were designed with the two-fold purpose of replacing the arthritic joint as well as restoring the joint stability that had been presumably lost as a result of rotator cuff pathology. It was also theorized that a prosthesis designed with an inherently stable fulcrum would permit the deltoid to elevate the humerus without assistance from the rotator cuff.[195, 281, 284–286]

The majority of constrained shoulder implants employ a fixed fulcrum or semifulcrum concentric ball-and-socket design. With the fixed-fulcrum implant, constraint is maximized by coupling of the humeral and scapular components whereas the ball-and-socket prosthesis is somewhat less restricted. The basic structure of the latter design emulates a total hip prosthesis in that it provides simple static congruity and architectural stability. Unfortunately, the constrained nature of these devices in a joint that normally affords an almost unlimited range of motion results in a high incidence of complications. These complications occur as stress is transferred to the prosthesis-

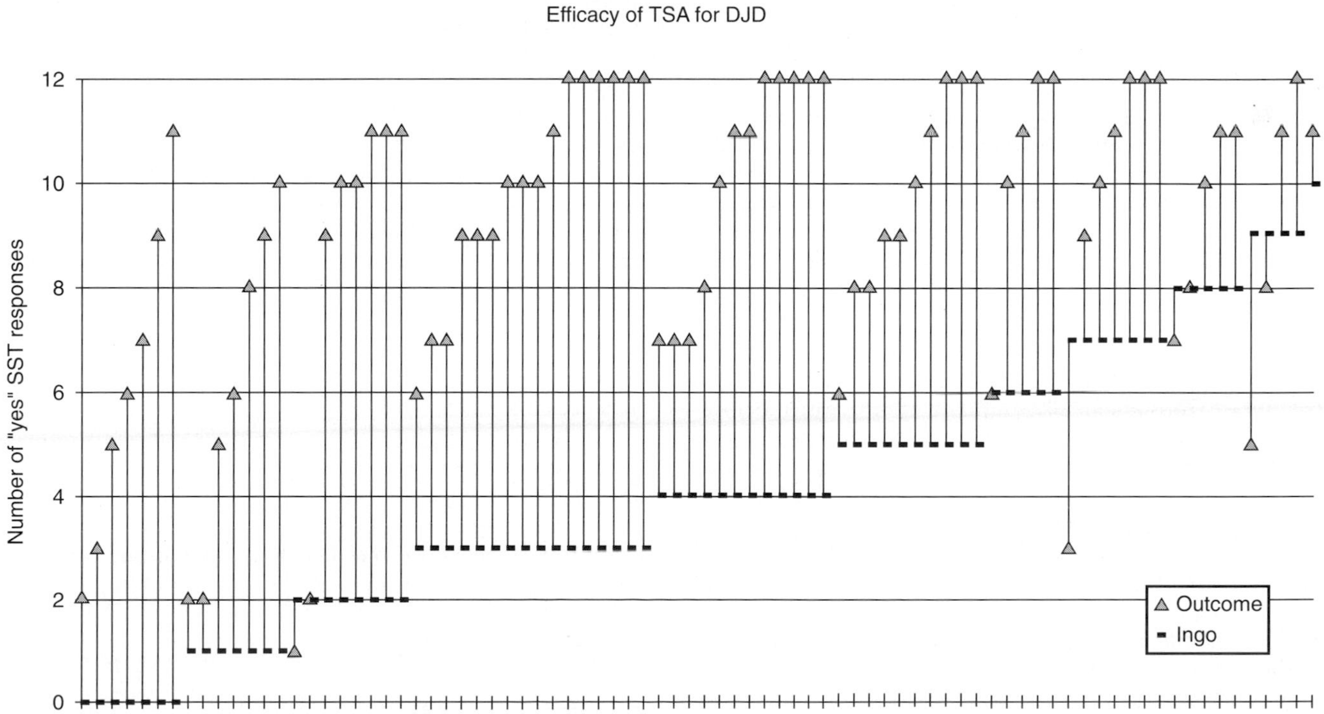

Figure 16–186

This Codman graph shows the efficacy of total shoulder arthroplasty for 82 patients with glenohumeral degenerative joint disease followed for at least 1 year. The ordinate indicates the number of the 12 SST questions answered "yes." Each patient is represented by a check mark on the abscissa. The ingo for each patient is indicated by the short horizontal line. The outcome for each patient is indicated by the arrow. For each patient, the efficacy is the height of the vertical line connecting the ingo to the outcome. The graph indicates that most, but not all, patients improved substantially after shoulder arthroplasty.

bone interface, and forces acting across the glenoid anchorage lead to loosening or mechanical failure.

Since their introduction, constrained total shoulder prostheses have met with limited success and have been associated with a uniformly high frequency of complications compared with unconstrained implants. In a retrospective review of 314 constrained total shoulder arthroplasties reported in 10 series from 1975 through 1992, the overall incidence of complications was approximately 36% with limited follow-up in a number of reports (10 ~ 103).[47, 84, 92, 115, 195, 200, 203, 207, 266] In many cases, the length of follow-up was not specified or was less than 1 year. Only three reports established minimum 2-year follow-up criteria for inclusion in the respective study.[47, 200, 286] Over a similar study period, but with much longer follow-up, a review of 32 reports of unconstrained shoulder implants revealed a mean complication rate of only 16%.[37, 43, 47, 49, 65, 81, 96, 110, 114, 120, 125, 141, 142, 159, 188, 218, 228, 232–234, 256, 257, 266, 277, 309, 340, 342, 352, 357]

In an analysis of 296 constrained shoulder replacements described in seven reports, complications were numerous and included a 25% overall incidence of reoperations (range of 4 to 54%) that were mainly the result of the biomechanical considerations noted earlier.[47, 92, 195, 200, 203, 207, 285] More specifically, 82% of the complications were attributed to the following three factors in order of frequency: (1) mechanical loosening, (2) instability, and (3) implant failure secondary to plastic deformation, fracture, or dissociation of the components. Although these three factors were the most common problems noted in the literature, other complications such as sepsis,[92, 203, 266] neurovascular injury,[115, 281] ankylosis,[200] and periprosthetic fractures[47, 195, 200, 203, 207, 266, 281, 284, 285] have also been described. In two studies, the number of failures were especially high with a revision rate exceeding 50% of the total cases.[207, 285] In 1979, Post and associates reported on their early experience with a constrained shoulder prosthesis.[284] Eight years later in 1987, Post reported extended follow-up of the original series.[281] In this later report, 47 complications were noted in a series of 50 constrained total shoulder arthroplasties performed over a 13-year period. The majority of these complications were significant and included 10 broken or plastically deformed humeral components, 19 episodes of glenohumeral component instability, and 15 cases of mechanical loosening. Chronologically, implant failure was the most common initial complication, and the frequency of this problem increased from 33 to 48% with increasing follow-up (10 ~ 103). The problem of mechanical failure was addressed by altering two parameters: changing the implant material from stainless steel to a cobalt-chrome alloy and improving the mechanical properties of the prosthesis by enlarging the humeral head and neck diameters. These implant modifications resulted in a substantial decrease in the rate of prosthetic failure but at the cost of an increasing incidence of prosthetic dissociation and aseptic loosening. In fact, these two problems alone accounted for 85% of the complications noted by Post in a series and have also been noted by other investigators to be a frequent source of complications.[195, 207, 281]

Focusing briefly on these two problems, controlled dissociation of the glenoid and humeral components was actually part of the engineering rationale that was designed to protect the component anchorage by limiting the peak moments acting on the implant-bone interface. As the applied torque reaches a critical threshold (17 Nm and 9 Nm for the Michael-Reese and Kolbel prostheses, respectively), an uncoupling of the glenoid and humeral components occur. Unfortunately, this complication is rarely rectified without revision surgery to reduce the assembly. As for the other major complication, symptomatic aseptic loosening of the prosthesis posed difficulties with revision surgery secondary to loss of bone stock. Consequently, reoperations were often fraught with an even higher incidence of early loosening and ultimately resulted in resectional arthroplasty or arthrodesis of the glenohumeral joint. The generally poor results after reoperation for this complication led Post to conclude that a loose glenoid component could not be corrected by revision surgery.[281]

In conclusion, our review of the literature indicates that complications such as mechanical impingement, aseptic loosening, instability, and implant failure are disturbingly common in most constrained shoulder replacements, and reoperation rates are unacceptably high in many cases. An ever-expanding fundamental knowledge of shoulder anatomy and biomechanics suggests that these failures reflect not only an error in design rationale but also an underestimation of the forces involved in glenohumeral kinematics. Biomechanical studies by Inman and associates,[170] and Poppen and Walker[279, 280] have determined that glenohumeral joint reactive forces approximate body weight during unrestricted active shoulder elevation. These compressive forces are greatly magnified with any additional load and increase linearly, reaching a maximum at 90 degrees of abduction. Clearly, the forces acting across the glenohumeral joint are impressive in magnitude and must be considered in the design of shoulder prosthesis if untoward complications are to be avoided. To this end, further investigation of joint kinematics, prosthetic limitations, material properties, and survivorship data influenced the evolution of constrained shoulder implants to more anatomically and physiologically unconstrained and semiconstrained prostheses. This same learning curve was observed with other joint replacement procedures in locations such as the knee and elbow where constrained arthroplasties were similarly characterized by unacceptable failure rates.

At the present time, the indications for constrained total shoulder replacement surgery are exceedingly rare and most investigators who have experience with this procedure reserve it strictly as a salvage operation. However, our analysis of the literature pertaining to constrained shoulder implants and the overwhelming number of complications associated with this type of prosthesis would lead us to question its efficacy even in this setting.

Complications of Unconstrained and Semiconstrained Total Shoulder Arthroplasty

Unconstrained and semiconstrained total shoulder arthroplasty has proved to be a highly successful procedure with good and excellent results in more than 90%

of shoulders evaluated at early and midterm follow-up.[5, 15, 16, 43, 72, 125, 159, 232, 233, 259] Despite this success, complications such as aseptic loosening, instability, implant longevity, sepsis, and periprosthetic fracture remain a concern as it does for prosthetic arthroplasty in other major joints. According to Neer and associates,[259] four specific issues must be considered at the time of unconstrained shoulder replacement surgery if complications are to be minimized: (1) humeral head or glenoid bone deficiency; (2) a defective rotator cuff; (3) a deficient deltoid; and (4) chronic instability. Recognition of these variables along with careful patient selection, surgical precision, and a fundamental understanding of shoulder anatomy and kinematics will minimize the complications associated with this procedure.

Our review of the literature pertaining to total shoulder arthroplasty yielded 32 reports involving a total of 1615 shoulders.[9, 10, 15, 16, 37, 43, 47, 49, 65, 81, 96, 110, 114, 120, 125, 141, 159, 188, 218, 228, 232–234, 256, 257, 266, 277, 309, 340, 342, 352, 357] These studies were published over a 19-year period from 1976 to 1995 and included at least 11 different unconstrained or semiconstrained prostheses. Although various implants were utilized, the Neer prosthesis accounted for 70% of these devices.[9, 10, 15, 16, 37, 43, 49, 65, 110, 125, 159, 188, 232, 256, 257, 266, 277, 342, 357]

Although traditional unconstrained and semiconstrained shoulder replacement based on the Neer system has proved more than satisfactory with numerous series reporting good and excellent results in most cases, the mean follow-up was only 42 months (range of 3 to 204 months), and 14 reports had less than a 2-year minimum follow-up. Furthermore, of the 18 reports that met the 2-year minimum evaluation period, only eight series (432 shoulders) had a mean follow-up that exceeded 4 years.[10, 16, 65, 84, 120, 159, 256, 257]

Aware of the potential shortcomings inherent in an analysis of complications associated with this duration of follow-up, our analysis revealed a mean overall complication rate of 16% (range of 0 to 62%) and included the following factors in order of frequency: component loosening, glenohumeral instability, rotator cuff tear, periprosthetic fracture, infection, implant failure including dissociation of modular prostheses, and deltoid weakness or dysfunction.[365]

COMPONENT LOOSENING

Although Péan is credited with performing the first artificial joint replacement of any type, it was not until after the independent pioneering work of McKee and Watson-Farrar,[234] and Charnley[63] in the 1950s that total joint replacement was firmly established. Early complications associated with these devices centered around implant fixation. In 1960, Sir John Charnley suggested that the factors governing component loosening were by no means clearly understood.[62] Although problems related to component anchorage and progressive loosening were greatly improved by Charnley's introduction of polymethyl methacrylate, an incomplete understanding of aseptic loosening persists to the present day and this complication remains a center of focus owing to its ongoing threat to implant longevity.

Symptomatic loosening of glenoid and humeral components occur with a combined incidence of 3.5% and are a major source of complications associated with total shoulder replacement surgery.[15, 43, 81, 125, 141, 159, 228, 233, 234, 256, 266, 309, 340, 342, 352, 357] In fact, prosthetic loosening has the distinction of being the most common problem encountered with total shoulder arthroplasty, representing nearly one third of all complications.[9, 10, 15, 16, 37, 43, 47, 49, 65, 81, 96, 110, 114, 120, 125, 141, 159, 188, 218, 228, 232–234, 256, 257, 266, 277, 309, 340, 342, 352, 357] Most clinical and radiographic loosening involves failure of the glenoid fixation, and this will occupy the central focus of the following discussion.

Kelleher and associates[185] pointed to the need for appropriate orientation of radiographs to evaluate the components in shoulder arthroplasty.

Glenoid Component Loosening

Glenoid component stability is determined by a complex interaction between intrinsic and extrinsic factors. Anatomic, biologic, and biomechanical factors are intrinsically important.

Ten factors contribute to implant stability and are affected by glenoid preparation, soft tissue balancing, wear debris, intercellular mediators of osteoclastic bone resorption, and the availability of glenoid bone-stock for prosthetic fixation. Important extrinsic factors include prosthetic design considerations such as articular surface geometry, glenohumeral conformity, biomaterials, and the glenoid keel or peg morphology. In a report, Neer reviewed 46 total shoulder arthroplasties that had current radiographic evaluation and more than 10-year follow-up and found no evidence of clinical loosening.[253] Although clinical loosening of the glenoid is infrequent, radiolucent lines at the bone-cement interface of the glenoid component are common with a frequency ranging from 30 to 96%.[15, 16, 47, 72, 159, 188, 259] As suggested by numerous authors,[81, 85, 124, 253] this variation is partially attributed to nonstandardized methods of measurement, inconsistent definitions, and limitations of conventional radiography.

In 1982, Neer and associates[259] reported a 30% incidence of radiolucencies around the glenoid component in a series of 194 shoulders. More than 90% of these radiolucent lines were observed in the initial postoperative radiographs and were attributed to poor cementing technique. Six years later an additional 214 implants were reviewed and were found to have almost the same incidence of loosening although the frequency of complete lines was much lower.[253] The authors emphasized that radiolucencies were not progressive during the period of follow-up and concluded that the clinical significance of these radiographic findings was unclear.

Offering a different perspective, other investigators have expressed concern that the appearance or progression of radiolucent zones may herald the onset of future problems related to symptomatic component loosening (Fig. 16–187).[8, 15, 47, 72, 81, 159, 184, 342, 359] A review of 350 shoulder replacements from five centers well known for their expertise in total shoulder arthroplasty revealed a 32% incidence (range of 10 to 96%) of progressive glenoid loosening.[15, 37, 47, 72, 159] One particular series from Sweden reported radiolucent zones around the glenoid component in 96% of 26 shoulders with a mean follow-

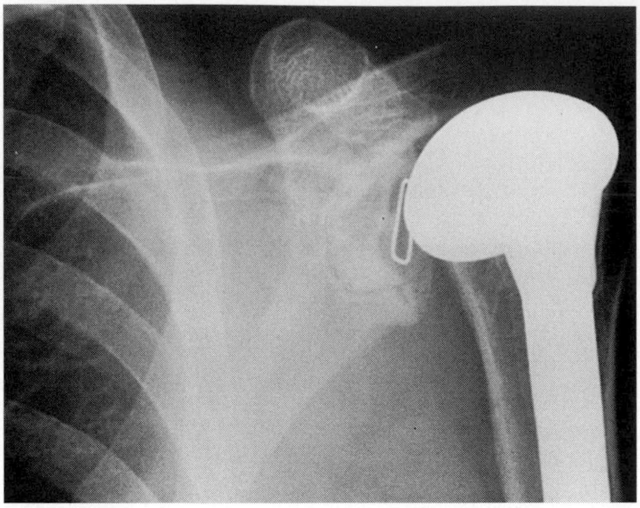

Figure 16–187

This anteroposterior radiograph shows a complete radiolucent line about the bone cement interface of a glenoid component. This finding was present at the 6-month follow-up but showed no progression on several subsequent radiographic examinations. (From Wirth MA and Rockwood CA: Complications of shoulder arthroplasty. Clin Orthop *307*:47–69, 1994.)

up of 47 months.[47] Disconcertingly, no radiolucencies were observed around the glenoid component in immediate postoperative radiographs, but with increasing follow-up, 25 of 26 shoulders had developed this interval change within 3 years after surgery. The development of these radiographic findings were associated with a slight decrease in function and a mild increase in pain.

In 1984, Cofield[72] reported improved shoulder motion and reliable pain relief in the majority of 73 Neer total shoulder arthroplasties with follow-up ranging from 2 to 6 years. Although clinical results were excellent and compared favorably with other reports in the literature, 82% of the cases demonstrated radiolucencies at the bone-cement interface and 11% had radiographic evidence of component loosening. More recently, Torchia and associates[342] analyzed 89 total shoulder replacement arthroplasties that included extended evaluations on patients included in the original report. At a mean follow-up of 12 years (range of 5 to 17 years), 75 glenoid components (84%) had developed radiolucencies at the bone-cement interface and 39 glenoid implants (44%) demonstrated definite radiographic loosening as defined by a shift in component position or the presence of a complete bone-cement radiolucent line at least 1.5 mm in diameter. Comparing the original and recent reports, radiographic component loosening had increased fourfold using established and consistently applied criteria over the extended study period. Even more concerning was the statistically significant association between radiographic glenoid implant loosening and pain ($P = .0001$). With increasing duration of follow-up, the number of patients reporting satisfactory pain relief declined from 92% to 82%.

The present concerns of aseptic glenoid component loosening have led to a variety of new innovations including cementless press-fitted, plasma sprayed, and tissue ingrowth glenoid implants. The literature on this subject includes 150 cases from six series with an average follow-up of 3.5 years.[81, 89, 114, 218, 233, 309] Deficiencies were noted in many of these reports due to an incomplete radiographic review, insufficient follow-up, and inconsistent reporting methods; however, some of the preliminary data were encouraging and suggested a lower incidence of both radiolucencies and subsequent component loosening. Bonutti and associates[34] have reported the use of arthroscopy to evaluate suspected glenoid loosening.

Although a number of different glenoid component designs were used in these studies, there is little published information specifically addressing the influence of glenoid morphology on implant stability. In 1988, Orr and colleagues utilized finite element analysis to examine several glenoid component design parameters.[265] The effect of keel geometry, metal backing, and superior constraints were assessed. The glenoid bone was modeled as a four-region homogeneous isotropic structure based on the material properties of the natural glenoid. For each of these regions, the yield strength, modulus of elasticity, and Poisson's ratio were calculated based on local bone density data from values in the literature. The authors concluded that keel geometry could be altered to approximate the stress distribution found in the natural glenoid and to improve the glenoid component stability. Also in 1988, Fukuda and associates performed a biomechanical analysis of stability and fixation strength in four different glenoid designs: the Neer-I, the Neer-II (Kirschner Medical Corp, Fairlawn, NJ), Cofield (Smith and Nephew Richards, Memphis, TN), and Gristina (Howmedica Inc., Rutherford, NJ) components.[131] The test results demonstrated less resistance to failure by pull-out in a direction perpendicular to the face of the glenoid for the Neer-I high-density polyethylene glenoid that did not have a metal backing. The clinical significance of this is unclear as suggested by Collins and associates, who suggested glenoid component loosening resulted more often from eccentric or off-center compressive loads in contrast to a pull-out mechanism of failure.[85] Furthermore, as suggested by Fukuda and colleagues, the fatigue testing did not consider the biologic stress shielding effect of metal-backed glenoid implants or the systemic response to metallic and polymeric wear debris.[131] In 1992, Friedman and associates studied the stress distributions of several glenoid component designs using two-dimensional finite element analysis.[129] It was hypothesized that adverse bone remodeling at the implant site would lead to aseptic loosening and that this would be minimized by reproducing the physiologic stress patterns across the natural glenoid. The analysis indicated that physiologic stresses were approximated when the subchondral bone was preserved.

The influence of fixation peg design on implant stability was evaluated by Giori and associates in a parametric study.[137] The parameters included the number and size of fixation pegs as well as the aspect ratio (length/diameter). Five peg geometries of various shapes and sizes were tested for sheer stability. The results of the study suggested that components with multiple small pegs created a more uniform stress distribution in the anchoring material and provided more sheer stability per unit volume than implants with fewer, but larger pegs.

Current concepts to enhance glenoid fixation and durability include preservation of the subchondral plate, concentric spherical reaming that ensures optimal bone support of the glenoid implant, diametral mismatching of the glenoid and humeral head to decrease eccentric loading, and the introduction of new glenoid designs and enhanced biomaterials.[85, 169, 323, 367] Although theoretically and biomechanically sound, these concepts must remain as a focus of ongoing basic science and clinical research to determine if this promising new technology will decrease the incidence of glenoid component failure.

Despite considerable success with total shoulder arthroplasty after the independent introduction of glenoid components by Kenmore,[189] Zippel,[370] and Neer[253] in the early 1970s, many problems remain unsolved (Fig. 16–188). An inability to resolve some of these issues and the apparent success with hemiarthroplasty have led some investigators to question the indications for glenoid resurfacing.[15, 47, 126, 359]

In 1974, Neer[251] reviewed 47 shoulder hemiarthroplasties with an average follow-up of 6 years. Twelve patients were followed for more than 10 years without evidence of progressive degenerative changes or resorption of the glenoid fossae. Pain relief and functional recovery was the rule leading Neer to conclude that there was little reason to treat osteoarthritis with a more extensive replacement that might increase complications and jeopardize prosthetic longevity.

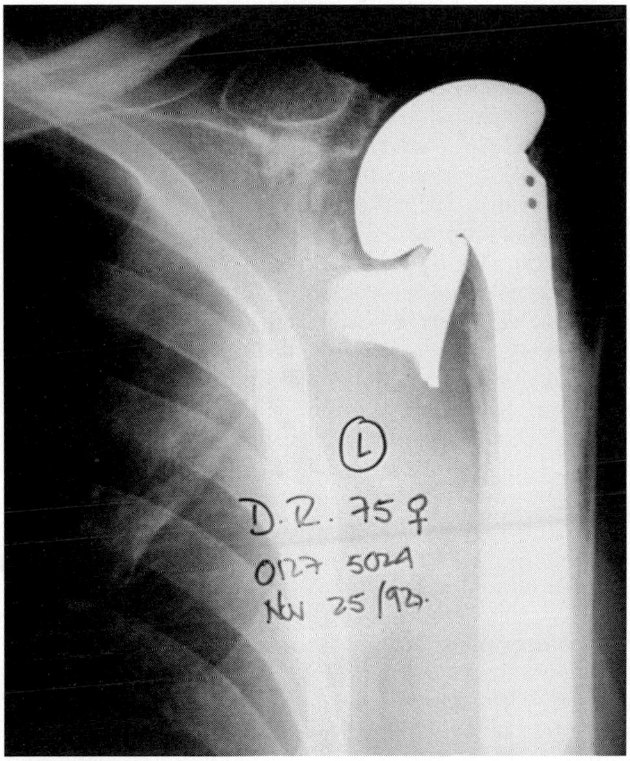

Figure 16–188

An anteroposterior radiograph made after the patient complained of an acute worsening of symptoms that had occurred when the shoulder "slipped out of place" while she was getting out of bed. Note the inferior dislocation of the metal-backed glenoid component. (Adapted from Wirth MA and Rockwood CA: Complications of total shoulder replacement arthroplasty. J Bone Joint Surg *78A*:603–616, 1996.)

After Neer's report in 1974, several studies have documented good and excellent results with hemiprosthetic replacement of the shoulder, but only a few have compared the results of hemiarthroplasty to total shoulder arthroplasty in a similar patient population, and no randomized prospective studies exist.[8, 37, 65, 184, 346] Interestingly, complications are less frequent with hemiarthroplasty of the shoulder and statistically significant differences in overall pain relief, function, and patient satisfaction compared with total shoulder arthroplasty have not been demonstrated.[8, 16, 37, 65, 71, 184, 188, 346]

Several authors have described an association between symptomatic glenoid loosening, glenohumeral instability, and irreparable rotator cuff deficiencies.[15, 85, 126, 159, 277] These issues, in conjunction with the limited follow-up in most total shoulder arthroplasty series, the prevalence of osteolysis about the bone-cement interface of glenoid components, current knowledge pertaining to material properties in the pathogenesis of prosthetic loosening, and the association of symptomatic glenoid component translation with glenohumeral instability, lead us to conclude that the current indications for total shoulder arthroplasty need further refinement.

Glenoid Wear After Hemiarthroplasty

Cofield and Edgerton[82] pointed to the potential for medial migration and progressive glenoid wear after hemiarthroplasty. They pointed out that revision to total shoulder arthroplasty almost always resolved the process and symptoms.

Rockwood and associates have reported successful results using hemiarthroplasty in patients with osteoarthritis and rheumatoid arthritis.[17, 173]

Humeral Component Loosening

Undeniably, difficulties with glenoid component fixation account for most complications related to aseptic loosening of total shoulder prostheses. In short- and mid-term follow-up studies, radiographic evaluations reveal a 5% incidence of implant subsidence or complete radiolucent lines measuring 2 mm or more about the humeral prosthesis.[15, 37, 43, 72, 78, 259] Complete radiolucent lines were more frequently observed in uncemented humeral components, but clinical findings associated with loosening were rare and accounted for symptoms in fewer than 2% of patients.[15, 16, 37, 43, 72, 78, 259]

In a long-term series with a mean follow-up of 12 years, 49% of 81 press-fit humeral components had shifted in position.[342] Furthermore, 93% of the humeral prostheses that demonstrated a change in position also demonstrated radiolucent lines at the prosthesis-bone interface. In contrast, radiolucent lines were present in less than 50% of the 41 prostheses that did not reveal a change in position. Consistent with previous studies, only one of eight cemented humeral components developed a radiolucent line at the bone-cement interface, and none demonstrated a change in position.[15, 43, 81, 125, 141, 234, 309] As opposed to the statistically significant correlation between symptoms and loosening of the glenoid prosthesis, loosening of the humeral component was not associated with pain.

GLENOHUMERAL INSTABILITY

Glenohumeral instability after total shoulder arthroplasty is rarely discussed in the literature despite a frequency that varies between 0 and 35%[16, 43, 65, 81, 141, 159, 228, 233, 234, 256, 266, 309, 342, 357] and the fact that it is the second leading cause of complications associated with prosthetic arthroplasty of this joint. From an extensive review of the literature, anterior, anterosuperior, or anteroinferior instability was found in 30 (43%) shoulders,[16, 114, 141, 228, 233, 240, 256, 357, 366] posterior instability in 14 (20%) shoulders,[8, 9, 15, 16, 43, 65, 81, 159, 256, 366] inferior instability in three (4%) shoulders,[125, 256] multidirectional instability in two (4%) shoulders, and an unspecified direction of instability in 21 (30%) shoulders[16, 65, 233, 234, 266, 309, 342] for an overall incidence of approximately 4%.

In the normal glenohumeral joint, stability is provided by a hierarchy of mechanisms that labor in concert to ensure a virtually unlimited range of motion and uncompromised function. Small loads are offset by passive means such as joint surface architecture,[45, 204, 244] finite joint volume,[223, 364] atmospheric pressures,[204, 244, 324] and the adhesion/cohesion of joint fluid.[324] Moderate loads are counterbalanced by the deltoid and rotator cuff musculature whose coordinated contractions resist displacing forces, and large loads are resisted by the capsulolabral structures and bone architecture.[223, 320, 324, 344, 351, 364, 366] Unfortunately, these complex interactions can become ineffective in shoulder arthroplasty, thus increasing the propensity for instability. This tendency increases the shoulder's dependence on precise soft tissue balancing and proper positioning of the prosthetic components to restore both rotational and translational components of normal shoulder kinematics. Although the diagnosis of a fixed dislocation should be obvious when the triad of history, physical examination, and radiographic studies are properly applied, the analysis of more subtle instability can be quite challenging when it presents as discomfort associated with a vague sense of shoulder dysfunction.

Anterior Instability

Anterior instability following shoulder replacement surgery is most commonly associated with malrotation of the humeral component, anterior deltoid dysfunction, or disruption of the subscapularis repair. Thirty shoulders with this complication were reported in the literature; four shoulders were managed expectantly with closed reduction and immobilization; 17 were treated by reoperation; and treatment was not specified for the remaining shoulders.[114, 141, 228, 233, 240, 357, 366]

In 1993, Moeckel and associates[240] described their findings and the results of reoperation in seven patients whose total shoulder arthroplasty had been complicated by anterior glenohumeral instability. At the time of surgery, all patients demonstrated a disruption of the subscapularis tendon repair that was mobilized and repaired. The anterior instability recurred in three shoulders (43%) but was successfully reconstructed with a secondary operative procedure in which a bone-Achilles tendon allograft was inserted as a static anterior restraint.

In our series, surgical exploration of three total shoulder arthroplasties with anterior instability revealed decreased retroversion of the humeral component ($\leq$ 20 degrees) in all shoulders, disruption of the subscapularis in two shoulders, and erosion of the anterior glenoid in one shoulder.[366] One of these patients had a massive irreparable tear of the rotator cuff and had a previous distal clavicle resection, coracoacromial ligament resection, and acromioplasty that rendered the coracoacromial arch as an incompetent restraint to anterior glenohumeral translation. Revision of these shoulders involved various techniques, including restoration of normal humeral component version, coracoacromial ligament reconstruction, and pectoralis major tendon transfer.

While inadequate retrotorsion of the humeral component may lead to an increased anterior translation of the humeral head, clinically obvious anterior subluxation or dislocation will usually not occur unless the subscapularis is deficient or previous surgery has compromised the stabilizing effect of an intact coracoacromial arch. In our experience, disruption of the subscapularis repair is usually attributed to surgical technique, poor tissue quality, inappropriate physical therapy, or the use of oversized components. The use of thick metal-backed glenoid components or excessively large humeral head implants may dramatically increase the lateral humeral offset that creates an internal rotation contracture of the shoulder and stresses the subscapularis repair during external rotation maneuvers.

Superior Instability

Progressive superior migration of the humeral head has been reported in association with dynamic muscle dysfunction, attenuation of the supraspinatus, failed rotator cuff repairs, and frank rupture of the rotator cuff.[15, 37, 39, 72] In one series, major cuff tears were present in 20% of all patients and in 29% of patients with proximal migration. The amount of proximal humeral migration was independent of the size of the rotator cuff defect but correlated positively with the association of cuff deficiency and poor preoperative function.[39] Similarly, the series of Boyd and associates[37] noted proximal humeral migration in 29 (22%) of 131 total shoulder arthroplasties with an average follow-up of 44 months. Rotator cuff tears were present in only seven shoulders in this subgroup, suggesting that proximal migration may be secondary to an imbalance in the force couple between a strong deltoid and a weak, poorly rehabilitated rotator cuff.

Although superior migration of the humeral head is well recognized in the literature, it does not appear to be directly related to the development of shoulder discomfort or impending failure after hemiarthroplasty. In fact, Boyd and associates[37] noted no increased pain with proximal migration of the humeral head, and we have also made this observation. However, our concern is related to the potential complication of glenoid component loosening as a result of progressive superior humeral migration. In this setting, the humeral head articulates with the superior portion of the glenoid component and results in eccentric loading of the component and progressive loosening over time. This observation was reported by Barrett and colleagues[15] who suggested that superior migration leads to eccentrically applied glenoid compressive forces, increased stress at the bone-cement interface, and eventual loosening of the glenoid component within the glenoid fossa. In 1988, Franklin and associates[124] reported an association between proximal humeral migration, incompletely reconstructible rotator cuff tears, and glenoid component loosening in seven cases of total shoulder arthroplasty. The amount of proximal humeral migration was closely correlated with the degree of glenoid loosening and superior tilting of the component. The translation of the glenoid component was referred to as a "rocking horse" glenoid, and the authors credited Gristina for first recognizing that eccentric loading would stress the glenoid anchorage.

From the preceding discussion of superior instability in conjunction with our experience during the last 20 years in performing humeral hemiarthroplasty for combined degenerative glenohumeral arthritis and irreparable rotator cuff tears, we can only conclude that humeral hemiarthroplasty is the procedure of choice for this condition.

Posterior Instability

Approximately 14 cases of posterior glenohumeral instability following total shoulder arthroplasty have been recorded in the literature.[9, 15, 43, 65, 81, 159, 256, 259] This complication is frequently associated with increased retrotilt of the glenoid component or excessive retroversion of the humeral prosthesis, posterior glenoid erosion, and soft tissue imbalance. Patients with long-standing arthritis of the glenohumeral joint usually demonstrate a characteristic wear pattern of the glenoid, and in most circumstances this can be predicted by the disease process. For example, central glenoid erosion is the usual pattern of wear in rheumatoid arthritis, whereas posterior glenoid deficiency characterizes long-standing osteoarthritis. Failure to recognize posterior glenoid erosion may lead to placement of the glenoid component in excessive retrotilt at the time of surgery, resulting in an increased propensity for posterior instability.[365] When the patient's physical examination demonstrates a marked restriction of external rotation, and radiographic examination reveals posterior glenohumeral subluxation, the physician should be wary of uneven posterior glenoid wear. In this situation, CT scans of both shoulders will precisely define the degree of posterior glenoid deficiency and will greatly facilitate preoperative planning. In most situations, minor deficiencies of the posterior glenoid can be compensated by decreasing the degree of humeral retroversion by the amount of glenoid retrotilt or by a careful reaming of the anterior glenoid.[253, 305] Occasionally, severe posterior glenoid deficiency will require bone grafting of the glenoid as described by Neer and Morrison.[257]

Patients who demonstrate posterior glenohumeral subluxation associated with long-standing osteoarthritis or a history of chronic posterior instability, whether recurrent or fixed, are at increased risk for posterior instability after shoulder replacement. Although proper placement of the humeral and glenoid components will minimize this tendency, the avoidance of this complication is also critically dependent on soft tissue balancing. In most patients, the shoulder demonstrates restricted external rotation with a tight and contracted anterior soft tissue envelope. In contrast, the posterior capsule is stretched and its volume is greatly increased due to chronic and progressive posterior displacement of the humeral head. Namba and Thornhill[245] have described the application of posterior capsulorrhaphy to the problem of intraoperative posterior instability.

The experience at the University of Texas Health Sciences Center at San Antonio with posterior glenohumeral instability following shoulder arthroplasty includes seven shoulders.[366, 367] Objective findings in these shoulders included increased retroversion of the humeral component ($\geq$ 80 degrees) in four shoulders, posterior glenoid erosion in four shoulders, and a nonunion of the greater tuberosity (Fig. 16–189). These shoulders were revised by restoring normal retroversion of the humeral component, sculpting or reaming the glenoid to re-establish proper glenoid version, and posterior capsulorrhaphy to address the asymmetric soft tissue pathology.

Inferior Instability

Inferior instability after shoulder arthroplasty usually occurs as a complication of treatment for acute proximal humerus fractures but has also been noted after total shoulder replacement in cases of prosthetic revision, chronic fractures, previous osteosynthesis, and uncomplicated rheumatoid or osteoarthritis.[114, 125, 126, 259] Many of the patients with this complication demonstrate inadequate active motion and lack the ability to raise the arm above the horizontal plane due to shortening of the humerus, which renders the deltoid ineffective. Authors reporting this complication emphasize the importance of re-establishing anatomic humeral length, which in turn restores the resting tension of the deltoid and rotator cuff.[71, 256, 259] This optimizes function by minimizing the tendency for inferior instability and subsequent weakness during elevation.

ROTATOR CUFF TEARS

Postoperative tearing of the rotator cuff is the third most frequent complication of total shoulder arthroplasty, with an incidence of 2%. Although this entity is considered a common complication after shoulder replacement surgery, symptoms are usually minimal and reflect the natural history of cuff disease in the general population. A review of several large series suggests that both nonoperative and operative treatment have been employed in the management of this complication; however, the benefits of surgical intervention are somewhat unclear because recurrent tearing of the cuff and insignificant improvement in function and motion have been noted in several cases.[5, 15, 16, 43, 120, 159, 188, 357]

In Neer's 1982 report,[259] patients with massive rotator cuff deficiencies fared quite well after shoulder arthroplasty. This series included two paraplegic patients, seven rheumatoid patients, and 10 patients with rotator cuff arthropathy whose shoulders were all graded as a successful result despite having massive rotator cuff tears. This experience led Neer to conclude that rotator cuff

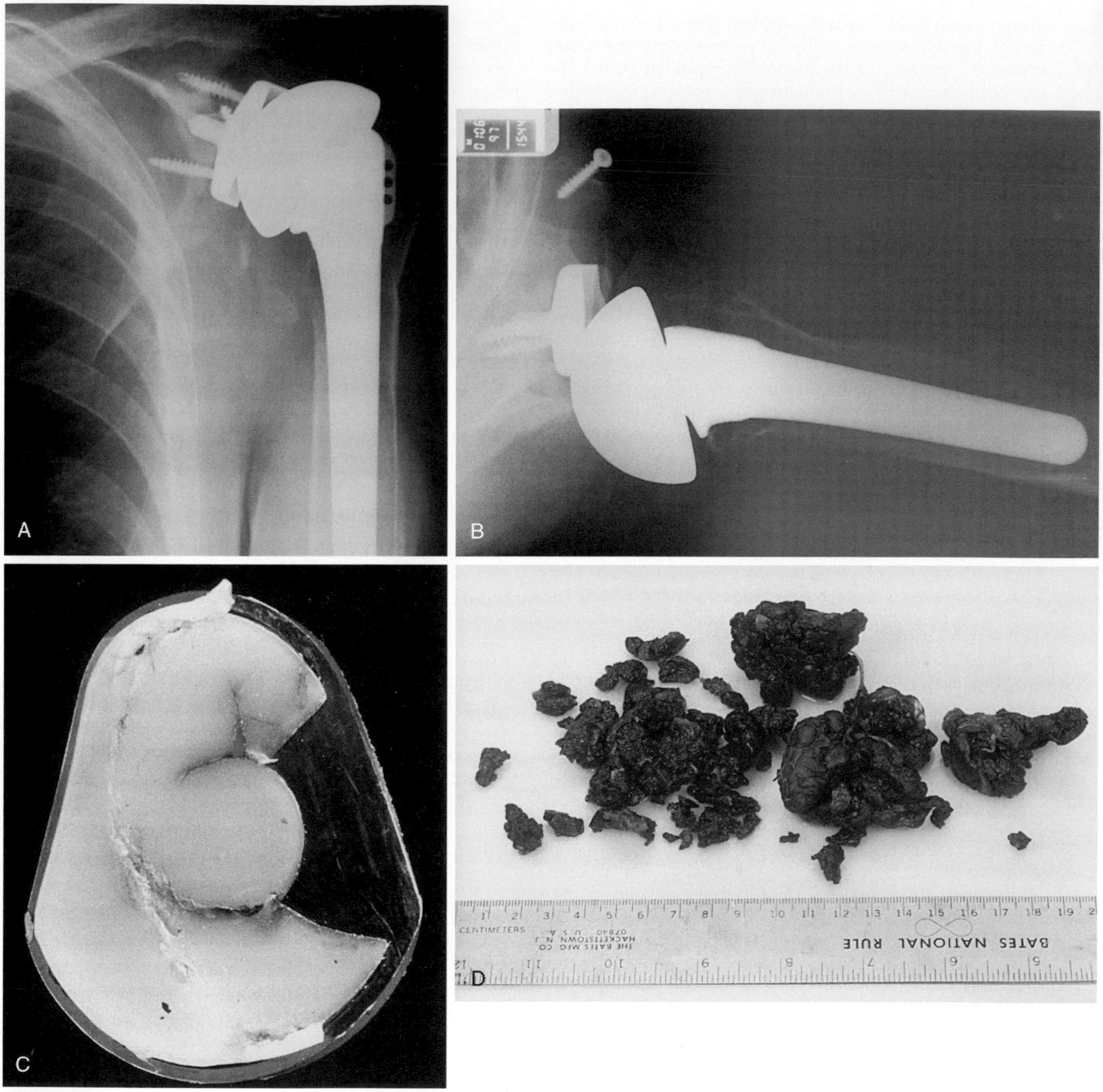

Figure 16–189

A, An anteroposterior radiograph of a 71-year-old man who had pain and a "mechanical clunk" with motion of the shoulder 2 years after operation. Narrowing of the glenohumeral articulation suggests metal-on-metal contact. *B*, This axillary lateral radiograph shows posterior subluxation of the humeral head from the glenoid. *C*, At the time of revision surgery, performed 36 months after the primary arthroplasty, the glenoid component was loose. This photograph shows the marked wear of the polyethylene insert. The marked wear of the metal glenoid tray is not apparent on this photograph. *D*, Metal-on-metal wear between the humeral head and the glenoid tray resulted in a proliferative metal synovial reaction. The volume of excised synovial tissue exceeded 240 cm^3.

deficiency was not a contraindication to unconstrained total shoulder arthroplasty as advocates of constrained arthroplasties had suggested.

In our experience, most patients with symptoms suggesting a chronic rotator cuff tear will respond to expectant management consisting of an anti-inflammatory agent, moist heat, and a physician-directed rehabilitation program that emphasizes strengthening of the deltoid, the remaining rotator cuff, and the scapular stabilizing musculature. We reserve reoperation of postoperative rotator cuff tears for patients with persistent symptoms and for those with obvious functional deficits after acute trauma.

PERIPROSTHETIC FRACTURES

Although a prevalence of less than 2% might appear as insignificant, periprosthetic shoulder fractures account for approximately 20% of all complications associated with total shoulder arthroplasty and often present difficult treatment challenges. We reviewed 14 reports describing 45 fractures of the glenoid or humerus associated with prosthetic replacement of the shoulder.[5, 9, 15, 33, 37, 38, 114, 144, 159, 188, 232, 256, 266, 342] In several of these articles the mechanism of injury, subsequent management, and final outcome were either omitted or not discussed in detail, making analysis difficult. Nonetheless, we reviewed the results according to three parameters: the type of fracture, the temporal relationship of the fracture to surgery, and the clinical outcome. The clinical outcome was graded as satisfactory or unsatisfactory. A satisfactory rating was characterized by clinical and radiographic bony union, minimal to no symptoms, and the absence of associated complications such as component loosening. Our analysis revealed humeral shaft or tuberosity involvement in 86% of these injuries[9, 15, 37, 124, 159, 188, 233, 266, 342] and glenoid fractures in an additional 12% of cases.[159, 188, 232] The division of fracture complications into intraoperative and postoperative groups identified the former group as the most frequently occurring injury with an incidence of 62%. According to the clinical outcome parameters, 87% of the intraoperative fractures that were diagnosed and stabilized at the time of injury were graded as satisfactory. With regard to fractures occurring in the postoperative period, only 54% healed uneventfully with expectant management.

In 1989, Hawkins and associates[159] reported two humeral shaft fractures and two glenoid fractures in a series of 70 total shoulder arthroplasties, all of which were sustained intraoperatively. The humeral shaft fractures occurred in elderly patients with rheumatoid arthritis. Overzealous reaming, impaction of the humeral component, and excess torque placed upon the humerus were all mentioned as mechanisms leading to fracture. The humeral shaft fractures were treated initially with cerclage wiring and postoperative immobilization, but both required reoperation. One was treated successfully with a long-stem revision humeral component while the second was treated with compression plating. This last patient subsequently refractured distal to the plate but was treated successfully with a humeral fracture brace.

Boyd and associates[38] reported seven patients who had a humeral fracture after either a total shoulder arthroplasty or a shoulder hemiarthroplasty. Trauma after a fall was the cause of fracture in six patients; and the final patient sustained injury in a motor-vehicle accident. Common to all injuries was a fracture pattern that involved the humeral shaft at the tip of the prosthesis. The initial treatment in four patients consisted of an Orthoplast or sugar-tong splint, whereas two patients were initially immobilized with only a sling and swathe. Both of these patients developed progressive loss of radial nerve function that necessitated early operative intervention. Surgical management of the fractures consisted of open reduction and internal fixation with a dynamic compression plate in two patients and revision shoulder arthroplasty with a long-stem humeral component in three patients. All operatively treated fractures healed at an average time of approximately 5 months after surgery. Of the two patients treated nonoperatively, one developed a nonunion but refused further treatment for medical reasons and the other eventually required revision surgery unrelated to the humeral fracture. In the latter patient, the humeral fracture united with the tip of the prosthesis protruding outside the humeral shaft. Apparently, persistent symptoms were attributed to glenoid component loosening, while the humeral malunion was asymptomatic. In five of six patients the authors noted a decrease in shoulder motion from pre-injury levels, but the extent of this was unclear because information specifying the range of shoulder motion prior to injury was not available. In conclusion, Boyd and associates[38] emphasized several factors that influenced the natural history of fractures adjacent to humeral prostheses. These factors included the advanced age of many of the patients, osteopenia or bone quality, rheumatoid arthritis, and associated deficiencies of the soft tissues. The authors also stressed that only one of seven fractures healed with immobilization alone, but the results of conservative fracture management could not be assessed in two patients owing to the development of a radial nerve palsy that prompted subsequent operative intervention. Moreover, by admission of the investigators, these seven cases probably did not represent all of the periprosthetic fractures that occurred during the 15-year period of their study.

Wright and Cofield[369] presented a similar series of nine fractures that had occurred at an average of 39 months after 499 arthroplasties with an average patient age of 70 years. The original indication for arthroplasty was either rheumatoid arthritis or old trauma. The authors concluded that long oblique and spiral fractures can be successfully treated nonoperatively if alignment is acceptable. Operative treatment is considered for transverse or short oblique fractures at the level of the distal tip of the prosthesis or for those associated with a loose prosthesis. Autogenous bone grafting is recommended with all surgeries.

In 1994, we presented the results of treatment of fractures adjacent to humeral prostheses at the University of Texas Health Science Center at San Antonio.[144] The series consisted of 12 humeral fractures, eight of which occurred as an intraoperative complication and four that resulted from postoperative trauma. Of the eight intraoperative humeral fractures, six occurred during primary shoulder arthroplasty and two occurred in revision procedures. In the primary arthroplasty group of six patients, fractures occurred during manipulation of the limb in two patients, reaming of the intramedullary canal in one patient, broaching of the canal in one patient, and insertion of the prosthesis in two patients. In the revision arthroplasty cases, both fractures occurred in areas of moderate to severe cortical thinning. Intraoperative fractures were managed with open reduction and internal fixation with simple cerclage wiring, or a long-stem prosthesis in conjunction with cerclage wiring (Fig. 16–190). All intraoperative fractures healed at an average of 8 weeks with a mean forward elevation at final follow-up of 122 degrees.

Four postoperative fractures occurred at an average of 14 months after the index arthroplasty. All of these injuries were managed with a fracture orthosis and resulted in bone union at an average of 9 weeks after injury. At final evaluation, the average forward elevation was 121 degrees.

The treatment of periprosthetic shoulder fractures is divided into two seemingly divergent schools of thought. Bonutti and Hawkins[33] advocated aggressive treatment of these injuries, which included open reduction and internal fixation, bone grafting, and postoperative immobilization in a spica cast for a minimum of 6 weeks. Similarly, Boyd and associates[38] reported an increased likelihood of nonunion after nonoperative treatment and suggested that fractures treated operatively would fare better.

Although one would expect uniform treatment guidelines based on the 11 patients in the reports of Bonutti and Hawkins[33] and Boyd and associates,[38] the results of the San Antonio experience involving 12 patients suggests an alternative and perhaps more conservative approach to the management of postoperative periprosthetic fractures. Of note, three patients in our series with fractures that extended distal to the tip of the prosthesis were managed with a fracture orthosis, and these fractures healed uneventfully. In all, five fractures that progressed to bone union were managed with an Orthoplast fracture brace, isometric exercises, and early range-of-motion rehabilitation. Our approach to intraoperative fractures was more aggressive because most of these injuries were treated with open reduction and internal fixation. Four intraoperative fractures were also managed by replacing the primary prosthesis with a long-stem revision component. Bone union was achieved in all cases without supplemental bone grafting or postoperative shoulder spica immobilization.

Although a meaningful comparison of various treatment modalities is difficult because of the few reported cases, we prefer to manage all intraoperative fractures by whatever means necessary to obtain a stable surgical construct. The purpose of this treatment is to restore stability to the limb, to create an environment that is favorable to fracture healing, and to allow unimpeded postoperative rehabilitation so that the functional result is not compromised by prolonged immobilization.

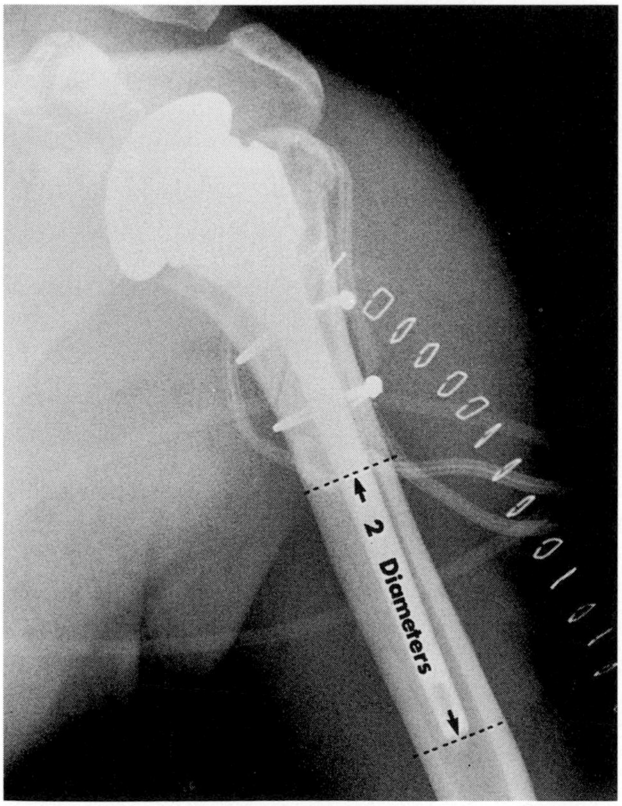

Figure 16–190

An anteroposterior radiograph demonstrating cerclage wire stabilization of a periprosthetic proximal humerus fracture. Note that the humeral stem bypasses the distal extent of the fracture by approximately two cortical diameters.

Intraoperative Periprosthetic Fractures

For the most part, intraoperative fractures of the humerus or glenoid arise from errors in surgical technique, many of which are avoidable. These surgical errors include inadvertent reaming, overzealous impaction, or manipulation of the upper extremity during exposure of the glenoid. Several points deserve emphasis.[33, 38, 144, 159] First, spiral fractures of the humerus are usually observed when the shoulder is externally rotated by using the upper extremity as a lever arm. This places the humerus at risk for fracture due to the magnitude of torsional stress generated by this maneuver. The torsional force imparted to the humerus can be minimized by performing a complete anterior and inferior capsular release and by using a bone hook on the humeral neck to deliver the proximal humerus out of the glenoid fossa. Occasionally, exposure is still less than optimal; however, this can be improved by continuing the inferior soft tissue release to the posteroinferior and posterior capsular structures. One must pay meticulous attention to detail while releasing the capsule from the glenoid in this region of the glenohumeral joint because of the close proximity of the axillary nerve as it passes through the quadrangular space. Second, if the arm is not extended off the side of the operating table, it is difficult to insert the trial prosthesis or medullary reamers and this may result in perforation or complete fracture of the proximal humerus. Third, after humeral head resection, the entry point of the trial stem or reamer should be superolateral in an eccentric location on the cancellous surface of the proximal humerus. This ensures that the trial stem or reamer will pass directly down into the medullary canal rather than medially where it may perforate the humeral neck or medial cortex. Finally, hand reaming is preferred to power instrumentation, because the latter may remove too much cancellous bone or increase the likelihood of perforating osteoporotic bone.

If intraoperative fractures occur, we have been pleased with the results of cerclage wiring and the use of a long-stem prosthesis if the situation warrants. For humeral fractures occurring proximal to the tip of the humeral prosthesis, simple cerclage wiring of the proximal humerus and implantation of a standard size of prosthesis is appropriate. Autogenous bone graft from the humeral head is used to make a slurry of cancellous bone, which is placed into the metaphyseal portion of the proximal humerus after the stem of the prosthesis is inserted to the level of the metaphyseal-diaphyseal junction. The trial prosthesis is then used in a piston fashion to work the slurry of autogenous bone into the fracture site or other areas of bone deficiency before placing the final prosthesis. For fractures occurring entirely distal to the prosthesis or for those occurring in the proximal portion of the humerus with distal extension beyond the tip of the prosthesis, we prefer to use a long-stem prosthesis that extends at least two humeral cortical diameters beyond the most distal extent of the fracture. This is accomplished by extending the deltopectoral incision into an extensile anterolateral approach to the humerus. The relatively straight, cylindrical anatomy of the humeral diaphysis is ideal for this method of intramedullary fracture fixation. There are several advantages of this form of treatment over dynamic compression plating or cerclage wiring alone. First, the need for secure screw purchase in bone, which is often of poor quality, is obviated. Second, bending and torsional loads are better tolerated and decrease the risk of implant failure. Third, a rigid and biomechanically sound surgical construct is usually ensured. Fourth, the extensile exposure and soft tissue dissection needed for plate fixation is avoided. Finally, the ever-present concern for stress shielding is minimized.

With regard to glenoid fractures, it is important to remember that glenoid component stability is affected by glenoid preparation, soft tissue balancing, and the availability of uncompromised glenoid bone stock for prosthetic fixation.[362] Scapular fractures adjacent to glenoid components may compromise implant stability and lead to symptomatic loosening. Bone grafting or revision glenoid components that are built up with a wedge to accommodate the defect can be used; however, if bone support cannot be ensured, resurfacing of the glenoid should not be performed. In this situation, the remaining glenoid is sculpted with a hand bur or glenoid reamer to match the radius of curvature on the head of the humeral component and the glenoid component is omitted.

Postoperative Periprosthetic Fractures

As a rule of thumb, our initial approach to management of postoperative periprosthetic fractures of the shoulder is more conservative than the usual methods of treatment recommended for similar fractures that occur during surgery. If a trial of expectant management is not contraindicated by the development of a radial nerve palsy or other ominous complication, one can proceed with a simple regime consisting of an Orthoplast fracture brace, isometric exercises for the entire upper extremity, and early motion as pain and swelling subside. In our experience at the University of Texas Health Science Center at San Antonio, satisfactory results are often obtained with this simple form of initial treatment. However, it cannot be overemphasized that one must do what is necessary in order to ensure that early functional rehabilitation is not delayed, because prolonged immobilization has been associated with poor results in our experience.

INFECTION

Infection after total shoulder arthroplasty is a rare but potentially devastating complication with a prevalence of about 1%.[321] The unique predilection for bacterial seeding of endoprostheses is the result of several factors, including bacterial adhesion, glycoprotein encapsulation, bacterial resistance to antibiotics, physical properties of the implant such as chemical composition and surface texture, and inhibiting factors from ion elusion. Of 39 cases reported in the literature, 18 had a mean interval of 17 months from the initial arthroplasty to the diagnosis of shoulder sepsis; 10 were classified as late infections and six as early infections, without specifying the exact time of occurrence.[47, 68, 81, 114, 120, 141, 205, 228, 233, 256, 266, 309, 342] In three shoulders the time of occurrence was not mentioned at all, thus making it impossible to determine the temporal relationship of the infection to the index arthroplasty.[81, 234, 309] In three reports,[68, 94, 205] the interval from the initial arthroplasty to the diagnosis of glenohumeral sepsis often exceeded a period of 12 months. An increased susceptibility to infection was correlated with host risk factors such as diabetes mellitus, rheumatoid arthritis, systemic lupus erythematosus, and remote sites of infection. Additionally, immunosuppressive chemotherapy, systemic corticosteroids, multiple steroid injections, and previous shoulder surgery were noted in 66% of patients from the combined series.[68, 94, 205] Although it is only speculation, the apparent increased risk of infection after local steroid injections may be attributed to the unique bursal anatomy of the shoulder. Inadvertent or purposeful injection of the subdeltoid, subscapular, or infraspinatus bursae, or the sheath of the long head of the tendon of the biceps may provide an avenue for intra-articular bacterial invasion.

The value of preoperative laboratory tests (i.e., WBC count, erythrocyte sedimentation rate, and C reactive protein), radioisotope scanning, and joint aspiration was difficult to ascertain because of rare and inconsistent reporting methods. Eighteen patients with infected shoulder arthroplasties from the series of Codd and associates[68] and five patients with septic shoulder arthroplasties treated at the University of Texas were combined for the purpose of analysis. Laboratory values for the preoperative erythrocyte sedimentation rate and WBC count averaged 55 mm and 11,260 WBCs, respectively. Radioisotope scans were interpreted as positive in 58% of shoulders, and positive culture joint aspirations were found in only 38% of shoulders.

A review of 39 infected shoulder arthroplasties reported in the literature revealed *Staphylococcus aureus* as the etiologic organism in three shoulders and *Candida parapsilosis* in one shoulder.[47, 68, 81, 114, 120, 141, 205, 228, 234, 256, 266, 309, 342] In the remaining shoulders, the infectious organism was not identified in the report. Our experience with five infected shoulder arthroplasties revealed *S. aureus* in three shoulders, *S. epidermidis* in one shoulder, and a mixed infection in one shoulder.

As with other joint replacement surgery, infections can present early or late, and optimal treatment depends on isolation of the pathogen through tissue or fluid specimens. Once the diagnosis has been made, several treatment options exist including antibiotic suppression, irrigation and débridement, reimplantation, resectional arthroplasty, arthrodesis, and amputation. The type of treatment depends on a host of factors, including the time interval from arthroplasty to the diagnosis of sepsis, the feasibility of implant removal as dictated by anesthetic risk, the pathogen's virulence and susceptibility to antibiotics, and implant stability.

The differential diagnosis of a draining wound in the early postoperative period after shoulder replacement surgery must include early infection despite negative cultures and the lack of obvious constitutional symptoms. In this scenario, we advocate early wound exploration with irrigation, débridement, and the judicious use of parenteral antibiotics. The prosthesis is retained if the infection is secondary to a gram-positive organism and the components are stable. For early infections with gram-negative organisms or late deep wound infections, we are currently advising thorough débridement of granulation tissue and scar and the removal of all biomaterials including cement. This is followed by a 6-week course of parenteral antibiotics as advised by infectious disease consultation. The majority of infected shoulder implants that we have treated are managed with resectional arthroplasty; however, other modes of treatment can be used, such as glenohumeral arthrodesis or two-stage revision arthroplasty.

In one report, 18 infected shoulder arthroplasties were managed with resectional arthroplasty in five shoulders and endoprosthetic reimplantation utilizing antibiotic-impregnated cement in 13 shoulders.[68] In the latter group, eight components were revised with a one-stage reimplantation, and five were managed with reimplantation at a second operation. Pain decreased in most patients; however, interestingly, the degree of pain relief was not significantly different in patients undergoing reimplantation compared with resectional arthroplasty alone. Not surprisingly, functional results in terms of range of motion and the ability to perform activities of daily living were much better in the reimplantation group. For this reason, it is important to convey to the patients that resectional arthroplasty of the shoulder is a salvage procedure that, at best, allows patients to achieve acceptable pain relief, the ability to perform simple activities of daily living, and resolves their infection.

Although the literature is somewhat limited, several reports substantiate infection about a joint replacement from transient bacteremia secondary to dental manipulation, urinary tract infections, pneumonia, and genitourinary instrumentation.[1, 260, 331, 332] Due to the variety of possibilities leading to secondary infection, we advocate prophylactic antimicrobial coverage that is individualized to each clinical situation.

NERVE INJURIES

Approximately 14 cases of peripheral nerve or brachial plexus complications associated with total shoulder arthroplasty have been recorded in the literature.[9, 15, 37, 120, 125, 141, 189, 232, 277, 342] Fortunately, most of these injuries involved neuropraxia and were managed expectantly with good results. However, in two cases, the mechanism of neural injury involved a laceration of the axillary nerve that occurred in heavily scarred surgical fields.[71] Although the majority of these complications involve the axillary nerve (six cases), injuries to the ulnar nerve (three cases), musculocutaneous nerve (two cases), median nerve (one case), and the brachial plexus (two cases) have also been reported. Seven of these injuries resolved completely; two exhibited incomplete recovery; and one demonstrated no recovery. The recovery status of the remaining four neurologic injuries was not mentioned.

Lynch and associates[213] reported on 18 shoulders with neurologic deficits out of 417 arthroplasties. Thirteen shoulders had injuries involving the brachial plexus, usually the upper and middle trunks. Eleven shoulders recovered well at 1 year. In most cases, traction was thought to be the cause of the injury.

IMPLANT-RELATED COMPLICATIONS

Occasionally, shoulder replacement surgery is complicated by the development of implant-related failure. From our analysis of the literature we conclude that the prevalence of this complication is approximately 0.7%, and 80% of these failures have been observed in uncemented metal-backed glenoid components. Dissociation of the polyethylene glenoid insert from its metal tray,[81, 107, 233] Driessnack and associates' fracture of the keel or metal glenoid backing,[81, 107, 218] fractured fixation screws,[218, 233] and subluxation or dislocation of polyethylene subacromial spacers [43, 65] have all been reported (Fig. 16–191).

Since their introduction in the late 1980s, modular total shoulder arthroplasty systems have been widely accepted for their ability to optimize soft tissue balancing, maximize proximal humeral metaphyseal and canal fit, facilitate glenoid revision, and permit hemiarthroplasty to total shoulder arthroplasty conversion. Although some complications of total shoulder replacement surgery have been decreased by changes in prosthetic design, improved component fixation, and the evolution of biomaterials, new problems have arisen that are unique to modular shoulder implants. In 1991, Cooper and Brems[88] described a case report of a patient with recurrent dissociation of a modular humeral component that was ultimately revised to a Neer II humeral component. In addition to this case report and another case that was referred to our institution, we are aware of 11 cases of humeral component dissociations.[32] With the exception of one episode, all dissociations occurred within 6 weeks of the index arthroplasty procedure. Unlike previous case reports involving disassembly of modular femoral components used in the hip, none of the shoulder component dissociations were associated with joint dislocation or subsequent reduction maneuvers.[273, 368] In fact, several of the patients in the report of Blevins and associates[32] were uncertain of when the dissociation occurred. Similarly, our patient was unaware of a specific event that correlated with disassembly of the humeral prosthesis but noted discomfort associated with shoulder dysfunction since the time of operation. At the time of revision surgery, the posterior aspect of the humeral collar was subsided in the metaphy-

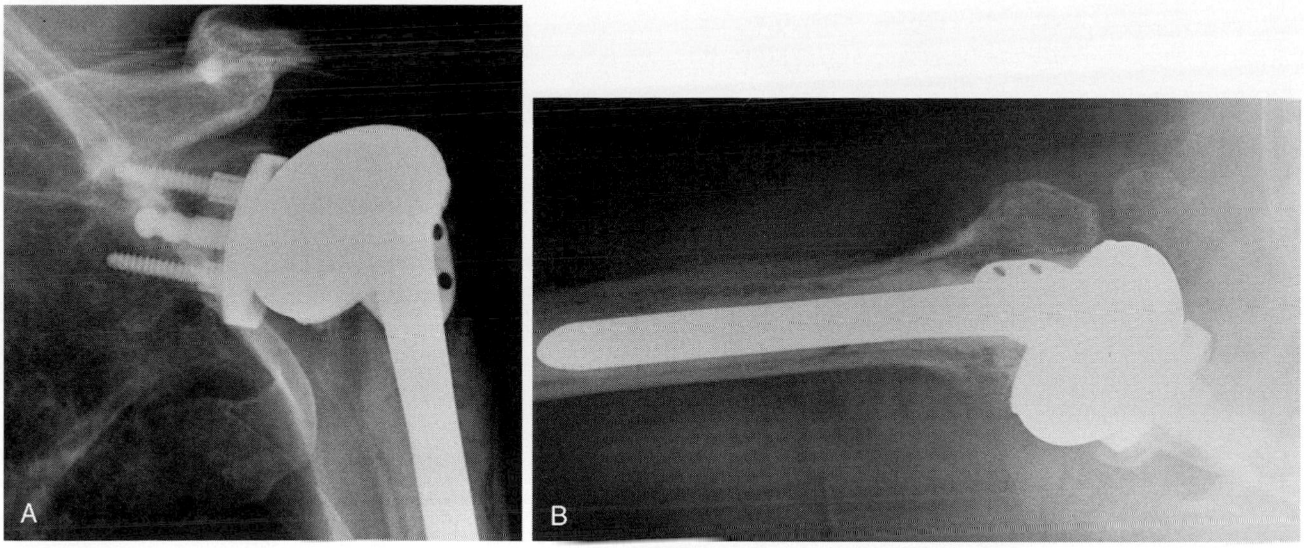

Figure 16–191

A and *B*, Radiographs of a patient who sustained a posterior shoulder dislocation that was complicated by dissociation of the polyethylene glenoid insert. Narrowing of the glenohumeral articulation suggests metal-on-metal contact.

seal bone of the proximal humerus and most likely precluded adequate seating of the Morse taper components during the initial arthroplasty procedure.

In the laboratory setting, biomechanical studies of Cooper and Brems[88] and Blevins and colleagues[32] have demonstrated that a volume of water, saline, or blood as little as 0.4 ml may be enough to prevent locking of the Morse taper. To minimize complications such as this, the Morse taper socket of the modular prosthesis must be thoroughly free of tissue or fluids that would preclude an adequate weld of the Morse taper fixation. Additionally, it is imperative to recognize soft tissue or bone encroachment that might become interposed between the humeral head and the collar.

DELTOID DYSFUNCTION

The technique of prosthetic replacement of the shoulder joint requires great familiarity with the anatomy and biomechanics of the shoulder. Critical to the final outcome of this procedure is maintenance of the deltoid origin and insertion, because loss of the deltoid through a failed repair or injury to the axillary nerve results in a catastrophic loss of shoulder function.[10, 94, 146, 256, 259, 357] Although optimal exposure is key to the ease at which total shoulder arthroplasty is accomplished, it is equally important to realize that the procedure can be performed through an extended deltopectoral approach without detaching the origin or insertion of the deltoid muscle.[302]

In Neer's 1982 series of total shoulder replacements, three different surgical exposures were utilized.[259] Initially, a short deltopectoral approach was employed that involved detachment of the anterior deltoid from the clavicle. The second approach was more superior and involved detachment of the middle deltoid, but both of these exposures were discontinued because they were found to weaken the anterior and middle portions of the deltoid, respectively. The third approach, which Neer has advocated since 1977, utilizes a long deltopectoral interval and preserves the origin and insertion of the deltoid. Maintenance of the deltoid in this fashion facilitates early postoperative rehabilitation and minimizes the problems associated with the first two operative exposures. In 1982, Neer and Kirby included deltoid detachment as a major cause of failed unconstrained shoulder arthroplasty (Fig. 16–192).[256] These authors observed consistent weakening and atrophy of the deltoid in all except three of 37 patients. Fibrotic and ischemic changes in the anterior deltoid were presumably the result of overzealous retraction in most cases, whereas previous surgical approaches denervated the anterior deltoid in five patients. Overall, severe compromise of deltoid function was observed in 92% of failed unconstrained total shoulder and humeral head arthroplasties.

One of us (CAR) has treated 36 patients who had a postoperative loss of deltoid muscle function after shoulder operations, including endoprosthetic replacement procedures.[277] Nine of these replacement procedures were primary operations, and three were revision procedures. Of these 12 patients, 10 lost function of the anterior or anterior and middle deltoid secondary to a failed repair, and two lost complete function of the deltoid as a result of axillary nerve denervation. Patients were evaluated using a standardized evaluation form proposed by the American Shoulder and Elbow Surgeons, which independently documents the patient's pain, range of motion, strength, stability, and function. All patients were significantly disabled with a mean forward elevation of only 33 degrees (range of 0 to 75 degrees). Additionally, several patients demonstrated painful anterosuperior dislocation of the glenohumeral joint with attempted elevation of the upper extremity. Functional limitations were severe with nine poor and three fair results based on 15 activities of daily living. Without question, loss of deltoid function to denervation or detachment was poorly tolerated and resulted in pain and functional impairment.[146]

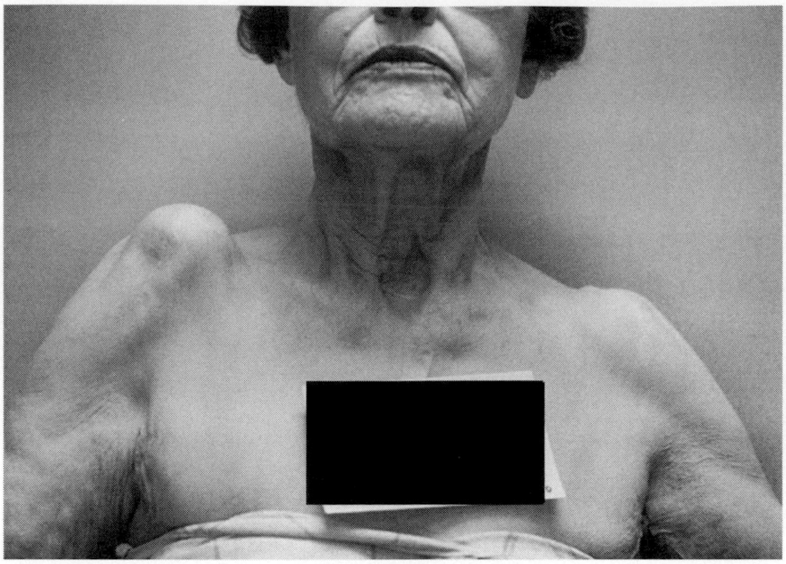

Figure 16–192

Appearance of the shoulder in a patient with loss of the anterior deltoid attachment following total shoulder replacement surgery. Note the anterior shoulder atrophy and the prominent humeral component.

REVISION SHOULDER ARTHROPLASTY

The number of shoulder replacement procedures performed in the United States has increased substantially in the past decade. Although widespread use of unconstrained total shoulder prosthetic designs has resulted in a marked decrease in complications, difficulties requiring reoperation are not uncommon. In a review of 22 shoulder arthroplasty series that reported this complication, the frequency of reoperation was 7%.[10, 37, 43, 47, 71, 81, 96, 114, 120, 124, 141, 159, 188, 218, 233, 234, 256, 277, 309, 340, 352, 357] Although many of these operations consisted of soft tissue procedures for postoperative complications such as rotator cuff tears and glenohumeral instability, approximately 46% involved removal or revision of prosthetic components. A stratification of the latter two subgroups revealed revision of the glenoid, humeral, or both components in 16 shoulders, glenohumeral resectional arthroplasty in 10 shoulders, glenoid component resection in seven shoulders, and glenohumeral arthrodesis in four shoulders. The treatment of several shoulders in these subgroups was not specified.

One of the greatest drawbacks in the surgical management of failed total shoulder prostheses is underestimating the technical demands and substantial complications that may occur with revision surgery of this magnitude. The literature reflects revision rates of 0 to 17% after shoulder arthroplasty, but publications that specifically address revision shoulder surgery are rare. In fact, we are aware of only two peer reviewed published articles that specifically address revision shoulder arthroplasty.[256, 259]

In 1982, Neer and Kirby[256] published a report on a series of 40 revision arthroplasties performed over a 9-year period. The index procedures included 31 hemiarthroplasties, six unconstrained total shoulder arthroplasties, and three constrained total shoulder replacements. The authors analyzed the index procedures and categorically assigned the causes of failure into one of three major groups: (1) general preoperative considerations such as neuromuscular problems, infection, or arthritis of adjacent joints, (2) surgical or prosthetic complications including deltoid detachment, tuberosity nonunion, and component loosening or breakage, and (3) postoperative considerations such as residual or recurrent instability and inadequate rehabilitation. More than one cause of failure was noted in almost every case.

According to Neer and Kirby, the most common causes of failure included deltoid scarring and detachment, loss of external rotation due to contracture of the subscapularis, prominence or retraction of the greater tuberosity, glenoid insufficiency, and inadequate postoperative rehabilitation.[256] The common denominator to all failed hemiarthroplasties and unconstrained total shoulder replacements was adhesions of the rotator cuff and deltoid that had occurred as a result of prolonged immobilization. Revision surgery consisted of unconstrained total shoulder replacement in 32 shoulders, glenohumeral arthrodesis in three shoulders, a fixed fulcrum constrained implant in one shoulder, and resectional arthroplasty and scar débridement in two shoulders each. It is important to emphasize that more than 80% of these revisions involved prostheses that had been originally inserted for displaced fractures and fracture-dislocations of the proximal humerus. The degree of surgical difficulty in revision surgery was greatly magnified by contracture and muscle scarring, associated tuberosity malunion, or nonunion, and bone loss with shortening of the humeral shaft. The results of the majority of these revisions were reported in another series and were found to be inferior to other diagnostic groups, prompting the authors to stress the importance of a successful primary procedure.[259]

In 1993, Caldwell and associates[57] reviewed 13 revision arthroplasties with an average follow-up of 36 months. Two total shoulder replacements and one hemiarthroplasty were revised for glenohumeral instability. Seven hemiarthroplasties were revised to total shoulder replacements secondary to glenoid arthropathy, and three total shoulder arthroplasties were revised due to glenoid component loosening. The results were considered satisfactory in only 62% of the cases, and five shoulders required seven reoperations. Glenoid loosening and incorrect version were regarded as the most frequent causes of revision surgery.

Wirth and Rockwood reviewed 38 failed unconstrained shoulder arthroplasties that were revised at the University of Texas Science Center at San Antonio between 1977 and 1993.[367] The initial indication for arthroplasty was acute trauma in 19 shoulders, osteoarthritis in 12 shoulders, post-reconstruction arthropathy in five shoulders, and rheumatoid arthritis in two shoulders. Five patients had undergone eight prior attempts at revision arthroplasty. Our analysis of these cases revealed findings that were similar to those of Neer and Kirby[256] in that failure was often multifactorial, making it difficult to associate failure with one specific factor in 70% of shoulders. Patients were divided into two groups, similar to those described by Neer and associates.[259] Shoulders in group I patients were characterized by infected prostheses, anterior deltoid dysfunction or axillary nerve injury, chronic intractable pain, severely limited range of motion, and poor function. These patients were treated with resectional arthroplasty, with the expectation that they would achieve only limited goals consisting of pain relief and the ability to perform simple activities of daily living (Fig. 16–193). Patients in group II were managed with a revision hemiarthroplasty or total shoulder replacement procedure. The most common complication leading to revision surgery was symptomatic glenohumeral instability (43%), which included posterior instability in eight shoulders, anterosuperior instability in six shoulders, and inferior instability in four shoulders. The instability was correlated with inadequate humeral length and soft tissue balancing in 12 shoulders, component malpositioning or subsidence in seven shoulders, asymmetric glenoid erosion in five shoulders, and failure of the subscapularis repair in two shoulders. Other causes of failure, listed in order of decreasing frequency, included: anterior deltoid insufficiency, glenoid component loosening, glenoid erosion, humeral component loosening, tuberosity detachment or malunion, bony or fibrous ankylosis, glenohumeral infection, and dissociation of a modular humeral component.

Twenty-five shoulders were followed between 2 and 9 years and included nine resectional arthroplasties. Seven of the nine shoulders (group I) obtained acceptable pain relief and were successful in achieving limited goal activities; the remaining two shoulders required additional proximal humeral resection.[94] The remaining 16 shoulders (group II) were graded according to Neer's rating system with five excellent, seven satisfactory, and four unsatisfactory results that compared favorably with the findings of Caldwell and associates.[57] Of the four shoulders with an unsatisfactory result, all demonstrated marked anterior deltoid weakness and dysfunction.

In summary, there are many different causes of failure of primary shoulder arthroplasty and the multifactorial nature of these problems makes analysis difficult. Revision shoulder arthroplasty represents a formidable challenge and requires a careful preoperative evaluation if satisfactory management is to be expected. We agree with Neer[259] that this is the most technically challenging of shoulder replacement procedures and emphasize that although pain relief is usually achieved, a functioning deltoid is required if more than limited goals are to be expected.

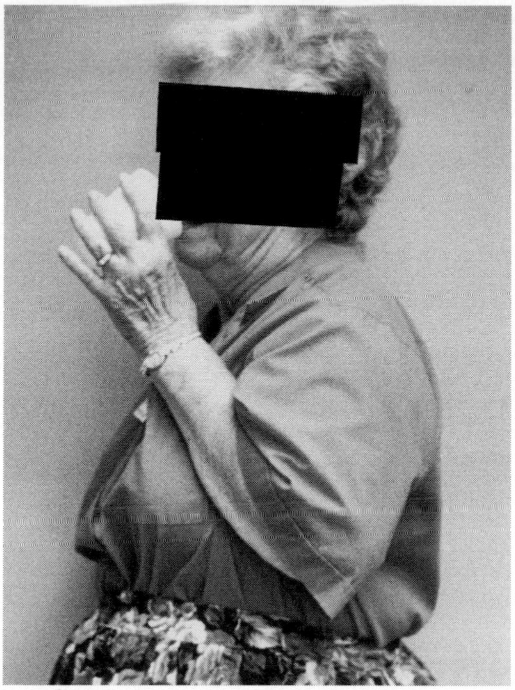

Figure 16–193

A 76-year-old patient demonstrating function of the upper extremity after a resectional arthroplasty of a failed constrained total shoulder prosthesis. Although simple activities of daily living can be performed by adducting the arm to the body for stability, shortening of the humerus significantly limits deltoid effectiveness in elevation of the arm.

Although major advances in total shoulder arthroplasty have been made in recent years, we would do well to remember that complications are an inescapable aspect of shoulder surgery and that these problems exert a substantial burden on the patient's health, function, and quality of life. It is with this in mind and in the spirit of Codman that we press on to carefully assess the interminable difficulties with the purpose of further advancement.

References and Bibliography

1. Adams MA, Weiland AJ, and Moore JR: Nonconstrained total shoulder arthoplasty: An eight year experience. Orthop Trans *10*:232–233, 1986.
2. Alasaarela EM and Alasaarela ELI: Ultrasound evaluation of painful rheumatoid shoulders. J Rheumatol *21*:1642–1647, 1994.
3. Amstutz HC: The DANA Shoulder Replacement. Rutherford, NJ: Howmedica, 1982.
4. Amstutz HC, Sew Hoy AL, and Clarke IC: UCLA anatomic total shoulder. Clin Orthop *155*:7–20, 1981.
5. Amstutz HC, Thomas BJ, Kabo JM, et al: The DANA total shoulder arthroplasty. J Bone Joint Surg *70A*:1174–1182, 1988.
6. Armbuster TG, Slivka J, Resnick D, et al: Extraarticular manifestations of septic arthritis of the glenohumeral joint. J Roentgenol *129*:667–672, 1977.
7. Arntz CT, Jackins S, and Matsen FA III: Surgical management of complex irreparable rotator cuff deficiency. J Arthroplasty *6*:363–370, 1991.
8. Arntz CT, Jackins S, and Matsen FA III: Prosthetic replacement of the shoulder for the treatment of defects in the rotator cuff

and the surface of the glenohumeral joint. J Bone Joint Surg *75A*:485–491, 1993.
9. Averill RM, Sledge CB, and Thomas WH: Neer total shoulder arthroplasty (Abstract). Orthop Trans *4*:287, 1980.
10. Bade HA III, Warren RF, Ranawat CS, and Englis AE: Long-term results of Neer total shoulder replacement. *In* Bateman JE and Welsh RP (eds): Surgery of the Shoulder. St. Louis: BC Decker and CV Mosby, 1984, p 294.
11. Baker GL, Oddis CV, and Medsger TA Jr: *Pasteurella multocida* polyarticular septic arthritis. J Rheumatol *14*:355–357, 1987.
12. Ballmer FT, Lippitt SB, Romeo AA, and Matsen FA III: Total shoulder arthroplasty: Some considerations related to glenoid surface contact. J Shoulder Elbow Surg *3*:299–306, 1994.
13. Ballmer FT, Sidles JA, Lippitt SB, and Matsen FA III: Humeral head prosthetic arthroplasty: Surgically relevant geometric considerations. J Shoulder Elbow Surg *2*:296–304, 1993.
14. Bankes MJ and Emery RJH: Pioneers of shoulder replacement: Themistocle Gluck and Jules Emile Pean. J Shoulder Elbow Surg *4*:259–262, 1995.
15. Barrett WP, Franklin JL, Jackins SE, et al: Total shoulder arthroplasty. J Bone Joint Surg *69A*:865–872, 1987.
16. Barrett WP, Thronhill TS, Thomas WH, et al: Non-constrained total shoulder arthroplasty for patients with polyarticular rheumatoid arthritis. J Arthroplasty *4*:91–96, 1989.
16a. Barton NJ: Arthrodesis of the shoulder for degenerative conditions. J Bone Joint Surg *54*(8):1759–1764, 1972.
17. Basamania CJ, Gonzales J, Kechele P, et al: Hemiarthroplasty vs Total Shoulder Arthroplasty in Patients with Rheumatoid Arthritis. 10th Open Meeting American Shoulder and Elbow Surgeons, New Orleans, 1994.
18. Bateman JE: Arthritis of the glenohumeral joint. *In* The Shoulder and Neck. Philadelphia: WB Saunders, 1978, pp 343–362.
19. Bayley JIL and Kessel L: The Kessel total shoulder replacement. *In* Bayley I and Kessel L (eds): Shoulder Surgery. New York: Springer-Verlag, 1982, pp 160–164.
20. Bechtol CO: Bechtol Total Shoulder. Memphis, TN: Richards Manufacturing Co., 1976.
21. Becker W: Arthrodesis of the shoulder joint (review of 47 cases). *In* The Arthrodesis in the Restoration of Working Ability. Stuttgart: Georg Thieme, Stuttgart, 1975, p 25.
22. Beddow FH and Elloy MA: The Liverpool Total Replacement for the Gleno-humeral Joint. *In* Joint Replacement in the Upper Limb. Institution of Mechanical Engineering Conference, London, 1977, pp 21–25.
23. Bodey WN and Yeoman PM: Prosthetic arthroplasty of the shoulder. Acta Orthop Scand *54*:900–903, 1983.
24. Bell S and Gschwend N: Clinical experience with total arthroplasty and hemiarthroplasty of the shoulder using the Neer prosthesis. Int Orthop *10*:217–222, 1986.
25. Beltran JE, Trilla JC, and Barjau R: A simplified compression arthrodesis of the shoulder. J Bone Joint Surg *57A*:538, 1975.
26. Benjamin A, Hirschowitz D, Arden GP, and Blackburn N: Double osteotomy of the shoulder. *In* Bayley I and Kessel L (eds): Shoulder Surgery. New York: Springer-Verlag, 1982, pp 170–175.
27. Benjamin A, Hirschowitz G, and Arden GP: The treatment of arthritis of the shoulder joint by double osteotomy. Int Orthop *3*:211–216, 1979.
28. Bennett WF and Gerber C: Operative treatment of the rheumatoid shoulder (Editorial). Curr Opin Rheumatol *6*:177–182, 1994.
29. Bigliani LU, Flatow EL, McCluskey GM, and Fisher RA: Failed prosthetic replacement in displaced proximal humerus fractures. Orthop Trans *15*:747–748, 1991.
30. Bigliani LU, Weinstein DM, Glasgow MT, et al: Glenohumeral arthroplasty for arthritis after instability surgery. J Shoulder Elbow Surg *4*:87–94, 1995.
31. Blauth W and Hepp WR: Arthrodesis of the shoulder joint by traction absorbing wiring. *In* Chapchal G (ed): The Arthrodesis in the Restoration of Working Ability. Stuttgart: Georg Thieme, 1975, p 30.
32. Blevins FT, Deng X, Torzilli PA, et al: Dissociation of Humeral Shoulder Arthroplasty Components. American Academy of Orthopaedic Surgeons 61st Annual Meeting, New Orleans, LA, 1994.
33. Bonutti PM and Hawkins RJ: Fracture of the humeral shaft associated with total replacement arthroplasty of the shoulder. J Bone Joint Surg *74A*:617–618, 1992.
34. Bonutti PM, Hawkins RJ, and Saddemi S: Arthroscopic assessment of glenoid component loosening after total shoulder arthroplasty. Arthroscopy *9*:272–276, 1993.
35. Bostrom C, Harms-Ringdahl K, and Nordemar R: Clinical reliability of shoulder function assessment in patients with rheumatoid arthritis. Scand J Rheumatol *20*:36–48, 1991.
36. Boyd AD Jr, Aliabadi P, and Thornhill TS: Postoperative proximal migration in total shoulder arthroplasty. Incidence and significance. J Arthroplasty *6*:31–37, 1991.
37. Boyd AD Jr, Thomas WH, Scott RD, et al: Total shoulder arthroplasty versus hemiarthroplasty. J Arthroplasty *5*:329–336, 1990.
38. Boyd AD Jr, Thornhill TS, and Barnes CL: Fractures adjacent to humeral prostheses. J Bone Joint Surg *74A*:1498, 1992.
39. Boyd AD Jr, Thornhill TS, Thomas WH, et al: Post-operative Proximal Migration in Total Shoulder Replacement: Incidence and Significance. American Shoulder and Elbow Surgeons Annual Meeting, New York, 1989.
40. Bradford DS, Szalapski EWJ, Sutherland DER, et al: Osteonecrosis in the transplant recipients. Surg Gynecol Obstet *159*:328–334, 1984.
41. Brems J: The glenoid component in total shoulder arthroplasty. J Shoulder Elbow Surg *2*:47–54, 1993.
42. Brems JJ: Rehabilitation following total shoulder arthroplasty. Clin Orthop *307*:70–85, 1994.
43. Brenner BC, Ferlic DC, Clayton ML, and Dennis DA: Survivorship of Unconstrained Total Shoulder Arthroplasty. Fourth International Conference of Surgery of the Shoulder, New York, 1989.
44. Brett AL: A new method of arthrodesis of the shoulder joint, incorporating the control of the scapula. J Bone Joint Surg *15*:969, 1933.
45. Brewer BJ, Wubben RC, and Carrera GF: Excessive retroversion of the glenoid cavity: A cause of non-traumatic posterior instability of the shoulder. J Bone Joint Surg *68*:724–731, 1986.
46. Brittain HA: Architectual Principles in Arthrodesis. Baltimore, MD: Williams & Wilkins, 1942.
47. Brostrom LA, Kronberg M, and Wallensten R: Should the glenoid be replaced in shoulder arthroplasty with an unconstrained DANA or St. Georg prosthesis? Ann Chir Gynaecol *81*:54–57, 1992.
48. Brownlee C and Cofield MD: Shoulder Replacement in Cuff Tear Arthropathy. Paper presented at American Shoulder and Elbow Surgeons Open Meeting, New Orleans, 1986.
49. Brumfield RH Jr, Schilz J, and Flinders BW: Total shoulder replacement arthroplasty: A clinical review of 21 cases (Abstract). Orthop Trans *5*:398, 1981.
50. Bryan JB, Schouder K, Tullos HS, et al: The axillary nerve and its relationships to common sports medicine shoulder procedure. Am J Sports Med *14*:113–116, 1986.
51. Buechel FF, Pappas MJ, and DePalma AF: "Floating socket" total shoulder replacement: Anatomical, biomechanical, and surgical rationale. J Biomed Mater Res *12*:89–114, 1978.
52. Burdge DR, Reid GD, Reeve CE, et al: Septic arthritis due to dual infection with *Mycoplasma hominis* and *Ureaplasma urealyticum*. J Rheumatol *15*:366–368, 1988.
53. Burkhead WZ: Musculocutaneous and axillary nerve position after coracoid graft transfer. *In* Post M, Morrey BF, and Hawkins RJ (eds): Surgery of the Shoulder. St. Louis: Mosby-Year Book, 1990, pp 152–155.
54. Burkhead WZ Jr and Hutton KS: Biologic resurfacing of the glenoid with hemiarthroplasty of the shoulder. J Shoulder Elbow Surg *4*:263–270, 1995.
55. Burkhead WZ, Scheinberg RR, and Box G: Surgical anatomy of the axillary nerve. J Shoulder Elbow Surg *1*:31–36, 1992.
56. Burri C: Indication, technique and results in prosthetic replacement of the shoulder joint. Acta Orthop Belg *51*:606–615, 1985.
57. Caldwell GL Jr, Dines D, Warren R, et al: Revision Shoulder Arthroplasty (Abstract). American Shoulder and Elbow Surgeons Annual Meeting, San Francisco, CA, 1993.
58. Campion GV, McCrae F, Alwan W, et al: Idiopathic destructive arthritis of the shoulder. Semin Arthritis Rheum *17*:232–245, 1988.
59. Carroll RE: Wire loop in arthrodesis of the shoulder. Clin Orthop *9*:185, 1957.
60. Chard MD and Hazleman BL: Shoulder disorders in the elderly (a hospital study). Ann Rheum Dis *46*:684–687, 1987.
61. Charnley J: Compression arthrodesis of the ankle and shoulder. J Bone Joint Surg *33B*:180–191, 1951.

62. Charnley J: Anchorage of the femoral head prosthesis of the shaft of the femur. J Bone Joint Surg *42B*:28–30, 1960.
63. Charnley J: Low Friction Arthroplasty of the Hip. New York: Springer-Verlag, 1979.
64. Charnley J and Houston JK: Compression arthrodesis of the shoulder. J Bone Joint Surg *46B*:614–620, 1964.
65. Clayton ML, Ferlic DC, and Jeffers PD: Prosthetic arthroplasty of the shoulder. Clin Orthop *164*:184, 1982.
66. Cockx E, Claes T, Hoogmartens M, and Mulier JC: The isoelastic prosthesis for the shoulder joint. Acta Orthop Belg *49*:275–285, 1983.
67. Codd TP, Pollock RG, and Flatow EL: Prosthetic replacement in the rotator cuff-deficient shoulder. Tech Orthop 8:174–83, 1994.
68. Codd TP, Yamaguchi K, and Flatow EL: Infected Shoulder Arthroplasties: Treatment with Staged Reimplantations vs. Resection Arthroplasty. American Shoulder and Elbow Surgeons 11th Open Meeting, Orlando, FL, 1995.
69. Codman EA: The Shoulder, Rupture of the Supraspinatus Tendon and Other Lesions In or About the Subacromial Bursa. Boston: Thomas Todd, 1934.
70. Cofield RH: Arthrodesis and resection arthroplasty of the shoulder. *In* McCollister EC (ed): Surgery of the Musculoskeletal System. New York: Churchill Livingstone, 1983, pp 109–124.
71. Cofield RH: Unconstrained total shoulder prostheses. Clin Orthop *173*:97–108, 1983.
72. Cofield RH: Total shoulder arthroplasty with the Neer prosthesis. J Bone Joint Surg *66A*:899–906, 1984.
73. Cofield RH: Shoulder arthrodesis and resection arthroplasty. Instr Course Lect *34*:268–277, 1985.
74. Cofield RH: Preliminary experience with bone ingrowth total shoulder arthroplasty. Orthop Trans *10*:217, 1986.
75. Cofield RH: Total shoulder arthroplasty with bone ingrowth fixation. *In* Kolbel R, Helbig B, and Blauth W (eds): Shoulder Replacement. Berlin: Springer-Verlag, 1987, pp 209–212.
76. Cofield RH: Subscapularis tendon transposition for large rotator cuff tears. Tech Orthop 3:58, 1989.
77. Cofield RH: Degenerative and arthritic problems of the glenohumeral joint. *In* Rockwood CA and Matsen FA III (eds): The Shoulder. Philadelphia: WB Saunders, 1990, pp 678–749.
78. Cofield RH: Complications of Shoulder Arthroplasty. ICL No. 317. American Academy of Orthopaedic Surgeons Annual Meeting, San Francisco, CA, 1993.
79. Cofield RH: Uncemented total shoulder arthroplasty: A review. Clin Orthop *66(A)*:899–906, 1994.
80. Cofield RH and Briggs BT: Glenohumeral arthritis. J Bone Joint Surg *61A*:668–677, 1979.
81. Cofield RH and Daly PJ: Total shoulder arthroplasty with a tissue-ingrowth glenoid component. J Shoulder Elbow Surg *1*:77–85, 1992.
82. Cofield RH and Edgerton BC: Total shoulder arthroplasty: Complications and revision surgery. Instr Course Lect *39*:449–462, 1990.
83. Cofield RH, Frankle MA, and Zuckerman JD: Humeral head replacement in glenohumeral arthritis. J Shoulder Elbow Surg 2:S13, 1993.
84. Cofield RH and Stauffer RN: The Bickel glenohumeral arthroplasty. *In* Conference on Joint Replacement in the Upper Limb. London: Institute of Mechanical Engineering, 1977, pp 15–25.
85. Collins D, Tencer A, Sidles J, and Matsen FA III: Edge displacement and deformation of glenoid components in response to eccentric loading. J Bone Joint Surg *74A*:501–507, 1992.
86. Collins DN, Harryman DT II, Lippitt SB, et al: The technique of glenohumeral arthroplasty. Tech Orthop *6*:43–59, 1991.
87. Compito CA, Self EB, and Bigliani LU: Arthroplasty and acute shoulder trauma: Reasons for success and failure. Clin Orthop *307*:27–36, 1994.
88. Cooper RA and Brems JJ: Recurrent disassembly of a modular humeral prosthesis: A case report. J Arthroplasty *6*:375–377, 1991.
89. Copeland S: Cementless total shoulder replacement. *In* Post M, Morrey BF, and Hawkins RJ (eds): Surgery of the Shoulder. St. Louis: Mosby-Year Book, 1990, pp 289–293.
90. Cornell CN and Ranawat CS: Survivorship analysis of total hip replacements. Results in a series of active patients who were less than fifty-five years old. J Bone Joint Surg *68A*:1430–1432, 1986.
91. Cosendai A, Gerster JC, Vischer TL, et al: Destructive arthroplasties associated with articular chondrocalcinosis. Clinical and metabolic study of 16 cases. Schweiz Med Wochenschr *106*:8–14, 1976.
92. Coughlin MJ, Morris JM, and West WF: The semiconstrained total shoulder arthroplasty. J Bone Joint Surg *61A*:574–581, 1979.
93. Cowell HR and Curtiss PH Jr: The randomized clinical trial (Editorial). J Bone Joint Surg *67A*:1151–1152, 1985.
94. Craviotto DF, Seltzer DG, Wirth MA, and Rockwood CA Jr: Resection Arthroplasty for Salvage of Failed Shoulder Arthroplasty. American Shoulder and Elbow Surgeons Annual Meeting, New Orleans, 1994.
95. Cruess RL: Osteonecrosis of bone: Current concepts as to etiology and pathogenesis. Clin Orthop 208:30–39, 1986.
96. Cruess RL: Shoulder resurfacing according to the method of Neer. J Bone Joint Surg *62B*:116–117, 1980.
97. Cruess RL: Corticosteroid-induced osteonecrosis of the humeral head. Orthop Clin North Am *16*:789–796, 1985.
98. Curran JF, Ellman MH, and Brown NL: Rheumatologic aspects of painful conditions affecting the shoulder. Clin Orthop *173*:27–37, 1983.
99. Cutler SJ and Ederer F: Maximum utilization of the life table method in analyzing survival. J Chron Dis *9*:699–712, 1958.
100. De Velasco Polo G and Cardoso Monterrubio A: Arthrodesis of the shoulder. Clin Orthop *90*:178, 1973.
101. Hawkins RJ, Bell RH, and Jallay B: Experience with the Neer total shoulder arthroplasty: a review of 70 cases. Orthop Trans *10*:232, 1986.
102. Dines DM, Warren RF, Altchek DW, and Moeckel B: Posttraumatic changes of the proximal humerus: Malunion, nonunion, and osteonecrosis. Treatment with modular hemiarthroplasty or total shoulder arthroplasty. J Shoulder Elbow Surg 2:121, 1993.
103. Dobbs HS: Survivorship of total hip replacements. J Bone Joint Surg *62B*:168–173, 1980.
104. Dorey F and Amstutz HC: Survivorship analysis in the evaluation of joint replacement. J Arthroplasty *1*:63–69, 1986.
105. Dorwart RH, Genant HK, Johnston WH, and Morris JM: Pigmented villonodular synovitis of synovial joints: Clinical, pathologic, and radiologic features. AJR Am J Roentgenol *143*:87–885, 1984.
106. Dorwart RH, Genant HK, Johnston WH, and Morris JM: Pigmented villonodular synovitis of the shoulder: Radiologic-pathologic assessment. AJR Am J Roentgenol *143*:886–888, 1984.
107. Driessnack RP, Ferlic DC, and Wiedel JD: Dissociation of the glenoid component in the Macnab/English total shoulder arthroplasty. J Arthroplasty 5:15–18, 1990.
108. Ellman MH and Curran JJ: Causes and management of shoulder arthritis. Compr Ther *14*:29–35, 1988.
109. Engelbrecht E and Heinert K: More than ten years' experience with unconstrained shoulder replacement. *In* Kolbel R, Helbig B, and Blauth W (eds): Shoulder Replacement. New York: Springer-Verlag, 1987, pp 85–91.
110. Engelbrecht E, Siegel A, Rottger J, and Heinert K: Erfahrungen mit der Anwendung von Schultergelenksendoprothesen. Chirurg *51*:794, 1980.
111. Engelbrecht E and Stellbrink G: Total Schulterendoprosthese Modell (St. Georg). Chirurg *47*:525–530, 1976.
112. Ennevaara K: Painful shoulder joint in rheumatoid arthritis: A clinical and radiological study of 200 cases with special reference to arthrography of the glenohumeral joint. Acta Rheum Scand Suppl *11*:1–108, 1967.
113. Epps CH Jr: Painful hematologic conditions affecting the shoulder. Clin Orthop *173*:38–43, 1983.
114. Faludi DD and Weiland AJ: Cementless total shoulder arthroplasty: Preliminary experience with thirteen cases. Orthopedics *6*:431–438, 1983.
115. Fenlin JM: Total glenohumeral joint replacement. Orthop Clin North Am *6*:565–583, 1975.
116. Fenlin JM, Frieman BG, and Allardyce TJ: Hemiarthroplasty in rotator cuff tear arthropathy. J Shoulder Elbow Surg *4*:S62, 1995.
117. Fenlin JM, Ramsey ML, Allardyce TJ, and Frieman BG: Modular total shoulder replacement. Design rationale, indications and results. Clin Orthop *307*:37–46, 1994.
118. Field LD, Zubinski SJ, Dines DM, et al: Hemiarthroplasty of the shoulder for rotator cuff arthropathy. J Shoulder Elbow Surg *4*:S62, 1995.

119. Figgie HE, Inglis AE, Goldberg VM, et al: An analysis of factors affecting the long-term results of total shoulder arthroplasty in inflammatory arthritis. J Arthroplasty *3*:123–130, 1988.
120. Figgie MP, Inglis AE, Figgie HI, et al: Custom Total Shoulder Arthroplasty for Inflammatory Arthritis. Fourth International Conference on Surgery of the Shoulder, New York, 1989.
121. Flatow EL, Bigliani LU, and April EW: An anatomical study of the musculocutaneous nerve and its relationship to the coracoid process. Clin Orthop *244*:166–171, 1989.
122. Fournie B, Railhac JJ, and Monod P: The enthesopathic shoulder. Rev Rhum Mal Osteoartic *54*:447–451, 1987.
123. Frank CB: Ligament healing: Current knowledge and clinical applications. J Am Acad Orthop Surg *4*:74–83, 1996.
124. Franklin JL, Barrett WP, Jackins SE, and Matsen FA III: Glenoid loosening in total shoulder arthroplasty; association with rotator cuff deficiency. J Arthroplasty *3*:39–46, 1988.
125. Frich LH, Moller BN, and Sneppen O: Shoulder arthroplasty with the Neer Mark-II prosthesis. Arch Orthop Trauma Surg *107*:110–113, 1988.
126. Frich LH, Sojbjerg JO, and Sneppen O: Shoulder arthroplasty in complex acute and chronic proximal humeral fractures. Orthopaedics *14*:949–954, 1991.
127. Friedman RJ: Glenohumeral translation after total shoulder arthroplasty. J Shoulder Elbow Surg *1*:312–316, 1992.
128. Friedman RJ, Hawthorne KB, and Genez BM: The use of computerized tomography in the measurement of glenoid version. J Bone Joint Surg *74A*:1032–1037, 1992.
129. Friedman RJ, LaBerge M, Dooley RL, and O'Hara AL: Finite element modeling of the glenoid component: Effect of design parameters on stress distribution. J Shoulder Elbow Surg *1*:261–270, 1992.
130. Friedman RJ, Thornhill TS, Thomas WH, and Sledge CB: Non-constrained total shoulder replacement in patients who have rheumatoid arthritis and class-IV function. J Bone Joint Surg *71A*:494–498, 1989.
131. Fukuda K, Chen C-M, Cofield RH, and Chao EYS: Biomechanical analysis of stability and fixation strength of total shoulder prostheses. Orthopedics *2*:141–149, 1988.
132. Galinat BJ, Howell SM, and Kraft TA: The glenoid posterior acromion angle: An accurate method of evaluating glenoid version. Orthop Trans *12*(727), 1988.
133. Garancis JC, Cheung HS, Halverson PB, and McCarty DJ: "Milwaukee shoulder"–association of microspheroids containing hydroxyapatite crystals, active collagenase, and neutral protease with rotator cuff defects. Arthritis Rheum *24*:484–491, 1981.
134. Gariepy R: Glenoidectomy in the repair of the rheumatoid shoulder. J Bone Joint Surg *59B*:122, 1977.
135. Gartland JJ: Orthopaedic clinical research: Deficiencies in experimental design and determinations of outcome. J Bone Joint Surg *70A*:1357–1364, 1988.
136. Gerard P, Leblanc JP, and Rousseau B: Une prothèse totale d'épaule. Chirurgie *99*:655–663, 1973.
137. Giori NJ, Beaupre GS, and Carter DR: The influence of fixation peg design on the shear stability of prosthetic implants. J Orthop Res *8*:892–898, 1990.
138. Glasson JM, Pollock RG, Djurasovic M, et al: Hemiarthroplasty for Glenohumeral Osteoarthritis in a Patient with an Intact Rotator Cuff: Results Correlated to Degree of Glenoid Wear. 12th Open Meeting of the American Shoulder and Elbow Surgeons, Atlanta, GA, 1996.
139. Green A and Norris TR: Imaging technique for glenohumeral arthritis and glenohumeral arthroplasty. Clin Orthop *307*:7–17, 1994.
140. Green A and Norris TR: Imaging techniques for glenohumeral arthritis and glenohumeral arthroplasty. Clin Orthop *307*:7–17, 1994.
141. Gristina AG, Romano RL, Kammire GC, and Webb LX: Total shoulder replacement. Orthop Clin North Am *18*:444–453, 1987.
142. Gristina AG and Webb LX: The trispherical total shoulder replacement. *In* Bayley I and Kessel L (eds): Shoulder Surgery. New York: Springer-Verlag, 1982, pp 153–157.
143. Gristina AG, Webb LX, and Carter RE: The monospherical total shoulder. Orthop Trans *9*:54, 1985.
144. Groh GI, Heckman MM, Curtis RJ, et al: Treatment of fractures adjacent to humeral prostheses. Orthop Trans *18*:1072, 1994–1995.
145. Groh GI and Rockwood CA: Loss of Deltoid Following Shoulder Operations: An Operative Disaster. Monterey, CA: Western Orthopaedic Association, 1992.
146. Groh GI, Simoni M, Rolla P, and Rockwood CA, Jr: Loss of the deltoid after shoulder operations: An operative disaster. J Shoulder Elbow Surg *3*:243, 1994.
147. Gschwend N: Is a Glenoid Component Necessary for Rheumatoid Patients? Second Congress of the European Shoulder and Elbow Society, Berne, Switzerland, 1988.
148. Habermeyer P and Schweiberer L: Corrective interventions subsequent to humeral head fractures. Orthopade *21*:148–157, 1992.
149. Halverson PB, Cheung HS, and McCarty DJ: Enzymatic release of microspheroids containing hydroxyapatite crystals from synovium and of calcium pyrophospate dihydrate crystals from cartilage. Ann Rheum Dis *41*:527–531, 1982.
150. Halverson PB, Cheung HS, McCarty DJ, et al: "Milwaukee shoulder"-association of microspheroids containing hydroxyapatite crystals, active collagenase, and neutral protease with rotator cuff defects. II. Synovial fluid studies. Arthritis Rheum *24*:474–483, 1981.
151. Halverson PB, Garancis JC, and McCarty DJ: Histopathological and ultrastructural studies of synovium in Milwaukee shoulder syndrome—basic calcium phosphate crystal arthropathy. Ann Rheum Dis *43*:734–741, 1984.
152. Halverson PB, McCarty DJ, Cheung HS, and Ryan LM: Milwaukee, shoulder syndrome: eleven additional cases with involvement of the knee in seven (basic calcium phosphate crystal deposition disease). Semin Arthritis Rheum *14*:36–44, 1984.
153. Harryman DT II, Sidles JA, Clark JM, et al: Translation of the humeral head on the glenoid with passive glenohumeral motion. J Bone Joint Surg *72A*:1334–1343, 1990.
154. Harryman DT, Sidles JA, Harris SL, et al: The effect of articular conformity and the size of the humeral head component on laxity and motion after glenohumeral arthroplasty. J Bone Joint Surg *77A*:555–563, 1995.
155. Harryman DT II, Sidles JA, Harris SL, and Matsen FA III: Laxity of the normal glenohumeral joint: A quantitative in-vivo assessment. J Shoulder Elbow Surg *1*:66–76, 1992.
156. Harryman DT II, Walker ED, Harris SL, et al: Residual motion and function after glenohumeral or scapulothoracic arthrodesis. J Shoulder Elbow Surg *2*:275–285, 1993.
157. Hauge MF: Arthrodesis of the shoulder: A simple elastic band appliance utilizing the compression principle. Acta Orthop Scand *31*:272, 1961.
158. Hawkins RJ and Angelo RL: Glenohumeral arthrosis: A late complication of the Putti Platt repair. J Bone Joint Surg *72A*:1193–1197, 1990.
159. Hawkins RJ, Bell RH, and Jallay B: Total shoulder arthroplasty. Clin Orthop *242*:188–194, 1989.
160. Hawkins RJ and Neer CS II: A functional analysis of shoulder fusions. Clin Orthop *223*:65–76, 1987.
161. Hawkins RJ, Neer CS II, Pianta RM, and Mendoza FX: Locked posterior dislocation of the shoulder. J Bone Joint Surg *69A*:9–18, 1987.
162. Hernigou P, Duparc F, and Filali C: Humeral retroversion and shoulder prosthesis. Rev Chir Orthop Reparatrice Appar Mot *81*:419–427, 1995.
163. Hinton MA, Parker AW, Drez DJ, and Altcheck D: An anatomic study of the subscapularis tendon and myotendinous junction. J Shoulder Elbow Surg *3*(4):224–229, 1994.
164. Hjelkrem M and Stanish WD: Synovial chondrometaplasia of the shoulder. A case report of a young athlete presenting with shoulder pain. Am J Sports Med *16*:84–86, 1988.
165. Hsu HC, Wu JJ, Chen TH, et al: The influence of abductor lever-arm changes after shoulder arthroplasty. J Shoulder Elbow Surg *2*:134–140, 1993.
166. Hucherson DC: Arthrodesis of the paralytic shoulder. Am Surg *25*:430, 1959.
167. Hughes GM, Biundo JJJ, Scheib JS, and Kumar P: Pseudogout and pseudosepsis of the shoulder. Orthop Grand Rounds *13*:1169–1172, 1990.
168. Huten D and Duparc J: L'arthroplastie prothetique dans les traumatismes complexes récents et anciens de l'épaule. Rev Chir Orthop *72*:517–529, 1986.
169. Iannotti J, Gabriel JP, Schneck SL, et al: The normal glenohumeral

relationships: An anatomical study of one hundred and forty shoulders. J Bone Joint Surg *74A*:491–499, 1992.
170. Inman VT, Saunders JBDCM, and Abbott LC: Observations on the function of the shoulder joint. J Bone Joint Surg *26A*:1–30, 1944.
171. Jacobson SR and Mallon WJ: The glenohumeral offset ratio: A radiographic study. J Shoulder Elbow Surg 2:141–146, 1993.
172. Jenkinson ML, Bliss MR, Brain AT, and Scott DL: Peripheral arthritis in the elderly: A hospital study. Ann Rheum Dis *48*:227–231, 1989.
173. Jensen K and Rockwood CA: Hemiarthroplasty vs total shoulder arthroplasty in patients with osteoarthritis of the shoulder. Orthop Trans *19*:821, 1995–96.
174. Jensen K and Rockwood CA Jr: The Value of Preoperative Computed Tomography in Shoulder Arthroplasty. Combined meeting of the New Zealand and Australian Orthopaedic Associations, Perth, Australia, 1996.
175. Jinnah RH, Amstutz HC, Tooke SM, et al: The UCLA Charnley experience: A long-term follow-up study using survival analysis. Clin Orthop *221*:164–172, 1986.
176. Johnson CA, Healy WL, Brooker AF Jr, and Krackow KA: External fixation shoulder arthrodesis. Clin Orthop *211*:219–223, 1986.
177. Jones L: Reconstructive operation for nonreducible fractures of the head of the humerus. Ann Surg 97:217, 1933.
178. Jones L: The shoulder joint–observations on the anatomy and physiology: With an analysis of a reconstructive operation following extensive injury. Surg Gynecol Obstet 75:433, 1942.
179. Jónsson E: Surgery of the Rheumatoid Shoulder with Special Reference to Cup Hemiarthroplasty and Arthrodesis. Lund, Sweden: Infotryck, 1988.
180. Jónsson E, Egund N, Kelly I, et al: Cup arthroplasty of the rheumatoid shoulder. Acta Orthop Scand 57:542–546, 1986.
181. Jonsson E, Lidgren L, and Rydholm U: Position of shoulder arthrodesis measured with Moire photography. Clin Orthop 238:117–121, 1989.
182. Kalamchi A: Arthrodesis for paralytic shoulder: Review of ten patients. Orthopedics *1*:204–208, 1978.
183. Kechele P, Basmania C, Wirth MA, et al: Rheumatoid shoulder: Hemiarthroplasty vs. total shoulder arthroplasty. J Shoulder Elbow Surg *4*:S13, 1995.
184. Kechle PR, Seltzer DG, Gonzalez JC, et al: Hemiarthroplasty vs. Total Shoulder Arthroplasty for the Rheumatoid Shoulder. American Shoulder and Elbow Surgeons 10th Open Meeting, New Orleans, LA, 1994.
185. Kelleher IM, Cofield RH, Becker DA, and Beabout JW: Fluoroscopically positioned radiographs of total shoulder arthroplasty. J Shoulder Elbow Surg *1*:306–311, 1992.
186. Kelly IG: Surgery of the rheumatoid shoulder. Ann Rheum Dis *49*:824–829, 1990.
187. Kelly IG: Shoulder arthroplasty in rheumatoid arthritis. Clin Orthop *307*:94–102, 1994.
188. Kelly IG, Foster RS, and Fischer WD: Neer total shoulder replacement in rheumatoid arthritis. J Bone Joint Surg *69B*:723–726, 1987.
189. Kenmore PI: A Simple Shoulder Replacement. Clemson University Biomaterials Symposium, 1973.
190. Kenmore PI, MacCartee C, and Vitek B: A simple shoulder replacement. J Biomed Mater Res *5*:329–330, 1974.
191. Kessel L and Bayley JL: The Kessel total shoulder replacement. *In* Shoulder Surgery. New York: Springer-Verlag, 1982, pp 160–164.
192. Klimaitis A, Carroll G, and Owen E: Rapidly progressive destructive arthropathy of the shoulder—a viewpoint on pathogenesis. J Rheum *15*:1859–1862, 1988.
193. Knight RA and Mayne JA: Comminuted fractures and fracture-dislocations involving the articular surface of the humeral head. J Bone Joint Surg *39A*:1343, 1957.
194. Kolbel R and Friedebold G: Schultergelenkersatz. Z Orthop *113*:452–454, 1975.
195. Kolbel R, Rohlmann A, and Bergmann G: Biomechanical considerations in the design of a semi-constrained total shoulder replacement. *In* Bayley I and Kessel L (eds): Shoulder Surgery. New York: Springer-Verlag, 1982, pp 144–152.
196. Kraft SM, Panush RS, and Longley S: Unrecognized staphylococcal pyarthrosis with rheumatoid arthritis. Semin Arthritis Rheum *14*:196–201, 1985.
197. Kronberg M, Brostrom LA, and Soderlund V: Retroversion of the humeral head in the normal shoulder and its relationship to the normal range of motion. Clin Orthop *253*:113–117, 1990.
198. Krueger FJ: Vitallium replica arthroplasty on the shoulder: A case report of aseptic necrosis of the proximal end of the humerus. Surgery *30*:1005–1011, 1951.
199. Laumann U and Schilgen L: Varisierende subkapitale Osteotomie in Verbindung mit Schulterarthrodese und Oberarmamputation bei Plexusparese. Z Orthop *115*:787, 1977.
200. Laurence M: Replacement arthroplasty of the rotator cuff deficient shoulder. J Bone Joint Surg *73B*:916–919, 1991.
201. Lee DH and Niemann KMW: Bipolar shoulder arthroplasty. Clin Orthop *304*:97–107, 1994.
202. Leslie BM, Harris JMI, and Driscoll D: Septic arthritis of the shoulder in adults. J Bone Joint Surg *71A*:1516–1522, 1989.
203. Lettin AWF, Copeland SA, and Scales JT: The Stanmore total shoulder replacement. J Bone Joint Surg *64B*:47–51, 1982.
204. Levick JR: Joint pressure-volume studies: Their importance, design and interpretation. J Rheumatol *10*:353–357, 1983.
205. Lichtman EA: Candida infection of a prosthetic shoulder joint. Skeletal Radiol *10*:176–177, 1983.
206. Linell EA: The distribution of nerves in the upper limb with reference to variabilities and their clinical significance. J Anat *55*:79–112, 1921.
207. Linscheid RL and Cofield RH: Total shoulder arthroplasty: Experimental but promising. Geriatrics *31*:64–69, 1976.
208. Lippitt SB, Harris SC, Harryman DT II, et al: In vivo quantification of the laxity of normal and unstable glenohumeral joints. J Shoulder Elbow Surg 3:215–223, 1994.
209. Lippitt SB, Harryman DT II, and Matsen FA III: A practical tool for evaluation function: The simple shoulder test. *In* Matsen FA III, Fu FH, and Hawkins RJ (eds): The Shoulder: A Balance of Mobility and Stability. Rosemont, IL: American Academy of Orthopaedic Surgeons, 1993, pp 510–518.
210. Louthrenoo W, Ostrov BE, Park YS, et al: Pseudoseptic arthritis: An unusual presentation of neuropathic arthropathy. 1990.
211. Lugli T: Artificial shoulder joint by Péan (1893). The facts of an exceptional intervention and the prosthetic method. Clin Orthop *133*:215–218, 1978.
212. Lusardi DA, Wirth MA, Wrutz D, and Rockwood CA Jr: Loss of external rotation after capsulorraphy of the shoulder. J Bone Joint Surg *75A*:1185–1192, 1993.
213. Lynch NM, Cofield RH, Silbert PL, and Hermann RC: Neurologic complications after total shoulder arthroplasty. J Shoulder Elbow Surg *5*:53–61, 1996.
214. Madhok R, Lewallen DG, and Wallrichs SL: Utilization of upper limb replacements during 1972–90: The Mayo Clinic experience. I Mech E 207, 1993.
215. Mallon WJ, Brown HR, Vogler JB, and Martinez S: Radiographic and geometric anatomy of the scapula. Clin Orthop 277:142–154, 1992.
216. Marks SH, Barnett M, and Calin A: Ankylosing spondylitis in women and men: A case control study. J Rheumatol *10*:624–628, 1983.
217. Marmor L: Hemiarthroplasty of the rheumatoid shoulder joint. Clin Orthop *122*:201–3, 1977.
218. Martin SD, Sledge CB, Thomas WH, and Thornhill TS: Total Shoulder Arthroplasty with an Uncemented Glenoid Component. American Shoulder and Elbow Surgeons 11th Annual Meeting, Orlando, FL, 1995.
219. Mason JM: The treatment of dislocation of the shoulder-joint complicated by fracture of the upper extremity of the humerus. Ann Surg *47*:672, 1908.
220. Matsen FA III: Early effectiveness of shoulder arthroplasty for patients with primary glenohumeral degenerative joint disease. J Bone Joint Surg *78A*:260–264, 1996.
221. Matsen FA III, Lippitt SB, Sidles JA, and Harryman DT II: Practical Evaluation and Management of the Shoulder. Philadelphia: WB Saunders, 1994, pp 1–242.
222. Matsen FA III, Smith KL, DeBartolo SE, and Von Oesen G: A comparison of patients with late-stage rheumatoid arthritis and osteoarthritis of the shoulder using self-assessed shoulder function and health status. Arthritis Care Res *10*:43–47, 1997.
223. Matsen FA III, Thomas SC, and Rockwood CA Jr: Anterior glenohumeral instability. *In* Rockwood CA Jr and Matsen FA III (eds): The Shoulder. Philadelphia: WB Saunders, 1990, pp 534–540.

224. Matsen FA III, Ziegler DW, and DeBartolo SE: Patient self-assessment of health status and function in glenohumeral degenerative joint disease. J Shoulder Elbow Surg *4*:345–351, 1995.
225. Matsunaga M: A new method of arthrodesis of the shoulder. Acta Orthop Scand *43*:343, 1972.
226. Mau H and Nebinger G: Arthropathy of the shoulder joint in syringomyelia. Z Orthop *124*:157–164, 1986.
227. May VR Jr: Shoulder fusion: A review of 14 cases. J Bone Joint Surg *44A*:65, 1962.
228. Mazas F and de la Caffiniére JY: Total arthroplasty of the shoulder: Experience with 38 cases (Abstract). Orthop Trans *5*:57, 1981.
229. Mazas F and de la Caffiniére JY: Une prothèse totale d'épaule non rétentive: A propos de 38 cas. Rev Chir Orthop *68*:161–170, 1982.
230. McCarty D: Crystals, joints, and consternation. Ann Rheum Dis *42*:243–253, 1983.
231. McCarty DJ, Halverson PB, Carrera GF, et al: "Milwaukee shoulder"—association of microspheroids containing hydroxyapatite crystals, active collagenase, and neutral protease with rotator cuff defects. I. Clinical aspects. Arthritis Rheum *24*:353–354, 1981.
232. McCoy SR, Warren RF, Bade HA, et al: Total shoulder arthroplasty in rheumatoid arthritis. J Arthroplasty *4*:105–113, 1989.
233. McElwain JP and English E: The early results of porous-coated total shoulder arthroplasty. Clin Orthop *218*:217–224, 1987.
234. McKee GK and Watson-Farrar J: Replacement of arthritis hips by the McKee-Farrar prosthesis. J Bone Joint Surg *48B*:245, 1966.
235. Medicare Hospital Utilization Data Bases: Consolidated Consulting Group, Fairfax, VA.
236. Medsger TA, Dixon JA, and Garwood VF: Palmar fasciitis and polyarthritis associated with ovarian carcinoma. Ann Intern Med *96*:424–432, 1982.
237. Milbrink J and Wigren A: Resection arthroplasty of the shoulder. Scand J Rheumatol *19*:432–436, 1990.
238. Mills KL: Severe injuries of the upper end of the humerus. Injury *6*:13, 1974.
239. Milne JC and Gartsman GM: Cost of shoulder surgery. J Shoulder Elbow Surg *3*:295–298, 1994.
240. Moeckel BH, Altchek DW, Warren RF, et al: Instability of the shoulder after arthroplasty. J Bone Joint Surg *75A*:492–497, 1993.
241. Moeckel BH, Dines DM, Warren RF, and Altcheck DW: Modular hemiarthroplasty for fractures of the proximal humerus. J Bone Joint Surg *74A*:884–889, 1992.
242. Mullaji AB, Beddow FH, and Lamb GHR: CT measurement of glenoid erosion in arthritis. J Bone Joint Surg *76B*:384–388, 1994.
243. Muller ME, Allgower M, Schneider R, and Willenegger H: Manual of Internal Fixation. New York: Springer-Verlag, 1979, pp 384–385.
244. Muller W: Uber den negativen Luftdruck im Gelenkraum. Dtsch A Chir *217*:395–401, 1929.
245. Namba RS and Thornhill TS: Posterior capsulorrhaphy in total shoulder arthroplasty: A case report. Clin Orthop *313*:135–139, 1995.
246. National Health Interview: National Center for Health Statistics, 1988.
247. National Hospital Discharge Survey: National Center for Health Statistics, 1984–1990.
248. National Hospital Discharge Survey: National Center for Health Statistics, 1990–1992.
249. Neer CS II: Articular replacement for the humeral head. J Bone Joint Surg *37A*:215–228, 1955.
250. Neer CS II: The rheumatoid shoulder. *In* Cruess RR and Mitchell NS (eds): Surgery of Rheumatoid Arthritis. Philadelphia: JB Lippincott, 1971, pp 117–125.
251. Neer CS II: Replacement arthroplasty for glenohumeral arthritis. J Bone Joint Surg *56A*:1–13, 1974.
252. Neer CS II: Unconstrained shoulder arthroplasty. Instr Course Lect *34*:278–86, 1985.
253. Neer CS II: Shoulder Reconstruction. Philadelphia: WB Saunders, 1990.
254. Neer CS II, Brown TH Jr, and McLaughlin HL: Fracture of the neck of the humerus with dislocation of the head fragment. Am J Surg *85*:252–258, 1953.
255. Neer CS II, Craig EV, and Fukuda H: Cuff-tear arthropathy. J Bone Joint Surg *65A*:1232–1244, 1983.
256. Neer CS II and Kirby RM: Revision of humeral head and total shoulder arthroplasty. Clin Orthop *170*:189–195, 1982.
257. Neer CS II and Morrison DS: Glenoid bone-grafting in total shoulder arthroplasty. J Bone Joint Surg *70A*:1154–1162, 1988.
258. Neer CS II and Rockwood CA: Fractures and dislocations of the shoulder. *In* Rockwood CA and Green DP (eds): Fractures in Adults. Philadelphia: JB Lippincott, 1984, pp 675–985.
259. Neer CS II, Watson KC, and Stanton FJ: Recent experience in total shoulder replacement. J Bone Joint Surg *64A*:319–337, 1982.
260. Nelson JP, Fitzgerald RH, Jaspers MT, and Little JW: Prophylactic antimicrobial coverage in arthroplasty patients (Editorial). J Bone Joint Surg *72A*:1, 1990.
261. Nguyen VD and Nguyen KD: "Idiopathic destructive arthritis" of the shoulder: A still fascinating enigma. Comput Med Imaging Graph *14*:249–255, 1990.
262. Norris T and Iannotti J: A Prospective Outcome Study Comparing Humeral Head Replacement and Total Shoulder Replacement for Primary Osteoarthritis of the Shoulder. 12th Open Meeting of the American Shoulder and Elbow Surgeons Meeting, Atlanta, GA, 1996.
263. Norris TR, Green A, and McGuigan FX: Late prosthetic shoulder arthroplasty for displaced proximal humerus fractures. J Shoulder Elbow Surg *4*:271–280, 1995.
264. Nussbaum AJ and Doppman JL: Shoulder arthroplasty in primary hyperparathyroidism. Skeletal Radiol *9*:98–102, 1982.
265. Orr TE, Carter DR, and Schurman DJ: Stress analyses of glenoid component designs. Clin Orthop *232*:217–224, 1988.
266. Pahle JA and Kvarnes L: Shoulder replacement arthroplasty. Ann Chir Gynaecol *74*(Suppl 198):85–89, 1985.
267. Pahle JA and Kvarnes L: Shoulder synovectomy. Ann Chirurg Gynaecol *198* (Suppl 75):37–39, 1985.
268. Parikh JR, Houpt JB, Jacobs S, and Fernandes BJ: Charcot's arthropathy of the shoulder following intraarticular corticosteroid injections. J Rheumatol *20*:885–887, 1993.
269. Pavlov PW: A fifteen year follow-up study of 512 consecutive Charnley-Müller total hip replacements. J Arthroplasty *2*(2):151–156, 1987.
270. Reference deleted.
271. Pearl ML and Lippitt SB: Shoulder arthroplasty with a modular prosthesis. Tech Orthop *8*(3):151–162, 1994.
272. Pearl ML and Volk AG: Retroversion of the proximal humerus in relationship to prosthetic replacement arthroplasty. J Shoulder Elbow Surg *4*:286–289, 1995.
273. Pellicci PM and Hass SB: Disassembly of a modular femoral component during closed reduction of the dislocated femoral component: A case report. J Bone Joint Surg *72A*:619–620, 1990.
274. Petersson CJ: Painful shoulders in patients with rheumatoid arthritis. Scand J Rheumatol *15*:275–279, 1986.
275. Petersson CJ: Shoulder surgery in rheumatoid arthritis. Acta Orthop Scand *57*:222–226, 1986.
276. Podgorski M, Robinson B, Weissberger A, et al: Articular manifestations of acromegaly. Aust N Z J Med *18*:28–35, 1988.
277. Pollock RG, Deliz ED, McIlveen SJ, et al: Prosthetic replacement in rotator cuff-deficient shoulders. J Shoulder Elbow Surg *1*:173–186, 1992.
278. Pollock RG, Higgis GB, Codd TP, et al: Total shoulder replacement for the treatment of primary glenohumeral osteoarthritis. J Shoulder Elbow Surg *4*:S12, 1995.
279. Poppen N and Walker P: Normal and abnormal motion of the shoulder. J Bone Joint Surg *58A*:195–201, 1976.
280. Poppen N and Walker P: Forces at the glenohumeral joint in abduction. Clin Orthop *135*:165–170, 1978.
281. Post M: Constrained arthroplasty of the shoulder. *In* Neviaser RJ (ed): Orthopaedic Clinics of North America. Philadelphia: WB Saunders, 1987, pp 455–462.
282. Post M: Shoulder arthroplasty and total shoulder replacement. *In* The Shoulder. Post M (ed). Lea & Febiger, Philadelphia, pp 221–278, 1988.
283. Post M and Haskell S: Michael Reese Total Shoulder. Memphis, TN: Richards Manufacturing Company, 1978.
284. Post M, Haskell SS, and Jablon M: Total shoulder replacement with a constrained prosthesis. J Bone Joint Surg *62A*:327, 1980.
285. Post M and Jablon M: Constrained total shoulder arthroplasty: long-term follow-up observations. Clin Orthop *173*:109–116, 1983.
286. Post M, Jablon M, Miller H, and Singh M: Constrained total shoulder joint replacement: A critical review. Clin Orthop *144*:135–150, 1979.
287. Pritchett JW and Clark JM: Prosthetic replacement for chronic unreduced dislocations of the shoulder. Clin Orthop *216*:89–93, 1987.

288. Putti V: Artrodesi nella tubercolosi del Ginocchio e della Spalla. Chir Organi Mov *18*:217, 1933.
289. Radosevich DM, Wetzler H, and Wilson SM: Health status questionnaire (HSQ) 2.0: Scoring comparisons and reference data. Health Outcomes Institute, Bloomington, MN, 1994.
290. Rand JA and Sim FH: Total shoulder arthroplasty for the arthroplasty of hemochromatosis: A case report. Orthopaedics *4*:658–660, 1981.
291. Raskob GE, Lofthouse RN, and Hull RD: Current concepts review: Methodological guidelines for clinical trials evaluating new therapeutic approaches in bone and joint surgery. J Bone Joint Surg *67A*:1294–1297, 1985.
292. Reeves B, Jobbins B, Dowson D, and Wright V: A total shoulder endo-prosthesis. N Engl J Med *1*:64–67, 1974.
293. Rhoades CE, Neff JR, Rengachary SS, et al: Diagnosis of posttraumatic syringohydromyelia presenting as neuropathic joints. Clin Orthop *180*:182–187, 1983.
294. Richard A, Judet R, and René L: Acrylic prosthetic reconstruction of the upper end of the humerus for fracture-luxations. J Chir *68*:537–547, 1952.
295. Richards RR, An K-n, Bigliani LU, et al: A standardized method for the assessment of shoulder function. J Shoulder Elbow Surg *3*:347–352, 1994.
296. Richards RR, Beaton D, and Hudson AR: Shoulder arthrodesis with plate fixation: function outcome analysis. J Shoulder Elbow Surg *2*:225–239, 1993.
297. Richards RR, Sherman RMP, Hudson AR, and Waddell JP: Shoulder arthrodesis using a pelvic-reconstruction plate—a report of eleven cases. J Bone Joint Surg *70A*:416–421, 1988.
298. Richards RR, Waddel JP, and Hudson AR: Shoulder arthrodesis for the treatment of brachial plexus palsy. Clin Orthop *198*:250–258, 1985.
299. Riggins RS: Shoulder fusion without external fixation: A preliminary report. J Bone Joint Surg *58A*:1007, 1976.
300. Roberts SNJ, Foley APJ, Swallow HM, et al: The geometry of the humeral head and the design of prostheses. J Bone Joint Surg *73B*:647–650, 1991.
301. Rockwood CA Jr: The technique of total shoulder arthroplasty. Instr Course Lect *39*:437–447, 1990.
302. Rockwood CA Jr: Personal communication, 1995.
303. Rockwood CA Jr, Jarman RN, and Williams GR: Complications of shoulder arthrodesis using internal fixation. Orthop Trans *15*:45, 1991.
304. Rockwood CA and Matsen RM: Global Shoulder Arthroplasty System. Warsaw, IN: DePuy Inc., 1994.
305. Rockwood CA Jr and Wirth MA: Global Total Shoulder Arthroplasty Video, Parts I and II. AAOS Individual Orthopaedic Instruction Video Award Winner, 1992.
306. Rodosky MW and Bigliani LU: Surgical treatment of nonconstrained glenoid component failure. Oper Tech Orthop *4*:226–236, 1994.
307. Rodosky MW, and Bigliani LU: Indications for glenoid resurfacing in shoulder arthroplasty (Review article). J Shoulder Elbow Surg *5*(3):231–248, 1996.
308. Rodosky MW, Weinstein DM, Pollock RG, et al: On the rarity of glenoid failure. J Shoulder Elbow Surg *4*:S13, 1995.
309. Roper BA, Paterson JMH, and Day WH: The Roper-Day total shoulder replacement. J Bone Joint Surg *72B*:694–697, 1990.
310. Rossleigh MA, Smith J, Straus DJ, and Engel IA: Osteonecrosis in patients with malignant lymphoma. Cancer *58*:1112–1116, 1986.
311. Rountree CR and Rockwood CA Jr: Arthrodesis of the shoulder in children following infantile paralysis. South Med J *58*:861, 1959.
312. Rowe CR: Re-evaluation of the position of the arm in arthrodesis of the shoulder in the adult. J Bone Joint Surg *56A*:913–922, 1974.
313. Rowe CR and Zarins B: Chronic unreduced dislocations of the shoulder. J Bone Joint Surg *64A*:494–505, 1982.
314. Rudicel S and Esdiale J: The randomized clinical trial in orthopaedics: Obligation of option? J Bone Joint Surg *67A*:1284–1293, 1985.
315. Russe O: Schulterarthrodese nach der AO-methode. Unfallheilkunde *81*:299, 1978.
316. Rutherford CS and Cofield RH: Osteonecrosis of the shoulder. Orthop Trans *11*:239, 1987.
317. Rybka V, Raunio P, and Vainio K: Arthrodesis of the shoulder in rheumatoid arthritis: A review of 41 cases. J Bone Joint Surg *61B*:155, 1979.
318. Rydholm U and Sjogren J: Surface replacement of the humeral head in the rheumatoid shoulder. J Shoulder Elbow Surg *2*:286–295, 1993.
318a. Saha AK, Bhattacharyya D, Dutta SK: Total shoulder replacement: A preliminary report. Calcutta: SK Sitcar, 1975.
319. Samilson RL and Prieto V: Dislocation arthroplasty of the shoulder. J Bone Joint Surg *65A*:456–460, 1983.
320. Schwartz RR, O'Brien SJ, Warren RF, and Torzilli PA: Capsular restraints to anterior-posterior motion in the shoulder. American Shoulder and Elbow Surgeons 4th Open Meeting, Atlanta, GA, 1988.
321. Schwyzer HK, Simmen BR, and Gschwend N: Infection following shoulder and elbow arthroplasty: Diagnosis and therapy. Orthopade *24*:367–375, 1995.
322. Sethi D, Naunton Morgan TC, Brown EA, et al: Dialysis arthropathy: A clinical, biochemical, radiological and histological study of 36 patients. Q J Med *77*:1061–1082, 1990.
323. Severt R, Thomas BJ, Tsenter MJ, et al: The influence of conformity and constraint on translational forces and frictional torque in total shoulder arthroplasty. Clin Orthop *292*:151–158, 1993.
324. Simkin PA: Structure and function of joints. *In* Schumacher HR (ed): Primer on the Rheumatic Diseases. Atlanta, GA: Arthritis Foundation, 1988.
325. Slawson SH, Everson LI, and Craig EV: The radiology of total shoulder replacement. Radiol Clin North Am *33*:305–318, 1995.
326. Smith-Peterson MN, Aufranc OE, and Larson CB: Useful surgical procedures for rheumatoid arthritis involving joints of the upper extremity. Arch Surg *46*:764–770, 1943.
327. Sneppen O, Fruensgaard S, Johannsen HV, et al: Total shoulder replacement in rheumatoid arthritis: proximal migration and loosening. J Shoulder Elbow Surg *5*:47–52, 1996.
328. Spencer R and Skirving AP: Silastic interposition arthroplasty of the shoulder. J Bone Joint Surg *68B*:375–377, 1986.
329. Steffee AD and Moore RW: Hemi-resurfacing arthroplasty of the shoulder. Contemp Orthop *9*:51–59, 1984.
330. Steindler A: Orthopedic Operations: Indications, Technique, and End Results. Springfield, IL: Charles C. Thomas, 1944, p 302.
331. Stinchfield FE, Bigliani LU, Neu HC, et al: Late hematogenous infection of total joint replacement. J Bone Joint Surg *62A*:1345–1350, 1980.
332. Sullivan PM, Johnston RC, and Kelley SS: Late infection after total hip replacement, caused by an oral organism after dental manipulation. J Bone Joint Surg *72A*:121–122, 1990.
333. Summers MN, Haley WE, Reveille JD, and Alarcon GS: Radiographic assessment and psychologic variables as predictors of pain and functional impairment in osteoarthritis of the knee or hip. Arthritis Rheum *31*:204–209, 1988.
334. Svend-Hansen H: Displaced proximal humeral fractures: A review of 49 patients. Acta Orthop Scand *45*:359, 1974.
335. Swanson AB: Implant resection arthroplasty of shoulder joint. *In* Swanson AB (ed): Flexible Resection Arthroplasty in the Hand and Extremities. St. Louis: CV Mosby, 1973, pp 287–295.
336. Swanson AB: Bipolar implant shoulder arthroplasty. *In* Bateman JE and Welsh RP (eds): Surgery of the Shoulder. St. Louis: CV Mosby, 1984, pp 211–223.
337. Swanson AB, deGroot G, Maupin BK, et al: Bipolar implant shoulder arthroplasty. Orthopedics *9*:343–351, 1986.
338. Swanson AB, deGroot Swanson G, Sattel AB, et al: Bipolar implant shoulder arthroplasty: Long-term results. Clin Orthop *248*:227–247, 1989.
339. Tanner MW and Cofield RH: Prosthetic arthroplasty for fractured and fracture-dislocations of the proximal humerus. Clin Orthop *179*:116–128, 1983.
340. Thomas BJ, Amstutz HC, and Cracchiolo A: Shoulder arthroplasty for rheumatoid arthritis. Clin Orthop *265*:125–128, 1991.
341. Tonino AJ and van de Werf GJIM: Hemiarthroplasty of the shoulder. Acta Orthop Belg *51*:625–631, 1985.
342. Torchia ME, Cofield RH, and Settergren CR: Total shoulder arthroplasty with the Neer prosthesis: Long-term results. Orthop Trans *18*(4):977, 1994–1995.
343. Tully JG Jr and Latteri A: Paraplegia, syringomyelia tarde and neuropathic arthrosis of the shoulder: A triad. Clin Orthop *134*:244–248, 1978.
344. Turkel SJ, Panio MW, Marshall JL, and Girgis FG: Stabilizing mechanisms preventing anterior dislocation of the glenohumeral joint. J Bone Joint Surg *63A*:1208–1217, 1981.

345. Uematsu A: Arthrodesis of the shoulder: Posterior approach. Clin Orthop *139*:169, 1979.
346. van Cappelle HGJ, and Visser JD: Hemiarthroplasty of the shoulder in rheumatoid arthritis. J Orthop Rheum *7*:43–47, 1994.
347. van Schaardenburg D, Van den Brande KJS, Ligthart GJ, et al: Musculoskeletal disorders and disability in persons aged 85 and over: A community survey. Ann Rheum Dis *53*:807–811, 1994.
348. Varian JPW: Interposition silastic cup arthroplasty of the shoulder. J Bone Joint Surg *62B*:116–117, 1980.
349. Wainwright D: Glenoidectomy in the treatment of the painful arthritic shoulder (Abstract). J Bone Joint Surg *58B*:377, 1976.
350. Ware JE, Snow KK, Kosinski M, and Gandek B: SF 36 Health Survey Manual and Interpretation Guide. Boston: New England Medical Center, The Health Institute, 1993.
351. Warren RF, Kornblatt IB, and Marchand R: Static factors affecting posterior shoulder instability. Orthop Trans *8*:1–89, 1984.
352. Warren RF, Ranawat CA, and Inglis AE: Total Shoulder Replacement Indications and Results of the Neer Nonconstrained Prosthesis. *In* The American Academy of Orthopaedics Surgeons, Symposium on Total Joint Replacement of the Upper Extremity. Inglis AE (ed). St. Louis: CV Mosby, 1982, pp 56–67.
353. Watson-Jones RW: Extra-articular arthrodesis of the shoulder. J Bone Joint Surg *15*:862, 1933.
354. Weigert M and Gronert HJ: Zur Technik der Schultergelenksarthrodese. Z Orthop *112*:1281, 1974.
355. Weiss APC, Adams MA, Moore JR, and Weiland AJ: Unconstrained shoulder arthroplasty. A five-year average follow up study. Clin Orthop *257*:86–90, 1990.
356. Wheble VH and Skorecki J: The design of a metal-to-metal total shoulder joint prosthesis. *In* Joint Replacement in the Upper Limb. Conference sponsored by the Medical Engineering Section of the Institution of Mechanical Engineers and the British Orthopaedic Association, London, 1977, pp 7–13.
357. Wilde AH, Borden LS, and Brems JJ: Experience with the Neer total shoulder replacement. *In* Bateman JE and Welsh RP (eds): Surgery of the Shoulder. St. Louis: BC Decker and CV Mosby, 1984, p 224.
358. Wilde AH, Brems JJ, and Boumphrey FRS: Arthrodesis of the shoulder: Current indications and operative technique. Orthop Clin North Am *18*:463–472, 1987.
359. Williams GR and Rockwood CA Jr: Massive rotator cuff defects and glenohumeral arthritis. *In* Friedman RJ (ed): Arthroplasty of the Shoulder. New York: Thieme Medical, 1994, pp 204–214.
360. Williams GR and Rockwood CA Jr: Hemiarthroplasty in rotator cuff deficient shoulders. J Shoulder Elbow *5*:362–367, 1996.
361. Winalski CS and Shapiro AW: Computed tomography in the evaluation of arthritis. Rheum Dis Clin North Am *17*:543–557, 1991.
362. Wirth MA, Basamania C, and Rockwood CA Jr: Fixation of glenoid component: Keel vs. pegs. Oper Tech Orthop *4*:218, 1994.
363. Wirth MA, Butters KP, and Rockwood CA Jr: The posterior deltoid-splitting approach to the shoulder. Clin Orthop *296*:92–98, 1993.
364. Wirth MA and Rockwood CA Jr: Traumatic instability: Pathology and pathogenesis. *In* Matsen FA (ed): The Shoulder: A Balance of Mobility and Stability. Chicago: American Academy of Orthopaedic Surgeons, 1993.
365. Wirth MA and Rockwood CA Jr: Complications of shoulder arthroplasty. Clin Orthop *307*:47–69, 1994.
366. Wirth MA and Rockwood CA Jr: Glenohumeral Instability Following Shoulder Arthroplasty. American Academy of Orthopaedic Surgeons 62nd Annual Meeting, Orlando, FL, 1995.
367. Wirth MA, Seltzer DG, Senes HR, et al: An analysis of failed humeral head and total shoulder arthroplasty. Orthop Trans *18*:977–978, 1994–1995.
368. Woolson ST and Potorff GT: Disassembly of a modular femoral prosthesis after dislocation of the femoral component: A case report. J Bone Joint Surg *72A*:624–625, 1990.
369. Wright TW and Cofield RH: Humeral fractures after shoulder arthroplasty. J Bone Joint Surg pp 1340–1346, 1995.
370. Zippel J: Vollstandiger Schullergelen Kersatz ans Kunstoff und Metall. Biomed Techink *17*:87, 1972.
371. Zippel J: Luxationssichere Schulterendoprothese Modell BME. Z Orthop *113*:454–457, 1975.
372. Zuckerman JD: Shoulder Arthroplasty—Costs/Results. Instructional course lecture No. 110 at the annual meeting of the American Academy of Orthopaedic Surgeons, Atlanta, GA, 1996.
373. Zuckerman JD and Cofield RH: Proximal humeral prosthetic replacement in glenohumeral arthritis. Orthop Trans *10*:231, 1986.
374. Zuckerman JD and Cuomo F: Glenohumeral arthroplasty: A critical review of indications and preoperative considerations. Bull Hosp Jt Dis *52*:21–30, 1993.
375. Zuckerman JD and Matsen FA III: Complications about the glenohumeral joint related to the use of screws and staples. J Bone Joint Surg *66(A)*:175–180, 1984.

ROBERT D. LEFFERT, M.D.

CHAPTER

17

Neurologic Problems

HISTORICAL REVIEW

The shoulder girdle is an anatomic area in which orthopedics, neurology, and neurosurgery, vascular surgery, and thoracic surgery all may be involved; however, patients with clinical problems in this area that do not lend themselves to an immediate diagnosis may fail to obtain relief because each specialist may assume that the problem relates to a different specialty. This is true particularly for neurologic problems, since they tend to be relatively uncommon, and the symptoms are often vague and difficult to interpret. The differential diagnosis may involve consideration of entities that are either rarely encountered or are totally unknown to the orthopedic surgeon.[5, 71]

The understanding of the function of the normal shoulder is dependent on anatomic and biomechanical considerations that are thoroughly covered in other chapters of this book. In addition, there are several useful references to which the reader is directed.[22, 34, 72, 84] In this chapter, the pertinent anatomy is illustrated by means of simple line drawings.

The study of abnormal shoulders, particularly those paralyzed by poliomyelitis, has provided much of the available information regarding the treatment of other neurologic problems. Poliomyelitis provided a continuous supply of patients with paralysis of virtually every muscle in the upper limb, and it was only natural that their patterns of motor loss should be studied. Probably the most intensive work on this subject is that of Duchenne, the 19th century anatomist whose masterful treatise *The Physiology of Motion* was translated by Kaplan in 1949.[22] This textbook should be consulted by anyone interested in this problem (Fig. 17–1). In the 20th century, the conservator of this material was Steindler, whose book *Kinesiology*[84] and contributions to the armamentarium of surgical procedures have been of great value. Many surgeons have contributed to our understanding of the reconstruction of the shoulder paralyzed by poliomyelitis, among them, Schottsteadt, Bost, Larsen, Ober, Harmon, Saha, and others[4, 28, 30, 51, 52, 59, 70, 72, 74, 83]

After the elimination of poliomyelitis as a cause of paralysis in people of the industrialized world, trauma to the brachial plexus and peripheral nerves became the most common basis for shoulder paralysis. Many of the lessons learned from the poliomyelitis experience were applied to these injuries. Seddon and the group that he inspired at the Royal National Orthopaedic Hospital in London contributed significantly to our knowledge.[6, 10, 43, 74, 100, 101]

Unfortunately, the relatively recent advances in techniques of nerve repair have not proved to be as dramatically beneficial to the restoration of adult shoulder function as they have been in the remainder of the limb. As techniques of surgical reconstruction and rehabilitation have become disseminated, they have allowed their application to the paralytic shoulder of muscular dystrophy and the stroke shoulder.[13, 40, 55] Suffice it to say that the need for work in this area continues.

CLINICAL PRESENTATION

When there has been a history of trauma to the area of the shoulder and a localized neurologic deficit exists, there should be little diagnostic confusion as to the cause. Nevertheless, when patients who have sustained multisystem trauma are first encountered, either in a life-threatening situation or under anesthesia when they cannot be properly examined, a potentially difficult situation can arise if a nerve injury is found after treatment. These difficulties can be minimized by a careful preoperative evaluation whenever possible, including a detailed neurologic examination.

The clinical picture generated by a neurologic problem about the shoulder may be complicated by the anatomic situation of the shoulder as a “waystation” through which the nerves and vessels to the upper limb must pass. Consequently, there may be local shoulder discomfort referred from lesions of the spinal cord or the cervical roots. In brachial plexus injuries or thoracic outlet syndrome (TOS), nerves have been affected by pathology in the region of the shoulder, yet the symptoms will be appreciated further distally in the arm or hand.

The anatomy of the brachial plexus is shown in Figure 17–2. In addition, since cervical radiculopathy may be

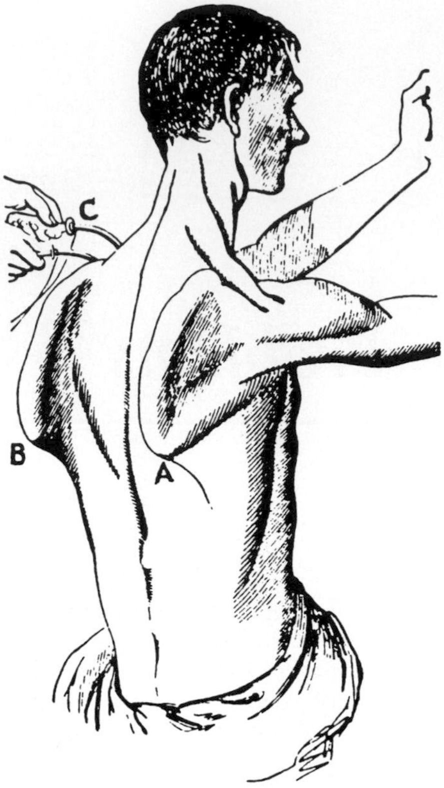

Figure 17–1

Reproduced from Duchenne's *Physiology of Motion,* showing on the right (*A*) the winging of the scapula caused by paralysis of the serratus anterior, and on the left (*B*) a similar deformity elicited experimentally by electrical stimulation of the deltoid. (From Duchenne GB: The Physiology of Motion [trans. EB Kaplan]. Philadelphia: WB Saunders, 1959.)

expressed as pain, paresthesias, or motor weakness in the limb, Figures 17–3 and 17–4 summarize the segmental distribution of the motor and sensory components of the nerve supply.

Pain that originates in the pleural or abdominal cavities may be perceived as pain in the shoulder girdle. Occasionally, a patient with cholecystitis may present with shoulder pain, and there are others whose intrapleural or cardiac problems can be diagnostic. Consider the patient who was recently brought into my office with the complaint that his frozen shoulders were symptomatic when he was walking against the wind or up stairs!

A general medical and family history is important when making a diagnosis. The presentation of painless, atraumatic weakness and atrophy about the shoulder girdle, especially bilaterally, in a patient in the first or second decades of life, should raise the possibility of an underlying neurologic disease, either neurogenic or myopathic. A positive family history may often be present in these cases.[1, 5, 23]

The physical examination must begin with the head and neck, since it is not at all uncommon for shoulder pain to come from discogenic radiculopathy. Foraminal closure tests, done by gently hyperextending the cervical spine and laterally flexing it to the affected side, may completely reproduce the patient's shoulder pain and exonerate this joint as the culprit. It should be remembered, however, that patients may have pathology and symptoms coming from both areas simultaneously, and each of them may require treatment.

The entire upper limb must be examined next, and a thorough manual muscle test and sensory examination must be recorded. The contralateral limb must also be examined for comparison, and, when indicated, particularly if a generalized neurologic condition is suspected, the lower extremities must be evaluated. The finding of hyperreflexia or pathologic plantar responses will indicate the presence of an upper motor neuron lesion. Because it is not unheard of for an intracranial or intraspinal lesion to present as a disability of the upper limb, and sometimes of the shoulder girdle, we must not neglect to examine the patient with this in mind. I am reminded of a personal case many years ago of a woman with a provisional diagnosis of an intractable frozen shoulder and reflex sympathetic dystrophy. She was found ultimately to have a brain tumor, which caused her inability to move the limb. I have now seen three relatively young women who had been thought to have TOS and who ultimately proved to have apical lung tumors.

RADIOGRAPHIC AND LABORATORY EVALUATION

In all patients in whom there is a problem of a neurologic disorder about the shoulder, or one further distally in the limb that is felt to originate proximally, it is most important to obtain plain radiographs of the shoulder and cervical spine in three planes (Fig. 17–5 *A* and *B*). This is important even in cases in which there is no known bony injury, such as brachial plexus trauma without clinically obvious fractures. In patients with traction injury we should look for displaced fractures of the cervical transverse processes, since they constitute presumptive evidence of avulsion of cervical nerve roots.[75] Patients with TOS may have cervical ribs or long transverse processes at C7 that may contribute materially to the problem of compression, although only about 20% of patients in whom I make the diagnosis of TOS do have such bony abnormalities. In some patients with TOS, an ununited or malunited clavicular fracture may be appreciated.[36] Occasionally, one may see a nerve lesion that has occurred as a result of a totally unsuspected bone tumor.

Chest x-rays, particularly in patients who smoke, are mandatory, because lesions of the apical pleura can present with pain in the shoulder (Fig. 17–6). When there is suspicion of pathology that cannot be clearly demonstrated by plain radiographs, tomography or computer-assisted tomography may be helpful. The use of magnetic resonance imaging (MRI) of the cervical spine has materially advanced the diagnosis of discogenic radiculopathy and many other lesions about the shoulder. MRI of the brachial plexus is now the most effective technique for imaging this area, although I find it more useful in the nontraumatic cases such as neoplasms.

Arthrography of the shoulder joint is particularly useful in the differential diagnosis of atrophy and weakness of the supraspinatus and infraspinatus. This finding may be

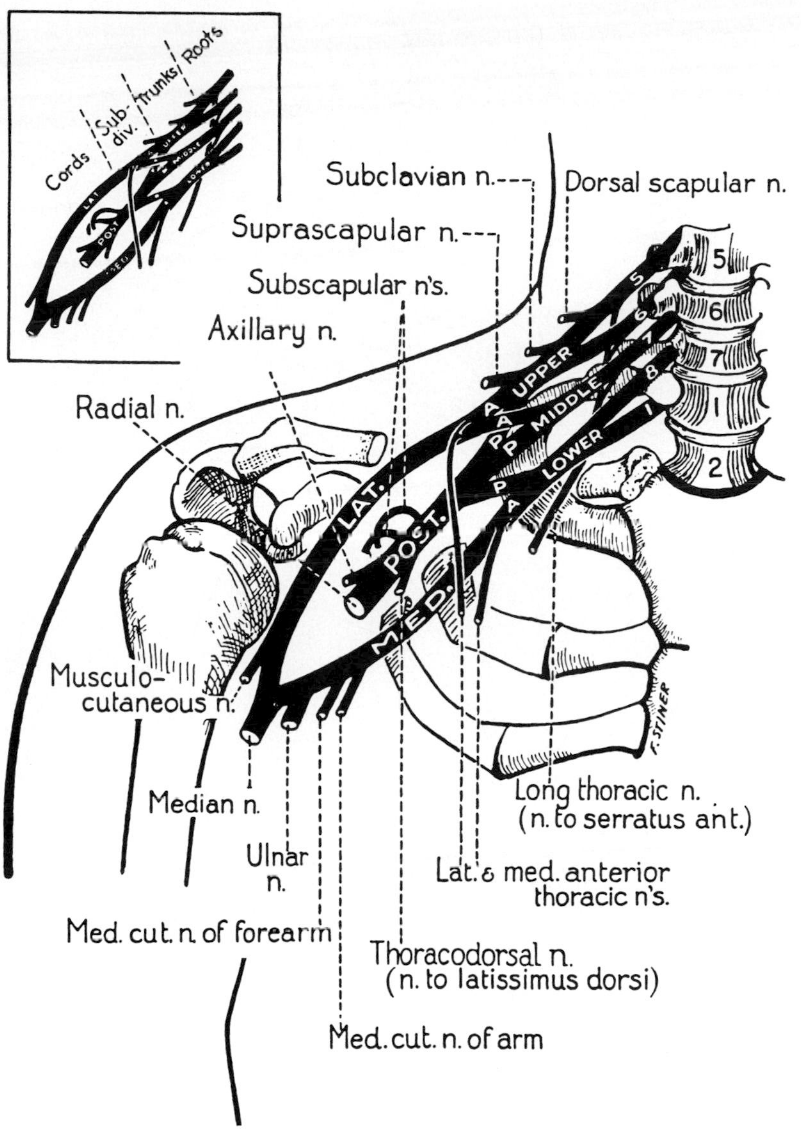

Figure 17–2

The brachial plexus. (From Haymaker W and Woodhall B: Peripheral Nerve Injuries. Philadelphia: WB Saunders, 1953, p 210.)

due to a lesion of the suprascapular nerve[62, 63] or a rotator cuff tear, and sometimes the two may coexist. Here, the MRI can be of great value, because it may reveal the presence of an unsuspected space-occupying lesion such as a ganglion compressing the suprascapular nerve. Although the relative cost of MRI is a consideration, it may also provide more information than plain arthrography. Nevertheless, a patient with severe atrophy thought to be due to a suprascapular nerve lesion ought to have an arthrogram or equivalent, and a patient with a cuff tear and an unexpectedly severe degree of atrophy should have an electromyogram (EMG).

Electrodiagnostic testing may be very helpful to refine the clinical diagnosis of a neurologic disorder about the shoulder in situations wherein there is a lower motor neuron lesion.[3, 11, 41, 49, 77, 80] Electromyography may reveal an extension of the pathologic process beyond the confines of a single peripheral nerve, as in the case of idiopathic brachial neuritis,[92] or may indicate that the observed neuropathy is part of a generalized peripheral neuropathy. Although a detailed consideration of the fine points of electromyographic theory and practice is probably not necessary for most orthopedic surgeons, a basic understanding of its applications and limitations is as necessary as the corresponding considerations of bone radiology. A general discussion of the pathology of nerve injury and electromyographic findings follows.

The use of nerve conduction velocity determination, an extension of the EMG, may help to further localize a specific lesion. The more proximal portions of the peripheral nervous system can be studied by use of the "late responses," including somatosensory evoked potentials and F responses. The specific applications are described within the sections devoted to particular entities.

Electromyography is also very useful in the identification of chronic myopathies such as muscular dystrophy.[41, 49] It may be difficult to precisely classify myopathies of an acute nature such as acute polymyositis on the basis of an EMG, but these disorders are not confined to the shoulder girdles, which are more likely to be affected by the localized facioscapulohumeral or limb girdle dystrophies (Fig. 17–7). In these cases, the diagnosis will have to include further study of muscle biopsies by means of electron microscopy and histochemistry. The study of

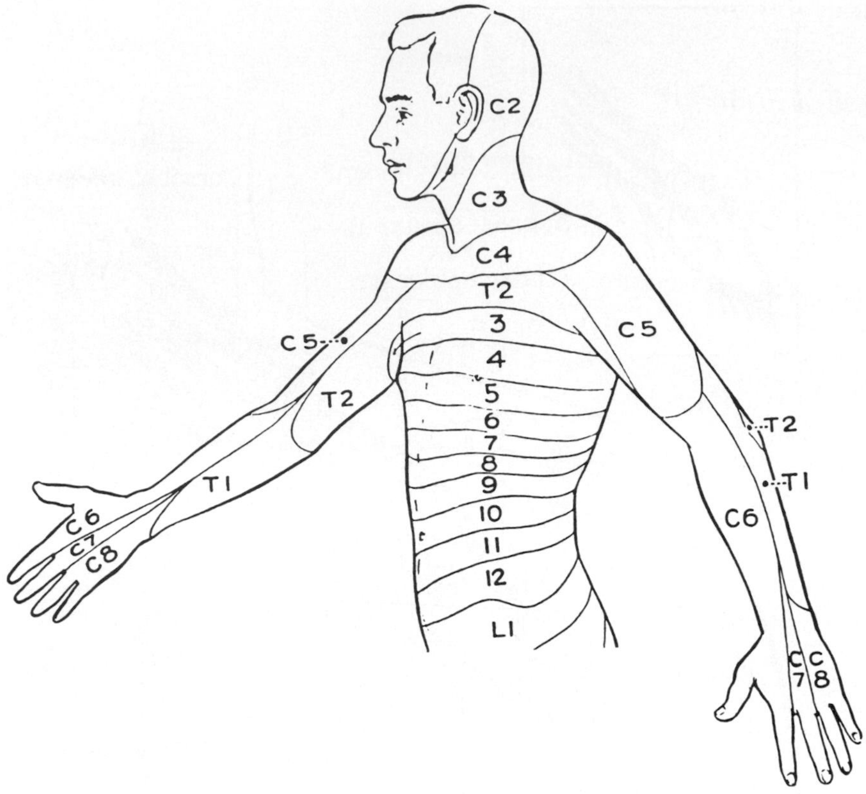

Figure 17–3

The dermatomes as depicted by Foerster in 1933. (From Haymaker W and Woodhall B: Peripheral Nerve Injuries. Philadelphia: WB Saunders, 1953, p 21.)

serum enzymes will also be an important part of the evaluation.[5, 56]

PATHOLOGY AND CLASSIFICATION

The classification of disorders of the nervous system that can affect the function of the shoulder, or that can be influenced by pathology in the region of the shoulder girdle, can be approached in several ways. It makes little sense to list as many diseases as possible for the sake of inclusiveness, since this is not a textbook of neurology. Rather, I will group these diseases according to the unique functional consequences that are addressed by the shoulder surgeon. No attempt will be made to be encyclopedic, although the more commonly encountered entities are included under the category in which the most pronounced manifestation belongs.

In addition, because of the varying pathology inherent in traumatic lesions of the peripheral nerves and their problems of prognostication, it will be necessary to discuss their specific classification.

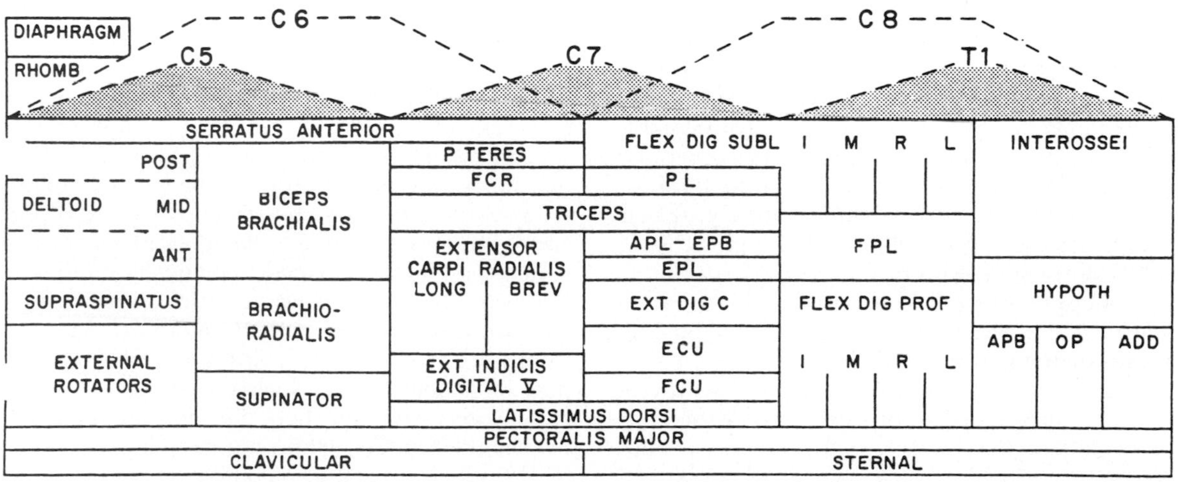

Figure 17–4

The segmental supply of the muscles of the upper limb as depicted by D'Aubigne. (From Leffert RD: Brachial Plexus Injuries. New York: Churchill Livingstone, 1985, p 76.)

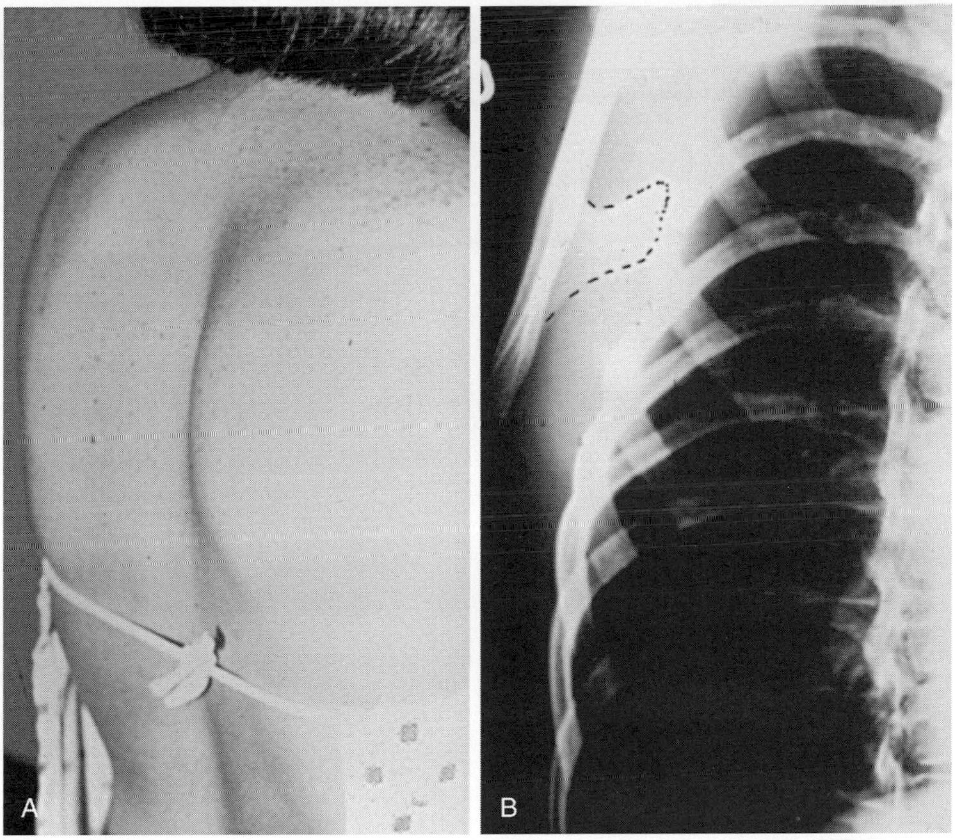

Figure 17–5

A, A 24-year-old woman referred with a diagnosis of a winged scapula that was thought to be due to an idiopathic serratus palsy. *B,* An axial view of the scapula showing the large osteochondroma that caused the problem. The patient had complete relief of the deformity after the lesion was removed.

Finally, we will complete this section of the chapter with a discussion of the differential diagnosis of organic and functional causes of dysfunction of the shoulder complex.

CLASSIFICATION OF NEUROLOGIC DISEASES THAT PRODUCE SHOULDER DYSFUNCTION

1. Upper Motor Neuron Diseases
   - Stroke
   - Head injury
   - Tumors of the brain and spinal cord
   - Cerebral palsy
   - Multiple sclerosis
2. Lower Motor Neuron Diseases
   - Idiopathic brachial neuritis
   - Infectious or idiopathic myelopathy or neuropathy
     - Poliomyelitis
     - Guillain-Barré syndrome
     - Motor neuron disease (progressive muscular atrophy)
     - Herpes zoster
     - Mononeuritis multiplex, metabolic, or other
     - Diffuse peripheral neuropathy
   - Brachial plexus injuries
     - Supraclavicular
     - Subclavicular
     - Infraclavicular
     - Open wounds
     - Postanesthetic palsy
     - Radiation neuropathy
   - Cervical radiculopathy, discogenic or due to spondylosis
     - Spinal cord tumors (intrinsic or extrinsic)
   - Compression neuropathy
     - Suprascapular nerve
     - Thoracic outlet syndrome
     - Quadrilateral space syndrome
   - Cranial nerve injury
     - Spinal accessory nerve
   - Peripheral nerve injuries

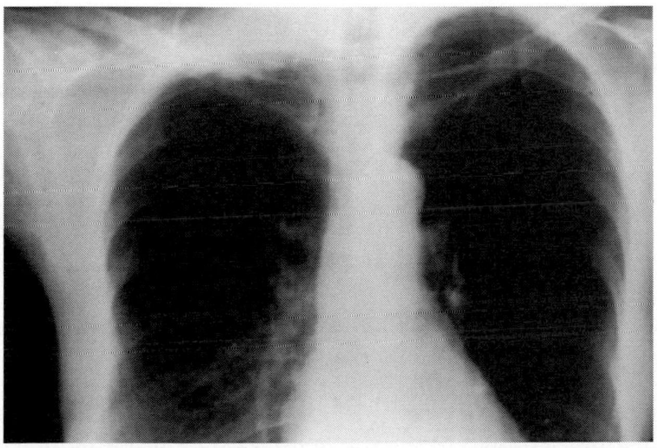

Figure 17–6

A chest radiograph of a 38-year-old woman with undiagnosed pain in the right shoulder. The patient smoked two packs of cigarettes a day.

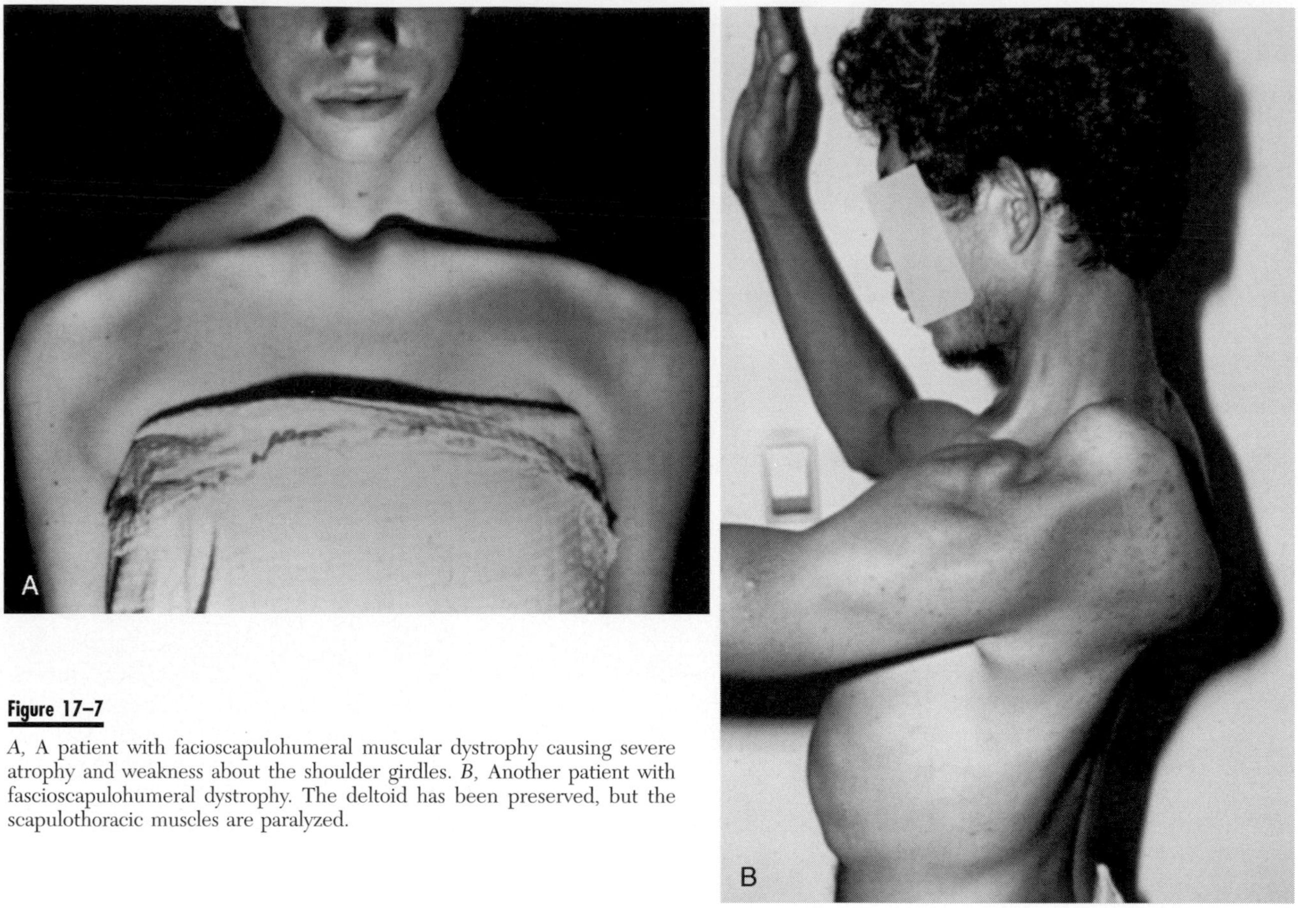

Figure 17–7

A, A patient with facioscapulohumeral muscular dystrophy causing severe atrophy and weakness about the shoulder girdles. *B*, Another patient with fascioscapulohumeral dystrophy. The deltoid has been preserved, but the scapulothoracic muscles are paralyzed.

Axillary
Musculocutaneous
Long thoracic
Suprascapular

3. Myopathies
    Muscular dystrophy
      X-linked: Duchenne, Becker,
      Autosomal recessive
        Limb girdle: scapulohumeral
        Childhood
        Congenital
      Autosomal dominant
        Fascioscapulohumeral
    Metabolic myopathies
    Inflammatory myopathies
      Polymyositis
      Dermatomyositis
    Endocrine myopathies
    Toxic and drug-induced myopathies
4. Mixed Pathology and Miscellaneous
    Reflex sympathetic dystrophy
      Shoulder-hand syndrome
    Arthrogryposis

CLASSIFICATION OF THE PATHOLOGY OF PERIPHERAL NERVE INJURIES

With the publication in 1934 of his seminal article, "Three Types of Nerve Injury," Seddon provided clinicians with a common language by which they could not only describe a nerve injury but also begin to understand the nature of the pathology and the basis for the prognosis, as well as formulate a rational treatment program.[73, 75]

The first grade of nerve injury, neurapraxia (non-action of nerve), describes the most benign situation. It commonly results from milder degrees of compression or traction and is clinically expressed in motor loss that may be quite profound, yet usually is accompanied by a partial sensory deficit and little or no disturbance of the sympathetic innervation. There is no evidence of wallerian degeneration, and the electrical changes are limited to a local conduction block with intact conduction distal to the lesion. An electromyographic examination will fail to demonstrate any spontaneous electrical activity at rest, thus there will be no fibrillations or sharp positive waves seen if the patient is still paralyzed at 3 weeks from onset. The circumstances under which these lesions occur vary from the "foot falling asleep" to crutch palsy and the milder tourniquet palsies. Many gunshot wounds involve "near-misses" of the nerves by bullets that generate shock waves in the tissues, and in these cases, it is the local stretch of the nerves that is expressed in a local conduction block without degeneration of the axon. Consequently, there is rapid recovery of function. This clinical picture was first described by the American Civil War neurologist, Silas Weir Mitchell in 1872[97] when he noted the speed with which many nerve injuries incurred in this manner recovered. In fact, the duration of the paralysis with neurapraxia may vary from moments to days to weeks, and the patient usually makes a complete recovery within 10 weeks but often in considerably less time. Although the more transient of these palsies may be solely attributed to local vascular compromise, the experiments of Denny-Brown and Brenner in 1944,[20] using spring clips to produce nerve compression, demonstrated degeneration of the myelin sheaths at the site of the lesion and edema of the axon above and below it. They characterized this lesion as one of ischemic demyelination.

The term axonotmesis was used by Seddon to describe the situation in which the damage to the nerve is confined to loss of continuity of the axon and the myelin sheath. Usually it results from a more severe crush or traction injury than the former circumstance, but the supporting stroma of the nerve including the Schwann sheath, endoneurium, and successively larger subdivisions of the nerve remain intact. This lesion-in-continuity results in complete loss of motor and sensory function below the level of the lesion that is indistinguishable from a complete transsection of the nerve, and wallerian degeneration does take place. The appropriate electrical changes of denervation are found after 3 weeks. However, because the Schwann sheaths and endoneurial tubes are intact, these lesions recover spontaneously with a rate of regeneration of the nerves that averages 1 inch/month or 1 mm/day. Because of the persistence of the supporting stroma that precludes loss of axonal material as well as confused reinnervation, the quality of neurologic recovery is excellent. Assuming that the temporarily denervated parts are protected from injury and contractures, functional recovery should follow suit.

For the clinician encountering a complete loss of motor and sensory function after an injury to a peripheral nerve, the dilemma is usually that of defining the more benign lesion of axonotmesis with its excellent prognosis from the situation in which there is complete division of all the structural elements of the nerve, axon, and Schwann sheath. This was called neurotmesis by Seddon. It requires surgical manipulation to re-establish the continuity of the peripheral nerve with fascicular alignment sufficiently correct to allow for regeneration and functional recovery. The electromyographic findings after the 3-week period needed for wallerian degeneration will be the same as for axonotmesis, with fibrillation potentials at rest, and, in the case of a complete lesion, no action potentials seen on attempted voluntary contraction.

In most cases, the history of the mode of injury will be helpful in making the correct diagnosis. For example, a patient with a nerve injury caused by a knife is much more likely to have sustained a laceration rather than a lesser degree of damage. Closed fractures, unless they involve extremely displaced or very sharp bone fragments, are less likely to cause lacerations of nerves, and since they are usually axonotmesis, have a relatively good prognosis for spontaneous recovery. However, they may cause severe injury by local compression or crushing of nerve.

At this point it would be well to consider those injuries to the nerves about the shoulder girdle that may occur during the course of surgical operations about the shoulder, and particularly, anterior repair. Richards, Waddell, and Hudson[64] studied these and concluded that if a brachial plexus deficit is present after anterior shoulder stabilization, there is a high likelihood of structural injury if function does not return rapidly. They found that the musculocutaneous nerve was at greatest risk and recommended early brachial plexus exploration in these situations. It should be noted that with misplacement of the anterior portal for arthroscopy it is possible to cause a plexus injury, and these injuries should be treated similarly, as should those lesions of the axillary nerve that can be incurred during the course of capsular shift procedures. The axillary nerve should be identified and can be palpated during the exposure for the capsular shift. The Bristow procedure puts the musculocutaneous nerve at particular risk, not only at the time of the original surgery but also in cases where a redo is necessary after this procedure has failed. Further discussion of this topic will continue under the headings of the individual nerves.

Although the classification of Seddon has been very useful, there are some situations in which additional descriptive terms are needed. For this reason, the classification advanced by Sunderland[86] is of use. It has five categories, the first, second, and fifth grade being equivalent to neurapraxia, axonotmesis, and neurotmesis as stated earlier. The fourth grade, according to Sunderland, describes the situation wherein all that remains in continuity of the nerve is the external or epifascicular epineurium, giving the false impression that the nerve is intact and will recover with time. This situation may be encountered clinically, but can be recognized if the nerve is carefully dissected under magnification, to reveal that there are really no intact elements beneath the epineurium. In these circumstances, nerve repair will be necessary. Finally, Sunderland's third degree of injury[87] represents the situation wherein the perineurium is intact, but the fascicles themselves have been disrupted. Although some degree of regeneration may occur, its quality is extremely poor, and such lesions usually require formal repair.

Having these considerations of the spectrum of pathology of the peripheral nerves in mind, the surgeon can approach a clinical problem with a better understanding of the diagnostic, and therefore, prognostic possibilities for a particular case. Knowledge of the mechanism of injury allows for an informed presumption of the state of the nerve.

DIFFERENTIAL DIAGNOSIS OF ORGANIC VERSUS FUNCTIONAL DISEASE OF THE SHOULDER JOINT COMPLEX

This area of evaluation is not only one of the most difficult but also has the greatest risk in terms of the consequences of misdiagnosis. Yet, we as clinicians are often called upon to make such distinctions, with the full knowledge that organic and functional disorders may coexist in the same patient and that there is no organic entity that cannot be mimicked by its counterpart in psychogenic or factitious disease. For this section, I have, as in my clinical practice over the past 17 years, relied heavily and drawn from the excellent chapter in *The Neurological Examination* by De Jong[19] entitled "Examination in Cases of Suspected Hysteria and Malingering."

If we are to differentiate between organic and nonorganic disorders as expressed about the shoulder girdle, a few definitions are essential. First, the term hysteria should be replaced by conversion reaction, because it describes the process whereby emotional disturbances are converted into physical symptoms and signs. It is a psychoneurosis in which the patient is unaware that the disability or symptoms are not the result of an alteration of anatomy or physiology, so that to the patient, they are real. This condition must be distinguished from malingering, which is a deliberate and willful, fraudulent imitation or exaggeration of illness. It is conscious and involves deception for the purpose of attaining a goal. Unfortunately, it must be stated, that these two entities may sometimes overlap, making a clean and precise diagnosis impossible. However, some useful generalizations may be articulated.

In cases of malingering, the symptoms rarely vary from time to time. A malingerer with pain may insist that the quality of the discomfort is always the same (usually excruciating) no matter what the time of day, degree of activity, or modalities used to treat it. The pain and disability often appear to be greater than one would expect from the situation. It should be noted, however, that this last curiosity is also to be found in patients with reflex sympathetic dystrophy.

Symptoms of malingerers may fail to fit a pattern consistent with an anatomic lesion and may present as completely bizarre. The patient may often not be able to give an exact description of just what the complaint is and may be evasive in answers to questions directed at clarification. He or she may, in addition, be sullen and uncooperative in the process.

The patient with a conversion reaction, by contrast, may appear honest, sincere, and cooperative in all aspects of treatment, including submitting to surgery. Unfortunately, either conversion reactions or malingering may follow trauma, including industrial situations, although in the latter case, if there are persistent symptoms associated with the process of attempting to secure compensation, appropriate inferences may usually be made. A history of the patient's activities of daily living, including questions regarding ability to sleep or engage in recreational activities in addition to employment, may prove to be extremely enlightening. The patient with organic pathology who is disabled is generally globally impaired.

Although there really is no foolproof process that one may use to detect nonorganic disease, there are observations within the routine, detailed neurologic examination that can be extremely helpful. Specifically, in the history taking, it is important to search for prior episodes similar to the present one or evidence of adjustment problems. The patient can be asked to re-enact the accident (if there was one), and occasionally a very naive malingerer may move the allegedly weak or paralyzed limb to demonstrate its former utility. (I have successfully used this maneuver on several occasions.)

The patient should be surreptitiously observed in the process of entering the room and disrobing as well as gesturing. Facial expression and vital signs must be assessed, particularly when the examination is likely to produce discomfort. A departure from what would be expected should be noted, particularly theatrical or dramatic gesturing in response to the physical examination. The examiner should appear sympathetic and nonjudgmental in approach but should consciously test the patient at all times. It is useful to exclude family, friends, lawyers, or rehabilitation counselors from the room for the examination, although they may return for any discussions that take place at the end of the session.

Hyperesthesia and tenderness may be found in both organic and functional disorders. In the latter, however, the patient may exhibit an inconstant response to stimulation in that he or she may wince and cry out when barely touched, only to hardly react to deep pressure over the same area when distracted. Mankoff's sign may sometimes be useful in differentiating between organic pain and malingered pain; in organic pain, pressure over a painful area usually causes an increase in pulse of from 20 to 30 beats/min, whereas the malingerer's pulse will remain unchanged.

Disturbances of sensibility are commonly found in nonorganic as well as organic neurologic disorders. Unfortunately, it is the rare patient who will succumb to the old "say yes when you feel my touch, and no when you don't" routine! Nevertheless, those patients with sensory deficits that do not conform to known anatomic distributions are suspect. The glove or stocking sensory loss found in peripheral neuropathies differs from that which is feigned or is a manifestation of a conversion reaction in that it does not have a sharply defined margin. Hemisensory loss involving the head, neck, and trunk, which changes at the midline, should be evaluated by proceeding from the anesthetic to the side with sensibility. Using this approach, in organic lesions, sensation begins to return slightly before the midline is reached. All sensory modalities may be lost with nonorganic disorders, and these may include vibration sense over the skull or sternum. However, since vibration is partially conducted through bone, such sharp midline changes cannot be attributed to organic lesions. In situations in which there is a hemisensory defect, the cutaneous reflexes may be compared on both sides. If they are retained on the anesthetic side, it cannot be truly anesthetic. Furthermore, an anesthetic area with a preserved psychogalvanic response (mediated by sweating) is inconsistent, since in organic anesthesia due to a nerve lesion, this response would be abolished.

The motor system must be carefully evaluated in all patients with reference to muscle bulk, tone, volume, strength, and coordination. The presumptive diagnostic impression can then be further clarified by means of electrodiagnostic testing. It would be rare to see changes of volume or contour in muscles apparently paralyzed or weakened by nonorganic disease, except in long-term situations in which disuse atrophy may supervene. However, it should be noted that significant psychopathology or factitious disorders may result in contractures and deformities if they are allowed to persist long enough.

The examiner should be aware of the variety of tricks that may be encountered during the course of detailed manual muscle testing. Patients may make little effort to contract muscles when asked to do so. The antagonist of the muscle or group under consideration should be observed and palpated, since it may be contracted in an effort to simulate weakness of the agonist. On passive movement there may be evidence of contraction of the agonists when the antagonists are moved.

The muscle contractions in nonorganic weakness may be poorly sustained or of the "give-way" variety. There may be absence of follow-through when the examiner withdraws pressure.

If the examiner drops the flail upper limb, particularly when the patient is lying supine on the examining table and the hand is above the face, it will gracefully and slowly glide away from the patient so that it will not strike him. A truly paralyzed limb will lack the motor control needed to avoid having the patient hit himself in the face. Of course, one must be very confident of the result before trying this particular maneuver, but it certainly has great appeal to the residents watching the examination!

Muscle testing should be done with the patient and the limb in different positions. For example, testing the power of forward flexion of the humerus with the patient supine and then prone may confuse the unsophisticated malingerer if the test is done in the context of asking the patient to first "push up" and then "push down," implying that these are really two different functions that employ different muscle groups. I would hasten to add, however, that for the patient with the residua of stroke, there will often be a bona fide difference in the responses elicited when the patient is sitting up or lying down.

Finally, one may ask the patient to exert maximal effort on one side, such as is involved in adducting the humerus tightly against the body. The examiner feels the contralateral adductors, and unless these muscles are truly paralyzed, they will be felt to contract, since it is extremely difficult to suppress this phenomenon. As a variant of this, a patient feigning total loss of power in a limb including the shoulder girdle will be unable to suppress the involuntary contraction of the latissimus dorsi when asked to inhale and then give a deep cough.

Stereotyped tests of coordination may convey the impression of significant ataxia or clumsiness of the upper limb, which may be totally abolished when at the end of the examination the patient is putting on his shirt. It is useful to have a mirror on the wall near the door to the examining room as the doctor exits.

As one becomes more experienced in the art of examination, these techniques and others can be smoothly integrated into the process of evaluation and should not be treated any differently from the standard neurologic examination. Remember, however, that a patient's problem rarely is totally clearly defined, and the last thing that a responsible examiner would want to do would be to dismiss a patient's complaints as nonorganic without having used every possible technique to make that diagnosis on as firm a basis as possible. When that has been done, however, there is the problem of what one writes in a report and what one tells the patient. No report should ever be written that cannot be read in open court or to the patient and his or her lawyer, because this will invariably come to pass if the opinion does not have a solid basis. When there are inconsistencies in the examination, or bizarre responses, I describe them as such and then comment that they do not, in my opinion, conform to known organic neurologic deficits. When a patient complains of pain, I do not presume to say that he or she does not feel it, only that I can find no evidence of organic pathology with which to diagnose the subjective complaint. Although there are numerous psychological tests and personality indices that have been used to define the malingerer from the psychoneurotic, I resist the temptation to enter this minefield, because little good can come to an orthopedic surgeon from such excursions. This is not to say that one should not avail oneself of the opinions of nonsurgical colleagues in neurology, psychiatry, or psychology for help in making a diagnosis of these very complex patients when it appears necessary.

METHODS OF TREATMENT OF KINESIOLOGIC ABNORMALITIES ABOUT THE SHOULDER

Because normal function of the shoulder joint complex depends on the smooth integration of nerve, muscle, bone, and joint, the treatment of its kinesiologic abnormalities must be based on knowledge of the functional status of each of these interrelated tissues. Only in this way can the varied pathologic entities be approached in a logical fashion, using available techniques of medical or surgical therapy as required. When, for example, there is muscle weakness about the shoulder caused by a generalized myopathy that can be treated, or that will recover spontaneously, then one must await the limit of improvement before proceeding to considerations of surgical therapy. However, it is important that the orthopedic surgeon be included in the assessment of such patients early in the course of the disease so that reasoned decisions can be made regarding the rehabilitation process. In this way, the patient will benefit from the combined knowledge and differing points of view of the various medical and surgical specialists who take care of him or her.

A thorough and complete consideration of the surgical treatment of all of the neuropathologic entities that can disturb the function of the shoulder girdle complex or impair the limb distally would require an encyclopedic presentation beyond the scope of this chapter. Instead, by describing the management of the more common entities, an attempt will be made to provide a working framework from which treatment plans can be established for the less common disorders that must be omitted due to limitations of space and time.

No matter what the original etiology of the motor deficit about the shoulder, the ultimate result will be a disturbance in the smooth and exquisitely balanced interaction of the force couples that provide a stable yet globally mobile base for the function of the upper limb.[34, 70, 84] Certain basic principles can be enumerated as common to the approach of any of the resultant kinesiologic disturbances. Nerves may require decompression and neurolysis when compressed, or with more severe degrees of injury, either direct repair or grafting. The classification of pathology of traumatic neuropathy and the manner in which it leads to therapeutic decisions has already been presented in the previous section devoted to classification.

When muscle power is permanently lost, either from nerve injury, neuropathy, direct trauma, or myopathy, then tendon transfer is an option. This technique preserves mobility more than any other and most closely simulates normal function. However, since no muscle is added to the limb by the operation, its total strength will remain less than normal. For the paralyzed glenohumeral joint when there are no available motors for transfer, arthrodesis provides useful and reasonably strong function within a limited range of motion, provided that the serratus and trapezius are intact.[18, 69, 82] In situations in which the scapular motors are deficient and the glenohumeral musculature is intact, then an entirely different set of problems exists.

It should be apparent that different avenues of therapeutic approach may be required for management of a single entity, depending on the stage or severity of the lesion. Finally, there are complex interrelations between the components of the shoulder girdle complex and neurologic dysfunction that may be expressed as secondary TOS or lesions of the brachial plexus that will require correction before the neurovascular dysfunction can be alleviated.[44, 47] An example of this situation would be a fracture of the clavicle with malunion or nonunion that compromises the costoclavicular space available to the neurovascular structures and thus creates a TOS.[36] In addition, the patient may have superimposed disuse atrophy of the trapezius muscle because of pain, and this will result in postural ptosis of the scapula, thus aggravating the compression. In a number of patients that I have observed with anterior instability of the glenohumeral joint, the symptoms of "dead arm syndrome" have been accompanied by physical findings consistent with the diagnosis of TOS. I believe that this association is more than coincidence and that many of the symptoms of what has been labeled "dead arm syndrome" are actually due to TOS.[46] The subject will be further discussed later.

Specific neurologic disorders for which functional restoration or significant improvement of shoulder dysfunction may be obtained by surgical treatment are as follows:

1. Spinal accessory nerve palsy
2. Muscular dystrophy
3. Serratus anterior palsy
4. Brachial plexus injuries:
    a. Supraclavicular
    b. Infraclavicular
    c. Subclavicular
5. Suprascapular nerve compression
6. Axillary nerve injury
7. Musculocutaneous nerve injury
8. TOS
9. Stroke shoulder

Spinal Accessory Nerve Palsy

The spinal accessory nerve, which leaves the jugular foramen at the base of the skull, passes obliquely through the sternomastoid muscle in its upper third and then across the posterior triangle of the neck to the trapezius. It is the major nerve supply to that muscle, and because it is quite superficially located, the nerve is vulnerable to injury. Unfortunately, this occurs not uncommonly as a result of surgical operations in posterior triangle of the neck. It may be damaged by traction with injury to the shoulder girdle (Fig. 17–8).

The nerve may be sacrificed intentionally during the course of radical neck dissection for cancer (Fig. 17–9), although recent appreciation of the disability that this can cause has prompted its preservation whenever possible. Inadvertent spinal accessory nerve lesions may also occur during the course of "minor surgical procedures" in the area, such as lymph node biopsy.[99] Often the patient does not realize that anything is wrong until days after the biopsy, when the pain from the surgery should have gone away, but the patient is unable to abduct the arm without pain. As one might imagine, the actual incidence of this complication is difficult to establish with certainty. Nevertheless, it is not rare, and often the diagnosis takes considerable time to establish. If by 3 months there is persistent and complete paralysis of the trapezius both clinically and electromyographically, the nerve should be surgically explored. If it appears to be caught in scar tissue, neurolysis should be done. An obvious discontinuity requires

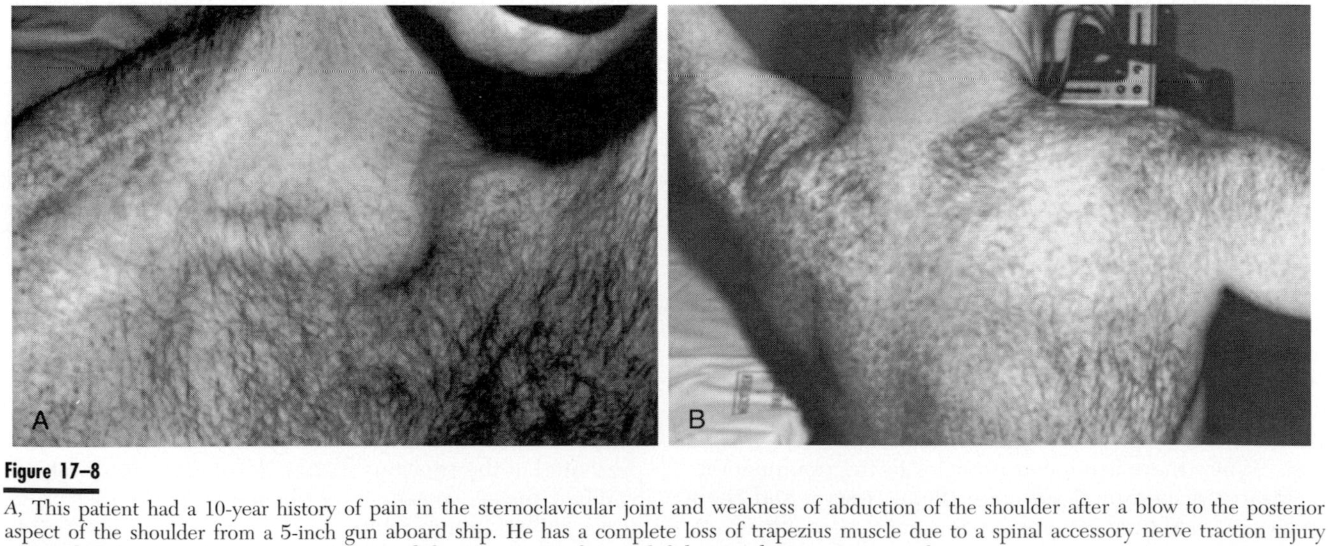

Figure 17–8

A, This patient had a 10-year history of pain in the sternoclavicular joint and weakness of abduction of the shoulder after a blow to the posterior aspect of the shoulder from a 5-inch gun aboard ship. He has a complete loss of trapezius muscle due to a spinal accessory nerve traction injury incurred at the time of sternoclavicular joint dislocation. *B,* Weakness of abduction due to trapezius palsy.

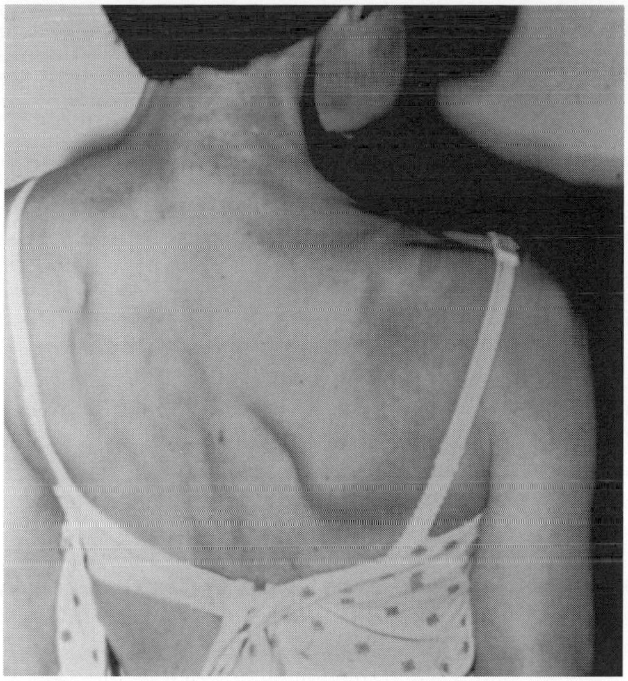

Figure 17–9

Complete loss of the trapezius muscle after radical neck dissection.

a suture, or graft if the gap cannot be closed without tension.[29]

For patients in whom the trapezius palsy is judged to be permanent, usually 6 months after attempted repair or injury without electromyographic evidence of recovery, the options for reconstruction are tendon transfer, scapular suspension, or fusion to the rib cage.

The tendon transfer of levator scapulae and rhomboids, the Eden-Lange procedure, has been favorably reported by Bigliani and associates.[9] A vertical incision is made halfway between the scapula and the vertebral spines along the length of the scapula so that the levator scapulae and the rhomboids may be detached. The levator is then reattached as far laterally on the spine of the scapula as it will reach. The infraspinatus is gently elevated from the posterior aspect of the body of the scapula, and the rhomboids are brought laterally to be attached to the bone about 4 or 5 cm from their original insertion on the medial border of the scapula. The limb is immobilized in a splint or sling for 6 weeks, after which gentle mobilization and strengthening exercises are begun. This operation has the greatest potential for maintaining mobility and providing near-normal function. It is particularly useful for elimination of the pain that these patients usually have in their shoulders with any type of activity that requires lifting. The patients in whom I have done the operation have been very enthusiastic about their increased function as a result of surgery. In consideration of the alternatives and their disadvantages, I would judge this to be my first choice in management of this entity, assuming that the anatomic prerequisites are present. Bigliani and associates' papers should be consulted for the specifics of technique and results.[9]

The operation of scapular suspension has been adapted from the polio era, when the Whitman procedure used fascial grafts from the vertebral spines to the medial aspect of the scapula. Dewar and Harris[21] transferred the levator scapulae insertion laterally to substitute for the upper trapezius and used fascial strips in place of the middle and lower parts of the muscle as was done in the Whitman operation. Because it has been my experience that static procedures subjected to heavy or even everyday loading over a long period of time have a high failure rate, I have not used this one despite the fact that part of it is dynamic since it does use the levator to substitute for the upper trapezius. In a patient in whom the upper trapezius had to be sacrificed because of a local malignancy yet the spinal accessory nerve and the lower two thirds of the muscle were preserved, our result of the levator transfer was functionally superb.

Another variant of scapulopexy was described by Ketenjian.[10] The procedure is done using the same vertical incision between the vertebrae and the medial border of the scapula, but in this case, the scapula is positioned in 30 degrees of abduction, which appears to be the optimal one for function of these arms in abduction. Four or five drill holes are made in the vertebral border of the scapula, through which either fascia lata, or Mersilene tape may be passed to subperiosteally encircle the subjacent ribs. Although at one time I was enthusiastic about the use of a Dacron artificial ligament for this purpose, in four cases it stretched after 2 to 3 years. I have, therefore, discontinued its use. The operation is contraindicated in patients with osteoporotic bone or those whose rib cages show the effects of heavy radiation, because the ribs are likely to fracture in these situations. When fascia lata is used, it is usually possible to begin gentle mobilization exercises at 6 weeks. The degree of motion that may be obtained with a solid suspension is surprisingly good, with forward elevation of 140 degrees being common in the postoperative patients (Fig. 17–10). Rotation and strength are adequate for most activities. However, the success of the Eden-Lange tendon transfer, and later failure of the scapular suspensions, has eliminated this procedure from my consideration.

For those patients in whom the aforementioned procedures have failed to provide adequate stability or range of motion, the salvage procedure that is most effective is the scapulothoracic fusion. Patients who have heavy demands on their shoulders may be best treated with it as the primary procedure. The same longitudinal incision is used, and the undersurface of the scapula as well as the underlying rib cage, usually four or five ribs, are decorticated. A generous amount of iliac crest graft is then placed between the scapula and the rib cage and augmented by sufficient allograft or bone substitutes to ensure an adequate fusion mass. The construct is secured by heavy nonabsorbable sutures through drill holes in the scapula and around the ribs. A compression plate may be used on the posterior surface of the scapula to act as a retention device when the sutures are passed through its holes before they are tightened. This protects the bone from splintering and distributes the stress over a greater area than that of the drill holes themselves. The fusion must be protected for 10 to 12 weeks with a shoulder spica, after which graduated exercises are begun. In a few

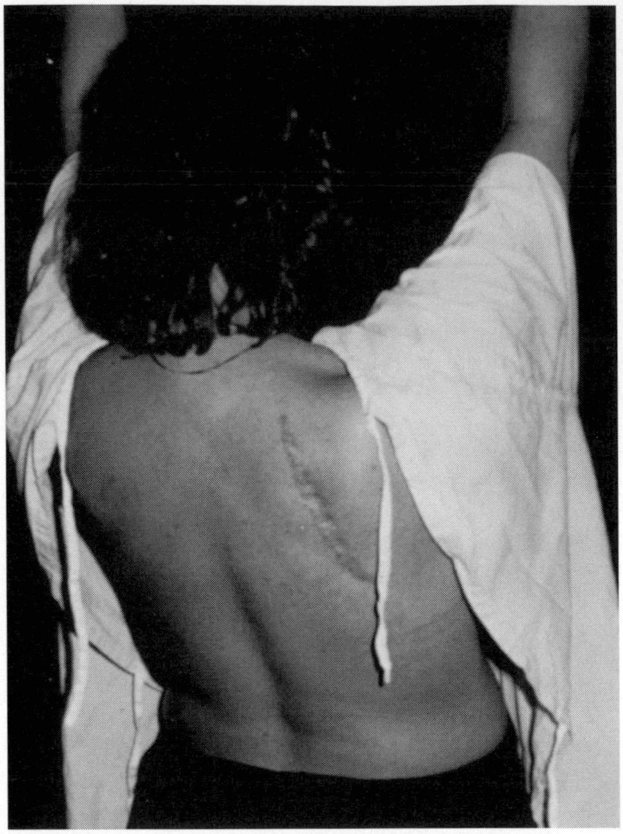

Figure 17–10

Postoperative appearance of a patient whose spinal accessory nerve was severed during a lymph node biopsy and who underwent scapular stabilization.

very reliable patients I have substituted a pelvic support brace for the plaster cast.

A less extensive method of achieving scapular fixation to the rib cage has been described by Spira.[82]

Muscular Dystrophy

Muscular dystrophy, particularly of the fascioscapulohumeral variety, often causes weakness about the shoulder girdle in a patient who is otherwise unimpaired.[1, 56] Although the affliction may be asymmetric, leaving one shoulder in comparatively good condition, the disease often progresses so that both shoulders are paralyzed and the patient is significantly handicapped. The deltoids and lateral rotators are less severely involved than are the scapular motors in some cases. Consequently, these patients may be considered for the same approach as those with irrevocably damaged spinal accessory nerves, and the same reconstructive techniques may be employed. It is most important in the care of patients with involvement of all limbs that they are mobilized and encouraged to get out of bed as quickly as possible lest their general condition deteriorates.

Brachial Plexus Injuries

The subject of injuries to the brachial plexus is an extremely complex one that will not be covered in its entirety in this chapter, although it is important when considering the neurologic lesions about the shoulder.[45] The anatomy is extremely complex.[32, 39, 85] Not only may shoulder function be severely compromised by the nerve injuries but also the nerves themselves may be injured by fractures and dislocations within the shoulder joint complex.[43] We will not discuss nerve surgery for obstetrical palsy in this chapter.[88]

Most closed brachial plexus injuries result from traction on the nerves that occurs when a motorcyclist falls and lands on his or her helmet and shoulder.[6] The forces that can be brought to bear on the soft tissues between these two points may be sufficient to either avulse individual nerve roots from the spinal cord or to rupture the nerves distally in the supraclavicular fossa. The former situation is one for which there is as yet no reliable surgical remedy, since the nerves cannot be predictably reimplanted into the spinal cord despite the intense interest and rare success in accomplishing this feat. In the case of distal rupture, however, some function may be regained by nerve grafting, particularly in the upper and intermediate trunk outflow.[53, 58, 76]

If confronted by a traction injury of the plexus with paralysis of the shoulder, the surgeon must ascertain whether there is a possibility of spontaneous recovery before considering the surgical options.[10] The clinical appearance of the shoulder may provide important insights into the localization and severity of the lesion. If, for example, the patient with a traction lesion and a flail shoulder has lost the function of the serratus anterior and rhomboids as well as the deltoid and rotator cuff, it is highly likely that root avulsion has occurred, since these two muscles are innervated by root collaterals, which originate immediately where the spinal nerve exits from the intervertebral foramen. Preservation of these two muscles with loss of glenohumeral control would infer that the lesion is beyond the branches that supply them, so that distal rupture is probably present. An electromyographic examination that includes the cervical paravertebral muscles would be extremely useful in defining the two types of injury, and it should be done at about 1 month from the time of injury.[11] Particularly if the patient has a flail and anesthetic arm, a computed tomography (CT) myelogram will help to clarify the issue, and this can be done in conjunction with the electrodiagnostic studies.[41, 101]

The questions that must be addressed about the shoulder are as follows:

1. What is the prognosis for spontaneous reinnervation of the paralyzed muscles, and in what time frame?
2. Can the outlook for recovery of the muscles be significantly enhanced by surgical manipulations of the nerves, and what are the time limits for neurologic reconstruction?
3. Would tendon transfer or arthrodesis be applicable in this situation? If so, how would these procedures affect the timetable or sequence of any other reconstructive procedures in the distal parts of the limb?

In general, these issues may be summarized as follows: For lesions of the upper trunk of the plexus that are determined to be root avulsions, the prognosis for spontaneous recovery of function is virtually nil, not only for the glenohumeral joint but also for the possibility of reconstruction by means of shoulder fusion, because the all-important serratus anterior will have been paralyzed, and no forward flexion of the fusion would be possible. Fortunately, the incidence of root avulsions at these levels is considerably less than that for the lower roots of the plexus. Although the trapezius would be intact unless the spinal accessory nerve has been injured as well, its function as a transfer will simply not duplicate all of the force couples about the shoulder to the point that will provide satisfactory function.

When the weakness is a result of distal rupture of the upper trunk, it usually occurs proximal to the origin of the suprascapular nerve, with the result that the power of lateral rotation is lost as well. Although that would seem relatively unimportant with the arm at the side, when the arm is brought into forward flexion, as it is for most functional activities, unless there is the stabilization conveyed by active lateral rotators, the arm will medially rotate and the hand will drop below the functional plane. In the absence of active control of the lateral rotatory components of the cuff, forward flexion and abduction will be severely compromised and reduced to shrugging of the shoulder or the ability to overcome the downward subluxation of the glenohumeral joint.

In evaluation of an individual patient with a plexus injury involving the shoulder, if the loss of motor power is incomplete, then the outlook is relatively good, particularly if there is no muscle that is totally paralyzed. However, it is mandatory that the passive range of motion be preserved by means of daily exercise, active when possible, and gentle passive range of motion by the patient when it is not, otherwise the joint will stiffen while awaiting full recovery. The prognosis for recovery of the shoulder is considerably better for the patient in whom the injury is confined to upper trunk as opposed to one in whom more roots, or the entire plexus is involved, since the incidence of nondegenerative or neurapractic lesions is much higher in the more restricted lesions.[6] In general, if there has been no evidence of either electromyographic or clinical recovery of the muscles by 9 months after an injury, then the outlook for meaningful recovery is poor.

The next question that must be addressed is whether the outlook for the nerves can be substantially improved by surgical manipulation of any type. Here it is most important to be critical in evaluation of the published reports of brachial plexus neural reconstructions. Function must be considered as the measure of success rather than an ability to shrug the shoulder or to overcome the inferior subluxation of the glenohumeral joint.[76] Although there have been some documented cases of significant functional improvement after surgery compared with the results of observation of the paralyzed shoulder in infants with obstetric paralysis,[26] the prognosis in the adult brachial plexus injury is considerably less favorable,[58] and most patients will not be able to raise their arms overhead as a result of surgical reinnervation of the shoulder musculature. In fact, in all cases, it is absolutely vital that the suprascapular nerve be repaired, otherwise the all-important lateral rotatory stability will be lacking. In my opinion, the results of repair of the upper trunk for the restitution of elbow flexion are significantly better than for shoulder function, and approximately 75% of these patients will be able to flex the elbow against gravity and resistance. The general consensus of opinion regarding the time frame in which surgery holds promise for reinnervation is that operation should be done within the first 6 months after the injury if at all possible, and a lapse of more than 1½ years makes it hardly worthwhile. Since most of the lesions are the result of traction injuries, direct suture of these distal ruptures will not be possible, and an autograft is usually required. The sural nerve is the most frequently used donor nerve, and the interval between surgical repair and the onset of observable recovery of elbow flexion is between 1 year and 18 months in successful cases (Fig. 17–11).

It is because of the poor functional results in the shoulder of the neural reconstructions in adult traumatic injury that peripheral reconstruction is, in my opinion, the mainstay of surgical therapy of these patients.[45] Despite the fact that within the first 2 decades of this century there were reports of repair of brachial plexus injuries, particularly in the neonatal population,[16, 27, 38, 78] the majority of the paralyzed shoulders accrued from poliomyelitis. For these patients, numerous attempts have been made to use the trapezius as a substitute for the multiple force couples that are necessary to control the glenohumeral joint.[8, 52] Some results have been encouraging, including a report by Karev.[37] For the most part, the transfer has not enjoyed wide popularity because of its biomechanical shortcomings. In 1906 Hildebrand[30] used the pectoralis major elevated and attached to the lateral third of the clavicle and acromion. Others such as Spitzy,[83] Mau,[51] and Ansart[4] used multiple transfers about the shoulder. Ober[59] in 1932 brought the long head of the triceps and the short head of the biceps to the acromion, and in 1950 Harmon[28] described multiple transfers for the combination of deltoid and lateral rotator paralysis. The latissimus dorsi and teres major were transferred for lateral rotation, as in the L'Episcopo[48] procedure for obstetric palsy, and the posterior deltoid was shifted anteriorly if this was available. The clavicular pectoralis major could be brought laterally to the acromion, and then the short head of the biceps and long head of the triceps were moved to the acromion. The long head of the biceps can similarly be shifted to the acromion as an aid to forward flexion of the humerus.

In 1967, the work of Saha[70] was particularly notable in terms of its analysis of the mechanics of tendon transfers for the shoulder paralyzed by poliomyelitis. Saha argued that these methods are equally applicable to the patient with a brachial plexus injury and that arthrodesis of the shoulder is, therefore, no longer required. I have not used the transfer that Saha has advocated for the totally flail shoulder, which includes the upper two digitations of the serratus anterior, the levator scapulae, and a modification of the trapezius transfer; however, I will comment that since the serratus and trapezius are both essential to the success of a shoulder fusion, and if the transfer were to fail, then, the only bridge to a salvage procedure would have been burned.

In my experience, arthrodesis of the flail glenohumeral

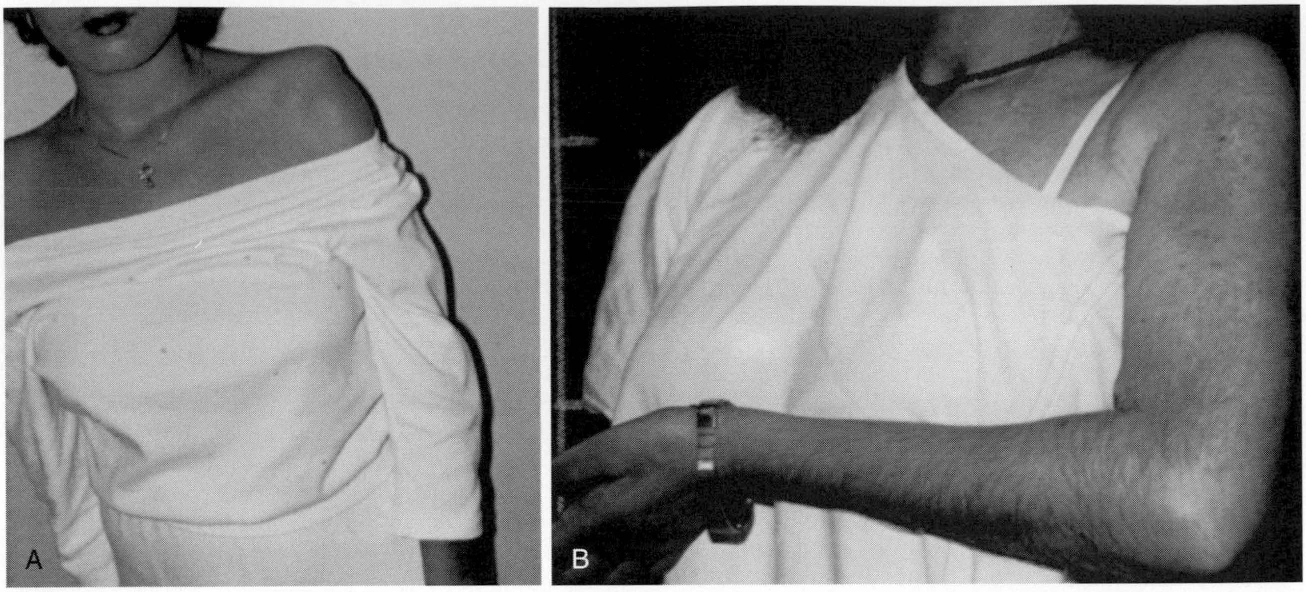

Figure 17–11

A, A 26-year-old woman with a flail, anesthetic arm after a motorcycle accident that caused a traction injury to the left brachial plexus. *B*, Eighteen months after an 11-cm sural nerve graft was done from the upper trunk to the musculocutaneous nerve and neurolysis of the remainder of the plexus. The patient regained finger flexion but had no intrinsic function.

joint due to brachial plexus injury can provide the patient with useful function that allows use of the limb as an assistive member and overcomes the often painful subluxation of the joint. It is an operative procedure that is well within the technical abilities of the average orthopedic surgeon, whereas most of the complex tendon transfers are best done by those who do them frequently, although, obviously even they are not so technically demanding that they cannot be attempted. As was previously stated, it is imperative that the trapezius and the serratus are functioning normally, because this is the minimal muscle pattern that will allow good function postoperatively. If the lesions of C5 and C6 are root avulsions, the upper serratus will have been denervated, thus compromising control.

Assuming these muscles are intact, the remaining considerations are of operative approach, choice of position for the fusion, and method of fixation.

Although I have previously used either anterior, lateral, or posterior approaches for fusion, I prefer the posterior approach because of the ease of dissection free of vital structures, lesser vascularity, and general lack of wound problems. However, in patients who are extremely thin, one must be careful about the placement of the plates and screws with reference to the surgical incision and potential pressure points.

The patient is placed in the lateral decubitus position, and the arm is supported on a sterile Mayo stand or on pillows on the chest and abdomen so that an assistant will not have to support it during the course of the procedure. The incision is made just caudad to and parallel to the spine of the scapula, then continues across the midacromial point and down the lateral aspect of the proximal third of the arm. If the axillary nerve function is already gone, there is no harm in transsecting the nerve in the approach; however, if sensation is unimpaired, it should be preserved. The bleeding from the circumflex humeral vessels may be annoying at this level. Hemostasis is assisted by the use of self-retaining retractors and the cutting cautery, and dissection is carried sharply down in the plane of the incision, detaching the deltoid to the level of the rotator cuff muscles. These muscles are then sectioned transversely in line with the joint, which is then opened so that the humeral head can be dislocated. The Fukuda retractor is used to position the head so that the cartilage of the glenoid can be cleared of all soft tissue attachments. Then, a 3- to 4-cm, straight osteotome removes the glenoidal joint surface perpendicular to the neck of the scapula down to bleeding bone. At this point, the position for fusion must be verified by palpation of the shaft of the humerus and the vertebral border of the scapula as well as its posterior surface. I generally aim for about 20 degrees of abduction, just enough to permit access to the axilla, 30 degrees of forward flexion, and 30 to 40 degrees of medial rotation. This combination should ultimately allow the patient to reach the opposite axilla, the midline, and both front and rear pants' pockets on the ipsilateral side as well as to get the arm to the horizontal position and the hand to the mouth. These recommendations are according to Rowe.[69]

Fixation of the fusion site is usually by means of a 10- to 14-hole pelvic reconstruction plate that is contoured to fit along the spine of the scapula, over the midline of the acromion, and laterally down the proximal shaft of the humerus. It is an advantage to translocate the humerus cephalad and to decorticate both the undersurface of the acromion and the upper surface of the humerus and greater tuberosity so that a secondary, extra-articular site for fusion can be obtained. Some of the cancellous screws can transfix the joint through the plate, whereas others may be introduced down the body of the scapula; the remaining ones will be cortical screws to the shaft of the humerus, for which one would hope to have at least two. Additional fixation through the glenohumeral fusion site can be obtained with cancellous screws on either side of the plate at the level of the joint. Usually there is no need for a supplementary bone graft; however, if needed, the resected humeral head is available.

Postoperative immobilization of the patient who is cooperative and reliable can be in the form of a light Orthoplast pelvic-support brace for 6 weeks, although I do not hesitate to use a shoulder spica in cases in which I have reason to doubt the patient's ability to protect the fusion. It should be noted that as in all things, there are definite advantages and disadvantages, and fusion of the shoulder is no exception. Some patients will continue to have pain in the shoulder despite a solid fusion, and in my experience this is more likely if there is neurogenic pain rather than that which comes from the traction of the inferiorly subluxating joint. Sleeping on the fused shoulder may be uncomfortable for some patients, and others may have an increased tendency to fracture the humerus if the arm is subjected to unusually violent stress. I have seen five such fractures in the last 24 years, and four of them healed with further immobilization. One, treated elsewhere, developed a nonunion that we treated successfully with bone grafting and the addition of a long plate. It is important for the resident orthopedic surgeon who sees a patient with a fractured humerus below a fusion to realize that unless the arm is immobilized in the prefracture position after a fracture, the alignment of the arm and its function may be severely restricted. In other words, if such a patient is given a sling, this will leave the patient unable to advance the arm away from the body, since it will have healed in internal rotation relative to its original position.

INFRACLAVICULAR BRACHIAL PLEXUS INJURIES

Fractures and fracture-dislocations in the region of the shoulder joint complex can produce injuries to the nerves and vessels that have a different mechanism from that described earlier. Rather than the indirect traction produced as the head and shoulder are forced apart, the plexus is compressed or locally injured in its infraclavicular portion as a result of pressure from the displaced bones or joints. Assuming that no sharp fracture fragments will lacerate the nerves, the amount of damage that can be inflicted is of a different order of magnitude compared with the supraclavicular injuries. The mode of injury is usually different as well, with fewer high-velocity situations. More of these patients are hurt in falls, or low-velocity vehicular accidents, and as reported by Leffert and Seddon[43] in 1965, their prognosis for recovery is usually very good. It is important to define this group of patients from the larger group of patients with supraclavicular injuries and their worse prognosis. However, one should realize that if there is evidence of injury to supraclavicular branches of the plexus such as the suprascapular nerve, or evidence of root avulsion such as in Horner's syndrome, then the prognosis is that of the supraclavicular injury even if it has been accompanied by a dislocated shoulder. For the most part, these patients with infraclavicular injuries will not require surgery on their nerves, although occasionally one will see a patient with a direct, blunt injury to the infraclavicular plexus that will benefit from local neurolysis. As in other injuries where recovery is anticipated, it is most important to maintain the range of motion of those joints that lack normal voluntary control by daily exercise and stretching.

SUBCLAVICULAR BRACHIAL PLEXUS INJURY

Direct injury to the subjacent nerves of the plexus by bone fragments resulting from a closed fracture of the clavicle is unusual on an acute basis, and when it does occur, it is usually the upper trunk and suprascapular nerve that are involved. When, however, the clavicle fails to heal, or does so with hypertrophic callus posteriorly, there is danger that the underlying nerves and vessels will be compressed.[36] The subclavian vein is also at risk and is a major consideration for the surgeon who must decompress the nerves, since they may become adherent to the callus. The onset of the neurologic deficit may be insidious, with weakness of the shoulder abductors, lateral rotators, and elbow flexors coming on gradually. In most cases, the clavicle has ceased to be painful and is presumed to have healed, yet the build-up of callus continues. Operative intervention should be preceded by CT scanning, angiography, and venography, and the surgeon should be prepared for the possibility of a major vascular complication. A high-speed air drill and burr facilitate the removal of the compressing bone, but the nerves and vessels must be shielded by malleable retractors. Attention may then be directed to the state of union of the clavicular fracture, which may require plating and bone grafting.[36] Of course, one would be well advised to avoid placing the grafts posteriorly so as to avoid a recurrence of nerve compression.

Suprascapular Nerve Palsy

As indicated earlier, the suprascapular nerve is not often injured acutely due to a closed fracture of the clavicle. However, its path from the upper trunk of the plexus to its eventual termination in the supraspinatus and infraspinatus leads through the unyielding confines of the notch in the scapula adjacent to the base of the coracoid process. Here it is separated from its accompanying artery by the transverse suprascapular ligament, which can cause compression resulting in pain and motor weakness[62] (Fig. 17–12). Clearly there is little problem in making the diagnosis when there has been a fracture that has distorted the bony confines of the notch and the patient subsequently has weakness and atrophy of the supraspinatus and infraspinatus.[81] It is in the chronic situation, particularly when there has not been a history of trauma and the patient presents with a history of loss of power and with vague pain in the posterior aspect of the shoulder and has only slight atrophy of the lateral rotators on physical examination, that the diagnosis must be entertained. It is valuable to obtain an electromyographic examination and to measure the velocity of nerve conduc-

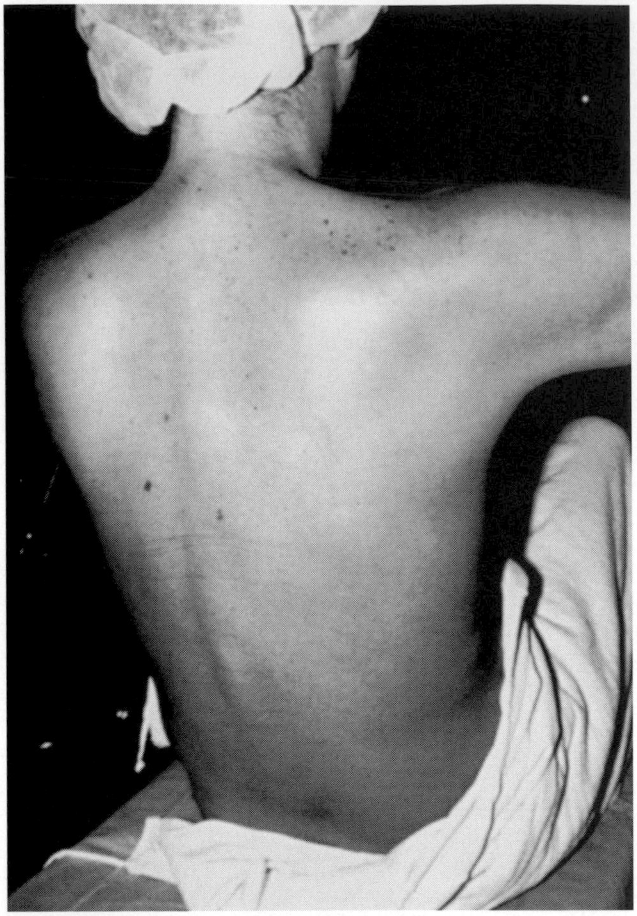

Figure 17–12

An idiopathic suprascapular nerve lesion resulted in atrophy and weakness of the supraspinatus and infraspinatus muscles.

tion (actually latency from stimulus at Erb's point to a response in the supraspinatus (normal range of 1.7 to 3.7 msec) to confirm the clinical diagnosis.[62]

In some cases there can be atrophy and weakness of the infraspinatus without involvement of the supraspinatus, and the EMG will confirm the clinical impression of the sparing of the supraspinatus. These have been explained by compression of the nerve by a ganglion[90] as it crosses the root of the spine of the scapula or by the spinoglenoid ligament before the innervation to the infraspinatus is given off. Where there is significant atrophy of the lateral rotators and weakness of abduction of the arm, the differential diagnosis of the rotator cuff tear may make arthography or MRI necessary as well.

The surgery of compression lesions of the suprascapular nerve in the notch is deceptively simple in description.[57] The approach is a transverse incision parallel to the spine of the scapula, splitting the fibers of the trapezius short of the medial border of the scapula to avoid injury to the spinal accessory nerve. The superior surface of the supraspinatus is then identified and retracted posteriorly so that the notch may be uncovered. This is actually a deep field in which exposure is difficult. It is helpful to palpate along the superior surface of the scapula to feel the base of the coracoid to assist in locating the notch. The suprascapular artery crosses above the ligament and must be gently retracted and either preserved or sealed, otherwise troublesome bleeding will obscure the field and make safe dissection impossible. The ligament is a thick and unyielding structure, and the nerve should be protected by a probe between the nerve and the ligament when the nerve is divided. The configuration of the notch has been the subject of considerable interest from an anatomic point of view.[63] If it is apparent that the bone itself is continuing to contribute to the compression, then the notch can be enlarged with a rongeur. An approach to the area that gives more easy access is that which either detaches part of the trapezius from the acromion and clavicle or splits its upper fibers.

The results of the surgery are generally good with reference to relief from pain, although severe atrophy of the muscles may not be reversed by surgery if it has been present for a long time.

In some cases, the infraspinatus alone will appear to be atrophied and weak. This may result from local compression at the level of the spinoglenoid ligament or it may occur from compression due to a ganglion arising in the posterior aspect of the glenohumeral joint. Since the advent of the MRI and its wide use in evaluation of shoulder disorders, this entity has gone from one that is a rare curiosity to one that should enter into the differential diagnosis.

The diagnostic tests that are appropriate to the patient with what is apparently isolated infraspinatus weakness should therefore include an MRI (particularly the axial cuts) and a needle electromyographic examination of both the infraspinatus and supraspinatus muscles. The determination of latency of response with stimulation in the supraclavicular fossa and pick-up at both muscles when compared with the sound side will complete the evaluation. A posterior approach to the glenohumeral joint can be easily extended to allow exploration of the area of the spinoglenoid ligament as well as any ganglia that may be visualized.

Finally, there is the question of whether patients who are suspected of having compression of the suprascapular nerve and who have normal electromyographic studies and no atrophy should have the nerve surgically explored. For most patients, the answer is negative. It is common that patients with rotator cuff tears, especially those that are extensive and of long duration, will present with atrophy of the cuff muscles. Most of them will not have nerve lesions and do not require EMGs. However, a patient with what appears to be a small tear and severe atrophy of the cuff muscles by MRI should have an EMG to rule out the possibility of a double lesion.

Axillary Nerve Injury

The axillary nerve, derived from the posterior cord, is a terminal branch representing C5 and C6. In its course behind the axillary artery, it lies on the subscapularis muscle and then proceeds posteriorly in intimate relationship to the inferior aspect of the glenohumeral joint to emerge from the quadrilateral space where it supplies the teres minor and the deltoid muscle. The anterior and middle deltoids are supplied by the anterior division of the nerve, which is subfascially applied to the muscle, while the posterior division supplies the posterior third of the muscle and ultimately becomes cutaneous to supply the skin on the lateral aspect of the arm over the deltoid. The relationships to the joint are most important with reference to the liability to injury. Fractures and fracture-dislocations are very likely to directly traumatize the nerve, since it becomes stretched across the humerus as it dislocates anteriorly and inferiorly.[17] This mechanism was well described and illustrated by the work of Milton[54] (Fig. 17–13). In fact, an examination of the anatomic relationships of the nerve to the joint leaves one wondering why the nerve is not injured whenever the joint dislocates. It is for this reason that the findings that Seddon and I published in 1965[43] were troublesome. Specifically, we found little or no recovery in six cases of isolated axillary nerve lesions accompanying dislocations and fractures in this region and stated that the prognosis for such lesions was poor. I now believe that the incidence of axillary nerve lesions with such skeletal injuries is considerably more common and that the prognosis for recovery is much better than we had stated. The reason for this change of opinion is not only the anatomic consideration but also the experience of specifically looking for evidence of nerve lesions in such patients examined right after their injuries, finding them, and then watching them go on to recovery, which is usually complete. Probably our spurious conclusion arose from the patient population selected for our study from two peripheral nerve injury centers located at the Royal National Orthopaedic Hospital in London and the Oxford Nerve Injury Center. There were, doubtless, many patients whose lesions were never diagnosed at the time of injury, or they spontaneously recovered and were therefore never referred to the Oxford Nerve Injury Center.

In addition to the possibility of injury to the nerve accompanying closed injury to the glenohumeral joint, it is extremely vulnerable in any operative procedure at the inferior aspect of the shoulder, such as one for capsular shift. One must also remember that the nerve runs horizontally 5 cm inferior to the acromion anteriorly, so that deltoid-splitting incisions must not be prolonged distally in case they divide the nerve and denervate all of the deltoid muscle anterior to the incision (Fig. 17–14). Finally, blunt injury to the deltoid from heavy falls on the shoulder or blows can injure the nerve in its course through the muscle.

Watson-Jones[95, 96] described 15 cases of dislocation of the shoulder with axillary palsy and reported a considerably brighter picture for recovery. Ten of these patients recovered spontaneously over 6 months, three between 6 and 12 months, and two remained permanently paralyzed.

The problem of when and how to explore the nerve after closed injury has been addressed by several authors, including Coene[17] from Narakas' clinic in Lausanne and Petrucci, Morelli, and Raimondi[61] from Legano in Italy.

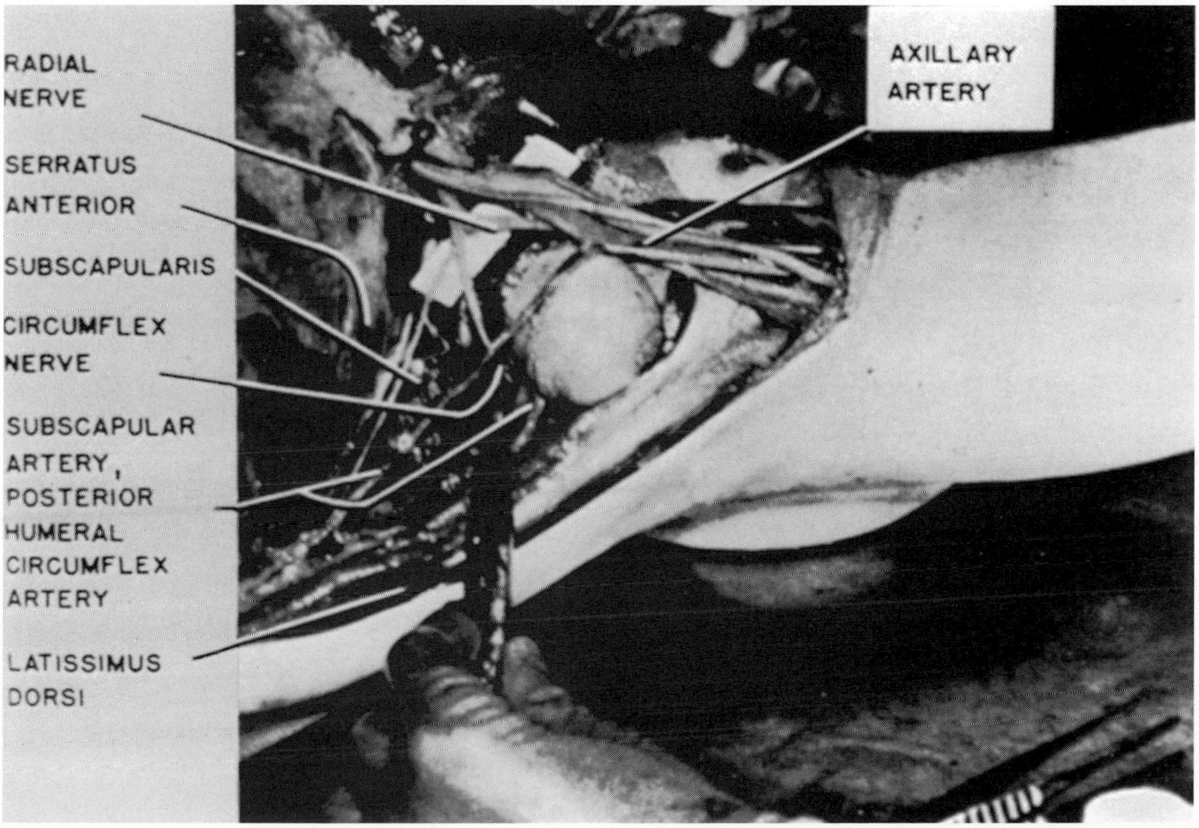

Figure 17–13

The axillary (circumflex) nerve stretched over the humeral head during experimental dislocation of the shoulder in a cadaver dissection. (From Milton GW: The mechanism of circumflex and other nerve injuries in dislocation of the shoulder and the possible mechanism of nerve injury during reduction of dislocation. Aust N Z J Surg 23:4, 1953.)

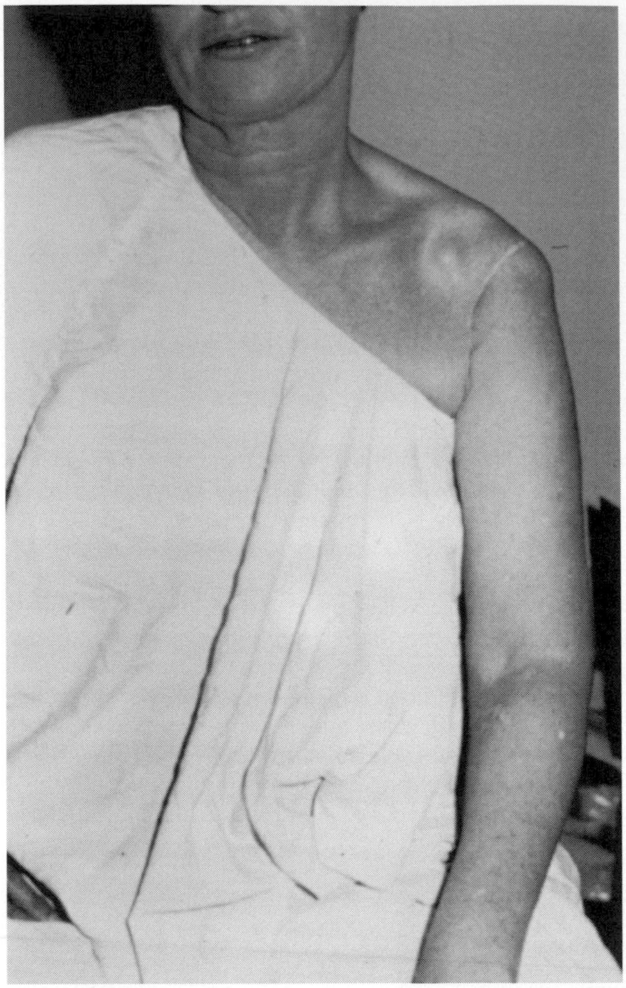

Figure 17–14

This patient had a misplaced deltoid-splitting incision that transected the axillary nerve and denervated the entire anterior deltoid muscle. The disability was severe, and the patient lost forward flexion of the humerus.

There is agreement that if there is no sign of recovery 3 to 4 months after an injury, then the nerve should be explored. Coene described the results of 54 operations, with recovery to at least M4 in 60% and at least M3 in more than 70% at 1 year after surgery. The Legano group reported on 21 patients and also had extremely favorable results. The reader is referred to their papers for the specifics of the anatomic and technical details.[17, 61]

It is well known that patients with complete paralysis of the deltoid may still, by trick and supplementary motions, be able to elevate their arms quite well. However, not all patients are able to use these mechanisms, and thus loss of the deltoid can be, as expected, quite disabling. For these patients the reconstructions are similar to those that have already been described for the brachial plexus injuries, with the same considerations of arthrodesis if all else is not possible. For the patient with denervation of the anterior deltoid due to a misplaced deltoid-splitting incision, a rotational transfer of the entire deltoid with excision of the denervated portion has been valuable on several occasions in my practice. In this procedure, the entire deltoid is carefully detached from all its osseous origins so that it may be rotated anteriorly on its neurovascular pedicle. Fortunately, the nerves and vessels may be safely mobilized to allow the posterior part of the muscle to occupy the lateral acromion, and the middle will now become the functional anterior part after the denervated portion has been excised. It is mandatory to ensure that the attachment to bone is secure. The tendinous origin of the muscle must have been preserved, and multiple nonabsorbable sutures through drill holes are recommended. Postoperatively the arm is immobilized in abduction of 60 degrees and forward flexion of about 20 degrees to take the stress off the repair for 6 weeks after which gentle passive range-of-motion exercises are begun. Active exercise is begun at 8 weeks. The loss of the function of the posterior deltoid is not usually noticed by the patients, but they must have a functioning rotator cuff for good function. The results in the four patients in whom I have done the procedure have been very gratifying, and all four patients have had significantly improved function.

Although I have used the clavicular head of the pectoralis major to substitute for the anterior deltoid, it has always been in combination with other transfers so that I cannot accurately assess its efficacy.

Musculocutaneous Nerve Injury

The musculocutaneous nerve is rarely injured in the absence of an open wound to the area. Nevertheless, it is at risk during surgery about the shoulder and particularly with procedures done for anterior instability of the glenohumeral joint.[64] Although it is stated that the nerve crosses obliquely to enter the coracobrachialis muscle 5 cm below the coracoid process, this safe interval may diminish because of the abducted position of the arm or because of anatomic variations that are not rare. The result is that unless the surgeon keeps the nerve in mind, there is the possibility of the patient awakening with paralysis of the biceps and brachialis and numbness along the radial aspect of the forearm.

There are two alternative techniques for anatomic approach to the area and considering the protection of the nerve during surgery. The first is not to take the conjoined tendon down from the coracoid but to incise part of its origin just below the bone and then gently retract the tendon. The other, which I no longer favor, is to do an osteotomy of the tip of the coracoid and to allow the muscle to retract medially. The osteotomy may be fixed by means of two heavy, nonabsorbable sutures.

The question that usually arises with reference to the musculocutaneous nerve is what to do if the patient awakens from anesthesia with total inability to flex the elbow after an operation in the region of the shoulder joint. The patient may be able to flex the elbow by means of the brachioradialis muscle even with profound weakness or complete paralysis of the biceps and brachioradialis (Fig. 17–15). The first thing that must be established is that there is a true lesion of the musculocutaneous nerve rather than a brachial plexus lesion due to plexus traction on the operating table, because the two entities can present in very similar fashion. Obviously, if the shoulder is weak in abduction and lateral rotation, elbow flexion is

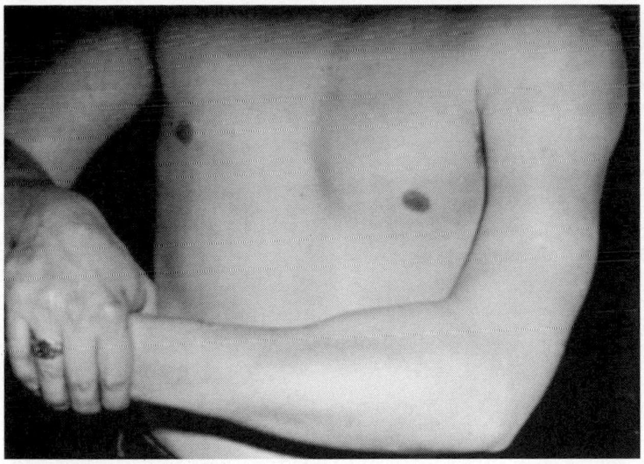

Figure 17–15

A patient after a closed injury to the brachial plexus that completely denervated the biceps and brachialis. Nevertheless, the patient had powerful elbow flexion using the brachioradialis.

deficient, and there is sensory loss over the lateral aspect of the arm, this would correspond more with a lesion of the upper trunk of the plexus than with a localized lesion of the musculocutaneous nerve due to injury in the operative field. The prognosis for anesthetic palsies is extremely favorable, and such patients usually recover within 6 weeks of their surgery, although some may take longer.[42] For the patient who appears to have a lesion of the musculocutaneous nerve after shoulder surgery, there is little indication for immediate reoperation unless it is known that the nerve has definitely been divided, in which case, every effort should be made to find and repair the nerve before the wound is closed. Otherwise, a short-term conservative approach with maintenance of range of motion for the elbow is taken for the first 3 weeks. At that time, unless there is definite evidence of beginning recovery, an electromyographic examination of the paralyzed muscles should be done. Failure to demonstrate the presence of voluntary action potentials, and the finding of fibrillations at rest, are indications of a degenerative lesion of the nerve but do not give any information as to whether this represents a neurotmesis or an axonotmesis. That will become evident within 3 months of the injury, since at the rate of regeneration of 1 inch per month one would expect a local traction lesion to have shown evidence of recovery by this time. If it has not recovered, then I believe that surgical exploration of the nerve should be done without delay, since the likelihood of an anatomic lesion requiring repair is extremely high.

LONG THORACIC NERVE PALSY

The nerve to the serratus anterior is derived from the C5, C6, and C7 nerve roots immediately after their exit from the intervertebral foramina. As root collaterals, they are often spared from the effects of traction injury when the entire plexus is affected, since root avulsions are less common at the upper parts of the plexus than at the lower roots. However, the nerve is heir to a number of poorly understood lesions that result in paralysis of the serratus anterior. Isolated serratus palsy may follow viral illnesses, immunizations, recumbence for a prolonged period of time, and unfortunately, lying on an operating table during the course of general anesthesia.[25] For cases in which a viral illness is involved Horowitz and Tocantins[31] have proposed an intriguing explanation of the pathomechanics that hinges on the anatomic location of the multiple bursae that they have described along the course of the nerve.

Open injury to the nerve is unusual except as a complication of surgical procedures done in the area of the axilla, and both breast surgery for cancer and surgery done to relieve TOS can produce paralysis. In the latter case, although minor degrees of weakness following transaxillary first rib resection are not uncommon, and have a good prognosis,[47] a complete paralysis has a poor outlook. I do not believe that surgical repair is practical and have no personal experience with trying to repair the nerve in this situation. I have done tendon transfers for several of these patients, and the results have been gratifying.

Closed trauma to the shoulder girdle or upper limb may cause a traction lesion of the long thoracic nerve, and when this is an isolated lesion, the prognosis is usually favorable. Some patients will become aware of the problem either because of significant pain in the shoulder with difficulty raising the arm, or they may suddenly realize that the scapula is winging because they are uncomfortable when they are seated in a chair with a high back. In any case, the loss of the stabilization that the serratus conveys to the scapula in forward elevation of the arm becomes a functional problem in many activities, since lifting weights is difficult, and the shoulder may become quite painful as a result. Some athletic activities, such as volleyball, may result in long thoracic nerve lesions because of chronic irritation of the nerve due to repetitive motions.

In my experience, if a patient has either a closed injury, or an atraumatic and essentially idiopathic one, the patient usually recovers from paralysis. However, if paralysis persists for 1 year without any evidence of either clinical or electromyographic recovery, then the prognosis is poor. One paper expressed the opinion that recovery may occur after as long as 2 to 3 years.[25] During the recovery period, there is little in the way of therapy that is effective, although some patients will get relief from the dragging, painful feeling in the shoulder by the use of a pelvic-support orthosis. Braces that attempt to hold the scapula to the rib cage are usually ineffective and very uncomfortable.

Some patients with permanent serratus palsies learn to live with their disability by altering their functional activities and do not desire reconstructive surgery to alleviate the weakness. Some of these people have been told that there is nothing that can be done for them, and others are simply frightened of surgery. Several surgical options are available, but I do not favor scapulopexy or scapulothoracic fusion, since it is possible to maintain the mobility of the scapula by means of tendon transfers. The pectoralis minor prolonged with a fascial graft to reach to the vertebral border of the scapula gives good function,[14]

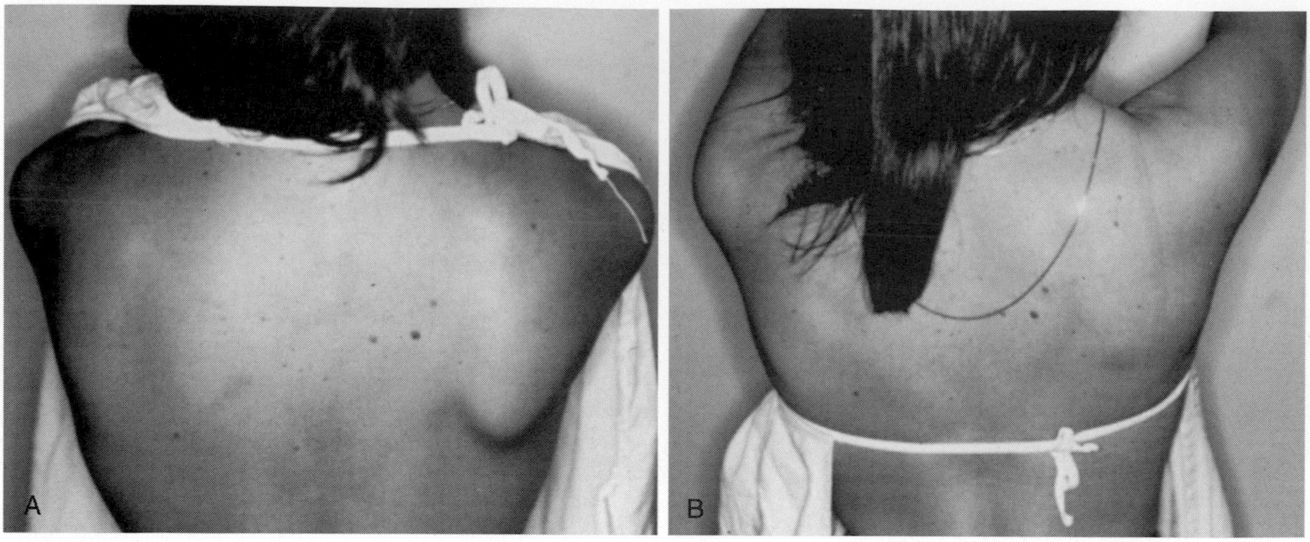

Figure 17–16

A, Serratus palsy after an injury to the long thoracic nerve during transaxillary first rib resection. *B,* Six months after pectoralis major transfer.

but since the mass of the pectoralis major muscle is much greater, the strength is correspondingly increased.[50] Fourteen patients whom we have followed up to 2 years after this transfer have had good results in terms of pain relief and loss of the winging as well as function (Fig. 17–16 *A* and *B*).

Thoracic Outlet Syndrome

TOS is a complex of signs and symptoms caused by compression of the nerves and vessels to the upper limb where they pass through the interval between the scalene muscles, over the first rib, and down into the axilla. There is a very significant relationship between the posture of the shoulder girdle and the production of symptoms that was well described by Todd in 1912.[91] He measured the inclination of the clavicle and the first rib in different age groups and both sexes and related the descent of the scapula to several factors, both normal and abnormal. He reasoned that the inverted U-shaped course of the first thoracic nerve root from the intervertebral foramen over the first rib results in traction on the nerve when for any reason the descent of the scapula is greater than normal. Scapular ptosis was, therefore, identified as a significant factor in the production of the symptoms of TOS. This theory predated the indictment of the anterior scalene muscle as the major etiologic factor. It has since been significantly neglected because concern then shifted to readily identifiable abnormalities such as cervical ribs. In my own experience, about 20% of the patients in whom I make the diagnosis of TOS have cervical ribs or abnormally long transverse processes at C7. Thus, any pathology in the region of the shoulder girdle, whether traumatic or atraumatic, that alters the posture of the scapula, can cause symptoms of TOS. In cases where there has been a fracture of the clavicle, the space between the clavicle and the first rib may be significantly diminished, leading to compression. Disuse of the shoulder due to pain or immobilization from any cause may result in atrophy of the trapezius, levator scapulae, and rhomboids. This, in turn, will result in ptosis of the scapula (Fig. 17–17).

There is an interesting relationship between anterior glenohumeral instability and the feeling of fatigue and aching in the arm that has been called "dead arm syndrome." As stated earlier, I believe that the symptoms in many of these patients are explainable on the basis of thoracic outlet compression.[46]

Because the symptoms are often vague, and the signs are subtle to the inexperienced examiner, there is a need for diagnostic criteria for TOS.

The history is often that of pain and paresthesias that extend from the lateral aspect of the neck into the shoulder, down the arm, and into the medial aspect of the forearm and hand to the little and ring fingers. Positional changes, particularly raising the hand above the head, tend to bring on symptoms that may be experienced at night and disturb sleep, or during the day with activities

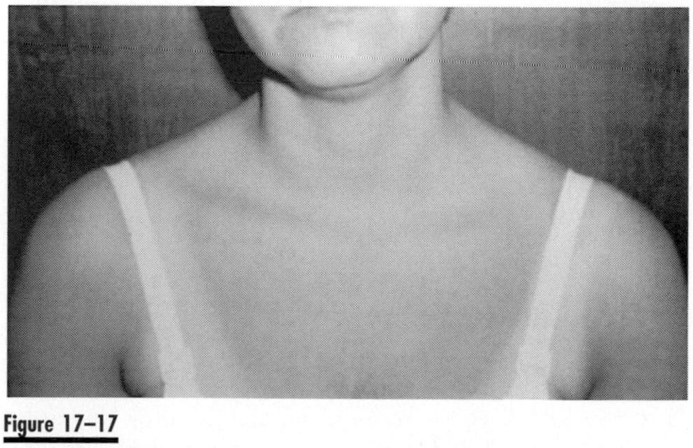

Figure 17–17

This patient had severe symptoms of thoracic outlet syndrome after blunt trauma to the left shoulder. Note the scapular ptosis. The patient was ultimately cured by transaxillary first rib resection and intensive postoperative muscle re-education after conservative therapy failed.

such as holding a blow-drier to the hair. Carrying heavy loads can provoke symptoms, and sometimes the pain will be felt in the chest. Some patients will have headaches.

The most important sign, in my experience, is the ability to reproduce the patient's symptoms by abducting and laterally rotating the arm at the shoulder while palpating the pulses at the wrist (Fig. 17–18). Although many patients will lose the palpable pulse with this maneuver, it is a normal finding that should not be considered as pathologic unless there is a concomitant reproduction of symptoms. The overhead exercise test, done by rapidly flexing and extending the fingers as the arms are held overhead, will cause aching and fatigue in the forearm and hand of patients with TOS within 20 to 30 seconds in a high percentage of cases. The classical Adson maneuver with the arm dependent while the patient turns the head to the affected side and hyperextends the neck, has a low yield in my experience. The neurologic findings are usually subtle, and motor loss, if present, tends to slight wasting and weakness of the interossei and hypothenar muscles as well as the profundi of the little and ring fingers. Sensory deficit, when present, is usually over the little and ring fingers and medial side of the forearm.

Although electrodiagnostic testing, particularly nerve conduction velocity determination, has been thought to be a reliable indicator of TOS,[93, 94] this has not stood the test of time.[98] Noninvasive vascular studies have not been of great value in making the diagnosis in my patients. Invasive studies such as arteriography and venography are rarely indicated unless there has been previous surgery in the area, or a large cervical rib is present.[35, 89] The diagnosis remains a clinical one, but it is most important that other conditions that can cause paresthesias, weakness, and numbness in the limb are sought and ruled out as well. Foremost among these are cervical radiculopathies and peripheral compression lesions of the median and ulnar nerves. It cannot be overemphasized that patients with apical lung tumors may present with very similar complaints.

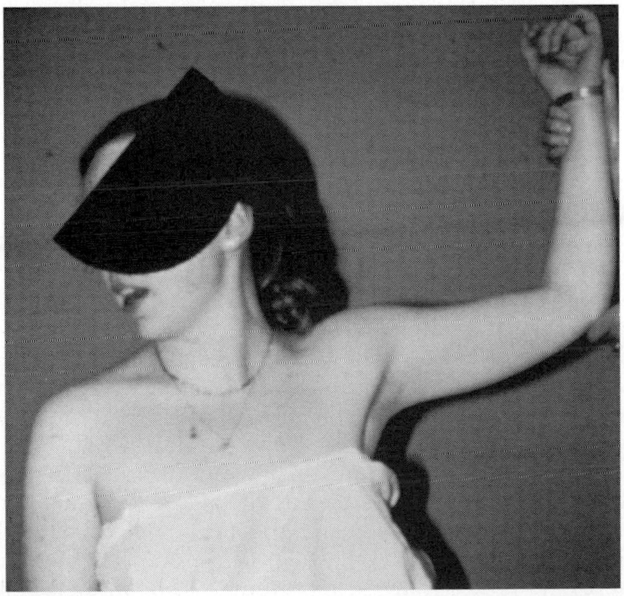

Figure 17–18

The Wright maneuver to elicit symptoms of thoracic outlet compression.

Treatment of the patient with TOS should be directed toward reversing the pathologic condition that appears responsible for the compression. When, for example, patients with ununited clavicular fractures have symptoms of TOS, they must usually undergo osteosynthesis before they will get relief.[36] Patients with paresthesias after apparently successful surgery who have scapular ptosis and muscle atrophy will usually get relief with muscle-strengthening exercises and postural re-education. When the patient is obese, weight reduction is indicated along with exercise. Emotional depression can negatively affect TOS, because it can be expressed physically in scapular ptosis. It should be dealt with either using psychotherapy or antidepressant medication.

Muscle strengthening and postural re-education remain the cornerstone of conservative management of the complex problem of TOS. Because compression may be caused by various anatomic and physiologic factors, the rehabilitation program must be adjusted to consider individual needs. Exercise programs must be introduced gently in order to avoid provocation of symptoms, and they must be carefully evaluated, since some of them will contain maneuvers that involve overhead positions, or shoulder bracing will actually exacerbate the symptoms.[60] The therapist must be in contact with the patient so that the program can be monitored closely. If a particular exercise causes significant pain, then it must be eliminated. Simply admonishing the patient to "stand up like a West Pointer, and get the shoulders back" is likely to result in frustration rather than relief. Sometimes the patient's activities of daily living or conditions of employment are causing aggravation of the condition, and these should be scrutinized so that appropriate adjustments may be made. In all, such a program should have a time limit, which in my patients is usually 3 or 4 months.

The indications for surgical intervention in TOS are as follows:

1. Failure to respond to a carefully supervised conservative program of muscle strengthening and postural reeducation exercises
2. Functionally significant muscle weakness or sensory loss in the hand
3. Intractable pain
4. Impending vascular catastrophe

The purpose of surgery in TOS is to relieve the compression of the neurovascular structures. A detailed description of all of the techniques that can be used to accomplish this end is beyond the scope of this chapter because most shoulder surgeons do not usually do this type of surgery; however, for those who are interested, there are a number of very informative references.[2, 15, 24, 66–68] The procedures may be summarized as follows:

1. Scalenotomy
2. Scalenectomy
3. First rib resection
4. Cervical rib resection
5. Combinations of the above

In addition, the anatomic approaches that have been used for these operations are:

1. Posterior
2. Supraclavicular
3. Subclavicular
4. Axillary

The transaxillary approach to and resection of the first rib, with the cervical rib if it is present, or any congenital bands that are found to be causing compression, is, in my experience, the most physiologic in that it does not cause significant damage to the important suspensory musculature of the scapula, trapezius, and rhomboids.[66–68] In addition, assuming that all goes well with the surgery and there are no complications, the blood loss is trivial, because no important muscles are divided. It is, however, a technically demanding procedure with little margin for error, thus it should not be done by the occasional operator. The results in patients who are carefully selected on the basis of the aforementioned criteria have, in my experience, been very favorable.

Stroke Shoulder

The so-called "stroke shoulder" is a painful and stiff shoulder that occurs in a patient who has had a cerebrovascular accident that affects the same side. It can be responsible for the inability of the patient to progress in a rehabilitation program and may be the major factor that prevents independence.[13, 55] Although it is a common occurrence, there are still a number of unanswered questions regarding the pathogenesis and treatment. Some of the patients have pre-existing disease of the shoulder involving either the articular surfaces or the soft tissues such as the rotator cuff, but the majority of them do not. The incidence of true thalamic pain syndrome in the general stoke population is not high enough to be responsible for the "stroke shoulder" nor is reflex sympathetic dystrophy, and these two entities are sufficiently distinct to be ruled out on the basis of clinical findings.

Quite commonly the patients exhibit downward subluxation of the glenohumeral joint that comes on in the initial flaccid period after the vascular accident, and it becomes manifest when the patient assumes the vertical position. The mechanism of the downward subluxation is debated. Basmajian and Bazant[7] theorized that in the normal shoulder, the obliquity of the glenoid and tightening of the upper capsule and coracohumeral ligament and the activity of the supraspinatus muscle combined to prevent downward drift. After a stroke, with flaccidity of the muscles, the obliquity of the scapula would be lost, and the scapula would rotate to allow the subluxation. Caillet stated that loss of the trapezius and serratus allowed this rotation.[12] The depressors of the humeral head may be spastic and contribute to the forces encouraging subluxation. A prospective study of stroke patients by Smith and associates[79] demonstrated that the subluxation occurred during the initial period of flaccidity, but there was no correlation with the degree of spasticity.

With time, the adductors and medial rotators of the glenohumeral joint become tight; the joint capsule contracts; and, if an arthrogram is done, the capsule appears contracted like that of the typical frozen shoulder in a high percentage of the patients.[65]

Although the problem of flaccidity of muscles would appear to allow making analogies with poliomyelitis, brachial plexus injuries, or specific peripheral nerve injuries to formulate treatment plans, it is most important to consider the problem of the stroke shoulder as distinct from these lower motor neuron lesions. In addition to the paralysis, the stoke patient may have to contend with spasticity, proprioceptive defects, and severe distortion of body image. The last of these problems may result in the hemiplegic patient no longer recognizing the affected side as belonging to him or her. Clearly, any of these factors may complicate treatment and seriously prejudice the ultimate functional result. Nevertheless, the stroke shoulder can serve as the prototype for treatment of the shoulders of patients with other upper motor neuron lesions, such as head injuries, degenerative lesions, and tumors since they have received the most study.

The overall objective of treatment is to maintain a functional range of motion that will, at minimum, allow for self-care. As soon as the stroke patient can cooperate, he or she may be taught self-ranging of the affected arm with the assistance of the well limb. Nurses and even the family can assist in this passive exercise, but it is most important that vigorous or forceful stretching be avoided lest soft tissues are injured. The physical therapist must be brought in as soon as the patient is medically stable. When the patient is in bed, pillows can support the arm to avoid contractures, and turning the patient to the prone position with the arm abducted and laterally rotated can also be beneficial. Since the emphasis of the rehabilitation program is to attain the vertical position as soon as possible, the shoulder will require support when the patient is sitting in a chair and eventually standing and walking. The use of the sling is controversial.[33] Although it can help to prevent downward subluxation, its uninterrupted use can result in the development of internal rotation and adduction contractures. Thus, it must be used judiciously and with exercises as described. These exercises can be begun with the patient in the supine position and in diagonal patterns, which are usually well tolerated if done gently.

Due to the effects of education about stroke rehabilitation, the number of stiff and painful stroke shoulders that are seen has diminished considerably, although they are still seen, particularly in patients who have left the hospital to go to nursing homes or their own homes and who have not regained voluntary control. Because the limb is considered to be "useless," it is neglected, and contractures quickly develop. These patients often have so much pain that it is not possible to treat them with even the most gentle manipulations by the therapist, and the only successful therapy will involve surgical release. This procedure, and its subsequent program of exercises, was described at Rancho Los Amigos Hospital.[13, 55] An anterior axillary incision is used, and the pectoralis major and subscapularis are released, while the capsule is left intact. At 2 days postoperatively, the exercise program is begun and must be continued indefinitely to prevent a recurrence. A light, plastic brace may be used to maintain the gain in passive motions. The results have been most satisfactory with reference to relief of pain.

Brachial Plexus Neuropathy

Finally, although the entity of idiopathic brachial neuropathy is not one that can be treated surgically, or in any meaningful manner other than by observation, it is most important that the physician who is responsible for care of patients with shoulder disorders be familiar with its clinical manifestations because of the great importance of differential diagnosis.[92] The disorder occurs about twice as frequently in men as in women, and particularly in persons in their 20s and 30s, although it may be seen in other age groups. The most common presenting symptom is that of severe pain that comes on with no apparent reason and that can vary in location but usually involves the shoulder. The pain may extend over the scapula and down the arm to the hand, and it may be bilateral, although this is not common. The pain is followed in days or weeks by loss of motor and sensory function in the limb. Rarely is the entire limb involved, and the distribution depends on the part of the plexus that is involved; however, the roots themselves are usually spared, as is the spinal cord. Most commonly the shoulder is affected, and particularly the long thoracic, axillary, and suprascapular nerves may be predilected, and they may appear to be involved singly or in combinations. The remainder of the plexus may also be involved, but it is unusual in the absence of shoulder dysfunction. The problem of differentiating a compression lesion that requires surgical exploration from a "forme fruste" of brachial neuritis can usually be solved by electrodiagnostic techniques.

The prognosis for recovery in this entity is good in that approximately 80% of the patients recover completely in 2 years, and 90% in 3 years, although some patients may be left with residual weakness. Recurrences do occur, but they are unusual, and sometimes they may be seen in the contralateral limb.[92]

The pathology is unclear, and although it has been characterized as an autoimmune disease, particularly in conjunction with immunizations with various sera and vaccines, it may occur after viral illnesses and in the absence of any of these factors. The treatment is supportive, and the use of narcotics to alleviate the pain is avoided whenever possible. Steroids have been used in empirical treatment, although they have not been shown conclusively to alter the course of the disease even though they are thought to help diminish the pain. When the discomfort is most severe, treatment is symptomatic, but range-of-motion exercises and an orthosis may be introduced as needed as soon as the patient can tolerate them.

References and Bibliography

1. Adams RD, Denny-Brown D, and Pearson CM: Diseases of Muscle, 2nd ed. New York: Harper & Row, 1962.
2. Adson AW and Caffey JF: Cervical rib: A method of anterior approach for relief of symptoms by section of the scalenus anterior. Ann Surg *85:*839, 1927.
3. Aminoff MJ: Electromyography in Clinical Practice. Menlo Park, CA: Addison-Wesley, 1978.
4. Ansart B: Die Myoplastik bei der Paralyse des Deltoideus. Z Orthop Chir *48:*57, 1927.
5. Asbury AK, McKhann GM, and McDonald WI (eds): Diseases of the Nervous System. Philadelphia: WB Saunders, 1986.
6. Barnes R: Traction injuries to the brachial plexus in adults. J Bone Joint Surg *31B:*10, 1949.
7. Basmajian JV and Bazant FJ: Factors preventing downward dislocation of the adducted shoulder joint. J Bone Joint Surg *41A:*1182, 1959.
8. Bateman JE: The Shoulder and Environs. St. Louis: CV Mosby, 1954.
9. Bigliani L, Perez-Sanz JR, and Wolfe IN: Treatment of trapezius paralysis. J Bone Joint Surg *67A:*871, 1985.
10. Bonney G: Prognosis in traction lesions of the brachial plexus. J Bone Joint Surg *41B:*4, 1959.
11. Bufalini C and Pescatori G: Posterior cervical electromyography in the diagnosis and prognosis of brachial plexus injuries. J Bone Joint Surg *51B:*627, 1969.
12. Caillet R: Shoulder in Hemiplegia. Philadelphia: FA Davis, 1980.
13. Caldwell CR, Wilson DJ, and Braun RM: Evaluation and treatment of the upper extremity in the hemiplegic stroke patient. Clin Orthop *63:*69, 1969.
14. Chavez JP: Pectoralis minor transplanted for paralysis of the serratus anterior. J Bone Joint Surg *33B:*2128, 1951.
15. Claggett OT: Presidential address: Research and prosearch. J Thorac Cardiovasc Surg *44:*153, 1962.
16. Clark LP, Taylor AS, and Prout TP: Study on brachial birth palsy. Am J Med Sci *130:*670, 1905.
17. Coene LNJEM: Axillary nerve lesions and associated injuries. Oegstgeest, Holland: Privately printed by de Kempenaer, 1985.
18. Cofield RH and Briggs BT: Glenohumeral arthrodesis, operative and long-term functional results. J Bone Joint Surg *61A:*668, 1979.
19. De Jong RN: The Neurological Examination, 3rd ed. New York: Hoeber, 1979.
20. Denny-Brown D and Brenner C: Lesions in peripheral nerves resulting from compression by spring clip. Arch Neurol Psychiatr *52:*1, 1944.
21. Dewar FP and Harris RI: Restoration of the function of the shoulder following paralysis of the trapezius by fascial sling and transplantation of the levator scapulae. Ann Surg *132:*1111, 1950.
22. Duchenne GB: The Physiology of Motion. Translated by EB Kaplan. Philadelphia: JB Lippincott, 1949.
23. Dyck PJ, Thomas PK, and Lambert EH: Peripheral Neuropathy. Philadelphia: WB Saunders, 1975.
24. Falconer MA and Li FWP: Resection of the first rib in costoclavicular compression of the brachial plexus. Lancet *1:*59, 1962.
25. Foo CL and Swann M: Isolated paralysis of the serratus anterior: A report of 20 cases. J Bone Joint Surg *65B:*552, 1983.
26. Gilbert A and Tassin JL: Obstetrical palsy: A clinical, pathologic, and surgical review. *In* Terzis J (ed): Microreconstruction of Nerve Injuries. Philadelphia: WB Saunders, 1987.
27. Gilmour J: Notes on the surgical treatment of brachial birth palsy. Lancet 2:696, 1925.
28. Harmon PH: Surgical reconstruction of the paralytic shoulder by multiple muscle transplantation. J Bone Joint Surg 32A:583, 1950.
29. Harris HH and Dickey JR: Nerve grafting to restore function of the trapezius muscle after radical neck dissection. Ann Otolaryngol *74:*880, 1965.
30. Hildebrand A: Uber eine neue Methode der Muskletransplantation. Arch Klin Chir *78:*75, 1906.
31. Horowitz MT and Tocantins LM: An anatomic study of the role of the long thoracic nerve and the related scapular bursae in the pathogenesis of local paralysis of the serratus anterior muscle. Anat Rec *71:*375, 1938.
32. Hovelacque A: Anatomie des Nerfs Craniens et Rachidiens et du Système Grand Sympathique. Paris: Doin, 1927.
33. Hurd MM, Farrell KH, and Waylonis GW: Shoulder sling for hemiplegia: friend or foe? Arch Phys Med Rehabil *55:*519, 1974.
34. Inman VT, Saunders JB de CM, and Abbott LC: Observations on the function of the shoulder. J Bone Joint Surg *26:*1, 1944.
35. Judy KL and Heyman RL: Vascular complications of thoracic outlet syndrome. Am J Surg *123:*521, 1972.
36. Jupiter J and Leffert RD: Non-union of the clavicle: Associated

complications and surgical management. J Bone Joint Surg *69A:*753, 1987.
37. Karev A: Trapezius transfer for paralysis of the deltoid. J Hand Surg *11B:*81, 1986.
38. Kennedy R: Suture of the brachial plexus in birth paralysis of the upper extremity. BMJ *1:*298, 1903.
39. Kerr AT: The brachial plexus of nerves in man, the variations in its formation, and its branches. Am J Anat *2:*285, 1918.
40. Ketenjian AV: Scapulocostal stabilization for scapular winging in fascioscapulohumeral muscular dystrophy. J Bone Joint Surg *60A:*476, 1978.
41. Kimura J: Electrodiagnosis in Diseases of Nerve and Muscle. Philadelphia: FA Davis, 1983.
42. Kwaan JHM and Rappaport I: Postoperative brachial plexus palsy. Arch Surg *101:*612, 1970.
43. Leffert RD, and Seddon HJ: Infraclavicular brachial plexus injuries. J Bone Joint Surg *47B:*9, 1965.
44. Leffert RD: Thoracic outlet and the shoulder. *In* Jobe F (ed): Symposium on Injuries to the Shoulder in the Athlete. Philadelphia: WB Saunders, 1983.
45. Leffert RD: Brachial Plexus Injuries. New York: Churchill Livingstone, 1985.
46. Leffert RD, and Gumley G: The relationship between dead arm syndrome and thoracic outlet syndrome. Clin Orthop *223:*20, 1987.
47. Leffert RD: Thoracic outlet syndrome. J Am Acad Orthop Surg *2:*317, 1994.
48. L'Episcopo JB: Restoration of muscle balance in the treatment of obstetrical paralysis. N Y State J Med *39:*357, 1939.
49. Marinacci AA: Applied Electromyography. Philadelphia: Lea & Febiger, 1968.
50. Marmor L and Bechtal CO: Paralysis of the serratus anterior due to electric shock relieved by transplantation of the pectoralis major muscle: A case report. J Bone Joint Surg *45A:*156, 1983.
51. Mau C: Kombinierte Muskelplastik bei Deltoideus Lahmung. Verh Dtsch Ges Orthop *22:*236, 1927.
52. Mayer L: Transplantation of the trapezius for paralysis of the abductors of the arm. J Bone Joint Surg *36A:*775, 1954.
53. Millesi H: Surgical treatment of brachial plexus injuries. J Hand Surg *2:*367, 1977.
54. Milton GW: Mechanism of circumflex and other nerve injuries in dislocations of the shoulder and the possible mechanisms of nerve injuries during reduction of dislocations. Aust N Z Surg *23:*25, 1953.
55. Mooney V, Perry J, and Nickel V: Surgical and non-surgical orthopaedic care of stroke. J Bone Joint Surg *49A:*989, 1967.
56. Morgan-Hughes JA: Diseases of striated muscle. *In* Asbury AK, McKhann GM, and McDonald WI (eds): Diseases of the Nervous System. Philadelphia: WB Saunders, 1986.
57. Murray JWG: A surgical approach for entrapment neuropathy of the suprascapular nerve. Orthop Rev *3:*33, 1975.
58. Narakas A: Brachial plexus injury. Orthop Clin North Am *12:*303, 1981.
59. Ober F: An operation to relieve paralysis of the deltoid. JAMA *99:*2182, 1932.
60. Peet RM, Hendricksen JD, Guderson TP, and Martin GM: Thoracic outlet syndrome: Evaluation of a therapeutic exercise program. Proc Mayo Clin *31:*281, 1956.
61. Petrucci FS, Morelli A, and Raimondi PL: Axillary nerve injuries—21 cases treated by nerve graft and neurolysis. J Hand Surg *7:*271, 1982.
62. Post M and Mayer J: Suprascapular nerve entrapment: Diagnosis and treatment. Clin Orthop *223:*126, 1987.
63. Rengachary SS, Burr D, Lucas S, et al: Suprascapular entrapment neuropathy: A clinical, anatomical and comparative study, Parts 1 and 2. Neurosurgery *5:*441, 1979.
64. Richards RR, Waddell JP, and Hudson AR: Shoulder arthrodesis for the treatment of brachial plexus palsy: A review of twenty-two patients. Orthop Trans *11:*240, 1987.
65. Rizk TEW, Christopher RP, Pinals RS, and Salazar JE: Arthrographic studies in painful hemiplegic shoulders. Arch Phys Med *65:*254, 1984.
66. Roos DB: Transaxillary approach to the first rib to relieve thoracic outlet syndrome. Ann Surg *163:*354, 1966.
67. Roos DB and Owens JC: Thoracic outlet syndrome. Arch Surg *93:*71, 1966.
68. Roos DB: Congenital anomalies associated with thoracic outlet syndrome: Anatomy, symptoms, diagnosis and treatment. Am J Surg *132:*771, 1976.
69. Rowe CR: Re-evaluation of the position of the arm in arthrodesis of the shoulder in the adult. J Bone Joint Surg *56A:*913, 1974.
70. Saha AK: Surgery of the paralyzed and flail shoulder. Acta Orthop Scand Suppl 97, 1967.
71. Sandifer P: Neurology in Orthopaedics. London: Butterworths, 1967.
72. Schottsteadt ER, Larsen LJ, and Bost FG: Complete muscle transposition. J Bone Joint Surg *37A:*897, 1955.
73. Seddon HJ: Three types of nerve injury. Brain *66:*237, 1943.
74. Seddon HJ: Reconstructive surgery of the upper extremity. *In* Poliomyelitis, Second International Poliomyelitis Congress. Philadelphia: JB Lippincott, 1952.
75. Seddon HJ: Surgical Disorders of the Peripheral Nerves. Baltimore: Williams & Wilkins, 1972.
76. Sedel L: Results of surgical repair of brachial plexus injuries. J Bone Joint Surg *64B:*54, 1982.
77. Sethi RJ and Thompson LL: The Electromyographer's Handbook, 2nd ed. Boston: Little, Brown, 1989.
78. Sharpe W: The operative treatment of brachial plexus paralysis. JAMA *66:*876, 1916.
79. Smith RG, Cruikshank JG, Dunbar S, and Akhtar AJ: Malalignment of shoulder after stroke. BMJ *284:*1224, 1982.
80. Smorto MP and Basmajian JV: Clinical Electroneuromyography, 2nd ed. Baltimore: Williams & Wilkins, 1979.
81. Solheim LF and Roaas A: Compression of the suprascapular nerve after fracture of the scapular notch. Acta Orthop Scand *49:*338, 1978.
82. Spira E: The treatment of dropped shoulder—a new operative technique. J Bone Joint Surg *30A:*229, 1948.
83. Spitzy H: Aussprache zur Deltoideuslahmung, Muskleplastik. Verh Dtsch Ges Orthop *22:*236, 1927.
84. Steindler A: Kinesiology of the Human Body Under Normal and Pathological Conditions. Springfield, IL: Charles C Thomas, 1955.
85. Stevens JH: Brachial plexus injuries. *In* Codman EA (ed): The Shoulder. Brooklyn, NY: G. Miller Medical Publishers, 1934.
86. Sunderland S: A classification of peripheral nerve injuries producing loss of function. Brain *74:*491, 1951.
87. Sunderland S: Nerves and Nerve Injuries, 2nd ed. New York: Churchill Livingstone, 1978.
88. Tassin JL: Paralysies obstetricales du plexus brachial: Evolution spontanée, résultâts des interventions réparatrices précoses. Thesis, Universite Paris VII, 1983.
89. Telford ED and Stopford JSB: The vascular complications of cervical rib. Br J Surg *18:*557, 1931.
90. Thompson RC, Schneider W, and Kennedy T: Entrapment neuropathy of the inferior branch of the suprascapular nerve by ganglia. Clin Orthop *166:*185, 1982.
91. Todd TW: The descent of the shoulder after birth. Anatomischer Anzeiger Centralblatt fur die gesamte wissenschaftlichje. Anatomie *14:*41, 1912.
92. Tsairis P, Dyck PJ, and Mulder DW: Natural history of brachial plexus neuropathy; report on 99 patients. Arch Neurol *27:*109, 1972.
93. Urschel HC, Paulson DL, and MacNamara JJ: Thoracic outlet syndrome. Ann Thorac Surg *6:*1, 1968.
94. Urschel HC, and Rossuk M: Management of thoracic outlet syndrome. N Engl J Med *286:*1140, 1972.
95. Watson-Jones R: Fracture in the region of the shoulder joint. Proc R Soc Med *29:*1058, 1930.
96. Watson-Jones R: *In* Wilson JN (ed): Fractures and Joint Injuries. Edinburgh: Churchill Livingstone, 1976.
97. Weir Mitchell S: Injuries of Nerves and Their Consequences. London: Smith, Edler, 1872.
98. Wilbourn AJ and Lederman RJ: Evidence for conduction delay in thoracic outlet syndrome is challenged. N Engl J Med *310:*1052, 1984.
99. Woodhall B: Trapezius paralysis following minor surgical procedures in the posterior cervical triangle. Ann Surg *136:*375, 1952.
100. Yeoman PM: Brachial plexus injuries. J Bone Joint Surg *47B:*187, 1965.
101. Yeoman PM: Cervical myelography in traction injuries of the brachial plexus. J Bone Joint Surg *50B:*25, 1968.

CHAPTER

18

HANS K. UHTHOFF, M.D.
JOACHIM F. LOEHR, M.D.

Calcifying Tendinitis*

Calcifying tendinitis of the rotator cuff is a common disorder of unknown etiology in which reactive calcification usually undergoes spontaneous resorption in the course of time with subsequent healing of the tendon. During the deposition of calcium, the patient may be either free of pain or suffer only a mild to moderate degree of discomfort, but the disease becomes acutely painful when the calcium is being resorbed.

HISTORICAL REVIEW

The subacromial-subdeltoid bursa as a source of painful shoulders was recognized by Duplay[33] as early as 1872, and he described the condition as scapulohumeral periarthritis, later also called Duplay's disease.[116] Numerous other nomenclatures have since been used. The bursal localization of calcific deposits was first described by Painter,[93] who was also the first to demonstrate the radiologic appearance of the disease, and by Stieda and colleagues.[11, 124] However, surgical explorations soon established that the calcification was primarily in the rotator cuff tendons.[25, 141] In his classic textbook on the shoulder, Codman[26] stated definitively: "The deposits do not arise in the bursa itself, but in the tendons beneath it." Wrede[141] gave a masterly description of the disease, including the pathologic changes of the tendon: "the cells resemble more and more chondrocytes, meanwhile the fibre arrangement of the tendon is lost."

The intratendinous localization of calcification has been repeatedly confirmed by later authors.[112, 113, 117] But this did not stop the proliferation of newer nomenclatures, and terms such as peritendinitis calcarea,[113] periarthropathy,[99] or calcified peritendinitis[32] are well known. In the English literature, calcific or calcified tendinitis is more generally accepted. We, however, prefer calcifying tendinitis, a term that to our knowledge was first used by Plenk[101] and later by de Sèze and Welfling[30] (tendinite calcifiante). This term denotes the evolutionary process that is directed to spontaneous healing, contrary to the other terms that imply a progressive deterioration.

ANATOMY

The anatomy of the shoulder has been dealt with in earlier chapters. A few aspects of the rotator cuff tendons relevant to calcifying tendinitis are discussed briefly in this section. The cuff tendons that blend with the capsule of the glenohumeral joint before insertion into bone consist of the supraspinatus in its most superior portion, the infraspinatus and teres minor posteriorly and posteroinferiorly, and the subscapularis anterior to the supraspinatus. The first three tendons insert into the greater tuberosity, whereas the subscapularis attaches to the lesser tuberosity. At the zone of the tendon where calcification takes place, we were unable to distinguish histologically between the deeper, more collagenous tendon and the joint capsule, a fact already noted by Codman.[26] Cells of the synovial layer were often inconspicuous.

The supraspinatus tendon is the most frequent site of cuff tendinopathies. It is 2 to 3 cm long, and it traverses the subacromial compartment that is rigidly limited by the coracoacromial arch above and the humeral head below. Codman[26] pointed out that the diseases in the supraspinatus tendon tend to occur in a specific area of the tendon: "about half an inch proximal to the insertion." He called this area the "critical portion," which was later renamed by Moseley and Goldie[85] as the "critical zone." The vascularity of this area has been repeatedly investigated because a possible hypoperfusion is believed to initiate degenerative changes that subsequently result in calcification or tear.

The rotator cuff tendons are regularly supplied by the suprascapular, anterior circumflex humeral, and posterior circumflex humeral arteries. In addition, contributions are received from the thoracoacromial, suprahumeral, and subscapular arteries in a descending order of frequency.[108] The vascularity of the cuff tendons, especially that of the supraspinatus, has been studied in many cadaver shoulders by microangiography simultaneously with histology.

*The first edition of this chapter has been done with Dr. Kiriti Sarkar who unfortunately is now deceased.

Moseley and Goldie[85] found that the supraspinatus was well supplied by a network of vessels coming from both the muscular and the osseous ends of the tendon, which anastomosed in the area of the "critical zone." They stated that there is "no evidence that the critical zone is much less vascularized than any other part of the tendinous cuff." On the other hand, microangiographic studies by Rothman and Parke[109] showed that the "critical zone" was markedly "undervascularized," and their histologic examinations corroborated this view. Although the supraspinatus tendon was most frequently involved, the infraspinatus and subscapularis tendons showed zones of hypovascularity as well. Brooks and associates[20] performed a quantitative histologic study of the cuff and concluded that supraspinatus and infraspinatus are equally hypovascular in their distal 15 mm and that the diameter of vessels decreases toward the bony insertion.

Rathbun and Macnab[102] documented in their cadaver study a zone of avascularity in the supraspinatus tendon near its bony insertion. This avascularity was dependent on the position of the arm. They showed that when Micropaque (barium sulfate) was injected into the vessels with the arm of the cadaver in the position of adduction, the "critical zone" did not fill. The nonfilling area sometimes extended up to the point of insertion. If the vessels of the contralateral shoulder of the same cadaver were injected after passive abduction, they filled completely throughout the tendon. Therefore, the authors postulated that the zone of avascularity was a "wring-out" effect resulting from pressure of the head of the humerus on the tendon. In a more recent study, Tillmann[126] documented that the zone of insertion of the supraspinatus is avascular.

Our histologic findings have been similar to those of previous authors. There is hardly an area in the supraspinatus tendon that is conspicuously devoid of vascular channels. However, we have observed that vascular channels, especially the larger ones, are abundant in the loose connective tissue underneath the bursa but are relatively scarce in the dense collagenous part close to the joint. Interestingly, this is already evident in the supraspinatus tendon of the fetus (Fig. 18–1), even before the fascicular arrangement of the tendon fibers has occurred.

Our histologic studies of cadaver tendons were supplemented by microangiographic studies that consistently showed an area of underfilling at the articular aspect of the tendon near its insertion, regardless of the position of the arm.[70]

It is obvious, then, that the question of reduced or lack of vascular perfusion in certain areas of cuff tendons is not entirely settled. Maneuvering the cadaveric arm to obtain optimal results through microangiography is not easy. Furthermore, it is doubtful that microangiography can reveal the entire vasculature up to capillary levels. However, it seems safe to assume that an anatomic as well as transient hypoperfusion exists in cuff tendons, particularly in the deeper portion of the supraspinatus.

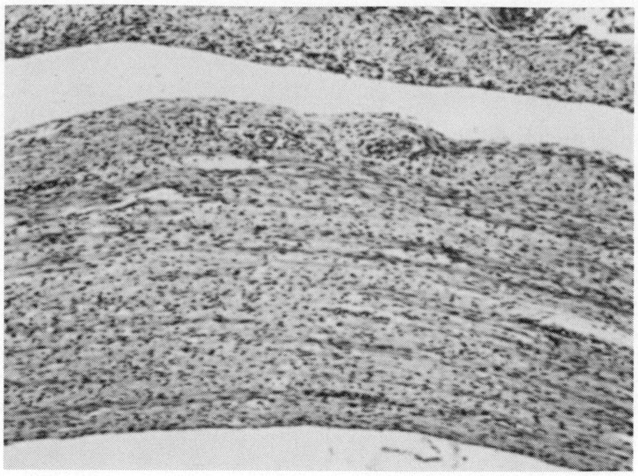

Figure 18–1

The supraspinatus tendon, close to the bony insertion, of a 20-week-old human fetus. Note the rather rich vascular supply in the part of the tendon close to the bursa. On the other hand, vessels are scarce in the articular part. (Goldner, original magnification, ×100.)

INCIDENCE

Reports on the overall incidence of tendon calcification vary tremendously. The variation depends not only on the clinical material used but also on the radiographic technique. Bosworth examined both shoulders of 6061 office workers and found an incidence of calcification of 2.7%.[15, 16] Welfling and colleagues[137] radiographed 200 shoulders of persons without any complaints and found calcifications in 15 (7.5%). Rüttimann[111] radiographed 100 individuals without symptoms and found an incidence of calcification of 20%.

The incidence of calcification in 925 painful shoulders reported by Welfling and collaborators[137] was 6.8%. When broken down by age groups, patients between 31 and 40 years had a 19.5% incidence of calcification. Evidently, the peak at this age did not correspond with the peak seen in patients with rotator cuff tears. They therefore concluded that both diseases represent different entities. Friedman radiographed the shoulders of 228 patients with a painful rotator cuff and found calcific deposits in 75 patients.[40] Fifty-four of the 75 individuals with calcification were between 30 and 49 years of age. Bosworth estimated that 35 to 45% of patients with calcareous deposits will eventually become symptomatic.[15, 16]

Plenk[101] found that 82% of the calcifications were located in the supraspinatus tendon. Bosworth[15, 16] found 90% in the supraspinatus and infraspinatus. DePalma and Kruper[28] reported an incidence of 74% when assessing the supraspinatus alone, whereas the incidence of simultaneous calcific deposits in the supraspinatus and other short rotators was 90%. In Bosworth's series[15, 16] calcifications in the supraspinatus occurred in 51%, in the infraspinatus in 44.5%, in the teres minor in 23.3%, and in the subscapularis in 3%. Obviously, deposits were sometimes seen in more than one tendon.

In general, authors agree that women are affected more often than are men. Bosworth[15, 16] reported an incidence of 76.7% in women; DePalma and Kruper[28] reported an incidence of 60.3%; Welfling and collaborators[137] reported an incidence of 62%; Lippmann[65] as well as Hartig and Huth[51] reported 64%; and, in our series of 127 patients, the incidence was 57%. A higher incidence in men (56%)

was reported by Friedman.[40] An even higher incidence was seen by Hsu and co-workers.[54] Of 82 patients, 61 men suffered from calcifying tendinitis. (74%).

The age distribution varies slightly among authors. Welfling and collaborators[137] found the highest incidence occurred in persons aged between 31 and 40 years, whereas DePalma and Kruper[28] found 36% of patients in the 40- to 50-year group. In our series, 53 patients (42%) were seen in the 40- to 49-year-old group. Welfling and coworkers[137] state that in their group of 925 individuals, no calcification was seen in patients older than 71 years, and McLaughlin[75] reported that no calcification was discovered in about 1000 older cadavers in an anatomy laboratory. It seems that men peak slightly later than do women. Lippmann[65] had similar results: the average age of women was 47 years and of men was 51 years. Hsu and associates[54] reported that 56 of 82 patients were older than 60 years. They conclude that the sex and age of patients with calcifying tendinitis is different in Asians. Nutton and Stothard[89] reported the presence of calcifying tendinitis in a 3-year-old child.

Occupation seems to play a role in calcifying tendinitis. In DePalma and Kruper's group,[28] 41% were housewives and 27% were professionals, executives, and salespersons. In our series, 43% were housewives, and 44% were persons who had a clerical job.

The right shoulder is usually affected more often than is the left shoulder. This difference amounted to 64% in Hartig and Huth's study,[51] to 57% in DePalma and Kruper's series,[28] and to 51% in our series. Bilateral involvement was found in 24.3% by Welfling and coworkers.[137] In DePalma and Kruper's series,[28] the difference was 13%. Of our patients, 17% came back with calcification of the opposite shoulder; this incidence increases with increasing length of the follow-up period.

The incidence of simultaneous calcifications around the hip in 23 patients radiographed in Welfling and associates'[137] series amounted to 62.5%, whereas the incidence was only 4% in control subjects.

All authors agree that calcifying tendinitis is not related to any generalized disease process, and Welfling and colleagues[137] rightly conclude that tendon calcification constitutes a disease entity on its own. Neither McLaughlin[75] nor Rüttimann[111] could find a correlation between tendon tear and calcific tendinitis. Partial tears occur mostly on the bursal side when the deposit ruptures into the bursa. Ruptures into the glenohumeral joint are said to occur extremely seldom.[47] Patte and Goutallier[94] observed two cases. Hsu and collaborators[54] found arthrographic evidence of rotator cuff tearing in 28% (23 patients). We did not record a single instance.

Most authors agree that no relationship exists between calcifying tendinitis and trauma.

CLASSIFICATION

Several classifications of calcifying tendinitis have been proposed. Bosworth[15, 16] divided the deposits into three categories according to their size and corresponding clinical significance: (1) small (up to 0.5 mm), (2) medium (0.5 to 1.5 mm), and (3) large (>1.5 mm). He believed that small deposits have little clinical significance, whereas deposits larger than 1.5 mm are likely to give rise to symptoms. DePalma[29] classified calcifying tendinitis into acute, subacute, and chronic, according to the degree and duration of symptoms. It has been suggested that some patients with the chronic form who have acute exacerbations should be classified in a separate category because they have a better prognosis. Patte and Goutallier[94] classified the deposits into localized and diffuse forms. Radiologically, the localized form is round or oval, dense, and homogeneous and lies close to the bursal wall; it tends to heal spontaneously. In contrast, the diffuse form is situated much deeper in the tendon, close to the bony insertion, and has radiologically a heterogeneous appearance. The diffuse form produces more symptoms and takes longer to disappear.

We have not used these classifications in the clinical management of our patients with calcifying tendinitis because they do not take into account the cyclic nature of the disease. It is, however, important to remember that radiologically visible calcifications in the cuff tendons may occur with diseases other than calcifying tendinitis. Dystrophic calcifications can be seen around the torn edges of the tendon after a complete tear.[140] Massive calcification, as seen in the Milwaukee shoulder or in cuff arthropathy with a complete tear, is associated with severe osteoarthritic changes in the glenohumeral joint and, to some extent, in the acromioclavicular joint.[1, 48, 73, 88] Dystrophic calcification associated with a tear indicates a poor prognosis and progressive degenerative changes and is not comparable with the spontaneous healing of the tendon in calcifying tendinitis. Moreover, dystrophic calcifications do not occur in mid-tendon but arise much closer to the bony insertion.

PATHOLOGY

As the etiology of calcifying tendinitis is still a matter of speculation, we believe that a careful study of its pathology is necessary before any logical assumptions can be made about the pathogenetic mechanism.

Under the light microscope, the calcific deposits appear multifocal, separated by fibrocollagenous tissue or fibrocartilage (Fig. 18–2). The latter consists of easily distinguishable chondrocytes, described by Archer and collaborators[6] as chondrocyte-like cells, within a matrix showing varying degrees of metachromasia (Fig. 18–3). The appearance of chondrocytes within the tendon substance near calcification was noted by Wrede[141] in 1912, by Harbin[49] in 1929, by Sandström and Wahlgren[113] in 1937, by Howorth[53] in 1945, and by Pederson and Key in 1951.[96] The ultrastructure of these chondrocytes shows that the cells often have a fair amount of cytoplasm containing a well developed endoplasmic reticulum, a moderate number of mitochondria, one or more vacuoles, and numerous cell processes (Fig. 18–4). The margin of the nucleus is indented. The cells are surrounded by a distinct band of pericellular matrix with or without an intervening lacuna.

The fibrocartilaginous areas are generally avascular. The intercellular substance is metachromatic, and gly-

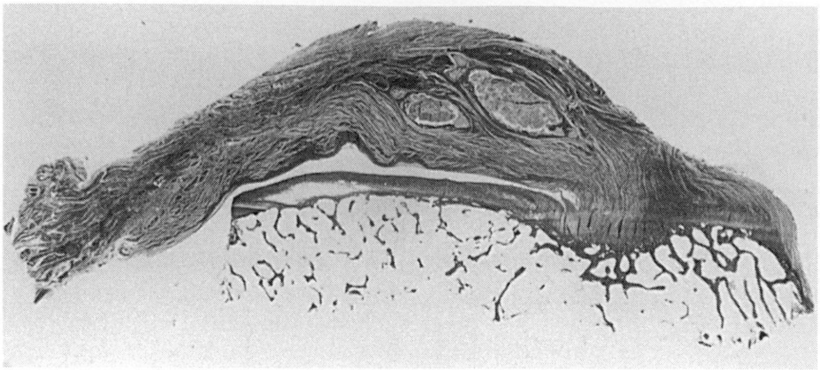

Figure 18–2

An autopsy specimen of a 45-year-old woman showing the typical location of multiple calcific deposits in the more superficial (bursal) part of the supraspinatus tendon. The bursal reaction is minimal. The deeper part is spared (Azan, original magnification, ×3.)

cosaminoglycan-rich pericellular halos around rounded cells are prominent.[6] Surprisingly, monoclonal collagen staining performed by Archer and colleagues[6] did not reveal the presence of collagen type II. In our studies using collagen type II monoclonal antibodies, we occasionally documented its presence. The difference in outcome may be due to differences in tissue preparation, source of monoclonal antibodies, and staining technique. In contrast to the fibrocartilage, the fibrocollagenous tissue abutting against the calcification may appear compressed, forming a pseudocapsule around the deposits. The neighboring tendon fibers may show thinning and fibrillation.

The calcium deposits may be loosely granular or appear in clumps. With the transmission electron microscope, aggregates of rounded structures containing crystalline material are found in a matrix of amorphous debris or irregularly fragmented collagen fibers (Fig. 18–5). When examined by scanning electron microscope, calcific deposits appear as rocky bulks engulfed in mortar.[39] The irregularly rectangular crystals are sometimes found within membrane-bound structures resembling matrix vesicles, also called calcifying globules.[3–5, 13] Infrequently, crystalline densities seem to be embedded between collagen fibers.

An examination by chemical methods, x-ray diffraction, and infrared spectrometry as well as thermogravimetry has shown that the crystals are carbonated apatite.[38] However, high-resolution transmission electron microscopy revealed that the crystals are much larger than the classic apatite crystals and have a different configuration.[131]

In 1915, Moschkowitz[81] identified the deposits within the tendon but stated that the deposits failed to evoke a cellular reaction. A few years before, however, Wrede[141] had already written that, although inflammation or vessels were notably absent around some deposits, "young mesenchymal cells, epithelioid cells, leukocytes, a certain number of lymphocytes and occasionally giant cells" were present at other sites of calcification. The presence of these cells is compatible with a resorptive activity at that stage. Indeed, the marked cellular reaction around calcific deposits—the "calcium granuloma"—was considered by Pederson and Key[96] as the characteristic lesion of calcifying tendinitis. The granulomatous appearance is imparted

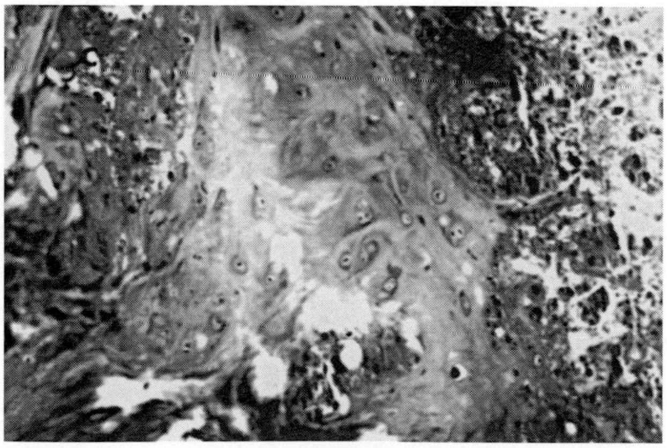

Figure 18–3

A fibrocartilaginous area between calcific deposits (C) shows typical chondrocytes. The appearance characterizes the formative phase. The deposits are partly in clumps and partly granular. (Toluidine blue, ×100.)

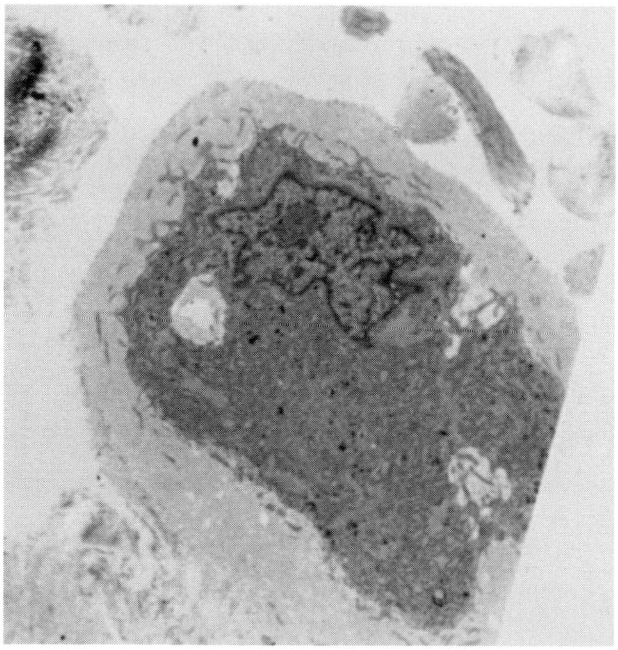

Figure 18–4

The ultrastructure of a chondrocyte surrounded by a pericellular matrix shows a nucleus with an indented margin and the cytoplasm containing a fairly extensive rough endoplasmic reticulum and vacuoles. (Uranyl acetate and lead citrate, ×6500.)

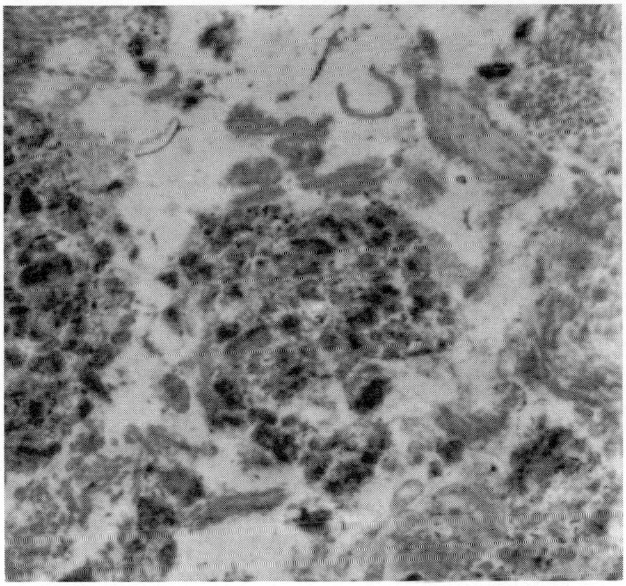

Figure 18–5

Rounded structures resembling matrix vesicles contain electron-dense crystalline structures. (Uranyl acetate and lead citrate, ×23,200.)

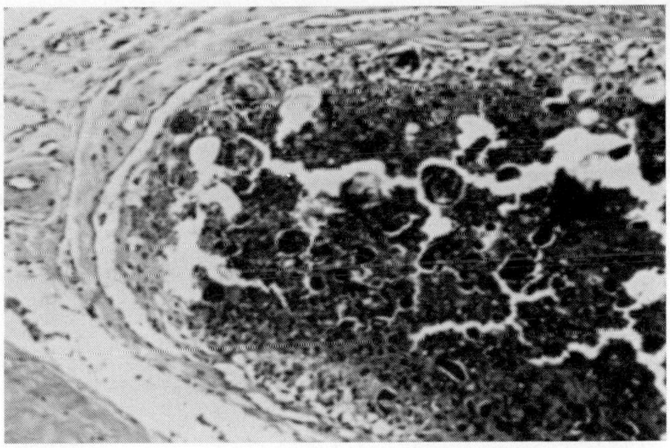

Figure 18–7

Capillary channels surround a calcific deposit. (Toluidine blue, ×100.)

by the presence of multinucleated giant cells (Fig. 18–6) and macrophages. Archer and co-authors[6] interpreted the presence of the latter two cell types as a resorption phenomenon. The cellular reaction is often accompanied by capillary or thin-walled vascular channels around the deposits (Fig. 18–7). The margin and the interior of the deposits are infiltrated by macrophages and a few leukocytes including polymorphonuclear cells and fibroblasts. Phagocytosed substance within macrophages or multinucleated giant cells can be easily discerned (Fig. 18–8). The ultrastructure of these cells shows electron-dense crystalline particles in cytoplasmic vacuoles (Fig. 18–9), but the crystals are slightly different in appearance from those in the extracellular deposits.[114] Some of the intracellular accumulations have a rounded aspect and are known as microspheroliths or psammomas (Fig. 18–10).

Small areas representing the process of repair can be found in the general vicinity of calcification, and these areas show considerable variation in appearance. Granulation tissue with young fibroblasts and newly formed capillaries contrasts with well-formed scars with vascular channels and maturing fibroblasts that are in the process of alignment along the long axis of the tendon fibers (Figs. 18–11 and 18–12). Using monoclonal antibodies against collagen type III, we were able to confirm collagen neoformation, which was most pronounced around vascular channels.

Calcific deposits in the wall of the subacromial bursa also tend to be multifocal (Fig. 18–13). A cellular reaction is seldom seen around the bursal deposits.[115]

PATHOGENESIS

Codman[26] proposed that degeneration of the tendon fibers precedes calcification. The fibers become necrotic, and dystrophic calcification follows. Degeneration of fibers of the rotator cuff tendons because of a "wear-and-tear" effect and aging has been postulated or demonstrated by many investigators. Obviously, these two causes are interrelated. It is reasonable to assume that the rotator

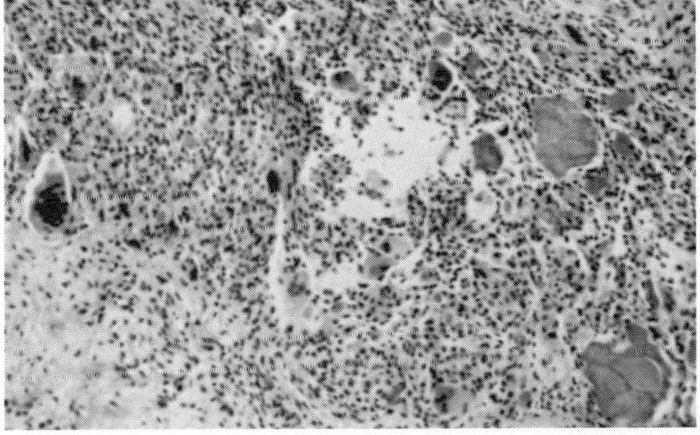

Figure 18–6

A "calcium granuloma" contains scattered small deposits of calcium, macrophages, and multinucleated giant cells. (Hematoxylin and eosin, ×100.)

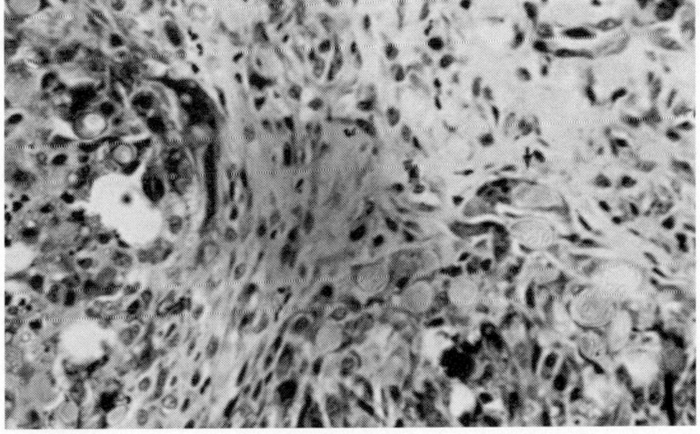

Figure 18–8

Macrophages and multinucleated giant cells contain a phagocytosed substance (*arrow*). (Toluidine blue, ×250.)

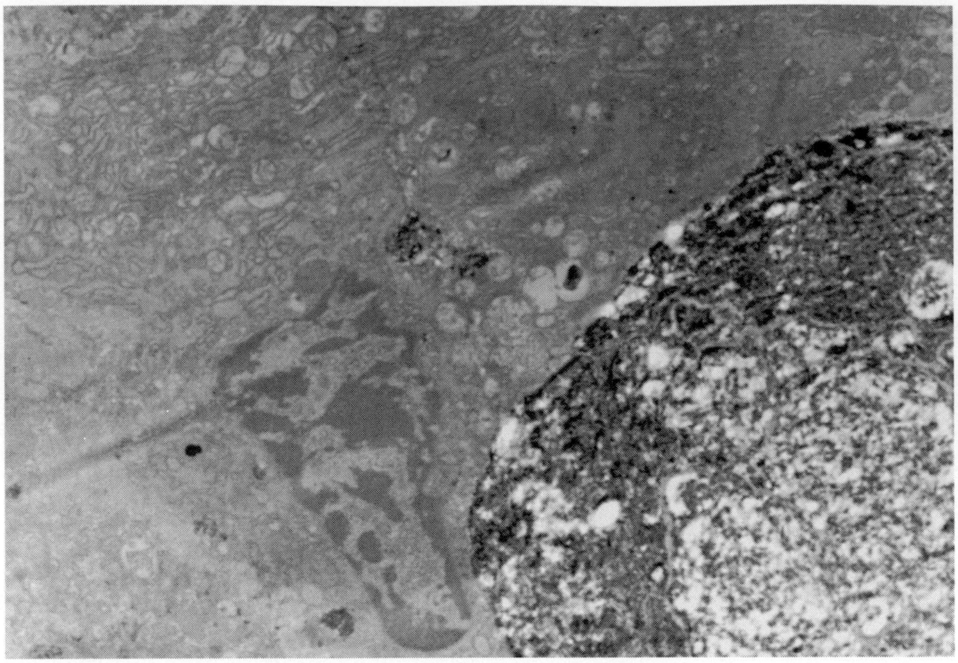

Figure 18–9

The ultrastructure of a macrophage shows apparently phagocytosed electron-dense material in the cytoplasm. (Uranyl acetate and lead citrate, ×11,500.)

cuff tendons suffer a "wear-and-tear" effect because the glenohumeral joint is not only a universal but probably also the most used joint in the body. Studies performed in Sweden seem to indicate that stress and strain induced by work involving the arm can lead to supraspinatus tendinitis.[52] However, there are no indications that even a worker engaged in heavy manual labor would develop calcifying tendinitis in time, and Olsson[91] has shown that the cuff tendons from the dominant arm show no more evidence of degeneration than do those from the contralateral arm.

Aging is considered to be the foremost cause of degeneration in cuff tendons. Brewer[18] believes that with aging there is a general diminution in the vascularity of the supraspinatus tendon along with fiber changes. The well-delineated bundles of collagen or the fascicles that constitute the distinctive architecture of the tendon show the most conspicuous age-related changes that begin at the end of the fourth or the fifth decade.[91] The majority of the fascicles undergo thinning and fibrillation, which are defined as a degenerative process characterized by splitting and fraying of the fibers. The thinned fascicles show irregular cellular arrangement, and the fragmented fibers are often hypocellular. The intervening connective tissue that carries the blood vessels between the fascicles may appear to be increased when contrasted with the volume of the fascicles. In our experience, it is difficult to ascertain the numerical decrease in vessels, but more vessels with thicker walls are consistently found in the cuff tendons of aged individuals.

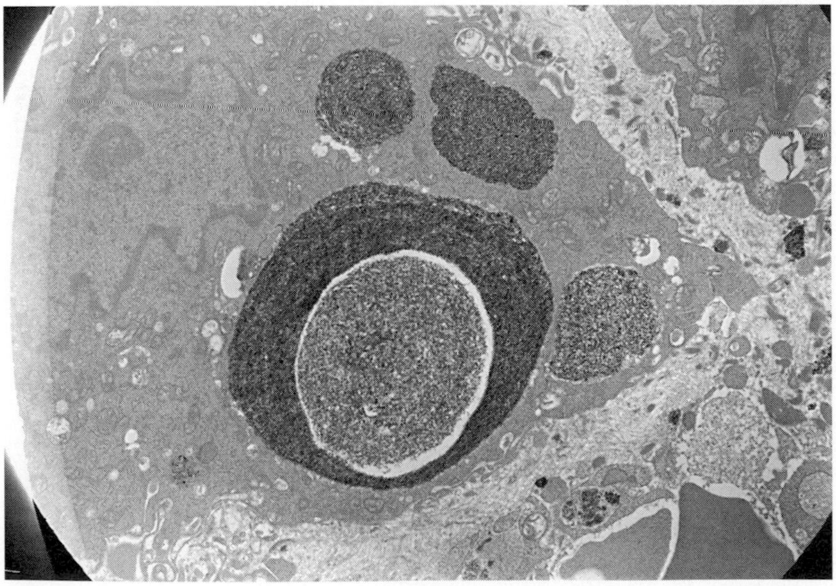

Figure 18–10

This electron microphotograph shows a psammoma inside a macrophage beside three smaller accumulations of electron-dense material. The multilayered structure of the psammoma is quite evident. (Uranyl acetate and lead citrate, ×14,500.)

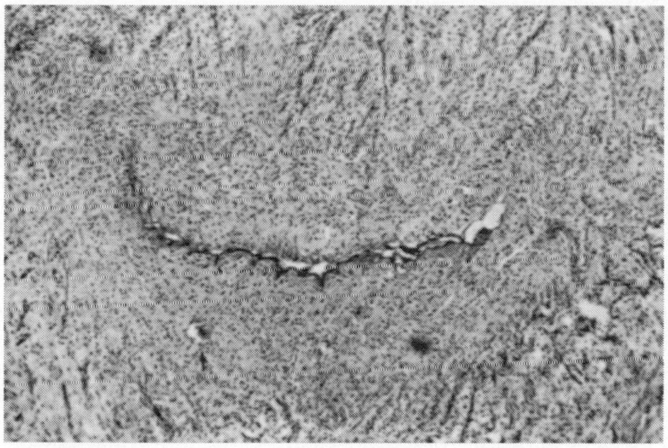

Figure 18–11

Granulation tissue is almost completely replacing the area that was occupied previously by calcific deposits. A speck of calcium is still visible (*arrow*). The central portion shows amorphous precipitate. (Hematoxylin and eosin, ×40.)

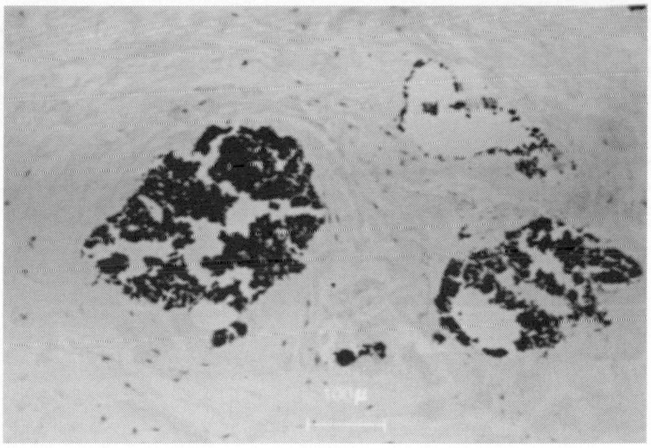

Figure 18–13

Multiple foci of calcific deposits in the wall of the subacromial bursa do not show any cellular reactions. (Hematoxylin and eosin, ×40.)

Since calcifying tendinitis seldom affects persons before the fourth decade, it can be argued that a primary degeneration of tendon fibers is responsible for the subsequent deposition of calcium. Following Codman's[26] suggestion of the degenerative nature of calcifying tendinitis, subsequent investigators have found ample histologic evidence for the sequence of degeneration, necrosis, and calcification.[42, 43, 77] According to McLaughlin,[75] the earliest lesion is focal hyalinization of fibers that eventually become fibrillated and get detached from the surrounding normal tendon. Continued motion of the tendon grinds the detached, curled-up fibers into a "wen-like substance," consisting of necrotic debris on which calcification occurs. This sequence of events was demonstrated experimentally by MacNab[72] in the course of investigations on the effects of interruption of vascular supply to the tendo Achilles of rabbits. Pedersen and Key,[96] who are also in favor of a degenerative calcification, state that "calcium is deposited in the necrotic collagenic tissue."

Mohr and Bilger[79] believe that the process of calcification starts with a necrosis of tenocytes with a concomitant intracellular accumulation of calcium, often in the form of microspheroliths, also known as psammomas. Contrary to Mohr and Bilger,[79] we never observed psammomas during the early phases of formation but we did observe them regularly during the phase of resorption (see Fig. 18–10). Our electron microscopic examinations leave no doubt that the electron-dense material is situated intracellular and not extracellular, as seen in pathologic conditions cited by these authors. Moreover, it is unfortunate that these authors do not distinguish between calcifications at the insertion and intratendinous calcifications (i.e., the site of calcifying tendinitis).

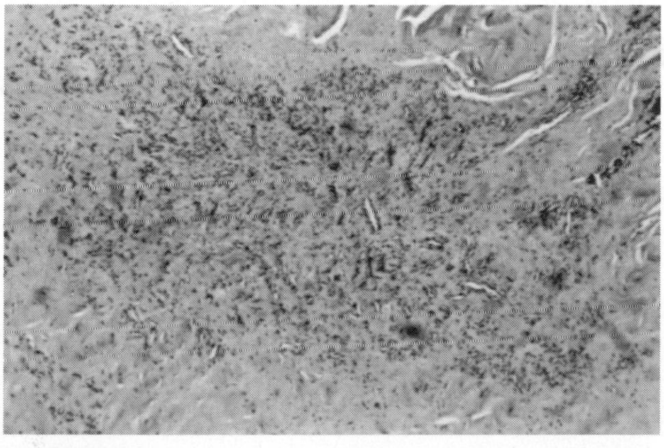

Figure 18–12

A scar represents the area of healing in the tendon. (Hematoxylin and eosin, ×40.)

Authors' Opinion

The aforementioned investigators failed to distinguish between fundamentally different histologic aspects of calcifying tendinitis and dystrophic calcification. Lippmann[65] observed that "The early deposit, located in a totally avascular bed, provokes no tissue reaction." He contrasted this with "the mechanism of absorption that primarily is dependent upon vascularity and inflammation." Moreover, Jones[56] deplored the fact that "proper assessment of the natural repair process in acute cases has not been made."

We would like to add that neither the self-healing nature of calcifying tendinitis nor the various aspects of its pathology are characteristic of a degenerative disease. We believe that the process of calcification is actively mediated by cells in a viable environment.[98, 104, 114, 128, 131–133] Moreover, there cannot be the slightest doubt that formation of the calcium deposit must precede its resorption. Consequently, we propose the following concept for the evolution of the disease, which can be divided into three distinct stages: (1) precalcific, (2) calcific, and (3) postcalcific (Fig. 18–14).

Precalcific Stage

In the precalcific stage, the site of predilection for calcification undergoes fibrocartilaginous transformation. This

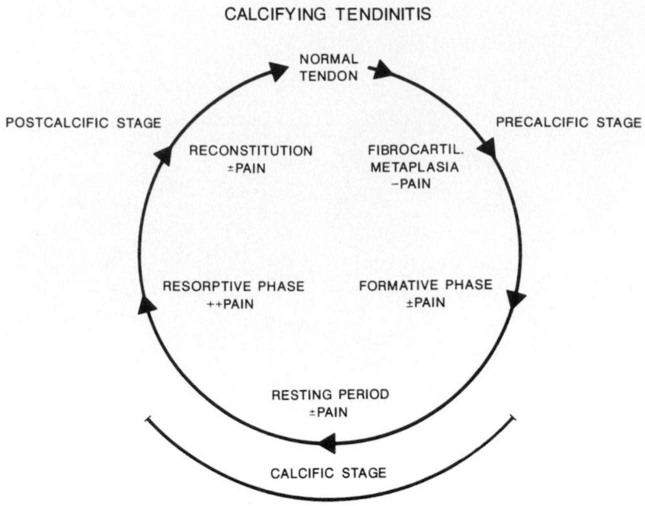

Figure 18–14

The evolution of calcifying tendinitis.

metaplasia of tenocytes into chondrocytes is accompanied by metachromasia, which is indicative of the elaboration of proteoglycan.

Calcific Stage

This stage is subdivided into the formative phase and the resorptive phase.

FORMATIVE PHASE

In the ensuing calcific stage, calcium crystals are deposited primarily in matrix vesicles that coalesce to form large areas of deposits.[114] For the convenience of description, we have used the term "formative phase" to describe the initial period of the calcific stage.[131] If the patient undergoes surgery at this stage, the deposit appears chalk-like (Fig. 18–15) and has to be scooped out for removal. At this time, the area of fibrocartilage with the foci of calcification is generally devoid of vascular channels. Septa of fibrocartilage separating the foci of calcification stain positively metachromatic. They do not consistently stain positively for collagen type II, which is known to be a component of fibrocartilage. These fibrocartilaginous septa are gradually eroded by the enlarging deposits.

RESORPTIVE PHASE

Following a variable period of inactivity of the disease process ("resting period" in the schema), the spontaneous resorption of calcium is heralded by the appearance of thin-walled vascular channels at the periphery of the deposit. Soon after, the deposit is surrounded by macrophages and multinucleated giant cells that phagocytose and remove the calcium. This is the last step in the calcific stage, which we have called the "resorptive phase." If an operation is performed at this stage, the calcific deposit is a thick, white, cream-like or toothpaste-like material (Fig. 18–16).

Postcalcific Stage

Simultaneously with the resorption of calcium, granulation tissue containing young fibroblasts and new vascular channels begins to remodel the space occupied by calcium. These sites stain positively for collagen type III. As the scar matures, fibroblasts and collagen eventually align along the longitudinal axis of the tendon. During this remodeling process, collagen type III is replaced by collagen type I. We have called this stage of tendon reconstitution "postcalcific." Figure 18–17 outlines the correlation between pathogenesis, morphologic findings, and symptoms during the various stages of calcifying tendinitis.

Although the pathogenesis of the calcifying process can be reasonably constructed from morphologic studies, it is difficult to determine what triggers the fibrocartilaginous transformation in the first place. Codman[26] suggested tissue hypoxia as the primary etiologic factor. This still remains an attractive hypothesis because of the peculiarity of the tendon vasculature and shoulder mechanics. We have found that there is an increased frequency of HLA-Al in patients with calcifying tendinitis, indicating that

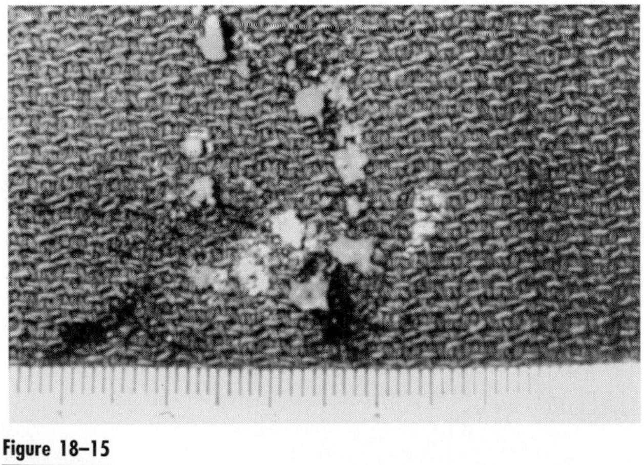

Figure 18–15

The calcium removed from a patient during the formative phase has a granular aspect.

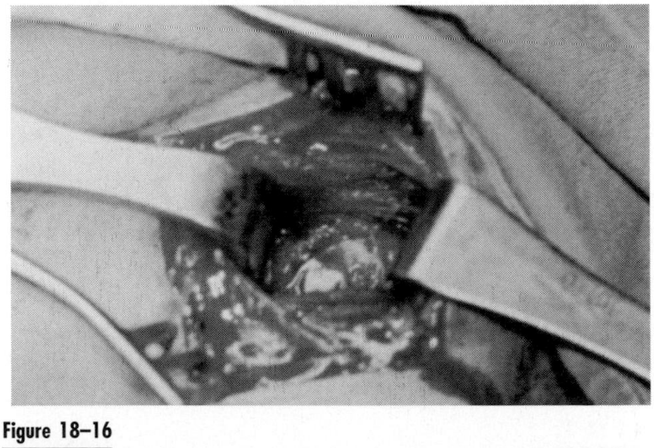

Figure 18–16

After opening a deposit, which was in the resorptive phase, a cream-like fluid spurted out under pressure; it can be seen in the wound margins.

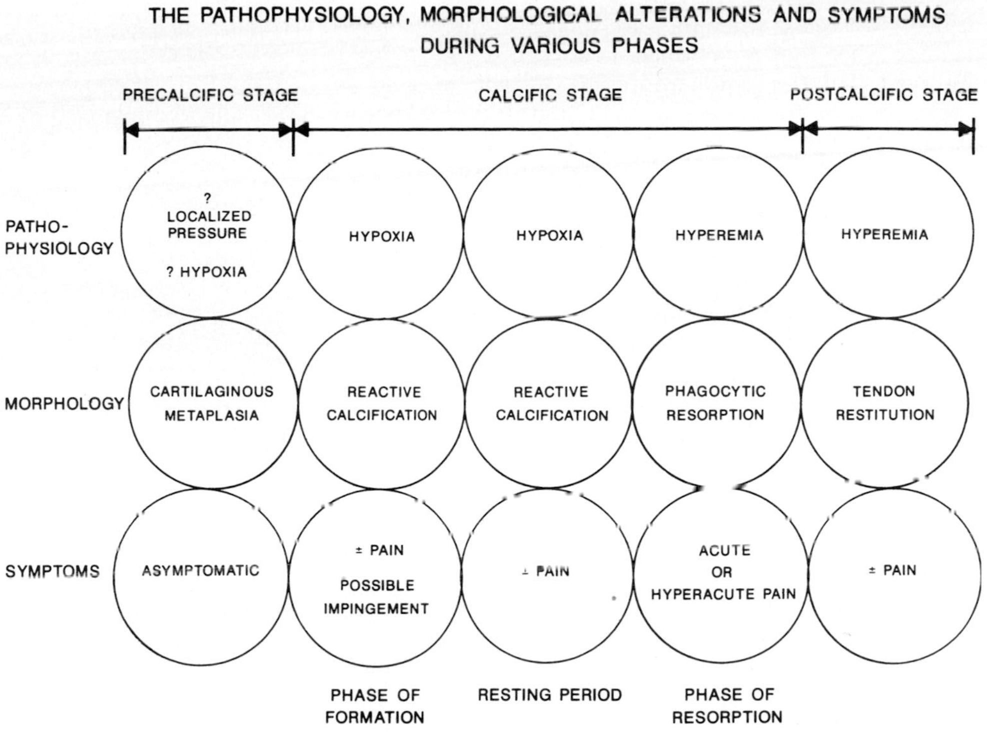

Figure 18–17

The pathophysiology, morphologic alterations, and symptoms are shown during various stages of calcifying tendinitis. In the course of evolution of the disease, the stages are likely to overlap each other.

these individuals may be genetically susceptible to the condition.[120] Factors that trigger the onset of resorption also remain unknown. Our phase of formation seems to be identical to Lippmann's[65] early phase of increment, whereas his late phase of increment is analogous to our phase of resorption.

CLINICAL PRESENTATION

Pain is the cardinal symptom of calcifying tendinitis[14, 57, 62, 123, 125]

We would like to emphasize strongly that an understanding of the pathogenetic mechanism of calcifying tendinitis is essential for the clinical evaluation and management of this disease entity. There is a tendency to assume that calcifying tendinitis, as most diseases, begins with acute symptoms and progresses to a chronic state. Others maintain that we deal with two separate disease entities. Our understanding of the disease is entirely to the contrary. We believe that the initial stage of formation of the deposit, which lacks a vascular and cellular reaction, is likely to cause few symptoms or nondebilitating discomfort because the intratendinous tissue tension is hardly raised by the deposit. Thus, the disease generally begins with chronic symptoms, if any at all. Larger deposits can lead to impingement against the coracoacromial ligament, a fact already observed by Baer[8] in 1907 during surgery. During the later phase of calcium resorption, on the other hand, exudation of cells along with vascular proliferation must enlarge the tissue space considerably and thus produce a raised intratendinous pressure that causes pain. The pain is probably further exacerbated as the increased volume of the tendon impinges on the unyielding structures that limit the subacromial compartment.

In fact, the subclinical nature of the formative phase of calcification has been recognized by many authors. Codman[26] stated that "the usual history is not acute pain at the beginning." Wilson[138] noted that many patients might know about a calcium deposit in one or both shoulders for months or years prior to an acute attack. Lippmann[65] stressed the well-known fact that early deposits are usually symptomless and that the acute pain signals "the onset of 'break-up' of the deposit." Pinals and Short[100] wrote: " . . . calcium deposition precedes rather than follows the development of an acute attack of calcific periarthritis and the attack is accompanied by disintegration and gradual disappearance of the deposit." Similarly, Gschwend and associates[47] believed that the calcification is often symptomless at the beginning, whereas its disappearance is associated with pain.

It is therefore evident that we are not dealing with two unrelated disease processes, an acute and a chronic calcific tendinitis, but a disease cycle. Lippmann[65] described a phase of increment followed by a short, self-limited phase of disruption. Each phase has its characteristics. During the phase of increment, the symptoms were described as being mild, the consistency of the deposit was said to be hard and chalky, and no inflammation was noted. During the phase of disruption, the pain was severe, the consistency allowed tapping, and radiographs showed a fluffy deposit. Lippmann[65] concluded that failure to identify the phase of the cycle resulted in crediting "useless therapeutic measures with magical healing power and, on the other hand, led to the performance of needless surgical procedures."

The clinical presentation depends on the acuteness of symptoms. Simon[121] believed that a definite relationship exists between the intensity of symptoms and their duration. The symptoms can last up to 2 weeks when they are acute, 3 to 8 weeks when they are subacute, and 3 months or more when they are chronic. Pendergrass and Hodes[97] observed that the acute symptoms subside in 1 to 2 weeks, even in the absence of treatment. It is also known that symptoms may change rapidly.

During the subacute and chronic phases, patients complain of pain or tenderness. They are usually able to localize the point of maximum tenderness. Irradiation of pain is the rule, the insertion of the deltoid being the most frequent site of pain referral. Referred pain was seen in 42.5% of the patients of De Sèze and Welfling.[30] The radiation of pain occurred more often into the arm than toward the neck. Wrede[141] and many authors after him found that clinical symptoms are often absent. Usually the range of motion is decreased by pain; the patients cannot sleep on the affected shoulder; and they often complain of an increase in pain during the night. A painful arc of motion between 70 and 110 degrees has been described by Kessel and Watson,[60] but they were unable to classify these patients into any of their three types of the painful arc syndrome (posterior, anterior, and superior). In 97 patients with this syndrome, they found 12 cases of calcification. Patients often have the sensation of catching when going through the arc of motion. This is most probably due to a localized impingement. This, in turn, leads to a loss of the scapulohumeral rhythm. Impingement between calcium deposit and coracoacromial ligament during abduction has already been noted by Baer[8] and by Wrede.[141] A further sign of long-standing symptoms of calcifying tendinitis is the atrophy of both spinati muscles. Although some authors have reported the presence of swelling and redness on clinical examination, we were never able to find these signs.

During the acute phase, the pain is so intense and excruciating that patients refuse to move their shoulders. De Sèze and Welfling[30] believe that this severe pain leads to a locking. Any attempt at mobilization of the glenohumeral joint will be resisted by the patient. Patients hold their arms close to their bodies in internal rotation.

Although we have described the involvement of the bursa in painful shoulder syndromes,[114] its involvement in various phases of calcifying tendinitis has not been documented in detail.

During the formative phase, the subacromial bursa is not the site of a widespread reaction. Only in the presence of impingement is a zone of hyperemia noted around the calcium deposit (Fig. 18–18). Carnett[21] noted that bursitis forms a minor and infrequent feature.

During the resorptive phase, bursitis is said to be a source of pain. However, during surgery, the bursal reaction is minimal and often limited to a localized hyperemia (Fig. 18–19). This reaction is usually not severe enough to cause a bursal thickening; in fact, the calcific deposit often shines through the deep or visceral layer of the bursa. Litchman and colleagues[66] also noted the absence of bursal inflammation. Many authors state that rupture of the deposit into the bursa causes a crystalline type of bursitis and consequently pain. We would like to emphasize again that only during the resorptive phase does the consistency of the deposit allow its rupture into the bursa. DePalma and Kruper[28] noted that deposits rupturing into the bursa are encountered in acute cases. De Sèze and Welfling[30] followed 12 patients with ruptures of the deposit into the bursa. Only eight patients showed symptoms. In our histologic specimens we could observe synovial cells resorbing calcium. No inflammatory reaction, in particular no leukocytes or lymphocytes, accompanied this resorptive process. It seems therefore probable that the edema and the proliferation of cells and vessels cause an increased intratendinous pressure that evokes pain rather than the localized bursal reaction. This impression seems to be confirmed by intraoperative observations during the acute phase. Key[61] reported: "In some hyperacute cases of short duration, the calcific material is thin or milklike in consistency and may be under such pressure that when the surface of the tendon is incised, the contents of the deposit may spurt out into the air." An identical observation has been made by Friedman.[40]

In 41 operated patients, we have correlated the symptoms with radiologic findings and with consistency of the deposit. Of 31 patients with chronic symptoms, 24 patients had radiographic signs compatible with formation, and 29 patients had chalk-like granular calcium deposits. Of 10 patients with acute symptoms, eight patients had

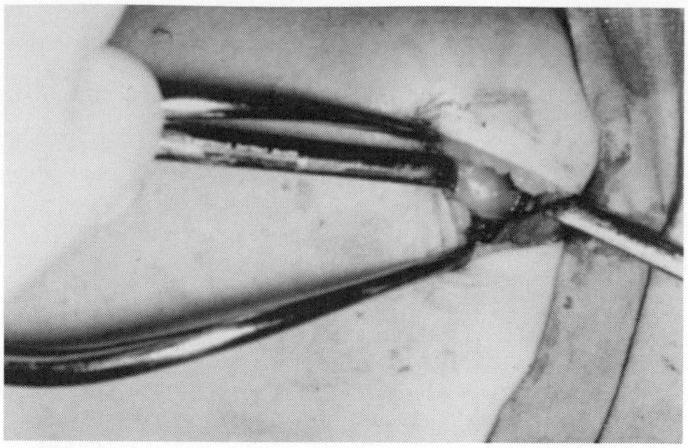

Figure 18–18

An intraoperative photograph after opening the bursal cavity. The whitish area of a deposit during the formation phase is surrounded by slight bursal hyperemia.

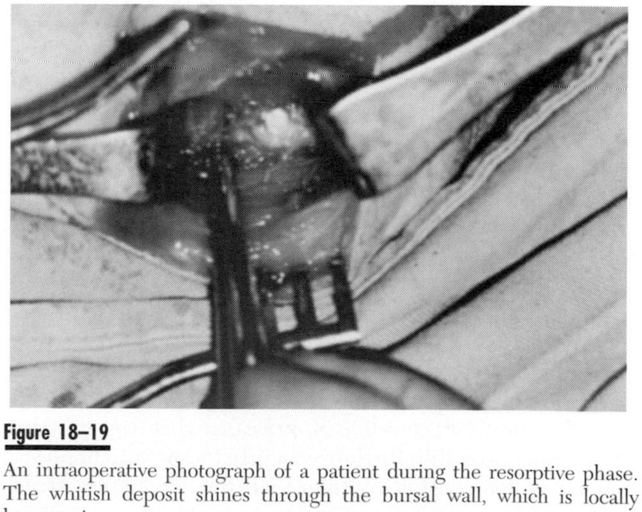

Figure 18–19

An intraoperative photograph of a patient during the resorptive phase. The whitish deposit shines through the bursal wall, which is locally hyperemic.

radiographic signs typical of resorption, and nine patients exhibited a toothpaste-like consistency of their deposit.

Should calcifying tendinitis be considered a systemic disease as Pinals and Short[100] have speculated? There is no good evidence despite the high incidence of calcifications occurring at other sites. With the exception of an increased incidence of HLA-Al in patients with calcifying tendinitis, all other laboratory tests are normal.[120] An associated illness was never reported,[66] and Gschwend and associates[47] were unable to prove an association with diabetes or gout, although this association had been repeatedly suspected by various authors but never documented. A relationship to occupation must be suspected, given the high incidence of clerical workers observed by us and other investigators. Litchman and colleagues,[66] on the other hand, stated that no relationship to occupation could be found. A possible correlation between stiff and painful shoulders and calcifying tendinitis has been suspected for approximately 90 years.[19, 24] We could only observe a single case of this syndrome. Lundberg[71] reported 24 patients with calcification among 232 patients with frozen shoulders. This finding does not point toward a strong correlation between calcifying tendinitis and frozen shoulder.

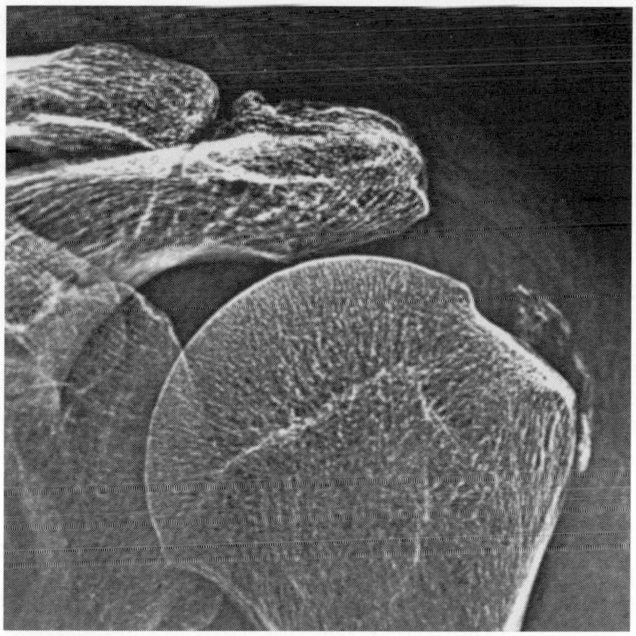

Figure 18–20

A xerogram of a calcium deposit in the resorptive phase. Note the presence of calcific material in the bursa.

RADIOLOGY

Calcium deposits in calcifying tendinitis are localized inside a tendon. They are usually not in continuity with the bone nor do they extend into the bone. DePalma and Kruper[28] observed extensions into bone in 8 of 136 patients. The only other occurrence has been reported by Toriyama and associates.[127] Calcium deposits close to bone must be clearly distinguished from stippled calcifications seen at the tendon insertion in cases of arthropathies.

In all cases of suspected calcification of tendons, a radiograph must be taken. The radiologic assessment is also important during follow-up examinations. It permits assessment of changes in density and in extent.

Initial radiographs should include an anteroposterior film in neutral rotation and also in internal and external rotation. Deposits in the supraspinatus are readily visible on films in neutral rotation, whereas deposits in the infraspinatus and teres minor are best seen in internal rotation. Calcifications in the subscapularis occur only in rare cases, and a radiograph in external rotation will show them well. Axillary views are rarely indicated. Scapular views, however, will help to determine whether a calcification causes an impingement. Ruptures into the bursa will show as a crescent-like shadow overlying the actual calcification and extending over the greater tuberosity, outlining well the extent of the bursa (Fig. 18–20).

The presence of calcium deposits, particularly in the acute or resorptive phase, is often barely visible on radiographs (Fig. 18–21). In these cases, xerography (see Fig. 18–20) or sonography is helpful.[27, 37, 51] We suspect that computerized radiography may give similar results. Loew and colleagues[69] reported their experience with magnetic resonance imaging in 75 patients. Calcifications appeared in T1-weighted images as in areas of decreased signal intensity, whereas T2-weighted images frequently showed a perifocal band of increased signal intensity compatible with edema.

Bursograms have not been shown to be of great value in our experience.[129] When arthrograms are performed, they show a distinct delineation between the deposit and the joint cavity. We believe that they are indicated only in exceptional cases, especially when a tear is suspected.

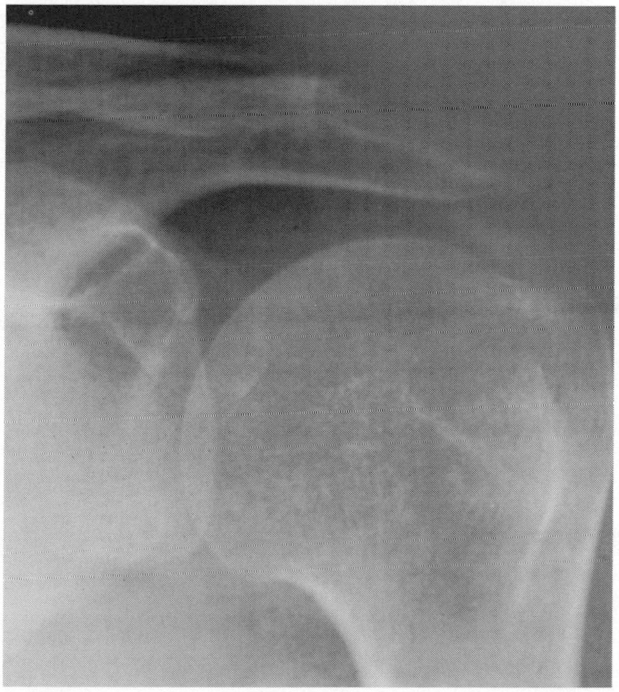

Figure 18–21

Calcifying tendinitis during the resorptive phase. The deposit is fluffy and ill defined.

Radiographs not only allow confirmation of the absence or presence of calcium deposits, they also permit proper localization. Furthermore, the extent, delineation, and density can be well appreciated.[134] Moreover, serial radiographs are helpful in the assessment of the evolution of the disease (Fig. 18–22).

DePalma and Kruper[28] described two radiologic types. Type I has a fluffy, fleecy appearance, and its periphery is poorly defined. This type is usually encountered in acute cases. An overlying crescent-like streak indicates a rupture of the deposit into the bursa, which occurs only in this type. Type II is more or less discrete and homogeneous. Its density is uniform, and the periphery is well defined. This type is seen in subacute and chronic cases. Moreover, DePalma and Kruper[28] reported that in 52% of their patients, the calcification was seen as a single lesion.

De Sèze and Welfling[30] observed that in the presence of acute pain, the deposit was less dense and the margins were not well defined. In chronic cases, on the other hand, the margins were well defined, and the calcification was dense. They described the following radiologic sequence in acute cases. First, a fluffy, ill-defined intratendinous deposit is followed in time by calcific material in the bursa only, and finally, no calcific material can be seen at all. We believe, however, that calcific material can often be seen in both the bursa and the tendon, that the calcific material disappears rather rapidly from the bursa, and that often a faintly visible shadow remains in the tendon for some time.

Our observations confirm those made by DePalma and Kruper[28] and by De Sèze and Welfling.[30] During the formative or chronic phase, the deposit is dense and well defined and of homogeneous density (see Fig. 18–22). During the resorptive or acute phase, the deposit is fluffy, cloud-like, and ill defined, and its density is irregular (see Fig. 18–19). Communications with the bursa have been observed only during the latter phase.

Most authors agree that radiologic evidence of degenerative joint disease is usually lacking. This, of course, holds true mostly for patients in the fourth and fifth decades of life. It is therefore not surprising that in the group of patients reported by Hsu and collaborators[54] the incidence of degenerative joint changes was higher. In three of our patients in the sixth decade, we observed acromioclavicular osteophytes.

Bony changes at the insertion of the supraspinatus into the greater tuberosity can sometimes be seen after resorption of the deposit. Whether this occurs more often after intraosseous extension of the calcium deposit into bone is difficult to confirm.

Calcifications seen in arthropathies have a quite different appearance. They are stippled and overlie the bony insertion. They are always accompanied by degenerative bony or articular changes. Moreover, the acromiohumeral compartment or interval is always narrowed. These calcium deposits constitute dystrophic calcifications; they must be distinguished clearly from the reactive intratendinous calcifications.

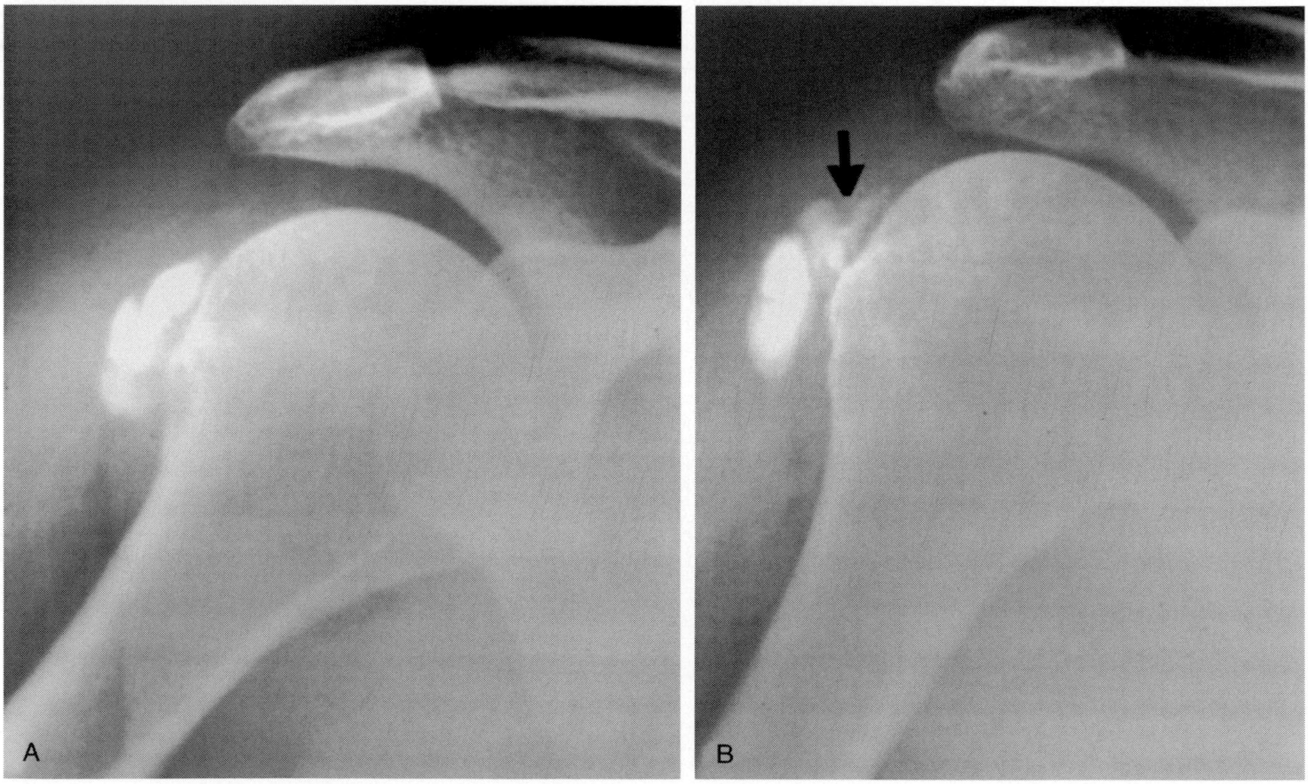

Figure 18–22

Calcifying tendinitis of the infraspinatus. At the time of the first consultation, symptoms were chronic. *A*, At that time the deposit was dense, homogeneous, and well defined. This aspect is typical of the formative phase. *B*, Four months later, the patient reported the spontaneous onset of acute pain. Note the beginning of resorption. The *arrow* points to an area of decreased density with irregular margins that is typical of the resorptive phase.

According to Hartig and Huth,[51] sonography is more sensitive than radiography in detecting calcium deposits (Fig. 18–23 *A* and *B*). In 90% of their 217 patients, the deposit could be visualized radiologically and 100% sonographically (as well as histologically).

LABORATORY INVESTIGATIONS

There are no abnormalities of calcium and phosphorus metabolism. Therefore, serum values are within normal limits. The alkaline phosphatase is also normal. There is no increase in the number of white blood cells, and the erythrocyte sedimentation rate is normal.

In our attempts to distinguish further between degenerative and reactive tendinopathies, we proceeded with tissue typing in 50 patients with calcifying tendinitis and compared the results with those of 36 patients with a tear of the rotator cuff and with 982 control patients.[120] HLA-Al was present in 50% of patients with calcifications, in 27.8% of patients with tears, and in 26.7% of controls. There is a statistically significant difference between patients suffering from calcifying tendinitis and those having a tear, the *P* value being .0025.

During screening of patients with calcifications, the serum glucose values and the level of uric acid and iron should be determined.

COMPLICATIONS

Although the calcification starts inside the tendon, it may extend into the muscle or bone. DePalma and Kruper[28] noted that in cases of osseous penetration, the point of entry was to be found at the sulcus, the interval between the articular cartilage and the tendon insertion. They observed that intraosseous deposits were always in continuity with intratendinous calcifications. In their experience, a bony involvement led to protracted symptoms; deposits in these patients were resistant to conservative measures, and they advocated surgical removal.

Bicipital tendinitis may complicate calcifying tendinitis. It occurred in 16 of 136 patients reported by DePalma and Kruper.[28]

As stated earlier, frozen shoulder may occur in association with calcification. It was seen by DePalma and Kruper[28] in 7 of 94 patients. They believed that frozen shoulder was caused by an inflammatory process whereby adhesions occur between the cuff and the humeral head.

Rupture of the deposit into the bursa cannot be regarded as a complication. Complete tears, however, must be included, and to our knowledge, they have been reported only by Patte and Goutallier,[94] who observed a rupture of the deposit into the glenohumeral joint, seen only in the type that they call diffuse calcification.

Complications from surgery must be of little importance, because they have not been reported. Careful attention must be paid to spare the axillary nerve during the splitting of the deltoid. Postoperative wound infection has not been seen by us, and all wounds healed without undue delay.

A recurrence of calcification after surgical removal has been observed by us in one of 127 operated patients. In other patients in whom the deposit was not completely removed, the spontaneous disappearance of the deposit was rather slow.

DIFFERENTIAL DIAGNOSIS

Here again we wish to insist on a proper distinction between reactive and dystrophic calcifications. In calcifying tendinitis, the major part of the deposit is situated inside the tendon without being either in continuity or in contact with bone. Dystrophic calcifications, on the other hand, are part of a degenerative process with concomitant radiologic evidence of osteoarthritis and a rotator cuff tear, leading to a narrowing of the interval between the humeral head and the acromion. These calcifications are small and stippled and sit just over the greater tuberosity.

TREATMENT

Treatment varies according to the training and expertise of the treating physician. In general, rheumatologists

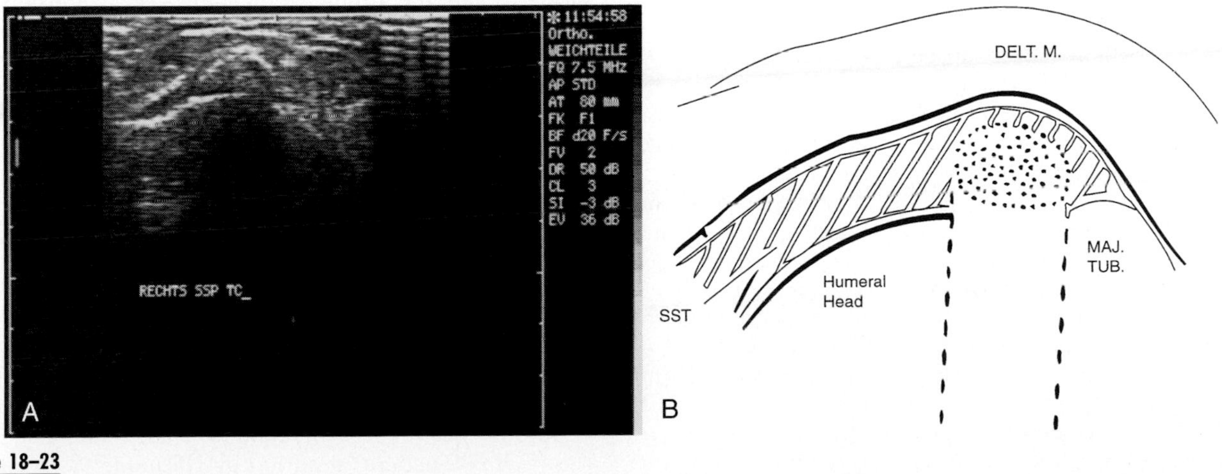

Figure 18–23

A, Ultrasonography of a calcific deposit in the supraspinatus tendon (coronal section, Siemens SI-400). *B*, Drawing of the ultrasonographic picture. (Delt.m., deltoid muscle; Maj.tub., greater tuberosity; ROM, range of motion. SST, supraspinatus tendon.)

seem to favor a conservative approach more often than do surgeons. The approach also depends on the acuteness of symptoms and on the patience of the physician and the patient. Some impatience is understandable, since no one knows how long the disease in its chronic phase will last or when the calcification will spontaneously disappear.

Nonoperative

The natural evolution of the deposit has been followed by Gärtner[41] in 235 patients over 3 years. Radiologically dense deposits disappeared in 33% in contrast with 85% of fluffy accumulations.

Gschwend and co-workers[47] estimate that at least 90% of patients are treated conservatively. In a series of 100 patients reported by Litchman and colleagues,[66] only one patient underwent surgery.

All authors agree about the need for adequate physiotherapy.[10, 76] Range of motion and pendulum exercises and, later on, muscle strengthening exercises are recommended. In acute cases, gentle attempts at mobilization are preceded by the local application of ice, whereas local heat is recommended in chronic cases. Infrared treatments should be understood as a local application of heat. Ultrasonography is said to be able to mobilize the calcium crystals, but no randomized study proving its value could be found by Griffin and Karselis.[45] Griffin and Karselis[45] observed pain relief, which is thought to result from a physiologic rise in tissue temperature. The main aim of physiotherapy is the decrease of muscle spasm and the prevention of stiffness. Relief of pain can sometimes be obtained by placing the arm on a pillow in abduction.[21] The treatment regimen outlined is indicated mainly in chronic cases. Whether pulsed ultrasound will have a positive effect on the dissolution of the calcium deposit remains to be seen.

EXTRACORPOREAL SHOCK WAVE THERAPY

Recently this technique, which is well established and known as lithotripsy in urology, has also been used in the treatment of calcific deposits. Loew and co-workers[67] stated in a preliminary study with five patients that all except one patient had a satisfactory result. Rompe and associates[107] reported later on a series of 40 patients in whom 1500 impulses were applied to the shoulder area under regional anesthesia during a single therapy session. Fifteen of these patients had no improvement after a relatively short follow-up period of 24 weeks; however, in 25 patients, a partial or complete disappearance of the calcific deposit was observed. A similar experience was reported by Loew and co-workers[68] in a follow-up paper on their initial study. Fourteen of 20 patients with "chronic, symptomatic calcifying tendinitis," who had a lithotripsy treatment, experienced improvement from symptoms, but again the follow-up time was only 12 weeks. They controlled their patients by a magnetic resonance imaging study, demonstrating no secondary changes to the rotator cuff or the underlying bone, although 14 of the 20 patients developed local hematomas after this therapy. Thirty per cent of their patients had an improvement of the constant score, and in seven patients the deposit disappeared completely.

This technique is still under trial, and one will have to wait for longer follow-up studies, a larger patient population, and reports from other centers before being able to comment on its indication and details of the technique.

NEEDLING AND LAVAGE

In acute cases, easing pain becomes a priority. Patterson and Darrach[95] and later Lapidus[63] recommended needling and injection of local anesthetics. Gärtner[41] followed 33 patients for 1 year after needling and observed a resorption of the deposit in 23 patients. Repeated perforations seem to decrease the intratendinous pressure. An additional lavage may also help to remove part of the deposit. Its effect on symptoms was studied by Pfister and Gerber[99] in 149 of 212 patients after 5 years. Sixty per cent were free of pain; 34% had a marked relief; and 6% were unchanged. Lavage can be effective only in the presence of radiologic evidence of resorption. The site of needle insertion is based on the site of maximum tenderness and radiographic localization. Although these injections had to be repeated in some patients twice or three times, Harmon[50] reported that they led to excellent results in 78.9% of more than 400 patients. DePalma and Kruper's[28] results were less good; they obtained 61% good, 22% fair, and 17% poor results.

Some authors suggest the addition of a corticosteroid preparation to local treatment. Gschwend and colleagues[47] note that its action is short, and its effect is exclusively symptomatic. Dhuly and associates[31] showed that corticosteroids inhibit vascular proliferation, local hyperemia, and macrophage activity. Lippmann[65] warns that corticosteroids abort the activity that produces disruption and that they return the deposit to a static phase. Harmon[50] believed that the addition of corticosteroids did not accelerate the process of resorption but did reduce the muscle spasm. Murnaghan and McIntosh[86] treated 27 patients with lidocaine (Xylocaine) injections alone and 24 with hydrocortisone and found no difference in results. During the acute phase, analgesics are absolutely necessary to calm the often excruciating pain. Nonsteroidal anti-inflammatory drugs are often recommended. No randomized study, however, could be found to document its salutary effect on the process of resorption.

RADIATION

In the past radiotherapy has enjoyed an important place in the treatment of calcifying tendinitis.[9, 17] Milone and Copeland[78] treated 136 patients with radiotherapy. They concluded that "patients with the acute syndrome experience the most favorable response." Of 54 patients in the acute phase, 49 patients had excellent and good results, whereas only 15 of 24 patients with chronic pain obtained the same degree of relief. Results in patients with chronic symptoms fell to 33% in Young's[142] and Chapman's series.[23] Of 609 patients reported by Harmon,[50] 79 received radiotherapy. Of these patients, 28 needed surgical excision at a later date. Plenk[101] concluded that radiotherapy was ineffective. In a series of 38 patients, Plenk radiated 21 patients and interposed a lead shield between the source of radiation and the shoulder in 17 patients. The calcium deposit disappeared in 67% of the shielded patients and in 44% of the radiated patients. Plenk gained the impression that in acute cases radiation delayed resorption in five out of nine patients, whereas in shielded patients the deposit persisted in only one out of eight patients. In this context, Gschwend and colleagues'[47] sarcastic remark that in acute cases any form of treatment is successful is noteworthy. "Therapy cannot hinder the success," they conclude. Whereas radiotherapy is not any more an acceptable mode of treatment in North America, a recent report from France recommends the use of "anti-inflammatory radiotherapy." Ollagnier and colleagues[90] reported 68% of good results in 47 patients. It seems that their assessment has been based mainly on pain relief.

Surgery

Bosworth[15, 16] expressed the opinion of many surgeons when he wrote that the quickest and most dependable way of relieving patients of large and troublesome deposits is by open surgery. Vebostad[135] obtained excellent and good results with surgery in 34 of 43 patients. Litchman and colleagues[66] believe that prolonged waiting in the chronic group leads to adhesive capsulitis and frozen shoulder. This view is not commonly shared. Gschwend and associates[47] formulated the following operative indications:

1. Progression of symptoms
2. Constant pain interfering with activities of daily living
3. Absence of improvement of symptoms after conservative therapy.

They reported excellent and good results in 25 of 28 subjects. Moseley[83] restricts the indication in recommending surgery for large deposits in the mechanical phase. He, like most other authors, is in favor of conservative treatment for acute cases. DePalma and Kruper[28] reported 96% good results and only 4% fair results after surgery. The time of recovery after surgery is surprisingly long. In DePalma and Kruper's[28] series, 53% recovered in 2 to 6 weeks, and in an additional 30%, recovery took 5 to 10 weeks. DePalma and Kruper gained the impression that the period of convalescence was longer in patients treated surgically than in conservatively managed persons. The observation of Carnett[21] is of equal interest: the postoperative pain clears up less rapidly in chronic than in acute cases. Our investigations showed that the postoperative symptoms persist for much longer periods than anticipated.[74]

SURGICAL TECHNIQUES

Arthroscopy

Arthroscopy has become a common tool in dealing with pathology in the shoulder. The main indication is not any more a purely diagnostic evaluation, but rather a therapeutic procedure for intra-articular changes or subacromial pathology.[2, 12, 22, 34, 35, 122]

Ark and co-workers[7] reported on their results with 23 patients undergoing arthroscopic surgery after a brief trial of conservative therapy. They felt that the advantages of arthroscopic surgery for calcifying tendinitis are a shorter time of rehabilitation, possibly a better functional result, and improved cosmetic appearance. Fifty per cent of their patients experienced full relief from pain after 26 months, with nine patients having occasional discomfort (41%), and two patients (9%) complaining about persistent pain. The pain relief in the successful group was instant in seven patients and gradual over 3 to 6 months in another four patients. An even higher success rate is reported by Molé and co-workers[80] in a multicenter study conducted by the French Society of Arthroscopy. Eighty-eight per cent of the patients had a complete disappearance of the calcific deposit, and 82 patients were satisfied with the result. There seemed to be a positive correlation between the removal of the calcific deposit and a good result. On the other hand, they could not find any correlation between the result obtained and the age of the patient or the location of the calcification within the tendon. Re and Karzel[103] felt that arthroscopic surgery was ideal for patients who failed to improve on conservative measures. They reported a good success with arthroscopic removal of the calcific deposit. Kempf[59] presented a classification of calcifications into four groups, stating that calcifications that are heterogenous, type D, are rather difficult to deal with because they might have multiple deposits that are very hard to find during either open or arthroscopic surgery.

The answer to the question whether an acromioplasty should always be performed at the time of surgical excision of a calcific deposit remains controversial.[44] Molé and collaborators[80] as well as Re and Karzel[103] reviewed their respective patients and could not demonstrate an improvement in results with an associated acromioplasty. Johnson[55] believed that acromioplasty was indicated only in patients in whom an associated pathology of the subacromial space such as a hooked or beaked acromion was present. The same applies to the exclusive resection of the coracoacromial ligament. His finding confirms the experience gained in subacromial impingement surgery in which no benefit of a simple ligament resection has been seen unless performed in association with an acromioplasty. In patients with a diffuse type D calcification, however, the French group[59, 64] suggests consideration of an acromioplasty, because it seems unlikely to them that removal of the deposit alone would be successful. A concomitant tear of the rotator cuff is a very rare finding.[54, 106] Nevertheless, a proper exploration is always indicated, and if a tear is found, a mini-open or conventional repair might be indicated.

Complications seem to be rare and are mainly reported as insufficient pain relief often secondary to unsuccessful removal of the calcific deposit.[44, 58] Rupture of the rotator cuff may be a sequela.

Authors' Preferred Technique

We consider patients complaining about persistent pain with an obvious calcific deposit candidates for arthroscopic surgery. All of these patients should have had a trial of physical therapy possibly associated with nonsteroidal anti-inflammatory medication, and with rarely more than one subacromial steroid injection.[110] The chief complaint of these patients is a chronic aching type of pain that is accentuated by activity and that occurs at night.

On radiographs most of the calcific deposits are located in the supraspinatus tendon (70%), and a shoulder series consisting of an anterior posterior view in neutral, internal, and external rotation and an axial view as well as a view in the plane of the scapula are obtained. Since ultrasonography (see Fig. 18–23 *A* and *B*) often permits a determination of the site of the deposit, we have reduced this to two anteroposterior views in internal and external rotation and to one view in the plane of the scapula. We consider calcific deposits that are dense and sharply demarcated as ideal, and these deposits should preferably be monolocular and not heterogeneous.

Arthroscopic Technique

The patient is placed in a beach chair position for surgery under general endotracheal anesthesia with an interscalene regional anesthesia in place for postoperative relief of pain. The portals used are placed posterior, anterolateral, and if needed anterolateral and posterolateral.

Initially, the glenohumeral joint is explored through the posterior portal with a 4.5-mm 30-degree tilt arthroscope. A vascular injection pattern of the rotator cuff tendons can occasionally be seen on the articular surface of the tendon, indicating an inflammatory response to the calcific deposit,[139] and this site may then be marked with a suture.

After drainage of the joint the scope is removed and introduced into the subacromial space, where a working cannula is introduced into the subacromial space through the anterolateral portal and the surface of the rotator cuff is palpated. In many cases a bursal leaf might be present requiring a partial resection with a full radius resector. The acromion is then inspected, as well as the coracoacromial ligament and the border of the acromioclavicular joint. The rotator cuff is examined methodically by palpating the cuff for any hardening, which is indicative of a calcific deposit. Needling can be performed, and usually an 18-gauge spinal needle will fill with the calcific material when withdrawn from the tendon. This can be observed through the scope in the subacromial space. Depending on the consistency of the deposit, the calcium might extrude as a paste but usually occurs in small flakes seen in sharply demarcated deposits that constitute the ideal indication for arthroscopic therapy. In some cases, the so-called "snow-storm" appearance might occur. Once the deposit is identified, we prefer to make a longitudinal incision in line with the direction of the fibers with the needle in the superficial part of the rotator cuff, avoiding any deep penetrating cuts. Palpation with the hook will usually then allow one to liberate the calcific deposit, and one is careful not to create a rotator cuff defect by utilizing large curettes or possibly knives and tissue cutters.

Careful irrigation of the subacromial space is then performed, because the calcific debris can act as an irritating agent in the subacromial bursa. Subacromial decompression is performed only if an associated pathology is present, such as an obvious acromial beak or signs of subacromial impingement, the same being true for associated acromioclavicular joint pathology with osteophytes.

Once the subacromial space has been drained, one may consider a reinspection of the glenohumeral joint to ensure that no rotator cuff rupture has occurred. Otherwise, the instruments are removed and the portal holes are closed with a skin suture after a Hemovac drain has been placed in the subacromial space.

Postoperative management consists of range-of-motion exercises 24 hours after the drain has been removed postoperatively. The exercises start with pendular exercises, then active-assisted exercises are begun after the third day and progress to active exercises as tolerated by the patient. Usually no arm sling is necessary, except for patient comfort at night.

Open Procedures

Discussing the surgical technique, Gschwend and colleagues[46, 47] recommend a muscle-splitting approach but warn against a deltoid detachment. They are in favor of a resection of the coracoacromial ligament. Vebostad[135] could not find an improvement in results when he added a partial resection of the acromion which, according to his description, seems to have consisted of an anterior acromioplasty. Occasionally, serial vertical tendon incisions become necessary when the deposit is not readily identifiable. Resch[105] recommends that an acromioplasty be performed in cases with radiologic or arthroscopic changes only. This recommendation is based on a series of 43 patients. In 1975, Vebostad[135] reported results of an isolated subtotal acromionectomy performed in five patients in whom the deposit could not be easily found during surgery. He obtained good and excellent relief of symptoms in four patients. Goutallier and colleagues[44] recommended an isolated anterior acromioplasty without removal of the calcium deposit in instances of "heterogeneous calcifications which infiltrate the tendon." Most of the 19 calcifications disappeared during the first postoperative year.

After surgery, early mobilization is recommended. If a sling is worn, it must be removed at regular intervals for exercises.

Authors' Preferred Method of Treatment

Our therapeutic approach is based mainly on the severity of symptoms. Of course, the radiologic aspect of the deposit will also be taken into consideration (Fig. 18–24).

Since it is our firm belief that symptoms during the formative phase are chronic or even absent and that the acute symptoms accompany the process of resorption, we will first state our management during the formative phase. Patients with subacute symptoms are classified as belonging to the formative phase unless the radiographs show evident signs of resorption.

SYMPTOM	THERAPY	EFFECTS
CHRONIC PAIN	CONSERVATIVE AVOID CORTISONE SURGERY, IF UNSUCCESSFUL AND IF INTERFERENCE WITH WORK AND ADL	MAINTENANCE OF ROM AND OF STRENGTH
ACUTE PAIN	NEEDLING AND LAVAGE SINGLE CORTISONE INJECTION PENDULUM AND ROM EXERCISES	DECOMPRESSION HYPEREMIA ↓ PHAGOCYTOSIS ↓ AVOIDANCE OF FROZEN SHOULDER
SUBSIDING PAIN	REST IN ABDUCTION ROM AND STRENGTHENING EXERCISES AVOID CORTISONE	RELIEVE STRETCH PRESSURE ↓ BLOOD FLOW ↑ AVOIDANCE OF FROZEN SHOULDER AND OF MUSCLE WEAKNESS

Figure 18–24

Outline of the treatment approach (ROM, range of motion).

FORMATIVE PHASE

During the formative phase, we favor a conservative approach. Surgical removal is the exception and is done only when an adequate conservative approach has failed and when the symptoms interfere with either work or the activity of daily living.

Conservative Measures

The patient is instructed to do a daily program of exercises to maintain the full mobility of the glenohumeral joint. We also instruct the patient to position the arm in abduction as often as possible. This can be achieved by placing the arm on the backrest of a chair or on a seat beside the patient. While lying down, a pillow should be placed in the axilla. Application of moist heat is also suggested if the symptoms are subacute. Diathermy may be included. Although ultrasound is used occasionally in our physiotherapy department and some patients have commented on its beneficial effect, we have seen no evidence that this treatment modality accelerates the disappearance of calcium deposits.

Local intrabursal corticosteroid injections are never done in the presence of chronic symptoms. Only in the presence of impingement causing subacute symptoms do we give one intrabursal corticosteroid injection mixed with lidocaine. Needling of dense, homogeneous deposits has never been attempted. Attempts at lavage have not been successful in our hands. This is not surprising, given the chalk-like consistency of the deposit.

Nonsteroidal anti-inflammatory drugs are not prescribed when the symptoms are chronic but are given for 1 week to 10 days when subacute symptoms are present. Analgesics are rarely indicated.

Patients are assessed clinically and radiologically every 4 weeks. In cases where the outcome of conservative treatment is not satisfactory and the patient meets our criteria for surgical intervention, the indication is discussed with the patient. If the patient consents, the removal of the calcium deposit is done on a short-stay basis in the hospital. A history and physical examination as well as all laboratory tests and radiographs (chest and affected shoulder) are taken 1 week before surgery. On the day of surgery, the patient is admitted to our short-stay unit and discharged the same day after surgery. Before being discharged, the patient will be seen by the physiotherapist to ensure that a proper postoperative exercise program is followed.

Surgical Technique

Removal of calcium deposits is done under general anesthesia. The patient is in a supine position, and a sandbag is placed under the affected shoulder. We make sure that the side of the patient to be operated on is as close to the edge of the table as possible. The arm is free-draped to ensure full mobilization of the arm during surgery. We use the skin incision recommended by Neer,[87] going from the acromion to the coracoid process. The deltoid fibers are bluntly separated. A stitch to protect the axillary nerve in the distal part near the deltoid splitting has not been found necessary. The deltoid muscle is not detached from the acromion. The bursa is then opened, and the edges are retracted with Army-Navy retractors. The bursal wall is inspected. The coracoacromial ligament is then identified and cleaned of all overlying soft tissues. Care is taken to visualize the posterior edge of the ligament. The state of the ligament is recorded. We have never observed a thickening, although it was described by Watson.[136] The narrowness of the interval between the rotator cuff and the ligament is then tested, usually using the little finger. Introduction of this finger is made easier through longitudinal traction of the arm. While the finger is in place, the arm is rotated and lifted in position between flexion and abduction. The undersurface of the acromion is also palpated. If the space between the ligament and the rotator cuff is "tight," it is usually necessary to proceed with an anterior acromioplasty, although this procedure is definitely an exception. An anterior acromioplasty makes the inspection of the rotator cuff and its covering bursal wall easy. External and internal rotation of the arm will permit inspection of the entire rotator cuff. If a bursal reaction is present, its localization and extent are recorded. It is usually limited to a hyperemic reaction around the calcific deposit, which shines through the bursal wall. The tendon is then incised in the direction of its fibers, and the calcific mass is curetted. We proceed then with a limited resection of the frayed tendon edges, which are usually sites of calcium encrustation. Sometimes more than one deposit is present, necessitating separate tendon incisions. A proper preoperative radiograph is very important to determine not only the location but also the number of deposits. If no calcium can be seen during inspection, small incisions are made at the site of suspected calcifications as determined by radiography.

After the deposit has been removed, a copious lavage is done. The shoulder is moved through its full range of motion; the tendon edges are approximated if necessary; and the wound is closed in layers. A sling is applied after surgery. We hasten again to add that this sling must be removed at least four times a day for pendulum and gentle passive range-of-motion exercises. The sling is removed completely after 3 days, and active exercises are started. We encourage patients to keep the arm in abduction as often as possible. If the postoperative pain is severe, local ice packs should be applied. We have never resorted to postoperative corticosteroid injections.

RESORPTIVE PHASE

Injection Technique

During the phase of resorption when the symptoms are acute or in the presence of subacute symptoms when radiographs indicate ongoing resorption, we attempt a lavage of the deposit using two 18-gauge needles. A local anesthetic (lidocaine 2% without epinephrine) is used to freeze the sites of needle placement, and 5 ml are injected into the bursa. The site of lavage is based on the site of tenderness and on radiographic localization. Lidocaine 2% is also used for lavage. In the outflow, calcium particles can easily be recognized. If the lavage is not successful, the needling usually helps to decrease the intratendinous pressure. At the end of lavage or needling, we only proceed with an intrabursal corticosteroid injection when the pain is excruciating. This injection will not be repeated.

The patient is instructed to apply ice and to do pendulum exercises. Analgesics are prescribed. Although we always instruct the patient to take nonsteroidal anti-inflammatory drugs for 1 week, we have no absolute proof of their beneficial effect. After the first treatment, the patient will be asked to report back 3 or 4 days later. As soon as the symptoms decrease, usually after 1 week, the patient is referred to physiotherapy for range-of-motion and strengthening exercises. Radiographs are taken 4 weeks after the first visit. They almost always show a considerable decrease in, if not disappearance of, the deposit. Ultrasound has not been used by us during the resorptive phase.

We have not observed a single case of frozen shoulder or adhesive capsulitis in patients treated in this fashion. One case with this syndrome, however, was seen in consultation. This patient had been treated with systemic corticosteroid medication and a sling for 6 weeks.

INDICATION FOR SURGERY

Although at the beginning of our intensive involvement with calcifying tendinitis we have operated during the acute phase, we feel now that surgery is not indicated at a time when nature attempts, and usually succeeds with, removal of the calcific deposit. This approach has already been advocated in 1970 by De Sèze and Welfling,[30] who stated that in the hyperalgic phase, the disease heals in general easily with supportive measures only.

CONCLUSION

The success of management of patients with calcifying tendinitis depends on a thorough understanding of the disease process. Obviously, formation of the deposit must precede its resorption. Moreover, clinical observations leave no doubt that spontaneous resorption usually takes place, the moment of the onset of resorption being the only question.

Factors responsible for the fibrocartilaginous metaplasia and ensuing calcification, as well as those triggering the resorptive process, are far from being known. Their elucidation should be the goal of future research.

Experimental reproduction of localized tendon calcification has not been too successful. Attempts were made at the level of the rotator cuff, using a plastic mold under the supraspinatus. This foreign body as well as the surgical trauma never led to changes compatible with calcifying tendinitis. Selye[119] published results obtained with his calciphylaxis model, which led to tendon calcification in only one strain of mice. However, there is no question that calciphylaxis constitutes a systemic metabolic disease and not a localized disease process. We have had the opportunity to examine specimens of tendon and ligament calcification of inbred tiptoe-walking Yoshimura (TWY) mice from the Japanese Research Council. The sections showed cartilaginous metaplasia in ligaments and tendons followed by calcification around chondrocytes.

References and Bibliography

1. Ali SY: Crystal induced arthropathy. *In* Verbruggen G and Veys EM (eds): Degenerative Joints, Vol 2. New York: Elsevier, 1985.
2. Altcheck DW, Warren RF, Wickiewicz TL, et al: Arthroscopic acromioplasty. J Bone Joint Surg *72-A*:1198–1207, 1990.
3. Anderson HC: Electron microscopic studies of induced cartilage development and calcification. J Cell Biol *35*:81–101, 1967.
4. Anderson HC: Vesicles associated with calcification in the matrix of epiphyseal cartilage. J Cell Biol *41*:59–72, 1969.
5. Anderson HC: Calcific diseases. Arch Pathol Lab Med *107*:341–348, 1983.
6. Archer RS, Bayley JI, Archer CW, and Ali SY: Cell and matrix changes associated with pathological calcification of the human rotator cuff tendons. J Anat *182*:1–11, 1993.
7. Ark JW, Flock TJ, Flatow EL, and Bigliani LU: Arthroscopic treatment of calcific tendinitis of the shoulder. J Arthroscopic Relat Surg 8:183–188, 1992.
8. Baer WS: The operative treatment of subdeltoid bursitis. Johns Hopkins Hosp Bull *18*:282–284, 1907.
9. Baird LW: Roentgen irradiation of calcareous deposits about the shoulder. Radiology *37*:316–324, 1941.
10. Bateman JE: The Shoulder and Neck. Philadelphia: WB Saunders, 1978.
11. Bergemann D and Stieda A: Über die mit Kalkablagerungen einhergehende Entzündung der Schulterschleimbeutel. Münch Med Wschr 52:2699–2702, 1908.
12. Bigliani LU, Morrison DS, and April EW: The morphology of the acromion and its relationship to rotator cuff tears. Orthop Trans *10*:228, 1986.
13. Bonucci E: Fine structure and histochemistry of "calcifying globules" in epiphyseal cartilage. Z Zellforsch *103*:192–217, 1970.
14. Booth RE Jr and Marvel JP Jr: Differential diagnosis of shoulder pain. Orthop Clin North Am 6:353–379, 1975.
15. Bosworth BM: Calcium deposits in the shoulder and subacromial bursitis: A survey of 12,122 shoulders. JAMA *116*:2477–2482, 1941.
16. Bosworth BM: Examination of the shoulder for calcium deposits. J Bone Joint Surg 23:567–577, 1941.
17. Brenckmann E and Nadaud P: Le traitement des calcifications périarticulaires de l'épaule par radio thérapie. Arch d'Electric Med *40*:27–29, 1932.
18. Brewer BJ: Aging of the rotator cuff. Am J Sports Med 7:102–110, 1979.
19. Brickner WM: Shoulder disability: Stiff and painful shoulder. Am J Surg *26*:196–204, 1912.
20. Brooks CH, Revell WJ, and Heatley FW: A quantitative histological study of the vascularity of the rotator cuff tendon. J Bone Joint Surg *74-B*:151–153, 1992.
21. Carnett JB: The calcareous deposits of so-called calcifying subacromial bursitis. Surg Gynecol Obstet *41*:404–421, 1925.

22. Caspari RB and Thal R: A technique for arthroscopic subacromial decompression. Arthroscopy 8:23, 1992.
23. Chapman JF: Subacromial bursitis and supraspinatus tendinitis: its roentgen treatment. Calif Med *56*:248–251, 1942.
24. Codman EA: On stiff and painful shoulders. Boston Med Surg J *154*:613–620, 1906.
25. Codman EA: Bursitis subacromialis, or periarthritis of the shoulder joint. Publications of the Mass Gen Hospital in Boston *2*:521–591, 1909.
26. Codman EA: The Shoulder. Boston: Thomas Todd, 1934.
27. Crass JR: Current concepts in the radiographic evaluation of the rotator cuff. Crit Rev Diagn Imaging *28*:23–73, 1988.
28. DePalma AF and Kruper JS: Long term study of shoulder joints afflicted with and treated for calcific tendinitis. Clin Orthop *20*:61–72, 1961.
29. DePalma A: Surgery of the Shoulder, 2nd ed. Philadelphia: JB Lippincott, 1973.
30. De Sèze S and Welfling J: Tendinites calcifiantes. Rhumatologie *22*:5–14, 1970.
31. Dhuly RG, Lauler DP, and Thorn GW: Pharmacology and chemistry of adrenal glucocorticosteroids. Med Clin North Am *57*:1155–1165, 1973.
32. Dieppe P: Crystal deposition disease and the soft tissues. Clin Rheum Dis 5:807–822, 1979.
33. Duplay S: De la périarthrite scapulohumérale et des raideurs de l'épaule qui en sont la conséquence. Arch Gen Med *513*:542, 1872.
34. Ellman H: Arthroscopic subacromial decompression: Analysis of one- to three year results. Arthroscopy 3:173–181, 1987.
35. Ellman H: Shoulder arthroscopy: Current indications and techniques. Orthopaedics *11*:45–51, 1988.
36. Ellman H: The Controversy of Arthroscopic vs. Open Approaches to Shoulder Instability and Rotator Cuff Disease. Fourth open meeting of the American Society of Shoulder and Elbow Surgeons. American Academy of Orthopaedic Surgeons, Atlanta, Georgia, 1988 Symposium.
37. Farin PU and Jaroma H: Sonographic findings of rotator cuff calcifications. J Ultrasound Med *14*:7–14, 1995.
38. Faure G and Daculsi G: Calcified tendinitis: A review. Ann Rheum Dis 42(Suppl) 49–53, 1983.
39. Faure G, Netter P, Malaman B, et al: Scanning electron microscopic study of microcrystals implicated in human rheumatic diseases. Scanning Electron Microsc 3:163–176, 1980.
40. Friedman MS: Calcified tendinitis of the shoulder. Am J Surg *94*:56–61, 1957.
41. Gärtner J: Tendinosis calcarea—Behandlungsergebnisse mit dem Needling. Z Orthop Ihre Grenzgeb *313*:461–469, 1993.
42. Ghormley JW: Calcareous tendinitis. Surg Clin North Am *4*:1721–1728, 1961.
43. Glatthaar E: Zur Pathologie der Periarthritis humeroscapularis. Dtsch Z Chir *251*:414–434, 1938.
44. Goutallier D, Duparc F, and Allain J: Treatment of Calcific Tendinopathies Through a Simple Acromioplasty. European Symposium of Shoulder, St. Etienne, France, 26–28 April 1996, pp 205–206.
45. Griffin EJ and Karselis TC: Physical agents for physical therapists. *In* Ultrasonic Energy, 2nd ed. Springfield, IL: Charles C Thomas, 1982.
46. Gschwend N, Patte D, and Zippel J: Die Therapie der Tendinitis calcarea des Schultergelenkes. Arch Orthop Unfallchir *73*:120–135, 1972.
47. Gschwend N, Scherer M, and Lohr J: Die Tendinitis calcarea des Schultergelenks. Orthopade *10*:196–205, 1981.
48. Halverson PB, McCarty DJ, Cheung HS, and Ryan LM: Milwaukee shoulder syndrome. Ann Rheum Dis *43*:734–741, 1984.
49. Harbin M: Deposition of calcium salts in tendon of supraspinatus muscle. Arch Surg *18*:1491–1512, 1929.
50. Harmon HP: Methods and results in the treatment of 2580 painful shoulders. With special reference to calcific tendinitis and the frozen shoulder. Am J Surg 95:527–544, 1958.
51. Hartig A and Huth F: Neue Aspekte zur Morphologie und Therapie der Tendinosis calacarea der Schultergelenke. Arthroskopie 8:117–122, 1995.
52. Herberts P, Kadefors R, Hogfors C, and Sigholm G: Shoulder pain and heavy manual labor. Clin Orthop *191*:166–178, 1984.
53. Howorth MB: Calcification of the tendon cuff of the shoulder. Surg Gynecol Obstet *80*:337–345, 1945.
54. Hsu HC, Wu JJ, Jim YF, et al: Calcific tendinitis and rotator cuff tearing: A clinical and radiographic study. J Shoulder Elbow Surg *3*:159–164, 1994.
55. Johnson LL: The subacromial space and rotator cuff lesions. *In* Johnson LL (ed): Diagnostic and Surgical Arthroscopy of the Shoulder. St. Louis-Baltimore: CV Mosby, 1993, pp 377–380.
56. Jones GB: Calcification of the supraspinatus tendon. J Bone Joint Surg *31-B*:433–435, 1949.
57. Jozsa L, Baliut BJ, and Reffy A: Calcifying tendinopathy. Arch Orthop Trauma Surg *97*:305–307, 1980.
58. Kempf JF: Arthroscopie de l'épaule. J Chir (Paris) *129*:271–275, 1992.
59. Kempf JF: Arthroscopic Treatment of Rotator Cuff Calcifications by Isolated Excision. European Symposium of Shoulder, St. Etienne, France, 26–28 April 1996, pp 206–209.
60. Kessel L and Watson M: The painful arc syndrome. J Bone Joint Surg *59-B*:166–172, 1977.
61. Key LA: Calcium deposits in the vicinity of the shoulder and other joints. Ann Surg *129*:737–753, 1949.
62. Kozin F: Painful shoulder and the reflex sympathetic dystrophy syndrome. *In* McCarty DJ (ed): Arthritis and Allied Conditions, 10th ed. Philadelphia: Lea & Febiger, 1985.
63. Lapidus PW: Infiltration therapy of acute tendinitis with calcification. Surg Gynecol Obstet *76*:715–725, 1943.
64. Levigne C: Are There Indications for Adjunct Acromioplasty in the Arthroscopic Treatment of Rotator Cuff Calcifications? European Symposium of Shoulder, St. Etienne-France, 26–28 April 1996, pp 208–209.
65. Lippmann RK: Observations concerning the calcific cuff deposit. Clin Orthop *20*:49–60, 1961.
66. Litchman HM, Silver CM, Simon SD, and Eshragi A: The surgical management of calcific tendinitis of the shoulder. Int Surg *50*:474–482, 1968.
67. Loew M and Jurgowski W: Initial experiences with extracorporeal shockwave lithotripsy (ESWL) in treatment of tendinosis calcarea of the shoulder. Z Orthop Ihre Grenzgeb *131*:470–473, 1993.
68. Loew M, Jurgowski W, Mau HC, and Thomsom M: Treatment of calcifying tendinitis of the rotator cuff with extracorporeal shock waves: A preliminary report. J Shoulder Elbow Surg *4*:101–106, 1995.
69. Loew M, Sabo D, Mau H, et al: MR Imaging of the Rotator Cuff with Calcifying Tendinitis. 6th International Congress on Surgery of the Shoulder (ICSS), Helsinki, Finland, June 1995, Abstract FH 060.
70. Lohr JF and Uhthoff HK: The microvascular pattern of the supraspinatus tendon. Clin Orthop *254*:35–38, 1990.
71. Lundberg J: The frozen shoulder. Acta Orthop Scand *119*:(Suppl):1–59, 1969.
72. Macnab I: Rotator cuff tendinitis. Ann R Coll Surg *53*:271–287, 1973.
73. McCarty DJ, Halverson PB, Carrera GF, et al: "Milwaukee Shoulder": Association of microspheroids containing hydroxyapatite crystals, active collagenase, and neutral protease with rotator cuff defects. I. Clinical aspects. Arthritis Rheum *24*:464–473, 1981.
74. McKendry RJR, Uhthoff HK, Sarkar K, and St George-Hyslop P: Calcifying tendinitis of the shoulder: Prognostic value of clinical, histologic and radiologic features in 57 surgically treated cases. Rheumatology 9:75–80, 1982.
75. McLaughlin HL: Lesions of the musculotendinous cuff of the shoulder. III. Observations on the pathology, course and treatment of calcific deposits. Ann Surg *124*:354–362, 1946.
76. McLaughlin HL: Selection of calcium deposits for operation—the technique and results of operation. Surg Clin North Am *43*:1501–1504, 1963.
77. Meyer AW: Chronic functional lesions of the shoulder. Arch Surg *35*:646–674, 1937.
78. Milone FP and Copeland MM: Calcific tendinitis of the shoulder joint. AJR Am J Roentgenol *85*:901–913, 1961.
79. Mohr W and Bilger S: Morphologische Grundstrukturen der kalzifizierten Tendopathie und ihre Bedeutung für die Pathogenese. Z Rheumal *49*:346–355, 1990.
80. Molé D, Kempf JF, Gleyze P, et al: Résultats du traitement arthroscopique des tendinopathies non-rompues de la coiffe des rotateurs. 2. Calcifications de la coiffe. Rev Chir Orthop Reparative Appat Mot *79*:532–541, 1993.

81. Moschkowitz E: Histopathology of calcification of the spinatus tendons associated with subacromial bursitis. Am J Med Sci *149*:351–361, 1915.
82. Moseley HF: Shoulder Lesions, 3rd ed. Edinburgh: Churchill Livingstone, 1960.
83. Moseley HF: The natural history and clinical syndromes produced by calcified deposits in the rotator cuff. Surg Clin North Am *43*:1489–1494, 1963.
84. Moseley HF: The results of nonoperative and operative treatment of calcified deposits. Surg Clin North Am *43*:1505–1506, 1963.
85. Moseley HF and Goldie I: The arterial pattern of the rotator cuff of the shoulder. J Bone Joint Surg *45-B*:780–789, 1963.
86. Murnaghan GF and McIntosh D: Hydrocortisone in painful shoulder. Controlled trial. Lancet *21*:798–800, 1955.
87. Neer CS II: Impingement lesions. Clin Orthop *173*:70–77, 1983.
88. Neer CS II, Craig EV, and Fukuda H: Cuff-tear arthropathy. J Bone Joint Surg *65-A*:1232–1244, 1983.
89. Nutton RW and Stothard J: Acute calcific supraspinatus tendinitis in a three year old child. J Bone Joint Surg *69-B*:148, 1987.
90. Ollagnier E, Bruyère G, Gazielly DF, and Thomas TH: Medical treatment of calcifying tendinopathies of the rotator cuff. European Symposium of Shoulder, St. Etienne, France, 26–28 April 1996, p 202.
91. Olsson O: Degenerative changes of the shoulder and their connection with shoulder pain. Acta Chir Scand *181*(Suppl):1–110, 1953.
92. Ozaki J, Fuijimoto S, Nakagawa Y, et al: Tears of the rotator cuff of the shoulder associated with pathological changes in the acromion. J Bone Joint Surg *70-A*:1224–1230, 1988.
93. Painter CF: Subdeltoid bursitis. Boston Med Surg J *156*:345–349, 1907.
94. Patte D and Goutallier D: Calcifications. Rev Chir Orthop *74*:277–278, 1988.
95. Patterson RL and Darrach W: Treatment of acute bursitis by needle irrigation. J Bone Joint Surg *19*:993–1002, 1937.
96. Pedersen HE and Key JA: Pathology of calcareous tendinitis and subdeltoid bursitis. Arch Surg *62*:50–63, 1951.
97. Pendergrass EP and Hodes PJ: Roentgen irradiation in treatment of inflammations. AJR Am J Roentgenol *45*:74–106, 1941.
98. Perugia L and Postacchini F: The pathology of the rotator cuff of the shoulder. Ital J Orthop Haematol *11*:93–105, 1985.
99. Pfister J and Gerber H: Behandlung der Periarthropathia humeroscapularis calcarea mittels Schulterkalkspülung: retrospektive Fragebogenanalyse. Z Orthop Ihre Grenzgeb *132*:300–305, 1994.
100. Pinals RS and Short CL: Calcific periarthritis involving multiple sites. Arthritis Rheum *9*:566–574, 1966.
101. Plenk HP: Calcifying tendinitis of the shoulder. Radiology *59*:384–389, 1952.
102. Rathbun JB and Macnab J: The microvascular pattern of the rotator cuff. J Bone Joint Surg *52-B*:540–553, 1970.
103. Re LP Jr and Karzel RP: Management of rotator cuff calcifications. Orthop Clin North Am *24*:125–132, 1993.
104. Remberger K, Faust H, and Keyl W: Tendinitis calcarea. Klinik, Morphologie, Pathogenese und Differentialdiagnose. Pathologe *6*:196–203, 1985.
105. Resch H: Calcific Tendinitis. European Symposium of Shoulder, St. Etienne, France, 26–28 April 1996, p 210.
106. Resch H and Beck E: Arthroskopie der Schulter. Berlin-Heidelberg-New York, Springer Verlag, 1991, pp 147–152.
107. Rompe JD, Rumler F, Hopf C, et al: Extracorporeal shock wave therapy for calcifying tendinitis of the shoulder. Clin Orthop *321*:196–201, 1995.
108. Rothman RH, Marvel JP Jr, and Heppenstall RB: Anatomic considerations in the glenohumeral joint. Orthop Clin North Am *6*:341–352, 1975.
109. Rothman RH and Parke WW: The vascular anatomy of the rotator cuff. Clin Orthop *41*:176–186, 1965.
110. Rowe CR: Injection technique for the shoulder and elbow. Orthop Clin North Am *19*:773–777, 1988.
111. Rüttimann G: Uber die Hüfigkeit röntgenologischer Veränderungen bei Patienten mit typischer Periarthritis humeroscapularis und Schultergesunden. Inaugural dissertation, Zurich, 1959.
112. Sandström C: Peritendinitis calcarea: Common disease of middle life: its diagnosis, pathology and treatment. AJR Am J Roentgenol *40*:1–21, 1938.
113. Sandström C and Wahlgren F: Beitrag zur Kenntnis der "Peritendinitis calcarea" (sog. "Bursitis calculosa") speziell vom pathologisch-histologischen Gesichtspunkt. Acta Radiol [Stockh] *18*:263–296, 1937.
114. Sarkar K and Uhthoff HK: Ultrastructural localization of calcium in calcifying tendinitis. Arch Pathol Lab Med *102*:266–269, 1978.
115. Sarkar K and Uhthoff HK: Ultrastructure of the subacromial bursa in painful shoulder syndromes. Virchows Arch *400*:107–117, 1983.
116. Schaer H: Die Duplay'sche Krankheit. Med Klin *35*:413–415, 1939.
117. Schaer H: Die Periarthritis humeroscapularis. Ergebn Chir Orthop *29*:211–309, 1936.
118. Seifert G: Morphologic and biochemical aspects of experimental extraosseous tissue calcification. Clin Orthop *69*:146, 1970.
119. Selye H: The experimental production of calcific deposits in the rotator cuff. Surg Clin North Am *43*:1483–1488, 1963.
120. Sengar DPS, McKendry RJ, and Uhthoff HK: Increased frequency of HLA-A1 in calcifying tendinitis. Tissue Antigens *29*:173–174, 1987.
121. Simon WH: Soft tissue disorders of the shoulder. Frozen shoulder, calcific tendinitis, and bicipital tendinitis. Orthop Clin North Am *6*:521–539, 1975.
122. Snyder SJ: Arthroscopic evaluation and treatment of the rotator cuff. *In* Snyder SJ (ed): Shoulder Arthroscopy. New York, McGraw-Hill, 1993.
123. Steinbrocker O: The painful shoulder. *In* Hollander JE (ed): Arthritis and Allied Conditions, 8th ed. Philadelphia: Lea & Febiger, 1972.
124. Stieda A: Zur Pathologie der Schultergelenkschleimbeutel. Arch Klin Chir *85*:910–924, 1908.
125. Thornhill TS: The painful shoulder. *In* Kelley WN, Harris ED, Shaun R, and Sledge CB (eds): Textbook of Rheumatology, 2nd ed. Philadelphia: WB Saunders, 1985.
126. Tillmann B: Rotatorenmanschettenrupturen. Operative Orthopädie und Traumatologie *4*:181–184, 1992.
127. Toriyama K, Fukuda H, Hamada K, and Noguchi T: Calcifying tendinitis of the infraspinatus tendon simulating a bone tumor. J Shoulder Elbow Surg *3*:165–168, 1994.
128. Uhthoff HK: Calcifying tendinitis, an active cell-mediated calcification. Virchows Arch *366*:51–58, 1975.
129. Uhthoff HK, Hammond DI, Sarkar K, et al: The role of the coracoacromial ligament in the impingement syndrome: A clinical, radiological and histological study. Int Orthop *12*:97–104, 1988.
130. Uhthoff HK, Loehr J, and Sarkar K: The pathogenesis of rotator cuff tears. *In* Takagishi N (ed): The Shoulder. Tokyo: Professional Postgraduate Services, 1986, pp 211–212.
131. Uhthoff HK, Sarkar K, and Maynard JA: Calcifying tendinitis. Clin Orthop *118*:164–168, 1976.
132. Uhthoff HK, Lohr J, Hammond I, and Sarkar K: Aetiologie und Pathogenese von Rupturen der Rotatorenmanschette. *In* Helbig B and Blauth W (eds): Schulterschmerzen und Rupturen der Rotatorenmanschette. Berlin: Springer-Verlag, 1986, pp 3–9.
133. Uhthoff HK and Sarkar K: Tendopathia Calcificans. Beitr Orthop Traumat *28*:269–277, 1981.
134. Uhthoff HK, Sarkar K, and Hammond I: Die Bedeutung der Dichte und der Schärfe der Abgrenzung des Kalkschattens bei der Tendinopathia calcificans. Radiologe *22*:170–174, 1982.
135. Vebostad A: Calcific tendinitis in the shoulder region: A review of 43 operated shoulders. Acta Orthop Scand *46*:205–210, 1975.
136. Watson M: The impingement syndrome in sportsmen. *In* Bateman JE and Welsh RP (eds): Surgery of the Shoulder. Philadelphia: BC Decker, 1984, pp 140–142.
137. Welfling J, Kahn MF, Desroy M, et al: Les calcifications de l'épaule. II. La maladie des calcifications tendineuses multiples. Rev Rheum *32*:325–334, 1965.
138. Wilson CL: Lesions of the supraspinatus tendon: Degeneration, rupture and calcification. Arch Surg *46*:307–325, 1943.
139. Wolf WB: Shoulder tendinoses. Clin Sports Med *11*:871–890, 1992.
140. Wolfgang GL: Surgical repairs of the rotator cuff of the shoulder. J Bone Joint Surg *56-A*:14–26, 1974.
141. Wrede L: Über Kalkablagerungen in der Umgebung des Schultergelenkes und ihre Beziehungen zur Periarthritis humeroscapularis. Langenbecks Arch Chir *99*:259–272, 1912.
142. Young BR: Roentgen treatment for bursitis of shoulder. AJR Am J Roentgenol *56*:626–630, 1946.

W.Z. (Biceps Buzzy) BURKHEAD, JR., M.D.
MICHEL A. ARCAND, M.D.
CRAIG ZEMAN, M.D.
PETER HABERMEYER, M.D.
GILLES WALCH, M.D.

CHAPTER

19

The Biceps Tendon

"Charlie Neer's never seen biceps tendinitis. Frank Jobe's never seen biceps tendinitis. I've never seen biceps tendinitis. You've been here from Dallas for 24 hours and you've seen a case of biceps tendinitis? I'm going to find you a dermatology residency at Duke and send you there on a bus!!! . . . or better still, I'm going to request that you contribute a chapter entitled 'The Biceps Tendon' for our new two-volume set entitled 'The Shoulder.'

CAR TO WZB
July 2, 1983, 1:15 p.m.
Audie Murphy VA

The day I thought my career ended.

The long head of the biceps brachii is the proverbial stepchild of the shoulder. It has been blamed for numerous painful conditions of the shoulder from arthritis to adhesive capsulitis. Kessell[129] described the tendon as "somewhat of a maverick, easy to inculpate but difficult to condemn." Lippmann[141] likened the long head of the biceps to the appendix: "An unimportant vestigial structure unless something goes wrong with it." Throughout time this tendon has been tenodesed, translocated, pulled through drill holes in the humeral head, and débrided with an arthroscope, often with marginal results.

Neer and Rockwood have, in the past, emphasized that 95 to 98% of patients with a diagnosis of biceps tendinitis have, in reality, a primary diagnosis of impingement syndrome with secondary involvement of the biceps tendon. They have condemned routine biceps tenodesis. Routine exposure of the biceps by the French surgeon, Patte, as well as arthroscopy, shed a new light on the pathophysiology of the long biceps tendon.[100] The advent of magnetic resonance imaging (MRI) used for diagnostic purposes around the shoulder allows clinicians to visualize this tendon through a noninvasive imaging modality. These new techniques have provided fundamental insight into shoulder pathology, which in turn has yielded important implications in the treatment of lesions of the long head of the biceps tendon.

A historical perspective of the treatment of lesions of the biceps tendon is presented in this chapter. The authors review the pertinent anatomy of the long head of the biceps tendon, attempt to explain the function of this tendon, and present a review of current concepts on the etiology, diagnosis, and management of these lesions.

HISTORICAL REVIEW

Hippocrates[110] was the first to call attention to the possibility of pathologic displacement of muscle and tendons in dislocations. Accurate depictions of the anatomy of the biceps region and intertubercular groove appeared in the 1400s (Fig. 19–1*A*). Traumatic injuries to the bicipital region are depicted in a German wound manikin in the 1500s (see Fig. 19–1*B*).

The first reported case of dislocation of the tendon of the long head of the biceps brachii muscle was in 1694 by Cowper in a book entitled *Myotoma Reformata*.[55] In his case, a woman who was wringing clothes felt something displace in her shoulder. Three days after the injury Cowper examined her and noticed a depression of the external part of the deltoid, accompanied by rigidity in the lower biceps and an inability to extend the forearm. The tendon was reduced by manipulation, and the patient immediately recovered the use of the arm. This miraculous recovery is seldom seen in practice. Recognition of this injury was accepted by Boerhaave and Bromfield.[30] Cowper's observation became subject to suspicion, however, because of his plagiarism of the Dutch anatomist Bidloo.[25] Before Cowper's description, most reported cases of biceps injury were undoubtedly a result of direct trauma, most likely as depicted in Figure 19–1*B*.

In 1803, Monteggia[179] reported a second case resembling that reported by Cowper, except that the dislocation was habitual. From that time until 1910, numerous additional clinical reports appeared.[97, 101, 212, 224, 225] It was not until 1841 that Soden[243] reported a case of biceps dislocation that was clinically proven at necropsy. Hueter[116] described clearly the signs and symptoms of lesions of this tendon.

However, there was a controversy. Jarjavey,[122] discussing cases in 1867, believed that most of the symptoms were related to subacromial bursitis and that simple luxa-

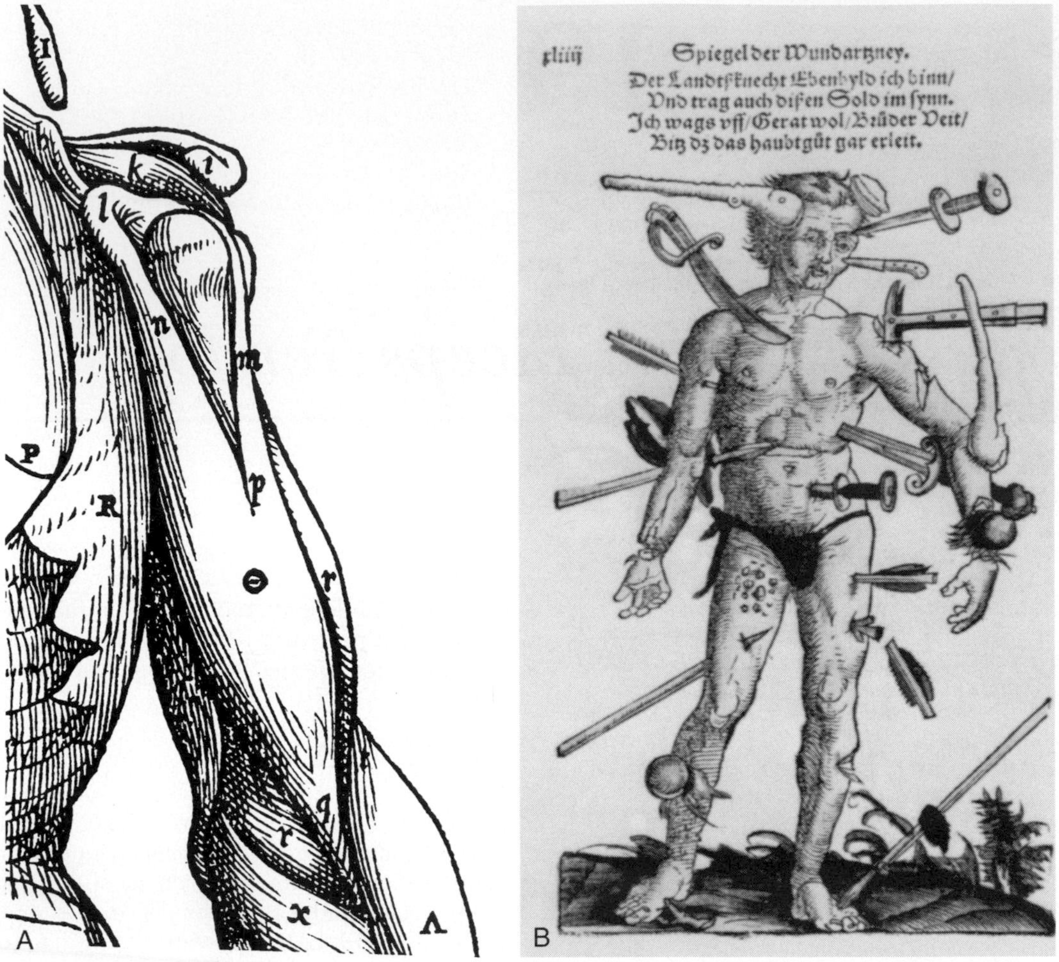

Figure 19–1

A, Close-up of the three tendons of the biceps brachii: short head (N), long head (M), and distal tendon (Q). (From the Sixth Plate of Muscles. Possibly by Jan Stevenz van Calcar [Flemish ca. 1499–1550]. From Vesalius A: De Humani Corporis Fabrica. Basel: Johames Oporinus, 1543.) *B*, Probable mechanism of injury to the biceps prior to Cowper's description. Notice the saber type of incision in the opposite shoulder. (Anonymous wound manikin, 1517. From von Gersdorff H: Feldthbuch der Wundartzney. Strasbourg: Hans Schotten, 1540. Reprinted with permission from Karp D: ARS Medica: Art, Medicine, and the Human Condition. Philadelphia, Copyright © 1985, the University of Pennsylvania Press.)

tion did not exist. Some authors[12, 30] believed that the lesion was secondary to arthritis or to concomitant problems. Callender[33] mentioned one case of recurrent dislocation in which the tendon could not be retained in the groove because of fibrous tissue. Duplay described "periarthrite scapulo-humerale."[66–68] It is evident from his work that this included tendinitis of the biceps.

McClellan[156] discussed the function of the biceps tendon:

Furthermore, the long tendon of the biceps muscle, which is lodged below the tuberosities, pierces the capsular ligament and passes over the head of the humerus to the top of the glenoid cavity, strengthens the upper anterior part of the joint and prevents the head of the humerus from being brought against the acromion, processing the normal upward movements of the arm. In fact it is mainly by the normal position of this tendon, assisted somewhat by atmospheric pressure, that the head of the humerus is retained in its natural position.

In 1910, Bera[23] believed that osteitis reduced the height of the lesser tuberosity and led to instability. In the 1920s, valuable contributions were made by Meyer.[163–170] He discussed his observations based on a total of 59 incidences of spontaneous dislocation of the long head of the tendon and on 20 examples of complete rupture. He was the first to describe the supratubercular ridge (Fig. 19–2), degenerative changes on the undersurface of the acromion, the acromioclavicular joint, and the coracoacromial ligament. Meyer concluded that attrition, particularly following the use of the extremity in abduction and external rotation, led to a gradual destruction of the capsule proximal to and in the region of the lesser tuberosity. Dislocation ensued as a consequence of the weakness of the capsule in this region.

According to Schrager,[234] Pasteur,[213] then a medical colonel at the military hospital at Val de Gras, recognized the condition of bicipital tendinitis in all its aspects, described it fully, and raised it to the status of a distinct clinical entity. In 1934, the specificity of the diagnosis of biceps tendinitis was questioned by Codman,[47] who wrote, "Personally, I believe that the sheath of the biceps is less

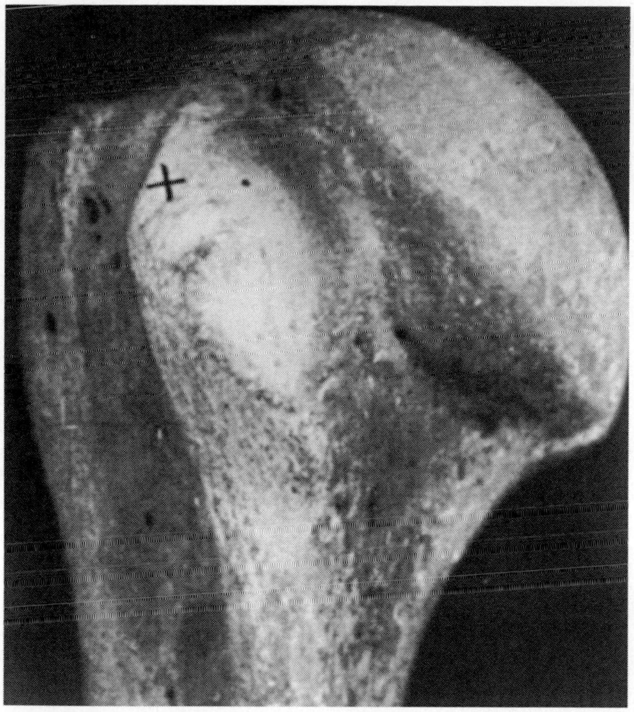

Figure 19–2

Original photograph of the supratubercular ridge taken by Meyer. (From Gilcreest EL: Dislocation and elongation of the long head of the biceps brachii: Analysis of six cases. Ann Surg *104:*118–138, 1936.)

apt to be involved than are other structures. I have never proved its involvement in a single case. I think that the substance of the tendon of the supraspinatus is most often involved." In the 1940s, Lippmann,[140, 141] Tarsy,[250] and Hitchcock and Bechtol[111] all believed that bicipital tendinitis was an important cause of shoulder pain, and these physicians individually described operations for the relief of symptoms. In 1950, DePalma[59] described degenerative changes in the biceps tendon that occurred with aging and reported on both operative and conservative management. Although he was grateful that more surgeons were recognizing the disorder (bicipital tendinitis), he felt that many were still reluctant to give this disorder the importance that it deserved. Based on gross and microscopic examination in 78 cases, DePalma concluded that bicipital groove tenosynovitis is the most common cause of the painful and stiff shoulder.

In 1972, Neer[186] described the anterior impingement syndrome, pointing to anterior acromial spurring with thickening and fibrosis of the coracoacromial ligament, as a cause of impingement wear on the rotator cuff and biceps tendon. Neer pointed out a close association between ruptures of the biceps tendon and rotator cuff tears.

While the pendulum has swung away from primary bicipital tendinitis and isolated biceps tendon instability during the past 25 years, several authors have published results for the diagnosis and treatment of isolated biceps tendinitis and dislocation. O'Donohue[201] reported on surgical techniques for treatment of the subluxating biceps tendon in the athlete. Neviaser and associates[198] recommended tenodesis of the biceps at the time of acromioplasty and excision of the distal clavicle as part of the four-in-one arthroplasty. In 1987, Post[221] presented a series of patients with primary bicipital tenosynovitis.

In the late 1980s and early 1990s, the frequent use of MRI and arthroscopy to visualize the long head of the biceps tendon has provided valuable insight into biceps pathology. In 1985, Andrews and associates[9] described tears in the superior labrum of the glenohumeral joint at its attachment to the biceps tendon. In 1990, Snyder and associates[241] first described the superolabral anterior to posterior (SLAP) lesion. He classified this lesion of the superior glenoid labrum and biceps anchor into four types. Walch classified both subluxations and dislocations of the biceps tendon in the early 1990s.[263, 264]

It has been almost 300 years since Cowper[55] described his first case, and controversy regarding the importance of this lesion still exists.

ANATOMY

The long head of the biceps brachii originates at the supraglenoid tubercle and the glenoid labrum in the most superior portion of the glenoid (Fig. 19–3). The tendon itself is approximately 9 cm long. At its origin the tendon presents a variable insertion type. It may be bifurcated or trifurcated, as well as presenting with a single insertion point.

In a study by Habermeyer and associates,[98] the biceps was found to originate off the supraglenoid tubercle in 20% of specimens studied. Its origin was off the superior posterior labrum in 48% of specimens studied, and 28% of the specimens studied had origins from both the tubercle and the labrum.

In a different study, Pal[209] showed that in 70% of specimens examined, the biceps tendon origin was mostly off the posterosuperior portion of the glenoid labrum. Usually only a small part of the tendon was attached to the supraglenoid tubercle in these specimens. However, in 25% of specimens, a major portion of the biceps tendon was attached to the supraglenoid tubercle.

A close association was noted between the glenoid

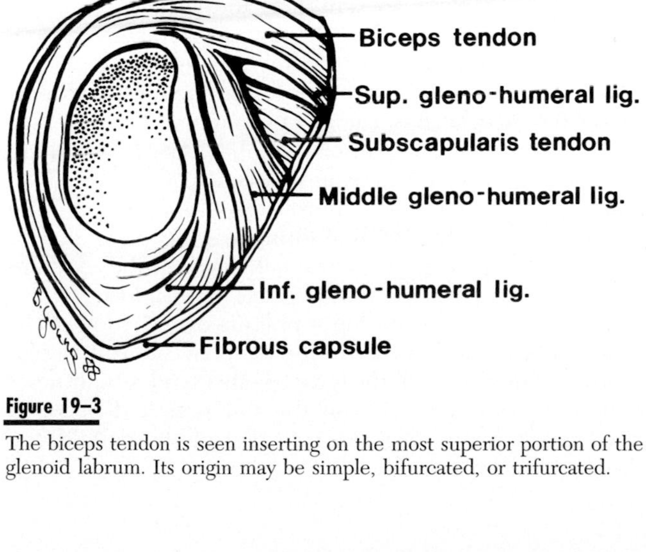

Figure 19–3

The biceps tendon is seen inserting on the most superior portion of the glenoid labrum. Its origin may be simple, bifurcated, or trifurcated.

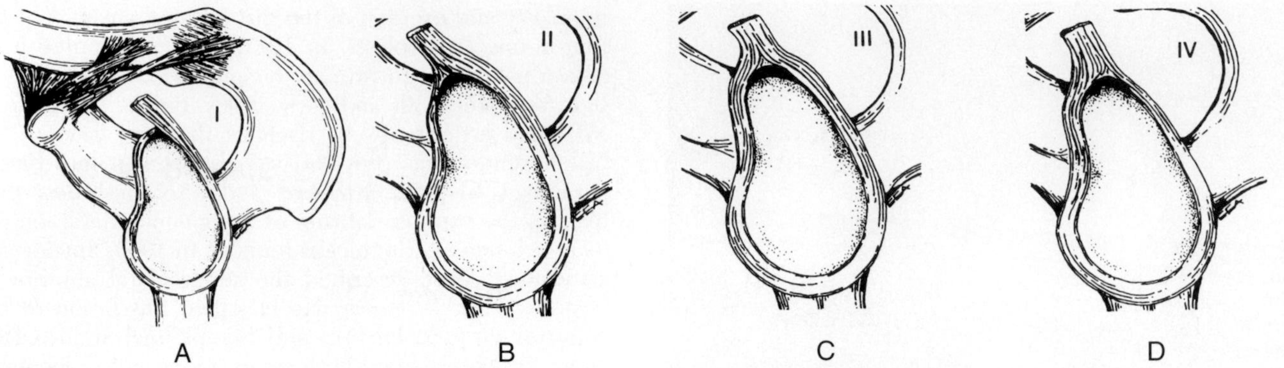

Figure 19–4

A, Type I: The labral attachment is entirely posterior, with no contribution to the anterior labrum (22%). *B,* Type II: Most of the labral contribution is posterior (33%). *C,* Type III: There are equal contributions to both the anterior and the posterior parts of the labrum (37%). *D,* Type IV: Most of the labral contribution is anterior, with a small contribution to the posterior labrum (8%). (From Vangsness CT Jr, Jorgenson SS, Watson T, and Johnson DL: The origin of the long head of the biceps from the scapula and glenoid labrum: An anatomical study of 100 shoulders. J Bone Joint Surg *76B*[6]:951–954, 1994.)

labrum and the biceps tendon, both grossly and histologically by Cooper and associates.[52] The primary attachment of the biceps tendon to the superior portion of the labrum was noted before it inserted onto the supraglenoid tubercle. Collagen fibers of the labrum and biceps tendon were found to be intimately blended in this area.

A study by Vangsness and associates[256] dissected 105 cadaveric shoulders to study the origin of the biceps tendon and the labrum and its relation to the supratubercular groove. They classified insertions into four types (Fig. 19–4). Type I occurred in 22% of the specimens and showed a labral attachment that was entirely posterior with no contribution to the anterior labrum. In type II, the labral contribution was mostly posterior with a small anterior band present. This occurred in 33% of their specimens. The type III insertion had an equal contribution in both the anterior and posterior labrum and was found in 37% of their specimens. Type IV origins occurred in 8% of specimens and mainly showed an anterior labral contribution to the biceps origin.

The cross-sectional characteristics of the long head of the biceps change during its course from the supraglenoid tubercle down to the musculotendinous junction. At its origin, the tendon measures 8.5 × 7.8 mm. In the area of strongest demand, the entrance to the bicipital sulcus, the tendon measured 4.7 × 2.6 mm. Finally, at its musculotendinous junction, the tendon measured 4.5 × 2.8 mm.[108] McGough and associates tested the tensile properties of the long head of the biceps tendon.[158] The average cross-sectional area was found to be 24.4 ± 3.1 mm^2. The cross-sectional area was reduced in the midsection and was the site where tensile failure occurred. The ultimate tensile strength and ultimate strain were 32.5 ± 5.3 Mpa and 10.1 ± 2.7% respectively, and the modulus of elasticity was calculated to be 241 ± 212 Mpa.

The course of this tendon is oblique over the top of the humeral head and down into the bicipital (intertubercular groove). Once out of the groove, the tendon continues down the ventral portion of the humerus and becomes musculotendinous near the insertion of the deltoid and the pectoralis major.

The angle formed by a line from the bottom of the groove to a central point on the humeral head is constant and corresponds with the retrotorsion angle measured from the epicondyles (Fig. 19–5).[98] This angle is important and can be used as a guide when placing a humeral head prosthesis. The bicipital tendon, although intra-articular, is extrasynovial. The synovial sheath reflects upon itself to form a visceral sheath that encases the biceps tendon (Fig. 19–6). The sheath is open, communicates directly with the glenohumeral joint, and ends in a blind pouch at the level of the bicipital groove.

The long head of the biceps muscle receives its blood supply from the brachial artery. Three arteries supply blood to the bicipital tendon. The distal portion of the tendon receives branches from the deep brachial artery. The proximal tendon also receives branches from the anterior circumflex humeral artery. In the intertubercular sulcus, a branch of the anterior circumflex humeral artery

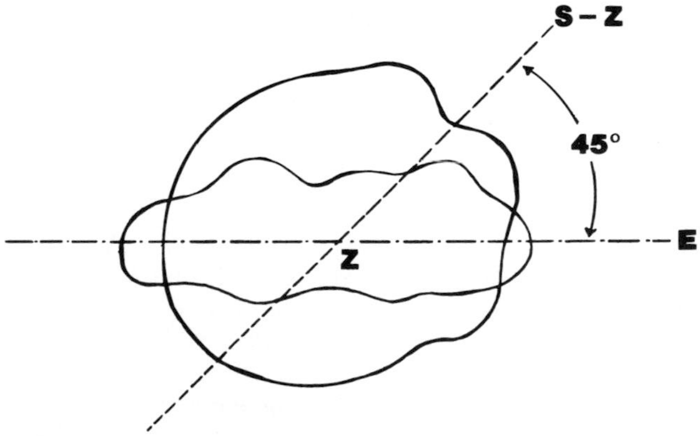

Figure 19–5

A line (S–Z) drawn through the center of the bottom of the bicipital groove, intersecting with a line drawn across the humeral condyles (E), accurately depicts the retroversion of the humeral head. (Redrawn from Habermeyer P, Kaiser E, Knappe M, et al: Functional anatomy and biomechanics of the long biceps tendon. Unfallchirurg *90*[7]:319–329, 1987.)

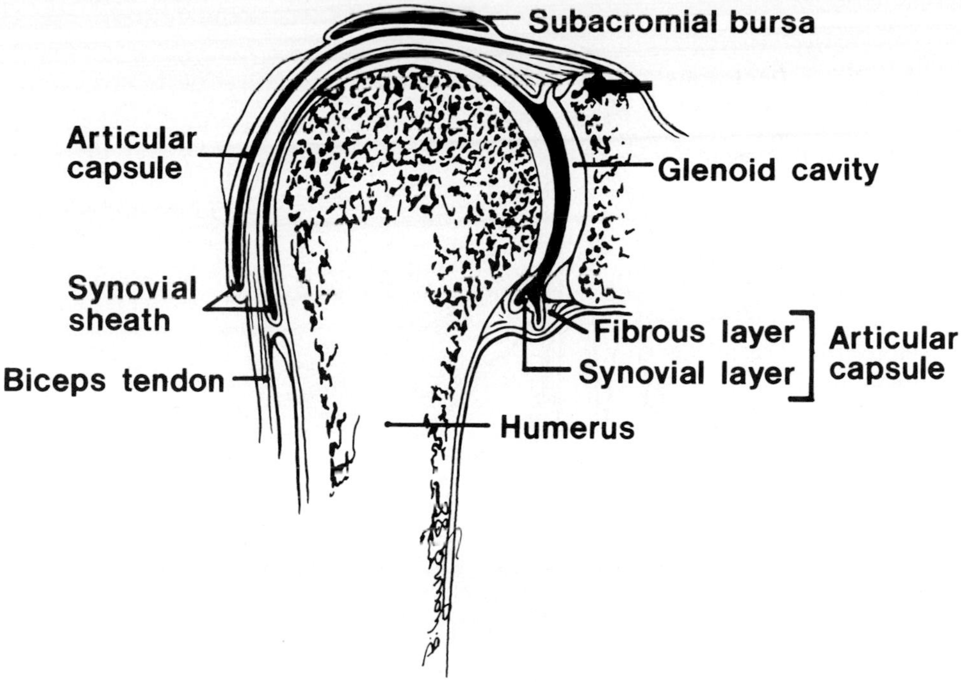

Figure 19–6

This figure illustrates both the insertion of the biceps onto the superior glenoid labrum as well as the supraglenoid tubercle *(black arrow)* and the reflection of the synovial sheath, which maintains the tendon as an extracapsular structure while it is on its intra-articular course.

gives rise to two small branches running in cranial and caudal directions.

The tendon of the long head of the biceps can be divided into two zones. The first is the traction zone in which the tendon of the biceps closely resembles a normal tendon and a sliding zone, which is the fibrocartilaginous portion of the tendon that is in contact with the bony groove. The density of intratendinous vessels in the traction zone is comparable with the vascularization of other tendons. In the sliding zone, the biceps tendon's vascularization is greatly decreased. In the part of the tendon upon which the humerus slides, there is an absence of vessels. This area has also been shown to consist of fibrocartilage.[133] The portion of the long head of the biceps inside the bicipital groove possesses a mesotendon that arises from the posterolateral portion of its groove.[98] Vascularization appears to play a minor rule in the pathogenesis of biceps tendon ruptures.

The biceps tendon has been classically described as having an intra-articular portion and a grooved portion. Experimental studies have shown that this type of classification is not 100% accurate. Because of the humeral head sliding on the biceps tendon, the position of the arm dictates the amount of intra-articular tendon present. The maximum amount of intra-articular tendon occurs with the arm in adduction and extension, whereas in extremes of abduction actually very little tendon resides inside the joint.

The long head of the biceps, along with the short head of the biceps, forms a common tendon before inserting onto the radial tubercle (Fig. 19–7). A third muscle belly has been described in some specimens. Mercer[162] and Gilcreest[83] measured the tensile strength of the biceps tendon as ranging from 150 to 200 lb. The blood supply of the muscle belly attached to the long head of the biceps is via the brachial artery.[98] The nerve supply to this muscle is via the musculocutaneous nerves arising from C5 to C7.

Soft Tissue Restraint

As the long biceps tendon courses from its origin on the superior glenoid labrum and supraglenoid tubercle to its muscular insertion, it is kept in its anatomic position by several structures. Among the most important of these structures are the capsuloligamentous tissues. These structures play a major role in retaining and stabilizing the long head of the biceps tendon in its groove. The supraspinatus, subscapularis, coracohumeral, and superior glenohumeral ligaments all play a vital role in stabilizing the biceps.

Rotator Interval

The rotator interval is the area between the supraspinatus and the subscapularis tendons. This triangular area, which contains both the coracohumeral and the superior glenohumeral ligaments, has as its medial boundary, the coracoid process.

In its anatomic position, the intra-articular portion of the biceps tendon runs underneath the coracohumeral ligament, which lies between and strengthens the interval between the subscapularis and the supraspinatus.

The rotator interval is an integral part of the cuff and the capsule and can be distinguished only by sharp dissection.[205] The most important retaining structure in this area is the portion of the shoulder capsule thickened by the coracohumeral ligament and the edges of the subscapularis and supraspinatus tendons that bridge the tuberosities in the uppermost portion of the sulcus (Figs.

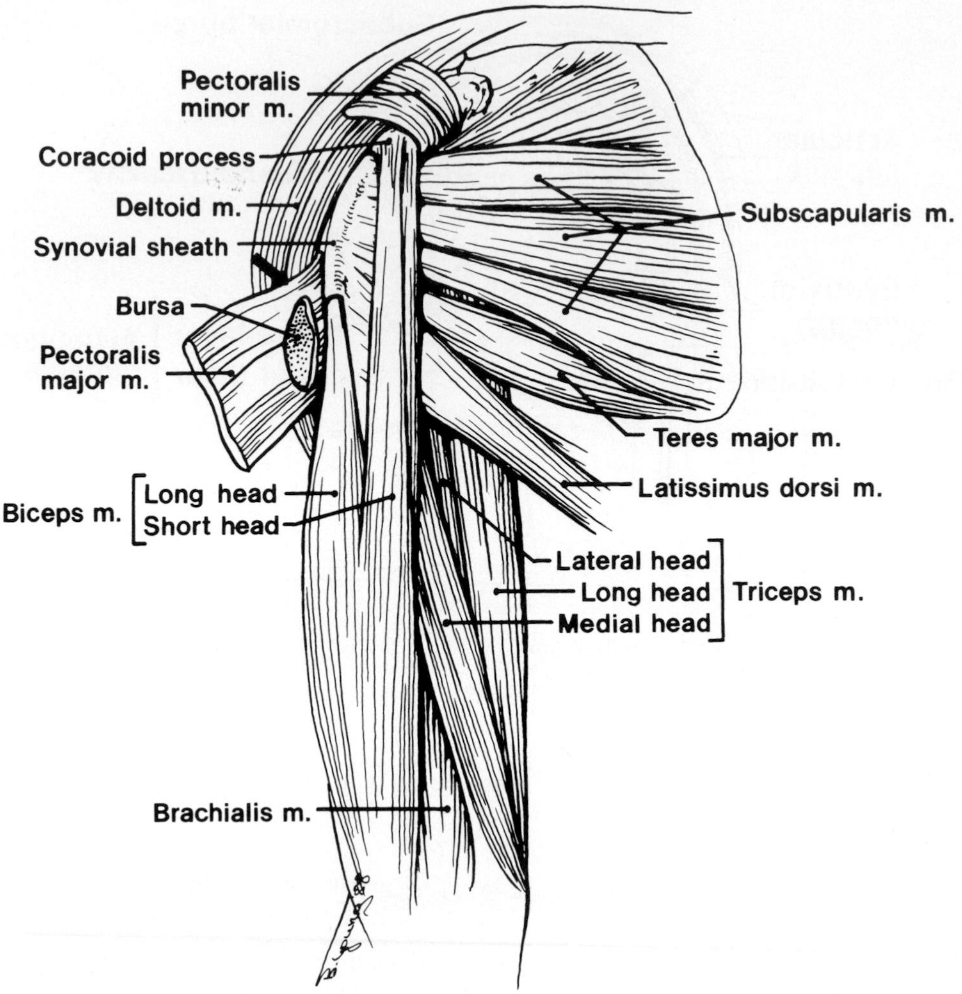

Figure 19–7

General anatomic relationships of the long head of the biceps. Note how the pectoralis major and falciform ligament *(large black arrow)* cross over the tendon and help to stabilize it after it exits the groove.

19–8 and 19–9). This portion of the capsule is the first and chief obstacle to medial dislocation of the tendon, and Meyer[163, 168] found that in all of his cases of dislocation it had been torn or stretched. Codman,[47] when commenting on Meyer's work, stated that in his opinion that "displacement of the tendon is a result of rupture at that portion of the musculotendinous cuff, which is inserted into the inner edge of the intratubercular notch."

The rotator interval contains two structures that are important in stabilization of the biceps tendon in the groove. The coracohumeral ligament has a broad thin origin on the coracoid. This origin is along the lateral border of the coracoid, and as the ligament passes laterally, it divides into two main bands. One band inserts onto the anterior edge of the supraspinatus tendon and the greater tuberosity. The other band inserts onto the

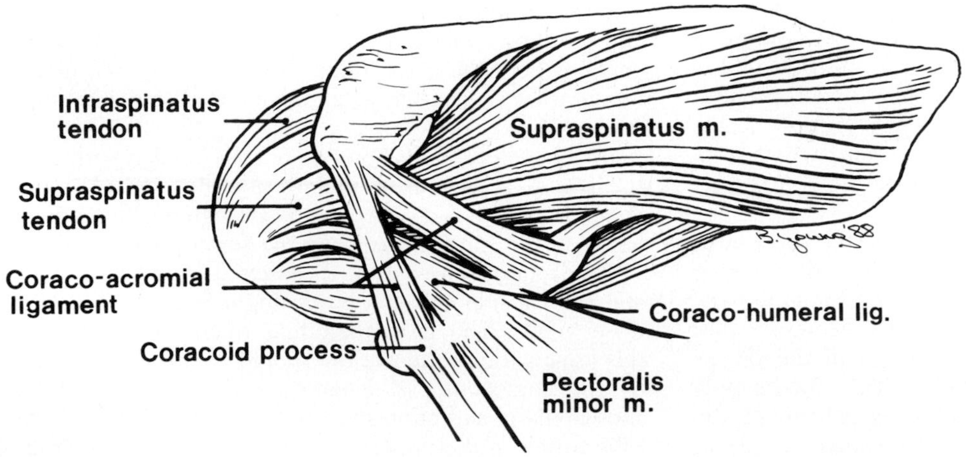

Figure 19–8

The coracohumeral ligament serves to reinforce the capsule in the rotator interval. The capsule, along with the edges of the supraspinatus and subscapularis, stabilizes the tendon as it leaves the sulcus.

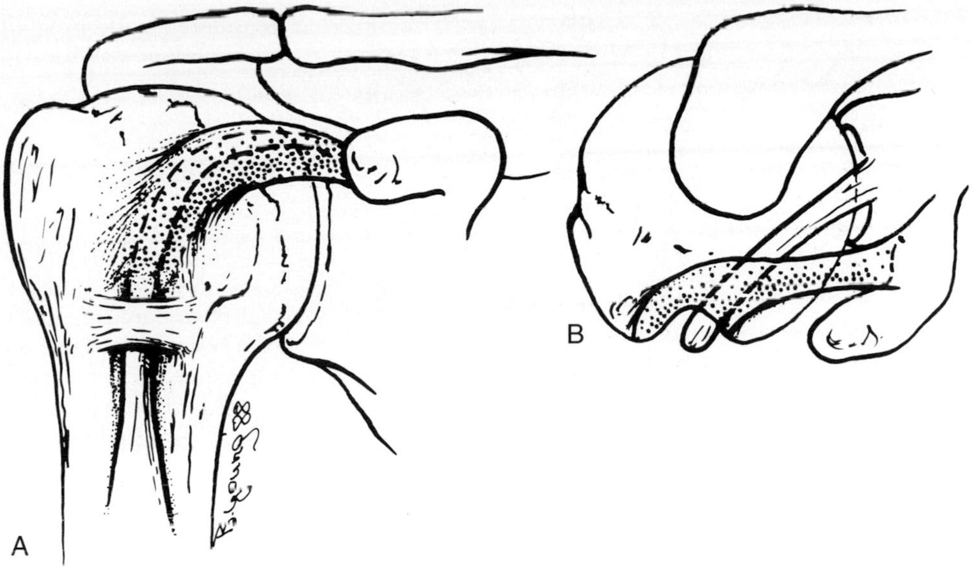

Figure 19–9

The coracohumeral ligament thickens the rotator interval; inserts on either side of the bicipital groove; and is an important stabilizer of the biceps tendon. (Modified from Paavolainen P, Slatis P, and Aalto K: Surgical pathology in chronic shoulder pain. *In* Bateman JE and Welsh RP [eds]: Surgery of the Shoulder. Philadelphia: BC Decker, 1984.)

superior border of the subscapularis, the transverse humeral ligament, and the lesser tuberosity (Figs. 19–10 and 19–11). The coracohumeral ligament has extensions that envelope the cuff tendons and blend into the superficial and deep layers of the supraspinatus and subscapularis tendons and into the articular capsule. This reinforces the capsule in the rotator interval at the border of the tendinous cuff.[48] The coracohumeral ligament is superficial to the shoulder capsule and overlies the biceps tendon.

The superior glenohumeral ligament is the second structure that adds stability to the biceps in the rotator interval. The superior glenohumeral ligament arises from the labrum adjacent to the supraglenoid tubercle, inserts onto the superior lateral portion of the lesser tuberosity, and is united to the medial aspect of the coracohumeral ligament. This structure crosses the floor of the rotator interval.[200] Along with the coracohumeral ligament, the superior glenohumeral ligament forms a reflection pulley

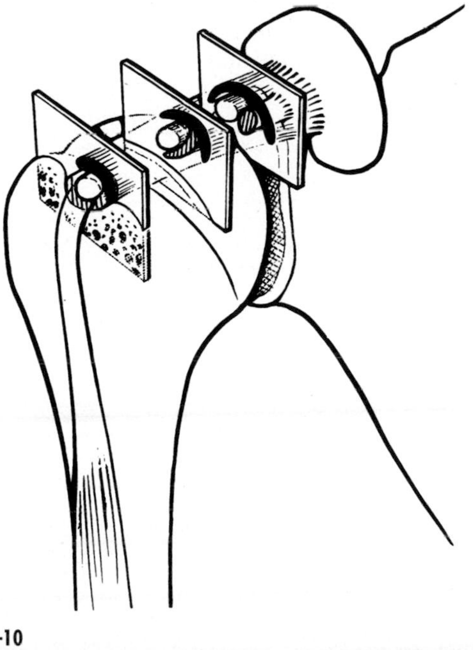

Figure 19–10

Schematic diagram showing the interelationship of the coracohumeral ligament, superior glenohumeral ligament, and long biceps tendon at several planes in the rotator interval. The long biceps tendon (white) is positioned centrally. The coracoacromial ligament (black) forms a crescent-shaped roof above it, and the superior glenohumeral ligament ("hatched area") forms a U-shaped trough. (From Habermeyer P and Walch G: The biceps tendon and rotator cuff disease. *In* Burkhead WZ Jr [ed]: Rotator Cuff Disorders. Media, PA: Williams & Wilkins, 1996, pp 142–159.)

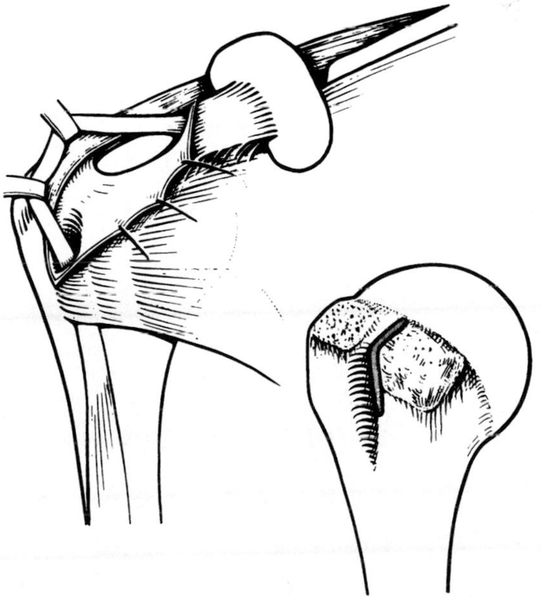

Figure 19–11

The rotator interval has been opened to demonstrate the common attachment of the coracohumeral ligament and superior glenohumeral ligament on the humeral head. (From Habermeyer P and Walch G: The biceps tendon and rotator cuff disease. *In* Burkhead WZ Jr [ed]: Rotator Cuff Disorders. Media, PA: Williams & Wilkins, 1996, pp 142–159).

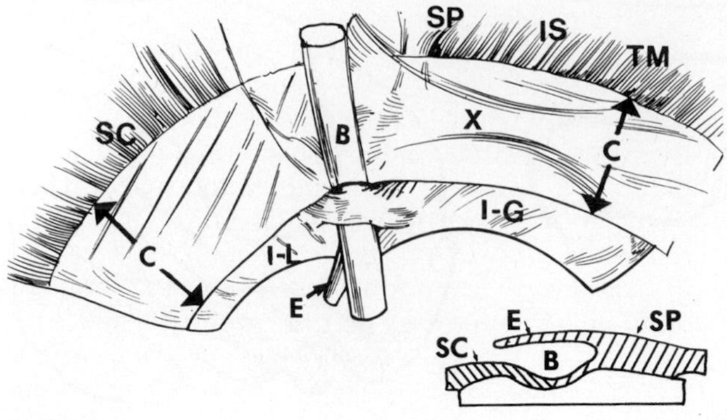

Figure 19–12

Drawing of the deep surface of the rotator cuff–capsule complex after it has been detached from the humerus. The diagram in the *inset* is a cross-section of the bicipital groove and related structures. Note the relationships of the capsule (C), subscapularis (SC), supraspinatus (SP), infraspinatus (IS), and teres minor (TM) tendons, as well as the confluence of the supraspinatus and subscapularis tendons proximal to their insertions on the lesser (I–L) and greater (I–G) tuberosities. In the *inset,* the complex sheath surrounding the biceps tendon (B) is shown diagrammatically in cross-section. The deep portion of this sheath is formed by the subscapularis tendon, and a slip (E) from the supraspinatus tendon forms a roof over the biceps tendon. The pericapsular band (X) is also shown. (From Clark JM and Harryman DT II: Tendons, ligaments, and capsule of the rotator cuff. Gross and microscopic anatomy. J Bone Joint Surg *74A*[5]:713–725, 1992.)

for the biceps tendon. This pulley is also in direct contact with the insertion of the subscapularis tendon. As can be seen by the descriptions of the superior glenohumeral ligament and the coracohumeral ligament, these structures blend together to form a sleeve above the entrance to the bicipital groove. This circular sleeve is comparable to the pulleys on the finger flexor tendons.[263] These structures prevent medial dislocation of the long biceps tendon. Although the superior glenohumeral ligament was considered to be insignificant previously, it appears to be an important stabilizer for the biceps tendon.

The Groove

The supraspinatus and subscapularis tendons fuse to form a sheath that surrounds the biceps tendon at the proximal end of the groove. Fibers from the subscapularis tendon pass below the biceps tendon to join with fibers from the supraspinatus to form the floor of the sheath (Fig. 19–12). The floor of the sheath is formed by the superior portion of the subscapularis and supraspinatus tendons. A slip from the supraspinatus forms the roof of the sheath along with the coracohumeral ligament. The deep portion of the sheath runs adjacent to the bone and forms a fibrocartilaginous lining in the groove that extends approximately 7 mm distal to the entrance of the groove.[48]

The transverse humeral ligament's role in providing stability of the biceps in its sulcus has been disputed by several authors.[163, 205] Traditional teaching showed that the biceps was kept in the sulcus by action of the transverse ligament (Fig. 19–13). Meyer[163] found that this structure was either too weak or often entirely absent. Paavolainen and associates[205] were unable to dislocate the biceps even after sectioning the intertubercular transverse ligament as long as the rotator cuff was intact.[205]

Once the tendon has entered the groove, the principal structure containing the tendon is the falciform ligament, a tendinous expansion from the sternocostal portion of the pectoralis major. It forms a margin with the deep aspect of the main tendon that stabilizes the biceps. The falciform ligament is attached to both lips of the groove and blends with the capsule at the shoulder joint.

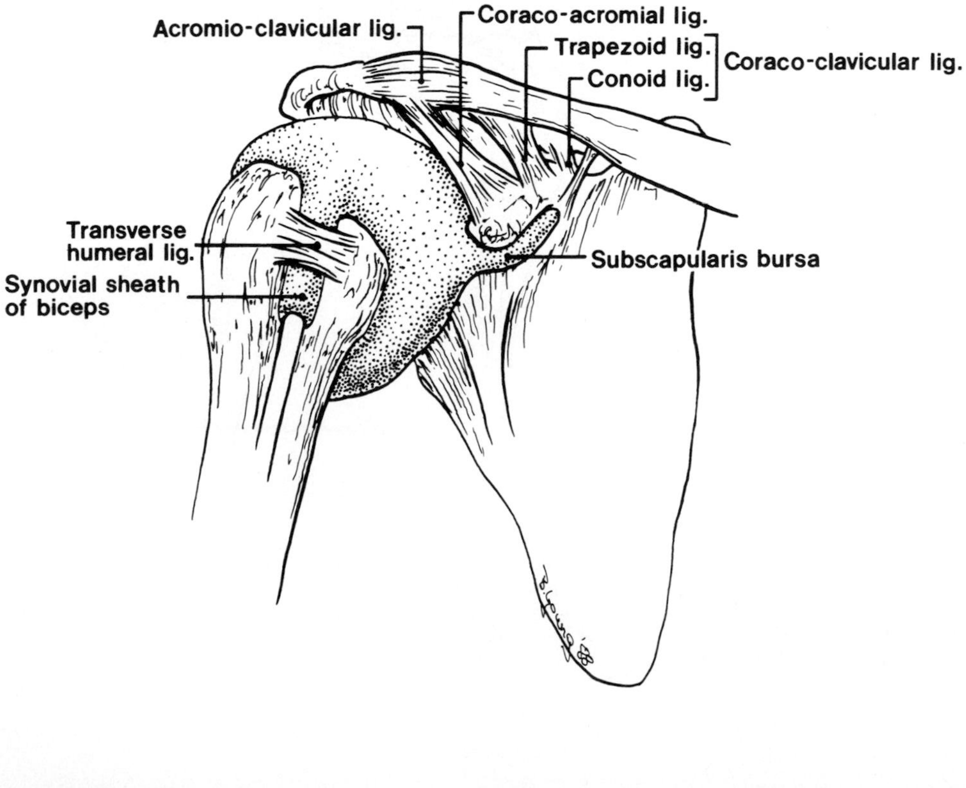

Figure 19–13

The ligaments around the shoulder. Meyer[163] found that the transverse ligament was too weak or entirely absent.

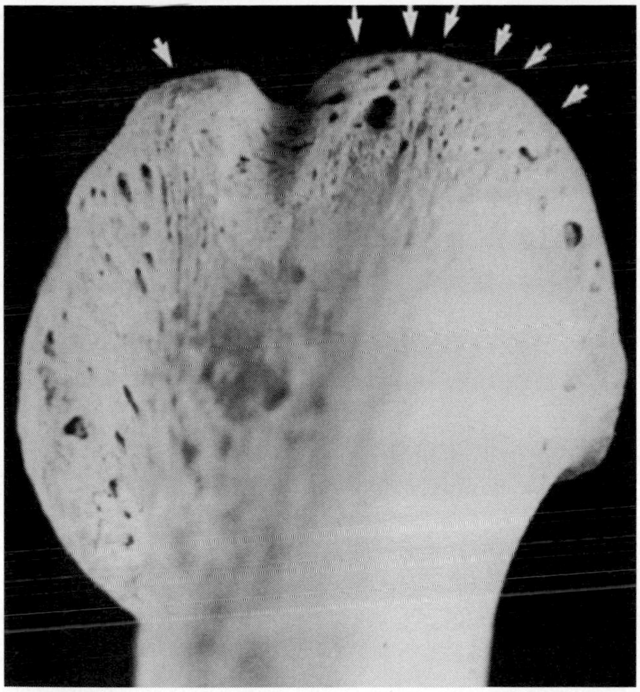

Figure 19–14

The bicipital groove is made up of the walls of the lesser tuberosity *(small arrow)* and the greater tuberosity *(multiple arrows)*. (From Cone RO, Danzig L, Resnick D, and Goldman AB: The bicipital groove: Radiographic, anatomic, and pathologic study. Am J Roentgenol *41:*781–788, 1983. Copyright © Am Roentgen Ray Society, 1983.)

Osseous Anatomy

The bicipital groove is formed between the lesser and greater tuberosities (Fig. 19–14). The medial wall is made up of the lesser tuberosity, whereas the lateral wall is the edge of the greater tuberosity. Cone and colleagues[49] have studied the bicipital groove. They measured the medial wall angle, width, and depth of the intertubercular groove (Fig. 19–15). The mean value for the medial wall angle was 56 degrees (range of 40 to 70 degrees). The width of the intertubercular sulcus was measured in two locations on the bicipital groove view. The top width was determined as the distance between the medial and lateral lips of the intertubercular sulcus. The middle width was measured between the walls of the intertubercular sulcus, a point equal to half of the depth of the sulcus. There was a wide difference between measurements, but the ratio of the width was constant at 1.6 from the top to the middle distances. The average depth of the groove was found to be 4.3 mm (range of 4 to 6 mm).

Variability of the medial wall angle was confirmed by studies by Hitchcock and Bechtol,[111] Habermeyer and associates,[98] and Cone and colleagues.[49] Hitchcock and Bechtol[111] found that the medial wall angle was 90 degrees in 10% of specimens, 75 degrees in 35%, 60 degrees in 34%, 45 degrees in 13%, 30 degrees in 6%, and 15 degrees in 2% (Fig 19 16). In Habermeyer's study,[98] as well as in Hitchcock and Bechtol's study,[111] the medial wall angle was correlated with the probability of subluxation of the long head of the biceps tendon. Cone and colleagues,[49] on the other hand, found that there was no correlation between the incidence of subluxation and low medial wall angles.

Vettivel and associates[260] found that the intertubercular sulcus of the humerus was related to handedness. In their study, the intertubercular sulcus was wider and had an acute medial wall angle on the side of the specimen's dominant arm. They believe that this was due to greater stress passing through the tendon in the dominant extremity, especially during manual activities.

Comparative Anatomy

Hitchcock and Bechtol,[111] using specimens from the Museum of Natural History in Chicago, have outlined the changes in relationship of the scapula and bicipital groove from the quadruped to the erect biped (Fig. 19–17). They described a progressive anteroposterior flattening of the thorax resulting in an increased angle that the scapula forms with the thorax and a relative lateral displacement of the scapula. Humans have a relatively short forearm

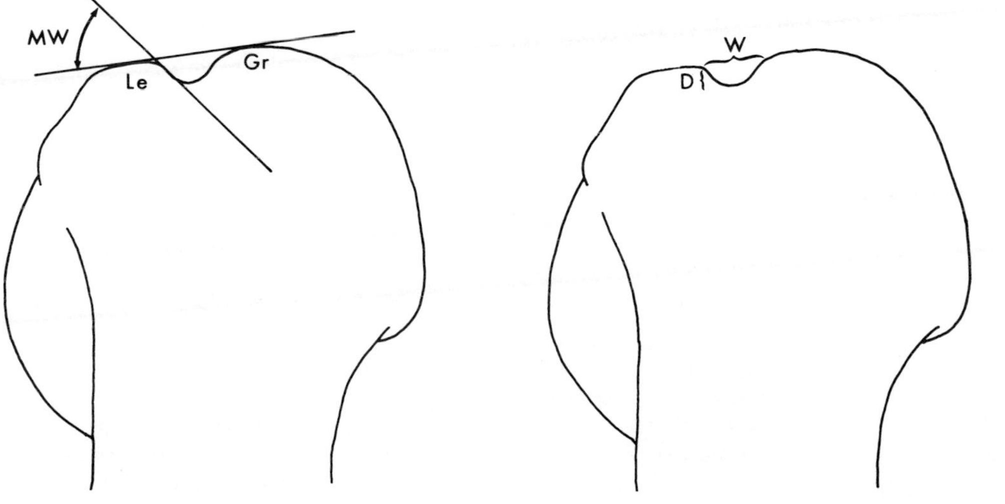

Figure 19–15

Measurements taken by Cone and associates, including the medial wall angle as well as the width and depth of the bicipital groove. (MW, medial wall angle; Le, lesser tuberosity; Gr, greater tuberosity; D, depth of groove; W, width of groove.) (From Cone RO, Danzig L, Resnick D, and Goldman AB: The bicipital groove: Radiographic, anatomic, and pathologic study. Am J Roentgenol *41:*781–788, 1983. Copyright © Am Roentgen Ray Society, 1983.)

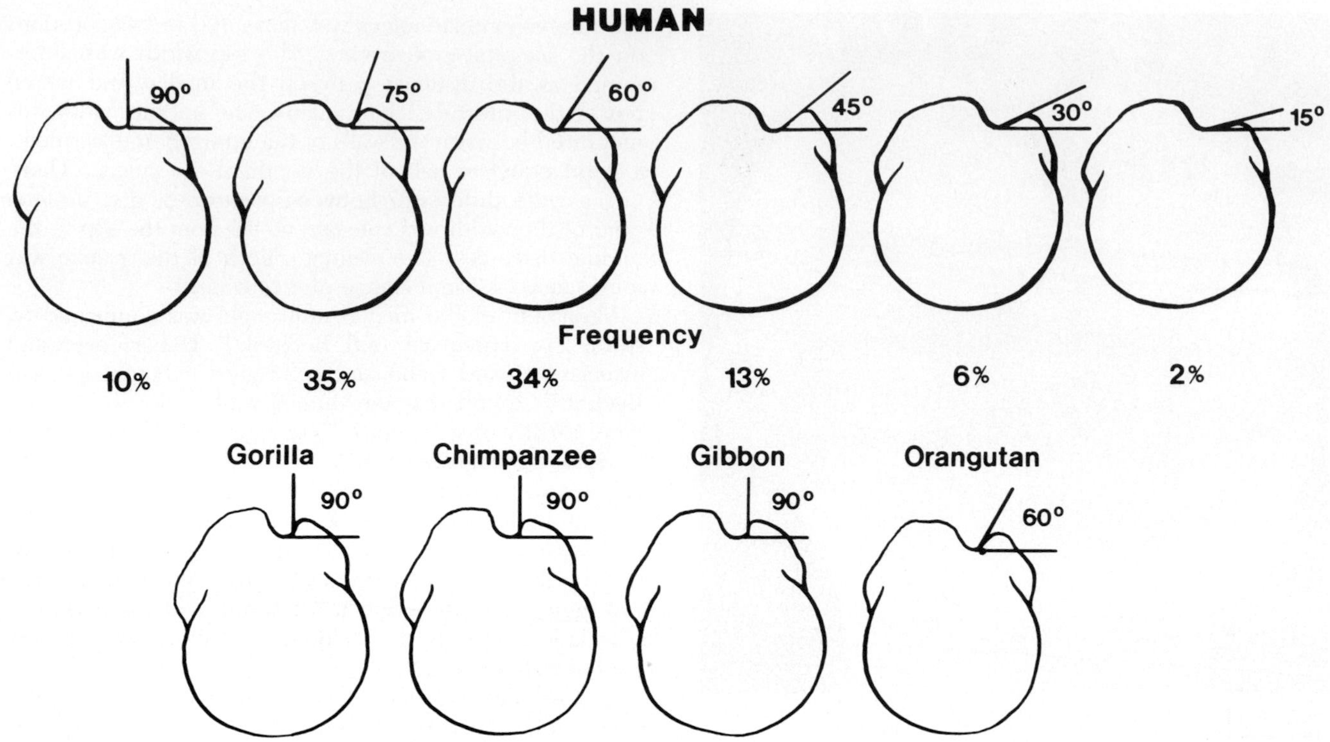

Figure 19–16

A, Humans are unique in having variations in the bicipital groove. *B*, The groove of the biceps in primates is constant within the species. (Modified and redrawn from Hitchcock HH and Bechtol CO: Painful shoulder. Observations on the role of the tendon of the long head of the biceps brachii in its causation. J Bone Joint Surg *30A*:263–273, 1948.)

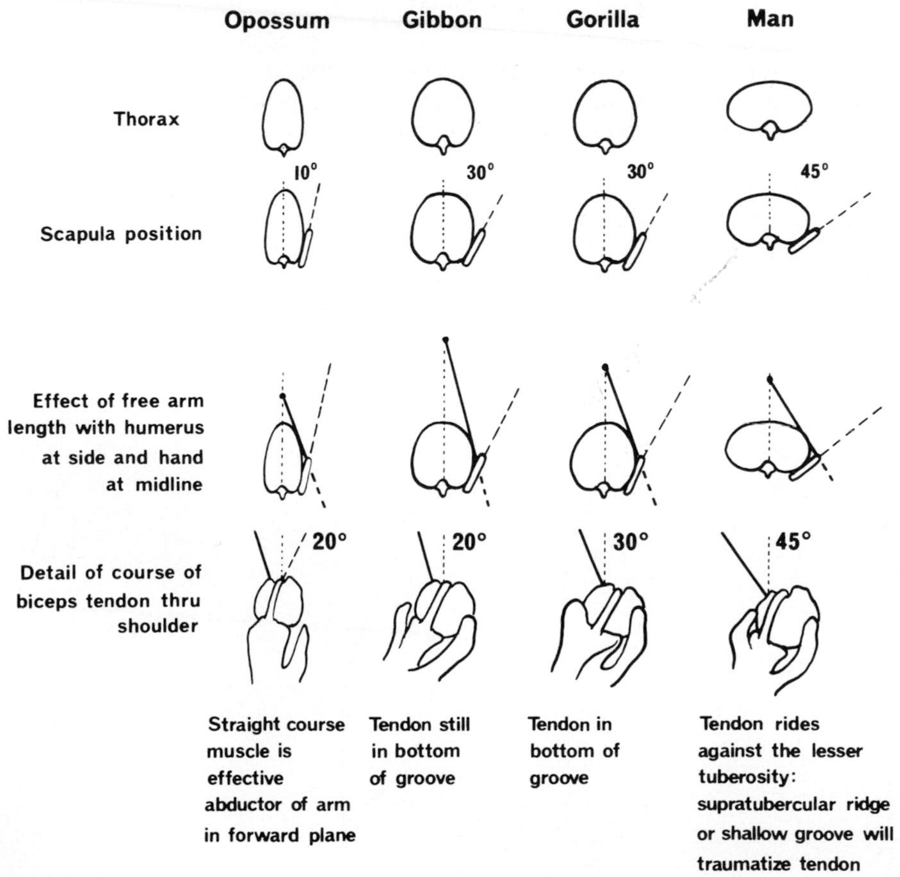

Figure 19–17

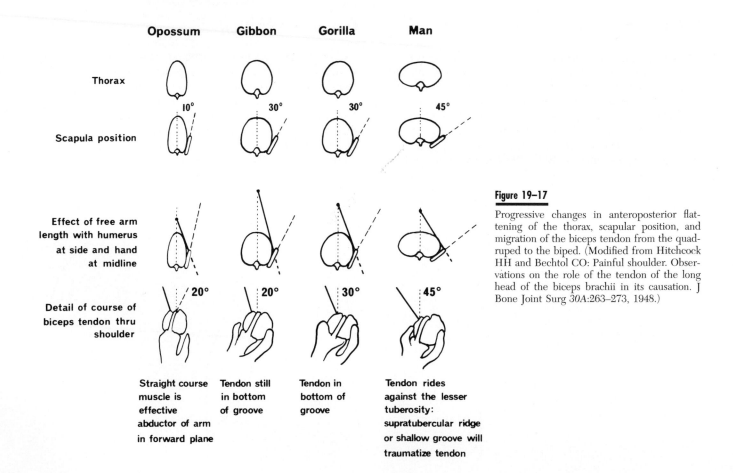

Progressive changes in anteroposterior flattening of the thorax, scapular position, and migration of the biceps tendon from the quadruped to the biped. (Modified from Hitchcock HH and Bechtol CO: Painful shoulder. Observations on the role of the tendon of the long head of the biceps brachii in its causation. J Bone Joint Surg *30A*:263–273, 1948.)

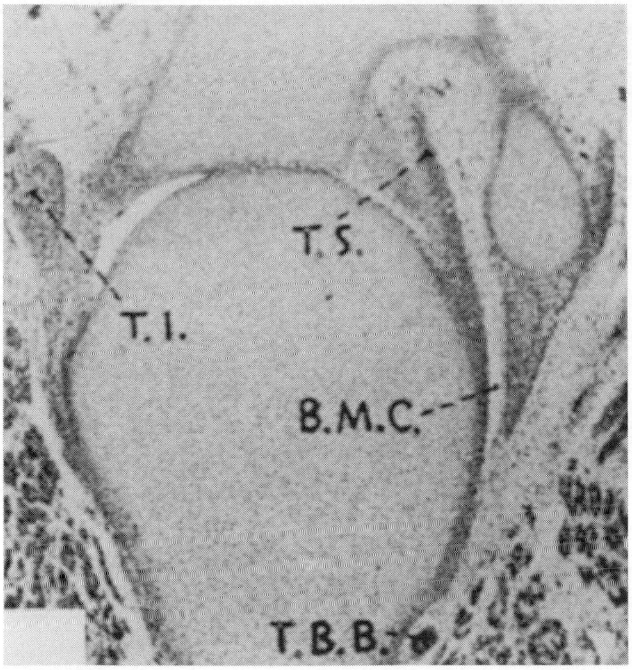

Figure 19–18

At approximately 7 weeks' gestation, the joint is well formed and the humeral head is spherical. The biceps tendon (TBB) is clearly seen in the groove. This picture is taken before rotation occurs; the biceps tendon will eventually assume a position less lateral than that shown here. The other structures in this picture are the tendon of the infraspinatus (TI), the subscapularis (TS), and the bursa of the coracobrachialis (BMC). (From Gardner E and Gray DJ: Prenatal development of the human shoulder and acromioclavicular joint. Am J Anat 92:219, 1953.)

and lateral scapula. This necessitates greater medial rotation of the humerus to enable the hand to reach the midline. The anteroposterior flattening of the thorax and the short forearm were compensated for, but only incompletely, by torsion of the humerus. In the quadruped opossum, the biceps tendon takes a straight course through the bicipital groove and is an effective abductor of the arm in the forward plane. However, in humans, the tendon is lodged against the lesser tuberosity, where a supratubercular ridge or shallow groove can traumatize the tendon. Humans are unique among the primates in presenting marked variations in the configuration of the bicipital groove (Fig. 19–18).

The human arm was derived from the foreleg of the quadruped. Although the forelimb was devised to bear weight in the quadruped, in humans the upper limb has moved away from the body. For its effective use it must move not only against its own weight but also against the weight of other objects. This short power arm has to act against a long lever arm, producing unfavorable mechanical conditions that can lead to tendinitis of the rotator cuff and biceps.

Developmental Anatomy

During the ninth week of gestation, the limbs undergo rotation. The upper limb rotates dorsally at the elbow. This rotation is reflected in the shoulder as humeral retroversion, which averages 35 degrees. This rotation, in essence, leaves the biceps tendon behind on the anterior aspect of the shoulder in the groove and requires that the biceps cross the joint obliquely at a 30- to 45-degree angle, rather than proceeding in a straight line laterally as in the quadrupeds.

The development of the glenohumeral joint is similar to that of other synovial joints in the human body. According to Gardner and Gray,[80] it involves two basic processes. Initially, an inner zone forms between the two developing bones of the joint, followed by the creation of cavities by enzymatic action. The inner zones often comprise three layers, a chondrogenic layer on either side of a looser layer of cells. The joint capsule and many of the intra-articular structures, such as the synovial membrane, the ligaments, the labrum, and the biceps tendon, form from this inner zone of tissue. Gluliani and associates[88] confirmed that the tendon of the long head of the biceps brachii arises in continuity with the anlage of the glenoid labrum. At approximately 7 weeks of gestation, the joint is well formed, the humeral head is spherical, and the tendons of the infraspinatus, subscapularis, and biceps as well as the glenoid labrum can be seen (see Fig. 19–18).

Pathologic Anatomy

Some authors believe that tenosynovitis is the chief cause of pain in bicipital tendinitis and leads to an altered tendon sheath gliding mechanism.[59–63] They describe gradual pathologic changes in the area of the biceps tendon, including, initially, capillary dilatation and edema of the tendon with progressive cellular infiltration of the sheath and synovium and the development of filmy adhesions between the tendon and the tendon sheath. In the chronic stage, there is fraying and narrowing of the biceps tendon with minimal to moderate synovial proliferation and fibrosis and, ultimately, replacement of the tendon fibers by fibrous tissue and organization of dense fibrous adhesions between the tendon passing through the bicipital groove and across the joint. The biceps tendon passes directly under the critical zone of the supraspinatus tendon. Claessens and Snoek[41] described microscopic changes consistent with a relatively avascular state, including atrophic irregular collagen fiber, fissurization and shredding of tendon fibers, fibrinoid necrosis, and a productive inflammatory reaction with an increase in fibrocytes (Fig. 19–19). Refior and associates found that the origin of the tendon and the portion of the tendon that exits the sulcus were sites of predilection for microscopic degeneration of the tendon (Fig. 19–20).[228] They believed that these areas are at the highest risk for rupture of the tendon. Macroscopic changes in cadaver studies by DePalma[59–63] and Claessens[40, 41] revealed tendinitis with shredding of the tendon fibers by osteophytes, adhesions between the synovial sheaths and between the tendon and its osteofibrous compartment, subluxation or dislocation of the tendon, and rupture of the tendon with retraction of the distal portion or adhesion of the distal portion to the sulcus. Although it was a common belief that the tendon, when it dislocates, always displaced medially to the lesser tuberosity riding over the subscapularis tendon

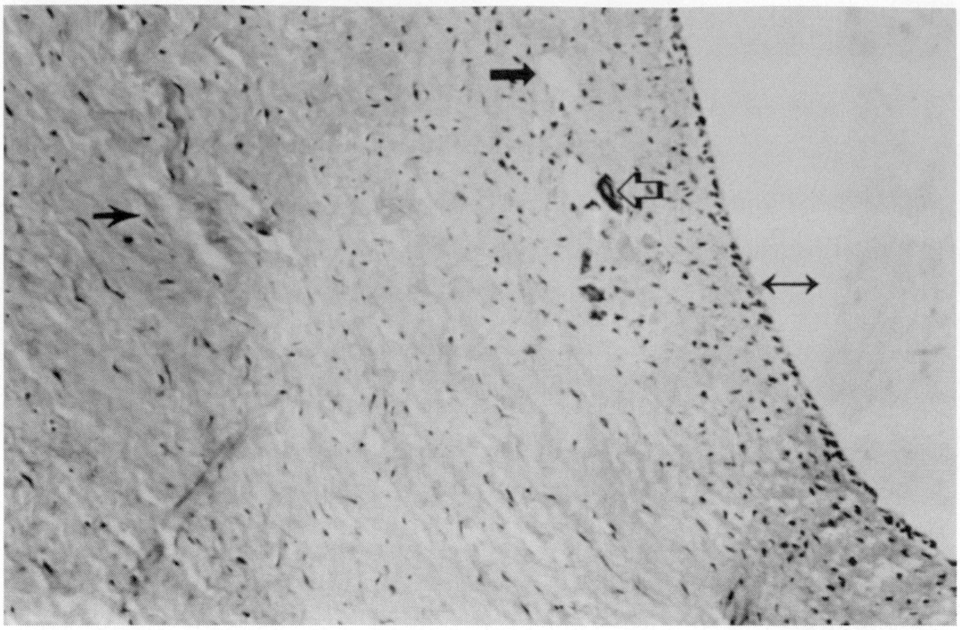

Figure 19–19

Pathology in a degenerative biceps tendon. The *double arrow* indicates the synovial membrane; the *open arrow* points to dystrophic calcification; the *closed arrow* marks total loss of fibers; the *arrowhead* indicates fissuring in the collagen with a disorderly collagen pattern. A productive inflammatory reaction with an increase in fibrocytes is seen in the lower right corner.

(Fig. 19–21*B*), Petersson,[215] in his study, found only one such case. In most cases in his series, internal degeneration of the subscapularis in the region of the lesser tuberosity had occurred, allowing the tendon to dislocate medially under the subscapularis (see Fig. 19–21*C*). Similar pathologic findings were described by DePalma (Fig. 19–22).

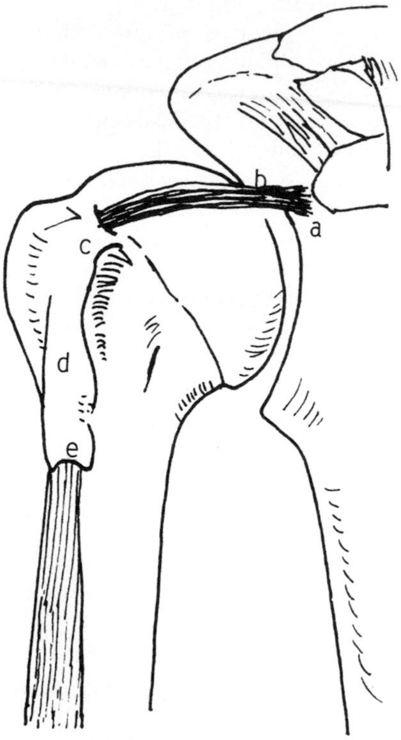

Figure 19–20

Areas of the long tendon of the biceps are examined histologically. *a,* Glenoid origin of the tendon; *b,* Proximal intra-articular region; *c,* Entrance to the bicipital groove; *d,* Bicipital groove; and *e,* Exit of the bicipital groove. Sites B and C are the most common sites of degeneration. (From Refior HJ and Sowa D: Long tendon of the biceps brachii: Sites of predilection for degenerative lesions. J Shoulder Elbow Surg *4*[6]:436–440, 1995.)

The biceps tendon and its enveloping synovial sheath are bound to be affected by inflammatory or infectious processes of the glenohumeral joint owing to their anatomic location and course. Tumorous conditions affecting the synovium of the shoulder may also involve the sheath of the tendon.[54] Therefore, tenosynovitis of the biceps accompanies septic arthritis of the shoulder as well as rheumatic inflammation, osteoarthritis, hemodialysis arthropathy,[249] and crystalline arthritis. The clinical syndrome in these cases is dominated by the articular pathology. In the past, biceps rupture has been reported to occur in conjunction with tuberculous and luetic infection.

OSSEOUS PATHOANATOMY

The shape of the groove has been implicated frequently in the pathogenesis of biceps tendon ruptures.[59–62, 98, 111] A shallow flattened groove (Fig. 19–23) is commonly associated with subluxation or dislocation of the biceps tendon, and a narrow groove with a sharp medial wall and an osteophyte at the aperture is associated with bicipital tendinitis and rupture (Fig. 19–24). Spurs on the floor of the groove may erode the tendon (Fig. 19–25). Although these groove abnormalities may contribute to bicipital tendon problems, it is more likely that some are changes in response to pathology of the soft tissues around the shoulder. In all of the degenerative conditions around the shoulder, soft tissue changes precede bony changes; that is, rotator cuff disorders, fibrosis, bursitis, and tendinosis or enesthopathy precede the formation of spurring in the anterior acromion. Synovitis and cartilage degeneration precede the spurs in the acromioclavicular joint. It seems logical that changes in the bicipital groove and its opening

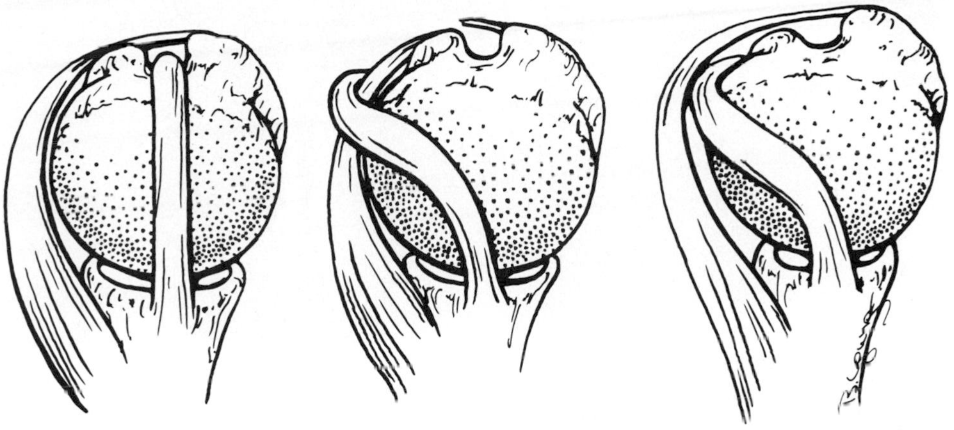

Figure 19–21

A, The normal relationship of the biceps tendon in the groove covered by the transverse ligament. *B*, Rupture of the transverse ligament and subluxation of the biceps tendon out of the groove, with the tendon lying anterior to the subscapularis muscle. *C*, Intratendinous disruption of the subscapularis found in the majority of cases by Petersson, in which the subscapularis insertion degenerates and the tendon subluxates beneath the muscle tendon belly. The subscapularis tendon may have an attachment to the greater tuberosity through the coracohumeral and transverse ligaments. (Modified from Petersson CJ: Degeneration of the gleno-humeral joint: An anatomical study. Acta Orthop Scand 54:277–283, 1983.)

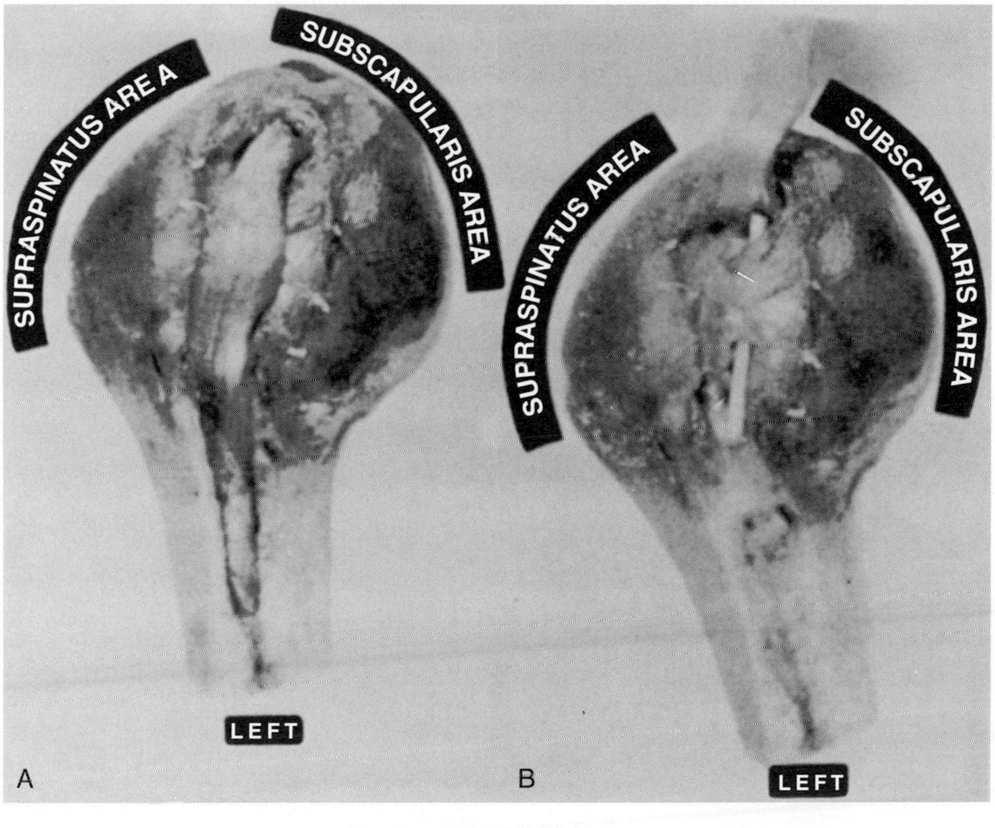

Figure 19–22

Obliteration of the bicipital groove by inflammation, with subluxation of the tendon lying in a fascial sling made by the insertion of the subscapularis. (From DePalma A: Surgery of the Shoulder, 2nd ed. Philadelphia: JB Lippincott, 1983.)

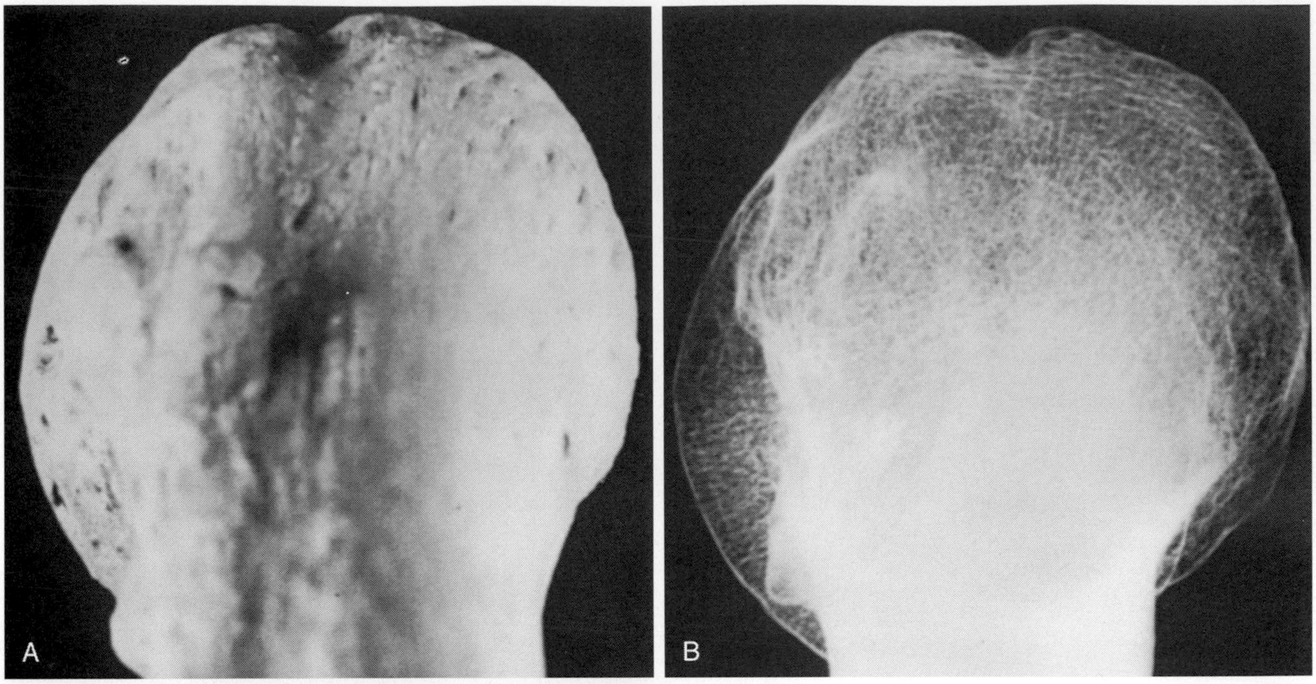

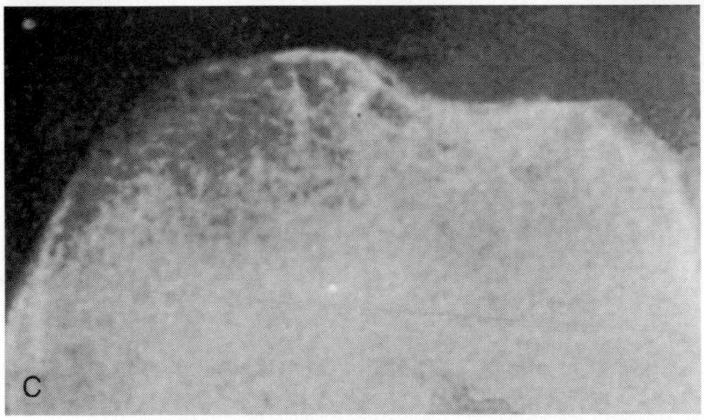

Figure 19–23

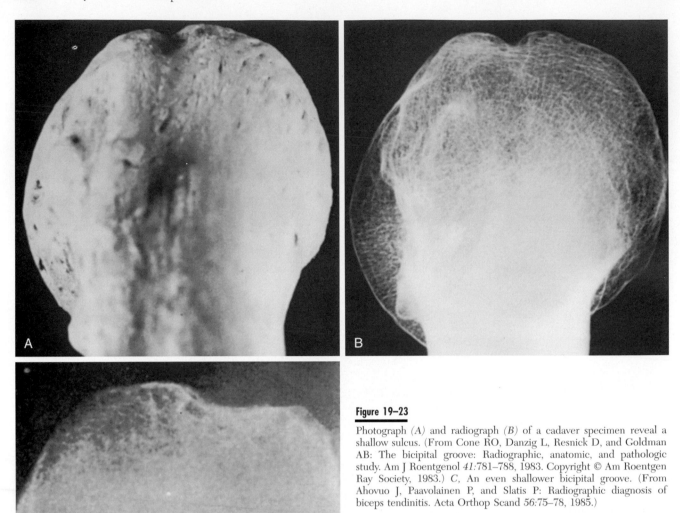

Photograph *(A)* and radiograph *(B)* of a cadaver specimen reveal a shallow sulcus. (From Cone RO, Danzig L, Resnick D, and Goldman AB: The bicipital groove: Radiographic, anatomic, and pathologic study. Am J Roentgenol *41*:781–788, 1983. Copyright © Am Roentgen Ray Society, 1983.) *C,* An even shallower bicipital groove. (From Ahovuo J, Paavolainen P, and Slatis P: Radiographic diagnosis of biceps tendinitis. Acta Orthop Scand *56*:75–78, 1985.)

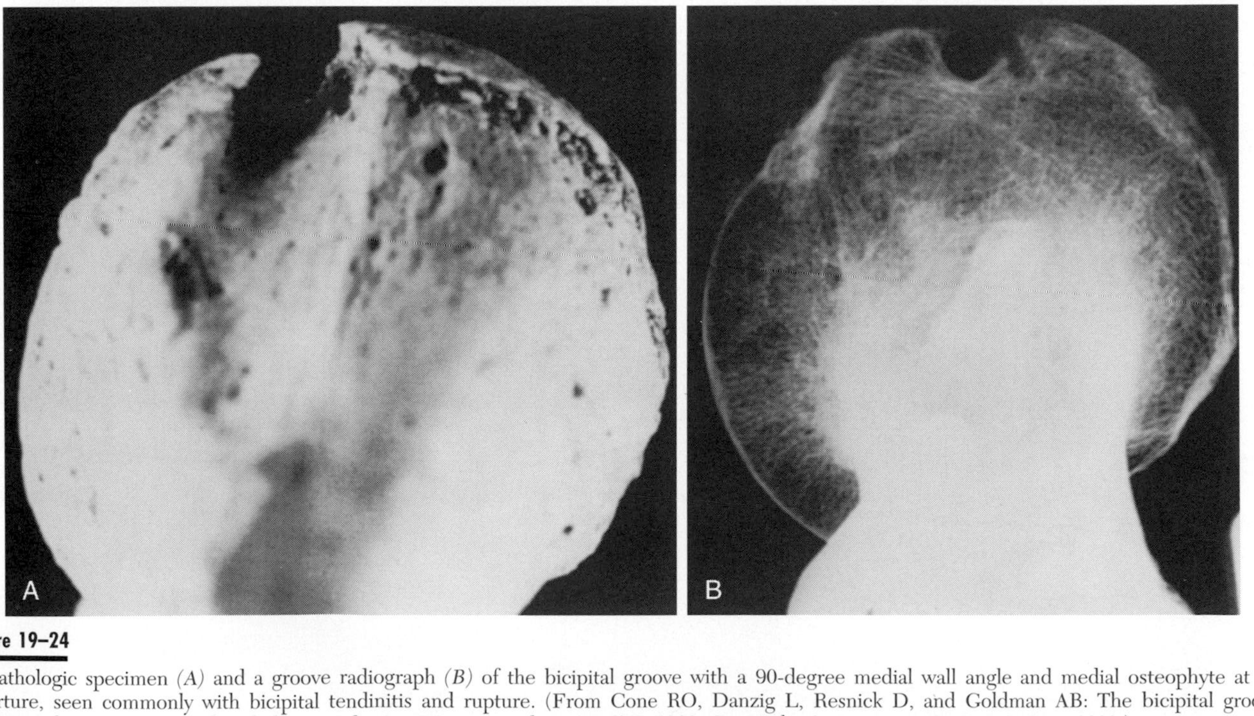

Figure 19–24

A pathologic specimen *(A)* and a groove radiograph *(B)* of the bicipital groove with a 90-degree medial wall angle and medial osteophyte at the aperture, seen commonly with bicipital tendinitis and rupture. (From Cone RO, Danzig L, Resnick D, and Goldman AB: The bicipital groove: Radiographic, anatomic, and pathologic study. Am J Roentgenol *41*:781–788, 1983. Copyright © Am Roentgen Ray Society, 1983.)

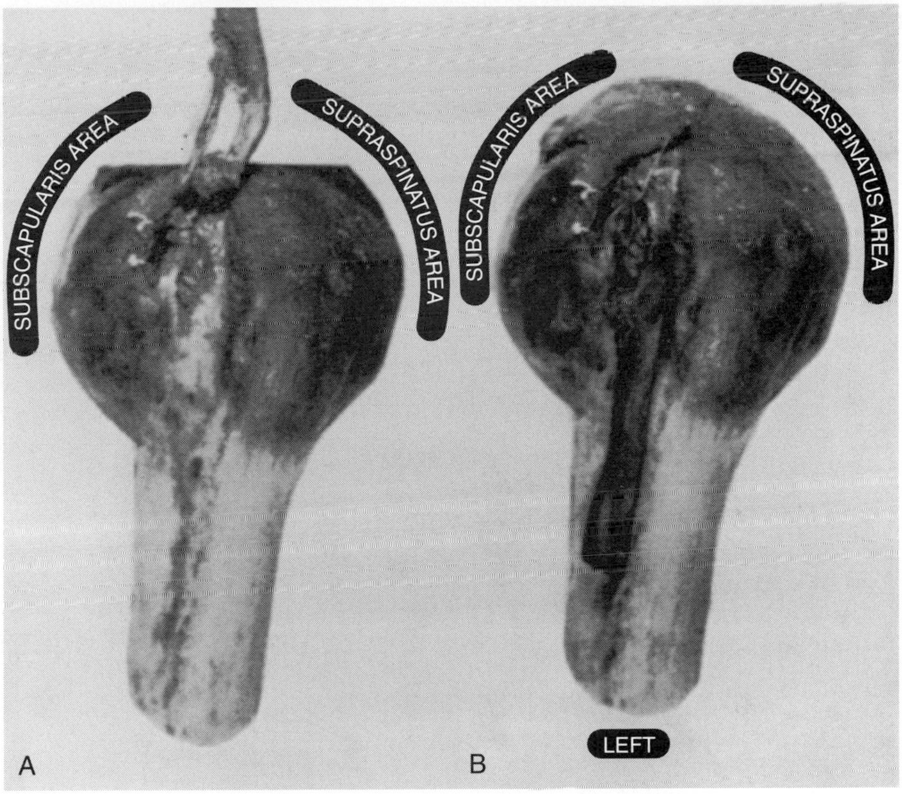

Figure 19–25

A, A large bony spur is seen in the floor of the groove. A corresponding defect is present in the biceps tendon. *B,* The tendon has been replaced in the groove. (From DePalma A: Surgery of the Shoulder, 2nd ed. Philadelphia: JB Lippincott, 1983.)

follow changes in the tendon, capsule, ligaments, and synovium around it.

Bony Anomalies

Bony anomalies and variations have been proposed as a cause of subluxation and tendinitis of the biceps tendon. The supratubercular ridge has been described by Meyer[163] as a ridge that extends forward and downward from the region of the articular cartilage to the upper and dorsal portions of the lesser tuberosity (Fig. 19–26). Its incidence, according to Cilley,[36] is 17.5% out of 200 humeri. The ridge, when present, decreases the depth of the sulcus and diminishes the effectiveness of the tuberosity as a trochlea. Meyer believed that the ridge pushed the biceps tendon against the transverse ligament, favoring dislocation.

In Hitchcock and Bechtol's[111] series, the supratubercular ridge was found to be markedly developed in 8% and moderately developed in 59%. Hitchcock and Bechtol[111] found a direct correlation with the supratubercular ridge and spurs on the lesser tuberosity (medial wall spurs). In their series, medial wall spurs were found in approximately 45% of patients with a supratubercular ridge. When there was no supratubercular ridge, only 3% of the humeri showed spurs on the lesser tuberosity (see Fig. 19–26*C*). They concluded that the spurs on the lesser tuberosity were spurs reactive to pressure from the biceps tendon being pressed up against the tuberosity by the supratubercular ridge.

A supratubercular ridge was found in approximately 50% of patients by Cone and colleagues[49] but did not correlate very well with the presence of bicipital groove spurs. They thought that the medial wall spur was related more to a traction enostosis (i.e., reactive bone formation at the site of a tendon or ligament insertion of the transverse humeral ligament). In one specimen, the transverse humeral ligament was completely ossified, converting the bicipital groove into a bony tunnel. They agree with DePalma that the presence of bony spurs on the floor of the bicipital groove is related to chronic bicipital tenosynovitis (Fig. 19–27).

FUNCTION OF THE BICEPS TENDON

Basmajian and Latif[14] characterized the actions of the biceps brachii muscle as flexion of the elbow joint when the forearm is in the neutral or supinated position. They found that it contributed very little to flexion at the elbow with the forearm in a pronated position. The biceps was also important in decelerating the rapidly moving arm such as occurs during forceful overhand throwing.

The function of the biceps at the elbow has been well worked out, and there is general agreement that the biceps brachii is a strong supinator of the forearm and a weak flexor at the elbow. Debate continues, however, regarding the exact function of the biceps at the shoulder level. Most anatomy textbooks regard the biceps as a weak flexor of the shoulder.[112] Studies on function of the biceps tendon can be divided into three broad categories: direct observation, electromyographic (EMG) studies, and biomechanical cadaver studies.

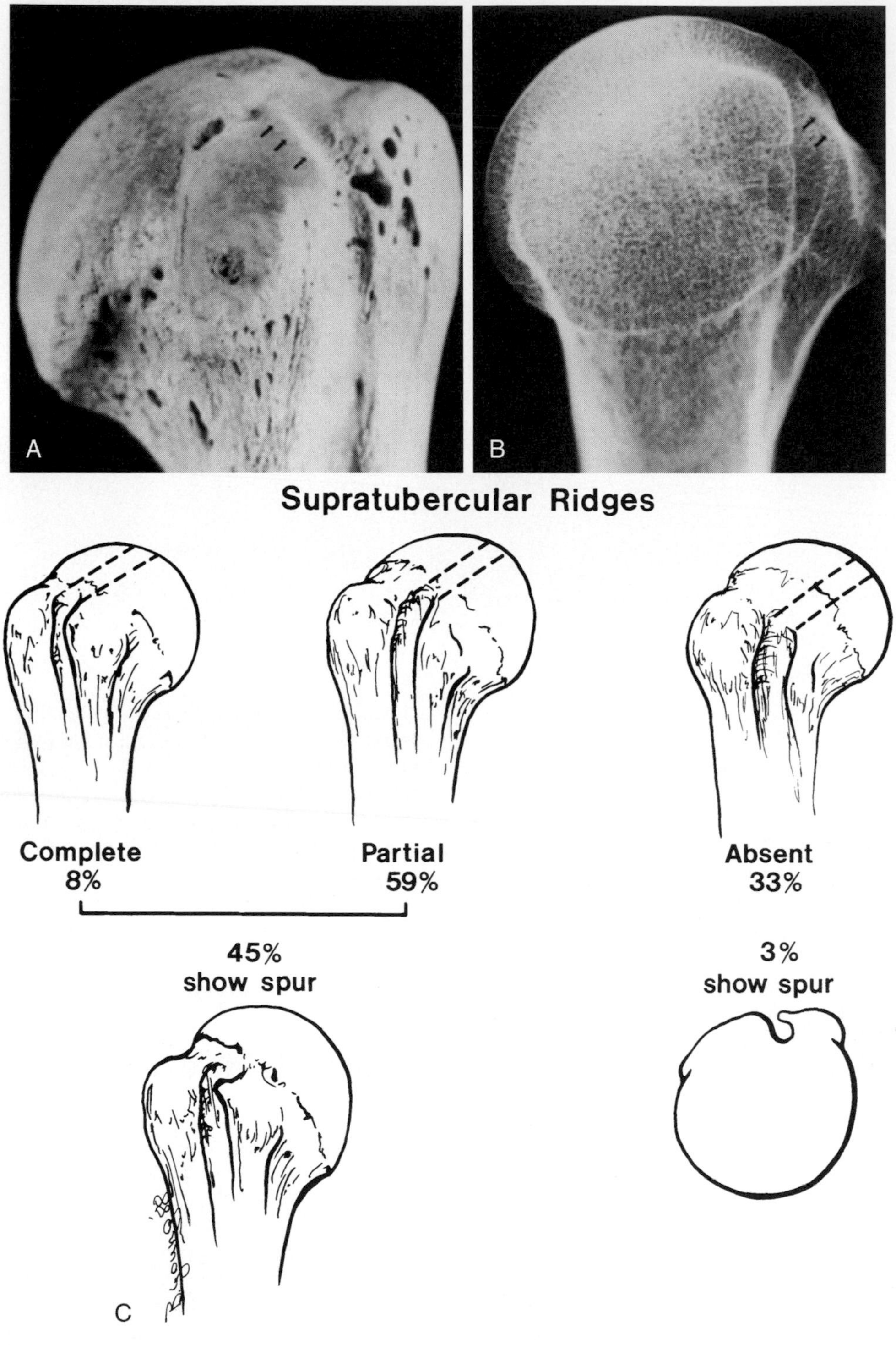

Figure 19–26

A, An externally rotated view of a cadaveric specimen showing the supratubercular ridge *(black arrows). B,* An internally rotated radiograph showing a prominent supratubercular ridge *(small black arrows).* (From Cone RO, Danzig L, Resnick D, and Goldman AB: The bicipital groove: Radiographic, anatomic, and pathologic study. Am J Roentgenol *41*:781–788, 1983. Copyright © Am Roentgen Ray Society, 1983.) *C,* This illustrates the presence of the supratubercular ridge (seen extending from the lesser tuberosity, altering the angle of the biceps tendon) and narrowing of the groove, both partial and complete in the specimens of Hitchcock and Bechtol. Medial wall spurs are much more common in specimens with supratubercular ridges. (Redrawn from Hitchcock HH and Bechtol CO: Painful shoulder. Observations on the role of the tendon of the long head of the biceps brachii in its causation. J Bone Joint Surg *30A*:263–273, 1948.)

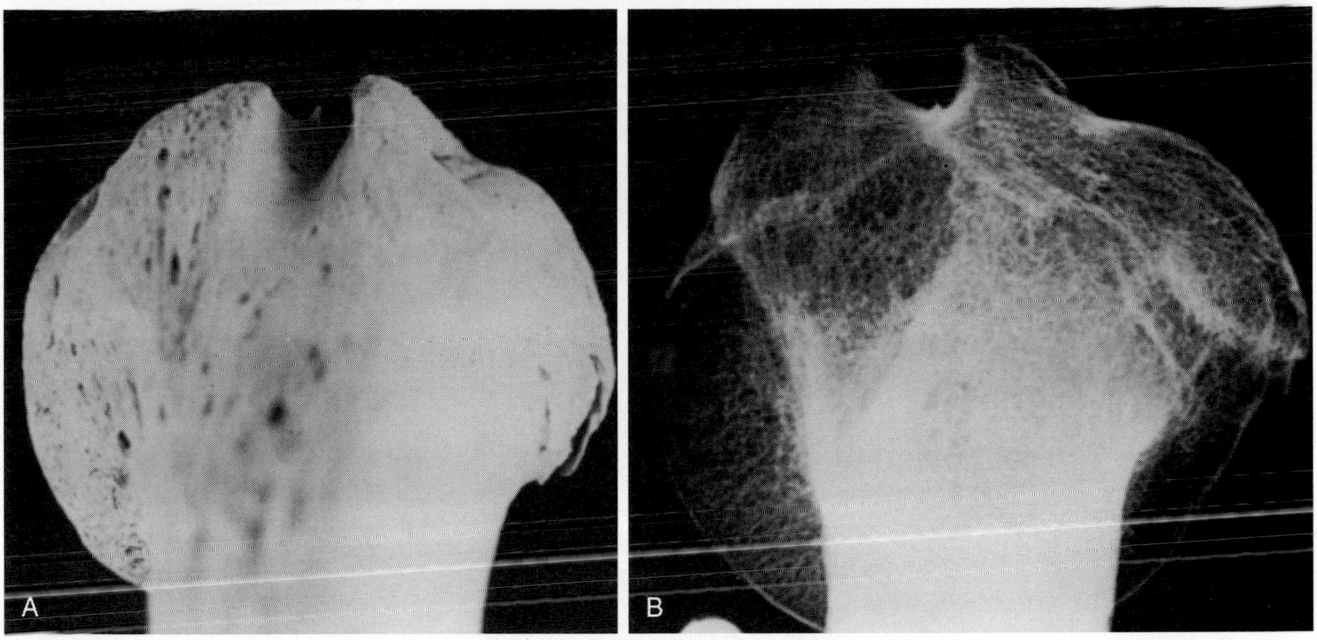

Figure 19–27

A, A bicipital groove floor spur thought by Cone and colleagues to be significant in biceps tendinitis as opposed to the medial wall spur, which was seen in several normal specimens. *B*, A groove radiograph of the same structure. (From Cone RO, Danzig L, Resnick D, and Goldman AB: The bicipital groove: Radiographic, anatomic, and pathologic study. Am J Roentgenol *41*:781–788, 1983. Copyright © Am Roentgen Ray Society, 1983.)

DIRECT OBSERVATION

Multiple investigators observed that the biceps tendon does not slide in the groove but, rather, the humerus moves on a fixed passive biceps tendon during shoulder motions.[111, 140, 141, 169] From adduction to complete elevation of the arm, the groove moves along the tendon for a distance of as much as 1½ inches. In order to facilitate this motion, the synovial pouch extends from the shoulder joint to line the intertubercular groove for a greater part of its extent (see Figs. 19–2 and 19–6). Below this bursa, the tendon glides through its peritendineum.

When the arm is in full external rotation, the tendon occupies the floor of the groove, and its more proximal portion exercises pressure on the humeral head. Therefore, it was originally believed that only in external rotation did the long head act directly on the shoulder as a head depressor and enhance somewhat the power of abduction of this joint. A vector diagram has been used by Lucas[146] to establish the resultant force of the biceps as that of depressing the head (Fig. 19–28). Figure 19–29 illustrates how the biceps acts as a static head depressor, preventing migration of the humeral head into the acromion by the pull of the deltoid.

Elevation of the arm in internal rotation causes minimal excursion of the tendon, whereas in external rotation, maximum excursion occurs. With the arm in the position of full abduction, 1.3 cm of tendon remained in the shoulder joint. Five centimeters of tendon is in the shoulder joint when the arm is depressed and externally rotated. This yields an overall excursion of 3.7 cm. Therefore, Lippmann believed that the tendon should not be considered to have two parts; that is, an intracapsular and a groove portion, because of this movement of the humeral head along the tendon (Fig. 19–30).

Rowe[233] states that in chronic rupture of the rotator cuff, the head depressor responsibility of the biceps tendon increases, and the tendon is often found to be hypertrophied. Bush[32] noted an increased depressor effect of the tendon when it was transplanted laterally for repairing cuff defects.

Andrews and colleagues[9] observed the biceps tendon and superior glenoid labrum complex arthroscopically during electrical stimulation of the biceps. They noted definite superior lifting of the labrum and compression of the glenohumeral joint. They observed that the biceps is in this respect a "shunt muscle of the shoulder" and does help to stabilize the glenohumeral joint during throwing. Its primary role during throwing, they agree, is still the deceleration of the elbow, and it is this sudden deceleration that leads to the tearing of the superior glenoid labral complex by the biceps tendon.

The authors have observed that during the treatment of four-part fractures, if a portion of the groove is maintained and the biceps returned to its groove, there is an increase in anteroposterior and inferosuperior stability. The replaced humeral head also seems to track more normally in the glenoid.

In a study by Itoi and Morrey,[120] the long head and short head of the biceps were shown to have similar function as anterior stabilizers of the glenohumeral joint with the arm in abduction and external rotation. It was further shown that as shoulder stability decreased due to sectioning of the inferior glenohumeral ligament, with the development of a Bankart lesion, that both heads of the biceps were shown to have increased stabilizing function to resist anterior displacement of the head. They concluded that strengthening of the biceps during rehabilitation for patients with chronic anterior instability should be included in conservative treatment of these lesions.

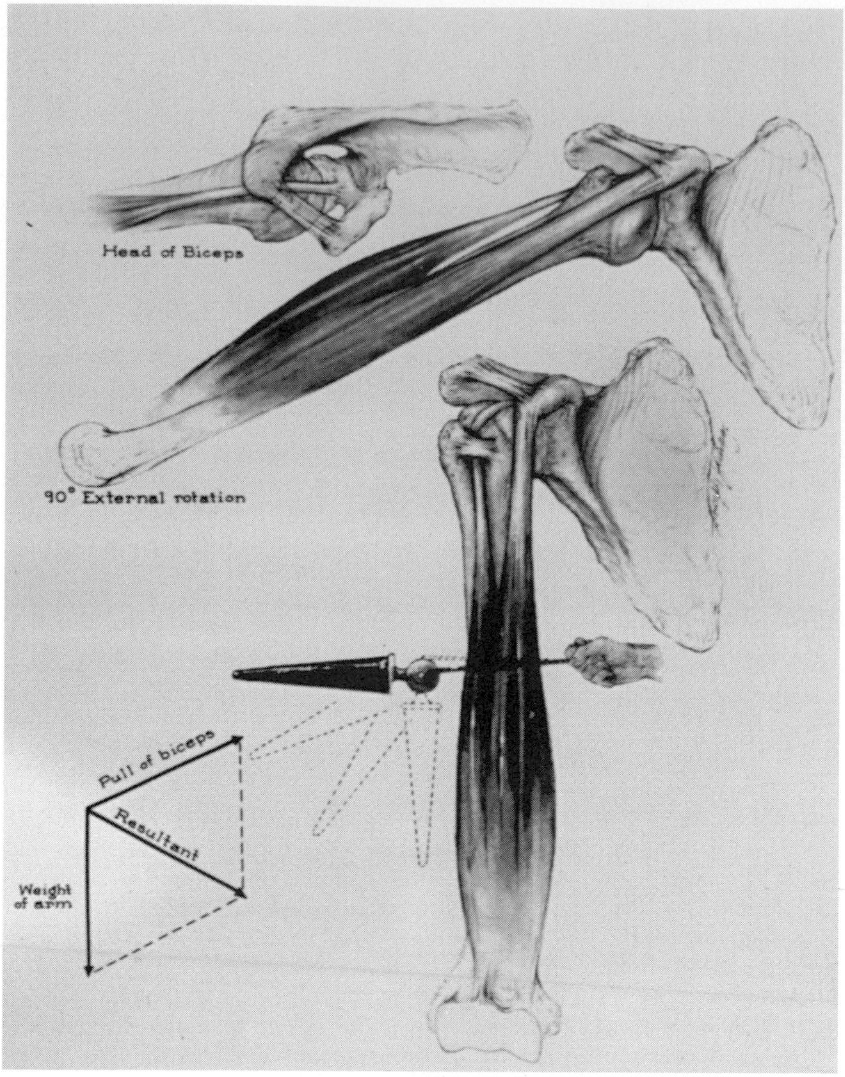

Figure 19–28

An artist's conception and vector diagram of the resultant force of the biceps tendon. (From Lucas DB: Biomechanics of the shoulder joint. Arch Surg *107*:425–432, 1973. Copyright © 1973, American Medical Association.)

Kumar also studied the stabilizing role of the biceps tendon. He was able to show that severing of the long head of the biceps tendon while both heads were tensed caused significant upwards migration of the humeral head. In this manner, the long head of the biceps is important in stabilizing the humeral head in the glenoid during powerful elbow flexion and forearm supination. He warned against the sacrifice of the intra-articular portion of the long head of the biceps tendon because of the danger of producing instability during forced elbow flexion and supination.

ELECTROMYOGRAPHIC EVALUATION

Basmajian and Latif[14] were pioneers in evaluating the musculoskeletal system, including the shoulder, with integrated function and dynamic spectrum EMG analysis. They reported that both heads of the biceps were active during shoulder flexion and that the long head was most active.[16] Habermeyer and associates[98] have performed EMG analysis, while Cybex testing was performed on normal individuals. Clear EMG activity was seen in the biceps during abduction, its peak being found at 132 degrees of abduction. Interestingly, Habermeyer and colleagues found that the muscle is active even with the arm in neutral rotation; that is, the biceps is active in abduction even when the arm is not externally rotated. In flexion, they found the main activity recorded during the first 90 degrees. The biceps was active in external rotation but not in internal rotation. The effectiveness of the long head of the biceps is greater in external rotation when its tension is maximal. In arm adduction and internal rotation, the long head was always inactive, whereas the short head was active in half of the cases of adduction and was only seldom active in internal rotation. The biceps was totally inactive in extension.

Laumann has divided by percentage the contribution of various muscles around the shoulder to shoulder flexion.[136, 137] Based on his work, he estimated that the biceps contributes approximately 7% of the power of flexion.

Furlani and colleagues studied EMG participation of the biceps in movements of the glenohumeral joint.[78] They found that in flexion of the shoulder with an extended elbow, both the long and short heads of the

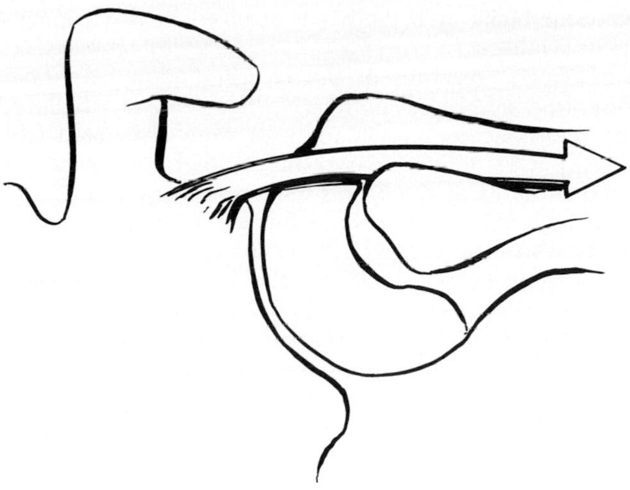

Figure 19–29

From this illustration it is evident that the biceps tendon is at least a static head depressor. Given the line of pull and the resultant vector, it is an active head depressor, although undoubtedly a weak one as is shown by the percentage of recruitment on electromyographic analysis. (Redrawn from Habermeyer P, Kaiser E, Knappe M, et al: Functional anatomy and biomechanics of the long biceps tendon. Unfallchirurg *90*[7]:319–329, 1987.)

biceps brachii were active in most cases, regardless of the presence or absence of resistance. In abduction without resistance, the biceps was inactive. The addition of resistance increased the activity of the biceps to 10%.

Ting and co-workers[251] have performed EMG analysis on the long head of the biceps in patients with rotator cuff tears. In all of their patients, an EMG record was expressed as a percentage of the activity recorded during maximal effort. They correlated their data with operative findings. During both shoulder abduction and flexion, four of five subjects tested demonstrated a significantly greater degree of EMG activity in the biceps tendon in the extremity with a torn cuff compared with that in the contralateral uninjured shoulder. In addition, all shoulders with compromised rotator cuffs proved to have a significantly larger tendon than did those of the controls, at the time of surgery, thus confirming Rowe's observations.[233] Ting and colleagues[251] suggested that the lateral head of the biceps may be a greater contributor to abduction and flexion in the compromised shoulder than in the normal shoulder. The concomitant enlargement of the tendon may indicate a use-induced hypertrophy. They, therefore, recommended not sacrificing the intracapsular portion of the tendon for graft material or tenodesing the tendon indiscriminately in the groove as a routine part of rotator cuff repair and acromioplasty.

The biceps' contribution to the shoulder during throwing has been evaluated by Jobe and associates[125] and also by Perry.[214] In these studies, the function of the biceps correlated with motion that occurred at the elbow but not in the shoulder. A relatively stable elbow position during acceleration was accompanied by marked reduction in the muscle's intensity. During follow-through, the need for deceleration of the rapidly extending elbow and pronating forearm was accompanied by peak action by the biceps. They showed no activity in the biceps muscle during the act of throwing, except when the elbow was active. Peak activity was only 36% of its maximum capacity. With a 9-cm^2 cross-section and only half of the muscle related to the long head, the humeral force is small. In Perry's words: "It seems doubtful that the long head (biceps tendon) is a significant stabilizing force at the glenohumeral joint." Glousman and associates,[89] on the other hand, have reported increased activity in the biceps during throwing in patients with unstable shoulders. Therefore, it seems that the biceps assumes more importance if the primary stabilizers are injured.

Yamaguchi and associates found little EMG activity of the biceps, even in patients with rotator cuff tears, when their elbows were flexed 100 degrees and in neutral rotation.[274] The biceps tendon does not appear to play a significant role in the stabilization of the humeral head under these circumstances.

EMG activity in patients with a less than 5-cm rotator cuff tear was found to be increased compared with healthy subjects studied by Ozaki and colleagues.[203] This increased activity could be compensating for the decreased function of the torn cuff. Ozaki and associates, like Ting and co-workers, postulate that this increased activity could be responsible for the hypertrophy of the long head of the biceps that often accompanies small and medium rotator cuff tears.[204] Patients with massive tears with dislocated biceps tendons had no similar increase in activity.

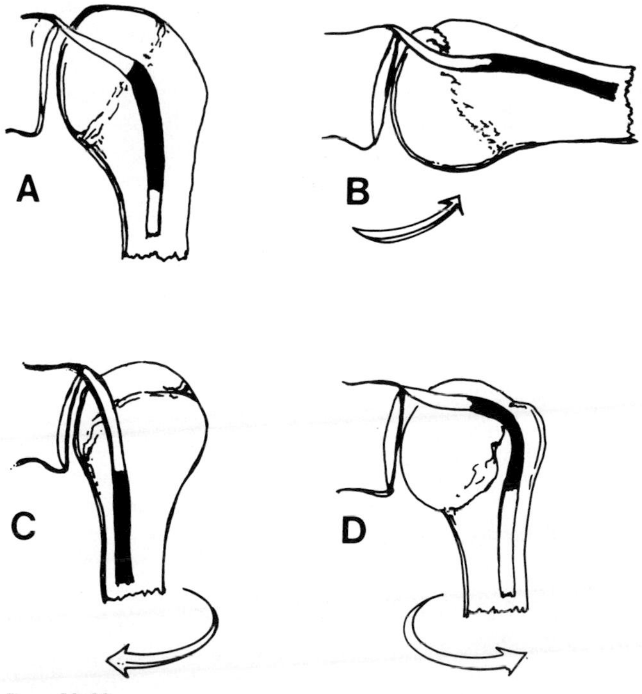

Figure 19–30

Lippmann found by direct observation under a local anesthetic that the biceps tendon slid freely in its sheath upon motion of the shoulder. Motion of the tendon in its groove appears only with motion of the shoulder joint. At any given position, a different amount of the biceps tendon can be found within the joint. (Modified from Lippmann RK: Bicipital tenosynovitis. N Y State J Med *90*:2235–2241, 1944. Copyright © by the Medical Society of the State of New York.)

Summary

It appears from a review of the literature that, based on the finding of consistent EMG activity with shoulder flexion and abduction independent of elbow flexion and given the resultant force of the biceps muscle, the biceps tendon does have a weak active head depressor effect. Based on its anatomic position, it serves as a superior checkrein to humeral head excursion and therefore at the very least acts as a static head depressor. As long as the tendon is located in its groove, the humeral head will slide up and down on the tendon and on the glenoid face in the normal fashion. With tears of the rotator cuff and medial subluxation of the biceps tendon, this checkrein effect is lost.

The tendon's activity seems to increase in pathologic states of the shoulder such as rotator cuff tears and shoulder instability, as evidenced by increased EMG activity as well as by observation of hypertrophy and resistance to translation. Based on these findings, the authors cannot recommend that it be routinely tenodesed at the time of acromioplasty or used as a free graft for performing rotator cuff repairs.

CLASSIFICATION OF BICIPITAL LESIONS

The classification of biceps lesions has historically been divided into biceps tendinitis and biceps instability. Biceps tendinitis was further divided into primary tendinitis, which was due to pathology of the biceps tendon sheath, and secondary biceps tendinitis, which had an associated lesion that caused the tendinitis. An example of this is rheumatoid arthritis or osteoarthritis or impingement causing bicipital tendinitis. More recently, an anatomic local classification has been offered by Walch.[265]

Primary biceps tendinitis has been likened to de Quervain's tenosynovitis by Lapidus.[136] Thickening and stenosis of the transverse ligament and sheath and narrowing of the tendon underneath the sheath were shown by this author. DePalma[59–63] showed that the severity of the process is governed by duration of the condition and by the age of the patient. Post[220] has found consistent inflammation within the intertubercular portion of the tendon with proliferative tenosynovitis, characterized by inflammation and irregularity of the walls of the groove. There appear to be no reports of inflammation of the intra-articular portion of the biceps. Codman[47] believed that primary biceps tendinitis was a rare entity, whereas DePalma thought that it was a common cause of stiff and painful shoulders.[59–63] In DePalma's series, 39% of cases had associated disorders. Crenshaw and Kilgore[56] were also proponents of primary biceps tendinitis, although 40% of their patients had an associated lesion. They conclude that whether the biceps tendon or its sheath is involved primarily or secondarily is not important, but that tenosynovitis is the chief cause of pain and limitation of motion in pericapsulitis.

Many authors believe that the pathology seen in the biceps is directly related to its intimate relationship with the rotator cuff.[61, 62, 186, 189, 220, 221] As they pass under the coracoacromial arch, both are involved in the impingement syndrome.

"Isolated" ruptures of the biceps tendon have been described by several authors.[51, 118, 168, 206] Neer believed that most biceps tendon ruptures were associated with supraspinatus tendon tears. Some studies have some isolated ruptures of the biceps tendon occurring in 25% of patients.[58] When CT arthrograms are performed on patients who have clinical criteria for isolated ruptures of the long head of the biceps, the incidence of isolated lesions decreases to 6%.[58] In an arthroscopically controlled study of isolated biceps tendon lesions, a 2.2% rate of isolated biceps ruptures was documented. These studies show the rarity of isolated ruptures of the long head of the biceps. Many authors have described bicipital groove osteophytes that were thought to cause ruptures of the long head of the biceps.[51, 118, 168, 206] Studies using CT scans have shown that depth and width of the bicipital groove do not have pathognomonic significance.[58]

Although primary bicipital tendinitis was recognized as a frequent cause of shoulder pain in the 1940s and 1950s, it is currently a diagnosis that is made much less frequently. Although we do not doubt the existence of this lesion, it is very uncommon. It should be considered as a diagnosis of exclusion.

Slatis and Aalto[240] have offered what appears to be a useful clinical classification of biceps lesions (Table 19–1). This classification is based on pathoanatomy and appears to have prognostic significance based on their review.

Slatis and Aalto Classification

TYPE A: IMPINGEMENT TENDINITIS

Type A is impingement tendinitis. This type is secondary to impingement syndrome and rotator cuff disease. The torn cuff exposes the biceps to the rigid coracoacromial arch and results in tendinitis (Figs. 19–31 and 19–32). This is the most frequent cause of biceps tendinitis.

TYPE B: SUBLUXATION OF THE BICEPS TENDON

Type B is called subluxation pathology. In this category, all pathologies of the biceps as well as subluxation and dislocation of the tendon are included (Fig. 19–33). In this group, lesions of the coracohumeral ligament allow the biceps tendon to gradually displace medially. This lesion can occur in an isolated fashion or it can be associated with tears of the supraspinatus and subscapularis. As the tendon slips in and out of its sulcus, it develops inflammation and fraying. The tendon can finally fully displace into a sling of ruptured cuff in early cases. In

Table 19–1 SLATIS AND AALTO CLASSIFICATION

TYPE A	Impingement tendinitis
TYPE B	Subluxation of the biceps tendon
TYPE C	Attrition is primary

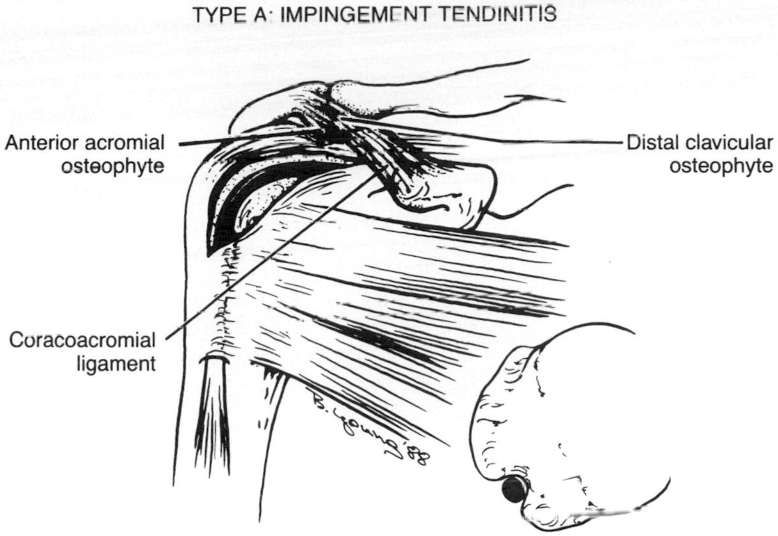

Figure 19–31

Type A impingement tendinitis. Rupture of the rotator cuff exposes the tendon to compression between the acromion above and the humeral head below. The tendon lies normally in its groove. (Modified from Paavolainen P, Slatis P, and Aalto K: Surgical pathology in chronic shoulder pain. *In* Bateman JE and Welsh RP [eds]: Surgery of the Shoulder. Philadelphia: BC Decker, 1984.)

more severe and later cases, the tendon may actually dislocate intra-articularly. The groove becomes shallower during this process as it fills with scar tissue.

TYPE C: ATTRITION TENDINITIS

Attrition tendinitis is the third category. These lesions are primary lesions of the biceps tendon that occur inside the canal. In this type of tendinitis, inflammation in the tight canal causes pain and degeneration of the biceps tendon (Fig. 19–34). These changes are associated with spurring and fraying of the tendon. Inflammation of the sheath causes formation of spurs and stenosis of the groove. This condition is thought to be extremely painful and rare.

Habermeyer and Walch's Classification

Habermeyer and Walch[100] classified lesions of the biceps tendon in a different manner (Table 19–2). They noted that the biceps tendon could be involved in pathology in different anatomic locations. In their classification, lesions of the biceps are affected either at: (1) their origin; (2) in the rotator interval; or (3) in association with rotator cuff tears.

ORIGIN LESIONS

Origin lesions are described as lesions affecting the attachment of the biceps tendon to the supraglenoid tubercle and to the superior glenoid labrum. These lesions can

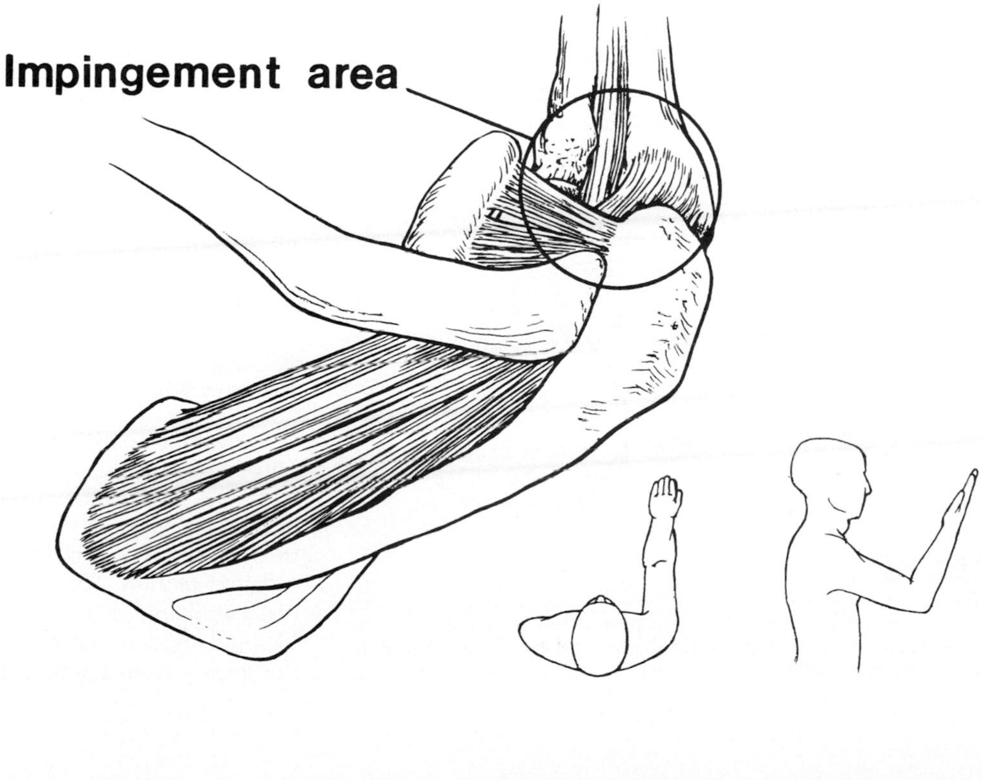

Figure 19–32

When the arm is forward flexed, the impingement area (i.e., the groove, biceps tendon, and anterior cuff) comes in contact with the coracoacromial arch. The longer the acromial process, the more likely the biceps will be involved. (Courtesy of Charles A. Rockwood, Jr., MD.)

TYPE B: SUBLUXATION

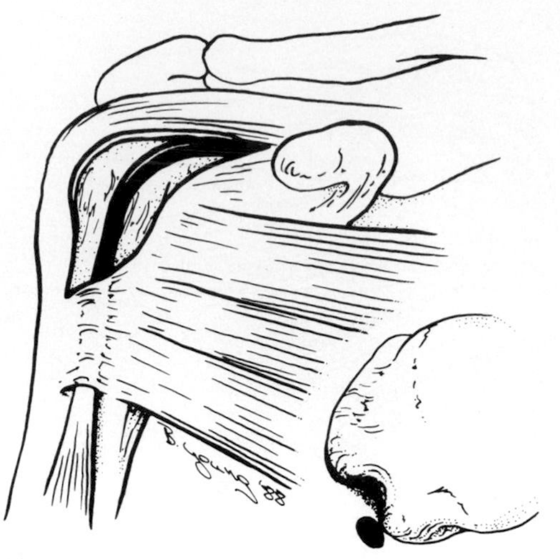

Figure 19–33

Type B subluxation of the biceps. A tear in the medial portion of the coracohumeral ligament causes subluxation and medial displacement of the tendon from the bicipital groove. Note the filling of the groove with fibrous tissue. (Modified from Paavolainen P, Slatis P, and Aalto K: Surgical pathology in chronic shoulder pain. *In* Bateman JE and Welsh RP [eds]: Surgery of the Shoulder. Philadelphia: BC Decker, 1984.)

involve the biceps origin from the superior labrum and spare the fibers coming off the supraglenoid tubercle or they can include lesions where the superior glenoid rim is avulsed off of the glenoid, pulling it away with the biceps tendon. These lesions have been observed to occur with the use of muscle stimulation. Biomechanical data by Grauer and associates[95] have shown that strain on the labrum from the working biceps is greatest when the arm is in overhead abduction.

TYPE C: ATTRITION TENDINITIS

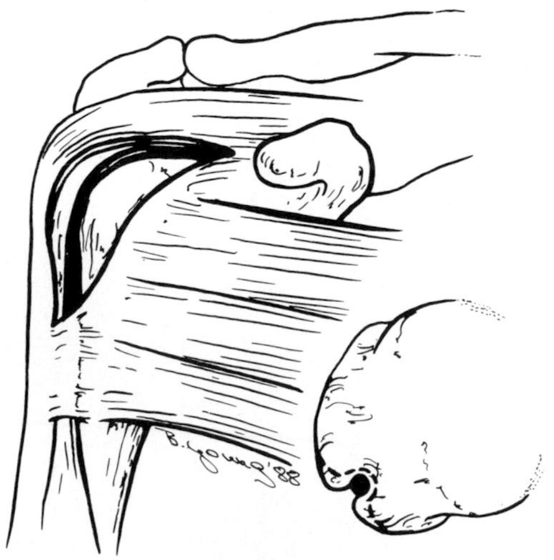

Figure 19–34

The cuff is exposed to show the pathology of constriction of the biceps tendon within the groove. Local formation of new bone and connective tissue causes stenosis of the bicipital groove, leading to attrition of the tendon of the long head of the biceps.

Lesions that affect the origin of the biceps tendon can occur in many different ways. These lesions have been described by Andrews and associates[9] as lesions of the anterior superior labrum in throwing athletes. These lesions are usually due to traction injuries in throwing athletes, especially during the release phase of throwing. They are associated with biceps tendon tears in 10% of cases.[9] These lesions can also be caused by falls on the outstretched arm with the shoulder in abduction and slight forward flexion.[241] Acute inferior traction as well as abduction-external rotation injuries can also cause this lesion.[99]

Snyder and colleagues[241] introduced the term SLAP (superior labrum anteroposterior) lesion in 1990. This author classified SLAP lesions into four basic types: A type I lesion is a lesion of the superior labrum. It shows marked fraying of the edges of the labrum, while the labral attachment to the glenoid is solid. This lesion does not really involve the biceps tendon. A type II lesion shows that the superior labral biceps complex is stripped from the underlying glenoid. This causes the labral biceps anchor to be unstable in the portion of the biceps origin that is not inserted onto the supraglenoid tubercle. Type III lesions show a bucket handle tear of the superior labrum in which the biceps tendon is not involved. Type IV lesions, on the other hand, show a bucket handle tear with splitting that extends into the biceps tendon.

Variations of SLAP lesions have also been described in association with complete ruptures of the long head of the biceps.[31, 99] SLAP lesions are covered more completely in Chapter 8.

INTERVAL LESIONS

Habermeyer and Walch[100] divided interval lesions into three types: biceps tendinitis, subluxation of the long head of the biceps tendon, and isolated ruptures.

Biceps Tendinitis

Biceps tendinitis is clinically characterized by chronic shoulder pain with tenderness over the bicipital groove and a positive result on Speed's test. When these criteria are used, 90% of all painful shoulders could be considered as having biceps tendinitis. A pathologic examination of biceps tendons in these shoulders rarely shows degenerative or microtraumatic lesions. These changes of the biceps tendon have been reported in only 5% of cases.

Primary Bicipital Tendinitis

This lesion, according to Habermeyer and Walch,[100] can only be diagnosed by arthroscopy. Findings of erythema and a vascular reaction around the long head of the biceps and in the groove is usually observed. For this diagnosis to be made, the shoulder must have a complete passive range of motion. The tendon should not be subluxated or dislocated out of its groove. Mechanical fraying of the bicipital tendon caused by osteophytes or narrowing of the groove from fracture is considered secondary.

Table 19–2 HABERMEYER AND WALCH'S CLASSIFICATION OF BICEPS LESIONS

I. ORIGIN	II. INTERVAL LESIONS	III. ASSOCIATED WITH RCT
	A. Biceps tendinitis	A. Tendinitis
	B. Isolated ruptures	B. Dislocation
	C. Subluxation	TYPE A: Extra-articular with a partial subscapular tear
	TYPE I: Superior	TYPE B: Extra-articular with intact subscapularis tendon
	TYPE II: At the groove	TYPE II: Intra-articular
	Type III: Malunion or nonunion of the lesser tuberosity	C. Subluxation with RCT
		D. Ruptured long head of the biceps with RCT

RCT, rotator cuff tear.

Subluxation of the Long Head of the Biceps Tendon

The definition of instability of the long head of the biceps tendon is poorly standardized and controversial.[65, 154, 201, 206, 216] Walch[263] defines subluxation of the long head of the biceps tendon as partial or incomplete loss of contact between the tendon and its bony groove. He defines dislocation as complete loss of contact between the tendon and its bony groove. Subluxation has been divided into three types by Walch.[263]

Superior Subluxation — Type I

This lesion occurs when the superior glenohumeral and the coracohumeral ligaments are partially or completely torn. The result of this tearing is that the long head of the biceps tendon above the entrance of the groove is subluxated superiorly. The subscapularis tendon is intact. The subscapularis tendon prevents a true dislocation of the tendon. The type I lesion is a discontinuity of the tendoligamentous rotator interval sling surrounding the long head of the biceps tendon, which allows the tendon to migrate superiorly.

Subluxation in the Groove—Type II

The lesion responsible for this type of subluxation is located inside the bony groove. The tendon slips over the medial rim of the bone of the groove and rides on the border of the lesser tuberosity. This lesion is caused by tearing of the outermost fibers of the subscapularis tendon, as well as some fibers that align the floor. The main criteria for type II biceps tendon subluxation is a partial rupture of the outer superficial tendinous portion of the subscapularis muscle. This lesion can involve the whole groove or only a portion of it.

Malunion and Nonunion of the Lesser Tuberosity—Type III

Fracture dislocation of the lesser tuberosity with malunion or nonunion can allow the biceps tendon to slip in and out of its groove. This lesion is seen after proximal humeral fractures. These patients have pain with internal rotation of the humerus.

Isolated Rupture of the Biceps Tendon Occurring in the Rotator Interval

Severe primary tendinitis of the tendon in the interval can cause weakening of the tendon and its eventual rupture in this area.

BICEPS TENDINITIS ASSOCIATED WITH ROTATOR CUFF TEARS

In this subgroup, patients have tendinitis of the biceps secondary to exposure of the biceps to the rigid coracoacromial arch. These patients have a rotator cuff tear but no dislocation or subluxation of the biceps tendon. The biceps is inflamed and painful and may appear hypertrophic when viewed through the arthroscope.

EXTRA-ARTICULAR DISLOCATION ASSOCIATED WITH SUBSCAPULARIS LESIONS (TYPE IA)

Extra-articular dislocation is combined with partial tear of the subscapularis tendon. This type of dislocation is when the biceps tendon is completely dislocated over the lesser tuberosity. Although there is superficial tearing of the subscapularis tendon, the deep portion of the subscapularis is intact. This allows the biceps tendon to line up over the lesser tuberosity and prevents the biceps from entering the joint. In this type of dislocation the outer layer of the subscapularis tendon is always torn. This is an evolutional type II subluxation.

EXTRA-ARTICULAR DISLOCATION OF THE LONG HEAD OF THE BICEPS TENDON ASSOCIATED WITH AN INTACT SUBSCAPULARIS (TYPE IB)

The biceps tendon can dislocate over an intact subscapularis tendon. This type is extremely rare. The long head of the biceps tendon is found lying superficial to the intact subscapularis tendon. An associated tear of the supraspinatus tendon is always seen. This was found in 3% of 70 patients with biceps dislocations.[199]

INTRA-ARTICULAR DISLOCATION OF THE LONG HEAD OF THE BICEPS TENDON (TYPE II)

Intra-articular dislocation of the long biceps tendon is combined with a complete tear of the subscapularis tendon. In this category, complete dislocation of the biceps is found in the intra-articular dislocation. This is usually in conjunction with extensive tearing of the rotator cuff. The subscapularis tendon is torn completely from its attachment on the lesser tuberosity, and this allows the biceps tendon to interpose itself into the joint. The biceps tendon is then opposed to the glenoid labrum and can be entrapped in the anterior joint space during rotational movements of the humerus. Subluxation of the biceps can also be associated with rotator cuff tearing.

RUPTURES OF THE BICEPS ASSOCIATED WITH A ROTATOR CUFF TEAR

The biceps can also rupture due to rotator cuff tears. Walch[264] has shown the frequency with which these lesions are associated. As has been stated earlier, an isolated rupture of the biceps tendon is rare. Most ruptures of the biceps tendon are associated with rotator cuff tears. This is usually due to impingement of the biceps and supraspinatus tendons in the area of the biceps sulcus.

TLC CLASSIFICATION

In an attempt to somehow simplify how to think about these complex lesions, the senior author (WZB) has developed the simple pneumonic TLC. The TLC System (Table 19–3) takes into account three distinct factors: (1) the status of the biceps tendon **(T)**; the anatomic location **(L)** of the pathologic process; and associated pathologic conditions of the rotator cuff **(C)**. With this classification there is "nothing to memorize" such as I, IIA, B, C, III, or IV. There are merely three items to remember when thinking about the biceps. TLC should be easy to recall because that is how the biceps should be handled.

INCIDENCE

In 1934, DePalma[59–63] stated that tenosynovitis of the long head of the biceps brachii muscle is the most common antecedent of painful and stiff shoulders. He believed that this was true of both younger and older age periods of life. In his 1954 series,[60] the lesion was encountered in 77 men and 98 women. The age of patients ranged from 16 to 69 years. The highest incidence was between the ages of 45 and 55. Bilateral involvement was observed in 8% of the cases. More severe lesions were found in the older decades of life, where more severe degenerative changes prevail. In 61.2% of the cases, the bicipital tenosynovitis was a localized pathologic process. In 38.8% of the cases, inflammation in the biceps tendon and sheath was part of a generalized and chronic inflammatory process. DePalma believed that bicipital tenosynovitis was the initiating agent in 80% of the cases of frozen shoulder.[59–63] Regardless of the cause, bicipital tenosynovitis was always a concomitant of the frozen shoulder.

Calcific tendinitis of the long head of the biceps brachii is uncommon.[230] This lesion has been described in two places. The first is the insertion of the biceps tendon into the supraglenoid tubercle and superior labrum. The second is in the distal portion of the groove near the musculotendinous junction. Calcific tendinitis was more frequent in a series by Goldman.[93] Nine cases of insertion tendinitis were seen in 119 cases of calcific tendinitis of the shoulder, compared with 11 of 19 for the more distal location.

Injuries to the superior labrum and biceps tendon complex occur infrequently. In a series by Andrews,[9] 10% of 73 throwing athletes had an incidence of associated partial tears of the biceps tendon and labral pathology. Burkhart and associates[31] have described two cases of complete tears of the biceps associated with SLAP lesions.

According to McCue[157] and O'Donohue,[201] biceps tendinitis and subluxation are common causes of anterior shoulder pain in throwing athletes. It is more common in football quarterbacks because of the weight of the ball and the need for additional pushing action and in softball pitchers because of forceful supinator strain with arm and forearm flexion.

Lapidus[136] identified 89 patients with tendinitis of the long head of the biceps in a total of 493 patients treated for shoulder pain (an incidence of 18%). Paavolainen, Slatis, and Aalto[206] reported on patients who failed to respond to conservative care and were referred to a shoulder center. A preoperative diagnosis of bicipital tendinitis was made prior to arthrotomy in 38 of 126 (30%) patients. Postoperatively with a direct inspection of the biceps tendon, the incidence was much higher, rising to 54% of the operative specimens and showing some evidence for biceps tendinitis. In patients with cuff ruptures, the incidence was 31 of 51 (60%) patients. If the rotator cuff was intact (no full-thickness tear), the incidence was approximately 50%. Although the cuff was "intact" at surgery, most of these cuffs did show some evidence of degeneration, edema, and signs of stage I and II impingement. Medial dislocation of the biceps tendon occurred in 12 of 51 cases with the cuff ruptured and 9 of 75 cases when the cuff was intact, yielding an overall incidence of dislocation of 17%. Frank ruptures of the biceps tendon were seen in 8 of the 126 patients, or 5%.

As bicipital tenosynovitis occasionally accompanies impingement syndrome, it remains a relatively common cause of anterior shoulder pain. However, as an isolated entity, that is, primary bicipital tenosynovitis, it is much less common.

Table 19–3 TLC

TENDON	Stable	Unstable	Tendinitis	Rupture
LOCATION	Origin	Interval	Groove	Musculotendinous junction
CUFF	Intact	Partial Tear	Complete Tear	Tendinosis

ETIOLOGY

Although the majority of biceps tendon dislocations occur secondarily, as the result of degeneration and attrition in the anterior acromion on the anterior cuff and coracohumeral ligament, acute traumatic dislocation of the tendon of the biceps has been described.[76, 80, 163–170, 186–189] In 1939, Abbott and Saunders presented six cases with operative findings.[1] Four cases occurred from falls with direct blows to the shoulder or from indirect force or falls on the outstretched hands. Two cases occurred during heavy lifting. All except one of these patients had a concomitant injury to the rotator cuff as well.

DePalma[59–62] and later Michele[171] divided the etiology of biceps tendinitis by the age group of the patient. In the younger age group, anomalies of the bicipital groove together with a repeated trauma are the major factors in initiating the syndrome. In the older age group, degenerative changes in the tendon are the predominant etiologic factor.

As with most other musculoskeletal problems, the etiology of biceps pathology is most likely multifactorial. Chief among the causes is the anatomic location of the tendon. The blood supply of the tendon has been studied by Rathbun and Macnab[227] and has been shown to be diminished, with a critical zone similar to that seen in the supraspinatus (Fig. 19–35). In abduction, there is a zone of avascularity in the intracapsular portion of the tendon that is felt to be caused by pressure from the head of the humerus, the so-called "wringing out" phenomenon. Occupational causes also exist because patients who do repetitive overhead lifting and throwing are more susceptible to ruptures, elongations, and dislocations of the biceps. Meyer reasoned that capsular defects leading to problems with the biceps resulted from repeated and continual use of the arm in a position of marked abduction and external rotation.[163–170] Borchers[27] and later DePalma[59–63] explained spontaneous ruptures within the groove on the basis of osteophytic excrescences, which eventually wear away the tendon. Etiologic factors based on the variations in the groove have been previously discussed.

The etiology of calcific deposits in the biceps may be active or passive. Hydroxyapatite deposition disease has been described and can occur in varied tendons throughout the body. The reader is referred to Chapter 18 for a detailed description of active calcification. In a study by Refior and Sowa,[228] a histologic analysis of the biceps tendon was performed and showed degeneration at the biceps origin and in the region where the biceps tendon exits the groove. They noted a kinking and destruction of the collagen fibers in both these areas. Whether this degeneration is responsible for inducing calcification in some susceptible patients is debatable.

SLAP lesions and lesions of the biceps and superior labrum can be caused by two mechanisms. The first mechanism is a fall on the outstretched hand that drives the humeral head up onto the labrum and the tendon. This lesion has been described by Snyder and associates.[241] Andrews[9] noted that excessive and forceful contraction of the biceps in throwing athletes, especially baseball pitchers and quarterbacks, can, in the deceleration phase of throwing, provide traction and avulsion of the biceps and superior labral complex. This mechanism of injury may also be responsible for some SLAP lesions seen.

Patients on dialysis with long-standing kidney failure can have shoulder pain and may have symptoms similar to those of biceps tendinitis. The etiology of this syndrome is often synovitis caused by deposition of amyloid-like substances. This is a rare cause of shoulder pain.[249] Another rare cause of bicipital pain and degeneration is a

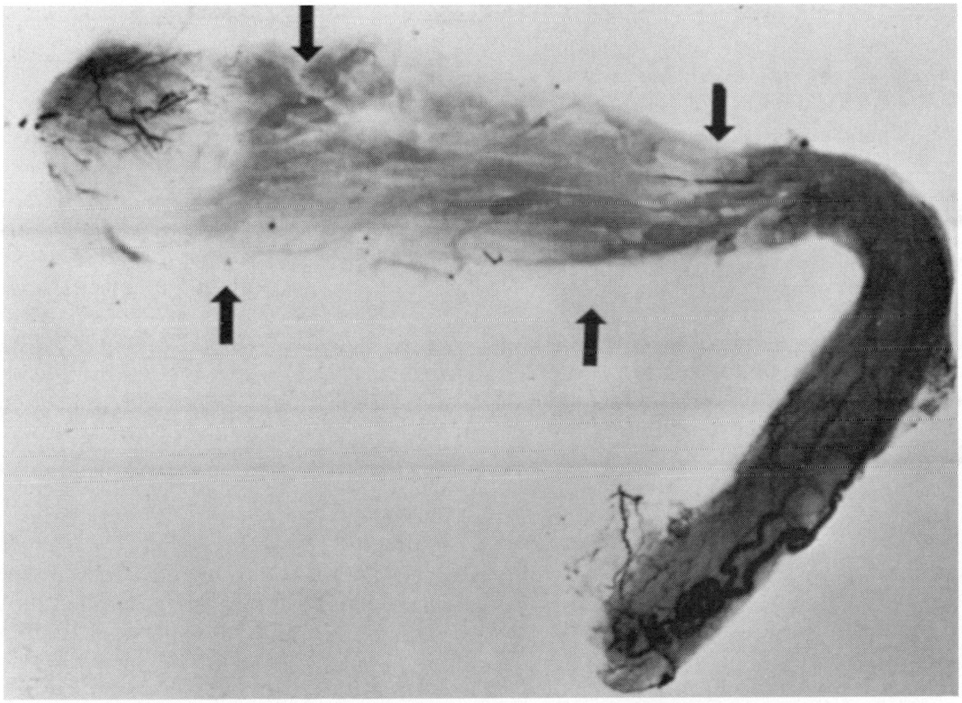

Figure 19–35

A zone of relative avascularity is seen in the biceps. (From Rathbun JB and Macnab I: The microvascular pattern of the rotator cuff. J Bone Joint Surg *52B*:540–553, 1970.)

tumoral condition, such as osteochondromatosis of the bicipital sheath.[57]

PREVENTION

Prevention of biceps injuries in workers and athletes entails the same type of preventive rehabilitation that is used in athletes for their rotator cuff (i.e., warm-up passive stretching, strengthening, and avoidance of painful activities during the time of symptoms). Strengthening should include all the muscles of the rotator cuff to improve the force couple and decrease impingement. The parascapular muscles should also be rehabilitated. A better balanced shoulder musculature will prevent or at least decrease the vicious circle of impingement tendinitis, irritation, and muscle weakness, which is followed by altered biomechanics, subluxation, and further impingement. Persons who do manual labor with heavy lifting or repetitive overhead work, such as carpenters, should probably spend as much time stretching before undertaking their jobs as football or baseball players spend before undertaking theirs. Stretching of the biceps tendon is maximal when the shoulder is fully extended and externally rotated and the elbow is fully extended as well.

Careful pre-employment screening and testing, including muscular strength, can help to identify shoulder problems before employees begin working. Deficits could be corrected with exercise before beginning a job that requires heavy lifting or overhead use of the arm. The scapular lateral outlet view and the 30-degree caudal tilt x-ray view may possibly be used to prevent people at risk for impingement from taking jobs that would put their shoulders at risk for injury.

Overhand athletes, especially pitchers and quarterbacks, should warm up and stretch the rotator cuff as well as the paraspinal and arm muscles before training sessions and competitions. They should be encouraged to strengthen the muscles of their upper extremity, especially the rotator cuff. Athletes should also be monitored closely to prevent overuse syndromes from developing. The use of a pitching rotation in young baseball pitchers can allow some of these players to rest adequately.

CLINICAL PRESENTATION OF BICIPITAL LESIONS

There is no substitute in any medical condition for an accurate history and physical examination. This is especially true of subtle lesions of the shoulder such as biceps tendinitis, instability, and impingement syndrome. In this section, the historical and specific clinical features of bicipital tendinitis and instability are presented; in the section on differential diagnosis, a more thorough history and physical examination of the shoulder are reviewed.

Patients with bicipital tendinitis usually present with chronic pain in the proximal anterior area of the shoulder. The pain sometimes extends down the arm into the region of the biceps muscle belly. It can, like pain from impingement syndrome, radiate to the deltoid insertion. Usually there is no radiation into the neck or distally beyond the biceps. In most cases, there is no history of major trauma, although, as has been stated previously, acute trauma can predispose to bicipital tendinitis rupture or dislocation. Typically, the patient is young or middle aged with a history of repetitive use of the arm in overhead activity. The pain is less intense at rest and worse with use. Neviaser[191] states that no significant pain occurs at night, whereas Simon[239] believes that nocturnal exacerbation is common. In the author's experience, all painful conditions of the shoulder are worse at night because of compression loading and because the supine position places the shoulder at or below the level of the heart. If a person rolls over on the involved shoulder, this action further increases the problem by decreasing the venous return from the upper extremity. The pain from calcific tendinitis of the biceps is of such great intensity that the patient often paces around at night.

Bicipital tendinitis is frequently seen in patients who participate in swimming, tennis, and golf and also in sports that involve throwing. In each of these activities, the rotation of the humerus at or above the horizontal level brings the tuberosities, intervening groove, biceps tendon, and rotator cuff in direct contact with the anterior acromion and the coracoacromial ligament.

Biceps instability is suggested by a pain pattern similar to the aforementioned. It is seen most commonly in throwing athletes. Motion is often accompanied by a palpable snap or pop at a certain position in the arc of rotation. The patient indicates pain in the front of the shoulder, which is usually reproduced by raising the arm up to 90 degrees. Biceps rupture appears frequently with acute pain and sometimes an audible pop in the shoulder. During the next several days, the patient will notice a change in contour of the arm and ecchymoses.

Clinical presentation of calcific tendinitis in the distal part of the long head of the biceps tendon presents with a picture of anterior shoulder pain in young and middle-aged adults. The pain of distal tendon involvement is usually referred to the anterior shoulder. The duration and severity of this pain can vary.

Physical Examination

Physical examination reveals point tenderness in the biceps groove, which is best localized with the arm in about 10 degrees of internal rotation.[155] With the arm in this position, the biceps tendon should be facing directly anteriorly and located 3 inches below the acromion (Fig. 19–36).[188] Point tenderness in this area (i.e., 3 inches below the anterior acromion) should move with rotation of the arm. It often disappears as the lesser tuberosity and groove rotate internally under the short head of the biceps and coracoid. The tenderness of subdeltoid bursitis is generally more diffuse and should not move with arm rotation. The tenderness seen with impingement is often diffuse and is accompanied by tenderness in the arm, acromion, coracoacromial ligament, and coracoid process. However, it does not move with rotation. This "tenderness in motion" sign is, in my (W.Z.B.) opinion, the most specific for bicipital lesions. It does not, however, differentiate biceps instability from tendinitis. Many authors

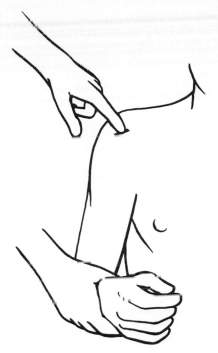

Figure 19–36

Matsen[155] has found that the biceps tendon can be palpated directly anteriorly with the arm in 10 degrees of internal rotation. This is the same position that is utilized in performing deAnquin's and Lippmann's tests (described in the text).

have stated that the biceps can be felt subluxating out of the groove. It is difficult to discern whether what one is feeling is actually a subluxating tendon or the muscle bundles of the deltoid rolling up underneath one's finger as it is pressed against the humerus. Anyone who has looked at the biceps surgically should have trouble thinking that he or she is actually palpating the tendon, especially in a well-muscled individual.

There may be a slight restriction of abduction and internal rotation. This loss of motion is usually due to pain and not to capsular constriction and should improve with local anesthetic injection. Pain is felt with abduction and internal rotation, abduction, and external rotation, and pain is resisted with forward flexion of the shoulder.

Several tests have been reported to aid in the diagnosis of biceps pathology. There are, however, no data as to the sensitivity or specificity of any of these tests on patients with shoulder pain. The most important question when performing provocative tests on any part of the musculoskeletal system is: "Does this maneuver specifically reproduce the patient's pain?" Selective injection with obliteration of pain is an extremely important part of clinical evaluation of the shoulder. There is no substitute for clinical experience, repeated examination, selective injection, and a cautious approach to anterior shoulder pain. Many poor results from surgery in this region come from a surgical procedure being performed too early or directed only at the biceps lesion. Repeated examination may show evolution of an impingement syndrome, adhesive capsulitis, or evidence of glenohumeral instability. The following tests have been described by authors in the past in isolating lesions in the biceps tendon:

1. *Speed's test* (Fig. 19–37).[87] The patient flexes the shoulder against resistance while the elbow is extended and the forearm is supinated. The pain is localized in the bicipital groove.
2. *Yergason's sign* (Fig. 19–38).[275] This test is performed with the patient's elbow flexed. The patient is asked to forcibly supinate against resistance. Pain referred to the front and inner aspect of the shoulder in the bicipital groove constitutes a positive sign. Post found an incidence of 50% positivity with this sign in patients with primary bicipital tendinitis.[221]
3. *Biceps instability test* (Fig. 19–39).[1] Dislocation of the tendon, complete or incomplete, may be differentiated from peritendinitis by the test of Abbott and Saunders.[1] After full abduction of the shoulder, the arm, which is held in complete external rotation, is slowly brought down to the side in the plane of the scapula. A palpable and even audible and sometimes painful click is noted as the biceps tendon, now forced against the lesser tuberosity, becomes subluxated or dislocated from the groove.
4. *Ludington's test* (Fig. 19–40).[147] In Ludington's test the patient is asked to put his or her hands behind the head. In this position of abduction and external rotation, the patient is asked to flex the biceps isometrically, and the pain is in the region of the bicipital groove in tendinitis. If the examiner's finger is in the groove at the time of the contraction, subluxation can sometimes be felt. Subtle differences in the contour of the biceps in cases of elongation are best noted in this fashion.
5. *DeAnquin's test* (Fig. 19–41).[247] The arm is rotated with the examiner's finger on the most tender spot. There is immediate pain as the tendon glides beneath the finger.
6. *Lippmann's test*.[140] Lippmann's test produces pain, and the tendon is displaced from one side to the other by the probing finger and released. This is done about 3 inches from the shoulder joint, with the elbow flexed at

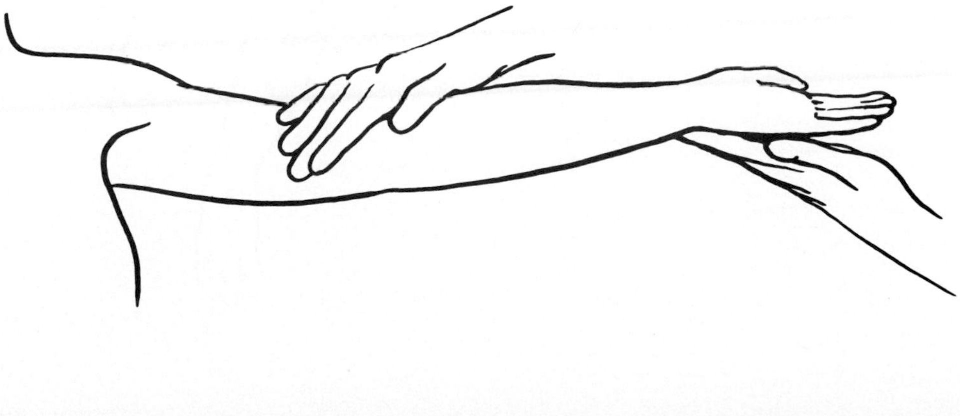

Figure 19–37

Speed's test. The biceps resistance test is performed with the patient flexing the shoulder against resistance, with the elbow extended and the forearm supinated. Pain referred to the biceps tendon area constitutes a positive result.

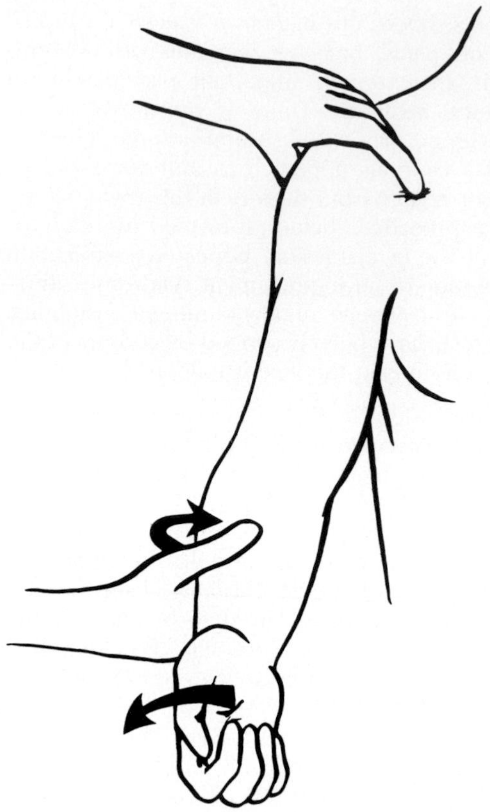

Figure 19–38

Yergason's sign. With the arm flexed, the patient is asked to forcefully supinate against resistance from the examiner's hand. Pain referred to the anterior aspect of the shoulder in the region of the bicipital groove constitutes a positive result.

a right angle. We are more often rolling up the deltoid muscle with this test, and the biceps is not palpated.

7. *Hueter's sign.*[116] Hueter's sign is positive when flexion of the supinated forearm (primarily a biceps function) is less forceful than flexion of the pronated forearm.

Physical examination in patients with complete biceps rupture is much less subtle because of the obvious deformity that develops (Fig. 19–42). There is a hollowness in the anterior portion of the shoulder accompanied by balling up of the biceps below the midbrachium. In these patients it is important to look specifically for cuff atrophy because tears of the biceps in the older population are frequently associated with attrition-type tears in the rota-

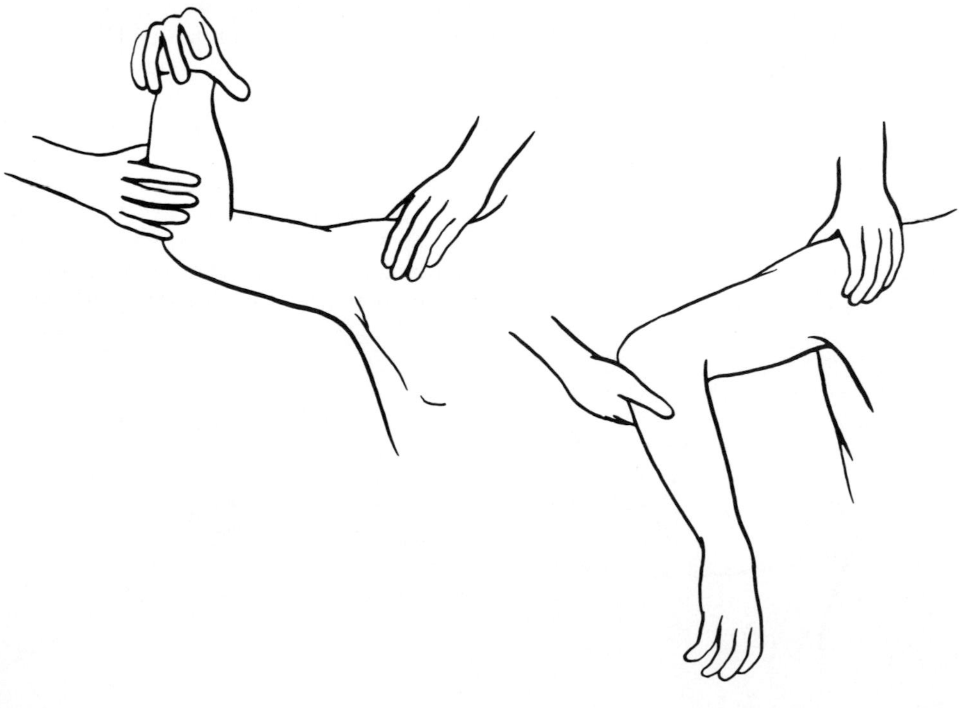

Figure 19–39

Biceps instability test (described by Abbott and Saunders). During palpation of the biceps in the groove while taking the arm from an abducted externally rotated position to a position of internal rotation, a palpable or audible painful click is noted as the biceps tendon is forced against or over the lesser tuberosity.

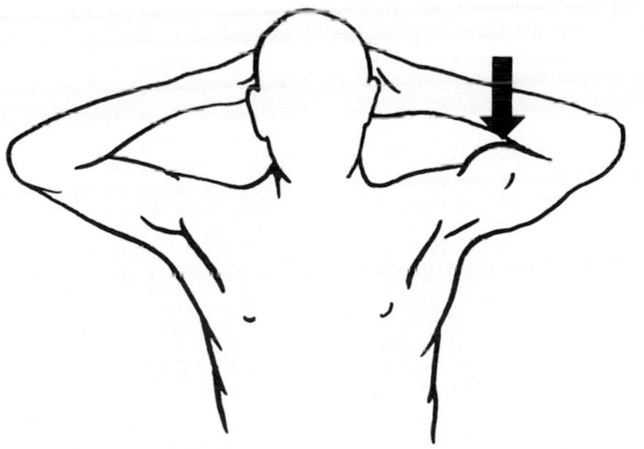

Figure 19–40

Ludington's test. The patient is asked to put his or her hands behind the head and flex the biceps. The examiner's finger can be in the bicipital groove at the time of the test. Subtle differences in the contour of the biceps are best noted with this maneuver. In this illustration the patient has a ruptured biceps at the left shoulder.

tor cuff preceding the biceps rupture. These may or may not have been symptomatic prior to the bicipital rupture, but it is not uncommon for the patient to have a history of being treated in the remote past for "bursitis."

ASSOCIATED CONDITIONS

The following are associated conditions and are discussed under the differential diagnosis:

1. Impingement syndrome
2. Adhesive capsulitis
3. Rheumatoid and osteoarthritis
4. Glenohumeral instability
5. Coracoid impingement syndrome
6. Thoracic outlet/brachial plexopathy/plexitis
7. Peripheral nerve entrapment, cervical radiculopathy
8. Dialysis patients
9. Rare tumors

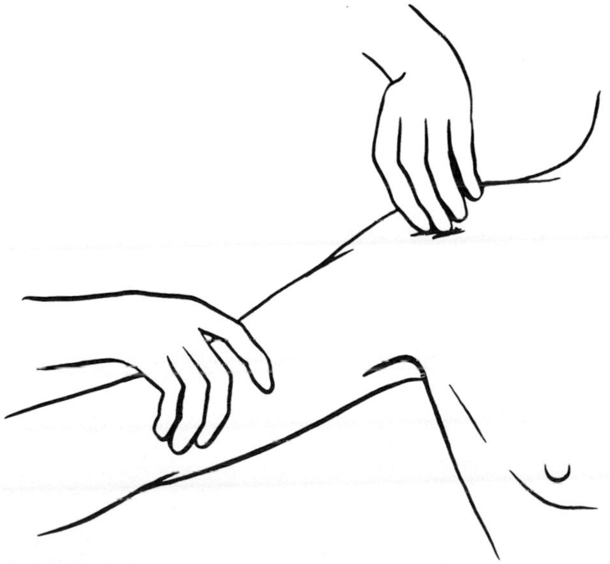

Figure 19–41

DeAnquin's test. The patient's arm is rotated while the examiner has his or her finger in the most tender spot in the bicipital groove. A positive result occurs in biceps tendinitis when the patient feels pain as the tendon glides beneath the finger.

Concomitant Injuries

One should remain alert for a wide range of lesions when evaluating a biceps rupture. Injuries include extensive damage to the rotator cuff and variable degrees of brachial plexus stretch, which are seen occasionally in association with biceps rupture and occur almost invariably as the result of a fall on the posteriorly outstretched arm in an elderly patient. Occasionally, there is an associated anterior dislocation of the shoulder. Humeral fractures and fracture dislocations can occur. The biceps can become interposed and block reduction of both fractures and dislocations.[115, 121, 159] An extensive area of ecchymoses of the chest associated with the injury should indicate to the examiner that the biceps tendon rupture is not an isolated injury. In isolated biceps ruptures, the swelling and ecchymoses should be limited to the brachium.

DIAGNOSTIC TESTS

Plain Film Radiology

Frequently, routine plain films of the shoulder are normal in biceps tendinitis. This has led to the development of special views for the bicipital groove and the use of other imaging techniques to evaluate this tendon.

FISK METHOD

In the Fisk method[75] (Fig. 19–43), the patient holds the cassette and leans over the table. The biceps groove is marked, and the central beam is perpendicular to the groove.

BICIPITAL GROOVE VIEW

In the bicipital groove view described by Cone and colleagues, the patient is supine with the arm in external rotation[49] (see Fig. 19–43*B*). The central beam is directed parallel to the coronal axis of the humerus and angled 15 degrees medially. The film cassette is held perpendicular to the superior aspect of the shoulder. Using the radiographs, the medial wall angle, the width, presence or absence of bicipital groove spurs, coexisting degenerative changes in the greater or lesser tuberosity, and the presence or absence of a supratubercular ridge can be determined (Fig. 19–44). In a study by Ahovuo[4] in which radiographic findings were correlated with the surgical findings, half of the patients with surgically proven bicipital tendinitis had degenerative changes in the walls of the groove. In patients with attrition tendinitis, the depth of the groove was 4.8 mm or more and its inclination was 58 degrees or more. A shallow groove was seen more frequently with bicipital dislocation.

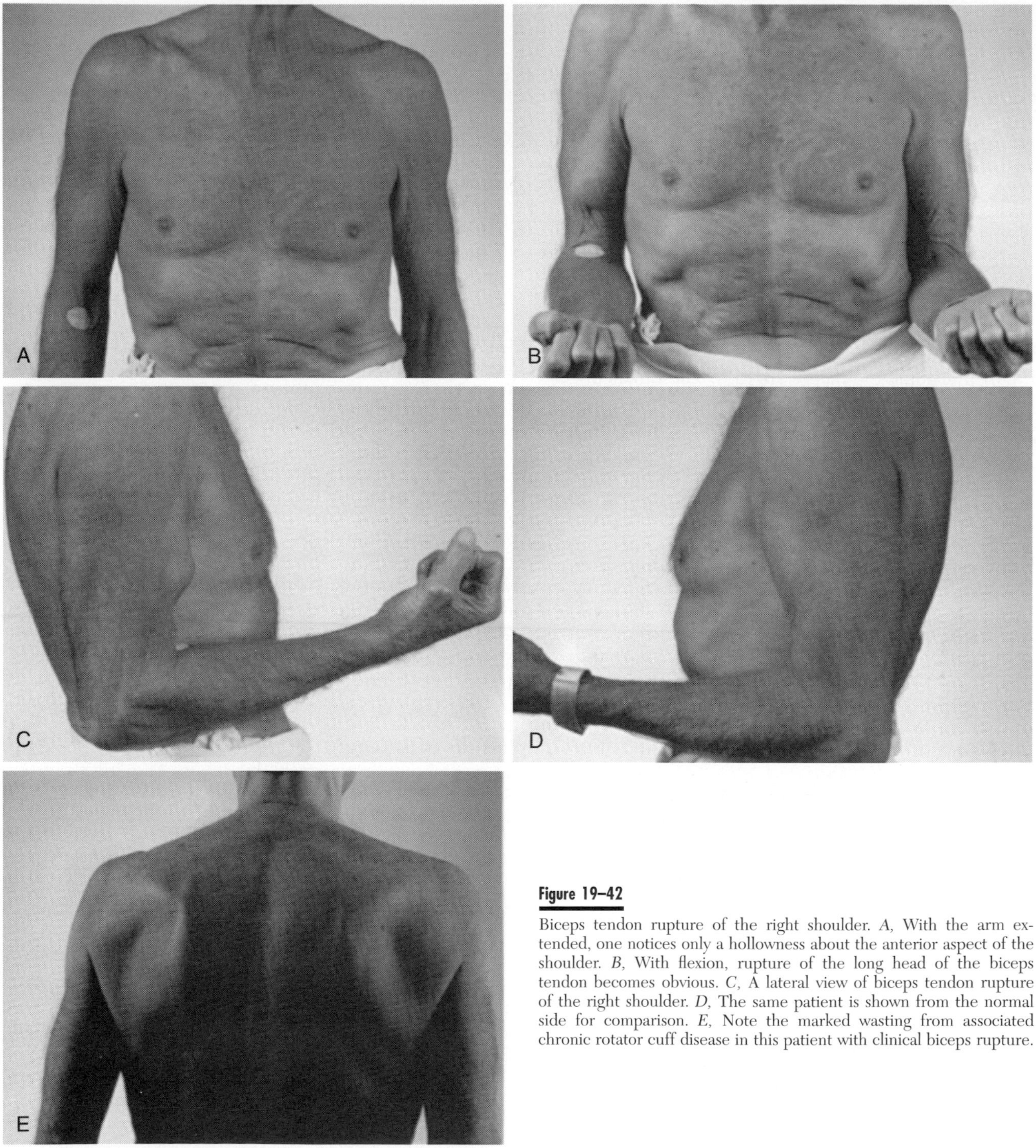

Figure 19–42

Biceps tendon rupture of the right shoulder. *A*, With the arm extended, one notices only a hollowness about the anterior aspect of the shoulder. *B*, With flexion, rupture of the long head of the biceps tendon becomes obvious. *C*, A lateral view of biceps tendon rupture of the right shoulder. *D*, The same patient is shown from the normal side for comparison. *E*, Note the marked wasting from associated chronic rotator cuff disease in this patient with clinical biceps rupture.

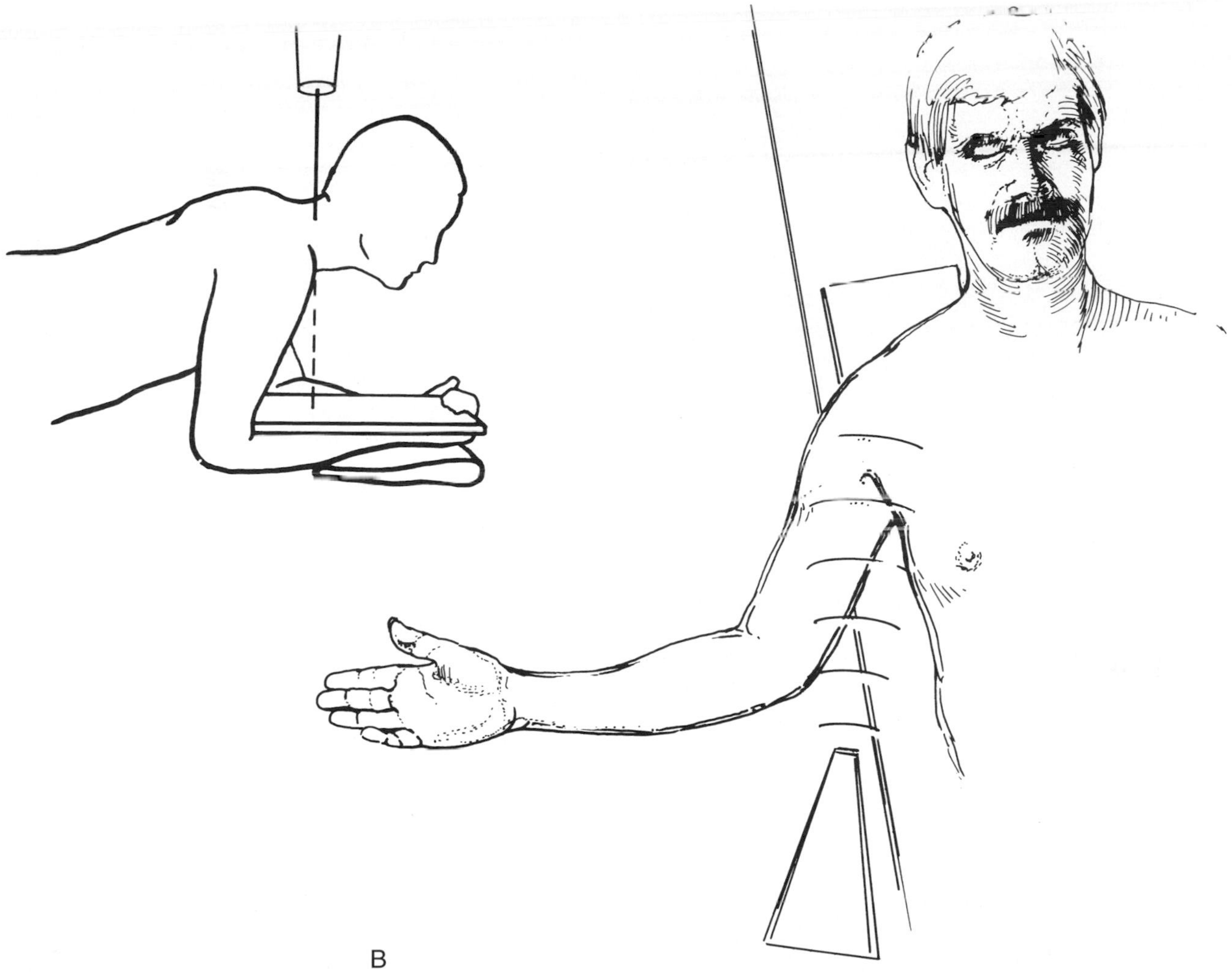

A

B

Figure 19–43

A, Fisk method. The patient holds the cassette while leaning over the table, bringing the bicipital groove perpendicular to the central beam of the x-ray. *B*, Bicipital groove view. The central beam is directed parallel to the coronal axis of the humerus and angled 15 degrees medially. The patient is supine with the arm in the externally rotated position.

Two additional views that are helpful in the differential diagnosis of biceps tendinitis are the caudal tilt view[231] radiograph and the outlet view of Neer and Poppen.[189] The caudal tilt radiograph is a standing anteroposterior view of the shoulder with a 30-degree caudal tilt to the x-ray beam (Fig. 19–45). With this technique, the degree of anterior acromial prominence or spurring can be appreciated. The outlet view is a trans-scapular radiograph done with a 10-degree caudal tilt. The easiest way to take this radiograph is with the patient standing with the spine of the scapula perpendicular to the cassette. The x-ray beam should be parallel to the spine but with a 10-degree caudal tilt (see Fig. 19–45*B*). These views should be done routinely to avoid the most common problem seen with biceps lesions today—failure to relieve the underlying cause of the bicipital lesion (i.e., coracoacromial arch impingement syndrome).

Arthrography

Shoulder arthrography can provide information on the state of the biceps tendon. Many shallow grooves contain a normal tendon.[4] Whether or not a shallow groove on plain films is associated with a dislocation of the biceps can be determined by an arthrogram. Sometimes the dislocation is obvious in the anteroposterior view (Fig. 19–46). In other patients, a groove view must be performed with the contrast instilled to make the diagnosis.[104, 106, 107] Second, in biceps tendinitis, there may be a loss of sharp delineation of the tendon.[104] In rheumatoid arthritis, irregularities in the sheath of the biceps tendon may be caused by synovitis. However, in the study by Ahovuo,[4] the arthrogram showed no difference in the filling of the tendon sheath between patients with surgically verified biceps tendinitis and those with a normal tendon. Arthrography in patients with biceps tendinitis may show that the cuff is intact and that the biceps is poorly outlined, has a thickened sheath, or is elevated at its origin.[193, 195] When adhesive capsulitis exists, the biceps sheath, like the subscapularis recess and dependent axillary fold, contracts (Fig. 19–47). The tendon and bicipital groove can also be assessed with computed tomographic (CT) arthrography (Fig. 19–48).

MRI with gadolinium injection is sometimes used to

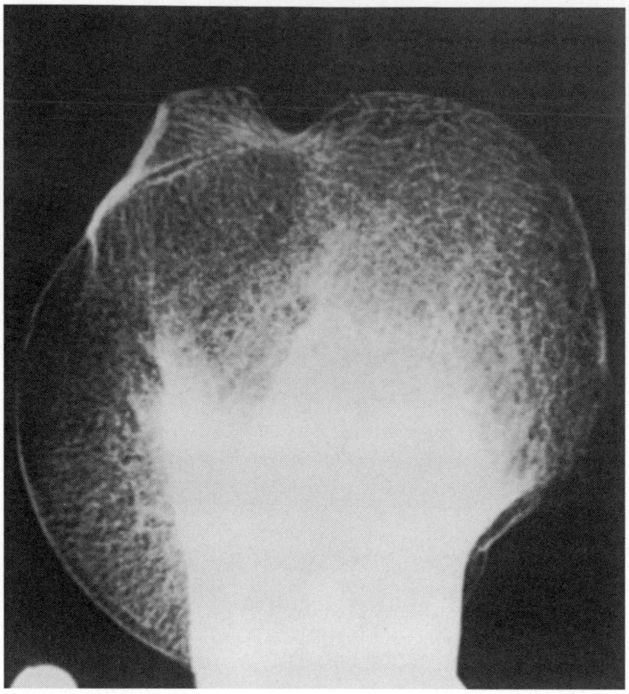

Figure 19–44

Normal bicipital groove projection. (From Cone RO, Danzig L, Resnick D, and Goldman AB: The bicipital groove: Radiographic, anatomic, and pathologic study. Am J Roentgenol *41:*781–788, 1983. Copyright © Am Roentgen Ray Society, 1983.)

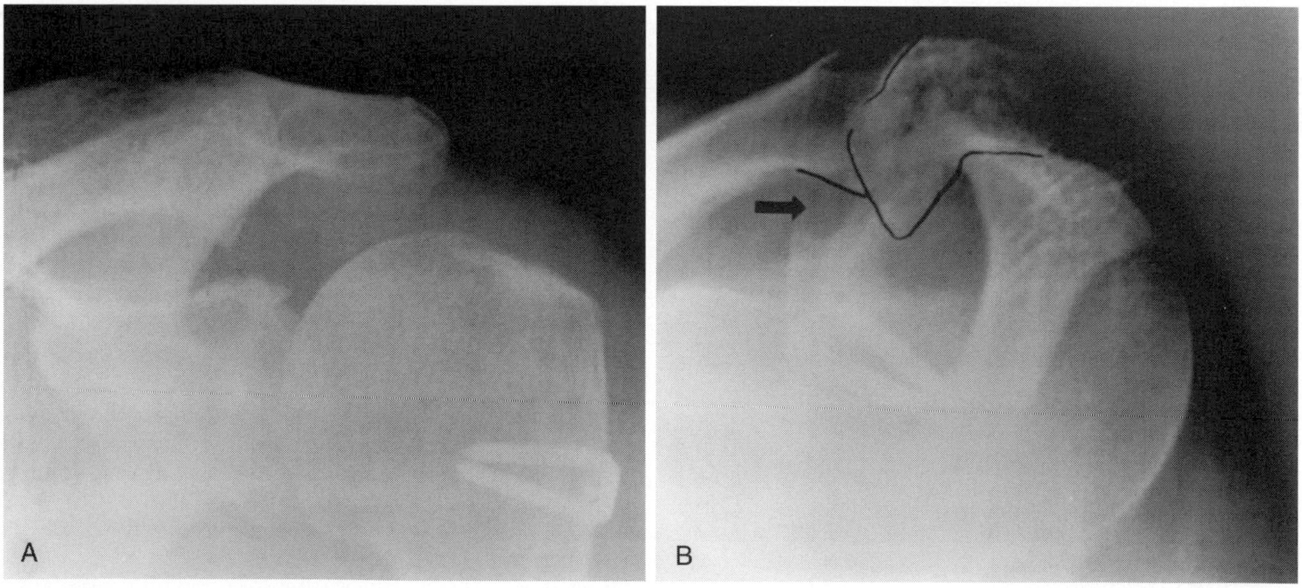

Figure 19–45

A, A 30-degree caudal tilt radiograph reveals anterior acromial spurring with the "shark's tooth" appearance. The patient had undergone a biceps tenodesis but continued to have pain after the surgery. His pain was completely relieved and function was greatly improved by acromioplasty and rotator cuff repair. *B,* An outlet view of the same patient demonstrating a type III acromion with marked inferior spurring and narrowing in the supraspinatus outlet. (The film is somewhat underexposed; the lines were added to aid in reproduction.)

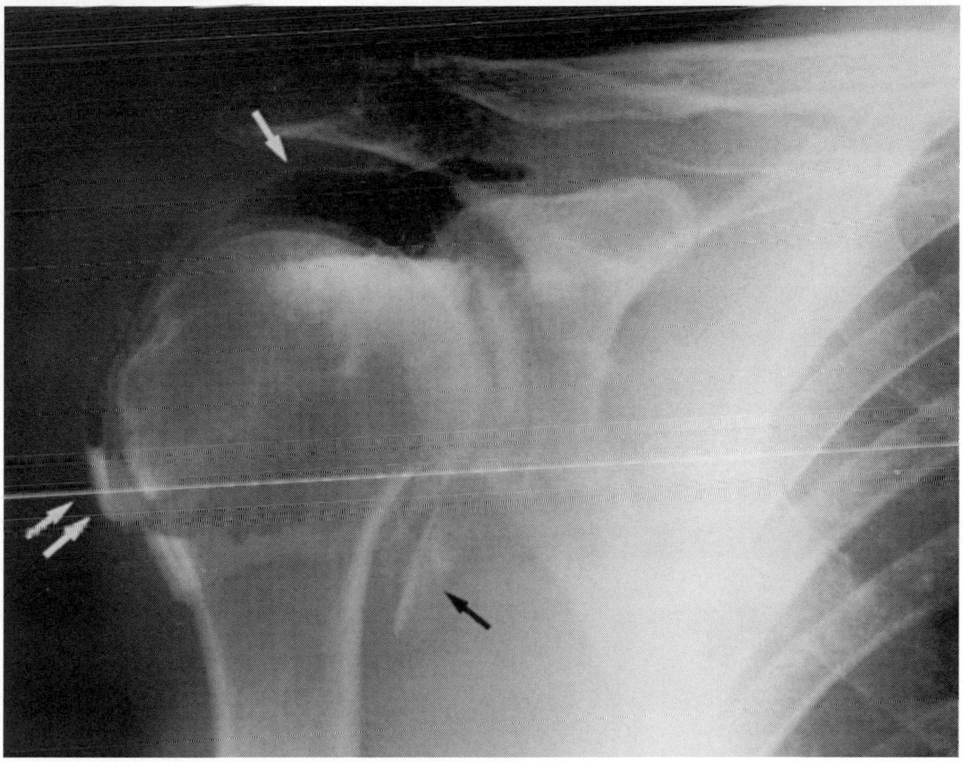

Figure 19–46

An anteroposterior arthrogram revealing medial dislocation of the biceps tendon, as indicated by the medial position of the biceps sheath *(black arrow)*. This patient also sustained a massive rupture of the rotator cuff at the time of the injury. Note the presence of air in the subacromial bursa *(single white arrow)* and contrast medium *(double white arrow)* in the subdeltoid bursa. (Courtesy of Guerdon Greenway, MD, and Robert Chapman, MD.)

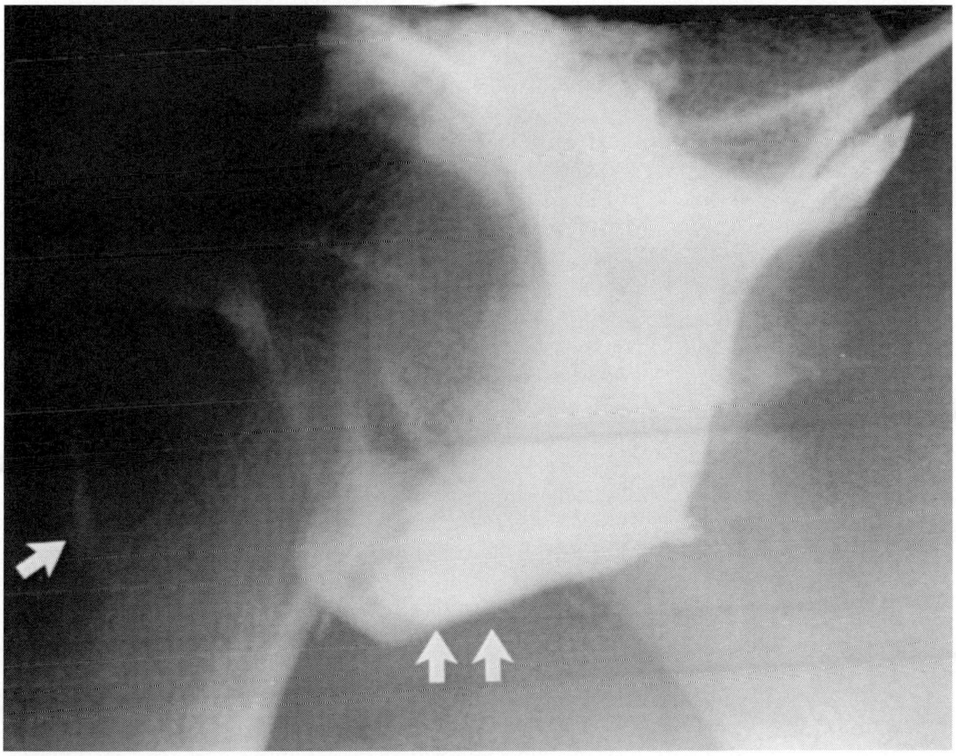

Figure 19–47

The arthrogram in adhesive capsulitis frequently will show nonfilling of the bicipital groove because of constriction in the bicipital sheath *(arrow)*. This is similar to the restriction that occurs in the axillary recess *(double arrows)*.

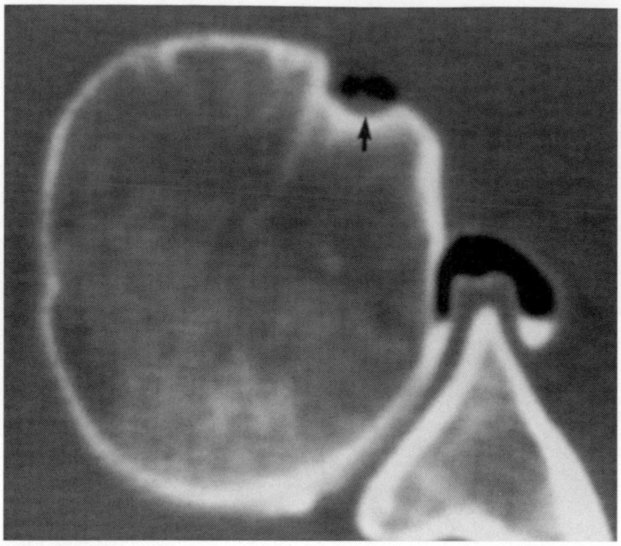

Figure 19–48

The bicipital tendon is seen *(black arrow)* seated in the groove on a computed tomography arthrogram.

evaluate the shoulder. This test can be used in much the same way as a CT arthrogram is used to assess the bicipital groove but also provides better imaging and contrast of soft tissues in the area. MRI can also be used to evaluate the superior labral biceps complex. A gadolinium arthrogram in this case is used to help identify superior labral avulsions and tearing in the bicipital attachment to the supraglenoid tubercle and the labrum.

Ultrasonography

The use of ultrasonography to evaluate the long head of the biceps has become popular.[4, 172] When comparing arthrography with sonography of the biceps, Middleton and colleagues[172] found that while sonography and arthrography were equally successful in facilitating the evaluation of the bony anatomy of the bicipital groove, sonography gave a superior image of the biceps tendon within the groove (Fig. 19–49). Not only can the tendon be visualized in the groove but also the intra-articular portion and that portion just distal to the groove can be visualized (see Fig. 19–49*B* and *C*). In Middleton's study, 16 patients were found to have biceps tendon sheath effusions or swelling detected by sonography (see Fig. 19–49*D*); 15 of these patients had associated pathologic conditions elsewhere in the joint. The majority of these were rotator cuff tears.

It has been previously documented that the biceps tendon sheath often does not fill when a rotator cuff tear is present.[191–198] This occurs either from an associated tendinitis and contracture of the capsule or from the fact that the dye leaks out of the joint through the tear in the supraspinatus before enough pressure is generated to force the dye into the bicipital groove. Since arthrograms often do not disclose a biceps tendon or sheath abnormality in many of the patients in which ultrasound was positive, Middleton and associates[172] concluded that sonography is the imaging method of choice in patients with suspected biceps tendon lesions.

An ultrasound subluxation test was able to detect subluxation in 12 of 14 (86%) patients who had surgically verified subluxation of the biceps tendon. Static scanning had a similar percentage of diagnoses for dislocations. The ultrasound examination failed or could not be performed in 6% of their patients. No false-positive results occurred.[72]

According to the author, the sonogram is an excellent noninvasive test for biceps and cuff lesions. It is, however, very examiner dependent, and, if equivocal, arthrography should be performed. A positive sonogram like the clinical entity of biceps rupture itself should also make one suspicious that rotator cuff pathology coexists.

Magnetic Resonance Imaging Scan

MRI scans can be used to visualize the normal biceps tendon, both intra-articularly and in its groove. For an optimal MRI evaluation, images should be obtained in the axial, oblique, and sagittal planes. The oblique and sagittal planes provide the best visualization of the intra-articular portion of the biceps tendon in the rotator interval.[253] The axial plane is best for showing the descending portion of the biceps in the groove. MRI is also useful to image the rotator cuff pathology that is frequently found in association with a biceps lesion.[128, 168]

Subluxations or dislocations can be visualized using MRI. Dislocation usually shows the tendon being displaced out of its groove and is seen lying medial to the lesser tuberosity (Fig. 19–50*A* and *B*). Subluxation can be identified where the tendon is noted to overlie the lesser tuberosity on some images. This test can also be used to visualize an intra-articular dislocation of the biceps. Care must be taken because osteophytes and scar tissue can resemble the presence of a tendon in the groove.[257]

Biceps tendinitis is a much more difficult diagnosis to make on MRI, but it can be suggested by certain criteria. Some of these criteria include fluid out of proportion to the intra-articular fluid in the shoulder. The presence of a large joint effusion and fluid surrounding the tendon can be a normal finding, but when there is little intra-articular fluid and a lot of fluid in the biceps sulcus, this may represent tendinitis (Fig. 19–51*A* and *B*). Thickening of the tendon and increased intensity on T1 and T2 images can suggest degenerative changes in the tendon that may be diffuse or that may be in segmental areas.[253]

SLAP lesions can be diagnosed through the use of MRI. Studies have shown that SLAP lesions can be evaluated using gadolinium-enhanced scanning as well as plain MRI scanning.[43] In gadolinium-enhanced scans, contrast can help to delineate lesions of the superior labrum and the biceps anchor. Gadolinium can be seen infiltrating under the labrum in type II SLAP lesions. Even with non–gadolinium-enhanced scans, changes in the superior labrum and subluxed bucket handle tears can be seen in the joint.

MRI scans are also useful when diagnosing biceps ruptures (Fig. 19–52*A* and *B*). A rupture is easier to diagnose than a partial tear, clinically and in MRI scan-

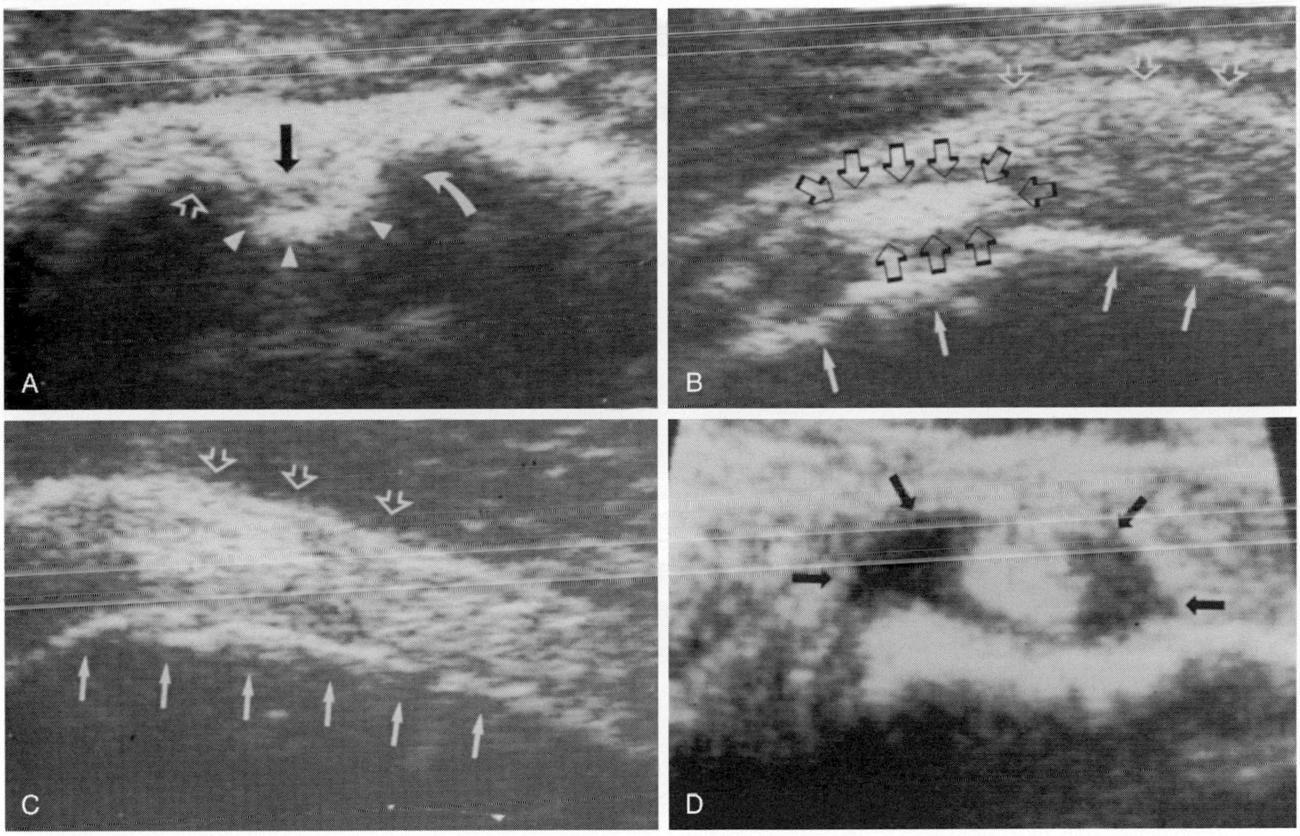

Figure 19–49

A, A transverse sonogram of the anterior aspect of the shoulder showing the bicipital groove *(arrowheads)* as a semicircular depression in the proximal part of the humerus formed by the lesser tuberosity medially *(open arrow)* and the greater tuberosity laterally *(curved arrow).* The biceps tendon is seen as an echogenic ellipse within the groove *(black arrow). B,* A sonogram perpendicular to the long axis of the intra-articular portion of the biceps tendon *(open black arrowheads),* seen between the subscapularis anteriorly and the supraspinatus posteriorly. The deep surface of the deltoid muscle is shown by *open white arrowheads* and the humeral head by *solid white arrows. C,* On longitudinal scans, the biceps tendon appears as an echogenic band sandwiched between the upper portion of the humeral head *(solid arrows)* and the lower portion of the deltoid *(open arrows). D,* A transverse sonogram of the distal part of the biceps tendon showing biceps sheath effusion *(arrows)* surrounding the biceps tendon. (From Middleton WD, Reinus WR, Tetty WG, et al: Ultrasonographic evaluation of the rotator cuff and biceps tendon. J Bone Joint Surg 68[3]:440–450, 1986.)

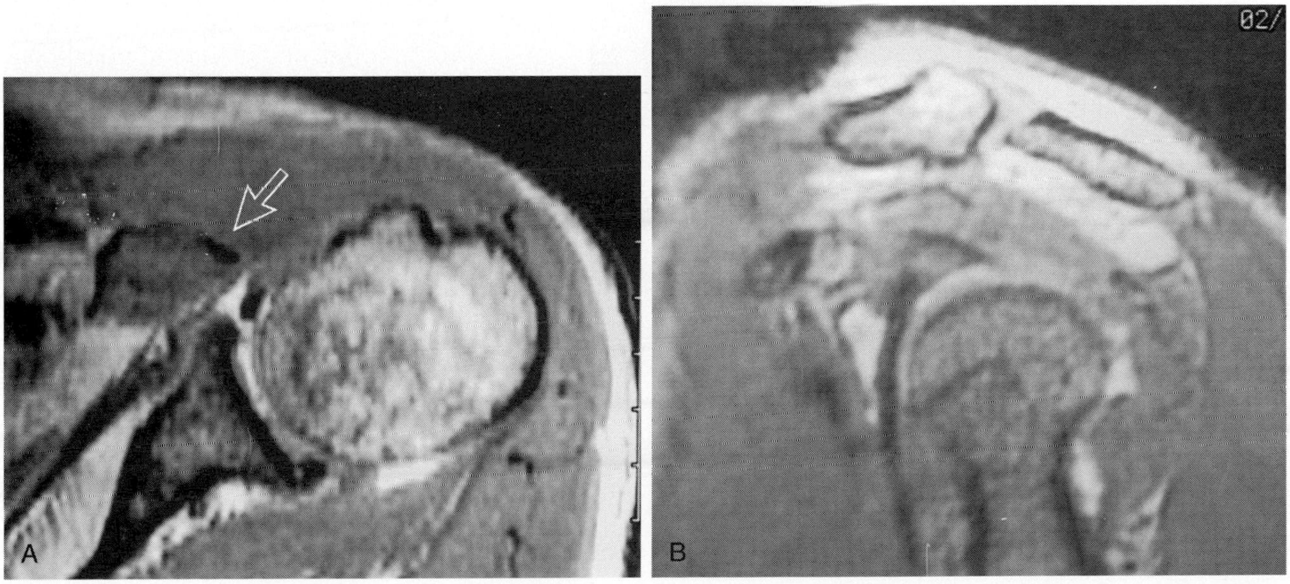

Figure 19–50

A, The biceps tendon *(open arrow)* is seen in an intra-articular position. Note the absent groove and the change in signal intensity of the subscapularis. *B,* Sagittal oblique magnetic resonance imaging reveals the biceps anterior to the humeral head.

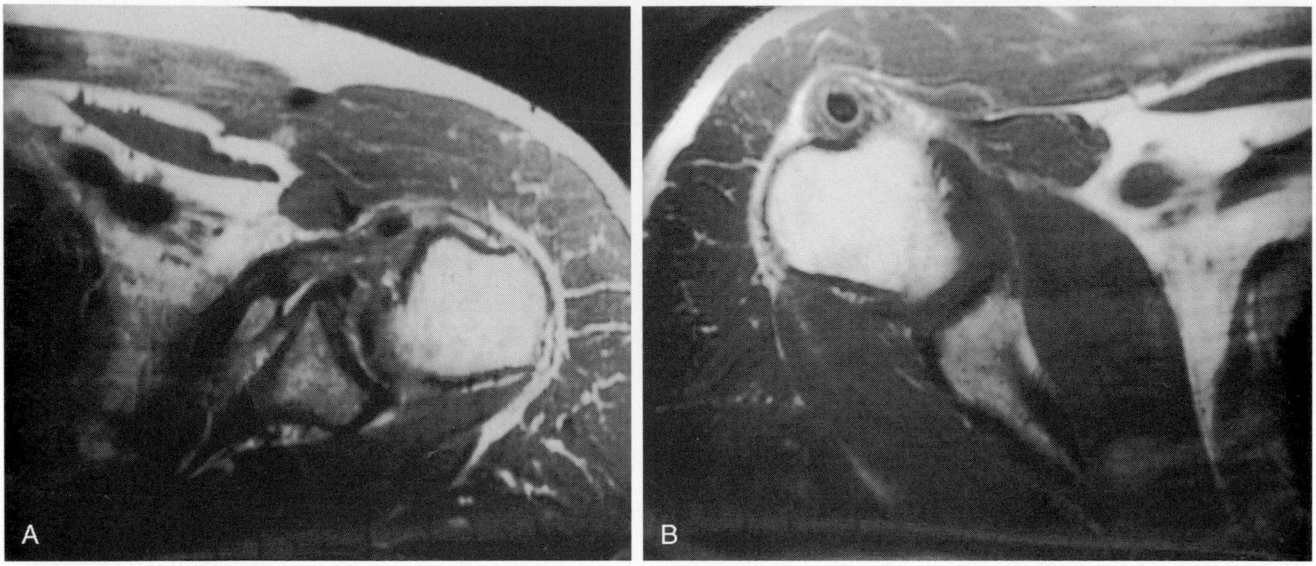

Figure 19–51

A, An axial plane T1-weighted magnetic resonance imaging scan reveals subluxation of the biceps within the substance of the subscapular sheath compared with the glenohumeral joint in the individual with surgically confirmed biceps tendinitis. *B,* An axial view of another individual with a T1-weighted image revealing tenosynovitis of the biceps with thick surrounding synovium.

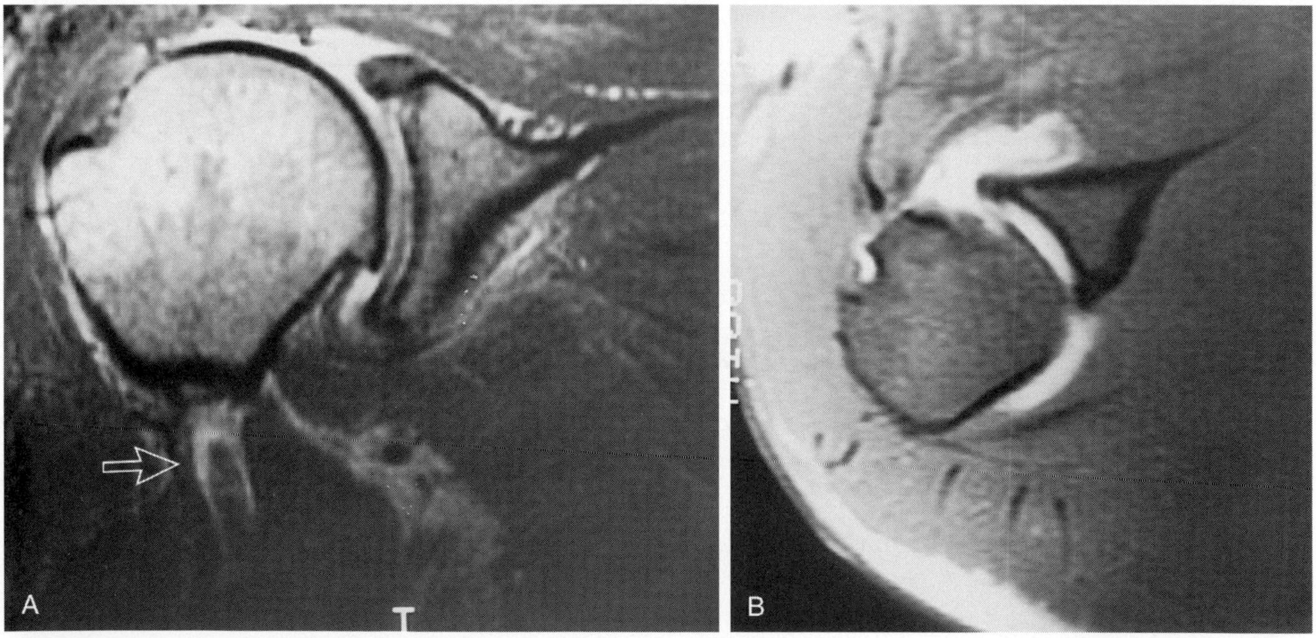

Figure 19–52

A, A coronal view magnetic resonance imaging (MRI) scan shows the location of the proximal biceps stump *(open white arrow)* to be at the distal end of the biceps groove. *B,* An axial view MRI scan of the same patient reveals an absent biceps from the groove. Note the medial osteophytic ridge.

ning. Ruptures are diagnosed by nonvisualization of the tendon at any point along its anatomic course. Sometimes an intra-articular stump can be visualized. Obviously, one must be careful to ensure that the biceps tendon is not dislocated in the groove before making the diagnosis of a biceps rupture. Other useful signs that can be seen on MRI that may help to diagnose ruptures include atrophy and retraction of the distal portion of the proximal part of the tendon. Tears are more difficult to diagnose. They can be inferred, however, by sudden changes in cross-sectional diameter of the tendon.[253] Longitudinal tears may be easier to see than transverse tears because they are seen on several cuts. Focal transverse partial lesions of the tendon can be missed or may be dismissed as artifact. MRI scans have been used to identify osteochondromatosis of the biceps sheath.[59]

Arthroscopy

Arthroscopy remains the best method for visualizing the biceps tendon in its intra-articular location (Fig. 19–53). It is also very useful when imaging other lesions that may be causing chronic anterior shoulder pain.[8, 9, 202, 270] Lesions of the biceps anchor and the superior labrum can be visualized and repaired using arthroscopy. Arthroscopy provides the examiner with both static as well as dynamic visualization of the biceps, thus helping to diagnose subtle cases of instability.

This technique can be used to evaluate numerous conditions that can cause anterior shoulder pain. Small bursal side tears can be seen along with lesions related to anterior instability, impingement syndrome, labral tears without instability, and bicipital tendinitis. Using the arthroscope, the subtle anterior and posterior glenoid labral tears and cartilaginous head defects can be visualized; these lesions are not always seen on CT scans or on MRI. A disadvantage of arthroscopy is that it is an invasive procedure that normally requires general anesthesia. As in all surgical procedures, there is a risk of infection and cartilage damage during insertion of the arthroscope. Extra-articular lesions of the biceps may not be appreciated using the arthroscope.

COMPLICATIONS

The most common complication of biceps tendon rupture or dislocation is, as has been emphasized previously, the failure to recognize a disruption of the rotator cuff. The majority of rotator cuff tears are secondary to chronic impingement wear and tendinitis. Some patients will sustain an acute massive cuff avulsion as the result of trauma. Although the results of cuff débridement and decompression are impressive in terms of pain relief and range of motion, if the patient is young (younger than 60 years of age) and wants to maintain a strong shoulder for use above the horizontal, an early diagnostic work-up and aggressive surgical approach are preferred.

Adhesive capsulitis can follow a number of painful conditions about the shoulder. Since biceps tendinitis has been previously associated with adhesive capsulitis, early recognition of this condition and treatment with anti-inflammatory agents, moist heat, and early, gentle patient-directed range-of-motion exercises may aid in preventing or shortening this process, which is often long and painful.

Nontreatment of biceps ruptures, especially in the elderly, is accepted by many patients and physicians. Very few of these individuals note any dysfunction related to the biceps rupture itself. Predictably, patients with bicipital rupture who have an intact brachialis muscle will have no decrease in flexion strength at the elbow. Loss of supination strength has been estimated by Warren and associates to be between 10 and 20% with Cybex testing.[266, 267]

Phillips and associates could not find a significant dif-

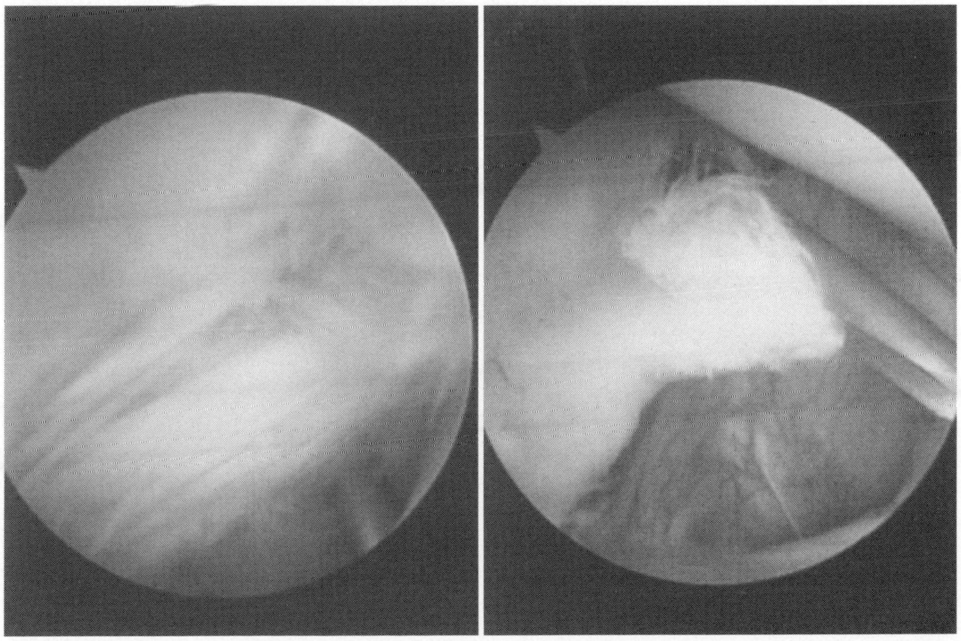

Figure 19–53

An arthroscopic view of the right shoulder reveals an intra-articular biceps with shredding of fibers secondary to the loss of the sling and chronic subluxation out of the proximal groove.

ference between patients who had operatively treated proximal biceps tendon ruptures compared with patients who had nonoperative treatment.[218] All of the patients in this study were middle-aged patients and older individuals. In this study, some patients who had objective weakness did not feel functionally impaired.

DIFFERENTIAL DIAGNOSIS

Because tendinitis of the long head of the biceps usually occurs secondary to another condition and primary bicipital tendinitis is a diagnosis of exclusion, the other clinical entities that can mimic or be associated with this entity must be remembered. These entities are impingement syndrome, adhesive capsulitis, rheumatoid arthritis, osteoarthritis, glenohumeral instability, coracoid impingement syndrome, thoracic outlet syndrome or brachial plexopathy/plexitis, peripheral nerve entrapment, and cervical radiculopathy.

One pertinent historical feature is the mechanism of injury. This should include the amount and direction of force applied, whether it was direct or indirect, and in what position the arm was at the time of application of the force. Was the onset insidious? Has there been a gradual loss of motion over several months? Had the patient engaged in any unusual overhead activity before the onset of symptoms? Has the patient had an injury to the shoulder before or been treated for "bursitis"? Has the patient engaged in activities that required overhead use of the arm such as swimming, throwing, or tennis? What makes the pain better; what makes the pain worse? Where does the patient feel the pain most in the shoulder? Does activity improve or exacerbate the painful phenomenon? Inspection for atrophy of the deltoid, infraspinatus, supraspinatus, and trapezius; swelling; and obvious biceps ruptures should be performed. The patient should be examined from the front, the side, and the back and a comparison with the other side should be made. The physical examination should include cervical spine range of motion and a detailed neurovascular examination, including deep tendon reflexes, sensation, strength testing, and specific physical tests for thoracic outlet syndrome. Range of motion of the shoulder should be examined. Both the active and passive ranges of forward flexion, abduction, external rotation, internal rotation, and extension should be noted. The relative contribution of glenohumeral and scapulothoracic joint motion should be assessed. Anterior apprehension testing as well as anterior, posterior, and inferior drawer test should be performed. The examiner should look for the impingement sign[186] and the impingement reinforcement sign of Hawkins.[107] The acromioclavicular joint is palpated, and a compression test or hug test, specific for acromioclavicular joint arthritis, is performed. Specific areas of point tenderness over the anterior acromion, coracoacromial ligament, and coracoid are noted. The biceps tendon is palpated in the groove, anteriorly at a position of approximately 10 degrees of internal rotation, 4 to 6 cm distal to the acromion (see Fig. 19–36). A helpful point in determining whether this is the tendon and groove area is to see if the point of tenderness moves with rotation of the humerus. A diffuse bursitis will not move, whereas an inflamed biceps will move. The point of tenderness of bicipital tendinitis may disappear completely underneath the coracoid upon marked internal rotation. The diagnosis of primary bicipital tendinitis must be reached by exclusion of the other, more common, causes of anterior shoulder pain.

MRI is a useful tool to differentiate between primary bicipital tendinitis and impingement syndrome. Along with plain radiographs that include a trauma series, a supraspinatus outlet view and a 30-degree caudal tilt view can be used to help diagnose impingement syndrome. The MRI scan can be used to demonstrate changes in the rotator cuff tendons, or it may show normal tendons and an increased signal in and around the biceps tendon, which would confirm primary bicipital tendinitis and more than likely exclude impingement type lesions.

Biceps Tendinitis Versus Impingement Syndrome

Biceps tendinitis usually occurs secondary to the impingement syndrome and only rarely exists as an isolated entity. To differentiate primary bicipital tendinitis from impingement tendinitis, selective injection with a local anesthetic is helpful. In patients with impingement syndrome without bicipital involvement, the pain is located more proximally, with tenderness primarily on the anterior acromion, coracoacromial ligament, and supraspinatus tendon insertion. The impingement sign and impingement reinforcement signs are positive. In patients with an impingement syndrome, the injection of lidocaine (Xylocaine) into the subacromial space usually relieves all of the patient's pain. In patients who have an associated bicipital tendinitis, there is pain distally in the groove; the subacromial injection does not relieve all of their pain, and they continue to have pain over the bicipital groove. Further injection of lidocaine into the sheath with obliteration of pain confirms the associated bicipital tendinitis. It is important to remember that the subdeltoid bursa, which covers the groove, is continuous with the subacromial bursa, and inadvertent injection into this area will anesthetize the subacromial bursa. Therefore, I (W.Z.B.) always inject the subacromial bursa first, doing it from the lateral or posterolateral corner of the acromion to avoid inadvertent injection of lidocaine into the groove. Only if subacromial injection has absolutely no effect on the patient's pain, while an isolated biceps injection relieves all pain and restores 100% of motion, will I (W.Z.B.) make a clinical diagnosis of primary bicipital tendinitis. A positive response to injection has been found to be a predictor of good long-term results.[24]

The technique of injection is described by Kerlan in which the patient is placed supine with the arm over the table.[128] The elbow is bent and the shoulder extended with the arm in external rotation, decreasing the distance from the groove to the surface. The biceps tendon is located anteriorly, and a mark is made on the skin. The area is prepared in a sterile fashion and injected. It is extremely important, especially if corticosteroids are used, that the injection be into the sheath and not into the tendon proper. The direction of the needle superiorly tangential to the tendon should hopefully eliminate this complication. There must be an easy flow of fluid; if any resistance is felt, the needle should be repositioned. Because of the anatomy of the sheath and its communication with the joint, I (W.Z.B.) use a very low volume of local anesthetic, only 2 to 3 ml of 1% lidocaine during the biceps ablation test.

Claessens and Snoek[41] thought that intra-articular injection of an anesthetic is important when differentiating rotator cuff tendinitis from bicipital tendinitis. Although this is true of bursal side lesions, undersurface tears of the rotator cuff will be anesthetized with this technique as well. Radiographs, sonography, and arthrography should be used to confirm one's clinical impression.

Anterior Shoulder Instability

The pain associated with anterior subluxation of the glenohumeral joint will be noted in the anterior portion of the shoulder. At the same time, patients may often have pain posteriorly from capsular stretching. The pain is episodic and associated with a palpable and audible clunk, such as has been described previously from medial dislocation in the biceps. The pain generally lasts for several days after a major subluxation episode. If the brachial plexus is inflamed and stretched, pain and paresthesias can be experienced transiently or in varying degrees for several weeks or months. The mechanism of injury described for both of these conditions is very similar in that they most commonly occur with forced abduction and external rotation. The differential diagnosis can be even more confusing if anterior shoulder instability and impingement syndrome coexist, which is not uncommon. A derangement in the glenohumeral joint leading to weakness in the short rotators and secondary impingement is seen frequently in patients with recurrent subluxation.

Historically, patients with pure instability have pain for only a few days after a subluxation episode unless impingement syndrome or brachial neuritis coexists. Therefore, it is relatively easy to differentiate this problem from pure bicipital tendinitis. When differentiating this problem from subluxation of the biceps tendon, provocative tests are helpful. In anterior shoulder instability, the maximum point of apprehension and clicking should be in 90 degrees of abduction and maximum external rotation (i.e., a positive apprehension sign). Pain in the anterior part of the shoulder occurs as the humeral head translates across the torn glenoid labrum. Pain can also be felt posteriorly at this time, secondary to cuff stretching. In the patient with a subluxating biceps tendon, the pain is not maximal until the arm is brought down from the position of maximum abduction and external rotation and the click occurs as the examiner begins to internally rotate the arm (i.e., the biceps instability test). Yergason's sign and Speed's sign should be negative in patients with anterior shoulder instability but positive if the biceps is inflamed. Special roentgenographic views for shoulder instability should be employed (see Chapter 5 on radiology of the shoulder). The CT arthrogram can be extremely helpful in demonstrating lesions of the anterior cartilaginous labrum in patients with instability. The biceps tendon can be visualized within its groove on CT arthrography.

MRI with gadolinium contrast can also be helpful in cases of instability, much in the same way as the CT arthrogram. Although this study is not as useful in demonstrating Bankart-type lesions, it can show findings similar to those seen on a CT arthrogram with this lesion. The disadvantage of using MRI is that bony lesions are not seen as well as they are on CT arthrograms. The MRI scan can also be used to visualize the biceps tendon and evaluate its position and whether or not it is inflamed.

If, after the aforementioned studies, the diagnosis remains unclear, an examination under anesthesia or arthroscopy can be performed. Examination under anesthesia can allow a physician to examine the patient's shoulder without the patient's muscles acting as secondary stabilizers. This examination can help to determine abnormal laxity and, when combined with glenohumeral arthroscopy, allows the surgeon to visualize directly the anterior labrum as well as the intra-articular portion of the biceps tendon. The aperture of the sulcus and the surrounding cuff tissue can be seen during arthroscopy. A Bankart lesion and a positive drive-through sign are both suggestive of glenohumeral instability as a cause of pain. This is especially true if no lesion can be noted on the intra-articular portion of the biceps tendon during arthroscopy. The biceps tendon can be pulled into the joint with a probe during arthroscopy so that a greater length of the tendon can be examined.

Glenoid Labrum Tears Without Instability

Glenoid labrum tears without instability, such as those that occur in the superior one third of the labrum in close proximity to the biceps, can demonstrate symptoms similar to those of subluxation of the biceps tendon. These superior labrum tears can occur in baseball players and other throwing athletes and frequently show symptoms very similar to those of a subluxating bicipital tendon or a rotator cuff tear (see Chapter 26 on shoulder injuries in athletes). An audible or palpable clunk occurs as the tear flips in and out of the joint impinging on the humeral head during rotation above the horizontal. A high index of suspicion for this lesion should be present if one is dealing with a throwing athlete with shoulder pain. These patients sometimes have more pain with release because of the deceleration effect of the biceps pulling on the torn labrum. CT arthrography will occasionally miss this lesion, and the best way to differentiate this problem from a subluxating biceps tendon is by glenohumeral arthroscopy.

MRI is useful in imaging this type of lesion. Studies using gadolinium-enhanced, as well as plain, MRI scans are both helpful in making this diagnosis. Arthroscopy can evaluate this lesion well.

Adhesive Capsulitis

Patients with adhesive capsulitis frequently have tenderness in the anterior aspect of the shoulder in the region of the bicipital groove and anterior portion of the subdeltoid bursa.

When evaluating patients with painful and stiff shoulders who have direct areas of point tenderness over the bicipital groove, I (W.Z.B.) will inject this area with lidocaine, initially without cortisone, to see what effect this has on motion. If one injects and infiltrates the tendon sheath with 2 to 3 ml of lidocaine and the patient's pain is obliterated but without an appreciable change in motion, one can be sure that one is dealing with an adhesive capsulitis or frozen shoulder and not just a painful stiff shoulder from biceps tendinitis. If injection into the biceps region eliminates pain and motion returns in full, a bicipital tendinitis exists. Whether it is part of the impingement syndrome can be determined by clinical examination and subacromial injection.

Glenohumeral Arthritis

Early arthritis of the glenohumeral joint frequently presents as anterior shoulder pain with limited range of motion. Since the biceps tendon is an intra-articular structure, it will be involved with any process within the joint. Inflammatory changes occur in the visceral layer of the synovium of the biceps recess as they do in the subscapular and axillary recess. Plain radiography may show spurring of the proximal humerus with a ring osteophyte and flattening of the glenoid. Prior to the development of obvious osseous spur formation, double-contrast arthrography can reveal thinning of the articular cartilage.

Coracoid Impingement Syndrome

Warren[266, 267] and Gerber[81] have described the role of the coracoid process in coracoid impingement syndrome. They have noted a similarity in its symptoms to biceps tendinitis and instability. Based on CT scan data, Gerber[81] has calculated the normal coracoid-to-humeral distance (8.6 mm) and noted that it is decreased in patients (average of 6.7 mm) with coracoid impingement. The syndrome has been described in patients with an excessively long or laterally placed coracoid process and in patients who have had bone block and osteotomy procedures for instability. Symptoms of coracoid impingement are dull pain in the front of the shoulder referred to the anterior, upper arm, occasionally extending down into the forearm. The pain is consistently brought about by forward flexion and internal rotation or by adduction or by internal rotation. In contrast with the more common type of impingement, forward flexion is most often painful between 120 and 130 degrees, rather than from 60 to 120 degrees. The diagnosis is established clinically by obliteration of the patient's pain by subcoracoid injection. The importance of considering this entity before performing surgery on the biceps tendon is pointed out by Dines and associates;[65] they report a series in which one third of their failures from biceps tenodesis were related to undiagnosed coracoid impingement syndrome.

Thoracic Outlet Syndrome

Thoracic outlet syndrome frequently presents with some anterior shoulder pain. It is generally associated with paresthesias in the distribution of the lower trunk of the brachial plexus (i.e., the ulnar two fingers). Neck pain, parascapular pain, and radiation into the pectorals are not uncommon. The body habitus may be asthenic with a long neck and round back or endomorphic with pendulous breasts. The shoulders slope forward and downward owing to rhomboid, levator, and trapezius weakness. Provocative tests for thoracic outlet syndrome, such as Wright's maneuver, Adson's test, or Roos' overhead grip test, will be positive whereas Yergason's test, Speed's test, and the impingement test are all negative or equivocal. Subacromial and bicipital injections should not alleviate pain completely. Cervical spine series looking specifically for cervical ribs as well as Doppler examination and EMGs are useful adjuncts to clinical testing. However, the diagnosis remains a clinical one.

Brachial Neuritis

Viral brachial plexitis (syndrome of Parsonage and Turner) is an extremely painful condition that frequently presents with anterior shoulder pain. Early in the course of this condition, which usually follows a viral illness, pain exceeds neurologic findings, and one may be fooled into thinking that one is dealing with an acute calcific tendinitis. Later, numbness and weakness with obvious atrophy become prominent. The course is variable.

Peripheral Nerve Entrapment/Cervical Radiculopathy

The common syndromes of peripheral nerve entrapment (i.e., carpal tunnel, ulnar neuritis, and posterior interosseous nerve entrapment) may all present with anterior shoulder pain that is referred and can potentially be confused with bicipital tendinitis. Cervical radiculopathy, especially C5 to C6, can also mimic primary shoulder lesions. A careful and repeated neurologic examination followed by EMG and nerve conduction velocity tests can help to distinguish these entities. In patients with persistent anterior shoulder pain, especially if there is typical neurogenic pain, while the work-up for primary shoulder pathology is negative and the neurologic examination is unrevealing, one must consider the possibility of a tumor in the apex, mediastinum, or diaphragm region.

Tumors

Osteochondromatosis has been described in the bicipital sheath. This lesion can cause chronic anterior shoulder pain in patients. The classical symptoms of catching may not be present when just the bicipital sheath is involved. If the rest of the shoulder joint is involved, classical symptoms may be present.

Dialysis Arthropathy

Arthropathy secondary to dialysis is a painful chronic shoulder condition found in patients on long-term dialysis. These patients have degeneration of the joint due to synovial inflammation and amyloid deposit. This condition is easily diagnosed because the patient is on dialysis and has radiologic signs of degeneration. This condition also seems to affect the biceps tendon and sheath, as well as the joint itself.

TREATMENT OF BICIPITAL LESIONS: REVIEW OF CONSERVATIVE TREATMENT

In 1773, Bromfield[30] discussed the technical aspects of reducing biceps tendon dislocation. Treatment of tendinitis was initially discussed by Schrager[234] in the 1920s. Recommendations during the 1920s and 1930s included morphine, sudden traction, diathermy, massage, faradization, light, and x-ray treatment. Milgram[174–177] and later Lapidus[136] were proponents of procaine hydrochloride (Novocaine) infiltration and aspiration of the calcific deposits in cases of acute calcific tendinitis.

DePalma[61] initially treated bicipital tenosynovitis conservatively with hydrocortisone injection directly into the tendon, under the transverse ligament, and noted improvement in 10 of 18 cases. He recommended, as a rule, three or four 1-ml injections into the tendon under the transverse ligament at weekly intervals. It is apparent now from data by Kennedy[127] that this interval is too frequent. The injection should only be made in the tendon sheath, and the tendon itself should not be directly injected. In conservatively treated patients he noted excellent results in 29%, good in 45%, fair in 9%, and poor in 16%.

Habermeyer and Walch[100] recommend conservative treatment for isolated tendinitis of the long head of the biceps tendon. They recommend a single intra-articular injection of cortisone and oral anti-inflammatory drugs in the acute stages of the disease. They recommended immobilization and local ice therapy combined with a conservative regimen of physical therapy. Physical therapy, including isometric and isokinetic strengthening of the rotator cuff, is the key in rehabilitating these patients.

Bicipital tendinitis secondary to impingement syndrome may respond to conservative treatment of the rotator cuff pathology. Subacromial injections of corticosteroids may help a patient with a large rotator cuff tear who refuses surgery. Since the intra-articular and subacromial spaces communicate, there is less need to inject the area of the biceps tendon specifically in these cases.

RESULTS OF NONOPERATIVE TREATMENT OF BICEPS RUPTURE

There is slight functional deficit after disruption of the long head of the biceps tendon. After a period of conservative care, including range of motion exercise, moist heat, and strengthening, most patients have relatively normal strength and flexion and only minimal loss of supination power.[114–118] Carroll and Hamilton[34] studied 100 patients who had a rupture of the biceps brachii as a result of forced extension. Follow-up function was ascertained by the patient's ability to lift weights. They believed that a patient could return to work earlier and suffer no residual disability from conservative treatment. When treated conservatively, the patients in their series returned to work on an average of 4 weeks. It was thought that a conservative approach should be adopted in treating this type of injury.

Warren,[266] using Cybex testing in 10 patients with chronic biceps rupture, failed to reveal any statistically significant loss of elbow flexion strength and only a 10% loss of elbow supination strength. Phillips and associates[218] confirmed some of Warren's findings. Cybex testing was used to assess the objective outcome of patients treated with long-term nonoperative therapy compared with patients treated with operative therapy. In 19 patients, no significant difference in supination or elbow flexion strength was found.

REVIEW OF OPERATIVE TREATMENT

Surgical treatment of the biceps tendon received little attention prior to Gilcreest[84] in 1926. He was the first to suggest suturing the stump of the tendon to the coracoid process and described intracapsular, intertubercular, and labral junction ruptures of the tendon. In 1939, Abbott and Saunders[1] reviewed six cases of surgical treatment of biceps dislocations. Their procedure involved stabilizing the biceps tendon, with half of the tendon drilled through drill holes, leaving the intracapsular portion intact. In their review, four of the six patients required re-operation for pain, and all patients had some pain, weakness, and limited range of motion, even after a second operation. Poor results from their procedure arose from two problem areas: (1) the procedure as described prevents the normal upward and downward motion of the humerus on the bicipital tendon; (2) too much attention was paid to the biceps lesion, while not enough attention was placed on the cuff rupture and impingement producing area. The one patient in their series who did have a good result had the biceps replaced into the groove and the fibrous roof reconstructed.

Lippmann[140, 141] recommended tenodesis of the long head of the biceps to the lesser tuberosity to shorten the course of frozen shoulder. He strongly believed, based on 12 operated cases, that periarthritis, or frozen shoulder, was caused by tenosynovitis of the long head of the biceps (Fig. 19–54).

In 1948, Hitchcock and Bechtol[111] described tenodesis of the biceps tendon within the groove with an osteal periosteal flap (Fig. 19–55). Hitchcock's name has become synonymous with tenodesis of the biceps tendon in the bicipital groove. According to the authors, extensive fixation of the long head of the biceps tendon to the floor of the intratubercular groove in the manner they described greatly expedites convalescence and promotes loss of pain and rapid functional recovery. However, they supplied no objective data to support this statement, describing

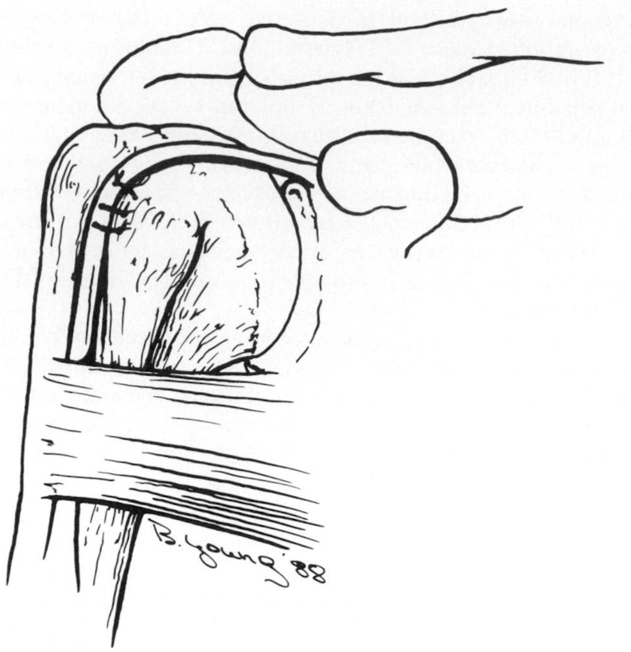

Figure 19–54

The Lippmann technique of suturing the biceps tendon to the lesser tuberosity for adhesive capsulitis.

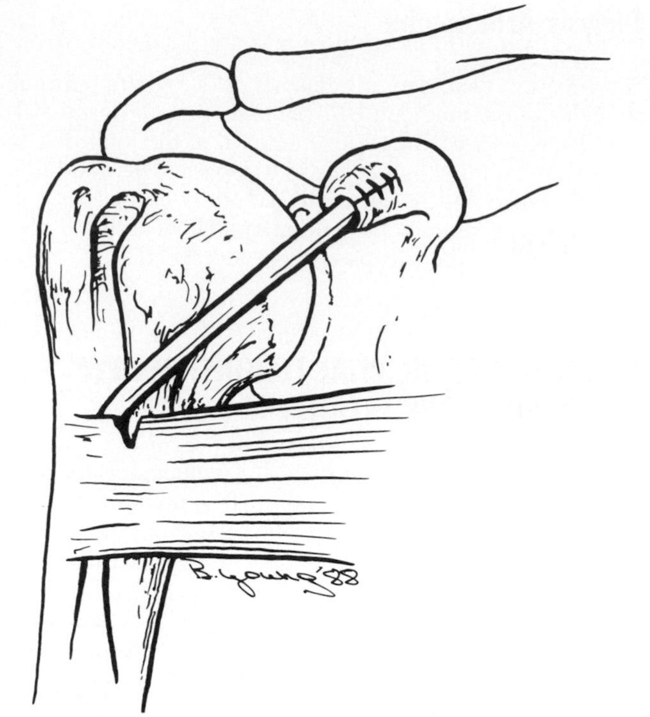

Figure 19–56

Tenodesis of the long head of the biceps to the coracoid process. This procedure was described initially by Gilcreest and was popularized by DePalma. It involves medial dissection and potential denervation of the deltoid if done through a deltoid-splitting approach. It also theoretically changes the long head from a static head depressor to an active head elevator. (Modified from Crenshaw AH and Kilgore WE: Surgical treatment of bicipital tenosynovitis. J Bone Joint Surg *45:*1496–1502, 1966.)

primarily case results and stating that, in 26 such cases, the results have been most satisfactory. The authors recognized the association of other lesions, such as ruptures of the rotator cuff. Their main concern was that peritendinitis of the biceps tendon not be overlooked and not the converse (i.e., overlooking rotator cuff pathology when biceps symptoms predominate).

In 1954, DePalma and Callery[60] reported on 86 cases of bicipital tenosynovitis treated operatively, the bulk of which were treated with suture of the long head of the biceps tendon into the coracoid process (Fig. 19–56). Shortly before publication several patients had tenodesis of the tendon in the groove, with a staple for fixation. The rationale cited for changing was that the three-prong staple provided firm fixation of the tendon and that tenodesis in the groove eliminated much of the dissection on the anterior aspect of the shoulder joint, necessary to expose the coracoid process. Of the 86 cases, only 59

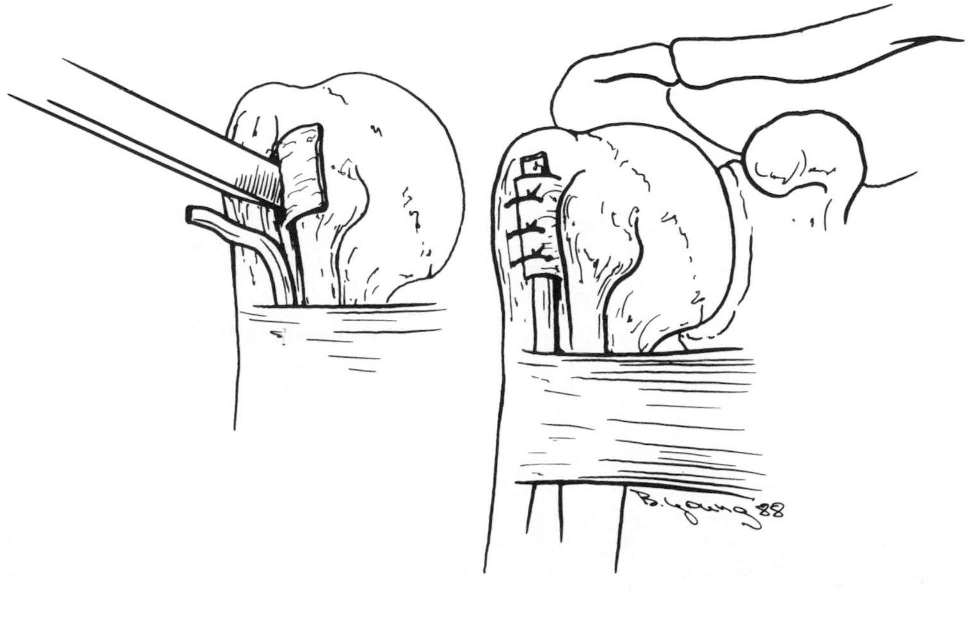

Figure 19–55

Hitchcock procedure. With an osteotome, a bed is made in the intertubercular groove by elevating a portion of the floor from the outside inward. The tendon is roughened and then sutured beneath this osteal periosteal flap with heavy nonabsorbable sutures. The transverse humeral ligament is laid down over the tendon and the osteal periosteal flap.

were available for follow-up, with an average of 27 months. Twenty-three were complicated by frozen shoulder. Excellent results were achieved in 64%, good results in 16%, fair results in 8%, and poor results in 10%; that is, 80% of the patients achieved an excellent or good result. An analysis of the poor results revealed errors in diagnosis, technique, and reflex sympathetic dystrophy.

Michele[171] in 1960 described the keystone tenodesis. In this technique, a rectangular block of bone, including the bicipital groove, is removed. The bone is decorticated. The bony trough is prepared for insertion and exit of the tendon by placement of two semilunar holes at the central poles at the sites of the remaining portions of the intertubercular sulcus. The tendon and sheath of the biceps are replaced into the defect, and the bone block is replaced in its original position. The periosteum is then sutured back to secure the bony block in place. Michele reported on 16 cases in which roentgenograms demonstrated persistence of the entrance and exit holes and "smooth gliding of the biceps through the holes." Maneuverability was complete in all directions and asymptomatic. There was no recurrence of symptoms.

In 1966, Crenshaw and Kilgore[56] reported on the surgical treatment of bicipital tendinitis. They used the Hitchcock procedure in most of their cases, performing a total of 65 Hitchcock procedures, five DePalma procedures, and three Lippmann procedures. Relief of moderate to severe pain was good in 90% of patients, whereas 2% of the patients continued to complain of "mild, nagging pain." Restoration of motion in their series was often disappointing, with only 85% of normal at follow-up. Interestingly, half of the patients who had good motion before surgery actually lost motion after the Hitchcock procedure. One has to wonder what the addition of an acromioplasty would have done to these results.

Keyhole tenodesis (Fig. 19–57) of the biceps origin was described by Froimson and Oh[77] for the treatment of rupture, instability, and tendinitis of the biceps in 1974. They reported on 12 shoulders in 11 patients, with an average follow-up of 24 months. They report satisfactory results in all of their patients but state that the patients with tenosynovitis enjoyed less than excellent results because of associated pericapsulitis. The advantages cited by the authors include: (1) The procedure avoids hardware and undue medial dissection; (2) The procedure removes the remnant of the biceps tendon, allowing motion of the humeral head and avoiding intra-articular derangement; and (3) The inherent stability of their method gives one confidence to begin early, gentle range of motion of both the shoulder and elbow.

Dines, Warren, and Inglis[65] commented on surgical treatment of lesions of the long head of the biceps in 1980. Seventeen patients had tenodesis of the long head of the biceps into the humeral head via the keyhole technique, and three had transfixion of the tendon into the coracoid. In addition, excision of the coracoacromial ligament was performed in 14 of their 20 patients. They had six failures out of the 20 patients (33%). Revision surgery was required for four of six patients. In four failures in the tendinitis group, three patients were found

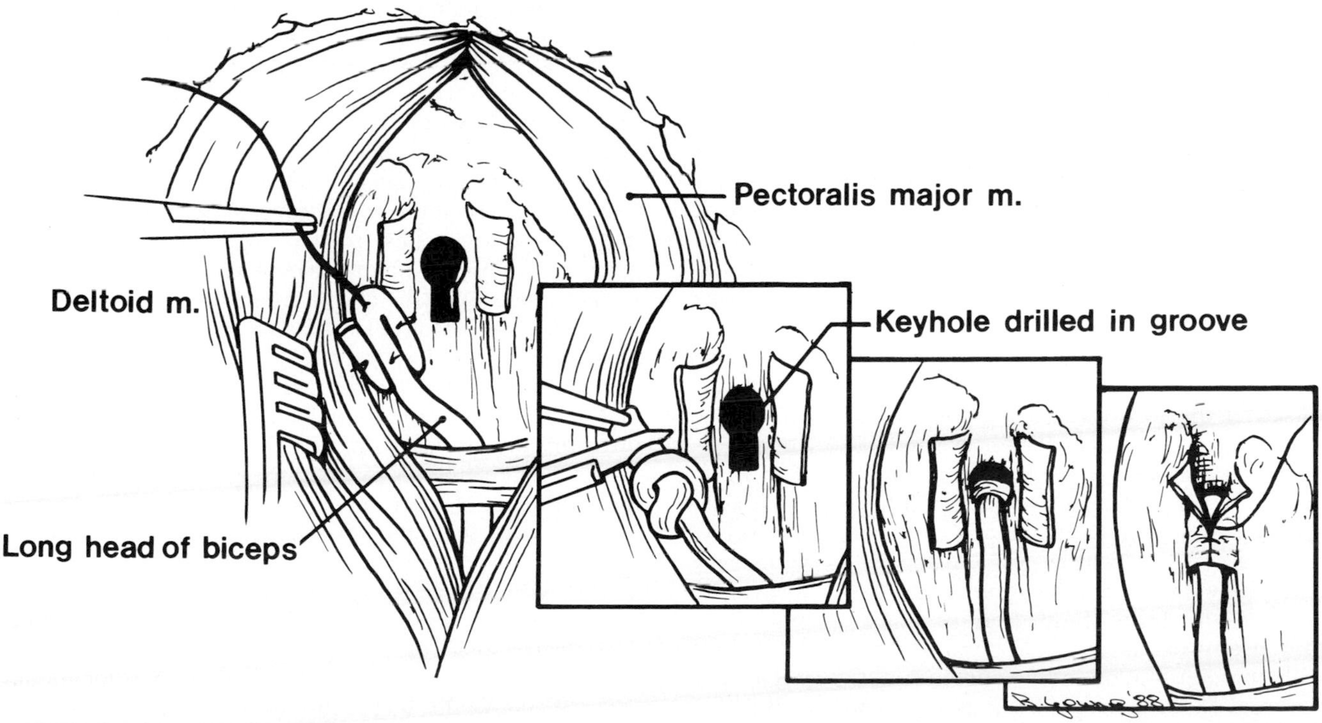

Figure 19–57

Keyhole tenodesis as described by Froimson. The biceps tendon is rolled into a thick ball in the proximal stump; this is sutured together in a knot. A keyhole is made in the groove using a dental bur. The tendon is then inserted into the keyhole, and the transverse ligament is repaired over the tendon with a nonabsorbable suture. Post has recommended marking the groove and the tendon with methylene blue before making an incision in the tendon in order to determine the normal tension of the tendon postoperatively. (Modified from Froimson AI and Oh I: Keyhole tenodesis of biceps origin at the shoulder. Clin Orthop *112*:245–249, 1974.)

to have an impingement syndrome. One had a typical anterior impingement, and two patients had coracoid impingement. The other patient was later noted to have glenohumeral instability. The patients who did well in their series were older patients, averaging 41 years of age. In those patients, excision of the coracoacromial ligament was part of the operation. However, it is their recommendation now that an acromioplasty as well as a coracoacromial ligament release be performed. In patients who were found to have coracoid impingement, coracoid osteotomy later relieved their pain. The most salient recommendation and lesson from this review is that at the time of surgical exposure, if biceps tenodesis is planned, the subacromial space and the inter-relation of the coracoacromial arch to the tendon must be observed. Careful preoperative evaluation as well as examination under anesthesia will reveal concomitant anterior instability. It was their impression that isolated inflammation of the long head of the biceps is an infrequent finding unless injury to the biceps tendon in the groove has occurred. The entity of the subluxating biceps tendon is still questionable in their opinion. They state, "The role of the biceps tendon in the production of shoulder pain is difficult to assess and easily overestimated. Biceps tendon inflammation may be a secondary manifestation of an impingement syndrome. Unless treated, the impingement syndrome surgery will not be successful."

O'Donohue[201] presented a series of 56 cases of biceps instability treated with the Hitchcock procedure. Of these cases, 71% reported excellent progress; 77% said they could throw satisfactorily; and 77% resumed their sport. They concluded that in the young, motivated athlete for whom throwing was important that this was a very worthwhile operation.

Neviaser[198] reported on the four-in-one arthroplasty for relief of chronic subacromial impingement. In his procedure all elements of the coracoacromial arch are addressed. The four-in-one arthroplasty includes anterior acromioplasty, excision of the coracoacromial ligament, excision of the distal clavicle, and biceps tenodesis. Eighty-six per cent of his 89 patients had no pain whatsoever, whereas 13% had pain only with excessive exercise. Motion was improved in 81%.

Most of the early studies showing good results of biceps tenodesis had very scant and short follow-up. Cofield[48] reviewed the long-term results of 51 patients in whom there were 54 shoulders with isolated biceps tenodesis. At 6 months 94% felt they had benefited from the procedure; however, satisfactory results fell to 52% at an average of seven years. Fifteen per cent underwent subsequent surgery, primarily cuff repairs and acromioplasty, and 33% continued to have moderate to severe pain. In another long-term study, Berleman and associates obtained approximately 70% good and excellent results without deterioration in the longer term. Ogilvie-Harris[202] reported on arthroscopic findings and treatment of biceps tendon lesions. The usual lesion consisted of fraying of the tendon, with loose fronds hanging down into the joint. The fraying appeared to be greatest at the point where the biceps tendon entered the groove. The arthroscopic procedure consisted of débridement of the tendon and in some cases, attempts at dilatation of the orifice. There were 46 patients with lesions of the biceps tendon in his series, some of whom had had previous rotator cuff repairs. The biceps tendon appeared to be adherent to the undersurface of the rotator cuff in these individuals. These adhesions were freed arthroscopically. Of patients with isolated lesions of the biceps tendon, "Three fourths of them did well with simple débridement." However, he admits that the follow-up was short, being only 24 months. Only four of nine patients who had the biceps tendon released from the undersurface of the rotator cuff had "relief of symptoms."

In 1987, Post[221] presented 21 patients in whom the diagnosis of primary tendinitis of the long head of the biceps was made. In his cases, he excluded any with associated impingement syndrome, rotator cuff pathology, recurrent anterior shoulder instability, and repeated biceps tendon subluxation. All patients in his series had marked tenderness over the long head of the biceps, a negative impingement sign, and little or no relief of pain with subacromial injection. Fifty per cent of the cases had a positive Yergason sign. Seventeen patients in his series underwent biceps tenodesis via the keyhole technique; four patients had a transfer to the coracoid process. In the transfer group there were two excellent and two good results. One patient required a manipulation under anesthesia. Of 17 patients who had tenodesis, there were 13 excellent results, two good results, and one failure. Two of these patients did require manipulation. The one patient who was considered a failure in this group developed symptoms and findings of an impingement syndrome postoperatively and eventually required a partial anterior acromioplasty. In the tenodesis group, there were 88.3% good and excellent results. On the basis of his experience, it is Post's conviction that primary biceps tendinitis does occur as an isolated entity. Also, when it does occur, it is observed in the intertubercular groove alone.

Habermeyer and Walch[100] believe that chronic bicipital tendinitis combined with a chronic subacromial impingement syndrome is best treated by subacromial decompression. They recommend biceps tenodesis only in patients younger than the age of 40 presenting with isolated biceps tendinitis that are refractory to conservative treatment. For subluxating or dislocating bicipital lesions, they recommend two types of reconstruction. If patients have underlying subacromial impingement, a procedure to address this disease is also performed.

The first technique to operatively repair instability is reconstruction of the rotator interval sling and the repair of the subscapularis tendon. The extensions of the supraspinatus and subscapularis tendon are formed into a lasso at the entrance of the groove to prevent it from resubluxating. The second technique is either a biceps tenodesis using some of the various previously mentioned techniques or to use the Walch tubularization technique (Fig. 19–58). In this technique the widened and damaged tendon is formed and fixed into a tube with a running suture. The groove is then deepened using an impactor, and the tendon is then relocated into the groove. The damaged rotator interval, subscapularis, and supraspinatus tendons are repaired. Berlemann and Bayley have reviewed biceps tenodesis with the keyhole technique

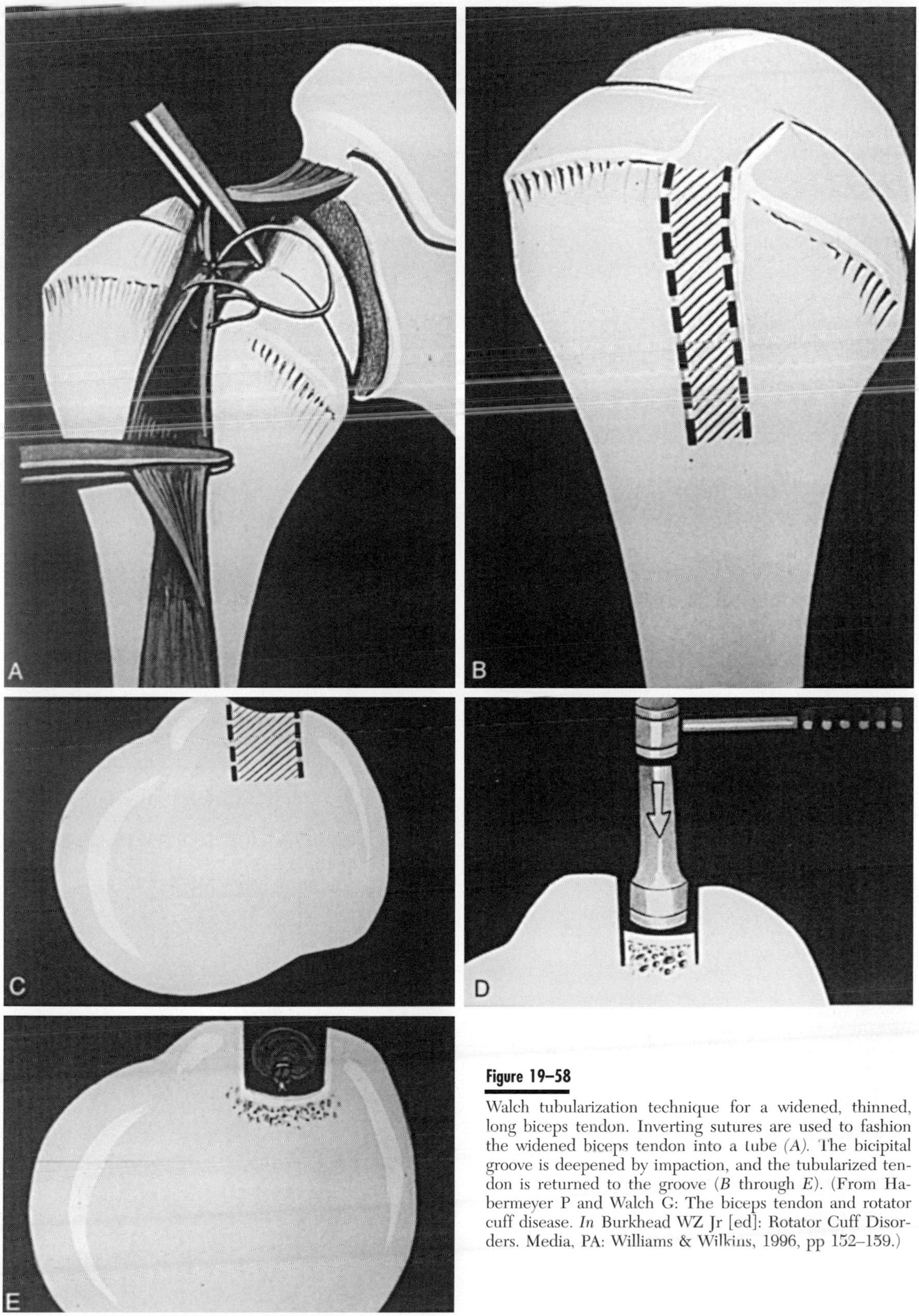

Figure 19–58

Walch tubularization technique for a widened, thinned, long biceps tendon. Inverting sutures are used to fashion the widened biceps tendon into a tube *(A)*. The bicipital groove is deepened by impaction, and the tubularized tendon is returned to the groove (*B* through *E*). (From Habermeyer P and Walch G: The biceps tendon and rotator cuff disease. *In* Burkhead WZ Jr [ed]: Rotator Cuff Disorders. Media, PA: Williams & Wilkins, 1996, pp 152–159.)

with approximately 65% good and excellent results. Multiple pathologies were encountered in most shoulders.[24]

Treatment of SLAP lesions is dependent on their type. Type I SLAP lesions are usually degenerative lesions that are often associated with rotator cuff or intra-articular pathology. Treatment of this lesion (as recommended by Field and Savoie,[74] Grauerand colleagues,[95] and Snyder and associates[241]) is treatment of the underlying abnormality and possibly shaving of the degenerated labrum. Type II SLAP lesions have been repaired using suture techniques as well as a tacking technique to re-establish the biceps anchor onto the glenoid edge.[99, 242] Type III lesions usually require débridement of the bucket handle tear.[241] The surgeon should also assess the patient for other associated pathology. Type IV lesions usually need a stabilization of the biceps anchor using either suturing techniques or a tacking technique similar to type II lesions. Resection of the bucket handle tear may be necessary.

Open operative treatment of synovial osteochondromatosis of the biceps tendon gives good results in the case report presented by Covall and associates.[53, 54] Débridement of the diseased synovium in hemodialysis-related shoulder arthropathy has given some good results according to Takenaka.[249]

AUTHOR'S (W.Z.B.) PREFERRED METHODS OF TREATMENT

The treatment of lesions of the biceps tendon, with the exception of acute traumatic rupture of the tendon in the young patient or in association with a massive cuff tear in an active patient, should be viewed as a continuum with prolonged (several months) conservative care and repeated evaluation. As long as the patient is making slow, gradual improvement, surgical intervention is not recommended. Surgical treatment is only indicated after a minimum of 6 months of conservative care. I have divided the treatment of chronic lesions using the classification of Paavolainen and associates.[205]

Impingement Tendinitis

Treatment of bicipital tendinitis when associated with coracoacromial arch impingement (enesopathy) closely

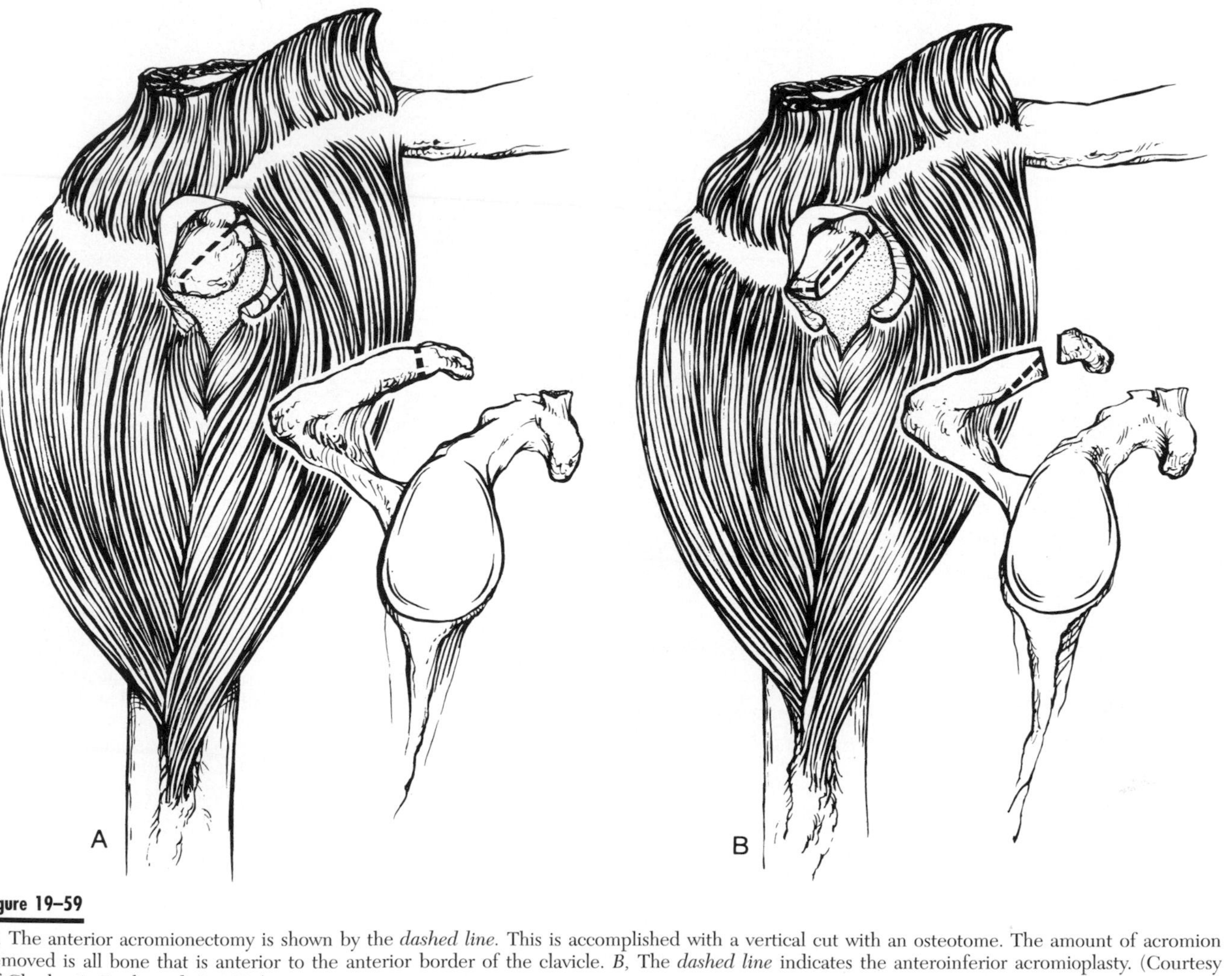

Figure 19–59

A, The anterior acromionectomy is shown by the *dashed line.* This is accomplished with a vertical cut with an osteotome. The amount of acromion removed is all bone that is anterior to the anterior border of the clavicle. *B,* The *dashed line* indicates the anteroinferior acromioplasty. (Courtesy of Charles A. Rockwood, Jr, MD.)

follows the treatment outlined by Neer in his original and follow-up articles. The stages and treatment of this clinical entity are well described in Chapter 15.

In stage II, if symptoms remain the same after 6 months of active conservative treatment, I (W.Z.B.) will sometimes employ glenohumeral arthroscopy to visualize the intra-articular portion of the biceps and glenoid labrum. The biceps tendon can be pulled into the joint with a probe and synovitis demonstrated if present. This obviates the need for opening the rotator interval, which prolongs recovery. Although good results from arthroscopic decompression have been reported in stage II impingement,[69] when biceps symptoms predominate, I (W.Z.B.) prefer an open approach (Fig. 19–59). In this technique the deltotrapezial fascia is taken down from the posterior corner of the acromioclavicular joint out to the anterolateral corner of the acromion. The distal clavicle is resected using a saw. A Rockwood two-step acromioplasty is then performed using a straight osteotome. The advantages of this double-cut approach are: (1) it ensures adequate removal of anterior bone, (2) it allows the surgeon to better appreciate the thickness of the acromion, and (3) it avoids leaving residual anteromedial and anterolateral acromion that can still impinge (Fig. 19–60).

When performing biceps tenodesis one of several methods is employed. Both the keyhole technique[69] and Mitek anchors, if proximal bone permits, provide secure fixation. With the Mitek technique, the proximal end is sutured into the rotator interval repair. I have used the technique described by Post in some situations, especially when the rupture has occurred low in the area of the groove.

Post[220] has offered a solution to one problem that I (W.Z.B.) have had previously when doing a biceps tenodesis, and that is, "Under what type of tension should the biceps be tenodesed?" Should this be done in elbow flexion, extension, and so forth? He recommends marking the biceps tendon and intertubercular groove with methylene blue after the bicipital groove is opened but before the intertubercular portion is cut so that after the tendon is cut, these adjacent areas can be matched again at the time of tenodesis.

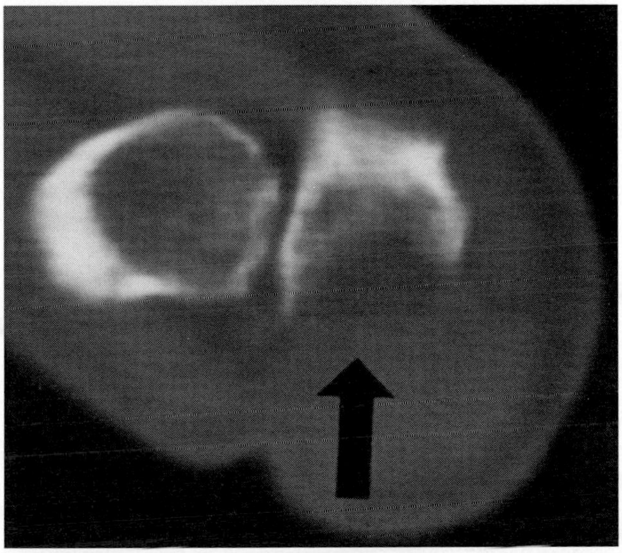

Figure 19–60

An anterior acromioplasty has been performed using a curved osteotome in a single oblique acromioplasty. This unfortunately left residual anterior acromion with residual coracoacromial ligament attached to the medial aspect *(arrow)*, as seen on this computed tomography scan. For this reason I recommend initially an anterior acromionectomy done with a straight osteotome (as taught by Rockwood).

In stage III impingement, by definition, a full-thickness tear exists in the rotator cuff. These patients generally have severe spurring of the anterior acromion and distal clavicle. Frequently, if the anterior cuff is involved, subluxation, hypertrophy, degenerative changes, or frank rupture of the biceps tendon may be present. In these patients, a formal open anterior acromioplasty and cuff repair is performed with reconstruction of the rotator cuff. If the biceps is dislocated, it is replaced in the groove, and after suturing the supraspinatus either tendon to tendon or tendon to bone, the rotator interval is closed and the edges of the subscapularis and coracohumeral ligament complex are sutured to the repaired supraspinatus, recreating the stabilizing effect at the aperture of the tuberosities (Fig. 19–61). The biceps tendon is not tenodesed unless severe attrition wear and eminent rupture is found. No attempt is made to repair chronic ruptures (> 6 weeks) of the tendon. The patient is informed preoperatively that he or she will continue to have a bulge in the lower portion of the brachium. The intra-articular portion is removed to prevent possible impingement in the joint.

Treatment of Biceps Instability

In my experience, surgically proven biceps instability is always related to a degenerative process in the cuff, restraining capsule, and coracohumeral ligament in the proximal portion of the groove. As with impingement tendinitis, primary attention should be placed on repair of the rotator cuff as well as on performing a thorough decompression of the coracoacromial arch. It has been well established that the main stabilizer of the biceps tendon is the musculotendinous cuff and the coracohumeral ligament. These structures can be injured acutely or by the mechanisms previously described, and a fixed or recurrent subluxation of the biceps tendon can occur. If the history of injury is acute and the patient is younger than 65 years of age, MRI scanning is recommended to diagnose this condition and to evaluate the status of the rotator cuff. If the biceps is dislocated, I (W.Z.B.) recommend early open reduction of the tendon with reconstruction of the fibrous roof, combined with an acromioplasty procedure (see Fig. 19–61). It is important to remember that once the diagnosis of a dislocated biceps tendon is made, a rotator cuff tear is also diagnosed. Whereas in the older (over 65 years) age group, this can be accepted and treated conservatively, younger (less than 50 years) patients will fare better if the tendon is replaced and the fibrous roof reconstructed.

Treatment of Isolated Biceps Lesions

These are patients in whom subacromial injection offers absolutely no improvement in the pain, but pain and motion consistently respond to local anesthetic injections into the bicipital groove region. These patients generally respond to the judicious use of rest, aspirin or nonsteroidal anti-inflammatory agents, moist heat, and gentle patient-directed exercises. The judicious use of corticosteroids by injection can also be helpful. The injection should be into the bicipital sheath and should require only minimal pressure on the syringe and a low volume of fluid; that is, 2 to 3 ml of lidocaine and 1 ml of water-soluble steroid should be used. The technique of injection has been described previously under the differential diagnosis. There have been numerous case reports of tendon ruptures temporally and causally related to corticosteroid injections. These include the patellar and Achilles' tendons, the flexor and extensor tendons of the hand, and the long head of the biceps. Although some tendons, especially those in the older patient with systemic disease or attrition tendinitis, may rupture as a result of the disease process, there is a strong suggestion that the use of injection into the tendon contributes to tendon degradation. Kennedy and Willis[127] have shown collagen necrosis as well as disorganization and loss of normal parallel collagen arrangement in Achilles' tendons injected with corticosteroids. This is accompanied by a 35% loss of failure strength at approximately 48 hours postinjection. The failure strength of the tendon returns at approximately 2 weeks; however, ultrastructural changes in the tendon persist for 6 weeks. Because of this, the patients are asked to avoid any strenuous activity for 3 weeks. In my (W.Z.B.) own experience, patients are injected at least at intervals and then only once or twice, or perhaps three times in unusual cases. Injections have been shown to be more efficacious than a placebo or naproxen (Naprosyn) in the treatment of chronic shoulder pain and are equivalent to the use of indomethacin (Indocin).[254, 255] Unfortunately, some patients with this problem cannot tolerate nonsteroidal anti-inflammatory agents in the doses required.

If the patient fails to respond to conservative care over a 6- to 12-month period, surgery is recommended. Since the results of isolated biceps tenodesis have not been spectacular in the long term and impingement syndrome has developed after biceps tenodesis, a subacromial decompression is routinely performed.

Treatment of Isolated Biceps Rupture in Patients Younger Than 50 Years of Age

In younger, active patients, particularly those involved in overhead sports or weight-lifting, or jobs requiring forceful supination, a sudden overload can result in an isolated biceps rupture. This may be within the muscle tendon junction, rather than the long head tendon. Physical examination and ultrasonography of the biceps should be able to isolate the point of rupture. Sonography or MRI of the rotator cuff should be used to determine the status of the rotator cuff. If the physical examination is consistent with an acute rupture and the sonogram is equivocal or negative, an arthrogram can be used. In

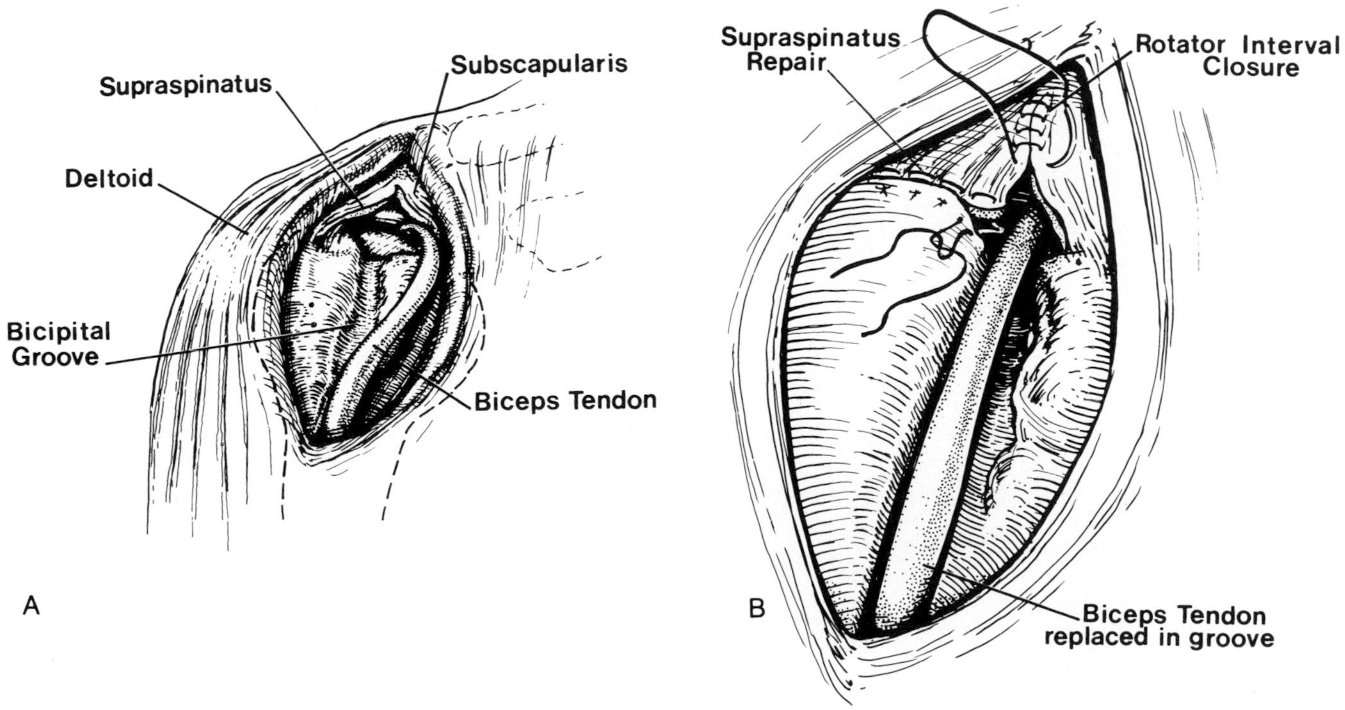

Figure 19–61

A, Rotator cuff tear and dislocated biceps tendon. *B*, The rotator cuff has been repaired into a bony trough, and the rotator interval has been closed with the tendon replaced in the groove.

these patients with high functional expectations, an early repair is the best alternative. If the rupture is musculotendinous or at the transverse ligament and sonography is negative for a cuff tear, early repair using a Bunnell-type weave suture through a deltopectoral incision is performed. This is the only group of patients in whom the use of the deltopectoral approach is recommended.

Treatment of Acute Bicipital Rupture in Patients Older Than 50 Years of Age

If the patient is inactive physically, graduated leave alone method (GLAM) technique of rest, anti-inflammatory medications, and moist heat are utilized. During this time, the patient is instructed in keeping the shoulder motion free with the use of passive exercises. If the patient is physically active, an early aggressive diagnostic work-up should be performed. This usually consists of an MRI scan; however, an arthrogram or sonography can be performed. One will generally find an "acute" cuff tear as well as the biceps tendon rupture. Many of these patients will have in reality an acute extension of a chronic tear or no extension at all. The two-incision approach in these cases is employed if the rupture is less than 6 weeks old (Fig. 19–62*A*). If a tear is present in the rotator cuff, an anterior acromioplasty with cuff repair and bicipital tenodesis is performed. The biceps tendon is exposed through a separate incision in the brachium (see Fig. 19–62*B*). The subcutaneous tissue is incised, and edema and old hemorrhage are evacuated. The tendon can be curled up in this area or stuck proximally, proximal to the pectoralis insertion. Using a suture-passer, passed down from above through the bicipital groove and into the lower wound, the tendon is advanced into the superior wound (see Fig. 19–62*C*). A biceps tenodesis in the groove is then performed.

Treatment of SLAP Lesions

Treatment of SLAP lesions is covered fully in Chapter 8.

Calcific Tendinitis

Calcific tendinitis is treated as described in Chapter 18.

Postoperative Care

Unless there is some tension on the cuff repair with the arm at the side, a Velcro elastic immobilizer is worn postoperatively for 3 weeks. The patient is encouraged to take the elbow out and gently flex and extend it passively with the opposite hand the night of the surgery. Gentle pendulum exercises are initiated on the first postoperative day. Passive flexion performed by the patient (with his other arm), nurse, or therapist is begun on the second postoperative day. Because holding on to a pulley handle requires some active contraction of the biceps, I (W.Z.B.) generally instruct a family member in gentle, passive forward flexion and external rotation. At 1 month, the pulley can safely be used and gentle, active elbow flexion begun. Strengthening of the repaired cuff, deltoid, and biceps generally begins at 2 months and becomes more vigorous at 3 months. Patients usually return to work at jobs that require moderate lifting at approximately 6 months.

SUMMARY

Inflammation of the biceps tendon often accompanies rotator cuff pathology. Because of its unique anatomic position and its close relationship with the coracoacromial arch, this tendon is susceptible to secondary injury and inflammation.

Biomechanically, the biceps tendon appears to function both as a dynamic and static head depressor. In the normal shoulder it contributes little to humeral head depression, while in the shoulder with a rotator cuff tear, the humeral head's primary stabilizer and increases the depressor role of the biceps have been demonstrated. Because of this, routine tenodesis of the biceps tendon or its use as a free graft in rotator cuff repair is not recommended.

Although the bicipital sheath is involved with the same inflammatory process as the rest of the synovium in adhesive capsulitis, biceps tendinitis is not the initiating factor in most cases of adhesive capsulitis. The loss of the gliding mechanism of the biceps is not the primary cause of loss of motion in this entity.

The biceps tendons primary restraint against dislocations are the coracohumeral ligament, superior glenohumeral ligament, and the rotator cuff, proximal to the groove. Because of its intimate relationship to the coracoacromial arch, whenever one considers the diagnosis of biceps pathology, one should also consider the diagnosis of impingement of the rotator cuff. Whenever possible, subluxation of the biceps should be treated with replacement of the tendon into the groove and reconstruction of the rotator cuff combined with subacromial decompression.

Isolated biceps tenodesis is not recommended. The addition of an anterior acromioplasty with excision of the coracoacromial ligament adds little morbidity to surgery on the biceps tendon and improves the results. Recognition that the diagnosis of isolated biceps tendon pathology is a diagnosis of exclusion, combined with long-term conservative care for painful conditions about the shoulder, can often obviate the need for surgery and improve the results if surgical procedures are required.

P.S. Charley, I still think that guy at the VA hospital needs a biceps tenodesis.

Acknowledgment

The Senior author would like to thank Karen Lozano very much for her valuable help and tremendous patience in preparing this manuscript. She is a jewel of a human being who makes me look much better than I really am.

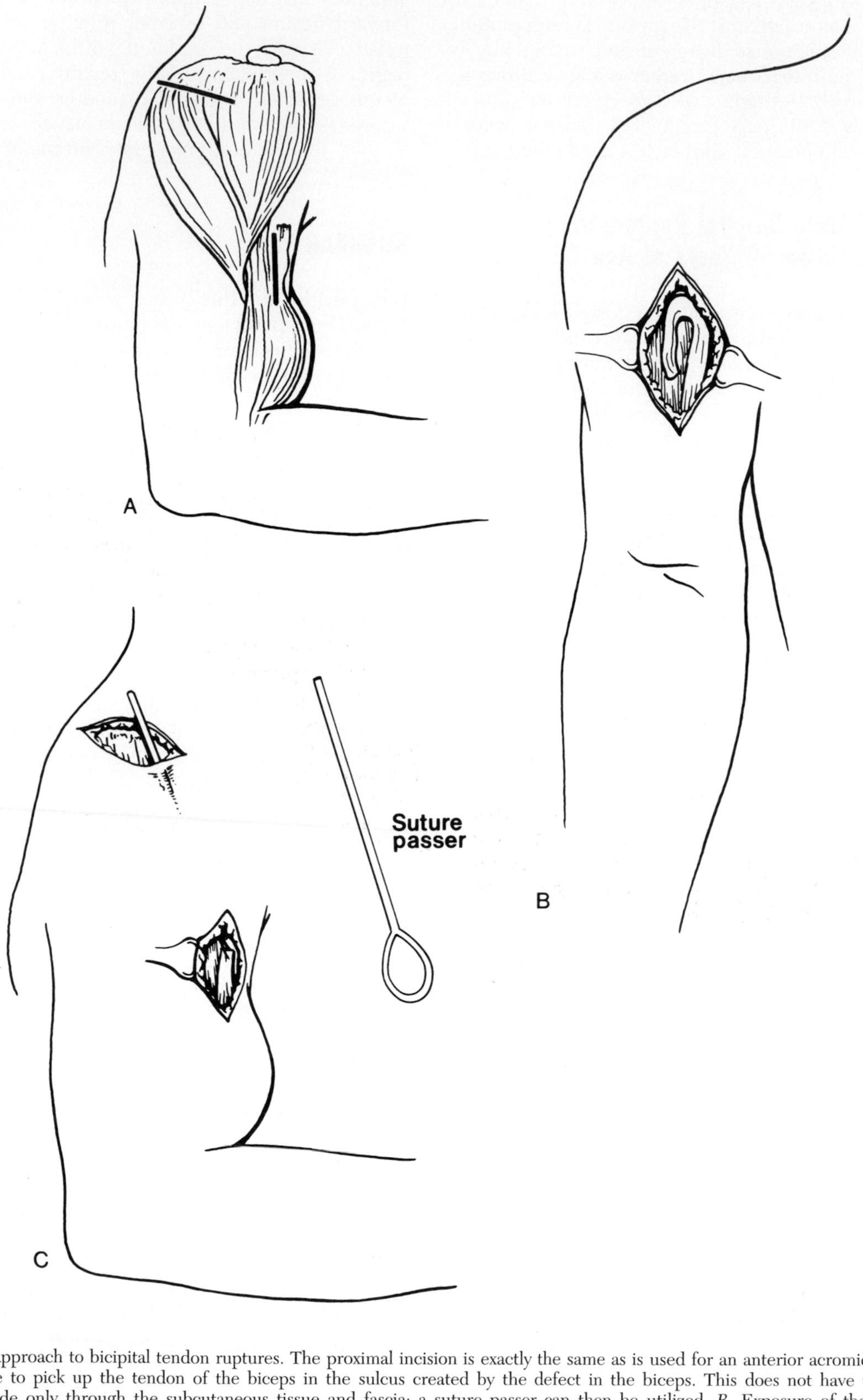

Figure 19–62

A, A two-incision approach to bicipital tendon ruptures. The proximal incision is exactly the same as is used for an anterior acromioplasty. The distal incision allows one to pick up the tendon of the biceps in the sulcus created by the defect in the biceps. This does not have to be a very long incision and is made only through the subcutaneous tissue and fascia; a suture passer can then be utilized. *B,* Exposure of the ruptured biceps tendon through the counterincision in the sulcus (magnified in this view). A 3-cm incision is all that is required to pick up the end of the tendon in this region. *C,* A suture passer is utilized to bring the tendon into the proximal wound for tenodesis or repair.

References and Bibliography

1. Abbott LC and Saunders LB de CM: Acute traumatic dislocation of the tendon of the long head of biceps brachii; report of 6 cases with operative findings. Surgery *6*:817–840, 1939.
2. Abbott LC and Lucas DB: The function of the clavicle: Its surgical significance. Ann Surg *140*:583–597, 1954.
3. Adams R: Abnormal Conditions of the Shoulder-Joint, Cyclopaedia of Anatomy and Physiology, Vol. 4. London: Longman, 1847–1849, p 595.
4. Ahovuo J: The radiographic anatomy of the intratubercular groove of the humerus. Eur J Radiol *2*:83, 1985.
5. Ahovuo J, Paavolainen P, and Slatis P: Radiographic diagnosis of biceps tendinitis. Acta Orthop Scand *56*:75–78, 1985.
6. Ahovuo J, Paavolainen P, and Slatis P: Diagnostic value of sonography in lesions of the biceps tendon. Clin Orthop *202*:184–188, 1986.
7. Anciaux-Ruyssen A and Claessens H: L'arthrographie de l'épaule. J Belge Radiol *39*:837, 1956.
8. Andrews J and Carson W: Shoulder joint arthroscopy. Orthopedics *6*:1157–1162, 1983,
9. Andrews J, Carson W, and McLeod W: Glenoid labrum tears related to the long head of the biceps. Am J Sports Med *13*:337 341, 1985.
10. Anglesio B: Osteotomia per omero varo. Arch Orthop *46*:417–428, 1930.
11. Ashurst J: The Principles and Practice of Surgery. Philadelphia: HC Lea, 1871, p 287.
12. Baer WS: Operative treatment of subdeltoid bursitis. Bull Johns Hopkins Hosp *18:*282–284, 1907.
13. Baker BE and Bierwagen D: Rupture of the distal tendon of the biceps brachii. J Bone Joint Surg *67*:414–417, 1985.
14. Basmajian JV and Latif MA: Integrated actions and function of the chief flexors of the elbow. J Bone Joint Surg *39A*:1106–1118, 1957.
15. Basmajian JV: Muscles Alive, 4th ed. Baltimore: Williams & Wilkins, 1978.
16. Basmajian JV: Muscles Alive, 5th ed. Baltimore: Williams & Wilkins, 1985.
17. Bateman JE: The Shoulder and Environs. St. Louis: CV Mosby, 1944.
18. Bateman JE: The Shoulder and Neck. Philadelphia: WB Saunders, 1978.
19. Bateman JE: The Shoulder and Neck, 2nd ed. Philadelphia: WB Saunders, 1978.
20. Becker DA and Cofield RH: Biceps brachii tenodesis for chronic tendinitis. Long term follow-up. Orthop Trans *210*:447, 1986.
21. Bedi SS and Ellis W: Spontaneous rupture of the calcaneal tendon in rheumatoid arthritis after local steroid injection. Ann Rheum Dis *29*:494–495, 1970.
22. Bennett GE: Shoulder and elbow lesions of professional baseball pitcher. JAMA *117*:510–514, 1941.
23. Bera A: Syndrome commun, rupture, elongation, luxation du tendon du long biceps. Paris, Thèse, 1910–1911.
24. Berlemann U and Bayley I: Tenodesis of the long head of biceps brachii in the painful shoulder: Improving results in the long term. J Shoulder Elbow Surg *4*:429–435, 1995.
25. Bidloo G: Anatomia Humani Corporis. Amstelodami, 1685.
26. Booth RE and Marvel JP: Differential diagnosis of shoulder pain. Orthop Clin North Am *6*:353–379, 1975.
27. Borchers E: Die ruptur der sehne des langen biceps kopfes. Beitr Klin Chir *90*:635–648, 1914.
28. Bossuet: Deux cas de luxation du tendon de la longue portion du biceps brachii. Bull Soc Anat Phys *28*:154, 1907.
29. Brickner WM: JAMA *69*:1237–1243, 1918.
30. Bromfield W: Chirgical Observations and Cases. London: 1773, p 76.
31. Burkhart SS and Fox DL: SLAP lesions in association with complete tears of the long head of the biceps tendon: A report of two cases. J Arthrop Rel Surg *8*:31–35, 1992.
32. Bush LF: The torn shoulder capsule. J Bone Joint Surg *57A*:256, 1975.
33. Callender GW: Dislocation of muscles and their treatment. BMJ July 13, 1878.
34. Carroll RE and Hamilton LR: Rupture of biceps brachii—a conservative method of treatment. J Bone Joint Surg *49A*:1016, 1967.
35. Gartland JP, Crues JV III, Stauffer A, et al: MR imaging in the evaluation of SLAP injuries of the shoulder. Findings in 10 patients. AJR Am J Roentgenol *159*:787–792, 1992.
36. Cilley: Quoted by Meyer AW. Arch Surg *17*:493–506, 1928.
37. Claessens II: De pijnlijke schouder. Belg T Geneesk 1050, 1956.
38. Claessens H and Anciauz-Ruyssen A: L'arthrographie de l'épaule. Acta Orthop Belg *3–4*:289, 1956.
39. Claessens H and Brosgol M: Rapport: Les lesions traumatiques des parties molles de l'épaule. Acta Orthop Belg *2*:97, 1957.
40. Claessens H and Biltris R: Diagnostic differentiel entre les lesions de la coiffe musculotendineuse et celles de la longue portion du biceps. J Belge Rheumatol Med Phys *20*:53, 1965.
41. Claessens H and Snoek H: Tendinitis of the long head of the biceps brachii. Acta Orthop Belg *38*:1, 1972.
42. Claessens H and Veys E: Les arthrites et l'arthrose de l'articulation scapulohumerale. J Belge Rheumatol Med Phys *72*:73, 1965.
43. Clark DD, Ricker JH, and MacCollum MS: The efficacy of local steroid injection in the treatment of stenosing tenovaginitis. Plast Reconstr Surg *51*:179–180, 1973.
44. Clark KC: Positioning in Radiography, Vol. 1, 9th ed. London. William Heinemann Medical Books, 1973.
45. Clark JM and Harryman DT: Tendons, ligaments and capsule of the rotator cuff. J Bone Joint Surg Am *74*:713–725, 1992.
46. Codman EA: The supraspinatus syndrome. Boston Med Surg J *150*:371–374, 1904.
47. Codman EA: The Shoulder. Boston: Thomas Todd, 1934.
48. Cofield RH and Becker D: Surgical Tenodesis of the Long Head of the Biceps Brachii for Chronic Tendinitis. Presented at the 53rd Annual Meeting of the American Academy of Orthopaedic Surgeons, New Orleans, Louisiana, February 21, 1986.
49. Cone RO, Danzig L, Resnick D, and Goldman AB: The bicipital groove: Radiographic, anatomic, and pathologic study. AJR Am J Roentgenol *41*:781–788, 1983.
50. Conti V: Arthroscopy in rehabilitation. Orthop Clin North Am *10*:709–711, 1979.
51. Cooper A: A Treatise on Dislocations and Fractures of the Joints. Boston: Lilly, Wait, Carter, & Hendee, 1832, p 407.
52. Cooper DE, Arnoczky SP, O'Brien SJ, et al: Anatomy, histology and vascularity of the glenoid labrum. An anatomical study. J Bone Joint Surg Am *74*:46–52, 1992.
53. Covall DJ and Fowble CD: Arthroscopic treatment of synovial chondromatosis of the shoulder and biceps tendon sheath. J Arthrop Rel Surg *9*:602–604, 1993.
54. Covall DJ and Fowble CD: Synovial Chondromatosis of the Biceps Tendon Sheath. Orthop Rev *23*:902–905, 1994.
55. Cowper W: Myotomia Reformata. London: 1694, p 75.
56. Crenshaw AH and Kilgore WE: Surgical treatment of bicipital tenosynovitis. J Bone Joint Surg *48A*:1496–1502, 1966.
57. Day BH, Govindasamy N, and Patnaik R: Corticosteroid injections in the treatment of tennis elbow. Practitioner *220*(1317):459–462, 1978.
58. Dejour D and Tayot O: La Rupture Isolée de la Longue Portion du Biceps. Lyons, France: Journées Lyonnaise de l'Epaule, 1993.
59. DePalma AF: Surgery of the Shoulder. Philadelphia: JB Lippincott, 1950.
60. DePalma AF and Callery GE: Bicipital tenosynovitis. Clin Orthop *3*:69–85, 1954.
61. DePalma AF: The painful shoulder. Postgrad Med *21*:368–376, 1957.
62. DePalma AF: Surgical anatomy of the rotator cuff and the natural history of degenerative periarthritis. Surg Clin North Am *43*:1507–1520, 1963.
63. DePalma AF: Surgery of the Shoulder, 2nd ed. Philadelphia: JB Lippincott, 1983.
64. Despates H: Gaz Hebd *15*:374–378, 1878.
65. Dines D, Warren RF, and Inglis AE: Surgical treatment of lesions of the long head of the biceps. Clin Orthop *164*:165–171, 1982.
66. Duplay S: Arch Gen Med *2*:513–542, 1872.
67. Duplay S and Reclus P: Traite de Chirurgie, Vol. 1. Paris: G. Masson, 1880–1882, p 825.
68. Duplay S: On scapulo-humeral periarthritis. (Paris Clinical Lectures.) Med Presse *69*:571–573, 1900.
69. Ellman H: Arthroscopic Subacromial Decompression. New Orleans: Society of American Shoulder and Elbow Surgeons, 1986.
70. Ennevaara K: Painful shoulder joint in rheumatoid arthritis: Clini-

cal and radiologic study of 200 cases with special reference to arthrography of the glenohumeral joint. Acta Rheumatol Scand (Suppl) 2:11–116, 1967.
71. Ewald: Traumatic ruptures usually due to arthritis deformans or other diseases of shoulder. Munch Med Wchnschr *74*:2214–2215, 1927.
72. Farin PU, Jaroma H, Harju A, and Soimakallio S: Medial displacement of the biceps brachii tendon: Evaluation with dynamic sonography during maximal external shoulder rotation. Radiology *195*:845–848, 1995.
73. McShane RB, Leinberry CF, and Fenlin JM Jr: Conservative open anterior acromioplasty. Clin Orthop *223*:137–144, 1987.
74. Field LD and Savoie FH: Arthroscopic suture repair of superior labral detachment lesions of the shoulder. Am J Sports Med *21*:783–790, 1993.
75. Fisk C: Adaptation of the technique for radiography of the bicipital groove. Radiol Technol *37*:47–50, 1965.
76. Freeland AE and Higgins RW: Anterior shoulder dislocation with posterior displacement of the long head of the biceps tendon. Arthrographic findings. A case report. Orthopedics *8*:468–469, 1985.
77. Froimson AI and Oh I: Keyhole tenodesis of biceps origin at the shoulder. Clin Orthop *112*:245–249, 1974.
78. Furlani J: Electromyographic study of the m. biceps brachii in movements at the glenohumeral joint. Acta Anat (Basel) *96*:270–284, 1976.
79. Gainer BJ, Piotrowski G, Truhl J, et al: The throw: Biomechanics and acute injury. Am Sports Med 8:114–118, 1980.
80. Gardner E and Gray DJ: Prenatal development of the human shoulder and acromioclavicular joint. Am J Anat *92*:219–276, 1953.
81. Gerber C, Terrier F, and Ganz R: The role of the coracoid process in the chronic impingement syndrome. J Bone Joint Surg *67B*:703–708, 1985.
82. Gerster AG: Subcutaneous injuries of the biceps brachii, with two new cases and some historical notes. N Y Med J *27*:487–502, 1878.
83. Gilcreest EL: Rupture of muscles and tendons, particularly subcutaneous rupture of the biceps flexor cubiti. JAMA *84*:1819–1822, 1925.
84. Gilcreest EL: Two cases of spontaneous rupture of the long head of the biceps flexor cubiti. Surg Clin North Am *6*:539–554, 1926.
85. Gilcreest EL: The common syndrome of rupture, dislocation and elongation of the long head of the biceps brachii: An analysis of one hundred cases. Surg Gynecol Obstet *58*:322–339, 1934.
86. Gilcreest EL: Dislocation and elongation of the long head of the biceps brachii. Analysis of six cases. Ann Surg *104*:118–138, 1936.
87. Gilcreest EL and Albi P: Unusual lesions of muscles and tendons of the shoulder girdle and upper arm. Surg Gynecol Obstet *68*:903–917, 1939.
88. Giuliani P, Scarpa G, Marchini M, and Nicoletti P: Development of scapulohumeral articulation in man, with special reference to its relation to the tendon of the long head of the biceps muscle of the arm. Arch Ital Anat Embriol *82*:85–98, 1977.
89. Glousman R, Jobe FW, Tibone JP, et al: Dynamic EMG analysis of the throwing shoulder with glenohumeral instability.
90. Godsil RD Jr and Linschied RL: Intratendinous defects of the rotator cuff. Clin Orthop *69*:181–188, 1970.
91. Goldman AB and Ghelman B: The double contrast shoulder arthrogram: A review of 158 studies. Radiology *127*:658–663, 1978.
92. Goldman AB: Shoulder Arthrography. Boston: Little, Brown, 1981, pp 239–257.
93. Goldman AB: Calcific tendinitis of the long head of the biceps brachii distal to the glenohumeral joint: Plain film radiographic findings. Am J Radiol *153*:1011–1016, 1989.
94. Goldthwait JE: An anatomic and mechanical study of the shoulder joint, explaining many of the cases of painful shoulder, many of the recurrent dislocations and many of the cases of brachial neuralgias or neuritis. Am J Orthop Surg *6*:579–606, 1909.
95. Grauer JD, Paulos LE, and Smutz WP: Biceps tendon and superior labral injuries. Arthroscopy *8*:488–497, 1992.
96. Green JS: Dislocation of the long head of the biceps flexor cubiti muscle. Virginia Med Monthly *4*:106, 1877–1878.
97. Guermonprez and Michel A: Posterior luxation of shoulder. Rupture of lesser tuberosity, rupture and luxation of tendon of long head of biceps. Recovery. Bull Soc Anat Paris 4:1890.
98. Habermeyer P, Kaiser E, Knappe M, et al: Functional anatomy and biomechanics of the long biceps tendon. Unfallchirurg *90*:319–329, 1987.
99. Habermeyer P, Brunner U, Treptow U, and Wiedemann E: Arthroskopische over-the top-naht zur behandlung von S.L.A.P. lasionen der schulter. Arthroskopie *6*:253–271, 1993.
100. Habermeyer P and Walch G: The biceps tendon and rotator cuff disease. *In* Burkhead WZ Jr (ed): Rotator Cuff Disorders. Media, PA: Williams & Wilkins, 1996, p 142.
101. Haenisch GF: Fortsch Rontgenstrahl *15*:293–300, 1910.
102. Ha'eri GB and Maitland A: Arthroscopic findings in the frozen shoulder. J Rheumatol *8*:149–152, 1981.
103. Ha'eri GB and Wiley AM: Advancement of the supraspinatus muscle in the repair of ruptures of the rotator cuff. J Bone Joint Surg *63A*:232–238, 1981.
104. Haggart GE and Allen HA: Painful shoulder: Diagnosis and treatment with particular reference to subacromial bursitis. Surg Clin North Am *15*:1537–1560, 1935.
105. Hall-Craggs EC: Anatomy as a Basis for Clinical Medicine. Baltimore: Urban & Schwartzberg, 1985, p 111.
106. Hammond G, Torgerson W, Dotter W, and Leach R: The painful shoulder. Am Acad Orthop Surg Instructional Course Lecture. St. Louis: CV Mosby, 1971, pp 83–90.
107. Hawkins RJ and Kennedy JC: Impingement syndrome in athletes. Am J Sports Med *8*:151–158, 1980.
108. Heikel HVA: Rupture of the rotator cuff of the shoulder. Acta Orthop Scand *39*:477–492, 1968.
109. Herberts P, Kadefors R, Andersson G, and Petersen I: Shoulder pain in industry: An epidemiological study on welders. Acta Orthop Scand *52*:299–306, 1981.
110. Hippocrates: Quoted by Duplay, Reclus, and Garrison.
111. Hitchcock HH and Bechtol CO: Painful shoulder. Observations on the role of the tendon of the long head of the biceps brachii in its causation. J Bone Joint Surg *30A*:263–273, 1948.
112. Hollinshead WH: Anatomy For Surgeons, Vol. 3. New York: Harper & Row, 1969, p 325.
113. Hollinsworth GR, Ellis RM, and Hattersley TS: Comparison of injection techniques for shoulder pain: Results of a double blind, randomized study. BMJ *287*:1339–1341, 1983.
114. Horowitz MT: Lesions of the supraspinatus tendon and associated structures. Investigation of comparable lesions in the hip joint. Arch Surg *38*:990–1003, 1939.
115. Howard HJ and Eloesser L: Treatment of fractures of the upper end of the humerus: An experimental and clinical study. J Bone Joint Surg *16*:1–29, 1934.
116. Hueter C: Zur Diagnose der Verletzungen des M. Biceps Brachii. Arch Klin Chir *5*:321–323, 1864; and also Grundriss der Chirurgie, Vol. 2, p 735.
117. Ingelbrecht: Arch Franco-Belges Chir *29*:922–923, 1926.
118. Inman VT, Saunders JB de CM, and Abbott LC: Observations on the function of the shoulder joint. J Bone Joint Surg *26*:1–30, 1944.
119. Inman VT and Saunders JB de CM: Observations on the function of the clavicle. Calif Med *65*:158–166, 1946.
120. Itoi E, Kuechle DK, Newman SR, et al: Stabilizing function of the biceps in stable and unstable shoulders. J Bone Joint Surg *75B*:546–550, 1993.
121. Janecki CJ and Barnett DC: Fracture dislocation of the shoulder with biceps interposition. J Bone Joint Surg *61A*:1–143, 1979.
122. Jarjavey JF: Luxation du tendon du biceps humeral et des tendons des peroniers lateraux. Gaz Hebd Med (Paris) *4*:325–327, 357–359, 387–391, 1867.
123. Jobe FW, Tibone JE, Perry J, et al: An EMG analysis of the shoulder in throwing and pitching: A preliminary report. Am J Sports Med *11*:3–5, 1983.
124. Jobe FW and Jobe CM: Painful athletic injuries of the shoulder. Clin Orthop *173*:117–124, 1983.
125. Jobe FW, Moines DR, Tibone JE, et al: An EMG analysis of the shoulder in pitching: A second report. Am J Sports Med *12*:218–220, 1984.
126. Jungmichel D, Winzer J, and Lippoldt G: Tendon rupture of the biceps muscle of the arm and its treatment with special reference to the key hole operation. Beitr Orthop Traumatol *33*:226–232, 1986.
127. Kennedy JC and Willis RB: The effects of local steroid injections on tendons: A biomechanical and microscopic correlative study. Am J Sports Med *4*:11–21, 1976.

128. Kerlan RK: Throwing injuries to the shoulder. *In* Zarins B, Andrews JR, and Carson WG (eds): Injuries to the Throwing Arm. Philadelphia: WB Saunders, 1985, p 114.
129. Kessel L and Watson M: The painful arc syndrome: Clinical classification as a guide to management. J Bone Joint Surg *59B*:166 172, 1977.
130. Kieft GJ, Bloem JL, Rozing PM, and Obermann WR: Rotator cuff impingement syndrome: MR imaging. Radiology *166*:211–214, 1988.
131. Killoran PJ, Marcove RL, and Freiberger RH: Shoulder arthrography. AJR Am J Roentgenol *103*:658–668, 1968.
132. Kneeland JB, et al: MR imaging of the shoulder: Diagnosis of rotator cuff tears. AJR Am J Roentgenol *149*:333–337, 1987.
133. Koltz I, Tillman B, and Lullmann Rauch R: The structure and vascularization of the biceps brachii long head tendon. Ann Anat *176*:75–80, 1994.
134. Kumar VP, Satku K, and Balasubramaniam P: The role of the long head of biceps brachii in the stabilization of the head of the humerus. Clin Orthop Rel Res *244*:172–175, 1989.
135. Lapidus PW: Infiltration therapy of acute tendinitis with calcification. Surg Gynecol Obstet *76*:715–725, 1943
136. Lapidus PW and Guidotti FP: Local injection of hydrocortisone in 495 orthopedic patients. Ind Med Surg *26*:234–244, 1957.
137. Laumann U: Decompression of the subacromial space: An anatomical study. *In* Bayley I and Kellel L (eds): Shoulder Surgery. Berlin: Springer-Verlag, 1982, pp 14–21.
138. Laumann U: Kinesiology of the shoulder joint. *In* Kolbel R, Bodo H, and Blauth W (eds): Shoulder Replacement. New York: Springer-Verlag, 1987.
139. Levitskii FA and Nochevkin VA: Plastic repair of the tendon of the long head of the biceps muscle. Vestn Khir Im I I Grek *130*:92–94, 1983.
140. Lippmann RK: Frozen shoulder, periarthritis, bicipital tenosynovitis. Arch Surg *47*:283–296, 1943.
141. Lippmann RK: Bicipital tenosynovitis. N Y State J Med *44*:2235–2240, 1944.
142. Lloyd-Roberts GC: Humerus varus. Report of a case treated by excision of the acromion. J Bone Joint Surg *35B*:268–269, 1953.
143. Logal R: Rupture of the long tendon of the biceps brachii muscle. Clin Orthop 2:217–221, 1976.
144. Loyd JA and Loyd HA: Adhesive capsulitis of the shoulder: Arthrographic diagnosis and treatment. South Med J *76*:879–883, 1983.
145. Lucas LS and Gill JH: Humerus varus following birth injury to the proximal humeral epiphysis. J Bone Joint Surg *29*:367–369, 1947.
146. Lucas DB: Biomechanics of the shoulder joint. Arch Surg *107*:425–432, 1973.
147. Ludington NA: Am J Surg *77*:358, 1923.
148. Lundberg BJ and Nilsson BE: Osteopenia in the frozen shoulder. Clin Orthop *60*:187–191, 1968.
149. Lundberg BJ: The frozen shoulder. Acta Orthop Scand *119*:1–59, 1969.
150. Lundberg BJ: The frozen shoulder: Clinical and radiographical observations, the effect of manipulation under general anesthesia, structure and glycosaminoglycans content of the joint capsule. Local bone metabolism. Acta Orthop Scand *119*:1–49, 1969.
151. Lundberg BJ: Glycosaminoglycans of the normal and frozen shoulder joint capsule. Clin Orthop *69*:279–284, 1970.
152. Macnab I: Rotator cuff tendinitis. Ann R Coll Surg Engl *53*:271–287, 1973.
153. Makin M: Translocation of the biceps humeri for flail shoulder. J Bone Joint Surg *59*:490 491, 1977.
154. Mariani EM and Cofield RA: The Tendon of the Long Head of the Biceps Brachii: Instability, Tendinitis and Rupture. Advances in Orthopaedic Surgery. Baltimore: Williams & Wilkins, 1988, pp 262–268.
155. Matsen F and Kirby R: Office evaluation and management of shoulder pain. Orthop Clin North Am *13*:45, 1982.
156. McClellan: Textbook of Surgery, 1892.
157. McCue FC III, Zarins B, Andrews JR, and Carson WG: Throwing injuries to the shoulder. *In* Zarins B, Andrews JR, and Carson WG (eds): Injuries to the Throwing Arm. Philadelphia: WB Saunders, 1985, p 98.
158. McGough R, Debski RE, Taskiran E, et al: Tensile Properties of the Long Head of the Biceps Tendon. Presented at American Shoulder and Elbow Surgeons Closed Meeting, 1995.
159. McLaughlin HL: Lesions of musculotendinous cuff of shoulder; observations on pathology, course and treatment of calcific deposits. Ann Surg 124:354, 1946.
160. McLaughlin HL: Dislocation of the shoulder with tuberosity fracture. Surg Clin North Am *43*:1615–1620, 1963.
161. Meagher DM, Pool R, and Brown M: Bilateral ossification of the tendon of the biceps brachii muscle in the horse. J Am Vet Med Assoc *174*:283–285, 1979.
162. Mercer A: Partial dislocations: Consecutive and muscular affections of the shoulder joint. Buffalo Med Surg J *4*:645–652, 1859.
163. Meyer AW: Spolia anatomica. Absence of the tendon of the long head of the biceps. J Anat *48*:133–135, 1913–1914.
164. Meyer AW: Anatomical specimens of the unusual clinical interest. II. The effect of arthritis deformans on the tendon of the long head of the biceps brachii. Am J Orthop Surg *13*:86–95, 1915.
165. Meyer AW: Unrecognized occupation destruction of the tendon of the long head of the biceps brachii. Arch Surg 2:130–144, 1921.
166. Meyer AW: Further observations upon use destruction in joints. J Bone Joint Surg *4*:491–511, 1922.
167. Meyer AW: Further evidences of attrition in the human body. Am J Anat *34*:241–267, 1924.
168. Meyer AW: Spontaneous dislocation of the tendon of the long head of the biceps brachii. Arch Surg *13*:109–119, 1926.
169. Meyer AW: Spontaneous dislocation and destruction of the tendon of the long head of the biceps brachii. Arch Surg *17*:493–506, 1928.
170. Meyer AW: Chronic functional lesions of the shoulder. Arch Surg *35*:646–674, 1937.
171. Michele AA: Bicipital tenosynovitis. Clin Orthop *18*:261, 1960.
172. Middleton WD, Remus WR, Totty WG, et al: Ultrasonographic evaluation of the rotator cuff and biceps tendon. J Bone Joint Surg *68*:440–450, 1986.
173. Middleton WD, et al: High resolution MR imaging of the normal rotator cuff. AJR Am J Roentgenol *148*:559–564, 1987.
174. Milgram JE: Pathology and Treatment of Calcific Tendinitis and Bursitis of the Shoulder. Scientific exhibit, American Academy of Orthopaedic Surgery, 1939 meeting.
175. Milgram JE: Bursitis—pathology and treatment of calcific tendinitis and bursitis by aspiration and vascularization. Med Rev Mex *125*:283–305, 1945.
176. Milgram JE: Shoulder anatomy. Instructional Courses Volume. American Academy of Orthopedic Surgeons, Chicago, January 1946, pp 55–68.
177. Milgram JE: Aspiration of bursal deposits (quoted by Crowe, Harold). Bull Am Acad Orthop Surg p 11, April 1963.
178. Minami M, Ishii S, Usui M, and Ogino T: A case of idiopathic humerus varus. J Orthop Trauma Surg *20*:175–178, 1975.
179. Monteggia GB: Instituzioni Chirurgiche. Milan: G. Truffi, T.V., 1829–1830, p 179; also Part II, 1803, p 334.
180. Monu JUV, Pope TL Jr, Chabon SJ, and Vanarthos WJ: MR diagnosis of superior labral anterior posterior (SLAP) injuries of the glenoid labrum: Value of routine imaging without intra-articular injection of contrast material. Am J Roentgenol *163*:1425–1429, 1994.
181. Moseley HF: Rupture of supraspinatus tendon. Can Med Assoc J *41*:280–282, 1939.
182. Moseley HF: Shoulder Lesions. Springfield, IL: Charles C Thomas, 1945, pp 58–65.
183. Moseley HF and Overgaard B: The anterior capsular mechanism in recurrent anterior dislocation of the shoulder: Morphological and clinical studies with special reference to the glenoid labrum and the glenohumeral ligaments. J Bone Joint Surg *44B*:913–927, 1962.
184. Moseley HF and Goldie I: The arterial pattern of the rotator cuff of the shoulder. J Bone Joint Surg *45B*:780–789, 1963.
185. Muller TH and Gohlke F: Synovial Chondromatosis of the Biceps Tendon. Presented at 6th International Congress on Surgery of the Shoulder, Helsinki, Finland and Stockholm, Sweden, June 27–July 4, 1995.
186. Neer CS II: Anterior acromioplasty for the chronic impingement syndrome in the shoulder. J Bone Joint Surg *54A*:41–50, 1972.
187. Neer CS and Marberry TA: On the disadvantages of radical acromionectomy. J Bone Joint Surg *63A*:416–419, 1981.
188. Neer CS II: Impingement lesions. Clin Orthop *173*:70–77, 1983.
189. Neer CS II and Poppen NK: Supraspinatus outlet. Orthop Trans J Bone Joint Surg *11*:234, 1987.

190. Neer CS: Less frequent procedures. *In* Neer CS II (ed): Shoulder Reconstruction. Philadelphia: WB Saunders, 1990, pp 426–427.
191. Neviaser JS: Adhesive capsulitis of the shoulder. A study of the pathological findings in periarthritis of the shoulder. J Bone Joint Surg 27:211–222, 1945.
192. Neviaser JS: Surgical approaches to the shoulder. Clin Orthop *91*:34, 1973.
193. Neviaser JS: Arthrography of the Shoulder. Springfield, IL: Charles C Thomas, 1975.
194. Neviaser JS, Neviaser RJ, and Neviaser TJ: The repair of chronic massive ruptures of the rotator cuff of the shoulder by use of a freeze-dried rotator cuff. J Bone Joint Surg *60A*:681, 1978.
195. Neviaser RJ: Lesions of the biceps and tendinitis of the shoulder. Orthop Clin North Am *11*:343–348, 1980.
196. Neviaser RJ and Nevaiser TJ: Lesions of the musculotendinous cuff of the shoulder: Diagnosis and management. In AAOS Instructional Course Lecture. St. Louis: CV Mosby, 1981, Vol 30, pp 239–257.
197. Neviaser TJ and Neviaser RJ: Lesions of the long head of the biceps tendon. Instr Course Lect *30*:250–257, 1981.
198. Neviaser TJ, Neviaser RJ, and Neviaser JS: The four in one arthroplasty for the painful arc syndrome. Clin Orthop *163*:107, 1982.
199. Nove-Josserand L: Subluxation et Luxation du Tendon du Long Biceps. Lyons, France: Journées Lyonnaise de l'Epaule, 1993.
200. O'Brien SJ, Arnoczky SP, Warren REF, and Rozbruch RS: Developmental anatomy of the shoulder and anatomy of the glenohumeral joint. *In* Rockwood CA and Matsen FA III (eds): The Shoulder, Vol 1. Philadelphia: WB Saunders, 1990.
201. O'Donohue D: Subluxating biceps tendon in the athlete. Clin Orthop *164*:26, 1982.
202. Ogilvie-Harris DJ and Wiley AM: Arthroscopic surgery of the shoulder: A general appraisal. J Bone Joint Surg *68B*:201–207, 1986.
203. Ozaki J: Repair of chronic massive rotator cuff tears with Teflon felt. *In* Burkhead WZ Jr (ed): Rotator Cuff Disorders. Media, PA: Williams & Wilkins, 1996, p 385.
204. Ozaki J: Personal communication, 1996.
205. Paavolainen P, Bjorkenheim JM, Slatis P, and Paukku P: Operative treatment of severe proximal humeral fractures. Acta Orthop Scand *54*:374–379, 1983.
206. Paavolainen P, Slatis P, and Aalto K: Surgical pathology in chronic shoulder pain. *In* Bateman JE and Welsh RP (eds): Surgery of the Shoulder. Philadelphia: BC Decker, 1984.
207. Packer NP, Calvert PT, Bayley JIL, and Kessel L: Operative treatment of chronic ruptures of the rotator cuff of the shoulder. J Bone Joint Surg *65B*:171–175, 1983.
208. Painter CF: Subdeltoid bursitis. Boston Med Surg J *156*:345–349, 1907.
209. Pal GP, Bhatt RH, and Patel VS: Relationship between the tendon of the long head of biceps brachii and the glenoid labrum in humans. Anat Rec *229*:278–280, 1991.
210. Pappas AM, Goss TP, and Kleinman PK: Symptomatic shoulder instability due to lesions of the glenoid labrum. Am J Sports Med *11*:279–288, 1983.
211. Parkhill CS: Dislocation of the long head of the biceps. Int J Surg *10*:132, 1897.
212. Partridge R: The case of Mr. John Soden. Communication to the Royal and Chirurgical Society of London, July 6, 1841.
213. Pasteur F: Les algies de l'épaule et la physiotherapie. La tenobursite bicipitale. J Radiol Electrol *16*:419–429, 1932.
214. Perry J: Muscle control of the shoulder. *In* Rowe C (ed): The Shoulder. New York: Churchill Livingstone, 1988, p 26.
215. Petersson CJ: Degeneration of the gleno-humeral joint: An anatomical study. Acta Orthop Scand *54*:277–283, 1983.
216. Petersson CJ: Spontaneous medial dislocation of the tendon of the long biceps brachii. Clin Orthop *211*:224–227, 1986.
217. Petri M, Dobrow R, Neiman R, et al: Randomized, double-blind, placebo-controlled study of the treatment of the painful shoulder. Arthritis Rheum *30*:1040–1045, 1987.
218. Phillips BB, Canale ST, Sisk TD, et al: Ruptures of the proximal biceps tendon in middle-aged patients. Orthop Rev 22:349–353, 1993.
219. Pinzur M and Hopkins G: Biceps tenodesis for painful inferior subluxation of the shoulder in adult acquired hemiplegia. Clin Orthop *206*:100–103, 1986.
220. Post M, Silver R, and Singh M: Rotator cuff tear: Diagnosis and treatment. Clin Orthop *173*:78–91, 1983.
221. Post M: Primary Tendinitis of the Long Head of the Biceps. Paper presented at the Closed Meeting of the Society of American Shoulder and Elbow Surgeons, Orlando, Florida, 1987.
222. Postacchini F and Ricciardi-Pollini T: Rupture of the short head tendon of the biceps brachii. Clin Orthop *124*:229–232, 1977.
223. Postacchini F: Rupture of the rotator cuff of the shoulder associated with rupture of the tendon of the long head of the biceps. Ital J Orthop Traumatol *12*:137–149, 1986.
224. Postgate J: Displacement of long tendon of biceps. Med Times (London) n.s. III: 615, 1851.
225. Pouteau C: Melanges de Chirurgie. Lyons: G. Regnault, 1760, p 433.
226. Quinn CE: Humeral scapular periarthritis. Observations on the effects of x-ray therapy and ultrasound therapy in cases of "frozen shoulder." Ann Phys Med *10*:64–69, 1967.
227. Rathbun JB and Macnab I: The microvascular pattern of the rotator cuff. J Bone Joint Surg *52B*:540–553, 1970.
228. Refior HJ and Sowa D: Long tendon of the biceps brachii: Sites of predilection for degenerative lesions. J Shoulder Elbow Surg *4*:436–440, 1995.
229. Resnick D: Shoulder arthrography. Radiol Clin North Am *19*:243–253, 1981.
230. Resnick D and Niwayama G: The shoulder. *In* Resnick D and Niwayana G (eds): Diagnosis of Bone and Joint Disorders, 2nd ed. Philadelphia: WB Saunders, 1988, pp 1733–1764.
231. Rockwood C, Burkhead W, and Brna J: Anterior acromial morphology in relation to the caudal tilt radiograph (unpublished).
232. Rothman RH and Parke WW: The vascular anatomy of the rotator cuff. Clin Orthop *41*:176–182, 1965.
233. Rowe CR (ed): The Shoulder. New York: Churchill Livingstone, 1988, p 145.
234. Schrager VL: Tenosynovitis of the long head of the biceps humeri. Surg Gynecol Obstet *66*:785–790, 1938.
235. Schutte JP and Hawkins RJ: Advances in shoulder surgery. Orthopedics *10*:1725–1728, 1987.
236. Seeger LL, Ruszkowski JT, and Bassett LW, et al: MR imaging of the normal shoulder: Anatomic correlation. AJR Am J Roentgenol *148*:83–91, 1987.
237. Sheldon PJH: A retrospective survey of 102 cases of shoulder pain. Rheum Phys Med *11*:422–427, 1972.
238. Simmonds FA: Shoulder pain: With particular reference to the "frozen" shoulder. J Bone Joint Surg *31B*:426–432, 1949.
239. Simon WH: Soft tissue disorders of the shoulder: Frozen shoulder, calcific tendinitis, and bicipital tendinitis. Orthop Clin North Am *6*:521–538, 1975.
240. Slatis P and Aalto K: Medical dislocation of the tendon of the long head of the biceps brachii. Acta Orthop Scand *50*:73–77, 1979.
241. Snyder SJ, Karzel RP, Del Pizzo W, et al: SLAP lesions of the shoulder. Arthroscopy *6*:274–279, 1990.
242. Snyder SJ: Repair of Type II SLAP Lesion Using Suture Anchors and Permanent Mattress Sutures. Ninth Annual San Diego Shoulder Meeting, San Diego, CA, 1992.
243. Soden J: Two cases of dislocation of the tendon of the long head of the biceps. Med Chir *24*:212, 1841.
244. Soto-Hall R and Haldeman KO: Muscles and tendon injuries in the shoulder region. Calif Western Med *41*:318–321, 1934.
245. Stanley E: Observations relative to the rupture of the tendon of the biceps at its attachment to the edge of the glenoid cavity. Med Gaz 3:12–14, 1828–1829.
246. Stanley E: Rupture of the tendon of the biceps at its attachment to the edge of the glenoid cavity. Med Gaz *3*:12, 1829.
247. Steindler A: Interpretation of pain in the shoulder. AAOS Instructional Course Lecture. Ann Arbor: JW Edwards, 1958, p 159.
248. Stevens HH: The action of short rotators on normal abduction of arm, with a consideration of their action on some cases of subacromial bursitis and allied conditions. Am J Med *138*:870, 1909.
249. Takenaka R, Fukatsu A, Matsuo S, et al: Surgical treatment of hemodialysis-related shoulder arthropathy. Clin Nephrol *38*:224–230, 1992.
250. Tarsy JM: Bicipital syndromes and their treatment. N Y State J Med *46*:996–1001, 1946.
251. Ting A, Jobe FW, Barto P, et al: An EMG Analysis of the Lateral Biceps in Shoulders with Rotator Cuff Tears. Third Open Meeting

of the Society of American Shoulder and Elbow Surgeons, California, 1987.
252. Treves F: Surgical Applied Anatomy. Philadelphia: HC Lea, 1883.
253. Tuckman GA: Abnormalities of the long head of the biceps tendon of the shoulder: MR imaging findings. Am J Radiol *163*:1183–1188, 1994.
254. Valtonen EJ: Subacromial triamcinolone, mexacetonide and methylprednisolone injections in treatment of supraspinatus tendinitis: A comparative trial. Scand J Rheumatol (Suppl) *16*:1–13, 1976.
255. Valtonen EJ: Double acting betamethasone (celestone chronodose) in the treatment of supraspinatus tendinitis: A comparison of subacromial and gluteal single injections with placebo. J Intern Med Res *6*:463–467, 1978.
256. Vangsness CT Jr, Jorgenson SS, Watson T, and Johnson DL: The origin of the long head of the biceps from the scapula and glenoid labrum. J Bone Joint Surg *76B*:951–954, 1994.
257. van Leersum M and Schweitzer ME: Magnetic resonance imaging of the biceps complex. MRI Clin North Am *1*:77–86, 1993.
258. Veisman IA: Radiodiagnosis of subcutaneous ruptures of the biceps tendons. Ortop Traumatol Protez *31*:25–29, 1970.
259. Verbrugge J, Claessens H, and Maex L: L'arthrographie de l'épaule. Acta Orthop Belg 3–4:280, 1956.
260. Vettivel S, Indrasingh I, Chandi G, and Chandi SM: Variations in the intertubercular sulcus of the humerus related to handedness. J Anat *180*:321–326, 1992.
261. Vigerio GD and Keats TE: Localization of calcific deposits in the shoulder. AJR Am J Roentgenol *108*:806–811, 1970.
262. Volkmann R: Luxationen der Muskeln und Sehnen. Billroth Pitha's Handb Allgemeinen Speciellen Chir 2:873, 1882.
263. Walch G: La Pathologie de la Longue Portion du Biceps. Conference d'Enseignement de la SOFCOT, Paris, 1993.
264. Walch G: Synthèse sur l'Epidémiologie et l'Ethiologie des Ruptures de la Coiffe des Rotateurs. Lyons, France: Journées Lyonnaise de l'Epaule, 1993.
265. Walch G: Posterosuperior glenoid impingement. *In* Burkhead WZ Jr (ed): Rotator Cuff Disorders. Media, PA: Williams & Wilkins, 1996, pp 193–198.
266. Warren RF: Lesions of the long head of the biceps tendon. AAOS Instr Course Lect *34*:204–209, 1985.
267. Warren RF, Dines DM, Inglis AE, and Pavlos H: The Coracoid Impingement Syndrome. Read at Second Meeting of the Society of American Shoulder and Elbow Surgeons, American Academy of Orthopaedic Surgery, New Orleans, February 19–20, 1986.
268. White JW: A case of supposed dislocation of the tendon of the long head of the biceps muscle. Am J Med Soc *87*:17–57, 1884.
269. White RH, Paull DM, and Fleming KW: Rotator cuff tendinitis: Comparison of subacromial injection of a long acting corticosteroid versus oral indomethacin therapy. J Rheumatol *13*:608–613, 1986.
270. Wiley AM and Older MW: Shoulder arthroscopy: Investigations with a fiberoptic instrument. Am J Sports Med *8*:31–38, 1980.
271. Winterstein O: On the periarthritis humero-scapularis and on the rupture of the long biceps tendon. Arch Orthop Unfallchir *63*:19–22, 1968.
272. Withrington RH, Girgis FL, and Seifert MH: A placebo-controlled trial of steroid injections in the treatment of supraspinatus tendinitis. Scand J Rheumatol *14*:76–78, 1985.
273. Wolfgang GL: Surgical repair of tears of the rotator cuff of the shoulder. J Bone Joint Surg *56A*:14–26, 1974.
274. Yamaguchi K, Riew KD, Galatz LM, et al: Biceps function in normal and rotator cuff deficient shoulders: An electromyographic analysis. Orthop Trans *18*:191, 1994.
275. Yergason RM: Rupture of biceps. J Bone Joint Surg *13*:160, 1931.

CHAPTER

20

DOUGLAS T. HARRYMAN II, M.D.
MARK D. LAZARUS, M.D.
RICHARD ROZENCWAIG, M.D.

The Stiff Shoulder

In order to attain the complete range of shoulder motion, four articulations and two bursal-lined interfaces of the shoulder girdle must have stable alignment, have smooth articular and motion plane surfaces, and must be free from contractures in the tissues about the joint. The musculotendinous units that interconnect the bones and joints of the shoulder girdle must retain flexibility and freedom of excursion to fully mobilize the extremity through its entire arc of motion. When joint surfaces are normal, are stably aligned, and have no skeletal block, a restriction in range is classified as *stiffness*. Stiffness may result from pathologic connections between motion interfaces, a contracture of the retaining soft tissue surrounding the articulations, or a shortened muscle-tendon unit excursion. As we will discuss, these sources of stiffness can occur independently of each other or in combination.

In our lifetime, all of us are likely to experience joint stiffness in response to injury or inflammation. Healing repairs our tissues and creates a stiffer construct which, over time, may relax with remodeling. Eventually, secondary to the natural aging process, we all become affected by stiffness as we lose our ability to gracefully jump, youthfully skip, or walk with a bounce.

How do we naturally prevent stiffness? Stretching our shoulders is as routine as rising in the morning and reaching for the heavens! Furthermore, as every aging athlete recognizes, mechanical traction on collagenous tissue increases and maintains flexibility and healthy joint motion. In contrast, disuse and immobilization allow an opportunity to develop ligamentous and musculotendinous contractures, adhesions between motion interfaces, and oxidative collagenous covalent cross-linked bonds.[79, 266] If disuse and immobilization are prolonged, tissue viscoelasticity may become lost, resulting in permanent motion restrictions that impair the function of the extremities. Prevention is the best way to resist *stiffness*, and *stretching* is our natural defense mechanism.

Not all motion restrictions about the shoulder are painful. They are poorly tolerated, however, when limitations interfere with athletics, daily activities, and hygiene.[22] When a person with shoulder stiffness presents to a practitioner, the challenge remains to determine the pathophysiology of the stiffness and, more important, the remedy. What structure will no longer glide or lengthen? Answering this question yields a method that we find useful in diagnosing, treating, and studying stiff shoulders.

CLASSIFICATION OF SHOULDER STIFFNESS

In 1923, Jones and Lovett, based on clinical examination, distinguished two principal types of shoulder stiffness.[144] In the latter half of the 20th century, five different investigators proposed a dichotomous nomenclature to separate clinical shoulder stiffness, each according to his or her own diagnostic criteria.[146, 168, 198, 241, 311] The two main clinical themes lending themselves to subgroup typing were the severity of stiffness and the presence or absence of an associated etiology. In their classification scheme, Reeves and Neviaser relied primarily on arthrographic criteria[198, 241]; Kay and Withers primarily divided stiffness according to the severity of restricted motion; and Lundberg sought the etiology.[146, 168, 311]

A loosely woven common thread among these classifications is the presence or absence of trauma. Reeves used the subgrouping "idiopathic frozen shoulder" and the "post-traumatic stiff shoulder" and related his arthrographic findings with the clinical descriptions provided by Jones and Lovett.[144, 241] Lundberg defined primary and secondary frozen shoulders as those in which there was no significant historical event contrasted with a history of trauma.[168] As Reeves and Matsen and associates have indicated, these categories of shoulder stiffness clearly present independent historical and clinical examination findings.[178, 241] Unfortunately, we typically find studies that group all shoulder stiffness together for an evaluation of a treatment regimen. Categorizing shoulder stiffness in this manner, therefore, is of great use in deciding a course of treatment. Studies on stiff shoulders that do not differentiate these types should, therefore, be read skeptically.

Definition of Shoulder Stiffness

In the late 18th century, Duplay in France and, soon after, Putnam in North America, described "scapulohumeral periarthritis," which encompassed a broad spectrum of pathologic conditions causing similar symptoms of painful shoulder stiffness and dysfunction.[75, 234] Rotator cuff tendinitis and tears, biceps tendinitis or tear, calcific deposits, acromioclavicular arthritis, and other painful conditions causing shoulder stiffness and dysfunction were often combined together under the term "periarthritis." Unfortunately, the term "periarthritis" is still in common usage today and has become synonymous with a wide range of affections of the shoulder.[10, 32, 52, 69, 106, 110, 145, 156, 237, 243, 315–317] Because of the lack of specific diagnostic criteria and persistent confusion surrounding the use of the term "periarthritis," some have recommended dropping the term.[243]

In 1934, Codman recognized a pattern of muscle spasm and glenohumeral stiffness and coined the term "frozen shoulder."[55] He said this entity was "difficult to define, difficult to treat and difficult to explain from the point of view of pathology."[55] He also "presumed" that the symptoms were related to tendinitis of the rotator cuff. Although this term fails to describe the pathologic process, it does provide a great description of the clinical picture. Like "periarthritis," Codman's "frozen shoulder" terminology is also a general descriptive term referring to shoulders that are stiff and painful.[50, 188, 213, 321] Authors continue to plead for an improved and more specific nomenclature to distinguish conditions of shoulder stiffness.[43, 44, 196, 203]

Zuckerman polled members of the American Shoulder and Elbow Society (ASES) to ensure the best consensus on the definition of frozen shoulder syndrome, after having defined it summarily as "a condition of uncertain etiology characterized by significant restriction of both active and passive shoulder motion that occurs in the absence of a known intrinsic shoulder disorder." The definition was accepted by the workshop committee at the 1992 symposia, "The Shoulder: A Balance of Mobility and Stability" and published by the American Academy of Orthopaedic Surgeons (AAOS).[321]

In 1945, Neviaser proposed the term "adhesive capsulitis,"[196] which he believed better described the underlying pathology. Neviaser identified a "chronic inflammatory process involving the capsule of the shoulder causing a thickening and contracture of this structure which secondarily becomes adherent to the humeral head." Today, this term is used synonymously with frozen shoulder even though very few, if any, at open or arthroscopic examination have identified an adherent nature of the capsule to the humeral head (discussed later). Neviaser should be credited with recognizing inflammation, thickening, and contracture of the capsule resulting in *capsular fibrosis*.

Authors' Preferred Classification

Matsen and associates combined Codman's original clinical observation of global motion restriction with today's best understanding of the documented pathophysiology affecting the glenohumeral joint and defined the syndrome as:

> An idiopathic global limitation of humeroscapular motion resulting from contracture and loss of compliance of the glenohumeral joint capsule.[178]

The authors prefer this interpretation while acknowledging that the common denominator between this definition and the one described earlier is that of *global* limitation of shoulder motion. This is a definition of exclusion.[289] Most stiff shoulders present after trauma or in association with a specific disease or with motion restrictions that occur only in particular directions. To avoid the risk of introducing additional divisions for shoulder stiffness, the authors have instead simply assigned stiff shoulders that are not idiopathic frozen shoulders to the "post-traumatic stiff shoulder" category. The authors define this group as:

> A limitation in humeroscapular motion presenting after an injury, low-level repetitive trauma or part of an accompanying condition which results in a contracture of structures participating in the glenohumeral or humeroscapular motion interfaces.

The authors, therefore, classify the stiff and nonarthritic shoulder as either a "frozen shoulder" or "post-traumatic stiff shoulder," a scheme first proposed by Reeves.[178, 241] As we will discuss later, the "post-traumatic" group can be easily subdivided further according to injury, disease process, or postsurgical stiffness. This system also nicely corresponds with the distinction suggested by Lundberg which separates stiffness into "primary" and "secondary" frozen shoulder syndrome.[167] Lundberg's secondary frozen shoulders were defined as those with a known intrinsic or extrinsic precursor typically causative of shoulder pain and dysfunction that leads ultimately to global stiffness.

PATHOPHYSIOLOGY

Investigators have asked, "Why is a frozen shoulder, frozen?"[10, 127] One answered humbly, we "Haven't got a clue!"[43] Although the etiology of stiffness that results in capsular fibrosis remains elusive, our understanding of its pathogenesis is increasing. Recent investigations have focused on the inflammatory cellular morphology and immunologic response, humoral mediators, and immunologic predisposition that provide insight into the pathogenesis of capsular fibrosis. Known immunologic disorders, such as collagen-vascular disease, inflammatory or infectious arthritides, and other common rheumatologic conditions (e.g., crystalline deposition), are generally excluded by appropriate laboratory tests.[128] Many plausible pathogenic mechanisms have been proposed during the last 60 years, yet none of the factors occasionally isolated and associated with the pathogenesis of one or a group of frozen shoulders have been found consistently (Table 20–1).[129]

Early investigators localized the "freezing" of frozen shoulder to the interface of the rotator cuff and subacromial space, hence the term "periarthritis."[55, 75, 76, 234] Little to no basic science supports involvement of this interface in the pathology of the primary frozen shoulder.

Table 20–1 PROPOSED PATHOGENIC MECHANISMS FOR PRIMARY FROZEN SHOULDER*

MECHANISM	DISORDER	PATHOLOGY	ETIOLOGY EXCLUDED BY
Autoimmume	Collagen-vascular disorders	Type IV reaction (to infarcted cuff tendon)	Absence of immune complexes and autoantibodies, no other affected joints
Inflammatory	Infectious arthritis	Viral, bacterial, or fungal infection	Absence of prodromal illness and systemic symptoms
Crystal arthropathy	CPPD disease and gout	Crystal deposition	Absence of recurrences, crystals, and inflammatory phases
Reactive arthropathy	Spondyloarthritides and ankylosing spondylitis	Seronegative arthritis	No systemic manifestations; normal joint fluid, no blood markers
Hemarthrosis	Hemoglobinopathies and trauma	Chemical irritation (hemosiderin)	No capsulitis or fibrositis with hemoglobinopathies
Paralytic	Suprascapular nerve palsy	Compression neuropathy	Absence of EMG or conduction abnormalities
Algodystrophy	Autonomic neuropathy	Neuropathic disturbance and hypervascularity	No sensory or vascular deficiency, stellate ganglion block not helpful
Degenerative	Rotator cuff tendon and degeneration/infarction	Microvascular infarction	Absence of tendon inflammation or infarction
Traumatic	Trauma and immobilization	Injury synovitis and tissue contracture	Brief shoulder stiffness after prolonged casting in the majority
Psychogenic	Hysteria and hypochondriasis	Depression, dependence, and chronic pain disorder	Similar MMPI between patients and controls
Fibrogenic	Cytokine induction of fibroplasia	Tissue contracture in response to cytokines, inflammatory cell products, and platelet-derived growth factor	No exclusion, current theory in text

CPPD, calcium-pyrophosphate disease; EMG, electromyogram; MMPI, Minnesota Multiphasic Personality Inventory.
*From Instr Course Lect *42*:248, 1993.

Riedel was the first to suggest that the basic pathology of shoulder stiffness may be localized to the joint capsule.[249] In the mid-20th century, Neviaser described the surgical, arthrographic, and histologic findings occurring in the synovium and subsynovial capsular regions of patients with painful shoulder stiffness.[196] Neviaser, on biopsy and histologic examination, identified perivascular infiltration, capsular thickening, contracture, and fibrosis.[196] He also identified a normal synovial layer.

Later in the same decade, Simmonds biopsied the hypervascular "tight inelastic tissue" around the joint and identified some focal necrosis that he attributed to tendon degeneration.[276] He postulated that this process led to chronic inflammation, especially around the biceps tendon, contracture, and tears of the rotator cuff.

Lundberg also did not find pathologic changes in the synovial cells lining the joint but identified an increase in the density of the capsular collagen and a pattern of glycosaminoglycan distribution that he likened to a repair reaction.[168] These observations pointed to inflammation of the capsule as an essential precursor of the process leading to stiffness, pain, and capsular fibrosis. McLaughlin, however, noted that in only 10% of his cases an "obvious inflammatory reaction involving the entire synovial lining of the shoulder joint and the biceps tendon sheath" was present and in the "great majority of cases neither clinical nor histologic evidences of inflammation were observed."[180] He concluded that perhaps "acute synovitis represents one phase in the life cycle of this condition."

Macnab studied the association between rotator cuff degeneration and painful stiffness.[171, 172] At open capsular release and biopsy, he identified round and lymphoid cell infiltrates and attributed them to an autoimmune response against degenerative collagen particles from hypovascular supraspinatus tendon.

The synovial or subsynovial inflammatory reaction histologically observed by Neviaser, Lundberg, and McLaughlin could represent a response to injury, an infectious agent, a chemical mediation, or an autoimmune reaction with cellular and humoral components. In an attempt to find immunologic clues, a study of 40 patients with frozen shoulders was undertaken by Bulgen and colleagues. They revealed that pretreatment increased circulating immune complex levels and C-reactive protein and decreased lymphocyte transformation to phytohemagglutinin and concanavalin-A relative to a control group.[39] The implications of these findings were impaired cell-mediated immunity and increased circulating immune complexes associated with an autoimmune process. Repeat testing after time and treatment showed that values tended to approach control levels. Bulgen and associates also determined serum immunoglobulin levels in 25 patients with frozen shoulder and in age- and sex-matched controls.[38, 41] Serum IgA levels were reduced significantly in the patients with a frozen shoulder, and this decrease persisted after clinical recovery. Lymphocyte transformation to phytohemagglutinin in 21 patients also showed significant depression. Despite early findings that indicated the presence of an immunologic basis for the disease, more recent reports have failed to support these findings or identify immunologic tests useful in diagnosis, treatment, or predicting outcome.[318]

Investigation has also centered on identifying a predisposition for stiffness using immunologic cellular markers. Initial research focused on the presence of certain histocompatibility antigens. For instance, the presence of the antigen HLA-B27 was reported as being more common in patients with frozen shoulder (42%) than in the controls (10%).[42] This result, however, was later refuted by the same authors.[41] As with other diseases, identifying a predisposition may be resolved only after genotypic analysis.[1, 292]

An association between a clinically frozen shoulder and Dupuytren's contracture was identified by Meulengracht and Schwartz in 18% of their patients.[182] More recent investigators likened the histologic changes in the glenohumeral capsule to Dupuytren's contracture in the palm and further noted that in the shoulder capsule, the inflammatory component was absent or localized to the synovial and subsynovial layers.[45, 113] Bunker and Anthony performed a manipulation and open excisional biopsy of the coracohumeral ligament and rotator interval capsule of patients who failed to improve with conservative treatment for frozen shoulder.[45] Tissue specimens revealed active fibroblastic proliferation amidst thick nodular bands of collagen accompanied by some transformation to a smooth muscle phenotype (myofibroblasts). These fibroblastic histologic features were very similar to those in Dupuytren's disease of the hand, with no inflammation and no synovial involvement! Fibrotic accumulation is most evident in later phases of the inflammatory response with collagen and matrix synthesis occurring after chemotactic and cellular responses have occurred; these findings, therefore, may reflect only one phase of the disease.[180, 297]

A proliferative pathologic repair by active fibroblasts occurs in response to inflammatory infiltration of connective tissue with mononuclear cells that produce polypeptide growth factors.[297] Rodeo and associates compared capsular tissue samples from patients undergoing arthroscopy who had adhesive capsulitis, nonspecific synovitis, or a normal capsule to determine specific cytokines involved in the inflammatory and fibroblastic response.[255] Their results indicate that cytokines such as transfroming growth factor (TGF)-β and platelet-derived growth factor (PDGF) and hepatocyte growth factor (HGF) are involved in the early inflammatory stages of adhesive capsulitis without relation to primary or secondary causes. PDGF is a mitogenic agent that causes fibroblastic cell proliferation and TGF-β increases extracellular matrix leading to capsular fibrosis.

In a closely related study, Hannafin and colleagues have attempted to correlate three histopathologic phases of fibroplasia found on biopsy of shoulders with adhesive capsulitis with the clinical examination and arthroscopic findings of the capsule. They hypothesized that the hypervascular synovitis provokes a progressive fibroblastic response in the adjacent capsule resulting in diffuse capsular fibroplasia, thickening, and contracture (Fig. 20–1).[113] Based on these immunohistochemical and histologic findings, these investigators have proposed an algorithm of pathology leading to capsular fibrosis (Fig. 20–2). Using this model, they believe investigators are poised to devise agents that may interrupt the cytokinetic connection and cellular mediated response leading to capsular fibroplasia.

NORMAL MOTION AND PATHOMECHANICS OF SHOULDER STIFFNESS

What determines the functional limit of shoulder range?[313] The answer to this question depends on our skeletal morphology, our articular surface area, and the flexibility of connecting capsule, ligaments, musculotendinous units, and integument. If a sphere were mapped about the shoulder to describe its range of motion, we could reach approximately one third of its inner surface with the tip of our elbow using humerothoracic range and one quarter using humeroscapular motion alone (Fig. 20–3). The sum of humerothoracic elevation is achieved from motion at two articulations in a ratio of glenohumeral and scapulothoracic range of approximately 2:1.[94, 139, 232]

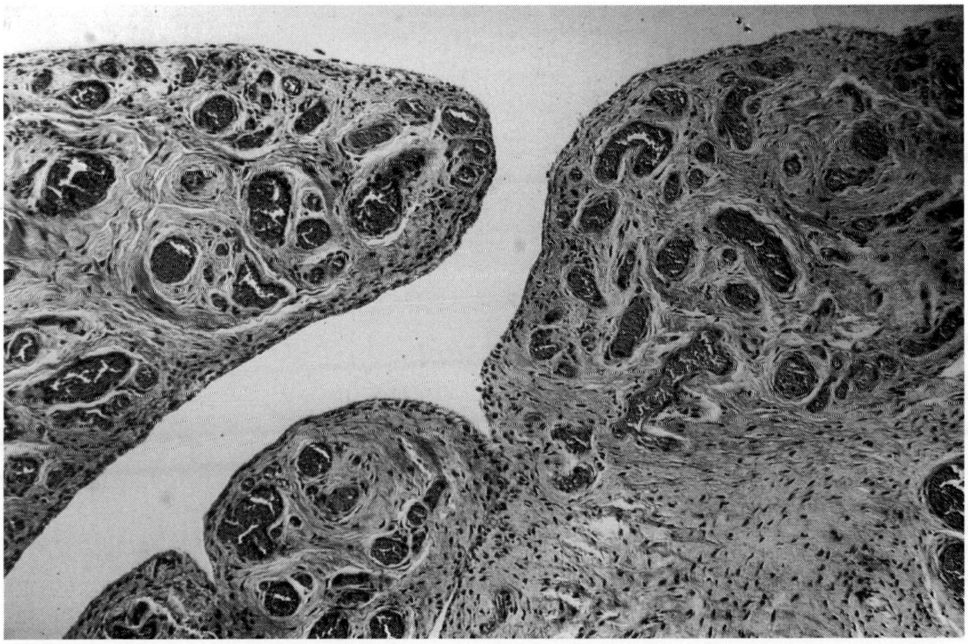

Figure 20–1

This capsular biopsy shows proliferation of synovial cells at the surface with underlying capsular fibroplasia. The capsular matrix is densely collagenous. There is evidence of neovascularization (red-cell–filled capillaries). The magnification of this section is 40×. The tissue was stained with hematoxylin and eosin. (Courtesy of S. Rodeo, M.D.[255])

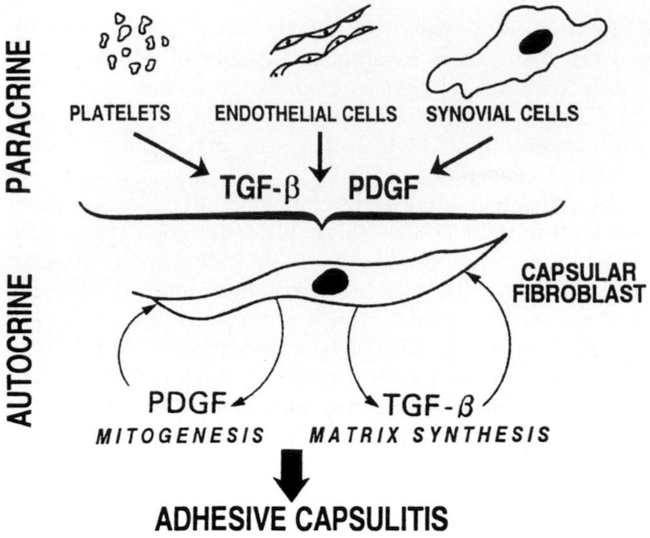

Figure 20–2

A theoretical algorithm leading to fibroplasia.[255] Transforming growth factor (TGF)-β and platelet-derived growth factor (PDGF), produced locally by synovial cells, platelets, and endothelial cells, stimulate capsular fibroblasts as a paracrine mechanism. Production of these cytokines by the capsular fibroblasts, in the setting of upregulation of TGF-β and PDGF receptors on the capsular fibroblasts, suggests that an autocrine mechanism may amplify the paracrine stimulation of these cells. (Courtesy of S. Rodeo, M.D.[255])

Defined further, humerothoracic motion occurs between the articular surfaces of the glenohumeral ball-and-socket joint and two major bursal-lined surfaces defined as the humeroscapular motion interface (HSMI) and the scapulothoracic motion interface (STMI).[178] In a glenohumeral joint with smooth articular surfaces, clinical shoulder stiffness occurs as a result of: (1) contractures shortening the length of the intra-articular capsule, ligaments, or muscle-tendon units; (2) adhesions along gliding surfaces such as the rotator cuff or biceps tendons; and (3) adhesions within the extra-articular humeroscapular or scapulothoracic motion interface.[178] Restrictions of these soft tissues may occur independently or in combination.

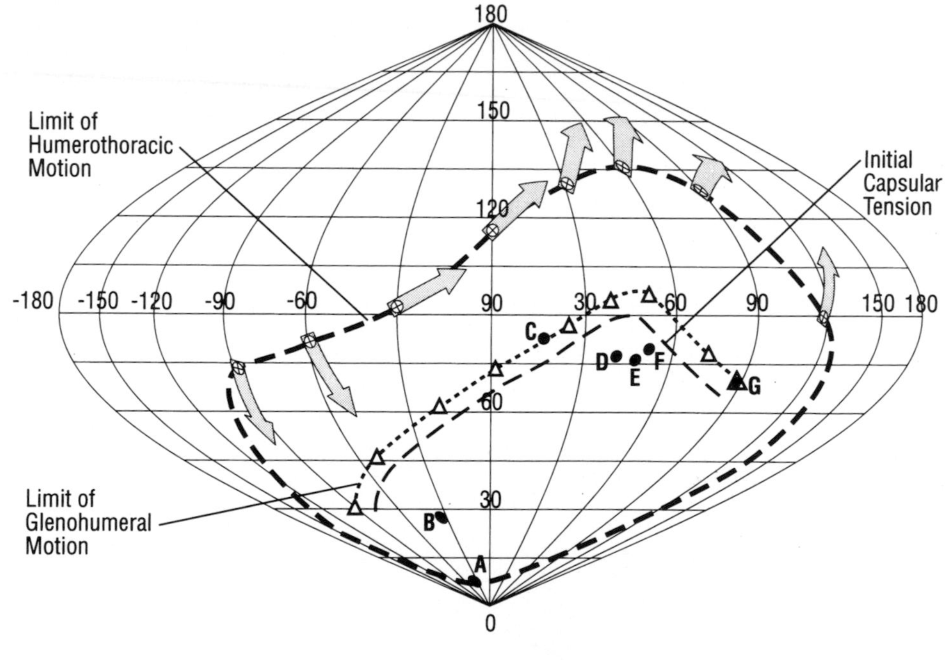

Figure 20–3

Global graphic diagram of shoulder motion. The outer *dashed line* is the limit of humerothoracic motion (in vivo glenohumeral plus scapulothoracic). The *dotted line* is the boundary of glenohumeral motion alone (in vivo after scapulothoracic fusion). The area between the outer *dashed line* and the *dotted line* represents the contribution of scapulothoracic motion. Inside the limit of glenohumeral motion, there is a second *dashed line,* which for lesser elevations without humeral rotation represents glenohumeral positions that do not result in capsular tension.[178, 257] (Modified from Harryman DT II, Lazarus MD, Sidles JA, and Matsen FA III: Pathophysiology of shoulder instability. *In* McGinty JB, Caspari RB, Jackson RW, and Poehling GG [eds]: Operative Arthroscopy, 2nd ed. Philadelphia: Lippincott-Raven, 1996, p 680.)

Points A, B, C, D, E, and F represent glenohumeral positions for routine daily activities.[228] Three of these positions, (C) lifting a gallon overhead, (F) washing the opposite shoulder, and (B) hand behind head (maximal rotation in mid-elevation), are performed at the end-range of glenohumeral motion, otherwise most activities are recorded in the functional midrange.

Point A: scratching the back; point B: tuck in shirt; point C: hand behind the head; point D: lifting a gallon to the top of the head; point E: place a coin on the shelf at shoulder height; point F: hand to mouth; point G: wash the back of the opposite shoulder.

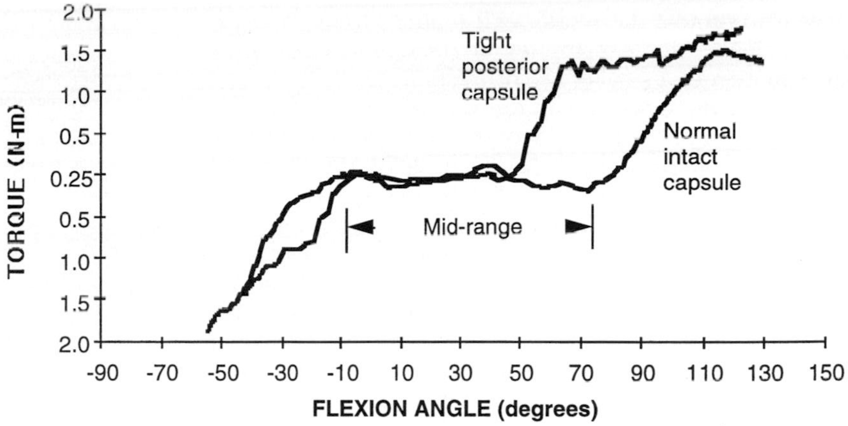

Figure 20–4

In the midrange of glenohumeral motion, the capsule and ligaments are not under tension. As the humerus is elevated (e.g., extreme flexion or extension), the cuff and capsule become tight near the end-range of motion where capsular torsion increases for each incremental degree of elevation. Torsional loads only become increased in the midrange of motion when a portion of the capsule is tight. (Modified from Harryman DT II, Lazarus MD, Sidles JA, and Matsen FA III: Pathophysiology of shoulder instability. *In* McGinty JB, Caspari RB, Jackson RW, and Poehling GG [eds]: Philadelphia: Lippincott-Raven, 1996, p 679.)

Glenohumeral Joint, Capsule, and Ligaments

The glenohumeral articular capsule remains lax while performing motions in the midrange. In cadaveric tests, Harryman and associates measured torsional resistance of the glenohumeral joint with an intact capsule and cuff tendon preparation.[119] In the midrange of glenohumeral motion, the capsular tissue remained essentially free of tension until the terminal degrees of range were approached (Fig. 20–4). The end-range, therefore, was defined by increased tension in the static restraints of the capsule and its ligaments. The majority of motions performed during work and activities of daily living are performed in humeroscapular positions away from the extremes of range (see Fig. 20–3).[123, 227]

Glenohumeral motion is limited by the length of the capsuloligamentous checkreins. In a biomechanical study of eight intact cadaveric shoulders, Romeo and colleagues measured the range of glenohumeral positions in which the capsular structures were "tension free."[257] Tension free was defined in the cadaver as the range of glenohumeral rotation exerting less than 0.5 Newton-meters of humeral torque with an intact capsule (see Fig. 20–3). Complete capsular division circumferentially about the glenoid increased the limits of tension-free elevation and internal and external rotation by a total average arc of only 20 degrees.[257] Nonarticular abutment did not result from increased over-rotation. Only a moderate increase in motion occurred after capsular division, presumably because the excursion of the rotator cuff tendons restrained glenohumeral rotation secondarily (Fig. 20–5).[247,257] Conversely, the capsule and its ligaments would

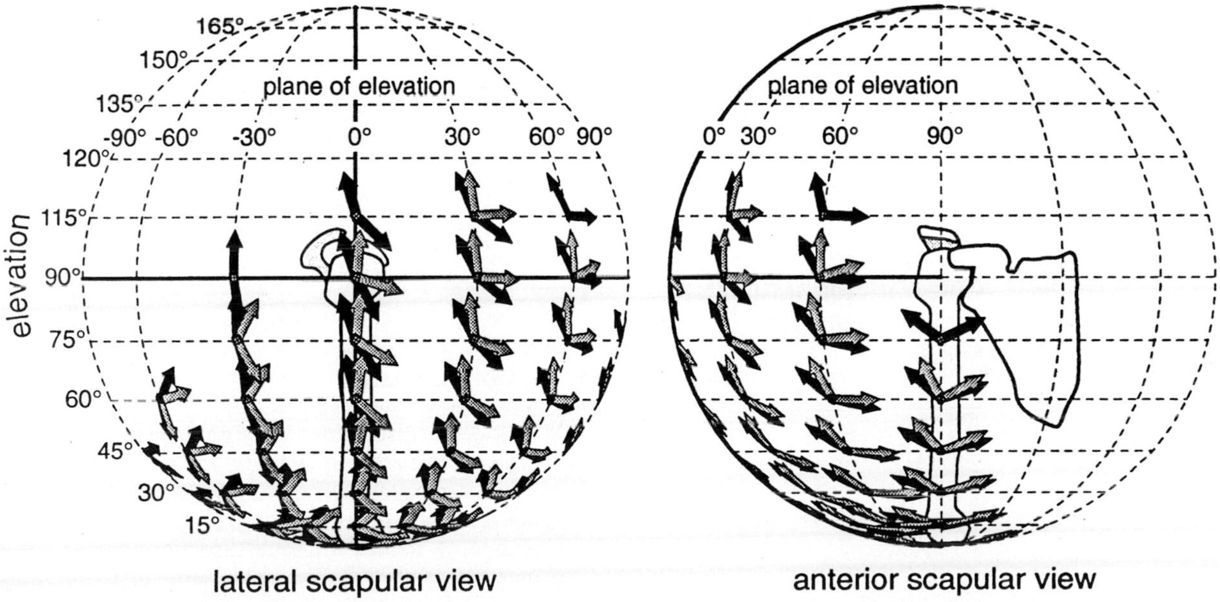

Figure 20–5

Global diagrams graphically summarizing the mean rotational data measured from eight cadaveric shoulders before and after capsular release. An increase in the motions of rotation and elevation before *(gray arrows)* and after *(black arrows)* total capsular release are depicted. Even after capsular release, only an average of approximately 20 degrees of gain in motion occurs, indicating that other soft tissue such as the intact rotator cuff secondarily restrains glenohumeral motion. (From Harryman DT II, Sidles JA, and Matsen FA III: Arthroscopic management of refractory shoulder stiffness. Arthroscopy *13*:133–147, 1997.)

appear to protect the rotator cuff tendons from excessive tensile loads at the extremes of rotation because they limit motion to a smaller arc of rotation.

Asymmetric tightness of the capsule or rotator cuff secondary to a contracture or surgical shortening may cause pathologic obligate translation of the humeral head.[120, 126, 178] Anatomically, the normal glenohumeral joint displays true ball-and-socket mechanics with the humeral head remaining centered within the glenoid fossa throughout its range.[98, 121, 232] In the cadaver, however, when the posterior capsule was surgically tightened, forward flexion caused consistent anterosuperior translation of the humeral head.[119] A posterior capsular contracture, therefore, may cause significant "impingement" with compression of the rotator cuff against the coracoacromial arch (Fig. 20–6). Clinically, a similar pathomechanical phenomenon (also called "capsular constraint") can also occur in shoulders after excessively tight anterior instability repairs (Fig. 20–7). Chronic asymmetric tightness can result in greater joint reaction forces directed to the opposite side of the glenoid and can cause excessive wear, posterior erosion, and osteoarthrosis.[126] Matsen has called this pathologic process capsulorrhaphy arthropathy.[178]

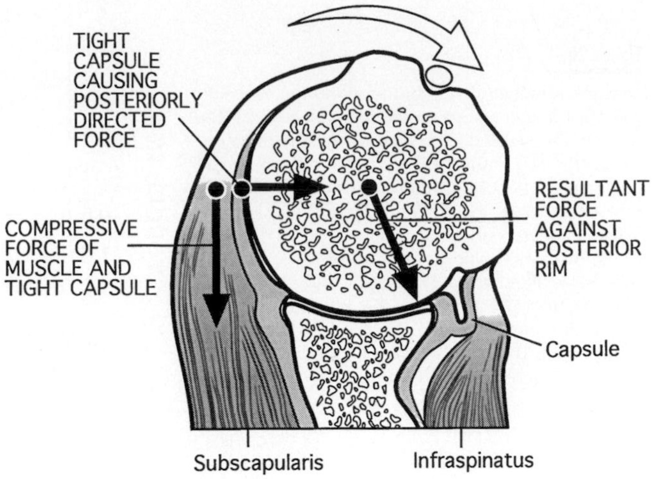

Figure 20–7

Rotation of the humeral head is associated with capsular tightening at the end-range of motion. The asymmetrically tight capsule opposes a load or displacement directed toward itself and attempts to translate the humeral head towards the opposite side of the glenoid. This stabilizing force is referred to as the "capsular constraint mechanism." The tense capsule also applies a load to compress the humeral head into the glenoid fossa. The resultant force vector is directed against the opposite side of the glenoid. (From Harryman DT II, Lazarus MD, Sidles JA, and Matsen FA III: Pathophysiology of shoulder instability. *In* McGinty JB, Caspari RB, Jackson RW, and Poehling GG [eds]: Operative Arthroscopy, 2nd ed. Philadelphia: Lippincott-Raven, 1996, p 686.)

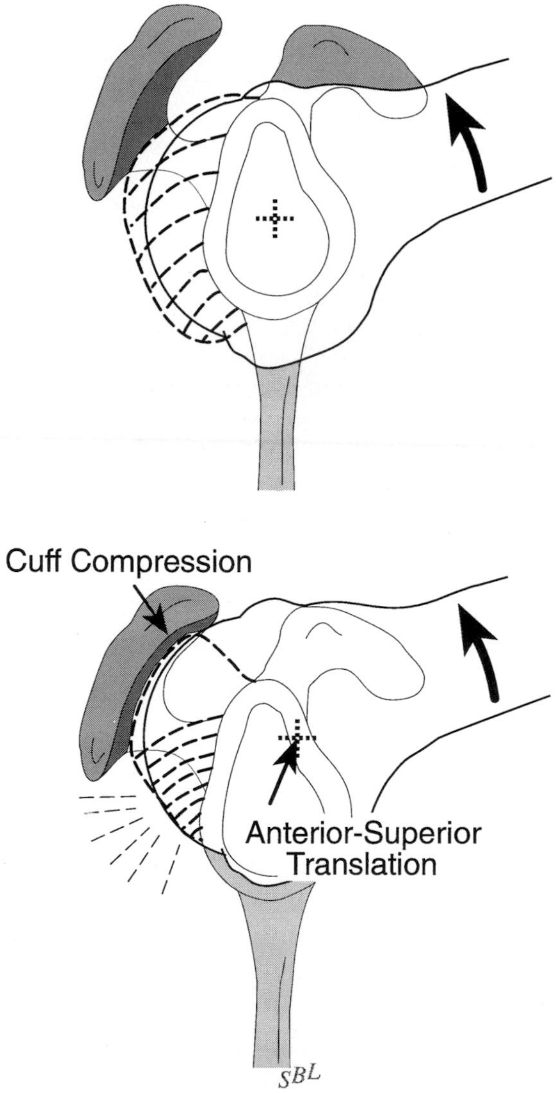

Figure 20–6

Tightness of the posterior capsular causes anterosuperior translation of the humeral head. The rotator cuff becomes entrapped between the humeral head and the coracoacromial arch. A posterior capsular contracture, therefore, may initiate or potentiate subacromial compression and abrasion of the rotator cuff. (Modified from Matsen FA III, Lippitt SB, Sidles JA, and Harryman DT II: Practical Evaluation of Management of the Shoulder. Philadelphia: WB Saunders, 1994, pp 19–109.)

A contracted capsule reduces the humeral head rotational motion.[119] In a cadaveric study, eight shoulders underwent posterior capsular plication. The ranges of forward elevation, internal rotation, and horizontal adduction became limited. The motions of external rotation with and without elevation, abduction, and adduction remained unaffected. Furthermore, tightening of the capsule increased the torque necessary to achieve an elevated position (see Fig. 20–4).[119] Releasing the tight capsule would be predicted to relieve this condition. The concept of releasing localized or generalized capsular contractures to increase range is not new and has been used clinically at open surgery for decades.[151, 178, 180, 190, 194, 207, 208]

A released capsule increases joint laxity, but increased laxity does not lead to instability. In the cadaver shoulder, Rhee and colleagues revealed increased anterior, posterior, and inferior translational laxity of the humeral head an average of 15 mm in each direction after a complete capsular release.[178, 247, 257] Clinical and experimental data have shown that releasing or surgically tightening the rotator interval capsule increases and decreases the posterior and inferior translational laxity, respectively (Fig. 20–8).[120, 207, 299] Lippitt and associates have shown that the humeral head, which is stabilized within the glenoid concavity by compressive loads and resistance to a displacing

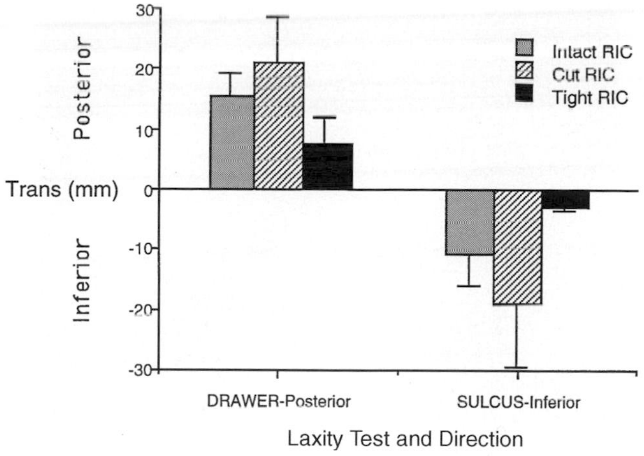

Figure 20–8

A tight rotator interval capsule (RIC) restricts normal joint laxity. Release of the RIC will increase translation and range in tight shoulders (see text). (From Harryman DT II, Lazarus MD, Sidles JA, and Matsen FA III: Pathophysiology of shoulder instability. *In* McGinty JB, Caspari RB, Jackson RW, and Poehling GG [eds]: Operative Arthroscopy, 2nd ed. Philadelphia: Lippincott-Raven, 1996, p 687.)

force, is augmented by increased depth and the presence of the labrum.[164, 178] Speer and associates and Harryman and co-workers have shown that detaching the labrum and capsular ligaments from the glenoid increased laxity but was inadequate to produce glenohumeral instability.[117, 280] Releasing the capsule and its ligaments in vivo, therefore, should increase laxity but not lead to instability.[118]

Specific regions of the glenohumeral joint capsule and their identified ligaments are responsible for limiting end-range rotations (Table 20–2). Early investigators found that the anterior capsular ligaments became taught at maximum external rotation.[286, 294] The anterosuperior capsule in the rotator interval that contains the coracohumeral ligament (CHL) and superior glenohumeral ligament (SGHL) assumes tension with humeral external rotation in the unelevated extremity.[91, 120, 299] The middle glenohumeral ligament (MGHL) and anterosuperior band

Table 20–2 CAPSULE AND LIGAMENTS LIMITING GLENOHUMERAL MOTIONS

CAPSULE AND LIGAMENTS	*GLENOHUMERAL MOTIONS*
Rotator interval capsule (RIC) Coracohumeral ligament (CHL) Superior glenohumeral ligament (SGHL)	Flexion, extension, adduction at low elevation, external rotation at low elevation
Middle glenohumeral ligament (MGHL)	External rotation at mid elevation
Inferior glenohumeral ligament (IGHL)	External rotation at high elevation
Inferior capsular sling (ICS)	Abduction and high elevation
Posteroinferior glenohumeral ligament (PIGHL)	Internal rotation at high elevation
Posterosuperior capsule (PSC)	Internal rotation at low elevation

of the inferior glenohumeral ligament (IGHL) become taught with maximal external rotation in midrange and full abduction, respectively.[287, 294] The inferior capsular sling becomes taut in full humeral elevation with tension shifting in orientation along cruciate lines (anterior and posterior) with external and internal rotation, respectively.[210, 299] The posterosuperior capsule becomes taut with internal rotation at the side, and tension is shifted inferiorly to the posteroinferior capsule with increasing angles of elevation.[119, 178]

A contracture of any given portion of the articular capsule will restrict range as though the end-range constraint were invoked prematurely (see Fig. 20–4). Pathologic contractures of isolated regions of the articular capsule have been identified[116, 122, 190, 194, 207, 213, 220, 290] or intentionally created[49, 78, 173, 192, 207, 219] at open or arthroscopic surgery that restrain motion. To eliminate clinical pathologic restrictions, authors have advocated specific open or arthroscopic surgical release of the contracted capsule and ligaments.[57, 95, 122, 151, 178, 190, 194, 207, 213, 220, 231, 267, 290, 300]

Humeroscapular Motion Interface

In 1934, Codman stated that, "The subacromial bursa itself is the largest in the body and the most complicated in structure and in its component parts. It is in fact, a secondary scapulohumeral joint, although no part of its surface is cartilage."[55] He also believed that the roughly hemispheric shape of the coracoacromial arch was "almost a counterpart in size and curvature of the articular surface of the true joint."

Matsen and Romeo have extended Codman's auxiliary joint concept and defined the humeroscapular motion interface (HSMI) as a set of sliding surfaces that include the deep sides of the deltoid, the acromion, the coracoid process and its tendons, and the superficial side of the humerus, rotator cuff, and long head of the biceps tendon and its sheath (Fig. 20–9).[178, 256] If pathologic conditions, such as adhesions secondary to trauma or surgery, spot-weld across or obliterate the humeroscapular motion interface, shoulder motion will be limited by the extent of involvement and by the location of pathology.

Romeo and associates measured humeroscapular motion in vivo in five normal shoulders.[178, 256] The relative motion of the proximal humerus to the deltoid, coracoid, and its tendons was measured using serial axial magnetic resonance imaging (MRI) views in sequential increments over the full range of external to internal rotation. The maximum average of interfacial sliding motion approached 3 cm (29.1 mm), which occurred at the level of the widest axial section of the humeral head. Interfacial motion varied depending on the site measured until no relative motion was present distally at the level of the deltoid tuberosity.

In clinical practice, humeroscapular stiffness following trauma, immobilization, or previous surgery is partly related to adhesions within the humeroscapular motion interface.[178] At repeat surgery, dense adhesions have been identified between the acromion and the bursal surface after rotator cuff repair and under the coracoid, conjoined tendon, and deltoid after an instability repair. Attempts to restore normal interfacial sliding motion after a surgical repair of the rotator cuff is difficult when shoulder stiffness is secondary to adhesions in the humeroscapular motion interface.[100]

The long head of the biceps tendon is unique in position about the shoulder. The root of the biceps is a structural extension of the glenohumeral articular surface forming part of the glenohumeral articular motion surface. Like a monorail system, the humeral head and its bicipital tendon groove move along the tendon rooted on the scapula to participate in relative humeroscapular motion. All glenohumeral motion is accompanied by gliding or rotation of the bicipital groove on the surface of the biceps tendon. If synovitis within the glenohumeral joint or tendon sheath is present, adhesions can spot-weld the long head of the biceps tendon to the cuff, capsule, or groove (Fig. 20–10).[116, 122, 213] Pasteur in 1932, followed by Lippmann, Neviaser, Hitchcock, Bechtol, and DePalma, reported peritendinous adhesions that caused a variable degree of motion impairment of the tendon within its groove in patients exhibiting frozen shoulder.[70, 133, 165, 196, 224] They recommended either a lysis of adhesions or excision of the biceps to restore motion.

Unrestricted humeral motion along the biceps tendon is essential to maintain the full range of glenohumeral motion. If this monorail assemblage is blocked, the range of glenohumeral motion will be limited.[178] Basta and colleagues used a mathematical model and a cadaveric shoulder instrumented with a 6-degree-of-freedom spatial sensor to experimentally verify the effect of limited biceps tendon excursion on glenohumeral motion.[11] They found that the bicipital groove translated 50 mm along the biceps tendon with maximal intra-articular tendon length (IATL) in external rotation and minimal IATL in maximal elevation.

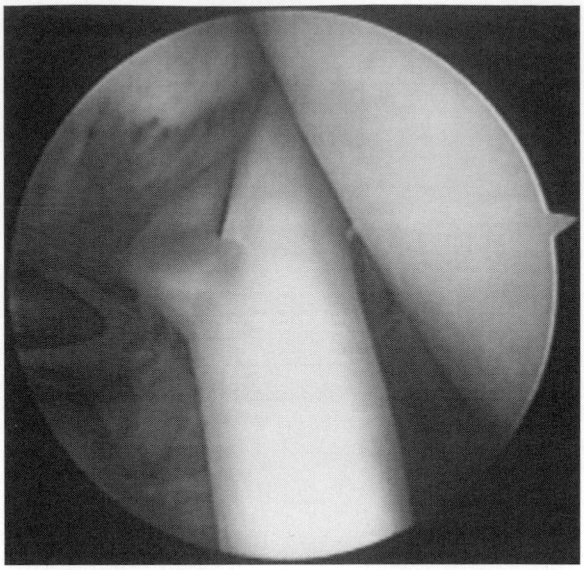

Figure 20–10

Arthroscopic glenohumeral joint view showing an intra-articular adhesion binding the biceps tendon to the contracted rotator interval. (From Harryman DT II: Shoulders: Frozen and stiff. Instr Course Lect *42*:247–257, 1993.)

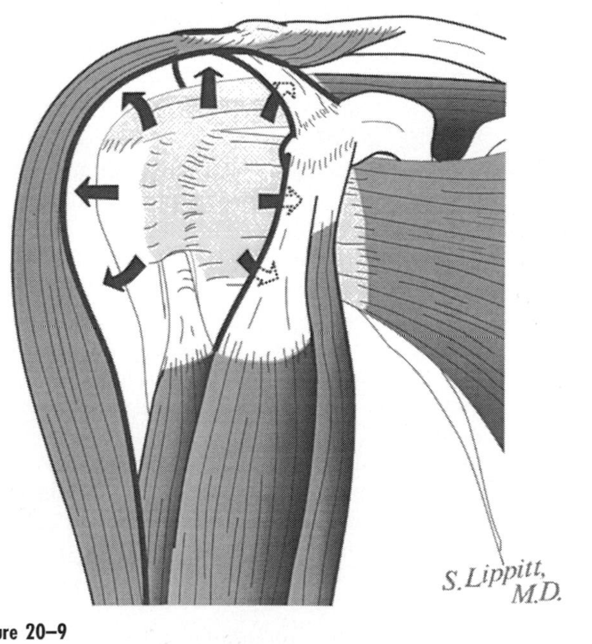

Figure 20–9

The humeroscapular motion interface (HSMI) is an important continuum of interfacial sliding surfaces that include the deep sides of the deltoid, the acromion, the coracoid process and its tendons, and the superficial side of the humerus, rotator cuff, long head of the biceps tendon, and its sheath. (Modified from Matsen FA III, Lippitt SB, Sidles JA, and Harryman DT II: Practical Evaluation of Management of the Shoulder. Philadelphia: WB Saunders, 1994, pp 19–109.)

A biceps tendon adhesed or tenodesed in situ within the bicipital groove after injury, inflammation, or surgical incorporation could potentially limit maximal recovery of significant useful glenohumeral motion. Basta and coworkers also performed a tenodesis of the biceps tendon in situ at three different angles of humeral rotation. Positions of tenodesis with increasing internal rotation demonstrated greater restriction in motion (Fig. 20–11).

Scapulothoracic Motion

Scapulothoracic motion is responsible for approximately one third of humerothoracic elevation (see Fig. 20–3).[94, 139] Poppen and Walker defined scapula motion according to the radiographic position of the glenoid, but this has limited usefulness for clinical examination.[232] Pearl designed a hand-held scapula locator to help determine the scapular plane, position, and motion of the shoulder.[228] Harryman and associates pinned electromagnetic sensors to the scapula and humerus in eight volunteers and recorded humerothoracic, scapulothoracic, and glenohumeral motions.[121] Scapular spine motion was described relative to thoracic anatomic axes in terms of plane of elevation, angle of elevation, and angle of rotation. The limits of scapulothoracic motion were determined: the maximum scapulothoracic elevation was 56 ± 8 degrees; the plane of maximal scapular elevation was 59 ± 10 degrees forward of the coronal plane (about 30 degrees forward of the nominal "plane of the scapula" determined radiographically), and the plane of scapular motion varied widely, ranging from +83 degrees (flexion) to −95 de-

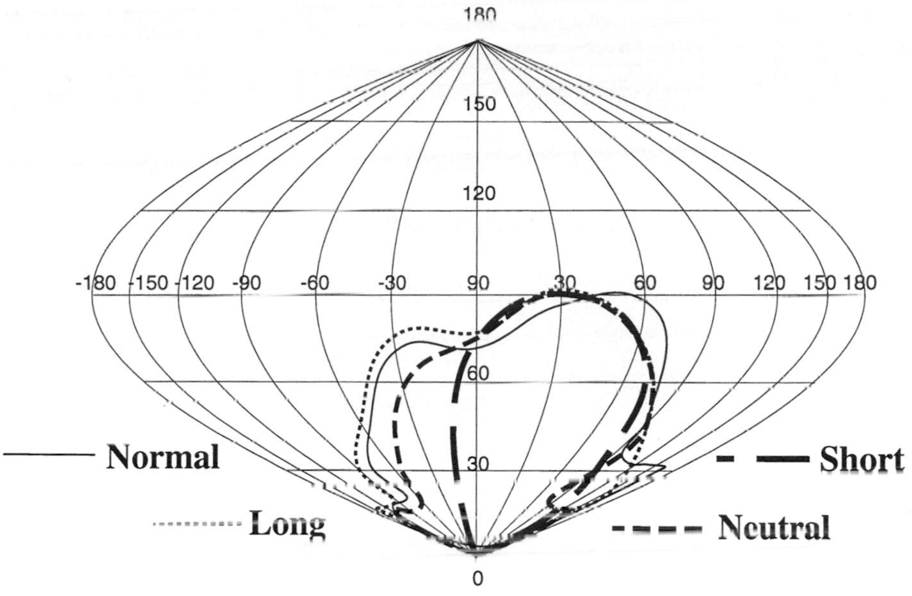

Figure 20–11

Tethering the intact biceps long head restricts glenohumeral motion. This global diagram shows the maximum limit of normal scapulohumeral motion in elevation and plane (humerus in maximal internal humeral rotation). The relative limits in plane and elevation for each in situ tenodesis preparation (short, neutral, long intra-articular biceps length) are exposed for comparative examination against the normal, nontenodesis preparation.

grees (extension) for low angles. They also found that scapular motion was constantly realigned on the thorax in response to load transfer from the torso to the extremity and vice versa (Fig. 20–12).

Since a loss of glenohumeral range (e.g., after shoulder fusion) can result in an accommodative increase in scapulothoracic range,[123] we would also predict that a contracture in the scapulothoracic musculature or a loss of scapulothoracic motion (e.g., after scapulothoracic fusion) may demand greater range from the glenohumeral joint. Although it is a challenge to clinically measure scapulothoracic motion accurately, Nicholson recorded excessive scapular upward rotation (elevation) during active attempts at humeral elevation in patients with frozen shoulder.[206]

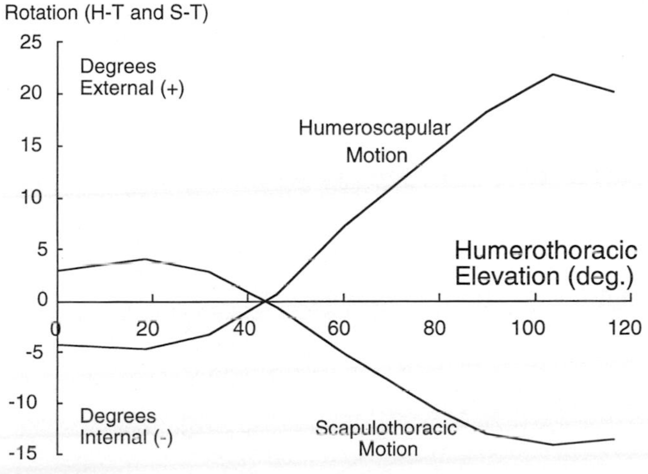

Figure 20–12

Graphic data from a subject with the transmitter fixed to the thorax and magnetic field oriented to anatomic axes. Spatial motion sensors were pinned to the scapula and humerus for tracking motion in three dimensions. The data show that glenohumeral and scapulothoracic motion is in constant balance, presumably to maintain the maximal efficiency in transfer of load from the extremity to the torso and vice versa.

DIAGNOSTIC CRITERIA

The frozen shoulder, or primary stiffness, implies glenohumeral contracture that occurs after minimal or no trauma and arises as a fibrotic process intrinsic to the glenohumeral joint capsule. A post-traumatic stiff shoulder, or secondary stiffness, is an extrinsic process that requires initiation from a traumatic precursor or other condition. Each of these diagnoses appear to have a different underlying pathology, history, and treatment. In addition, they may not be mutually exclusive. Although a post-traumatic stiff shoulder may originate as an extracapsular process, subsequent capsular contracture may soon develop. On the rare occasion, inflammation and adhesions have been identified in the subacromial bursa in association with an idiopathic frozen shoulder.[116]

Idiopathic Frozen Shoulder

A lack of consensus regarding the nomenclature and classification has in part originated with the confusion surrounding the necessary and sufficient diagnostic criteria for what we could call the frozen shoulder and the post-traumatic stiff shoulder. Many authors have suggested criteria that often refer to guidelines of measured range. These motion arcs have been defined in terms of humerothoracic planes of elevation (coronal abduction or sagittal flexion) and humeroscapular arcs of rotation (internal and external rotation). Traditional measurements assess humerothoracic motion between the arms and the thorax along anatomic axes, and some have attempted to isolate glenohumeral motion while stabilizing the scapulothoracic articulation to exclude motion.

On review of the literature, we might easily conclude that a restricted motion of approximately 50% is a reasonable mean among investigators who cite humerothoracic or scapulohumeral motion criteria.[22, 36, 146, 166, 168, 198, 200, 235, 236, 253] Yet, it is more than a challenge; if not impossible to

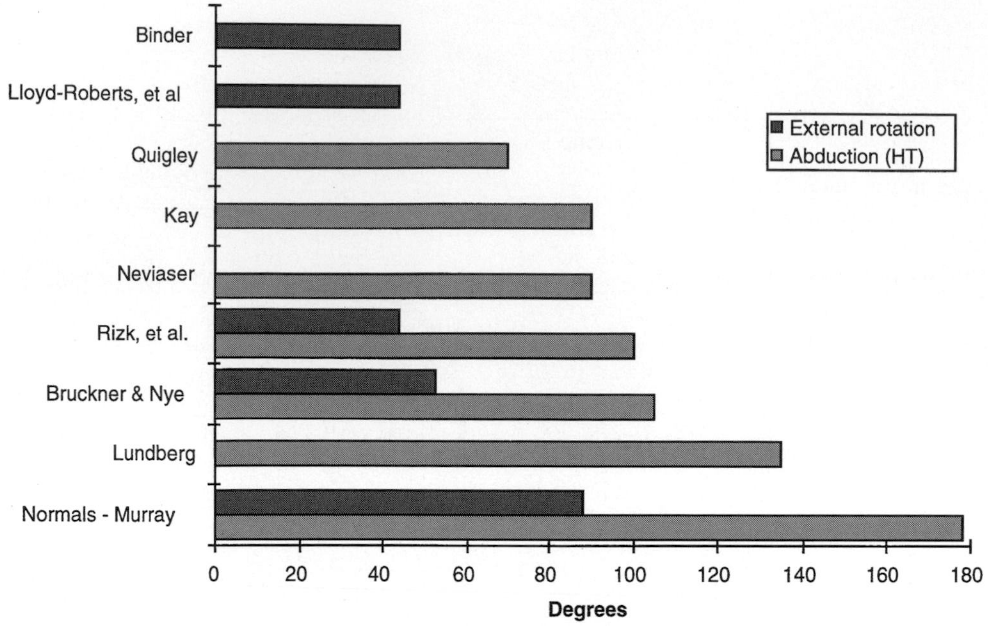

Figure 20–13

Investigators have recommended specific thresholds of limited motion to diagnose a frozen shoulder. The most frequent motion criteria have been set according to abduction in the coronal plane or the degree of external rotation (all motions adjusted to humerothoracic range relative to normal controls defined by Murray and associates[189]).

reconcile the minimum motion criteria, various authors have included a given set of diagnostic criteria for a frozen shoulder (Fig. 20–13). These criteria lead to some confusion since the percentage loss in range is clearly a measure of severity. Some authors define restrictive motion in a single motion arc and others in multiple planes. For example, Neviaser, Kay, Binder and associates, and Lloyd-Roberts included criteria that described on the average, a 50% limitation relative to normal in abduction or external rotation.[22, 146, 166, 198, 200] In contrast, Rizk set four motion criteria including combined abduction, forward elevation, and external and internal rotation with relative percentages of normal ranging from 55 to 80%![253]

Since motion restrictions are typically isolated to the scapulohumeral articulation, precise quantification of glenohumeral range should be attempted. Pearl suggested[229] elevating the humerus in the scapular plane 45 degrees to assume the midpoint of joint motion and capsular laxity and from there performing maximal external and internal rotation to assess the degree of restricted motion isolated to the glenohumeral joint (Fig. 20–14). An arc of rotation-restricted to less than 50% correlated significantly with a frozen shoulder as defined by conventional measures of humerothoracic elevation and external and internal rotation. The present authors have not attempted to define a specific threshold for measured ranges but instead rely on historical presentation and on examination of patterns of motion restriction and radiographic criteria. Similar to others,[40, 159] we have combined multiple measured ranges of standard examination mathematically into a composite ratio to allow meaningful comparisons between groups of patients (see Examination).

Other descriptive criteria have been deemed essential to diagnose a frozen shoulder. Kessel's criteria were unique in that no threshold of limited range was specified but instead required symptoms of spontaneous onset with progressive loss of glenohumeral motion, no identifiable associated illness, and normal radiographs.[149] Bruckner and Nye and Lloyd-Roberts have included symptomatic night pain for a duration of 1 and 3 months, respectively.[36, 166] Neviaser's criteria demand an ancillary arthrogram in addition to historic and clinical findings.

Our necessary and sufficient diagnostic criteria[178] for an idiopathic frozen shoulder embody some familiar features to those described by Kessel[149] and include:

1. A history of restricted shoulder motion *without* previous major injury or reconstructive surgery
2. An examination with *global* stiffness (i.e., restricted

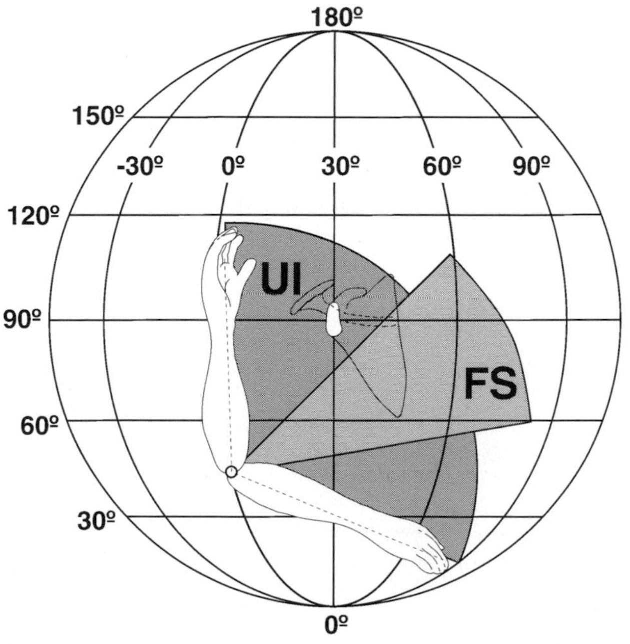

Figure 20–14

Global diagram showing humeral elevation of 45 degrees in the plane of the scapula (30-degree humerothoracic plane). The shaded rotational range measures the uninvolved (UI) side against the affected side limited by a frozen shoulder (FS). (Courtesy of M. Pearl, M.D.[229])

motion in all directions not accompanied by loss of strength, stability, or joint smoothness)

3. Plain radiographs with *normal* cartilaginous joint space and no focal periarticular abnormalities (osteopenia may be seen)

If uniform criteria such as these are applied to define the idiopathic frozen shoulder, then other investigators can correctly differentiate clinical entities grouped under the general guise of "scapulohumeral periarthritis," "frozen shoulder," or "adhesive capsulitis."[8] From this foundation, all of us can begin to study this anatomic affectation and its impact on functional performance.

Post-Traumatic Stiff Shoulder

The earliest description of shoulder stiffness occurring after trauma was recorded by Malgaigne, who wrote in regard to minor nondisplaced extracapsular fractures about the shoulder.[175] In 1859 he said,

> . . . there remains long afterwards a stiffness, and a difficulty in moving the shoulder; and however great care may be taken, the motion of elevation of the arm will always remain limited; at least I have in no case seen it perfectly restored, even after the lapse of from eleven to fifteen months.

We can only hope that his observations on outcome of this condition were premature! Reeves coined the term the *post-traumatic stiff shoulder*[241] and referred to the clinical presentation described by Robert Jones and Lovett in 1923.[144, 241]

Less controversy and confusion surrounds the nomenclature of this clinical entity; however, some people, like Neviaser and Neviaser, have introduced an alternate classification.[203] They included stiffness, which originated from trauma but was not associated with capsular contracture under the heading "the stiff and painful shoulder." Other classification alternatives, such as Kay's "early capsulitis" and Wither's "irritative capsulitis," border on being related to a post-traumatic stiff shoulder by virtue of less severe restrictions in motion but clearly were not defined for association with trauma.[146, 311] Lastly, the division of secondary frozen shoulders described by Lundberg includes all presentations of post-traumatic stiff shoulders.[168]

Some shoulder stiffness is typical after intrinsic injuries to the soft tissues or the articulations surrounding the shoulder. Restriction in shoulder motion has been reported after simple contusions, glenohumeral subluxations, dislocations, fracture-dislocations, acromioclavicular joint injury, clavicle and scapula fractures, and especially subcapital fractures of the humerus in the elderly.[60, 103] Partial restrictions in motion may also occur in association with soft tissue injury.

Reports of partial motion loss in specific patterns are more frequent in recent literature. These patterns are most often seen post-traumatically, usually after low-level, repetitive trauma. Neer recognized an asymmetric presentation associated with repetitive injury that he called "impingement syndrome" and encouraged therapeutic stretching in forward elevation, internal rotation, and cross-body adduction.[191] Thomas and associates reported three cases presenting atraumatically with stiffness in forward flexion and internal rotation, yet the inferior recess and joint capacity on arthrogram was normal and no specific lesion was identified at arthroscopy.[288] Ticker and associates reported the findings of nine patients who had painful stiffness and a discrete loss of forward elevation and internal rotation in abduction. At arthroscopy, these patients were found to have a thickened posterior capsule.[290] In a recent review of the senior author's first 30 patients from an ongoing prospective study of refractory shoulder stiffness, 11 patients experienced partial restriction in motion that was attributed to a posterior capsular contracture.[122] In each of these patients, an associated pathology was identified with seven having a partial-thickness rotator cuff tear. In an unpublished review of 90 patients who went on to surgical capsular release, the presenting degree of stiffness after an injury (60 shoulders), as opposed to those with an idiopathic onset (30 shoulders), was significantly less for the motions of flexion, external rotation at the side, and external and internal rotation in 90 degrees of abduction (Table 20–3).

Surgical procedures are widely recognized as a cause of shoulder stiffness. Anterior or posterior capsulorrhaphy, inferior capsular shift, and rotator cuff repairs are typical examples of iatrogenic tightening of the glenohumeral capsule that produce predictable limitations in motion.[126, 193, 211, 219] Repair of a defect in the supraspinatus or infraspinatus tendons often limits motions such as internal rotation and cross-body adduction.[178, 322] Major trauma requiring surgery to repair soft tissue tears or reconstruction of the proximal humerus often results in combined intra-articular and extra-articular adhesions.[98] Bush and Hansen have advocated incorporating the intact biceps tendon into rotator cuff reconstructions, which would be expected to cause motion restriction.[47, 114] The degree of stiffness and direction of limited range may reflect the presence of adhesions in the extra-articular humeroscapular motion interface, contractures in musculotendinous units, and fibrosis of the articular capsule.

Our necessary and sufficient diagnostic criteria[178] for a post-traumatic stiff shoulder (or post-surgical) include:

1. A history of injury or repetitive low-level trauma or

Table 20–3 COMPARATIVE MOTION RANGES OF FROZEN AND POST-TRAUMATIC STIFF SHOULDERS

NO. OF PATIENTS (117)	NONINJURED (49)	INJURED (68)	ANOVA DUNN
Motions			
FE	104 ± 20	118 ± 30	$P = 0.007$
ERS	13 ± 20	32 ± 25	$P < 0.0001$
ERA	37 ± 24	56 ± 29	$P = 0.0004$
IRA	12 ± 18	32 ± 19	$P < 0.0001$
IRB	6 ± 3	6 ± 3	NSD
XBA	25 ± 7	24 ± 8	NSD

FE, forward elevation; ERS, external rotation at side; ERA, external rotation in abduction; IRA, internal rotation in abduction; IRB, internal rotation up the back; XBA, cross-body adduction; NSD, no significant difference.

surgery with onset of stiffness that functionally restricts use of the extremity

2. An examination with limited shoulder motion in a specific direction, multiple directions, or globally
3. Radiographs with a normal cartilaginous joint space

In shoulders that become symptomatic after an injury, pronounced restrictions in shoulder motion may occur asymmetrically or globally. Although the history, examination, and management of the post-traumatic stiff shoulder may be different from that of idiopathic frozen shoulder, the long-term symptoms of post-traumatic stiffness and their progression have yet to be described but may not be appreciably different. Motion losses in isolated directions may progress to global limitations in motion depending on the severity of the injury or on the length of disability. We are unaware if stiffness of this type recovers without intervention or if a loss in range becomes accepted by adaptation.

Although the post-traumatic stiff shoulder may present less homogeneity than the idiopathic frozen shoulder in regard to a historical mechanism or severity, the recommended diagnostic criteria are easily applied to both categories at all levels of expertise and do not require special ancillary tests. Additional specific diagnostic criteria for studies of certain post-traumatic subgroups such as the posterior capsular contracture or postsurgical stiff shoulder are easily formulated. It is worthwhile recognizing that almost all cases of shoulder stiffness fit the basic criteria described, and wide application would allow meaningful comparison for prospective evaluation and treatment.

EPIDEMIOLOGY

In order to determine the exact incidence of a specific type of shoulder stiffness in the general population, investigators must prospectively define the entity with specific diagnostic criteria and establish age- and sex-matched controls.[40, 188] Small but significant differences in measured shoulder range have been established for adults in early or later age groups.[54, 189] Clarke and associates found slightly greater shoulder range for women than for men, but data from Murray and co-workers neither confirmed this finding nor noted differences in side or dominance.[54, 189]

Studies with stringent diagnostic criteria for frozen shoulder have defined the incidence of frozen shoulder in the general population at slightly greater than 2%. Reliable data were collected by Lundberg, who sampled a local hospital patient population, and by Bridgman who reviewed 600 outpatients.[32, 168] Pal and associates found a 5% incidence, and Sattar discovered a 3% incidence of clinical signs and symptoms of frozen shoulder in 75 and 100 nonpatient controls, respectively.[221, 264] In a study that included 100 geriatric inpatients, Chard found a 3% prevalence of painful stiff shoulders.[51] An accurate incidence of idiopathic frozen and post-traumatic stiff shoulders in a cross-section of a specified general population has yet to be determined.

FACTORS THAT PREDISPOSE THE SHOULDER TO STIFFNESS

Age Prevalence

The bulk of adults who present with a stiff shoulder, whether idiopathic or post-traumatic in origin, are generally between 40 and 60 years of age (Fig. 20–15).[36, 115, 178, 187, 188, 242] It is unusual to develop an idiopathic frozen shoulder in patients younger than 40 years of age unless insulin-dependent diabetes has been present since childhood. In a large study, Lundberg noted a slightly higher mean age for men (55) compared with women (52).[168] A difference in age according to sex, or type of stiffness, however, has not been evident in the senior author's unpublished data from 126 patients presenting with refractory shoulder stiffness. Our mean age was 50 years for both the diabetic and nondiabetic patients and 50 years for either sex. The mean ages between post-traumatic and idiopathic subclassifications were 49 and 50 years, respectively.

Injuries

Almost all patients who develop "idiopathic" shoulder stiffness can associate a minor traumatic incident contemporary with the onset of symptoms typically remembered upon questioning.[55, 72, 179] Of course, distinct trauma of a fracture, rotator cuff tear, or surgical procedure, for example, is easily documented and classified within the post-traumatic category.

A significant number of patients who present with painful stiffness after a rotator cuff strain or a repetitive overuse injury are often diagnosed with "impingement syndrome." On closer inspection, the history and physical examination of these patients typically fit within the post-traumatic classification, and these patients are suffering from a contracture of the posterior capsule.[116, 119, 122, 178, 290]

Surgical Trauma

Although stiffness after shoulder surgery is expected and typically addressed after surgical procedures are performed in the vicinity of the shoulder girdle, postoperative therapy to recover motion may be neglected or resisted by the patient who undergoes other types of surgery. Common examples include axillary node and cervical neck dissections that are known causes of impaired shoulder motion postoperatively, especially when combined with radiation therapy.[225, 277] Cardiac catheterization in the axilla, coronary artery bypass grafting with sternotomy, and thoracotomy may also restrict shoulder range because of severe pain after the procedure.[230, 274] It is important, therefore, to assist our surgical colleagues with a rehabilitation program to prevent a prolonged disability in these patients.

Immobility

After a minor strain, injury, surgery, or other painful source, it may seem logical to rest and immobilize the

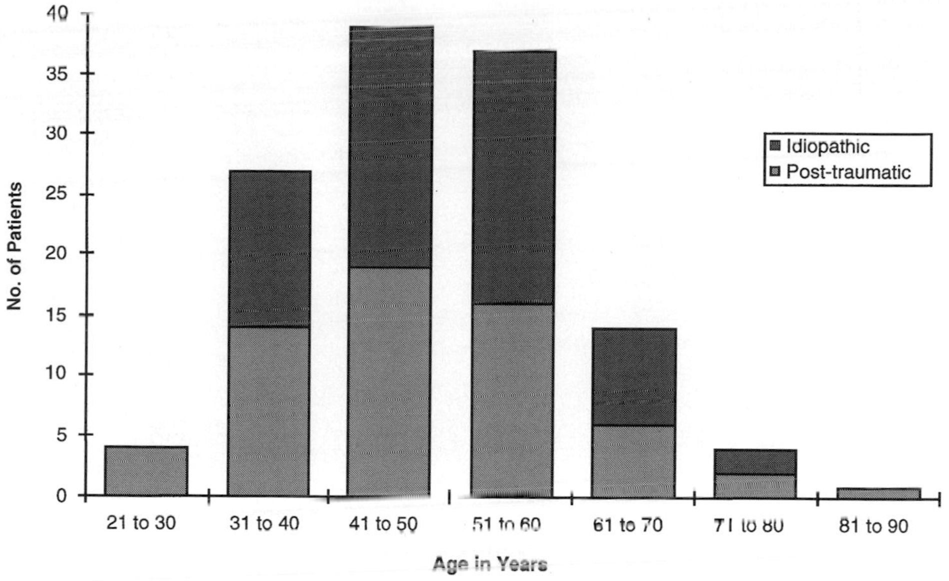

Figure 20–15

Graph depicting the age of presentation for 126 patients with a frozen (64) or post-traumatic stiff shoulder (62) as defined by our diagnostic criteria.[178] There were no differences in the mean age between these two diagnoses.

part, especially when inflammation may be involved. Yet, in the adult, when the shoulder is immobilized, it is at risk of becoming stiff.[66, 109, 143, 200, 278, 297] Bruckner and Nye performed a prospective study to evaluate the factors that placed neurologic patients (mostly after subarachnoid hemorrhage) at greater risk of adhesive capsulitis.[36] Over 6 months of observation, 25% of these patients developed a frozen shoulder. They identified five risk factors that could be linked primarily to a significant period of immobility of the affected upper extremity.

The majority of patient referrals for shoulder stiffness to an orthopedic specialist are subsequent to a recommended rest period imposed by the referring physician. In a review of patients referred to Binder and colleagues, 75% of the patients were told to rest the shoulder instead of prescribing gentle exercises to maintain mobility.[21] Only one half of these patients received advice in regard to the care of their painful shoulder after an initial assessment from their primary care physician.

In summary, the authors agree with Neviaser who in 1949 wrote, "I believe we can accept the fact that disuse and inactivity play a very important part in the etiology."[196] It is important, therefore, to educate those in our profession who, in turn, can pass along to the primary care gatekeepers that in order to prevent shoulder stiffness an early gentle full-range stretching program is indicated after injury. Similarly, surgeons must recognize that stiffness after procedures about the shoulder girdle is best avoided by an early rehabilitation program.[178, 179]

Diabetes Mellitus

Patients with diabetes mellitus are at much greater risk for developing limited joint motion, not only in the shoulder but also to an extent in all joints.[258] The incidence of frozen shoulder among diabetics averages approximately 10 to 20% but may be as high as 35%.[32, 92, 162, 168, 184, 221, 222, 264, 315] Diabetics who have been insulin dependent for many years show a much greater frequency of frozen shoulder and, in up to 42%, present with bilateral shoulder involvement.[32, 92, 184] Patients with diabetes of childhood onset may present with symptoms of stiffness in the fifth decade of life, but if adult-onset diabetics are included (type I plus type II diabetes mellitus), then the age of presentation is similar to that of the general population (Fig. 20–16).

Insulin-dependent diabetics affected by joint stiffness in the hands and other major articulations are categorized with limited joint motion syndrome.[258] High circulating blood glucose levels may actually accelerate "aging" of certain proteins in the body by triggering a series of chemical reactions that form and accumulate irreversible cross-links between adjacent protein molecules.[37, 134, 174] This pathway, which leads to diffuse arthrofibrosis, is termed nonenzymatic glycosylation. Diabetics who have cheiroarthropathy (a waxy thickening and induration of the skin associated with flexion contractures of the fingers) and a frozen shoulder have a higher incidence of retinopathy and bilateral shoulder involvement (77%).[92] Rarely, shoulder stiffness has been reported to antedate diabetic symptoms,[268] and joint stiffening is found more commonly in those with skin changes.[275] Lastly, the longer that a patient has been taking insulin, the higher is the risk of developing shoulder stiffness,[184] and the resistance is greater to all treatment modalities.[92, 264]

Lequesne found 17 patients with glucose intolerance out of 60 new patients who presented with an idiopathic frozen shoulder.[162] Therefore, the attentive clinician should inquire into the family history of all patients who have been newly diagnosed with frozen shoulder, and consideration should be given for an oral glucose tolerance test in those affected. Because of the refractory nature of shoulder stiffness in the long-term insulin-dependent diabetic, early intervention has been considered appropriate to prevent progressive disability.[92, 213, 264]

Cervical Disease

Degeneration of the cervical intervertebral disks between C5-C6 and C6-C7 has been noted to be more frequent

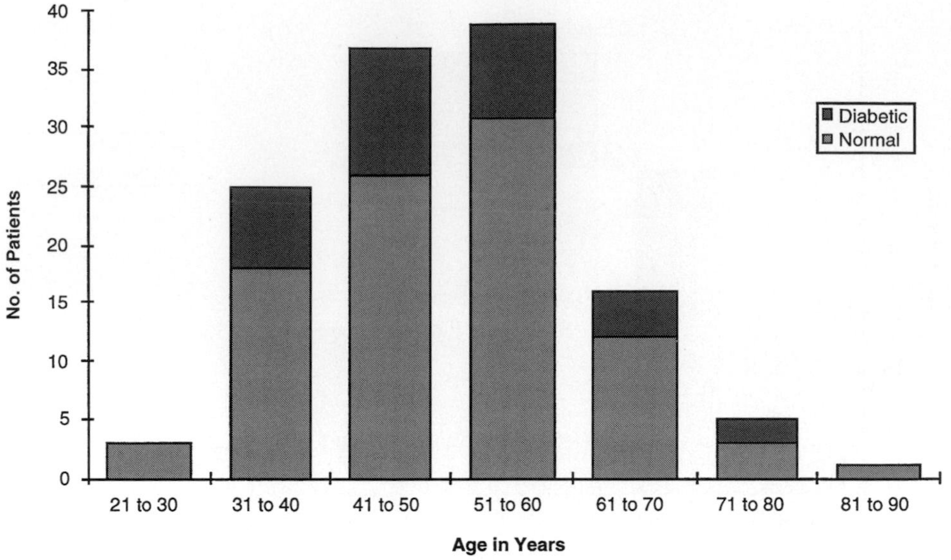

Figure 20–16

Graph depicting the age of presentation for 126 patients with shoulder stiffness divided by those with or without diabetes.[178] There were no differences in the mean age between patients with diabetes (32) and those without diabetes (92).

in patients with periarthritic shoulder stiffness than in a similarly age-matched control group.[316] The peak age incidence of frozen shoulder and cervical disk degeneration is similar.[145] In other studies, patients with degenerative disk disease of the cervical spine were noted to develop a frozen shoulder more frequently.[103, 168, 180] Lastly, patients with symptomatic cervical radiculitis and a painful shoulder, with or without a fixed joint contracture, experienced less pain and regained pain-free range when cervical traction was added to exercises.[53]

Thyroid Disorders

The rare presentation of bilateral frozen shoulders has been reported in both hyperthyroidism and hypothyroidism.[29, 182, 284, 315] Because of potential activation within the sympathetic nervous system, Wohlgethan has postulated that hyperthyroidism, frozen shoulder, and shoulder-hand syndrome are linked disorders.[312] Resolution of shoulder stiffness has occurred after thyroidectomy and stabilization of the thyroid hormone level.[218, 312]

Cardiac Disease

For many years, clinicians have been keen to associate ischemic heart disease and shoulder stiffness.[5, 85, 179, 315] Also, a frozen shoulder has been reported to persist years after a coronary artery occlusion.[5] On review of 133 consecutive cases of myocardial infarction, Ernstene and Kinell found 17 whose original presenting complaint was unrelenting pain in the shoulder region.[85] Because of this relationship, a good cardiac examination is justified to rule out an unrecognized coronary thrombosis. Similarly, shoulder-hand syndrome, an autonomic dystrophy, can be a sequel to myocardial infarction in 10 to 30% of cases.[183] Lastly, frozen shoulder may also be triggered by a cardiac catheterization through the brachial artery, but the genesis may likely be a consequence of the postsurgical discomfort.[230]

Pulmonary Disorders

Saha reported that frozen shoulder was more frequent in those afflicted with emphysema and chronic bronchitis, but he was unable to correlate the severity or the duration of illness with the presentation.[261] In 1959, Johnson reported that the incidence of frozen shoulder was 3.2% among pooled populations in sanitoria patients with tuberculosis.[143] In patients undergoing treatment for tuberculosis, Good and associates associated cases of frozen shoulder and the use of isoniazid therapy.[99]

Neoplastic Disorders

Bronchogenic carcinoma and Pancoast's tumors of the lung parenchyma have been known to cause deep shoulder aching and a neuritic type of pain.[84, 131] Other occult neoplastic tumors, masked by symptoms attributed to a frozen shoulder, include chest wall tumors and primary or metastatic carcinoma of the humerus.[68, 179, 197]

Neurologic Conditions

Riley and colleagues documented a 13% incidence of frozen shoulder in patients with Parkinson's disease compared with a 1.7% rate in age-matched controls.[250] They also highlighted that in 8% of the patients surveyed, the first symptom of Parkinson's disease was shoulder stiffness, which could occur up to 2 years before the onset of generalized symptoms! Brachial neuritis, a painful neuritic condition, also known as Parsonage-Turner syndrome, has also been associated with frozen shoulder.[20]

After a stroke or other cause of hemiplegia, painful shoulder stiffness can occur and may lead to a frozen shoulder.[25, 105] It was postulated by Griffin that "careless handling of the paralyzed upper limb at any time after the onset of hemiplegia can precipitate shoulder injury and pain."[105] Bruckner and Nye found a 25% incidence of frozen shoulder in neurosurgical patients who had suffered subarachnoid hemorrhage.[illegible] They found that subsequent development of adhesive capsulitis was associated with impaired consciousness, hemiparesis, intravenous infusion, older age, and depression.

Patients with cerebral hemorrhage and cerebral tumors have also been shown to be at increased risk of developing a frozen shoulder.[36, 316] Even compressive neuropathies such as thoracic outlet syndrome and palsy of the accessory nerve or suprascapular nerve have been associated with the onset of a frozen shoulder.[34, 152, 225]

Personality Disorders

In 1934, Codman described four patients with frozen shoulder who "were a little run-down without anything particular the matter."[55] This "run-down" condition may predispose an individual to develop chronic shoulder stiffness.[212, 235] Coventry dubbed some individuals with the "periarthritic personality," which was a character disposition susceptible to a frozen shoulder and in whom treatment was more difficult.[61] A person with this personality was characterized as hyperemotional and unable to tolerate pain. He went on to say that "they expect someone else to get them well and refuse to take the initiative in the recovery, a manifestation of their passivity." Many years later, however, Wright and Haq found no evidence of a characteristic personality disorder when using the Maudsley Personality Inventory on testing 186 patients who had a frozen shoulder compared with controls.[315] Fleming and associates also profiled the personality type of 56 patients with a frozen shoulder using the Middlesex Hospital Questionnaire and found that women had significantly greater anxiety levels compared with controls.[93]

Tyber treated 55 patients with painful shoulder syndromes using lithium and amitriptyline and found a significantly greater prevalence of depression that responded along with shoulder pain to these medications.[295] He entertained the theory that "a painful shoulder syndrome may be a clinical entity of psychogenic origin." In response to Tyber, Sullivan recommended that the physician "should not be detracted from giving proper and early treatment to the painful shoulder."[283]

Although it may be reasonable to say that patients with chronically painful shoulder stiffness may over time lose their tolerance to cope with chronic pain, especially when treatment measures are unsuccessful, the mental health of patients with shoulder stiffness appears to be normal. Matsen and Harryman reviewed their combined unpublished data collected at the University of Washington Shoulder Clinic for results of the mental health score on the SF-36 health status questionnaire for 295 patients with a frozen shoulder (175) or post-traumatic stiff shoulder (120). We found that our patients with frozen shoulder scored within 95% and post-traumatic patients with stiff shoulder scored within 88% of the mean for normal age-matched controls. Although these patients in pain may appear depressed, anxious, or passive aggressive, we believe that they are no different than the general population facing stressful circumstances. Of course, psychological evaluation and management are best left to our consulting specialists so that we can focus on functional evaluation and effective treatment.

DIAGNOSTIC EVALUATION

History

CLINICAL PRESENTATION OF IDIOPATHIC FROZEN SHOULDER

For a frozen shoulder, there are three stages that classically characterize the disease although their nomenclature and description vary among authors.[129, 187, 188] A patient with an idiopathic frozen shoulder may present with typical complaints and physical findings for this diagnosis, but the practitioner's clinical acumen is challenged to discriminate the exact stage or appropriate duration of symptoms or findings at presentation. Initial bilateral presentation of shoulder stiffness may be a clue to systemic disease, yet even with unilateral presentation, a prudent physician should consider the possibility of frequently associated diseases in the differential diagnosis (Table 20–4). Reports of bilateral involvement range from 10% in the general population to as high as 40% for those with insulin-dependent diabetes.[22, 242]

A frozen shoulder rarely recurs in the same shoulder unless an injury or disease process predisposes the joint to repeat episodes of stiffness.[72, 109, 150, 168, 182, 188] In patients without diabetes, up to 20% of patients may develop a frozen shoulder on the opposite side.[169, 251, 263]

Painful Phase: "Freezing"

As mentioned previously, the clinical presentation of frozen shoulder is segmented into three phases. The *painful phase* begins when a patient initially notices the onset of aching pain, which often begins at night and persists during the day.[129, 187, 188] Sudden jolts or attempts at rapid motion exponentially punctuate the chronic discomfort. Typically, there is no precipitating incident, but occasionally the patient recalls a specific event like a trivial injury, a flu shot, or a head cold that settled into the neck. As symptoms progress, fewer extremity positions remain comfortable and those that are tolerable typically leave the arm dependent at the side in a medially rotated resting position. The ache is unrelated to activity and may be worse at rest, especially at night. Lying on or turning over on the affected shoulder prevents sleep or soon awakens the afflicted person. Reeves wrote that this phase lasts somewhere between 2 and 9 months.[242]

Patients will often hold their shoulder in a position of adduction and humerothoracic internal rotation, because this is the neutral isometric position of relaxed tension for the inflamed glenohumeral capsule, biceps, and rotator cuff. In addition, because of nonspecific pain, patients are often treated with a period of immobilization, further placing the arm in an adducted and internally rotated position. Decreased motion, however, further worsens the stiffening process of all mobile units.

Table 20–4 DIFFERENTIAL DIAGNOSES OF SHOULDER STIFFNESS (INCLUDING ASSOCIATED DISEASES)

EXTRINSIC CAUSES		*INTRINSIC CAUSES*

Neurologic
Parkinson's disease
Autonomic dystrophy (RSD)
Intradural lesions
Neural compression
  Cervical disk disease
  Neurofibromata
Foraminal stenosis
Neuralgic amyotrophy
Hemiplegia
Head trauma
Muscular
Poliomyositis
Cardiovascular
Myocardial infarction
Thoracic outlet syndrome
Cerebral hemorrhage
Infectious
Chronic bronchitis
Pulmonary tuberculosis
Metabolic
Diabetes mellitus
Thyroid disease
Progressive systemic sclerosis (scleroderma)
Paget's disease
Neoplastic
Pancoast tumor
Lung carcinoma
Metastatic disease
Inflammatory
Rheumatologic disorders (see Table 20–1)
Polymyalgia rheumatica
	Trauma
	Surgery
	  Axillary node dissection, sternotomy, thoracotomy
	Fractures
	  Cervical spine, ribs, elbow, hand, etc.
	Medications
	Isoniazid, phenobarbitone
	Congenital
	Klippel-Feil
	Sprengel's deformity
	Glenoid dysplasia
	Atresia
	Contractures
	  Pectoralis major
	  Axillary fold
	Behavioral
	Depression
	Hysterical paralysis
	Referred Pain
	Diaphragmatic irritation
	Gastrointestinal disorders
	  Esophagitis
	  Ulcers
	  Cholecystitis
		Bursitis
		Subacromial
		Calcific tendinitis
		Snapping scapula
		Biceps Tendon
		Tenosynovitis
		Partial or complete tears
		SLAP lesions
		Rotator Cuff
		Impingement syndrome
		Partial rotator cuff tears
		Complete rotator cuff tears
		Instability-Glenohumeral
		Recurrent dislocation anterior and posterior
		Chronic dislocation
		Arthritides
		Glenohumeral and acromio-clavicular
		  Osteoarthritis
		  Rheumatoid
		  Psoriatic
		  Infectious
		  Neuropathic
		Trauma
		Fractures
		  Glenoid
		  Proximal humerus
		Surgery
		  Postoperative shoulder, breast, head, neck, chest
		Miscellaneous
		Avascular necrosis
		Hemarthrosis
		Osteochondromatosis
		Suprascapular nerve palsy

SLAP, superior labral anterior-posterior.

Progressive Stiffness Phase: "Frozen"

The phase of progressive stiffness is said to last between 3 and 12 months, which ultimately gives rise to what was classically described by Codman[55] as a frozen shoulder.[129, 242] Stiffness progresses to the extent that shoulder motion becomes limited in all planes. Pain is usually less than in the initial inflammatory phase and is often much more focused.

Activities of daily living are severely restricted (Fig. 20–17). Common complaints, therefore, are the inability to tuck in a shirt, fasten a bra, scratch the back, wash the top of the opposite shoulder, reach away from the body, or reach overhead. Inability to sleep comfortably on the side is a universal complaint, possibly related to decreased glenohumeral laxity.

During this stage, the diagnosis of frozen shoulder is made more easily. The history, therefore, must be directed towards ruling out associated conditions (see Table 20–4). The patient should be questioned specifically about glucose tolerance and a family history of diabetes mellitus. A history of neck stiffness or paresthesias in the upper extremity may be a clue to the presence of underlying cervical disk disease. The presence of pulmonary or cardiac symptoms should be sought.

As time passes, pain diminishes and only a narrow comfort zone exists, albeit within severely restrictive limits. Specifically, patients often feel little or no pain while using the shoulder within its permitted range. Any attempts to reach outside of the restricted range or sudden movements that demand shock absorption (e.g., hammering) are associated with pain. Once the degree of stiffness has plateaued, a steady state exists during which the patient gets no worse and no better, in a word—frozen! Although this phase is said to last anywhere between 3 and 12 months, it can become refractory and last much longer.[116, 122, 213, 300]

Resolution Phase: "Thawing"

The final stage of the idiopathic frozen shoulder is the *resolution* or *thawing* phase, characterized by a slow gain

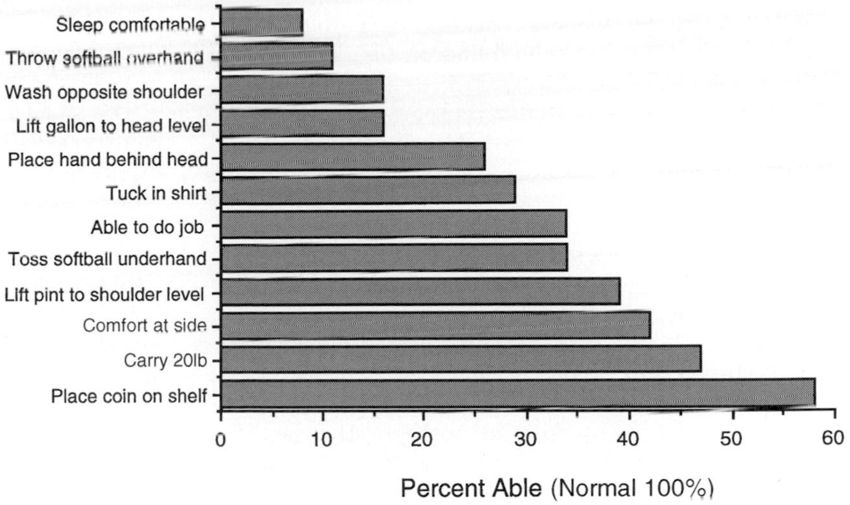

Figure 20–17

Shoulder function as depicted on the Simple Shoulder Test self-assessment examination for the first 30 patients of a prospective study who presented with recalcitrant shoulder stiffness.[122]

in motion and comfort.[30, 129] This stage can be as short as 4 weeks, especially with aggressive operative treatment. However, for most patients treated nonoperatively, months to years may be required to achieve functional motion and comfort. Typically, motion slowly improves over 12 to 42 months. Several authors, however, have demonstrated a significant number of patients with persistent symptoms lasting for as long as 6 years to as many as 10 years from the onset of disease (Fig. 20–18 and see natural history).[54, 263, 272] The challenge always remains recovery of full range and normal function. With or without aggressive treatment the patient's symptoms typically resolve, but often motion restrictions persist.[22, 129]

CLINICAL PRESENTATION OF POST-TRAUMATIC STIFF SHOULDER

By definition, the patient with a post-traumatic stiff shoulder will have a history of a significant antecedent trauma. Common etiologic factors are a proximal humeral fracture, severe soft tissue contusion, or rotator cuff injury. Most often there is a history of prolonged immobilization after the traumatic event, including a lengthy postoperative immobilization. For simplicity and because anatomic features may be similar to trauma, we also include patients with stiffness after a surgical procedure. Prior operative reports are essential in understanding limitations, and the symptoms before and after surgery should be noted.

Patients who develop shoulder stiffness after a rotator cuff strain typically display a pattern of restricted asymmetric range on forward elevation, internal rotation, and cross-body adduction.[116, 178, 290] The presentation is often confused with what has been called "impingement syndrome," but many of these patients do not exhibit subacromial roughness and crepitation on examination. Motion restrictions are related to contracture of the posterior capsule[119] which, because of pain, becomes stretched infrequently. On repetitive elevation, the rotator cuff or biceps tendons may become abraded leading to subacromial roughness.[178] A shoulder that has sustained a severe eccentric load to the rotator cuff may have in-

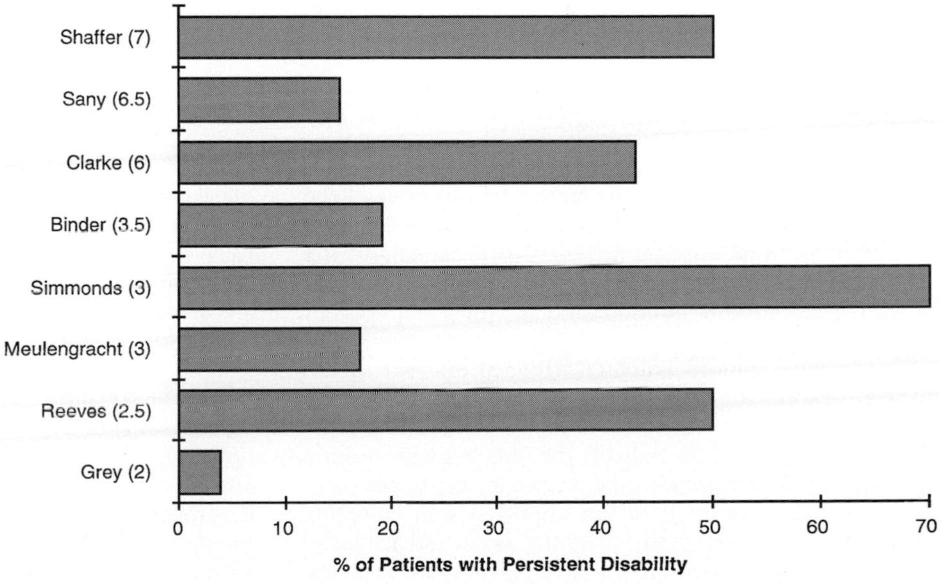

Figure 20–18

A graph showing the percentage of patients with persistent symptoms in studies that have more than 2 years of follow-up (years in parentheses after the first author). Symptoms typically extend well beyond the normal length of time expected for complete recovery.

curred a partial tendon fiber disruption. Partial rotator cuff tears, which are typically found on the deep surface of the supraspinatus or infraspinatus, are notoriously painful and often result in posterior capsular contractures.[122]

In shoulders that become symptomatic after an injury, a moderate degree of stiffness or asymmetric restrictions in shoulder motion may progress to global stiffness (see examination below). Although the history, examination, and nonoperative management of post-traumatic shoulder stiffness may be no different from that for an idiopathic frozen shoulder, the natural history of symptoms is often appreciably different because of associated damage (see Natural History and Predicting Outcome).

Postsurgical stiffness is either intentional by design or an inadvertent consequence of postoperative healing. Some surgical procedures are planned to limit glenohumeral or scapulothoracic range. For example, the Putti-Platt procedure used to correct anteroinferior shoulder instability shortens the capsule and imbricates the subscapularis tendon, intentionally limiting external rotation to prevent the shoulder joint from attaining a potentially unstable position.[219] Hawkins and Angelo have shown, however, the deleterious long-term effect of causing excessive asymmetric tightness, which can ultimately result in destructive capsulorrhaphy arthropathy.[126] Other procedures such as anterior or posterior capsular shifts for instability, rotator cuff repair, and prosthetic arthroplasty may also cause intrinsic tightening of the articular capsule and rotator cuff.

Open shoulder surgery almost always violates the motion plane external to the joint. Upon healing, adhesions between the external surface of the rotator cuff and proximal humerus and the deep surface of the deltoid, coracoacromial arch, and conjoined tendon (the so-called humeroscapular motion interface) are often identified.

If limited motion results after a surgical procedure, examination will either reveal a specific pattern of exaggerated stiffness or that of global restriction. Anterior surgical approaches that imbricate the anterior capsule and subscapularis effectively limit external rotation, whereas stiffness after rotator cuff surgery is typically global but with an accentuated posterior capsular stiffness pattern.

Examination

The examination of a patient with a painful stiff shoulder begins with both shoulders exposed. The positions of the head, neck, torso, and shoulder girdles are checked for proper alignment and symmetry. Note especially the height of each shoulder, looking for a spasmodically elevated or weak droopy shoulder and the muscular contour for localized atrophy.

The cervical spine is palpated for local tenderness and muscle spasm, starting at the occiput and continuing down the spinous processes and along paracervical muscles. It is important to palpate the musculature around the supraclavicular region and scapulae, especially near the posterosuperior angle of the scapular spine. Palpation should also be performed while the neck and shoulder are put through range of motion. A complete cervical examination includes signs for radiculopathy and a thorough neurologic and vascular examination of both upper extremities.

The shoulder examination begins with observation and palpation. Patients with chronic painful stiffness typically experience tenderness diffusely about the subacromial region, biceps tendon, and on applied pressure toward the deltoid insertion. Most report persistent discomfort around the deltoid tuberosity, even without application of local pressure.

In patients with shoulder stiffness, it is preferable to test the strength of the rotator cuff and deltoid with the arm at the side. A steady gentle force is applied to resist a patient's attempt to isometrically rotate internally and externally, abduct, forward elevate, extend, and adduct. If range will accommodate, the supraspinatus and the deltoid may also be tested against resistance in elevation. Isolated weakness in specific rotations may be indicative of a rotator cuff tear, and an ultrasound or arthrogram may be indicated (see Chapter 15). It is also important to test the strength of the distal musculature in the upper arm, forearm, and hand after examining these areas for swelling, texture, and color changes. Most patients with insidious onset of global stiffness do not exhibit signs of weakness but do experience moderate discomfort on forceful contraction. Although a rotator cuff tear and a frozen shoulder never coexist (by definition), stiffness is commonly seen with partial cuff tears (see Arthroscopic Treatment) and, much less frequently, is associated with full-thickness tears. The prevalence of a post-traumatic stiff shoulder in patients with a rotator cuff tear is unknown to the authors.

Active range of motion is observed from the anterior and posterior vantages, and six standard motion arcs are recorded. These are the standard ranges laid down by ASES.[9] Passive range is also checked at the end-point of each range to assess glenohumeral and scapulothoracic contributions to total humerothoracic range.

The six ranges of the ASES that are typically measured include (Fig. 20–19*A–E*): (1) forward elevation (sagittal plane), (2) external rotation at the side, (3) external rotation in coronal plane abduction, (4) internal rotation in coronal plane abduction (use maximum abduction if unable to assume 90 degrees), (5) cross-body adduction (measure span between the antecubital fossa and the opposite shoulder), and (6) internal rotation up the back (record tip of thumb at the highest spinous process). Some investigators also include abduction in the coronal or scapular plane, but since this measurement also requires external rotation to achieve the maximum arc and thus combine two motions, this measurement has not been included in the ASES standard examination. Ranges are always recorded for both extremities.

Clinical analysts have proposed alternate methods to simplify measurement of shoulder motion and to characterize the quantity of motion in a single factor. One author suggested a simple modification of the conventional shoulder wheel to provide the therapist, patient, and physician with an objective assessment of the shoulder range.[7] Other investigators have calculated a single number based on two to six measured ranges.[40, 116, 122, 159] These measures often prove useful in monitoring a

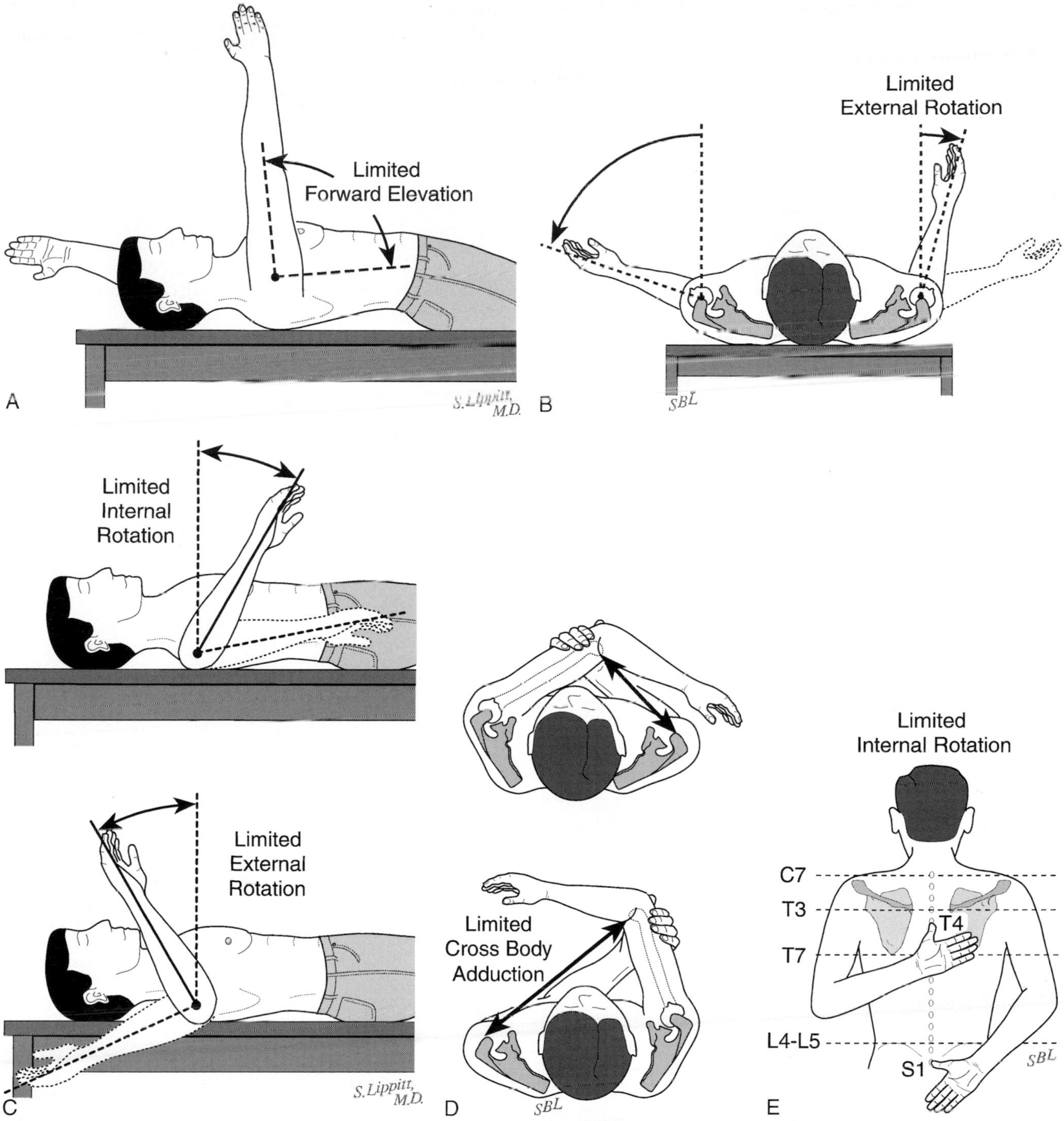

Figure 20–19

A, Active humerothoracic elevation is performed supine in the sagittal plane with comfortable rotation. A goniometer is placed in line with the humerus and long axis of the thorax for measurement. *B,* Active external rotation at the side is easily performed supine with the elbow one handbreadth from the thorax. A goniometer is placed in line with the forearm and perpendicular to the surface of the table. *C,* Active external and internal rotation in coronal plane abduction is performed supine. A goniometer is placed in line with the forearm and perpendicular to the surface of the table. *D,* Active assisted cross-body adduction is performed supine with the opposite unaffected extremity pulling the elbow toward the opposite shoulder. The distance between the antecubital fossa and the opposite shoulder is recorded in centimeters. *E,* Active internal rotation up the back is performed in the upright position. The highest spinous process reached with the thumb tip is recorded.

patient's progress or response to treatment and afford simple comparison. Combined measures, however, do not allow independent characterization of an isolated or specific group of motions (see later).

In order to accommodate all future combinations of independently measured motion arcs, we recommend recording six active motions at each visit and comparing these measurements with those of the opposite extremity (Fig. 20–20*A, B*). Each motion measured for the symptomatic shoulder is divided by the range of the asymptomatic shoulder to yield a ratio in which unity indicates functional symmetry with the opposite side. Graphics for a particular range (see Fig. 20–20*A, B*) or stiffness ratio (Fig. 20–21) can be generated to show patients their progress or final assessment relative to others. The mean ratios of total capsular stiffness (TCS), posterior capsular stiffness (PCS), or anterior capsular stiffness (ACS) for a specific shoulder can be calculated by combining the ratios for specific ranges and dividing by the total number as shown:

Stiffness ratio (SR) is the symptomatic range/asymptomatic range

TCS:

$$TCS_{SR} = (FE_{SR} + ERS_{SR} + ERA_{SR} + IRA_{SR} + IRB_{SR} + XBA_{SR})/6$$

PCS:

$$PCS_{SR} = (FE_{SR} + IRB_{SR} + XBA_{SR})/3$$

ACS:

$$ACS_{SR} = (ERS_{SR} + ERA_{SR})/2$$

Note that no range is ever recorded as 0 degrees,

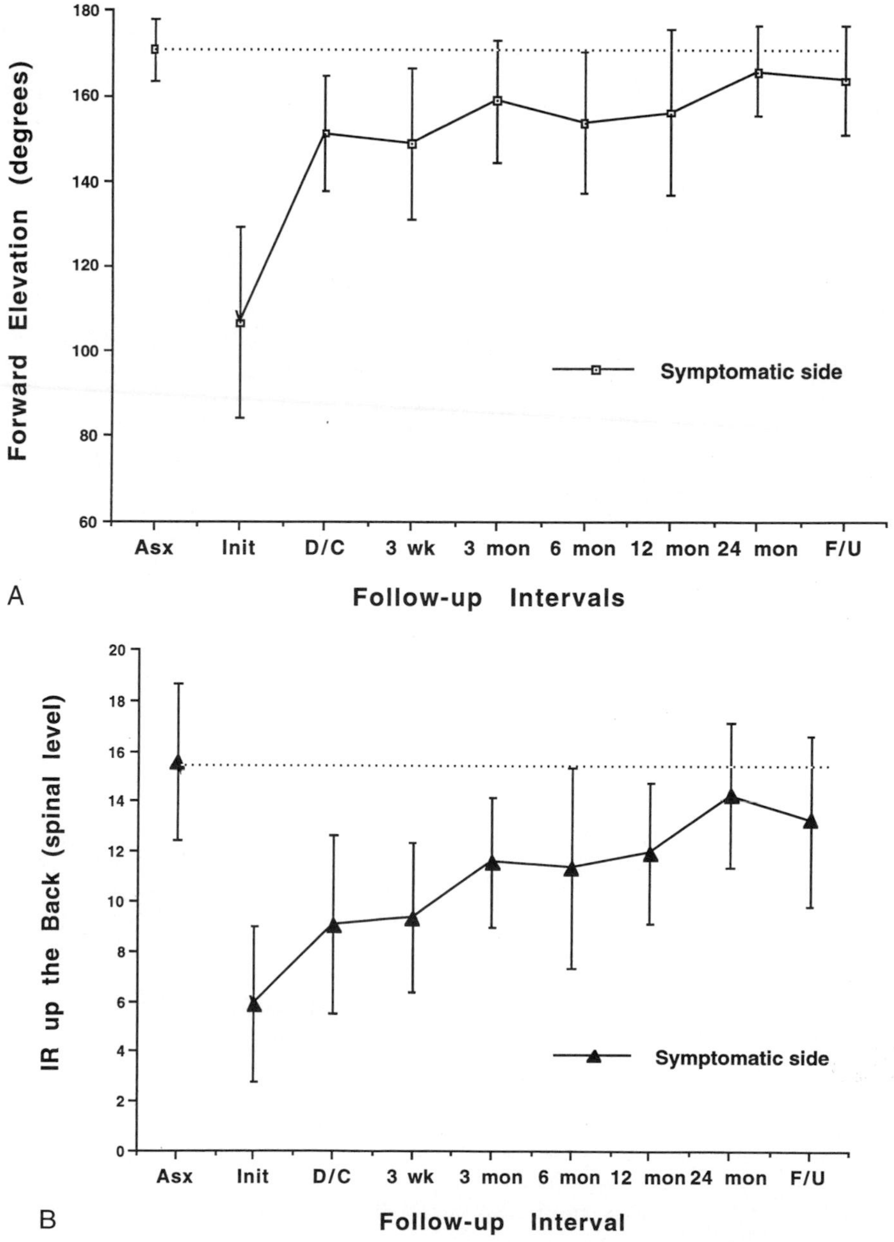

Figure 20–20

A, Marked improvement in the range of forward elevation occurred with arthroscopic capsular release. Range recovered rapidly for the motion of forward elevation compared with five other measured ranges (contrast with internal rotation up the back, see *B*). Thirty patients with a 2-year follow-up (meal ± 1 SD). (Asx, asymptomatic side; Init, range prior to release; D/C, range at hospital discharge; F/U, range at longest follow-up.) (From Harryman D II, Sidles J, and Matsen F III: Arthroscopic management of refractory shoulder stiffness. Arthroscopy *13*:133–147, 1997.) *B,* Compare the rate of improvement after arthroscopic capsular release for internal rotation up the back against forward elevation *(A)*. Internal rotation was improved least after release but slowly increased by the 2-year follow-up (mean ± 1 SD). (Asx, asymptomatic side; Init, range prior to release; D/C, range at hospital discharge; F/U, range at longest follow-up.) (From Harryman DT II, Sidles JA, and Matsen FA III: Arthroscopic management of refractory shoulder stiffness. Arthroscopy *13*:133–147, 1997.)

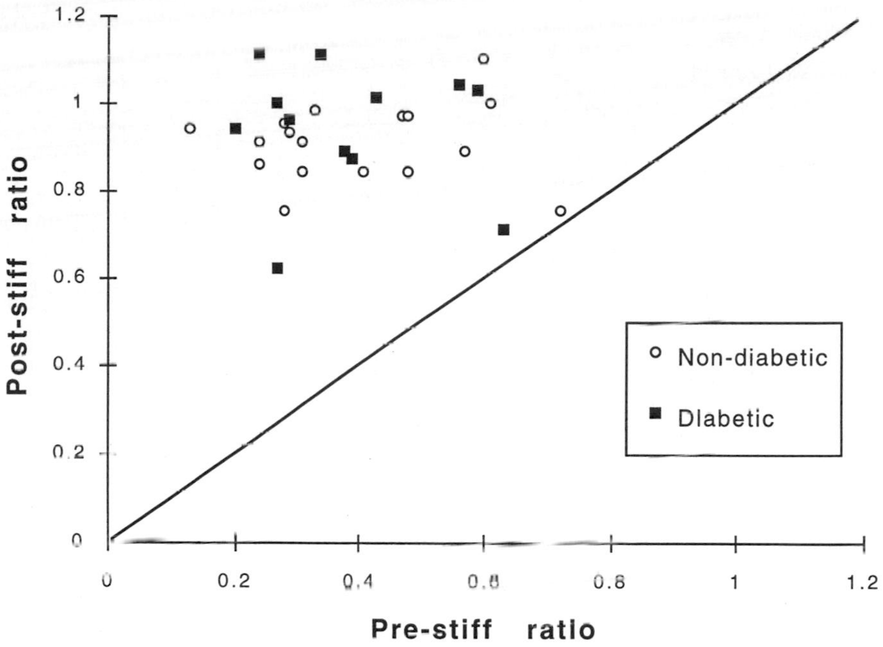

Figure 20–21

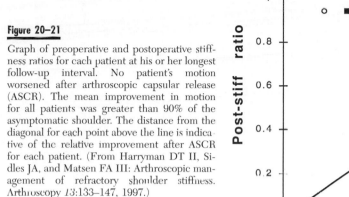

Graph of preoperative and postoperative stiffness ratios for each patient at his or her longest follow-up interval. No patient's motion worsened after arthroscopic capsular release (ASCR). The mean improvement in motion for all patients was greater than 90% of the asymptomatic shoulder. The distance from the diagonal for each point above the line is indicative of the relative improvement after ASCR for each patient. (From Harryman DT II, Sidles JA, and Matsen FA III: Arthroscopic management of refractory shoulder stiffness. Arthroscopy *13*:133–147, 1997.)

instead 1 degree is recorded to avoid numerators that yield a meaningless number. When the SR is unity, range is symmetric. These ratios could also be used for studies of bilateral stiffness but require the use of normal age-adjusted means[54, 189] for comparison, otherwise improvement after release will appear excessive relative to the opposite side.

Individual ranges and combined ratios were used to test whether differences in the severity of stiffness or the pattern of stiffness could be characterized among stiffness in groups separated by pathology. Patients with an idiopathic frozen shoulder typically have global restrictions in range. With two notable exceptions, a post-traumatic stiff shoulder often exhibits decreases in motion for all ranges. These exceptions are: (1) the postsurgical stiff shoulder after anterior reconstructions for instability, and (2) the post-traumatic posterior capsular contracture after a rotator cuff strain or partial rotator cuff tear.

One-hundred and seventeen patients with refractory shoulder stiffness have been enrolled prospectively into a specific management protocol (Fig. 20–22). A complete evaluation that included the six ranges listed earlier were measured for each patient at their initial visit. Patients were separated according to established diagnostic criteria,[178] into those with a frozen shoulder (49) and those with post-traumatic stiff shoulder (68). Patients who developed stiffness after an injury had significantly less overall stiffness ($P < .02$; TCS = 0.48) than did those who developed stiffness insidiously (TCS = 0.38). Patients who developed stiffness after an injury had significantly less restriction in flexion or external rotation at the side or in abduction for external and internal rotation (see Table 20–3). No significant differences were noted for the range of internal rotation up the back and cross-body adduction, although these groups were distinctly different. Although we are unable to explain why these latter motions were similar whereas all other motions were strikingly distinct, it may be attributed to a significant scapulothoracic contribution associated with measuring these motions.[15]

Clarke and associates measured the shoulder motion of normal individuals and those with painful stiff shoulders.[54] They compared the motion of stiff shoulders to that of age- and sex-matched normal control shoulders and expressed the reduction in range for movement of the stiff shoulder as a percentage of the control population. Their method provides an opportunity to relate the severity of restricted range in patients who suffer from bilateral shoulder stiffness.

Supplementary Clinical Assessment

BLOOD TESTS

After a thorough history and physical examination, the clinician must decide whether hematologic tests are necessary. The routine patient with shoulder stiffness does not need laboratory studies for diagnosis or management.[24, 251] A blood count, differential smear, and an erythrocyte sedimentation rate (ESR), however, should be requested when a recent change in the patient's health status has occurred. Lequesne found an abnormal glucose tolerance test result in 28% of new patients with a frozen shoulder; therefore, this test should be considered especially when there is a positive family history of diabetes.[162] In a prospective study of 50 patients with a diagnosis of primary frozen shoulder, Bunker and Esler measured the serum lipid levels and compared them with age-matched and sex-matched controls.[46] They found significantly elevated fasting serum triglyceride and cholesterol levels in the frozen shoulder group. If the history, physical examination, and routine radiographs point to a musculoskeletal condition localized to the shoulder, there is less need to order additional ancillary tests or consultations.

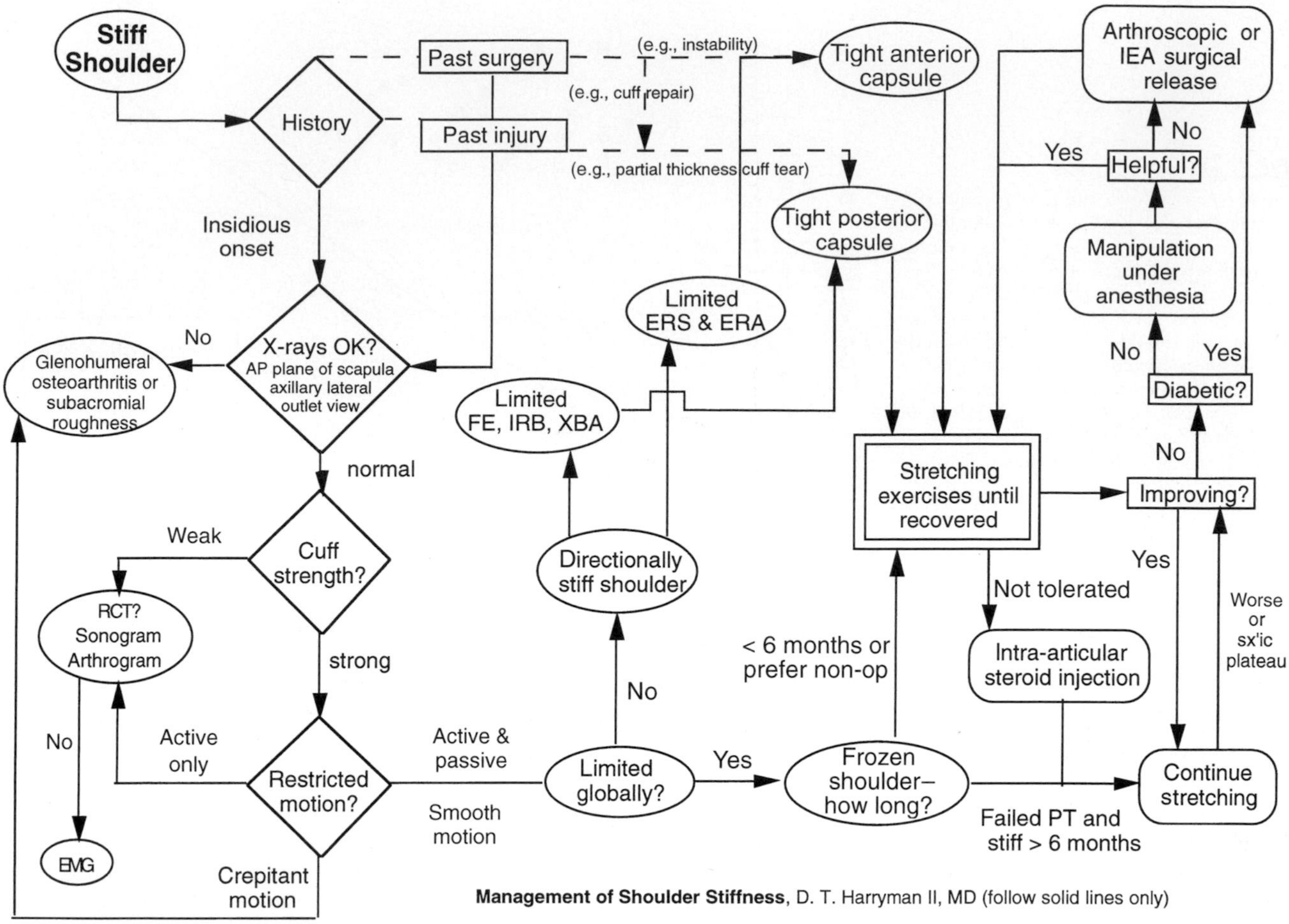

Figure 20–22

Evaluation and treatment algorithm for the stiff shoulder.

Investigators have searched for specific blood indices or markers that would be useful to predict the severity of disease and to monitor the progression or outcome of treatment. As in osteomyelitis or other chronic inflammation, we might expect an elevated ESR. A few reports have indicated that the ESR was elevated in up to 20% of patients with a frozen shoulder with some response to treatment.[22, 89, 182, 237, 259] In clinical practice and in more recent studies, however, the ESR has not proved to be reliable or useful when evaluating or monitoring the response to anti-inflammatory drugs or steroid agents.[149, 318] Bulgen and associates reported on the immune status of 40 patients who were diagnosed with frozen shoulder.[39] They found that pretreatment increased immune complex levels and decreased cellular-mediated indicators compared with a control group. Eight months after being diagnosed, each patient was retested, and values tended to approach control levels. Others have studied the presence of the HLA-B27 histocompatibility antigen in patients with a frozen shoulder, but on extended review, the marker is identified no more frequently than in the control group.[254, 269, 279, 318]

NONINVASIVE IMAGING

Routine Radiographs

Radiographs are essential to diagnose a frozen or post-traumatic stiff shoulder.[178] Plain radiographs are needed to rule out abnormalities in the bone (e.g., tumor) or in the local soft tissues (e.g., calcific deposit or heterotopic ossification). The history and physical examination may provide clues that are often helpful in the examination of the plain radiographs. For example, narrowing of the clear space between the subchondral surface of the humeral head and the glenoid may, in addition to the examination, be a clue of early degenerative arthritis.[81]

It is important to obtain at least two orthogonal views of the joint to rule out occult fractures, loose bodies, humeral head displacement and blocking osteophytes. In our clinic, we have seen patients referred with shoulder stiffness only to find a posterior dislocation on the axillary radiograph! The shoulder screening series at the University of Washington includes:

1. An anteroposterior radiograph perpendicular to the plane of the scapula with the humerus positioned in 35 degrees of external rotation (relative to the plane of the scapula)
2. The same view with internal rotation to the body
3. A true axillary view

Combined with the history and physical examination, these three views provide all the information necessary to classify shoulder stiffness (see Diagnostic Criteria).

Routine shoulder radiographs in patients with shoulder stiffness are typically normal.[22] Decreased bone density of the humeral head, however, is a fairly frequent finding on x-rays of patients with frozen shoulder syndrome and may be related to prolonged disuse.[22, 169, 245] Lundberg found approximately 50% loss of bone in a short period of time in 74 cases of frozen shoulder.[169] He attributed this loss in bone mass to an inflammatory process because the degree of loss could not be explained by disuse and immobilization alone. Radiographic changes in bone structure may often be seen postoperatively, such as after an acromioplasty. Narrowing of the subacromial space has been observed in patients who have stiffness associated with rotator cuff disease.[22]

When sentinel clues on the history and physical examination indicate potential risk in regions extrinsic to the shoulder, it is important to obtain routine cervical spine films (e.g., radicular symptoms/signs), a chest x-ray (e.g., cough or chest pain), or radiographs of the entire humerus (e.g., bone pain or tenderness below the deltoid tuberosity). If symptoms are unrelenting, atypical, or unresponsive, a high index of suspicion for systemic disease is necessary.

Bone Scans

In shoulder stiffness, a bone scan is particularly useful to rule out a neoplastic disorder or an autonomic dystrophy; however, it has not proved to be useful in the diagnosis, management, or prognosis of a frozen shoulder. Binder and colleagues used diphosphonate scans and found that 90% of their patients with a frozen shoulder had increased uptake on the symptomatic side, and almost a third demonstrated a 50% increase over baseline activity on the unaffected side.[23] They did not find an association between bone scan activity and the severity of disease, duration of symptoms, arthrographic findings, or ultimate outcome.

Most investigators have reported the use of radionuclide scanning in the frozen shoulder using technetium 99m (^{99m}Tc) pertechnetate or methylene diphosphonate uptake. Shoulder pain and an increased ^{99m}Tc pertechnetate have been related as opposed to a ^{99}Tc methylene diphosphonate scan.[282] Although a bone scan may not show differences in uptake between a frozen shoulder or an autonomic reflex dystrophy, it has proved to be useful to separate these conditions because the hand, the wrist, and the entire limb may show increased uptake in the latter.[154] Lastly, Wright and associates found that 4 of 10 patients with adhesive capsulitis who demonstrated a rapid response to corticosteroid injections with resolution of symptoms also had positive bone scans, but this association has not been duplicated.[314]

Magnetic Resonance Imaging and Ultrasound

In recent years, MRI has been used in clinical assessment of the stiff shoulder. Emig and colleagues reported on the characteristics of MRI in 10 patients diagnosed with a frozen shoulder compared with normal shoulders.[82] In those diagnosed with a frozen shoulder, they found a combined thickness of greater than 4 mm in the joint capsule and synovium. They did not note significant differences in the volume of intra-articular fluid seen on the MRI scan or on the thickness of the rotator cuff and rotator interval capsule. In another study that used MRI, Bernageau and associates did find an increased thickness of the rotator cuff as well as synovitis and bursitis in patients undergoing hemodialysis who had chronic shoulder stiffness for more than 6 months.[18]

A few investigators have reported on the use of dynamic sonography in the evaluation of adhesive capsulitis.[90, 260, 265, 270] Ryu and colleagues noted that the main sonographic feature of adhesive capsulitis was a constant limitation of the sliding movement of the supraspinatus tendon against the scapula.[260] They reported 91% sensitivity, 100% specificity, and an accuracy of 92% against arthrography as the gold standard for diagnosis. Because of the noninvasive method and accuracy in detecting adhesive capsulitis, they claimed that "dynamic sonography is a reliable technique for the diagnosis for this condition."

Considering the sufficient and necessary diagnostic criteria, we have not found it useful to request an MRI or a sonographic examination to make the diagnosis of a frozen or post-traumatic stiff shoulder. We do, however, recognize the clinical advantage of identifying partial or complete rotator cuff tears in patients who present with shoulder stiffness.[170, 177] These imaging studies fail to provide additional clinical information beneficial in classifying, treating, or predicting outcome.

ARTHROGRAPHY

Intra-Articular Pressure Measurement

Since a great deal of confusion has surrounded the nomenclature and diagnostic criteria used to describe the painful stiff shoulder, clinicians and investigators have searched for a simple diagnostic test that would assist in classification. It seems reasonable to consider closer examination of the capsule by indirect imaging methods because the joint capsule is visibly contracted in most stiff shoulder conditions. Murnaghan reminds us that the use of arthrography in shoulder stiffness is not a routine adjunct in the diagnosis or necessary in prescribing a treatment.[187, 188] The senior author only uses arthrography in patients with shoulder stiffness and rotator cuff weakness in whom ultrasonography has been difficult to perform or inconclusive. In these cases, ultrasonography requires a certain degree of mobility and may be less useful to visualize small tears in the rotator cuff tendons.

In 1957, after Neviaser revealed the contracted nature of the articular capsule, Kernwein and associates performed arthrographic studies in 12 patients with adhesive capsulitis.[148] On open biopsy they found that the capsule and coracohumeral ligament were very contracted, thickened, and inelastic with the presence subacute inflammation. Later, Neviaser described arthrographic findings of adhesive capsulitis that included decreased joint capacity; obliteration of the reflected axillary fold; and variable filling of the bicipital tendon sheath.[197] Other studies employing arthrography added more findings, such as frequent obliteration of the subscapularis bursa, poor visualization of the biceps sheath, a joint capacity of less than 10 to 12 ml, dye filling short of the humeral neck, a moth-eaten appearance to the capsular insertion on the humerus, and the observation of escaping dye through the ruptured subscapularis bursa and axillary recess after manipulation.[2, 130, 167, 168, 199, 201, 241, 244, 305] Arthrography has also been used to demonstrate the presence and location of joint capsule disruption during pressure injection and manipulation under anesthesia.[2, 86, 168, 241, 279] Recently, in an attempt to enhance arthrography, injection of air and contrast were touted superior to contrast alone for reasons of improved visualization along the margins of the joint and capsule, and improved tolerance in terms of patient comfort.[97, 291]

Lundberg and others showed a positive correlation between arthrographic contraction of the axillary pouch and range of motion.[130, 168, 198, 204, 241] A legitimate correlation can only be accomplished, however, by controlling for a defined volume of contrast medium or measurement of the intra-articular pressure during injection. Lundberg claimed that a normal range of motion could be detected in a shoulder joint that on arthrography showed a greatly decreased capacity and complete obliteration of the axillary pouch and subscapularis bursa.[168] Although contracture of the axillary pouch has been well documented,[197, 262] the extent of posterior capsule distention has not been assessed in the post-traumatic stiff shoulder even though contracture of the posterior pouch has been seen clinically in relative isolation.[116, 122, 290] Itoi and colleagues found only mild correlation between external and internal rotation with anterior capsular and axillary pouch filling of the dye, respectively.[140]

Intra-articular volume and pressure measurement have also been correlated with the restriction of shoulder range.[168, 198, 241] Resnick and associates observed a gradual increase in pressure on arthrographic fluid injection in normal individuals with a rapid increase in pressure for patients diagnosed with adhesive capsulitis.[246] They found that in a healthy shoulder, the intra-articular pressure in a resting position is less than 0 mm Hg. With dynamic contraction and elevation, pressure typically rose to above 90 mm Hg with the arm overhead, whereas patients with a contracted shoulder or a defect in the rotator cuff peaked in the range of 60 mm Hg. The early rise in pressure with elevation of the extremity[124] and a marked increase in pressure on continuous intra-articular fluid injection point to a decrease in compliance of the capsular containment.[209, 241, 246]

Proponents of arthrography claim its usefulness in standardizing classification and in selecting patients for clinical research.[167, 180, 196, 204] Reeves and Neviaser explain the use of arthrographic findings to differentiate between a true frozen shoulder and a post-traumatic or painful stiff shoulder.[203, 241] We have found that our diagnostic criteria are sufficient to differentiate these conditions.[178] No correlation between arthrographic findings and treatment outcome has been found.[23, 167] As seen with intra-articular injection studies, the presence of a contracted joint volume does not mitigate against clinical findings of a frozen shoulder.[168, 197] Lastly, many of these diagnostic injection studies were combined with steroids and manipulation in the treatment of the stiff shoulder (see Treatment; brisement, steroids).

ARTHROSCOPY

Many reports illustrate how arthroscopy has been used in cases of shoulder stiffness to: (1) evaluate pathologic changes to the glenohumeral joint and subacromial space, (2) recognize problems associated with shoulder stiffness (e.g., a tendon or labral tear), and, (3) determine the local effects of closed manipulation.[30, 108, 123, 202, 213–215, 231, 300, 307–309] We should, however, keep in mind what Neviaser and Neviaser have written: "arthroscopy is *not* a means of establishing a diagnosis."[202]

The arthroscopic findings of a frozen shoulder begin outside the joint on introduction of the trocar through the posterior capsule. Generally, insertion of the trocar is swift and simple. Shoulders with a contracted and fibrotic capsule, however, typically require additional insertional force.[122, 202, 213] On entry, the contracted space not only restricts visibility but also the ability to maneuver about the joint. In early phases, a mild to moderate red inflammatory synovitic carpet of variable thickness is evident especially under the rotator interval capsule, along the biceps tendon root, superior labrum, and posterior capsule (Fig. 20–23).[71, 108, 116, 122, 204, 308]

Neviaser described four arthroscopic stages of adhesive capsulitis and proposed that these stages could be used to guide treatment planning.[202] Their stages are: (1) a mild erythematous synovitis, (2) acute synovitis with adhesions in the dependent folds of the synovial lining, (3) maturation of adhesions with less reactive synovitis, and (4) chronic adhesions without synovitis. Other arthroscopists have found the articular surface free from capsular adhesions and have rarely identified adhesions in the recesses or dependent fold.[108, 122, 213, 308] These clinical observations detract from the "adhesive" nature of the

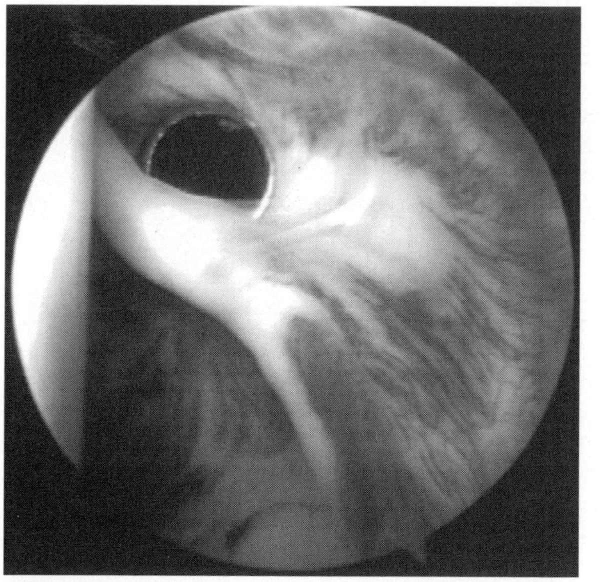

Figure 20–23

Arthroscopic view of inflamed hypervascular synovial proliferation along the biceps tendon root, rotator interval capsule, and posterosuperior capsule. Note that the proximal biceps tendon and root are adherent to the undersurface of the synovium and deep capsular layer under the rotator cuff (note the synovium fails to wrap around the biceps as in a mesosynovium).

capsular process and lend credence to the proliferative fibrosis leading to capsuloligamentous contractures.

The arthroscopic findings immediately after a successful manipulative release have been noted to include: an intra-articular hemarthroses, avulsion of the inferior capsule usually adjacent or peripheral to the labrum (Fig. 20–24), tears in the rotator interval capsule with occasional labral avulsions, or capsular tears anterosuperiorly or anteroinferiorly.[77, 122, 202, 213, 214, 231, 296]

Arthroscopists are also quick to point out the usefulness in identifying associated intra-articular pathology that had not been identified by means of a history or clinical examination.[122, 213, 231] Arthroscopy affords the opportunity to recognize these pathologies and direct proper rehabilitation once stiffness has resolved or to surgically address when appropriately indicated.

EXAMINATION UNDER ANESTHESIA

There are occasions when a clinical history, age of presentation, or examination fail to fit the diagnostic criteria, yet particular elements seem appropriate to a frozen or post-traumatic stiff shoulder. For example, an apprehensive or sensitive patient might present with a fixed restraint and have no restriction in shoulder range, but muscle spasm or an inability to actively relax prevents an adequate passive motion examination. These patients typically are younger than 40 years of age, and some have had previous surgery. For these patients we consider an examination after administration of a regional or general anesthetic to eliminate inhibitory painful or anxious reflexes. In our experience, we have found some without any motion restrictions and a stable shoulder or, rarely, a partial limitation and severe grinding secondary to articular damage with associated anterior or posterior instability. Appropriate rehabilitation exercises or further surgical treatment is then arranged.

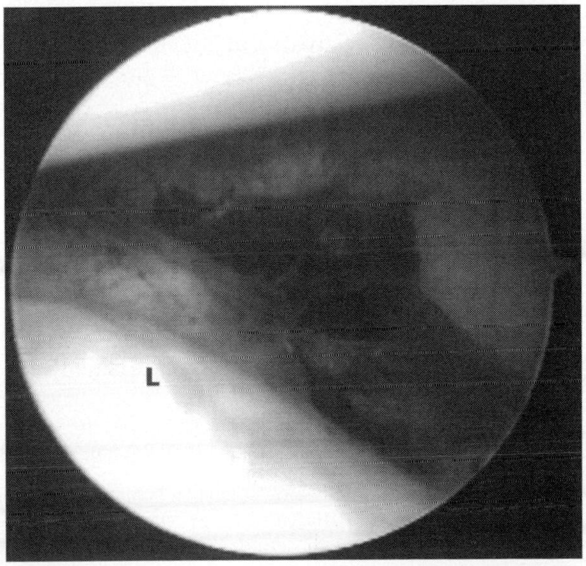

Figure 20–24

The contracted inferior capsule was avulsed during the manipulation away from the inferior peripheral articular labrum (L). Inferior capsular tears are often found to extend anterior and posterior through the recesses.

NATURAL HISTORY OF SYMPTOMS AND OUTCOME

For any diagnosis, treatment decisions are based on a known course for a disease. Effective treatment is begun only when it is believed to positively change the natural history of the disease. The natural history of idiopathic or post-traumatic frozen shoulder, however, is not entirely known and remains controversial. The majority of "natural history" long-term follow-up reports were performed in conjunction with the evaluation of the patient's response to a particular treatment regimen.

For years, much of the literature has referred to the idiopathic frozen shoulder as a self limiting disease.[55, 242, 263, 302] Even these studies, however, describe the process as lasting 12 to 18 months prior to resolution.[104, 109, 168, 310, 311] Others have described residual pain or stiffness many years after a frozen shoulder that may or may not be significantly disabling.[22, 104, 242, 272] Differentiation of these outcomes is critical when deciding on the appropriate treatment. If indeed frozen shoulder is a process that will resolve independent of treatment, only palliative treatment is necessary and patients should be encouraged to accommodate their temporary disability.[155] If, however, frozen shoulder is a debilitating, long-standing, and sometimes permanent process, aggressive treatment should begin immediately upon diagnosis.

Most patients cannot tolerate a debilitating chronically painful extremity during productive years of life and are concerned about the possibility of developing permanent dysfunction. Patients not only expect the physician to diagnose the condition but also to prognosticate how long it will take to recover. Studies with follow-up of more than 2 years and as long as 7 years have consistently demonstrated persistent symptoms in a large percentage of patients (see Fig. 20–18). Meulengracht and associates followed 65 patients for 3 years and found that 23% had persistent pain and limitation of shoulder motion.[182] Reeves followed 41 patients for more than 4 years and identified residual stiffness in more than 60% with 12% of this group displaying severe restriction in motion.[241]

Typically, a discrepancy may exist between a patient's perspective of functional limitation and that of measured motion restrictions by the physician. At a 3½-year follow-up, Binder and associates found an objective motion restriction in 16 of 40 patients, yet only a few recognized symptomatic functional impairment.[22] This result was quite different from the findings of Shaffer and colleagues. They followed 68 patients with frozen shoulder for approximately 7 years. On objective motion measurement, 30% were restricted when compared with the opposite unaffected side; however, after lodging the patient's perspectives, 50% complained of persistent pain or stiffness.[272]

Some prospective studies intended to demonstrate a particular benefit of one treatment over another, only to find that either all or none of the treatment regimens shortened the duration, thus concluding that patients would have recovered with or without intervention.[12, 40, 63, 72] Again in stark contrast, other authors, who performed comparative studies to demonstrate the benefit of one treatment over another, suggested that early presentation and early treatment results in early recovery.[22, 128, 242] Lastly, Helbig and co-workers and Harryman and colleagues observed that the degree of disability and the duration of symptoms prior to treatment in patients without diabetes had no influence on the final outcome, but that treatment appeared to effectively abbreviate the disease course.[122, 130]

Regression analyses have been performed to assess significant variables that would best prognosticate the course of disease. Dominant arm involvement has been reported as a good prognostic indicator, whereas patient occupation, ability to work, duration of stiffness, associated injuries, and the treatment program used did not achieve statistical significance when analyzed against other outcome measures.[22, 54, 122] The finding of an associated intrinsic pathology such as a partial-thickness rotator cuff tear[122] or insulin-dependent diabetes of more than 10 years would tend to indicate a poorer prognosis.[92, 142, 184]

TREATMENT

The choice of treatment for shoulder stiffness should always be aligned according to the duration and severity of symptoms in order to avoid undertreatment or overtreatment. Since shoulder stiffness often develops in response to a known variety of initiating factors, it is important to consider the potential cause or underlying disease and the appropriate timing of treatment in the context of the patient's needs, risk factors, and tolerance. Two examples follow.

Treating the Source of the Pain

If a patient develops a frozen shoulder subsequent to painful cervical radiculitis, it is most appropriate primarily to address the herniated cervical disk to eliminate the source of pain while encouraging a gentle shoulder stretching program instead of first manipulating the shoulder to restore full range. The symptoms in the neck will likely prevent adequate shoulder rehabilitation.

Treating the Stiffness

If a patient has a small rotator cuff tear and secondarily developed shoulder stiffness, it is important to treat the shoulder stiffness as the primary problem in order to fully recover range of motion before considering a rotator cuff repair. A rotator cuff tear may improve with rehabilitation alone, and a repair is often a "shoulder-tightening" procedure that may result in increased stiffness postoperatively.

These examples enumerate cases with a recognizable "cause and effect" of shoulder stiffness. After the physician has exhausted the differential diagnosis, however, we are frequently left with idiopathic stiffness which, on its own, must always be treated aggressively to prevent progression of disease. A specific plan that follows an appropriate algorithm and presents the least risk to the patient is best (see Fig. 20–22).

In the painful phase of shoulder stiffness, it is often beneficial to reduce discomfort using methods that do not involve narcotics. Ice or heat, rest or activity, support or traction, electrical or ultrasonic stimulation, chiropractic mobilization, and many other "modalities" have been used to reduce pain, but few have shown significant benefit relative to another.

In the review of treatment that follows, there are six major groups of therapeutic approaches, each of which includes a variety of therapeutic regimens. These six treatment categories consist of:

1. Supportive treatment, including observation and passive external modalities such as immobilization, heat, ice, diathermy, ultrasound, transcutaneous electrical nerve stimulation (TENS), massage, and others
2. Medications given orally, topically, and parenterally (local and intra-articular), such as nonsteroidal anti-inflammatory agents, analgesics, narcotics, neuroleptics, enzymatic preparations, and corticosteroids
3. Stretching exercises or traction, applied by the patient, mechanically by a device, or by an assistant; typically consisting of gentle stretching, with or without muscle activity along with daily functional activities
4. Injections of fluid, arthrographic dye, or medications (e.g., long-acting anesthetic agents with or without corticosteroids) for the purpose of joint distention to release capsular contracture (brisement)
5. Manipulative therapy with or without anesthesia to release adhesions or contracted structures
6. Surgical release of adhesions or contracted structures by open or arthroscopic means

Prophylaxis

The primary method of treatment for either a frozen or post-traumatic stiff shoulder is the same–prevention! The initial challenge is to avoid the natural tendency of most treating physicians to immobilize the extremity until comfort returns. The period of enforced immobilization, while provisionally somewhat comforting to the patient, will prolong and worsen the capsular contracture, delay diagnosis of an underlying condition, and may begin a self-propagating spiral of unrelenting shoulder pain, immobilization, and predictable motion losses in all ranges. We recommend instituting a gentle active-assisted range of motion program that intends to push the patient's limits immediately upon presentation.

ANALGESICS

Nonsteroidal anti-inflammatory drugs or salicylates and even nonsalicylate analgesics such as acetaminophen are said to be effective in alleviating the painful distress of shoulder stiffness.[21, 35, 251] The degree of relief from stiff shoulder conditions has been used frequently to test and compare a wide range of nonsteroidal anti-inflammatory medications.[28, 74, 87, 101, 138]

Analgesics and suitable anti-inflammatory agents can be given systematically or applied locally.[205] Binder found that patients experienced greater pain relief using nonsalicylate analgesics as opposed to nonsteroidal agents.[21] Lee and associates were able to show that patients who did exercises regularly demonstrated greater improvement when analgesics were added.[158] The use of analgesics, therefore, should be combined with an early gentle stretching exercise program.

INJECTIONS

Injections are often offered as an attempt to directly suppress or potentially eliminate the irritative source of the pain. Because an inflammatory phase is part of the pathophysiologic evolution of these painful conditions, the use of corticosteroids has been often advocated. Their use is not without risk or morbidity (see later). The literature is extremely controversial as to the benefit of this treatment.

Periarticular Injections

Well-localized painful periscapular areas are defined as "trigger" or "tender points." Trigger point injections are generally performed about the subscapularis tendon and the periscapular musculature to reduce symptoms of myofascial pain or fibrositis.[293] Some clinicians inject these painful sites with local anesthetics such as lidocaine or bupivacaine admixed with a steroid such as hydrocortisone. The effectiveness of these treatments is unknown to the authors.

Injections in other sites at the point of maximum tenderness about the shoulder and the periarticular region have been tried and found to be unsuccessful in providing long-term benefit or pain relief.[135, 186] On the other hand, Steinbrocker and Argyros reported rather surprising results with 85% restoration of function in 95% of 42 patients after multiple injections into the supraspinatus tendon, subdeltoid bursa, bicipital tendon, and joint capsule.[281] No control group, however, was provided.

Paired Injections

A paired injection refers to a "shot-gun" method of delivering local anesthetic and steroid in the subacromial bursa and another inside the joint in attempt to eliminate "pain and inflammation." Using comparative treatment regimens, studies by Richardson and Bulgen failed to show a significant difference or improvement of pain relief and increase in shoulder movement at follow-up examination after paired injections with deposition of steroids.[40, 248] Possibly, an inaccurate injection location is responsible for the poor response. It is rare to find a physician who is absolutely confident in accurate localization of deposition. Richardson monitored attempts at intra-articular injections using radiopaque dye and noted that the majority of physicians were unsuccessful in delivering the fluid into the shoulder joint.[248] Weiss and associates recommended routine use of arthrography in order to deliver an intra-articular dose of steroids.[305]

In England, Dacre and associates compared the use of local steroids against physiotherapy in a prospective randomized observer-blind trial to assess cost and efficacy of conventional nonoperative therapy for the painful stiff shoulder. Their results show that local steroid injections were as effective as physiotherapy alone or in combination. They provided rapid treatment and were less expensive. In the uncomplicated case, a local steroid injection was the most cost-effective treatment.[63]

Patients referred to our clinic are often relieved when we assure them that our primary treatment will not involve repetitive steroid injections. We believe that steroid injections are overused and that patients should not be treated with an exhaustive series of injections to reduce pain. We recognize that other investigators, however, have found injections of methylprednisolone to be significantly beneficial.[259]

Intra-Articular Injections

MacNab proposed an autoimmune hypothesis for the frozen shoulder whereby the degenerative tendon of the supraspinatus released proteinaceous fragments that invoke an inflammatory foreign body response in the glenohumeral joint.[171, 172] Assuming that this is true, steroids may suppress the painful inflammatory response. On the other hand, the deleterious effects of intra-articular steroid on tendon metabolism and articular hyaline cartilage are well documented.[65, 147, 285]

Studies that evaluate the response to intra-articular injections generally combine the injection with other treatment modalities and rarely compare the efficacy of deposition steroids alone. Williams compared repetitive intra-articular injections of hydrocortisone acetate against serial stellate ganglion blocks, but all patients were also instructed on an exercise program and given analgesics.[310] At follow-up, the investigators were unable to demonstrate improvement in half of the patients who received steroids, and there were no significant differences in treatment groups. In a combined comparative treatment study, Lee and associates failed to show a benefit by combining intra-articular hydrocortisone injections with exercises compared with heat and exercises; however, overall, they found that patients improved more than those who used analgesics alone.[159]

Cyriax found no benefit in intra-articular hydrocortisone injections, and Quin reported that his experience with these injections in the treatment of frozen shoulder was not encouraging.[62, 238] Quin went on to say, however, that "a local injection of hydrocortisone may give some relief of pain in cases of frozen shoulder, but it has very little affect in restoring movement."[238]

Some investigators are advocates of intra-articular steroid injections for painful shoulder stiffness.[135, 141, 236, 288, 305] Hollingworth and colleagues were able to demonstrate that intra-articular steroid injections were advantageous over trigger point injections.[135] They reported that one quarter of the patients with frozen shoulder received benefit from an intra-articular injection, whereas none of the other patients who received the other treatment were relieved. Thomas and associates demonstrated 50% improvement in pain scores after intra-articular injection and only a 13% increase in range of motion.[288] Steroid injections have not been shown to improve the rate of recovery in shoulder range.[167, 238]

There is a small but substantial risk of infection with intra-articular injections. Over the past 8 years, we have seen six cases of chronic sepsis referred to our practice after steroid and arthrographic injection. In some of these cases, the only treatment possible was shoulder fusion. Seradge reported a case of fatal clostridial myonecrosis that occurred after an intra-articular injection of steroids to the shoulder.[271] With these data in mind, it behooves the practitioner to prepare the skin and handle the procedure as though it were surgical.

At the University of Washington, we have found the occasional patient who is unable to tolerate physical therapy exercises solely because of intractable pain. Occasionally, these patients are relieved adequately after an intra-articular steroid injection to tolerate an exercise program (see Fig. 20–22). If a steroid injection appears indicated, remember that use of steroids in diabetic patients often causes blood glucose fluctuations and may incur greater risk of infection. We do not advocate *routine* use of intra-articular steroid injections for treatment of shoulder stiffness.

Physiotherapy

Physiotherapy in the form of gentle, firm stretching exercises in various planes of motion has been proved to be effective in the relief of pain and recovery of range of motion in up to 90% of patients with chronic frozen shoulder.[223] In 226 frozen shoulders treated with stretching exercises alone, Watson-Jones found that only 5% failed to regain satisfactory range within 6 months.[302] He recommended 3 minutes of active stretching each hour. The clinically effective therapeutic advantage of performing passive stretches in abduction in addition to active exercises was confirmed by Nicholson in the treatment of painfully stiff shoulders.[206]

Occasionally, therapy has been demonstrated inadequate to relieve symptomatic stiffness and has been shown to actually exacerbate the condition. Rizk and associates reported on patients who received physical therapy along with other modalities, and only 60% achieved the ability to sleep pain free after 5 months' duration.[251] Up to one third of Hazleman's patients who were treated by physiotherapy alone experienced an increase in their pain, and only one half of this group significantly improved by exercises.[128]

Other therapeutic modalities such as the application of ice packs or ice massage, microwaves, short waves, and heat lamps have not proved to be particularly beneficial in any specific phase of shoulder stiffness. Often, however, heat is applied to increase the extensibility of tight capsular tissues before range of motion stretching therapy.[161] A double-blind trial designed to test the efficacy of ultrasound for patients with tendinitis, bursitis, and adhesive capsulitis of the shoulder found little or no benefit when combined with range-of-motion exercises or nonsteroidal anti-inflammatory medications.[73] Although ultrasound also provides an increase in temperature that should augment tissue flexibility, these treatments did not offer any specific advantage over heat and therapeutic exercises in a short-term follow-up study performed by Quin.[237]

Therapeutic exercises are often combined with stimuli in an attempt to overload and distract the mind away from painful sensations. Echternach demonstrated a significant improvement in the recovery of motion in a comparative study using "audio analgesia" as an adjunct to mobilization in the chronic frozen shoulder.[80] They also reported a reduction in the number of treatments necessary for recovery. Similarly, Rizk used TENS to diminish pain as opposed to exercises alone and found a significant improvement and early recovery of shoulder range.[251]

In most patients, the physiotherapy can be successfully performed as a strictly home-based program. At our institution, we refer to this program as Jackins' Program, after our therapist Sarah Jackins. A single instructional visit to a physical therapist is often adequate, with monthly visits to the physician and therapist to determine whether symptoms and range of motion are improving. At each visit the patient should demonstrate the motions and the range recorded by the same examiner. A comparison is made with the values from the previous visit and with the opposite side. Ongoing encouragement from the family, physician, and therapist is valuable!

We stress daily and frequent home therapy exercises using Jackins' exercise program.[178] The four cornerstones of the Jackins' home-based stretching exercising program are patient motivation, frequency, consistency, and the four quadrants of capsular stretch. We recommend five repetitions of each exercise five times every day of the week. This exercise program must be performed gently against the limits of tolerance. We favor frequency over forcefulness and avoid the "no pain, no gain" regimen.

Short periods of exercise with increased frequency have proved to be therapeutic.[22, 167, 178, 302] Leffert and others have emphasized that the patient must assume primary responsibility and tolerate the discomfort that comes along with the exercise program in order to recover fully.[61, 160, 178, 180, 196]

We do not recommend performing any light-resistance strengthening or a muscle-toning exercise program until the patient has recovered functional range and comfort.[178]

Distention Arthrography or Brisement

Intra-articular fluid injection has been used: (1) to evaluate intra-articular pressure, (2) to measure joint compliance in response to a fluid challenge, and (3) to measure the capacity and maximum limit to progressively increased intra-articular pressures until the contracted glenohumeral capsule ruptures. Symptomatic relief and data from these experiments have received wide attention as an option in the treatment of the frozen and post-traumatic stiff shoulder. On literature review of these methods, most studies profess an extremely low risk and a high benefit ratio.[2, 57, 58, 86, 185, 216, 217, 226, 241, 273]

In 1931, Lundberg reported that Payr was the first to describe the use of "brisement," a distensive capsular stretching and rupturing technique.[168, 226] Since then, brisement has become a common outpatient procedure used in surgical and radiographic suites and even office practice. In review of the literature, only a single study did not find a significant improvement in the degree of pain or increase in motion at a follow-up at 1 to 3 months. Corbeil and associates ran a double-blind, prospective study of 45 patients with adhesive capsulitis to compare the therapeutic efficacy of nondistensive and distention arthrography in combination with intra-articular steroid injection.[59] Initially, they found 80% of the patients experienced diminution in nocturnal pain under both treatment regimens. During the initial months, range of motion was significantly improved, but after 3 months there was no significant difference between the two treatment regimens in the degree of pain or range of motion.

The procedure is performed by insufflating the glenohumeral joint with incremental injections of fluid, progressively increasing the intra-articular pressure to greater than 800 mm Hg and up to a maximum of 1500 mm Hg.[108, 124, 241, 261] During the initial injection phase, an arthrogram is often obtained to confirm intra-articular installation of fluid. Some authors instill a volume of approximately 60 to 100 ml followed by a manipulation to render a hydrostatic distention of the joint capsule.[58] Reeves identified that disruption occurs at the weakest point in the capsule, namely, the subcoracoid bursa or the biceps tendon sheath.[241]

Sharma and associates compared the results of brisement against manipulation under anesthesia and found significantly better results after distention.[273] In distinct opposition, Reeves, when analyzing time until resolution of disease, found that distention arthrography compared unfavorably with manipulation under anesthesia.[240, 241] Reeves also compared the results of this procedure with those diagnosed with a frozen and post-traumatic stiff shoulder.[240] In the post-traumatic stiff shoulder, Reeves found less severe joint restriction and a poorer response to serial distention, as opposed to 67% recovery by 6 months after treatment in those with a frozen shoulder. A reputable cadre of investigators have performed distention arthrography and claim that hydraulic distention is relatively noninvasive, simple to perform, and an effective mechanism in achieving symptomatic lasting relief in adhesive capsulitis.[86, 252, 273, 279]

Andrén and Lundberg noted that good results associated with joint distention are seen primarily in patients without severe restriction in motion and in those in whom moderate joint distention was successful prior to rupture.[2] They also found that relief from pain may occur without improvement in motion and that the procedure may be repeated at a later date to achieve additional improvement in function. Older demonstrated that, although distention arthrography alone did not seem to provide relief of pain, it did serve as an adjunct to range-of-motion exercises.[216, 217]

Like Corbeil and associates, the authors employed distention arthrography and failed to find lasting benefit. Our patients with severe motion restrictions eventually returned for further treatment. Since in a frozen shoulder the *entire* capsule is involved by the inflammatory process and subsequent capsular fibrosis, a treatment that has been found only to rupture the anterior bursa and not specifically reduce inflammation or lengthen the contracted capsule seems an unlikely answer to severe tissue contractures.

Prolonged Traction

Kottke and colleagues explained that the attachments between collagen fibers show high resistance to suddenly applied tension, but that they relax or creep when exposed to prolonged tension.[153] Applying this logic to the awake patient, Rizk and associates exerted prolonged traction using a pulley and weights to the affected upper extremity in 28 shoulders with adhesive capsulitis. In this group they compared 28 shoulders that were treated by heat and therapeutic exercises. Although both groups demonstrated improvement in range of motion, the increase was significantly greater in those who were treated with progressive abduction traction while pain was controlled with TENS.[251]

Neurologic Blockade

In 1941, Wertheim and Rovenstine were the first to report on the use of a suprascapular nerve block for relief of shoulder pain.[306] Later, Koppell and Thompson explained that the suprascapular nerve not only supplied motor but also sensory innervation to the external rotators and the shoulder joint.[152] They hypothesized that the suprascapular nerve might be the source of pain in patients with frozen shoulder and performed a suprascapular block in 20 cases with substantial pain relief in the majority within 24 hours. Because of the dramatic response to these blocks, they surmised that the suprascapular nerve was inflamed and the apparent source of pain in these conditions. Surgical decompression of the suprascapular was also performed. In more recent reports from the anesthesiology literature, other authors have recommended a suprascapular block with a local anesthetic and steroid to relieve pain.[48, 64, 102]

Wassef studied the use of suprascapular nerve blocks to manage a frozen shoulder associated with reflex sympathetic dystrophy.[301] He not only found a significant increase in comfort with an improvement in the patient's tolerance to deep pressure to the shoulder joint but also an improved passive range of motion when blocks were repeated twice weekly for a total of two to four treatments. This treatment, however, has not been proved to offer any advantage over other treatment modalities.

Isolated Alternative Methods

ULTRASOUND

Ultrasound is widely used to treat patients with painful shoulder conditions, but its use may not be justified. In a prospective study, ice and ultrasonic applications were compared in a series of patients with the frozen shoulder syndrome, and no significant advantage of one treatment over the other was appreciated.[112] In a double-blind comparison, patients with painful shoulder stiffness (not exclusive to adhesive capsulitis), were randomized in three treatment groups: ultrasound, conventional therapeutic exercises, and nonsteroidal anti-inflammatory drugs plus exercises.[73] Ultrasound offered no benefit over the other methods.

INTRA-ARTICULAR PROTEIN INSTILLATION

Leardini and colleagues performed intra-articular injections of hyaluronic acid into painful shoulders diagnosed with either osteoarthritis or adhesive capsulitis.[157] Although short in follow-up, the authors reported rapid and significant improvement in joint mobility and comfort. The results, however, were not compared with those in a control group. Enzymes such as α-chymotrypsin and hylase have also been injected into the shoulder, but the beneficial results are obscured by the combination with physiotherapy.[6, 17]

SALMON-CALCITONIN

In a prospective study that included 50 cases of frozen shoulder separated into three etiologic groups, Waldburger and associates demonstrated a statistically significant effect on pain reduction in patients treated with early mobilization associated with subcutaneous salmon-calcitonin injection when compared with physiotherapy alone.[298] This improvement was noted only in patients with post-traumatic frozen shoulders and not in those that were idiopathic or neurologic in origin.

ROENTGEN THERAPY

In surprisingly large series,[3, 26, 33, 125, 320] radiation proved to be effective in eliminating pain from shoulder stiffness in up to 70%, but the long-term risks were not considered. Quin compared radiation therapy with ultrasound or heat and physiotherapy and did not find a treatment advantage.[237] In a prospective study of 233 patients with periarthritis, Hassenstein identified improvement in only 26%. The authors agree with Coventry who, in 1953, surmised that radiotherapy did not have much effect on chronic forms of frozen shoulder.[61] Radiotherapy is no longer used in the United States for the treatment of idiopathic frozen shoulder. Radiation is used occasionally in association with shoulder stiffness secondary to heterotopic ossification to prevent a recurrence of ectopic bone after surgical resection (see later, Open Surgical Release).

ACUPUNCTURE

In patients with frozen shoulder who had received conventional physiotherapy treatment with limited success, six acupuncture treatment sessions were required to achieve an excellent response and complete recovery.[83] Lin and associates randomly divided 150 patients with a frozen shoulder into three treatment groups treated using electroacupuncture (EAP), regional nerve block (RNB), and a combination of both treatments.[163] They found that the combined EAP and RNB method had significant high pain control with a long duration and better range of motion than that of EAP or RNB alone.

OTHER MODALITIES

Common modalities such as massage and electrophysiotherapy or more atypical experiences like hyperbaric oxygen and magnetotherapy have been tried.[4, 27, 67, 107] Taken together, these studies of isolated alternative methods that attempt to compare and evaluate the effect of one treatment against another lack rigid diagnostic criteria and a control population. None of these treatments would fit into a standard treatment algorithm.

Operative Treatment

When a patient with a stiff shoulder remains symptomatic, failing a minimum 6 months of appropriate nonoperative treatment, manipulative or surgical intervention is usually considered. All patients should be aware that no treatment cures all cases, and more aggressive methods incur a greater risk of morbidity. Also, although we discuss each of these procedures as separate treatment entities, in fact they are frequently combined to provide for maximum restoration of motion.

It is reasonable again to review that of those patients who continue to have a significant loss of shoulder motion, fewer than 5 to 20% remain functionally disabled with persistent symptomatic impairment.[22, 54, 242, 263, 276] Often, many of these refractory cases are insulin-dependent diabetics. For recalcitrant frozen shoulders, aggressive surgical release by open or arthroscopic methods may be the only option.[116, 122, 160, 170, 177–179, 213, 231, 267, 300]

For all surgical procedures, we recommend the use of an interscalene brachial plexus block as either the primary anesthetic or as an adjunct to a general anesthesia. This regional long-lasting anesthetic, which is typically used by trained anesthesiologists,[239] allows the patient to tolerate an extremity connected to a continuous passive motion device immediately after the procedure. As an additional benefit, for as long as 6 to 8 hours after completion of the procedure, the surgeon can return to the patient to demonstrate the full range of motion achieved postoperatively. The block is generally effective for 12 hours or more when long-acting bupivacaine is combined with epinephrine and has proved to be useful in all postsurgical care of the shoulder. At our institution in 1989, we experimented with an indwelling interscalene block in a series of patients, but we discontinued its routine use because improvement in range after hospital discharge was no more rapid than in patients treated without indwelling catheters postoperatively. Pollock and associates, however, have found a significant advantage in recovered motion with the use of indwelling catheters in a larger series of patients.[231]

Manipulation Under Anesthesia

For well over a century, manipulation under anesthesia has been the primary mode of treatment recommended for a persistent frozen shoulder.[75, 234] Although the effectiveness of this treatment was presumably documented by several studies,[109, 111, 130, 311] others have denounced its use.[52, 66, 70, 160, 181] Why does this discrepancy arise? Could it be that because Lundberg noted no change in the time course of disease after manipulation that some clinicians decided to oppose the procedure?[168] This is unlikely, because if we review the reports of those who shun manipulation, we recognize that they cite complications that deterred their favor of the method.

Manipulation is primarily indicated for patients who are worsening after at least 3 months of an appropriate nonoperative exercise regimen or failure to respond after a 6-month exercise program (see Fig. 20–22).[116, 122, 150, 168] Kessel and associates suggested that patients who were symptomatic for more than 6 months prior to manipulative treatment achieved a greater degree of improvement than did those who had a shorter duration of symptoms.[150] Manipulation is generally contraindicated in patients with severe osteopenia of the humerus and long-term diabetes mellitus (greater than 20 years).[116, 122, 142]

Complications of manipulation do occur, although the cumulative reported risk of an inadvertent event is less than 1%. Reported complications of the procedure include subscapularis and rotator cuff rupture,[70] surgical neck and humeral shaft fracture,[233] and dislocation.[52] Other injuries such as a proximal humerus fracture and acute shoulder dislocation have been reported.[111, 236] In our own personal series, we have also treated a patient who was referred with a complete brachial plexus palsy after manipulation that resulted in an anterior/inferior dislocation. The reported rate of recurrent stiffness is between 5 and 20%; however, most of the studies reporting results followed patients for only about 6 months.[288, 302, 311] Janda and Hawkins have described an unacceptably high rate of recontracture after manipulation in patients with long-term insulin-dependent diabetes.[142]

The immediate effects of manipulation to structures about the shoulder have been observed at open and arthroscopic surgery. At open surgery, Neviaser and DePalma separately recorded tears in the subscapularis muscle and tendon along with disruption of the anterior and inferior capsule. Tears have also been observed in the supraspinatus tendon and the long head of the biceps tendon.[66, 180, 240]

The technique of shoulder manipulation is typically performed under interscalene brachial plexus block or a general anesthetic, but it has been performed as an outpatient and with a local injection combined with hydrostatic distention.[58] The standard technique is performed by applying a constant controlled force to the proximal humerus while holding the scapula stable. Sudden force causes greater risk to normal structures.[130] Most authors recommend an initial abduction force[111, 235]; however, Charnley recommended against this maneuver prior to obtaining external rotation in order to avoid a shoulder dislocation.[52] A crepitant disruptive release of the articular capsule is considered to be a good prognostic sign, because immediate full motion is usually recovered.[115, 150, 236] Increased force should not be applied if a crepitant release does not ensue under constantly applied force.[116, 168] If the recovered motion is not symmetric to the opposite side or recurs in a short time postoperatively, then repeat manipulation may be necessary and indicated[109, 115, 130] (see the authors' preferred method and Fig. 20–22).

After a completed manipulation, many authors have recommended injecting the shoulder with a corticosteroid to diminish early healing of the capsular disruption and to diminish local inflammation and pain associated with the procedure.[111, 115, 116, 122, 130] Quigley demonstrated in more than 100 cases that no medication other than codeine was required in the immediate postmanipulation period to control pain.[236] Thomas and associates randomly allocated 30 patients with frozen shoulders into two groups, one with manipulation and steroid use and the other with intra-articular steroids alone.[288] They found that the group treated by manipulation and steroid injection retained significantly greater movement (40% versus 13%) and less pain at follow-up (80% versus 47%) than did those treated by steroid injection alone. Weiser performed manipulation under local anesthetic with three to five multiple treatment sessions with 60% full recovery.[304]

The reported results of shoulder manipulation alone or in combination with steroid injection are extremely variable, with a range of 25% to as many as 90%, significantly improved by 3 months after manipulation, and on average of 70% improved by 6 months.[19, 56, 109, 111, 115, 130, 132, 146, 166, 168, 236, 238, 240, 288, 303, 304]

Manipulation may also be performed under local anesthesia after infiltrating the glenohumeral joint with a substantial volume of local anesthetic.[96, 167, 304] Some of these authors also recommend subacromial injection and arthrographic visualization before and after manipulation. These reports claim a successful relief of pain and recovered motion in approximately two thirds of patients; however, a greater percentage were relieved of discomfort alone.

There are a variety of recommended post-manipulation management regimens. After successful manipulation, systemic steroids have been given but are not recommended because of the potential side effects and lack of lasting benefit.[14, 166, 182] Some authors put the extremity into immediate passive motion. As an alternative to passive motion, Neviaser described attaching the arm to the bed, similar to that originally described by Codman, in a position of abduction and external rotation.[55, 200] Although the use of prolonged traction may stretch out residual contractures and promote range, it may require significant narcotic analgesia.[55, 204] While still under regional interscalene block, our patients are instructed on a four-quadrant capsular stretching program (refer to Jackins' stretching program). Re-manipulation can be performed while the patient observes the postoperative gain in range without pain inhibition. We recommend a single-day hospital stay, whereas Neviaser has recommended a 3- to 5-day inpatient visit.[116, 122, 200] Neviaser also suggests after discharge that the patient maintain the abducted and externally rotated position at night for 3 weeks to eliminate stiffness.[200]

Open Surgical Release

Codman originally described open release of adhesions in the subacromial and subdeltoid bursa.[55] Neviaser found it necessary to perform an arthrotomy through an anterior axillary approach in patients whose stiffness recurred after a manipulation under anesthesia.[200] He, like his father, recommended the release of periarticular adhesions and the tightly contracted articular capsule from the humeral head, especially in the location of the axillary fold.[196, 200]

Lippman asserted that an open lysis of adhesions about the long head of the biceps tendon would liberate the shoulder from restricted motion.[165, 276] Continuing in this mode, Simmonds performed complete excision of the biceps long head tendon in cases of intractable frozen shoulder with no improvement in range of motion.[276] He also noted that there were no intra-articular adhesions between the articular capsule and the surface of the joint.

In patients who failed to improve after a gentle manipulation, Harmon performed soft tissue release of contracted tissues about the joint in eight patients and found similar results to closed manipulation in all except two cases of intractable stiffness.[115] Alternatively, Harmon treated 30 cases of shoulder stiffness with excision of the acromion and the acromioclavicular joint. In all cases he found restoration of active abduction to 160 degrees or more by 3 months after surgery.

McLaughlin described release of the biceps tendon and subscapularis as a treatment for shoulder contracture.[180] Leffert recommended surgical release of those structures responsible for restricted motion when a patient failed to improve after 6 months of a nonoperative therapeutic regimen.[160] Matsen and Kirby found that surgical release of the capsule was safer than a closed manipulation for those patients with recalcitrant stiffness and osteoporosis that did not respond to 6 months of home exercise therapy.[177] In a study, Kieras and Matsen reported on open release in the management of refractory frozen shoulder in 12 patients, four of whom were insulin-dependent diabetics.[151] The duration of preoperative symptoms and treatment averaged 16 months. The average flexion improved from 73 degrees (range from 20 to 95) to 132 degrees (range of 90 to 150). The average external rotation improved from 3 degrees (range of 5 to 25) to 45 degrees (range of 15 to 60). Pain was decreased or eliminated in all patients at 2-year follow-up. There were no complications, and all patients returned to work.

In 1957, Kernwein and Sneed performed open release of the capsule and coracohumeral ligament in 4 of 12 patients with adhesive capsulitis and found that these tissues were markedly thickened and inelastic.[148] In 1987 and in 1990, Nobuhara and Ikeda reported on dysfunctional range in shoulders having a tight rotator interval capsule, which was remarkably relieved in 21 shoulders by a local release of this contracture.[207, 208] Ozaki and associates treated 17 of 365 patients who had recalcitrant chronic adhesive capsulitis, and at operation the major tether restricting glenohumeral movement was identified as a contracture of the coracohumeral ligament within the rotator interval capsule.[220] Release of this contracted structure relieved pain and restored motion of the shoulder in all patients. They also noted that the long head of the biceps was inflamed and stenosed beneath the contracted coracohumeral ligament and rotator interval capsule. In contrast, Becker and Cofield did not find a strong association between chronic bicipital tendinitis and the frozen shoulder syndrome in their study, which looked at surgical findings and the long-term results of biceps tenodesis.[16]

In patients who developed severe stiffness and a marked internal rotation contracture after a stroke, Braun and associates performed excision of the subscapularis tendon and incision of the pectoralis major insertion while preserving the anterior capsule.[31] Of 13 patients who were treated in this way, 14% were not improved but 10 patients regained 90 degrees of abduction and 20 degrees of external rotation and complete pain relief within 2 months postoperatively. This aggressive form of treatment, however, would not be indicated in refractory stiffness of idiopathic origin, because severely disabling permanent functional deficits after chronic insufficiency of the subscapularis can be avoided by other methods.[319]

Our current indication for open surgical release includes cases that cannot be managed by arthroscopic capsular release and subacromial lysis of adhesions. Often, the indication is the post-traumatic surgical stiff shoulder. For example, the patient with stiffness after a Putti-Platt repair may have severe intra-articular and extra-articular postsurgical contractures and is best managed by open release of the humeroscapular motion interface, subscapularis tendon lengthening, and release of the contracted articular capsule. The advantages of an open surgical release include: (1) access to the entire humeroscapular motion interface, (2) lengthening of musculotendinous subscapularis contractures, and (3) excision of heterotopic ossification or bone spurs (Fig. 20–25).[116, 151]

Open surgical release also has significant disadvantages and risks. It can be technically difficult to get a complete

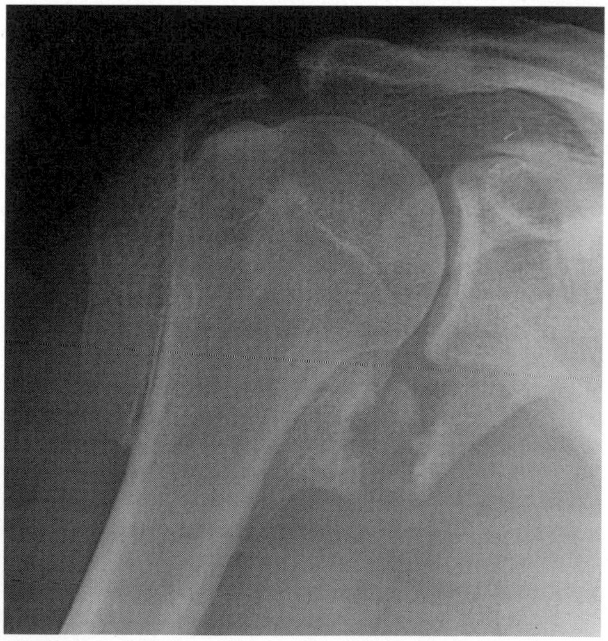

Figure 20–25

An x-ray of a patient with severe shoulder stiffness secondary to heterotopic ossification associated with a head injury. This is best treated by complete capsular release, excision of heterotopic ossification, and lysis of adhesions in the humeroscapular motion interface and subscapularis tendon lengthening.

posterior capsule release by open means. Postoperative pain and the need to protect a repaired or lengthened subscapularis tendon inhibits the patient from performing an unrestricted full-range stretching program necessary to maintain all the motion achieved under anesthesia. Lastly, extended hospitalization may be necessary for pain control.

As an alternative to open releases of contracted tissues, Baumann offers a method of denervating the ventral aspect of the shoulder capsule to cause an immediate and progressive decrease or total elimination of shoulder pain.[13] He reported on 20 shoulders treated with 85% of patients having painless mobilization with total rehabilitation of joint function. This experience, however, has not been duplicated.

Arthroscopic Surgical Release

Although some surgeons do not advocate using the arthroscope to manage shoulder stiffness,[202] others have performed synovectomy or release of contracted capsule and adhesions in the glenohumeral joint and subacromial space with documented effectiveness.[30, 57, 122, 213, 231, 267, 300]

Early reports that employed arthroscopic methods in the treatment of the stiff shoulder generally combined an examination of the glenohumeral joint with joint distention to stretch the tight capsular constraints and manipulation. In 1980, Wiley was the first to report this procedure in 10 patients, all of whom were relieved of their symptom. In 1981, Hsu and Chan performed a prospective study in 75 patients and demonstrated that arthroscopic distention or manipulation combined with physiotherapy was significantly better than physiotherapy alone.[136, 309] The latter recommended arthroscopic distention over manipulation, because it was controllable and provided valuable insight into intra-articular pathology.

The earliest report of actually using arthroscopic equipment to perform a partial arthroscopic surgical release of a contracted articular capsule was first described by Conti in France in 1979.[57] He divided the rotator interval capsule using a trocar and forceps, instilled a corticosteroid, and performed a gentle manipulation of the shoulder. Sixteen of 18 patients fully recovered within 3 weeks and two other patients recovered by 3 to 6 months. Using a similar technique, Ogilvie-Harris and Wiley reported arthroscopic "freeing-up" with a blunt instrument and in some cases cutting of the anterior capsule in a controlled manner to improve movement of recalcitrant stiffness in patients with a frozen shoulder.[214] Eleven of the 81 patients were diabetic and in those, results were less satisfactory.

Ogilvie-Harris and associates compared manipulation to arthroscopic release in patients with resistant frozen shoulder.[213] Arthroscopic division of tight structures was performed in four steps that included: (1) resection of the inflammatory synovium in the rotator interval, (2) division of the anterior/superior glenohumeral ligament and anterior capsule, (3) division of the subscapularis tendon, and (4) division of the inferior capsule. At 2- to 5-year follow-up, patients with arthroscopic division had significantly better pain relief and restoration of function compared with those who underwent arthroscopy and manipulation. Patients with diabetes initially did worse, but the final outcome was similar to patients without diabetes. These authors suggest that those with diabetes may benefit from early intervention.

Pollock and associates found that arthroscopy served as a useful adjunct to manipulation under anesthesia in the resistant frozen shoulder.[231] They performed a manipulation under interscalene brachial plexus block anesthesia followed by an arthroscopic examination, sectioning the coracohumeral ligament and débriding the glenohumeral joint as well as the subacromial space. Twenty-five of 30 shoulders treated in this manner yielded satisfactory results (83%); however, satisfactory results were only obtained in 64% of a subgroup of patients with diabetes mellitus.

Segmuller and associates reported a short-term (13.5 months) follow-up study of arthroscopic inferior capsulotomies performed with cutting diathermy.[267] More than 50% of their patients were found to have persistent stiffness of internal rotation during the longest examination, yet 88% of patients were satisfied with their outcome and 87% had good to excellent results by Constant score.

A more aggressive and complete release of chronic refractory capsular contractures of the shoulder has been reported in separate studies by Harryman and associates and Warner and colleagues.[122, 300] The advantage of their arthroscopic procedure included complete capsular release of the anterior/inferior and posterior capsule to free up the full range of global motions about the shoulder. Selective arthroscopic capsulotomy was performed in a portion of cases for those having isolated anterior or posterior capsular contracture. The subscapularis tendon was not released in any of these cases, and yet significant improvements in all contracted ranges was achieved (see Fig. 20–21). Morbidity was minimal as opposed to the open surgical procedure, and early pain relief was achieved with few recurrent cases of refractory stiffness. Each investigator reported one complication that included an anterior dislocation[300] immediately postoperatively with subsequent recovered stability and excellent motion and a complete axillary nerve palsy,[122] which also fully recovered at follow-up examination.

Harryman and associates demonstrated a remarkable improvement in six of nine health status scores on the SF-36 general health survey and an excellent recovery of function on all questions of the Simple Shoulder Test.[122] Warner and associates showed similar results using the Constant score.[300] Harryman and colleagues reported no differences among all outcome measures between diabetic and nondiabetic patients; however, three patients who developed recurrent refractory stiffness were insulin-dependent diabetics.[122] In summary, arthroscopic capsular release was deemed safe and effective in the management of refractory idiopathic global capsular fibrosis as well as post-traumatic posterior capsular fibrosis.[290, 300]

The arthroscope can also be useful in the post-traumatic stiff shoulder, including the postsurgical stiff shoulder. In a few cases, arthroscopic release of both capsular contracture extra-articular adhesions in the humeroscapular motion interface has been employed, but an inadequate number of procedures have been performed for comparison to open management. An alternative approach to the management of severe extra-articular adhesions associated with global capsular fibrosis in the posttraumatic and postsurgical shoulder has been developed. In a group of five patients, the senior author performed an arthroscopic release of contracted capsule combined with an open anterior axillary approach for release adhesions within the entire humeroscapular motion interface. The advantage of combining these procedures has been realized in the immediate postoperative rehabilitation and improved access to the posterior capsule compared with open release alone. A full unrestricted aggressive stretching program can be utilized because there are no restrictions to motion and no tendon repairs left to be protected. The early results have been encouraging.

Combined Modes of Treatment

A consensus exists among authors who have written about the current management for the stiff shoulder in that the initial treatment should consist of gentle range-of-motion exercises using a patient-managed program of stretching exercises in conjunction with analgesics.[21, 129, 137, 160, 188, 321] If this initial program is unsuccessful in improving comfort or range of motion, then several treatment options may be considered next. There is no agreement, however, as to the next best step along a treatment algorithm. A nonsurgical option such as an injection of steroids or arthrography with distention is often preferred prior to more aggressive manipulative or surgical options.[88, 279] For patients in whom this treatment has been unsuccessful or for those investigators who have not found brisement to be advantageous,[59] manipulative treatment has been the next step. Many recommend that shoulder manipulation be reserved for shoulders that have not responded to 6 months of consistent exercises and demonstrate persistent symptomatic stiffness.[52, 116, 168, 177, 195, 200] Although there are some orthopedists who condemn this procedure because of the rare complication, the overall morbidity is low.

For a patient with recalcitrant stiffness in whom manipulation may be contraindicated, an arthroscopic or open surgical alternative is considered next depending, of course, on the patient's pathology and the surgeon's experience with the technical approach. For most clinicians, an arthroscopic or open release is preferred for a recalcitrant idiopathic frozen or post-traumatic stiff shoulder.[52, 116, 122, 168, 177, 195, 200]

No matter what method is selected for a given patient, it is important to consider the patient's medical and psychological profile, the functional impact of delayed recovery on earning potential, and the most economic and effective approach. It is imperative that investigators collect long-term follow-up data since the functional and objective restrictions of chronic shoulder stiffness persist for years after the onset of disability.[54] Finally, in patients who have recovered from shoulder stiffness or in those who are at greater risk for shoulder stiffness, it is fundamental that a preventive stretching exercise program be the primary goal.[116, 129, 187, 188]

AUTHORS' PREFERRED TREATMENT

Nonoperative Treatment

Once a thorough history and physical examination have been completed and other treatable conditions frequently associated with painful shoulder stiffness have been addressed, then a simple nonoperative program should begin. Our initial management includes a trial of analgesics, anti-inflammatory medications, and therapeutic stretching exercises for 3 to 6 months (see indications below and Fig. 20–22). We initiate the Jackins' Stretching Program even if patients say they "had therapy" and especially when they are unable to recall or demonstrate their previous exercise regimen.[176]

JACKINS' EXERCISE PROGRAM

Our preferred stretching program consists of four basic passive or active-assisted stretching exercises performed by the patient.[178] Each exercise is completed five times during five sessions a day with each session lasting 5 minutes. Before stretching, it is often helpful to apply heat to the stiff shoulder to increase flexibility and relax tight musculature.

Jackins recommends that three of the four exercises be performed supine, but they can also be performed standing or sitting[178] (see Jackins' stretching program in Chapter 15; see Fig. 15–81 to 91). In each direction, a push against the firm end-point of range is maintained for a minimum count of 10. Severe pain should be avoided. After all the stretching exercises are finished, pain should subside to the previous baseline and gradually diminish after regular daily sessions. If pain and stiffness worsen with exercise, it is preferable to reduce the intensity of the stretch but not the frequency.

The contralateral extremity is used to assist each motion described below. Humeral elevation should be performed close to the sagittal plane while allowing the limb to rotate as necessary to achieve maximum range. Alternatively, this motion may be duplicated with the use of a pulley, especially when it is impossible to assist elevation with the opposite extremity. External rotation is performed supine by placing a cane between the hands while the elbow is held close to the body and then applying pressure to rotate the affected extremity away from the body. Alternatively, while standing, external rotation is assisted by placing the arm against a door jam and twisting the body away from the arm. To perform the cross-body stretch in either the supine, sitting, or standing position, the affected extremity is grasped behind the elbow and pulled across the chest towards the opposite shoulder. It is best to begin with the elbow low and then stretch to a higher level in a cross-body (horizontal) adduction motion. Internal rotation is performed by putting the hand behind the buttock and pulling the wrist up the back with the opposite extremity, or by using a towel to connect the hands similar to drying the back. Alternatively, a door handle may be grasped behind the buttock and with a deep knee bend an internal rotation stretch is applied.

If the pain becomes unbearable and exercises are not

tolerated in any direction or if painful stiffness increases even with regular exercises, it is often useful to inject the glenohumeral joint with 7 ml of a local, long-acting anesthetic (bupivacaine 0.05%) and 1 ml of a repository steroid (40 mg of methylprednisolone). Our experience with intra-articular steroid agrees with previous studies that quote effective pain reduction but no long-term advantage.[115] We use it solely to enable the patient to perform the stretching regimen with greater comfort (see Fig. 20–22).

We do not begin to advance isometric strengthening exercises until the majority of motion and comfort has been restored. The use of the symptomatic extremity in all daily activities speeds rehabilitation along.[115] Every patient must assume responsibility for his or her own 7-day-a-week exercise program.[100] Generally, it is unnecessary for a patient to see a therapist more than once a week to follow progress, receive encouragement, and ensure that stiffness and pain are not increasing.

EXAMINATION UNDER ANESTHESIA AND MANIPULATIVE RELEASE

Our indications for an examination under anesthesia (EUA) with gentle manipulation under anesthesia (MUA) are the following:

1. Inability to perform any stretching exercises due to severe pain usually after a failed attempt with local intra-articular anesthetic and steroid instillation (diagnostically useful to determine if stiffness actually exists)
2. Increasing painful global stiffness after 12 weeks of regular Jackins' exercises (usually after intra-articular steroid injection)
3. Absolutely no improvement in comfort with global stiffness after 18 to 24 weeks of regular Jackins' exercises (consideration for specific postsurgical stiffness with manipulation only in directions that would not stress a repair—see later).

The purpose of the EUA portion of this procedure is to confirm that the apparent restrictions in range are true physical boundaries and are not established solely by pain, fear of instability, muscular spasm, or even hysterical psychosis! All of these examples have presented as "stiffness" in our clinic and have initially deceived us. For example, a patient with frank instability may voluntarily or involuntarily hold the extremity tight at the side, never relaxing enough for an adequate examination. Often we are suspicious because the patient's age, history, or body language fails to fit typical patterns (see Table 20–4). Under anxiolytic relaxation or even an anesthetic paralyzing agent, the fixed physical restriction miraculously disappears.

If stiffness develops after a surgical repair, manipulation can be performed but extreme caution must be exercised! The manipulator must remember that the procedure incurs a definite potential risk of disruption of the repair. We prefer not to perform manipulation until the repair has had adequate time to heal (e.g., approximately 12 weeks for tendon to bone).

Consider the "not too unusual" example of stiffness occurring after a rotator cuff repair. If a patient is unable to approach 140 degrees of elevation after 8 to 12 weeks of therapy, it is reasonable to consider an examination and gentle manipulation under anesthesia. What about the cuff repair? The manipulative motion of forward elevation or external rotation in mid-elevation relaxes tension on the rotator cuff repair. We would not recommend manipulation in internal rotation or cross-body motion. Typically, we resort to an arthroscopic capsular release to relieve a recalcitrant tight capsule and release subacromial adhesions in patients with stiffness after a rotator cuff tear (see later, Arthroscopic Release).

The patient and surgeon should agree preoperatively whether to proceed with surgical intervention or return to a nonoperative supportive regimen if manipulation fails to gain a satisfactory result. An MUA is *contraindicated* and a surgical release is considered when:

1. A gentle manipulative force is inadequate to recover a functional range
2. No improvement or a worsening in range or comfort occurs after a previous manipulation
3. The patient has significant osteopenia, a rotator cuff tear or long-term insulin-dependent diabetes mellitus (e.g., more than 20 years)

EXAMINATION AND MANIPULATION TECHNIQUE

The purpose of the MUA portion of this procedure is to perform a traumatic capsular and extra-articular adhesion lysis. We prefer to manipulate the shoulder under an interscalene block anesthetic for the reasons previously discussed. With the patient supine, we compare the passive range of motion between the stiff extremity and the opposite side in five arcs previously described in the physical examination section. If the patient is awake, we can also add internal rotation up the back with the patient sitting. These ranges are our passive reference motions used for later comparison.

A gentle manipulative force is applied to the stiff extremity in the following order. We begin by elevating the extremity using a "two-finger" force applied in the sagittal plane while allowing free rotation. Brute force should be avoided or serious injury will occur! Force is applied to the humerus close to the shoulder to diminish the lever arm. With constant pressure, this stretch usually results in palpable and audible release of contractures associated with disruption of the inferior capsule.[70, 115, 196] If a crepitant give does not occur, manipulation is discontinued and the surgeon may proceed with an arthroscopic or open capsular release (see later).

If full forward elevation is successfully achieved, we proceed with the MUA. With the arm elevated at shoulder level, the humerus is then adducted without controlling rotation under the chin and across the body by pushing with a "two-finger" force to release the posteroinferior capsule. Next, the arm is abducted to the coronal plane with the arm elevated at shoulder level. In this position, internal rotation is applied to stretch the posterior capsule and soft tissues. Next, the arm is slowly lowered toward the side holding internal rotation and extending the elbow and pronating the forearm as required in the supine position. If the patient can sit up, internal rotation up the back works even better.

The arm is returned to the abducted position, and external rotation is performed to release the anteroinferior capsule. Each position should be held until the range is comparable with the normal opposite side. Once symmetric external rotation is obtained in abduction, the elbows are slowly lowered together to the side matching full external rotation to release the anterior capsule. If symmetric range to the opposite side is obtained, an intra-articular steroid (40 mg of methylprednisolone) is injected to end the procedure (unless contraindicated). If persistent asymmetry exists, the surgeon should then proceed to an arthroscopic or open capsular release if planned preoperatively (see Fig. 20–22).

AFTERCARE

The freed extremity is placed in a wrist gauntlet and connected immediately to a continuous passive motion device. We ask the therapist to work with each patient after the procedure and again in the morning to remind or re-teach the patient how to perform his or her own assisted exercise program prior to discharge. The magnitude of motion after manipulation and the prognosis for recovery is better for patients who are motivated to do their exercises.

If the patient initially recovers excellent motion but gradually loses the recovered range in the first 3 to 4 weeks after manipulation, repeating the procedure immediately has proved to be effective in our hands. Manipulations repeated later than 3 to 4 weeks after an index MUA are less successful.

Surgical Treatment

Only patients who have failed a satisfactory nonoperative treatment course and an attempt at manipulation (unless contraindicated) should be considered for surgical release. Noncompliance with an exercise program is *not* an indication for surgical treatment. Patients who are intolerant of exercises or motivated insufficiently to perform them will rarely improve with nonoperative or operative treatment!

Some patients should not be treated surgically! Contraindications include significant depression, autonomic dystrophy, poor health, and those who defy improvement for secondary gain. Although the indications for open and arthroscopic surgical release are similar, there are unique aspects to each; and, in special cases, we have even found it useful to combine these methods. Patients who are sensitive to fluid challenges (e.g., a diabetic with cardiac or renal insufficiency), may not be able to tolerate fluid extravasation that occurs during the arthroscopic release. Patients with a contracted articular capsule and extensive extra-articular adhesions, such as those with a post-traumatic or postsurgical stiff shoulder (e.g., after percutaneous pin treatment of humeral fractures) may require an arthroscopic capsular release and an open extra-articular release to lyse adhesions in the humeroscapular motion interface. Specific advantages inherent to the open and arthroscopic procedures are described later.

OPEN RELEASE

The major advantage of an open surgical release is the opportunity to safely palpate and visualize adhesions outside the joint. When rotating the extremity and palpating between tissue planes, it becomes easier to identify tight bands that restrict motion. For example, it is not unusual to find adhesions between the subscapularis, the coracoid, and the conjoined tendon that prevent full excursion.

Although an accurate release of the contracted articular and rotator interval capsule, the glenohumeral and coracohumeral ligaments, the biceps, and the subscapularis tendons can be accomplished under direct vision, significant disadvantages of this approach exist. In tight shoulders, we often encounter difficulty releasing the contracted posterior capsule via the open approach. The other major disadvantage of the open surgical procedure is the postoperative pain that may inhibit early passive and active-assisted motion and prevent a timely hospital discharge.

Open capsular release, combined with an arthroscopic release, is our procedure of choice for the post-traumatic and, more typically, the postsurgical stiff shoulder. Recall that the post-traumatic stiff shoulder contains both capsular and extracapsular fibrosis; therefore, surgical release must be directed toward both the capsule and the humeroscapular motion interface.

Technique

The procedure begins with a careful examination under anesthesia, which is directed at accurately defining directions of motion restriction. We recommend the same measurements as during the initial examination (see Physical Examination). In addition, similar measurements are recorded for the normal shoulder. For a post-traumatic stiff shoulder, we do *not* begin with a gentle manipulation under anesthesia. The dense adhesions that form within the humeroscapular motion interface are resistant to manipulation.

The choice of surgical approach depends on the original cause of stiffness. If the inciting event was previous surgery, we use the prior incision as the approach for open release, because the bulk of the surgical adhesions are likely to be within this approach. If a superior, deltoid-splitting approach was previously used, the deltoid is again divided in the same plane. The deltoid split should extend proximally to the acromion process and distally to just proximal to the palpable subdeltoid reflection of the subacromial bursa, as the axillary nerve is distal to this reflection.[15] Splitting the deltoid without incision from the acromion usually provides sufficient exposure. A self-retaining retractor is placed deep to the deep deltoid fascia, usually revealing a hypertrophic and thickly adhesed subacromial bursa. A complete subacromial bursectomy is performed, and scar tissue between the bursal surface of the rotator cuff and the coracoacromial arch is excised. By rotating the arm, adhesions deep to the deltoid are excised, again taking care not to stray distal to the subdeltoid bursal reflection. A periosteal elevator or flat retractor is passed into the supraspinatus and infraspinatus fossae, breaking adhesions between the superficial surface of these muscles and the overlying deltoid. When the humeroscapular motion interface is free enough to pass a finger deep to the conjoined tendon anteriorly and to the quadrangular space posteriorly, the procedure is completed. Upon completion, the bursal surface of the rotator cuff should be inspected for tears.

Since aggressive motion therapy will start immediately postoperatively, deltoid closure for deltoid-splitting approaches must be secure. We recommend heavy, nonabsorbable suture with adequate purchase in both superficial and deep layers of deltoid fascia. If possible, the deltoid should not be detached from the acromion during exposure, thus no acromial repair will require protection. If the deltoid is partially removed from the acromion, it should be securely repaired to drill holes in the acromion.

For a post-traumatic stiff shoulder that occurred secondary to a fracture or soft-tissue contusion, we prefer an anterior axillary incision followed by a standard deltopectoral approach. This approach allows access to the humeroscapular interface, the subscapularis tendon, and the glenohumeral capsule, if a capsular procedure is necessary.

The procedure begins with mobilization of the humeroscapular motion interface. This technique can often be quite challenging because the dense scar prevents accurate identification of the interface. Since this plane is defined as a "motion interface," it can be identified by visualizing motion of the rotator cuff tendons. Specifically, we use a test that we refer to as the "roll-no roll test."[116, 178] Simply by rotating the humerus, the plane between the underlying rotator cuff and the overlying deltoid and conjoined tendon is identified. As motion improves, identification of this interval is facilitated. Often the thick scar requires sharp dissection and excision. As an alternative, the interface can be identified by entering the subacromial space, thus defining the subdeltoid plane. An interface scar includes the thickened subacromial bursa, which should be excised. Excision of scar tissue between the conjoined tendon and the underlying subscapularis is more challenging, owing to the close proximity of the axillary nerve and major neurovascular structures. Adhesion resection is best accomplished by externally rotating the humerus and presenting the adhesions to the lateral aspect of the conjoined tendon. With excision, further external rotation is permitted, presenting more adhesions. Dissecting medial to the conjoined tendon should be avoided. The goal of release should be excision of all scar, leaving the humeroscapular motion interface both free and completely smooth. Interface release is complete when the surgeon can pass a finger over all surfaces of the rotator cuff and palpate the axillary nerve both anteriorly on the superficial surface of the subscapularis and posteriorly as it exits the quadrangular space. The entire bursal surface of the rotator cuff should then be visualized and palpated to ensure that the cuff is intact.

Open release is also a surgical option for the recalcitrant primary frozen shoulder, as initially proposed by McLaughlin.[179, 180] The primary indication for open release in the idiopathic frozen shoulder is failure to improve on an appropriate nonoperative treatment program for a minimum of 6 months and failure to achieve normal motion after a gentle manipulation under anesthesia.

The procedure is performed through a low axillary incision and deltopectoral approach. The clavipectoral fascia is divided just lateral to the conjoined tendon and muscle. This split is continued proximally up to but not through the coracoacromial ligament. The humeroscapular motion interface is then mobilized. In the primary frozen shoulder, any interface adhesions are usually easily mobilized by finger dissection, unlike in the post-traumatic stiff shoulder. The axillary nerve should be palpated deep to the conjoined tendon in order to precisely localize it. We then place a modified Balfour retractor deep to the anterior deltoid and conjoined tendon to enhance exposure.

Attention is then given to division of the subscapularis tendon and entrance to the glenohumeral joint. Although the primary frozen shoulder is mainly a capsular problem, we recommend that subscapularis lengthening be considered.

There are three options for lengthening of the subscapularis. The simplest choice, and the author's preferred option, is division of the subscapularis tendon from its insertion on the lesser tuberosity with subsequent repair of the tendon to the humeral articular margin. The technique begins by passing a small elevator into the joint and behind the combined subscapularis and anterior capsule, protecting the long head of biceps tendon. The thick upper-rolled border of the subscapularis is then identified. Using sharp dissection, the upper-rolled border is excised from the lesser tuberosity, and care is taken not to leave any subscapularis tendon attached. Subscapular release is then carried distally, always ensuring that the complete tendon is included in the release. As the subscapularis is divided, the anterior capsular insertion is exposed. Using sharp dissection, the anterior capsule is released from its attachment at the humeral articular margin. The capsule remains united with the deep surface of the subscapularis. Approximately at the level of the anterior humeral circumflex vessels, the subscapularis attachment becomes muscular. By passing a small Darrach retractor deep to the vessels and subscapularis muscle, the inferior capsule can be exposed while protecting the axillary nerve. The inferior capsule is then released from its humeral insertion. Upon closure, the subscapularis is repaired to drill holes placed at the humeral articular margin. This technique will gain approximately 1 cm in subscapularis length, which will correlate with a gain in rotation of approximately 20 degrees.[118, 178]

By placing a Fukuda humeral head retractor into the joint, the anterior glenoid rim is exposed. With sharp dissection, the anterior capsule is incised just lateral to its labral insertion. The incision is carried through the superior, middle, and superior band of the inferior glenohumeral ligaments. While protecting the axillary nerve, the inferior capsule is incised. Since the subscapularis tendon with the associated lateral aspect of anterior glenohumeral capsule will be repaired on closure, we believe that an incision into the capsule itself constitutes the actual release. Care must be taken to ensure that the incision remains lateral to the glenoid labrum, preserving the labral attachment and its contribution to glenohumeral stability.

The second option for subscapularis lengthening and open release is a coronal z-plasty of the combined subscapularis and anterior capsule, as described by Neer (Fig. 20–26).[192, 193] A small elevator is passed through the rotator interval and deep to both the subscapularis tendon and the anterior capsule. This maneuver will help to gauge the combined thickness of the anterior structures. Using sharp dissection, the superficial surface of the subscapularis tendon is longitudinally divided just medial to its insertion at the lesser tuberosity. When one half of the combined thickness of the tendon/capsule is incised, the superficial flap is elevated medially to the level of the anterior glenoid labrum, at which point the anterior capsule is longitudinally incised. While protecting the axillary nerve with a small Darrach retractor, the incision is carried through the inferior capsule, always preserving the glenoid labral attachment. On closure, the medial edge of capsule is repaired to the lateral edge of the coronal split using heavy nonabsorbable suture. Two centimeters of length and hence 40 degrees of rotation can be gained by this technique.

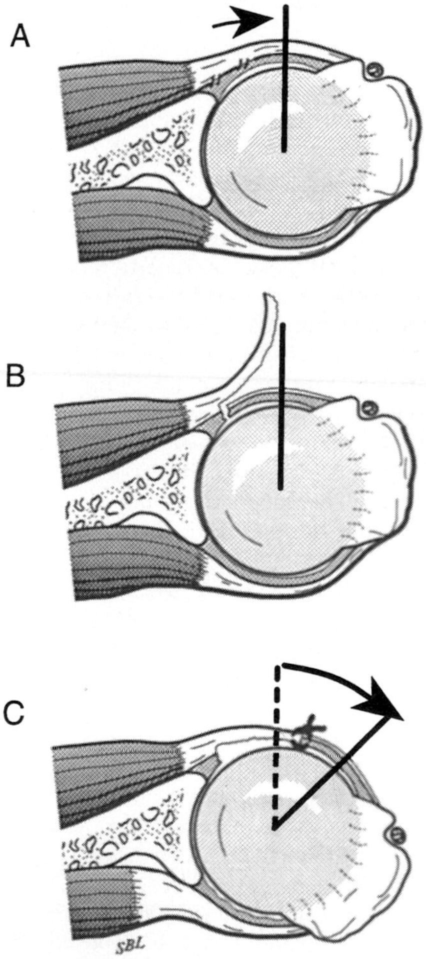

Figure 20–26

A, Contracted subscapularis and anterior capsule limit external rotation. *B,* The subscapularis tendon is incised from the lesser tuberosity laterally. The capsule is incised from the labrum medially. *C,* At the conclusion of the procedure, the lateral end of the subscapularis tendon is sutured to the medial end of the capsule, resulting in a substantial lengthening of these structures. As a rule of thumb, each centimeter of length gained by this procedure increases external rotation by approximately 20 degrees. (From Matsen FA III, Lippitt SB, Sidles JA, and Harryman DT II: Practical Evaluation of Management of the Shoulder. Philadelphia: WB Saunders, 1994.)

The final option for lengthening of the anterior capsule and subscapularis is an inside-out lengthening. Although this technique is the least desirable of the three choices, it is the only one that can be chosen in retrospect, after a subscapular and capsular incision has already been made. The anterior capsule is incised just lateral to the glenoid labrum as earlier. If at that point it becomes clear that a subscapularis lengthening is necessary, the anterior capsule is divided from the deep surface of the subscapularis from medial to lateral to 1 cm from the subscapularis and capsular arthrotomy incision, leaving the natural union between these structures intact. By repairing the medial capsular edge to the humeral articular margin through bone tunnels, a lengthening of 2 cm (40 degrees) can be achieved.

Unfortunately, tendon lengthening methods can be a dreadful disadvantage to the stiff shoulder because of the weakened subscapularis integrity and repair that must be protected from a forceful stretch for 6 to 8 weeks. In a review of 35 patients diagnosed with postoperative subscapularis insufficiency, three patients had previous subscapularis lengthening for severe refractory global shoulder stiffness.[319] In two cases, the subscapularis tendon integrity could not be restored.

The most difficult technical aspect of the procedure is release of the posterior capsule. With the lip of the Fukuda retractor placed behind the posterior glenoid rim, the hole in the retractor provides access to the posterior capsule. A long-handled scalpel is inserted through the retractor, and the posterior capsule is incised just lateral to the posterior labrum. By moving the Fukuda retractor superior and inferior or rotating the handle, the entire posterior capsule is released.

Prior to subscapularis repair, regardless of the lengthening technique, the subscapularis requires mobilization on all surfaces (a 360-degree release). Release of the coracohumeral ligament is an important component of this mobilization. By applying traction to the subscapularis, the coracohumeral ligament becomes taut at its coracoid origin. Using either sharp dissection or heavy scissors, the coracohumeral ligament is released from the coracoid. Adhesions in the subcoracoid recess and subscapular attachments to the anterior glenoid must be completely incised. The superficial surface was cleared of adhesions during the initial humeroscapular interface release. Finally, the more dangerous inferior release is accomplished, using a finger to palpate and protect the axillary nerve during scar incision. After release, the lengthened subscapularis is repaired with heavy, nonabsorbable suture. Intraoperative external rotation is noted and set as the limit during postoperative rehabilitation.

Aftercare

The patient is placed into a continuous passive motion machine in the recovery room. The shoulder is gently put through range of motion at the bedside daily, and a global capsular stretching program is begun immediately (refer to stretching program in Chapter 15; see Figs. 15–81 to 91). We will usually keep a patient in the hospital for 1 to 2 days postoperatively in order to ensure maintenance of motion prior to the patient's discharge. Pollock and associates have reported the use of continuous interscalene block in order to provide persistent pain relief and enhance the early postoperative program.[231] Patients are encouraged to use the arm for all activities of daily living, and their overhead reaching is limited. If a subscapularis lengthening was performed, internal rotation against resistance, as in closing a door, is restricted for the first 6 weeks postoperatively.

The most important aspect of the postoperative regimen is ensuring concentration on motion *only*. Too often, patients are referred to supervised physical therapy with orders to "evaluate and treat." This vague recommendation will likely lead to a generalized program, including modalities, weight training, and resistance exercises. These exercises not only take time away from the real beneficial stretching program but may also be detrimental. Therapists should be encouraged to concentrate only on motion exercises. Use of a pulley, in addition to the program as outlined, can be of some benefit. Therapists and patients should also be encouraged to use general aerobic conditioning as part of the postoperative program. Strengthening exercises are only begun when motion is symmetric in all directions.

Results. In a study performed in our institution, 12 patients ranging in age from 33 to 62 years were treated by open surgical release. In this group four patients were insulin-dependent diabetics. All patients failed to improve after a well-supervised rehabilitation program. The duration of preoperative symptoms and treatment averaged 16 months. The average flexion improved from 73 degrees (range of 20 to 95) to 132 degrees (range of 90 to 150). The average external rotation improved from 3 degrees (range of 5 to 25) to 45 degrees (range of 15 to 60). Pain was decreased or eliminated in all patients at 2-year follow-up. There were no complications, and all patients returned to work.

ARTHROSCOPIC RELEASE AND MANIPULATION UNDER ANESTHESIA

Conventional management strategies often fail to yield consistent or prompt return of comfort and function. During the past 5 years, we have employed an approach to the evaluation and management of glenohumeral stiffness using arthroscopic release of capsular contractures for the most refractory shoulder stiffness.

The main advantages of this approach include the following:

1. An accurate release of the contracted capsular structures
2. Increased mobility of musculotendinous units without compromising their integrity
3. Less pain postoperatively by avoiding an open incision
4. An opportunity to identify other intrinsic pathology that may have initiated or contributed to the pain leading to shoulder stiffness
5. Aggressive active and passive motion can be encouraged immediately

The objective of an arthroscopic capsular release is a direct intra-articular capsular release, including the anterior glenohumeral ligaments, the rotator interval capsule, the coracohumeral ligament, and the posterior and inferior capsule. Subacromial release of the bursal adhesions can also be accomplished.

In certain cases, an arthroscopic capsular release is absolutely contraindicated. These include:

1. Patients unable to understand or cooperate with a stretching motion program
2. Patients who cannot tolerate the surgical stress of a fluid challenge (e.g., renal or cardiac failure)

A relative contraindication includes patients with reflex sympathetic dystrophy or cervical radiculopathy because pain may significantly restrict rehabilitation exercises.

Technique of Arthroscopic Capsular Release

Before starting arthroscopy, 1 ml of 1:1,000 dilution injectable epinephrine is added to each 3-liter bag of saline. The tools required for the procedure include: one or two smooth diaphragm cannulas (5.5-mm outer diameter), a capsular elevator, a straight and 20-degree–angled capsular release forceps (Smith-Nephew-Dyonics-Acufex), and a motorized synovial resector blade.

We perform the procedure in the half-sitting beach chair position. A roll is placed adjacent to the vertebral border of the scapula to provide greater access to the posterior shoulder. The anatomy of the bony shoulder is marked on the skin along with the posterior soft spot and the lateral subacromial portal. The posterior incision is made slightly superior to the standard posterior portal to allow space for a second inferior posterior portal.

A blunt, tapered-tip trocar is advanced to penetrate the stiff posterior capsule. On removal of the trocar, the synovial "string" sign confirms intra-articular placement of the scope. If a manipulation was attempted before arthroscopy, blood may be present and lavage required to visualize the biceps tendon and rotator interval. The arthroscope is advanced superior to the biceps tendon to place an anterosuperior portal through the rotator interval. The degree of synovitis and pathologic findings seen about the biceps, labrum, capsule, and ligaments are recorded. The arthroscope is then switched to the anterior portal. Capsular release proceeds according to the following steps (Fig. 20–27).

1. Posterior Capsular Resection

The posterosuperior capsule is viewed by looking through the anterior portal. Again, the degree of synovitis is recorded prior to synovectomy with a motorized synovial resector blade to visualize the capsule. The posterior capsule should always be released first because fluid extravasation is limited posteriorly by the intact rotator cuff musculature, which is not the case after releasing the anterior rotator interval capsule.

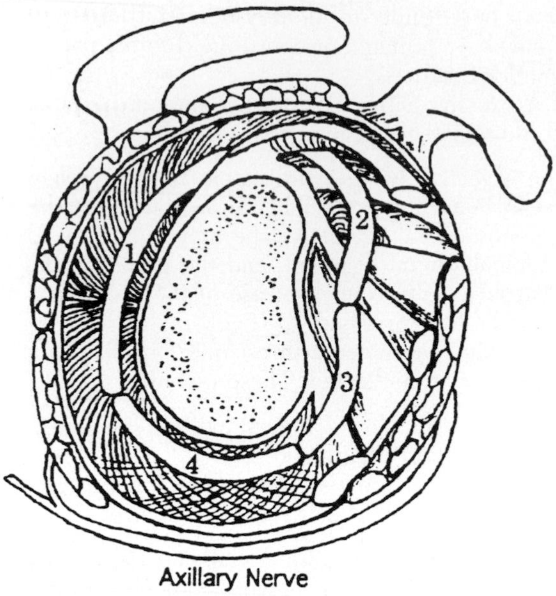

Figure 20–27

A diagram depicting the typical sequence of performing capsular release about the glenohumeral joint: (1) posterosuperior, (2) anterosuperior, (3) anteroinferior, and (4) posteroinferior. (From Harryman DT II, Sidles JA, and Matsen FA III: Arthroscopic management of refractory shoulder stiffness. Arthroscopy *13*:133–147, 1997.)

Capsular forceps are placed inside the joint through a posterior diaphragmmed cannula. The cannula is partially withdrawn outside the joint, and the forceps are opened to capture the capsule in the jaw at the edge of the portal. The capsule is lifted toward the joint away from the rotator cuff muscle fibers and sectioned approximately 1 cm peripheral to the labrum. Closed capsular forceps are advanced outside the capsule to separate the muscular fibers from the capsule. Capsular resection is continued into the superior recess avoiding the biceps root, labrum, and tendon.

Next, the scope is angled to view the capsule inferior to the posterior portal. The technique described earlier is used to transect the posterior capsule. Often, it is useful to switch to a 70-degree scope to view more of the posteroinferior recess. It is wise to discontinue this portion of the release when it becomes too difficult to see the tip of the forceps. Cutting posteroinferiorly without seeing the tip risks bleeding or injury to the axillary nerve (Fig. 20–28)!

2. Anterosuperior Capsular Resection

Next, the scope is switched to the posterior portal and the capsular forceps are placed into the joint through the cannula in the rotator interval. The cannula is withdrawn, and the superior glenohumeral ligament is transected. The labrum and root of the biceps tendon must remain intact. Next, the forceps are directed inferiorly to resect across the rotator interval capsule. The subcoracoid recess is often contracted or obliterated by synovitis. All attachments along the upper rolled border of the subscapularis tendon should be resected.

After release of the posterosuperior, anterosuperior, and rotator interval capsule, improved laxity and visibility results. Fluid insufflation pressure, however, must be minimized whenever possible to prevent excessive extravasation.

Next, the middle glenohumeral ligament is resected where it crosses the subscapularis tendon (Fig. 20–29). The superior band of the inferior glenohumeral ligament can be visualized and released by switching to a 70-degree arthroscope to continue anteroinferior capsular transection. The range of external rotation at the side and in abduction should be examined intermittently to check whether the degree of external rotation is symmetric to the opposite side recorded prior to the release. Our intraoperative goal is to achieve a minimum of 40 degrees of external rotation with the arm at the side.

3. Anteroinferior Capsular Resection

In shoulders that are still restricted in external rotation in the abducted position, a second anterior cannula is placed. We prefer one anterosuperior portal for viewing and a second anteroinferior portal for the capsular release forceps. The arm is internally rotated to relax the anterior capsule to visualize the superior border of the inferior glenohumeral ligament. Elevation of the capsule from the subscapularis with a capsular elevator helps to navigate the turn along the inferior recess adjacent to the anteroinferior glenoid rim. Then resection along the subscapularis with an angled capsular forceps is more easily accomplished. Again, do not resect capsule if visibility is poor or when the tip of the forceps cannot be seen!

4. Posteroinferior Capsular Resection

The 30-degree scope is switched to the posterior portal and angulated inferiorly with the humerus externally rotated. A second posterior cannula is placed 2 cm inferior

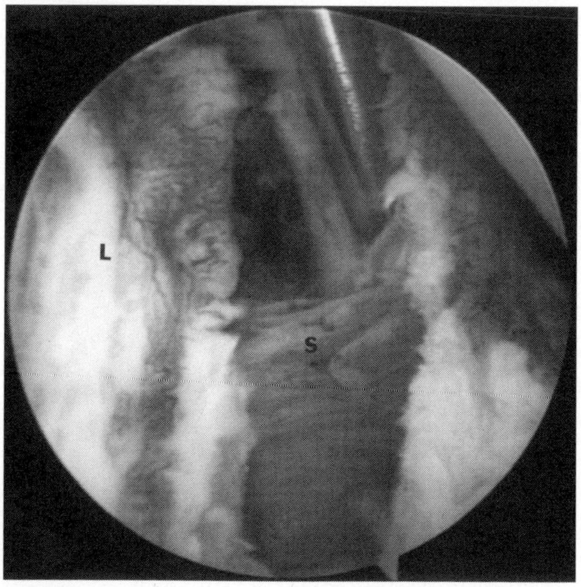

Figure 20–28

Axillary nerve adjacent to the probe after a complete posterior to anterior release of the inferior capsule peripheral to the glenoid labrum (L). Note that no protective tissue separates the divided capsule from the nerve posteroinferiorly. Anteroinferiorly, the muscular border of the subscapularis (S) muscle is interposed between the joint capsule and the axillary nerve. Inferior capsular release is best performed near the glenoid labrum to increase the margin of safety. (From Harryman DT II, Sidles JA, and Matsen FA III: Arthroscopic management of refractory shoulder stiffness. Arthroscopy *13*:133–147, 1997.)

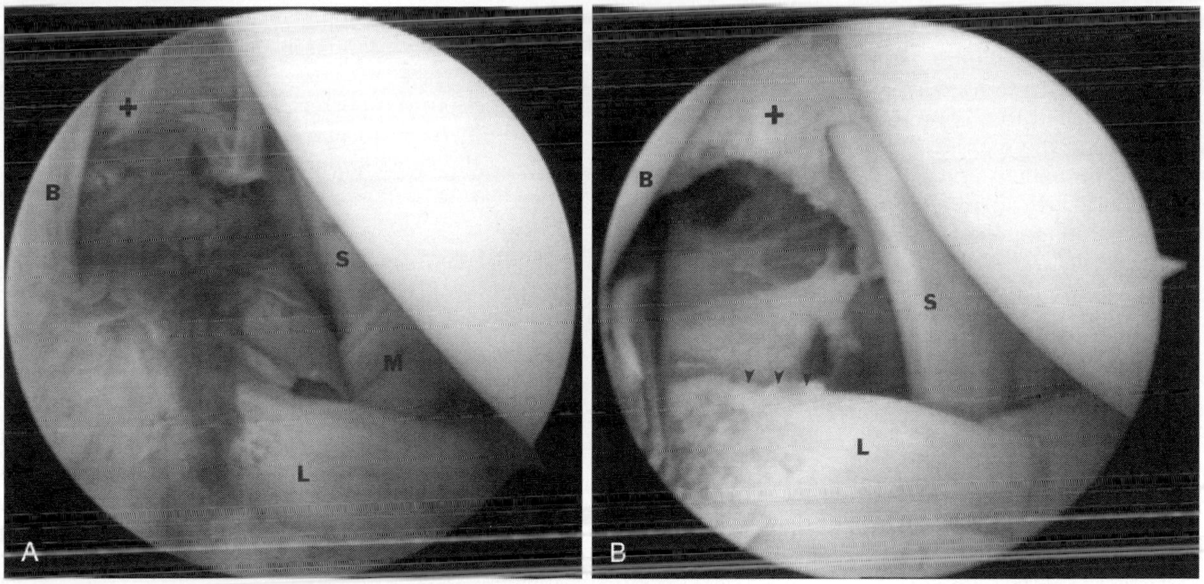

Figure 20–29

A, Arthroscopic view of the contracted rotator interval capsule, which is covered by synovitis. The tight superior glenohumeral ligament (+) is immediately adjacent to the biceps tendon *(B)*. The tip of the anterior cannula is positioned against the labrum (L) at the junction with the thickened middle glenohumeral ligament (M) that crosses the upper rolled border of the subscapularis tendon (S). *B,* The same arthroscopic view as earlier after complete transection and widening of the rotator interval capsule. Only a remnant of the superior glenohumeral (+) and middle glenohumeral *(arrowheads)* ligaments are visible. The biceps tendon (B) and labrum (L) are intact to the glenoid. Note that the humeral head has dropped inferiorly to expose the superior border of the subscapularis tendon (S). The middle and inferior glenohumeral ligaments are no longer visible because they have been divided and debrided. (From Harryman DT II, Sidles JA, and Matsen FA III: Arthroscopic management of refractory shoulder stiffness. Arthroscopy *13*:133–147, 1997.)

to the initial posterior portal. The cannula is advanced into the joint at the inferior extent of the previous posteroinferior capsule resection. After insertion of the forceps, the cannula is retracted outside the capsule. The straight forceps are advanced outside the capsule to free it from muscle or the axillary nerve. The jaws of the forceps are opened and retracted until the cutting jaw is inside the capsule.

Inferior resection continues anteriorly along the inferior recess adjacent to the labrum. Rotating angled capsular forceps afford access to the inferior capsule to help connect with the previous anteroinferior transection pathway.

5. Glenohumeral Clean-up and Subacromial Examination

A motorized shaver is inserted inside the joint to thoroughly remove residual synovitis and resected debris, as well as to widen the capsular margins. The shaver and scope are switched, and the process is repeated taking special care in the posterior and inferior recess (Fig. 20–30).

The arthroscope is inserted into the subacromial space to visualize the bursal side of the cuff. Generally, no surgical release or débridement is necessary for idiopathic frozen shoulders. In stiffness of post-traumatic or postsurgical origin, adhesions are released sharply with capsular forceps and resected with a motorized shaver. The coracoacromial arch is left untouched unless otherwise indicated by significant roughness or by the presence of an inferior directed bony protrusion.

After Release

Arthroscopic release is followed with an intra-articular injection of methylprednisolone (40 mg). It is unnecessary to put steroids in the subacromial space because they are contiguous after release of the rotator interval. After arthroscopy, the portals are closed and bulky dressings are applied.

Although extravasated fluid prevents immediate full range, postoperative motion is measured and a gentle

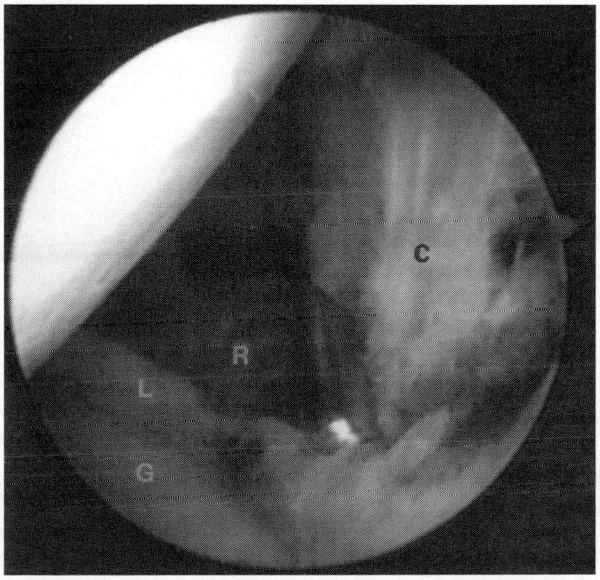

Figure 20–30

Posterior capsule (C) incompletely released with exposure of the internal surface of the rotator (R) cuff musculature. The capsule is transected widely inferior to the capsule and peripheral to the glenoid (G) and labrum (L). The inflamed synovium and residual capsule was excised.

manipulation is performed. In this way symmetric motion to the opposite side can be more reasonably ensured and a "fully aware" patient can participate. The released extremity is attached to a continuous passive motion device. Later during the same day, a repeat manipulation is performed at the patient's bedside while the interscalene block is still effective to free up residual adhesions and to allow the patient to assist and observe with his or her recovered motion.

Before being discharged from the hospital, the patient is reminded how to perform the Jackins' exercise program. Discharge from the hospital occurs the following day or after the patient achieves a minimum of 140 degrees of elevation and 40 degrees of external rotation.

Results of Arthroscopic Capsular Release

Ninety patients with refractory shoulder stiffness were treated according to a prospective algorithm between 1991 and 1996 (see Fig. 20–22). We have reviewed the results of the first 30 patients who failed at least 6 months (mean of 28, range of 6 to 131 months) of concerted nonoperative management for unilateral refractory shoulder stiffness.[122] The follow-up averaged 33 months (range of 12 to 56).

Motion and strength were prospectively documented according to the ASES' standard examination. Functional outcome measures were patient-assessed using the Simple Shoulder Test before and after surgery.

Before surgery, active range of motion of the affected shoulder averaged 41% of the opposite asymptomatic side. By the first day after surgery, motion was improved to a mean of 78% (range of 58% for internal rotation to 89% in forward elevation). An additional 15% of motion was gained after the patient was discharged from the hospital. Forward elevation and external rotation demonstrated the most rapid recovery, and internal rotation proved to be the most difficult to recover (see Fig. 20–20*A, B*) The final motion averaged 93% of the opposite side. Almost all patients recovered satisfactory motion and comfort, often as early as 3 months after release. Three long-term diabetic patients did not improve significantly by initial release (see Fig. 20–21).

All SST parameters and six of nine SF-36 health status scores were improved significantly. For example, only 6% of patients were able to sleep comfortably on their side, and 35% could place 1 lb on a shelf at shoulder height before surgery. After surgery, 73% were able to sleep comfortably on the affected side and 83% were able to place 1 lb on a shelf at shoulder height. There were no differences among all outcome measures between diabetic or nondiabetic patients.

COMBINED OPEN AND ARTHROSCOPIC RELEASE

Since patients with a post-traumatic stiff shoulder may have secondary capsular contracture, and since both open and arthroscopic release have benefits and drawbacks, we have performed combined open and arthroscopic releases in select patient groups. The advantages of combining the procedures are:

1. Ability to adequately release the humeroscapular motion interface
2. Access to the posterior capsule
3. Ability to perform a complete release without having to incise the subscapularis or rotator cuff
4. Decreased postoperative pain and faster rehabilitation

The primary indication for a combined arthroscopic and open release is the postsurgical stiff shoulder, primarily after anterior acromioplasty or rotator cuff repair. These patients usually have had a prior deltoid-splitting incision and have severe scar formation of the humeroscapular motion interface. In addition, these individuals often have associated posterior capsular contracture, particularly after rotator cuff repair. Neither open nor arthroscopic release will adequately mobilize these shoulders. Combined release is also indicated for long-standing post-traumatic stiff shoulders, in which secondary capsular contracture can be expected. Finally, the combined technique is indicated for shoulder stiffness after proximal humeral fractures, where associated capsular contracture is usually evident.

Technique

A thorough examination under anesthesia is done in order to define specific motion restrictions and assign likely locations of pathology. Glenohumeral arthroscopy is accomplished next, and a selective arthroscopic capsular release is performed, attending to those regions identified by the history and examination as likely to have capsular contracture. An open capsular release, performed through the prior deltoid-splitting incision, is accomplished next. Symmetric motion to the unaffected side is necessary before the procedure is completed.

Aftercare

The same care is required as after arthroscopic capsular release.

SUMMARY

The initiating etiology of capsular fibrosis still remains a mystery, but active investigations in cellular and molecular physiology may yield many clues in the near future. When treating the stiff shoulder, the physician must understand the major types of shoulder stiffness, their presentation, pathologic mechanism, and the location affecting function. We recommend the use of these simple definitions:

Frozen shoulder: An idiopathic global limitation of humeroscapular motion resulting from contracture and loss of compliance of the glenohumeral joint capsule

Post-traumatic stiff shoulder: A limitation in humeroscapular motion presenting after an injury, low-level repetitive trauma, or part of an accompanying condition that results in a contracture of structures participating in the glenohumeral or humeroscapular motion interfaces.

Differentiation of stiffness into defined groups helps to customize an individual's treatment within a logical framework. Investigators are also able to establish homogeneous treatment groups for analysis.[188] Classification is practically useful in planning treatment, because many shoulders that become stiff are treated best by corrective measures that address an intra- or extra-articular pathologic process contributing to the stiffness. In many stiff shoulders, addressing the stiffness alone is akin to misunderstanding the pathogenesis and is more likely to fail.

Examination of the patient and the pathologic site at open or arthroscopic surgery along with tissue biopsies has helped to distinguish *fibrosis* as the common lesion causing mechanical stiffness and clinical manifestations of shoulder stiffness. The authors suggest attaching a specific descriptor to the term *fibrosis,* which is associated with the pattern of clinical presentation or anatomic site of pathology. Terminology such as *global capsular fibrosis, posterior capsular fibrosis,* or *interfacial fibrosis* would accurately describe distinct clinically diagnosable entities and reflect recognizable pathophysiology.

The management and recovery from a stiff shoulder depends on motivating a patient to actively participate in nonoperative management. The Jackins' Exercise Program leads to early resumption of functional activities. For those patients who present with chronic or progressive global stiffness, manipulation may be indicated. Only patients with stiff shoulders refractory to nonsurgical treatment should be considered for surgical release by open or arthroscopic means. If necessary, operative management combined with an aggressive rehabilitation program can provide significant relief of pain and restoration of shoulder motion.

Once we clearly understand the initiating factors and find a method to inhibit the cascade of events that lead to capsular and interfacial fibrosis, then we will be able to suppress or eliminate its disabling progression. For now, our best effort is prevention by stretching mobilization.

References and Bibliography

1. Aitman TJ and Todd JA: Molecular genetics of diabetes mellitus. Baillieres Clin Endocrinol Metab 9:631–56, 1995.
2. Andrén L and Lundberg BJ: Treatment of rigid shoulders by joint distention during arthrography. Acta Orthop Scand *36*:45–53, 1965.
3. Angiolini G, Pasquinelli V, and Putti C: La roentgenterapia nella cura della periartrite della spalla. Minerva Med *56*:504–508, 1965.
4. Arenberg AA: [Oxygen therapy of brachio-scapular periarthritis]. Vestn Khir Im I I Grek *107*:126–127, 1971.
5. Askey JM: The syndrome of painful disability of the shoulder and hand complicating coronary occlusion. Am Heart J *22*:1–12, 1941.
6. Awad T, Losada M, and Losada A: [Treatment of scapulo-humeral periarthritis with alpha-chymotrypsin and rehabilitation]. Rev Med Chil *5*:372–376, 1967.
7. Bansil CK: Modification to the conventional wheel for measuring the range of movements of the shoulder joint. Med J Zambia 9:111–113, 1975.
8. Barnbeck F and Hierholzer G: [Analysis of the collective term "periarthritis humeroscapularis"]. Aktuelle Traumatol *21*:49–52, 1991.
9. Barrett WP, Franklin JL, Jackins SE, et al: Total shoulder arthroplasty. J Bone Joint Surg *69-A*:865–872, 1987.
10. Baslund B, Thomsen BS, and Jensen EM: [Humero-scapular periarthrosis]. Ugeskr Laeger *153*:170–173, 1991.
11. Basta J, Harryman II DT, and Sidles JA: Is biceps glide essential to glenohumeral motion? 64th Annual Meeting American Academy Orthopaedic Surgeons, San Francisco, CA, Feb. 16, 1997.
12. Baum J: Joint pain. It isn't always arthritis. Postgrad Med *85*:311–321, 1989.
13. Baumann F: Ventral capsular denervation: An operative treatment of periarthropathia humero-scapularis. Arch Orthop Trauma Surg *98*:13–17, 1981.
14. Bayley JIL and Kessel L: Treatment of the frozen shoulder by manipulation: a pilot study. *In* Shoulder Surgery. Berlin and Heidelberg: Springer-Verlag, 1982, pp 118–123.
15. Beals TC, Lazarus MD, and Harryman II DT: Useful boundaries of the subacromial bursa. Orthop Trans *19*:367, 1995.
16. Becker DA and Cofield RH: Tenodesis of the long head of the biceps brachii for chronic bicipital tendinitis. Long-term results [see comments]. J Bone Joint Surg Am *71*:376–381, 1989.
17. Bellmann H, Zacharias J, Hasert V, et al: [Use of hylase "Dessau" in periarthritis humero-scapularis (Duplay syndrome)]. Zentralbl Chir *94*:1288–1304, 1969.
18. Bernageau J, Bardin T, Goutallier D, et al: Magnetic resonance imaging findings in shoulders of hemodialyzed patients. Clin Orthop *304*:91–96, 1994.
19. Biermer SM: Manipulation in the treatment of frozen shoulder (Letter). Orthopedics *12*:356, 1989.
20. Billey T, Dromer C, Vedrenne C, et al: [Parsonage-Turner syndrome complicated by sympathetic dystrophy syndrome with adhesive capsulitis of the shoulder. A propos of 2 cases]. Rev Rhum Mal Osteoartic *59*:765–767, 1992.
21. Binder A, Hazleman BL, Parr G, and Roberts S: A controlled study of oral prednisolone in frozen shoulder. Br J Rheumatol *25*:288–292, 1986.
22. Binder AI, Bulgen DY, Hazleman BL, and Roberts S: Frozen shoulder: a long-term prospective study. Ann Rheum Dis *43*:361–364, 1984.
23. Binder AI, Bulgen DY, Hazleman BL, et al: Frozen shoulder: an arthrographic and radionuclear scan assessment. Ann Rheum Dis *43*:365–369, 1984.
24. Bland JH, Merrit JA, and Boushey DR: The painful shoulder. Semin Arthritis Rheum *7*:21–47, 1977.
25. Bohannon RW, Larkin PA, Smith MB, and Horton MG: Shoulder pain in hemiplegia: Statistical relationships with five variables. Arch Phys Med Rehabil *67*:514–516, 1986.
26. Bollini V: [Roentgen therapy of painful shoulder. Indications and results]. Minerva Ortop *22*:367–370, 1971.
27. Bosch-Olives V, Llurba-Llurba J, and Peinado-Visteur A: [Electrophysiotherapy in the treatment of a frozen shoulder]. Rev Esp Reum Enferm Osteoartic *12*:149–156, 1967.
28. Boussina I, Gunthner W, and Mart'i Mo-R: Double-blind multicenter study comparing meclofenamate sodium with indomethacin and placebo in the treatment of extra-articular rheumatic disease. Arzneimittelforschung *33*:649–652, 1983.
29. Bowman CA, Jeffcoate WJ, Pattrick M, and Doherty M: Bilateral adhesive capsulitis, oligoarthritis and proximal myopathy as presentation of hypothyroidism. Br J Rheumatol *27*:62–64, 1988.
30. Bradley JP: Arthroscopic treatment for frozen capsulitis. Oper Tech Orthop *1*:248–252, 1991.
31. Braun RM, West F, Mooney V, et al: Surgical treatment of the painful shoulder contracture in the stroke patient. J Bone Joint Surg *53A*:1307–1312, 1971.
32. Bridgman JF: Periarthritis of the shoulder and diabetes mellitus. Ann Rheum Dis *31*:69–71, 1972.
33. Bronzini C: [Roentgenotherapeutic methods in Duplay's disease]. Minerva Radiol *13*:630–632, 1968.
34. Brown C: Compressive, invasive referred pain to the shoulder. Clin Orthop *173*:55–62, 1983.
35. Bruckner FE: Frozen shoulder (adhesive capsulitis) (Editorial). J R Soc Med *75*:688–689, 1982.
36. Bruckner FE and Nye CJ: A prospective study of adhesive capsulitis of the shoulder ("frozen shoulder") in a high risk population. Q J Med *50*:191–204, 1981.
37. Bucala R, Makita Z, Koschinsky T, et al: Lipid advanced glycosylation: pathway for lipid oxidation in vivo. Proc Natl Acad Sci U S A *90*:6434–6438, 1993.
38. Bulgen D, Hazleman B, Ward M, and McCallum M: Immunological studies in frozen shoulder. Ann Rheum Dis *37*:135–138, 1978.

39. Bulgen DY, Binder A, Hazleman BL, and Park JR: Immunological studies in frozen shoulder. J Rheumatol *9*:893–898, 1982.
40. Bulgen DY, Binder AI, Hazleman BL, et al: Frozen shoulder: prospective clinical study with an evaluation of three treatment regimens. Ann Rheum Dis *43*:353–360, 1984.
41. Bulgen DY and Hazleman BL: Immunoglobulin-A, HLA–B27, and frozen shoulder (Letter). Lancet *2(8249)*:760, 1981.
42. Bulgen DY, Hazleman BL, and Voak D: HLA-B27 and frozen shoulder. Lancet *1(7968)*:1042–1044, 1976.
43. Bunker TD: Frozen shoulder (Editorial). Lancet *1(8420)*:87–88, 1985.
44. Bunker TD: Time for a new name for 'frozen shoulder' (Editorial). BMJ *290(6477)*:1233–1234, 1985.
45. Bunker TD and Anthony PP: The pathology of frozen shoulder. A Dupuytren-like disease. J Bone Joint Surg *77B*:677–683, 1995.
46. Bunker TD and Esler CN: Frozen shoulder and lipids. J Bone Joint Surg *77B*:684–686, 1995.
47. Bush LF: The torn shoulder capsule. J Bone Joint Surg Am *57*:256–259, 1975.
48. Carron H: Relieving pain with nerve blocks. Geriatrics *33*:49–57, 1978.
49. Caspari RB, McIntyre L, and Savoie FH: Arthroscopic Management of Multidirectional Instability. 13th Annual Arthroscopy Association of North America, Orlando, Florida, April, 1994.
50. Champion GD, Saxon JA, and Kossard S: The syndrome of palmar fibromatosis (fasciitis) and polyarthritis. J Rheumatol *14*:1196–1198, 1987.
51. Chard MD and Hazleman BL: Shoulder disorders in the elderly (a hospital study). Ann Rheum Dis *46*:684–687, 1987.
52. Charnley J: Periarthritis of the shoulder. Postgrad Med J *35*:384–388, 1959.
53. Cinquegrana OD: Chronic cervical radiculitis and its relationship to "chronic bursitis." Am J Phys Med *47*:23–30, 1968.
54. Clarke GR, Willis LA, Fish WW, and Nichols PJ: Preliminary studies in measuring range of motion in normal and painful stiff shoulders. Rheumatol Rehabil *14*:39–46, 1975.
55. Codman EA: The Shoulder. Boston: Todd, 1934, pp 216–224.
56. Connolly J, Regen E, and Evans OB: Management of the painful, stiff shoulder. Clin Orthop *84*:97–103, 1972.
57. Conti V: Arthroscopy in rehabilitation. Orthop Clin North Am *10*:709–711, 1979.
58. Coombes WN: Distension-manipulation for the treatment of adhesive capsulitis (frozen shoulder syndrome) (Letter). Clin Orthop *188*:309–310, 1984.
59. Corbeil V, Dussault RG, Leduc BE, and Fleury J: [Adhesive capsulitis of the shoulder: A comparative study of arthrography with intra-articular corticotherapy and with or without capsular distension]. Can Assoc Radiol J *43*:127–130, 1992.
60. Cotta H and Correll J: [The post-traumatic frozen shoulder]. Unfallchirurgie *8*:294–306, 1982.
61. Coventry MB: Problem of the painful shoulder. JAMA *151*:177–185, 1953.
62. Cyriax J and Trosier O: Hydrocortisone and soft tissue lesions. BMJ 2:966–968, 1953.
63. Dacre JE, Beeney N, and Scott DL: Injections and physiotherapy for the painful stiff shoulder. Ann Rheum Dis *48*:322–325, 1989.
64. Dangoisse MJ, Wilson DJ, and Glynn CJ: MRI and clinical study of an easy and safe technique of suprascapular nerve blockade. Acta Anaesthesiol Belg *45*:49–54, 1994.
65. Darlington LG and Coomes EN: The effects of local steroid injection for supraspinatus tears. Rheumatol Rehabil *16*:172–179, 1977.
66. De Seze S: Les épaules douloureuses et les épaules bloquées. Concours Med *96*:5329–5357, 1974.
67. Degen IL: [Magnetotherapy of brachio-scapular periarthritis]. Ortop Travmatol Protez *34*:66–68, 1974.
68. Demaziére A and Wiley AM: Primary chest wall tumor appearing as frozen shoulder: Review and case presentations. J Rheumatol *18*:911–914, 1991.
69. Denham RH Jr and Dingley AF Jr: Conservative management of periarthritis of the shoulder. J Indiana State Med Assoc *62*:376–379, 1969.
70. DePalma AF: Loss of scapulohumeral motion (frozen shoulder). Ann Surg *135*:193–204, 1952.
71. Detrisac DA and Johnson LL: Arthroscopic shoulder anatomy. Thorofare, NJ: Slack, Inc, 1986, pp 111–113.
72. Dickson JA and Crosby EH: Periarthritis of the shoulder: An analysis of two hundred cases. JAMA *99*:2252–2257, 1932.
73. Downing DS and Weinstein A: Ultrasound therapy of subacromial bursitis. A double blind trial. Phys Ther *66*:194–199, 1986.
74. Duke O, Zecler E, and Grahame R: Anti-inflammatory drugs in periarthritis of the shoulder: A double-blind, between-patient study of naproxen versus indomethacin. Rheumatol Rehabil *20*:54–59, 1981.
75. Duplay ES: De la periarthrite scapulo-humérale et des radeurs de l'épaule qui en sont la conséquence. Arch Gen Med *20*:513–542, 1872.
76. Duplay ES: De la périarthrite scapulo-humérale. Rev Frat Trav Med *53*:226, 1896.
77. Duralde XA, Jelsma RD, Pollock RG, et al: Arthroscopic treatment of resistant frozen shoulder. Arthroscopy *9*:345, 1993.
78. duToit GT and Roux D: A 24-year study of the Johannesburg stapling operation. J Bone Joint Surg *36-A*:1–12, 1956.
79. Dyer DG, Dunn JA, Thorpe SR, et al: Accumulation of Maillard reaction products in skin collagen in diabetes and aging. J Clin Invest *91*:2463–2469, 1993.
80. Echternach JL: Audio analgesia as an adjunct to mobilization of the chronic frozen shoulder. Phys Ther *46*:839–846, 1966.
81. Ellman H, Harris E, and Kay SP: Early degenerative joint disease simulating impingement syndrome: Arthroscopic findings. Arthroscopy *8*:482–487, 1992.
82. Emig EW, Schweitzer ME, Karasick D, and Lubowitz J: Adhesive capsulitis of the shoulder: MR diagnosis. AJR Am J Roentgenol *164*:1457–1459, 1995.
83. Ene EE and Odia GI: Effect of acupuncture on disorders of musculoskeletal system in Nigerians. Am J Chin Med *11*:106–111, 1983.
84. Engleman RM: Shoulder pain as a presenting complaint in upper lobe bronchogenic carcinoma: Report of 21 cases. Conn Med *30*:273–276, 1966.
85. Ernstene AC and Kinell J: Pain in the shoulder as a sequel to myocardial infarction. Arch Intern Med *66*:800–806, 1940.
86. Esposito S, Ragozzino A, Russo R, et al: [Arthrography in the diagnosis and treatment of idiopathic adhesive capsulitis]. Radiol Med *85*:583–587, 1993.
87. Famaey JP and Ginsberg F: Treatment of periarthritis of the shoulder: A comparison of ibuprofen and diclofenac. J Intern Med Res *12*:238–243, 1984.
88. Fareed DO and Gallivan WR Jr: Office management of frozen shoulder syndrome. Treatment with hydraulic distension under local anesthesia. Clin Orthop *242*:177–183, 1989.
89. Fearnley ME and Vadasz I: Factors influencing the response of lesions of the rotator cuff of the shoulder to local steroid injection. Ann Phys Med *10*:53–63, 1969.
90. Fernandes MS and Pinto AC: Ombros dolorosos. Acta Med Port *3*:229–234, 1990.
91. Ferrari DA: Capsular ligaments of the shoulder. Anatomical and functional study of the anterior superior capsule. Am J Sports Med *18*:20–24, 1990.
92. Fisher L, Kurtz A, and Shipley M: Association between cheiroarthropathy and frozen shoulder in patients with insulin dependent diabetes mellitus. Br J Rheumatol *25*:141–146, 1986.
93. Fleming A, Dodman S, Beer TC, and Crown S: Personality in frozen shoulder. Ann Rheum Dis *35*:456–457, 1976.
94. Freedman L and Munro RR: Abduction of the arm in the scapular plane: Scapular and glenohumeral movements. A roentgenographic study. J Bone Joint Surg *48*:1503–1510, 1966.
95. Galinat BJ and Howell SM: The containment mechanism: The primary stabilizer of the glenohumeral joint. Ortho Trans *11*:458, 1987.
96. Gilula LA, Schoenecker PL, and Murphy WA: Shoulder arthrography as a treatment modality. AJR Am J Roentgenol *131*:1047–1048, 1978.
97. Goldman AB and Ghelman B: The double contrast shoulder arthrogram: A review of 158 studies. Radiology *127*:655–663, 1978.
98. Goldman RT, Koval KJ, Cuomo F, et al: Functional outcome after humeral head replacement for acute three and four part proximal humeral fractures. J Shoulder Elbow Surg *Jan/Feb*:81–86, 1995.
99. Good AE, Green RA, and Zarafonetis CJD: Rheumatic symptoms during tuberculosis therapy: manifestation of isoniazid toxicity? Ann Intern Med *63*:800–807, 1965.

100. Gore DR, Murray MP, Sepic SB, et al: Shoulder-muscle strength and range of motion following surgical repair of full-thickness rotator cuff tears. J Bone Joint Surg *68*:266–272, 1986.
101. Gotter G: Comparative evaluation of tenoxicam and piroxicam in the treatment of humeroscapular periarthritis. Eur J Rheumatol Inflamm 9:95–97, 1987.
102. Grabovoi AF, Grishko AI, Rodichkin VA, et al: [Blockade of the suprascapular nerve in the complex treatment of humero-scapular periarthritis]. Vestn Khir *136*:65–66, 1986.
103. Greinemann H: [The painful frozen shoulder (author's transl)]. Unfallchirurgie *6*:239–244, 1980.
104. Grey RG: The natural history of "idiopathic" frozen shoulder. J Bone Joint Surg Am *60*:564, 1978.
105. Griffin JW: Hemiplegic shoulder pain. Phys Ther *66*:1884–1893, 1986.
106. Gudushauri ON and Goguadze DM: [Ambulatory treatment of humero-scapular periarthritis, humeral epicondylitis and radial styloiditis by local injections of hydrocortisone]. Ortop Travmatol Protez *8*:24–26, 1975.
107. Gusarova SA: [Massage in humeroscapular periarthosis]. Med Sestra *48*:36–38, 1980.
108. Ha'eri GB and Maitland A: Arthroscopic findings in the frozen shoulder. J Rheumatol *8*:149–152, 1981.
109. Haggart GE, Digman RJ, and Sullivan TS: Management of the "frozen" shoulder. JAMA *161*:1219–1222, 1956.
110. Haguenauer JP and Bouvier M: [Scapulo-humeral periarthritis of the "frozen shoulder" type following cervical lymph node 'evidement']. Rhumatologie *18*:231–235, 1966.
111. Haines JF and Hargadon EJ: Manipulation as the primary treatment of the frozen shoulder. J R Coll Surg Edinb *27*:271–275, 1982.
112. Hamer J and Kirk JA: Physiotherapy and the frozen shoulder: A comparative trial of ice and ultrasonic therapy. N Z Med J *83(560)*:191–192, 1976.
113. Hannafin JA, DiCarlo ED, Wickiewicz TL, and Warren RF: Adhesive capsulitis: capsular fibroplasia of the glenohumeral joint. J Shoulder Elbow Surg *3(S)*:5, 1994.
114. Hansen PE: Biceps transfer intra-position grafting in massive rotator cuff tears. *In* Burkhead WZ (ed): Rotator Cuff Disorders. Baltimore: Williams & Wilkins, 1996, pp 349–355.
115. Harmon PH: Methods and results in the treatment of 2580 painful shoulders. Am J Surg *95*:527–544, 1958.
116. Harryman II DT: Shoulders: Frozen and stiff. Instr Course Lect *42*:247–257, 1993.
117. Harryman II DT, Ballmer FP, Harris SL, and Sidles JA: Arthroscopic labral repair to the glenoid rim. J Arthroscopy *10*:20–30, 1994.
118. Harryman II DT, Lazarus MD, Sidles JA, and Matsen III FA: Pathophysiology of shoulder instability. *In* McGinty JB, et al (eds): Operative Arthroscopy. Philadelphia: JB Lippincott, 1996, pp 677–693.
119. Harryman II DT, Sidles JA, Clark JM, et al: Translation of the humeral head on the glenoid with passive glenohumeral motion. J Bone Joint Surg *72-A*:1334–1343, 1990.
120. Harryman II DT, Sidles JA, Harris SL, and Matsen III FA: The role of the rotator interval capsule in passive motion and stability of the shoulder. J Bone Joint Surg *74-A*:53–66, 1992.
121. Harryman II DT, Sidles JA, and Matsen III FA: Laxity of the normal glenohumeral joint: A quantitative in vivo assessment. J Shoulder Elbow Surg *1*:66–76, 1992.
122. Harryman II DT, Sidles JA, and Matsen III FA: Arthroscopic management of refractory shoulder stiffness. Arthroscopy *13*:133–147, 1997.
123. Harryman II DT, Walker ED, Harris SL, et al: Residual motion and function after glenohumeral or scapulothoracic arthrodesis. J Shoulder Elbow Surg *2*:275–285, 1993.
124. Hashimoto T, Suzuki K, and Nobuhara K: Dynamic analysis of intraarticular pressure in the glenohumeral joint. J Shoulder Elbow Surg *4*:209–218, 1995.
125. Hassenstein E, Nusslin F, Hartweg H, and Renner K: [Radiation therapy of humeroscapular periarthritis (author's transl)]. Strahlentherapie *155*:87–93, 1979.
126. Hawkins RJ and Angelo RL: Glenohumeral osteoarthrosis: A late complication of the Putti-Platt repair. J Bone Joint Surg *72-A*:1193–1197, 1990.
127. Hazleman BL: Why is a frozen shoulder frozen? Br J Rheumatol *29*:130, 1990.
128. Hazleman BL: The painful stiff shoulder. Rheum Phys Med *11*:413–421, 1972.
129. Hazleman BL: Frozen shoulder. *In* Watson MS (ed): Surgical Disorders of the Shoulder. New York: Churchill Livingstone, 1991, pp 167–179.
130. Helbig B, Wagner P, and Dohler R: Mobilization of frozen shoulder under general anesthesia. Acta Orthop Belg *49*:267–274, 1983.
131. Herbut PA and Watson JS: Tumor of the thoracic inlet producing the Pancoast Syndrome. A report of seventeen cases and a review of the literature. Arch Pathol *42*:88–103, 1946.
132. Hill JJ Jr and Bogumill H: Manipulation in the treatment of frozen shoulder. Orthopedics *11*:1255–1260, 1988.
133. Hitchcock HH and Bechtol CO: Painful shoulder. J Bone Joint Surg *30-A*:263–273, 1948.
134. Hogan M, Cerami A, and Bucala R: Advanced glycosylation end products block the antiproliferative effect of nitric oxide. Role in the vascular and renal complications of diabetes mellitus. J Clin Invest *90*:1110–1115, 1992.
135. Hollingworth GR, Ellis RM, and Hattersley TS: Comparison of injection techniques for shoulder pain: results of a double blind, randomised study. BMJ *287(6402)*:1339–1341, 1983.
136. Hsu SY and Chan KM: Arthroscopic distension in the management of frozen shoulder. Int Orthop *15*:79–83, 1991.
137. Hulstyn MJ and Weiss AP: Adhesive capsulitis of the shoulder. Orthop Rev 22:425–433, 1993.
138. Huskisson EC and Bryans R: Diclofenac sodium in the treatment of painful stiff shoulder. Curr Med Res Opin *8*:350–353, 1983.
139. Inman VT, Saunders JB, and Abbott LC: Observations on the function of the shoulder joint. J Bone Joint Surg *26*:1–30, 1944.
140. Itoi E and Tabata S: Range of motion and arthrography in the frozen shoulder. J Shoulder Elbow Surg *1*:106–112, 1992.
141. Jacobs LG, Barton MA, Wallace WA, et al: Intra-articular distension and steroids in the management of capsulitis of the shoulder. BMJ *302(6791)*:1498–1501, 1991.
142. Janda DH and Hawkins RJ: Shoulder manipulation in patients with adhesive capsulitis and diabetes mellitus: A clinical note. J Shoulder Elbow Surg 2:36–38, 1993.
143. Johnston JTH: Frozen shoulder syndrome in patients with pulmonary tuberculosis. J Bone Joint Surg *41*:877–882, 1959.
144. Jones R and Lovett RW: Orthopedic Surgery. New York: William and Wood, 1923, p 59.
145. Kamieth H: Radiology of the cervical spine in shoulder periarthritis. Z Orthop Ihre Grenzgeb *100*:162–167, 1965.
146. Kay NR: The clinical diagnosis and management of frozen shoulders. Practitioner *225(1352)*:164–167, 1981.
147. Kennedy JC and Willis RB: The effects of local steroid injections on tendons: A biomechanical and microscopic correlative study. Am J Sports Med *4*:11–21, 1976.
148. Kernwein GA, Rosenberg B, and Sneed WA: Arthrographic studies of the shoulder. J Bone Joint Surg *39*:1267–1279, 1957.
149. Kessel L: Disorders of the Shoulder. New York: Churchill Livingstone, 1982, p 82.
150. Kessel L, Bayley I, and Young A: The upper limb: the frozen shoulder. Br J Hosp Med *25*:334–339, 1981.
151. Kieras DM and Matsen III FA: Open release in the management of refractory frozen shoulder. Orthop Trans *15*:801–802, 1991.
152. Koppell HP and Thompson WAL: Pain and the frozen shoulder. Surg Gynecol Obstet *109*:92–96, 1959.
153. Kottke FJ, Pauley DL, and Ptak RA: The rationale for prolonged stretching for correction of shortening of connective tissue. Arch Phys Med Rehabil *47*:345–352, 1966.
154. Kozin F: Two unique shoulder disorders. Adhesive capsulitis and reflex sympathetic dystrophy syndrome. Postgrad Med *73*:207–210, 1983.
155. Lapidus PW and Guidotti FP: Common shoulder lesions—report of 493 cases. Calcific tendinitis, tendinitis of long head of biceps frozen shoulder, fractures and dislocations. Bull Hosp Jt Dis *29*:293–306, 1968.
156. Laumann U: The so-called "periarthritis humeroscapularis"—possibilities of an operative treatment. Arch Orthop Trauma Surg 97:27–37, 1980.
157. Leardini G, Perbellini A, Franceschini M, and Mattara L: Intra-articular injections of hyaluronic acid in the treatment of painful shoulder. Clin Ther *10*:521–526, 1988.

158. Lee M, Haq AM, Wright V, and Longton E: Periarthritis of the shoulder: A controlled trial of physiotherapy. Physiotherapy *59*:312–315, 1973.
159. Lee PN, Lee M, Haq AM, et al: Periarthritis of the shoulder: trial of treatments investigated by multivariate analysis. Ann Rheum Dis *33*:116–119, 1974.
160. Leffert RD: The frozen shoulder. Instr Course Lect *34*:199–203, 1985.
161. Lehmann JF, Warren CG, and Scham SM: Therapeutic heat and cold. Clin Orthop *99*:207–245, 1974.
162. Lequesne M, Dang N, Bensasson M, and Mery C: Increased association of diabetes mellitus with capsulitis of the shoulder and shoulder-hand syndrome. Scand J Rheumatol *6*:53–56, 1977.
163. Lin ML, Huang CT, Lin JG, and Tsai SK: [A comparison between the pain relief effect of electroacupuncture, regional nerve block and electroacupuncture plus regional nerve block in frozen shoulder]. Acta Anaesthesiol Sin *32*:237–242, 1994.
164. Lippitt SB, Vanderhooft JE, Harris SL, et al: Glenohumeral stability from concavity—compression: A quantitative analysis. J Shoulder Elbow Surg *2*:27–35, 1993.
165. Lippman RK: Frozen shoulder; periarthritis; bicipital tenosynovitis. Arch Surg *47*:283–296, 1943.
166. Lloyd-Roberts GC and French PR: Periarthritis of the shoulder. BMJ *1*:1569–1571, 1959.
167. Loyd JA and Loyd HM: Adhesive capsulitis of the shoulder: Arthrographic diagnosis and treatment. South Med J *76*:879–883, 1983.
168. Lundberg BJ: The frozen shoulder: Clinical and radiographical observations. The effect of manipulation under general anesthesia. Structure and glycosaminoglycan content of the joint capsule. Local bone metabolism. Acta Orthop Scand *119* [Suppl]:1–59, 1969.
169. Lundberg BJ and Nilsson BE: Osteopenia in the frozen shoulder. Clin Orthop *60*:187–191, 1968.
170. Mack LA, Gannon MK, and Kilcoyne RF: Sonographic evaluation of the rotator cuff: Accuracy in patients without prior surgery. Clin Orthop *234*:21–27, 1988.
171. Macnab I: The painful shoulder due to rotator cuff tendinitis. R I Med J *54*:367–374, 1971.
172. Macnab I: Rotator cuff tendinitis. Ann R Coll Surg Engl *53*:271–287, 1973.
173. Magnuson PB and Stack JK: Recurrent dislocation of the shoulder. JAMA *123*:889–892, 1943.
174. Makita Z, Radoff S, Rayfield EJ, et al: Advanced glycosylation end products in patients with diabetic nephropathy [see comments]. N Engl J Med *325*:836–842, 1991.
175. Malgaigne JF: Treatise on Fractures. Philadelphia: JB Lippincott, 1859, p 419.
176. Matsen III FA and Arntz CA: Subacromial impingement. *In* Rockwood CA and Matsen III FA (eds): The Shoulder, Vol 2. Philadelphia: WB Saunders, 1990, pp 629–638.
177. Matsen III FA and Kirby RM: Office evaluation and management of shoulder pain. Orthop Clin North Am *13*:453–475, 1982.
178. Matsen III FA, Lippitt SB, Sidles JA, and Harryman II DT: Practical Evaluation of Management of the Shoulder. Philadelphia: WB Saunders. 1994, pp 19–109.
179. McLaughlin HL: On the "frozen" shoulder. Bull Hosp Jt Dis *12*:383–393, 1951.
180. McLaughlin HL: The "frozen shoulder." Clin Orthop *20*:126–131, 1961.
181. Melzer C, Wallny T, Wirth CJ, and Hoffmann S: Frozen shoulder—treatment and results. Arch Orthop Trauma Surg *114*:87–91, 1995.
182. Meulengracht E and Schwartz M: The course and prognosis of periarthritis humeroscapularis with special regard to cases with general symptoms. Acta Med Scand *143*:350–360, 1952.
183. Minter WT: The shoulder-hand syndrome in coronary disease. JAMA *56*:45–49, 1967.
184. Morén-Hybbinette I, Moritz U, and Shersten B: The clinical picture of the painful diabetic shoulder—natural history, social consequences and analysis of concomitant hand syndrome. Acta Med Scand *221*:73–82, 1987.
185. Morency G, Dussault RG, Robillard P, and Samson L: [Distention arthrography in the treatment of adhesive capsulitis of the shoulder]. Can Assoc Radiol J *40*:84–86, 1989.
186. Murnaghan GF and McIntosh D: Hydrocortisone in painful shoulder—a controlled trial. Lancet *2*:798–801, 1955.
187. Murnaghan JP: Adhesive capsulitis of the shoulder: current concepts and treatment. Orthopaedics *11*:153–158, 1988.
188. Murnaghan JP: Frozen shoulder. *In* Rockwood CA and Matsen III FA (eds): The Shoulder, Vol 2. Philadelphia: WB Saunders, 1990, pp 837–862.
189. Murray MP, Gore DR, Gardener GM, and Mollinger LR: Shoulder motion and muscle strength of normal men and women in two age groups. Clin Orthop *192*:268–273, 1985.
190. Neer II CA, Satterlee CC, Dalsey RM, and Flatow EL: The anatomy and potential effects of contracture of the coracohumeral ligament. Clin Orthop *280*:182–185, 1992.
191. Neer II CS: Anterior acromioplasty for the chronic impingement syndrome in the shoulder. J Bone Joint Surg *54-A*:41–50, 1972.
192. Neer II CS: Shoulder Reconstruction. Philadelphia: WB Saunders, 1990, pp 328, 421–427.
193. Neer II CS and Foster CR: Inferior capsular shift for involuntary inferior and multidirectional instability of the shoulder. J Bone Joint Surg *62-A*:897–907, 1980.
194. Neer II CS, Satterlee CC, Dalsey RM, and Flatow EL: On the value of the coracohumeral ligament release. Ortho Trans *13–2*:235–236, 1989.
195. Nelson CL and Burton RI: Upper extremity arthrography. Clin Orthop *107*:62–72, 1975.
196. Neviaser JS: Adhesive capsulitis of the shoulder. J Bone Joint Surg *27*:211–222, 1945.
197. Neviaser JS: Arthrography of the shoulder joint. J Bone Joint Surg *44A*:1321–1330, 1962.
198. Neviaser JS: Arthrography of the Shoulder. Springfield, IL: Charles C. Thomas, 1975, pp 60–66.
199. Neviaser JS: Adhesive capsulitis and the stiff and painful shoulder. Orthop Clin North Am *11*:327–331, 1980.
200. Neviaser RJ: Painful conditions affecting the shoulder. Clin Orthop *173*:63–69, 1983.
201. Neviaser RJ: Radiologic assessment of the shoulder: Plain and arthrographic. Orthop Clin North Am *18*:343–349, 1987.
202. Neviaser RJ and Neviaser TJ: Arthroscopy of the shoulder. Orthop Clin North Am *18*:361–372, 1987.
203. Neviaser RJ and Neviaser TJ: The frozen shoulder: Diagnosis and management. Clin Orthop *223*: 59–64, 1987.
204. Neviaser TJ: Adhesive capsulitis. Orthop Clin North Am *18*:439–443, 1987.
205. Newton DR: The management of non-articular rheumatism. Practitioner *208(243)*:64–73, 1972.
206. Nicholson GG: The effects of passive joint mobilization on pain and hypomobility associated with adhesive capsulitis of the shoulder. Orthop Sports Phys Ther *6*:238–246, 1985.
207. Nobuhara K and Ikeda H: Rotator interval lesion. Clin Orthop *223*:44–50, 1987.
208. Nobuhara K, Sugiyama D, Ikeda H, and Makiura M: Contracture of the shoulder. Clin Orthop *254*:105–110, 1990.
209. Nobuhara K, Supapo AR, and Hino T: Effects of joint distention in shoulder diseases. Clin Orthop *304*:25–29, 1994.
210. O'Brien SJ, Neves MC, Arnoczky SP, et al: The anatomy and histology of the inferior glenohumeral ligament complex of the shoulder. Am J Sports Med *18*:449–456, 1990.
211. Obremskey WT: Follow-up of the Inferior Capsular Shift Procedure for Atraumatic Multidirectional Instability. Univ Wash Res Rep *4*:45, 1994.
212. Oesterreicher W and van Dam G: Social psychological researches into brachialgia and periarthritis. Arthritis Rheum *7*:670–683, 1964.
213. Ogilvie-Harris DJ, Biggs DJ, Fitsialos DP, and MacKay M: The resistant frozen shoulder. Manipulation versus arthroscopic release. Clin Orthop *319*:238–248, 1995.
214. Ogilvie-Harris DJ and Wiley AM: Arthroscopic surgery of the shoulder: A general appraisal. J Bone Joint Surg *68B*:201–207, 1986.
215. Ogilvie-Harris DJ and D'Angelo G: Arthroscopic surgery of the shoulder. Sports Med *9*:120–128, 1990.
216. Older MWJ: Distension arthrography of the shoulder Joint. *In* Bayler L and Kessel L (eds): Shoulder Surgery. Berlin and Heidelberg: Springer-Verlag, 1982, pp 123–127.
217. Older MWJ, McIntyre JL, and Lloyd GJ: Distension arthrography of the shoulder joint. Can J Surg *19*:203–207, 1976.

218. Oldham BE: Periarthritis of the shoulder associated with thyrotoxicosis. N Z Med J 29:766–770, 1959.
219. Osmond Clarke H: Habitual dislocation of the shoulder. The Putti-Platt operation. J Bone Joint Surg *30-B*:19–25, 1948.
220. Ozaki J, Nakagawa Y, Sakurai G, and Tamai S: Recalcitrant chronic adhesive capsulitis of the shoulder. Role of contracture of the coracohumeral ligament and rotator interval in pathogenesis and treatment. J Bone Joint Surg *71A*:1511–1515, 1989.
221. Pal B, Anderson J, Dick WC, and Griffiths ID: Limitation of joint mobility and shoulder capsulitis in insulin and non-insulin dependent diabetes mellitus. Br J Rheumatol *25*:147–151, 1986.
222. Pal B, Griffiths ID, Anderson J, and Dick WC: Association of limited joint mobility with Dupuytren's contracture in diabetes mellitus. J Rheumatol *14*:582–585, 1987.
223. Parsons JL, Shepard WL, and Fosdick WM: DMSO–an adjuvant to physical therapy in the chronic frozen shoulder. Ann N Y Acad Sci *141*:569–571, 1967.
224. Pasteur F: Les algies de l'épaule et la physiotherapie. J Radiol Electrol *16*:419–426, 1932.
225. Patten C and Hillel AD: The 11th nerve syndrome. Accessory nerve palsy or adhesive capsulitis? Arch Otolaryngol Head Neck Surg *119*:215–220, 1993.
226. Payr E: Gelenk-"Sperren" und "Ankylosen"; über die "Schultersteifen" verschiedener Ursache und die sogenannte "Periarthritis humero-scapularis", ihre Behandlung. Zbl Chir 58:2993, 1931.
227. Pearl ML, Harris SL, Lippitt SB, et al: A system for describing positions of the humerus relative to the thorax and its use in the presentation of several functionally important arm positions. J Shoulder Elbow Surg *1*:113–118, 1992.
228. Pearl ML, Jakins S, Lippitt SB, et al: Humeroscapular positions in a shoulder range-of-motion examination. J Shoulder Elbow Surg *1*:296–305, 1992.
229. Pearl ML, Wong K, and Frank C: Restriction of glenohumeral motion in patients with frozen shoulders. J Shoulder Elbow Surg 5:524, 1996.
230. Pineda C, Arana B, Martinez-Lavin M, and Dabague J: Frozen shoulder triggered by cardiac catheterization via the brachial artery. Am J Med *96*:90–91, 1994.
231. Pollock RG, Duralde XA, Flatow EL, and Bigliani LU: The use of arthroscopy in the treatment of resistant frozen shoulder. Clin Orthop *304*:30–36, 1994.
232. Poppen NK and Walker PS: Normal and abnormal motion of the shoulder. J Bone Joint Surg *58-A*:195–201, 1976.
233. Post M: The Shoulder. Philadelphia: Lea & Febiger, 1978, pp 281–284.
234. Putnam JJ: The treatment of a form of painful periarthritis of the shoulder. Boston Med Surg J *107*:536–539, 1882.
235. Quigley TB: Checkrein shoulder. A type of "frozen shoulder." N Engl J Med *250*:188–192, 1954.
236. Quigley TB: Indications for manipulation and corticosteroids in the treatment of stiff shoulders. Surg Clin North Am *43*:1715–1720, 1969.
237. Quin CE: Humeroscapular periarthritis. Observations on the effects of x-ray therapy and ultrasonic therapy in cases of "frozen shoulder." Ann Phys Med *10*:64–69, 1969.
238. Quin CE: Frozen shoulder: Evaluation of treatment with hydrocortisone injections and exercises. Ann Phys Med *8*:22–29, 1965.
239. Ready LB: Anesthesia for shoulder procedures. *In* Rockwood CA and Matsen III FA (eds): The Shoulder, Vol 1. Philadelphia: WB Saunders, 1990, pp 246–257.
240. Reeves B: Arthrographic changes in frozen and post-traumatic stiff shoulders. Proc R Soc Med *59*:827–830, 1966.
241. Reeves B: Arthrography of the Shoulder. J Bone Joint Surg *48-B*:424–435, 1966.
242. Reeves B: The natural history of the frozen shoulder syndrome. Scand J Rheumatol *4*:193–196, 1975.
243. Refior HJ: [Clarification of the concept humeroscapular periarthritis]. Orthopade *24*:509–511, 1995.
244. Resnick D: Shoulder arthrography. Radiol Clin North Am *19*:243–253, 1981.
245. Resnick D: Shoulder pain. Orthop Clin North Am *14*:81–97, 1983.
246. Resnik CS, Fronek J, Frey C, et al: Intra-articular pressure determination during glenohumeral joint arthrography. Preliminary investigation. Invest Radiol *19*:45–50, 1984.
247. Rhee YG, Harryman II DT, and Sidles JA: Translational Laxity of the Glenohumeral Joint. 61st AAOS Annual Meeting, Orlando, Feb 24 1994.
248. Richardson AT: The painful shoulder. Proc R Soc Med *68*:731–736, 1975.
249. Riedel R: Die Versteifung des Shultergelenkes durch Hangenlassen des Armes. Munschen Med Wschr *63*:1397, 1916.
250. Riley D, Lang AE, Blair RD, et al: Frozen shoulder and other shoulder disturbances in Parkinson's disease. J Neurol Neurosurg Psychiatry *52*:63–66, 1989.
251. Rizk TE, Christopher RP, Pinals RS, et al: Adhesive capsulitis (frozen shoulder): A new approach to its management. Arch Phys Med Rehabil *64*:29–33, 1983.
252. Rizk TE, Gavant ML, and Pinals RS: Treatment of adhesive capsulitis (frozen shoulder) with arthrographic capsular distension and rupture. Arch Phys Med Rehabil *75*:803–807, 1994.
253. Rizk TE and Pinals RS: Frozen shoulder. Semin Arthritis Rheum *11*:440–452, 1982.
254. Rizk TE and Pinals RS: Histocompatibility type and racial incidence in frozen shoulder. Arch Phys Med Rehabil 65:33–34, 1984.
255. Rodeo SA, Hannafin JA, Tom J, et al: Immunolocalization of Cytokines in Adhesive Capsulitis. Twelfth Open Meeting of the American Shoulder and Elbow Surgeons, February 25, 1995.
256. Romeo AA, Loutzenheiser TD, Rhee YG, and Harryman II DT: The Humeroscapular Motion Interface. ASES Tenth Specialty Day Meeting, New Orleans, 1994.
257. Romeo AA, Rhee Y-G, and Harryman II DT: Capsuloligamentous Restraint to Glenohumeral Motion. 61st Annual AAOS Meeting, New Orleans, 1994.
258. Rosenbloom AL: Limitation of finger joint mobility in diabetes mellitus. J Diabetic Comp *3*:77–87, 1989.
259. Roy S and Oldham R: Management of painful shoulder. Lancet *1(7973)*:1322–1324, 1976.
260. Ryu KN, Lee SW, Rhee YG, and Lim JH: Adhesive capsulitis of the shoulder joint: Usefulness of dynamic sonography. J Ultrasound Med *12*:445–449, 1993.
261. Saha NC: Painful shoulder in patients with chronic bronchitis and emphysema. Am Rev Respir Dis *94*:455–456, 1966.
262. Samilson RL, Raphael RL, Post L, et al: Arthrography of the shoulder joint. Clin Orthop *20*:21–32, 1961.
263. Sany J, Cillens JP, and Rousseau JR: Evolution lointaine de la retraction capsulaire de l'épaule. Revue Rhum *49*:815–819, 1982.
264. Sattar MA and Luqman WA: Periarthritis: Another duration-related complication of diabetes mellitus. Diabetes Care *8*:507–510, 1985.
265. Sattler H: Zum stellenwert der arthrosonographie der schulter in der rheumatologischen diagnostik. Untersuchungstechnik, befunde und ihre interpretation. Z Rheumatol *52*:90–96, 1993.
266. Schollmeier G, Uhthoff HK, Sarkar K, and Fukuhara K: Effects of immobilization on the capsule of the canine glenohumeral joint. A structural functional study. Clin Orthop *304*:37–42, 1994.
267. Segmuller HE, Taylor DE, Hogan CS, et al: Arthroscopic treatment of adhesive capsulitis. J Shoulder Elbow Surg *4*:403–408, 1995.
268. Seibold JR: Digital sclerosis in children with insulin-dependent diabetes mellitus. Arthritis Rheum 25:1357–1361, 1982.
269. Seignalet J, Sany J, Caillens JP, and Lapinski H: [Lack of association between HLA-B27 and frozen shoulder (author's transl)]. Semin Hop *57(41–42)*:1738–1739, 1981.
270. Sell S, Zacher J, Konig S, and Goethe S: Sonographie bei entzundlich-rheumatischen gelenkerkrankungen. Ultraschall Med *14*:63–67, 1993.
271. Seradge H and Anderson MG: Clostridial myonecrosis following intra-articular steroid injection. Clin Orthop *147*:207–209, 1980.
272. Shaffer B, Tibone JE, and Kerlan RK: Frozen shoulder: A long-term follow-up. J Bone Joint Surg *74A*:738–746, 1992.
273. Sharma RK, Bajekal RA, and Bhan S: Frozen shoulder syndrome: A comparison of hydraulic distension and manipulation. Int Orthop *17*:275–278, 1993.
274. Shaw DK, Deutsch DT, and Bowling RJ: Efficacy of shoulder range of motion exercise in hospitalized patients after coronary artery bypass graft surgery. Heart Lung *18*:364–369, 1989.
275. Sherry DD, Rothstein RRL, and Petty RE: Joint contractures preceding insulin-dependent diabetes mellitus. Arthritis Rheum 25:1362–1364, 1982.

276. Simmonds FA: Shoulder pain with particular reference to the frozen shoulder. J Bone Joint Surg *31*:834–838, 1949.
277. Simon L, Pujol H, Blotman F, and Pelissier J: [Aspects of the pathology of the arm after irradiation of breast cancer]. Rev Rhum Mal Osteoartic *43*:133–140, 1976.
278. Simon WH: Soft tissue disorders of the shoulder. Orthop Clin North Am *6*:521–539, 1975.
279. Simon WH: Soft tissue disorders of the shoulder. Frozen shoulder, calcific tendinitis, and bicipital tendinitis. Orthop Clin North Am *6*:521–539, 1975.
280. Speer KP, Deng X, Borrero S, et al: Biomechanical evaluation of a simulated Bankart lesion. J Bone Joint Surg *76A*:1819–1826, 1994.
281. Steinbrocker O and Argyros TG: Frozen shoulder: Treatment by local injections of depot corticosteroids. Arch Phys Med Rehabil *55*:209–213, 1974.
282. Stodell MA, Nicholson R, Scot J, and Sturrock RD: Radioisotope scanning in painful shoulder syndromes. Ann Rheum Dis *38*:496, 1979.
283. Sullivan JD: Painful shoulder syndrome. Can Med Assoc J *111*:505, 1974.
284. Summers GD and Gorman WP: Bilateral adhesive capsulitis and Hashimoto's thyroiditis (Letter). Br J Rheumatol *28*:451, 1989.
285. Sweetnam R: Corticosteroid arthropathy and tendon rupture. J Bone Joint Surg *51-B*:397–398, 1969.
286. Symeonides PP: The significance of the subscapularis muscle in the pathogenesis of recurrent anterior dislocation of the shoulder. J Bone Joint Surg *54-B*:476–483, 1972.
287. Terry GC, Hammon D, France P, and Norwood LA: The stabilizing function of passive shoulder restraints. Am J Sports Med *19*:26–34, 1991.
288. Thomas D, Williams RA, and Smith DS: The frozen shoulder: A review of manipulative treatment. Rheumatol Rehabil *19*:173–179, 1980.
289. Thomas T, Gazielly D, Bruyere G, and Alexandre C: Considerations about a unique clinical pattern: flexion block of the shoulder. Rev Rhum Engl Ed *62*:249–254, 1995.
290. Ticker JB, Beim GM, and Warner JJP: Recognition and Treatment of Refractory Posterior Capsular Contracture of the Shoulder. 63rd annual meeting of the American Academy of Orthopaedic Surgeons, 1996, p 103.
291. Tielbeek AV and van Horn JR: Double-contrast arthrography of the shoulder. Diagn Imaging *52*:154–162, 1983.
292. Todd JA: Genetic analysis of type 1 diabetes using whole genome approaches. Proc Natl Acad Sci U S A *92*:8560–8565, 1995.
293. Travell JG and Simmons DG: Myofascial Pain and Dysfunction: Trigger Point Manual. Baltimore: Williams & Wilkins, 1983, pp 410–424.
294. Turkel SJ, Panio MW, Marshall JL, and Girgis FG: Stabilizing mechanisms preventing anterior dislocation of the glenohumeral joint. J Bone Joint Surg *63-A*:1208–1217, 1981.
295. Tyber MA: Treatment of the painful shoulder syndrome with amitriptyline and lithium carbonate. Can Med Assoc J *111*:137–140, 1974.
296. Uitvlugt G, Detrisac DA, Johnson LL, et al: Arthroscopic observations before and after manipulation of frozen shoulder. Arthroscopy 9:181–185, 1993.
297. Wahl S and Renstrom P: Fibrosis in soft-tissue injuries. *In* Leadbetter WB, Buckwalter JA, and Gordon SL (eds): Sports-Induced Inflammation. Chicago: AAOS, 1989.
298. Waldburger M, Meier JL, and Gobelet C: The frozen shoulder: Diagnosis and treatment. Prospective study of 50 cases of adhesive capsulitis. Clin Rheumatol *11*:364–368, 1992.
299. Warner JJ, Deng XH, Warren RF, and Torzilli PA: Static capsuloligamentous restraints to superior-inferior translation of the glenohumeral joint. Am J Sports Med *20*:675–685, 1992.
300. Warner JJP, Allen A, Marks P, and Wong P: Arthroscopic release for chronic, refractory adhesive capsulitis of the shoulder. J Bone Joint Surg *78A*:1808–1816, 1996.
301. Wassef MR: Suprascapular nerve block: A new approach for the management of frozen shoulder. Anaesthesia *47*:120–124, 1992.
302. Watson-Jones R: Simple treatment of stiff shoulders. J Bone Joint Surg *45B*:207, 1963.
303. Weiser HI: [Mobilization under local anesthesia for painful primary frozen shoulder]. Harefuah *90*:215–219, 1976.
304. Weiser HI: Painful primary frozen shoulder mobilization under local anesthesia. Arch Phys Med Rehabil *58*:406–408, 1977.
305. Weiss JJ and Ting YM: Arthrography-assisted intra-articular injection of steroids in treatment of adhesive capsulitis. Arch Phys Med Rehabil *59*:285–287, 1978.
306. Wertheim HM and Rovenstine EA: Suprascapular nerve block. Anesthesiology *2*:541–545, 1941.
307. Wiley AM: Arthroscopic examination of the shoulder. *In* Bayley J and Kessel L (eds): Shoulder Surgery. Berlin and Heidelberg: Springer-Verlag, 1982, pp 113–118.
308. Wiley AM: Arthroscopic appearance of frozen shoulder. Arthroscopy 7:138–143, 1991.
309. Wiley AM and Older MWJ: Shoulder arthroscopy. Investigations with a fiberoptic instrument. Am J Sports Med *8*:31–38, 1980.
310. Williams NE, Seifert MH, Cuddigan JHB, and Wise RA: Treatment of capsulitis of the shoulder. Rheumatol Rehabil *14*:236, 1975.
311. Withers RJW: The painful shoulder: Review of one hundred personal cases with remarks on the pathology. J Bone Joint Surg *31*:414–417, 1949.
312. Wohlgethan JR: Frozen shoulder in hyperthyroidism. Arthritis Rheum *30*:936–939, 1987.
313. Woo SL-Y, McMahon PJ, Debski RE, et al: Factors limiting and defining shoulder motion: What keeps it from going farther? *In* Matsen III FA, Fu FH, and Hawkins RJ (eds): The Shoulder: A Balance of Mobility and Stability. Chicago: American Academy of Orthopaedic Surgeons, 1993, pp 141–157.
314. Wright MG, Richards AJ, and Clarke MB: 99mTc pertechnetate scanning in capsulitis. Lancet 2(7947):1265–1266, 1975.
315. Wright V and Haq AM: Periarthritis of the shoulder. I. Aetiological considerations with particular reference to personality factors. Ann Rheum Dis *35*:213–219, 1976.
316. Wright V and Haq AM: Periarthritis of the shoulder. II. Radiological features. Ann Rheum Dis *35*:220–226, 1976.
317. Xie KY, Zhao GF, and Lu JM: Treatment of 103 cases of periarthritis of the shoulder by acupoint laser irradiation. J Tradit Chin Med *8*:265–266, 1988.
318. Young A: Immunological studies in the frozen shoulder. *In* Bayley J and Kessel L (eds): Shoulder Surgery. Berlin and Heidelberg: Springer-Verlag, 1982, pp 110–113.
319. Ziegler DW, Harryman II DT, and Matsen III FA: Subscapularis Insufficiency in the Previously Operated Shoulder. American Shoulder and Elbow Surgery Twelfth Open Meeting, Atlanta, GA, 1996.
320. Zilberberg C and Leveille-Nizerolle M: La radiographie anti-inflammatoire dans 200 cas de periarthrite scapulo-humerale. Sem Hop Paris *52*:909–911, 1976.
321. Zuckerman JD and Cuomo F: Frozen shoulder. *In* Matsen III FA, Fu FH, and Hawkins RJ (eds): The Shoulder: A Balance of Mobility and Stability. Chicago: American Academy of Orthopedic Surgery, 1993, pp 253–268.
322. Zuckerman JD, Leblanc JM, Choueka J, and Kummer F: The effect of arm position and capsular release on rotator cuff repair. A biomechanical study. J Bone Joint Surg Br *73*:402–405, 1991.

CHAPTER

21

MICHAEL A. CAUGHEY, MBChB, FRACS
PETER WELSH, MBChB, FRCSC

Muscle Ruptures Affecting the Shoulder Girdle

Injury to muscle structures is exceedingly common, yet many of these injuries remain poorly described and ill defined. Most injuries are not identified as the cause of significant long-term disability unless they involve a complete disruption of the muscle or its attachments. Fortunately, this complication is much less common than when a rupture involves the tendon; for example, in rotator cuff tears. Interference with function, particularly diminution of strength, has previously been the major means of confirming muscular injury, combined with palpable deficiency or major atrophy of the muscle substance. The exact pathologic process, however, has seldom been defined because muscle strains and minor disruptions rarely require the surgical exposure that allows documentation of pathology. Recently, computed tomography (CT) and magnetic resonance imaging (MRI) have provided methods not hitherto possible of visualizing muscle injuries. Whereas in the past relatively few muscle injuries of the shoulder girdle have been described, these will undoubtedly be recorded more often and more precisely in the future.

Brickner and Milch[4] described muscle ruptures as being caused by: (1) active contraction of a muscle, (2) contraction of an antagonist, (3) increase of tearing over cohesive power, (4) asynchronic contraction, or (5) the additional muscular force of another muscle.

Basically, however, one may consider most significant muscle ruptures as occurring when an actively contracting muscle group is overloaded by the application of a resisting load or external force that exceeds tissue tolerance. When this occurs, the muscle fibers are torn and the muscle sheath is disrupted, leading to a palpable defect in the muscle. The defect can heal only by the formation of scar tissue. Effective surgical repair of muscle injury is very difficult to accomplish.

GENERAL PRINCIPLES OF RUPTURE OF THE MUSCULOTENDINOUS UNIT

The classic experiments done by McMaster[40] demonstrated the relative strengths of a muscle, tendon, and bone preparation. He suspended the gastrocnemius of the amputated limb of an adult rabbit. A wire was passed through the femur, and increasing weight was attached to the os calcis until rupture occurred. Between 10 kg and 21 kg of weight, the unit ruptured. In the seven preparations successfully tested, rupture occurred at the insertion with associated bony avulsion in three uses, two ruptured at the origin again with bony avulsion, whereas the others ruptured through either the muscle belly or the musculotendinous junction. McMaster could produce a rupture of the tendon midsubstance only after 50% of its substance has been divided. The normal tendon appears to be the strongest component of the musculotendinous unit, a finding that was confirmed by Cronkite.[8]

The site of rupture may be influenced by the rate of loading. In 1971 Welsh and co-workers,[77] while testing a tendon-bone system in the rabbit, found that lower rates of loading were associated with rupture at the tendon-bone junction. At higher rates, the tendon broke at the site of clamping while the strength of the tendon-bone junction was found to be more secure.

Similar studies have been undertaken in stimulated muscle.[18] The energy absorbed by the muscle before disruption was twice as great with pre-stimulation. Indeed, Safran and associates[64] have demonstrated experimentally that rabbit muscle preconditioned with isometric stimulation developed more tension and required a greater change in length before failure occurred.

Another point to note is that muscles that cross two joints are subject to stretch at each joint and are therefore more vulnerable to injury. Likewise, muscles with a higher percentage of type 2 fibers are also more susceptible.[17]

Other factors that should be considered include the mechanism of injury, which may well influence the site of rupture. For example, in rupture of the pectoralis major, McEntire and associates[39] noted that direct trauma more commonly resulted in muscle belly rupture, whereas indirect trauma was more likely to produce rupture distally. Similarly, although rupture of the long head of the biceps is common and rupture at the insertion is well recognized, rupture of the biceps muscle belly is exceedingly rare. However, as many as 48 complete belly ruptures were described by Heckman and Levine[28] in parachutists in whom the injury was caused by direct trauma from the static line.

The site of rupture is also influenced by anatomic factors peculiar to the shoulder. Rupture occurs most commonly in the tendons of the long head of the biceps and the rotator cuff. The intra-articular course of the former and impingement and impaired vascularity of the latter predispose them to rupture.

The role of anabolic steroids in predisposing to muscle rupture also bears consideration, especially in bodybuilding, weightlifting, and throwing athletes.[76, 79] In 1992, Miles and co-workers[43] conducted experiments on 24 male rats, using anabolic steroids and exercise as variables. Biomechanical tests revealed stiffer tendons in the group of rats receiving stanozolol intramuscularly, compared with rats not receiving steroid injections. In addition, "The energy at the time when the tendon failed, the toe-limit elongation, and the elongation at the time of first failure were all affected significantly."[43] Examination via electron microscope revealed alterations in the size of collagen fibrils in rats receiving stanozolol compared with the control group. In a similar study, Wood and associates[79] found that the crimp pattern of collagen was shorter and the angle between collagen fibrils was longer in tendons of rats treated with anabolic steroids. On the basis of the aforementioned results, it can be speculated that steroids play a role in altering both the structure and the pattern of collagen fibrils, in turn causing a stiffer and weaker musculotendinous junction that is more likely to rupture.

Clinically, rupture of the quadriceps tendon mechanism above the knee has been seen in power-lifting professionals who have been using anabolic steroids. Similarly, the authors have seen rupture of the pectoralis major at the musculotendinous junction in weight-training athletes indulging in a high intake of steroids.

Overall, however, ruptures of the muscles of the shoulder girdle are uncommon. The literature does not abound with reports of such involvement. In this chapter a comprehensive overview of the subject is presented with an account of lesions of the pectoralis major, deltoid, triceps, biceps, serratus anterior, coracobrachialis, and subscapularis muscles.

RUPTURE OF THE PECTORALIS MAJOR

Historical Review

Rupture of the pectoralis major, first described by Patissier[58] in 1822, is a relatively rare injury. In 1972, comprehensive review of the literature by McEntire and colleagues[39] revealed only 45 cases, to which they added 11 more. However, only 22 of the 56 patients had undergone surgical exploration, and one case of rupture was confirmed at autopsy. Thus, actual confirmation of the lesion was lacking in 33 patients, and cases of congenital absence of the pectoralis major may have been represented in this group. Since then, 88 additional cases have been published in the literature, of which at least 54 cases have been confirmed surgically.

Anatomy

The pectoralis major arises in a broad sheet as two distinct heads—an upper clavicular head and a lower sternocostal head—that spread to a complex trilaminar insertion along the lateral lip of the bicipital groove. A portion of the sternocostal head spirals on itself to produce the round appearance of the anterior axillary fold, with the result that the lowermost fibers are inserted most proximally on the humerus and in a crescent into the capsule of the shoulder joint. McEntire and associates[39] attribute the infrequency of complete ruptures of the pectoralis major to the layered form of the muscle and its complex insertion.

Classification

Pectoralis major ruptures may be classified according to the extent and the site of rupture. Type 1 ruptures consist of a contusion or sprain; type 2 are partial ruptures; and type 3 are complete ruptures of the muscle origin, muscle belly, musculotendinous junction, or tendon, or avulsion of the insertion.

Most cases are undoubtedly partial, but 40 of the 54 cases reported since 1972 that came to surgery were complete. In these reports the predominant lesion was an avulsion from the humerus in 36 cases. Avulsion from the musculotendinous junction occurred in nine cases; tendinous ruptures accounted for three cases; and only one case involved rupture of the muscle itself.

Incidence and Mechanisms

Rupture of the pectoralis major is relatively rare, and only 144 cases have been reported in the world literature. However, McEntire and colleagues[39] were able to add 11 cases from the Salt Lake City region; they believed that the injury occurs more commonly than reports indicate. The problem has been reported exclusively in males. Although the injury has occurred in patients ranging in age from newborns to 72 year olds, the majority occur between the ages of 20 and 40.

Rupture of the pectoralis major follows extreme muscle tension or direct trauma, or a combination of both. Of the 56 cases reviewed by McEntire and co-workers,[39] excessive muscle tension caused 37 injuries and direct trauma caused nine injuries. A combination of the two mechanisms was the cause in four cases, and spontaneous rupture was reported in three instances. In the more recent literature, excess tension injury was the cause in 78 patients, and direct injury occurred in three cases. A typical mechanism of injury is weightlifting, in particular bench presses, which accounted for four of the nine cases reported by Zeman and associates[80] and 9 of 19 cases reported by Kretzler and co-workers.[31]

Wolfe and associates,[78] supported by cadaver and clinical studies, provide an explanation for the high rate of injury with bench pressing. Their patients describe the rupture occurring when the bar is at its lowest point with the shoulders extended to 30 degrees. At this point the fibers of the lowest portion of the sternal head become disproportionately stretched. Elliot and associates[13] have shown by electromyogram (EMG) studies that the pectoralis major muscle is maximally activated at the initiation of the lift with the humerus in the extended position. Wolfe and associates[78] believe that the application of maximal loads to the inferior fibers that are stretched to an extreme mechanical disadvantage produces rupture of these fibers. Continued loading then increases the tension on the remaining fibers of the sternal head, which fail. This may account for the increased incidence of rupture of the sternal head during weightlifting. Another common mechanism of injury is when a person attempts to break a fall, resulting in severe force applied to a maximally contracted pectoralis major muscle.

There also appears to be a correlation between the mechanism of injury and the site of rupture. Direct trauma causes tears of the muscle belly, whereas excessive tension causes avulsion of the humeral insertion or disruption at the musculotendinous junction. Wrestlers have a propensity to disrupt the muscle at its upper sternoclavicular portion.

Clinical Presentation

In the case of an acute injury, a history of excessive muscle stress, a direct blow, or a crush, injury of the shoulder region is associated with severe, sharp, and often burning pain and a tearing sensation at the site of rupture. This is a major and severe injury that is accompanied by significant swelling and ecchymosis. Immediate shoulder dysfunction is apparent.

The physical findings depend on the site of rupture. If the muscle is injured in its proximal part, the swelling and ecchymosis are usually noted on the anterior part of the chest wall on the involved side. The muscle belly retracts toward the axillary fold, causing a prominent bulge. Rupture in the distal part may cause swelling and ecchymosis in both the arm and the chest; the body of the muscle bulges on the chest, causing the axillary fold to become thin (Fig. 21–1). There is tenderness at the site of rupture, and a visible or palpable defect is usually present. Zeman and co-workers[80] described one patient in whom the tendon felt intact through to its humeral insertion. At surgery, however, a complete tear was found at the musculotendinous junction (Fig. 21–2), with an overlying fascial layer giving the impression of an intact tendon. These authors cautioned that the lack of a palpable defect in the axilla is not a reliable sign of continuity of the pectoralis major muscle. Resisted adduction and internal rotation of the arm are weak and are accompanied by accentuation of the defect and pain. Indeed, in cases presenting late this is the predominant sign, with the palpable defect confirmatory of the pathologic process involved.

X-Ray and Laboratory Evaluation

X-rays generally fail to reveal any bone abnormality, but loss of the normal pectoralis major shadow has been described as a reliable sign of rupture. Soft tissue shadowing is visible when a significant hematoma is present, whereas ultrasound may be useful when confirming the site of rupture. More recently, the authors have found that MRI is beneficial in acute pectoralis major ruptures. However, in chronic ruptures, MRI has proved less effective because respiratory artefact has impaired definition to some extent. Undoubtedly, improvement in resolution

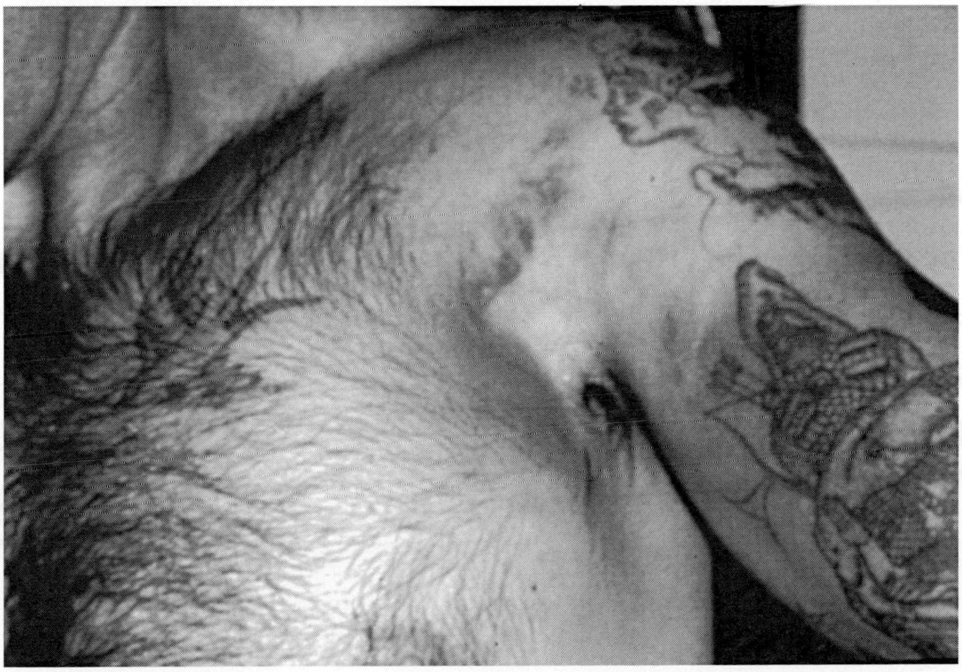

Figure 21–1

Rupture of the pectoralis major in a 30-year-old weightlifter. (Courtesy of J. J. Brownlee, M.D.)

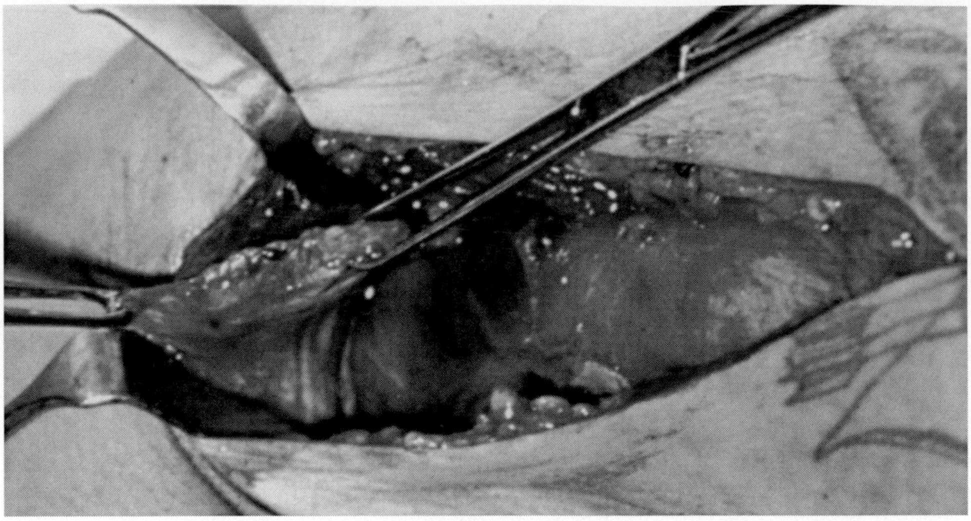

Figure 21–2

Findings at surgery in the case shown in Figure 21–1. The pectoralis major tendon is avulsed from its humeral insertion *(right)*.

will prove MRI to be the most useful investigative tool for defining the exact pathology of this injury.

Complications

The most sinister documented complication of pectoralis major rupture is sepsis involving the associated hematoma. Noted in three reported cases,[47, 54, 58] sepsis directly caused the death of one patient and led to death from pneumonia of a second patient. A patient described by Pai and Simison[54] was remarkable in presenting a temperature of only 37.5°C and a white blood cell count of 11,500/cm^3 despite 1500 ml of frank pus being drained. Beta-hemolytic streptococcus was cultured. Pseudocyst formation, which occurred in a hematoma, has been described by Ronchetti,[63] and associated neuromuscular injuries have also been reported. Kawashima and associates[30] described a patient with a crush injury and total rupture of the pectoralis major at the musculotendinous junction with hypoesthesia of the C6–C8 and T1 dermatomes of the affected extremity. Several associated muscle injuries have also been described; these injuries include rupture of the anteromedial portion of the adjacent deltoid, pectoralis minor rupture, and rotator cuff tears. Additional injuries in one patient included a fractured humerus and compound fractures of both forearm bones. Purnell[62] has described myositis ossificans in a patient seen 4 months after rupture, and Smith[68] reported the development of a rhabdomyosarcoma 10 years after rupture of the pectoralis major at the same site.

Treatment

METHODS

Partial ruptures of the pectoralis major or lesions of the muscle belly respond to conservative treatment with initial icing and rest to control the hematoma. The early application of heat and ultrasound and a program of shoulder-mobilizing exercises (both passive and active assisted) help to restore shoulder function. Unresisted stretching exercises should be included early in the rehabilitation program, but resisted strengthening should await a 6-week recovery with restoration of good shoulder mobility and settling of all pain.

SURGICAL TREATMENT

A complete rupture of the pectoralis major demands early surgical treatment in the active athlete. Results of late repair, although they may be satisfactory, are not as good as when primary repair is undertaken.[11]

Tendinous avulsion can be repaired by anatomic reattachment with heavy sutures through drill holes in the humeral cortex. When some tendon remains attached to the humerus, Orava and co-workers[52] have described an effective method of treatment by end-to-end repair of the tendons, reinforcing the repair with retention sutures into bone. The authors have used bone anchors and have had very satisfactory results.

Tears of the musculotendinous junction can be sutured directly; however, the shredding of tissue structure associated with muscle substance tears offers poor substance for repair, and only imperfect results can be anticipated with this injury.

RESULTS OF TREATMENT

In 1970, Park and Espiniella[55] reviewed 31 patients reported in the literature. Surgical treatment produced an excellent result in 80% of patients, and 10% had good results. This finding compared most favorably with the good results reported in only 58% of patients who were treated nonoperatively. These authors stated that in the nonoperative group, varying degrees of weakness of adduction and internal rotation were present. However, over time the teres major, subscapularis, deltoid, and latissimus dorsi slowly take over the function of the pectoralis major. Three cases have been reported of wrestlers returning to successful careers after nonoperative treatment. However, Gudmundsson[23] reported that normal power is rarely achieved in these instances. More recently, Zeman and colleagues[80] described nine athletes who had ruptures of the pectoralis major. Surgical treatment was undertaken in four cases; all patients had excellent results. In the five patients treated nonoperatively, residual weakness was present in all cases; one professional boxer could not return to boxing, and two weightlifters had good results but were not entirely happy because of persistent weakness.

Kretzler and Richardson[31] undertook repair in 16 of 19 patients, and 13 patients reported a full return of strength. This study included two patients who underwent repair as late as 5½ years after an injury. Although full strength was not achieved in these patients, significant improvement was reported. One patient improved in horizontal adduction strength from 50 to 80% and the other from 60 to 84%. The authors believe that with diligent freeing of adhesions and firm fixation to the humerus, late repair is worthwhile.

Scott and associates[66] recommended conservative treatment on the basis that late repair is possible for patients in whom dynamometry indicates persistent weakness. However, they believed that all four cases tested with dynamometry, one of which underwent repair, were complete ruptures of just the sternocostal head and that these would be expected to perform better than total ruptures. Wolfe and colleagues[78] tested six patients who had chronic tears, including four with complete tears. In the four patients with complete tears the peak torque in horizontal adduction was 74% of the normal side, and performance with repetitive testing showed 60% of the normal side at low speed and 76% of the normal side at high speed. Late repair yielded satisfactory results. The authors recommend acute repair for complete tears in patients who require their upper extremity and high-tension activities or sports.

Jones and Matthews[29] classified the outcomes in the literature into one of three gradings, depending on range of movement, power, and pain. If the results of those who had operations within 1 week of injury are compared with a combined group of patients who had delayed or no operation, the results of early operation are much better ($P < .001$).

Authors' Preferred Treatment

We use early surgical treatment for major avulsions at the musculotendinous junction or tendinous insertion in all except sedentary patients. We treat ruptures of the muscle belly or partial lesions nonoperatively.

RUPTURE OF THE DELTOID

Historical Review

The deltoid muscle is probably the single most important muscular structure in the shoulder girdle. Satisfactory function of the shoulder cannot be anticipated if this muscle is irrevocably injured or its nerve supply is compromised. Luckily, rupture of the deltoid muscle itself is a relatively uncommon clinical entity. First described by Clemens[6] in 1913 in a railway worker, reports in the literature have been sparse since then. In 1919, Davis[10] reported one case in which the deltoid became detached after suppuration of its bony origin owing to osteomyelitis of the clavicle. Gilcreest and Albi[22] described two further cases in 1939. In 1972, McEntire and co-workers[39] described a case associated with a rupture of the pectoralis major. In 1975, Samuel and associates[65] described a single case and in 1976, Pointud and colleagues[59] described a further case, both reported in the French literature. Both patients had received multiple injections of steroids—in the first case, 18 injections for a frozen shoulder, and in the second case, approximately 12 per year for several years in association with a rotator cuff tear. In the latter case the patient also received radiotherapy, and this treatment, combined with injections of steroids in direct contact with the deltoid, resulted in disruption of the middle third of the deltoid. Management was conservative.

The authors recently encountered a 79-year-old man with a rupture of the central third of the deltoid from its origin in association with a long-standing rotator cuff tear. The man collapsed due to a bleeding duodenal ulcer and fell heavily onto his left shoulder. When examined 6 months after the injury, the man was unable to abduct beyond 20 degrees actively, and when he attempted abduction, there was a marked defect over the upper aspect of the middle third of the deltoid and the humeral head could be easily palpated through it. MRI confirmed a complete tear of the supraspinatus, infraspinatus, and long head of biceps and disruption of the middle third of the deltoid. At surgery, a thickened band of fibrous tissue was found to bridge the gap between the deltoid origin and the retracted muscle belly. This was advanced and double breasted to provide a satisfactory repair (Fig. 21–3*A–D*). Excellent exposure for repair of the cuff was possible through the defect.

The literature does not abound with reports of deltoid rupture. Indeed, the rarity of this type of injury was exemplified in the Mayo Clinic series of 1014 cases of musculotendinous ruptures described by Anzel and colleagues,[3] in which no cases were unveiled.

Anatomy

The deltoid is a multipennate muscle arising from the outer aspect of the anatomic "horseshoe" formed by the spine of the scapula, the acromion, and the outer end of the clavicle. It enfolds the shoulder and encloses the rotator cuff, inserting on the outer aspect of the humerus. The motor supply from the axillary or circumflex nerve reaches the muscle posteriorly on its undersurface.

Mechanism

Minor strains of the deltoid are common in athletic activity, particularly in throwing sports. The anterior deltoid may be injured in the acceleration phase of throwing,

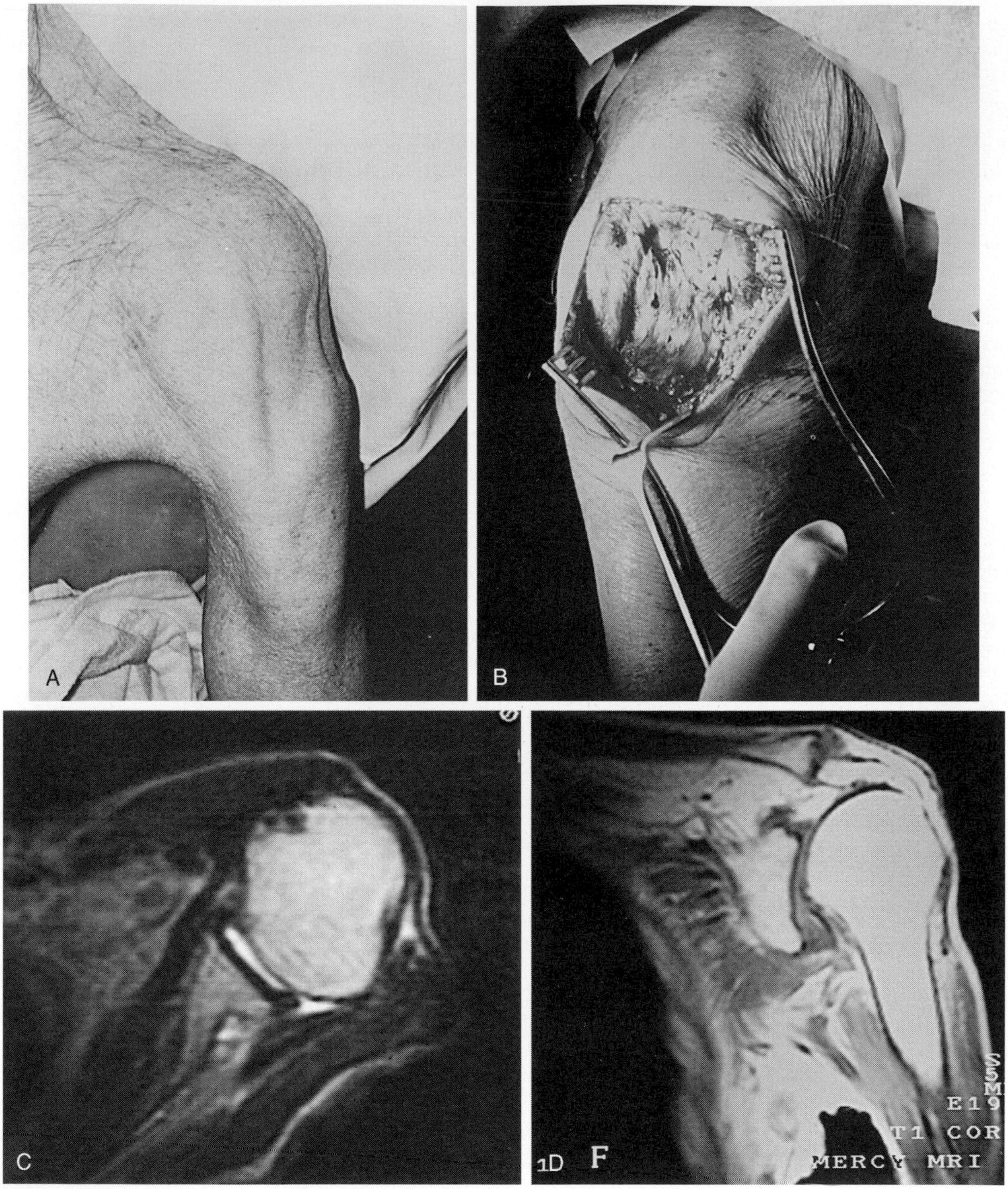

Figure 21–3

A, 79-year-old man 8 months after avulsion of the middle third of the deltoid at its origin. *B*, Muscle tissue inferiorly below a broad band of scar tissue that provides some continuity with the site of origin. *C* and *D*, Transverse and longitudinal magnetic resonance imaging images confirm the deltoid disruption and demonstrate a sizable rotator cuff tear with proximal migration of the humerus.

when a forward body movement and a forcible contraction are simultaneously applied to an already stretched musculotendinous unit. In the follow-through phase at the end of forward motion of the arm, the posterior deltoid must restrain the shoulder and is vulnerable to injury.

Complete traumatic disruption of the deltoid, as the literature reviewed indicates, is rare. Indeed, trauma to the deltoid most commonly seen in clinical practice is associated with misguided shoulder surgery. This is true particularly if the deltoid is detached from the acromion, resulting in dehiscence. The posterior approach to the shoulder, releasing the deltoid from the spine of the scapula, is a major culprit in this regard.

In those instances in which traumatic rupture of the deltoid is incurred, rupture inevitably involves the application of a major external force to an already maximally contracted deltoid muscle.

Clinical Presentation

Examination findings vary with the site of rupture. If the avulsion occurs from the origin, there is a loss of the normal deltoid contour with weakness of abduction, flexion, or extension, depending on the involved part. If the rotator cuff is also deficient, contraction of the remaining deltoid will cause the humeral head to protrude in the direction of the deltoid deficiency.

If the lesion is located near the deltoid insertion, a defect may be palpable, with an associated mass that becomes firmer upon contraction of the deltoid muscle.

Methods of Treatment

Minor strains and partial lesions of the deltoid muscle can be handled nonoperatively. Local icing in the acute phase followed by heat, mobilization of the shoulder, stretching, and gentle strengthening over 6 weeks will usually restore the shoulder to full activity.

In the management of complete disruptions, there is no published experience to guide us. If such an injury is observed, consideration should be given to prompt surgical exploration in an effort to try to restore the structure anatomically. However, unless the injury is an avulsion from bone, the repair is likely to be weak. Midsubstance muscle injuries are difficult to suture effectively.

Delay in the repair with retraction and scarring makes the situation even more difficult. In 1919, Davis[10] first reported the management of a chronic defect of the anterior deltoid with a broad graft of fascia from the thigh. He recommended retaining a thick layer of subcutaneous fat to prevent adhesion formation between the rotator cuff and the fascial implant. Clearly, the late salvage of this injury is not satisfactory; if deltoid ruptures are to be dealt with satisfactorily, early identification and prompt surgical repair are mandatory.

Postoperative care after such surgery is vital. Abduction or flexion splinting to relieve the tension on the repair is maintained for 6 weeks or so before mobilization is commenced, and a strengthening program is not introduced for 6 to 8 weeks after intervention.

Authors' Preferred Treatment

We carry out early surgical treatment in cases involving a complete disruption of one third or more of the deltoid substance. Tears and strains of lesser degrees are treated nonoperatively. The problem of compromise of the deltoid origin by previous surgery is a difficult one. When an acromionectomy has been performed, reconstruction is not possible because the important anterolateral deltoid has lost its origin. With symptomatic failure of deltoid reattachment after acromioplasty, we consider re-exploration, mobilization of the superficial and deep aspects of the muscle, and repair back to the acromion. Postoperative protection is necessary to avoid active flexion and passive extension.

RUPTURE OF THE TRICEPS

Historical Review

In 1868, Partridge[56] reported the first case of rupture of the triceps in a patient who fell partly on the roadway and partly on the sidewalk, striking the left arm just above and behind the elbow joint. He observed a 3/4-inch–long depression and a slight wound above and behind the elbow, in addition to tenderness over the triceps tendon. The arm was held extended and quiet for 1 week, after which passive motion commenced. Only eight more cases were reported during the next 100 years before Tarsney[72] added seven cases, clarifying the mechanism of injury and emphasizing the importance of the presence of avulsed bony fragments on the lateral radiograph when confirming the diagnosis. Although Tarsney described one patient with the combination of triceps rupture and fracture of the radial head, it was Levy and colleagues[34] who drew attention to this combination in 1978. In 1982 Levy and associates[35] reported on 16 patients with triceps rupture, of whom 15 had associated radial head fractures and one had a fracture of the capitellum.

Anatomy

The triceps muscle consists of two aponeurotic laminae. The long head arising from the inferior glenoid neck and the lateral head from the humerus converge to form the superficial lamina, which commences at about the middle of the muscle and covers its lower half. The tendon inserts into the posterior part of the upper surface of the olecranon.

The medial head lies deep and arises from a broad origin on the humerus, inserting both directly into the olecranon and indirectly via the superficial lamina formed from the other two heads. A few fibers are inserted into the posterior capsule of the elbow joint to retract it during extension.

Incidence and Mechanisms

Rupture of the triceps mechanism is a rare injury, and only 49 cases have been reported in the literature. Patients with renal osteodystrophy are at greater risk of sustaining triceps rupture with bony avulsion.[15, 60] The condition may result from either indirect injury or a direct blow. Of the 39 cases in which the mechanism of injury is known, 29 (74%) resulted from an indirect injury (the application of excessive tension to the muscle fibers), seven (18%) from a direct blow, and three (8%) from a combination of both. The usual cause of injury is a fall onto the outstretched hand. This mechanism was evident in 8 of 15 cases collected by Tarsney[72] and in 13 of 16 cases presented by Levy and co-workers[35] in which the mechanism was known. One of the present authors (M.A.C.) has had personal experience with an indirect injury resulting from a vigorous fend in a rugby game. The resisted extension resulted in a combination of partial muscle and tendon rupture as well as bony avulsion, producing a complete disruption of the triceps mechanism.

Most direct injuries are a result of the elbow striking a fixed object, but crush injury is also described.[45] There appears to be no correlation between the mechanism of injury and the site of disruption of the triceps.

Clinical Presentation

The patient gives a history of a direct blow or indirect injury, as described earlier. Particularly with an indirect injury, the patient may report a tearing sensation about the elbow. Pain, swelling, and weakness of elbow extension are commonly noted.

On examination a palpable defect is present, usually in the triceps tendon, and there is associated swelling and often bruising. The patient exhibits an inability to actively extend the elbow when the rupture is complete. When a fracture of the radial head has also occurred, tenderness and swelling are present over the fracture site and may dominate the clinical picture.[35]

X-Ray Evaluation

Radiographs may be helpful in confirming triceps avulsion. In six of seven patients described by Tarsney and in 12 of 16 patients in Levy's series, avulsion fragments from the olecranon were present. X-rays are also important in excluding associated injuries. Radial head fracture is a common associated finding,[35] and fracture of the distal radius and ulna has also been reported.[32]

Complications

Levy and colleagues[35] emphasized the association of radial head fractures with triceps rupture, which was present in 15 of 16 of their patients. Hence they recommended that all patients with a radial head fracture be carefully assessed to exclude injury to the triceps tendon.

A most unusual complication described in 1987 by Brumbuck[5] involved avulsion of the origin of the lateral head of the triceps with an associated compartment syndrome. Partial ulnar nerve palsy following a direct blow that resulted in rupture of the triceps tendon has also been described.[2] A year later, tenderness was still present over the ulnar nerve with hypoesthesia of the ulnar distribution; at surgery, the nerve was found to be enclosed in a bed of adhesions. Transposition of the ulnar nerve was carried out.

Methods of Treatment

In complete rupture of the triceps tendon, experience with nonoperative treatment is limited. In 1962, Preston and Adicoff[60] described a patient with hyperparathyroidism who had suffered avulsion of the quadriceps tendons bilaterally and rupture of the triceps tendon with an avulsed bone fragment. The elbow was not immobilized, and in the 14 months after injury the patient was described as having little disability with ordinary activity. In a case described by Anderson and Le Cocq[2] in which a 27-year-old woman had struck the triceps region against the gearshift of her car, the result was poor. After 1 year she still lacked 10 degrees of extension and had tenderness over the rupture site. Her triceps strength was reduced by approximately one half. Exploration revealed a completely ruptured tendon that had healed by scarring in an elongated position. After scar excision and tendon shortening, she achieved an excellent result with almost normal power. Sherman and co-workers[67] described a 24-year-old patient (a bodybuilder) who was examined 3 months after injury. Resisted extension of the arm was markedly weak compared with the opposite side. Cybex testing revealed a 42% extensor deficit at 60 degrees per second. After surgical repair at 6 months, normal function was eventually achieved. A patient described by Tarsney[72] was originally treated with a plaster cast with the elbow flexed to 90 degrees. Although the patient regained some active extension initially, at 4 months she had increased weakness. An examination confirmed a palpable defect and loss of extension of the elbow. Delayed repair resulted in a return of full motion and power. In 1992, O'Driscoll[51] reported on a patient with complete intramuscular rupture of the long head of the triceps that was treated nonoperatively. The patient's isometric strength was normal, but endurance testing was reduced by 5 to 10%. Nonoperative treatment was recommended for all except those who required significant endurance strength in elbow extension.

Authors' Preferred Treatment

We prefer surgical treatment for both early and late injuries. Although there has been some variation in our method of repair, fixation via drill holes in the olecranon using heavy suture material is effective. In one patient treated by the authors, the avulsed fragment was large enough to fix with Kirschner wires and a tension band wire, with supplementary sutures in the damaged tendon and muscle yielding sound fixation. The arm is immobilized in a cast at 30 degrees for a period of 4 weeks prior to mobilization.

RUPTURE OF THE BICEPS

Lesions of the biceps tendon have been discussed in detail in Chapter 19. This section focuses on rupture of the biceps muscle.

Historical Review

In documenting the history of biceps muscle rupture, we have had difficulty in confirming the site of the lesion. While reviewing the predominantly European literature, Gilcreest noted that of the 81 cases of biceps rupture, only 15 had come to surgery. Difficulty in locating the site of rupture clinically is highlighted by the comments made in 1935 by Haldeman and Soto-Hall,[24] who noted this problem in recent tears of the biceps.

The hematoma produced by a tear in the upper part of the tendon gravitates downward through the sheath to the region of the belly where it presents. The ecchymosis and tenderness suggest that the tear took place at the musculotendinous junction. This occurred in two cases in which we exposed the belly of the biceps muscle and then had to carry the incision upward to find the tear in the bicipital groove.

Many of the early cases of "muscle rupture" are likely to have been tears of the long head. In 1900, Loos[36] believed that 19.5% of ruptures of the biceps were actually ruptures of the long head and 43.6% occurred at the musculotendinous junction of the long head, whereas 15.1% were total muscle ruptures and 21.8% were partial muscle ruptures. In 1922 Gilcreest[20] stated, "According to most writers, about 66% are believed to occur in the muscle substance." Clearly these figures for muscle rupture are much too high; certainly, however, there are well documented muscle ruptures in the earlier literature. In 1937, Conwell[7] described a 38-year-old man who sustained a traction injury to the limb while holding a drill handle. Operation revealed a complete rupture of both bellies of the biceps in the middle third, with the margins of the rupture being quite smooth, as if cut by a knife.

In 106 biceps ruptures in 100 patients, Gilcreest[20] diagnosed complete rupture of the entire muscle in six, partial rupture in one, complete rupture of the muscle of the long head in three, and partial rupture in five. There was one complete rupture of the muscle of the short head and one partial rupture.

In 1941, Tobin and associates[73] described ruptures of the biceps muscle occurring in parachutists. In 1978, Heckman and Levine[28] reported on 48 parachutists with ruptures of the biceps muscle, making this by far the largest series in the literature.

Incidence and Mechanisms

Rupture of the biceps muscle was thought to be a rare injury. The lesion was overdiagnosed in the early literature for the reasons stated earlier, and the figures are therefore misleading. In the older literature, indirect injury from traction applied to a contracting biceps muscle is described. More recently, reports in the literature involve examples of direct injury in military parachutists.[28, 73] In the period from 1973 to 1975, Heckman and Levine[28] encountered more than 50 patients with closed transection of the biceps in a population of 40,000 paratroopers undertaking a total of over 10,000 parachute jumps each year.

The mechanism of injury is essentially the same for all parachutists. A 2-cm–wide woven nylon strap (the static line) is attached to the paratrooper's pack and the aircraft. The paratrooper jumps, and when a force of 6.33 kg/cm (80 lb/in^2) is applied to the casing of the parachute, it comes free, allowing the parachute to open. If the static line is positioned incorrectly in front of the arm, a severe force may be applied over the biceps, especially if the arm is simultaneously abducted after push-off.

Clinical Presentation

The patient gives a history of direct or indirect injury, as described earlier. A tearing or popping sensation in the arm often accompanies indirect injury, followed by severe pain, swelling, and loss of strength. Gilcreest[21] states that the pain is more intense with muscle ruptures than with tendon ruptures. A visible and palpable defect in the muscle may also be present (Fig. 21–4), particularly if the patient is seen early, before a significant hematoma and swelling occur. Gilcreest also states that the humerus may be felt beneath the skin in the defect, presumably with the brachialis interposed. There is often extensive ecchymosis and pronounced bruising. Weakness is present, and its severity depends on the extent of rupture. In the paratroopers described by Heckman and Levine, the skin always showed some degree of contusion or abrasion but had no laceration. These authors stated that although immediate, marked local hemorrhage and swelling occur, the defect may be difficult to appreciate immediately and the degree of the injury may not be recognized. After

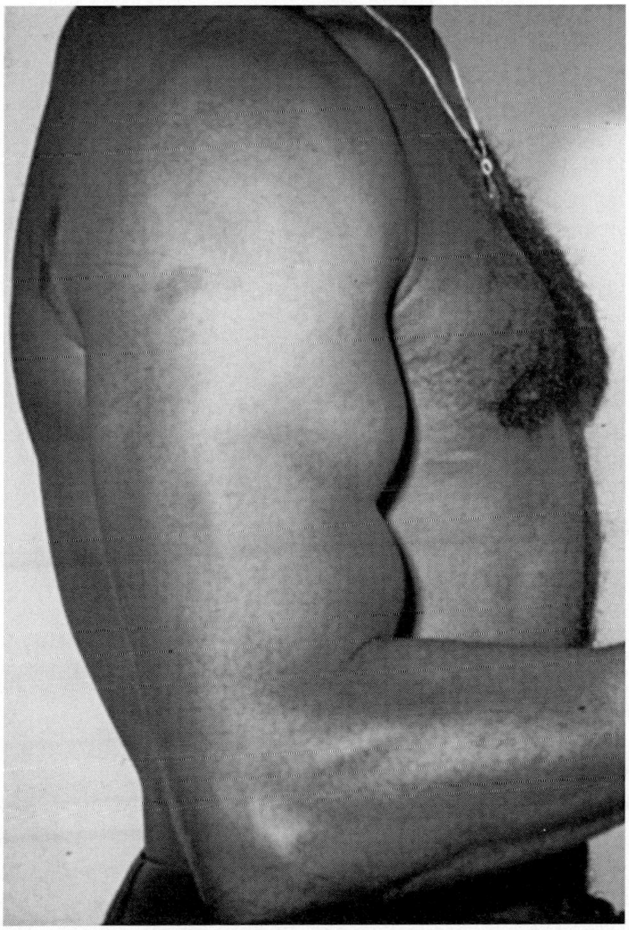

Figure 21–4
Biceps muscle rupture in a weightlifter.

the acute hematoma and swelling subside, however, the severity of the injury can more readily be appreciated.

X-Ray Evaluation

In Heckman and Levine's series,[28] radiographs at the time of injury were negative, except in one patient with an associated scapular neck fracture. Recent literature has offered numerous reports that support the authors' predictions regarding the usefulness of both ultrasound and MRI in confirming biceps ruptures.[14, 37, 41, 61, 74, 75] The superior soft tissue contrast resolution of these diagnostic tools compared with that of radiography not only allows for confirmation of a diagnosis but can also portray the extent of the muscle injury.

Complications

Musculocutaneous nerve injury was common in Heckman and Levine's series.[28] Although none of their patients showed alteration in sensation with respect to the distribution of the lateral cutaneous nerve of the forearm, EMG studies were positive in 9 of 11 patients studied. On follow-up, 1 year later, two patients had normal EMGs, six had signs of re-establishment of the nerve supply to the muscle, and one had persistent denervation. Two patients showed denervation of only one head of the biceps at 3 and 4 months after injury and were expected to recover. The authors concluded that there was frequently contusion of the musculocutaneous nerve but rarely permanent paralysis of the muscle.

The results of inadequately treated ruptures of the biceps muscle were well documented by Heckman and Levine.[28] They evaluated 28 male paratroopers an average of 19 months after injury. Twenty-five patients displayed weakness of the arm and fatigue, especially with activity requiring rapid, repeated elbow flexion. Seventeen patients complained of an unsightly cosmetic defect, and 12 patients experienced pain, generally when using the muscle. The maximum force generated by elbow flexion at 90 degrees was measured with an ergometer as 53% of that of the controls.

Methods of Treatment

Heckman and Levine[28] treated 20 patients whom they allocated to one of two treatment regimens. Ten patients underwent acute surgical repair within 72 hours of injury. Through an anteromedial approach, the muscle was explored. The typical lesion found in all cases was transection of the belly with an intact fascial envelope, with the space within the fascia being filled with blood. The hematoma was evacuated, and the muscle belly was reapproximated with double right-angled sutures of heavy catgut reinforced with a U-shaped flap of biceps fascia. The elbow was then immobilized in acute flexion for 4 weeks and at 90 degrees for an additional 2 weeks. The second group of 10 patients was treated by aspiration and splinting. It appeared to the authors that the intrafascial hematoma was the primary obstruction to closure of the muscle gap. Since it was seen at surgery that the hematoma could be aspirated with a 16-gauge needle and the muscle gap closed with acute elbow flexion, this treatment method was utilized. After aspiration, the elbow was immobilized in a cast in acute flexion for 6 weeks; range-of-motion exercises were then begun.

At follow-up 8.8 months after surgery or 7.1 months after aspiration, the muscle power was virtually identical—76.5% of normal and 77% of normal, respectively. Both were superior to the 53% of normal found in the original, untreated group. One patient in the surgical group developed a deep wound infection that required débridement, intravenous antibiotics, and secondary wound closure. In view of the equal strength of the two groups and the lack of complications with aspiration and splinting, this latter treatment was favored.

Delayed treatment gives only fair results. Heckman and Levine[28] undertook repair in six patients at 4 to 18 months. The musculocutaneous nerve was intact in the base of the wound in all cases. Scar tissue was noted to be denser in those operated on later. At 6 months, three of five patients showed improved power (an average of 42% of normal power improving to 57%), and the appearance was somewhat improved.

Interestingly, Leighton and associates,[33] expanding on previous work by Agins and associates,[1] revealed differences between complete repair of dominant and nondominant extremities after operative treatment for distal biceps tendon ruptures. Testing of dominant extremities showed a full return in forearm supination strength as well as elbow flexion strength. In nondominant repaired extremities, a 14% supination strength deficit and a 14% flexion strength deficit (both corrected for dominance) were noted from that of expected values. Endurance differences were not significant. Leighton and associates[33] suggested that although dominant extremities are more likely to achieve normal function after repair, nondominant extremities may require intense rehabilitation in order to achieve maximal strength.

Authors' Preferred Treatment

For patients seen with biceps rupture in the acute phase, we prefer aspiration of the hematoma and immobilization of the elbow in acute flexion for 6 weeks. For subacute ruptures, we favor open repair and immobilization in acute flexion for 4 weeks and flexion at 90 degrees for 2 weeks. When there is a significant delay before presentation, we base the decision to repair the muscle on the patient's occupation, functional deficit, and concern regarding cosmesis. The prognosis in such cases is guarded.

RUPTURE OF THE SERRATUS ANTERIOR

Although traumatic winging of the scapula secondary to long thoracic nerve injury is not uncommon, there being several hundred cases reported in the English literature, rupture of the serratus anterior muscle is extremely uncommon. Fitchet[16] was the first to report on injury to the serratus anterior muscle; in 1930 he described five cases, although the diagnosis was not confirmed surgically in any, nor was electrodiagnostic equipment available to exclude injury to the long thoracic nerve. In 1940, Overpeck and Ghormley[53] reported on five additional cases of suspected serratus anterior muscle rupture. They believed that the severity of the pain was helpful in differentiating muscle rupture from long thoracic nerve palsy in that trauma to the muscle produced more severe pain than that seen with involvement of the nerve alone. Again, the cases were not confirmed surgically or electrodiagnostically.

In 1981, Hayes and Zehr[27] provided the first report of a surgically proven traumatic avulsion of the serratus anterior muscle. Their patient, a 25-year-old man who was driving an all-terrain vehicle that rolled over, sustained a mild cerebral contusion, a fractured jaw, and an injury to the right shoulder that resulted in a displaced fracture of the inferior angle of the scapula. The exact mechanism of injury was uncertain. He was treated in a sling, and at 2 weeks winging of the scapula was noted. The winging persisted; when he returned to work as a carpenter several months later, he noted that the arm tired easily and was weak, particularly when he was working with the arm in front or overhead. He was also troubled by a grating sensation under the scapula. These symptoms persisted, and after 9 months he underwent exploration. The findings included rupture of both the rhomboideus major and serratus anterior muscles. The tendinous attachment of the serratus anterior to the separated inferior pole fragment remained intact. The inferior pole was excised, and both muscles were reattached to the freshened border of the scapula with No. 1 silk sutures. A Velpeau sling was used postoperatively, and the shoulder was protected for 6 weeks. Full strength was regained; there was no further winging of the scapula; and the patient returned to his former occupation. Hayes[26] has subsequently treated a second patient who rolled a car over and sustained a similar avulsion of the inferior pole of the scapula. He experienced pain and weakness in his work as a welder and greatly improved after repair.

In 1986, a third case of rupture of the serratus anterior was described by Meythaler and colleagues[42] in a 64-year-old man with severe rheumatoid arthritis. His injury occurred with two episodes of rolling over in bed with the shoulder flexed and abducted. Winging of the scapula was evident clinically, along with marked infrascapular swelling and ecchymoses that extended along the lateral chest wall. Nerve conduction studies were normal in the long thoracic nerve, as was electromyography. Treatment was conservative, with rest followed by an intensive physiotherapy program. After 16 weeks the patient was independent in activities of daily living, but the winging persisted. In this case, several predisposing factors existed. Gross restriction of glenohumeral joint movement resulted in increased stresses on the serratus anterior, which was already weakened by chronic prednisone therapy and type 2 muscle atrophy associated with rheumatoid arthritis. Salicylate-induced coagulopathy may have contributed to the hematoma.

From the limited experience with disruption of the serratus anterior muscle reported in the literature, the authors advocate surgical repair in all except elderly and debilitated patients.

RUPTURE OF THE CORACOBRACHIALIS

In 1939, Gilcreest and Albi[22] stated that they were unable to find any recorded case of rupture of the coracobrachialis in the literature. However, they reported a single case that was due to direct violence, and at operation they discovered a rupture of the belly of the muscle. The patient had experienced considerable impairment of function in the arm; he was reported to make a complete recovery postoperatively. In 1941, a second case was described by Tobin and colleagues[73] involving a parachutist with a direct injury caused by his static line. No cases were included in a series of 1412 muscle ruptures reported by Anzel and co-workers[3] from the Mayo Clinic. This lesion appears to be rare. Acute repair is recommended in young, active patients.

RUPTURE OF THE SUBSCAPULARIS

In 1835, Smith[69] first reported an isolated tear of the subscapularis tendon in a cadaver. Speed[70] reported two patients in whom rupture of the subscapularis tendon had been diagnosed clinically but did not come to surgery. Gilcreest and Albi[22] reported one rupture found at operation, but no details of the site of rupture were available.

Partial rupture of the subscapularis in association with anterior dislocation of the glenohumeral joint is well documented.[12, 25, 46, 71] The part of the muscle that appears particularly vulnerable is the lower quarter, where the insertion may be directly from muscle into bone.[12, 71] Of 45 patients operated on for recurrent anterior dislocation, Symeonides reported six ruptures of the lower quarter of the subscapularis; in 24 patients, there were partial ruptures of the muscle at various other points. Partial rupture of the subscapularis muscle has also been produced in cadavers from anterior dislocation of the shoulder.[12, 71] The presence of the muscle injury has been used as a rationale for immobilization in internal rotation after acute anterior dislocation of the shoulder.

McAuliffe and Dowd[38] reported a case of complete avulsion of the subscapularis insertion in a 54-year-old woman after she fell directly onto the shoulder. It was not possible to dislocate the shoulder under general anesthesia. Following reattachment at the fragment with nylon sutures, the patient regained full movement and returned to her normal activities in 3 months.

In the recent literature three larger studies have been published on isolated rupture of the subscapularis tendon. In 1991, Gerber and Krushell[19] reported on 16 men, three of whom had undergone previous surgery. The average age of the patients was 51 years. The injury was caused by violent external rotation of the adducted arm in seven cases and by violent hyperextension in six cases. Two injuries occurred in motor vehicle accidents, and only one was associated with an anterior dislocation. All patients complained of pain anteriorly, which was troublesome at night, and all had pain and weakness when the arm was used above and below the shoulder level. The authors describe the "lift-off" test, which was abnormal in 12 of 13 patients tested. One patient had limitation of internal rotation such that the test was not possible. Weakness of internal rotation was reduced in 13 of 14 patients tested, and increased passive external rotation was increased in 10 of 16 patients. The long head of the biceps was dislocated medially in nine patients and ruptured in two patients. Ultrasound, CT arthrography, and MRI scanning all correctly predicted the surgical diagnosis. The authors recommend ultrasound examination first and the addition of MRI in questionable cases. All 16 patients underwent surgery, mainly by the recommended deltopectoral approach, taking care to protect the axillary and musculocutaneous nerves because the tendon stump was mobilized. Early results of repair were very encouraging.

In 1994, Nove Josserand and associates[50] published a report on 21 cases of isolated subscapularis rupture, all of which were confirmed surgically. Also in the French literature, Nerot and colleagues[48] reported on 25 rotator cuff tears that predominantly involved the subscapularis. Where coracohumeral impingement is evident, the authors advise a high index of suspicion of subscapularis rupture. In summary, a significant number of isolated subscapularis ruptures have been reported in the recent literature, and it is apparent that the lesion is more common than was previously thought.

Rupture of the subscapularis after first-time dislocation of the shoulder predisposes to recurrent instability. Neviaser and associates[49] evaluated 37 patients older than 40 years of age who sustained rotator cuff tears with primary anterior dislocations of the shoulder. Eleven patients from this group developed anterior instability due to rupture of the subscapularis tendon and anterior capsule. Stability was restored with repair of the capsule and subscapularis. In 1993, Moeckel and colleagues[44] addressed the problem of instability in a review of 236 total shoulder replacements from the Hospital for Special Surgery. Ten patients developed instability, seven of them anteriorly. This instability was due to rupture of the subscapularis tendon. Despite repair, three patients continued to have instability.

In 1994, Patten[57] reported on the MRI findings in nine patients with surgically confirmed rotator cuff tears that predominantly or exclusively involved the subscapularis tendon. The contours of the subscapularis tendon were poorly defined, and the tendon itself was of abnormally high signal intensity on T2-weighted images. Discontinuity and frank retraction of the tendon were evident in seven patients (78%). Thickening of the distal portion of the tendon was present in three cases and calcification in one case. Five patients had medial dislocation of the tendon.

CONCLUSION

Muscle ruptures are not common, yet they can produce substantial disability after a direct or indirect injury to the shoulder or arm. Surgical repair is difficult because of the problem of suturing muscle tissue directly; however, repair in the acute phase is to be commended whenever possible. Such repair can be further assisted by immobilization in a position that approximates the edges of the torn muscle. Careful protected exercise programs can then be initiated to further ensure optimal rehabilitation.

Acknowledgment

The authors wish to thank Chris Duggan for his diligent research of the literature and great assistance in preparation of this chapter.

References and Bibliography

1. Agins HJ, Chess J, Hoekstra D, and Teitge R: Rupture of the distal insertion of the biceps brachii tendon. Clin Orthop *233:*34–38, 1988.
2. Albo A: Ruptured pectoralis major tendon: A case report on delayed repair with muscle advancement. Acta Orthop Scan *65:*652–653, 1994.
2a. Anderson KJ and Le Cocq JF: Rupture of the triceps tendon. J Bone Joint Surg *39A:*444–446, 1957.
3. Anzel H, Covey KW, Weiner AD, et al: Disruption of muscles and tendons: An analysis of 1,014 cases. Surgery *45:*406–414, 1959.
4. Brickner WM and Milch H: Ruptures of Muscles and Tendons. International Clinics, Vol II, Series 38–7, 97.
5. Brumbuck RJ: Compartment syndrome complicating avulsion of the origin of the triceps muscle: A case report. J Bone Joint Surg *69A:*1445–1447, 1987.
6. Clemens H: Traumatische Hemie des M. Deltoideus. Dtsch Med Wochenschr *39:*2197, 1913.
7. Conwell HL: Subcutaneous rupture of the biceps flexor cubiti; report of one case. J Bone Joint Surg *10:*788–790, 1928.
8. Cronkite AE: The tensile strength of human tendons. Anat Rec *64:*173–186, 1936.
9. Danielsson L: Ruptur av.m. pectoralis major en brottningsskada. Nord Med *72:*1089, 1964.
10. Davis CB: Plastic repair of the deltoid muscle. Surg Clin *3:*287–289, 1919.
11. Delport HP and Piper MS: Pectoralis major rupture in athletes. Arch Orthop Trauma Surg *100:*135–137, 1982.
12. DePalma AF, Cooke AJ, and Prabhaker M: The role of the subscapularis in recurrent anterior dislocations of the shoulder. Clin Orthop *54:*35, 1967.
13. Elliot BC, Wilson GJ, and Kerr GK: A biomechanical analysis of the sticking region in the bench press. Med Sci Sports Exerc *21:*450–462, 1989.
14. Falchook FS, Zlatkin MB, Erbacher GE, et al: Rupture of the distal biceps tendon: Evaluation with MR imaging. Acta Orthop Belg *59:*426–469, 1993.
15. Farrar FL and Lippert FG: Avulsion of the triceps tendon. Clin Orthop *161:*242, 1981.
16. Fitchet SM: Injury of the serratus magnus (anterior) muscle. N Engl J Med *303:*818–823, 1930.
17. Garrett WE Jr, Califf JC, and Bassett FH III: Histochemical correlates of hamstring injuries. Am J Sports Med *12:*98–103, 1984.
18. Garrett WE Jr, Safran MR, Scaber AV, et al: Biomechanical comparison of stimulated and nonstimulated skeletal muscle pulled to failure. Am J Sports Med *15:*448–454, 1987.
19. Gerber C and Krushell RJ: Isolated rupture of the tendon of the subscapularis muscle. Clinical features in 16 cases. J Bone Joint Surg *73B:*389–394, 1991.
20. Gilcreest EL: Rupture of muscles and tendons, particularly subcutaneous rupture of biceps flexor cubiti. JAMA *84:*1819–1822, 1922.
21. Gilcreest EL: The common syndrome of rupture, dislocation and elongation of the long head of the biceps brachii; analysis of 200 cases. Surg Gynecol Obstet *58:*322–324, 1934.
22. Gilcreest EL and Albi P: Unusual lesions of muscles and tendons of the shoulder girdle and upper arm. Surg Gynecol Obstet *68:*903–917, 1939.

23. Gudmundsson B: A case of agenesis and a case of rupture of the pectoralis major muscle. Acta Orthop Scand *44*:213–218, 1973.
24. Haldeman K and Soto-Hall R: Injuries to muscles and tendons. JAMA *104*:2319–2324, 1935.
25. Hauser FDW: Avulsion of the tendon of subscapularis muscle. J Bone Joint Surg *36A*:139–141, 1954.
26. Hayes JM: Personal communication, 1988.
27. Hayes JM and Zehr DJ: Traumatic muscle avulsion causing winging of the scapula. J Bone Joint Surg *63A*:495–497, 1981.
28. Heckman JD and Levine MI: Traumatic closed transection of the biceps brachii in the military parachutist. J Bone Joint Surg *60A*:369–372, 1978.
29. Jones MW and Matthews JP: Rupture of pectoralis major in weight lifters: A case report and review of the literature. Injury *19*:219, 1988.
30. Kawashima M, Sato M, Torisu T, et al: Rupture of the pectoral major: Report of 2 cases. Clin Orthop *109*:115–119, 1975.
31. Kretzler HH Jr and Richardson AB: Rupture of the pectoralis major muscle. Am J Sports Med *17*:453–458, 1989.
32. Lee MLH: Rupture of triceps tendon. BMJ 2:197, 1960.
33. Leighton MM, Bush-Joseph CA, and Bach BR Jr: Distal biceps brachii repair: Results in dominant and nondominant extremities. Clin Orthop *317*:114–121, 1995.
34. Levy M, Fishel RE, and Stern GM: Triceps tendon avulsion with or without fracture of the radial head—a rare injury. J Trauma *18*:677–679, 1978.
35. Levy M, Golderg I, and Meir I: Fracture of the head of the radius with a tear or avulsion of the triceps tendon. J Bone Joint Surg *64B*:70–72, 1982.
36. Loos: Beitr Z Klin Chir *29*:410, 1900.
37. Lozano V and Alonso P: Sonographic detection of the distal biceps tendon rupture. J Ultrasound Med *14*:389–391, 1995.
38. McAuliffe TB and Dowd GS: Avulsion of the subscapularis tendon: A case report. J Bone Joint Surg *69A*:1454, 1987.
39. McEntire JE, Hess WE, and Coleman S: Rupture of the pectoralis major muscle. J Bone Joint Surg *54A*:1040–1046, 1972.
40. McMaster PF: Tendon and muscle ruptures. Clinical and experimental studies and locations of subcutaneous ruptures. J Bone Joint Surg *15*:705–722, 1933.
41. Mayer DP, Schmidt RG, and Ruiz S: MRI diagnosis of biceps tendon rupture. Comput Med Imaging Graph *16*:345–347, 1992.
42. Meythaler JM, Reddy NM, and Mitz M: Serratus anterior disruption: A complication of rheumatoid arthritis. Arch Phys Med Rehabil *67*:770–772, 1986.
43. Miles J, Grana W, Egle D, et al: The effect of anabolic steroids on the biomechanical and histological properties of rat tendon. J Bone Joint Surg *74A*:411–422, 1992.
44. Moeckel BH, Altchek DW, Warren RF, et al: Instability of the shoulder after arthroplasty. J Bone Joint Surg *75A*:492–497, 1993.
45. Montgomery AH: Two cases of muscle injury. Surg Clin *4*:871, 1920.
46. Moseley HF and Overgaard B: The anterior capsular mechanism in recurrent anterior dislocation of the shoulder. J Bone Joint Surg *44B*:913, 1962.
47. Moulonguet G: Rupture spontanée du grand pectoral chéz un vieillard. Enorme hematome. Mort Bull Mem Soc Anat Paris *94*:24–28, 1924.
48. Nerot C, Jully JL, and Gerard Y: Rotator cuff ruptures with predominant involvement of the subscapular tendon. Chirurgie *291*:103–106, 1993–94.
49. Neviaser RJ, Neviaser TJ, and Neviaser JS: Anterior dislocation of the shoulder and rotator cuff rupture. Clin Orthop *291*:103–106, 1993.
50. Nove Josserand L, Levigne C, Noel E, and Walch G: Isolated lesions of the subscapularis muscle. A propos of 21 cases. Rev Chir Orthop Reparatrice Appar Mot *80*:595–601, 1994.
51. O'Driscoll SW: Intramuscular triceps rupture. Can J Surg *35*:203–207, 1992.
52. Orava S, Sorasto A, Aalto K, and Kvist H: Total rupture of the pectoralis major muscle in athletes. Int J Sports Med *5*:272–274, 1984.
53. Overpeck DO and Ghormley RK: Paralysis of the serratus magnus muscle. JAMA *114*:1994–1996, 1940.
54. Pai VS and Simison AJ: A rare complication of pectoralis major rupture. Aust N Z J Surg *65*:694–695, 1995.
55. Park JY and Espiniella JL: Rupture of pectoralis major muscle: A case report and review of literature. J Bone Joint Surg *52A*:577–581, 1970.
56. Partridge: A case of rupture of the triceps cubiti. Med Times Gaz *1*:175–176, 1868.
57. Patten RM: Tears of the anterior portion of the rotator cuff (the subscapularis tendon): NR imaging findings. Am J Roentgenol *162*:351–354, 1994.
58. Patissier P: Traite des Maladies des Artisans. Paris: 1922, pp 162–164.
59. Pointud P, Clerc D, Manigand G, and Deparis M: Rupture spontanée du deltoide. Nouv Presse Med *6*:2315–2316, 1976.
60. Preston FS and Adicoff A: Hyperparathyroidism with avulsion of three major tendons. N Engl J Med *266*:968–971, 1962.
61. Ptasznik R and Hennessy O: Abnormalities of the biceps tendon of the shoulder: sonographic findings. AM J Roentgenol *164*:409–414, 1995.
62. Purnell R: Rupture of the pectoralis major muscle: A complication. Injury *19*:284, 1988.
63. Ronchetti G: Rottura sottocutanea parziale del muscolo grand pettorale con formazione di pseudocistie ematica. Minerva Chir *14*:22–28, 1959.
64. Safran MR, Garrett WE Jr, Seaber AV, et al: The role of warm-up in muscular injury prevention. Am J Sports Med *16*:123–129, 1988.
65. Samuel J, Levernieux J, and de Sèze S: A propos dun cas de rupture du deltoide. Rev Rhum Mal Osteoartic *42*:769–771, 1975.
66. Scott BW, Wallace WA, and Barton MA: Diagnosis and assessment of pectoralis major rupture by dynamometry. J Bone Joint Surg *74B*:111–113, 1992.
67. Sherman OH, Snyder SJ, and Fox JM: Triceps avulsion in a professional body builder: A case report. Am J Sports Med *12*:329, 1984.
68. Smith FC: Rupture of the pectoralis major muscle: A caveat. Injury *19*:282–283, 1988.
69. Smith HG: Pathological appearances of seven cases of injury of the shoulder joint with remarks. Am J Med Sci *16*:219–224, 1835.
70. Speed K: Personal communication to Gilcreest, 1939.
71. Symeonides PP: The significance of the subscapularis muscle in the pathogenesis of recurrent anterior dislocation of the shoulder. J Bone Joint Surg *54B*:476–483, 1972.
72. Tarsney FF: Rupture and avulsion of the triceps. Clin Orthop *83*:177–183, 1972.
73. Tobin WJ, Cohen LJ, and Vandover JT: Parachute injuries. JAMA *117*:1318–1321, 1941.
74. Tomczak R, Friedrich JM, Haussler MD, and Wallner B: (Sonographic diagnosis of diseases of the bicep muscle of arm). Rontgenpraxis *45*:145–149, 1992.
75. Van Leersum M and Schweitzer ME: Magnetic resonance imaging of the biceps complex. Magn Reson Imaging Clin North Am *2*:77–86, 1993.
76. Visuri T and Lindholm H: Bilateral distal biceps tendon avulsions with use of anabolic steroids. Med Sci Sports Exerc *26*:941–944, 1994.
77. Welsh RP, Macnab I, and Riley V: Biomechanical studies of rabbit tendon. Clin Orthop *81*:171–177, 1971.
78. Wolfe SW, Wickiewicz TL, and Cavanaugh JT: Ruptures of the fectoralis major muscle. An anatomic and clinical analysis. Am J Sports Med *20*:587–593, 1992.
79. Wood T, Cooke P, and Goodship A: The effect of exercise and anabolic steroids on the mechanical properties and crimpmorphology of the rat tendon. Am J Sports Med *16*:153–158, 1988.
80. Zeman SC, Rosenfeld RT, and Lipscomb PR: Tears of the pectoralis major muscle. Am J Sports Med *7*:343–347, 1979.

Bibliography

Albo A: Ruptured pectoralis major tendon: A case report on delayed repair with muscle advancement. Acta Orthop Scan *65*:642–643, 1994.

Bach BR Jr, Warren RF, and Wickiewicz TL: Triceps rupture: A case report and literature review. Am J Sports Med *15*:285–289, 1987.

Bach NR, Warren RF, and Fronck K: Disruption of the lateral capsule of the shoulder: A cause of recurrent dislocation. J Bone Joint Surg *70B*:74, 1988.

Bakalim G: Rupture of the pectoralis major muscle: A case report. Acta Orthop Scan *36*:274–279, 1965.

Bayley I, Fisher K, Tsitsui H, and Matthews J: Functional biofeedback

in the management of habitual shoulder instability, Proceedings of the 3rd International Conference on Surgery of the Shoulder. Fukuoka, Japan, Oct. 28–30, 1986.
Bennett BS: L Triceps tendon ruptures. J Bone Joint Surg *44A*:741–774, 1962.
Berson BL: Surgical repair of pectoralis major rupture in an athlete. Am J Sports Med 7:348–351, 1979.
Blondi J and Bear TF: Isolated rupture of the subscapularis tendon in an arm wrestler. Orthopaedics *11*:647–649, 1988.
Borchers E and Iontscheff P: Die Subkutane Ruptur des grossen brustmuskels ein wenig bekanntes aber typishes Krankheitsbild. Zentralbl Chir *59*:770–774, 1932.
Bowerman JW and McDonnell EJ: Radiology of athletic injuries; baseball. Radiology *116*:611, 1975.
Brownlee JJ: Rupture of the pectoralis major: A case report. Proceedings of the New Zealand Orthopaedic Association, Oct. 1987.
Buck JE: Rupture of the sternal head of the pectoralis major: A personal description. J Bone Joint Surg *45B*:224, 1963.
Butters AC: Traumatic rupture of the pectoralis major. BJM *2*:652–653, 1941.
Cougard P, Petitjean D, Hamoniere G, and Ferry C: Rupture traumatique complète du muscle grand pectoral. Rev Chir Orthop *71*:337–338, 1985.
Coughlin EJ and Baker DM: Management of shoulder injuries in sport. Conn Med *29*:723–727, 1965.
de Rouguin B: Rupture of the pectoralis major muscle: Diagnosis and treatment: A propos of 3 cases. Rev Chir Orthop Reparatrice Appar Mot *78*:248–250, 1992.
Dragoni S, Giombini A, Candela V, and Rossi F: Isolated partial tear of subscapularis muscle in a competitive water skier: A case report. J Sports Med Phys Fitness *34*:407–410, 1994.
Dunkelman NR, Collier F, Rook JL, Nagler W, and Brennan NJ: Pectoralis major muscle rupture in windsurfing. Arch Phys Med Rehabil *75*:819–821, 1994.
Egan TM and Hall H: Avulsion of the pectoralis major tendon in a weight lifter: Repair using a barbed staple. Can J Surg *30*:434, 1987.
Guerterbock P: Zerreissung der Sehn des M.triceps brachii. Arch Klin Chir *265*:256–260, 1981.
Hayes WM: Rupture of the pectoralis major muscle: Review of the literature and report of two cases. J Int Coll Surg *14*:82–88, 1950.
Heimann W: Uber einige subkutane Muskel-und Sehnenverletzungen van den oberen Gliedmassen. Monatschr Unfallh *15*:266–279, 1908.
Holleb PD and Bach BR Jr: Triceps brachii injuries. Sports Med *10*:273–276, 1990.
Jens J: The role of subscapularis muscle in recurring dislocation of the shoulder. J Bone Joint Surg *46B*:780, 1964.
Kehl T, Holzach P, and Matter P: Rupture of the pectoralis major muscle. Unfallchirurg *90*:363–366, 1987.
Kingsley DM: Rupture of pectoralis major: Report of a case. J Bone Joint Surg *28*:644–645, 1946.
Knaack WHL: Die subkutanen Verletzungen der Muskeln Veroffentl. Geb Mil Sanitatswesens *16*:1–123, 1900.
Kuniichi A and Takehiko T: Muscle belly tear of the triceps. Am J Sports Med *12*:484, 1984.
Lage J de A: Ruptura do musculo grande pectoral. Rev Hosp Clin *6*:37–40, 1951.
Law WB: Closed incomplete rupture of pectoralis major. BJM *2*:499, 1954.
Letenneur M: Rupture sous-cutanée du muscle grand pectoral: Guérison complète en quinze jours. Gaz de Hop *35*:54, 1862.
Lindenbaum BL: Delayed repair of a ruptured pectoralis major muscle. Clin Orthop *109*:120–121, 1975.
Liu J, Wu JJ, Chang CY, Chou YE, and Lo WE: Avulsion of the pectoralis major tendon. Am J Sports Med *20*:366–368, 1922.
MacKenzie DB: Avulsion of the insertion of the pectoralis major muscle. S Afr Med J *60*:147–148, 1981.
McKelvey D: Subcutaneous rupture of the pectoralis major muscle. BJM *2*:611, 1928.
Mandl F: Ruptur des Musculus pect. maor. Wien Med Wochenschr *75*:2192, 1925.
Malinovski I: Rare case of rupture of the pectoralis major at its attachment with process of the humerus. Voyenno Med J *153*:136–138, 1885.
Manjarris J, Gershuni DH, and Moitoza J: Rupture of the pectoralis major tendon. J Trauma *25*:810–811, 1985.
Marmor L, Bechtol CO, and Hall CB: Pectoralis major muscle function of sternal portion and mechanism of rupture of normal muscle: Case reports. J Bone Joint Surg *43A*:81–87, 1961.
Maydl K: Veber Subcutane Muskel-urd Sehrerserrissungen, sowie Rissferacturer mit Berucksichligung de analogen, dirche directe Gewalt enstandenen und offerien verletzungen. Dtsch Z Chir *17*:306–361, 1882; *18*:35–139, 1883.
Mendoza Lopez M, Cardoner Parpal JC, Sanso Bardes F, and Coba Sotes J: Lesions of the subscapular tendon regarding two cases in arthroscopic surgery (published erratum appears in Arthroscopy 1994). Arthroscopy *9*:671–674, 1993.
Newmark H III, Olken SM, and Halls J: Ruptured triceps tendon diagnosed radiographically. Australas Radiol *29*:60–63, 1985.
Nikitin GD, Linnik SA, and Filippov KV: Allotendoplasty in rupture of the pectoralis major muscle. Ortop Travnatol Protez *9*:47–48, 1987.
O'Donoghu DH: Injuries to muscle tendon unit. Am Surg *29*:190–200, 1963.
Pantazopoulos T, Exarchov B, Stavrov Z, et al: Avulsion of the triceps tendon. J Trauma *15*:827–829, 1975.
Parkes M: Rupture of the pectoralis major muscle. Ind Med *12*:226, 1943.
Penhallow D: Report of a case of ruptured triceps due to direct violence. N Y Med J *91*:76–77, 1910.
Pirker H: Die Verletzungen durch Muskelzug. Ergebn d Chir u Orthop *25*:553–634, 1934.
Pulaski EJ and Chandlee BH: Ruptures of the pectoralis major muscle. Surgery *10*:309–312, 1941.
Pulaski EJ and Martin GW: Rupture of the left pectoralis major muscle. Surgery *25*:110–111, 1949.
Recht J, Docquier J, Soete P, and Forthomme JP: Avulsion-fracture of the subscapular muscle. Acta Orthop Belg *57*:312–316, 1991.
Redard P, cited by Deveny P: Contribution à l'étude des ruptures musculaires. Thesis No. 423:12, Paris 1878.
Regeard A: Étude sur les ruptures musculaires. Thesis No. 182:51, Paris, 1880.
Rijnberg WJ and Van Ling B: Rupture of the pectoralis major muscle in body-builders. Arch Orthop Trauma Surg *112*:104–105, 1993.
Rio GS, Respizzi S, and Dworzak F: Partial rupture of the pectoralis major muscle in athletes. Int J Sports Med *11*:85–87, 1990.
Schechter LR and Gristina AG: Surgical repair of rupture of the pectoralis major muscle. JAMA *188*:1009, 1964.
Searfoss R, Tripi J, and Bowers W: Triceps brachii rupture: Case report. J Trauma *16*:244–245, 1976.
Smart A: Rupture of pectoralis major. Guy's Hosp Gaz *2*:61, 1873.
Solokoff L and Hough AJ Jr: Pathology of rheumatoid arthritis and allied disorders. *In* McCarthy DJ (ed): Arthritis and Allied Conditions: A Textbook of Rheumatology, 10th ed. Philadelphia: Lea & Febiger, 1985, pp 571–592.
Stimson H: Traumatic rupture of thc biceps brachii. Am J Surg *29*:472–476, 1935.
Thielemann FW, Kley U, and Holz U: Isolated injury of the subscapular muscle tendon. Sportverlets-Sportschaden *6*:26–28, 1992.
Tietjen R: Closed injuries of the pectoralis major muscle. J Trauma *20*:2623–2624, 1980.
Urs ND and Jani DM: Surgical repair of rupture of the pectoralis major muscle: A case report. J Trauma *16*:749–750, 1976.
Von Eiselberg A: Cited by Mandl (reference 53).
Weinlechner J: Uber subcutane Muskel, Sehnen und Knochenrisse. Wien Med Blatter *4*:1561–1565, 1881.

CHAPTER

22

ERNEST U. CONRAD III, M.D.

Tumors and Related Conditions

The management of musculoskeletal tumors is a broad and complex topic that represents approximately 10% of all orthopedic diagnoses.[145] This chapter emphasizes the initial assessment and evaluation because of the typical delay and difficulty of reaching an accurate diagnosis. The classification, staging, and imaging of these lesions represents, in a broad sense, many of the improvements achieved in the last 10 to 15 years. A review of the salient radiographic and clinical features of the more common lesions is included without an in-depth discussion of any one particular lesion. The principles of biopsy and surgical resection, the definition and significance of surgical margins, and the classification of resections and reconstructions are all discussed. Most of the surgical reconstructive techniques (e.g., allografts, arthrodesis, and arthroplasty) presented have only short follow-up to date and should be considered accordingly. Many biologic findings relevant to musculoskeletal tumors have occurred in the last 4 to 5 years and are discussed briefly.

HISTORICAL REVIEW

The term "sarcoma" was used by Abernethy in the 19th century to describe tumors that have a "firm and fleshy feel." Sarcoma refers to malignancies of mesenchymal, or connective tissue, origin. In that early period, sarcomas were lesions of the extremities and were confused with osteomyelitis and other conditions. Even the most accomplished professors of surgery demonstrated little interest in the recognition of sarcomas as malignancies distinct from carcinomas, and consequently, there was little prior work involving their classification or treatment.

An exception to that rule was Samuel W. Gross (1837 to 1884), a well-known surgeon, pathologist, and anatomist at the Jefferson Medical College in Philadelphia, who authored one of the first works that attempted to deal with the classification of various sarcomas, their salient features, and indications for treatment and prognosis. Gross was one of the first persons in the world to identify sarcomas as a distinctly different group of tumors from carcinomas.[81] With the discovery and development of radiographs (1893), various lesions of bone were beginning to attract attention. Gross was one of the first to appropriately identify sarcomas as locally invasive, extremity tumors, with frequent metastases to the lungs and infrequently demonstrating lymphatic or hepatic metastases. These unusual lesions were associated with a history of trauma in half of the cases and, according to Gross, required radical amputation or resection. In retrospect, his description of these first cases is remarkable for its clinical accuracy.

The scientific and technical developments in radiology, surgery, and medicine in the early 20th century resulted in significant advances in orthopedics, which were reflected in improvements in the care of fractures, infections, and tumors. At that time, pathologists and surgeons such as John Ewing (New York), Ernest A. Codman (Boston), and James Bloodgood (Baltimore) became interested in various tumors of bone.[107] The treatment for sarcomas varied greatly during those early years, but the management of these unusual and difficult tumors gradually became more uniform as lesions were recognized histologically and radiographically as distinct entities. Surgical treatment also improved with the developments in pathology and radiology. Aggressive ablative surgery for sarcomas was first recommended by Gross in his classic article on sarcomas[1] and was followed by various reports in the early 20th century of various innovative surgical techniques.[82, 104] Linberg's classic article in 1928 regarding interscapulothoracic resections[108] for malignancies of the shoulder joint reported on aggressive surgery for skeletal tumors. Since those early reports, dramatic advances in imaging, chemotherapy, pathology, and surgical techniques have resulted in improved survival and allowed more limb-sparing surgery.

In the 20th century, Dallas B. Phemister (University of Chicago, 1882 to 1951) was one of the first surgeons in North America to demonstrate a special interest in limb-sparing or "limb salvage" surgery as we know it today.[152] Phemister reviewed the American College of Surgeons' records for osteosarcoma in 1938 and found that only 4 of 86 extremity cases (4.6%) were treated with a limb-sparing resection.[152] Other reports of limb-sparing surgery at that time described variable results in terms of morbidity and mortality.[140, 152] The popularity of "limb salvage" surgery reached its zenith in the past 6 to 7 years, only to taper off to a more conservative approach, emphasizing the need for appropriate tumor resections and good functional results.

The specialty of musculoskeletal oncology has crystallized from improvements in radiographic "staging" studies, chemotherapy, pathology, and surgery. One of the most significant developments has involved the evolution of a classification system for sarcomas of bone and soft tissue that allows the assessment of a patient's prognosis based on the stage of the tumor and the proposed treatment.[44, 158] It is one of the only systems that appropriately reflect a patient's prognosis based on the most significant determinants of that prognosis: a tumor's stage and its surgical and "adjuvant" treatment. It is a system that is useful for chemotherapists, surgeons, radiation therapists, radiologists, and pathologists in the diagnosis and treatment and also the assessment of treatment results.

Limb-sparing procedures, when properly executed, involve innovative reconstructive techniques to achieve an arthroplasty or arthrodesis associated with reasonable functional results. The indications for and assessment of these procedures in terms of functional results and tumor recurrence are discussed briefly. Although the true worth of some of these procedures, in many cases, remains to be determined, the value of an accurate classification system for sarcomas and the coordinated multidisciplinary treatment of musculoskeletal neoplasms is obvious. Sarcomas are unusual tumors that require complex treatment. Their rarity and complexity have been major reasons for their haphazard treatment in the past. Recent advancements in the description of the molecular phenotypes of these tumors and in the assessment of their corresponding grade allow more accuracy in both tumor subtyping and in decisions regarding the treatment of high-grade tumors.

ANATOMY

Many anatomic considerations are involved in the treatment of musculoskeletal tumors. In the shoulder girdle these considerations are amplified by the proximity of the brachial plexus and major vessels of the upper extremity to the humerus, scapula, and chest wall. The implications of these anatomic points involve many aspects of the treatment and prognosis of shoulder neoplasms.

While the evaluation of musculoskeletal tumors frequently refers to the various anatomic compartments of the region involved, the exact anatomy of the compartments about the shoulder remains poorly defined. The compartments of the shoulder include the deltoid compartment, the posterior scapular compartment (supraspinatus, infraspinatus, teres minor, and teres major), the subscapular compartments (subscapularis), the anterior pectoral compartment (pectoralis minor and major), the anterior humeral compartment (biceps and coracobrachialis), the lateral humeral compartment (brachialis), the posterior humeral compartment (medial, lateral, and long head of the triceps), and the intra-articular compartment of the glenohumeral joint.

Compartments at the level of the humeral head and the proximal and mid-diaphysis are seen in Figure 22–1. Little work has been done on the true containment or integrity of these compartments, and their boundaries are theoretical. Although they are anatomically based, their actual potential for containment remains untested.

There are many anatomic clues that are helpful in making the initial diagnosis in patients presenting with an unknown musculoskeletal lesion. For instance, Ewing's sarcoma typically occurs in the shaft or diaphysis of the humerus; it rarely occurs in the metaphysis of a long bone. On the other hand, the epicenter of an osteogenic sarcoma rarely occurs in the shaft and usually occurs in the metaphysis. Similarly, whether a lesion is intra-articular or extra-articular is important for several reasons. Intra-articular tumors are very unusual because most lesions have their epicenter in bone or in the soft tissues outside a joint. An intra-articular lesion is more likely to represent a degenerative, traumatic, or other nontumorous diagnosis. The fact that a tumor might involve a joint primarily or secondarily is significant from the treatment point of view, because it requires a more complex, extra-articular resection. Secondary involvement of a joint by an intraosseous malignancy is usually a late phenomenon associated with a longer diagnostic delay or a more aggressive lesion and a worse prognosis[44, 191] (see the section on Staging and Classification of Tumors).

Difficult locations for neoplasms in the shoulder girdle include those of the brachial plexus or lesions involving the axillary brachial vessels. Both the plexus and the axillary vessels are contained within their own sheaths, which can eventually be penetrated or infiltrated by an aggressive lesion. Primary tumors of the brachial plexus (neurosarcomas) are usually manifested by a brachial plexus nerve deficit on clinical examination. Any patient who presents with distinct peripheral nerve symptoms associated with a shoulder mass should be assumed to have nerve involvement until demonstrated otherwise. A biopsy of that type of lesion is therefore very likely to involve that nerve and result in further nerve loss. Lesions involving the axillary or brachial vessels require magnetic resonance imaging (MRI) and arteriography in order to define the precise extent of involvement.

The shoulder girdle is unique in that it has one of the largest and most well-defined muscle compartments in the body in the deltoid muscle. To function normally, the shoulder is dependent on a well-innervated deltoid and rotator cuff in addition to adequate glenohumeral stability. The deltoid, like most muscle compartments, has anatomic subdivisions (acromial, clavicular, scapular), but grossly it is a well-defined muscle that is easily resectable, although extremely difficult to reconstruct functionally. Perhaps the most important anatomic consideration involved in the treatment of shoulder tumors is the anatomy of the axillary nerve and its relationship to the deltoid and placement of shoulder incisions, biopsies, and so forth. Injuries to the axillary nerve during tumor resections or biopsy may result in almost total loss of deltoid function. Thus, the location of the axillary nerve at the time of biopsy and at the time of resection has great

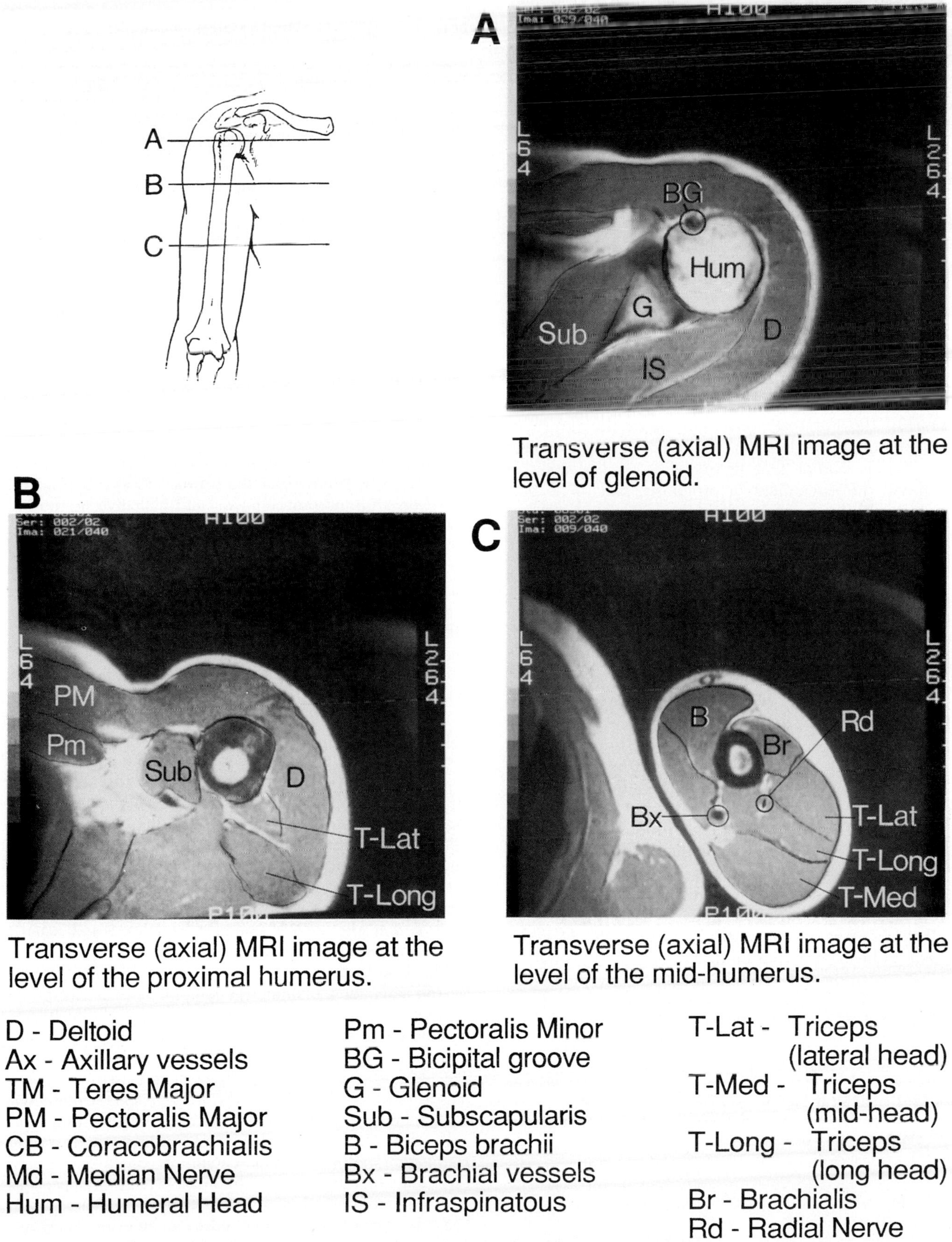

Figure 22–1

Shoulder anatomy on axial magnetic resonance imaging.

significance. In general, the functional prognosis for tumors of the shoulder girdle is much better if the axillary nerve, deltoid, and rotator cuff are preserved. Whereas glenohumeral joint mechanics can be replaced by shoulder arthroplasty, reconstruction of the deltoid or rotator cuff is much more difficult.

STAGING AND CLASSIFICATION OF TUMORS

Staging

The early classification system for musculoskeletal tumors was popularized by Lichtenstein according to basic histologic categories.[105] It was useful in identifying general trends in diagnosis and prognosis, but this descriptive histologic system had limited significance for determining adjuvant treatment (e.g., chemotherapy, radiation therapy) and prognosis.

One of the greatest contributions to the improved treatment of sarcomas today has been the development of a staging system that assists with the selection of treatment, the assessment of prognosis, and the evaluation of results. Such a classification system was introduced by Enneking in 1980,[44] adopted by the Musculoskeletal Tumor Society, and subsequently accepted, with modifications, by the NIH Sarcoma Consensus Study Group as the staging system for all sarcomas.[158] It represents a combined assessment of the histologic, or "surgical," grade (G), the anatomic site of primary disease (T), and the presence or absence of metastases (M). Surgical grading is based on the histologic assessment, identifying a lesion as benign (C_0), low-grade malignant (G_1), or high-grade malignant (G_2) (Tables 22–1 and 22–2).

The original concept of the staging system as devised by Enneking represented a departure from the staging system of the American Joint Committee for Cancer Staging and End-Results,[3] originally designed for the evaluation of various carcinomas. Enneking thought that system correlated poorly with the natural history of sarcomas. He described the salient features of sarcomas with reference to their distinction from carcinomas and the significance of those features regarding staging.[3, 44, 158]

Most sarcomas, in contrast with carcinomas, were described as having a similar natural history, one of progressive local invasion and eventual hematogenous pulmonary metastasis. The surgical treatment of sarcomas of the extremities is significantly different from that of lesions of the head and neck, retroperitoneum, trunk, and abdomen. Appropriate surgery with or without radiation therapy remains the definitive treatment of the primary disease for most sarcomas. However, surgery must be combined with systemic chemotherapy to be curative. Chemotherapy or radiation therapy without surgery is rarely, if ever, curative for the primary lesion. It remains, however, an important adjuvant and palliative method of treatment.

The extent of disease in the Enneking system is defined by the "anatomic setting." Compartmentalization, or compartmental escape, is an important characteristic of sarcomas in contrast to previous classification systems and other tumors (carcinomas). It was postulated that the anatomic site (T) was the greatest factor in the prognosis because it represented a composite of the following characteristics: anatomic site, rate of growth, and delay in diagnosis. The primary extent of disease is limited by the natural boundaries of the anatomic compartment in which the lesion is located. A lesion located in the anterior thigh is contained by the fascial envelope of the quadriceps compartment until progressive growth causes it to extend beyond the natural boundary. When that occurs, the patient has a worse prognosis and a higher risk of metastatic disease, reflecting a more aggressive tumor. Lesions that occur in poorly compartmentalized anatomic sites (e.g., groin, popliteal fossa, perivascular space) are, by the nature of that site, poorly compartmentalized and usually associated with a worse prognosis.

The histologic grading system proposed for sarcomas by the Enneking system was simplified to a two-grade system, that of high-grade versus low-grade histology. No allowance for intermediate-grade histology was made because there was no intermediate surgical treatment. This system required the pathologist to classify all sarcomas as either high-grade or low-grade lesions, which contradicts most classical sarcoma grading systems that typically described high-, low-, and intermediate-grade histology. Grading remains a topic of controversy today, especially for soft tissue sarcomas, which do occur as intermediate-grade lesions in certain cases. The system has subsequently been modified to include intermediate-grade soft tissue tumors. The basic concept, however, remains a valid one, and intermediate-grade soft tissue tumors remain a treatment paradox regarding the indications for chemotherapy. Tumor grading should not be

Table 22–1 SURGICAL STAGING SYSTEM: BENIGN TUMORS*

STAGE	GRADE	SITE
1	Latent (G_0)	Intracapsular (T_0)
2	Active (G_0)	Intracapsular (T_0)
3	Aggressive (G_0)	Intracompartmental (T_1) or Extracompartmental (T_2)

*From Enneking WF, Spanier SS, and Goodman MA: A system for the surgical staging of musculoskeletal sarcoma. Clin Orthop *153*:105–120, 1980.

Table 22–2 SURGICAL STAGING SYSTEM: MALIGNANT BONE TUMORS*

STAGE	GRADE	SITE
IA	Low grade (G_1)	Intracompartmental (T_1)
IB	Low grade (G_1)	Extracompartmental (T_2)
IIA	High grade (G_2)	Intracompartmental (T_1)
IIB	High grade (G_2)	Extracompartmental (T_2);
III	Any grade (G_1 or G_2 with regional or distant metastases [M_1])	any site (T_1 or T_2)

*From Enneking WF, Spanier SS, and Goodman MA: A system for the surgical staging of musculoskeletal sarcoma. Clin Orthop *153*:105–120, 1980.

based on the histologic type alone. The theory that some histologic diagnoses always represent high-grade lesions and a worse prognosis, regardless of their histologic grade, is not generally acceptable.

In the original Enneking staging system, the prognosis for a patient with regional lymph node involvement was believed to be as poor as that for the patient with pulmonary metastasis. Therefore, either lymph node metastasis or pulmonary metastasis was represented by stage III disease.

The strength of the Enneking staging system is its simplicity. By emphasizing high-grade versus low-grade histology and by limiting the number of tumor stages (IA, IB, IIA, IIB, III), this system is simple enough to be used by a wide group of specialists and to allow for a variety of treatments. The Enneking system employs a subtly but significantly different numbering system for benign and malignant disease. Benign disease is denoted as grade 1, 2, or 3, depending on whether it is a latent, active, or aggressive tumor (see Table 22–1). A latent benign lesion does not show active growth. An active lesion shows active growth but is confined within the compartment defined by the surrounding natural boundaries. An aggressive lesion has the potential to penetrate or violate natural boundaries, such as cortical bone, periosteum, or fascial compartments, and to remain locally aggressive without metastasizing. Theoretically, only malignant tumors (by definition) have the ability to metastasize: A contradiction in terms is presented by the ability of histologically "benign" giant cell tumors to "metastasize" to the lung in a few cases. Other aggressive benign tumors (chondroblastoma) have also demonstrated lung metastases in a small number of cases.

Malignant tumors are denoted as stage I or II (see Table 22–2), depending on whether the histology is high grade or low grade, and as A or B, depending on whether the lesion is intracompartmental or extracompartmental. Thus, a IA lesion is malignant, low grade, and intracompartmental. A IIA lesion is high grade and intracompartmental, and IIB is high grade and extracompartmental (see Table 22–2). Grade III lesions are metastatic regardless of the grade or anatomic site of the lesion. The system is somewhat different for soft tissue.

The anatomic or surgical site classification (T) defines the primary lesion in relationship to its position in the anatomical compartment of origin. Tumors are described as encapsulated (T0), intracompartmental (T1), or extracompartmental (T2). This designation is based on the Enneking compartmental theory that describes an anatomic compartment as a space or potential space defined by natural boundaries (Table 22–3).[44] Tumors contained within an anatomic compartment may violate the boundaries of the compartment with growth—usually a sign of an aggressive benign or malignant tumor. Active benign tumors are typically well encapsulated (T0) and intracompartmental, whereas aggressive benign lesions may be poorly encapsulated but remain intracompartmental (T1). Low-grade malignant lesions are typically intracompartmental (T1), whereas extracompartmental lesions (T2) usually represent high-grade malignancies. Extracompartmental tumors may extend from one compartment into another or from one compartment into a surrounding extrafascial plane, or they may arise within a poorly compartmentalized, extracompartmental space. Poorly compartmentalized anatomic spaces include perivascular areas such as the subsartorial space of the common femoral artery, the popliteal fossa, the antecubital fossa, or the midhand, midfoot, axilla, or groin (see Table 22–3).

Table 22–3 SURGICAL SITES (T)*

INTRACOMPARTMENTAL	*EXTRACOMPARTMENTAL*
Intraosseous	Soft tissue extension
Intra-articular	Soft tissue extension
Superficial to deep fascia	Deep fascial extension
Parosseous	Intraosseous or extrafascial
Intrafacial compartments	Extrafascial planes or spaces
Ray of hand or foot	Mid- and hindfoot
Posterior calf	Popliteal space
Anterolateral leg	Groin–femoral triangle
Anterior thigh	Intrapelvic
Midthigh	Midhand
Posterior thigh	Antecubital fossae
Buttocks	Axilla
Volar forearm	Periclavicular
Dorsal forearm	Paraspinal
Anterior arm	Head and neck
Posterior arm	
Periscapular	

*From Enneking WF, Spanier SS, and Goodman MA: A system for the surgical staging of musculoskeletal sarcoma. Clin Orthop *153*:105–120, 1980.

The stage of the lesion and the surgical margin of the procedure are associated with a certain local recurrence rate as described in the work of Enneking (see the section on Surgical Margin). These recurrence rates are based on an extensive retrospective review of the literature and reflect the risk of local recurrence following surgical resection without the use of adjuvant treatment. A benign aggressive (stage 3) lesion treated with a wide margin has a recurrence rate of 10% or less. This recurrence reflects surgical treatment alone and does not reflect the lower recurrence rate associated with surgery and adjuvant treatment, as is performed for most malignant conditions. High-grade malignant tumors (IIB), such as the typical osteosarcoma, require at least a wide surgical margin that includes a surrounding cuff of normal tissue in order to avoid a local recurrence.

After careful anatomic staging of the tumor, the appropriate surgical procedure can be predicted by considering the grade of the lesion and the extent of involvement at the primary site (stage). The difficulty of that resection will also become apparent from this evaluation. A patient's prognosis and risk for local recurrence can similarly be assessed by considering the grade of the tumor and the surgical margin achieved at the time of the surgical procedure. This "articulation" or correlation of the tumor "stage" and the "surgical margin" allows an assessment of the risk of local recurrence as a result of the procedure and margin achieved.

Thorough initial evaluation and staging, before treatment, remain the crucial ingredients for a successful outcome. Without these initial studies and an adequate and accurate biopsy, a successful treatment plan is unlikely. A universally accepted staging classification system is important in order to direct patient care and to adequately assess clinical results regarding disease-free status. This initial staging philosophy remains one of the major contributions of the Enneking staging system to patient care.

The staging evaluation involves an assessment by various radiographic studies to determine the precise anatomic extent of primary disease, in addition to whether or not regional or distant metastases have occurred. Typical staging studies include plain radiographs, technetium bone scan, computed tomographic (CT) scans, MRI scans, and other studies that better define a lesion's location. A total body bone scan is the best study to assess the extent of the primary bone lesion and the possibility of metastatic disease.[86, 190, 191] CT scans are excellent for visualizing cortical geography and bone involvement at the primary site on a two-dimensional plane.[44] CT scanning of the lung is routinely carried out in most institutions to assess possible pulmonary metastasis, and it is a more sensitive method than plain radiographs.

MRI scans are indicated for evaluating soft tissue disease, intramedullary bony disease, and spinal or pelvic lesions.[202] The soft tissue or neurovascular margins are best assessed by the MRI scan, because it is much more sensitive than the CT scan for evaluating soft tissue margins. MRI does image the peripheral inflammatory "reactive zone" with a bright signal that may or may not contain a tumor. Similarly, the radiologist may over-read soft tissue margins when interpreting malignancies such as osteosarcoma and Ewing's sarcoma[202] because of the inability to distinguish inflammation from a tumor on the MRI scan.

Classification of Tumors

Although the histologic classification of tumors has limitations in predicting the prognosis and directing treatment, it does serve a purpose in identifying tumor or sarcoma subtypes and their general tendencies. Knowledge of a tumor's histologic type and the age of the patient is quite helpful when making a reliable tentative diagnosis in many patients, especially when the x-ray appearance is added to that information. The most common lesions of bone, cartilage, and soft tissue are described here in order to discuss their general histologic, radiographic, and clinical characteristics. The clinical scenario of patient age, type of radiographic abnormality, and type of tissue involvement can, in many cases, lead to a significant and limited differential diagnosis.

BENIGN OSSEOUS LESIONS

Osteoid Osteoma

Benign osseous lesions of the shoulder are uncommon. Osteoid osteoma and osteoblastoma occur in the proximal humerus or scapula in 10 to 15% of cases and, when they do occur, favor the proximal humerus or glenoid.[57, 92] Osteoid osteoma typically displays the classic symptom of night pain, which is relieved by salicylates. Radiographically, it is characterized by a large area of reactive bone surrounding a small lucent "nidus." On technetium bone scan, it has impressive increased activity, and the central nidus can be visualized as a distinct cortical hole on CT scanning or tomography. Histologically, this lucent nidus is a well-demarcated, small area of immature, very active osteoblastic tissue. Preoperative localization is an extremely important strategy in order to avoid intraoperative difficulties in locating these lesions and thus in minimizing local recurrences.

Osteoblastoma

Some clinicians regard osteoblastoma as a larger version of osteoid osteoma ("giant osteoid osteoma") typified by a large lucent area of osteoblastic tissue surrounded by a thin, sclerotic, reactive rim of bone.[57] Radiographically, osteoblastoma is typically seen as a lucent lesion that has expanded the overlying cortex into a thin rim. As with osteoid osteoma, osteoblastoma may be difficult to localize radiographically and requires careful preoperative imaging in order to avoid recurrences. Osteoblastoma, unlike osteoid osteoma, also occurs in an aggressive (stage 3) form that is less well-defined radiographically, has a high recurrence rate, and may have a histologic appearance that is difficult to distinguish from low-grade osteosarcoma. Technetium bone scanning and CT scans are good imaging techniques for both of these lesions. Plain x-ray tomography may also be an effective diagnostic tool for localizing many osteoid osteomas.

Myositis Ossificans

Myositis ossificans is a benign, reactive, bone-forming process occurring intramuscularly or in the "areolar tissues" (tendon, ligament, capsule, fascia) adjacent to bone. It may occur with or without a history of trauma and, in the latter instance, may be referred to as pseudomalignant myositis ossificans of soft parts.[143] The pseudomalignant form is typically seen as a symptomatic enlarging soft tissue mass that develops in the second decade of life, occurring in the shoulder in 15% of cases. The typical radiographic appearance is an osseous density in soft tissue that demonstrates a peripheral radiographic maturity or margination of the mass, separated from the adjacent cortical bone by a narrow zone of uninvolved soft tissue. This characteristic histologic margination or zonation phenomenon (peripheral maturity) reflects the fact that the more active (immature) osteoblastic tissue is located centrally in the lesion, in contrast to other neoplasms that have their most active histologic area peripherally. Isotope scans of myositis ossificans demonstrate a high uptake peripherally that may continue for 8 to 12 weeks or until spontaneous maturation occurs. Excision before that time is associated with a high recurrence rate.

In some patients, myositis ossificans may be confused with osteosarcoma or a soft tissue sarcoma, which does not demonstrate the same zonation or peripheral margination phenomenon, nor does it have the same radiographic characteristics. When there is confusion about the proper diagnosis, optimal management includes a complete radiographic evaluation and careful clinical observation rather than a hasty or premature excision or biopsy (which may be difficult to interpret).[30] The radiographic differential diagnosis for myositis ossificans includes extraosseous or parosteal osteosarcoma, synovial sarcoma, vascular lesions, and calcification of soft tissue secondary to necrosis or inflammation.

MALIGNANT OSSEOUS LESIONS

Osteosarcoma

Osteosarcoma is the most common primary sarcoma of bone (excluding multiple myeloma). It represents the most common primary sarcoma occurring in the shoulder, followed by Ewing's sarcoma and chondrosarcoma. In the past, it has typically occurred in the adolescent age group, although a significant percentage of patients are young adults in their third decade of life.

Classic osteosarcoma is a high-grade, aggressive tumor that occurs in the metaphyseal bone, typically as a stage IIB lesion, usually with an extraosseous soft tissue component at presentation.[77, 91, 105] The typical patient presents with intrinsic bone pain at night that is frequently unrelated to activity. The average duration of symptoms at presentation is 3 to 6 months, which reflects the subtle nature of the preliminary symptoms and the need for early recognition of intraosseous pain and night pain as warning symptoms.[49]

Approximately 10 to 15% of all osteosarcomas occur in the proximal humerus, whereas 1 to 2% occur in the scapula or clavicle.[34, 46, 91, 105] The typical radiograph for osteosarcoma has a sunburst or osteoblastic pattern, with penetration of the adjacent cortex (Fig. 22–2*A*). Osteosarcomas usually have increased activity on bone scan (Fig. 22–2*B*), and a soft tissue mass is seen on CT (see Fig. 22–2*C*) and MRI (see Fig. 22–2*D*). Arteriography is no longer the technique of choice for evaluating soft tissue involvement but may be obtained to evaluate major vessel involvement or for intra-arterial chemotherapy (see Fig. 22–2*E*). Variants of osteosarcoma other than the classic type include telangiectatic (vascular) osteosarcoma,[130] secondary osteosarcoma (Paget's disease or radiation-induced), and various low-grade lesions such as periosteal and parosteal osteosarcoma.[46, 207, 208] The basic histologic criterion for the diagnosis of classic osteosarcoma includes a malignant stroma-producing (spindle cells) tumor or immature, neoplastic osteoid.[34, 91, 105] The overall prognosis for osteosarcoma at 5 years of follow-up is approximately 70% with appropriate chemotherapy and surgery.[142] Prognostic factors for survival remain debatable; however, histologic necrosis at resection and the size of the tumor are probably the most significant variables.[35]

BENIGN CARTILAGINOUS LESIONS

Osteochondroma

The incidence of cartilaginous tumors in the shoulder is second only to those occurring about the pelvis.[49] Solitary osteochondroma or exostosis is the most common benign tumor of the shoulder; approximately one fourth of all exostoses occur in the proximal humerus. Osteochondromas actually represent a developmental abnormality arising from the peripheral growth plate and are typically active, benign (stage 2) lesions during skeletal growth. The plain radiograph is usually diagnostic in demonstrating a smooth excrescence of metaphyseal cancellous bone that is confluent and continuous with normal metaphyseal bone (Fig. 22–3). Exostoses may appear as pedunculated, stalk-like lesions or as flat, sessile lesions. Concern regarding a possible secondary chondrosarcoma may arise in adult patients who present with pain, an enlarging soft tissue mass, or intraosseous bony erosions. Evidence of a thickened cartilaginous cap (> 1 cm) on a CT scan, in association with a soft tissue mass, pain, or radiographic evidence of possible malignant degeneration, suggests a secondary chondrosarcoma. The risk of a secondary chondrosarcoma arising out of an exostosis is approximately 1% per lesion, although rates as high as 10 to 30% have been referred to in the literature regarding secondary malignancy in patients with multiple hereditary exostoses.[183]

Exostoses are typically diagnosed in the skeletally immature. An enlarging or symptomatic exostosis should be considered with caution in the skeletally mature because parosteal osteosarcoma is an alternative diagnosis in that situation. The treatment for solitary exostosis involves an excision through the base of the lesion. In the sessile form, care should be taken to excise the cartilaginous cap in order to avoid a recurrence. The most common complication of an exostosis is an iatrogenic or surgical injury to the adjacent growth plate or neurovascular structures at the time of excision. An adequate surgical exposure should be emphasized, especially for proximal humeral and proximal femoral lesions, which are usually large and adjacent to the major neurovascular bundle of that extremity.

The diagnosis of secondary chondrosarcoma, arising out of an exostosis, is unusual and best made on a preoperative CT scan (of a thickened "cap" or enlarging soft tissue mass) and not by biopsy. Cartilage histology is very difficult to interpret, and thus the diagnosis of a secondary malignancy is best made clinically and radiographically. The transition from benign to malignant is usually a protracted one involving relatively subtle histologic changes. The finding of a cartilage cap thicker than 1 cm should serve as a warning of at least a low-grade chondrosarcoma.

Chondroblastoma

Chondroblastoma, or Codman's tumor, is an unusual benign, cartilaginous tumor that occurs in the proximal humeral epiphysis (25% of cases) as a round or oval lesion containing fine calcifications surrounded by a reactive bony margin.[31, 89, 101] It occurs in the skeletally immature, and histologically it consists of aneurysmal tissue, "chicken wire" calcifications, and immature "paving stone" chondroblasts. Chondroblastoma occurs as an active, benign stage 2 lesion, although it also has a more aggressive stage 3 form. Treatment usually involves an extensive intralesional curettage that results in a large subchondral defect of the humeral head, requiring autogenous bone graft to prevent subchondral and cartilaginous collapse. The radiographic appearance of this epiphyseal lesion is usually typical and involves adolescents or young

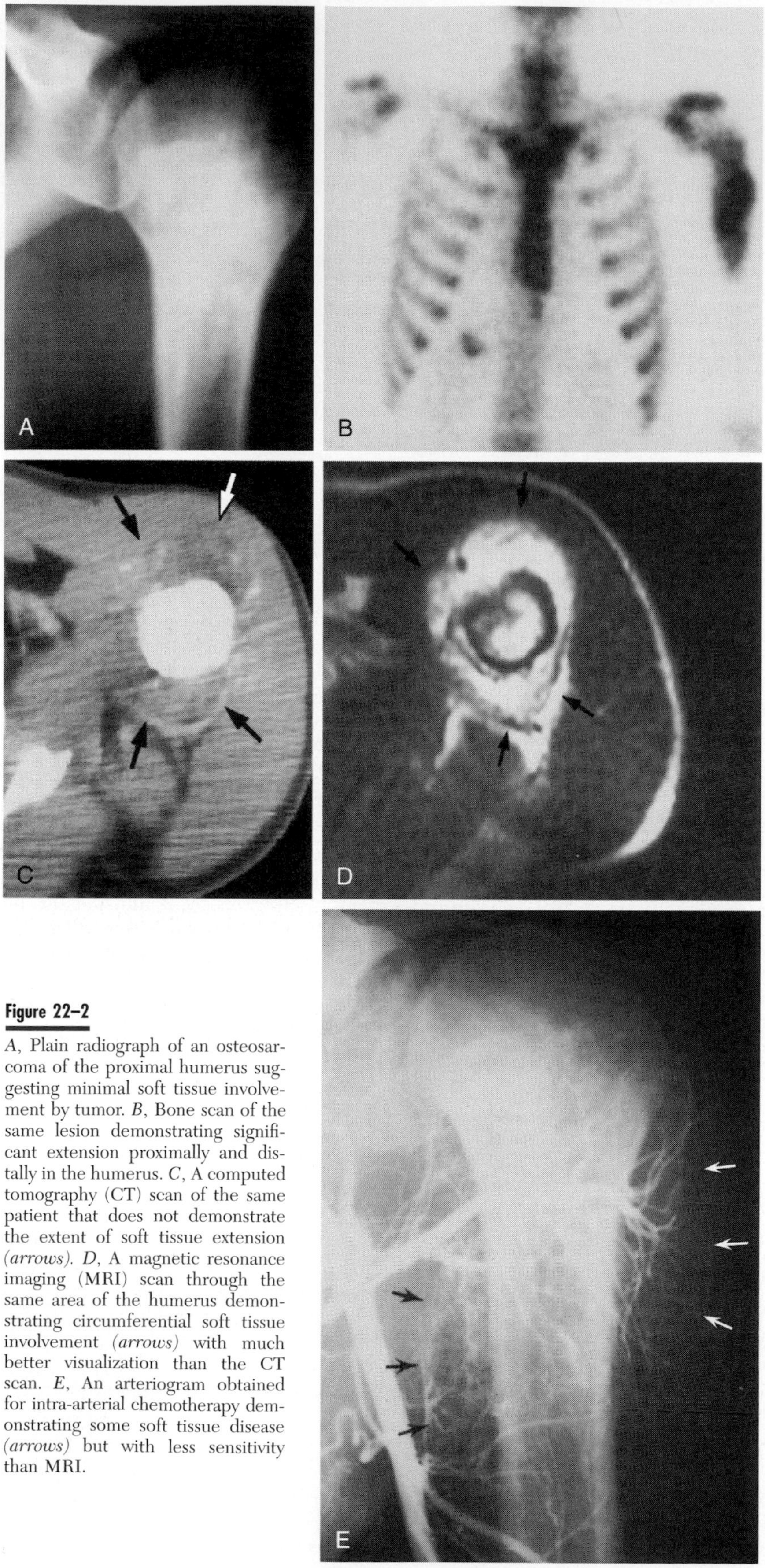

Figure 22–2

A, Plain radiograph of an osteosarcoma of the proximal humerus suggesting minimal soft tissue involvement by tumor. *B*, Bone scan of the same lesion demonstrating significant extension proximally and distally in the humerus. *C*, A computed tomography (CT) scan of the same patient that does not demonstrate the extent of soft tissue extension *(arrows)*. *D*, A magnetic resonance imaging (MRI) scan through the same area of the humerus demonstrating circumferential soft tissue involvement *(arrows)* with much better visualization than the CT scan. *E*, An arteriogram obtained for intra-arterial chemotherapy demonstrating some soft tissue disease *(arrows)* but with less sensitivity than MRI.

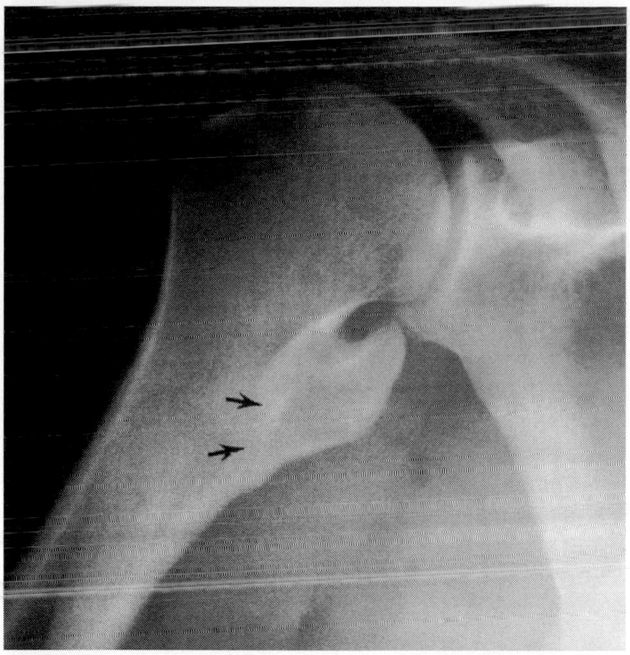

Figure 22–3

Osteochondroma of the proximal humerus demonstrating "confluence" of normal metaphyseal bone into the lesion *(arrows)*.

adults. The differential diagnosis includes a simple cyst, eosinophilic granuloma, osteomyelitis, or aneurysmal bone cyst.

Periosteal Chondroma

Periosteal chondroma is another benign cartilaginous lesion of the proximal humerus and is usually located just proximal to the deltoid insertion of the lateral humeral shaft. It typically presents as a minimally symptomatic or asymptomatic mass that is radiographically a sessile lesion with a distinct, well-defined margin of reactive cortex underlying the radiolucent cartilaginous mass.[31] Marginal excision results in a cortical defect of the humerus that may or may not require bone grafting. The differential diagnosis includes periosteal osteosarcoma, which does not have the well-defined underlying sclerotic cortex. Periosteal osteosarcoma is a more aggressive intracortical lesion that may extend into the medullary canal in a small percentage of cases.

Enchondroma

Solitary enchondroma is a benign, central cartilaginous lesion that is most commonly found in the small tubular bones of the hand but also occurs in the proximal humerus in 10 to 15% of cases.[9, 50, 90] As a benign lesion, enchondromas are asymptomatic and require no treatment. When they occur adjacent to a joint that is symptomatic for degenerative reasons, the clinical assessment of bone pain related to the enchondroma may be difficult. This scenario is not uncommon, and it makes the initial evaluation of intraosseous cartilage tumors difficult, because intrinsic bone pain is an important symptom suggestive of a low-grade malignancy. Thus, the ability to distinguish intraosseous from intra-articular symptoms is a difficult but necessary challenge. The typical radiographic appearance of a benign enchondroma is that of a central lucent lesion with a well-defined bony margin and intrinsic calcifications. Figure 22–4 represents such a lesion in a 35-year-old woman with rotator cuff symptoms and a heavily calcified benign cartilage lesion.

MALIGNANT CARTILAGINOUS LESIONS

Chondrosarcoma

Chondrosarcoma may arise de novo as a primary chondrosarcoma, or it may arise out of a pre-existing benign cartilage lesion, which is then referred to as a secondary chondrosarcoma. Secondary chondrosarcoma occurs in young adults, accounts for approximately 25% of all chondrosarcomas, and may be found in patients with a pre-existing enchondroma, osteochondroma, multiple enchondromatosis (Ollier's disease),[100, 101, 186] or multiple hereditary exostosis.[70] The radiographic evidence of a secondary, or low-grade, chondrosarcoma arising out of such a lesion includes enlarging radiolucent areas within the lesion or endosteal cortical erosions along the cortical margins (Fig. 22–5). Technetium bone scans are typically moderately "hot" for both enchondroma and low-grade chondrosarcoma and are not helpful in distinguishing one from the other. The microscopic evaluation of cartilage lesions is not diagnostic in a large percentage of cases. Histologic characteristics suggestive of malignancy include cellularity, pleomorphism, and evidence of mitotic activity, such as double-nucleated lacunae. These are subtle findings, and the histologic evidence for low-grade chondrosarcoma versus enchondroma is frequently in-

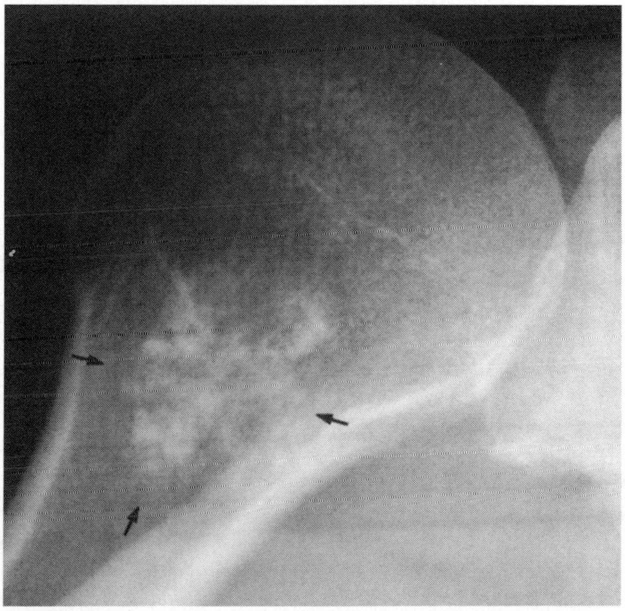

Figure 22–4

A plain radiograph of a 35-year-old woman with rotator cuff symptoms and an incidental benign enchondroma. There is no involvement or erosion of the endosteal cortical surface *(arrows)*.

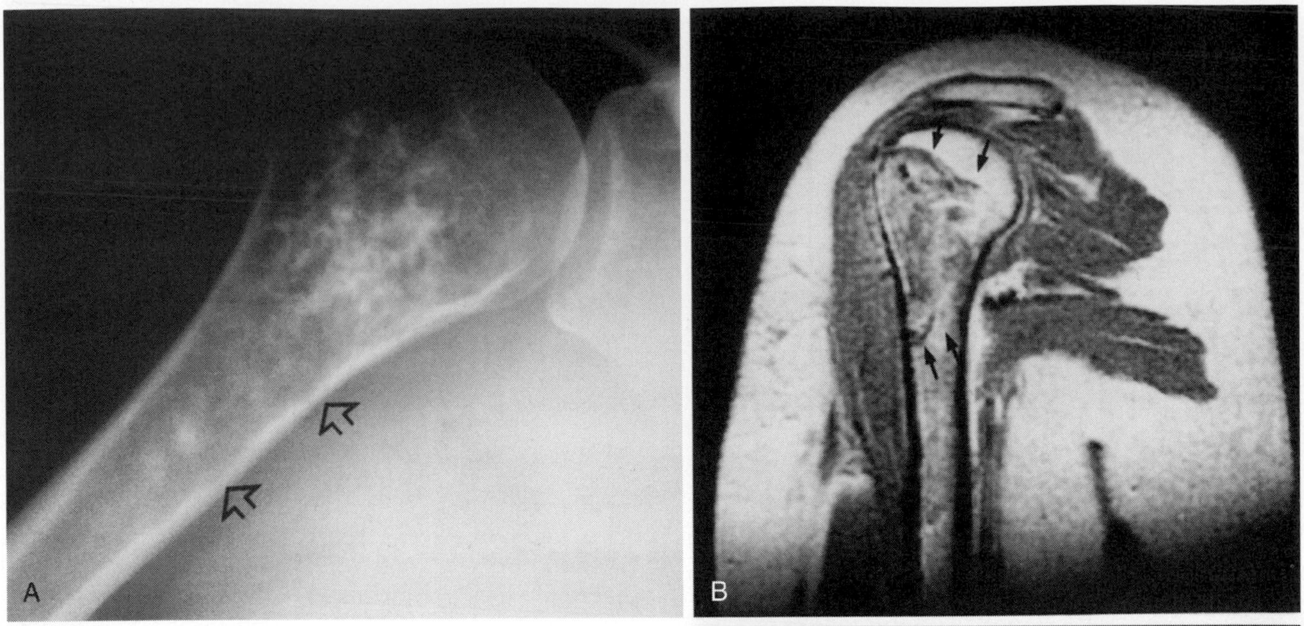

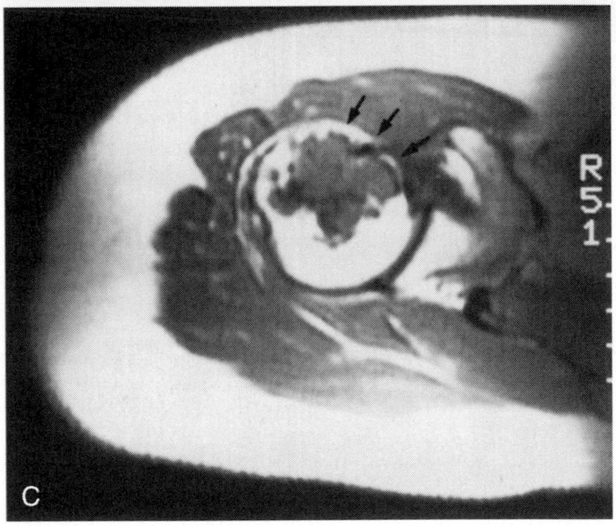

Figure 22–5

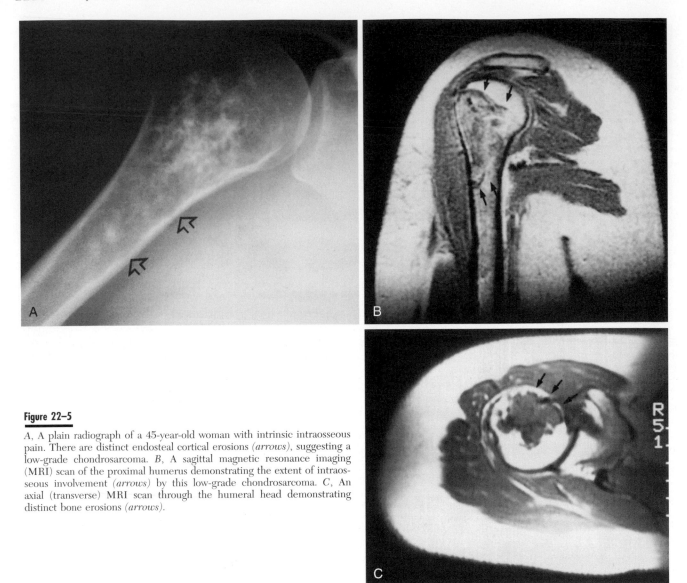

A, A plain radiograph of a 45-year-old woman with intrinsic intraosseous pain. There are distinct endosteal cortical erosions *(arrows)*, suggesting a low-grade chondrosarcoma. *B*, A sagittal magnetic resonance imaging (MRI) scan of the proximal humerus demonstrating the extent of intraosseous involvement *(arrows)* by this low-grade chondrosarcoma. *C*, An axial (transverse) MRI scan through the humeral head demonstrating distinct bone erosions *(arrows)*.

complete and inconclusive.[50, 100] This confusion has led to the use of the term "grade one-half chondrosarcoma" to describe cartilage tumors that are histologically borderline between low-grade chondrosarcoma and benign enchondroma. In most patients, the diagnosis of low-grade chondrosarcoma is best made radiographically by assessing whether there is evidence for endosteal erosions created by active cartilaginous tumor growth. Low-grade, or secondary, chondrosarcomas are unique among intraosseous tumors in the difficulty in interpreting their light microscopic picture.

Primary chondrosarcoma is more commonly seen in the middle decades of life, and the incidence in the shoulder is second to that of the pelvis or hip joint.[12, 59, 74, 116, 157] These tumors typically present as intraosseous lesions with a poorly defined margin and faint intrinsic calcifications. Less commonly, a primary chondrosarcoma may arise from the surface of a bone or joint. Its clinical and radiographic appearance is very subtle, and a diagnostic delay of 6 to 12 months is not uncommon. Approximately two thirds of primary chondrosarcomas are also low grade and may present as benign, encapsulated cartilage lesions. High-grade lesions are more invasive, have a higher metastatic rate, and usually occur in long-standing lesions as a "dedifferentiated" chondrosarcoma.[26, 30, 69, 123] As a general rule, low-grade chondrosarcomas may be treated surgically with curettage and grafting, whereas high-grade tumors deserve a surgical resection and subsequent reconstruction.

Synovial Dysplasias

Cartilaginous loose bodies typically arise out of a proliferative synovium, in a reactive metaplastic process known as synovial chondromatosis (or osteochondromatosis).[134] It most commonly affects large joints (knee, elbow, shoulder, hip) in young adults and results in multiple small, cartilaginous, intra-articular loose bodies as the process matures. In the few cases where the nodules form a compact mass of cartilage, it may be confused with a low-grade, periarticular or juxta-articular chondrosarcoma. An intra-articular location favors the benign diagnosis of synovial chondromatosis; determining the intra-articular versus extra articular location is somtimes one of the preoperative goals. In such cases, MRI or CT scans with or without arthrography might pinpoint the exact site of involvement. Synovial chondromatosis is typically a slowly progressive, degenerative disease that leads ultimately to joint destruction. It requires an aggressive total synovectomy to prevent persistence or recurrence, and in older patients with degenerative disease it is well treated with joint excision and replacement. A few cases in the literature associate malignant transformation with long-standing synovial chondromatosis, which occurs over a prolonged period.[137]

Another disease associated with proliferating synovium is pigmented villonodular synovitis.[159] It is usually associated with a boggy, inflammatory synovitis, with or without bony erosions, in adolescents or young adults. It is histologically an aggressive synovial-histiocytic process that defies description as inflammatory or neoplastic. Treatment requires aggressive complete synovectomy for the diffuse form of the disease. Various forms of radiation therapy have been used in some centers with acceptable early clinical results.[196] As a general rule, the long-term prognosis for synovial sarcoma is poor, with a high local recurrence rate and incidence of lung metastasis.

MISCELLANEOUS INTRAOSSEOUS TUMORS

Simple Bone Cyst

Simple bone cysts, or unicameral bone cysts, occur most commonly in children between the ages of 4 and 12. Figure 22–6 demonstrates a simple cyst in the humerus of an 8 year old. Although the lesion appeared somewhat expansile, suggesting an aneurysmal bone cyst, the cortices remained intact; clear fluid was aspirated; and the cyst healed after the injection of intraosseous steroids. Simple bone cysts present as well-defined, central, radiolucent lesions arising in the metaphysis adjacent to the physis (active) and, with maturation, migrate distally into the diaphysis (latent). They typically involve the proximal humerus (50%), contain straw-colored fluid, and may be confused with an aneurysmal bone cyst.[60, 80, 113, 140, 144, 179]

Pressure measurement of the cyst, aspiration, and intraosseous steroid injection constitute the treatment of choice. The result is complete healing of the cystic area in approximately 50% of cases and partial healing in 45%. Approximately three fourths of patients require multiple injections.[179] Complete repair following injection is most common in more inactive cysts with a lower pressure. Varying results in more recent reports have cast some doubt on the efficacy of steroid injections for simple bone cysts, especially when associated with a venogram at the time of the injection of dye into the lesion.[80] Recurrence or persistence of the cyst after surgical curettage and bone grafting occurs in approximately 30% of cases. This relatively high local recurrence rate may be lowered by the addition of a liquid nitrogen freeze to the curettage.[184] There is some diagnostic overlap between aneurysmal and simple cysts in children, because some simple cysts can have hemorrhagic fluid and yet do not contain aneurysmal tissue.

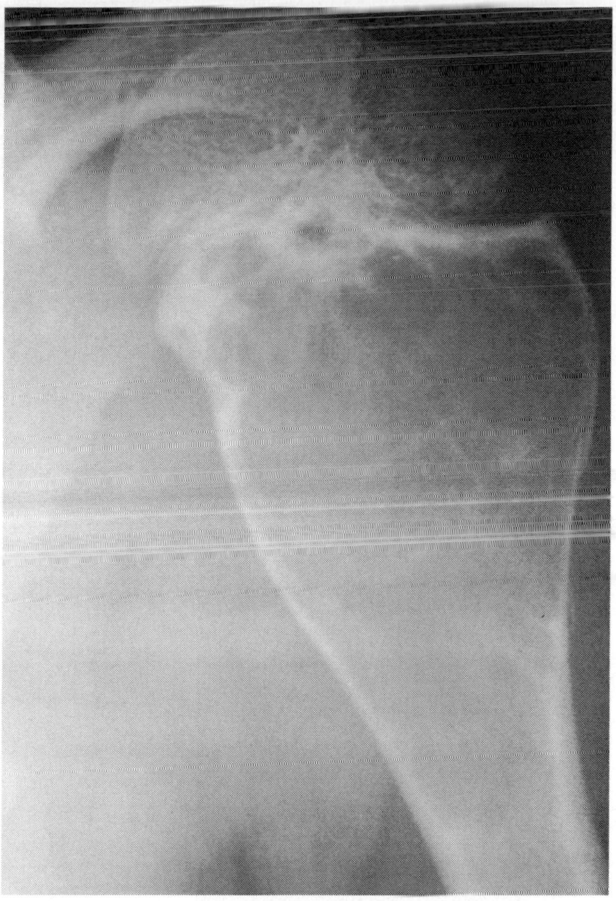

Figure 22–6

A simple cyst in an 8-year-old boy that is centrally located and juxtaepiphyseal (active).

Aneurysmal Bone Cyst

Aneurysmal bone cyst, nonossifying fibroma, and fibrous dysplasia are all benign lesions that also may occur in the shoulder. Aneursymal bone cysts are not uncommon in the proximal humerus, but because of their widespread occurrence as a “secondary” lesion engrafted upon other tumors (simple cyst, giant cell tumor, chondroblastoma), the true incidence is unknown. The radiographic hallmark is that of a lucent, expansile metaphyseal lesion. Treatment includes curettage and bone grafting,[10, 47] which is associated with a recurrence rate of 20 to 30%. Aneurysmal bone cysts can have an aggressive appearance and should have a careful biopsy prior to curettage in order to exclude the possibility of a telangiectatic osteosarcoma.

Fibrous Dysplasia

Fibrous dysplasia is a congenital dysplasia of bone that frequently surfaces as a painful lesion secondary to pathologic fractures, microfracture, or the subtle, intrinsic, diaphyseal weakness resulting from pathologic bone. The typical plain radiograph demonstrates a ground-glass density with cortical thickening. Figure 22–7*A* and *B* are the plain radiograph and CT scan, respectively, of the humerus of a 20-year-old woman with severe polyostotic

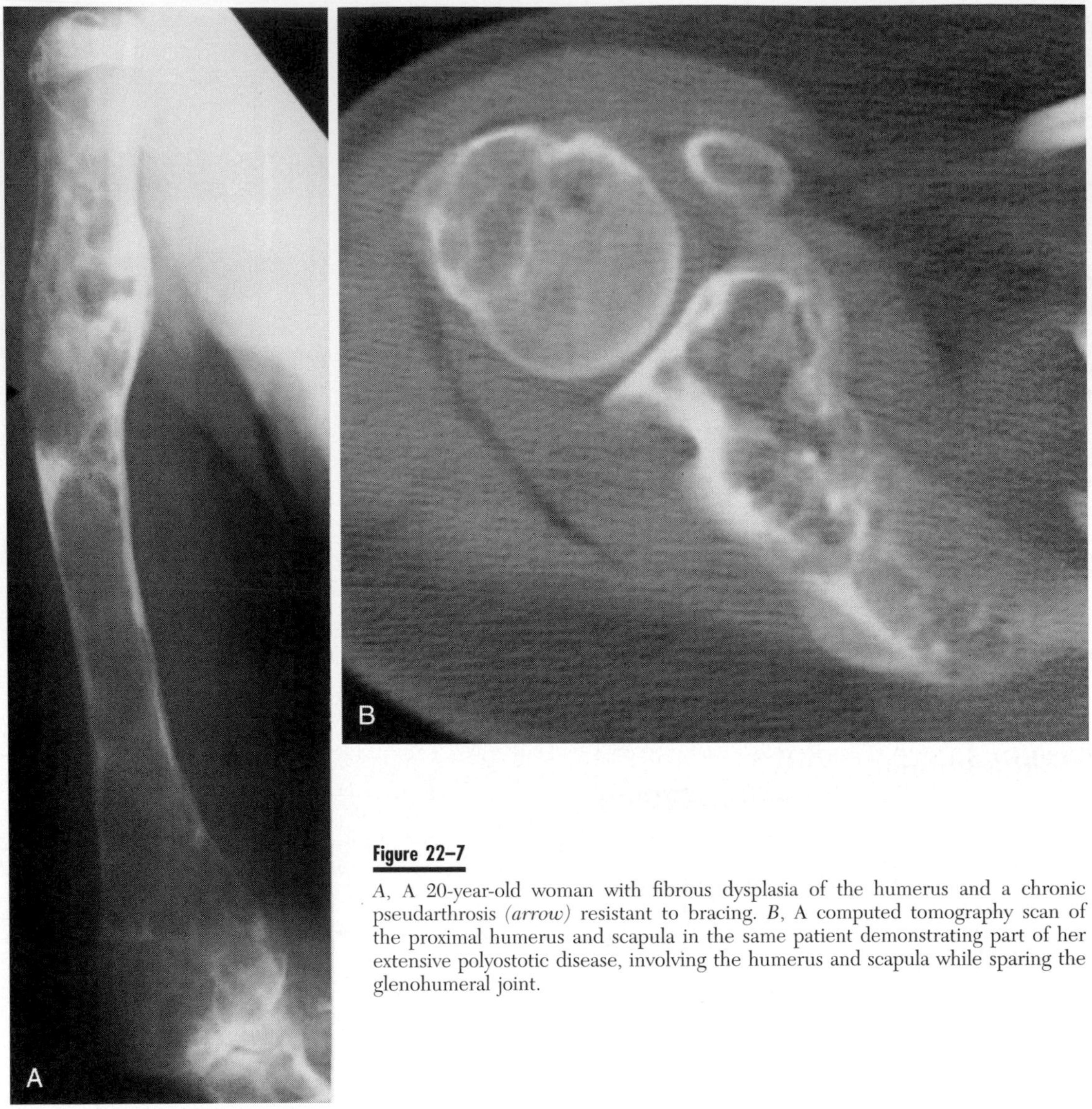

Figure 22–7

A, A 20-year-old woman with fibrous dysplasia of the humerus and a chronic pseudarthrosis *(arrow)* resistant to bracing. *B*, A computed tomography scan of the proximal humerus and scapula in the same patient demonstrating part of her extensive polyostotic disease, involving the humerus and scapula while sparing the glenohumeral joint.

fibrous dysplasia. She had a history of chronic pseudarthroses (see Fig. 22–7A) that had persisted despite bracing. When associated with symptoms or pathologic fracture, diaphyseal involvement usually requires intramedullary fixation rather than bone grafting, because cancellous bone grafting is consistently "consumed" by the dysplastic process and is ineffective in resolving the weakened dysplasia process. Histologically, fibrous dysplasia demonstrates a furnace of dysplastic bone activity with a similar, impressive increased activity on the bone scan.[84, 85, 94, 106, 200]

Nonossifying Fibroma

Nonossifying fibroma is a benign fibrous lesion that appears radiographically as an eccentric, well-defined, lucent lesion that has a scalloped border abutting the adjacent cortex (Fig. 22–8). It is more commonly found in the lower extremity than in the upper extremity. When the lesion is smaller than 2 cm, it may be referred to as a fibrous cortical defect. When larger than 3 cm or occupying more than half of the transverse diameter of the bone, these lesions are at risk for a pathologic fracture. The majority of nonossifying fibromas probably heal spontaneously and require no treatment. Treatment is reserved for those lesions with atypical radiographs (requiring biopsy) or for symptomatic or larger lesions (> 3 cm) that require treatment to prevent a pathologic fracture.[4]

Giant Cell Tumor

Giant cell tumor of bone is a common lesion in young adults that occurs primarily in the distal femur or proximal tibia (60 to 70%) and also in the proximal humerus in 5 to 10% of cases. It is a radiolucent, epiphyseal or metaphyseal tumor that most usually has a distinct bony margin and is frequently associated with extensive subchondral bone erosion. It is typically a stage 2 active lesion (60% of cases) but also shows up as a more aggressive, benign stage 3 tumor in 20% of cases. The treatment alternatives for giant cell tumor include curettage with or without local adjuvant treatment versus marginal resec-

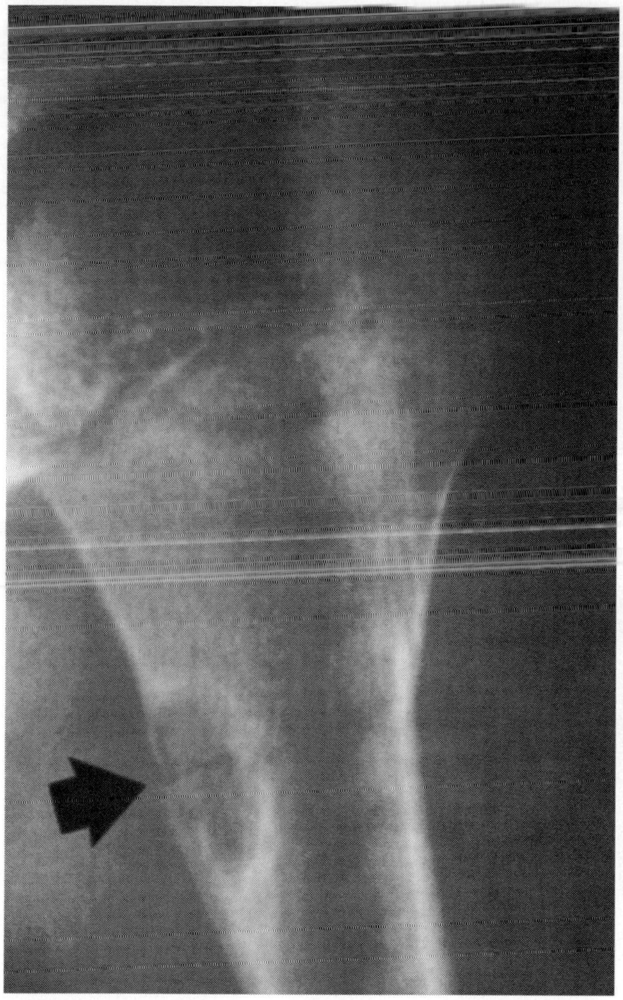

Figure 22–8

A small eccentric, juxtacortical, nonossifying fibroma that presented as a pathologic fracture *(arrow)*.

tion. The local recurrence rate after curettage alone is 20 to 30% for active lesions versus 5% after marginal resection.[23, 28, 32, 76, 132] Local adjuvants used in conjunction with curettage include the application of phenol, bone cement (cementation), or liquid nitrogen freeze (cryotherapy). Histologically, "benign" giant cell tumor has demonstrated a potential for pulmonary metastasis in a very small percentage of cases.[28, 77, 112, 122, 124, 126, 150, 151] The radiographic differential diagnosis in an adult includes aneurysmal bone cyst, metastatic adenocarcinoma, lymphoma, chondrosarcoma, and osteomyelitis.

RETICULOENDOTHELIAL TUMORS

Tumors of reticuloendothelial origin include a category of intraosseous lesions that arise from marrow stem cells and lesions of similar histology. They are also referred to as round cell or small, blue cell tumors. This category of tumors or abnormalities includes diagnoses such as leukemia, lymphoma,[203] neuroblastoma, histiocytosis, rhabdomyosarcoma, Ewing's sarcoma, infection, and, in adults, multiple myeloma and metastatic adenocarcinoma.

Multiple Myeloma

Multiple myeloma is the most common primary malignancy of bone and typically occurs in the middle decades of life, involving the shoulder girdle in 5 to 10% of cases.[38, 77] The most common site of involvement is in the axial skeleton, but a significant number of patients develop multiple distinct lesions in the extremities that may require surgical stabilization to prevent impending fracture if medical treatment has failed. In patients presenting initially with a solitary intraosseous myeloma or plasmacytoma of the shoulder, biopsy is indicated for diagnostic reasons. Elevated serum calcium levels, anemia, serum protein electrophoresis, or a distinctly cold bone scan may suggest the diagnosis of myeloma prior to biopsy in a patient with a solitary lesion or unknown diagnosis. The overall prognosis is poor; however, newer treatment involving aggressive chemotherapy and plasma cell antibodies offers hope for the future. Figure 22–9*A* is the plain radiograph of a 42-year-old man in apparent good health but experiencing shoulder pain. Coronal (see Fig. 22–9*B*) and transverse (see Fig. 22–9*C*) MRI scans demonstrate a suprascapular soft tissue lesion that extends anteriorly and posteriorly to the scapula. The preoperative diagnosis was a probable soft tissue sarcoma. Open biopsy was diagnostic for multiple myeloma with extensive bone disease. The patient died suddenly 1 week after the biopsy, with an undocumented serum calcium level. All patients with the diagnosis of myeloma need to have careful evaluation of their serum electrolytes for the possibility of hypercalcemia.

Ewing's Sarcoma

The second most common intraosseous malignancy in adolescence is that of Ewing's sarcoma, an aggressive marrow cell tumor that appears as a permeative diaphyseal tumor which is poorly marginated and typically associated with a large, soft tissue mass.[6, 51] Figure 22–10*A* demonstrates such a "permeative" lesion in the humeral diaphysis on a 16 year old with a typically hot bone scan (see Fig. 22–10*B*) and an associated soft tissue mass (see Fig. 22–10*C*). Ewing's sarcoma today is primarily treated with aggressive chemotherapy and surgical resection or radiation therapy, depending on the size and location of the primary lesion.

MISCELLANEOUS DYSPLASIAS

Gaucher's Disease

Gaucher's disease is an uncommon metabolic disorder of the reticuloendothelial system and glucocerebroside-glycolipid metabolism affecting the liver, spleen, and bone marrow.[75] The disease has an increased incidence in the Jewish population and occurs most commonly in the first 3 decades of life and without sexual preference. Patients typically experience pain secondary to bone involvement and marrow infiltration, which occurs most commonly in the femoral head, with a high degree of bilaterality. The disease in many ways represents a form of avascular necrosis of the femoral head. The humeral head is the second most common site of involvement, and radio-

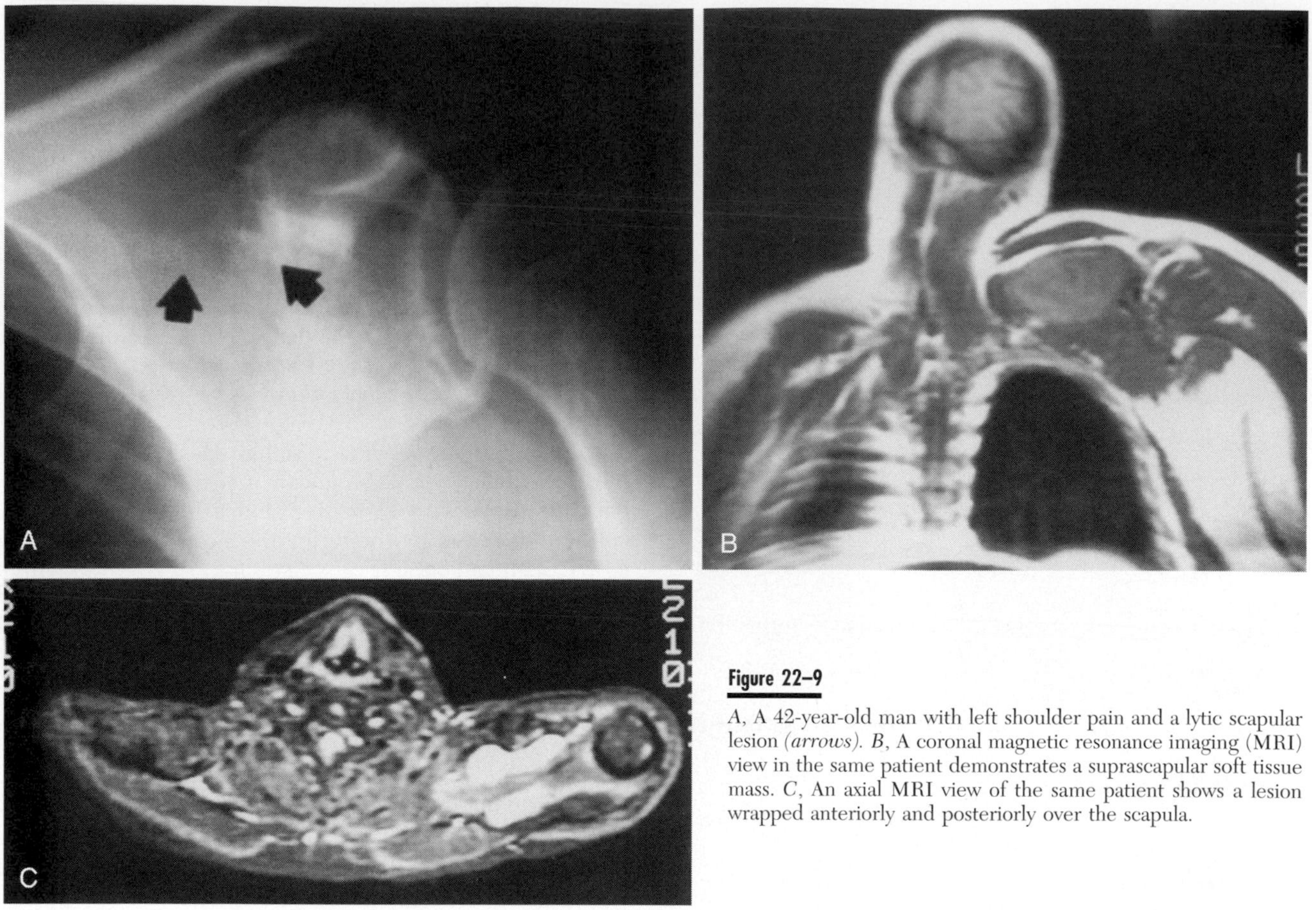

Figure 22–9

A, A 42-year-old man with left shoulder pain and a lytic scapular lesion *(arrows)*. *B*, A coronal magnetic resonance imaging (MRI) view in the same patient demonstrates a suprascapular soft tissue mass. *C*, An axial MRI view of the same patient shows a lesion wrapped anteriorly and posteriorly over the scapula.

graphic changes include osteopenia, diaphyseal or medullary expansion, or cortical erosions. The differential diagnosis includes osteomyelitis in the acute setting and round cell tumors in the nonacute setting. Surgical treatment involves internal fixation for fracture prophylaxis, joint replacement for adults, when appropriate, and the appropriate management of pediatric femoral head necrosis in children.

Paget's Disease

Paget's disease (osteoporosis circumscripta, osteitis deformans) occurs after the fourth decade and has a slight preponderance in men.[97] Geographically, it appears to have a higher incidence in Great Britain, Europe, Australia, and the United States, while relatively rare in India and most parts of Asia. Paget's disease occurs most commonly in the pelvis, skull, lumbosacral spine, femur, and humerus. It can occur in a polyostotic or a monostotic form usually manifested at the time of presentation. The typical radiographic picture shows cortical thickening and rarefaction, followed by pathologic microfracture and diaphyseal bowing (Fig. 22–11*A*). The differential diagnosis in an adult includes metastatic adenocarcinoma, osteosarcoma, and osteomyelitis. Patients should be assessed by evaluating serum alkaline phosphatase and urinary hydroxyproline levels, total body bone scan, and a CT scan or MRI scan.

Patients with Paget's disease undergoing orthopedic surgery should, in general, be pretreated. Paget's disease itself is best managed medically with diphosphonates or calcitonin. Sarcoma arising out of Paget's disease is associated with a history of progressive pain and a bony lytic lesion (see Fig. 22–11*B*) associated with a soft tissue mass. "Pagetoid sarcoma" is a rare variant of osteosarcoma and has been associated with a 5-year mortality of 80 to 90%.[156] Paget's sarcoma is best managed by a radical surgical margin because of the diffuse nature of the process of Paget's disease and the difficulty in assessing the extent of sarcomatous changes.

Figure 22–11*A* and *B* demonstrates the early and late radiographs of Paget's disease in the proximal humerus. The lytic lesion, combined with a history of increasing arm pain, serves notice of an early secondary osteosarcoma that showed up 3 months later with a more impressive lytic lesion of the proximal humerus (see Fig. 22–11*C*). Paget's disease affected the full humerus, and the bone scan (see Fig. 22–11*D*) was of little help in demarcating bony margins or osseous involvement by this secondary, or pagetoid, osteosarcoma.[105] MRI and CT scans again demonstrate the soft tissue and bony extent of disease in the proximal humerus (see Fig. 22–11*E*,*F*).

BENIGN SOFT TISSUE TUMORS

Lipoma

Lipomas may occur intramuscularly or within normal fat planes of the axilla or the subscapular or other perivascu-

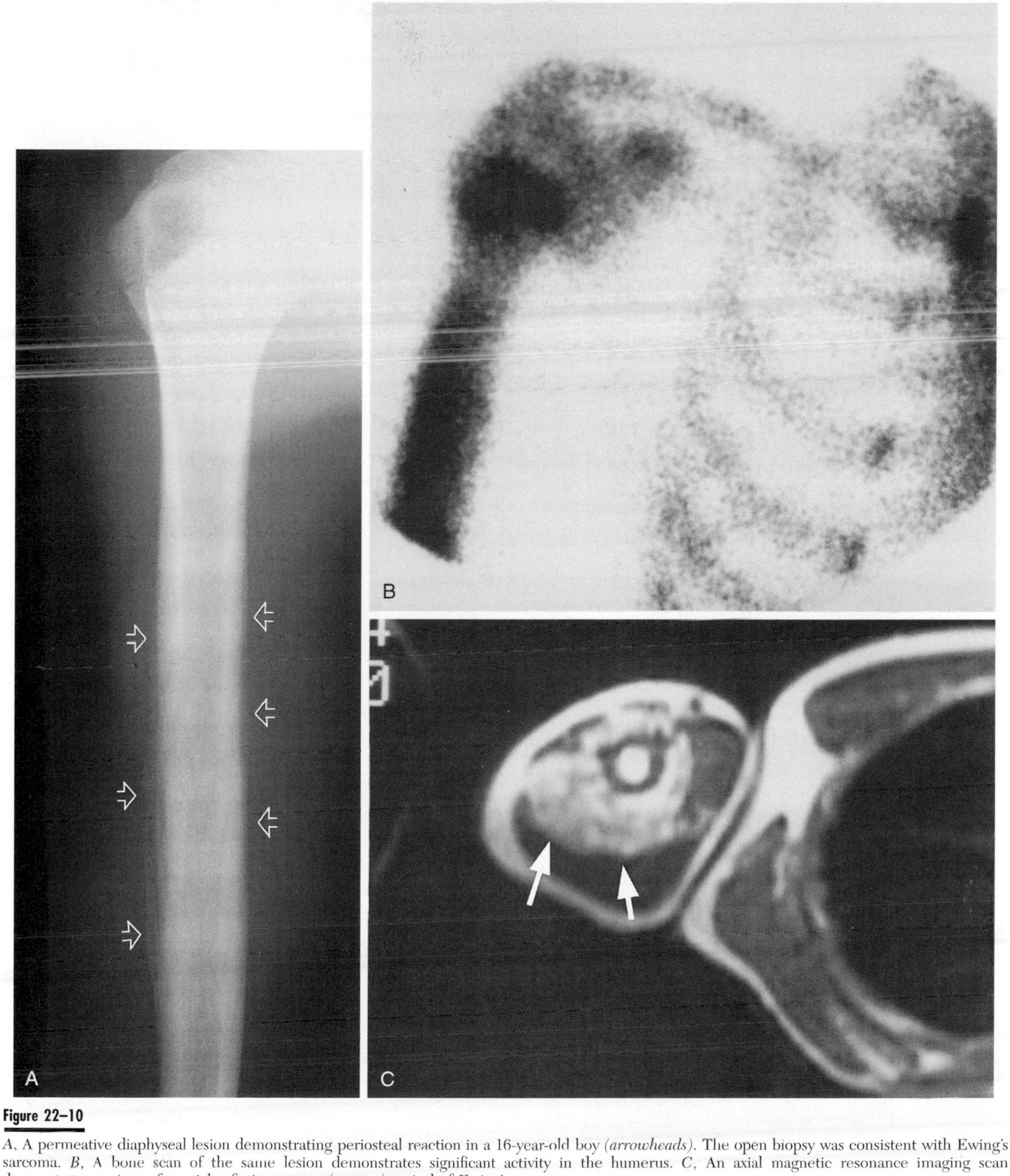

Figure 22–10

A, A permeative diaphyseal lesion demonstrating periosteal reaction in a 16-year-old boy *(arrowheads)*. The open biopsy was consistent with Ewing's sarcoma. *B*, A bone scan of the same lesion demonstrates significant activity in the humerus. *C*, An axial magnetic resonance imaging scan demonstrates a circumferential soft tissue mass *(arrows)* typical of Ewing's sarcoma.

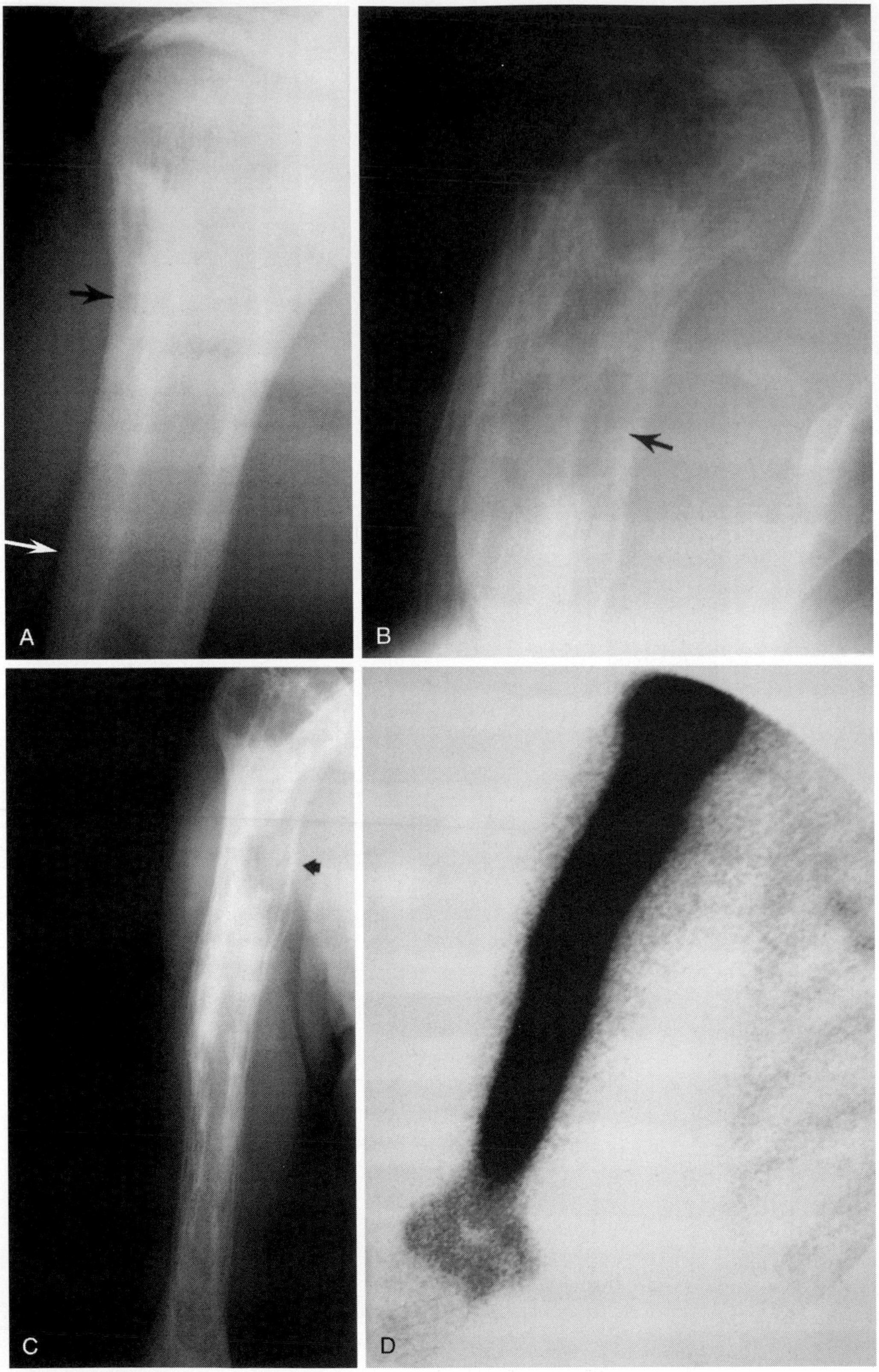

Figure 22–11

A, Early Paget's disease of the proximal humerus demonstrating cortical thickening and rarefaction *(arrows)*. *B*, The same patient presented years later with shoulder pain and a lytic lesion of the humerus *(arrow)* consistent with a secondary osteosarcoma. *C*, Several months later, this lytic process has become larger *(arrow)* and is associated with a large soft tissue mass (sarcoma). *D*, Bone scanning demonstrates intense humeral activity without distinguishing involvement by Paget's disease from sarcomatous changes.

Illustration continued on opposite page

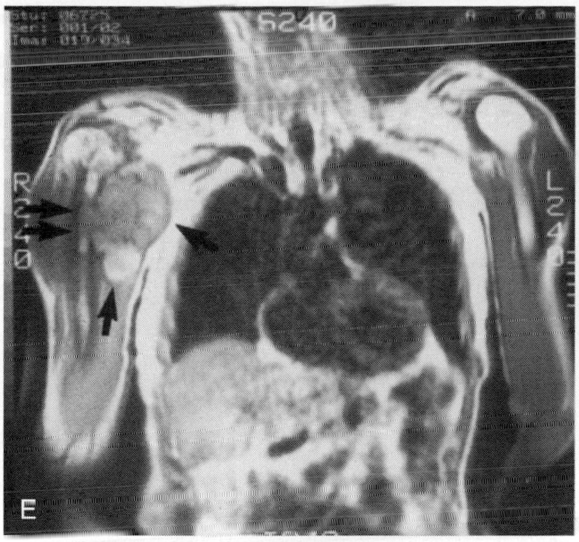

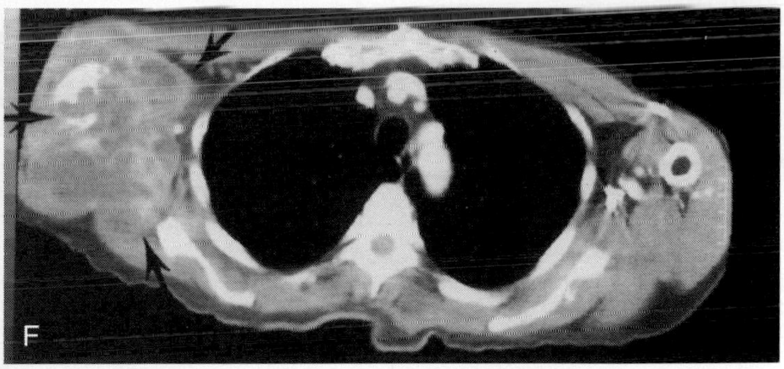

Figure 22–11 *Continued*

E, A coronal magnetic resonance imaging scan shows a large soft tissue mass arising out of the proximal humerus *(double arrows)* and extending into the axilla. *F*, A computed tomography scan also demonstrates this secondary osteosarcoma with gross destruction of the proximal humerus *(arrows)*.

lar spaces. They frequently appear in the anterior deltoid as a large, soft, nontender, intramuscular mass.[54] A few lipomas may be tender or firm or have an equivocal history of a change in size. On an MRI or CT scan, a benign lipoma usually has a uniform, fatty consistency. Clinically, a liposarcoma has a firmer, denser consistency than does a lipoma. If a lipoma feels very dense or firm clinically, an MRI scan should be done for further evaluation. If the MRI scan demonstrates areas of distinctly different density, a biopsy should precede marginal excision to exclude the possibility of a liposarcoma.

Hemangioma

Hemangiomas typically appear as "enlarging" intramuscular lesions in a child or young adult and are best visualized by an MRI scan. If they are intimately involved with a major vessel, they should also be evaluated with an arteriogram. These lesions do not usually pose diagnostic or surgical problems, with the exception of large hemangiomas or hemangiomatosis of the skeletal muscle. These are aggressive, congenital lesions that are frequently unresectable because of extensive neurovascular and soft tissue involvement.[2, 62] Many of these extensive lesions result in amputations for painful, dysvascular, or infected extremities. Most of these lesions are best diagnosed by open biopsy after an MRI scan, CT scan with contrast, or arteriography. Well-localized lesions are more easily resected than the more extensive congenital lesions. Embolization has had mixed results in halting the progression of disease.

Fibromatosis

Fibromatosis (desmoid) is a locally aggressive (stage 2 or 3) lesion found in young children, teenagers, and young adults. These lesions have a firm consistency on clinical examination and may be associated with osseous erosions or invasion of a neurovascular bundle. Many of these lesions suffer a local recurrence because of inadequate preoperative staging, underestimation of their potential for local recurrence, and an inadequate surgical margin. The literature reveals considerable confusion and contradiction regarding the natural history of fibromatosis. Spontaneous regression as described in some publications is unusual except in some congenital forms, and the natural history for lesions in adolescents is progressive growth and recurrence after marginal resections. These lesions rarely demonstrate pulmonary metastasis, and chemotherapy is not usually efficacious, although indications for chemotherapy do exist.[52, 63, 65, 162] The congenital form of the disease is referred to as a congenital fibrosarcoma primarily because of its very impressive histologic cellularity. The adolescent version is best referred to as aggressive fibromatosis and behaves as an active aggressive lesion. Preoperative and postoperative MRI studies are mandatory in these patients in order to assess fully soft tissue involvement. Bone scans should also be carried out if there is any doubt about secondary bone involvement. The essence of treatment for fibrous dysplasia remains adequate resection and radiation therapy.

SOFT TISSUE SARCOMAS

Soft tissue sarcomas occur in the upper extremity in approximately one third of all cases. They are frequently misdiagnosed initially as benign lesions and suffer a contaminated marginal resection before a definitive biopsy. Soft tissue sarcomas are characterized by four fairly typical clinical characteristics. They usually have a firm consistency, are deep to the superficial muscular fascia, are larger than 5 cm, and are nontender (Table 22–4). Ade-

Table 22–4 SARCOMA: SIGNS AND SYMPTOMS*

BONE	SOFT TISSUE
Bone pain	Firm mass
Night pain	Nontender mass
Pain (unrelated to joint motion)	Large (5 cm) or enlarging
Tender, soft tissue mass	Deep or subfascial

*From Enneking WF, Spanier SS, and Goodman MA: A system for the surgical staging of musculoskeletal sarcoma. Clin Orthop *153*:105–120, 1980.

quate staging prior to biopsy is important for soft tissue sarcomas, just as it is for bone sarcomas (Fig. 22–12). Open biopsy is preferred in such lesions rather than needle biopsy in order to diagnose both the histologic type and the histologic grade of the lesion.

The most common soft tissue sarcoma in adults is malignant fibrous histiocytoma (MFH), which occurs most often in older adults (50 to 70 years).[25, 65, 211] Liposarcoma[64, 160, 188] typically occurs in the lower extremities in young adults as a large lesion with a histology ranging from low-grade to high-grade or pleomorphic. Synovial sarcoma[215] is a less common lesion associated with faint, soft tissue calcifications, a juxta-articular location, and a high metastatic rate. Fibrosarcoma, rhabdomyosarcoma,[131] leiomyosarcoma, clear cell sarcoma, and epithelioid lesions are other, less common soft tissue malignancies.[66] Regardless of the tissue type, the grade of the lesion and the anatomic location of the primary tumor are the most significant factors determining prognosis and treatment. Soft tissue sarcomas of intermediate-grade

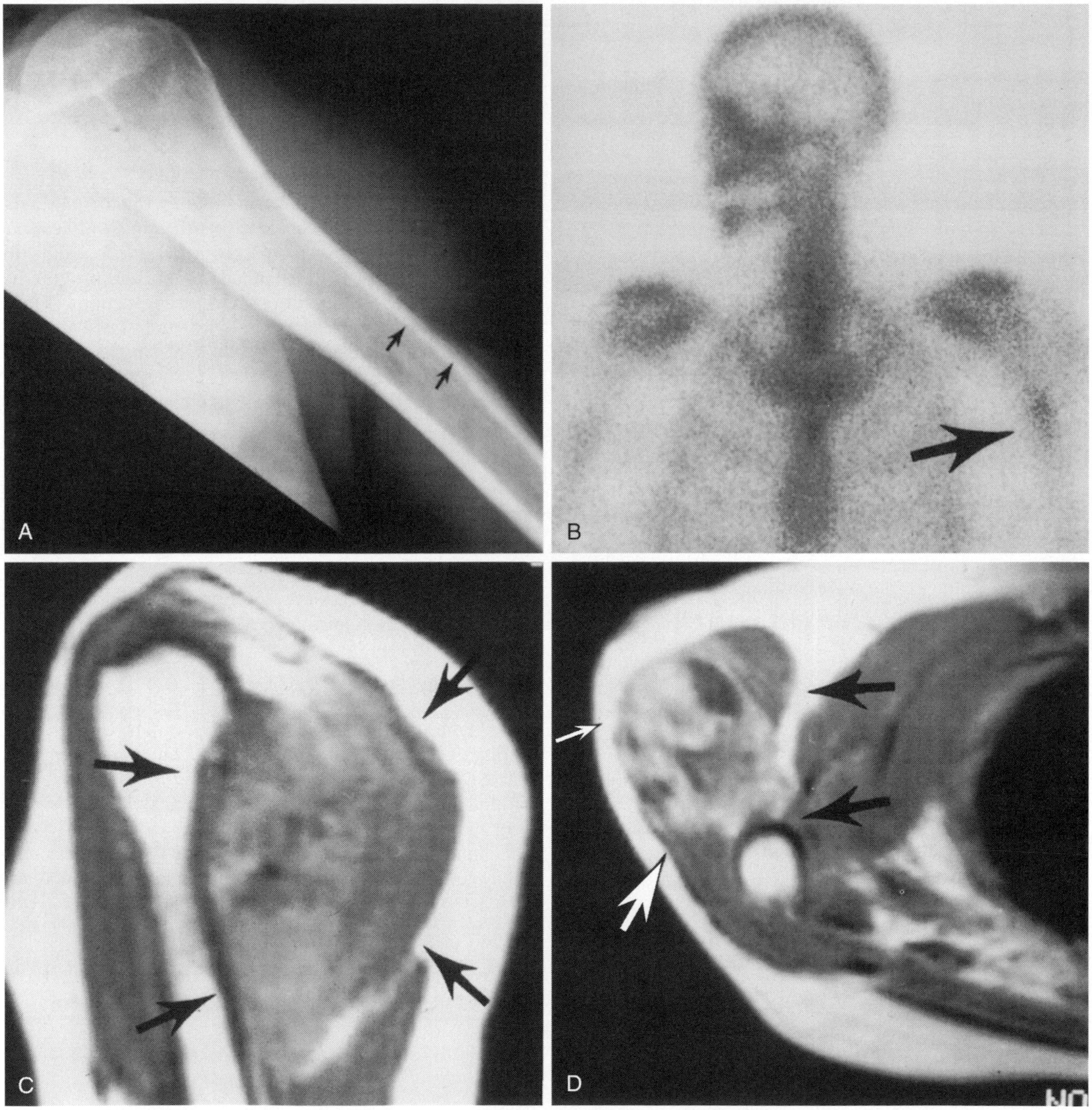

Figure 22–12

A, A plain radiograph of a 55-year-old woman with a large soft tissue sarcoma at the deltoid. Cortical irregularity at the deltoid insertion *(arrows)* is suggestive of bone invasion. *B*, The bone scan demonstrates distinct bone involvement at the deltoid tubercle with increased uptake *(arrow)*. *C*, A sagittal magnetic resonance imaging (MRI) scan shows a large mass *(arrows)* abutting against the proximal humerus. *D*, An axial MRI scan also suggests posterior humeral cortical invasion by a large deltoid malignant fibrous histiocytoma *(arrows)*.

histology are problematic to treat because of a variable prognosis and response to chemotherapy. There has been some early experience with flow cytometry in identifying more active (aneuploid) tumors, and this knowledge may prove helpful in the future in subclassifying or grading intermediate-grade tumors. Synovial sarcoma, epithelioid sarcoma, and rhabdomyosarcoma are characterized as soft tissue sarcomas with a high incidence (10 to 20%) of regional lymph node metastasis and a poor prognosis,[40, 45, 109, 168, 169, 173, 193, 201] but survival is generally recognized as being closely related to an individual tumor's histologic grade.[175]

INCIDENCE OF NEOPLASMS

Malignant tumors arising within the musculoskeletal system are rare and account for 0.5 to 0.7% of all malignancies.[94] They are relatively more common in children, representing 6.5% of all cancers in children. Although there is little apparent sexual or racial predilection in the incidence of soft tissue sarcomas, osteosarcoma and Ewing's sarcoma have demonstrated a slight male preference (1.3 to 1.0).[33, 88] Approximately 4500 new cases of soft tissue sarcoma occur in the United States each year, with an incidence of 1.8 per 100,000, or approximately 18 cases per million. The number of new bone and cartilage or skeletal malignancies is similar. Various sources estimate 1000 to 2000 new cases of osteosarcoma occur annually in the United States.[24, 34, 172] The true incidence of most of these tumors remains somewhat speculative.

The most common tumor of the adult musculoskeletal system is metastatic adenocarcinoma, most commonly from the kidney, lung, breast, or prostate.[56] The most common primary malignancy of bone is multiple myeloma, a plasma cell malignancy usually diagnosed by the medical oncologist rather than the orthopedic surgeon.[77] Multiple myeloma has an incidence that is approximately twice that of osteosarcoma. Exclusive of multiple myeloma, the most common primary malignant tumor of bone is osteosarcoma. If both benign and malignant primary lesions of the musculoskeletal system are included, cartilaginous tumors are the most common primary lesion (benign and malignant) of the skeletal system.[33]

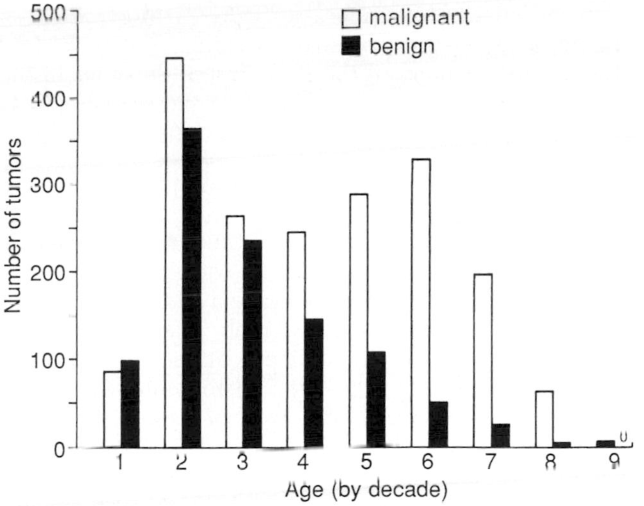

Figure 22–13

Distribution of musculoskeletal tumors by age.

Age is a very important characteristic in the occurrence and distribution of tumors. The overall distribution of tumors by age in decades (Figs. 22–13 and 22–14) demonstrates the preponderance of benign tumors in the skeleton of the growing child; 58% of all benign lesions occur in the second and third decades. Malignant tumors of the skeleton have a peak incidence in adolescents and middle-aged adults.[34, 56, 172] Osteosarcoma and Ewing's sarcoma are the most common malignant bone tumors in adolescents. In adults, osteosarcoma and chondrosarcoma occur with an incidence second to multiple myeloma and metastatic adenocarcinoma. Osteosarcoma represents approximately 40% of all primary malignancies of bone; chondrosarcoma accounts for 20%; and Ewing's sarcoma accounts for 12.5%.[34, 56, 172]

The incidence of tumors by anatomic location is best estimated by review of the works of Enneking[56] and Dahlin.[34] The overall incidence of primary sarcomas in the shoulder is approximately 15%.[34, 56] Lesions of the shoulder are the third most common overall site for sarcomas, behind the hip-pelvis (1) and the knee (distal femur and proximal tibia) (2). In general, one third of all

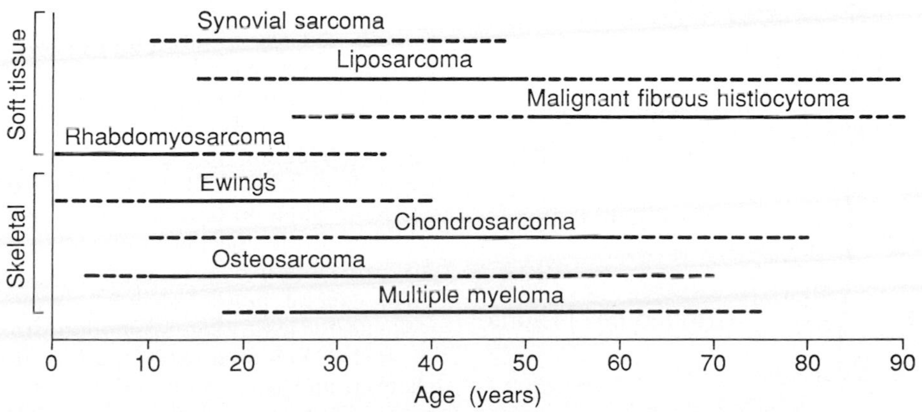

Figure 22–14

Sarcomas versus age. (Adapted from Enzinger FM and Weiss SW: Soft Tissue Tumors. St. Louis: CV Mosby, 1983.)

sarcomas affect the upper extremity.[169] Most shoulder tumors occur in the proximal humerus (68.6 to 71.5%) (Fig. 22–15). Tumors of the shoulder girdle occur in the clavicle (6 to 10% of all cases) and in the scapula (18 to 24%) to a much less common degree.[34, 56]

CLINICAL PRESENTATION

Despite the refinement and developments in the field of musculoskeletal oncology, patients with musculoskeletal malignancies, in general, experience a 3- to 6-month history of symptoms before an accurate diagnosis is made. The challenge for the general practitioner is to predict the diagnosis based on the initial history, physical examination, and plain radiographs. Most of these lesions have a subtle onset, and their initial diagnosis requires attention to certain details and an understanding of a few hallmark signs. The patient's initial assessment remains the first and crucial step to a successful evaluation and treatment plan. In fact, in 70 to 80% of cases, it is possible to correctly diagnose and recognize most malignancies based on the initial history, physical examination, and plain radiographs.[56]

Patients with an intraosseous malignancy almost always have pain. The challenge to the physician is to distinguish between the pain of malignancy and the other more common types of musculoskeletal pain secondary to degenerative joint disease, overuse, inflammatory joint disease, trauma, sepsis, and so forth. The hallmark symptom of an intraosseous malignancy is that of pain at night or pain at rest (see Table 22–4). Any patient who experiences a symptom of significant pain at night should be very carefully assessed radiographically at the time of the first evaluation. Patients who experience significant pain at night should routinely have a technetium bone scan in addition to plain radiographs in order to evaluate their symptoms further. Some patients with inflammatory or degenerative joint disease will complain of pain at night, but, in general, pain at night as a prominent symptom is very suggestive of a possible tumor.

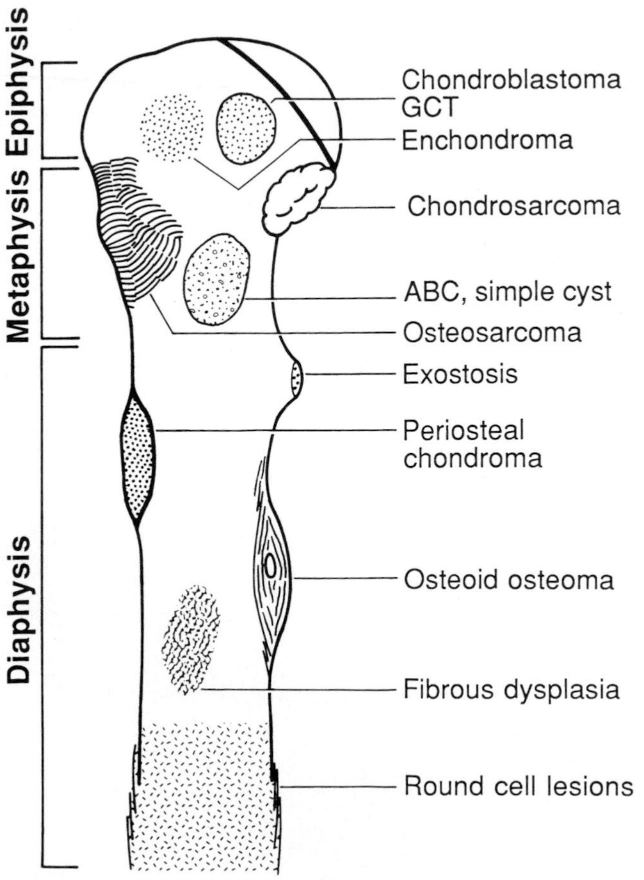

Figure 22–15

Common tumors of the proximal humerus.

Other pertinent findings in the history that may be helpful include a strong family history for malignancy (adenocarcinoma or sarcoma) or a history of a previous malignancy in the patient that may now be metastatic to the skeleton. Weight loss and general malaise may be significant symptoms for metastatic disease, and the physician should initiate a work-up to further evaluate the patient's general health. It is unusual, however, for a patient to have generalized symptoms or metastatic disease as the initial symptom of a sarcoma.

Musculoskeletal neoplasms present a clinical challenge to the orthopedist in the determination of whether a patient has intraosseous pain or intra-articular pain. This is not readily apparent in the early diagnosis of most intraosseous tumors. A careful physical examination can sometimes elicit findings consistent with joint tenderness, impingement, or weakness, thus suggesting some sort of intra-articular process. It is unusual for sarcomas to extend into a joint, and the presence of joint findings or symptoms is more consistent with trauma, degenerative disease, or some other non-neoplastic process. In general, intra-articular processes are exacerbated by physical activities and joint motion (see the section on physical examination). Similarly, some patients present with referred pain that may lead to the erroneous diagnosis of shoulder pain that has really originated from the cervical spine or hip pain that originates in the lumbar spine. The challenge of determining whether a particular patient's problem is intraosseous or intra-articular requires a careful musculoskeletal evaluation that is usually best accomplished by an orthopedist.

A careful orthopedic examination is important when evaluating all patients but is vital when evaluating the patient with difficult symptoms. Every adult patient who is evaluated specifically for a possible neoplasm should have a careful general examination of the head and neck, cardiopulmonary status, abdomen, spine, breasts (women), prostate (men), and also an examination for lymphadenopathy. This sort of general examination is most appropriate for adults older than 35 to 40 years of age who are more likely to have a metastatic adenocarcinoma. In addition to the specific examination to evaluate patients for a possible neoplasm, all patients should have a complete general musculoskeletal examination in order to evaluate for joint range of motion, strength, stability, and so forth. Regional adenopathy should be routinely checked on examination and will be found to be present with many tumors. It is usually an inflammatory phenomenon, reactive to the tumor. However, adenopathy involving lymph nodes larger than 1 cm should be evaluated further by MRI, and a biopsy should be performed before definitive resection of the primary tumor is attempted.

Patients with an aggressive intraosseous malignancy usually have bone tenderness and a mass. The primary site may be deep and well-covered by muscle and may be difficult to palpate. Usually, careful palpation will demonstrate the presence or absence of any soft tissue mass. However, low-grade intraosseous lesions may not involve the soft tissues. The ability to elicit joint findings is more suggestive of an intra-articular, traumatic, inflammatory, or degenerative process. Thus, joint tenderness or stiffness can be a very helpful finding. Extension of an intraosseous malignancy medially toward the major neurovascular bundle, which is close to the humerus, may preclude limb-sparing surgery and is associated with a worse prognosis. The extent of involvement of the soft tissues on physical examination is an important finding to follow in addition to radiographic imaging. Clinical involvement of the soft tissues can yield important information for the directing of the MRI scan and other studies. In general, the soft tissue mass produced by an intraosseous malignancy is relatively subtle as an early clinical finding and requires some attention on examination. If osseous sarcomas present with a large soft tissue mass, more care should be taken when evaluating the extent of soft tissue involvement if limb-sparing surgery is planned.

Soft tissue sarcomas most commonly have a history of a mass. Most soft tissue sarcomas, in contradistinction to intraosseous malignancies, are not painful. All soft tissue lesions should be carefully evaluated for the four characteristics of a soft tissue sarcoma: nontender mass, firm consistency, deep or subfascial location, and larger than 5 cm in size (see Table 22–4). There are exceptions to these characteristics, but as a general rule, they are very reliable guidelines in the initial evaluation of various soft tissue lesions. The most reliable clinical sign for a soft tissue sarcoma is the consistency or density of the lesion. For instance, the most common soft tissue tumor in an adult is a lipoma, which may be large, deep in location, and nontender; however, its consistency will usually indicate whether it is malignant. Lipomas are typically very soft with the consistency of normal fat, whereas liposarcomas are usually firm. The ability to distinguish the consistency of a soft tissue mass can be a somewhat subtle but important finding. Anything with a consistency more dense than normal fat should be evaluated carefully. Lipomas that feel firmer than normal fat or larger than 10 cm should be evaluated by MRI; intramuscular lesions that are firmer than normal muscle should also be evaluated by MRI. If a soft tissue mass is felt to be cystic, it is reasonable and advisable to attempt careful aspiration in the clinic in order to document whether that lesion contains fluid. Repeated or multiple aspirations are not advised and will only lead to contamination of a possible soft tissue sarcoma.

In summary, all patients with a possible musculoskeletal neoplasm (or an unknown diagnosis) should have a complete general examination and musculoskeletal examination emphasizing the joints and the soft tissues. Always put your hand on the patient and consider the possibility of a mass when examining a patient with a difficult problem. Always consider the challenges of referred pain. The size of any soft tissue mass should be carefully measured and recorded in the chart in order to give an objective finding for further follow-up. It is also helpful to take a photograph in the clinic for future reference. The most common omission in the general physical examination for patients without a known tumor diagnosis is failure to detect an obvious primary site of involvement for an adenocarcinoma (e.g., prostate, abdominal mass, prostatic mass). The most common mistake on the initial orthopedic examination is a failure to detect the true location of the abnormality (referred pain) or to detect a soft tissue mass.

Routine clinical follow-up for a patient with a malignancy is important in order to detect progressive disease at an early stage. After the immediate postoperative evaluation, patients with high-grade sarcomas are generally followed every 3 months for 2 years, every 6 months for another 2 years, and every year thereafter. Frequent clinical follow-up is important in order to detect metastatic or recurrent disease at an early stage, thus enhancing further treatment. Frequent follow-up is also advisable in patients with undiagnosed skeletal pain. This is most appropriate in the adult who has significant joint symptoms and normal-appearing plain radiographs. If the plain radiographs are not consistent with the patient's symptoms, a total body technetium bone scan is well indicated in order to rule out a possible neoplasm. On the other hand, most patients who have a small (< 5 cm) soft tissue mass can be followed without biopsy or MRI without significant danger of missing a possible malignancy. Similarly, intraosseous lesions that appear benign on plain x-rays or lesions that are picked up incidentally in the evaluation of a patient with intra-articular shoulder pathology can easily be followed if the plain radiographs are well demarcated and the lesions are obviously benign. If the initial plain radiographs are equivocal, a bone scan and CT or MRI scan are indicated to determine if the lesion is active and a biopsy needs to be done or if it can be followed clinically. For instance, most low-grade, calcified, or cartilaginous intraosseous lesions can be safely followed at 6-month intervals.

X-RAY AND LABORATORY EVALUATION

The orthopedist's interpretation of the initial plain radiographs is an important step in the early diagnosis of most musculoskeletal tumors. When dealing with intraosseous or skeletal lesions, the orthopedist should have a system for evaluating the initial plain radiographs and formulating the initial diagnosis. Every bone lesion has a characteristic location, margin, and density that typify it radiographically. These three radiographic characteristics are important in describing a lesion's growth rate and intrinsic density.[56] These concepts originated in a different format from that of Jaffee,[95] who first posed the questions: "What is the lesion's density?"; "What is it doing to bone?"; "What is the bone doing to it?"; and "What is its location?" when evaluating radiographs. This approach helps to focus attention on a lesion's growth rate, its degree of activity, and thus, its malignant potential. With these three characteristics in mind, the initial plain radiographs can be interpreted with the correct diagnosis in most cases.

Location

Where is the lesion located? Is it in the epiphysis, metaphysis, or diaphysis? Are there multiple metastatic sites or one primary site of involvement? For example, an aggressive metaphyseal tumor in an adolescent is very likely to be an osteosarcoma, whereas a diaphyseal lesion is much more likely to be a Ewing sarcoma. Whether the lesion is central or eccentric with the bone is also important information. Nonossifying fibroma is almost always eccentric, whereas cartilaginous lesions (enchondroma) are usually centrally located.

Margin

The margin of the lesion on plain radiographs is the best reflection of that lesion's growth rate at the time of the initial evaluation. It refers to the margin or interface between the lesion and surrounding normal bone. If a tumor is slow growing, it will have a distinct or sclerotic margin that demonstrates the ability of the surrounding normal bone to react to it, thus marginating, or walling off, that lesion. A sclerotic or distinct peripheral bony margin indicates a slow-growing or benign lesion and is not usually seen with malignant or aggressive benign tumors. This type of margin reflects the ability of bone to respond to a slowly growing tumor. At the other end of the spectrum is the lesion that is not well marginated and does not have a sclerotic rim of reactive bone around it. This reflects a more rapidly growing tumor that enlarges at a rate that is faster than normal bone can react to it. The best example of an aggressive lesion that infiltrates or percolates through bone is the permeative lesion of Ewing's sarcoma or any intramedullary round cell tumor or small blue cell tumor of bone. Round cell tumors occur more commonly in children, and the differential diagnosis includes lymphoma, leukemia, Ewing's sarcoma, rhabdomyosarcoma, neuroblastoma, histiocytosis, Wilms' tumor, or acute osteomyelitis. In contrast, the differential diagnosis for round cell tumors in adults includes metastatic carcinoma, Ewing's sarcoma, multiple myeloma, lymphoma, or osteomyelitis.

Density

The intrinsic density of a lesion within bone or soft tissue is another piece of information that contributes to the initial diagnosis. Is the lesion making bone, cartilage (calcifications), fibrous dysplasia (ground-glass density), or soft tissue (clear)? A truly cystic (or fluid-filled) lesion is most likely to be a benign or infectious lesion in bone or soft tissue, and this cystic nature may be determined clinically or demonstrated by the staging studies.

Thus, the complete assessment of the patient with a musculoskeletal lesion involves a careful evaluation of both the clinical and radiographic findings. The complex anatomy and frequency of referred pain make many diagnoses in the shoulder a challenge. A knowledge and an awareness of typical symptoms, physical findings, and radiographic clues for sarcomas are essential for successful treatment.

Appropriate initial radiographs for evaluating most patients include a well-exposed, properly positioned film. Accepting poor-quality radiographs can lead to disaster. It is essential that a well-exposed radiograph of the shoulder be obtained in all patients, especially those with persistent symptoms who may be failing conservative treatment for what is believed to be an intra-articular glenohumeral problem. There is no doubt that the best initial staging diagnostic study for evaluating a possible intraosseous malignancy is a technetium bone scan. The best staging study for a soft tissue lesion is an MRI scan. CT scans are routinely used for ruling out lung metastasis in addition to initial plain chest radiographs for all patients who have probable soft tissue or bone malignancies.

The staging studies involved with assessing a high-grade intraosseous lesion, such as an osteosarcoma, include bone scan, MRI of the extremity, CT of the extremity, and CT of the lung. An MRI scan is indicated in order to assess the degree of soft tissue involvement and the neurovascular bundle margin before and after biopsy and induction chemotherapy. The CT scan of the extremity remains a good study to assess the degree of bony cortical involvement. A total body bone scan be carried out in all patients with musculoskeletal malignancies in order to assess the presence of distant bone metastases and to assess the extent of primary disease. Diagnostic strategies for evaluation of possible skeletal metastases have been reviewed.[170]

Possible tumor involvement of the neurovascular bundle and brachial plexus is best assessed by MRI, whereas arteriography is now reserved specifically for lesions located adjacent to a major vessel. Arteriography has also been used in the past to assess the extent of soft tissue involvement by sarcomas, but it has been more or less replaced at present by MRI scans. Other modalities for assessing the extent of soft tissue sarcomas have included gallium scans, which have generally been considered of inferior resolution quality compared with MRI scans.

The assessment of possible chest wall involvement by shoulder lesions remains a difficult task. It is best assessed by CT, MRI, and bone scans. If there is rib uptake on the bone scan, bony chest wall involvement is obvious. It is somewhat unusual for proximal humeral malignancies to have chest wall involvement. However, soft tissue lesions that have extended from the brachial plexus, axilla, or scapula may well develop chest wall involvement.

Metabolic imaging using radioisotopes such as fluorodeoxyglucose, et cetera, have received greater attention over the last several years. Such studies are potentially useful in grading tumors (high grade versus low grade), assessing the response to chemotherapy, and assessing patients for residual minimal disease.

Laboratory

In general, laboratory studies for sarcomas are not of great assistance in making the initial diagnosis. The most common exception is the serum alkaline phosphatase, which is frequently elevated in osteosarcoma or in Paget's disease.[102] Measurement of serum acid phosphatase or prostatic specific antigen levels and a urinalysis (microscopic hematuria) are helpful in the evaluation of possible malignancies of the prostate or kidney.[149] A hematocrit, white blood cell count, and erythrocyte sedimentation rate (ESR) are well indicated in evaluating for possible sepsis, although both the white blood cell count and the ESR may be nonspecifically elevated with various tumors and the hematocrit may be nonspecifically low. Any patient who has plasmacytoma or multiple myeloma in his or her differential diagnosis should have serum calcium and serum electrolytes checked preoperatively in order to detect hypercalcemia. In addition, those patients should undergo a serum and urine protein electrophoresis study in order to evaluate their immunoglobulin profile.[93]

Routine laboratory studies (e.g., liver enzymes) are checked in the routine follow-up of patients with a musculoskeletal malignancy; however, it is unusual for a sarcoma to metastasize to the liver, and thus liver enzymes are rarely elevated secondarily to tumor. Elevated liver enzymes can occur for other reasons (hepatitis) and are included in routine follow-up blood work for that reason. It is useful to evaluate liver enzymes and complete blood counts in all sarcoma patients in order to assess a patient's general medical health.

COMPLICATIONS OF TUMORS

Pathologic Fractures

One of the most significant complications of a musculoskeletal tumor is that of pathologic fracture, the majority of which are secondary to metastatic adenocarcinoma. Approximately one third of all diagnosed cases of breast, pulmonary, thyroid, renal, and prostatic carcinoma include skeletal metastases.[11, 67, 83, 210] Although the most common site for metastasis is the axial skeleton, approximately 25% of all metastases are located in the shoulder girdle.

Surgery may be indicated to obtain a primary diagnosis by open biopsy or to achieve internal fixation for fracture prophylaxis. Patients with an established tumor diagnosis and lytic lesions representing bone metastases should, in general, be treated with chemotherapy and radiation therapy first, if the evidence indicates that that particular lesion is likely to respond to that treatment. Metastatic lesions that are generally considered to be resistant to radiation therapy or chemotherapy or those lesions that have failed similar previous treatment should be treated surgically (e.g., renal cell carcinoma). Surgical stabilization or internal fixation is indicated in any patient with an impending or completed pathologic fracture who can tolerate a general anesthetic and has a life expectancy of at least 1 month. Coaptation splinting, as an alternative to surgery, does a relatively poor job of relieving fracture symptoms in the humerus because of persistent rotational instability. Figure 22–16 shows a pathologic fracture of the proximal humerus in a 65-year-old patient with extensive metastatic disease. His pain was unrelieved with coaptation bracing, and he was treated surgically with methyl methacrylate and short Ender rods placed through the fracture site. His poor medical status and limited life expectancy (several months) dictated this more conservative surgical procedure rather than the usual treatment of hemiarthroplasty. Even patients with widespread metastatic disease can benefit greatly from a careful but aggressive approach to the management of pathologic fractures versus impending fractures.

Intraosseous sarcomas that result in a pathologic fracture represent less than 10% of all sarcomas, and although they present a challenge, they are no longer considered to be an absolute indication for immediate amputation. Another problem seen is that of fractures occurring after a poorly designed biopsy, thus emphasizing the need for careful biopsy procedures. Another problem with Ewing's sarcoma arises in patients who develop a late fracture in a diaphyseal lesion that has been previously irradiated. Such lesions should be stabilized prophylactically with an intramedullary rod to prevent possible fracture if there is any evidence of an impending fracture. Fractures through irradiated bone are unlikely to heal and should be internally fixed or resected as soon as possible. Fibrous dysplasia represents another example of pathologic bone that may require intramedullary fixation to prevent repeated fractures and progressive deformity. Intramedullary fixation is the method of choice because of its biomechanical superiority. Plating with screws is vastly inferior to intramedullary fixation of impending or completed pathologic diaphyseal lesions.

DIFFERENTIAL DIAGNOSIS

The shoulder girdle is an area that presents a challenge to the diagnosis of many different conditions. Its close relationship with the cervical spine and brachial plexus can present a formidable challenge in distinguishing cervical spine problems from shoulder problems. The complexity of the soft tissue anatomy of the glenohumeral joint and the difficulty of distinguishing intra- from extra-articular diagnoses is significant, even for the most skilled orthopedist. The confusion that may arise can delay the diagnosis for various musculoskeletal tumors for a significant period of time.

The differential diagnosis for various musculoskeletal lesions includes those lesions identified in Table 22–5. Although the categories of trauma, tumor, infection, and

Table 22–5 DIFFERENTIAL DIAGNOSIS OF MUSCULOSKELETAL LESIONS

1. Trauma (subtle, bony, acute, or chronic)
2. Tumor (benign or malignant, primary or metastatic)
3. Infection (bacterial, viral, fungal, or venereal)
4. Inflammatory disease (rheumatoid arthritis, gouty arthropathy, collagen vascular disease, PVNS)
5. Degenerative disease (osteoarthritis)
6. Dysplasias (fibrous dysplasia, Paget's disease, multiple hereditary exostoses, neurofibromatosis)
7. Hematologic disorders (hemophilia, histiocytosis, myeloproliferative disorder)
8. Metabolic disorders (osteomalacia, rickets, hyperparathyroidism, renal osteodystrophy)

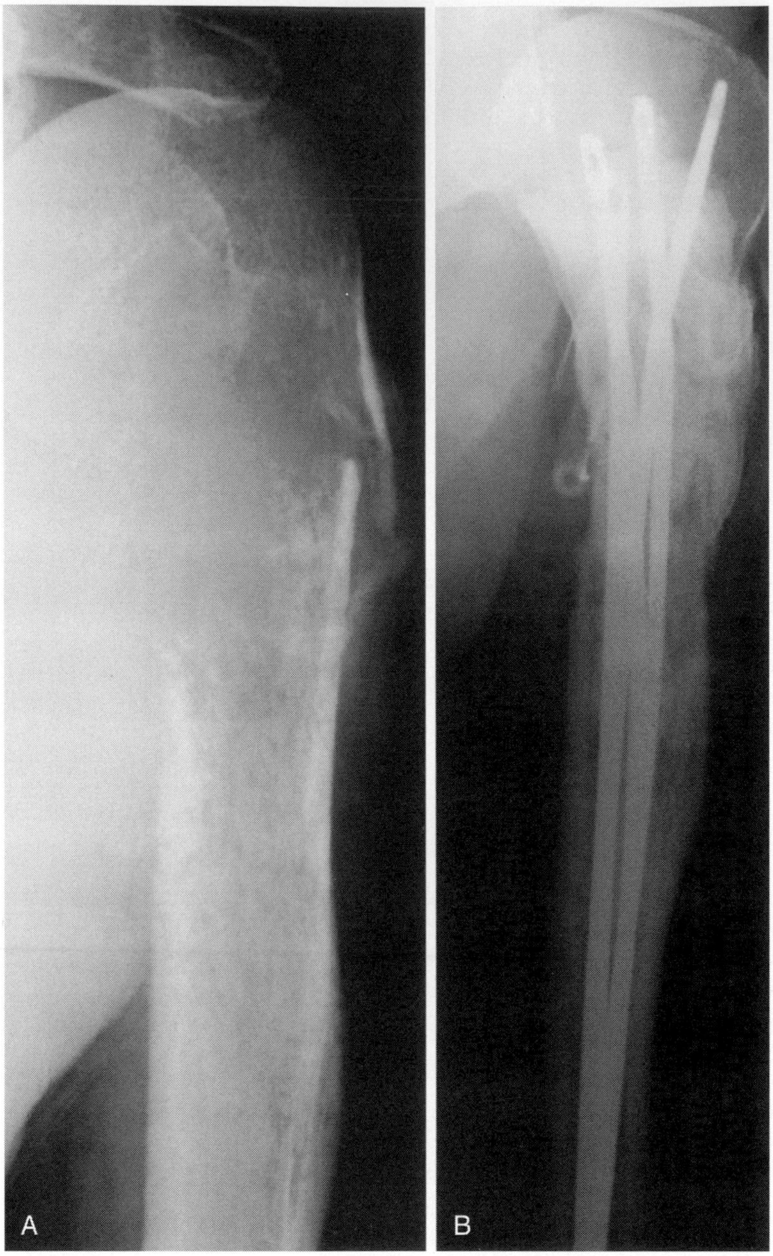

Figure 22–16

A, Metastatic adenocarcinoma of the lung in a 65-year-old man with extensive metastatic disease and a pathologic fracture. *B*, A conservative surgical stabilization in this patient involved cementation and placement of a rod through the fracture site.

inflammatory or degenerative disease include the diagnosis in most cases, various dysplastic, hematologic, or metabolic problems are important and require a more extensive evaluation. Certainly the process of separating out difficult problems starts with an accurate and thorough history and physical examination.

Trauma as the cause of lesions of the musculoskeletal system obviously often includes a history of an injury, but "incidental" trauma is also frequently associated with sarcomas, although no causal relationship has been demonstrated. Chronic injuries or stress fractures are often a more subtle and challenging diagnosis but are less common in the shoulder than in the lower extremity. Figure 22–17 demonstrates a degenerative condition of the sternoclavicular joint in an area that does not easily lend itself to imaging techniques; this degenerative lesion with an apparent soft tissue mass could be misinterpreted as a possible neoplasm of the proximal clavicle. An understanding of the pathology of the sternoclavicular joint is of great assistance in interpreting diagnostic studies of this area.

Infections are a common problem in healthy young children who suffer from acute hematogenous osteomyelitis or septic arthritis. In fact, the differential diagnosis for any lesion in a child should always include infection as a possible cause. Acute hematogenous osteomyelitis is an unusual problem in adults, because adults usually develop osteomyelitis secondary to traumatic wounds, surgical complications, or chronic decubiti. Tuberculous or fungal infections are an even greater diagnostic and treatment challenge and a culture should be taken in all suspected infections. In general, tuberculous infections have an unimpressive amount of reactive bone on the radiographs and a chronic history. Whenever an infectious

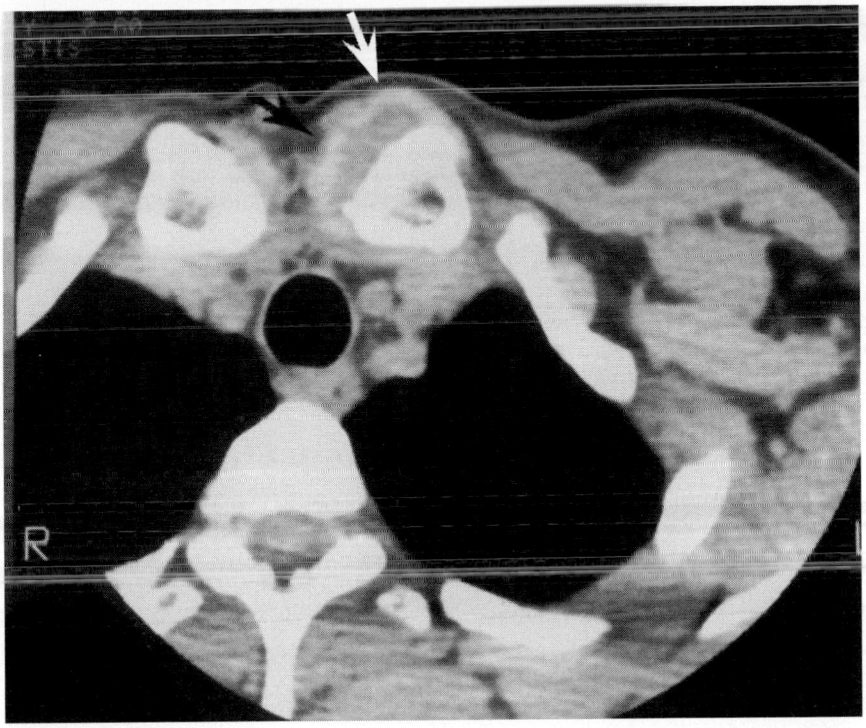

Figure 22–17

A computed tomography scan of the sternoclavicular joint in a patient with degenerative joint disease, an effusion, and a soft tissue mass consisting of redundant synovium *(arrows)*. This area is difficult to image and could be misinterpreted as a neoplasm.

problem is being considered, a biopsy specimen should be sent in addition to abundant, appropriate cultures. Some necrotic soft tissue tumors contain pus and strongly resemble a soft tissue abscess. The old adage "always biopsy an infection and culture a tumor" remains good advice as a general rule in the evaluation of any lesion.

Inflammatory and degenerative disease is usually associated with typical findings on plain radiographs such as a joint space narrowing, subchondral sclerosis, and cyst formation. Clinically, it can be very difficult to distinguish inflammatory or degenerative disease from a subtle neoplasm. The differential diagnosis can also be difficult in children, in whom pauciarticular juvenile rheumatoid arthritis in its initial presentation can be very difficult to distinguish from septic arthritis or other soft tissue tumors.

The most common dysplasias of bone masquerading as neoplasms include fibrous dysplasia in children and Paget's disease in adults. These are usually polyostotic "tumors" that actually represent dysplasias of bone. Fibrous dysplasia and Paget's disease can frequently be diagnosed by plain x-rays and bone scans, as can many of the polyostotic syndromes. Both fibrous dysplasia and Paget's disease may require intramedullary fixation in order to treat chronic, pathologic, painful, and weak long bones. Secondary malignancies are unusual and associated with increasing pain and obvious x-ray changes. Other dysplasias include multiple hereditary exostoses and enchondromatoses.

Hematologic disorders (excluding myeloma) that may masquerade as tumors occur most commonly in children or young adults with the various histiocytoses, hemophilia, and other blood dyscrasias. The least aggressive form of histiocytosis is that of eosinophilic granuloma, which is truly the "great imitator" in children, because it can masquerade as a tumor. Eosinophilic granuloma occurs in the diaphysis and is usually seen as a solitary lesion in a healthy child. However, it may occur as multiple lesions, and when diagnosed in a young child (2 years or younger), there is always the concern that the initial lesion may signal the presence of other lesions in the more severe form of the syndrome, such as Hand-Schüller-Christian disease (older children) or Letterer-Siwe disease (infants). Similarly, classic hemophilia or factor 8 deficiency, although uncommon, may show up initially as a solitary knee effusion (septic knee). Therefore, it is important to obtain an accurate history, and questions should be asked specifically about previous bleeding problems in other family members in order to make the diagnosis.

Metabolic disorders in adults can also be difficult diagnoses to make. Adult patients with osteomalacia may present with a stress fracture, a hot bone scan, equivocal staging studies, and a risk factor in their history (e.g., renal disease, gastrointestinal malabsorption). Syndromes of renal osteodystrophy, osteomalacia, and osteoporosis are unlikely to show up as a problem of the upper extremity, but they remain an important part of any complete differential diagnosis. Patients with osteomalacia frequently appear with diffuse manifestations of their disease (e.g., vertebral fractures, osteopenia) and may require a full metabolic work-up: serum calcium, PO_4, serum and urinary hydroxyproline, vitamin D, parathyroid hormone levels, bone scan, densitometry, and a tetracycline-labeled iliac crest biopsy.

BIOPSY, RESECTIONS, RECONSTRUCTIONS, AND THE MANAGEMENT OF SPECIFIC LESIONS

Biopsy

The management and treatment of any malignancy begins with a sound histologic diagnosis. Biopsy is recommended for all suspicious abnormalities of bone and soft tissue, although, as previously discussed, biopsies of low-grade cartilage and fatty tumors are usually not indicated. Although every institution has its own experiences and prejudices regarding biopsy for sarcomas, nevertheless open, or incisional, biopsy is regarded by most as the standard method.[194] Incisional biopsy is an operative technique that involves incising a small wedge-shaped piece of tissue from the tumor for histologic evaluation. Its primary advantage over a closed, or needle, biopsy is the acquisition of a larger, more adequate specimen, which is especially important in the face of challenging diagnoses of sarcoma. However, open or incisional biopsies do carry a risk of tumor contamination from postoperative hemorrhage. It is important that the surgical principles of incisional biopsy be strictly observed in the shoulder, just as in any other anatomic site. A dissecting hematoma after any biopsy can easily contaminate otherwise normal tissue and expand the necessary margin for resection, or it can contaminate nearby major neurovascular structures such as the brachial plexus or brachial vessels and thus preclude the possibility of a limb salvage type of resection. Needle biopsies have become a preferred technique in most medical centers with an established sarcoma program. This technique is now preferred for both soft tissue and osseous lesions.

Mankin and colleagues, under the auspices of the Musculoskeletal Tumor Society,[120] carried out a retrospective comparison of 329 cases of sarcomas on which biopsies were performed in a referring (primary or secondary) hospital versus those done in a setting where there was experience with sarcomas. The study concluded that biopsy-related problems were three to five times more frequent in the outside referring hospital compared with the treatment center. The referring hospitals without sarcoma experience had a higher incidence of major diagnostic errors, nonrepresentative biopsies, wound complications, treatment alterations, changes in results, and changes in final results. Last, the incidence of unnecessary amputations was 4.5% of all the cases. This sort of study may be prejudiced in favor of the tertiary institutions by the fact that most patients presented as difficult cases that had been referred for treatment, but the study does emphasize a high complication rate for biopsies and the need for careful planning and execution. Higher complications and diagnostic errors do occur in less experienced centers, reflecting the complexity of the diagnosis and treatment of sarcomas. The best management for all patients with sarcomas is to have the biopsy carried out in an experienced center where the definitive treatment will be rendered.[61] A follow-up review of biopsy complications in sarcoma patients suggests that biopsy complications have increased. The best surgical approach for a biopsy of the proximal humerus has traditionally been through the anterior substance of the deltoid (Fig. 22–18). The deltopectoral groove should be avoided, because any hematoma after the biopsy might enter the groove, spread proximally into the axilla, and lead to considerable proximal contamination. Approaching malignant lesions through the anterior deltoid requires resection of that portion of the deltoid with the definitive procedure but minimizes the risk of contamination; thus this is the traditional site for an incisional biopsy of the proximal humerus. Tumor contamination after the biopsy is a significant problem even in experienced hands and should observe the following principles of technique.[194]

PLACEMENT OF THE INCISION

When biopsying lesions in the extremities, the surgeon should use a longitudinal (not transverse) incision, usually 4 to 5 cm in length (see Fig. 22–18). The incision should be placed in the line of the proposed future definitive resection or so that it does not contaminate the lines of a possible future amputation. Around the scapula or clavicle, as in the pelvic girdle, an oblique or transverse incision is appropriate; however, as a general rule, all extremity tumors should be biopsied through a longitudinal incision.

CONTAMINATION BY TUMOR HEMATOMA

If possible, always perform a biopsy of a tumor at its most superficial and accessible site. An incisional biopsy technique should involve as little soft tissue dissection as possible. A marginal, or excisional, biopsy should be reserved only for obviously benign lesions (e.g., lipoma) or for small (2 to 3 cm) lesions. Similarly, always biopsy the lesion away from a major neurovascular bundle or joint in order to avoid contaminating those structures and thus

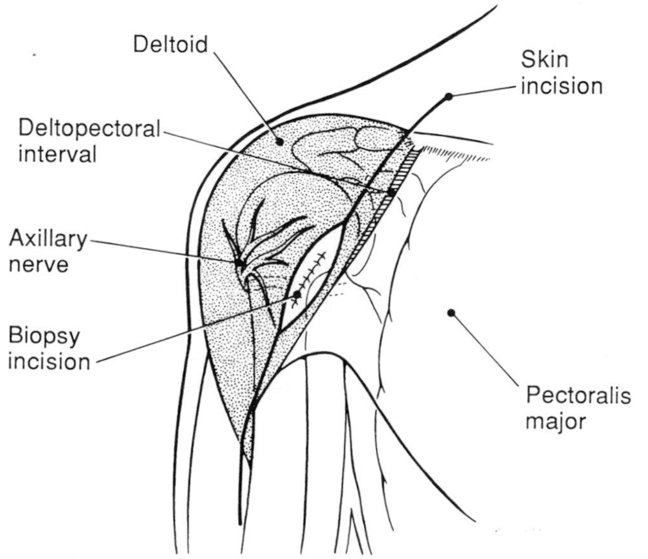

Figure 22–18

Biopsy of the proximal humerus.

precluding a need for limb-sparing surgery. This precaution is especially important in the proximal humerus and shoulder because of the proximity of the brachial vessels and brachial plexus.

Before wound closure, strict hemostasis should be carefully accomplished. The use of a tourniquet is not possible in the shoulder and, even in areas where one is used, should be released before wound closure to achieve hemostasis. Very vascular malignant lesions (e.g., angiosarcoma, myeloma, hypernephroma, or Ewing's sarcoma) in the shoulder may prove to be a challenge regarding hemostasis. In those situations, packing the wound with various coagulant materials in addition to a pressure dressing may prove helpful in enhancing hemostasis. The use of surgical drains or the practice of leaving the wound open after an open biopsy is associated with a higher incidence of wound contamination or infection and is not an accepted method of management. After achieving hemostasis, the surgeon should meticulously close the biopsy wound and carefully close the deep and superficial layers to prevent late wound dehiscence. The skin is best closed with a subcuticular closure in order to minimize skin contamination and enable a smaller ellipse of skin to be excised with the main tumor specimen at the time of the definitive resection.

ADEQUACY OF THE SPECIMEN

Prior to awakening the patient, it is important to wait for the pathologist to confirm the adequacy of the specimen by frozen section under the microscope. Although it may not be possible to make a definitive diagnosis by frozen section in every case, it is possible to determine whether the specimen has diagnostic or lesional tissue and thus whether it is an adequate specimen. Bacterial and fungal cultures should be obtained routinely, in addition to sending tissue for special stains, electron microscopy, flow cytometry,[117] or immunohistochemistry. As a general rule, it is advisable to biopsy infections and culture tumors. If there is some doubt about the location of a biopsy site in the extremity, pelvis, or spine, an intraoperative radiograph with an appropriate marker should be taken before the biopsy. In many cases of osteogenic sarcoma, it is not necessary to biopsy the bone to obtain adequate tissue. A biopsy of a bone lesion can frequently be obtained from its soft tissue extension, thus avoiding fenestration of that bone and the complications of postoperative fracture and further contamination from osseous bleeding.

OPEN VERSUS CLOSED BIOPSY

The alternatives to an incisional, or open, biopsy include a marginal, or excisional, biopsy, or closed needle biopsy. Excisional biopsy is not an accepted method for any lesion that may be malignant. It is an acceptable biopsy technique only when used to excise a small lesion (< 3 cm) or to excise a lesion that is obviously benign (e.g., lipoma). The marginal excisional biopsy of a small lesion produces little more contamination than an incisional biopsy and thus is an adequate technique for that size of lesion. Marginal excision of a tumor, however, is best indicated for benign lesions. Small (< 5 cm) soft tissue sarcomas do exist in the upper extremity, and if there is concern or confusion about a lesion, a consultation with a specialist before the biopsy is the appropriate approach.[48]

Needle biopsy is the recommended method for use on most tumors.[15, 136, 180] The disadvantage is the small size of the specimen and the difficulty of assessing whether a lesion is high grade or low grade.[8, 15] The attraction of a needle biopsy is that it avoids the operative setting and is achievable in the clinic, giving a quick diagnosis that may be useful in initiating preoperative chemotherapy if a lesion is obviously high grade. The disadvantage remains that of sampling error, which has been reported in approximately 25 to 30% of cases.[194] Needle biopsy is the preferred method for biopsying osteosarcoma when the radiographs are typical, and only a tissue diagnosis (malignant stroma or osteoid) is required. It has the advantage of a small bony fenestration, minimizing both the potential for postbiopsy hemorrhage and the risk of pathologic fracture. The best indications for a needle biopsy include the following:

1. **To achieve a "tissue and grade" diagnosis** (i.e., metastasis, recurrence, or confirming an otherwise classic presentation). In experienced medical centers, needle biopsy is now a relatively reliable method for grading soft tissue sarcomas.
2. **For cystic lesions or abscesses**. Cystic lesions are usually not malignancies, and in children, a needle biopsy is a good way to quickly rule out possible infections. It is the preferred method of diagnosing and treating many cystic lesions. If purulent drainage is not obvious, beware of soft tissue sarcomas with central necrosis; a definitive open biopsy should accompany any surgical drainage procedure.
3. **Vertebral or pelvic tumors**. Needle biopsy is an appropriate technique for vertebral and pelvic lesions, thus avoiding a more extensive open biopsy. Most of these lesions are biopsied with CT guidance in the radiology department.

The instruments required for needle biopsy are not complex. Needle biopsy for soft tissue sarcomas typically involves the use of a trocar cutting needle that delivers a small strip of tissue. Larger trephine or bone marrow needles (3 to 5 mm in diameter) are used for bone lesions. The skinny needle technique for soft tissue tumors uses a 22-gauge needle for a cytologic smear; this smear requires interpretation by an experienced cytopathologist.

Immediately proceeding with the definitive resection following an open biopsy is a treatment alternative that offers the advantage of minimizing the risk of postbiopsy hematoma and contamination. It requires appropriate intraoperative precautions, such as a change in gowns, gloves, instruments, and the operative drapes, between the biopsy and the definitive resection. The issue of whether or not it is prudent to proceed with a definitive surgical resection immediately after the frozen section histologic diagnosis depends on the lesion involved and on the confidence level of the pathologist giving the diagnosis. This course of action requires careful planning and a confident, well-informed pathologist at the time of the frozen section biopsy. It is not a reasonable alternative for patients who are candidates for preoperative adjuvant therapy or when the differential diagnosis includes radiosensitive tumors, such as lymphomas, which are not treated with resection. When there is doubt regarding whether a lesion is malignant or benign, high grade or low grade, treatment should be delayed until a definitive diagnosis is reached.

Biopsies are a challenging aspect of sarcoma management, reflecting both the rarity and the complexity of diagnosing and treating these lesions. Although the biopsy appears to be a technically small operative procedure, it represents a significant hurdle to the achievement of an appropriate and successful treatment plan. The complexities of the diagnosis of most sarcomas require that this significant, initial step in the treatment be carried out in a center experienced in the management of sarcomas.[61] Biopsy is recommended for all tumors, except when dealing with low-grade chondrosarcoma (versus enchondroma) and lipomatous soft tissue tumors.

Table 22–6 SURGICAL MARGINS*

SURGICAL MARGIN	SURGICAL PROCEDURE	RESULT
Intralesional	Piecemeal debulking or curettage	Leaves macrosopic tumor
Marginal	Excision of the tumor and pseudocapsule through the reactive zone	Leaves microscopic tumor
Wide	Excision of the tumor, pseudocapsule, reactive zone, and a cuff of normal tissue	Risk of leaving microscopic tumor
Radical	Extracompartmental procedure removes the tumor, pseudocapsule, reactive zone, and entire compartment	Minimal risk of residual microscopic tumor

*From Enneking WF, Spanier SS, and Goodman MA: A system for the surgical staging of musculoskeletal sarcoma. Clin Orthop *153*:105–120, 1980.

Surgical Resections About the Shoulder Girdle

SURGICAL MARGIN

Appropriate surgery remains the definitive treatment for most sarcomas at their primary site. The surgical treatment is best described by separately defining the tumor resection part of the procedure and the reconstructive part of the procedure. These two aspects of any surgical procedure for a tumor are potentially conflicting in their objectives, and great care should be taken to ensure that the resection is not minimized or compromised to facilitate the reconstructive part of the procedure and thus enhance function. The resection must take precedence over the reconstruction to accomplish a cure. It is imperative that these two procedures remain separate in principle. In some institutions, different surgeons carry out these two parts of the procedure in order to achieve that goal.

When discussing the probable success of a procedure in terms of local tumor control, the resection procedure is best defined by the surgical margin achieved. The surgical margin describes the efficacy of the procedure in terms of possible future tumor recurrence.[98] Assessing and describing the surgical margin requires a cooperative effort by both the surgeon and the pathologist, who must immediately review the surgical specimen. The four fundamental types of margins are intracapsular, marginal, wide, and radical (Table 22–6 and Fig. 22–19).

An intracapsular, or intralesional, surgical margin describes an inadequate margin resulting from a resection that violates the tumor's pseudocapsule and runs through the tumor, leaving gross residual tumor. It involves a partial and incomplete excision of tumor. In general, debulking procedures such as this are grossly inadequate and not indicated for any tumor.

A marginal surgical margin (see Fig. 22–19) involves a plane of dissection through the reactive zone located between the tumor and normal tissue. The reactive zone refers to areolar tissue surrounding the tumor that is compressed and inflamed by tumor invasion and enlargement. Although it is located outside a tumor's pseudocapsule, it potentially contains foci of microscopic tumor, and thus a dissection through this plane is associated with a high recurrence rate, especially when dealing with high-grade malignant tumors. This reactive or inflammatory zone usually demonstrates a significant decrease in activity with appropriate chemotherapy.

A wide margin (see Fig. 22–19) involves a surgical procedure that excises the tumor, its pseudocapsule, the surrounding reactive zone, and a cuff of normal tissue. The dissection remains outside the zone of reactive tissue, and thus the tumor specimen contains a cuff of normal tissue around its entire circumference. There are no specifications or requirements for the thickness of this cuff of normal tissue. According to this system, however, it is generally believed that a wide margin extends at least 1 to 2 cm.

A radical margin (see Fig. 22–19) involves an en bloc excision of tumor, its pseudocapsule, reactive zone, and the entire compartment within which it is contained.

A malignant intraosseous tumor of the proximal humerus treated with a radical surgical margin requires an excision of the entire humerus. A similar lesion of the deltoid treated with a radical surgical margin would involve a procedure that includes a total excision of the deltoid compartment from origin to insertion. The surgical margin is defined by its worst or closest margin. If a specimen has primarily a wide margin but is marginal in one aspect, it is described as marginal and not as a wide margin. Each particular surgical margin may be achieved by local resection or by amputation (see Fig. 22–19). Determination of the surgical margin is the critical step that allows the surgeon to integrate the surgical treatment with the staging system and thus outline treatment and assess clinical results. By assessing the surgical margin and the stage of the lesion, a prediction of local recurrence can be made based on past experience (Table 22–7).

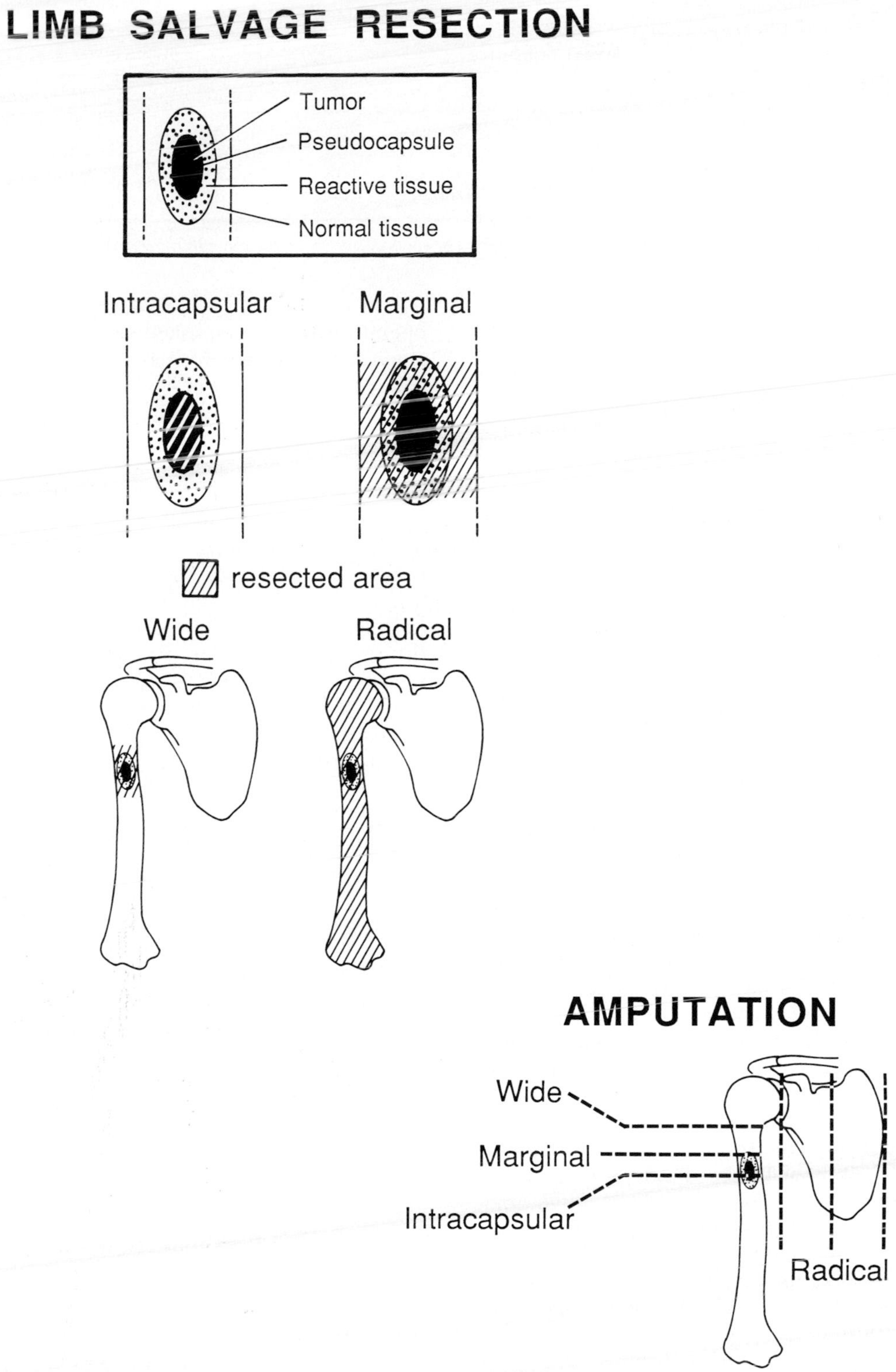

Figure 22–19

Surgical margins.

Table 22–7 RECURRENCE RATE BY SURGICAL MARGIN VERSUS STAGE*

	STAGE						
	Benign			Malignant			
SURGICAL MARGIN	1	2	3	IA	IB	IIA	IIB
Intracapsular	0%	30%	50%	90%	90%	100%	100%
Marginal	0%	0%	50%	70%	70%	90%	90%
Wide	0%	0%	10%	10%	30%	50%	70%
Radical	0%	0%	0%	0%	0%	10%	20%

*Adapted by permission from Enneking WF: Musculoskeletal Tumor Surgery. New York: Churchill Livingstone, 1983, p 99.

LIMB SALVAGE SURGERY

The surgical treatment of high-grade sarcomas of bone may involve amputation or limb salvage. In the skeletally immature with significant remaining growth potential, amputation is preferable to resection, although expandable prostheses are also available. These are metallic arthroplasties that have an extendible screw mechanism that can be lengthened at intervals to allow for skeletal growth. Limb salvage surgery is a reasonable alternative to amputation when a wide surgical margin is achievable and when enough soft tissue is preserved to allow a reasonably good functional result. In most cases, the functional criteria for limb-sparing surgery are stricter than the criteria for tumor control. Sufficient functional muscle mass is required to obtain a reasonable functional result and to avoid wound complications.[192]

Limb salvage, or limb-sparing, resections of the shoulder girdle are generally indicated for neoplasms that have no major neurovascular involvement and have enough remaining bone stock proximally and distally to allow a reasonable reconstruction. In addition, adequate soft tissue coverage and deltoid function are required in order to avoid wound complications and achieve sufficient functional results.[1, 41, 53, 55, 111, 139, 152] The most common restrictions for effective limb salvage involve the adequacy of nerve involvement or soft tissue coverage.

Patients with soft tissue sarcomas or bony sarcomas of the proximal humerus with considerable soft tissue extension are challenging limb salvage candidates. The brachial neurovascular structures and glenohumeral joint are not infrequently involved by tumor, and careful preoperative staging is essential before deciding on a surgical plan or attempting limb salvage procedures. High-grade malignant tumors of the proximal humerus typically present as extracompartmental lesions (IIB) and require a wide surgical resection to achieve a cure. Patients who undergo marginal resections for high-grade malignancies are at risk for local recurrences in most cases, no matter how efficacious their adjuvant chemotherapy. Thus, a typical IIB osteosarcoma of the proximal humerus requires a wide surgical margin for an adequate margin. In fact, many if not most resections for osteosarcoma involve a marginal margin at some part of the resected specimen. That marginal margin remains an adequate margin if the patient has had an adequate response to preoperative chemotherapy. Determining appropriate surgical candidates and the feasibility of a wide surgical resection preoperatively is accomplished by the preoperative staging studies. Most osteosarcomas show up as IIB lesions with soft tissue involvement by the tumor. The amount of soft tissue involvement and the proximity of the medial neurovascular bundle present a preoperative challenge to determining candidates for limb salvage. Another preoperative challenge for high-grade sarcomas involves the assessment of the extent of bone disease and whether disease extends into the glenohumeral joint. If the joint is involved, an extracapsular or extra-articular resection is indicated with resection of the glenoid en bloc with the capsule of the glenohumeral joint and the remainder of the proximal humerus. Preoperative tasks include assessing distant, metastatic disease and determining the extent of bone and soft tissue margins with the planned resection.[139]

The primary site of a tumor to some extent predicts certain resection and reconstruction tendencies. High-grade sarcomas of the proximal humerus are likely to have a close relationship to the medial neurovascular bundle (brachial plexus or brachial artery or vein) axillary nerve, deltoid, or the glenohumeral joint. Chest wall involvement with these tumors is less common and usually occurs as a late finding after involvement of the medial neurovascular structures. Obviously, the best limb salvage candidates are those with primary bone tumors with minimal extraosseous extension. Soft tissue sarcomas of the shoulder region are easily resected when located in the deltoid, but deltoid resection precludes arthroplasty as a reasonable alternative because of the subsequent loss of active abduction. The following classification system is useful for describing these different resections and the various reconstructive principles (Fig. 22–20).

Type 1—Short Proximal Humeral Resection

Type 1 resections, short proximal humeral resections, are proximal to the deltoid insertion of the humerus (see Fig. 22–20). These resections are intra-articular; that is, the bone resection includes the humeral head and the proximal plane of resection goes through the glenohumeral joint. These resections may or may not involve an en bloc resection of the abductor mechanism. The abductor mechanism refers to the rotator cuff, deltoid muscle, and its (axillary) innervation. The sacrifice of any part of this composite results in significantly weakened abduction and a significant change in the expectation of postoperative

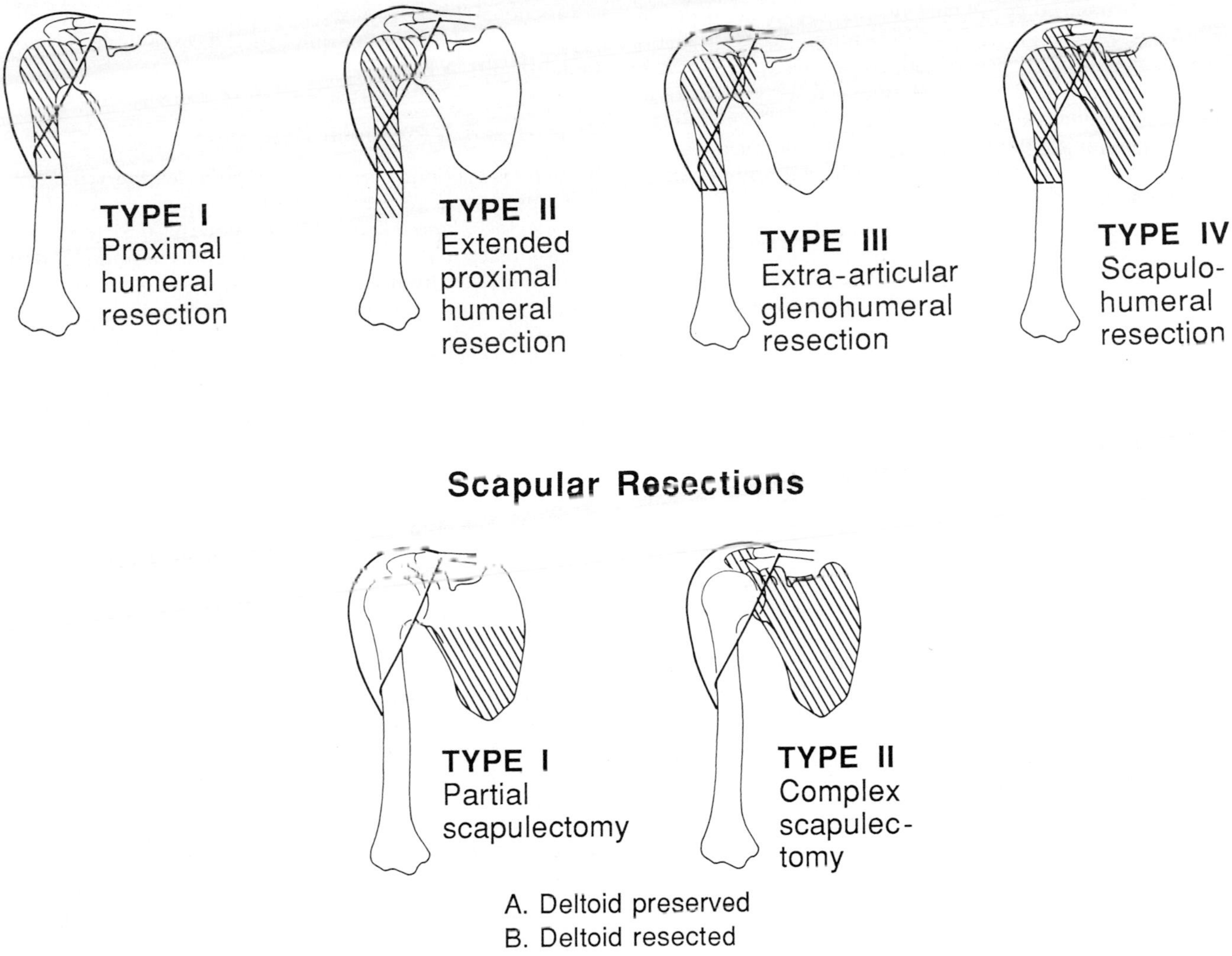

Figure 22–20

Classification of shoulder resections.

function (see various reconstructive procedures). Axillary nerve injury or resection is a common consideration because of its strategic location at the inferior and posterior humeral neck.

The deltoid muscle inserts into the humerus at approximately 10 to 14 cm from the articular surface of the proximal humeral head. Removal of the deltoid insertion from the humerus involves a reconstructive procedure with greater complications and a longer rehabilitation period than a procedure without detachment of the deltoid insertion. Such deltoid resections for shoulder tumors are in fact rarely indicated in today's sarcoma environment. Thus, bone resections distal to the deltoid insertion are associated with more complications or more limited functional results. If the deltoid and rotator cuff with their respective innervations are preserved, good active abduction can be achieved postoperatively and a better functional result can be expected following after the reconstruction. Sacrifice of the rotator cuff, the deltoid, its innervation, or vascular supply leads to a significant reduction in potential shoulder abduction. There is a great difference between resections of the proximal humerus that include the deltoid muscle, axillary nerve, or rotator cuff and those that do not. Proximal humeral resections including a part of the abductor mechanism are referred to in this classification system as type 1B humeral resections (see Fig. 22–20). Resections of the humerus that do not sacrifice a part of the abductor mechanism are referred to as type 1A resections. This subclassification of A (preservation or an active abductor mechanism) and B (resection or sacrifice of a part of the abductor mechanism) is also used to classify the other resection types as described.

Type 2—Long Proximal Humeral Resections

Type 2 resections (see Fig. 22–20) refer to proximal humeral resections where the distal osteotomy is made distal to the deltoid insertion. This type usually includes proximal humeral resections longer than 12 cm. They are referred to as 2A or 2B, depending on whether or not they spare or include (respectively) the abductor mechanism with the resection. Type 1 or type 2 resections of the proximal humerus may be reconstructed with an arthroplasty or an arthrodesis, depending on whether or not the potential for active abduction remains following the resection. Type 2, or long humeral resections, have a longer rehabilitative period and a greater overall incidence of complications or more limited functional results because of the long bone reconstruction and the need for reattachment of the deltoid.

Type 3—Glenohumeral Resections

Type 3 resections of the proximal humerus extend to the glenoid side of the glenohumeral joint in an extra-articular or extracapsular fashion (see Fig. 22–20). The proximal bone resection is through the base of the glenoid or scapular neck. If enough bone stock remains in the glenoid area, an arthroplasty or an arthrodesis may be achieved, depending on the competency of the abductor mechanism. Without a good abductor mechanism, an arthrodesis is preferable, but adequate bone stock must exist in the lateral scapula, either at the acromion or at the remaining scapular neck or glenoid area. Type 3 resections are typically carried out for a high-grade malignancy of the proximal humerus or humeral head with intra-articular invasion, as can occur with osteosarcoma or chondrosarcoma. The indications for type 3 glenohumeral resections represent relatively rare indications.

Type 4—Scapulohumeral Resections

Type 4 resections refer to scapulohumeral resections of the proximal humerus and scapula (see Fig. 22–20), including the classic Tikhoff-Linberg procedure that involves a full scapular resection with a resection of the humeral head.[68, 108, 114, 121] An extended Tikhoff-Linberg resection refers to a full scapular resection with a lengthy proximal humeral resection. The resection may or may not include a portion of the deltoid or abductor mechanism (A or B). Modifications of the original Tikhoff-Linberg involve a subtotal scapular resection en bloc with an extra-articular resection of the proximal humerus. These large resections are typically carried out for high-grade lesions of the proximal humerus with glenohumeral joint involvement. One criterion for a Tikhoff-Linberg procedure, as with any limb-sparing surgery, is a lack of involvement of the neurovascular structures (brachial artery, vein, and brachial plexus). The procedure involves a large scapular resection that is usually left without reconstruction.

Scapulohumeral resections are an example of a limb-sparing procedure that results in very limited postoperative function. They are accepted well by the patient when the functional limitations are fully discussed before surgery. Postoperatively, patients typically have varying degrees of proximal humeral stability and a well-innervated, functional hand and elbow. Elbow motion depends on the degree of postoperative humeral stability. In this setting, where the surgical alternative is an amputation, many patients are satisfied with this limited degree of function. Patients frequently prefer to retain the extremity even with limited functional expectations. When the patient is well informed preoperatively and a functional hand persists postoperatively, the patient's subjective evaluations are quite good despite limited functional results.[68, 108, 114, 121]

Types 1 and 2—Scapular Resections

Scapular resections may be classified as partial type 1 or complex type 2 resections, depending on whether they include the glenoid (complex) or not (partial) (see Fig. 22–20). Partial resections of the scapula are associated with relatively high functional results postoperatively, compared with the more restricted functional performance after complex or complete resections of the scapula.[21, 127, 206] This classification system does not include other, less common resections about the shoulder such as various partial or intercalary resections of the humerus that may or may not involve reconstruction. These resections are associated with excellent function postoperatively when there is preservation of the surrounding neurovascular structures and the abductor mechanism. Partial resections of the humerus may be undertaken for less aggressive benign lesions, such as periosteal chondroma or chondroblastoma. Generally, these partial resections lead to superior functional results. Partial resections of the scapula and clavicle are also unusual and may be undertaken for malignant or benign lesions.[179, 180] Partial and complete scapular resections are associated with surprisingly good functional results even in the absence of reconstruction.

Reconstructive Procedures of the Shoulder

There are three basic choices for reconstruction after limb-sparing resections of the shoulder: arthroplasty, arthrodesis, or a flail shoulder (Fig. 22–21). A flail shoulder is defined as a shoulder that lacks functional motor power and stability. It is functionally inferior to arthroplasty or arthrodesis but superior to a painful arthroplasty or arthrodesis. The flail shoulder, such as the shoulder that results following a Tikhoff-Linberg procedure, constitutes an acceptable result for the patient who has undergone a large scapulohumeral resection for an aggressive tumor and who is satisfied with limited shoulder and elbow function. Elbow motion is limited by instability of the proximal humerus and thus stabilization of the proximal humerus significantly enhances function of both the elbow and the hand. Multiple techniques have been attempted in the past to stabilize the remaining humerus to the chest wall. The original technique of using an intramedullary rod sutured to a proximal rib was discontinued because of migration of the rod into the wound flaps.[21] In addition, suspension of the midhumerus to the remaining clavicle to achieve some degree of stability has also been carried out. The best method of stabilization involves reattachment of any remaining proximal musculature to the proximal humerus. Although a flail shoulder is not functionally attractive, it does allow a generous tumor resection and is usually associated with a predictable relief of pain. It remains a viable alternative following large resections and for the complications of a painful, infected, or failed

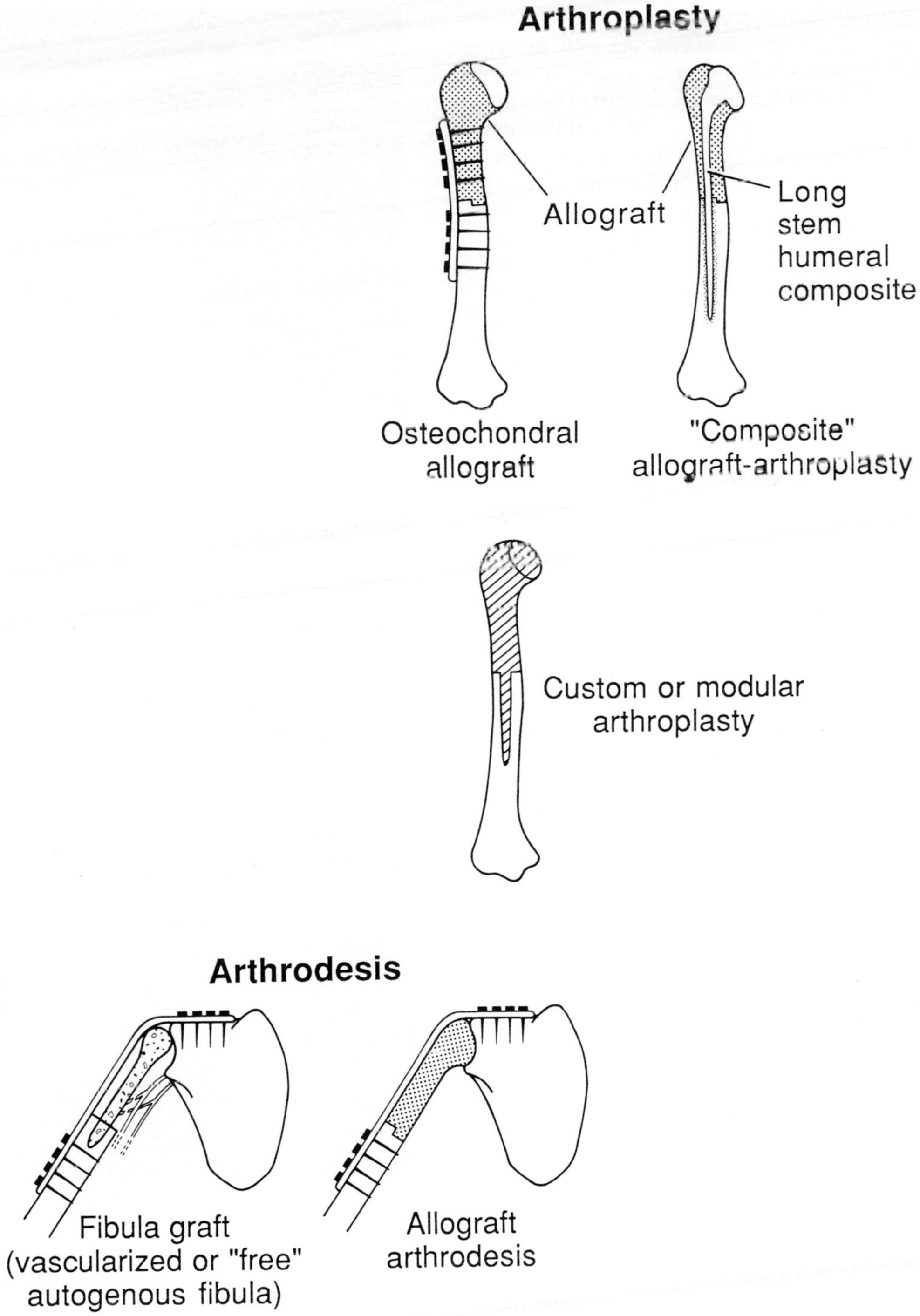

Figure 22–21

Reconstruction alternatives.

arthroplasty or arthrodesis. However, a flail joint is unstable, in the true sense of the word, and an attempt should be made to limit instability by soft tissue reconstruction whenever possible.[68, 108, 114, 121, 146]

The choice of arthroplasty versus arthrodesis after shoulder resections should be considered carefully with the patient before surgery. A patient's personality, vocation, lifestyle, and handedness all affect the decision, and all these factors should be taken into account. In general, an arthroplasty requires active abduction and glenohumeral stability, both of which require a competent, functional abductor mechanism. What constitutes a functionally competent abductor mechanism is a source of some debate. The abductor mechanism has three basic anatomical components: the deltoid muscle, the rotator cuff muscles (supraspinatus, infraspinatus, and teres minor), and their respective blood supply (circumflex and suprascapular vessels) and innervation (axillary and suprascapular nerves). Resections or injuries to the axillary nerve after resection or biopsy of the humerus are not uncommon, and the loss of deltoid function has significant functional consequences. A well-innervated deltoid is the minimum requirement for a functional, stable arthroplasty. Loss of rotator cuff function has, in the past, required a constrained or semiconstrained arthroplasty, which is associated with greater complications, and may have served as an indication for an arthrodesis.[154] Newer reconstructive procedures have achieved functional arthroplasties using various unconstrained prostheses with oversized humeral components instead of constrained glenohumeral designs.[129] These techniques and others have improved results significantly over the previous high failure rates in earlier series (50%), but they lack long-term follow-up.[7, 79, 141, 153]

Currently, the techniques of arthroplasty employ metallic, ceramic, or osteochondral allograft implants.[20, 72, 93, 99, 153, 163, 176, 177, 189, 213] The increasing use of allograft transplantation[118, 119, 148] has had two major effects on the reconstruction of humeral resections. First, it has increased the length of the proximal humerus that can be reconstructed, thus expanding the indications for limb salvage procedures. Previously, resections were limited to those that could be reconstructed by an autogenous fibular graft or a customized long-stem humeral component. It is now possible to replace resections within 8 cm of the distal humerus. Second, allograft reconstructions may be a more reasonable reconstructive alternative in younger patients because of their potential as a biologic structure. An allograft reconstruction offers the advantages of enhanced soft tissue attachment to the graft, bone union to the remaining humerus, and the potential for the transplantation of viable cartilage. The relative complications of an allograft versus a prosthetic reconstruction have not yet been demonstrated to be significantly different.

Arthroplasty reconstructions after tumor resections involve the choice of an allograft,[153] a metallic[14] or ceramic[14, 176, 185, 189] prosthesis, or the combination of an allograft and a prosthesis, referred to as a "composite" reconstruction (Fig. 22–22).[161] This "composite" reconstruction involves an allograft that is fixed with a long-stem humeral component through the graft and cemented into the remaining humeral bone stock. Composite proximal humeral allografts are the preferred type of allograft reconstruction because of the relatively high (50%) failure rate with osteochondral grafts. It can be cemented or press fitted into the allograft or the remaining humerus. With this type of reconstruction, reattachment of the deltoid or rotator cuff to the allograft represents a distinct advantage compared with reattachment to metallic prostheses. Thus, there is the potential for enhanced stability, strength, motion, and function. However, the preliminary results for transplanted allograft rotator cuff and other allograft ligaments show a high failure rate.[79]

The greatest challenge after a proximal humeral hemiarthroplasty reconstruction with an allograft is in the reconstruction of the surrounding soft tissues. Great care has to be taken in reconstructing the glenohumeral joint capsule, the rotator cuff, and the deltoid insertion at the time of transplantation. The processes of bone ingrowth and remodeling, soft tissue attachment, graft fixation, revascularization, and cartilage survival remain areas of active research and clinical investigation. Graft fractures, infection, rejection, and instability remain serious potential complications that occur in 20 to 30% of all patients.[118, 119, 148]

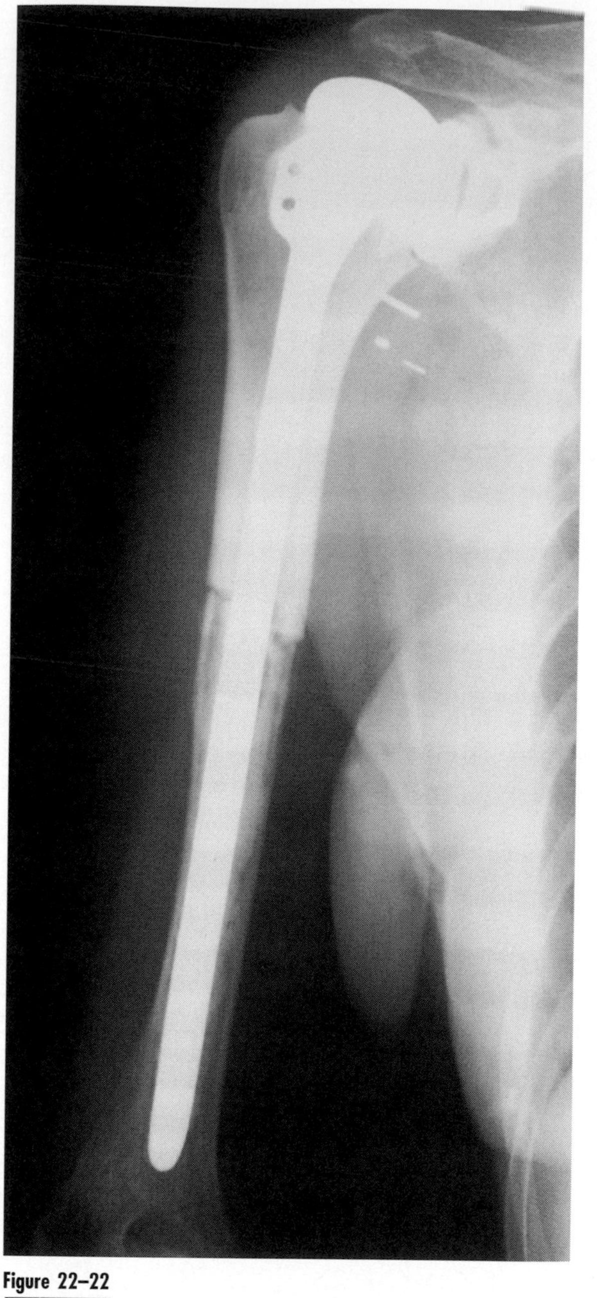

Figure 22–22

"Composite" reconstruction of the proximal humerus.

The reconstructive alternative to allograft transplantation lies with a custom prosthetic implant of acceptable metals or ceramics.[14, 20, 72, 93, 99, 153, 161, 163, 176, 177, 185, 187, 189, 213] Prosthetic implants offer the advantage of strength and custom fit and are an excellent alternative, especially in older patients. To date, the functional results of arthroplasties in the proximal humerus are excellent for both composite reconstructions and metallic implants.[14, 161, 185, 187] As yet, no studies have described comparative differences in function, infection, and revision surgery for these procedures. Newer modular prosthetic designs provide the attractive alternative of a readily available implant that can be customized to the resection defect intraoperatively without delay. These are newer designs with as yet little clinical follow-up, but they appear to have significant application in reconstructing the humerus after tumor resections.[161]

When the deltoid muscle is sacrificed by resection, the best reconstructive choice is an arthrodesis. As a technique, arthrodesis has changed significantly. An arthrodesis after tumor resection may be achieved with various bone graft materials, including free or vascularized autogenous fibular grafts or allograft transplantation.[27, 20, 71, 171, 209] Resections of 5 to 6 cm or less may use autogenous cancellous grafts from the iliac crest, with or without some shortening of the humerus itself.[17, 18, 197, 209] The remaining humerus should be buttressed against the acromion and may or may not be offset from the glenoid with autogenous grafts. Resections of the humerus up to 20 cm in length may be reconstructed with a vascularized autogenous fibular graft. Free (nonvascularized) autogenous fibular grafts may be used for defects less than 12 cm.[182] Nonvascularized fibular grafts longer than 12 cm are associated with a high incidence of graft fractures.[17]

Frozen allograft is a reasonable alternative graft material for shoulder arthrodesis. However, its use has been reported in several series with short follow-up, and there may be some potential problems with the increased risk of nonunion or loss of fixation following nonunion.[213] The use of postoperative radiation therapy or chemotherapy has deleterious effects on the bone union of any reconstruction. Patients with high-grade lesions needing arthrodesis are immediately at even higher risk for nonunion and fracture if they receive postoperative radiation therapy. Most surgeons consider postoperative radiation therapy a contraindication to an allograft arthrodesis.

Internal fixation of an arthrodesis is best achieved with the use of a long-angled custom plate that enables patients to avoid prolonged postoperative immobilization and has enhanced fixation and positioning of the fusion. Such long-angled plates are required for long humeral resections, whereas shorter, more conventional plates may be used for shorter humeral resections.[29] Newer implants to enhance fixation of the proximal humerus to the scapula are currently being evaluated clinically.

The use of a long-angled plate with adequate purchase of the scapula and remaining humerus has improved postoperative function by avoiding immobilization with a postoperative shoulder spica cast. Proper positioning of the plate on the scapular spine, acromion, and lateral border of the humerus is crucial to achieve proper positioning of the arm and adequate postoperative function. Intraoperative positioning remains a demanding part of the procedure and significantly affects the rotational position of the arm by its orientation proximally and distally. When such a plate is used, at least eight cortices are required for adequate distal humeral fixation. Likewise, the scapular fixation requires four to five good scapula screws to prevent failure of fixation proximally. Careful positioning of the plate at the acromion is necessary in order to avoid prominence and wound complication. Spica cast immobilization is not required postoperatively if adequate fixation is achieved, as it is in most cases.[29] Postoperatively, patients may use a sling with a soft bolster under the elbow. They begin exercises to improve rhomboid and periscapular strength 6 weeks after surgery and may carefully begin abduction exercises at 8 weeks.[29]

The greatest functional disadvantage in an arthrodesis is the restriction of rotation inherent in the procedure. Most patients are happy with the functional results and obtain adequate abduction (70 to 80 degrees) postoperatively. Limited abduction after arthrodesis usually reflects prolonged immobilization, poor rehabilitation, or a persistent or painful nonunion. The abduction that does occur after arthrodesis is at the scapulothoracic interval and is powered by the rhomboids and other scapular muscles. Patients who are not candidates for an arthroplasty are frequently good candidates for an arthrodesis, because their alternative reconstructive choice is usually a flail shoulder.[27, 29, 71, 171]

Scapular resections are unusual procedures that may involve partial or complex resections.[21, 36, 127, 147, 174, 178, 206] Complex scapular resections in this classification system (see Fig. 22–18) involve a portion of the glenoid. There is some experience with the prosthetic replacement of the scapula after total scapulectomy.[39] Reconstruction with a scapular prosthesis requires humeral head replacement to articulate with the prosthetic glenoid. According to the most recent report of this procedure, the ideal indication for such a prosthesis is a partial scapulectomy.[39] Eckhard and colleagues[39] report a series of eight patients treated with endoprosthetic replacement of the scapula for various malignant or benign aggressive lesions. The follow-up on these patients was limited (20 months' mean follow-up), and 50% achieved acceptable (good to excellent) functional results. As yet, scapular prosthetic replacement remains a somewhat experimental procedure for which only early, short-term clinical results have been reported. Partial and complete scapulectomies achieve remarkably good functional results without reconstructive procedures beyond soft tissue closure.

Management of Specific Lesions

AGGRESSIVE BENIGN BONE TUMORS

The surgical treatment of active or aggressive bone tumors presents a greater challenge when the tumor occurs adjacent to significant structures such as a major nerve or vessel, a joint or joint surface, or active growth plate. Aggressive benign lesions of bone presenting with significant subchondral bone loss frequently present the greatest challenge in preserving a functional joint.

Aggressive and active benign tumors are typified in the adult by benign giant cell tumor of bone, which occurs in the proximal humerus in 15 to 20% of cases. The choice of treatment for such a lesion includes resection versus intralesional curettage. The latter is usually associated with the use of a local adjuvant to enhance the opportunity to kill the tumor. Various local adjuvants that have been used in the recent past include the application of liquid nitrogen (cryosurgery) or phenol (phenolization), the placement of methyl methacrylate (cementation), and various forms of cauterization. Wide surgical resection offers the lowest risk of tumor recurrence but, to some extent, diminishes joint function. For that reason, the slightly less effective intralesional procedures are preferred when associated with a relatively low rate of recurrence tumor (10%). Experience with curettage and cryosurgery has demonstrated a lower recurrence rate (<10%) compared with other forms of local adjuvant treatment and may represent the preferred intralesional treatment.[28, 77]

Surgical resection is more effective at controlling tumor and is the preferred method for more aggressive or recurrent lesions. Reconstructions after humeral head resection usually involve an allograft or a custom or modular arthroplasty. Thus, a larger resection that enhances tumor control requires a larger, more complicated reconstruction.

Aggressive benign soft tissue tumors are best exemplified by aggressive fibromatosis in young adults and are lesions that also require a wide surgical margin to minimize the risk of recurrence. Lesions that are juxtaposed to a major neurovascular structure may be treated with a marginal surgical margin in addition to radiation therapy. Radiation therapy appears to be efficacious in minimizing the recurrence rate after marginal resections, despite controversy to the contrary.

LOW-GRADE MALIGNANCIES OF BONE

Chondrosarcoma

Chondrosarcoma represents the most common low-grade malignancy of bone. It occurs frequently in the proximal humerus and presents a clinical challenge in interpreting the source of pain (intra-articular versus extra-articular) and early radiographic signs of malignancy. The definitive treatment for low-grade chondrosarcoma is usually an intralesional curettage. Chemotherapy and radiotherapy have no added benefit in the treatment of an intermediate- or low-grade intraosseous lesion such as chondrosarcoma. Patients who develop a local recurrence after surgery can also be treated surgically for the local recurrence, but if multiple occurrences appear, restaging and adjuvant therapy should be considered.

The appropriate surgical treatment for a low-grade intraosseous chondrosarcoma that is well contained within the cortices of the proximal humerus is intralesional curettage with or without cryosurgery. The functional results of an intralesional procedure are grossly superior to that of a resection and reconstruction. Control of tumor is better with resection than with any intralesional procedure, although it is usually not required. Most chondrosarcomas that are intraosseous in the proximal humerus are low grade and may be treated with curettage alone. A significant proportion of those patients develop a local recurrence over 5 to 10 years; thus curettage should include some type of adjuvant treatment in order to optimize tumor control.

The resection of a chondrosarcoma involving the glenohumeral joint necessitates an extra-articular resection of the shoulder. This is a more difficult procedure that requires a total shoulder arthroplasty. The risk of a contaminated surgical margin is higher with this procedure; however, the alternative tumor procedure is either an inadequate, contaminated resection or a forequarter amputation.

Intermediate- or high-grade chondrosarcomas are less common and require a wide surgical margin and appropriate arthroplasty reconstruction. These higher-grade malignancies cannot be reasonably treated using intralesional procedures with or without local adjuvant because of an increased risk of local recurrence and metastatic disease. Results of chemotherapy for high-grade chondrosarcoma are quite limited, but chemotherapy is nonetheless indicated.

HIGH-GRADE MALIGNANCIES OF BONE

Osteosarcoma

High-grade malignant lesions of bone, such as osteosarcoma, are best treated with preoperative (induction) chemotherapy, reassessment of the response to chemotherapy (restaging), surgical resection, and postoperative chemotherapy.[35, 142, 166, 195] Osteosarcoma of the proximal humerus is usually best reconstructed with composite allograft reconstruction. Postoperative chemotherapy is tailored or adjusted, depending on the degree of necrosis in the surgical tumor specimen. This type of treatment was first developed in the Sloan Kettering T10 methotrexate protocol and has become the standard treatment for osteosarcoma in many centers.[35, 166, 192] Controlled studies specifically evaluating the true significance of preoperative chemotherapy, the significance of the histologic response to that preoperative therapy, and the effect of postoperative tailoring of chemotherapy have demonstrated statistical significance with the degree of histologic necrosis.[35] We do not know how much of a histologic response to chemotherapy is required to improve survival. We do not know which tumor types respond to which drugs. We do not know which drug combinations are more efficacious (cisplatinum versus methotrexate). We do not know if the intra-arterial administration of chemotherapy has a greater effect on tumor. There are proponents for many of these theories but very few well-controlled studies.[35]

Adequate evidence does exist to demonstrate improved survival with the addition of chemotherapy to surgery.[13] There has been little experience with radiation therapy in the primary treatment of osteosarcoma, and such therapy does not have a significant role in the curative treatment of osteosarcoma in most centers today. Although there has been a significant increase in survival with more aggressive chemotherapy, many of the significant studies have yet to be carried out.[22, 96, 138, 214] In addition, the protocols for managing metastatic pulmonary disease remain to be written. Although it is apparent that pulmonary resection aids survival, its integration with chemotherapy has been poorly defined.[19, 73, 78, 128, 181]

Ewing's Sarcoma

The treatment of Ewing's sarcoma today is somewhat similar to the treatment of osteosarcoma in that preoperative induction chemotherapy is delivered after a histologic diagnosis is obtained with an appropriate biopsy.[78, 135, 165, 199, 204, 212] Placement of the biopsy is very important in Ewing's sarcoma because of the high risk of pathologic fracture after radiation therapy. Although the treatment of Ewing's sarcoma 10 years ago involved the combination of chemotherapy and radiation therapy, several studies documenting a high local recurrence rate, especially with large tumors (>10 cm), have led to a greater emphasis on surgical treatment of the disease.[165] Thus, lesions that are surgically resectable, especially when larger than 8 to 10 cm, are frequently treated with preoperative chemotherapy, restaging, and surgical resection. A wide surgical margin should be the goal of surgical resection, and surgical margins are more difficult to assess with Ewing's sarcoma. If a marginal surgical resection results, postoperative radiation therapy is indicated. Patients with Ewing's sarcoma typically present with a large soft tissue mass that usually demonstrates an impressive shrinkage with reasonable response to chemotherapy.[165, 204] Patients who do not demonstrate this shrinkage of the inflammatory border of the soft tissue part of Ewing's sarcoma probably have lesions that are not responding well to chemotherapy and should be reassessed very carefully, both pre- and postoperatively. The total treatment protocol for Ewing's sarcoma usually involves approximately 12 months of treatment (chemotherapy).

Amputation may be indicated for treatment of young patients with Ewing's sarcoma with significant growth potential remaining if they present with a lesion in the lower extremity.[205] The alternative is to treat that patient with chemotherapy and radiation therapy, which will usually result in physeal arrest and a discrepancy in leg length. There is significant experience with morbidity after the radiation treatment of lower extremity lesions in young children with Ewing's sarcoma.[103, 135, 199, 212] In addition, these patients represent one of the highest risks for secondary sarcomas, such as osteosarcoma, arising from their radiation field.[115, 142] In the upper extremity, Ewing's sarcoma not infrequently occurs in the proximal humerus, and a surgical resection of the humerus is usually indicated for most patients with an intercalary allograft reconstruction.

SOFT TISSUE SARCOMAS

Soft tissue sarcomas may present as high-grade, low-grade, or intermediate-grade neoplasms. Low-grade and intermediate-grade soft tissue sarcomas with adequate surgical margins are best treated with a surgical resection and postoperative radiation therapy. Worrisome surgical margins may serve as an indication for preoperative radiation therapy. High-grade soft tissue sarcomas have been treated in the past with preoperative radiation therapy followed by surgical resection and chemotherapy.[5] Local recurrence has not been a significant problem (<10%), whereas pulmonary metastases have posed a problem (10 to 30%). The institution of preoperative radiation therapy usually delays surgical resection by approximately 7 to 8 weeks. Chemotherapy in that setting is given postoperatively and is usually not possible until 2 to 3 weeks after resection or 10 to 12 weeks after the institution of treatment. Because of this delay in chemotherapy and the real problems of pulmonary metastases, chemotherapy may be given preoperatively in order to assess the histologic response and treat systemic disease. Postoperative therapy is adjusted according to the histologic response and is given 2 to 3 weeks after surgery. Radiation therapy is indicated for marginal surgical margins and is integrated with postoperative chemotherapy.

AUTHOR'S PREFERRED METHODS OF TREATMENT

Biopsy

The biopsy of musculoskeletal tumors will always represent the initial and probably one of the most important steps in the evaluation and treatment of these challenging lesions. The biopsy site should always be placed in the line of a possible future resection and should not be executed before an adequate clinical evaluation and diagnostic radiographic staging studies have been completed. When the staging studies and the clinical presentation of the patient are suggestive of a particular lesion, a needle biopsy is the preferred method. A fairly reliable, tentative diagnosis can be made after staging studies have been completed. This can then be easily confirmed with a needle biopsy. Thus, most classic osteosarcomas have a fairly typical x-ray and can be easily diagnosed with a needle biopsy. However, when a lesion's diagnosis is still uncertain, even after initial staging studies, an open biopsy provides the best diagnosis. In that situation, the more generous the biopsy specimen, the easier will be the diagnosis. Providing enough of a biopsy specimen without contaminating an extremity remains a challenge even for the experienced oncology surgeon. In general, the biopsy should be executed by the surgeon who will carry out the definitive resection.

Surgical Choices

In terms of treatment choices, three different categories of lesions remain a challenge in today's setting: (1) aggressive benign lesions, such as giant cell tumor; (2) low-grade malignant lesions, such as chondrosarcoma; and (3) high-grade malignant lesions, such as osteosarcoma or Ewing's sarcoma.

Giant cell tumor, in many cases, is a difficult lesion to treat because it is locally aggressive and destructive to the adjacent joint. It is a difficult tumor to grade histologically and radiographically, and the specific indications for various surgical treatments are nebulous. In most cases, curettage is indicated for all benign tumors. Curettage supplemented with liquid nitrogen freezing (cryosurgery) may be a better method of treatment in terms of controlling tumor. Aggressive recurrent lesions will not be resolved with curettage alone and require curettage with liquid nitrogen freezing or a wide surgical resection. The experience with curettage and liquid nitrogen has been good regarding tumor control and function of the extremity.[28, 77] It requires very careful intraoperative monitoring of the patient for both embolic precautions and protection of the soft tissues and neurovascular structures. It should be carried out only by someone experienced in the technique and is best combined with a subchondral bone graft and internal fixation or cementation of the remaining bone defect. Patients should be advised of the risks and benefits of cryosurgery versus wide resection in the treatment of a giant cell tumor. Resection is clearly indicated for benign tumors that recur after multiple attempts at curettage. In many clinical settings, either procedure is a reasonable alternative.

Low-grade malignancies are typified by low-grade chondrosarcomas, which are difficult lesions to define histologically. Microscopically, a low-grade chondrosarcoma is defined by increased cellularity, binucleated lacunae, and microscopic bone resorption, in addition to the clinical radiographic picture of endosteal cortical resorption and bone destruction. Most of these low-grade lesions are located at the metaphyseal-diaphyseal junction in intramedullary or cancellous bone. In general, surgical treatment is indicated only in the symptomatic patient (intraosseous pain). Biopsy is unreliable as a diagnostic procedure for this problem. When there is doubt about the diagnosis, the patient is much better off being followed carefully with repeat x-rays every 3 to 6 months and a repeat CT scan or MRI scan. Low-grade chondrosarcomas of the extremities (secondary chondrosarcoma) constitute a very low-grade malignancy in the typical case, with very little threat of pulmonary metastasis. They can be comfortably followed clinically with little or no risk to the patient. Biopsy of such a low-grade cartilaginous lesion is frequently difficult to interpret and may result in an equivocal histologic diagnosis regarding the malignant grade or potential. Thus, the diagnosis of benign versus low-grade malignant is best made in the clinical setting rather than in the pathology department. This is a rare exception to the general rule of relying on the histologic evaluation of all musculoskeletal lesions in order to define their true nature.

The treatment of a low-grade malignancy (chondrosarcoma) is similar to that of an aggressive benign lesion (giant cell tumor). Curettage alone will be associated with a very high (70 to 80%) recurrence rate for low-grade malignancies, although that recurrence may take 5 to 10 years to show up. Thus, curettage alone is really, in the strict sense of the word, an inadequate form of treatment. Lesions that have failed to respond to previous curettage procedures should be treated with a resection in order to minimize multiple recurrences and wider contamination. For most patients, curettage with freezing (cryosurgery) is indicated prior to resection.

High-Grade Tumors and Preoperative Chemotherapy

High-grade malignancies in the shoulder have a distribution similar to those in other sites, with the most common lesions being osteosarcoma and Ewing's sarcoma. Most patients with a high-grade malignancy of bone or soft tissue are best treated with chemotherapy before surgical resection in order to minimize local recurrence and to attempt to evaluate tumor response. The Sloan Kettering T10 protocol of preoperative chemotherapy was the first to use methotrexate-based therapy in high dosages (combination of methotrexate, cisplatin, and doxorubicin [Adriamycin]) given before surgical resection and then tailored postoperatively according to the histologic response of the tumor specimen. It has been effective in significantly improving the 5-year survival rate for osteosarcoma in several different clinical studies. Five-year survival went from 25 to 30% previously to a current rate of approximately 50 to 60%. Other improvements in treatment (e.g., radiology, pathology, surgery) have also contributed to this improved survival rate. The chemotherapy protocols are complex and demand a multidisciplinary setting with real communication between the chemotherapist and the surgeon. Preoperative chemotherapy is also used for Ewing's sarcoma; that is, preoperative chemotherapy followed by surgery and then by maintenance chemotherapy. When a patient with Ewing's sarcoma appears to have a lesion that will have a close or marginal surgical margin, the alternative treatment choice for that patient is chemotherapy and radiation therapy without surgery or chemotherapy with preoperative radiation therapy and surgical resection. The pendulum has more or less swung away from radiation therapy and toward surgical resection for Ewing's sarcoma because of higher recurrence rates after radiation therapy of the primary site alone. Ewing's sarcomas smaller than 8 to 10 cm may be reasonably treated with chemotherapy and radiation therapy in some settings. However, lesions larger than 8 to 10 cm require surgical resection and chemotherapy with or without radiation therapy as the definitive treatment of their primary disease. There are many experienced musculoskeletal tumor surgeons who believe that radiation therapy has no role at all in the treatment of Ewing's sarcoma, especially in the young child with a juxtaepiphyseal lesion that should be treated with an amputation in order to maximize survival. The dilemma of when to use radiation therapy for Ewing's sarcoma persists; however, higher local recurrence rates and greater morbidity in young patients have resulted in little enthusiasm for radiation therapy as the treatment for primary disease, especially in the skeletally immature.

Soft tissue sarcomas are also best treated with preoperative chemotherapy, surgery, and further postoperative chemotherapy. The benefit of preoperative chemotherapy for soft tissue sarcomas is the early systemic treatment of a systemic disease, the minimization of local recurrences, and the opportunity to evaluate the tumor specimen for response to chemotherapy. Most patients who present with a soft tissue sarcoma have microscopic circulating tumor cells in their bloodstream. A delay in the institution of systemic chemotherapy may represent a deleterious delay in systemic treatment. This explains a significant pulmonary metastasis rate despite adequate local control with any treatment. Protocols that call for radiation therapy before surgical resection and chemotherapy for soft tissue sarcomas usually result in a 6-week delay in the institution of chemotherapy and a higher wound complication rate.[16] At the University of Washington, we have therefore elected to give preoperative chemotherapy to all high-grade soft tissue sarcomas followed by restaging and surgical resection after three cycles of chemotherapy. If the surgical margin is marginal, patients also receive postoperative radiation therapy interposed with their postoperative chemotherapy. There are other similar protocols elsewhere that have replaced preoperative radiation therapy with preoperative chemotherapy.

Much has been written and proclaimed about limb-sparing procedures.[43, 155] In fact it is relatively easy to carry out a limb-sparing procedure in the current context of preoperative chemotherapy and to have adequate local control without recurrence at the primary tumor site. It is a much greater challenge, however, to carry out limb-sparing procedures and have a good or excellent functional result after that procedure. Thus, soft tissue involvement may be more important than bone and joint involvement. A good functional result requires well-innervated muscle, adequate soft tissues, and a stable joint. If the soft tissues, strength, and stability of the reconstruction are inadequate, the emotional and financial investment in limb-sparing surgery is probably not warranted. When appropriately carried out, limb-sparing procedures do not increase a patient's risk for local recurrence or diminish the patient's chances for survival.[192] These procedures should, however, be very carefully planned and coordinated in the treatment of all patients. Surgical complications need to be limited enough to enable the resumption of chemotherapy within 2 to 3 weeks after surgery.

Because of the emotional effect of losing an extremity, most patients are naturally drawn to the idea of limb salvage surgery. The responsibility of outlining the true risks and benefits of such a procedure rests with the surgeon, who will transmit his or her own prejudices. The gold standard for comparison is an amputation, and all rehabilitation time should be compared with the limited recovery time of an upper or lower extremity amputation (6 months). These comparisons and differences should be well thought out beforehand so that a clear picture can be presented to the patient. In the final analysis, tumor control should be emphasized, and any attempt at limb salvage should stress stabilization and mobilization in order to maximize functional results. These are challenging problems that require challenging treatments, and only experience and a carefully coordinated team approach will meet that challenge.

All of these treatment protocols are logistically complex and demand a close relationship between the chemotherapist, surgical oncologist, and radiation therapist. The specialized treatment of these patients also requires a clinical nurse specialist to serve as a clinical coordinator and a source of continuity for patients. It is very difficult to treat sarcoma patients only occasionally and do it well.

References and Bibliography

1. Albee FH: The treatment of primary malignant changes of bone by radical resection and bone graft replacement. JAMA *107*:1693, 1936.
2. Allen PW and Enzinger FM: Hemangioma of skeletal muscle. Cancer 29:8, 1972.
3. American Joint Committee for Cancer Staging and End-Results Reporting: Manual for Staging of Cancer. Chicago. AJC, 1977.
4. Arata MA, Peterson HA, and Dahlin DC: Pathologic fractures through non-ossifying fibromas. J Bone Joint Surg *63A*:980–988, 1981.
5. Azzarelli A, Quagliuolo V, Casali P, et al: Preoperative doxorubicin plus ifosfamide in primary soft-tissue sarcomas of the extremities. Cancer Chemother Pharmacol *31* (Suppl):210–212, 1993.
6. Bacci G, Picci P, Gherlinzoni F, et al: Localized Ewing's sarcoma of bone: Ten years' experience at the Istituto Ortopedico Rizzoli in 124 cases treated with multimodal therapy. Eur J Cancer Clin Oncol *21*:163–173, 1985.
7. Barrett WP, Franklin JL, Jackins SE, et al: Total shoulder arthroplasty. J Bone Joint Surg *69A*:865–872, 1987.
8. Barth RJ Jr, Merino MJ, Solomon D, et al: A prospective study of the value of core needle biopsy and fine needle aspiration in the diagnosis of soft tissue masses. Surgory *112*:536–543, 1992.
9. Bauer HC, Brosjo O, Kreicbergs A, et al: Low risk of recurrence of enchondroma and low-grade chondrosarcoma in extremities: 80 patients followed for 2–25 years. Acta Orthop Scand *66*:283–288, 1995.
10. Belsecker JL, Marcove RC, Huvos AG, and Moke V: Aneurysmal bone cysts: A clinicopathologic study of 66 cases. Cancer *26*:615, 1970.
11. Berrettoni BA and Carter JR: Mechanisms of cancer metastasis to bone. Curr Conc Rev *68A*:308–312, 1986.
12. Bjornsson J, Unni KK, Dahlin DC, et al: Clear cell chondrosarcoma of bone: Observations in 47 cases. Am J Surg Pathol *8*:223–230, 1984.
13. Bleyer WA, Haas JE, Feigl P, et al: Improved 3-year disease-free survival in osteogenic sarcoma: Efficacy of adjunctive chemotherapy. J Bone Joint Surg *64B*:233–238, 1982.
14. Bos G, Sim FH, Pritchard DJ, et al: Prosthetic proximal humeral replacement: The Mayo Clinic experience. *In* Enneking WF (ed): Limb Salvage in Musculoskeletal Oncology. (Bristol-Myers/Zimmer Orthopaedic Symposium.) New York: Churchill Livingstone, 1987, p 61.
15. Broders AC: The microscopic grading of cancer. *In* Pack GT and Arrel IM (eds): Treatment of Cancer and Allied Diseases. New York: PB Hoeber, 1964.
16. Bujko K, Suit HD, Springfield DS, et al: Wound healing after preoperative radiation for sarcoma of soft tissues. Surg Gynecol Obstet *176*:124–134, 1993.
17. Burchardt H, Busbee GA III, and Enneking WF: Repair of experimental autologous grafts or cortical bone. J Bone Joint Surg *57A*:814–819, 1975.
18. Burchardt H, Jones H, Glowczewskie F, et al: Freeze dried allogenic segmental cortical bone grafts in dogs. J Bone Joint Surg *60A*:1081–1090, 1978.
19. Burgers JMV, Breur K, van Dobbenburgh OA, et al: Role of metastatectomy without chemotherapy in the management of osteosarcoma in children. Cancer *45*:1664–1668, 1980.
20. Burrows HJ, Wilson JN, and Scales JT: Excision of tumors of humerus and femur, with restoration by internal prostheses. J Bone Joint Surg *57B*:140, 1975.
21. Burwell HN: Resection of the shoulder with humeral suspension for sarcoma involving the scapula. J Bone Joint Surg *47B*:300, 1965.
22. Campanacci M, Bacci G, Bertoni F, et al: The treatment of osteosarcoma of the extremities: Twenty years' experience at the Istituto Ortepedico Rizzoli. Cancer *48*:1569–1581, 1981.
23. Campanacci M, Baldini N, Boriani S, and Sudanese A: Giant-cell tumor of bone. J Bone Joint Surg *69A*:106–114, 1987.
24. Cancer Patient Survival. Report No. 5, U S Dept. of Health, Education and Welfare. Publication No. (NIH) 77–992, 1976.
25. Capanna R, Bertoni F, Bacchini P, et al: Malignant fibrous histiocytoma of bone: The experience at the Rizzoli Institute: Report of 90 cases. Cancer *54*:177–187, 1984.
26. Capanna R, Bertoni F, Bettelli G, et al: Dedifferentiated chondrosarcoma. J Bone Joint Surg *70A*:60–69, 1988.
27. Cofield R: Glenohumeral anthrodesis. J Bone Joint Surg *61A*:673, 1979.
28. Conrad EU III, Enneking WF, and Springfield DS: Giant cell

tumor treated with curettage and cementation. *In* Limb Salvage in Musculoskeletal Oncology. New York: Churchill Livingstone, 1987, p 626.
29. Conrad EU and Enneking WF: Shoulder arthrodesis following tumor resection. Presented to AAOS, February 1986.
30. Dahlin DC and Beaubout JW: Dedifferentiation of low-grade chondrosarcomas. Cancer *28*:461–466, 1971.
31. Dahlin DC and Ivins JC: Benign chondroblastoma: A study of 125 cases. Cancer *30*:401–413, 1972.
32. Dahlin DC, Cupps RE, and Johnson EW Jr: Giant cell tumor: A study of 195 cases. Cancer *25*:1061–1070. 1970.
33. Dahlin DC: Bone Tumors: General Aspects and Data on 6,221 Cases, 3rd ed. Springfield, IL: Charles C Thomas, 1978, pp 3–17.
34. Dahlin DC: Bone Tumors: General Aspects and Data on 6,221 Cases, 3rd ed. Springfield, IL: Charles C Thomas, 1978, pp 156–175.
35. Davis AM, Bell RS, Goodwin PJ: Prognostic factors in osteosarcoma: A critical review. J Clin Oncol *12*:423–431, 1994.
36. DeNancrede CBG: The end results after total excision of the scapula. Ann Surg *50*:1, 1909.
37. DeSantos LA, Murray SA, and Ayaler AG: The value of percutaneous needle biopsy in the management of primary bone tumors. Cancer *43*:735–744, 1979.
38. Durie BGM and Salmon SE: A clinical staging system for multiple myeloma. Correlation of measured myeloma cell mass with presenting clinical features, response to treatment and survival. Cancer *36*:842–854, 1975.
39. Eckardt JJ, Eilber FR, Jinnah RH, and Mirra JM: Endoprosthetic replacement of the scapula, including the shoulder joint, for malignant tumors: A preliminary report. *In* Enneking WF (ed): Limb Salvage in Musculoskeletal Oncology. New York: Churchill Livingstone, 1987, pp 542–553.
40. Eilber FR, Eckhardt J, and Morton DL: Advances in the treatment of sarcomas of the extremity: Current status of limb salvage. Cancer *54*:2695–2701, 1984.
41. Eilber FR, Morton DL, Eckardt JJ, et al: Limb salvage for skeletal and soft tissue sarcomas. Cancer 53:2579, 1984.
42. Eiselsberg A: Zur Heilung Groesserer. Defects der Tibia Durch Gestielte Haut-Periost-KnochenLappen. Arch Klin Chir *55*:435, 1897.
43. Enneking WF, Dunham W, Gebhardt MC, et al: A system for the functional evaluation of reconstructive procedures after surgical treatment of tumors of the musculoskeletal system. Clin Orthop *286*:241–246, 1993.
44. Enneking WF, Spanier SS, and Goodman MA: A system for the surgical staging of musculoskeletal sarcoma. Clin Orthop *153*:106, 1980.
45. Enneking WF, Spanier SS, and Malawer MM: The effect of the anatomic setting on the results of surgical procedures for soft parts sarcoma of the thigh. Cancer *47*:1005–1022, 1981.
46. Enneking WF, Springfield DS, and Gross M: The surgical treatment of parosteal osteosarcoma in long bones. J Bone Joint Surg *67A*:125–135, 1985.
47. Enneking WF: Aneurysmal bone cysts. *In* Musculoskeletal Tumor Surgery. New York: Churchill Livingstone, 1983, pp 1513–1530.
48. Enneking WF: Biopsy. *In* Musculoskeletal Tumor Surgery. New York: Churchill Livingstone, 1983, pp 185–201.
49. Enneking WF: Cartilaginous lesions in bone. *In* Musculoskeletal Tumor Surgery. New York: Churchill Livingstone, 1983, pp 875–997.
50. Enneking WF: Enchondroma. *In* Musculoskeletal Tumor Surgery. New York: Churchill Livingstone, 1983, pp 878–892.
51. Enneking WF: Ewing's sarcoma. *In* Musculoskeletal Tumor Surgery. New York: Churchill Livingstone, 1983, pp 1345–1380.
52. Enneking WF: Fibromatosis. *In* Musculoskeletal Tumor Surgery. New York: Churchill Livingstone, 1983, pp 760–773.
53. Enneking WF: Functional evaluation of reconstruction after tumor resection. Proceedings of the Second International Workshop on the Design and Application of Tumor Prostheses for Bone and Joint Reconstruction, Vienna, 1983.
54. Enneking WF: Lipoma. *In* Musculoskeletal Tumor Surgery. New York: Churchill Livingstone, 1983, pp 1225–1240.
55. Enneking WF: Modified system for functional evaluation of surgical management of musculoskeletal tumors from limb salvage. *In* Enneking WF (ed): Musculoskeletal Oncology. New York: Churchill Livingstone, 1987.
56. Enneking WF: Musculoskeletal Tumor Surgery. New York: Churchill Livingstone, 1983, pp 1–60.
57. Enneking WF: Osseous lesions originating in bone. *In* Musculoskeletal Tumor Surgery. New York: Churchill Livingstone, 1983, pp 1021–1123.
58. Enneking WF: Periosteal chondroma. *In* Musculoskeletal Tumor Surgery. New York: Churchill Livingstone, 1983, pp 913–919.
59. Enneking WF: Primary chondrosarcoma. *In* Musculoskeletal Tumor Surgery. New York: Churchill Livingstone, 1983, pp 945–964.
60. Enneking WF: Simple cyst. *In* Musculoskeletal Tumor Surgery. New York: Churchill Livingstone, 1983, pp 1494–1513.
61. Enneking WF: The issue of the biopsy (Editorial). J Bone Joint Surg *644*:1119–1120, 1982.
62. Enneking WF: Vascular lesions. *In* Musculoskeletal Tumor Surgery. New York: Churchill Livingstone, 1983, pp 1175–1190.
63. Enzinger FM and Weiss SW: Fibromatoses. *In* Soft Tissue Tumors. St. Louis: CV Mosby, 1983, p 45.
64. Enzinger FM and Weiss SW: Liposarcoma. *In* Soft Tissue Tumors. St. Louis: CV Mosby, 1983, p 242.
65. Enzinger FM, and Weiss SW: Malignant fibrohistiocytic tumors. *In* Soft Tissue Tumors. St. Louis: CV Mosby, 1983, p 166.
66. Enzinger FM and Weiss SW: Rhabdomyosarcoma. *In* Soft Tissue Tumors. St. Louis: CV Mosby, 1983, p 338.
67. Fidler IJ and Hart IR: Biological diversity in metastatic neoplasms: Origins and implications. Science *217*:998–1003, 1982.
68. Francis KC and Worcester JN Jr: Radical resection for tumors of the shoulder with preservation of a functional extremity. J Bone Joint Surg *44A*:1423–1429, 1962.
69. Frassica FJ, Unni KK, Beaubout JW, and Sim FH: Differentiated chondrosarcoma. A report of the clinicopathological features and treatment of 78 cases. J Bone Joint Surg *68A*:1197, 1986.
70. Garrison RC, Unni KK, McLeod RA, et al: Chondrosarcoma arising in osteochondroma. Cancer *49*:1890–1897, 1982.
71. Gebhardt MC, McGuire MH, and Mankin HJ: Resection and allograft arthrodesis for malignant bone tumors of the extremity. *In* Enneking WF (ed): Lung Salvage in Musculoskeletal Oncology. New York: Churchill Livingstone, 1987.
72. Gebhart MJ, Lane JM, McCormack RR, and Glasser D: Limb salvage in bone sarcomas—Memorial Hospital experience. Orthopaedics *8*:262, 1985.
73. Giritsky AS, Etcubanas E, and Mark JBD: Pulmonary resection in children with metastatic osteosarcoma. J Thorac Cardiovasc Surg *75*:354–362, 1978.
74. Gitellis S, Bertoni F, Chieti PP, et al: Chondrosarcoma of bone. J Bone Joint Surg *63A*:1248–1256, 1981.
75. Goldblatt J, Sacks S, and Beighton P: The orthopaedic aspects of Gaucher disease. Clin Orthop *137*:208, 1978.
76. Goldenberg RR, Campbell CJ, and Bonfiglio M: Giant-cell tumor of bone: An analysis of two hundred and eighteen cases. J Bone Joint Surg *52A*:619–663, 1970.
77. Goodman MA: Plasma cell tumors. Clin Orthop *204*:87–92, 1986.
78. Goorin AM, Deloney MJ, Lack EE, et al: Prognostic significance of complete surgical resection of pulmonary metastases in patients with osteogenic sarcoma: Analysis of 32 cases. J Clin Oncol *2*:425–430, 1984.
79. Gore DR, Murray MP, Sepic MS, and Gardner GM: Shoulder-muscle strength and range of motion following surgical repair of full-thickness rotator-cuff tears. J Bone Joint Surg *68A*:266, 1986.
80. Griffith M, Betz RR, Mardjetko S, et al: Review of Treatment of Unicameral Bone Cysts. Presented at American Association of Orthopaedic Surgeons, Annual Meeting, Atlanta, Georgia, February 8, 1988.
81. Gross SW: Sarcoma of the long bones: Based upon a study of one hundred and sixty-five cases. Clin Orthop *18*:17–57, 1975.
82. Hardin CA: Interscapulothoracic amputations for sarcomas of the upper extremity. Surgery *49*:355, 1961.
83. Harrington KD: Metastatic disease of the spine. Curr Conc Rev *68A*:1110–1115, 1986.
84. Harris WH, Dudley HR Jr, and Barry RJ: The natural history of fibrous dysplasia: An orthopaedic, pathological and roentgenographic study. J Bone Joint Surg *44A*:207–233, 1962.
85. Henry A: Monostotic fibrous dysplasia. J Bone Joint Surg *51B*:300–306, 1969.
86. Hudson TM, Schakel M, Springfield DS, et al: The comparative value of bone scintigraphy and computed tomography in determin-

ing bone involvement by soft-tissue sarcomas. J Bone Joint Surg *66-A*:1400–1407, 1984

87. Huvos AG, Rosen G, Dabska M, and Marcove RC: Mesenchymal chondrosarcoma: A clinicopathologic analysis of 35 patients with emphasis on treatment. Cancer *51*:1230–1237, 1983.
88. Huvos AG: Bone Tumors: Diagnosis, Treatment and Prognosis. Philadelphia: WB Saunders, 1979.
89. Huvos AG: Chondroblastoma. *In* Bone Tumors: Diagnosis, Treatment and Prognosis. Philadelphia: WB Saunders, 1979.
90. Huvos AG: Osteochondroma and enchondromas. *In* Bone Tumors: Diagnosis, Treatment and Prognosis, Philadelphia: WB Saunders, 1979, pp 139–170.
91. Huvos AG: Osteogenic sarcoma. *In* Huvos AG (ed): Bone Tumors. Philadelphia: WB Saunders, 1979, pp 47–93.
92. Huvos AG: Osteoid osteoma. *In* Bone Tumors: Diagnosis, Treatment and Prognosis. Philadelphia: WB Saunders, 1979, pp 8–46.
93. Imbriglia JE, Negr CS, and Dick HM: Resection of the proximal one half of the humerus in a child for chondrosarcoma. J Bone Joint Surg *60A*:262, 1978.
94. Jaffe HL: Fibrous dysplasia. *In* Tumors and Tumorous Conditions of the Bones and Joint. Philadelphia: Lea & Febiger, 1958, pp 117–142.
95. Jaffe HL: Tumors and Tumorous Conditions of the Bone and Joints. Philadelphia: WB Saunders, 1979.
96. Jaffe N, Prudich J, Knapp J, et al: Treatment of primary osteosarcoma with intra-arterial and intravenous high-dose methotrexate. J Clin Oncol *1*:428–431, 1983.
97. Kanis JA and Gray RE: Long term follow-up observations on treatment in Paget's disease of bone. Clin Orthop *217*:99–125, 1987.
98. Klapp R: Ueber Einen Fall Ausgedehnter Knochev-transplantation. Dtsch Ztschr Chir *54*:576, 1900.
99. Koelbel R, Rohlmann A, and Bergmann G: Biomechanical considerations in the design of a semi-constrained total shoulder replacement. *In* Bayley I and Kessel L (eds): Shoulder Surgery. Berlin: Springer-Verlag, 1982.
100. Kreicbergs A, Boquist L, Borssen B, and Larsson SE: Prognostic factors in chondrosarcoma: A comparative study of cellular DNA content and clinicopathologic features. Cancer *50*:577–583, 1982.
101. Lane JM, Hurson B, Boland PJ, and Glasser DB: Osteogenic sarcoma, ten most common bone and joint tumors. Clin Orthop *204*:93–110, 1986.
102. Levine AM and Rosenberg SA: Alkaline phosphatase levels in osteosarcoma tissue as related to prognosis. Cancer *44*:2291–2293, 1979.
103. Lewis RJ, Marcove RC, and Rosen G: Ewing's sarcoma: Functional effects of radiation therapy. J Bone Joint Surg *59A*:325–331, 1977.
104. Lexer E: Die Gesamte Widerherstellungs Chirurgie. Leipzig: Barth, 1931.
105. Lichtenstein L: Bone Tumors, 4th ed. St. Louis: CV Mosby, 1972.
106. Lichtenstein L: Polyostotic fibrous dysplasia. Arch Surg *36*:874–898, 1938.
107. Lichtenstein L: Preface to the First Edition. General Remarks, Classification of Primary Tumors of Bone. *In* Bone Tumors. St. Louis: CV Mosby, 1959, pp 6–34.
108. Linberg BF: Interscapulothoracic resection for malignant tumors of the shoulder joint region. J Bone Joint Surg *10*:344, 1928.
109. Lindberg RD, Martin RG, Romsdahl MM, and Barkley HT Jr: Conservative surgery and postoperative radiotherapy in 300 adults with soft-tissue sarcomas. Cancer *47*:2391–2397, 1981.
110. Linder L: Reaction of bone to the acute chemical trauma of bone cement. J Bone Joint Surg *59A*:82, 1977.
111. Lugli T: The facts of an exceptional intervention and the prosthetic method. Clin Orthop *133*:215–218, 1978.
112. Malawer MM, Dunham WK, Zaleski T, and Zielinski CJ: Cryosurgery in the Management of Benign (Aggressive) and Low Grade Malignant Tumors of Bone: Analysis of 40 Consecutive Cases. Presented at the meeting of the American Academy of Orthopedic Surgeons (AAOS), New Orleans, February 1986.
113. Malawer MM, McKay DW, Markle B, et al: Analysis of 40 Consecutive Cases of Unicameral Bone Cysts Treated by High Pressure Renograffin Injection and Intracavitary Methylprednisolone Acetate: Prognostic Factors and Hemodynamic Evaluation. 52nd Annual Meeting, American Academy of Orthopaedic Surgeons, Las Vegas, Nevada, 1985.
114. Malawer MM, Sugarbaker PH, et al: The Tikhoff-Linberg procedure and its modifications. *In* Atlas of Extremity Sarcoma. Philadelphia: JB Lippincott, 1984, pp 205–226.
115. Mameghan H, Fisher RJ, O'Gorman-Hughes D, et al: Ewing's sarcoma: Long-term follow-up in 49 patients treated from 1967 to 1989. Int J Radiat Oncol Biol Phys *25*:431–438, 1993.
116. Mankin HJ, Cantley KD, Lipielo L, et al: The biology of human chondrosarcoma. I. Description of the cases, grading, and biochemical analyses. J Bone Joint Surg *62*:160–176, 1980.
117. Mankin HJ, Connor JF, Schiller AL, et al: Grading of bone tumors by analysis of nuclear DNA content using flow cytometry. J Bone Joint Surg *67A*:404–413, 1985.
118. Mankin HJ, Doppelt SH, Sullivan TR, and Tomford WW: Osteoarticular and intercalary allograft transplantation in the management of malignant tumors of bone cancer. Cancer *50*:613–630, 1982.
119. Mankin HJ, Fogelson FS, Thrasher AA, et al: Massive resection and allograft transplantation in the treatment of malignant bone tumors. N Engl J Med *294*:1247–1255, 1976.
120. Mankin HJ, Lange TA, and Spanier SS: The hazards of biopsy in patients with malignant primary bone and soft-tissue tumors. J Bone Joint Surg *61A*:1121–1127, 1982.
121. Marcove RC, Lewis MM, and Huvos AG: En bloc upper humeral-interscapular resection: The Tikhoff-Linberg procedure. Clin Orthop *124*:219–228, 1977.
122. Marcove RC, Lyden JP, Huvos AC, and Bullough PB: Giant cell tumor treated by cryosurgery. A report of twenty-five cases. J Bone Joint Surg *55*:1633–1644, 1973.
123. Marcove RC, Mike V, Hutter RVP, et al: Chondrosarcoma of the pelvis and upper end of femur. J Bone Joint Surg *54*:561–572, 1972.
124. Marcove RC, Stovell P, Huvos AC, et al: The use of cryosurgery in the treatment of low and medium grade chondrosarcoma: A preliminary report. Clin Orthop *122*:147–156, 1977.
125. Marcove RC, Weis LD, Vaghaiwall MR, et al: Cryosurgery in the treatment of giant cell tumors of bone. A report of 52 consecutive cases. Cancer *41*:957–969, 1978.
126. Marcove RC: A 17-year review of cryosurgery in the treatment of bone tumors. Clin Orthop *163*:231–233, 1982.
127. Marhade G, Monastryrski J, and Steuner B: Scapulectomy for malignant tumors, function and shoulder strength in five patients. Acta Orthop Scand *56*:332, 1985.
128. Martini N, Huvos AG, Mike V, et al: Multiple pulmonary resections in the treatment of osteogenic sarcoma. Ann Thorac Surg *12*:271–280, 1971.
129. Matsen FA III: Personal communication, January 1988.
130. Matsuno T, Unni KK, McLeod RA, and Dahlin DC: Telangiectatic osteosarcoma. Cancer *38*:2538–2547, 1976.
131. Maurer HM, Moon T, Donaldson M, et al: The intergroup rhabdomyosarcoma study. Cancer *40*:2015, 1977.
132. McDonald DJ, Sim FH, McLeod RA, and Dahlin DC: Giant-cell tumor of bone. J Bone Joint Surg *68A*:235–242, 1986.
133. McKenzie DH: The fibromatoses: A clinicopathologic concept. BMJ *4*:777, 1972.
134. Milgram JW: Synovial osteochondromatosis. J Bone Joint Surg *59A*:792–901, 1977.
135. Miser J, Kinsella T, Tsokos M, et al: High response rate of recurrent childhood tumors to etoposide (VP16), ifosfamide (IFOS0, and mesna (MES) uroprotection. Proc Soc Clin Oncol 5:209, 1986.
136. Moore TM, Meyers MH, Patzakis MJ, et al: Closed biopsy of musculoskeletal lesions. J Bone Joint Surg *61*:375–380, 1979.
137. Mullins F, Berard CW, and Eisenberg SH: Chondrosarcoma following synovial chondromatosis. Cancer *18*:1180, 1965.
138. Murray JA, Jessup K, Romsdahl M, et al: Limb salvage surgery in osteosarcoma: Early experience at M.D. Anderson Hospital. Proceedings of NIH Consensus Development Conference on Limb-Sparing Treatment of Adult Soft Tissue Sarcomas and Osteosarcoma. U S Dept. of Health and Human Services. Public Health Services. NIH Cancer Treatment Symposia, Vol 3, 1985.
139. National Institutes of Health, Consensus Development Panel: Limb-sparing treatment of adult soft-tissue sarcomas and osteosarcomas. JAMA *254*:1791–1794, 1985.
140. Neer CS, Francis KC, Kiernan HA, et al: Current concepts in the treatment of solitary unicameral bone cysts. Clin Orthop *97*:40–51, 1973.
141. Neer CS, Watson KC, and Stanton FJ: Recent experience in total shoulder replacement. J Bone Joint Surg *64A*:319–337, 1982.

142. Nicholson HS, Mulvihill JJ, and Byrne J: Late effects of therapy in adult survivors of osteosarcoma and Ewing's sarcoma. Med Pediatr Oncol *20*:6–12, 1992.
143. Ogilvie-Harris DJ, Hans CB, and Fornasier VL: Pseudomalignant myositis ossificans: Heterotopic new bone formation without a history of trauma. J Bone Joint Surg *62-A*:1274–1283, 1980.
144. Oppenheimer WL and Galleno H: Operative treatment versus steroid injection in the management of unicameral bone cysts. J Pediatr Orthop *4*:1–7, 1984.
145. Orthopaedic Practice in the U.S. 1986–1987. American Academy of Orthopaedic Surgeons, Department of Professional Affairs, Chicago, 1987.
146. Pack GT, McNeer G, and Coley BL: Interscapulo-thoracic amputation for malignant tumors of the upper extremity. Surg Gynecol Obstet *74*:161, 1942.
147. Papaioannou AN and Francis KD: Scapulectomy for the treatment of primary malignant tumors of the scapula. Clin Orthop *41*:125, 1965.
148. Parrish FF: Treatment of bone tumors by total excision and replacement with massive autologous and homologous grafts. J Bone Joint Surg *48A*:968–990, 1966.
149. Paulson DF, Perez CA, and Anderson T: Cancer of the kidney and ureter. *In* DeVita VT, Hellman S, and Rosenberg SA (ed): Cancer: Principles and Practice of Oncology, 2nd ed. Philadelphia: JB Lippincott, 1985, pp 895–905.
150. Persson BM and Wouters HW: Curettage and acrylic cementation in surgery of giant cell tumors of bone. Clin Orthop *120*:125–133, 1976.
151. Persson BM, Ekelund L, Lovdahl R, and Gunterberg B: Favourable results of acrylic cementation for giant cell tumors. Acta Orthop Scand *55*:209–214, 1984.
152. Phemister DB: Conservative bone surgery in the treatment of bone tumors. Surg Gynecol Obstet *70*:355, 1940.
153. Poppen NK and Walker PS: Forces at the glenohumeral joint in abduction. Clin Orthop *135*:165–170, 1978.
154. Post M, Haskell SS, and Jablon M: Total shoulder replacement with a constrained prosthesis. J Bone Joint Surg *62A*:327–335, 1980.
155. Pstma A, Kingma A, De Ruiter JH, et al: Quality of life in bone tumor patients comparing limb salvage and amputation of the lower extremity. J Surg Oncol *51*:47–51, 1992.
156. Price CHG and Golde W: Paget's sarcoma of bone: A study of eighty cases. J Bone Joint Surg *51B*:205–224, 1969.
157. Pritchard DJ, Lunke RJ, Taylor WF, et al: Chondrosarcoma: A clinicopathologic and statistical analysis. Cancer *45*:149–157, 1980.
158. Proceedings of NIH Consensus Development Conference on Limb-Sparing Treatment of Adult Soft Tissue Sarcomas and Osteosarcoma. U S Dept. of Health and Human Services, Public Health Services, NIH Cancer Treatment Symposia, Vol 3, 1985.
159. Rao A, Srinvasa V, and Vincent J: Pigmented villonodular synovitis (giant-cell tumor of the tendon sheath and synovial membrane): A review of eighty-one cases. J Bone Joint Surg *66A*:76–94, 1984.
160. Reszel PA, Soule EH, and Coventry MB: Liposarcomas of the extremities and limb girdles: A study of 222 cases. J Bone Joint Surg *48A*:229, 1966.
161. Rock M: Intercalary allograft and custom Neer prosthesis after en block resection of the proximal humerus. *In* Enneking WF (ed): Limb Salvage in Musculoskeletal Oncology. (Bristol-Myers/Zimmer Orthopaedic Symposium.) New York: Churchill Livingstone, 1987, p 586.
162. Rock MG, Pritchard DJ, Reiman HM, et al: Extra-abdominal desmoid tumors. J Bone Joint Surg *66A*:1369–1374, 1984.
163. Rock MG, Sim FH, and Chao EYS: Limb salvage procedures for primary bone tumors of the shoulder. *In* Bateman JE and Welsh RP (eds): Surgery of the Shoulder. Philadelphia: BC Decker, 1984.
164. Rosen G, Caparros B, Huvos AC, et al: Preoperative chemotherapy for osteogenic sarcoma: Selection of postoperative adjuvant chemotherapy based upon the response of the primary tumor to preoperative chemotherapy. Cancer *49*:1221–1230, 1982.
165. Rosen G, Caparros B, Nirenberg A, et al: Ewing's sarcoma. Ten-year experience with adjuvant chemotherapy. Cancer *47*:2204–2213, 1981.
166. Rosen G: Neoadjuvant chemotherapy for osteogenic sarcoma. A model for treatment of malignant neoplasm. *In* Recent Results in Cancer Research, Vol 103. Berlin: Springer-Verlag, 1986, pp 48–157.
167. Rosenberg SA, Fyle MW, Conkle D, et al: The treatment of osteosarcoma. II. Aggressive resection of pulmonary metastases. Cancer Treat Rep *63*:753–762, 1979.
168. Rosenberg SA, Kent H, Cost J, et al: Prospective randomized evaluation of the role of limb sparing surgery, radiation therapy, and adjuvant chemoimmunotherapy in the treatment of adult soft tissue sarcomas. Surgery *84*:62–69, 1978.
169. Rosenberg SA, Suit FD, and Baker LH: Sarcoma of soft tissue. *In* DeVita VT, Hellman S, and Rosenberg SA (eds): Cancer: Principles and Practice of Oncology, 2nd ed. Philadelphia: JB Lippincott, 1985, pp 1243–1293.
170. Rougraff BT, Kneisl JS, and Simon MA: Skeletal metastases of unknown origin. A prospective study of a diagnostic strategy. J Bone Joint Surg *75A*:1276–1281, 1993.
171. Rowe CR: Re-evaluation of the position of the arm in arthrodesis of the shoulder in the adult. J Bone Joint Surg *56A*:913, 1974.
172. Rubin P: Clinical Oncology, 6th ed. American Cancer Society, 1983.
173. Rydholm A: Management of patients with soft-tissue tumors: Strategy developed at a regional oncology center. Acta Orthop Scand Suppl *203*:3–76, 1983.
174. Ryerson EW: Excision of the scapula: Report of a case with excellent functional result. JAMA *113*:1958, 1939.
175. Saddegh MK, Lindholm J, Lundberg A, et al: Staging of soft-tissue sarcomas. Prognostic analysis of clinical and pathological features. J Bone Joint Surg *74B*:495–500, 1992.
176. Salzer M, et al: A bioceramic endoprosthesis for the replacement of the proximal humerus. Arch Orthop Trauma Surg *93*:169, 1979.
177. Salzer M, Zweymueller K, Locke H, et al: Further experimental and clinical experience with aluminum oxide endoprosthesis. J Biomed Mater Res *10*:847, 1976.
178. Samilson RL, Morris JM, and Thompson RW: Tumors of the scapula: A review of the literature and an analysis of 31 cases. Clin Orthop *58*:105, 1968.
179. Scaglietti O, Marchetti PG, and Bartolozzi P: The effects of methylprednisolone acetate in the treatment of bone cysts. Results of three years follow-up. J Bone Joint Surg *61*:200–204, 1970.
180. Schajowicz F and Derquie JC: Puncture biopsy in lesions of the locomotor system: Review and results in 4050 cases, including 941 vertebral punctures. Cancer *21*:5331–5487, 1968.
181. Schaller RT Jr, Haas J, Schaller J, et al: Improved survival in children with osteosarcoma following resection of pulmonary metastases. J Pediatr Surg *17*:546–550, 1982.
182. Schauffler RM: Transplant of the upper extremity of the fibula to replace the upper extremity of the humerus. J Bone Joint Surg *8*:723, 1926.
183. Schmale GA, Conrad EU III, and Raskind WH: The natural history of hereditary multiple exostoses. J Bone Joint Surg *76A*:986–992, 1994.
184. Schreuder HWB, Conrad EU III, Bruckner JD, et al: The treatment of simple bone cysts in children with curettage and cryosurgery. J Pediatr Orthop *17*(6), 1997.
185. Sekera J, Ramach W, Pongracz N, et al: Experience with ceramic and metal implants for the proximal humerus in cases of malignant bone tumor. *In* Enneking WF (ed): Limb Salvage in Musculoskeletal Oncology (Bristol-Myers/Zimmer Orthopaedic Symposium.) New York: Churchill Livingstone, 1987, p 211.
186. Shapiro F: Ollier's disease: An assessment of angular deformity, shortening, and pathological fracture in twenty-one patients. J Bone Joint Surg *64A*:95–103, 1982.
187. Shibata T: Reconstruction of skeletal defects after the Tikhoff-Linberg procedure using aluminum ceramic endoprosthesis and stabilization of the shoulder. *In* Enneking WF (ed): Limb Salvage in Musculoskeletal Oncology (Bristol-Myers/Zimmer Orthopaedic Symposium.) New York: Churchill Livingstone, 1987, p 553.
188. Shiu MH, Castro EB, Hajdu SI, and Fortner JG: Results of surgical and radiation therapy in the treatment of liposarcoma arising in an extremity. AJR Am J Roentgenol *123*:577, 1975.
189. Sim FH, Chao EYS, Prichard DJ, and Salzer M: Replacement of the proximal humerus with a ceramic prosthesis: A preliminary report. Clin Orthop *146*:161, 1980.
190. Simon MA and Bos GD: Epiphyseal extension of metaphyseal osteosarcoma in skeletally immature individuals. J Bone Joint Surg *62-A*:195–204, 1980.
191. Simon MA and Hecht JD: Invasion of joints by primary bone sarcomas in adults. Cancer *50*:1649–1655, 1982.

192. Simon MA, Aschliman MA, Thomas N, and Mankin HJ. Limb-salvage treatment versus amputation for osteosarcoma of the distal end of the femur. J Bone Joint Surg *68A*:1331–1337, 1986.
193. Simon MA, Spanier SS, and Enneking WF: The management of soft tissue tumors of the extremities. J Bone Joint Surg *60*.317, 1976.
194. Simon MA: Biopsy of musculoskeletal tumors. J Bone Joint Surg *64A*:1253–1257, 1982.
195. Simon MA: Current concepts review: Causes of increased survival of patients with osteosarcoma: Current controversies. J Bone Joint Surg *66A*:306–310, 1984.
196. Sledge CB, Atcher RW, Shoetkeoff S, et al: Intra-articular radiation synovectomy. Clin Orthop *182*:37–40, 1984.
197. Smith WS and Struhl S: Replantation of an autoclaved autogenous segment of bone for treatment of chondrosarcoma. Long-term follow-up. J Bone Joint Surg *70A*:70, 1988.
198. Springfield D: Liposarcoma. CORR *289*:50–57, 1993.
199. Springfield DS and Pagliarulo C: Fractures of long bones previously treated for Ewing's sarcoma. J Bone Joint Surg *67A*:477–481, 1985.
200. Stewart MJ, Gilmer WS, and Edmonson AS: Fibrous dysplasia of bone. J Bone Joint Surg *44B*;302–318, 1962.
201. Suit HD, Proppe KH; Mankin HJ, et al: Preoperative radiation therapy for sarcoma of soft tissue. Cancer *47*:2267–2274, 1981.
202. Sundaram M, McGuire MH, Herbold DR, et al: Magnetic resonance imaging in planning limb-salvage surgery for primary malignant tumors of bone. J Bone Joint Surg *68-A*.809–819, 1986.
203. Sweet D, Mass DP, Simon MA, and Shapiro CM: Histiocytic lymphoma of bone: Current strategy for orthopaedic surgeons. J Bone Joint Surg *63A*:79–84, 1981.
204. Thomas PRM, Perez CA, Neff JR, et al. The management of Ewing's sarcoma: Role of radiotherapy in local tumor control. Cancer Treat Rep *68*:703–710, 1984.
205. Toni A, Neff JR, Sudanese A, et al: The role of surgical therapy in patients with nonmetastatic Ewing's sarcoma of the limbs. Clin Orthop *286*:225–240, 1993.
206. Turnbull A, Blumencranz P, and Fortner J: Scapulectomy for soft tissue sarcoma. Can J Surg *21*:37, 1981.
207. Unni KK, Dahlin DC, and Beabout JW: Periosteal osteogenic sarcoma. Cancer *37*:2467–2485, 1976.
208. Unni KK, Dahlin DC, McLeod RA, et al: Interosseous well-differentiated osteosarcoma. Cancer *40*:1337–1347, 1977.
209. Weiland AJ, Daniel RK, and Riley CH: Application of the free vascularized bone graft in the treatment of malignant or aggressive bone tumors. Johns Hopkins Med J *140*:85, 1977.
210. Weiss L and Gilbert HA: Bone Metastases. Boston: GK Hall, 1981.
211. Weiss SW and Enzinger FM: Malignant fibrous histiocytoma: An analysis of 200 cases. Cancer *41*:2250–2266, 1978.
212. Wilkins RM, Pritchard DJ, Burgert EO, and Unni KK: Ewing's sarcoma of bone—experience with 140 patients. Cancer *58*:2551–2555, 1986.
213. Wilson PD and Lance EM: Surgical reconstruction of the skeleton following segmental resection for bone tumors. J Bone Joint Surg *47A*:1629, 1965.
214. Winkler K, Beron C, Kotz R, et al: Neoadjuvant chemotherapy for osteogenic sarcoma: Results of a cooperative German/Austrian study. J Clin Oncol 2:617–624, 1984.
215. Wright PH, Sim FH, Soule EH, and Taylor WF: Synovial sarcoma. J Bone Joint Surg *64A*:112–122, 1982.

CHAPTER

23

ROBIN R. RICHARDS, M.D., F.R.C.S.(C.)

Sepsis of the Shoulder: Molecular Mechanisms and Pathogenesis

General principles in the pathogenesis of shoulder sepsis are similar to those pertaining to all intra-articular infections. There are three fundamental pathways for infection to enter a joint: (1) spontaneous hematogenous seeding via the synovial blood supply, (2) contiguous spread from adjacent metaphyseal osteomyelitis via the intra-articular portion of the metaphysis, and (3) penetration of the joint by trauma, therapy, or surgery (Fig. 23–1). Susceptibility to infection is determined by the adequacy of the host defenses. Spontaneous bacteremia, trauma, and surgery are common opportunities for infection. Shoulder infection is uncommon, however, because of normal defense mechanisms, the use of antibiotic prophylaxis, and a good local blood supply.

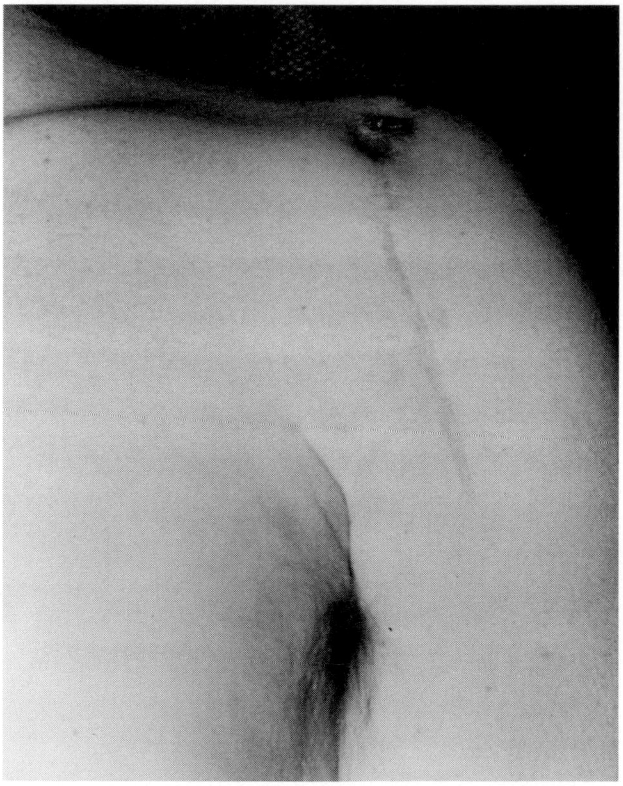

Figure 23–1

Sinus communicating with a prosthetic shoulder joint. This patient developed a chronic low-grade infection after undergoing a total shoulder arthroplasty.

Certain patient groups with immune system depression or aberrations are at increased risk for infection. Patients with rheumatoid disease manifest a spontaneous and somewhat cryptic sepsis in joints.[65, 80] Diabetics, infants, children, the aged, patients with vascular disease, drug abusers, and patients with human immunodeficiency virus (HIV) are at increased risk to specific organisms, as are patients with hematologic dyscrasia and neoplastic disease. Joint infection requires a threshold inoculum of bacteria and is facilitated by damaged tissue, foreign body substrata, the acellularity of cartilage surfaces, and the presence of receptors. Total joint arthroplasty is at potential risk because of the presence of metallic and polymeric biomaterials and the decreased phagocytic ability of macrophages in the presence of methyl methacrylate. Biomaterials and adjacent damaged tissues and substrata are readily colonized by bacteria in a polysaccharide biofilm that is resistant to macrophage attack and antibiotic penetration.[44, 55, 58, 64] With antibiotic prophylaxis, published infection rates of total joint arthroplasty are low—1 to 5%, depending on the device and the location.[26, 28, 60, 103, 139] However, once infected, biomaterials and damaged tissues are exceedingly resistant to treatment.

Clinical infection in normal or immunosuppressed patients involves the maturation of an inoculum of known pathogens (e.g., *Staphylococcus aureus* or *Pseudomonas aeruginosa*) or the transformation of nonpathogens (*S. epidermidis*) to a septic focus of adhesive, "slime-producing," virulent organisms. This transformation occurs in the presence of, and is potentiated by, the surface of biomaterials[54, 55, 57, 58, 64, 136] or damaged tissue[100] and is also particularly virulent on acellular, susceptible, and defenseless cartilage matrix surfaces.[144]

HISTORY

Experiences in shoulder infection have paralleled those of other large joints, although with less frequency. The work of outstanding scientists, such as Louis Pasteur (1822 to 1895), Joseph Lister (1827 to 1912), and Robert Koch (1843 to 1910), in the last quarter of the 19th century, ushered in the modern age of bacteriology and an early understanding of intra-articular sepsis. Koch's experiments with culture media at the Berlin Institute for Infectious Disease verified the role of the tubercle bacillus in musculoskeletal infection. In 1893, Péan attempted to reconstruct the tuberculous shoulder of a 30-year-old man using a prosthetic replacement made of platinum and rubber.

The latter part of the 19th century also saw the development of the concept of antisepsis. Lister maintained that sepsis was the main obstacle to significant advances in surgery. He documented a dramatic drop in cases of empyema, erysipelas, hospital gangrene, and surgical infection through the use of antiseptic techniques. Although the popularization of antiseptic technique in the surgical theater greatly reduced the rate of complication owing to infection, it was not until the 1930s that specific antimicrobial therapy was discovered. In 1935, a German bacteriologist, Gerhard Domagk, discovered that sulfonamides protected mice against fatal doses of hemolytic staphylococci. Sulfonamides were soon employed for infections in patients with excellent results.

Although the history of bacteriology and subsequent antiseptic techniques in surgery and the development of antibiotics are well documented, very little of the early literature relates specifically to infections about the shoulder. In Codman's book, *The Shoulder*, published in 1934, infection of the shoulder and, in particular, osteomyelitis of the proximal humerus were considered very rare lesions.[25] Codman cited a report by King and Holmes in 1927 in which a review of 450 consecutive symptomatic shoulders evaluated at the Massachusetts General Hospital revealed five cases of tuberculosis of the shoulder, one luetic infection of the shoulder, three unspecified shoulder infections, and two cases of osteomyelitis of the proximal humerus. The rarity of tubercular lesions of the shoulder was documented through the results of four large series of tuberculosis involving the musculoskeletal system (Townsend, 21 of 3244 cases; Whitman, 38 of 1833 cases; Young, 7 of 5680 cases; Billroth, 14 of 1900 cases). As microbial culturing and identification techniques developed in the early 20th century, streptococcal and staphylococcal species were more frequently identified as the causative agents in shoulder infection.

SEPTIC ANATOMY OF THE SHOULDER

A review of shoulder anatomy reveals specific structural relationships that are intimately linked to the pathogenesis of joint sepsis and osteomyelitis. The circulation of the proximal humerus and periarticular structures (particularly the synovium) and the intricate system of bursae about the shoulder are critical factors.

Classically, diverse, age-dependent presentations of hematogenous osteomyelitis and septic arthritis of the shoulder (and other large joints such as the hip and knee) have been attributed to the vascular development about the growth plate and epiphysis. The most detailed studies of the vascular development in this area have been done on the proximal femur but are analogous to the same development about the proximal humerus. Experimental work by Trueta[141] demonstrated that, before 8 months of age, there are direct vascular communications across the growth plate between the nutrient artery system and the epiphyseal ossicle. This observation was believed to account for the frequency of infection involving the epiphyseal ossicle and subsequent joint sepsis in infants. At some point between 8 months and 18 months of age (an average of 1 year), the growth plate forms a complete barrier to direct vascular communication between the metaphysis and epiphysis. The last vestiges of the nutrient artery turn down acutely at the growth plate and reach sinusoidal veins. At this point the blood flow "slows down," creating an ideal medium for the proliferation of pathogenic bacteria.[142] In addition, there is evidence that the afferent tracts of the metaphyseal vessels have no or insufficient phagocytizing properties.[134]

In the adult shoulder, the intra-articular extent of the metaphysis is located in the inferior sulcus and is intracapsular for approximately 10 to 12 mm.[24] Infection of the proximal metaphysis, once established, may gain access to the shoulder joint via the haversian and Volkmann canals at the nonperiosteal zone (Fig. 23–2). With obliteration of the growth plate at skeletal maturity, anastomoses of the metaphyseal and epiphyseal circulation are again established.

In his study of the vascular development of the proximal femur, Chung did not find evidence of direct communications between the metaphyseal and epiphyseal circulation across the growth plate in any age group.[22] Chung's work demonstrated a persistent extraosseous anastomosis between metaphyseal and epiphyseal circulation on the surface of the perichondral ring. He found no evidence of vessels penetrating the growth plate in the infant population and attributed apparent changes in the arterial supply with age to enlargement of the neck and ossification center.

Branches of the suprascapular artery and the circumflex scapular branch of the subscapular artery from the scapular side of the shoulder anastomose with the anterior and posterior humeral circumflex arteries from the humeral side of the shoulder. This anastomotic system supplies the proximal humerus by forming an extra-articular and extracapsular arterial ring. Vessels from this ring traverse the capsule and form an intra-articular synovial ring. This fine anastomosis of vessels in the synovial membrane is located at the junction of the synovium and the articular cartilage over an area that has been called the transition zone.[122] This subsynovial ring of vessels was first described by William Hunter in 1743 and named the circulus articuli vasculosus.[73] At the transitional zone, synovial cells become flattened over this periarticular vascular fringe. Fine arterioles at this boundary acutely loop back toward the periphery. Again, blood flow at this level may be slowed, which provides a site for the establishment of an inoculum of pathogenic organisms. Rather than hemodynamic changes, however, it is more probable that receptor-specific, microbe-to-cell surface interactions potentiate the infectious process.

Another consideration in the septic anatomy of the

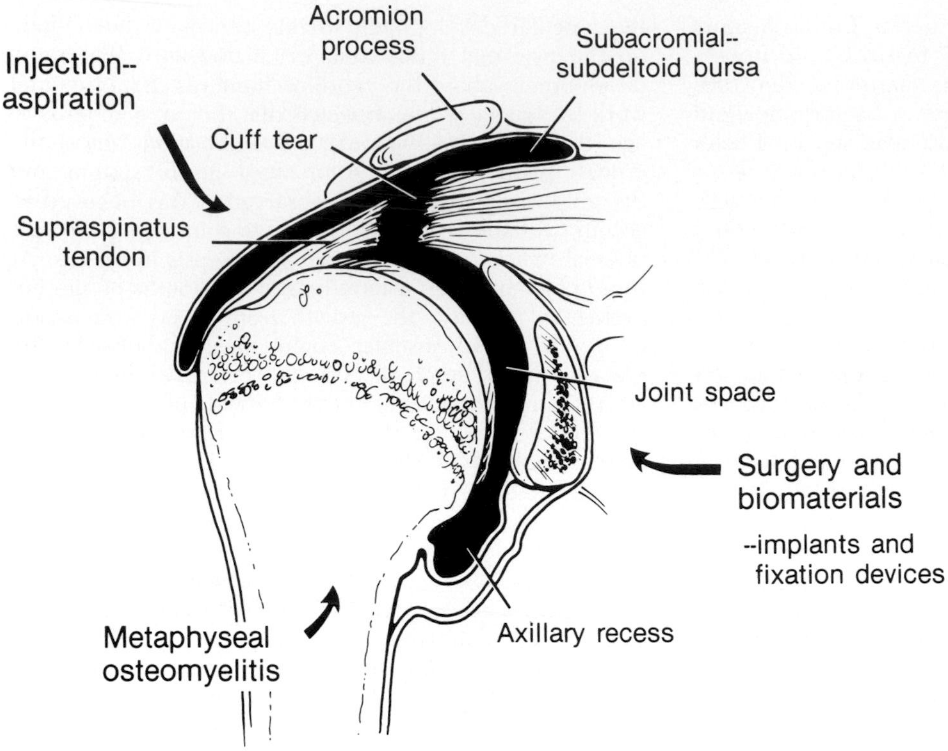

Figure 23–2

Routes of infection for intra-articular sepsis.

shoulder is the communication between the joint space and capsule and the system of bursae about the shoulder. Anteriorly, there is direct communication between the capsule and the subscapular bursa located just below the coracoid process. Posteriorly, the capsule communicates with the infraspinatus bursa. A third opening in the capsule occurs at the point at which the tendon of the long head of the biceps enters the shoulder. From the transverse humeral ligament to its entry into the shoulder capsule, the tendon of the long head of the biceps is enveloped in folds of synovium. Intentional or inadvertent injection of the subscapular bursa, the infraspinatus bursa, or the tendon of the long head of the biceps provides the potential for intra-articular bacterial inoculation. Injection of the subdeltoid or subacromial bursa in the presence of a rotator cuff tear (degenerative or traumatic) provides another potential setting for bacterial contamination of the joint.

Ward and Eckardt reported on four subacromial/subdeltoid bursa abscesses.[149] Three of the four patients were chronically ill and debilitated and in these patients the bursal abscesses coexisted with clinically diagnosed mild to resolving glenohumeral pyarthrosis. The symptoms and signs of these abscesses were minimal in all four patients. Ward and Eckardt found that computed tomography (CT) or magnetic resonance imaging (MRI) may help to detect abscesses and plan treatment.

Microanatomy and Cell Biology

The articular cavity is unique because the surface of hyaline cartilage, although noncrystalline, is essentially acellular and consists of horizontally arranged collagen fibers in proteoglycan macromolecules. The boundaries of joint cavities are composed of a richly vascularized cellular synovial tissue. Recent studies indicate that collagen fibers and the glycoprotein matrix, rather than the synovium, are the target substrata for microbial adhesion and colonization.[132, 144]

Synovial cells are somewhat phagocytic and appear to combat infection as part of the inflammatory response. Microscopic examination of infected joints in a rabbit animal model indicated predominant colonization of cartilaginous, rather than synovial, surfaces.[144] Receptors for collagen have been identified on the cell surfaces of certain strains of *S. aureus*.[132] The infrequent occurrence of bacteria on synovial tissue may reflect innate resistance of synovial cells to colonization, the lack of appropriate synovial ligands, or functional host defense mechanisms at a synovial level.[12]

The synovial intima consists of several layers of cells designated types A and B.[16] Type A cells are predominant and have phagocytic qualities. Type B cells have pinocytic characteristics. The subintimal vascularized layer contains fibroadipose tissue, lymphatic vessels, and nerves.[122] Ultrastructural studies of the synovial subintimal vessels reveal that gaps between endothelial cells are bridged by a fine membrane.[122] There is no epithelial tissue in the synovial lining and, therefore, no structural barrier (basement membrane) to prevent the spread of infection from synovial blood vessels to the joint. The synovial lining in the transition zone is rarely more than three or four cell layers thick, which places the synovial blood vessels in a superficial position and makes them susceptible to damage from relatively minor trauma.

Intra-articular hemorrhage caused by trauma, combined with transient bacteremias, may be implicated as a factor in the pathogenesis of joint sepsis. Random hematogenous seeding allows bacterial penetration of synovial vessels, producing an effusion consisting primarily of neutrophils that release cartilage-destroying lysosomal enzymes.[16] Staphylococci also release enzymes and toxins that destroy tissue matrix and cells.

Articular (hyaline) cartilage varies from 2 to 4 mm in thickness in the large joints of adults. This avascular, aneural tissue consists of a relatively small number of cells and chondrocytes and an abundant extracellular matrix. The extracellular matrix contains collagen and a ground substance composed of carbohydrate and noncollagenous protein and has a high water content. The chondrocytes are responsible for the synthesis and degradation of matrix components and are therefore ultimately responsible for the biomechanical and biologic properties of articular cartilage. Collagen produced by the chondrocytes accounts for more than one half of the dry weight of adult articular cartilage (type II). Individual collagen fibers, with a characteristic periodicity of 640 Å, vary from 300 to 800 Å in diameter, depending on their distance from the articular surface.[122]

The principal component of the ground substance produced by chondrocytes is a protein polysaccharide complex called proteoglycan. The central organizing molecule of proteoglycan is hyaluronic acid. Numerous glycosaminoglycans (mainly chondroitin sulfate and keratin sulfate) are covalently bound from this central strand. Glycosaminoglycans carry considerable negative charge. The highly ordered array of electronegativity on the proteoglycan molecule interacts with large numbers of water molecules (small electric dipole). Approximately 75% of the wet weight of articular cartilage is water, the majority of which is structured by the electrostatic forces of the proteoglycan molecule.[122]

The structure of articular cartilage varies relative to its distance from the free surface. For purposes of description, the tissue has been subdivided into zones that run parallel to the articular surface. Electron microscopy of the free surface reveals a dense network of collagen fibers (40 to 120 Å in diameter) that is arranged tangentially to the load-bearing surface and at approximately right angles to each other. This dense, mat-like arrangement, the lamina obscurans, is approximately 3 μm thick. No cells have been identified in this layer.[122, 143]

Zone 1 contains large bundles of collagen fibers that are approximately 340 Å thick and lie parallel to the joint surface and at right angles to each other (Fig. 23–3).[122, 143] This zone, the lamina splendins, has little or no intervening ground substance and contains the highest density of collagen. Chondrocytes in zone 1 are ellipsoid in shape and are oriented parallel to the articular surface. They

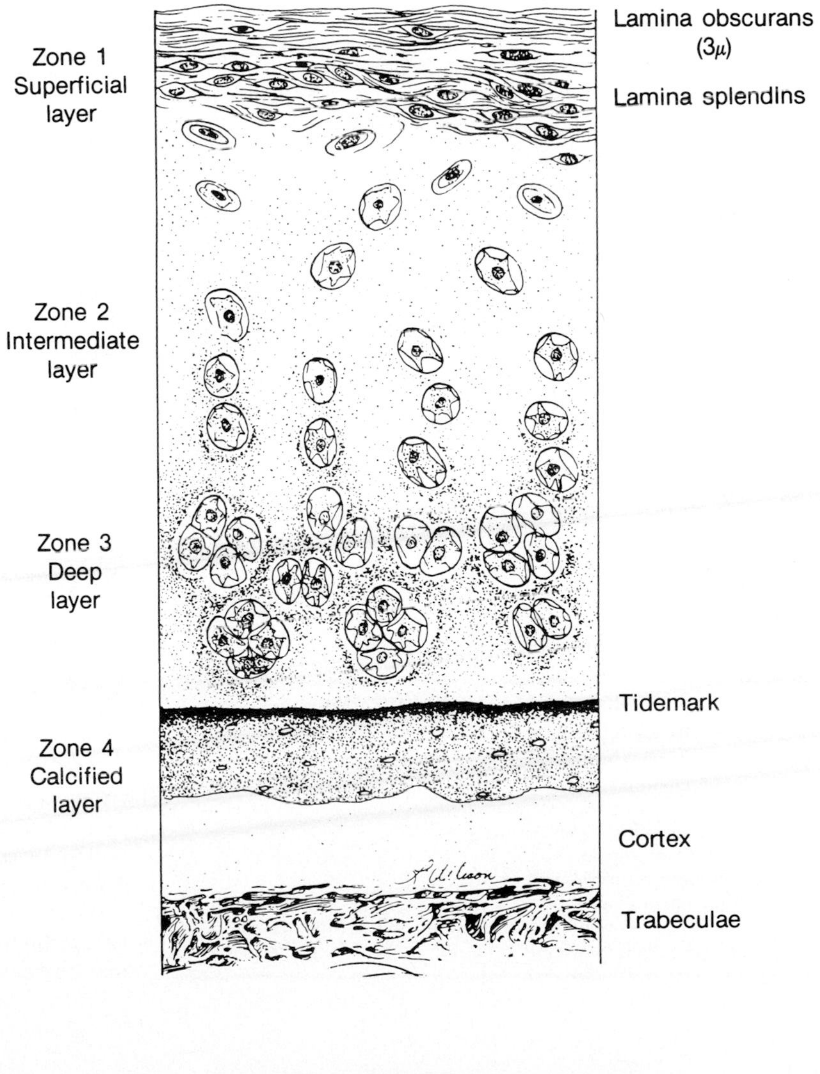

Figure 23–3

The zones of adult articular cartilage. (Modified with permission from Turek SL: Orthopaedics: Principles and Their Application. Philadelphia: JB Lippincott, 1977.)

show little electron microscopic evidence of metabolic activity.

In zone 2, the collagen consists of individual, randomly oriented fibers of varying diameters. The chondrocytes in zone 2 tend to be more spherical and larger than those of zone 1, with abundant mitochondria and extensive endoplasmic reticulum, suggesting greater metabolic activity. The proteoglycan:collagen ratio in zone 2 is much higher than that near the surface.

In zone 3, the collagen fibers are thicker, often in the range of 1400 Å, and tend to form a more orderly meshwork that lies radial to the articular surface. The chondrocytes in zone 3 are larger and tend to be arranged in columns, often appearing in groups of two to eight cells. The cells are noted to have enlarged Golgi complexes, many mitochondria, and an extensively developed endoplasmic reticulum, indicating a high degree of metabolic activity.

Bone is a composite structure incorporating calcium hydroxyapatite crystals in a collagen matrix grossly similar to synthetic composites or to partially crystalline polymers. Devitalized bone provides a passive substratum for bacterial colonization and the ultimate incorporation of its proteinaceous and mineral constituents as bacterial metabolites.[57, 59, 134] *S. aureus* binds to bone sialoprotein, a glycoprotein found in joints, and it produces chondrocyte proteases that hydrolyze synovial tissue.[127]

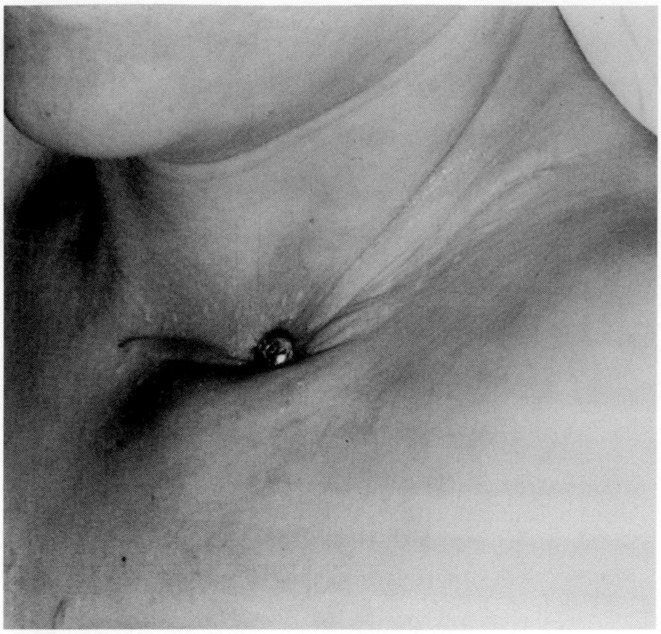

Figure 23–4

Internal fixation visible over the clavicle. The patient had a clavicular nonunion that was treated with internal fixation and bone grafting. Infection occurred resulting in a wound breakdown and exposure of the internal fixation. The patient was treated by removal of the internal fixation and dressing changes. The wound healed with this treatment, and there has been no recurrence of drainage over 6 years. Infection is not uncommon in the area of the clavicle and the acromioclavicular joint due to the thin soft tissue envelope that overlies the clavicle and the acromioclavicular joint.

CLASSIFICATION

Intra-articular sepsis may be classified in order of pathogenesis and frequency as: (1) direct hematogenous, (2) secondary to contiguous spread from osteomyelitis, or (3) secondary to trauma, surgery, or intra-articular injection (Fig. 23–4 and Table 23–1). Most joint infections are caused by hematogenous spread, although direct contamination is not uncommon with trauma. Inoculation of the joint with bacteria can occur in association with intra-articular injection of steroid, local anesthetic, or synthetic joint fluid.

Osteomyelitis of the humerus may spread intra-articularly, depending on the age of the patient, the type of infecting organism, and the severity of infection. Osteomyelitis of the clavicle or scapula is uncommon, although it does occur after surgery and internal fixation, from retained shrapnel fragments, or in heroin addicts.[14, 46, 85, 92, 133, 155]

Hematogenous osteomyelitis, although common in children,[98] is uncommon in adults until the sixth decade or later and is usually associated with a compromised immune system. Intravenous drug use is associated with the development of osteomyelitis in adults. Direct spread from wounds or foreign bodies, including total joint and internal fixation devices, is the most common etiology for shoulder sepsis in adults. Gowans and Granieri have noted the relationship between intra-articular injections of a hydrocortisone acetate in the subsequent development of septic arthritis.[53] Kelly and associates noted that two of their six patients had a history of multiple intra-articular injections of corticosteroid.[83]

Table 23–1 CLASSIFICATION OF OSTEOMYELITIS AND INTRA-ARTICULAR SEPSIS

Hematogenous
Contiguous spread
Osteomyelitis
Soft tissue sepsis
Vascular insufficiency
Direct inoculation
Trauma with or without a foreign body or biomaterials
Surgery with or without a foreign body or biomaterials

INCIDENCE AND PATHOGENIC MECHANISMS OF SEPTIC ARTHRITIS AND OSTEOMYELITIS

Surfaces as Substrata for Bacterial Colonization

The pathogenesis of bone and joint infections is related, in part, to preferential adhesive colonization of inert substrata whose surfaces are not integrated with healthy tissues composed of living cells and intact extracellular polymers such as the articular surface of joints or damaged bone (Fig. 23–5).[13, 59, 67, 125, 135, 151]

Almost all natural biologic surfaces are lined by a cellular epithelium or endothelium. Exceptions are intra-articular cartilage and the surface of teeth. Mature enamel is

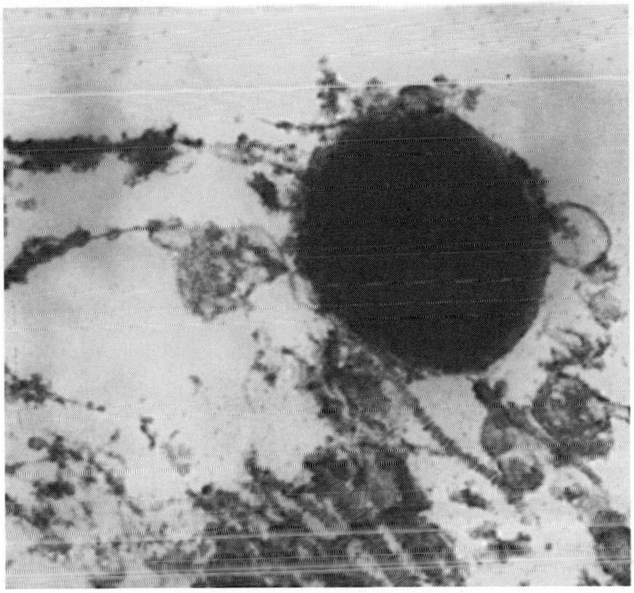

Figure 23–5

A photoelectromicrograph of rabbit articular cartilage illustrating direct bacteria-to-collagen fiber contact. (From Voytek A, Gristina AG, Barth E, et al: Staphylococcal adhesion to collagen in intra-articular sepsis. Biomaterials 9:107–110, 1988, by permission of the publishers, Butterworth & Co, Ltd. Copyright © 1988.)

the only human tissue that is totally acellular; it is primarily composed of inorganic hydroxyapatite crystals (96% by weight), with a small amount of water (3%) and organic matrix (<1%).[6] Proteins in the organic matrix are distributed between the hydroxyapatite crystals, forming a framework that strengthens the enamel by decreasing its tendency to fracture or separate. These proteins are unique among mineralized tissue because they are not a fibrous collagen protein like that found in bone, dentin, and cementum or in cartilage but are similar to the keratin family of proteins.[6]

Cartilage and enamel are readily colonized by bacteria because they lack the protection by natural desquamation or by intact extracapsular polysaccharides that is provided by an active cellular layer. Their acellular surfaces are similar to many of those in nature for which bacteria have developed colonizing mechanisms. Certain strains of *S. aureus* adhere to specific sites on collagen fibrils, a process that is mediated by specific surface receptor proteins. Dissimilarities in surface structure are probably responsible for the specificity of the colonization of bacterial species on these surfaces.

Enamel is mostly crystalline and inorganic, and cartilage is organic and noncrystalline. Enamel contains no collagen, whereas collagen is ubiquitous in cartilage and bone. *S. aureus* is the natural colonizer of cartilage but not of enamel, because it contains collagen receptors.[69, 70, 137] The specificity of colonization is also modulated in part by lectins and the host-derived synovial fluid, blood, and serum, conditioning films of protein, and polysaccharide macromolecules.

The colonization of teeth by *S. mutans* and other organisms is a natural polymicrobial process and may be symbiotic or slowly destructive; for joint cartilage, bacterial colonization is unnatural and rapidly destructive.[45] The acellular cartilage matrix and inanimate biomaterial surfaces offer no resistance to colonization by *S. aureus* and *S. epidermidis*, respectively. The observed invasion and gradual destruction of the cartilage over time supports clinical observations of the course of untreated septic arthritis (Fig. 23–6).[69, 99, 129, 130] Several strains of *S. aureus* produce collagenase, which, along with host-originated inflammatory products, is probably the main cause of progressive cartilage destruction.[95, 99, 122] The acellular cartilaginous surfaces of joints are particularly vulnerable to sepsis because they allow direct exposure to bacteria from open trauma, surgical procedures, or hematogenous spread. This mechanism parallels previous observations on the mechanism of osteomyelitis, which suggest that the adhesion of bacteria to dead bone or naked cartilage (surfaces not protected by living cells) via receptors and extracellular polysaccharides is a factor in pathogenesis.[37, 39, 131]

Intra-Articular Sepsis

The articular cavity is a natural dead space that becomes a major closed abscess and media bath for bacteria. In this avascular and acellular space, host defense mechanisms are at a disadvantage. Synovial cells are not actively antibacterial, although they are somewhat phagocytic. White blood cells must be delivered to the area and lack a surface for active locomotion. Under such conditions it is expected that phagocytic action is impaired, especially against encapsulated organisms.

Spontaneous intra-articular sepsis of the shoulder is derived from random hematogenous bacterial seeding. Synovial vasculature is abundant, and the vessels lack a limiting basement membrane. Bacteremia, especially *Neisseria gonorrhoeae*, increases the risk of intra-articular spread. Contiguous spread from adjacent and intracapsular metaphyseal osteomyelitis also occurs. Surgery,

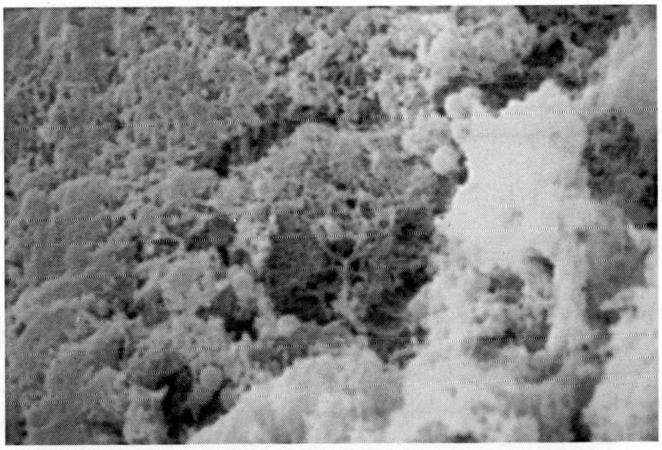

Figure 23–6

A photoelectromicrograph of articular cartilage at 7 days demonstrates destructive changes occurring beneath matrix-enclosed cocci. (From Voytek A, Gristina AG, Barth E, et al: Staphylococcal adhesion to collagen in intra-articular sepsis. Biomaterials 9:107–110, 1988, by permission of the publishers, Butterworth & Co, Ltd. Copyright © 1988.)

arthroscopy, total joint replacement, aspirations, and steroid injections also can result in direct inoculation of bacteria into the intra-articular space. The presence of foreign bodies from trauma or after surgery (stainless steel, chrome cobalt alloys, ultra-high molecular weight polyethylene, and methyl methacrylate) increases the possibility of infection by providing a foreign body nidus for colonization, allowing antibiotic-resistant, slime-enclosed colonization to occur.[55, 57, 59] The presence of a foreign body also lowers the size of the inoculant required for sepsis and perturbs host defense mechanisms.

Septic arthritis of the shoulder complex most frequently involves the glenohumeral joint. The acromioclavicular and sternoclavicular joints are occasionally infected in specific patient groups or after steroid injections in arthritis. Direct contamination from open wounds is also possible. Sternoclavicular sepsis is more common in drug addicts and usually involves gram-negative organisms, specifically *P. aeruginosa*. The involvement of *S. aureus*, *Escherichia coli*, *Brucella*, and *N. gonorrhoeae* has also been reported.[102]

Septic arthritis of the shoulder represents up to 14% of all septic arthritis cases.[94] In earlier studies, the incidence was 3.4%.[83] A more elderly population, increased trauma, and the common use of articular and periarticular steroids may be factors in this epidemiology (Fig. 23–7). The primary causal organism of shoulder sepsis also appears to have changed from pneumococcal to staphylococcal *(S. aureus)*. The shift in causal organisms involved in intra-articular sepsis is probably a result of antibiotic use and increased diagnostic accuracy. Sepsis in immunocompromised patients may be polyarticular as well as polymicrobial. Ten per cent of septic arthritis involves more than one joint and is likely to occur in children. Viral infections commonly involve more than one joint.

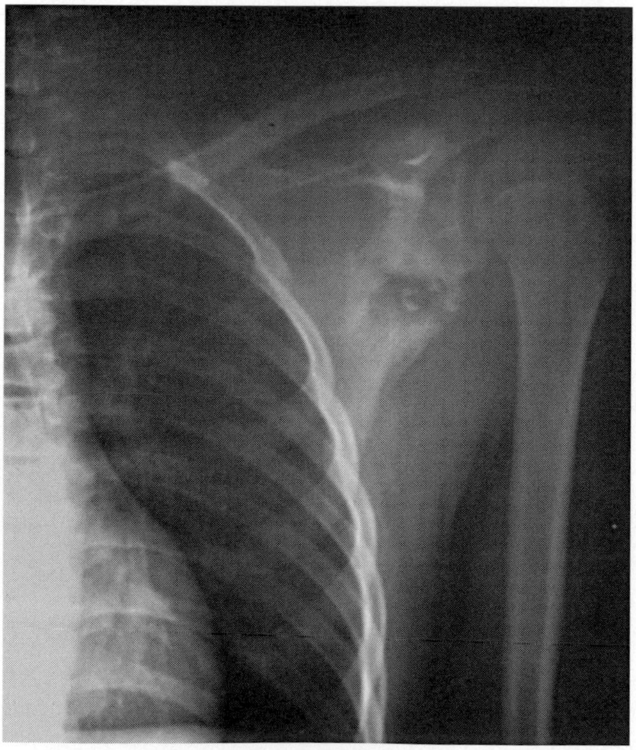

Figure 23–7

Staphylococcal osteomyelitis of the scapula secondary to closed trauma and hematologic seeding with abscess formation. The shoulder joint is not involved. (From the Department of Radiology, Wake Forest University Medical Center, Winston-Salem, NC.)

Table 23–2 FREQUENCY OF JOINT INVOLVEMENT IN INFECTIOUS ARTHRITIS (%)*†

	BACTERIAL (SUPPURATIVE)			
JOINT	Children‡	Adults§	MYCOBACTERIAL‖	VIRAL
Knee	41	48	24	60
Hip	23	24	20	4
Ankle	14	7	12	30
Elbow	12	11	8	20
Wrist	4	7	20	55
Shoulder	4	15	4	5
Interphalangeal and metacarpal	1.4	1	12	75
Sternoclavicular	0.4	8	0	0
Sacroiliac	0.4	2	0	0

*From Mandell L, Douglas KG Jr, and Bennett JE (eds): Principles and Practice of Infectious Diseases, 2nd ed. New York: John Wiley, 1985, p 698.

†More than one joint may be involved; therefore, the percentage exceeds 100%.

‡Compiled from Nelson and Koontz[104] and Jackson and Nelson.[75]

§Compiled from Kelly and colleagues,[82] Argen and colleagues,[4] and Gifford and associates.[46]

‖Compiled from Smith and Sanford[128] and Medical Staff Conference.[96]

Osteomyelitis

Hematogenous osteomyelitis accounts for 80 to 90% of osteomyelitis in children. Contiguous osteomyelitis is more common in adults, secondary to surgery and direct inoculation. In persons older than 50 years of age, contiguous osteomyelitis and disease related to vascular insufficiency are predominant.

Osteomyelitis in children is usually caused by one organism and by mixed organisms (*S. aureus* and gram-negative and anaerobic bacteria) in adults. Of the bones of the shoulder, the humerus is most frequently involved in osteomyelitis. The clavicle is occasionally involved in drug addicts by hematogenous spread. The scapula is rarely involved; usually infection occurs by direct inoculation or contiguous spread (Table 23–2).

MICROBIAL ADHESION AND INTRA-ARTICULAR SEPSIS

An understanding of microbial adhesion is required for complete clinical and therapeutic insights in joint sepsis. Studies of bacteria in marine ecosystems indicate that they tend to adhere in colonies to surfaces or substrata. The number of bacteria that can exist in a given environment is related directly to stress and nutrient supply.[72, 154] Since surface attachment, rather than a floating or suspension population, is a favored survival strategy, it is the state of the major portion of bacterial biomasses in most natural environments[72, 115] and is a common mode of microbial life in humans.

Bacterial attachment to surfaces is influenced by proteinaceous bacterial receptors and by an extracapsular exopolysaccharide substance within which bacteria aggregate and multiply.[27, 37] Once bacteria have developed a biofilm-enclosed, adhesive mode of growth, they become more resistant to biocides,[115] antiseptics,[93] antibiotics,[51] antagonistic environmental factors,[27, 72] and host defense systems.[8, 52, 151] Free-floating, nonadhesive bacteria or microbes that lack a well developed outer layer or exopolysaccharide are more susceptible to host-clearing mechanisms[8, 121] and to lower concentrations of antibacterial agents.[51]

Gibbons and van Houte[45] first described the significance of this adhesive phenomenon in the formation of dental plaque. In diseases such as gonococcal urethritis,[150] cystic fibrosis,[153] and endocarditis, bacterial colonization and propagation occur along endothelial and epithelial surfaces. The association between bacterial growth on biomaterial surfaces and infection was first described in 1963,[56] with the adhesive colonization of biomaterials first being reported in 1979.[58]

Microbial adhesion and associated phenomena also explain the foreign body effect, an increased susceptibility to infection experienced in the presence of a foreign body. Infections centered on foreign bodies are resistant to host defenses and treatment and tend to persist until the infecting locus is removed.[59] Foreign bodies include implanted biomaterials, fixation materials, prosthetic monitoring and delivery devices, traumatically acquired penetrating debris and bone fragments,[54] and compromised tissues.[54, 55, 59]

Molecular and Atomic Mechanisms in Adhesion

Initial bacterial attachment or adhesion depends on the long-range physical forces characteristic of the bacterium, the fluid interface, and the substratum. Specific irreversible adhesion, which occurs after initial attachment, is based on time-dependent adhesin-receptor interactions and on extracapsular polysaccharide synthesis.[38, 45, 77, 136]

Biomaterial surfaces present sites for environmental interactions derived from their atomic structures (Fig. 23–8).[140] Metallic alloys have a thin (100 to 200 Å) oxide layer that is the true biologic interface.[1, 79] The surfaces of polymers and metals are modified by texture, manufacturing processes, trace chemicals, and debris and also by host-derived ionic, polysaccharide, and glycoproteinaceous constituents (conditioning films). The finite surface structure of conditioning film in a human host has not been defined for any biomaterials but is specific for each individual biomaterial, type of tissue cell, and local host environment.[1, 7, 28]

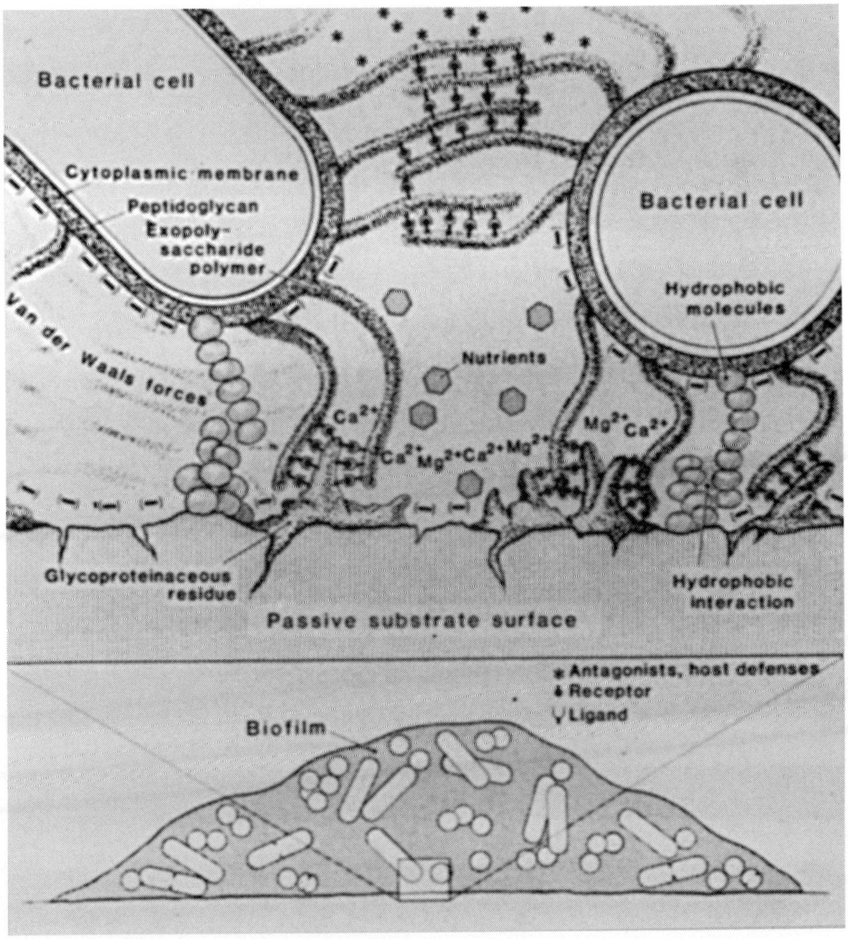

Figure 23–8

Mechanism of bacterial adherence. At specific distances the initial repelling forces between like charges on the surfaces of bacteria and substrate are overcome by attracting van der Waals forces, and there are hydrophobic interactions between molecules. Under appropriate conditions extensive development of exopolysaccharide polymers occurs, allowing ligand-receptor interaction and proteinaceous binding of the bacteria to the substrate. (From Gristina AG, Oga M, Webb LX, and Hobgood CD: Adherent bacterial colonization in the pathogenesis of osteomyelitis. Science *228*:990–993, 1985. Copyright © 1985, American Association for the Advancement of Science.)

Biomaterial surfaces may also act as catalytic hot spots for molecular and cellular activities.[1, 57, 79, 87] Tissue cells and matrix macromolecules also provide substrata for bacterial colonization. Bacteria have developed adhesins or receptors that interact with tissue cell surface structures (Fig. 23–9). Intermediary macromolecules or lectins may also play a role. Cells (endothelial) are more susceptible to bacterial colonization when their extramembranous outer polysaccharide glycocalyx has been traumatized or damaged by toxins.

Subsequent to or concomitant with initial attachment, fimbrial adhesins (*E. coli*) and substratum receptors may interact, as in bacteria-to-tissue cell pathogenesis or for the glycoproteinaceous conditioning films that immediately coat implants.[7, 21] The production and composition of the extracellular polysaccharide polymer, which tends to act like a glue, is a pivotal factor.[20, 154] The bacterial extracapsular exopolysaccharides may bind to surfaces or to surface absorbates and may act to consolidate microbial and polymicrobial environments.[118]

After colony maturation, cells on the periphery of the expanding biomass may separate or disaggregate and disperse, a process that is moderated by colony size, nutrient conditions, and hemodynamic or mechanical shear forces; in natural environments disaggregation is a survival strategy. In humans, however, it is involved in the pathogenesis of septic emboli. Disaggregation (dispersion) and its parameters may explain the phenomenon of intermittent or short-term "bacterial showers" or disseminated bacterial emboli.

BACTERIAL PATHOGENS

The following organisms are involved in septic arthritis and osteomyelitis of the shoulder and are listed in order of frequency.[81]

Bacteria: *S. aureus*, *S. epidermidis*, *Streptococcus* group B, *E. coli*, *P. aeruginosa*, *Haemophilus influenzae* type B, *N. gonorrhoeae*, *Mycobacterium tuberculosis*, and *Salmonella* and *Pneumococcus* species

Fungi: *Actinomyces*, *Blastomyces*, *Coccidioides*, *Candida albicans*, and *Sporothrix schenckii*

H. influenzae type B is most frequently isolated in children younger than 2 years of age and is rarely found in children older than 5 years of age. Group B *Streptococcus*, gram-negative bacilli, and *S. aureus* are common infecting organisms in the neonatal period. *S. aureus* is most common in adults; *N. gonorrhoeae* is common in adults younger than 30 years of age.[42] β-Hemolytic streptococci are the most common streptococci in adults and children; however, group B is more common in neonates and diabetics. Hematogenous septic arthritis in infants is primarily streptococcal, whereas hospital-acquired infections are primarily staphylococcal but may also feature *Candida* and gram-negative organisms, especially in infants.[120]

Gram-negative bacilli are found in approximately 15% of joints, especially in association with urinary tract infections or debilitating disease. *E. coli*, *P. aeruginosa*, and

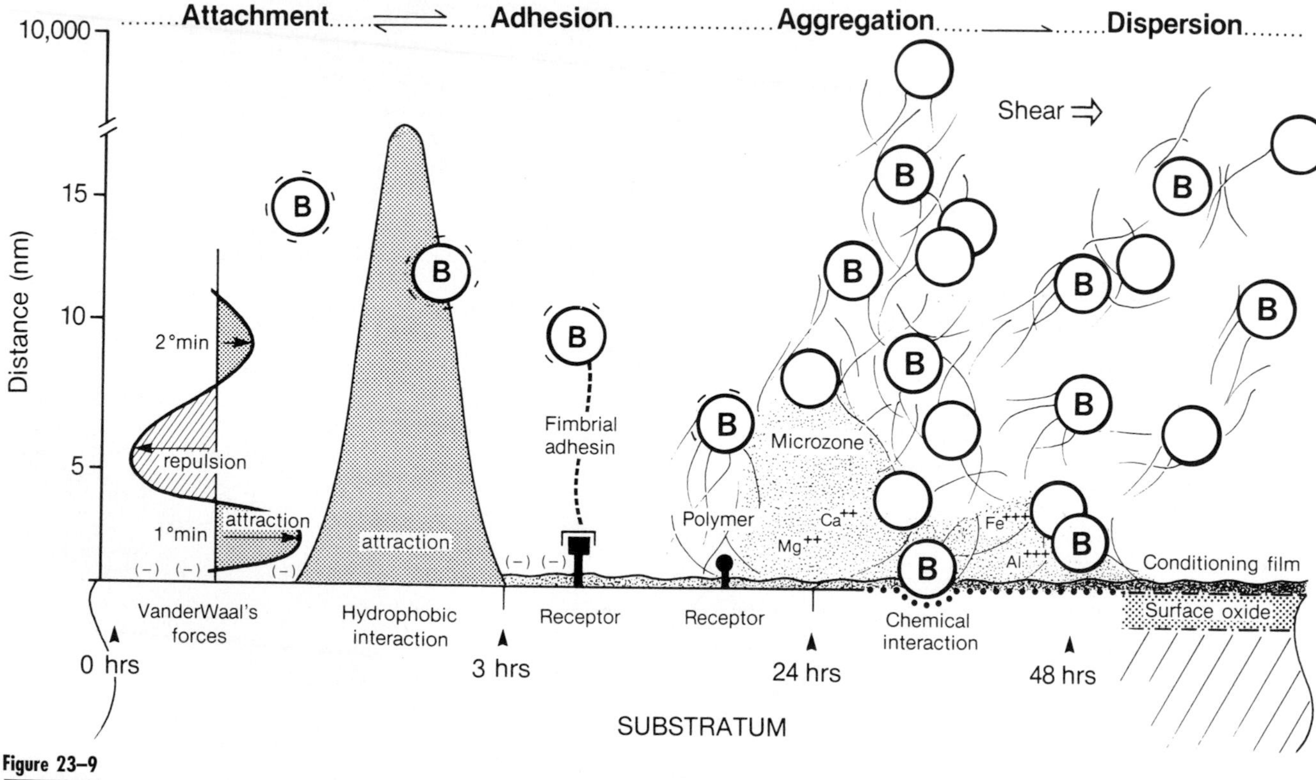

Figure 23–9

Molecular sequence in bacterial (B) attachment, adhesion, aggregation, and dispersion at the substratum surface. A number of possible interactions may occur, depending on the specificities of the bacteria or substratum system (graphics, nutrients, contaminants, macromolecules, species, and materials). (From Gristina AG: Biomaterial-centered infection: Microbial adhesion versus tissue integration. Science 237:1558–1595, 1987. Copyright © 1987, American Association for the Advancement of Science.)

other gram-negative bacilli have been isolated more frequently in the last decade, along with group A streptococci and an occasional appearance by group B and G streptococci. Pneumococcal arthritis is now unusual.

M. tuberculosis involves the knee, hip, ankle, and wrist more frequently than the shoulder. *M. marinum* is found in marine environments.

Coccidioides immitis involves the knee more frequently than the shoulder. *Blastomyces* usually spreads from osteomyelitis to the intra-articular space. *C. albicans* may spread via the hematogenous route in debilitated patients or directly from steroid injections.

S. aureus is often the major pathogen in biometal, bone, joint, and soft tissue infections and is the most common pathogen isolated in osteomyelitis when damaged bone or cartilage acts as a substratum.[23, 57, 59] The predominance of *S. aureus* in adult intra-articular sepsis[19, 111] may be explained by its ubiquity as a tissue pathogen seeded from remote sites, its natural invasiveness and toxicity, and its receptors for collagen, fibronectin, fibrinogen, and laminin. *S. epidermidis* is most frequently involved when the biomaterial surface is a polymer or when a polymer is a component of a complex device (extended-wear contact lenses,[125] vascular prostheses,[151] an artificial heart,[64] and total joint prostheses[57]).

Studies of chronic adult osteomyelitis have revealed polymicrobial infections in more than two thirds of cases.[17, 23, 59] The most common pathogens isolated included *S. aureus* and *S. epidermidis* and *Pseudomonas*, *Enterococcus*, *Streptococcus*, *Bacillus*, and *Proteus* species. Polymicrobial infections, therefore, appear to be an important feature of substratum-induced infections, are probably present more often than is realized, and should be regarded as a poor prognostic sign for total joint revision surgery.[61] Polymicrobial infection is a feature of chronic intra-articular sepsis and sinus formation and may be a feature of HIV infection with suppression of host defense mechanisms.[61, 62]

In summary, *S. aureus* is the most common organism in septic infections and is usually spread via hematogenous seeding. *S. epidermidis* is the principal organism in biomaterial-related infections, especially those centered on polymers. Mixed (polymicrobial), gram-negative, and anaerobic infections are probably more common than past studies have indicated and are frequently associated with open wounds and sinus tracts.

CLINICAL PRESENTATION

Symptoms and Signs

Pain, loss of motion, and effusion are early signs of infection.[19] Shoulder effusion is difficult to detect and often missed. Motion is painful, and the arm is adducted and internally rotated. X-rays may show a widened glenohumeral joint space and later signs of osteomyelitis (Fig. 23–10). Systemic signs include fever, leukocytosis, and sedimentation rate changes. The symptoms of immunosuppressed and rheumatoid patients may be muted.

The sternoclavicular joint may be involved and should be suspected in unilateral enlargement without trauma in patients younger than 50 years of age. Gonococcal and staphylococcal infections have been reported.[102] Intravenous drug addicts are susceptible to infection by gram-negative organisms, especially *P. aeruginosa* and *Serratia marcescens*. The acromioclavicular joint is rarely involved in sepsis but may be contaminated by steroid injections. Wound infection is not uncommon after surgical resection of the distal clavicle for osteoarthritis, probably due to the proximity of the joint to the overlying skin and lack of an intervening muscle layer.

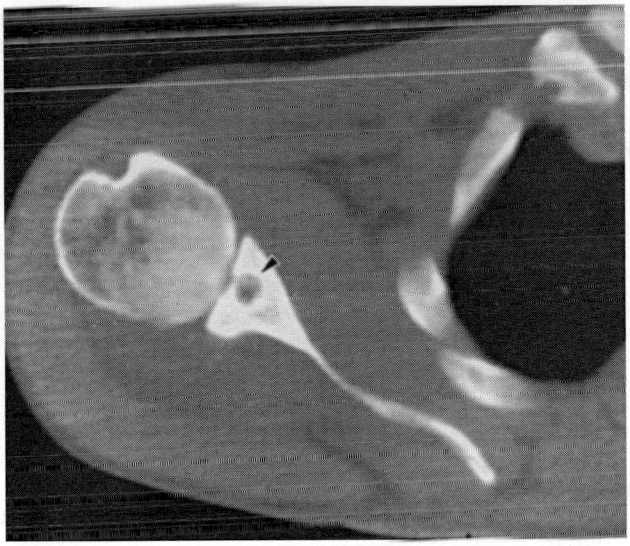

Figure 23–10

Staphylococcal osteomyelitis of the scapula. The *arrow* indicates an abscess secondary to infection caused by intra-articular steroid injection. (Courtesy of Mark Warburton, M.D., High Point, NC.)

Gabriel, Thometz, and Jaradeh reported on a 5-week-old male infant who had a brachial plexus neuropathy and paralysis of the upper extremity secondary to septic arthritis of the glenohumeral joint and osteomyelitis of the proximal part of the humerus.[40] They point out that pseudoparalysis of a limb associated with sepsis is a well-documented phenomenon. Similarly muscular spasm associated with pain caused by infection can lead to apparent weakness. True nerve paralysis associated with osteomyelitis is uncommon, and documentation by electrodiagnostic studies is rare. Permanent weakness persisted in their patient even though the glenohumeral joint and proximal humerus were surgically drained. The possible causes of plexus neuropathy associated with infection include ischemic neuropathy from thrombophlebitis of the vasa nervorum, arterial embolism, hyperergic or hypersensitivity reactions, and local compression due to abscess formation.

TOTAL SHOULDER REPLACEMENT

Sepsis after total joint replacement of the shoulder is rare (<0.5%) because of antibiotics, excellent blood supply, and the axial gradient or proximal location of the shoulder. Symptoms of infection include pain, loss of motion, and subluxation. Pain relief is so universal after total shoulder replacement that infection should be suspected if pain, radiographic joint distention, and, later, a widening around the cement, especially about the humerus, are present.

RHEUMATOID ARTHRITIS

Patients with chronic rheumatoid arthritis are susceptible to spontaneous septic arthritis.[65, 80] Because the active destructive process of the rheumatoid arthritis masks the septic condition, detection of infection is often delayed. The onset of septic arthritis should be suspected when the clinical course of the rheumatoid patient worsens acutely, especially if the disease is long term. When infection is present, the patient experiences a sudden aggravation of pain and swelling and increased temperature in the joint. Sudden chills may also occur. The physician should emphasize to patients with chronic rheumatoid arthritis (and to himself or herself) that a sudden exacerbation of symptoms warrants investigation.

Differential Diagnosis

Aspiration of the joint is essential; however, it is often possible to diagnose septic arthritis from the external appearance of the joint. Roentgenograms are not very useful in the early diagnosis because septic arthritis does not significantly alter the bone destruction owing to rheumatoid arthritis and because bone and joint radiographic changes are delayed.

Other acute arthritic disorders may imitate or mask sepsis, including gout, pseudogout, rheumatic fever, juvenile rheumatoid arthritis, and the oligoarthritic syndromes. Trauma and tumours may cause adjacent joint effusions and must be considered.

LABORATORY EVALUATION

Culturing and analysis of synovial fluid is critical for diagnosis. Aspiration of the joint should always be performed when sepsis is suspected. X-ray control is indicated if the approach is difficult or about total joints. The injection of saline or simultaneous arthrogram of the glenohumeral joint may be helpful in certain cases. When the results of cultures are negative and the diagnosis is difficult to make, an arthroscopic biopsy can be useful. In expert hands, frozen sections and touch preparations may be helpful at surgery but tend to give only an indication of pyogenic versus granulomatous or traumatic lesions. A synovial biopsy and culture for acid-fast organisms and fungi should be performed in patients with chronic monarticular arthritis, especially those with tenosynovitis. The leading infectious cause of chronic monarticular arthritis is atypical mycobacteria, such as *M. kansasii*, followed closely by *Sporothrix schenckii*. The occurrence of *M. tuberculosis* is rare today.[10, 126, 133]

Viral infection must be considered when bacteria cannot be identified. Smith and Percy report that viral arthritis is associated with rubella, parvovirus, mumps, hepatitis B, and lymphocytic choriomeningitis.[127] For a person who presents with multiple joint involvement and systemic manifestations consistent with a viral infection, serologic confirmation of the infection should be obtained because it is not usually possible to isolate the virus from joint fluid.

Synovial Fluid Analysis

If septic arthritis is suspected, the synovial fluid should be examined. The following findings indicate septic arthritis: the leukocyte count is usually more than 50,000 cells; the glucose level tends to be low (however, this is not a reliable indication of sepsis); and more than 75% of the cells are polymorphonuclear. These findings are beyond the range compatible with uncomplicated rheumatoid arthritis.[148]

In bacterial infections, aspiration may yield 10 ml or more of fluid. Synovial joint fluid is usually opaque or brownish, turbid, and thick but may be serosanguineous in 15% of cases with poor mucin clot. Proteins are elevated, primarily because of an elevated white blood cell count (usually greater than 50,000 and often as great as 100,000, and primarily composed of neutrophils).[148] One half of adults and a lower percentage of children will have a joint fluid glucose level of 40 mg less than serum glucose drawn at the same time.[75, 124, 147] These findings are more common later in infection. Polymorphonuclear leukocytes are dominant (90%). Counts over 100,000 per mm^3 are typical of staphylococcal and acute bacterial infection. Monocytes are more predominant in mycobacterial infections. Rheumatoid, rheumatic, and crystalline joint diseases also elevate leukocytes, but the presence of these diseases does not exclude concomitant sepsis. Crystal examination is needed to rule out gout or pseudogout.

The results of Gram stains are positive approximately 50% of the time, but false-positive results do occur.[146] Methylene blue-stained smears are more sensitive.[126] Positive joint cultures occur in 90% of established bacterial septic arthritis cases and in 75% of patients with tubercular arthritis.[146] Blood cultures should also be obtained, and the results are positive in approximately 50% of patients with acute infection. Depending on the type of systemic disease and organism, distant sites such as gastrointestinal, genitourinary, respiratory, and central nervous systems should also be cultured.[126] Some prosthesis-centered infections are difficult to detect unless tissues are biopsied and vortexed and homogenates are prepared for culture (Table 23–3).

Culture specimens should be taken for gram-positive, gram-negative, aerobic, and anaerobic bacteria, mycobacteria, and fungi. In approximately two thirds of cases, the causative organism may be identified by Gram staining. Laboratory technique and media selection should be based on the type of antibiotic given to the patient and on the special nutrient requirements of suspected bacteria. Use of blood agar is routine; chocolate agar is the best medium for culturing *Neisseria* and *Haemophilus* species. Thayer-Martin media may be used to isolate gonococcal organisms, but since it contains vancomycin and colistin methanesulfonate, *Haemophilus* species or other mixed flora will not grow on it.[119] Sabouraud's medium is specific for fungi. An egg-glycerol-potato and

Table 23–3 SYNOVIAL FLUID FINDINGS IN ACUTE PYOGENIC ARTHRITIS*

JOINT FLUID EXAMINATION	NONINFLAMMATORY FLUIDS	INFLAMMATORY FLUIDS	
		Noninfectious	Infectious
Color	Colorless, pale yellow	Yellow to white	Yellow
Turbidity	Clear, slightly turbid	Turbid	Turbid, purulent
Viscosity	Not reduced	Reduced	Reduced
Mucin clot	Tight clot	Friable	Friable
Cell count (per mm^3)	200–1000	3000 → 10,000	10,000 → 100,000
Predominant cell type	Mononuclear	PMN†	PMN†
Synovial fluid/blood glucose ratio	0.8–1.0	0.5–0.8	<0.5
Lactic acid	Same as plasma	Higher than plasma	Often very high
Gram stain for organism	None	None	Positive‡
Culture	Negative	Negative	Positive‡

*From Schmid FR: Principles of diagnosis and treatment of bone and joint infections. *In* McCarty DJ (ed): Arthritis and Allied Conditions: A Textbook of Rheumatology. Philadelphia: Lea & Febiger, 1985, p 1638.

†PMN, polymorphonuclear leukocyte.

‡In some cases, especially in gonococcal infection, no organisms may be demonstrated.

synthetic agar combination is used to culture mycobacteria.[119] Centrifugation is recommended for detection of mycobacteria (which are less frequently present) if sufficient fluid can be obtained. The magnitude of anaerobic septic arthritis has been underestimated in the past.[35]

Radiographic, Ultrasound, Computed Tomography, Magnetic Resonance Imaging, and Isotope Techniques

X-rays and CT scans of the septic shoulder may indicate changes ranging from widening to subluxation and from bone destruction to new bone formation (Figs. 23–11 to 23–13).[145] Arthrography may be useful for identifying rotator cuff tears,[5] which are present in many patients with septic arthritis. Ultrasound is useful in assisting aspiration and in assessing the infected shoulder joint.[49] Positive technetium bone scanning has been reported in 75 to 100% of septic arthritis cases, but technetium, gallium, and indium scans are not consistent.[43, 97, 156] Schmidt and colleagues found that the results of technetium bone scans performed on children with septic arthritis were frequently negative.[120] Indium scans may be more accurate indicators of sepsis, but conclusive data are lacking. Indium scintigraphy for osteomyelitis should be preceded by a positive result on a technetium scan. If the result of an indium scan is negative, infection is unlikely. A positive result on an indium scan increases the specificity of diagnosis. Indium uptake should be evaluated against the normal reticuloendothelial background.[156] False-negative results can occur in neonates and during the acute phase of osteomyelitis.[41]

Gupta and Prezio found that the specificity of nuclear scintigraphy using ^{99m}Tc phosphonates, ^{67}Ga citrate or ^{111}In-labeled leukocytes for diagnosing musculoskeletal infection could be improved if two nucleotide studies were used in conjunction.[66] The main limitation of scintigraphic investigations is their limited spacial resolution, making the results inexact. Furthermore, such studies may take hours to days to complete.

CT is useful in identifying small early lytic lesions caused by osteomyelitis that might be obscured in ordinary x-rays. Diagnosis of sternoclavicular joint sepsis and clavicular osteomyelitis infections may be improved using

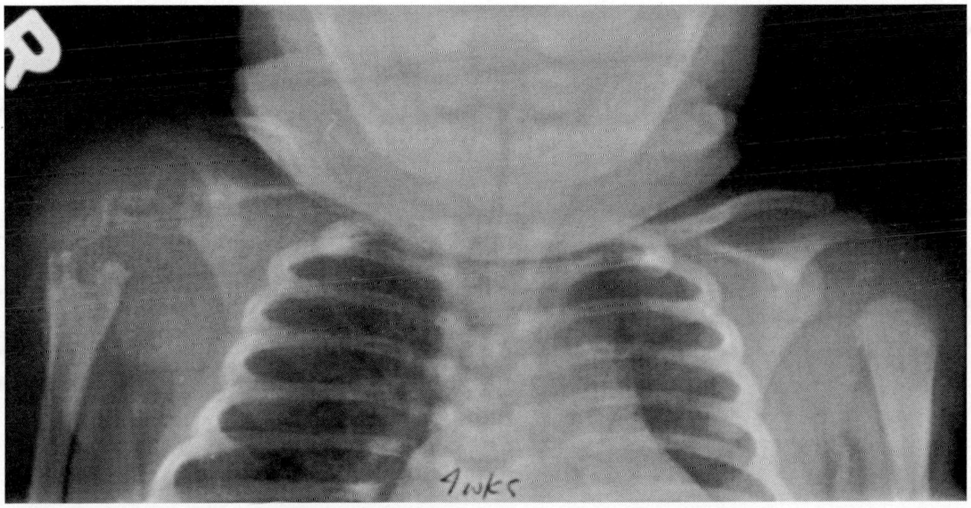

Figure 23–11

Septic arthritis of the right shoulder with destruction and widening of the proximal humerus. Also note healing of a right clavicle fracture. Organism: β-hemolytic streptococci. (From the Department of Radiology, Wake Forest University Medical Center, Winston-Salem, NC.)

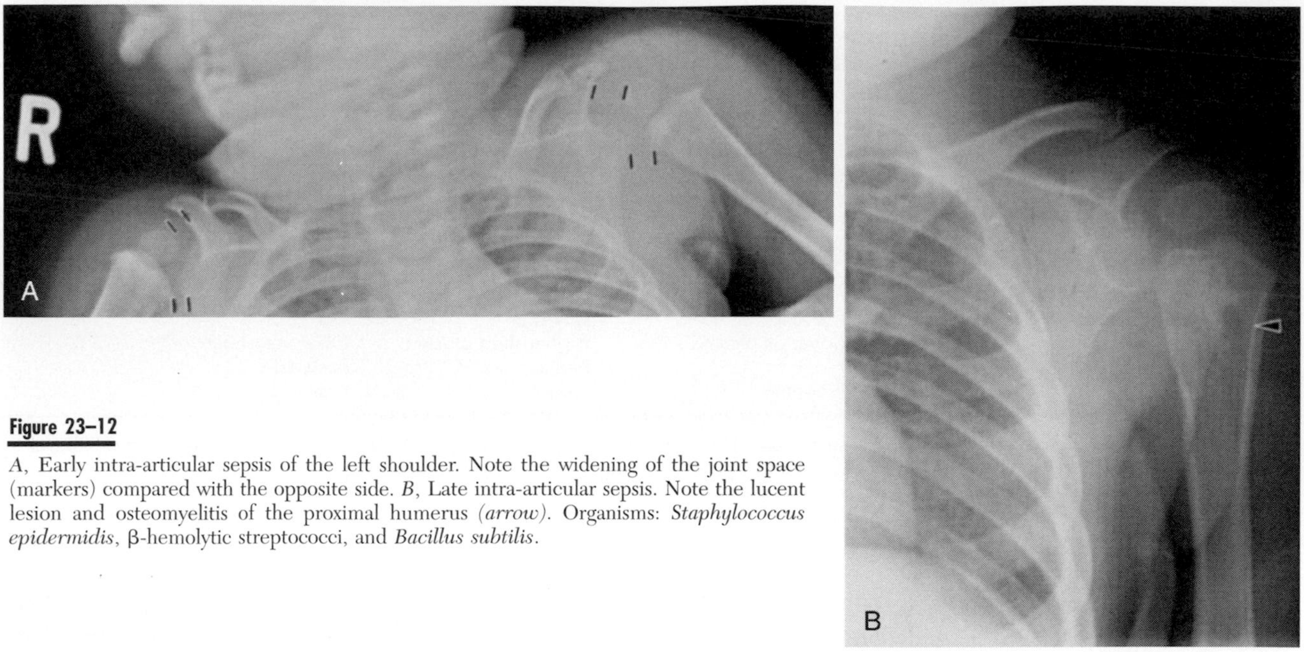

Figure 23–12

A, Early intra-articular sepsis of the left shoulder. Note the widening of the joint space (markers) compared with the opposite side. *B*, Late intra-articular sepsis. Note the lucent lesion and osteomyelitis of the proximal humerus *(arrow)*. Organisms: *Staphylococcus epidermidis*, β-hemolytic streptococci, and *Bacillus subtilis*.

CT, because it overcomes the tissue overlap problem that occurs with ordinary x-rays; however, CT does not offer much advantage in imaging the humerus.

MRI may facilitate differentiation of acute from chronic osteomyelitis and may help to detect evidence of active infection in the presence of chronic inflammation or post-traumatic lesions.[11, 138] Early changes of osteomyelitis cause fluid, inflammatory cell, and exudate accumulation in the marrow producing a focus of low signal intensity within bright, fatty marrow. In chronic osteomyelitis, large areas of abnormal or low signals with MRI may indicate an area of possible sequestration and hyperemia, especially along sinus tracts.[29] Capsular distention of articular cartilage and fluid-filled spaces are clearly visible on MRI, as are damaged surfaces, loose bodies, and avascular regions. MRI can be sensitive in early detection and specific for the localization and identification of sequestra.[36, 68, 117]

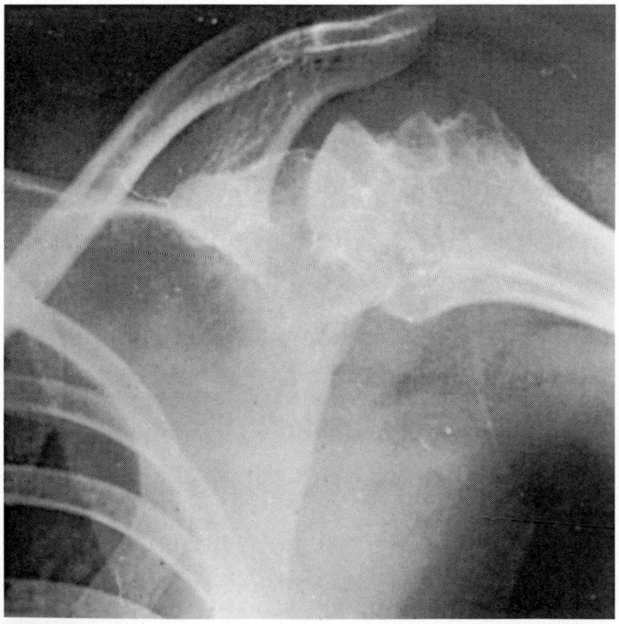

Figure 23–13

Cystic lesions in the humeral head consistent with tuberculosis sicca in a 19-year-old woman. (From DePalma AF [ed]: Surgery of the Shoulder, 3rd ed. Philadelphia: JB Lippincott, 1983.)

De Boeck, Noppen, and Desprechins reported on the usefulness of MRI in detecting pyomyositis.[30] MRI was useful in excluding other pathologic processes such as infectious arthritis, osteomyelitis, hematoma, thrombophlebitis, and malignant tumor. Itokazu and associates reported on the usefulness of MRI in diagnosing osteomyelitis associated with suppurative arthritis of the knee.[74] They report on a patient with septic arthritis of the knee with a normal radiograph and bone scan. MRI confirmed the presence of an osteomyelitic lesion with associated subperiosteal abscess formation. The early MRI finding in osteomyelitis consists of decreased signal intensity of the bone marrow on the T1-weighted image and increased signal intensity on the T2-weighted image, reflecting a decrease in marrow fat and an increase in water content and intramedullary pressure. Abnormalities remained in the marrow of the patient 1 year after surgery due to marrow fibrosis.

Egerman and associates reported on septic sacroiliitis associated with pyelonephritis in a 17-year-old pregnant patient with a history of illicit drug use.[34] CT and MRI were both helpful in making the diagnosis. MRI is helpful in pregnant patients becuase it provides a highly sensitive method of detecting skeletal infection without exposing the fetus to ionizing radiation.

Hopkins, Li, and Bergman assessed the role of gadolinium-enhanced MRI in providing diagnostic information beyond that given by nonenhanced MRI in the evaluation of musculoskeletal infectious processes.[71] They found that gadolinium-enhanced MRI was a highly sensitive technique that was especially useful in distinguishing abscesses from surrounding cellulitis or myositis. Lack of contrast enhancement ruled out infection with a high degree of certainty. However, these authors point out that contrast enhancement cannot be used to reliably distinguish infectious from noninfectious inflammatory conditions. In their study, gadolinium-enhanced MRI was found to have a very high sensitivity (89 to 100%) and accuracy (79 to 88%) in the diagnosis of various infectious lesions in the musculoskeletal system. However, the specificities (46 to 88%) were not as high. Tehranzadeh, Wang, and Mesgarzadeh have reported on the use of MRI in diagnosing osteomyelitis.[138] In several comparative studies MRI has been more advantageous in detecting the presence and determining the extent of osteomyelitis over scintigraphy, CT, and conventional radiography.

COMPLICATIONS

Inadequately treated intra-articular sepsis or osteomyelitis may result in recurrent infection, contiguous spread, bacteremia, distant septic emboli, anemia, septic shock, and death. Delayed diagnosis with adequate treatment may result in joint surface destruction, contractures, subluxation, arthritis, and growth aberrations (Fig. 23–14).[110] Inflammation, bacterial products, and lysosomal enzymes break down cartilage.[84] Within weeks, bacterial antigens stimulate destructive inflammation that may persist after the infection is treated. Bacterial endotoxins are chemotactic, and bacterial proteolytic enzymes further destroy surfaces. Increased intra-articular pressure also causes ischemia. Thrombotic events are also stimulated by burgeoning infection, further destroying the joint and adjacent bone. Long-term complications of chronic osteomyelitis include amyloidosis, nephrotic syndrome, and epidermal carcinoma.

TREATMENT

Most clinicians agree that systemic antibiotic therapy should begin immediately after the diagnosis of septic arthritis, but there is less agreement on subsequent therapy. In internal medicine, repeated needle aspiration is recommended as a primary treatment[82, 147]; however, the author believes that immediate arthrotomy is the treatment of choice, especially for the shoulder.[78, 113]

In general, the literature suggests that treatment of septic arthritis with repeated needle aspiration and appropriate intravenous antibiotics may be adequate except for the hip. However, conclusive studies of initial surgical drainage versus needle aspiration are lacking. A retrospective study comparing 55 infected joints treated by needle aspiration with 18 joints treated surgically concluded that 60% of surgically treated patients had sequelae, whereas 80% of medically treated patients recovered completely.[48] The author questions these data. Most orthopedic surgeons believe that the anatomy of the shoulder and the nature of shoulder sepsis demand surgical treatment. Septic arthritis that does not respond to medical management in 7 days should be surgically drained. Sternoarticular infections in drug abusers usually involve bone and joint. For these patients, needle aspiration has not been useful in establishing the diagnosis. However, surgical drainage has been useful in providing the pathogen. It also allows débridement of necrotic bone and permits drainage of abscesses, which are often present.[9, 114, 134]

Gelberman and associates reported a satisfactory outcome in eight of ten patients with septic arthritis of the

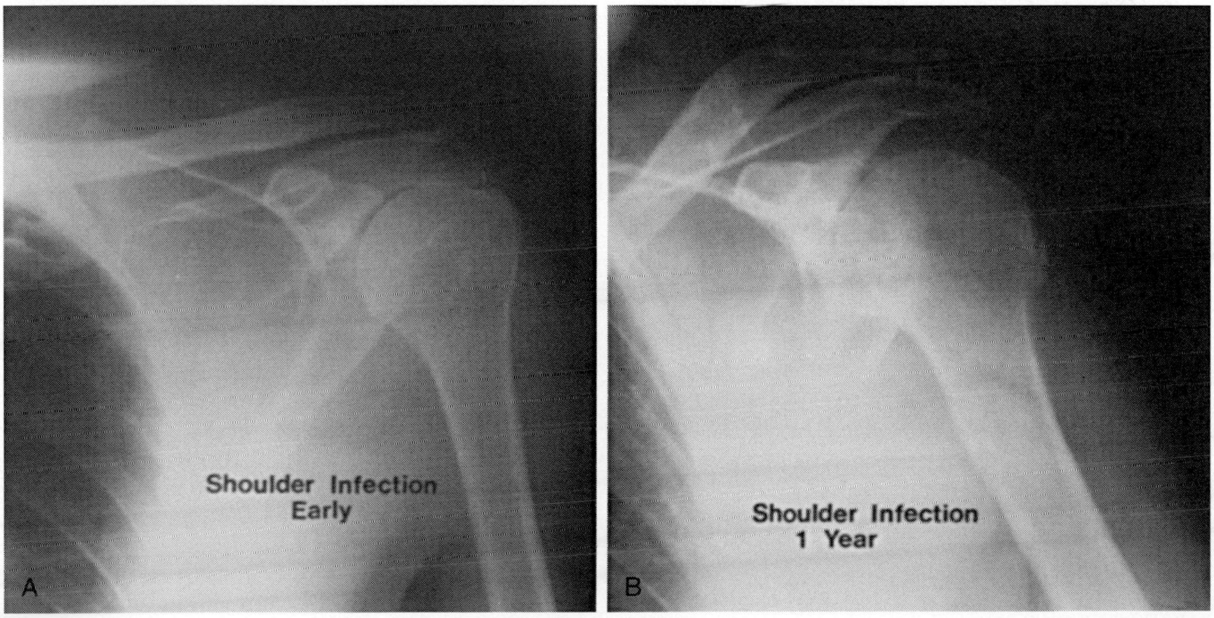

Figure 23–14

Hematogenous osteomyelitis secondary to intra-articular sepsis. *A*, Minimal lucency of proximal humerus at 2 weeks after probable onset of infection. *B*, After arthrotomy, antibiotic treatment, and resolution of infection, the x-ray reveals periosteal new bone formation and joint contracture. Organism: *Staphylococcus aureus*.

shoulder when treatment was begun 4 weeks or less after symptoms appeared.[42] Six of the eight satisfactory results from Gelberman's series were in patients who had either infection with *Streptococcus* or coagulase-negative *Staphylococcus*. Gelberman attributed poor results in eight patients due to delay in diagnosis, although six of the poor results were in patients who were infected with *S. aureus*.

Leslie, Harris, and Driscoll reviewed 18 cases of septic arthritis of the shoulder in adults.[88] The patients ranged in age from 42 to 89 years. All except one patient had at least one serious associated disease. Eight patients had an injection or aspiration of the shoulder before the development of their infection. The diagnosis was delayed in 17 of the 18 patients. At the time of admission to hospital the erythrocyte sedimentation rate was always elevated but the body temperature and white blood cell count were not. After treatment the functional result was usually poor. Only five patients regained forward flexion to 90 degrees or more. Eight patients had no active motion of the glenohumeral joint and two patients died. Arthrotomy appeared to have resulted in a better result than did repeated aspiration.

Smith and Piercy report that the characteristics of patients with bacterial arthritis for whom a poor outcome is expected include persons older than 60 years of age, preexisting rheumatoid arthritis, infection in the shoulder, duration of symptoms before treatment for more than 1 week, involvement of more than four joints, and persistently positive cultures after a 7-day course with appropriate antibiotic therapy.[127]

A retrospective study of a 10-year period at the Bowman Gray School of Medicine revealed 17 septic shoulders in 16 patients.[139] Patients with gonococcal infections were excluded from the study. The patients' ages ranged from 26 days to 72 years (average age of 33 years). The causative organism was *S. aureus* in five patients, group B *Streptococcus* in two patients, *Pneumococcus* in three patients, multiple organisms in one patient, *Proteus* in one patient, and *Haemophilus* in one patient. Three patients had obvious clinical infection with negative cultures owing to treatment, technique, and timing.

Ten patients with septic shoulder (treated by different physicians) underwent arthrotomy; one patient was treated by arthrocentesis; and another patient was treated initially with aspirations, but later an arthrotomy was performed for osteomyelitis of the glenoid. Total joints were involved in two patients. Both infections were delayed and due to seeding from distant sites; one was associated with repeated local trauma. One total joint infection was resolved by removal of the component and resulted in a nonpainful pseudarthrosis. A second patient had chronic drainage and a greatly decreased range of motion, even after débridement.

One patient treated with aspirations and intravenous antibiotics died of septic shock. Five patients developed chronic drainage or osteomyelitis. Underlying shoulder pathology significantly delayed diagnosis and treatment of shoulder sepsis in four patients.

All patients received intravenous antibiotics, and the treatment lasted from 7 days to 4 weeks. All patients received at least 3 weeks of antibiotic therapy, including oral and intravenous administration. All children had complete resolution and excellent function at several months follow-up. Complete resolution of symptoms occurred with the treatment provided in nine of the 16 patients. We suggest early active motion and therapy as tolerated. Predisposing factors included rheumatoid arthritis, previous surgery, steroid injections, trauma, burns, and septic emboli from distant infections. CT scans were positive 60% of the time.

Intra-articular sepsis should be treated swiftly.[130] Variables that influence the selection of treatment methods include the duration of infection, host immune status, types of infecting organisms, and presence of foreign bodies or adjacent osteomyelitis. The most critical factors in treatment are the infecting organism and the presence of a foreign body.

Osteomyelitis of the proximal metaphysis may either precede or be secondary to septic arthritis of the glenohumeral joint (Fig. 23–15). Therefore, drilling of the metaphysis has been recommended for pediatric septic glenohumeral arthritis to rule out osteomyelitis and to allow adequate decompression of the bone. Diagnosed osteomyelitis should be surgically treated.

Leslie, Harris, and Driscoll noted that five of six patients who had rotator cuff tears had a marked discrepancy between active and passive shoulder motion.[88] They noted that the poor functional results recorded in these six patients may have been more of a reflection of the rotator cuff tear than of damage to the articular cartilage as a result of infection.

Immobilization is usually recommended for septic arthritis. However, Salter and colleagues' study of septic arthritis in a rabbit model indicated that the use of continuous passive motion was superior to immobilization or to intermittent active motion.[116] Possible explanations for these results include prevention of bacterial adhesion, enhanced diffusion of nutrients, improved clearance of lysosomal enzymes and debris from the infected joints, and stimulation of chondrocytes to synthesize the various components of the matrix.

The majority of children do well after treatment for septic shoulder arthritis. In a study of nine children with glenohumeral arthritis, Schmidt and associates suggested surgical treatment with exploration of the biceps tendon sheath.[120] Growth center damage is possible. The prognosis for adults with septic arthritis of the shoulder is poor, but shoulders treated within 4 weeks or less of the onset of symptoms may do well. Poor results are associated with delayed diagnosis, virulent (gram-negative) infecting organisms, persistent pain, drainage, osteomyelitis, and destruction of the joint.

Gonococcal septic arthritis may be polyarticular.[47] Fever is low grade, usually below 102°F. Articular and periarticular structures are swollen, stiff, and painful, followed by desquamation of skin over the joints. During septicemia, a macular rash or occasionally a vesicular rash occurs in one third of patients but is also caused by *Neisseria meningitidis*, *Haemophilus*, and *Streptobacillus*.[18, 123] Organisms are not common in joint fluid and, therefore, are not isolated in most cases. The general picture of gonococcal septic arthritis is less acute than staphylococcal infection. Gonococcal arthritis responds well to systemic

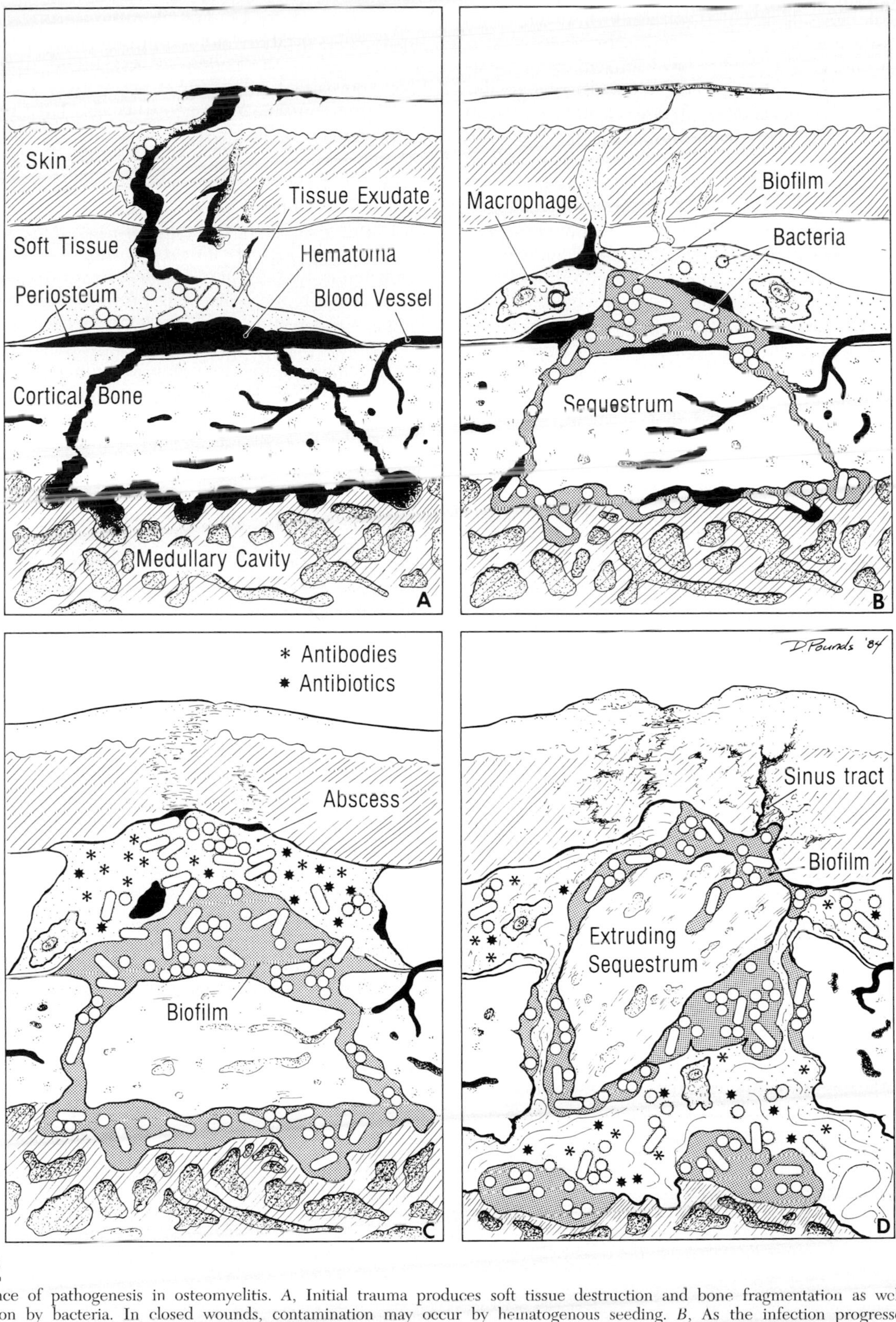

Figure 23–15

The sequence of pathogenesis in osteomyelitis. *A*, Initial trauma produces soft tissue destruction and bone fragmentation as well as wound contamination by bacteria. In closed wounds, contamination may occur by hematogenous seeding. *B*, As the infection progresses, bacterial colonization occurs within a protective exopolysaccharide biofilm. The biofilm is particularly abundant on the devitalized bone fragment, which acts as a passive substratum for colonization. *C*, Host defenses are mobilized against the infection but are unable to penetrate or be effective in the presence of the biofilm. *D*, Progressive inflammation and abscess formation eventually result in the development of a sinus tract and, in some cases, ultimate extrusion of the sequestrum that is the focus of the resistant infection. (From Gristina AG, Barth E, and Webb LX: Microbial adhesion and the pathogenesis of biomaterial-centered infections. *In* Gustilo RB, Gruninger RP, and Tsukayama DT [eds]: Orthopaedic Infection. Diagnosis and Treatment. Philadelphia: WB Saunders, 1989, pp 3–25.)

antibiotic therapy and needle aspiration; however, in refractory cases, the authors have used arthrocentesis.

Antimicrobial agents used to treat joint infections generally achieve levels intra-articularly equal to or greater than serum levels except for erythromycin and gentamicin (Table 23–4). Intra-articular antibiotics are generally not advocated and may cause sterile abscesses. The authors do, however, use bacitracin in irrigating solutions at surgery. Rarely, carefully monitored intra-articular aminoglycosides may be indicated. In osteomyelitis, antibiotic penetration into bone is unreliable.[108] Clindamycin achieves higher bone levels than cephalothin or methicillin.[107] When healthy (non-sequestrated) bone in children is being treated, delivery of antibiotics to the infected site is likely. The opposite situation exists in adults, the aged, vascularly compromised patients, and patients with chronic osteomyelitis, sequestration, and sinus formation. Animal studies have suggested that antibiotic combinations (e.g., oxacillin and aminoglycosides) may be more effective in osteomyelitis.[108] The new quinolone group of antibiotics under evaluation for treatment of bone and joint infections may be useful because of its broad spectrum of activity against staphylococci, *Pseudomonas* species, and gram-negative bacteria.[31] These agents achieve excellent local levels in living and dead bone. The emergence of mutant strains may occur but can be reduced by intelligent use of quinolones in combination with other antibiotics.

Mader, Landon, and Calhoun report that antibiotic selection should be based on in vitro sensitivity testing and that the drug exhibiting the highest bactericidal activity with the least toxicity and lowest cost should be chosen.[90] Surgical treatment must convert an infection with dead bone to a situation with well-vascularized tissues that are readily penetrated by blood-borne antibiotics. The length of antibiotic therapy is empiric and depends on the clinical response of the patient. Four to 6 weeks of treatment has become a standard length for empiric reasons. Dirschl and Almekinders report that combined intravenous and oral antibiotic therapy has become accepted as a standard treatment for osteomyelitis in children.[33] The duration of intravenous antibiotic therapy ranges from 3 to 14 days in various series. Adequate serum concentrations of the oral antibiotic must be documented before the patient is discharged from hospital. Close outpatient follow-up is imperative, and treatment should be continued for 4 to 6 weeks. Treatment should be prolonged if the erythrocyte sedimentation rate does not fall below 20 mm/hr after 6 weeks.

Oral therapy of osteomyelitis in adults has lagged behind that of children, although studies are available demonstrating that the results generally are good. Oral antibiotic therapy has obvious economic advantages over intravenous therapy and as such is very desirable. The route of antibiotic delivery is probably not important as long as the infecting organism is susceptible to the antibiotic and the antibiotic is delivered to the tissues in adequate concentration to eradicate infection. The serum bactericidal titer is used as a method of determining adequacy of therapy. This titer is defined as the maximum dilution of the patient's serum that will kill more than 99.9% of the infecting organisms in vitro. The serum bactericidal titer is useful in ensuring adequate antimicrobial activity, absorption, and compliance.

Staphylococci may persist after nafcillin therapy owing to selection of cell wall–deficient organisms, requiring the use of an antistaphylococcal agent such as clindamycin.[3] Intravenous therapy is generally continued for more than 3 weeks in septic arthritis and for more than 4 to 6 weeks in osteomyelitis and is monitored by systemic signs, white blood cell count, and sedimentation rates.[109, 126] Serum levels greater than or equal to 1:8, minimum inhibitory concentration (MIC), and minimum bactericidal concentration (MBC) are suggested.[89] Oral antibiotics may be used after intravenous therapy as required.[89, 107]

Surgical débridement is the mainstay of treatment for septic arthritis and osteomyelitis of the shoulder. The logic is as follows: (1) toxic products, damaged tissue, and foreign bodies must be removed to prevent damage and to treat infection effectively; and (2) laboratory studies have shown that the MIC and MBC levels needed to treat surface-adherent bacterial populations are 10 to 100 times higher than those for suspension populations.[63, 76, 86, 110] These findings suggest that it is possible to clear a

Table 23–4 EMPIRIC ANTIBIOTIC THERAPY FOR SEPTIC ARTHRITIS*

AGE	PREFERRED	ALTERNATIVE
< 2 Months: no organism on stain	Oxacillin and aminoglycoside	Cefazolin and aminoglycoside
2 Months–5 years: no organism	Nafcillin and chloramphenicol	Cefuroxime
5–15 Years: no organism	Nafcillin or oxacillin	Cefazolin or vancomycin
>40 Years: no organism	Nafcillin ± aminoglycoside	Cefazolin ± aminoglycoside
<2 Months: gram-positive cocci	Oxacillin or nafcillin	Cephalothin or cephapirin
<2 Months–40 years: gram-negative bacilli	Aminoglycoside	Cefotaxime
>2 Months: gram-positive cocci	Nafcillin or oxacillin	Cefazolin, cephalothin, vancomycin, clindamycin
2 Months–5 years: gram-negative coccobacilli	Cefotaxime or ampicillin and chloramphenicol	Chloramphenicol alone; trimethoprim/sulfamethoxazole
15–40 Years: gram-negative cocci	Treat for *Neisseria gonorrhoeae*	
>40 Years: gram-negative bacilli	Ticarcillin plus aminoglycoside	Cefotaxime ± aminoglycoside

*American Medical Association, Division of Drugs and Toxicology: Anti-microbial therapy for common infectious diseases. *In* Drug Evaluations Annual 1995, Chicago, Illinois, pp 1277–1282.

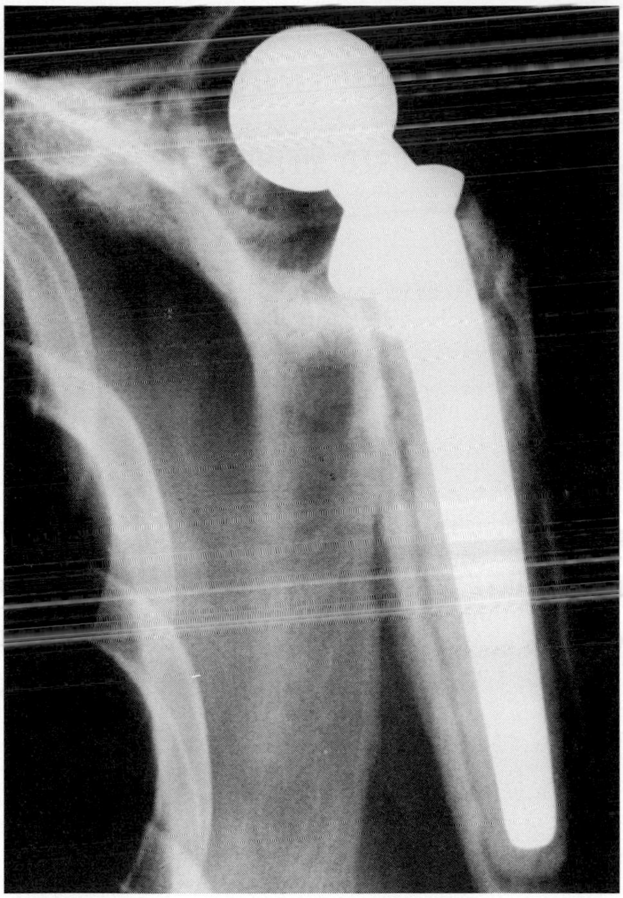

Figure 23–16

Infected total shoulder arthroplasty (radiograph of patient shown in Fig. 23–1). The glenoid and humeral cement mantles are surrounded by large radiolucent lines. There is some reactive periostitis of the medial humerus.

bacteremia or bacteria suspended in synovial fluid but very difficult to sterilize an infected cartilaginous joint surface or sequestrum covered with debris without administering toxic levels of antibiotics.

Antibiotic-impregnated beads (gentamicin or tobramycin) may be indicated in certain cases of osteomyelitis and articular sepsis.[15, 39, 50] We suggest their removal at 6 to 12 weeks. Studies suggest that eventually these methyl methacrylate surfaces may provide a substratum for resistant organisms.[152] Closed suction and irrigation may be used for short periods (<3 days) if necessary in special cases in septic joints, provided the system does not allow retrograde contamination. However, the literature does not indicate a definite advantage with this treatment, and it is seldom required in de novo joint sepsis because adequate antibiotic levels can be achieved systemically.

Open wounds involving joints are by definition contaminated, even though bacteria are not always detected. Type 3 open fractures, especially those involving joints, have a very high rate of infection. There are indications that these should be treated with a combination of cefazolin and gentamicin.[108] Topical or local antibiotics may be used in the future for damaged tissue or chronic infections in certain population groups because these infections require higher antibiotic levels than can be achieved via the bloodstream. A biodegradable, resorbable, antibiotic-loaded substrate placed in a surgically débrided musculoskeletal site may be even more effective than methyl methacrylate beads. Intravenous amphotericin B remains the preferred drug in patients with deep systemic fungal infections.[33]

Infection After Shoulder Arthroplasty

Infection occurs in less than 1% of cases after total joint arthroplasty of the shoulder (Figs. 23–16 and 23–17).[60, 103] Parallels in hip surgery indicate that early infection may be treated with irrigation and débridement if it is due mainly to an infected hematoma. This is rarely the case, however, and removal of components is usually required. All damaged tissue and methyl methacrylate should be removed if possible. The prognosis for revision total joint arthroplasty after infection is poor.[101] A fusion may be required (Fig. 23–18). Some patients may have surprisingly good function 1 year after removal of components without fusion. Resection, rather than fusion, is preferred by some authors as our standard salvage method for failed, infected shoulders and elbows. The author prefers arthrodesis as a method of reconstruction after removal of prosthetic components. Delayed bone grafting may be required as a result of the extent of bone loss after removal of the prosthetic components.

The author has minimal experience with the reimplantation of a prosthesis after a prosthetic infection. It is possible that removal of the prosthesis and insertion of

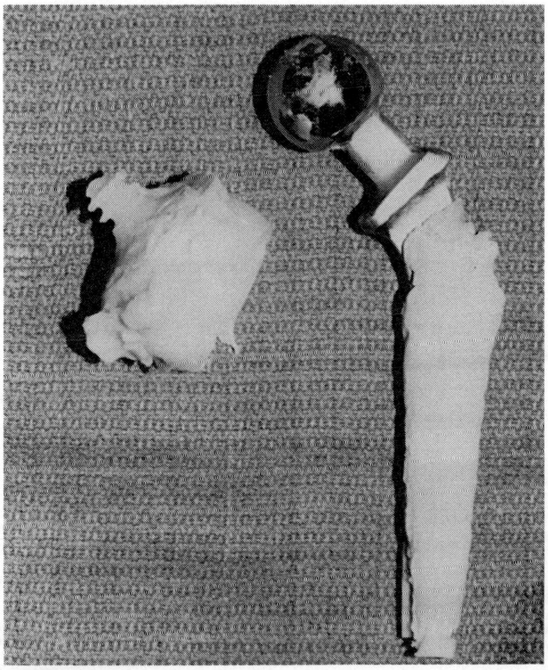

Figure 23–17

An infected total shoulder arthroplasty (same patient) shown in Figures 23–1 and 23–16. Both the humeral and glenoid components were removed. It was not difficult to remove the infected arthroplasty components because they were surrounded by purulent debris and a prolific membrane.

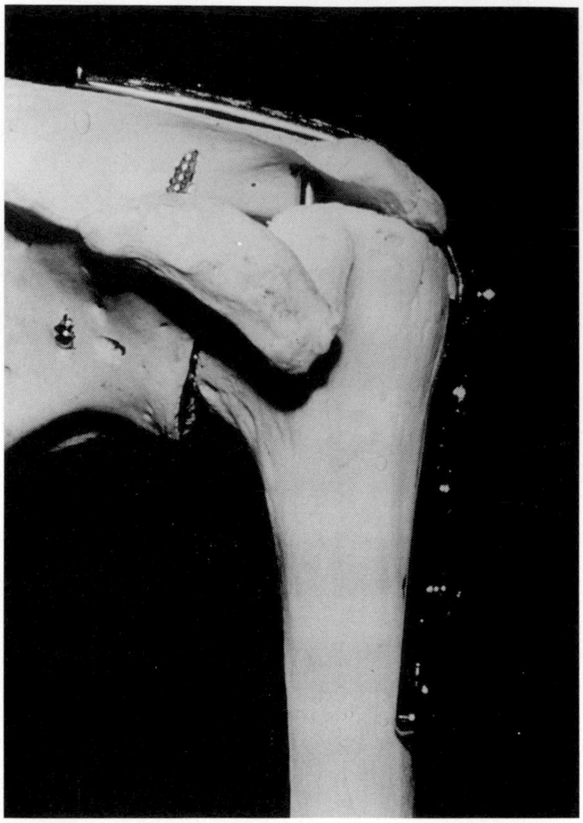

Figure 23–18

Shoulder arthrodesis using plate fixation. (From Richards RR, Waddell JP, and Hudson AR: Shoulder arthrodesis for the treatment of brachial plexus palsy. Clin Orthop *198*:250–258, 1985.) Shoulder arthrodesis is the preferred method of treatment in patients with chronic glenohumeral sepsis and destruction of articular cartilage. If there is bone loss following removal of a shoulder arthroplasty of a tumor, curettage and bone grafting may have to be combined with internal fixation. Depending on the adequacy of the débridement and the health of the surrounding soft tissues, it may be necessary to stage débridement and bone grafting in order to obtain a solid arthrodesis.

cement-impregnated beads or the immediate reimplantation of a prosthesis with antibiotic-impregnated cement may salvage some arthroplasties after infection develops. This type of treatment is best attempted for infections due to organisms of low virulence, such as *S. epidermidis*. The author does not recommend reimplantation of a prosthesis after infection with gram-negative bacilli or any other organism of high virulence.

Prophylaxis

Antibiotic prophylaxis is effective because bacteria are cleared before they establish slime-shielded, surface-adherent, rapidly growing populations at sites deep within bone or on biomaterials. The author suggests using antibiotic prophylaxis, such as cefazolin, 1 g intravenously at anesthesia and repeated at 4 hours.[106] The use of prophylactic antibiotics is suggested for all implant surgery, including both prosthetic and internal fixation of fractures, and trauma. Antibiotics may be varied, depending on the special conditions of each case and patient.[108] Treatment for 24 hours in clean cases is believed sufficient. Clean air, laminar flow, and ultraviolet light are also effective based on local cost:benefit ratios.

AUTHOR'S PREFERRED METHODS OF TREATMENT

The shoulder joint is capacious and anatomically complicated. For this reason, open surgical drainage rather than aspiration or arthroscopic drainage is indicated. We use an anterior deltopectoral approach. The deltoid and coracoid are not detached. Infected surfaces are débrided of adhesins, clots, and debris. Surgical lavage with antibiotics is an appropriate technique. In most cases, the wound may be loosely closed and a large Hemovac is inserted for 24 hours to remove postsurgical accumulations. In cases of chronic sepsis or infection by gram-negative organisms, the wound is left open. Adequate intra-articular concentrations of antibiotics can be achieved by intravenous and intramuscular administration.[105] The duration of antibiotic treatment varies, depending on the host and organism; 3 weeks of intravenous therapy followed by 3 weeks of oral treatment is a reasonable base. The patient's response is the key to duration of treatment.

In summary, intra-articular shoulder sepsis is becoming increasingly frequent in adults. Shoulder anatomy is unique in that bursae communicating with the joint provide a pathway for bacteria for which cartilage is the target substratum. Successful treatment depends on the immune system response, the type of infecting organism, and early surgical débridement.

References and Bibliography

1. Albrektsson T: The response of bone to titanium implants. Crit Rev Biocompat *1*:53–84, 1985.
2. American Medical Association, Division of Drugs and Toxicology: Anti-microbial therapy for common infectious diseases. *In* Drug Evaluations Annual 1995. Chicago, IL: American Medical Association, 1995, pp 1277–1282.
3. Antibiotics for osteomyelitis. Lancet *1*:153–154, 1975.
4. Argen RJ, Wilson DH Jr, and Wood P: Suppurative arthritis. Arch Intern Med *117*:661–666, 1966.
5. Armbuster G, Slivka J, Resnick D, et al: Extraarticular manifestations of septic arthritis of the glenohumeral joint. AJR Am J Roentgenol *129*:667–672, 1977.
6. Avery JK (ed): Oral Development and Histology. Baltimore: Williams & Wilkins, 1987.
7. Baier RE, Meyer AE, Natiella JR, et al: Surface properties determine bioadhesive outcomes: Methods and results. J Biomed Mater Res *18*:337–355, 1984.
8. Baltimore RS and Mitchell M: Immunologic investigations of mucoid strains of *Pseudomonas aeruginosa*: Comparison of susceptibility to opsonic antibody in mucoid and nonmucoid strains. J Infect Dis *141*:238–247, 1980.
9. Bayer AS, Chow AW, Louie JS, et al: Gram-negative bacillary septic arthritis: Clinical, radiologic, therapeutic, and prognostic features. Semin Arthritis Rheum *7*:123–132, 1977.
10. Berney S, Goldstein M, and Bishko F: Clinical and diagnostic features of tuberculous arthritis. Am J Med *53*:36–42, 1972.
11. Berquist TH, Brown M, Fitzgerald R, et al: Magnetic resonance imaging: Application in musculoskeletal infection. Magn Reson Imaging *3*:219, 1985.
12. Bhawan J, Das Tandon H, and Roy S: Ultrastructure of synovial membrane in pyogenic arthritis. Arch Pathol *96*:155–160, 1973.

13. Birinyi LK, Douville C, Lewis SA, et al: Increased resistance to bacteremic graft infection after endothelial cell seeding. J Vasc Surg *5*:193–197, 1987.
14. Broadwater JR and Stair JM: Sternoclavicular osteomyelitis: Coverage with a pectoralis major muscle flap. Surg Rounds Orthop 2:47–50, 1988.
15. Buccholz HW and Gartmann HD: Infektionsprophylaxe und operative Behandlung der schleichenden tiefen Infektion bei der totalen Endoprothese. Chirurg *43*:446–452, 1972.
16. Bullough PG and Vigorita VJ: Atlas of Orthopaedic Pathology. Baltimore: University Park Press, 1984, p 94.
17. Burch KK, Fine G, Quinn EL, and Eisses JF: *Cryptococcus neoformans* as a cause of lytic bone lesions. JAMA *231*:1057–1059, 1975.
18. Cabot RC (ed): Case records of the Massachusetts General Hospital: An obscure general infection. Boston Med Surg J *197*:1140–1142, 1927.
19. Calhoun J, Cantrell J, and Mader J: Septic Shoulders. Paper 28. The Society of American Shoulder and Elbow Surgeons, 4th Open Meeting, Atlanta, Georgia, February 7, 1988.
20. Calleja GB, Atkinson B, Garrod DR, et al: Aggregation. Group report. *In* Marshall KC (ed): Microbial Adhesion and Aggregation. Berlin: Springer-Verlag, 1984, pp 303–321.
21. Christensen CD, Simpson WA, and Beachey EH: Adhesion of bacteria to animal tissues: Complex mechanisms. *In* Savage DC and Fletcher M (eds): Bacterial Adhesion, Mechanisms and Physiological Significance. New York: Plenum Press, 1985, pp 279–305.
22. Chung SMK: The arterial supply of the developing proximal end of the human femur. J Bone Joint Surg *58A*:961–970, 1976.
23. Cierny G, Couch L, and Mader J: Adjunctive Local Antibiotics in the Management of Contaminated Orthopaedic Wounds. *In* Final Program. American Academy of Orthopaedic Surgeons, 53rd Annual Meeting, New Orleans, Louisiana, 1986, p 86.
24. Clemente C (ed): Gray's Anatomy of the Human Body, 5th ed. Philadelphia: Lea & Febiger, 1985.
25. Codman EA: The Shoulder. Rupture of the Supraspinatus Tendon and Other Lesions in or About the Subacromial Bursa, 2nd ed. Malabar, FL: Robert E. Kreiger, 1984.
26. Cofield RH: Total shoulder arthroplasty with the Neer prosthesis. J Bone Joint Surg *66A*:899–906, 1984.
27. Costerton JW, Geesey GG, and Cheng K-J: How bacteria stick. Sci Am *238*:86–95, 1978.
28. Dankert J, Hogt AH, and Feijen J: Biomedical polymers: Bacterial adhesion, colonization, and infection. Crit Rev Biocompat 2:219–301, 1986.
29. David R, Barron BJ, and Madewell JE: Osteomyelitis, acute and chronic. Radiol Clin North Am *25*:1171–1201, 1987.
30. De Boeck H, Noppen L, and Desprechins B: Pyomyositis of the adductor muscles mimicking an infection of the hip. Diagnosis by magnetic resonance imaging: A case report. J Bone Joint Surg *76A*:747–750, 1994.
31. Desplaces N and Acar JF: New quinolones in the treatment of joint and bone infections. Rev Infect Dis *10*(Suppl 1):S179–S183, 1988.
32. DePalma AF (ed): Surgery of the Shoulder, 3rd ed. Philadelphia: JB Lippincott, 1983.
33. Dirschl DR and Almekinders LC: Osteomyelitis: Common causes and treatment recommendations. Drugs *45*:29–43, 1993.
34. Egerman RS, Mabie WC, Eifrid M, et al: Sacroiliitis associated with pyelonephritis in pregnancy. Obstet Gynaecol *85*:834–835, 1995.
35. Fitzgerald RH, Rosenblatt JE, Tenney JH, and Bourgault A-M: Anaerobic septic arthritis. Clin Orthop *164*:141–148, 1982.
36. Fletcher BD, Scoles PV, and Nelson AD: Osteomyelitis in children: Detection by magnetic resonance. Radiology *150*:57–60, 1984.
37. Fletcher M: Adherence of marine micro-organisms to smooth surfaces. *In* Beachy EH (ed): Bacterial Adherence. Receptors and Recognition, series B, Vol 6. London: Chapman & Hall, 1980, pp 347–374.
38. Fletcher M: Effect of solid surfaces on the activity of attached bacteria. *In* Savage DC and Fletcher M (eds): Bacterial Adhesion: Mechanisms and Physiological Significance. New York: Plenum Press, 1985, pp 339–362.
39. Flick AB, Herbert JC, Goodell J, and Kristiansen T: Noncommercial fabrication of antibiotic-impregnated polymethylmethacrylate beads. Technical note. Clin Orthop *223*:282–286, 1987.
40. Gabriel SB, Thometz JG, and Jaradeh S: Septic arthritis associated with brachial plexus neuropathy. J Bone Joint Surg *78A*:103–105, 1996.
41. Garnett ES, Cockshott WP, and Jacob J: Classical acute osteomyelitis with a negative bone scan. Br J Radiol *50*:757, 1977.
42. Gelberman RH, Menon J, Austerlitz S, and Weisman MH: Pyogenic arthritis of the shoulder in adults. J Bone Joint Surg *62A*:550–553, 1980.
43. Gentry LO: Osteomyelitis: Options for diagnosis and management. J Antimicrob Chemother *21*(Suppl):115–128, 1988.
44. Gibbons RJ and Van Houte J: Dental caries. Annu Rev Med *26*:121–136, 1975.
45. Gibbons RJ and Van Houte J: Bacterial adherence and the formation of dental plaques. *In* Beachey EH (ed): Bacterial Adherence: Receptors and Recognition, Series B, Vol 6. London: Chapman & Hall, 1980, pp 63–104.
46. Gifford DB, Patzakis M, Ivler D, and Swezey RL: Septic arthritis due to Pseudomonas in heroin addicts. J Bone Joint Surg 57-A:631–635, 1975.
47. Goldenberg DL: Gonococcal arthritis. *In* McCarty DJ (ed): Arthritis and Allied Conditions. A Textbook of Rheumatology, 10th ed. Philadelphia: Lea & Febiger, 1985, pp 1651–1661.
48. Goldenberg DL and Reed JI: Bacterial arthritis. N Engl J Med *312*:764–771, 1985.
49. Gompels BM and Darlington LG: Septic arthritis in rheumatoid disease causing bilateral shoulder dislocation: Diagnosis and treatment assisted by grey scale ultrasonography. Ann Rheum Dis *40*:609–611, 1981.
50. Goodell JA, Flick AB, Hebert JC, and Howe JG: Preparation and release characteristics of tobramycin-impregnated polymethylmethacrylate beads. Am J Hosp Pharm *43*:1454–1460, 1986.
51. Govan JRW and Fyfe JAM: Mucoid *Pseudomonas aeruginosa* and cystic fibrosis: Resistance of the mucoid form to carbenicillin, flucloxacillin and tobramycin and the isolation of mucoid variants in vitro. J Antimicrob Chemother *4*:233–240, 1978.
52. Govan JRW: Mucoid strains of *Pseudomonas aeruginosa*: The influence of culture medium on the stability of mucus production. J Med Microbiol *8*:513–522, 1975.
53. Gowans JDC and Granieri PA: Septic arthritis, its relation to intra-articular injections of hydrocortisone acetate. N Engl J Med *261*:502–504, 1959.
54. Gristina AG and Costerton JW: Bacteria-laden biofilms: A hazard to orthopedic prostheses. Infect Surg *3*:655–662, 1984.
55. Gristina AG and Costerton JW: Bacterial adherence to biomaterials and tissue. The significance of its role in clinical sepsis. J Bone Joint Surg *67A*:264–273, 1985.
56. Gristina AG and Rovere GD: An in vitro study of the effects of metals used in internal fixation on bacterial growth and dissemination. J Bone Joint Surg *45A*:1104, 1963.
57. Gristina AG, Hobgood CD, and Barth E: Biomaterial specificity, molecular mechanisms and clinical relevance of *S. epidermidis* and *S. aureus* infections in surgery. *In* Pulverer G, Quie PG, and Peters G (eds): Pathogenesis and Clinical Significance of Coagulase-Negative Staphylococci. Stuttgart: Fischer Verlag, 1987, pp 143–157.
58. Gristina AG, Kolkin J, Leake E, et al: Bacteria and Their Relationship to Biomaterials. First World Biomaterials Conference, Final Programme Book of Abstracts, p 2.39. Vienna, European Society for Biomaterials, 1980.
59. Gristina AG, Oga M, Webb LX, and Hobgood CD: Adherent bacterial colonization in the pathogenesis of osteomyelitis. Science *228*:990–993, 1985.
60. Gristina AG, Romano RL, Kammire GC, and Webb LX: Total shoulder replacement. Orthop Clin North Am *18*:445–453, 1987.
61. Gristina AG, Webb LX, and Barth E: Microbial adhesion, biomaterials, and man. *In* Coombs R and Fitzgerald R (eds): Infection in the Orthopaedic Patient. London: Butterworth Press, 1989, pp 30–42.
62. Gristina AG, Barth E, and Myrvik Q: Materials, microbes and man. The problem of infection associated with implantable devices. *In* Williams DF (ed): Current Perspectives on Implantable Devices. London: JAI Press, 1989.
63. Gristina AG, Hobgood CD, Webb LX, and Myrvik QN: Adhesive colonization of biomaterials and antibiotic resistance. Biomaterials *8*:423–426, 1987.
64. Gristina AG: Biomaterial-centered infection: Microbial adhesion versus tissue integration. Science *237*:1558–1595, 1987.

65. Gristina AG, Rovere GD, and Shoji H: Spontaneous septic arthritis complicating rheumatoid arthritis. J Bone Joint Surg *56A*:1180–1184, 1974.
66. Gupta NC and Prezio JA: Radionuclide imaging in osteomyelitis. Semin Nucl Med *18*:287, 1988.
67. Hamill RJ, Vann JM, and Proctor RA: Phagocytosis of *Staphylococcus aureus* by cultured bovine aortic endothelial cells: Model for postadherence events in endovascular infections. Infect Immun *54*:833–836, 1986.
68. Hendrix RW and Fisher MR: Imaging of septic arthritis. Clin Rheum Dis *12*:459–487, 1986.
69. Holderbaum D, Spech T, Ehrhart L, et al: Collagen binding in clinical isolates of Staphylococcus aureus. J Clin Microbiol *25*:2258–2261, 1987.
70. Holderbaum D, Hall GS, and Ehrhart LA: Collagen binding to *Staphylococcus aureus*. Infect Immun *54*:359–364, 1986.
71. Hopkins KL, Li KC, and Bergman G: Gadolinium-DTPA-enhanced magnetic resonance imaging of musculoskeletal infectious processes. Skeletal Radiol *24*:325–330, 1995.
72. Hoppe HG: Attachment of bacteria. Advantage or disadvantage for survival in the aquatic environment. *In* Marshall KC (ed): Microbial Adhesion and Aggregation. New York: Springer-Verlag, 1984, pp 283–301.
73. Hunter W: Of the structures and diseases of articulating cartilage. Philos Trans R Soc Lond *42*:514–521, 1743.
74. Itokazu M, Wenyi Y, Ooshima Y, and Matsunaga T: Suppurative knee arthritis following acute osteomyelitis of the femur detected by magnetic resonance. Chin Med J (Engl) *108*:704–707, 1995.
75. Jackson MA and Nelson JD: Etiology and medical management of acute suppurative bone and joint infections in pediatric patients. J Pediatr Orthop *2*:313, 1982.
76. Jennings R, Myrvik Q, Naylor P, et al: Comparative in vitro activity of LY146032 against biomaterial-adherent *Staphylococcus epidermidis*. *In* Abstracts of the Annual Meeting of the American Society for Microbiology, Washington, DC, 1988, p 18.
77. Jones GW and Isaacson RE: Proteinaceous bacterial adhesins and their receptors. Crit Rev Microbiol *10*:229–260, 1984.
78. Karten I: Septic arthritis complicating rheumatoid arthritis. Ann Intern Med *70*:1147–1151, 1969.
79. Kasemo B and Lausmaa J: Surface science aspects on inorganic biomaterials. Crit Rev Biocompat *2*:335–380, 1986.
80. Kellgren JH, Ball J, Fairbrother RW, and Barnes KL: Suppurative arthritis complicating rheumatoid arthritis. BMJ *1*:1193–1200, 1958.
81. Kelly PJ and Fitzgerald RH Jr: Bacterial arthritis. *In* Braude AI, Davis CE, and Fierer J (eds): Infectious Diseases and Medical Microbiology, 2nd ed. Philadelphia: WB Saunders, 1986, pp 1468–1472.
82. Kelly PJ, Martin WJ, and Coventry MD: Bacterial (suppurative) arthritis in the adult. J Bone Joint Surg *52A*:1595–1602, 1970.
83. Kelly PJ, Conventry MB, and Martin WJ: Bacterial arthritis of the shoulder. Mayo Clin Proc *40*:695–699, 1965.
84. Klein RS: Joint infection, with consideration of underlying disease and sources of bacteremia in hematogenous infection. Clin Geriatr Med *4*:375–394, 1988.
85. Krespi YP, Monsell EM, and Sisson GA: Osteomyelitis of the clavicle. Ann Otol Rhinol Laryngol *92*:525–527, 1983.
86. Ladd TI, Schmiel D, Nickel JC, and Costerton JW: Rapid method for detection of adherent bacteria on Foley urinary catheters. J Clin Microbiol *21*:1004–1006, 1985.
87. Lehninger AL: Principles of Biochemistry. New York: Worth Publishers, 1982.
88. Leslie BM, Harris JM, and Driscoll D: Septic arthritis of the shoulder in adults. J Bone Joint Surg *71A*:1516–1522, 1989.
89. Luskin RL and Kabins SA: Antimicrobial therapy in orthopaedic patients. *In* Post M (ed): The Shoulder. Surgical and Nonsurgical Management, 2nd ed. Philadelphia: Lea & Febiger, 1988, pp 108–138.
90. Mader JT, Landon GC, and Calhoun J: Antimicrobial treatment of osteomyelitis. Clin Orthop *295*:87–95, 1993.
91. Mandell GL, Douglas RG Jr, and Bennett JE (eds): Principles and Practice of Infectious Diseases, 2nd ed. New York: John Wiley, 1985.
92. Manny J, Haruzi I, and Yosipovitch Z: Osteomyelitis of the clavicle following subclavian vein catheterization. Arch Surg *106*:342–343, 1973.
93. Marrie TJ and Costerton JW: Prolonged survival of Serratia marcescens in chlorhexidine. Appl Environ Microbiol *42*:1093–1102, 1981.
94. Master R, Weisman MH, Armbuster TG, et al: Septic arthritis of the glenohumeral joint. Unique clinical and radiographic features and a favorable outcome. Arthritis Rheum *10*:1500–1506, 1977.
95. McCarty DJ (ed): Arthritis and Allied Conditions. A Textbook of Rheumatology, 10th ed. Philadelphia: Lea & Febiger, 1985.
96. Medical Staff Conference: Arthritis caused by viruses. California Med *119*:38–44, 1973.
97. Merkel KD, Brown ML, DeWanjee MK, and Fitzgerald RH: Comparison of indium-labeled leukocyte imaging with sequential technetium-gallium scanning in the diagnosis of low-grade musculoskeletal sepsis. J Bone Joint Surg *67A*:465–476, 1985.
98. Morrey BF and Bianco AJ: Hematogenous osteomyelitis of the clavicle in children. Clin Orthop *125*:24–28, 1977.
99. Morrissy RT: Bone and joint sepsis in children. *In* American Academy of Orthopaedic Surgeons Instructional Course Lectures. 55th Annual Meeting of the American Academy of Orthopedic Surgeons, Atlanta, Georga, February 4–9, 1988.
100. Neihart RE, Fried JS, and Hodges GR: Coagulase-negative staphylococci. Southern Med J *81*:491–500, 1988.
101. Neer CS and Kirby RM: Revision of humeral head and total shoulder arthroplasties. Clin Orthop *170*:189–195, 1982.
102. Neer CS and Rockwood CA Jr.: Fractures and dislocations of the shoulder. *In* Rockwood CA and Green DP (eds): Fractures in Adults, Vol 1. Philadelphia: JB Lippincott, 1984, pp 675–721.
103. Neer CS, Watson KC, and Stanton FJ: Recent experience in total shoulder replacement. J Bone Joint Surg *64A*:319–337, 1982.
104. Nelson JD and Koontz WC: Septic arthritis in infants and children: A review of 117 cases. Pediatrics *38*:966–971, 1966.
105. Nelson JD: Antibiotic concentrations in septic joint effusions. N Engl J Med *284*:349–353, 1971.
106. Neu HC: Cephalosporin antibiotics as applied in surgery of bones and joints. Clin Orthop *190*:50–64, 1984.
107. Norden CW: Osteomyelitis. *In* Mandell G, Gordon D, and Bennett J (eds): Principles and Practice of Infectious Diseases, 2nd ed. New York: John Wiley, 1985, pp 704–711.
108. Norden C: Experimental osteomyelitis. IV. Therapeutic trials with rifampin alone and in combination with gentamicin, sisomicin, and cephalothin. J Infect Dis *132*:493–499, 1975.
109. Norden CW: A critical review of antibiotic prophylaxis in orthopedic surgery. Rev Infect Dis *5*:928–932, 1983.
110. O'Meara PM and Bartal E: Septic arthritis: process, etiology, treatment outcome: A literature review. Orthopedics *11*:623–628, 1988.
111. Patzakis MJ, Wilkins M, and Moore TM: Use of antibiotics in open tibial fractures. Clin Orthop *178*:31–35, 1983.
112. Post M: The Shoulder: Surgical and Nonsurgical Management. Philadelphia: Lea & Febiger, 1988.
113. Rimoin DL and Wennberg JE: Acute septic arthritis complicating chronic rheumatoid arthritis. JAMA *196*:617–621, 1966.
114. Roca RP and Yoshikawa TT: Primary skeletal infections in heroin users: A clinical characterization, diagnosis and therapy. Clin Orthop *144*:238–248, 1979.
115. Ruseska I, Robbins J, and Costerton JW: Biocide testing against corrosion-causing oil-field bacteria helps control plugging. Oil Gas J *10*:253–264, 1982.
116. Salter RB, Bell RS, and Keeley FW: The protective effect of continuous passive motion in living articular cartilage in acute septic arthritis: An experimental investigation in the rabbit. Clin Orthop *159*:223–247, 1981.
117. Sartoris DJ and Resnick D: Magnetic resonance imaging for musculoskeletal disorders. Western J Med *148*:102–109, 1988.
118. Savage DC and Fletcher M (eds): Bacterial Adhesion: Mechanisms and Physiological Significance. New York: Plenum Press, 1985.
119. Schmid FR: Principles of diagnosis and treatment of bone and joint infections. *In* McCarty DJ (ed): Arthritis and Allied Conditions. A Textbook of Rheumatology. Philadelphia: Lea & Febiger, 1985, pp 1627–1650.
120. Schmidt D, Mubarak S, and Gelberman R: Septic shoulders in children. J Pediatr Orthop *1*:67–72, 1981.
121. Schwarzmann S and Boring JR III: Antiphagocytic effect of slime from a mucoid strain of Pseudomonas aeruginosa. Infect Immun *3*:762–767, 1971.
122. Scott JT (ed): Copeman's Textbook of the Rheumatic Diseases, 6th ed, Vol 1. New York: Churchill Livingstone, 1986.

123. Sharp JT: Gonococcal arthritis. *In* McCarty DJ (ed): Arthritis and Allied Conditions. A Textbook of Rheumatology, 9th ed. Philadelphia: Lea & Febiger, 1979, pp 1353–1362.
124. Sharp JT, Lidsky MD, Duffey J, and Duncan MW: Infectious arthritis. Arch Intern Med *139*:1125–1130, 1979.
125. Slusher MM, Myrvik QN, Lewis JC, and Gristina AG: Extended-wear lenses, biofilm, and bacterial adhesion. Arch Ophthalmol *105*:110–115, 1987.
126. Smith JW: Infectious arthritis. *In* Mandell GL, Douglas RG Jr., and Bennett JE (eds): Principles and Practice of Infectious Diseases. New York: John Wiley & Sons, 1985, pp 697–704.
127. Smith JW and Piercy EA: Infectious arthritis. Clin Infect Dis *20*:225–231, 1995.
128. Smith JW and Sanford JP: Viral arthritis. Ann Intern Med *67*:651–659, 1967.
129. Smith RL and Schurman DJ: Comparison of cartilage destruction between infectious and adjuvant arthritis. J Orthop Res *1*:136–143, 1983.
130. Smith RL, Schurman DJ, Kajiyama G, et al: The effect of antibiotics on the destruction of cartilage in experimental infectious arthritis. J Bone Joint Surg *69A*:1063–1068, 1987
131. Speers DJ and Nade SML: Ultrastructural studies of adherence of Staphylococcus aureus in experimental acute haematogenous osteomyelitis. Infect Immun *49*:443–446, 1985
132. Speziale P, Raucci G, Visai L, et al: Binding of collagen to *Staphylococcus aureus* Cowan 1. J Bacteriol *167*:77–81, 1986.
133. Srivastava KK, Garg LD, and Kochhar VL: Tuberculous osteomyelitis of the clavicle. Acta Orthop Scand *45*:668–672, 1974.
134. Steigbigel NH: Diagnosis and management of septic arthritis. *In* Remington JS and Swartz MN (eds): Current Clinical Topics in Infectious Diseases. New York: McGraw-Hill, 1983, pp 1–29.
135. Stern GA and Lubniewski A: The interaction between *Pseudomonas aeruginosa* and the corneal epithelium. Arch Ophthalmol *103*:1221–1225, 1985.
136. Sugarman B and Young EJ (eds): Infections Associated with Prosthetic Devices. Boca Raton, FL: CRC Press, 1984.
137. Switalski LM, Ryden C, Rubin K, et al: Binding of fibronectin to *Staphylococcus* strains. Infect Immun 42:628–633, 1983.
138. Tehranzadeh J, Wang F, and Mesgarzadeh M: Magnetic resonance imaging of osteomyelitis. Crit Rev Diagn Imaging *33*:495–534, 1992.
139. Toby EB, Webb LX, Voytek A, and Gristina AG: Septic arthritis of the shoulder. Orthop Trans *11*:230, 1987.
140. Tromp RM, Hamers RJ, and Demuth JE: Quantum states and atomic structure of silicon surfaces. Science *234*:304–309, 1986.
141. Trueta J: The normal vascular anatomy of the human femoral head during growth. J Bone Joint Surg *39B*:358–394, 1957.
142. Trueta J: The three types of acute hematogenous osteomyelitis: A clinical and vascular study. J Bone Joint Surg *41B*:671–680, 1959.
143. Turek SL: Orthopaedics. Principles and Their Application. Philadelphia: JB Lippincott, 1977.
144. Voytek A, Gristina G, Barth E, et al: Staphylococcal adhesion to collagen in intra-articular sepsis. Biomaterials *9*:107–110, 1988.
145. Waldvogel FA, Medoff G, and Swartz MN: Osteomyelitis. Clinical Features, Therapeutic Consideration, and Unusual Aspects. Springfield, IL: Charles C Thomas, 1971.
146. Wallace R and Cohen AS: Tuberculous arthritis. A report of two cases with review of biopsy and synovial fluid findings. Am J Med *61*:277–282, 1976.
147. Ward JR and Atcheson SG: Infectious arthritis. Med Clin North Am *61*:313–329, 1977.
148. Ward J, Cohen AS, and Bauer W: The diagnosis and therapy of acute suppurative arthritis. Arthritis Rheum *3*:522–535, 1960.
149. Ward WC and Eckardt JJ: Subacromial/subdeltoid bursa abscesses: An overlooked diagnosis. Clin Orthop *288*:189–194, 1993.
150. Watt PJ and Ward ME: Adherence of Neisseria gonorrhoeae and other Neisseria species to mammalian cells. *In* Beachey EH (ed): Bacterial Adherence. Receptors and Recognition, series B, Vol 6. London. Chapman & Hall, 1980, pp 251–288.
151. Webb LX, Myers RT, Cordell AR, et al: Inhibition of bacterial adhesion by antibacterial surface pretreatment of vascular prostheses. J Vasc Surg *4*:16–21, 1986.
152. Webb LX, Naylor P, and Gristina AG: Unpublished data.
153. Woods DE, Bass JA, Johanson WG Jr, and Straus DC: Role of adherence in the pathogenesis of *Pseudomonas aeruginosa* lung infection in cystic fibrosis patients. Infect Immun *30*:694–699, 1980.
154. Wrangstadh M, Conway PL, and Kjelleberg S: The production and release of an extracellular polysaccharide during starvation of a marine *Pseudomonas* sp. and the effect thereof on adhesion. Arch Microbiol *145*:220–227, 1986.
155. Wray TM, Bryant RE, and Killen DA: Sternal osteomyelitis and costochondritis after median sternotomy. J Thorac Cardiovasc Surg *65*:227–233, 1973.
156. Wukich DK, Abreu SH, Callaghan JJ, et al: Diagnosis of infection by preoperative scintigraphy with indium-labeled white blood cells. J Bone Joint Surg *69A*:1353–1360, 1987.

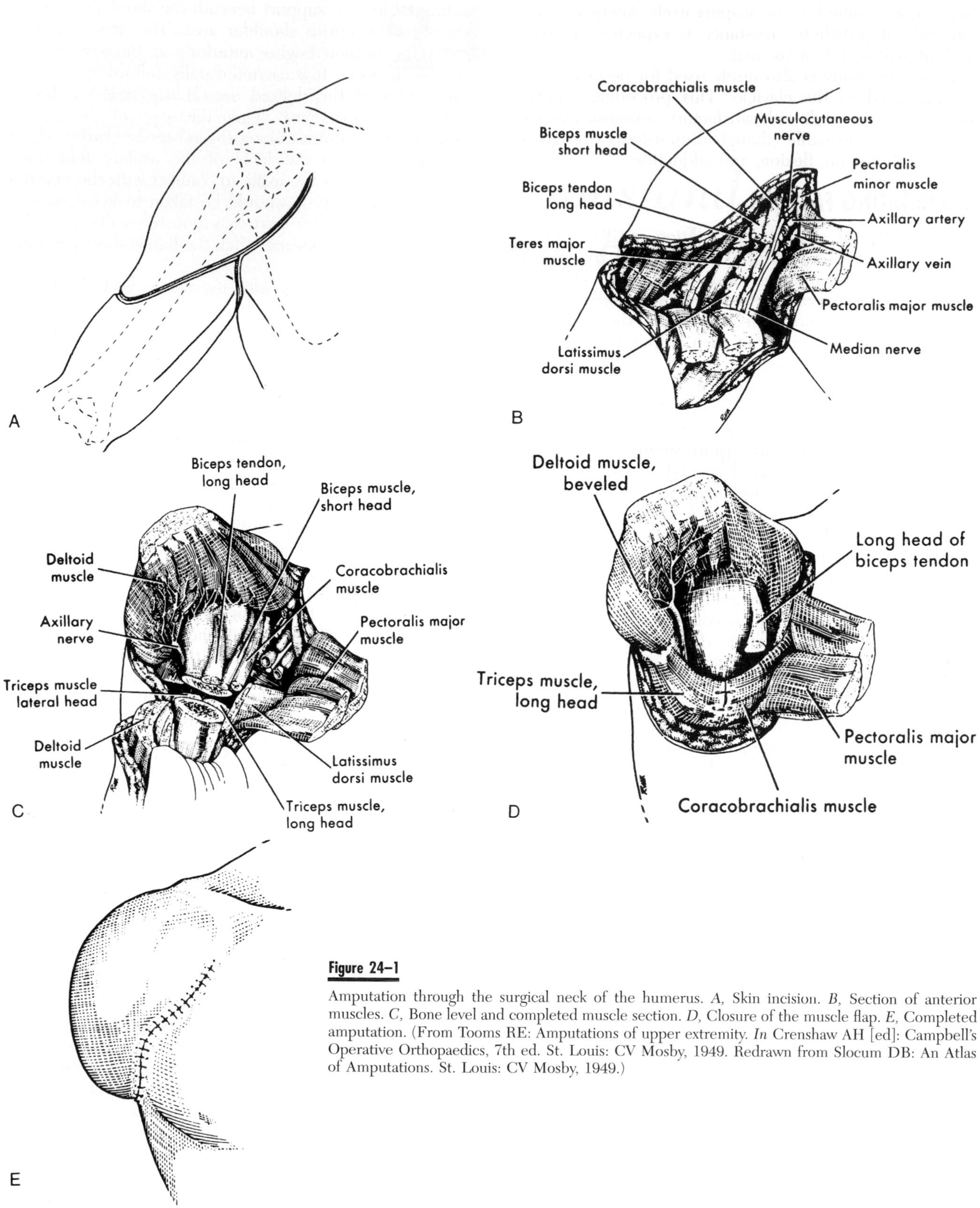

Figure 24–1

Amputation through the surgical neck of the humerus. *A,* Skin incision. *B,* Section of anterior muscles. *C,* Bone level and completed muscle section. *D,* Closure of the muscle flap. *E,* Completed amputation. (From Tooms RE: Amputations of upper extremity. *In* Crenshaw AH [ed]: Campbell's Operative Orthopaedics, 7th ed. St. Louis: CV Mosby, 1949. Redrawn from Slocum DB: An Atlas of Amputations. St. Louis: CV Mosby, 1949.)

years, described and illustrated his technique, which established the standard of the day. Baron Larrey was a skilled anatomist and an expert surgical technician; it has been said that he amputated more limbs than any surgeon before or since. He described performing 200 thigh amputations in one 24-hour period while accompanying Napoleon during the battle of Borodino. (A modified illustration of his shoulder disarticulation technique is shown in Figure 24–2.)

The patient is positioned supine with support under the affected shoulder, allowing complete access to the shoulder and shoulder girdle area. The incision begins anteriorly at the coracoid process and continues along the anterior border of the deltoid muscle, then is carried transversely across the proximal lateral humerus at the level of the deltoid muscle insertion (Fig. 24–3*A*). It is then continued superiorly along the posterior border of the muscle to end at the posterior axillary fold, where the two ends of the incision are joined with a second incision passing across the axilla. The cephalic vein is identified in the deltopectoral groove and ligated. The deltoid and pectoralis major muscles are separated anteriorly. The deltoid is then retracted laterally; the pectoralis major is divided at its humeral insertion and reflected medially.

The interval between the coracobrachialis and the short head of the biceps is opened to expose the neurovascular bundle (see Fig. 24–3*B*). The axillary artery and vein are doubly ligated independently of each other and then sectioned. The thoracoacromial artery, just proximal to the pectoralis minor muscle, is identified, ligated, and divided. The vessels then retract superiorly under the pectoralis minor muscle. The median, ulnar, musculocutaneous, and radial nerves can then be identified, drawn gently distally into the wound, ligated with a circumferential suture, and sectioned under mild tension. They then retract beneath the pectoralis minor muscle.

The coracobrachialis and short head of the biceps are then sectioned near their insertions on the coracoid process (see Fig. 24–3*C*). The deltoid muscle is freed from its insertion on the humerus and reflected superiorly to expose the capsule of the shoulder joint. The teres major and latissimus dorsi muscles are divided at their insertions, and the arm is placed in internal rotation to expose the short external rotator muscles, the posterior aspect of the shoulder joint, and the adjacent fascia. All of these structures are divided.

The arm is then rotated into full external rotation, and the anterior aspect of the joint capsule, the remaining shoulder capsule, and the subscapularis muscle are sectioned (see Fig. 24–3*D*). The triceps muscle is divided near its insertion, and the limb is severed from the trunk by dividing the inferior capsule of the shoulder joint. The

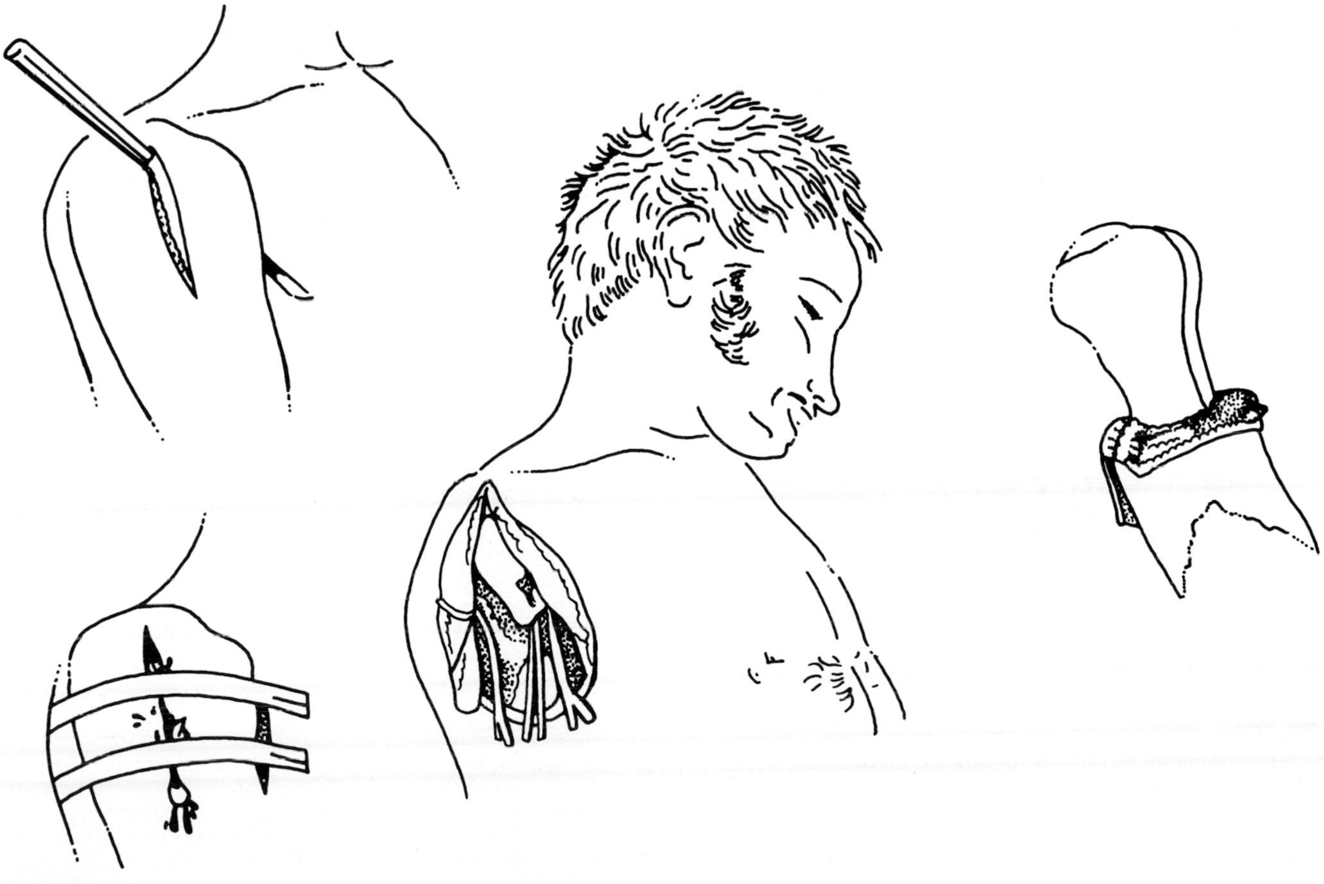

Figure 24–2

Modified illustration of shoulder disarticulation, which was performed by Baron Larrey and described in 1797. (Redrawn from Larrey DJ: Memoire sur les Amputations des Membres à La Suite des Coups de Feu Etaye de Plusieurs Observations. Paris: Du Pont, 1797.)

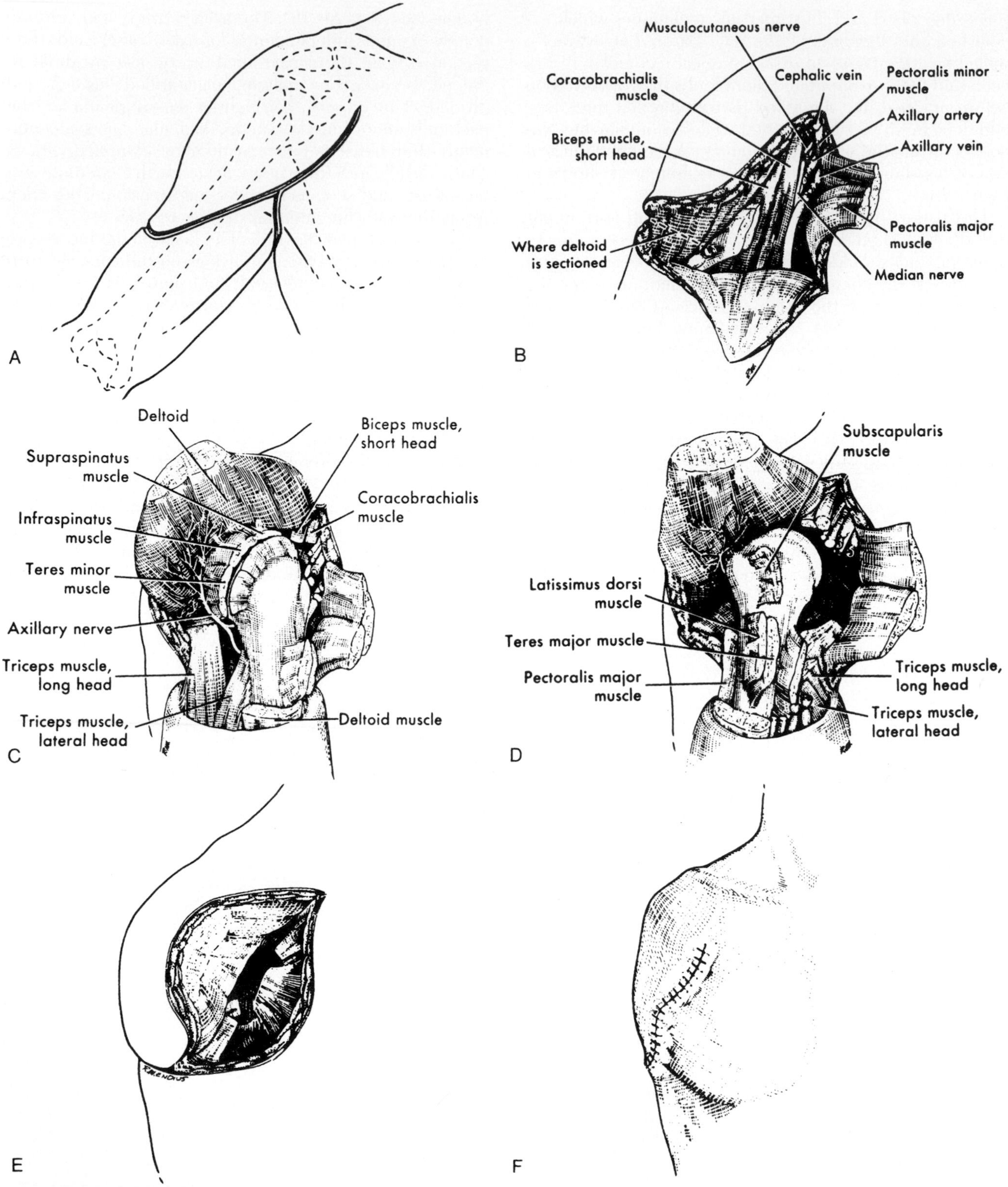

Figure 24–3

Disarticulation of the shoulder. *A,* Incision. *B,* Exposure and section of the neurovascular bundle. *C,* Reflection of the deltoid; the arm is placed in internal rotation; section of the supraspinatus, infraspinatus, and teres minor tendons and of the posterior capsule; section of the coracobrachialis and biceps at the coracoid. *D,* The arm is placed in external rotation; subscapularis and anterior capsule section. *E,* Suture of muscles in the glenoid cavity. *F,* Completed amputation. (From Tooms RE: Amputations of upper extremity. *In* Crenshaw AH [ed]: Campbell's Operative Orthopaedics, 7th ed. St. Louis: CV Mosby, 1987. Redrawn from Slocum DB: An Atlas of Amputations, St. Louis: CV Mosby, 1949.)

cut ends of all muscles are reflected into the glenoid cavity and sutured there to help fill the hollow left by the removal of the humeral head (see Fig. 24–3*E*).

The deltoid muscle flap is then brought down inferiorly to permit suturing just below the glenoid (see Fig. 24–3*F*). The closure is accomplished without tension using optimal wound closure technique. Drains, either suction or through-and-through or both, are inserted and closure is carried out in layers. Compression dressings are applied to assist in eliminating any residual dead space. Scar adhesions about the site of surgery can be painful and can complicate both cosmetic and functional prosthetic fit. Drains are usually removed in 48 hours, and the effective compression dressings are reapplied.

Forequarter Amputation

This radical procedure involves the surgical removal of the entire upper limb in the interval between the scapula and the thoracic wall. Its primary indication is the presence of malignant tumors about the shoulder girdle. Because such tumors often invade the regional lymph nodes and chest wall, the operation is considered essentially a life-saving salvage procedure. The surgery may control intractable pain for a time, although in present neoplastic management pain is best handled by a variety of medical techniques. Open ulceration and infection can further require careful planning to obtain skin and soft tissue coverage.

Most forequarter amputations performed today in Western countries are carried out by surgical services specializing in neoplastic diseases. The management of connective tissue malignant tumors of the limbs has been changing dramatically over the past decade and continues to change. In those few cases in which forequarter amputation seems to be indicated, the management team should consist of oncologists, plastic and reconstructive surgeons, and orthopedic or general surgeons. The surgery itself—except in unusual circumstances of trauma or tumor—is not complicated when carried out with the standard accepted techniques that have been used successfully for most of this century. Occasionally, staged procedures and skin or composite grafts are required to achieve wound closure.

ANTERIOR APPROACH

The incision begins at a point 4 cm lateral to the sternoclavicular articulation at a point corresponding to the lateral border of the sternocleidomastoid muscle insertion (Fig. 24–4*A*). It follows the entire anterior aspect of the clavicle and passes over the top of the shoulder to the spine of the scapula. At this point, the arm is flexed over the chest to rotate the scapula forward and outward so that its bony contour is outlined in greater relief. The posterior aspect of the upper incision then proceeds down over the spine to its vertical border, which it follows distally to the angle of the scapula. The lower portion of the ellipse starts in the middle third of the clavicle and passes downward in the groove between the deltoid and the pectoral muscles to the anterior axillary fold. The arm is abducted, and the incision is continued across the axilla at the level of the junction of the skin of the arm with the axillary skin. As the incision passes the posterior axillary fold, it continues medially across the back to join the upper incision at the angle of the scapula. The head is bent toward the normal side so that the sternocleidomastoid muscle may be better outlined, and the pectoralis major muscle is severed from its clavicular insertion. The dissection starts at the lateral border of the insertion and proceeds close to bone to the lateral border of the sternocleidomastoid muscle. The pectoralis major muscle is then reflected downward and medially. If further exposure is needed, the humeral insertion of the pectoralis major may be divided. The upper border of the clavicle is exposed by sectioning the superficial layer of the deep fascia along the upper border of the clavicle as far medially as the sternocleidomastoid muscle. Further dissection beneath the clavicle is carried out by means of the finger or a blunt curved dissector. The external jugular vein, which emerges just above the clavicle at the lateral border of the sternocleidomastoid, may be sectioned and ligated if it is in the way.

The clavicle is now divided by a Gigli or reciprocating power saw at the lateral border of the sternocleidomastoid muscle. It is not desirable to section the clavicle more medially because of the danger of injuring the veins that hug its medial inch. The clavicle is sectioned at or near the acromioclavicular joint, and the freed portion is removed (see Fig. 24–4*B*). If the humeral insertion of the pectoralis major muscle has not already been sectioned, this is done. This whole muscle may then be reflected downward, and the entire shoulder girdle may be retracted outward and downward so that the axillary and subclavian region is in full view. The axillary fascia is sectioned; the pectoralis minor is severed from its coracoid insertion; and the costocoracoid membrane that lies between the pectoralis minor and the subclavius is divided (see Fig. 24–4*D*). The second layer of deep fascia up to the level of the omohyoid muscle, the periosteum at the back of the clavicle, and the subclavius are divided to complete the exposure of the neurovascular bundle. The subclavian artery is isolated, sectioned, and doubly ligated. The blood in the extremity is emptied into the general circulation by elevation; the subclavian vein is then clamped, cut, and doubly ligated. The brachial plexus is identified, and each trunk is carefully ligated circumferentially. The nerves are sectioned one by one at the cranial end of the incision and allowed to retract. The latissimus dorsi muscle and all remaining soft tissues binding the shoulder girdle to the anterior chest wall are sectioned, and the limb falls freely backward.

SECTION OF THE POSTERIOR MUSCLES

The arm is placed across the chest and held with gentle downward traction. The posterior incision is deepened through the fascia, and the skin is retracted medially. The remaining muscles fixing the shoulder girdle to the scapula are divided as they are encountered from above downward. The muscles holding the scapula to the thorax are divided (see Fig. 24–4*E*). The incision starts at the inser-

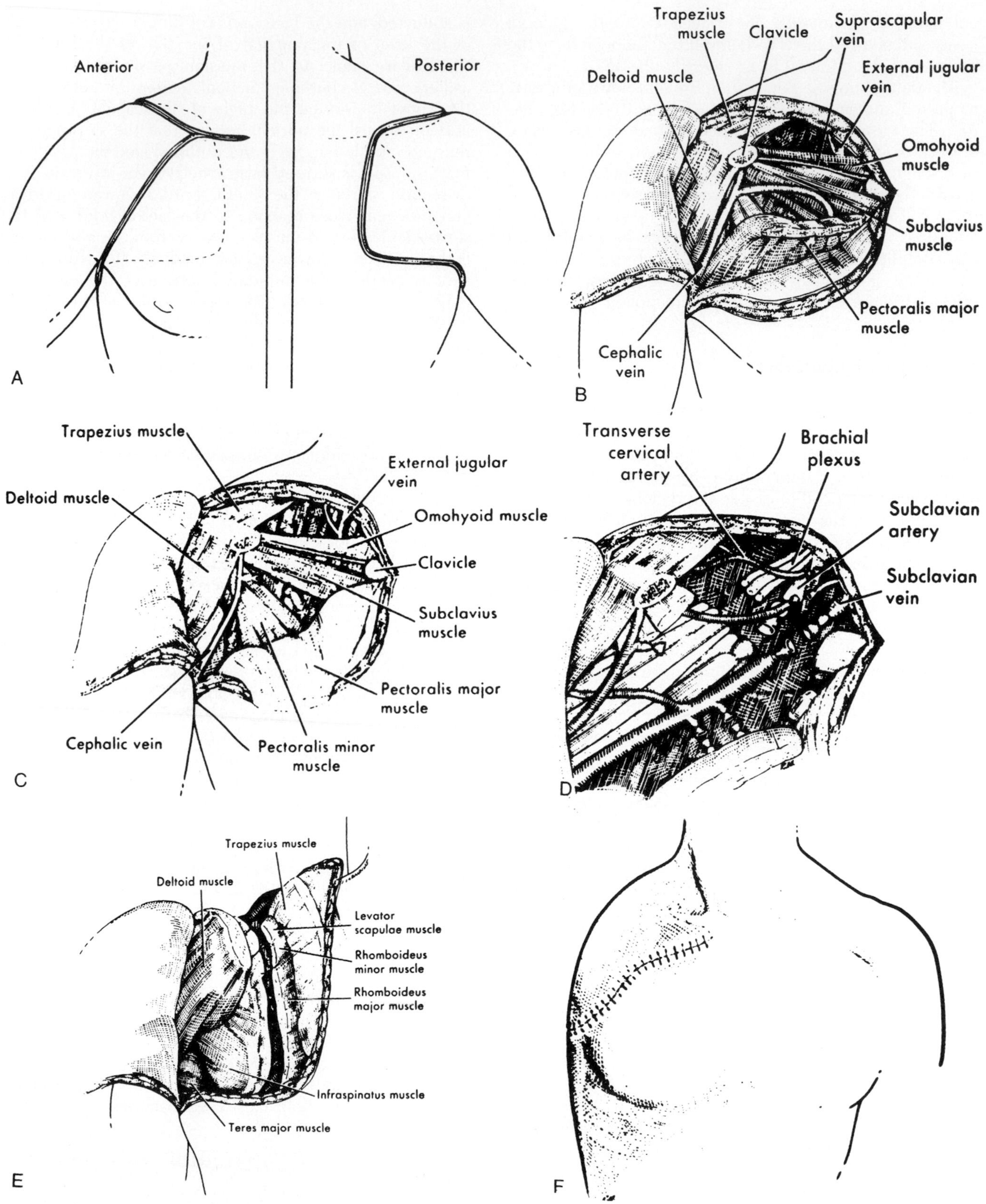

Figure 24–4

Forequarter amputation through the anterior approach. *A,* Incision. *B,* Resection of the clavicle. *C,* Lifting of the pectoral lid. *D,* Section of the vessels and nerves after incision through the axillary fascia and insertion of the pectoralis minor, the costocoracoid membrane, and the subclavius. *E,* Section of supporting muscles of the scapula. *F,* Completed amputation. (From Tooms RE: Amputations of upper extremity. *In* Crenshaw AH [ed]: Campbell's Operative Orthopaedics, 7th ed. St. Louis: CV Mosby, 1987. Redrawn from Slocum DB: An Atlas of Amputations. St. Louis: CV Mosby, 1949.)

tion of the trapezius to the clavicle and acromion and is carried downward along the upper border of the spine of the scapula. After sectioning, each muscle is retracted medially. The muscles along the superior angle of the vertebral border of the scapula—the omohyoid, levator scapulae, rhomboideus major and minor, and serratus anterior—are sectioned by placing double clamps near their insertions and cutting between the clamps from above downward. The extremity is removed, and hemostasis is controlled with meticulous care.

CLOSURE

Careful inspection is made to ensure that all malignant tissue has been removed. If the pectoralis major has not, of necessity, been removed, it should be sutured to the trapezius muscle. Closure is accomplished in layers, with all remaining muscular structures grouped over the lateral chest wall to provide as much padding as possible. The skin flaps are brought together and tailored to form an accurate approximation. The wound is closed with interrupted sutures (see Fig. 24–4*F*), and adequate drainage is accomplished. Dry dressings are applied, and a snug pressure dressing is placed over the lateral chest wall. The drains are removed in 48 to 72 hours, and the sutures are removed between the 10th and 14th days.

POSTERIOR APPROACH

Littlewood, in 1922, described a technique of forequarter amputation requiring two incisions and approaching the shoulder area from the posterior aspect (Fig. 24–5). This posterior approach is considered technically easier. We have used the conventional (Berger) anterior approach for cases under our care over the years but recognize the advantages of the two-incision technique, especially in atypical cases.

The patient is positioned on the uninvolved side near the edge of the operating table (see Fig. 24–5). Two incisions are required—one posterior (cervicoscapular) and one anterior (pectoroaxillary). The posterior incision is made first. Beginning at the medial end of the clavicle, the incision extends laterally for the entire length of the bone, carries over the acromion process to the posterior axillary fold, continues along the axillary border of the scapula to a point inferior to the scapular angle, and finally curves medially to end 2 inches from the midline of the back. From the scapular muscles an entire full-thickness flap of skin and subcutaneous tissue is elevated medially to a point just medial to the vertebral border of the scapula.

Next, the trapezius and latissimus dorsi muscles are identified and divided parallel with the scapula. The same is done to the levator scapulae, the rhomboideus major and minor, and the scapular attachments of the serratus anterior and the omohyoid. As the dissection progresses, vessels are ligated when necessary, especially the branches of the transverse cervical and transverse scapular arteries. The soft tissues are then freed from the clavicle, and the bone is divided at its medial end. The subclavius muscle is also divided.

The extremity is then allowed to fall anteriorly, thus placing the subclavian vessels and the brachial plexus under tension and making their identification easier. The cords of the plexus are clamped close to the spine, and the subclavian artery and vein are clamped, doubly ligated, and divided.

The anterior incision is then begun at the middle of the clavicle. It curves inferiorly just lateral to but parallel with the deltopectoral groove, extends across the anterior axillary fold, and finally carries inferiorly and posteriorly to join the posterior axillary incision at the lower third of the axillary border of the scapula. As the final step in the operation, the pectoralis major and minor muscles are divided and the limb is removed. The skin flaps are trimmed to allow a snug closure, and their edges are sutured with interrupted sutures of nonabsorbable material. Effective through-and-through and suction drains are inserted to eliminate accumulation of fluid. Firm chest wall pressure dressings are required. Drains can be removed after 48 hours.

Surgical variations, based on the nature and extent of the pathologic process, may indicate the need for regional lymph node resection and for soft tissue removal at the chest wall when the tumor has extended into these structures. Skin grafts, including composite tissues, may be necessary to obtain primary or secondary closure.

Interscapulothoracic Resection

Intercalary shoulder resection (the Tikhor-Linberg technique) achieves a massive removal of the musculoskeletal elements of the shoulder girdle, including the scapula, the lateral three fourths of the clavicle, and a portion of the proximal humerus, with extensive removal of all adjacent muscles. The neurovascular structures that supply the arm and the hand are preserved. Excessive skin is often left after this radical resection. The remaining connecting soft tissues across the former shoulder joint consist only of the axillary vessels and the brachial plexus, together with the axillary skin. Closure of the soft tissues, including the skin, is individualized according to the nature of the malignancy for which the surgery is performed. It is necessary to stabilize the proximal humerus to the remaining medial stump of the clavicle or the chest wall in order to prevent excessive drooping and telescoping of the arm.

This operation is rarely used in surgical practice today. A patient's refusal to allow formal amputation can, however, justify its use. The authors' experience is limited to two patients (both male), one with chondrosarcoma of the shoulder girdle and one with reticulum sarcoma. The latter patient achieved a 5-year survival and, in fact, is alive and well 12 years after the surgery; he has retained quite a remarkable degree of function of the elbow, forearm, and hand. An avid tennis player, he manages a competitive game as a bimanual athlete.

The operation is carried out with the patient in the full lateral position and lying on the uninvolved side. The entire upper extremity, chest, and neck are prepared and draped so that the arm, shoulder, and shoulder girdle are free for manipulation and positioning. The incision resembles a tennis racquet—the "handle" extends from

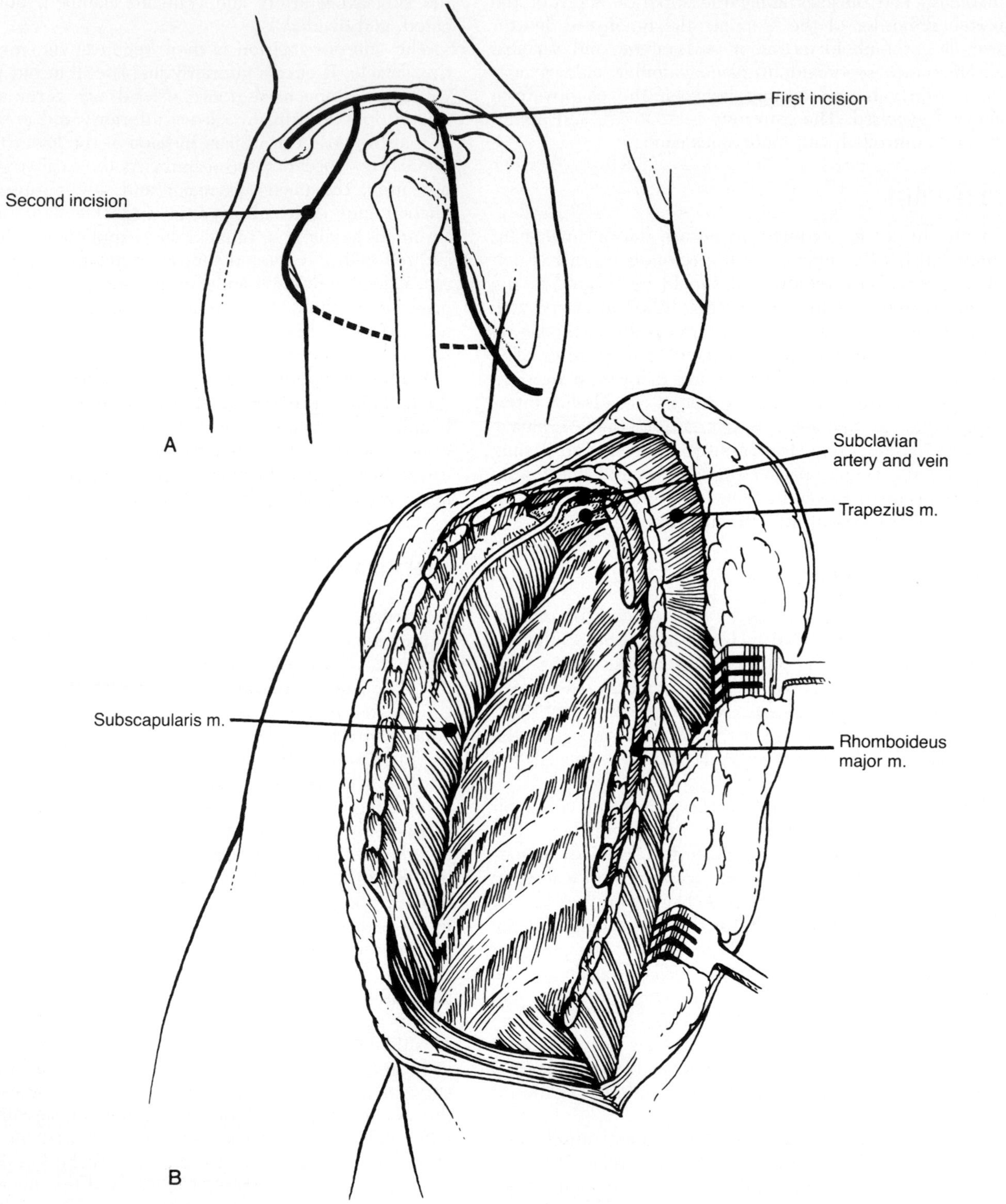

Figure 24–5

Forequarter amputation through the posterior approach (the Littlewood technique). (Redrawn from Littlewood H: Amputations at the shoulder and at the hip. BMJ *1*:381, 1922.)

the medial third of the clavicle laterally, while the anterior limb extends downward along the deltopectoral groove to the midpoint of the medial edge of the biceps, proceeds distally for 7 to 8 cm, then curves upward to cross the lateral surface of the arm at or just below the mid-deltoid level (Fig. 24–6). From this point, the posterior limb of the "racquet" curves from the mid-deltoid area downward and medially toward the inferior angle of the scapula, where it again curves upward to join the original clavicular incision near the acromioclavicular joint.

Deeper dissection can be carried out from either an anterior or a posterior approach. We have utilized a combination of both approaches. In effect, this dissection combines the classical anterior technique of forequarter amputation with the posterior approach (Littlewood) technique of this surgery. The brachial plexus is preserved, as are major vessels. It is necessary to ligate the transverse cervical, suprascapular, circumflex scapular, circumflex humeral, and thoracoacromial arteries. With the scapulothoracic muscles detached and the deltoid, biceps, and triceps sectioned, the humerus can be transected at or below the surgical neck at the level of election. The biceps, triceps, and deltoid muscles are attached to the thoracic wall, and the trapezius suspends the arm as firmly as possible without compromising neurovascular integrity. The wound is drained both by suction and through-and-through drains, which are removed in 48 hours. Soft compression dressings and a Velpeau-like sling support are used postoperatively.

The skin and soft tissue resection is modified to accommodate the removal of the neoplasm. The arm should be supported until sufficient scarring has occurred at the operative site to provide some stability. No attempt is made to regain a semblance of shoulder function. Rehabilitation concentrates on the neck and trunk muscles and on the arm distal to the site of amputation of the humerus. An adequate degree of hand, wrist, forearm, and elbow function can be achieved. Cosmesis is also surprisingly good, considering the massive tissue resection. The defect in the shoulder girdle and shoulder contour can be concealed with a light, modern prosthetic cosmetic restoration, using currently available materials—particularly the urethanes—that provides a more normal appearance of the shoulder area under clothing.

Scapulectomy

In 1864 Syme described excision of the scapula for primary bone tumors. The operation is used for isolated neoplasms of the scapula, a condition that is rarely seen. Neglected, slow-growing osteocartilaginous tumors arising in the scapula may cause functional compromise sufficient to warrant excision of the scapula, which is usually accom-

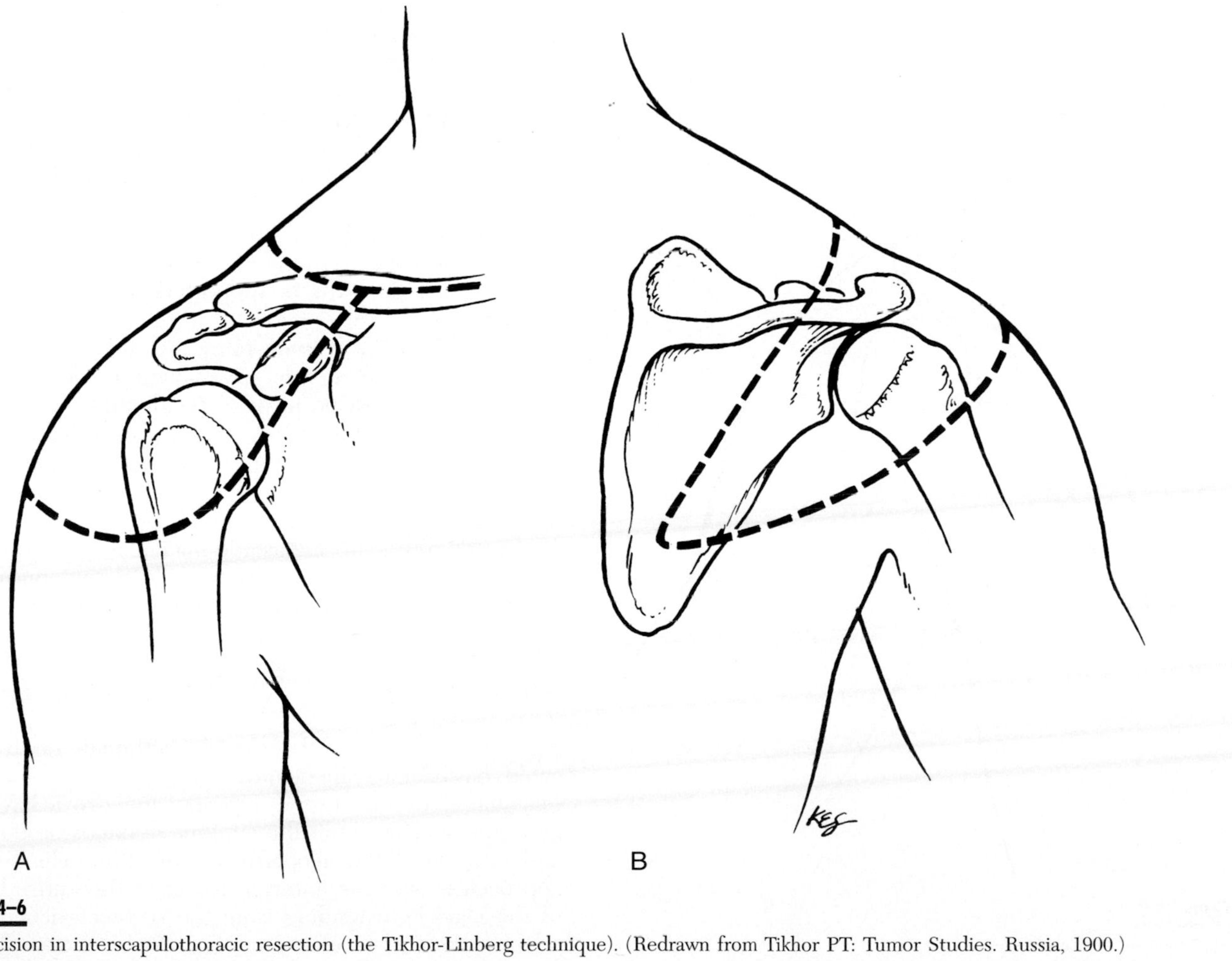

Figure 24–6

Skin incision in interscapulothoracic resection (the Tikhor-Linberg technique). (Redrawn from Tikhor PT: Tumor Studies. Russia, 1900.)

panied by adjuvant chemotherapy and radiation. A general description of the operative technique is presented here in the realization that there is literally no standard operative approach. When the tumor has extended beyond the confines of the bone, the surgery may require excision of lymph nodes in the complicated chains surrounding the shoulder girdle. Scapulectomy following a biopsy should include wide resection of the biopsy site, including skin and deep tissues.

The operation is carried out with the patient in the prone position, supported under the affected shoulder. The arm is draped free to allow movement of the humerus and scapula as the dissection proceeds. Regardless of the nature and type of the incision, adequate access to the entire superior border of the scapula is mandatory.

The classical incision begins laterally at the tip of the acromion and extends posteriorly directly below the acromion spine to its midportion, then gently curves distally across the body of the scapula to its inferior angle (Fig. 24–7). The nature of the pathologic process will determine the management of muscles and, specifically, those muscles that should be resected. Detaching the latissimus dorsi from the inferior angle allows the scapula to be tilted upward and outward, thus affording free access to the subscapular space.

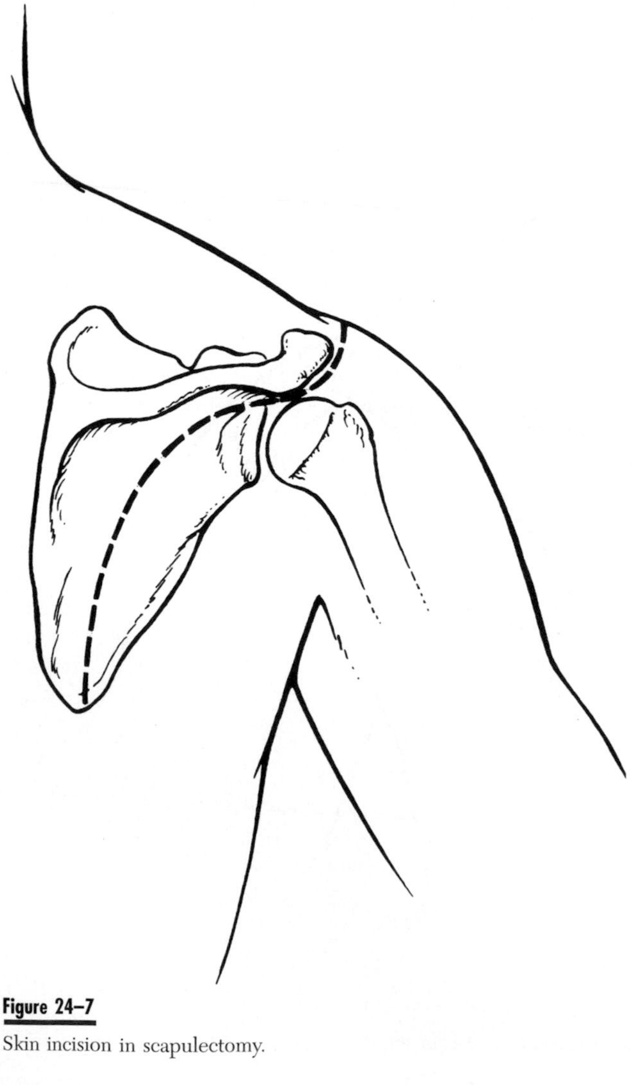

Figure 24–7

Skin incision in scapulectomy.

The vertebral border of the scapula is then freed, and the remaining insertions of the inferior and middle trapezius are detached from the spine of the scapula, exposing the rhomboids for division. The superior trapezius is divided from the scapular spine, the acromion, and the distal clavicle. The levator scapulae is sectioned. The superficial cervical and descending scapular vessels are identified and ligated. The suprascapular vessels and nerves are exposed; and, as the scapula is lifted further laterally from the thorax, the brachial plexus and axillary vessels come into view. It is important to remove the supraspinatus and infraspinatus and the serratus anterior along with the scapula itself. The nature and extent of the pathologic process will dictate whether it is possible to preserve the acromion and the continuity of the superior trapezius-deltoid suspensory system.

The axillary border of the scapula is then approached with transection of the deltoid from the spine of the scapula and from the acromion. The teres major and the long head of the triceps muscles are transected; the subscapular artery is identified and ligated; and the underlying axillary and radial nerves are carefully preserved. The disarticulation of the acromioclavicular joint and detachment of the coracoclavicular ligaments or division of the clavicle just medial to the coracoclavicular ligaments allows the scapula to be further freed from the chest. The pectoralis minor, coracobrachialis, and short head of the biceps muscles can then be detached from the coracoid process, and the rotator cuff can be transected by external and internal rotation of the humerus. It may be appropriate to modify the level of section of the rotator cuff so that after removal of the scapula, the distal cuff can be sutured about the distal clavicle to suspend and stabilize the humerus and to preserve a more cosmetic shoulder outline. The wound is closed in layers over adequate drainage systems. Compression dressings are applied, and the arm is supported in a Velpeau-type dressing.

Variations of the scapulectomy technique are the rule rather than the exception. Even with modern imaging systems, it may not be possible to identify the extent of the tumor until surgery. In general, oncologists prefer other nonoperative and surgical methods of treatment of neoplasms involving the scapula. Similarly, scapulectomy to control intractable pain caused by a tumor can be unsuccessful. Finally, metastatic malignancy involving the scapula is not an indication for scapulectomy; nonsurgical management is considered to be the treatment of choice.

Claviculectomy

En bloc resection of the clavicle, although rarely indicated, has occasionally been recommended for a localized malignancy or for chronic osteomyelitis. To a large degree, the specific surgical technique depends on the type and location of the neoplasm or infection. The surgical approach is over the anterior aspect of the entire length of the clavicle, extending from the sternoclavicular joint to the acromioclavicular joint (Fig. 24–8). Biopsy sites, if

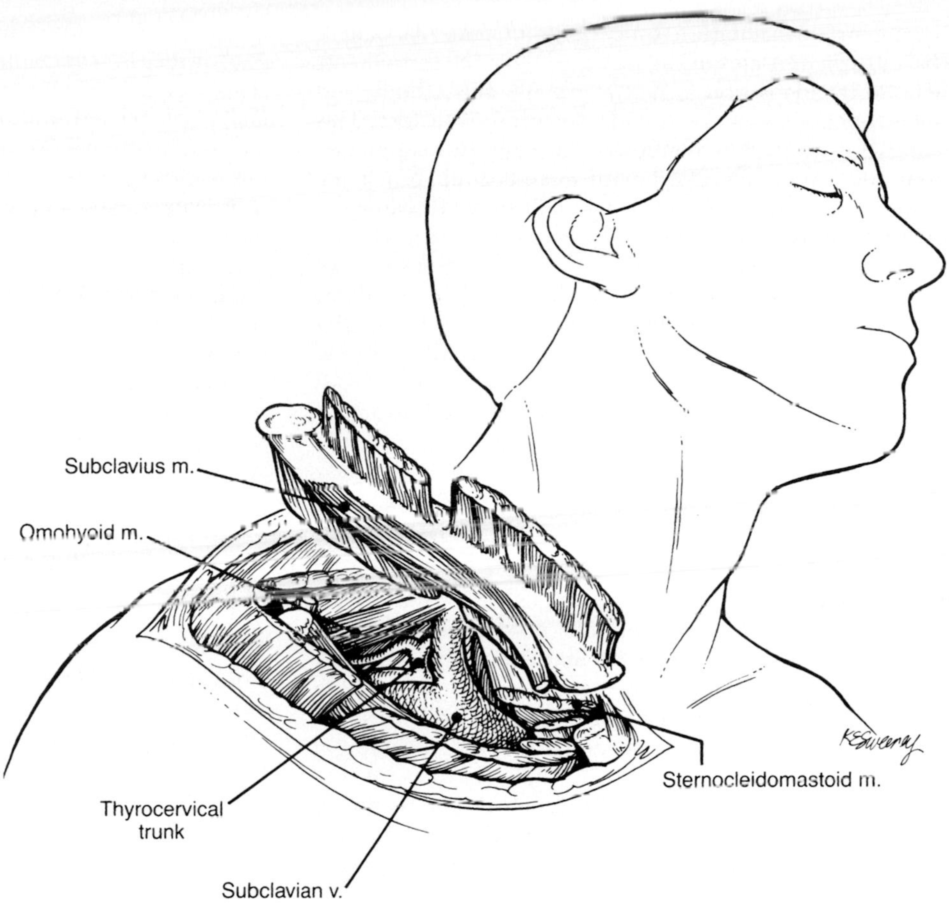

Figure 24–8

Claviculectomy. (Redrawn from Lewis MM, Ballet FL, Kroll PG, and Bloom N. En bloc clavicular resection, operative procedure and postoperative testing of function. Clin Orthop 193:214, 1985.)

present, are widely excised. Dissection is carried down to the deltoid insertion, which is divided from the clavicle, leaving an intact proximal muscular cuff. The conoid and trapezoid ligaments are divided near their clavicular attachment, and the sternocleidomastoid muscle is carefully sectioned, avoiding injury to the external jugular vein. The omohyoid muscle is retracted, and the pectoralis major is incised. The clavicle is then elevated, leaving the subclavicular muscle attached to the clavicle. The sternoclavicular capsule, sternohyoid muscle insertion, and costoclavicular ligament are all excised. Immediately adjacent vascular structures are carefully protected, and the branches of the transverse cervical artery are ligated. The clavicle is then removed.

Closure in layers, eliminating dead spaces, is carried out over drainage. Compression dressings and a sling are applied, and drains are removed within 24 to 48 hours. The shoulder and the arm are mobilized as early as is consistent with wound healing.

Technical variations, based on the site and nature of the tumor, individualize the surgery to such a degree that each case must be planned surgically as a specific technical challenge. Reported series usually include only three or four cases. We have not had occasion to perform this resection-amputation.

PROSTHETIC REHABILITATION

Shoulder area amputations present the most difficult challenge for functional restoration by external prosthetic replacement. Many unilateral amputees reject a functional prosthesis because of the weight, the limitations of dexterity, the difficulty positioning the terminal device where it is needed, the slowness of the prosthesis, and the inability to use these prosthetic devices without undue mental involvement. The requirements of providing a functional terminal device and the control to rapidly position that terminal device in space are rarely met with current prosthetic devices. Although the functional gain is less than ideal, the cosmetic deformity of shoulder level amputations should not be underestimated. Shirts and jackets drape awkwardly on the side of the shoulder disarticulation or forequarter amputation, exaggerating the cosmetic deformity. Often, a lightweight cosmetic substitute or merely a prosthetic shoulder cap to recreate the normal shoulder contour can meet a patient's goals better than a heavier, functional prosthesis. The remaining limb, whether initially dominant or not, rapidly accommodates to permit most basic activities associated with daily life.

Bilateral shoulder amputations create just the opposite functional demand. The handicap is so severe that prostheses, even though uncomfortable, heavy, and functionally crude compared with normal limbs, provide sufficient critically needed function to justify the training, discomfort, and inconvenience associated with their use. Children born with amelia of both upper limbs rapidly learn to use their legs and feet to substitute. Remarkable skill can be achieved. Lower limb joints, particularly the hips, ankles, and feet, develop abnormally large ranges of movement to facilitate a wide range of foot placement. The intrinsic muscles of the feet as well as the tarsal joints respond by adaptation to perform many grasp, hook, and pinch functions that are usually not present in feet. This adaptive substitution continues through the amputee's adult life. Although fitted with cosmetic or functional upper limb prostheses, the individual usually discards the artificial limbs in the home and work setting and uses them only for social purposes.

Adults who sustain bilateral shoulder level amputations, and in particular the elderly, often cannot develop the lower limb functional response seen in children. Some substitution can occur, although under most circumstances such a severely disabled individual requires constant attendant help.

Types of Prostheses

Prostheses for shoulder level amputees are of four types: (1) body powered, (2) externally powered, (3) hybrid combinations of body powered and externally powered, and (4) cosmetic. The amputee is often best served by a hybrid combination of body powering and external powering with interchangeable terminal devices, including a cosmetic hand.

The simplest artificial substitute is a nonfunctional, strictly cosmetic device (Fig. 24–9). Modern designs are light, usually fabricated of urethanes or similar synthetics, with light internal or external frame rigidity (when necessary) supplied by graphite, light metals, or semi-rigid thermoplastics. The shoulder cap of the prosthesis is contoured to correspond with the opposite shoulder shape. Light shoulder strap suspension stabilizes the limb and prevents it from slipping off. The elbow is simple and nonfunctional and permits stable positioning at various angles by the opposite limb. The hand can be individually constructed to match the remaining hand. The psychological advantage of a cosmetic prosthesis often plays a very important and integral part in physical rehabilitation.

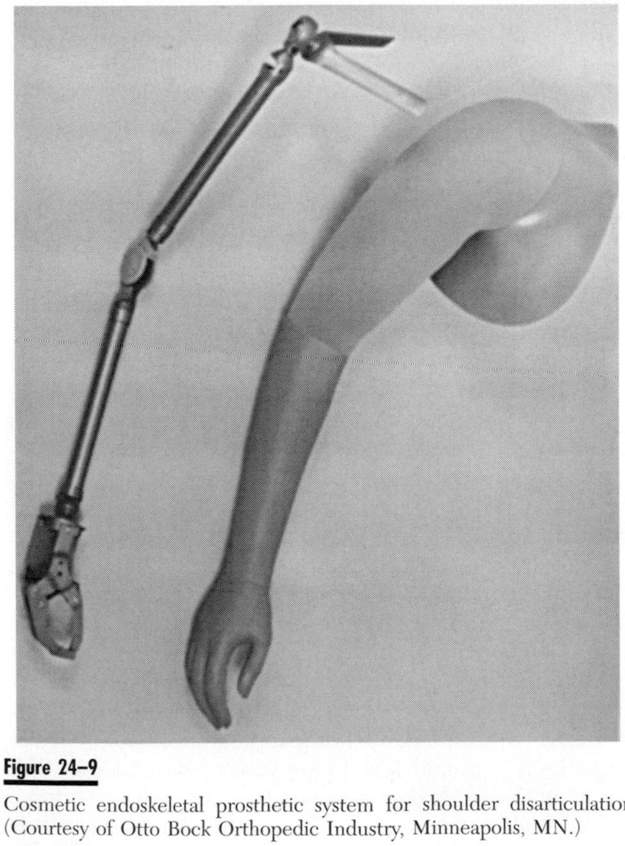

Figure 24–9

Cosmetic endoskeletal prosthetic system for shoulder disarticulation. (Courtesy of Otto Bock Orthopedic Industry, Minneapolis, MN.)

These cosmetic limbs vary tremendously in cost. While simply recreating the shape and contour can be relatively cost effective, the most elegant and detailed cosmesis can be quite expensive. They are obtained through regular prosthetic sources with the services of a cosmetic restoration artist, who is responsible for the shape, texture, and surface detail, including color. Most major population centers in the United States, Canada, and Europe can provide these services. Contact with these skilled professionals is made in cooperation with conventional professional prosthetists.

This passive cosmetic replacement is not entirely without function. The hand can assist in stabilizing objects on a table or workbench. In general, the active unilateral amputee will use a cosmetic prosthesis only for special social occasions and not in the course of daily work and living activities. In these instances, one should not overlook the possibility that a simple shoulder cap can improve the thoracic contours, help clothing fit better, and help the patient feel less conspicuous (Fig. 24–10 *A–C*).

BODY-POWERED FUNCTIONAL PROSTHESES

A substitute limb that can perform useful functions poses a difficult engineering challenge. It requires articulation at the elbow and should permit a degree of positioning of the terminal device (wrist/hand) (Fig. 24–11). Some degree of shoulder abduction and elbow rotation is also required if positioning of the hand or hook is to operate within a significant range of usefulness. Suspending the limb and attaching it sufficiently to the body to provide stability dictates the use of a large shoulder cap, which is usually made of semi-flexible materials, and additional straps around the trunk and across the opposite shoulder. Activation of the hand or hook is accomplished by opposite shoulder movement using a shoulder loop attached to cabling, either light, housed metal or nylon. The prosthesis can be either pre-positioned and then locked or, in the case of the elbow, cable controlled (Fig. 24–12).

For years prosthetic engineers have attempted to simplify this prosthesis. Attempting to duplicate, even to a small degree, the unbelievably complex motor and sensory function of the upper limb frustrates such engineering attempts. As a result, even with present technology, the body-powered limbs are rather crude, uncomfortable, and severely limited in function. More often, such limbs are designed for a special purpose, such as working at a bench or desk. When the zone of functional activity of the terminal device is confined to a relatively small area, it is more feasible to accommodate design, thus making the prosthesis more acceptable (Figs. 24–13 to 24–16).

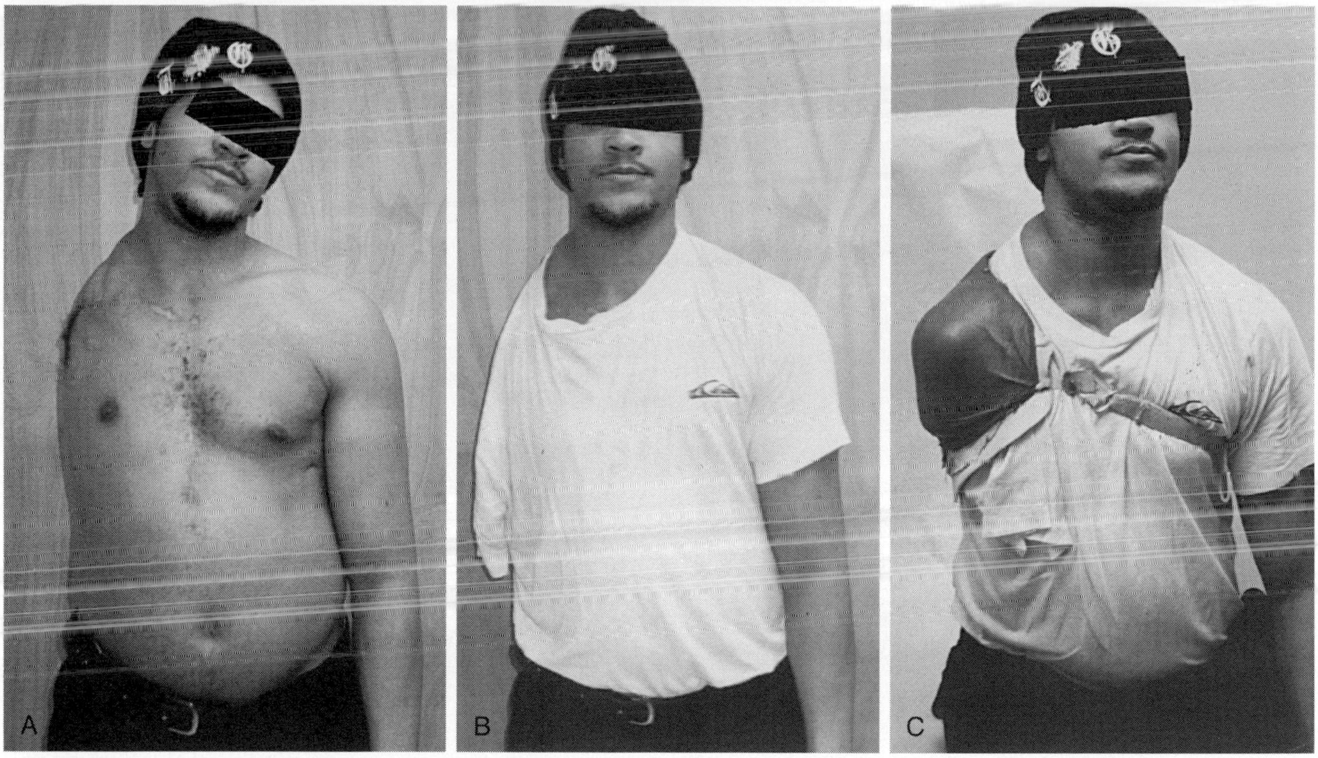

Figure 24–10

A, Dramatic loss of shoulder contour following forequarter amputation. *B*, Clothing drapes awkwardly exaggerating the cosmetic deformity. *C*, A simple shoulder cap prosthesis recreates a more normal shoulder contour and improves the fit of clothing worn over the shoulder cap. (*A–C*, Courtesy of Prosthetics Research Study, Seattle, WA.)

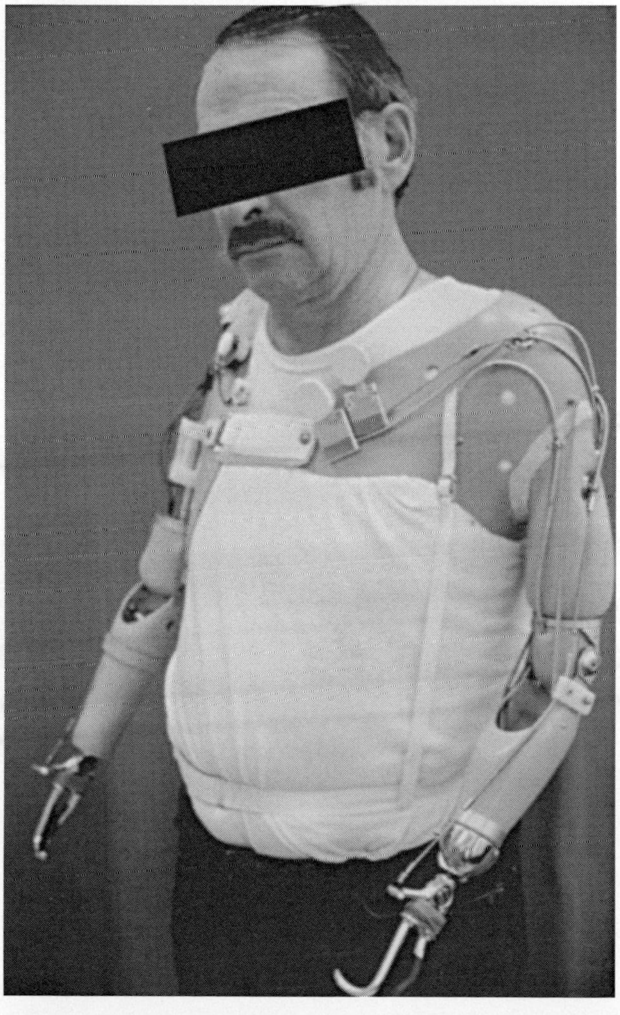

Figure 24–11

A cable-operated left arm with a positive-locking cable-operated elbow, positive-locking wrist rotation unit, positive-locking wrist flexion unit, and cable-operated split hook. The elbow lock is controlled by a tether to a waist belt. The locks of the two wrist components are controlled by the two nudge controls on the anterior panel of the socket. (Courtesy of Dudley S. Childress, Ph.D., Prosthetics Research Laboratory, Northwestern University and the Orthotics and Prosthetics Clinical Services Department, Rehabilitation Institute of Chicago.)

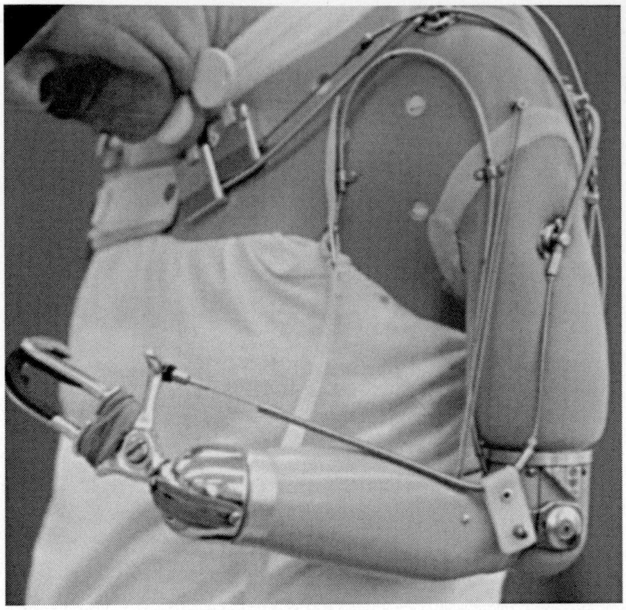

Figure 24–12

The patient is releasing the lock of the wrist flexion unit. (Courtesy of Dudley S. Childress, Ph.D., Prosthetics Research Laboratory, Northwestern University and the Orthotics and Prosthetics Clinical Services Department, Rehabilitation Institute of Chicago.)

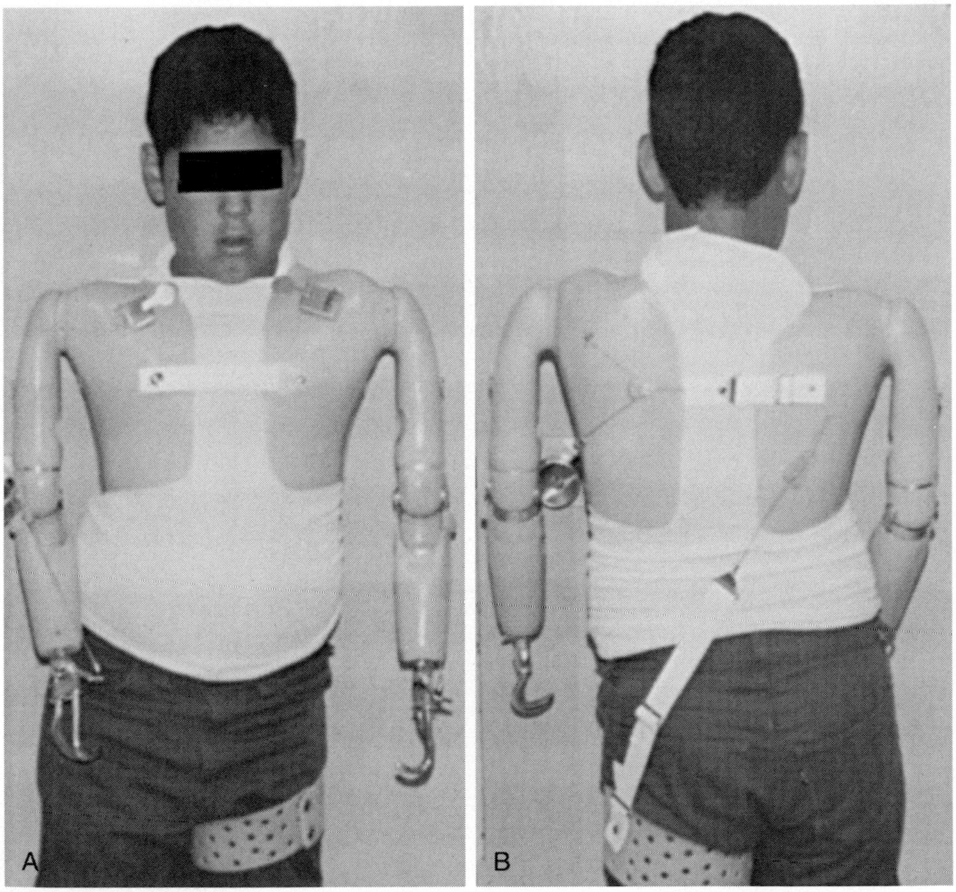

Figure 24–13

A body-powered prosthesis for bilateral phocomelia. (Courtesy of Alpha Orthopedic Appliance Co., Los Angeles, CA.)

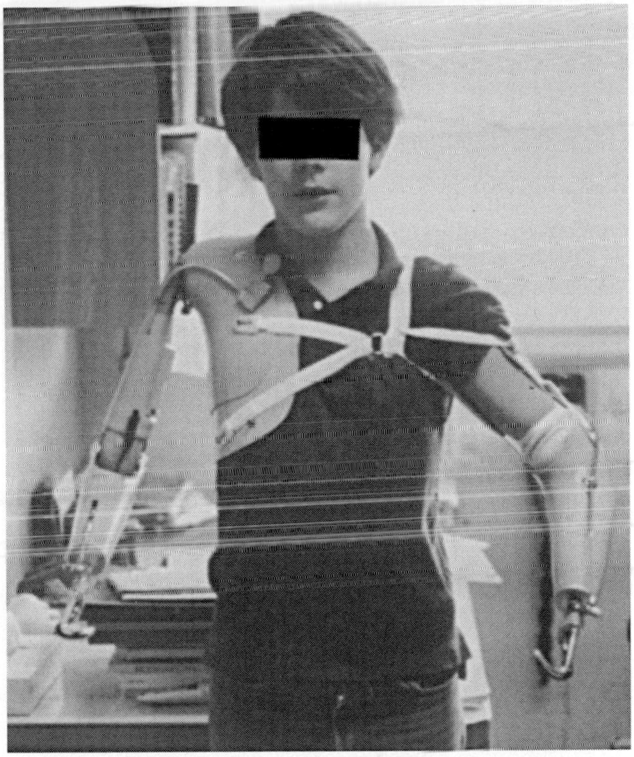

Figure 24–14

Prosthetic management for bilateral upper limb amputation. Right shoulder disarticulation and left below-elbow prostheses. (Courtesy of Eric Baron, C.P.O., University of California, Child Amputee Prosthetics Project, Los Angeles, CA.)

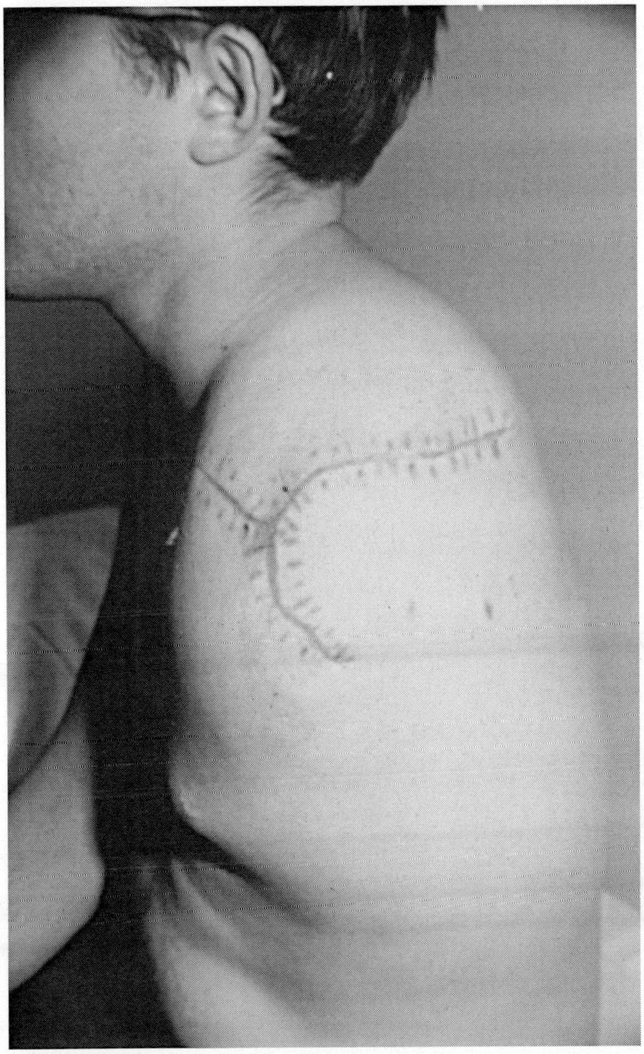

Figure 24–15

A forequarter amputee ready for prosthetic fitting.

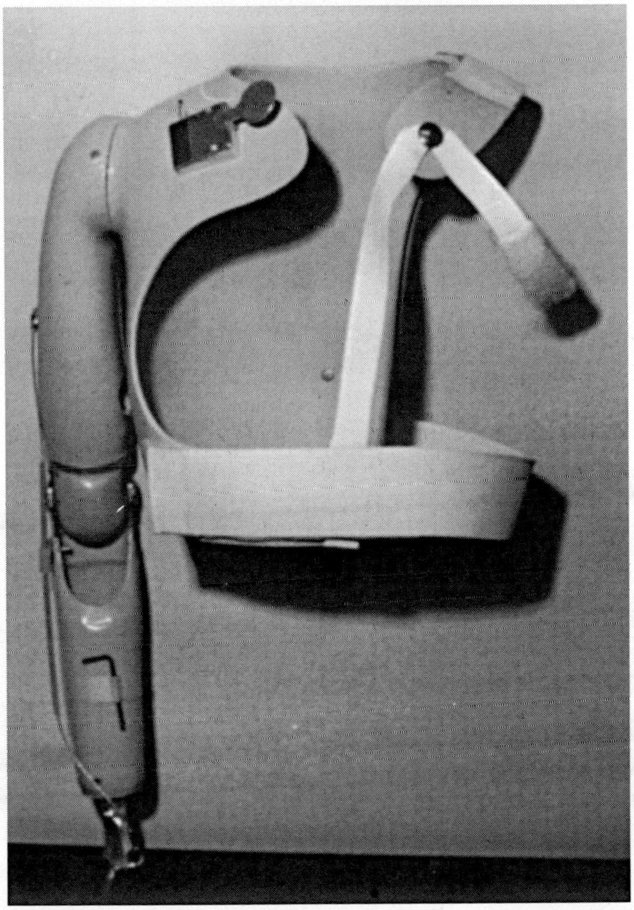

Figure 24–16

A body-powered forequarter amputation prosthesis. (Courtesy of Alpha Orthopedic Appliance Co., Los Angeles, CA.)

EXTERNALLY POWERED PROSTHESES

For the reasons just outlined, prosthetic engineers have turned to external power sources. After the thalidomide experience, which produced a significant number of bilateral shoulder disarticulations, prosthetic engineers sought to activate prosthetic substitutes by using compressed gas or electricity. Although useful in the past, the compressed gas systems have been discarded for lighter, more responsive electrical power systems. In the last decade, battery technology and improved microsystems have led to smaller, lighter, and more durable devices. The current state of electronic technology has allowed considerable ingenuity in myoelectric control in which currents generated by body muscles or switches activated by small body motions control the electrical motors that in turn move the prosthesis. A number of such prosthetic systems have been developed and are commercially available worldwide.

With amputations about the shoulder, it is often most practical to seek active elbow and terminal-device control only. The shoulder joint and forearm rotation are usually both positioned manually with the opposite limb. The elbow can be positioned actively by the amputee through electrical means and then stabilized in the locked position (Fig. 24–17). The terminal device is usually then operated actively through electric signals (Fig. 24–18). In the authors' opinion, the prosthesis developed at the University of Utah (the Utah Arm) represents the current state of the art for this approach (Fig. 24–19). The elbow of this device can be controlled electrically, and the terminal

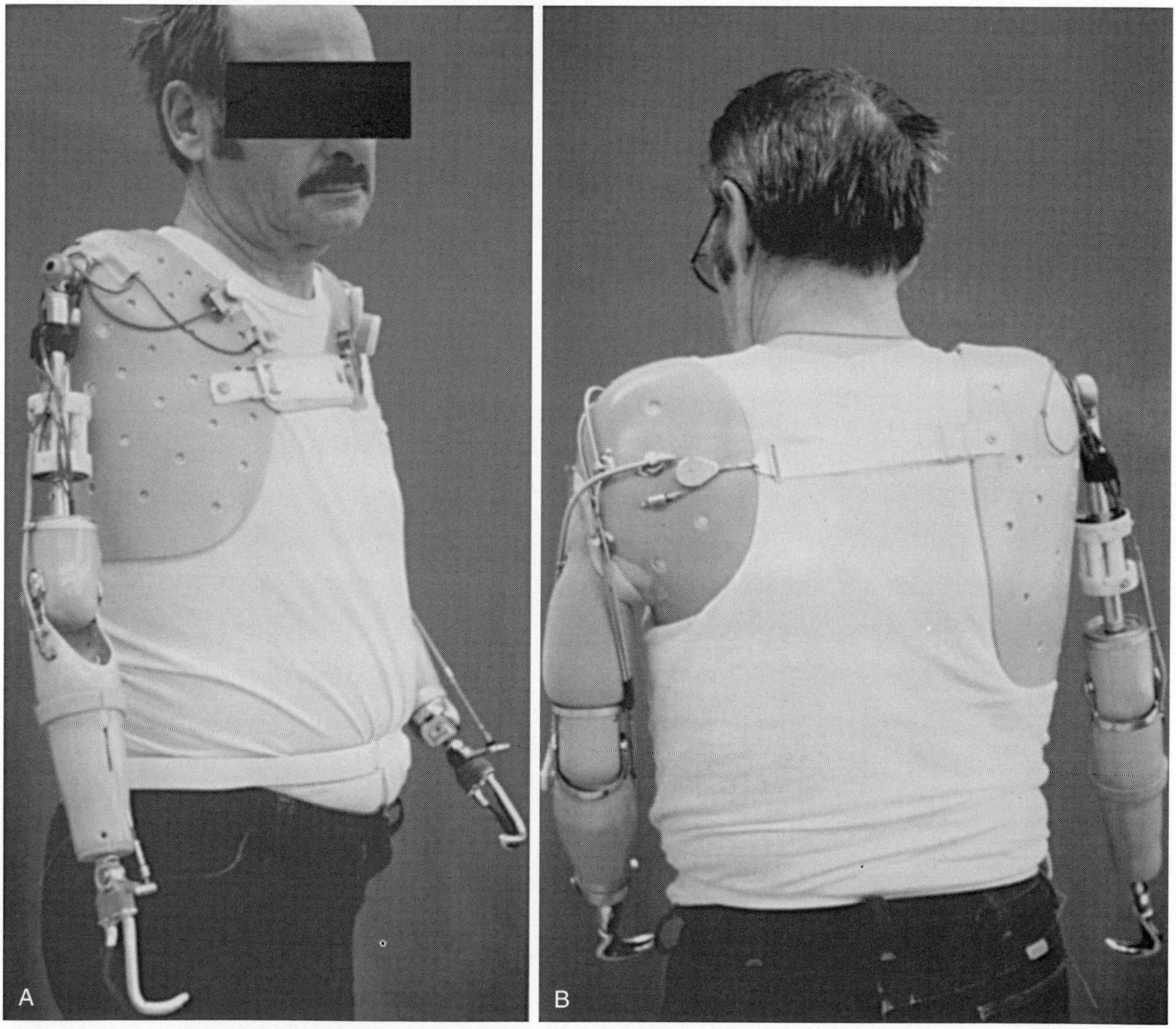

Figure 24–17

A patient with a right shoulder disarticulation electrically powered prosthesis. The powered components are the Hosmer electric elbow and the NY/Hosmer Prehension Actuator. Both components are controlled by chin-actuated push switches near the anterosuperior border of the socket. The shoulder, turntable, and forearm rotation joints are all manually positioned friction joints. The crepe band around the forearm provides surface friction for rotation against objects. (Courtesy of Dudley S. Childress, Ph.D., Prosthetics Research Laboratory, Northwestern University and the Orthotics and Prosthetics Clinical Services Department, Rehabilitation Institute of Chicago.)

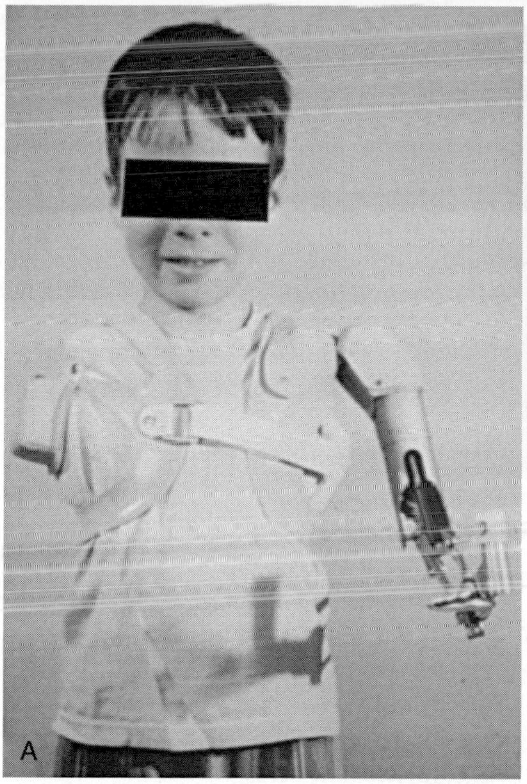

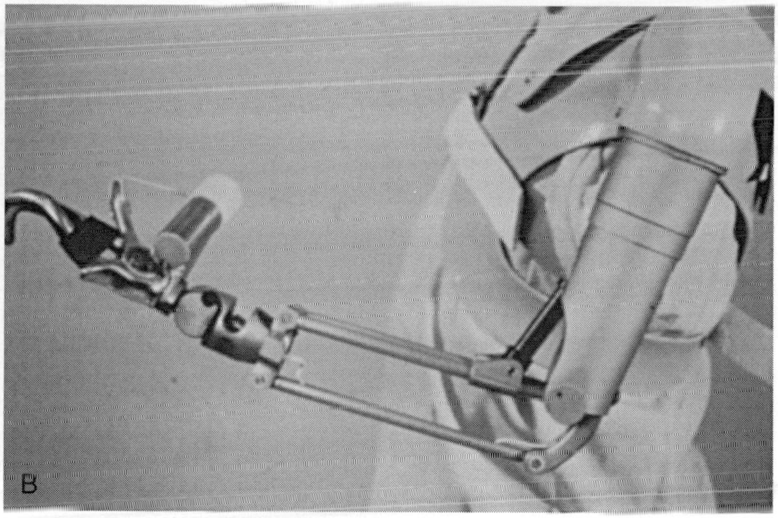

Figure 24–18

A, Child provided with a noncommercial prosthesis—the NU/Michigan Feeder Arm—with parallelogram linkage in the forearm (kinematic coupling of the elbow and wrist). *B*, The prehensor is the electrically powered Michigan Hook. (Courtesy of Dudley S. Childress, Ph.D., Prosthetics Research Laboratory, Northwestern University and the Orthotics and Prosthetics Clinical Services Department, Rehabilitation Institute of Chicago.)

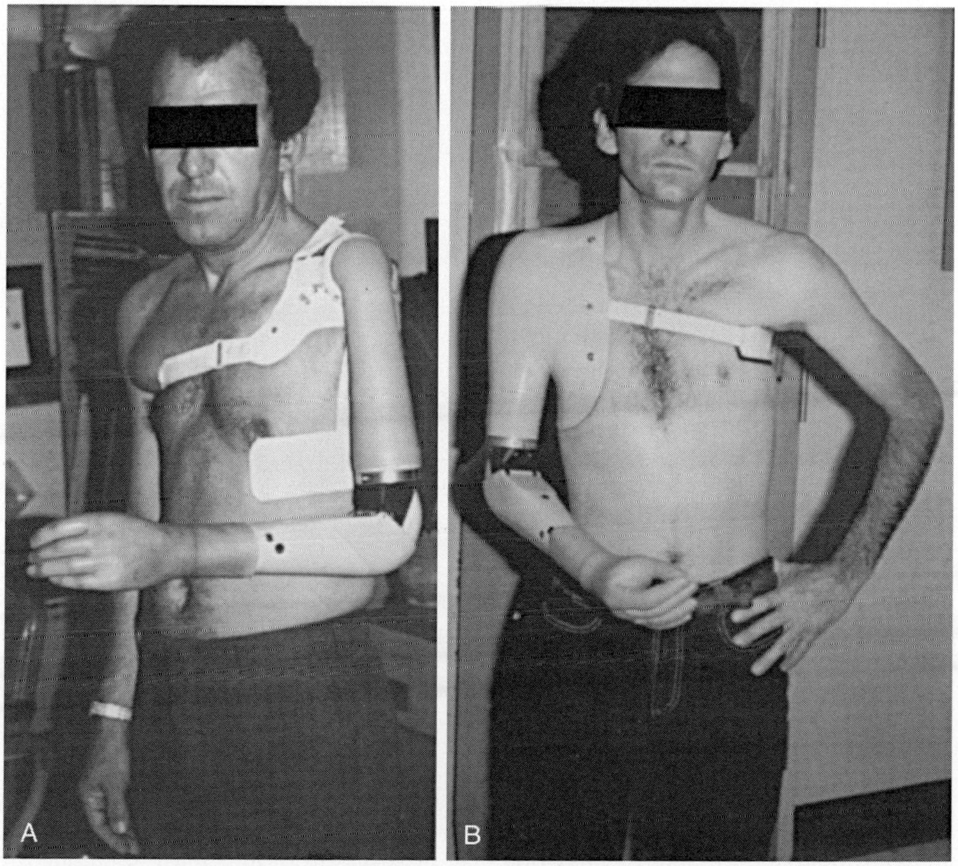

Figure 24–19

Myoelectrical prostheses for proximal humerus/shoulder disarticulation amputations (Utah Arm). (Courtesy of Eric Baron, C.P.O., University of California, Child Amputee Prosthetics Project, Los Angeles, CA.)

device can be operated electrically or by body power. Hybrid limbs are also commonly worn (i.e., partially body powered and partially powered by electricity). This combination has been particularly successful in the young, vigorous amputee. Even with the lightest materials, weight is still the usual limiting factor.

Recent advances have incorporated "proportional control" into externally powered prosthetic systems. Originally the response from the prosthetic limbs was "on" and "off," similar to a light switch. The elbow moved up or down or the terminal device opened or closed at one set speed. Proportional control acts like a dimmer light switch, grading the output response according to the intensity of the input. This has given the amputee the ability to move the prosthetic limb more naturally. Another development has been in augmenting traditional body-powered systems. Patients with shoulder level amputations often lack the shoulder excursion to effectively use cable control systems and lack muscles in the residual limb to signal myoelectric sensors. Other electrical switching systems now take advantage of small body motions from the chin, chest expansion, or a change in shoulder/pelvic distance to provide the human input. Although these body motions do not usually have the excursion to power a traditional cable system, they can signal proportional electrical switches to control an externally powered prosthesis (Fig. 24–20).

Despite these technical advances, in order to be successful, functional prostheses require a high degree of motivation on the part of the amputee. With one remaining functional upper limb, most acts of daily living can be accomplished by the normal arm with increasing skill as training proceeds. Even after being fitted with a state-of-the-art prosthesis, users tend to gradually discard the prosthetic limb as their opposite normal limb becomes more functional. The cosmetic substitute then becomes the limb of choice.

Special Considerations

POSTURAL ABNORMALITIES

Normally, the weight of the arm and the muscle activity associated with shoulder/arm function keep the shoulders appropriately level. Unilateral hypertrophy of an upper limb, including the shoulder girdle, occurs in certain occupations and is also seen in some sports. Some people are born with a degree of asymmetry of shoulder level, which involves relatively minor postural abnormalities and does not require special clothing.

When the arm is removed and the clavicle and scapula remain, the shoulder girdle elevators are unopposed by the weight of the arm and by those muscles passing across the shoulder that tend to depress the shoulder and arm. The consequence of this imbalance is an upward elevation described as "hiking" of the shoulder girdle. This "high shoulder" tends to accentuate the cosmetic loss, even when the individual is wearing a cosmetic shoulder filler or a cosmetic limb. Abnormal shoulder elevation can be countered by corrective exercises that begin as soon as they are tolerated after the amputation. The wearing of a prosthesis with its dependent weight also diminishes shoulder "hike." In most circumstances, the shoulder girdle elevation is inevitable; however, its degree can be minimized by appropriate physical measures.

Removal of the entire upper limb in the growing skeleton routinely results in a sharp scoliosis of the dorsal spine at the mid and upper dorsal levels. Muscular imbalance is considered to be the cause of the deformity. It may be seen to a slighter degree in the adult but is confined primarily to the growing skeleton. The combined postural deformity of upper dorsal spine scoliosis and elevation of the shoulder girdle produces asymmetry of the head and neck on the trunk, with the head appearing to be placed asymmetrically as the person stands.

In general, no corrective splinting or orthotic device successfully counteracts the postural changes associated with shoulder level amputation. Neck and shoulder-girdle exercises offer the most effective prophylaxis and treatment. The postural deficits are particularly evident with forequarter amputation. Soft, light polyurethane cosmetic restoration, either as part of a cosmetic prosthesis or separately used with the empty sleeve, will counter to some degree the unsightly upper body contour.

AMPUTATION FOR SEVERE BRACHIAL PLEXUS INJURY

Management of the severe brachial plexus injuries is complex, emotional, and individual. The decision to amputate all or part of the dysfunctional limb should be carefully thought out and discussed. In the authors' opinion, it is not appropriate to perform or encourage amputation at an early stage. Education, support, and visitor programs with other brachial plexus injury patients tend to be most helpful. The patients need time to adapt to the injury, learn the advantages and disadvantages of retaining a nonfunctional arm, and come to terms with the hope of neurologic recovery and the practical reality of the injury.

The reason for performing an amputation, the specific level of amputation, and the expected goals can vary considerably in the incomplete plexus injury. Setting specific goals for function, cosmesis, and prosthetic use before the surgery can be very helpful for both the patient and the surgeon. Occasionally, above-elbow amputation is elected to manage a totally dysfunctional arm after a complete brachial plexus avulsion. The advantages involve unloading the weight from the shoulder and scapulothoracic joints, and removing a paralyzed arm that hinders function because it gets in the way. The necessity for shoulder arthrodesis is controversial and should be individualized. One clinical series found a slightly better rate of return to work in the group of patients with above-elbow amputation without shoulder arthrodesis. In the authors' opinion, shoulder arthrodesis makes sense only if the patient has motor control of the scapulothoracic joint and not of the glenohumeral joint. If both are flail, fusion is probably not beneficial; and if both joints have motor control, arthrodesis is not needed.

Prosthetic expectations in these patients should be very limited, because prosthetic fitting adds weight to a dysfunctional shoulder girdle, often defeating one of the

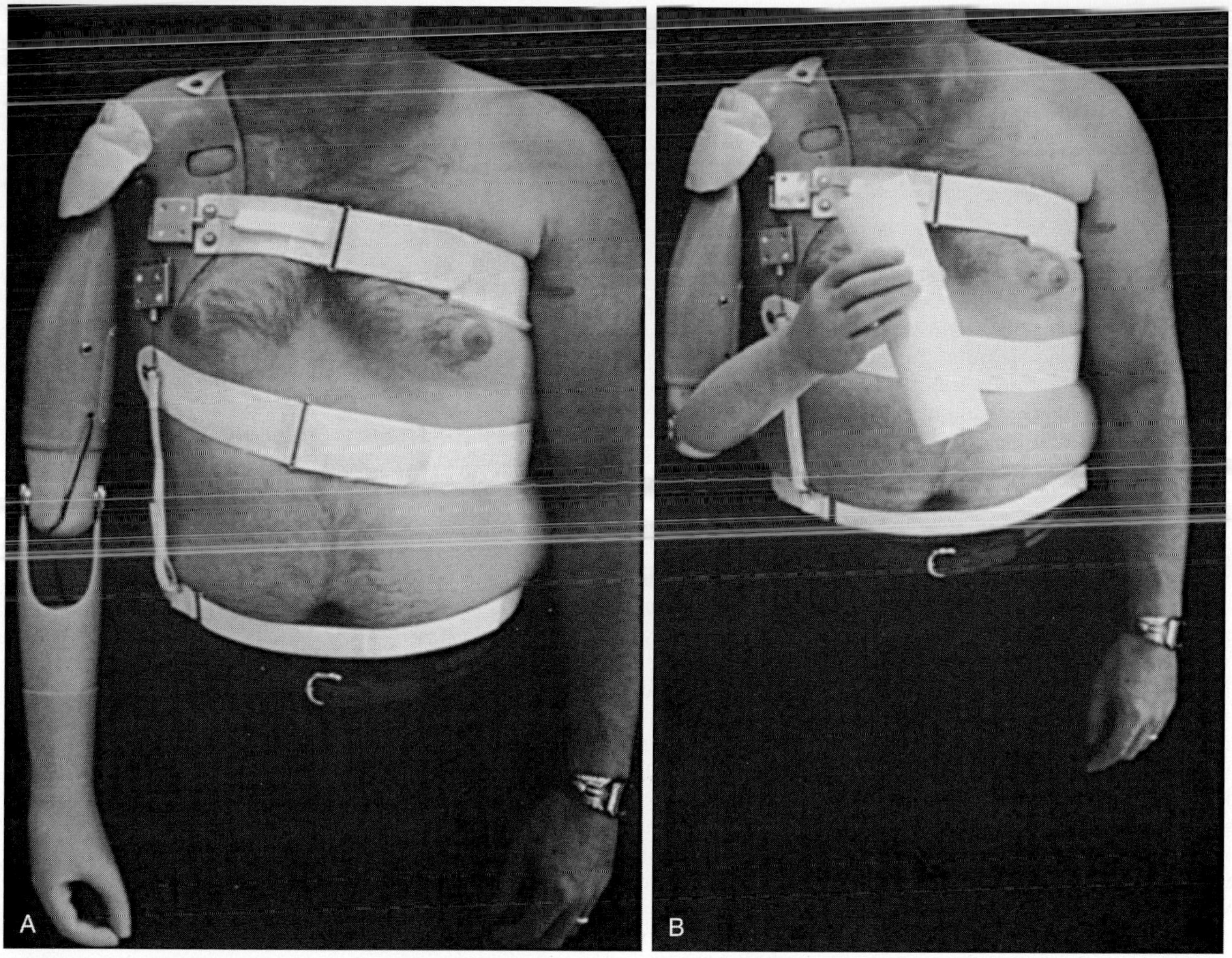

Figure 24–20

A switch-activated unilateral shoulder disarticulation prosthesis. Two four-state (Off-Function 1–Off-Function 2) switches control an electric elbow and an electric hand. Both switches are attached to the exterior of the anterior panel of the socket. The switch for the elbow is connected to a waist belt so that elevation of the shoulder moves the switch through its four states. The switch for the hand is connected to the chest strap and is operated by chest expansion. (Courtesy of Dudley S. Childress, Ph.D., Prosthetics Research Laboratory, Northwestern University and the Orthotics and Prosthetics Clinical Services Department, Rehabilitation Institute of Chicago.)

original goals of the amputation. A very lightweight, cosmetic prosthesis is often desired and indicated to help restore body image.

PAIN

All amputees with acquired amputations have a sense that all or part of the missing limb is still present. This phantom sensation is not always described in terms of pain and is not always bothersome to the amputee. True phantom pain, a sensation that occurs in the missing limb and is described in terms of pain, does occur after some amputations. Unfortunately, phantom pain seems to be encountered in a higher percentage of persons with shoulder level amputations than with lower limb amputations. This is particularly true with limb loss caused by trauma. Avulsion of the arm can cause severe traction trauma to nerve trunks and nerve roots up to their spinal origin. Likewise, painful neoplasms that require shoulder area amputation tend to “carry over” established pain patterns after ablation.

There is no direct surgical relief for these painful phenomena, either at the time of amputation or subsequently. Careful, meticulous isolation and ligation of nerve trunks followed by sharp knife sectioning below the level of ligature has proved to be the most effective method of handling nerves at the time of surgery. The sectioned nerves should retract well under remaining muscles and are thus protected by soft tissues. Nerve cautery and injection of the nerve ends with a long-acting local anesthetic or with tissue-destroying chemicals (e.g., phenol or absolute alcohol) have been ineffective. The transected nerve will always form a neuroma, but these neuromas tend not to be symptomatic if they retract into the deeper tissue, away from areas of pressure, scarring, and pulsating vessels. Because of this, the authors believe that the nerves should not be ligated together with the vessels.

The incidence of phantom pain in lower extremity

amputations seems to be reduced by the use of perioperative epidural anesthesia. The use of axillary or intrascalene blocks to provide perioperative analgesia can lessen the perioperative opioid requirements. There is early evidence that blocking the sensory pathways in the perioperative period may decrease the incidence of long-term phantom pain, although this has not yet been proved conclusively.

When pain remains a serious problem, the best management is nonsurgical. Central neural surgery, particularly, should be avoided. High nerve division or tractotomy are almost routinely unsuccessful and, in fact, may aggravate the pain patterns. Local physical measures, including massage, cold, exercise, neuromuscular stimulation by external electrical currents, acupuncture, and regional sympathectomy, may under certain circumstances have a place in therapy when the pain is intractable. A technique that has gained some acceptance and success is the use of transcutaneous electrical nerve stimulators (TENS), either incorporated into a prosthesis or as an isolated unit. The TENS system can be worn by the amputee at night and even during the day with the battery pack attached to the belt or inside a pocket. We have used this TENS system with moderate short-term success, but patients rarely continue to use the TENS system for more than 1 year. Pharmacologic treatment has been reasonably successful with several oral agents, including amitriptyline, carbamazepine (Tegretol), phenytoin (Dilantin), and more recently mexiletine. The appropriate use of an intravenous lidocaine challenge has been predictive of a favorable response to oral mexiletine. Unfortunately, we have not found good indicators to predict who will respond to treatment with amitriptyline, carbamazepine, or phenytoin. Psychological support can be beneficial, particularly when personality problems seem to accentuate the occurrence of pain. The individual needs patience and reassurance that the discomfort will decrease over time, especially when a supportive social environment is present.

References and Bibliography

1. Abbott LC and Lucas DB: The function of the clavicle; its surgical significance. Ann Surg *140:*583–599, 1954.
2. Anderson-Ranberg F and Ebskov B: Major upper extremity amputation in Denmark. Acta Orthop Scand *59:*321–322, 1988.
3. Bach S, Noreng MF, and Tjellden NU: Phantom limb pain in amputees during the first 12 months following limb amputation, after preoperative lumbar epidural blockade. Pain *33:*297–301, 1988.
4. Bauman PK: Resection of the upper extremity in the region of the shoulder joint. Khirurg Arkh Velyaminova *30:*145–149, 1914.
5. Berger P: Amputation du membre supérieur dans la contiguité du tronc (des articulation de l'omoplate). Bull Mem Soc Nat Chir *9:*656, 1883.
6. Blumenfeld I, Schortz RH, Levy M, and Lepley JB: Fabricating a shoulder somatoprosthesis. J Prosthet Dent *45:*542–544, 1981.
7. Bogacki W and Spyt T: Interscapular-thoracic amputation of the arm. Nowotwory *30:*261–264, 1980.
8. Burgess EM: Sites of amputation election according to modern practice. Clin Orthop *37:*17–22, 1964.
9. Burton DS and Nagel DA: Surgical treatment of malignant soft-tissue tumors of the extremities in the adult. Clin Orthop *84:*144–148, 1972.
10. Chappell PH: Arm amputation statistics for England 1958–88: An exploratory statistical analysis. Int J Rehabil Res *15:*57–62, 1992.
11. Copland SM: Total resection of the clavicle. Am J Surg *72:*280, 1946.
12. DeNancrede CBG: End-results of total excision of the scapula for sarcoma. Ann Surg *50:*1–22, 1909.
13. DePalma AF: Scapulectomy and a method of preserving normal configuration of the shoulder. Clin Orthop *4:*217–224, 1954.
14. Elizaga AM, Smith DG, Sharar SR, et al: Continuous regional analgesia by intraneural block: Effect on postoperative opioid requirements and phantom limb pain following amputation. J Rehabil Res Dev *31:*179–187, 1994.
15. Fanous N, Didolkar MS, Holyoke ED, and Elias EG: Evaluation of forequarter amputation in malignant diseases. Surg Gynecol Obstet *142:*381–384, 1976.
16. Fisher A and Meller Y: Continuous postoperative regional analgesia by nerve sheath block for amputation surgery—a pilot study. Anesth Analg *72:*300–303, 1991.
17. Flor H, Elbert T, Knecht S, et al: Phantom-limb pain as a perceptual correlate of cortical reorganization following arm amputation. Nature *375*(6531):482–484, 1995.
18. Grimes OF and Bell HG: Shoulder girdle amputation. Surg Gynecol Obstet *91:*201, 1950.
19. Guerra A, Capanna R, Biagini R, et al: Extra-articular resection of the shoulder (Tikhoff-Linberg). Ital J Orthop Traumatol *11:*151–157, 1985.
20. Haggart GE: The technique of interscapulothoracic amputation. Lahey Clin Bull *2:*16, 1940.
21. Hall CB and Bechtol CO: Modern amputation technique in the upper extremity. J Bone Joint Surg *45A:*1717, 1963.
22. Ham SJ, Hoekstra HJ, Schraffordt KH, et al: The interscapulothoracic amputation in the treatment of malignant diseases of the upper extremity with a review of the literature. Eur J Surg Oncol *19:*543–548, 1993.
23. Hardin CA: Interscapulothoracic amputations for sarcomas of the upper extremity. Surgery *49:*355, 1961.
24. Harty M and Joyce JJ: Surgical approaches to the shoulder. Orthop Clin North Am *6:*553–564, 1975.
25. Hau T: The surgical practice of Dominique Jean Larrey. Surg Gynecol Obstet *154:*89, 1982.
26. Herberts P: Myoelectric signals in control of prostheses: Studies on arm amputees and normal individuals. Acta Orthop Scand *124* (Suppl):1–83, 1969.
27. Janecki CJ and Nelson CL: En bloc resection of the shoulder girdle: Technique and indications. J Bone Joint Surg *54A:*1754–1758, 1972.
28. Knaggs RL: Mr. Littlewood's method of performing the interscapulothoracic amputation (Letter to the editor). Lancet *1:*1298, 1910.
29. Kneisl JS: Function after amputation, arthrodesis, or arthroplasty for tumors about the shoulder. J South Orthop Assoc *4:*228–236, 1995.
30. Kochhar CL and Strivastava LK: Anatomical and functional considerations in total claviculectomy. Clin Orthop *118:*199, 1976.
31. Larrey DJ: Memoire sur les Amputations des Membres à La Suite des Coups de Feu Etaye de Plusieurs Observations. Paris: Du Pont, 1797.
32. Levinthal DH and Grossman A: Interscapulothoracic amputations for malignant tumors of the shoulder region. Surg Gynecol Obstet *69:*234, 1939.
33. Lewis MM, Ballet FL, Kroll PG, and Bloom N: En bloc clavicular resection, operative procedure and postoperative testing of function. Clin Orthop *193:*214, 1985.
34. Littlewood H: Amputations at the shoulder and at the hip. BMJ *1:*381, 1922.
35. Luiberg BE: Interscapulothoracic resection for malignant tumors of the shoulder joint region. J Bone Joint Surg *10:*344–349, 1928.
36. Malawer MM, Buch R, Khurana JS, et al: Postoperative infusional continuous regional analgesia—a technique for relief of postoperative pain following major extremity surgery. Clin Orthop *266:*227–237, 1991.
37. Mansour KA and Powell RW: Modified technique for radical transmediastinal forequarter amputation and chest wall resection. J Thorac Cardiovasc Surg *76:*358–363, 1978.
38. Marcove RC: Neoplasms of the shoulder girdle. Orthop Clin North Am *6:*541–552, 1975.
39. McLaughlin J: Solitary myeloma of the clavicle with long survival after total excision: Report of a case. J Bone Joint Surg *55B:*357, 1973.

40. McLaurin CA, Sauter WF, Dolan DM, and Harmann GR: Fabrication procedure for the open-shoulder above-elbow socket. Artif Limbs *13*:46–54, 1969.
41. Melzack R: Phantom limbs. Sci Am *266*:120–126, 1992.
42. Moseley HF: The Forequarter Amputation. Edinburgh: E. and S. Livingstone, 1957, p 49.
43. Nadler SH and Phelan JT: A technique of interscapulo-thoracic amputation. Surg Gynecol Obstet *122*:359, 1966.
44. Neff G: Prosthetic principles in bilateral shoulder disarticulation or bilateral amelia. Prosthet Orthot Int *2*:143–147, 1978.
45. Oible JH: Napoleon's Surgeon. London: William Heinemann Medical Books, 1970.
46. Ojemann JG and Silbergeld DL: Cortical stimulation mapping of phantom limb rolandic cortex: Case report. J Neurosurg *82*:641–644, 1995.
47. Pack GT: Major exarticulations for malignant neoplasms of the extremities: Interscapulothoracic amputation, hip joint disarticulations and interilioabdominal amputation: A report of end results in 228 cases. J Bone Joint Surg *38A*:249, 1956.
48. Pack GT and Baldwin JC: The Tikhor-Linberg resection of shoulder girdle. Surgery *38*:753–757, 1955.
49. Pack GT and Crampton RS: The Tikhor-Linberg resection of the shoulder girdle: Indications for its substitution for interscapulothoracic amputation, recent data on end-results of the forequarter amputation. Clin Orthop *19*:148, 1961.
50. Pack GT, Ehrlich HE, and Gentil F: Radical amputations of the extremities in the treatment of cancer. Surg Gynecol Obstet *84*:1105–1116, 1947.
51. Pack GT, McNeer G, and Coley BL: Interscapulo-thoracic amputations for malignant tumors of the upper extremity: A report of thirty-one consecutive cases. Surg Gynecol Obstet *74*:161, 1942.
52. Rorabeck CH: The management of the flail upper extremity in brachial plexus injuries. J Trauma *20*:491–493, 1980.
53. Roth JA, Sugarbaker PH, and Baker AR: Radical forequarter amputation with chest wall resection. Ann Thorac Surg *37*:432–437, 1984.
54. Salzer M and Knahr K: Resection of malignant bone tumors. Recent Results Cancer Res *54*:239–256, 1976.
55. Sauter WF: Prostheses for the child amputee. Orthop Clin North Am *3*:483–494, 1972.
56. Slocum DB: Atlas of Amputations. St. Louis: CV Mosby, 1949.
57. Spar I: Total claviculectomy for pathological fractures. Clin Orthop *129*:236, 1977.
58. Sperling P and Rloding H: Interthoracoscapular amputation (forequarter amputation). Zentralbl Chir *106*:340–343, 1981.
59. Sturup J, Thyregod HC, Jensen JS, et al: Traumatic amputation of the upper limb: The use of body-powered prostheses and employment consequences. Prosthet Orthot Int *12*:50–52, 1988.
60. Syme J: Excision of the Scapula. Edinburgh: Edmonton and Douglas, 1864.
61. Tikhor PT: Tumor Studies (Monograph). Russia, 1900.
62. Tooms RE: Amputation surgery in the upper extremity. Orthop Clin North Am *3*:383–395, 1972.
63. Trishkin VA, Saakian AM, Stoliarov VI, and Kochnev VA: Interscapulothoracic amputation in treating malignant tumors of the upper extremity and shoulder girdle. Vestn Khir Im I Grek *124*:75–78, 1980.
64. Turnbull A, Blumencranz P, and Fortner J: Scapulectomy for soft tissue sarcoma. Can J Surg *24*:37–38, 1981.
65. Ye Q, Zhao H, and Shen J: Modified en bloc resection procedure for malignant tumor of the shoulder girdle. Chung Kuo I Hsueh Ko Hsueh Yuan Hsueh Pao Acta Academiae Medicinae Sinicae *16*:378–382, 1994.
66. Zachary LS, Gottlieb LJ, Simon M, et al: Forequarter amputation wound coverage with an ipsilateral, lymphedematous, circumferential forearm fasciocutaneous free flap in patients undergoing palliative shoulder-girdle tumor resection. J Reconstr Microsurg *9*:103–107, 1993.
67. Zancolli E, Mitre HJ, Bick M, et al: Interscapulo-cleidothoracic disarticulation. Indications and technique. Prensa Med Argent *52*:1122–1126, 1965.

CHAPTER

25

FRANK W. JOBE, M.D.
JAMES E. TIBONE, M.D.
MARILYN M. PINK, PhD., P.T.
CHRISTOPHER M. JOBE, M.D.
RONALD S. KVITNE, M.D.

The Shoulder in Sports

Mobility of the shoulder in sports is a double-edged sword that enables athletic performance but also leaves the shoulder vulnerable to injury. As clinicians, we want to allow the individual to perform optimally while minimizing the chance of injury or effectively treating the injury if it occurs. The purpose of this chapter is to discuss information that the clinician may want to know about the shoulder in order to allow optimal performance, while minimizing or treating the injury. This is accomplished by first discussing the biomechanics of sport, then the continuum of instability and impingement, followed by principles in prevention and rehabilitation and common surgical procedures for shoulder problems.

BIOMECHANICS

In order to minimize injury or effectively treat injury, one must understand the tissues at risk for a given sport. In the past, athletic activities involving the arm tended to be grouped as "overhead" or "overhand" sports, possibly because much of the initial research was done on the baseball pitcher. The findings of the pitcher were then frequently extrapolated into all "overhead" sports. We now realize that the pitcher is a paradigm unto itself. In addition, research in swimming has proved that a swimmer has tissues at risk and mechanics of injury that are specific to each of the four competitive strokes: the freestyle, butterfly, backstroke, and breaststroke. The golfer (although technically not an "overhead" sport because shoulder elevation rarely exceeds 90 degrees) also has specific mechanics that a clinician must understand in order to be of help to the athlete. Thus, the specific mechanics of each sport need to be understood by the clinician. In order to communicate this, the mechanics of the shoulder in the baseball pitcher and the freestyle swimmer are discussed.

Baseball Pitch

The phases of the baseball pitch that leave the shoulder most at risk for injury are late cocking, acceleration, and deceleration (Fig. 25–1).

LATE COCKING

During the late cocking phase, the humerus is moving toward maximal external rotation. As it moves into external rotation, the cuff muscles are rotated posteriorly (Fig. 25–2). In the pitcher with a normal shoulder, this is done in the scapular plane. The scapular plane allows not only for maximal congruency of the humeral head and glenoid, but it also allows for the least twisting of the anterior capsule,[21] the least risk of anterior subluxation of the humeral head, and the least chance of the posterior cuff to abut against the posterior or superior glenoid rim. Figure 25–3 demonstrates how the humeral head can more easily subluxate anteriorly when in the coronal plane, and Figure 25–4*A* and *B* reveals the abutment and fraying of the posterior cuff undersurface on the posterosuperior glenoid rim.

During the late cocking phase, the infraspinatus and teres minor are quite active as they externally rotate the humerus and provide a posterior restraint to the anterior subluxation.[7] The upper portion of the subscapularis also demonstrates high activity as it helps to control the degree of external rotation and forms part of the "anterior wall" to help prevent anterior subluxation of the humeral head (see Fig. 25–2). Once the humerus is maximally externally rotated, the subscapularis is rotated more superiorly and can offer some superior compression of the head to prevent superior migration of the humeral head.[38] At this point, the supraspinatus is rotated more posteriorly and cannot afford the superior compression.

The serratus anterior is firing during late cocking as it upwardly rotates and anchors the scapula for the humerus. The levator scapula is functioning at the opposite corner to allow for synchronous scapular motion.

ACCELERATION

During acceleration, the humerus internally rotates approximately 100 degrees in 0.05 second in order to contribute to the momentum of the ball upon release.[8] Very high angular velocities and torques have been suggested to occur during this phase.[8, 12, 28] All of the scapular muscles are quite active as they form a stable base for the

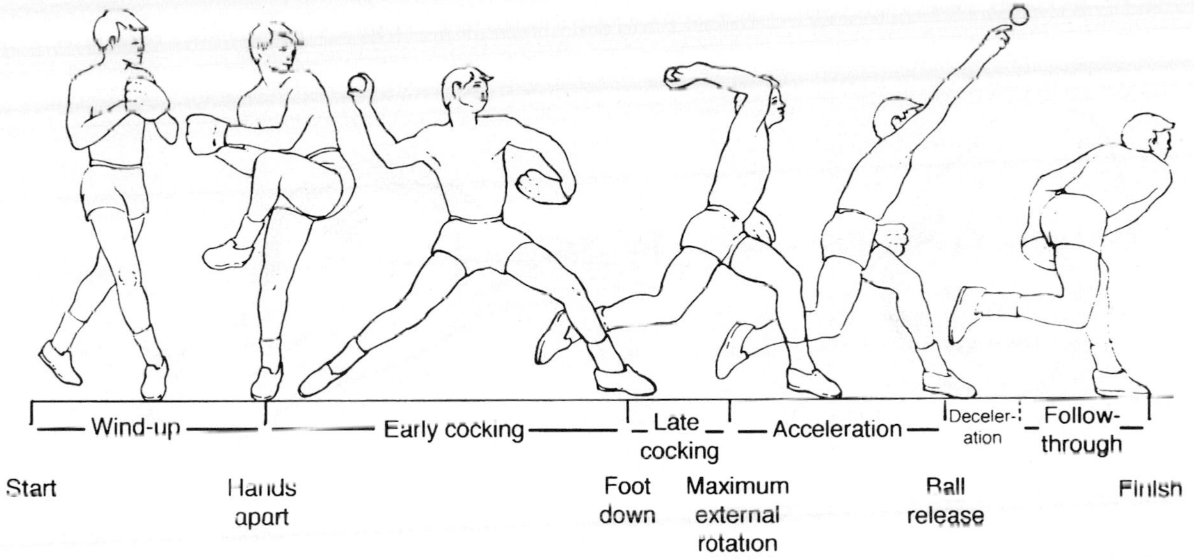

Figure 25–1

Phases of the baseball pitch. (From Pink MM and Perry J: Biomechanics. *In* Jobe FW, et al [eds]: Operative Techniques in Upper Extremity Sports Injuries. St Louis, MO: Mosby-Year Book, 1996.)

humeral rotation. Of the internal rotators, the subscapularis reveals the most electrical activity followed by the latissimus dorsi.[7] In that the subscapularis inserts close to the axis of rotation, it helps to keep the humeral head centered on the glenoid while it assists with internal rotation. If the subscapularis were not functioning, the humeral head could be levered anteriorly as the latissimus dorsi rotates the humerus from a more distal attachment. Thus, to prevent injury, the clinician would want to ensure that the pitcher has a stable scapular base (i.e., strong scapular muscles) and excellent strength of the subscapularis.

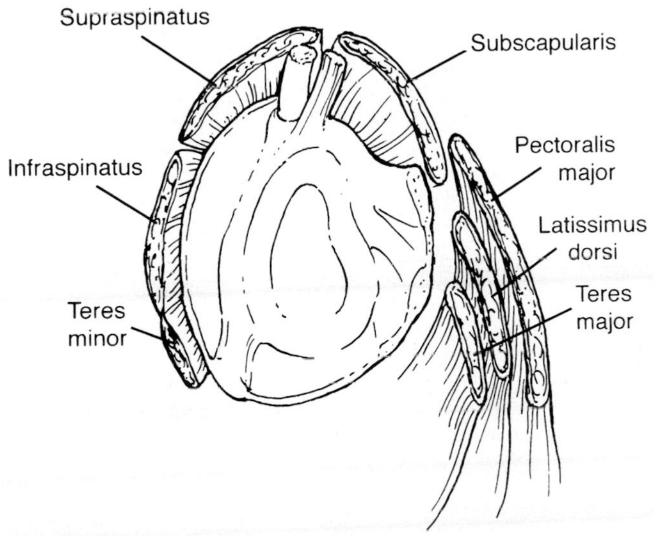

Figure 25–2

Position of the tendons and ligaments around the glenohumeral joint in the position of 90 degrees of abduction and 90 degrees of external rotation. With maximal external rotation, the muscles are rotated even more. (From Pink MM and Perry J: Biomechanics. *In* Jobe FW, et al [eds]: Operative Techniques in Upper Extremity Sports Injuries. St Louis, MO: Mosby-Year Book, 1996.)

DECELERATION

During the deceleration phase, the excess kinetic energy that was not transferred to the ball is dissipated by controlled deceleration of the upper extremity. Once again, high forces and torques have been suggested.[12, 28]

The teres minor not only demonstrates the highest level of activity of all the glenohumeral muscles but also functions eccentrically. The intensity of firing of the teres minor is clinically relevant in that many ball players note posterior cuff pain that can be isolated to the teres minor and reproduced in a deceleration motion. Thus, it appears that the teres minor may be vulnerable during the deceleration phase and the clinician may want to strengthen this muscle in an arc of motion that is similar to the deceleration phase of the pitch (Fig. 25–5).

Freestyle Swimming

Approximately half of competitive swimmers will experience shoulder pain that is severe enough to prevent them from swimming for 3 weeks or more at some point in their swimming career.[34] Factors that have commonly been thought to influence this high rate of shoulder dysfunction include the extremely high number of shoulder revolutions, the extremes of shoulder range of motion (ROM) necessary for each revolution, and the generalized state of joint laxity in swimmers.

A recent study investigated some of these characteristics as well as clinical signs of shoulder pathology in 350 competitive swimmers and age-, race-, and gender-matched controls (Pink, unpublished data). The swimmers demonstrated significantly more generalized joint

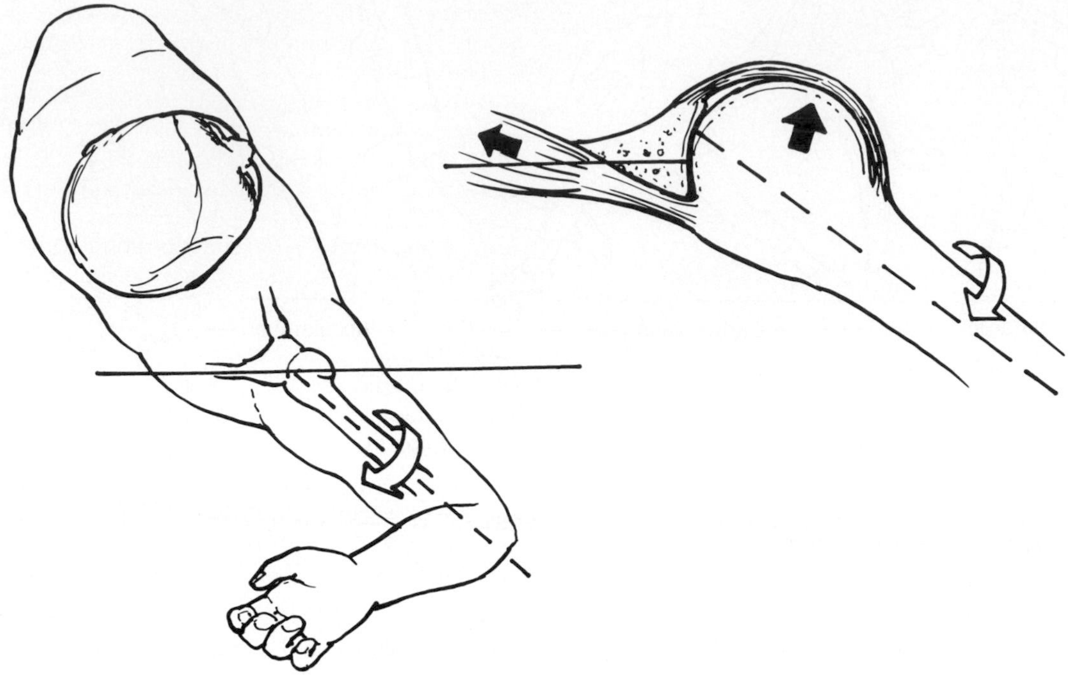

Figure 25–3

Anterior subluxation and resultant anatomic damage with the arm in the coronal plane.

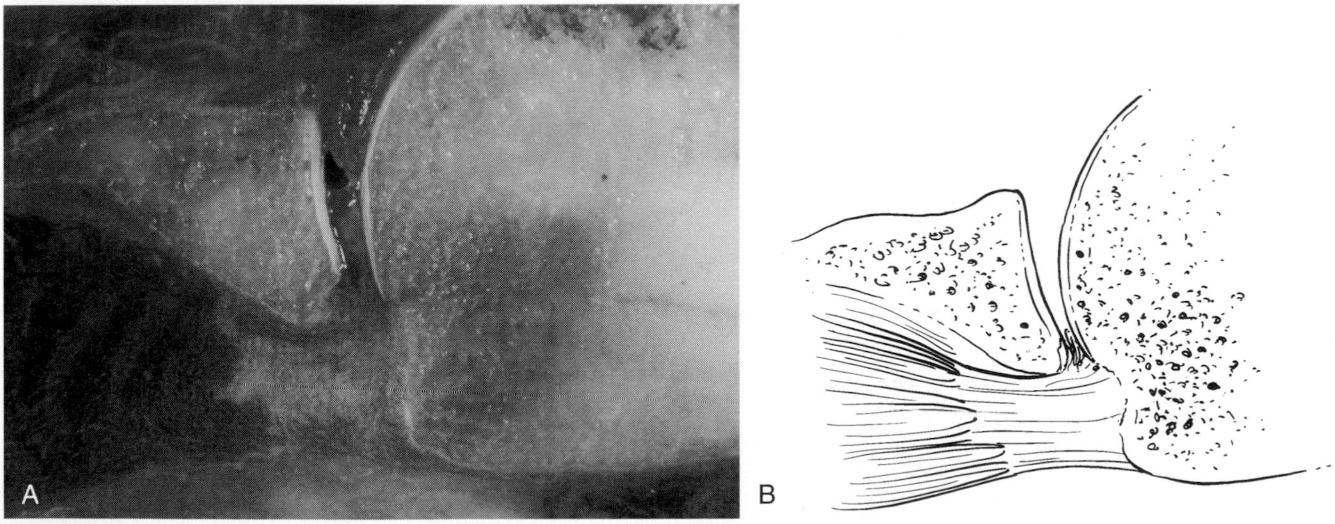

Figure 25–4

Impingement of the rotator cuff on the posterosuperior glenoid labrum during humeral abduction and maximal external rotation. *A*, Cross-section from a cadaver. *B*, Schematic of *A*. (From Jobe CM, et al: Theories and concepts. *In* Jobe FW, et al [eds]: Operative Techniques in Upper Extremity Sports Injuries. St Louis, MO: Mosby-Year Book, 1996.)

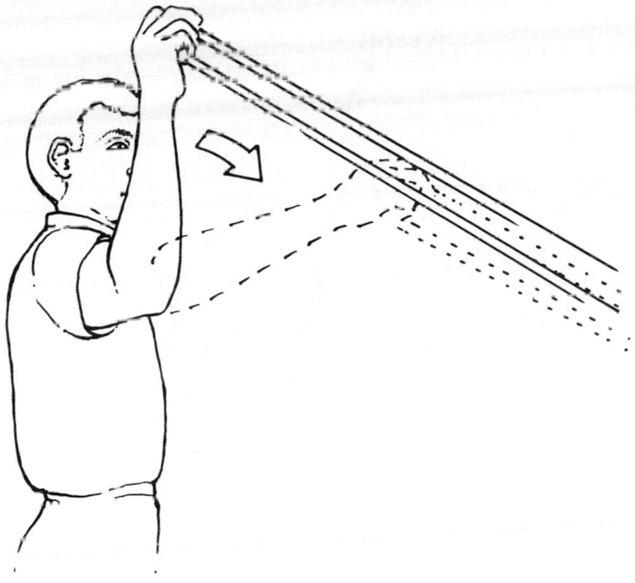

Figure 25–5

Deceleration exercise for the teres minor. (From Pink MM, et al: Injury prevention and rehabilitation in the upper extremity. *In* Jobe FW, et al [eds]: Operative Techniques in Upper Extremity Sports Injuries. St Louis, MO: Mosby-Year Book, 1996.)

laxity than did the nonswimmers. There was an increased prevalence of classic impingement as measured by the Hawkins and Neer tests in the swimmers when compared with the control group even though both groups reported no pain during their functional activities. It is interesting to note that there were significantly more positive results on the Hawkins test than were found on the Neer test. Yet, the swimmers did not exhibit any more shoulder instability as measured by the relocation test than did the controls. Thus, the problem involving the swimmer's shoulder appeared not to be related to the anterior subluxation that can be found in the pitcher.

One of the common positions of pain in the swimmer is the position that the hand enters the water. This position is somewhere between the Neer and Hawkins tests for impingement (Fig. 25–6*A–C*). Cadaver cross-sections of these two impingement tests were done by one of the authors (C.M.J.) (Figs. 25–7 and 25–8). During the Neer test, the impingement appears to be on the undersurface of the cuff on the anterosuperior glenoid rim. During the Hawkins test, the cuff appears to be compressed between the acromion and the glenoid rim. Thus, the impingement in the swimmer's shoulder may be more closely related to the classic impingement with some additional rubbing on the cuff's undersurface.

One of the muscles in the swimmer's shoulder that appears to be quite vulnerable to fatigue is the serratus anterior. In an underwater electromyographic study of the freestyle stroke, the serratus anterior in swimmers with pain-free shoulders was constantly firing above 20% of the maximum manual muscle test (MMT).[29] At this intensity, the muscle is vulnerable to fatigue if no rest is provided.[25] And, indeed, in swimmers with painful shoulders, the muscle activity in the serratus anterior was significantly depressed (Fig. 25–9).[32] If the serratus anterior were not functioning, the swimmer would be susceptible to the nonoutlet type of impingement that was described by Neer.[27] Thus, a clinician would want to be certain that the serratus anterior not only demonstrates normal strength but also has good endurance.

The subscapularis is the other shoulder muscle that may be vulnerable to fatigue during the freestyle stroke in that it also constantly fires above 20% MMT in swimmers with normal shoulders (Fig. 25–10).[29] The constant firing of the subscapularis is easily understood when one realizes that the humerus is always in internal rotation during the stroke. The arm is positioned in neutral rotation during mid-recovery; however, that is as far into "external rotation" that it moves. Therefore, the clinician would want to check the strength and endurance of this muscle along with the serratus anterior.

With this biomechanics information as a background, one can begin to see the value of understanding the normal mechanics of individual sports and the relationship of the mechanics to instability and impingement that will be elaborated on next. Hopefully this will also enable the clinician to see the logic behind the surgical programs and rehabilitative principles described subsequently.

IMPINGEMENT AND INSTABILITY

As Neer noted in his early writings, his observations that led to the theories of outlet and nonoutlet impingement were based on an older, athletic population.[27] We now realize that the mechanics of impingement in the younger, overhead athletic population may be different. At this point, we shall proceed to develop the concept of impingement and instability in the baseball pitcher.

Instability Continuum

As already mentioned, anterior instability in the baseball pitcher can lead to undersurface fraying of the posterior cuff (see Fig. 25–4). In addition to cuff pathology, there may be skeletal damage to both the labrum and the humeral head.

The instability is caused by several factors. One of these factors is the microtrauma from the repetitive event of throwing. Fatigue or weakness of the anterior wall muscles (the subscapularis, pectoralis major, latissimus dorsi, and teres major) contribute to the potential for instability as does stretching of the anterior structures such as the capsule and the glenohumeral ligaments. In addition, if the arm moves into the coronal plane (instead of the scapular plane) when abducted and externally rotated, the humeral head is levered anteriorly (see Fig. 25–3). This is called "hyperangulation." Each of these factors can contribute to one another until instability occurs (Fig. 25–11).

GROUPS OF INSTABILITY

In developing a scheme for classification of impingement/instability, the first divisor tends to be age (Fig. 25–12). The population older than 35 years of age has a tendency

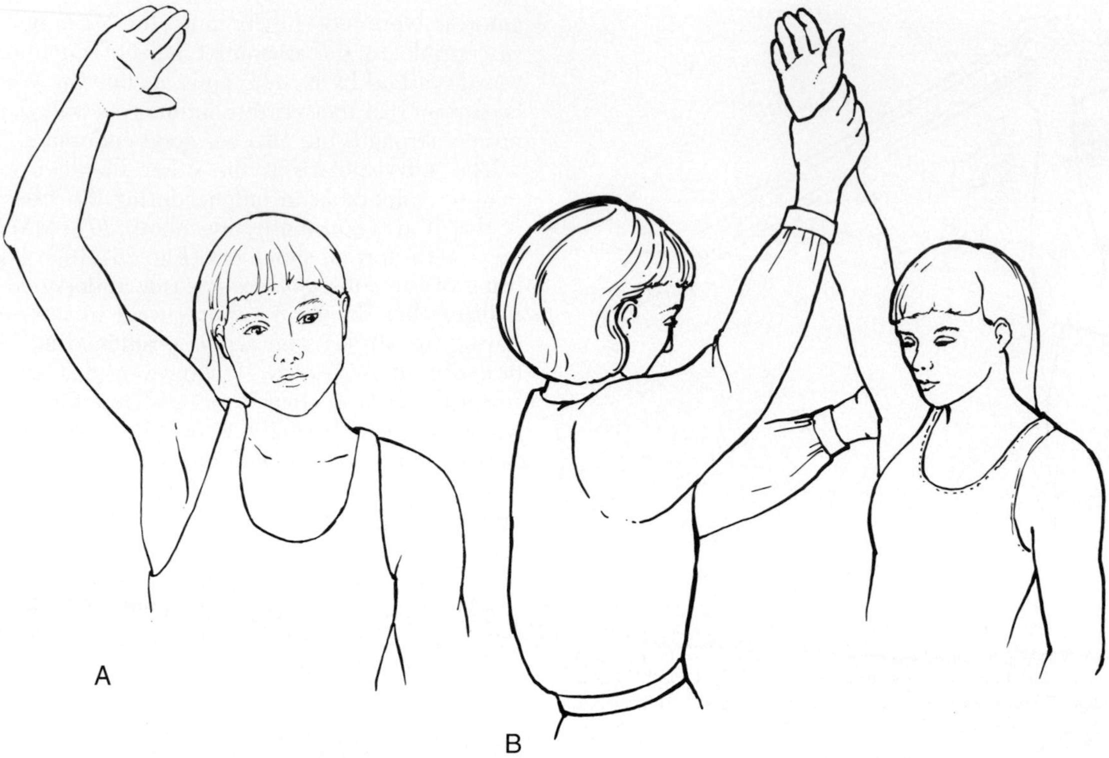

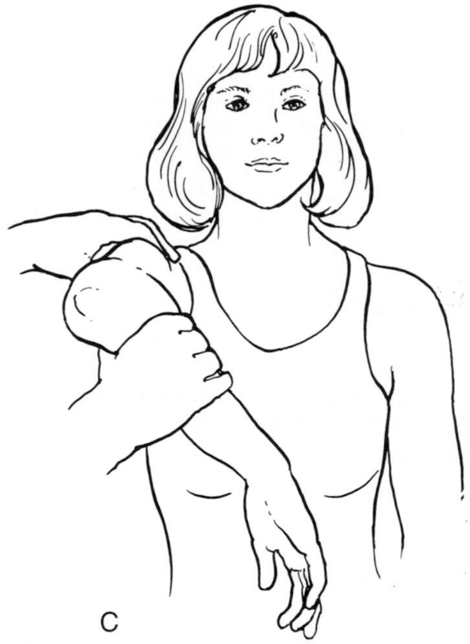

Figure 25–6

Hand entry during the freestyle swim stroke is between that of the Neer and Hawkins impingement tests. *A*, Hand entry position during freestyle swimming. *B*, Neer impingement test. *C*, Hawkins impingement test. (From Jobe CM, et al: Theories and concepts. *In* Jobe FW, et al [eds]: Operative Techniques in Upper Extremity Sports Injuries. St Louis, MO: Mosby-Year Book, 1996.)

toward the classic type of impingement that was described by Neer, and the population younger than 35 years of age has a tendency toward impingement due to instability. The algorithm for impingement/instability can be further divided into the following groups:

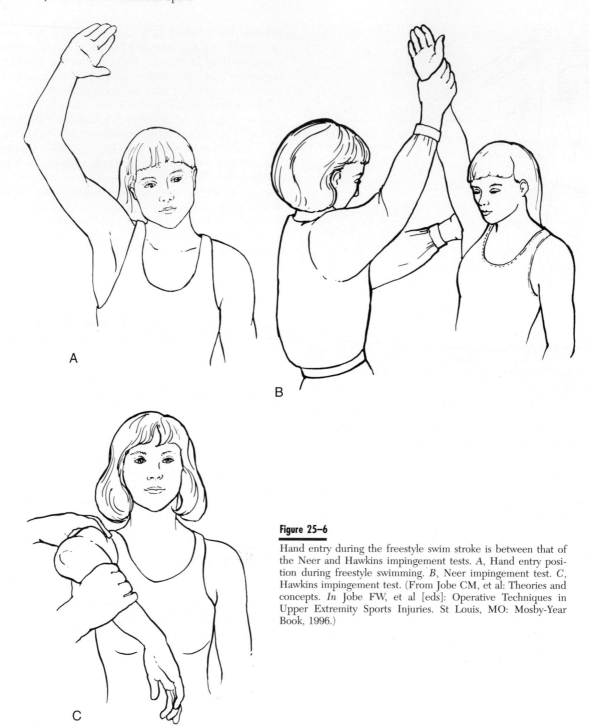

Group I. Group I instability is typically found in the older (i.e., older than 35 years of age) professional or recreational athlete or the older, nonathletic individual. It is rarely found in the younger population but should be kept in mind. This group is subdivided into group IA and IB. Group IA encompasses patients with pure isolated impingement on the acromial process or on the coracoacromial ligament. No instability is present. These patients demonstrate positive Hawkins' or Neer's impingement signs. An arthroscopic examination is likely to reveal lesions on the bursal surface of the rotator cuff and may reveal additional pathologic factors such as subacromial spurs. The glenohumeral joint may or may not have evidence of arthritis but does not show signs of instability. This group is analogous to outlet impingement. Group IB demonstrates instability and impingement of the undersurface of the rotator cuff.

Group II. Group II patients are the younger population who demonstrate instability with impingement secondary to repetitive trauma. Many young throwing athletes fall into this group. The clinical examination frequently elicits positive impingement signs, and the result of the relocation test is positive

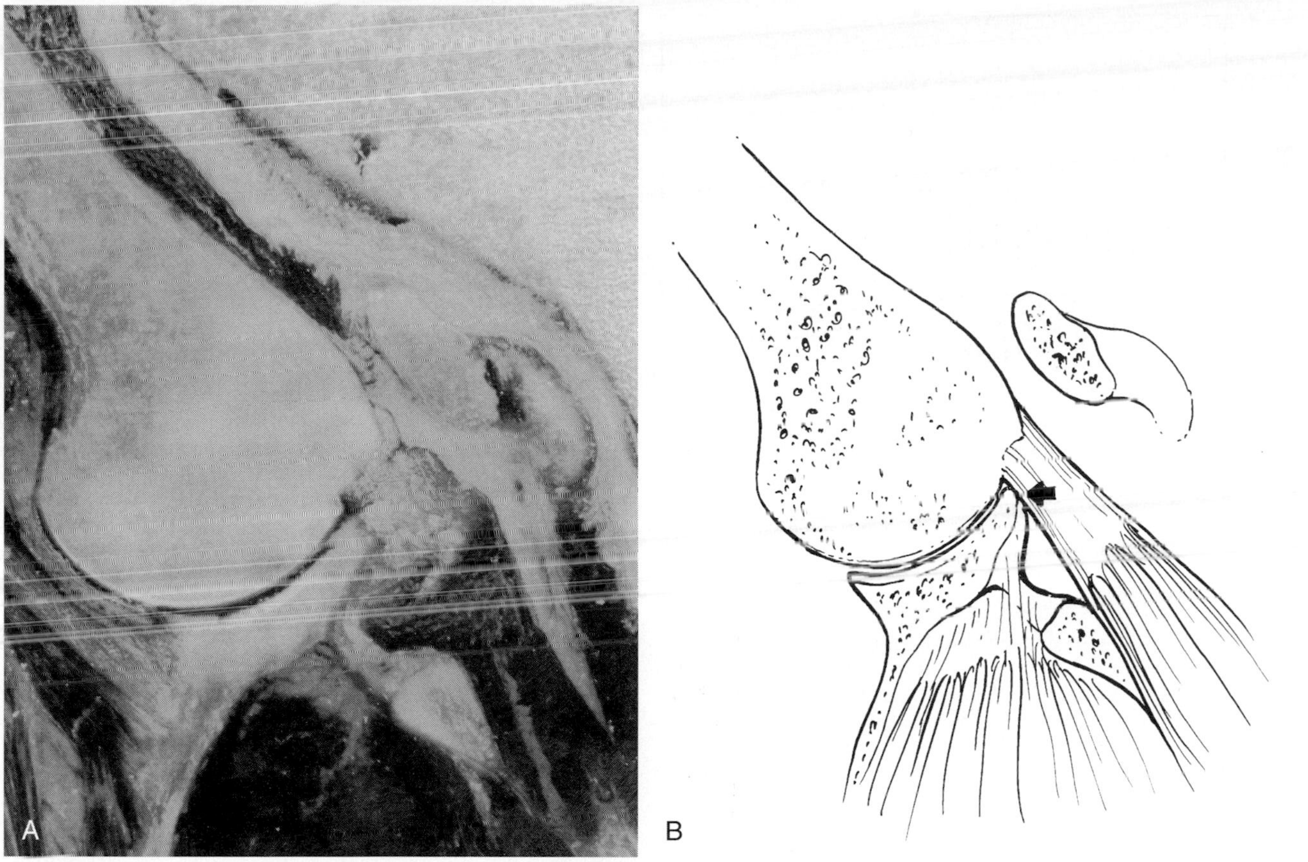

Figure 25–7

Impingement of the rotator cuff on the anterosuperior glenoid labrum during maximal humeral flexion and forceful internal rotation. *A*, Cross-section of a cadaver. *B*, Schematic of *A*. (From Jobe CM, et al: Theories and concepts. *In* Jobe FW, et al [eds]: Operative Techniques in Upper Extremity Sports Injuries. St Louis, MO: Mosby-Year Book, 1996.)

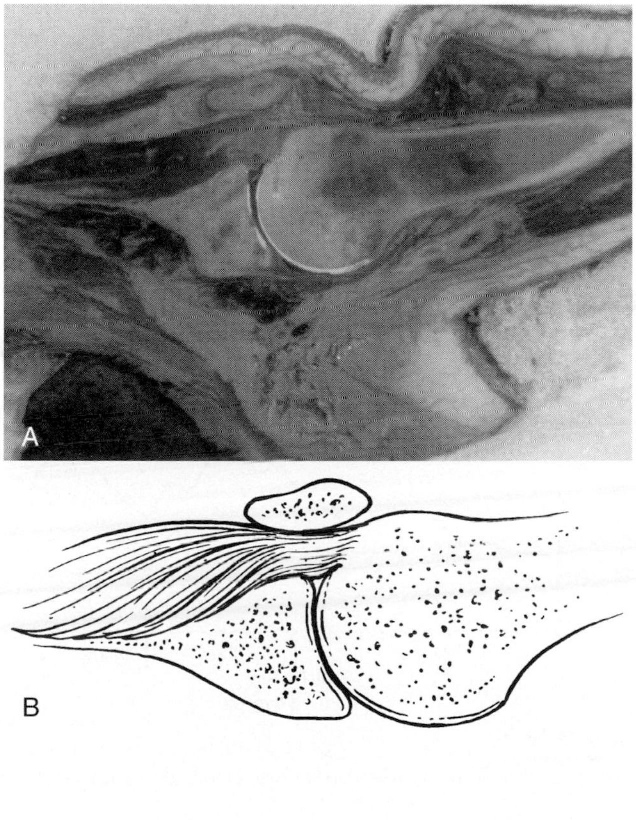

Figure 25–8

Impingement of the rotator cuff between the acromion and glenoid rim during the Hawkins test. *A*, Cross-section of a cadaver. *B*, Schematic of *A*.

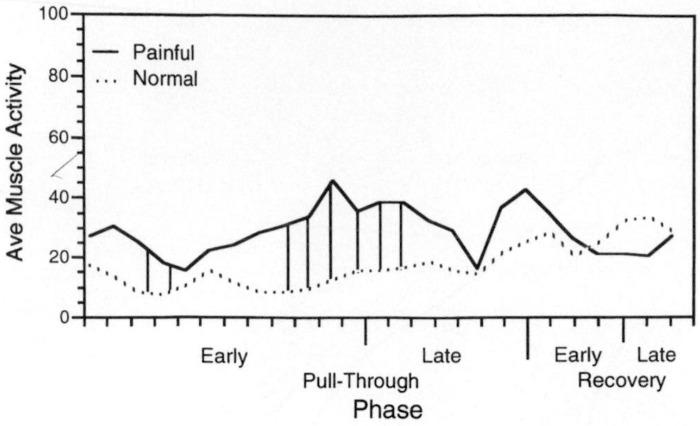

Figure 25–9

Muscle activity of the serratus anterior in swimmers with normal and painful shoulders. Vertical lines show periods of significant differences. (From Pink MM and Perry J: Biomechanics. *In* Jobe FW, et al [eds]: Operative Techniques in Upper Extremity Sports Injuries. St Louis, MO: Mosby-Year Book, 1996.)

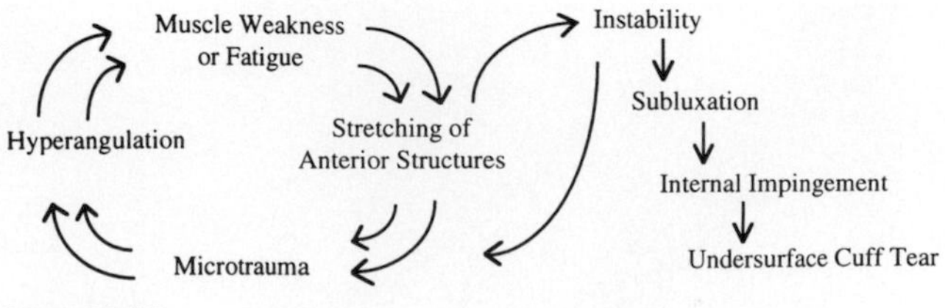

Figure 25–11

Instability continuum. (Modified from Jobe CM, et al: Theories and concepts. *In* Jobe FW, et al [eds]: Operative Techniques in Upper Extremity Sports Injuries. St. Louis, MO: Mosby-Year Book, 1996.)

(Fig. 25–13). When under anesthesia, members of this group may also demonstrate excessive anterior translation of the humeral head. There is a pass-through sign in which the arthroscope is easily passed beneath the head of the humerus along the anterior glenoid rim. The lesions of repetitive trauma are clearly evident along the posterosuperior labrum or the anteroinferior capsule. An enlarged bare spot on the posterior humeral head is also common. The glenohumeral ligaments, especially the inferior glenohumeral ligament, are lax or noticeably attenuated when the humerus is externally rotated. In addition, tears on the undersurface of the supraspinatus and infraspinatus are commonly encountered.

Group III. The group III category of shoulder dysfunction also commonly includes young, throwing athletes. The clinical examination demonstrates generalized ligamentous laxity (i.e., elbow and knee recurvation, hyperextensibility of the fingers and thumb), which is the differentiating factor between groups II and III. Shoulder instability is evident, as demonstrated by a positive result on the relocation test.

Arthroscopically, the humeral head can easily be displaced, sometimes by merely palpating it with the probe. Because of the ligamentous laxity, the arthroscope can be easily passed between the humeral head and the anterior glenoid labrum in the pass-through test. There may be humeral head lesions, such as that seen in group II patients, but they are less severe.

Group IV. The patients in group IV have experienced a traumatic event, such as a fall onto the outstretched arm, or direct trauma, such as sliding into a base under a tag with the arm forcibly hyperabducted and externally rotated. This singular traumatic event renders the shoulder unstable but without impingement. This group may also include patients who have had only partial dislocations. These patients have not developed an apprehension sign but do sometimes have a positive result on the relocation test. Arthroscopically, these patients show evidence of a Bankart lesion from the traumatic event and sometimes erosion of the posterior humeral head caused by the instability. This erosion is not a true Hill-Sachs lesion in that the humeral head has never actually dislocated.

Prevention of Injury

When discussing preventative exercise programs, once again the mechanics of the sport and the mechanism of pathology is important to understand. In the thrower, it is important to have as much static stability as possible, a stable scapular base, strong posterior checkreins for the humeral head, and a strong anterior wall.

STATIC STABILITY

The static stabilizers include the labrum, capsule, and glenohumeral ligaments. The ligament of most concern when the arm is elevated to 90 degrees and beyond is the inferior glenohumeral ligament. It is very easy to overstretch the capsule and ligaments. As a matter of fact the mere repetitive act of throwing can overstretch them. Furthermore, because these structures have no contractile elements, once they are overstretched, there is not a good noninvasive treatment. The clinician would therefore need to be very selective and careful about stretching the arm and would want to have a specific reason and goal with any stretch.

The one area that may be tight in the thrower is the posterior capsule. If it is too tight, it can push the humeral head anteriorly and therefore contribute to instability. One would want to consider stretching the posterior capsule while in the scapular plane (Fig. 25–14).

Because of the tendency for generalized ligamentous laxity in the thrower, any shoulder stretch to tissues other than the posterior structures could be detrimental. As a rule, stretching of the anterior or inferior structures is not recommended.

DYNAMIC STABILITY

The dynamic stabilizers include the scapular muscles and the rotator cuff. If there are scapular asymmetries noted

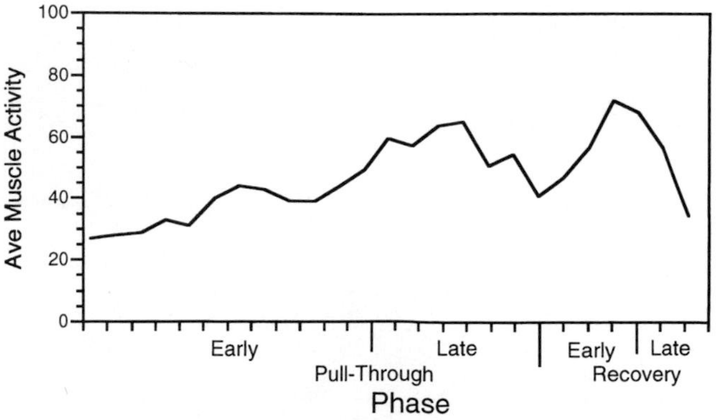

Figure 25–10

Muscle activity of the subscapularis in swimmers with normal shoulders.

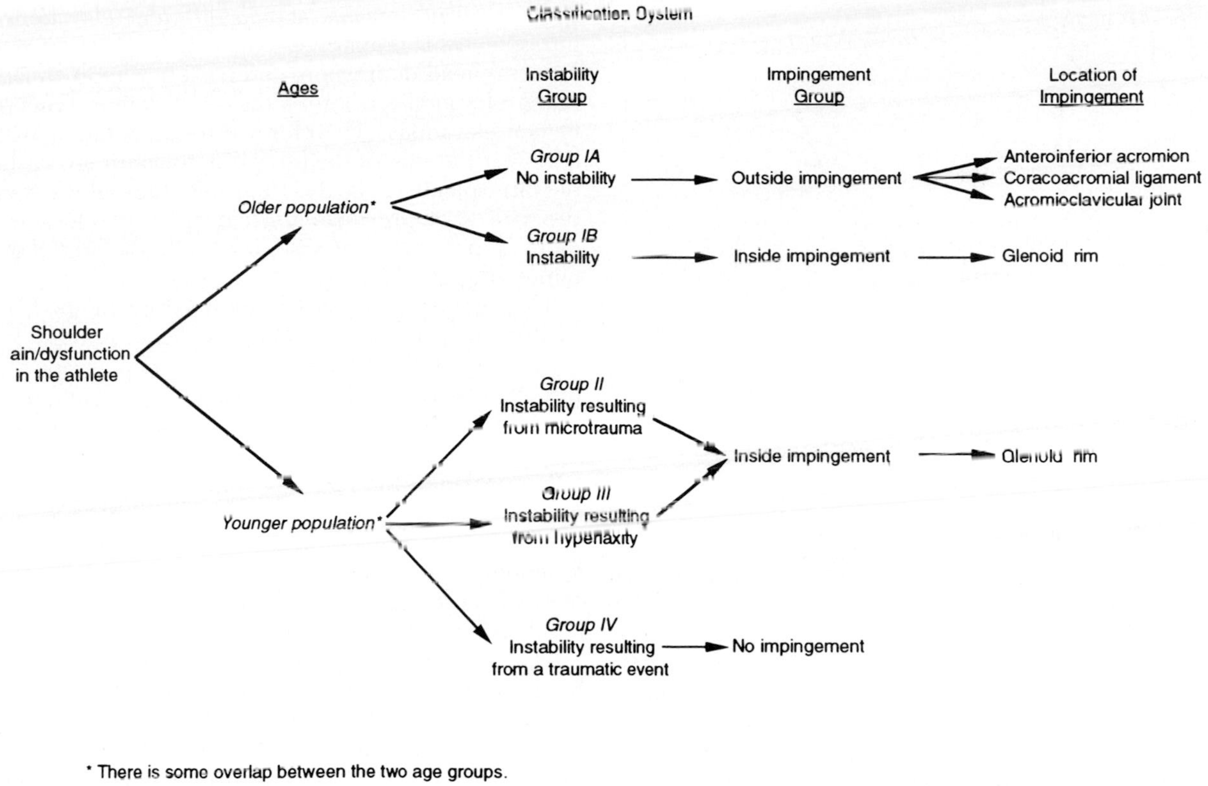

Figure 25–12

Classification system for shoulder pain and dysfunction in the overhead athlete. (From Jobe CM, et al: Theories and concepts. *In* Jobe FW, et al [eds]: Operative Techniques in Upper Extremity Sports Injuries. St Louis, MO: Mosby-Year Book, 1996.)

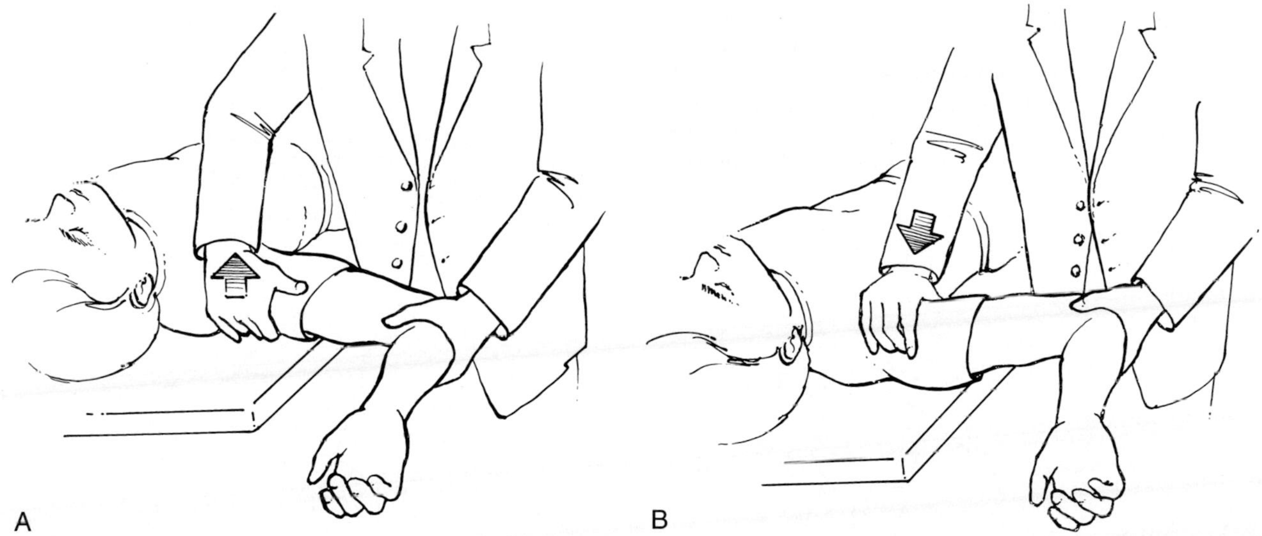

Figure 25–13

Relocation test: The patient is supine with the arm off the table at 90 degrees of abduction and maximum external rotation. *A*, The examiner grasps the humeral head posteriorly and pushes anteriorly. The examiner sometimes feels sliding (subluxation) of the humeral head, and this sliding typically elicits pain located at the posterior joint line. *B*, The examiner grasps the humeral head anteriorly and pushes posteriorly to relocate the head and lift the rotator cuff off the posterior labrum. If the patient feels pain in the first half of the test, *A*, the pain is usually relieved in the second half of the test. (From Jobe CM, et al: Theories and concepts. *In* Jobe FW, et al [eds]: Operative Techniques in Upper Extremity Sports Injuries. St Louis, MO: Mosby-Year Book, 1996.)

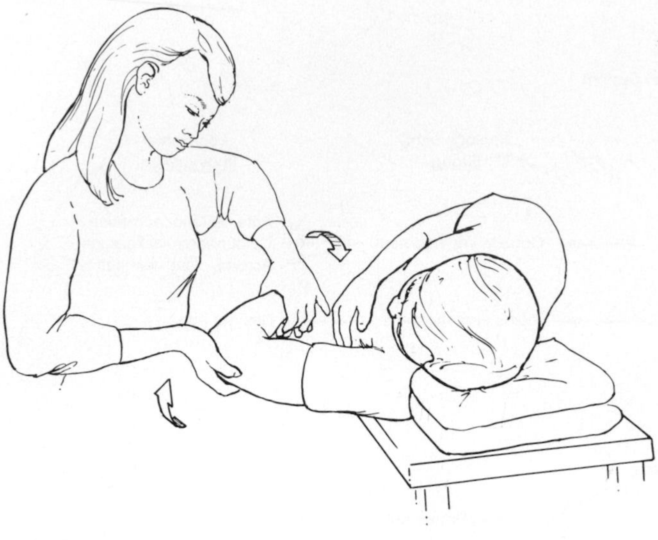

Figure 25–14

Posterior capsule stretch. (From Pink MM, et al: Injury prevention and rehabilitation in the upper extremity. *In* Jobe FW, et al [eds]: Operative Techniques in Upper Extremity Sports Injuries. St Louis, MO: Mosby-Year Book, 1996.)

during bilateral arm motion, quite likely the serratus anterior is the culprit. If the serratus anterior is deficient, one will notice shoulder hiking as the upper trapezius tries to substitute for the serratus anterior. However, no muscle can effectively substitute and allow for controlled motion at the inferior border of the scapula. For that reason, winging and asynchronous motion will occur.

The serratus anterior has several functions. It can both protract and upwardly rotate the scapula. The upper fibers tend to be the protractors, while the lower fibers tend to be the upward rotators.[17] The breadth of this large, flat muscle reminds us of the multiple directions of the muscle fibers. The multiplicity of function and anatomy lends itself to multiple exercises. Elevation above 120 degrees in all three planes (frontal, coronal, and scapular) is an optimal position to exercise the serratus anterior.[26] The push-up with a plus is also an excellent exercise (Fig. 25–15).

The teres minor and the infraspinatus are the posterior checkreins that help to hold the humeral head back. We now know that these two muscles possess distinct mechanical advantages at two different elevations. The infraspinatus is primarily responsible for external rotation, humeral head depression, and posterior approximation at lower elevations, whereas the teres minor functions at higher elevations. Therefore, external rotation with the arm near the side of the body is optimal for strengthening the infraspinatus (Fig. 25–16), while external rotation with the arm at approximately 70 degrees of elevation is a more appropriate exercise for strengthening the teres minor (Fig. 25–17).

The supraspinatus is the most easily fatigued of the rotator cuff muscles.[2, 15] One excellent exercise for the supraspinatus is scapular plane elevation (scaption).[36] If this exercise is used for a preventative program, it can be done with external rotation and the arm can be elevated above the head. However, if it is being used for a rehabilitative program, the elevation should be kept well below 90 degrees in order to avoid impingement (Fig. 25–18). In the normal shoulder, the humeral head depressors are functioning in synchrony and keep the humeral head clear of the coracoacromial arch, and the arm can safely be elevated above the head.

The subscapularis can be a difficult muscle to exercise because the latissimus dorsi and pectoralis major are also glenohumeral internal rotators. The clinician has to be certain that the subscapularis is functioning during an exercise along with these two large muscles. All three of these muscles have been considered anterior wall muscles; however, because the subscapularis inserts closest to the axis of rotation, it functions best to protect the

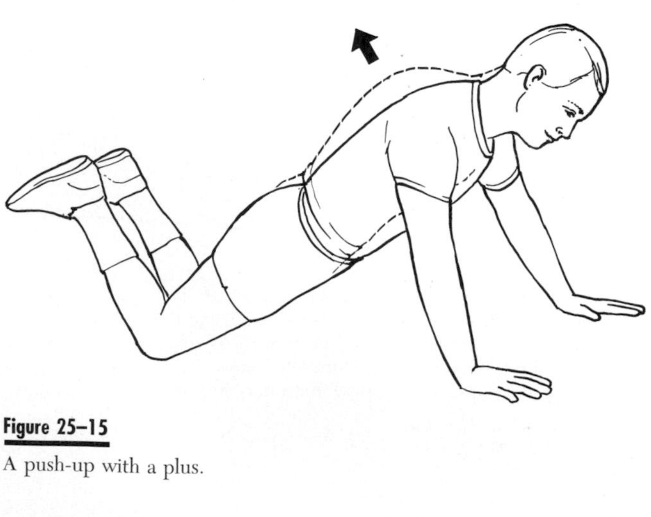

Figure 25–15

A push-up with a plus.

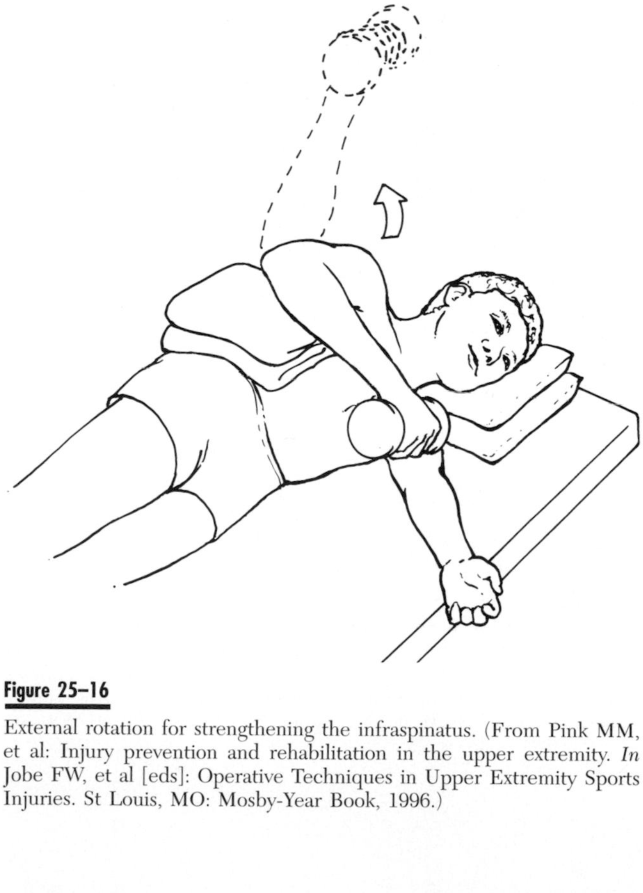

Figure 25–16

External rotation for strengthening the infraspinatus. (From Pink MM, et al: Injury prevention and rehabilitation in the upper extremity. *In* Jobe FW, et al [eds]: Operative Techniques in Upper Extremity Sports Injuries. St Louis, MO: Mosby-Year Book, 1996.)

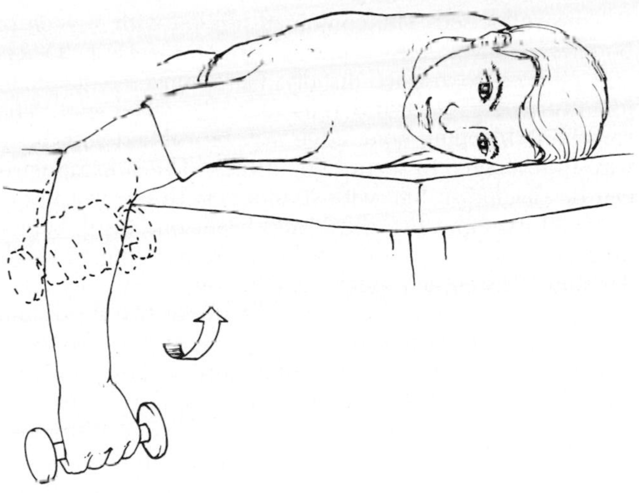

Figure 25–17

External rotation for strengthening the teres minor. (From Pink MM, et al: Injury prevention and rehabilitation in the upper extremity. *In* Jobe FW, et al [eds]: Operative Techniques in Upper Extremity Sports Injuries. St Louis, MO: Mosby-Year Book, 1996.)

glenohumeral joint from anterior subluxation. Experience has shown that internal rotation on an isokinetic device at high speeds for a prolonged time is a good way to activate the subscapularis (Fig. 25–19). If such a device is not available, elevation in all three planes as well as the military press will activate the subscapularis.[36]

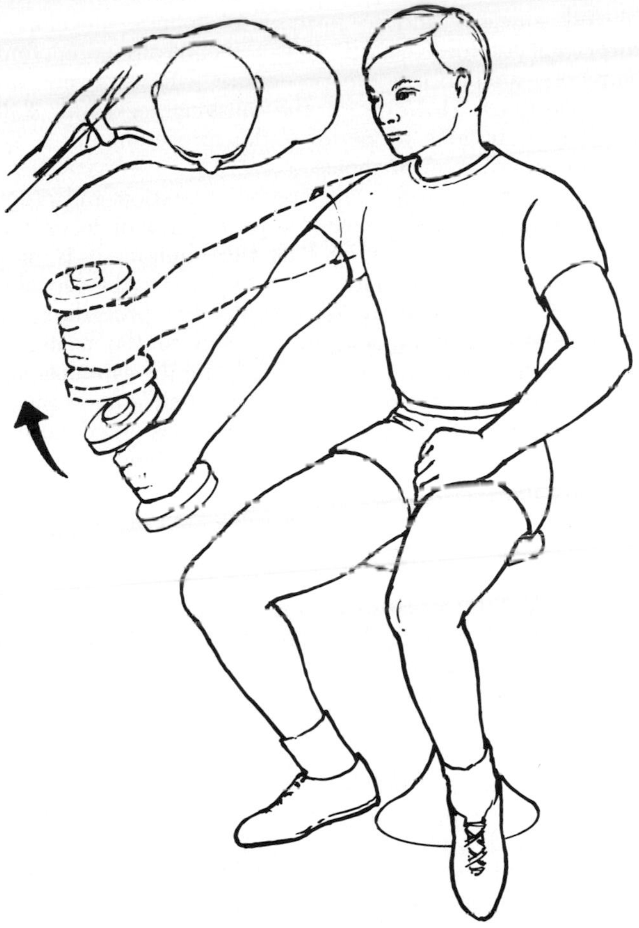

Figure 25–18

Scaption with humeral internal rotation (see also *inset*).

Surgical Procedures

BRISTOW OPERATION

For many years, the Bristow operation (designed by Helfet and modified by May) has been popular as a treatment for anteriorly dislocating shoulders. A detailed description is included here because it is still the procedure of choice in certain conditions. Within the last 10 years, other procedures have been developed, and indications for the Bristow operation have been narrowed considerably. The primary indication for the Bristow procedure is a shoulder with a large amount of bone loss to the anterior rim or a large Hill-Sachs lesion on the humeral head.

The Bristow procedure has not been successful in subluxing shoulders or in hyperelastic patients. The tendency of this procedure to produce posterior dislocation precludes its use in hyperelastic patients. Better procedures have been developed for many patients who would have been candidates for this operation in the past. The evolution of these newer techniques allows us to be more exacting in our selection of patients.

The Bristow procedure results in a loss of 6 to 10 degrees of humeral external rotation. This renders it unsatisfactory in the treatment of the dominant arm of a thrower. Even a minimal decrease in motion usually prevents the patient from returning to high-level participation.

The Bristow procedure has also been criticized because of complications such as screw loosening, migration or breakage, neurovascular injuries, nonunion of the trans-

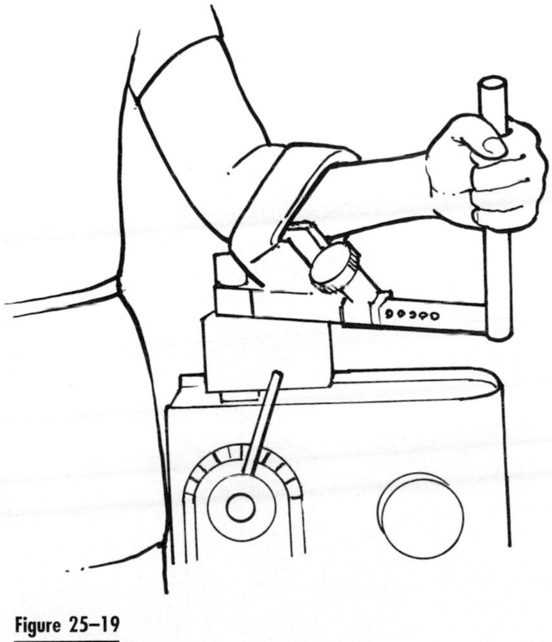

Figure 25–19

Humeral rotation on an isokinetic device.

ferred coracoid, and so forth. Our opinion, developed over the last few years, is that a technically competent surgeon can perform the procedure without significant complications. However, if the surgeon lacks the skill or the equipment to perform this procedure, it is an inappropriate surgical choice.

The choice between the Bristow operation and other soft tissue procedures may be purely academic as the surgeon's skills develop and as the equipment is now available which allows him or her to perform the capsulolabral reconstructions. In the capsulolabral procedure, no muscles are removed and no changes in the anatomic relationship occur. An athlete treated with the capsulolabral procedure will be able to throw and perform overhead activities and will not risk the complications noted earlier. Indeed, we anticipate that as the range of indications narrows for the Bristow procedure and widens for the capsulolabral reconstruction, the former will go out of vogue.

The Magnuson-Stack and Putti-Platt procedures are not recommended for the athlete's dominant throwing arm under any circumstances. These procedures can tighten the shoulder to such an extent that the athlete is left with limited mobility.

Technique

The following is a detailed description of the Bristow procedure. The procedure is easily performed supine with an arm board. A folded towel is placed under the scapula. Using a modified axillary approach (Fig. 25–20), the deltopectoral interval is identified and developed with the cephalic vein retracted laterally. The clavipectoral fascia is likewise incised. The conjoined tendon with ¼ inch of bone is removed with a curved osteotome (Fig. 25–21) and allowed to retract distally. Care must be taken to identify and protect the musculocutaneous nerve. The remaining bleeding bone edge may be rubbed with bone wax, if necessary, to secure hemostasis. The subscapularis can be divided in line with its fibers with electrocautery between its upper two thirds and lower one third, beginning just medial to the bicipital groove (Fig. 25–22). Anatomic dissections performed in our laboratory have shown that the interval between the upper two thirds and the lower one third lies in the internervous plane between the upper and lower subscapular nerves. This is a safe interval for dissection, therefore, because the branches of the upper subscapular nerve supply innervate the upper two thirds of the subscapularis muscle and the lower subscapular nerve innervates the lower one third of the muscle.[22]

The capsule is separated from the subscapularis and incised in line with the subscapular interval. A blunt-tipped, three-pronged retractor is placed anteriorly on the scapular neck so that the following steps can be performed without damage to cartilage (Fig. 25–23). The anterior glenoid rim is débrided down to bleeding bone. Using a 3.2-mm drill, a hole is created across the glenoid, parallel to the joint (Fig. 25–24). The depth is then measured with a depth gauge. The bony block height is added to the depth, and 5 mm is subtracted. The block is then shaped to fit snugly against the prepared surface and is secured in position with the appropriately sized malleolar screw (Fig. 25–25).

The inferior capsular flap is now pulled up and sutured

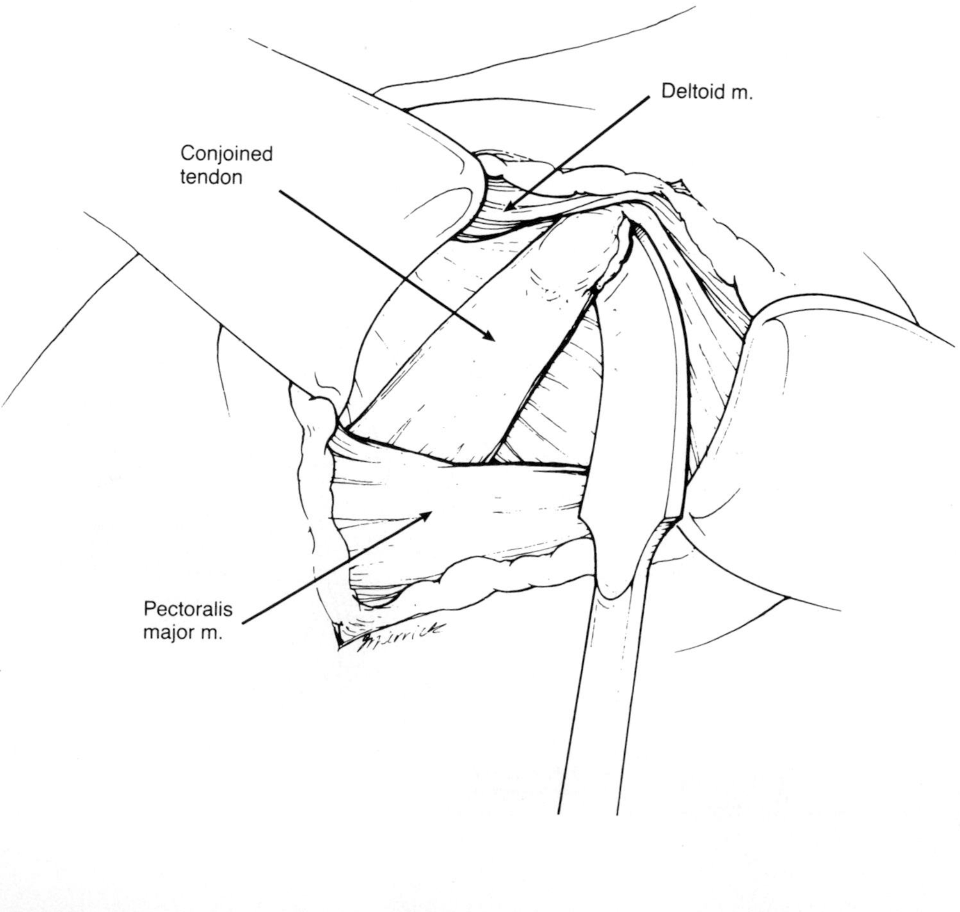

Figure 25–20

The deltopectoral interval is identified.

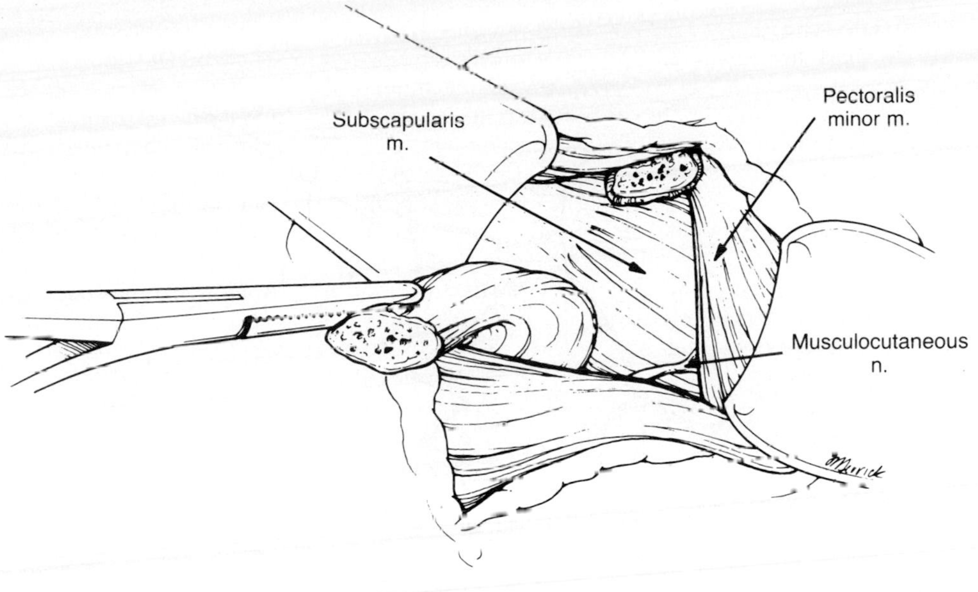

Figure 25–21

The conjoined tendon with ¼ inch of bone is removed with a curved osteotome.

to the superior capsular flap just lateral to the bony block (Fig. 25–26). Incising the inferior capsule at the glenoid rim may facilitate a tighter capsular closure if there is marked anteroinferior capsular redundancy. The shoulder is put through its range of motion. If it appears too tight, the conjoined tendon can be partially released in a controlled fashion to allow additional motion. Bleeding is controlled, and the muscles are allowed to return to their anatomic position. The wound is closed in the usual manner.

Postoperatively, the arm is placed in a sling; Codman's exercises begin the next day. Motion is encouraged out of the sling within the middle of the shoulder's range. Care is taken to avoid forced abduction and external rotation until healing progresses. Light weights are used in mid-range only to regain strength. Strong abduction and external rotation should be avoided lest the screw is dislodged; also the use of the biceps against resistance is avoided. The bony block heals after 3 months, and more vigorous stretching and strengthening can be initiated.

The purpose of this procedure is to reinforce the middle and inferior capsule and the glenohumeral ligament system. By transferring the tip of the coracoid process with the attached conjoined tendon, the inferior portion of the subscapularis muscle is effectively tethered during abduction and external rotation of the arm. The superior

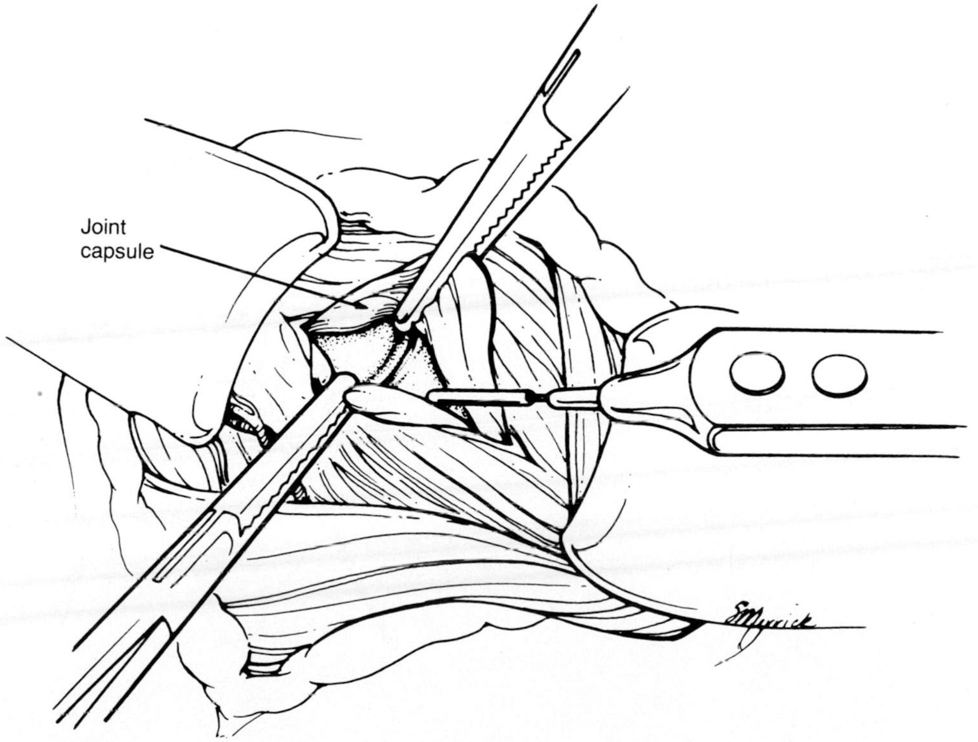

Figure 25–22

The subscapularis muscle is divided between its upper two thirds and lower one third with an electrocautery.

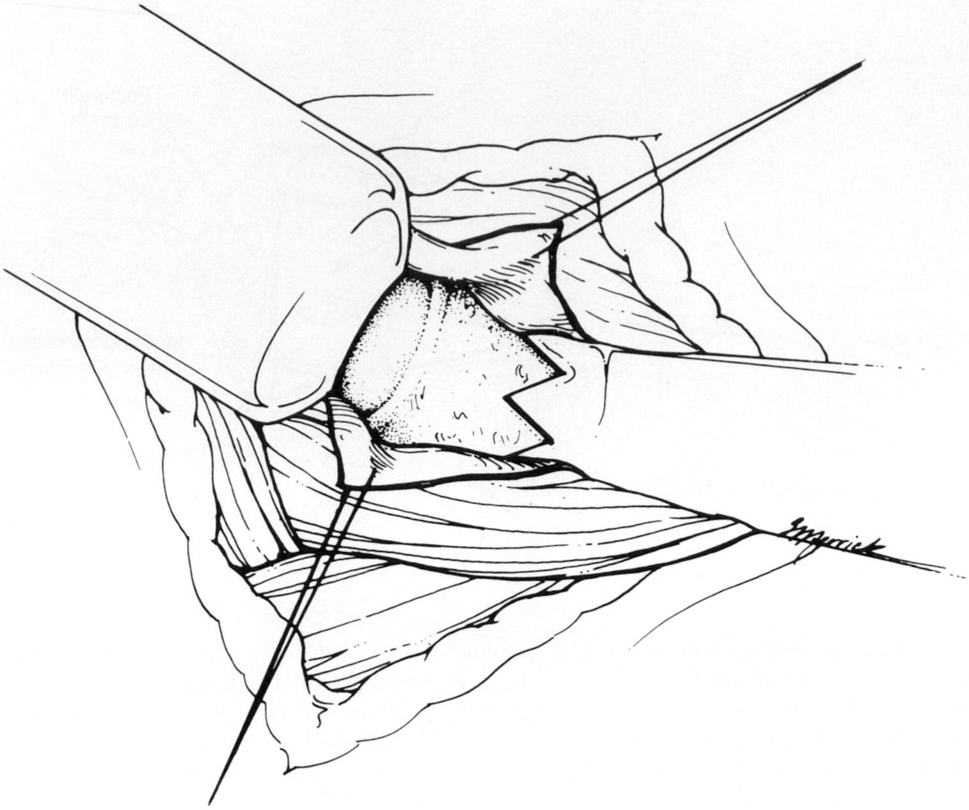

Figure 25–23

A blunt-tipped, three-pronged retractor is placed anteriorly on the scapular neck.

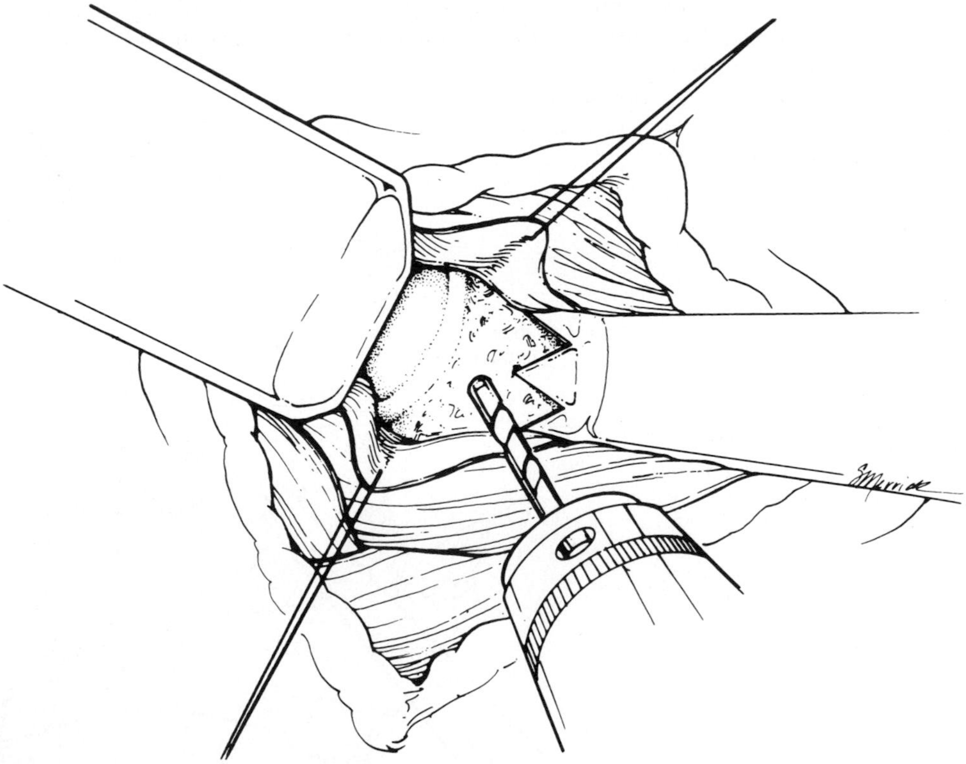

Figure 25–24

A 3.2-mm drill is used to create a hole across the glenoid, parallel to the joint.

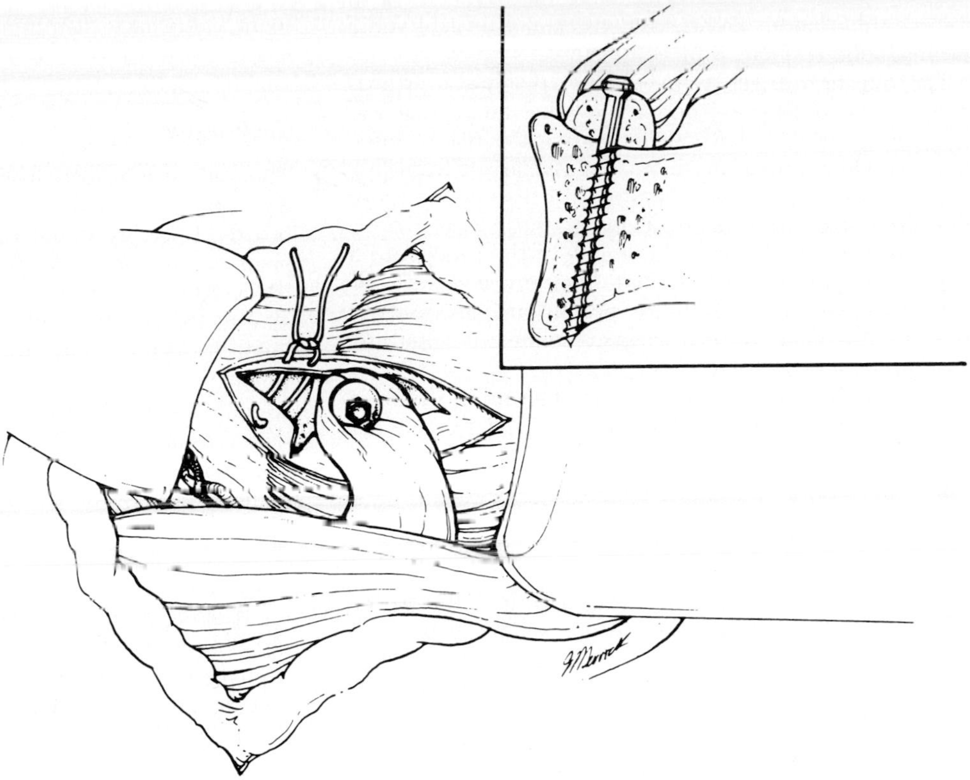

Figure 25–25

The bone block is secured in position with the appropriate size of malleolar screw.

excursion of this portion of the subscapularis muscle tendon unit is prevented, thus providing stability.

ARTHROSCOPY

Any discussion of sports medicine raises the question of the proper place of arthroscopy in the management of shoulder problems. When properly used, the arthroscope is an invaluable tool that provides capabilities, especially in diagnosis, not afforded by other tools.

As with arthroscopy of other joints, shoulder arthroscopy can be divided into three main groups of procedures: (1) diagnostic, (2) removal of unwanted materials, and (3) reconstruction of various structures.

The arthroscopic examination can be extremely valuable and can confirm the exact nature of the disease. For example, is a subluxing shoulder secondary to labral detachment or a stretched capsule? Is there any rotator cuff disease? Arthroscopy is superior to magnetic resonance imaging and other radiographic techniques in its degree of resolution in viewing intra-articular structures. In cases of instability, arthroscopy allows positioning of the shoulder to

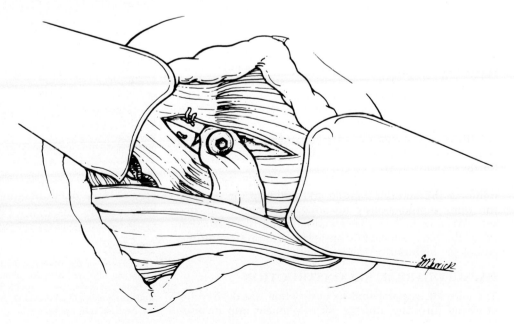

Figure 25–26

The inferior capsular flap is pulled up and sutured to the superior capsular flap just medial to the bony block.

observe subluxation. These positions cannot be achieved in the magnetic resonance imaging gantry.

The question arises as to whether diagnostic arthroscopy can be performed under the same anesthesia with the open procedure without increasing the risk of infection. We believe that any increased risk arises from fluid extravasation into the surrounding soft tissues. We therefore limit diagnostic arthroscopy in these cases to the posterior portal only, limit the length of the procedure to a maximum of 5 minutes, and then proceed with the operative procedure. If more portals are necessary, if more time is needed, or if excessive edema is noted, the open procedure is delayed.

Not only is diagnostic arthroscopy helpful in the treatment of the injured shoulder in the athlete, but also arthroscopic removal of unwanted materials can often be the definitive procedure. Materials to be removed may include a torn labrum, loose bodies, rheumatoid synovium, pus from pyarthrosis in the joint or in its subacromial bursa, and so forth. If the material removed was formerly part of a stabilizing structure (e.g., labrum), the patient must be cautioned that although one symptomatic problem has been addressed (torn labral fragment), a second problem (an instability) may be unmasked and may require a second surgery. Parenthetically, we do no more rotator cuff débridement than is necessary for visualization of tears. Also, sometimes a labral débridement can be done with an accessory posterior lateral portal without disturbing the anterior tissues where an incision may later need to be made.

Arthroscopic repair of superior labral (SLAP) lesions seems to be the treatment of choice. Such lesions have become amenable to repair with the refinement of arthroscopic techniques. Using bioabsorbable tacks, or any number of suture anchors available today, these lesions can be anchored securely to the glenoid rim, stabilizing the biceps anchor and the superior labrum. Not only does this address the labral pathology, but it may also eliminate glenohumeral joint laxity that can be associated with such lesions.

With regard to arthroscopic reconstructions, we regard them as techniques in development. The success rate of stapling, in the best of hands, is 80% compared with 95% and better for the anterior capsulolabral reconstruction (ACLR) procedure, which is an open procedure. The apparent advantage of reduced early postoperative morbidity following arthroscopy is less striking when one considers that these open procedures are among the least painful in shoulder surgery. Moreover, the length of time of postoperative immobilization is much less when open stabilization procedures are performed. Therefore, arthroscopic procedures do not shorten the recovery time for these individuals.

The ideal procedure for all athletes will repair and reinforce the anterior capsule and build up the anterior rim while simultaneously adjusting the laxity of the capsule. We now believe that a capsulolabral reconstruction offers the most satisfactory answer to the problem of the pathologic high-performance shoulder.[19]

CAPSULOLABRAL RECONSTRUCTION

The anterior capsulolabral reconstruction was devised for overhead throwing athletes with dominant arm involvement, who have documented anterior instability and in whom conservative treatment has failed.

Technique

The patient is placed supine on the operating table with the arm positioned on a Parker table or on two arm boards. To create stability and prominence of the humeral head, two or three folded surgical towels are placed along the vertebral border and under the scapula. This will elevate the scapula and provide room to sublux the humeral head posteriorly for access to the anterior glenoid. Below the level of the coracoid, a 6- to 8-cm skin incision is made in line with a midaxillary skinfold in the relaxed skin tension lines. The skin is undermined in all directions, exposing the deltopectoral fascia and interval. Meticulous hemostasis is required for proper visualization. The anterior deltoid, cephalic vein, pectoralis major, and deltopectoral groove are identified (Fig. 25–27). The deltopectoral fascia is split in line with the cephalic vein and freed along its pectoral border. Using Goulet retractors, the deltopectoral groove is opened while retracting the cephalic vein laterally with the deltoid and the pectoralis major medially. The lateral border of the conjoined tendon is identified and freed from surrounding tissues (Fig. 25–28). The conjoined tendon is retracted medially with a long, narrow Richardson retractor. The superior border of the subscapularis is identified by the recess; the inferior

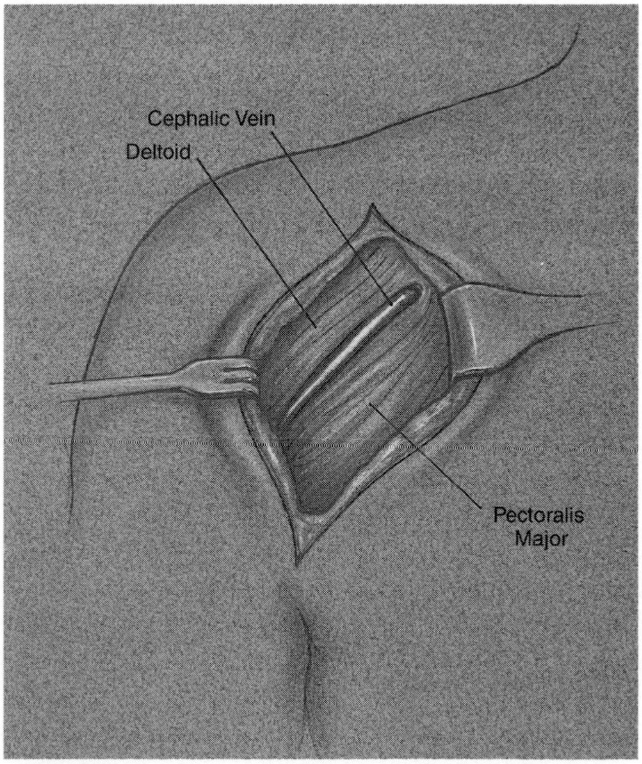

Figure 25–27

The incision of the right shoulder is in the skin lines of the shoulder extending into the axilla for about ½ inch. The proximal end of the incision begins over the coracoid. The margins of the skin are mobilized so that the deltoid and pectoralis major can be identified, and if present the cephalic vein can be seen.

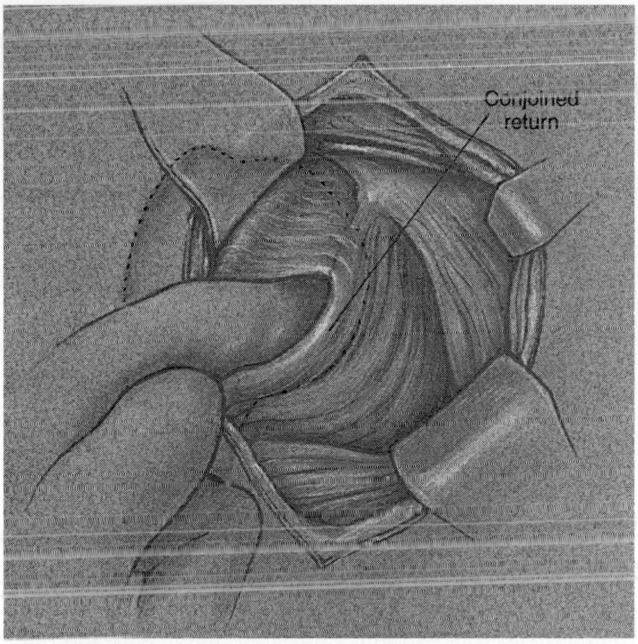

Figure 25–28

The conjoined tendon is identified and freed on its lateral aspect up to the coracoid so that it can be retracted medially.

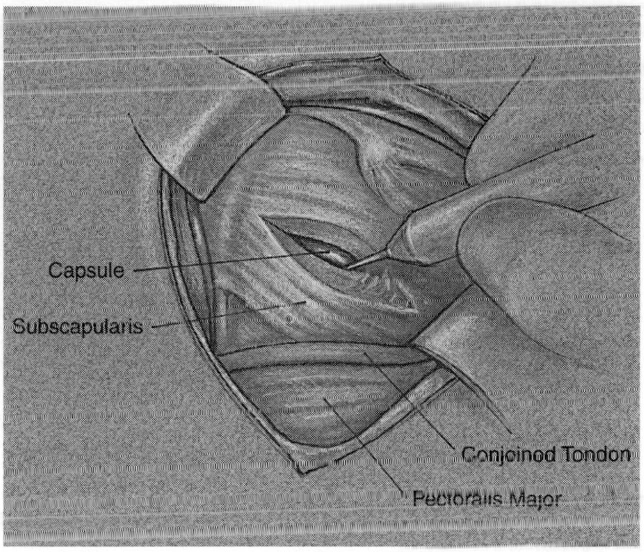

Figure 25–29

The subscapularis tendon is exposed. The superior and inferior borders are noted, and the upper two thirds and the lower one third are identified so that the muscle can be split longitudinally in the direction of its fibers. A coagulation bovie is used for this purpose.

border is identified by the anterior humeral circumflex vessels. Internal and external rotation of the humeral head helps to delineate the superior and inferior margins. At this point, the rotator interval is examined and judgement is made as to whether it needs to be closed as part of the procedure.

With the arm in external rotation (protecting the long head of the biceps) and using coagulating electrocautery, the subscapularis tendon is split in line with its fibers at its lower third (Fig. 25–29). Kocher clamps are then placed on the superior and inferior margins of the subscapularis to provide tension while the dissection progresses. Using a No. 15 surgical blade, the interval between the capsule and the subscapularis is sharply defined (Fig. 25–30). This is most easily accomplished at the myotendinous junction where the tendon and capsule are less adherent. Meticulous dissection to define this interval is paramount. By lifting the superior and inferior edges, the interval may be more readily identified near the muscle border. Further separation superiorly, inferiorly, and medially is obtained by using a soft tissue elevator. Improved exposure to the capsule is obtained by placing a blunt-tip, three-pronged pitchfork retractor onto the glenoid neck, then a modified self-retaining, long-tonged Gelpi retractor is placed beneath the superior and inferior margins of the cut subscapularis muscle and tendon, laterally. Better exposure to the joint capsule and the underlying glenohumeral joint can now be appreciated.

Near the center of the humeral head, a transverse capsulotomy is made parallel to the split in the subscapularis at approximately midjoint level (Fig. 25–31) and extended medially toward the bony glenoid rim, creating a superior and inferior flap. The capsulotomy is extended onto the neck of the glenoid and the flaps are elevated subperiosteally (Fig. 25–32). Examination at this time will determine whether the labrum is severely damaged, or whether a Bankart lesion is present. At this time, the capsule can also be evaluated for the amount of redundancy that needs to be corrected. It has been our experience that if the redundancy is mainly capsular and the labrum is in excellent condition, then the majority of the procedure can be directed toward a capsular shift leaving the labrum in place. Whether or not bone anchors are used is a decision made at that time. Generally, however, the labrum is damaged and sometimes pulled away from the bone. We have found that it is not of prime impor-

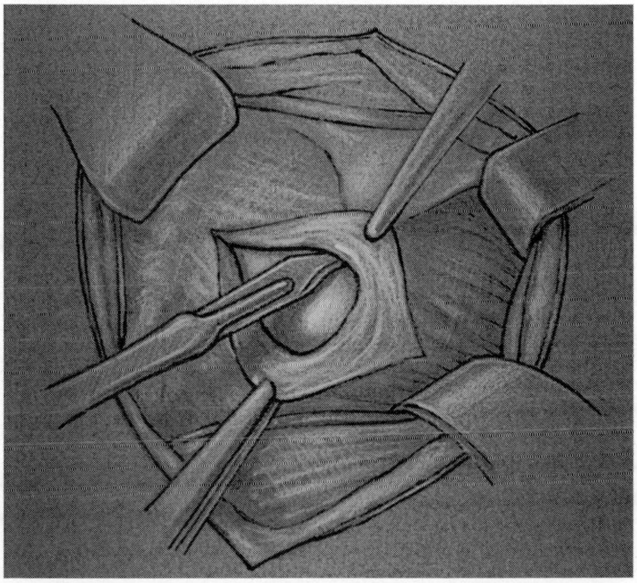

Figure 25–30

The split is carried down to the capsule. A knife is then used to separate the capsule from the subscapularis. The sharp section is used laterally, and the blunt section is used medially under the muscle.

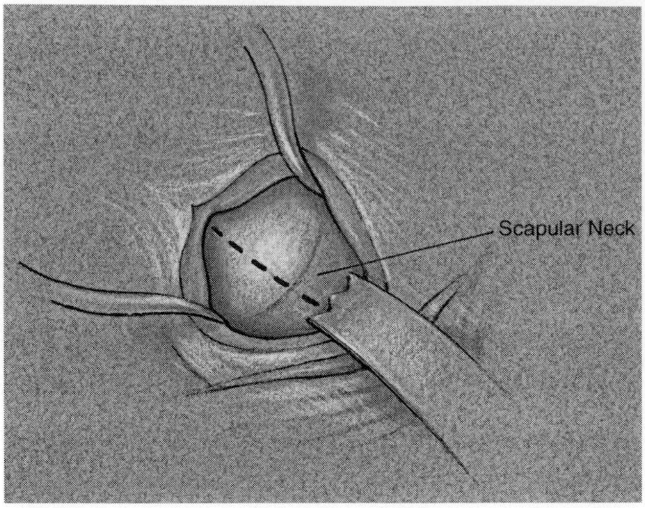

Figure 25–31

The capsule is split longitudinally in the same direction as the subscapularis.

tance to save a damaged labrum. It can be trimmed or removed without compromising the end result.

Care is taken as the glenohumeral joint is approached that all of the structures are carefully cleaned and separated so that at the time of closure there is no confusion as to which structures are approximated. To aid in this identification, a stay suture is placed both in the superior flap and in the inferior flap at the margin of the joint. This gives a reference point so that as a capsular shift is carried out, no medialization of the capsule is inadvertently executed that might compromise the end result by making the capsule too tight thus preventing full range of motion after the repair.

With the stay sutures in hand, a two-pronged humeral head retractor can be positioned in the joint. The points of the retractor should be situated on the posterior rim, and care is taken not to injure the articulating cartilage of the glenoid fossa. In the proper position the retractor can be used as a lever to push the head posteriorly and laterally. By changing the pressure on this retractor as well as the pressure on the pitchfork retractor, appropriate changes in the position of the capsule can be made for good exposure.

After the capsule has been sufficiently cleaned and elevated from the glenoid, a half-size single point retractor is placed on the inferior neck of the glenoid. This enhances visualization immensely. The neck of the glenoid is then cleaned so that good material is present (usually some bleeding bone is desirable) and then drill holes are placed for the bone anchors. We have usually placed them at about 3:00 to 3:30 position, 4:00 to 4:30 position, and 5:00 to 5:30 position on the right shoulder. The drill holes are made parallel to the articulating cartilage about 2 or 3 mm away from the glenoid surface (Figs. 25–33 and 25–34). Many bone anchor systems are available at the present time. We have had the most experience with the Mitek* devices, and we commonly use the two-pronged device with a No. 2 suture. These devices are placed in position, and care is taken to aim the inferior one slightly cephalad so that there is no risk of the tip going through the posterior cortex.

The inferior flap of the capsule is then pulled superiorly. A great deal of care is used to avoid medialization, and sutures are placed through the flap so that it can advance a predetermined amount (Fig. 25–35). The amount, of course, is determined by the amount of hyper-

*Mitek Surgical Products, Norwood, Massachusetts.

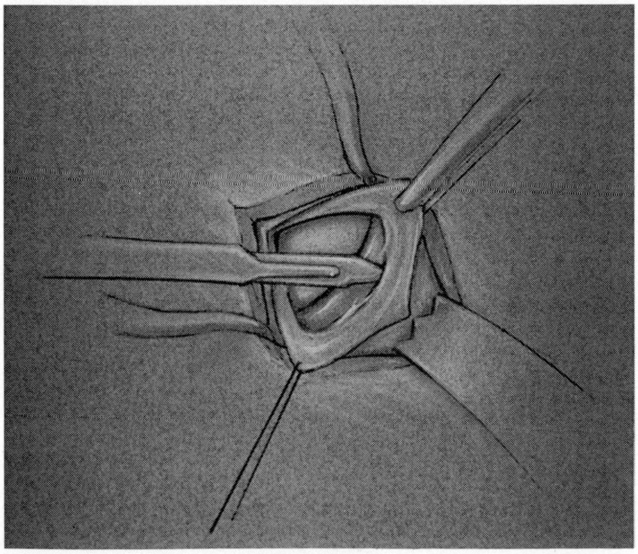

Figure 25–32

The incision is carried down onto the neck of the glenoid and elevated subperiosteally at that point. The labrum can be examined and removed if necessary or left in place.

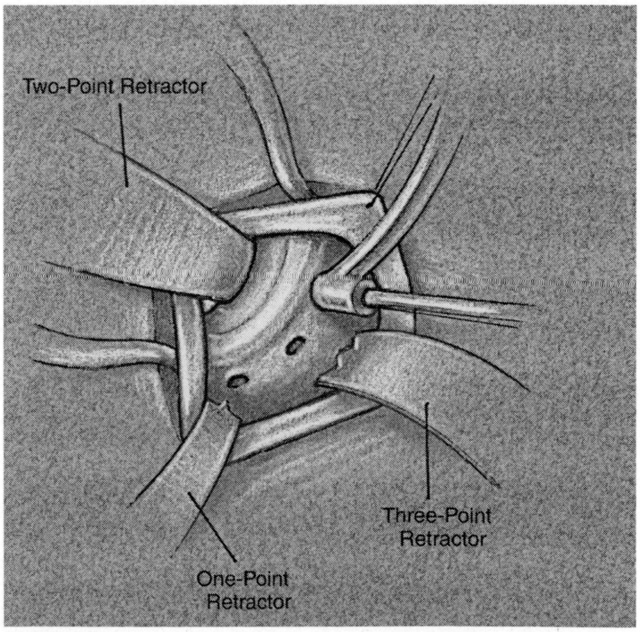

Figure 25–33

The anterior inferior rim of the glenoid is prepared, and three holes are placed next to the margin of the glenoid for placement of the bone anchors. Note the three retractors in place.

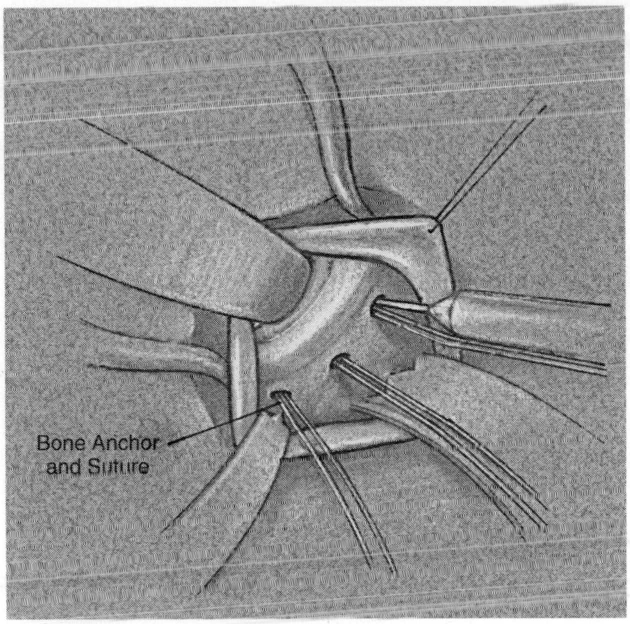

Figure 25–34

The bone anchors with No. 2 sutures are in position.

laxity and how much stretching was noted preoperatively. If the patient is an overhand athlete, it is very important that the capsule is not pulled too tight. If the capsule is too tight, the athlete will never regain his or her full range of motion.

When the capsule is properly positioned, one knot is placed in each of the three sutures and the superior flap is pulled down on top. The same sutures are used to secure it into position. Occasionally this flap will not reach all the way to the third anchor, but it usually reaches to the second anchor. With these sutures in place, the knots cannot be tied until the two-pronged humeral head retractor is removed. When this is accomplished, the sutures are tied (Fig. 25–36). At this point a judgement needs to be made as to how tight the overlap should be. It has been our custom to position the shoulder in the throwing position and see how much tightness is necessary with the arm at 90 degrees and full external rotation. Sometimes only a very small amount of flap overlap is necessary, and a single suture is usually placed just to keep the overlap in position. This leaves some portion of the split unsutured near the humeral head, which is helpful in regaining the capacity of the joint once range of motion is carried out.

When this has been accomplished, the retractors are removed and the subscapularis is closed with absorbable sutures (Fig. 25–37). The wound is usually washed with an antibiotic solution, and closure is carried out with an absorbable suture for the subcutaneous tissue and a 4–0 clear subcuticular nylon for the skin.

Postoperative Rehabilitation Program

The patient is immobilized in an abduction brace for 2 weeks. The postoperative position is important. To regain full range of motion afterwards, the shoulder is typically placed in 90 degrees of abduction, 30 degrees of forward flexion, and 45 degrees of external rotation. This is the optimal position for the throwing athlete because it positions the shoulder in external rotation and prevents tightening of the anterior and inferior capsule. If there is

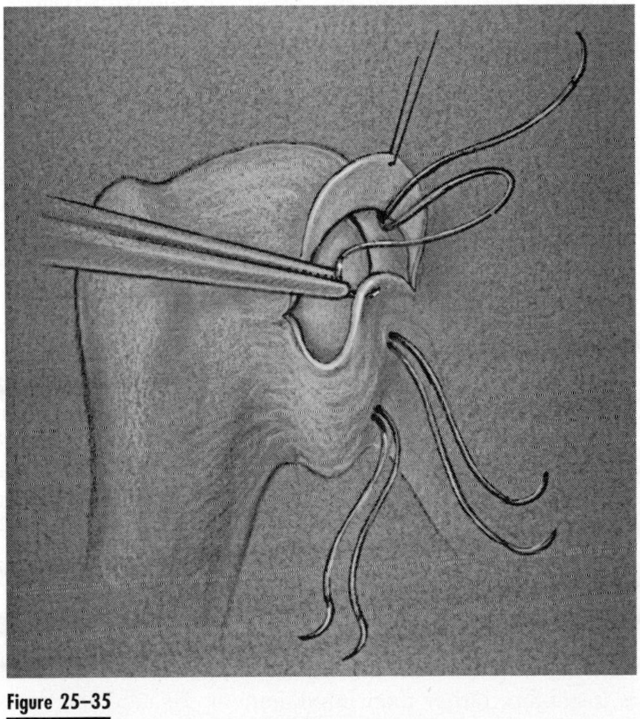

Figure 25–35

The inferior flap is pulled superiorly, and care is taken that no medialization is carried out so that overtightening of the capsule is avoided.

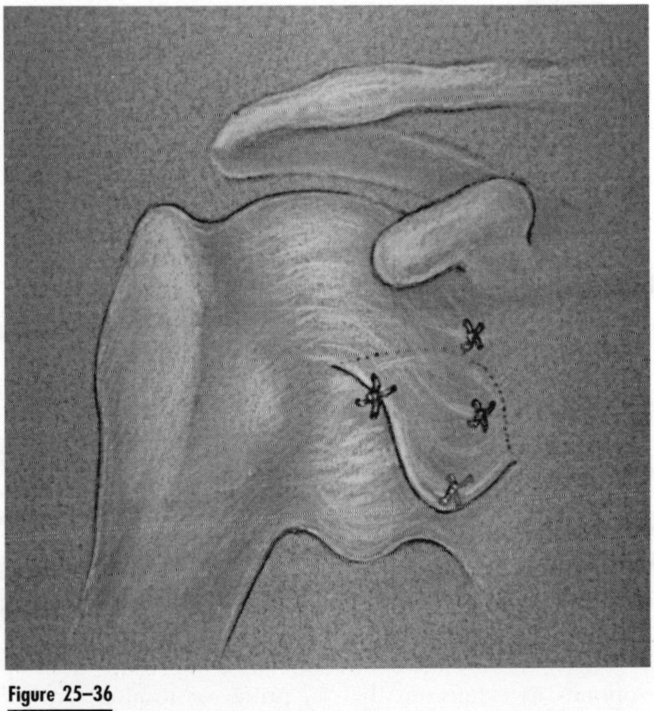

Figure 25–36

The superior flap is pulled over the top, and an adjustment is made according to the predetermined need.

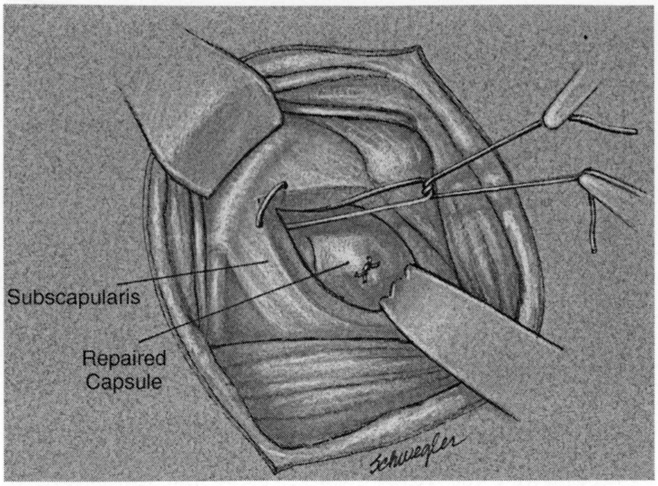

Figure 25–37

The subscapularis tendon is closed with absorbable sutures over the repair.

concern about excessive connective tissue laxity in a patient, a sling may be worn instead of the abduction brace.

During this immediate postoperative period, the patient removes the sling or splint for active and active-assisted elevation exercises. On the first day, the patient lifts the arm up and out of the splint. Active elbow flexion and extension and wrist motion begin on the first postoperative day. The patient begins to squeeze a ball or an egg-shaped plastic exerciser immediately.

As soon as the splint or sling is discarded, wand exercises are added for elevation and multiple-angle isometric exercises for internal rotation, external rotation, abduction, flexion, and extension.

Isotonic-resisted exercises begin by the third week. The first group of exercises includes active-resisted internal and external rotation with the arm at the side using elastic resistance bands or tubing. Active shoulder extension may be performed either prone or standing while bending forward at the waist. The patient extends the arm, with the elbow straight, to the plane of the trunk. The patient should not go beyond this plane. When horizontal adduction is added 1 or 2 weeks later, the patient starts in the supine position with the humerus supported so that the exercise begins in the scapular plane and the ending position does not extend beyond this plane.

The second phase of the rehabilitation program emphasizes progressive strengthening, beginning with the shoulder rotators. The patient moves from elastic band resistance of increasing difficulty to side-lying external rotation with free weights. The therapist must take care to position the arm during internal rotation with a bolster under the lateral chest wall. The patient also performs the supraspinatus exercise in a pain-free range only (see Fig. 25–18). The clinician continues strengthening the anterior deltoid. Elevation above 110 degrees can be included once the patient is able to do so with no pain.

Active horizontal abduction (with the same position options as extension; that is, prone or leaning forward from the waist) is limited to the plane of the trunk. Scapular adduction and trunk rotation can mimic some degree of horizontal abduction, making it appear that more horizontal abduction is accomplished than is really the case.

By the third postoperative month, eccentric rotator cuff exercises, vigorous elbow and wrist strengthening, and the military press exercise with the arms in front of the chest are all part of the program. For the serratus anterior, the patient can begin with modified hands-and-knees push-ups with a plus (see Fig. 25–15). The upper extremity ergometer can also be used to strengthen the serratus anterior if the seat is set back far enough to allow for exaggerated scapular protraction. The ergometer is set at a low resistance.

Isokinetic training is begun when the patient is able to lift 5 to 10 lb in external rotation and 15 to 20 lb in internal rotation without pain or swelling. At about 4 months after surgery (and if isokinetic testing has verified that the involved shoulder has at least 70% of the strength of the uninvolved shoulder), the third phase—sport-specific rehabilitation—begins. For a detailed explanation of various sports-specific rehabilitation programs, please see Chapter 7F in "Operative Techniques in Upper Extremity Sports Injuries."[20] The speed of the throw will progress to about three fourths of the maximum speed at about 7 months after surgery; full speed is not a reasonable goal until almost 1 year after surgery. It is important not to advance the patient too quickly with the throwing program. The time is necessary to allow adequate healing of the reconstructed tissues and adaptation for the stresses placed on them during throwing.

POSTERIOR SHOULDER PROBLEMS

Instability

Athletes very rarely suffer a posterior shoulder dislocation. Commonly, they present with repeated episodes of posterior shoulder subluxation. This occurs in one of two ways: (1) from overuse, which stretches out the posterior capsule, or (2) from a singular traumatic episode that results in subluxation with stretching of the posterior capsule, which then recurs with repeated use of the shoulder. For example, a pitcher will stress his posterior capsule repeatedly in the follow-through phase of throwing. If he overthrows, does not warm up properly, or limits his follow-through by poor lower body mechanics, he can injure the posterior capsule, which will lead to repeated subluxation. Another example is a quarterback who falls on his outstretched hand while being tackled and immediately feels a pulling sensation in the posterior aspect of his shoulder. He may or may not feel that his shoulder came out of the joint. When he recovers from this acute injury, he notices that he has posterior pain with throwing and cannot throw with the same velocity. On examination he may have pain over the posterior shoulder joint, but he may also present with pain over the biceps and rotator cuff tendons, as in a typical impingement syndrome. It may take a number of examinations on different occasions to ascertain that the problem is instability rather than impingement. Usually, the position of pain is in both forward flexion at 90 degrees and internal rotation. It may also be possible to sublux the shoulder in this position. If this is not possible, the patient should be positioned supine with the affected shoulder over the edge of the examination table; an attempt is made, while grasping the humeral head, to sublux the humeral head posteriorly. This is usually done by positioning the arm in forward flexion and then applying a posterior longitudinal thrust to the arm, thus attempting to sublux the shoulder. It must be remembered that the athlete in this group may be able to voluntarily sublux his shoulder posteriorly. He can often demonstrate the instability on a clinical examination. As the patient performs this maneuver, there is usually an audible "clunk." This can be confusing, because the audible "clunk" occurs with the reduction maneuver. These athletes, unlike voluntary subluxers, are usually not psychologically disturbed and do not use their shoulder instability for secondary gain. They can be treated exactly the same as the athlete who cannot voluntarily dislocate his shoulder.

Occasionally, in the well-muscled athlete, the instability cannot be defined in the clinical examination. Examination under anesthesia, as well as arthroscopy, will usually be necessary to determine the correct diagnosis. The examination under anesthesia usually reveals increased anterior/posterior translation compared with the normal shoulder. The arthroscopic findings are usually not striking, because the only findings include capsular stretching or minor posterior labral damage. The major value of arthroscopy is the assessment of the anterior glenohumeral ligaments and the labrum in order to determine the major direction of instability.

Pathologic findings with posterior shoulder instability are different from those found with anterior instability. The true reverse Bankart lesion is usually seen in less than 5% of the cases, usually in athletes involved in contact sports with a traumatic injury. The labrum may be shallow and poorly developed, but it is almost always intact and not torn away from the posterior glenoid. The capsule is usually redundant. The initial management of these athletes is conservative, with an extensive physical therapy program. The physical therapist is instructed to strengthen the external rotators, namely the infraspinatus and the teres minor, as well as the posterior deltoid. Biofeedback may have a place in this form of instability, as described by Beall and associates.[3] The exercise program generally lasts for at least 6 months. Coaches work on follow-through technique to allow the leg muscles to accept some of the stress that the athlete has been placing on the posterior shoulder.

With a conservative program, approximately two thirds of the athletes note subjective improvement. The instability is often not eliminated, but the functional disability is improved so that the athlete can perform without a problem.[16]

Management of athletes with recurrent posterior shoulder subluxation who do not respond to conservative care is controversial. The results of surgical reconstruction for posterior instability have been disappointing in the past.[14, 31] Recent articles, however, have more promising results.[5, 11, 13]

POSTERIOR CAPSULORRHAPHY

Our recommended procedure in athletes with posterior shoulder subluxation is a posterior capsulorrhaphy. Initially the capsulorrhaphy was performed by stapling, but in the last 10 years, a suture technique has been developed. The patient is placed on the operating table in the lateral decubitus position with the involved shoulder superior and draped free. The patient is held in position with a Vacupack, supporting posts, and kidney rests. The operating table is placed in a slight reverse Trendelenburg position. The peroneal nerve should be protected where it crosses the neck of the fibula on the inferior leg. A diagnostic arthroscopy is usually performed to confirm the pathology and direction of instability. The patient is left in this position while the surgeon performs the posterior capsulorrhaphy. A saber incision is made on the superior aspect of the shoulder, beginning just posterior to the acromioclavicular joint and continuing posteriorly toward the posterior axillary fold (Fig. 25–38). This incision is usually 10 cm in length. The subcutaneous tissues are undermined to expose the deltoid. The deltoid is split (Fig. 25–39) from an area on the spine 2 to 3 cm medial to the posterolateral corner of the acromion, distally approximately 5 cm. The deltoid should not be split below the level of the teres minor because the axillary nerve, which enters the deltoid at the inferior border of the teres minor, might be damaged. It is usually not necessary to reflect the deltoid from the spine or acromion, except occasionally in a well-muscled individual. The teres minor and infraspinatus are encountered below the fascia, deep to the deltoid. The interval between these muscles is not always apparent (Fig. 25–40). An important landmark is the raphe between the two heads of the infraspinatus,

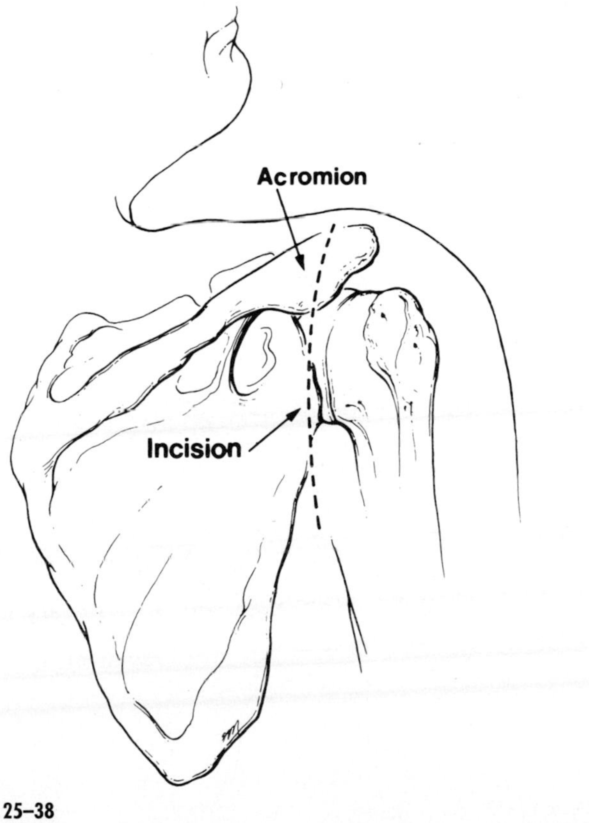

Figure 25–38

The incision is made superiorly, beginning posterior to the acromioclavicular joint and directed toward the posterior axillary fold.

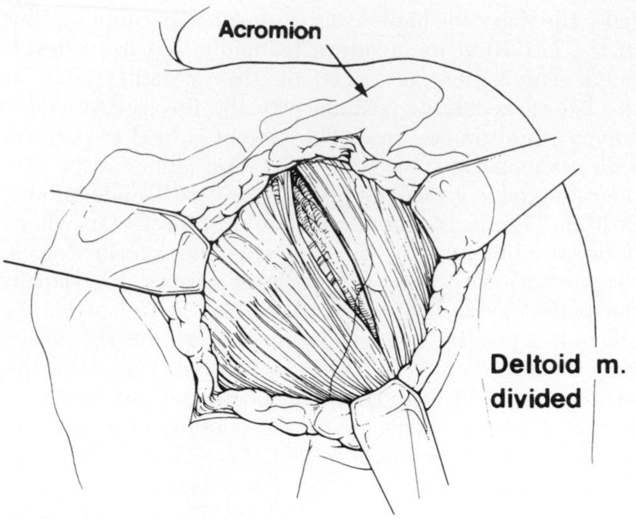

Figure 25–39

The deltoid is split 2 to 3 cm medial to the posterolateral corner of the acromion.

which is a bipennate muscle. This raphe should not be confused with the interval between the teres minor and the infraspinatus, which is usually below the equator of the humeral head. The interval between the two heads of the infraspinatus is developed by blunt dissection. Retractors are placed to expose the posterior shoulder capsule. Care must be taken not to split the infraspinatus more than 1.5 cm medially to the glenoid, in order to avoid damage to the branch of the suprascapular nerve leading to the infraspinatus (Fig. 25–41).[33]

The capsule needs to be freed from the muscles; this must be done by sharp dissection laterally since the capsule is adherent to the tendons of the teres minor and infraspinatus. Medially, this can be done with a periosteal elevator. Once the capsule is sufficiently freed from the overlying muscles, a transverse arthrotomy is made into the posterior capsule from lateral to medial, down to, but not into, the labrum. The joint is inspected. Two capsular flaps are developed by T-ing the capsule parallel to the glenoid and just adjacent to the labrum. These are tagged with the suture to control the flaps. The inferior capsular flap must be carefully developed because of the close proximity of the axillary nerve. If the labrum is intact, as is usually the case, the sutures can be placed directly into the labrum. (If the labrum is torn, it needs to be reflected so that suture anchors can be inserted and sutures passed through the ligamentous labrum complex, as is done in a capsulolabral reconstruction anteriorly.) The inferior capsule is then advanced superiorly and medially and attached to the glenoid labrum with No. 1 Ethibond sutures (Fig. 25–42). This usually eliminates the posterior as well as any inferior instability. The superior capsular flap is then sutured over the inferior flap by advancing it inferiorly and medially (Fig. 25–43). There may still be a transverse gap in the capsule laterally; this is closed with interrupted mattress sutures. The two heads of the infraspinatus fall together and do not usually need any sutures. The deltoid fascia, which has been split, is then repaired (Fig. 25–44).

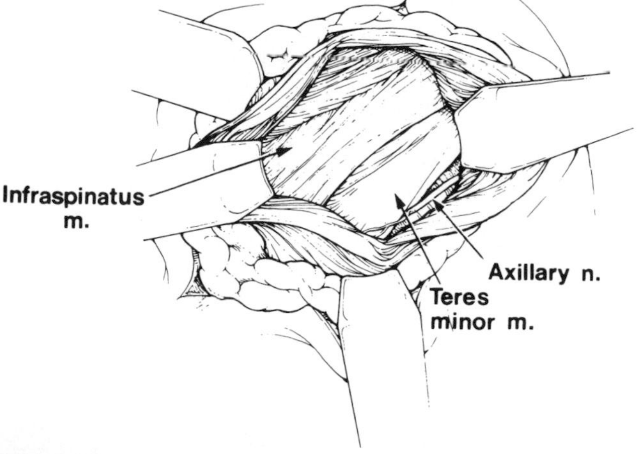

Figure 25–40

The teres minor and infraspinatus muscles are exposed; the axillary nerve enters the deltoid below the teres minor.

Postoperatively, the patient's arm and shoulder are immobilized in a position of 30 degrees of abduction, slight extension, and neutral rotation for 3 weeks.

POSTOPERATIVE REHABILITATION PROGRAM

Isometric exercises are begun in the immediate postoperative period for the deltoid and the rotator cuff muscles. After 3 weeks of isometric exercise, active and active-assisted range of motion is begun. The emphasis is on elevation in the scapular plane of the body and on regaining rotation. For the first 4 to 6 weeks postoperatively, no motion is performed in the sagittal plane (i.e., forward flexion) to avoid placing increased stress on the newly repaired posterior capsule and soft tissues. At 6 weeks, forward flexion is allowed. At 12 weeks, resistance beyond 90 degrees of elevation can be added to increase strength and endurance. Attention should be focused on regaining synchrony of the scapular rotators, rotator cuff, and deltoid. When this is firmly re-established, the athlete may return to his sport. The athlete will usually require another 6 months to develop the endurance necessary to return to competitive throwing.

Posterior shoulder repair can allow an athlete to return to his former throwing ability. Many athletes with posterior instability have little functional disability other than in their sport. The difficulty of returning to competitive throwing should not be underestimated; however, with careful surgical selection and meticulous rehabilitation, return is possible.

Posterior Lesions

Throwing athletes commonly have posterior glenoid spurs visible on x-ray. These spurs may or may not be sympto-

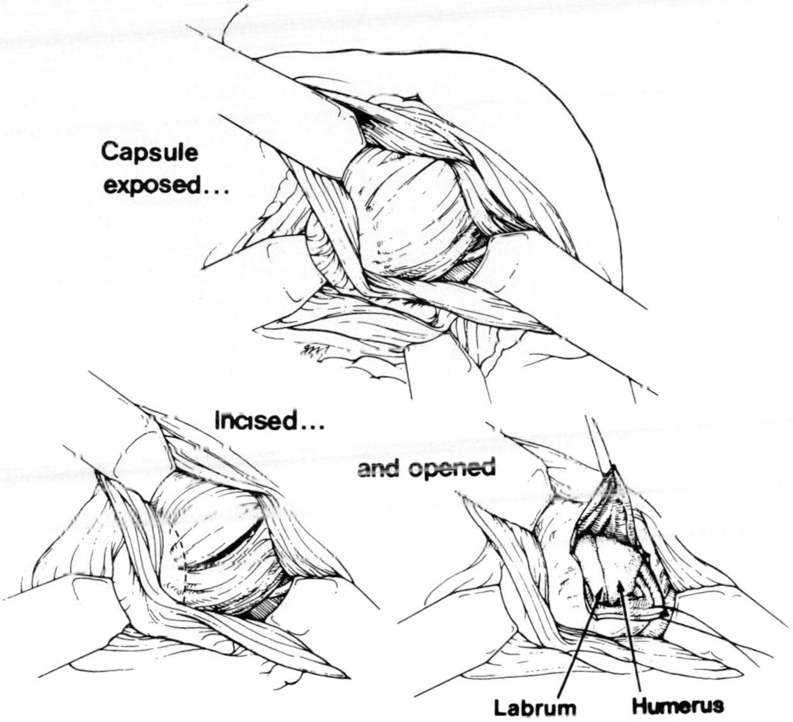

Figure 25–41

The capsule is exposed; a transverse arthrotomy is made in the posterior capsule from lateral to medial. Two capsule flaps are developed by "T-ing" the capsule parallel to the glenoid and adjacent to the labrum.

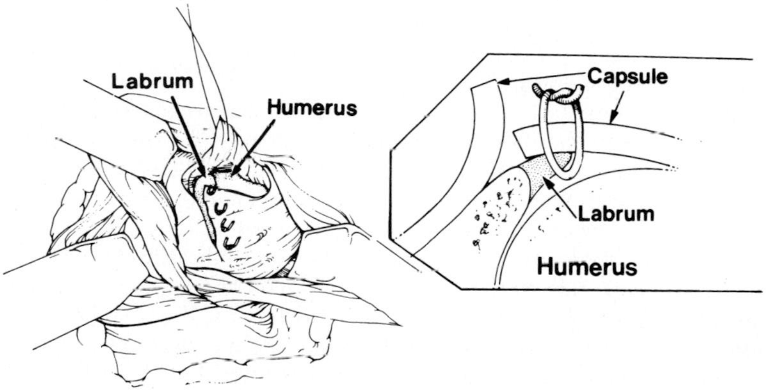

Figure 25–42

The inferior capsular flap is advanced superiorly and medially and attached to the labrum.

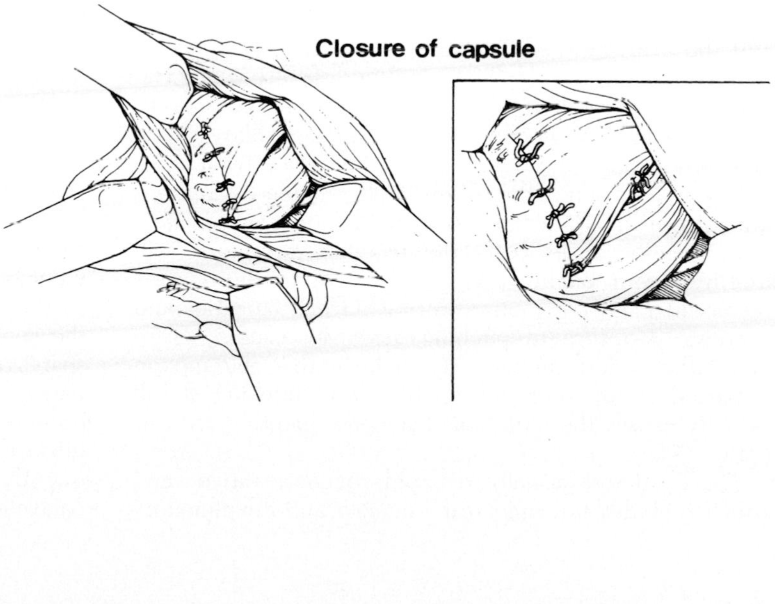

Figure 25–43

The superior flap is sutured over the inferior flap by advancing it inferiorly and medially. The lateral split in the capsule is closed with interrupted mattress sutures.

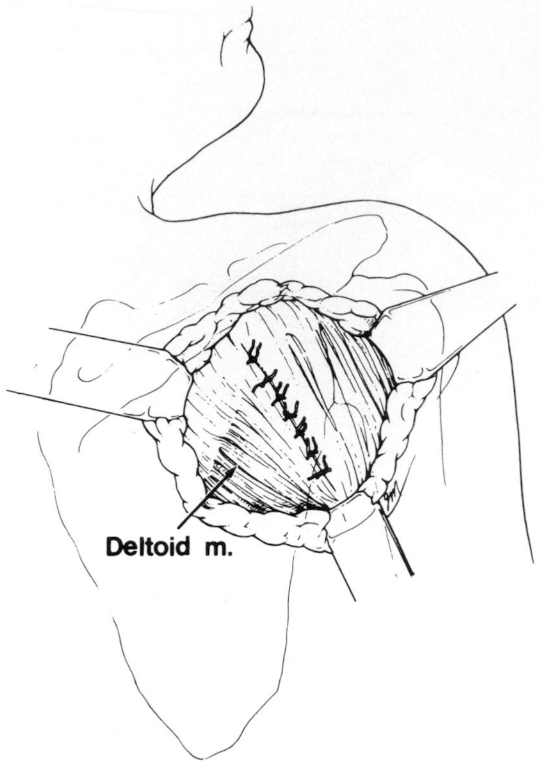

Figure 25–44

The deltoid fascia, which has been split, is repaired.

matic. Bennett described calcification in the posterior aspect of the shoulder.[4] He thought that these lesions were caused by a traction phenomenon at the insertion of the long head of the triceps in the posterior inferior glenoid. The symptom complex included pain referred to the posterior deltoid. It should be noted that not every pitcher in his study had the lesion. The site of the lesions were not related to the symptoms.

Occasionally, such lesions are noted in asymptomatic shoulders. Symptoms may develop gradually with increasing severity or, alternatively, may have a sudden onset. Bennett described an x-ray view to demonstrate the calcification or spur: an anteroposterior view of the glenohumeral joint with the machine tilted 5 degrees cephalad and the arm positioned in both abduction and external rotation, as in the cocking position of throwing. The scapula is then rotated to a position that shows the exostosis on the inferior glenoid. A conventional axillary lateral view often shows the bone spur in this area as well.

In our experience the lesion itself is often asymptomatic. However, when there is a fracture in the spur or a fibrous union at its base, the resultant symptoms will interfere with pitching. Generally, rest in these cases results in pain-free motion during normal activities and exercise. A return to pitching, however, causes severe pain after a few innings. We believe that the motion imparted to the spur during the act of pitching at full velocity causes the irritation that consequently produces pain.

These athletes usually respond to conservative care, which includes not only rest but also anti-inflammatory medication and steroid injections. Athletes whose pain prevents them from throwing effectively have responded to an operative approach with resection of the spur either arthroscopically or through the same deltoid-splitting approach described earlier. By exposing the capsule between the infraspinatus and the teres minor, the capsule is opened and the spur is identified and removed. The athlete can usually return to competitive throwing about 6 months after surgery. Lombardo and colleagues reported four cases with successful return to competition after removal of the spur.[23] The etiology process is probably a traction phenomenon on the posterior glenoid. It is now believed that the Bennett lesion is really a traction injury to the posterior inferior capsule.[9]

NEUROLOGIC PROBLEMS

Quadrilateral Space Syndrome

Cahill and Palmer described the quadrilateral space syndrome in 1983.[6] The axillary nerve function is compromised by fibrous bands in the quadrilateral space. The compromise of the function occurs when the athlete abducts and externally rotates the arm as in the cocking maneuver in throwing. The patient presents with posterior shoulder pain usually in the area of the teres minor muscle. The pain is exacerbated in the abducted and externally rotated position. There may or may not be tenderness directly in this area. The neurologic examination is usually normal, and electromyographic studies are not helpful. The diagnosis is usually confirmed by an arteriogram of the subclavian and axillary artery systems. With the shoulder in the neutral position, the posterior humeral circumflex artery is visualized. Upon repeated injections with the arm in abduction and external rotation, the artery is seen to no longer be patent. It is also helpful to perform comparative studies on both arms to look for anatomic variations. Rest and cortisone injections may prove to be helpful in the athlete with this condition. If the symptoms persist, however, an operative decompression of the quadrilateral space is indicated. The standard approach is through a deltoid-splitting incision and taking down the teres minor muscle. However, the authors of this chapter have found that the quadrilateral space can be approached through a vertical incision approaching the quadrilateral space below the deltoid and not releasing the teres minor.

Suprascapular Nerve Entrapment

In the general population, suprascapular nerve entrapment occurs most often in the suprascapular notch area. In the athlete, however, the nerve is often entrapped in the spinoglenoid notch or just distal to the notch. This spares the supraspinatus muscle function. The athlete may present with what appears to be tendinitis. On closer examination, however, the surgeon notices atrophy of the infraspinatus muscle. This condition is seen most frequently in high-level, hard-throwing pitchers. Surgical treatment of suprascapular nerve entrapment at the spinoglenoid notch has been variable, and return of muscle function is not always good. However, if the infraspinatus muscle is not completely denervated, some athletes have been able to return to throwing by maximizing whatever infraspinatus function that they have left.

VASCULAR PROBLEMS

Axillary Artery

Occlusion of the axillary artery typically occurs when the arm is brought overhead. Most likely it is the second portion of the axillary artery, occluded by pressure of the overlying pectoralis minor muscle. This occlusion can be observed in normal individuals and can be demonstrated by angiography. Tullos and associates described the occlusion of the axillary artery during pitching.[37] They thought that the transient occlusion in the axillary artery was due to stretching of the pectoralis minor that occurred with each pitch. In rare cases, there is sufficient local trauma over time to produce minimal damage and subsequent thrombosis. The axillary vein may also be involved. The clinical presentation includes various signs and symptoms that are often nonspecific. The diagnosis is difficult to make, and the athlete may complain of fatigue and muscle ache, lack of endurance, or intermittent paresthesia. He may report increased fatigue and loss of control. If there are no objective findings, the symptoms may be dismissed as minor psychosomatic. An arteriogram is usually necessary to confirm the diagnosis. Vascular surgery relieves the blockage by either excision with reanastomosis or with a bypass graft. In one well known case, a professional baseball pitcher developed progression of the thrombosis that resulted in a cerebral vascular accident and subsequent partial paralysis.

Aneurysm of the Subclavian and Axillary Arteries and Veins or Their Branches

More recently, a number of athletes have been found to have developed an aneurysm of a branch of the axillary artery or subclavian artery. In addition to the vascular occlusion symptoms mentioned earlier, these players sometimes present with embolic phenomenon in the hand distal to the aneurysm. This is thought to represent fragments of the thrombosis in the aneurysm.[10, 18, 24, 30, 35] Again, this diagnosis is confirmed by angiography, and the treatment is surgery on the vasculature. Thrombosis on the axillary vein was originally described by Paget in 1875 and by van Schroether in 1884.[1] This condition has been called "effort thrombosis" because of the association with a forceful event that produces injury to the vein. It usually occurs in active athletic individuals and is proceeded by strenuous effort or repetitive action. The athlete presents with pain and swelling in the arm. Objectively there may be venous distention involving the upper limb with secondary cyanosis. A venogram will confirm the diagnosis. The treatment is usually conservative involving rest and elevation. Anticoagulation is used in the initial phases to avoid progression of the thrombosis. After the initial episode, the athlete may continue to complain of external claudication. Vogel and Jensen reported on a college swimmer suffering from effort thrombosis of the subclavian vein.[39] They believed that there was an unusual presentation of thoracic outlet syndrome, although various provocative maneuvers did not cause any alteration in the radial pulse. A venogram revealed complete occlusion of the subclavian vein in the area of the first rib. Treatment consisted of therapy with intravenous streptokinase, heparin, and warfarin sodium (Coumadin). After 4 months, the first rib was removed and the patient became asymptomatic. Vogel and Jensen thought that the most likely site of compression at the subclavian vein was between the first rib and the clavicle in the costal clavicular area. A less likely mechanism of compression would be the tendons of the pectoralis minor, or the head of the humerus could also compress the axillary vein on its anterior aspect with shoulder abduction.

SUMMARY

The shoulder is challenged to its extremes during overhead sports. This challenge entails allowing the mobility that is necessary to play the sport while having a baseline of stability in order to prevent injury. Although the concept of balancing the stability and mobility is not new, the clinical understanding of these components has advanced. We now have a clearer understanding of the biomechanics that contribute to injury, and therefore we have been able to refine our treatments.

This subject is far from closed. As new research continues to define the shoulder's function, our medical approach shall also improve.

References and Bibliography

1. Adams JT and DeWeese JA: "Effort" thrombosis of the axillary and subclavian veins. J Trauma *11*:923–929, 1971.
2. Bain AM: Supraspinatus tendinitis. Physiotherapy 57:17–20, 1971.
3. Beall SM, Diefenbach G, and Allen A: Electromyographic biofeedback in the treatment of voluntary posterior instability of the shoulder. Am J Sports Med *15*:175–178, 1987.
4. Bennett GE: Elbow and shoulder lesions of baseball players. Am J Surg 98:484–488, 1959.
5. Bigliani LU, Pollock RG, McIlveen SJ, et al: Shift of the posteroinferior aspect of the capsule for recurrent posterior glenohumeral instability. J Bone Joint Surg *77A*:1011–1020, 1995.
6. Cahill BR and Palmer RE: Quadrilateral space syndrome. J Hand Surg *8*:65–69, 1983.
7. DiGiovine NM, Jobe FW, Pink M, and Perry J: An electromyographic analysis of the upper extremity in pitching. J Shoulder Elbow Surg *1*:15–25, 1992.
8. Feltner M and Dapena J: Dynamics of the shoulder and elbow joints of the throwing arm during a baseball pitch. Int J Sports Biomech *2*:235–259, 1986.
9. Ferrari JD, Ferrari DA, Coumas J, and Pappas AM: Posterior ossification of the shoulder: The Bennett lesion. Etiology, diagnosis, and treatment. Am J Sports Med *22*:171–175, 1994.
10. Fields W, Lemak N, and Ben-Menachem Y: Thoracic outlet syndrome: Review and reference to stroke in a major league pitcher. AJNR Am J Neuroradiol 7:73–78, 1986.
11. Fronek J, Warrer RF, and Bowen M: Posterior subluxation of the glenohumeral joint. J Bone Joint Surg *71A*:206–216, 1989.
12. Gainor BJ, Piotrowski F, Puhl J, et al: The throw: Biomechanics and acute injury. Am J Sports Med 8:114–118, 1980.

13. Goss TP and Costello G: Recurrent symptomatic posterior glenohumeral subluxation. Orthop Rev *17*:1024–1032, 1988.
14. Hawkins RJ, Koppert G, and Johnston G: Recurrent posterior instability (subluxation) of the shoulder. J Bone Joint Surg *66A*:169–174, 1984.
15. Herberts P and Kadefors R: A study of painful shoulder in welders. Acta Orthop Scand *47*:381–387, 1976.
16. Hurley JA, Anderson TE, Dear W, et al: Posterior shoulder instability: Surgical vs non-surgical results. Orthop Trans *11*:458, 1987.
17. Inman VT, Saunders JB de CM, and Abbott LC: Observations on the functions of the shoulder joint. J Bone Joint Surg *26*:1–30, 1944.
18. Itoh Y, Wakano K, Takeda T, and Murakami T: Circulatory disturbances in the throwing hand of baseball pitchers. Am J Sports Med *15*:264–269, 1987.
19. Jobe FW, Giangarra CE, Glousman RE, et al: Relationship of Instability and Impingement in Throwing Athletes: Review of the Anterior Capsulolabral Reconstruction. Paper presented at ASES, Las Vegas, Nevada, February, 1989.
20. Jobe FW, Pink MM, Glousman RE, et al: Operative Techniques in Upper Extremity Sports Injuries. St. Louis, MO: Mosby-Year Book, 1996.
21. Johnston TB: The movements of the shoulder-joint: A plea for the use of the 'plane of the scapula' as the plane of reference for movements occurring at the humero-scapular joint. Br J Surg *25*:252–260, 1937.
22. King W and Perry J: Personal communication, 1989.
23. Lombardo SJ, Jobe FW, Kerlan RK, et al: Posterior shoulder lesions in throwing athletes. Am J Sports Med *5*:106–110, 1977.
24. McCarthy W, Yao J, Schafer M, et al: Upper extremity arterial injury in athletes. J Vasc Surg *9*:317–327, 1989.
25. Monad H: Contractility of muscle during prolonged static and repetitive dynamic activity. Ergonomics *28*:81–89, 1985.
26. Moseley JB, Jobe FW, Pink M, et al: EMG analysis of the scapular muscles during a shoulder rehabilitation program. Am J Sports Med *20*:128–134, 1992.
27. Neer CS II: Anterior acromioplasty for the chronic impingement syndrome in the shoulder: A preliminary report. J Bone Joint Surg *54A*:41, 1972.
28. Pappas AM, Zawacki RM, and Sullivan TJ: Biomechanics of baseball pitching: A preliminary report. Am J Sports Med *13*:216–222, 1985.
29. Pink M, Perry J, Browne A, et al: The normal shoulder during freestyle swimming: An electromyographic and cinematographic analysis of twelve muscles. Am J Sports Med *19*:569–576, 1991.
30. Reekers J, den Hartog B, Kromhout J, et al: Traumatic aneurysm of the posterior circumflex humeral artery: A volleyball player's disease? J Vasc Interv Radiol *4*:405–408, 1993.
31. Rowe C and Zarins B: Recurrent transient subluxation of the shoulder. J Bone Joint Surg *63A*:863–871, 1981.
32. Scovazzo ML, Browne A, Pink M, et al: The painful shoulder during freestyle swimming: An electromyographic and cinematographic analysis of twelve muscles. Am J Sports Med *19*:577–582, 1991.
33. Shaffer BS, Conway JE, Jobe FW, et al: Infraspinatus splitting incision in posterior shoulder surgery. An anatomic and electromyographic study. Am J Sports Med *22*:113–120, 1994.
34. Stocker D, Pink M, and Jobe FW: Comparison of shoulder injury in collegiate- and master's level swimmers. Clin J Sport Med *5*:4–8, 1995.
35. Sugawara M, Ogino T, Minami A, and Ishii S: Digital ischemia in baseball players. Am J Sports Med *14*:329–334, 1986.
36. Townsend H, Jobe FW, Pink M, and Perry J: Electromyographic analysis of the glenohumeral muscles during a baseball rehabilitation program. Am J Sports Med *19*:264–272, 1991.
37. Tullos HS, Erwin WD, Woods WG, et al: Unusual lesions of the pitching arm. Clin Orthop *88*:169, 1972.
38. Turkel SJ: Stabilizing mechanisms preventing anterior dislocation of the glenohumeral joint. J Bone Joint Surg *63A*:1208–1217, 1981.
39. Vogel CM and Jensen JE: 'Effort' thrombosis of the subclavian vein in a competitive swimmer. Am J Sports Med *13*:269–272, 1985.

CHAPTER

26

JAMES O. SANDERS, M.D.
KIT M. SONG, M.D.

Fractures, Dislocations, and Acquired Problems of the Shoulder in Children

FRACTURES OF THE PROXIMAL HUMERUS

Developmental Anatomy

The proximal humerus forms as a cartilaginous anlage at approximately 5 weeks' gestation. During weeks 6 to 7, the glenohumeral joint forms by cavitation between the humerus and the scapula. By the beginning of the fetal period, the components of the shoulder region are adult in configuration and then progressively enlarge and mature. Although unlikely to be ossified on ultrasound by 38 weeks' gestation,[104] the proximal humeral ossification center is visible by ultrasound in 40%[79] at term and very commonly by 42 weeks' gestation. It generally does not appear on plain x-rays until 6 months of age.[79, 109] The upper humerus ossifies from three separate centers, representing the head appearing at 6 months, the lesser tuberosity appearing in the fifth year, and the greater tuberosity appearing in the second to third year. The tuberosities unite at 5 years of age, fuse with the head between 7 and 14 years of age, then subsequently fuse to the shaft by 19 years of age.[109, 130] Dameron reports earlier physeal closure at 14 to 17 years of age in girls and 16 to 18 years of age in boys.[31]

GROWTH

The proximal physis overall accounts for 80% of the growth of the humerus; however, this is not constant. Before the age of 2, less than 75% of growth occurs here, increasing to 85% at age 8, and remaining constant at 90% after age 11.[15, 116, 117] According to Stahl and Karpman[144] very little growth of the proximal humeral physis occurs beyond the skeletal age of 14, whereas Bortel and Pritchett indicate substantial growth remaining in boys until the skeletal age of 16.[15, 116, 117] The physeal shape is unique, with an inferior concavity, the apex of which is somewhat posteromedial. The epiphyseal contour remains essentially the same throughout growth, thus injury does not cause significant deformity.[12] This is unlike the proximal femur, in which the relative size and shape of the bone change as skeletal maturation occurs.

Surgical Anatomy

The physis peaks with an apex somewhat posteromedial. The articular surface covers both the epiphysis as well as a portion of the proximal medial metaphysis. The physeal contour turns distally in its most medial part so that the articular cartilage does not directly oppose metaphyseal bone but always lies over the epiphysis.[109] The joint capsule of the proximal humerus extends to the metaphysis, making a portion of the metaphysis intra-articular.[34] The periosteum is strongest posteromedially.

The humeral head's vascularity comes from the anterolateral ascending branch of the anterior circumflex artery,[50] which runs parallel to the lateral aspect of the biceps tendon and enters the humeral head where the proximal end of the intertubercular groove meets the tuberosity. The posterior circumflex artery vascularizes only a small portion of the greater tuberosity and a small inferior portion of the head.[60]

Fractures involving the proximal humeral physis tend to occur through the zone of hypertrophy adjacent to the zone of provisional calcification,[34, 129] although undulations through other zones occur. Fractures in this region rarely disturb physeal growth because this region is distal to the proliferating cells. The large amount of growth from the proximal humeral physis makes its remodelling potential superb.[12, 31, 105]

Because the proximal humeral physis is asymmetric, and the apex of the physis is somewhat posteromedial with a strong posteromedial periosteum, most fractures in this region show anterior and lateral displacement with the shaft fragment protruding through weaker anterolateral periosteum. The strong posteromedial periosteum remains attached distally, often with a metaphyseal bone fragment in older children. Occasionally, the periosteum of this region, along with the biceps tendon, can become interposed between the displaced metaphyseal fragment and the remaining epiphyseal fragment, making reduction difficult.[2, 5, 12, 31, 34, 85, 98, 159]

Displaced fractures above the pectoralis major have marked abduction of the proximal fragment with external rotation by the rotator cuff attachment.[31, 33] The distal fragment is pulled proximally by the deltoid and medially by the pectoralis major. Displaced fractures between the pectoralis major and the deltoid insertions show adduction of the proximal fragment from the pectoralis major and shortening by pull of the deltoid on the distal fragment, whereas diaphyseal fractures below the deltoid insertion have abduction of the long proximal fragment by the deltoid with shortening and medial displacement of the distal fragment by the pull of the biceps and triceps.[33] These anatomic factors should be remembered during fracture reduction.

Incidence

Fractures of the proximal humerus represent less than 5% of children's fractures,[4, 31, 58, 60, 65, 80, 87, 157, 167] and the incidence ranges from 1.2 to 4.4 per 10,000 per year.[9, 167] This is the fourth most common epiphyseal fracture reported in a large series from the Mayo Clinic.[124] These fractures are most common in infants and adolescents, and the highest peak is at 15 years of age, which probably reflects participation in sports and high-energy activities.[34, 61, 80, 124] Proximal humeral physeal fractures represent 1.9% to 6.7% of physeal injuries and are one of the more common birth fractures[84, 103, 114, 115, 119, 140] Fractures in the neonate and early childhood period are commonly the Salter-Harris type I injuries. By contrast, while children from 5 to 11 years of age may sustain physeal fractures, metaphyseal fractures are more common. This is most likely due to the rapid growth phase occurring in the metaphyseal area in this age group, leading to relative weakness.[34] In the adolescent, 75% of these fractures are Salter-Harris type II with type I fracture occurring in approximately 25%.[34]

Proximal humeral fractures can also occur through the unicameral bone cysts found most often in the proximal metaphysis (Fig. 26–1). Thirty-eight per cent of simple bone cysts are localized to the proximal humerus,[49] and a pathologic fracture is likely if more than 85% of the transverse plane on both the anteroposterior and lateral x-rays[1] is involved. Cysts that are small with surrounding cortical bone may heal without surgery if they are protected for an extended time.[6] The prognosis is best in patients who are older than 10 years of age and who have cysts farther from the physis.[6, 107] The fallen leaf sign is pathognomonic but occurs in only 20% of cysts.[148] Growth arrest has been reported in treated and untreated proximal humerus simple cysts.[59, 102, 107] Fractures through unicameral cysts are unlikely to speed the cyst's healing.[1, 6, 48, 72] Steroid injections are an effective treatment,[23, 24, 26, 29, 30, 41, 42, 121, 126, 131, 133–135] but the reason for their efficacy is unknown. It may be related to prostaglandin suppression of the high prostaglandin E_2 (PGE_2) levels found in cysts.[139] Methylprednisolone also has a direct effect on synovial cells, possibly indicating an effect on the cyst's cellular component.[169] Repeated steroid injections result in more than 90% healing with few complications. When this fails, bone grafting usually succeeds. They may also heal with osteotomy[146] and forceful injection of saline.[141]

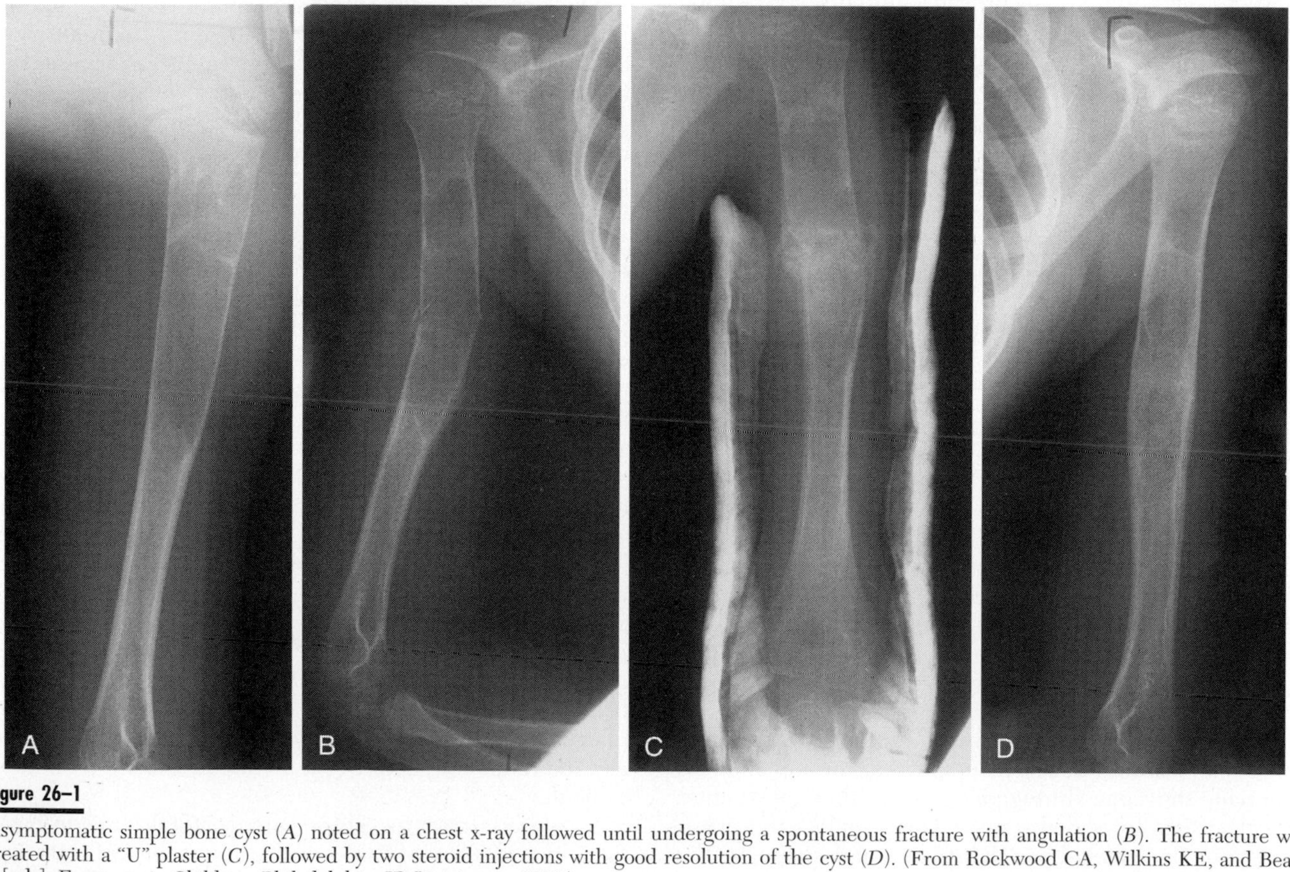

Figure 26–1

Asymptomatic simple bone cyst (*A*) noted on a chest x-ray followed until undergoing a spontaneous fracture with angulation (*B*). The fracture was treated with a "U" plaster (*C*), followed by two steroid injections with good resolution of the cyst (*D*). (From Rockwood CA, Wilkins KE, and Beaty J [eds]: Fractures in Children. Philadelphia: JB Lippincott, 1996.)

Mechanism of Injury

BIRTH INJURIES

Birth injuries may occur as the arm becomes hyperextended or rotated while the child is passing through the birth canal.[34, 53, 55, 57, 84, 97, 140] Although shoulder dystocia is strongly associated with macrosomia, it is difficult to predict prepartum.[25, 47, 69] Anatomic studies on stillborn infants produce Salter-Harris type I fractures. These fractures reduce without biceps tendon interposition unless it is manually forced into the site. In these studies by Dameron and Reibel, the metaphysis could not be displaced posteriorly by closed manipulation.[34] However, with the humerus extended and adducted, the metaphysis could be displaced anteriorly with relative ease with the top of the metaphysis penetrating the periosteum just lateral to the biceps tendon. Only after resecting the posterior periosteum could the metaphysis be displaced posteriorly. The physeal shape with its metaphyseal high point posterior and medial to the center and a stronger posterior periosteum attached to the periphery of the epiphysis causes the anterior displacement.

OLDER CHILDREN

In older children, falls, particularly from horses,[80] are the most common cause followed by traffic accidents and sports.[75] Falls from horses account for a large portion of proximal humerus fractures.[80] Although much older literature reports the most common mechanism as a fall on an outstretched hand, which transmits forces through the arm and drives the metaphysis anteriorly and laterally,[2, 16, 64, 69] better studies indicate that a direct blow to the posterior aspect to the shoulder is the most common mechanism.[94, 105, 142] Williams identified six potential mechanisms of injury causing proximal humeral fractures in children, which represent forced extension, flexion, lateral rotation, or medial rotation singly or in combination.[165]

Proximal humeral physeal slipping has been reported from gymnastics with humeral weight-bearing,[32] as a complication of radiotherapy,[38] and from pituitary gigantism.[122] Repetitive pitching can cause physeal stress injuries[91, 154, 155] (Fig. 26–2). The fracture may also result from child abuse.[46] Proximal humeral fractures are also reported with myelomeningocele.[92] Perhaps this is related to upper extremity weight-bearing or neuropathy from Arnold-Chiari malformations and syringomyelia.

Classification

Fractures may be physeal or metaphyseal. *Physeal involvement* is classified by the Salter-Harris classification. In younger patients, the fractures are predominantly Salter-Harris type I whereas older patients have predominantly Salter-Harris type IIs (Fig. 26–3). Taken together, most physeal fractures are Salter-Harris type IIs.[115] Salter-Harris type II fractures may have an additional anterorlateral fragment.[20] Salter-Harris type III fractures are reported with[28, 52] and without[150, 166] associated shoulder dislocations. Salter-Harris type IV fractures have not been reported. Dameron and Reibel[34] classified the fractures based on the Salter-Harris type and the age of the patient as 0 to 5 years, 5 to 11 years, or 11 to 17 years. The classification of metaphyseal fractures is by their displacement and by their relationship to the surrounding muscles

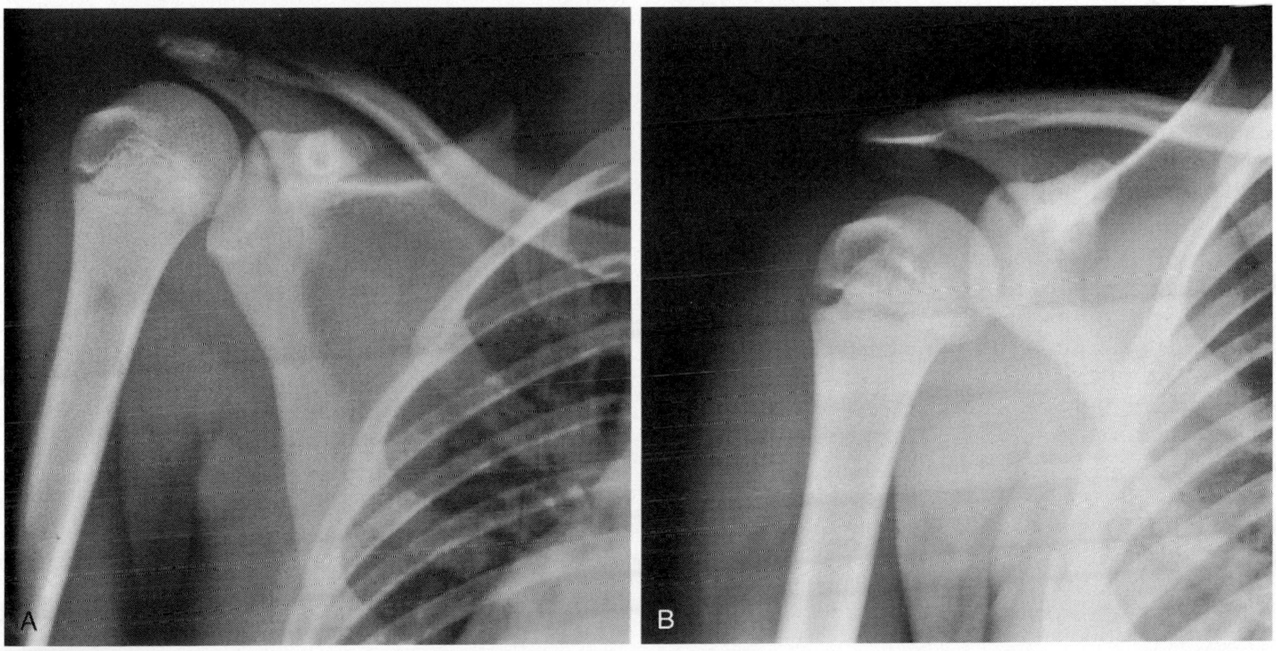

Figure 26–2

This 13-year-old Little League baseball pitcher complained of right shoulder pain for 2 weeks' duration. *A,* This original anteroposterior radiograph shows a suggestion of widening at the lateral physis. *B,* The patient was allowed to continue pitching and demonstrates displacement of this proximal humeral stress fracture.

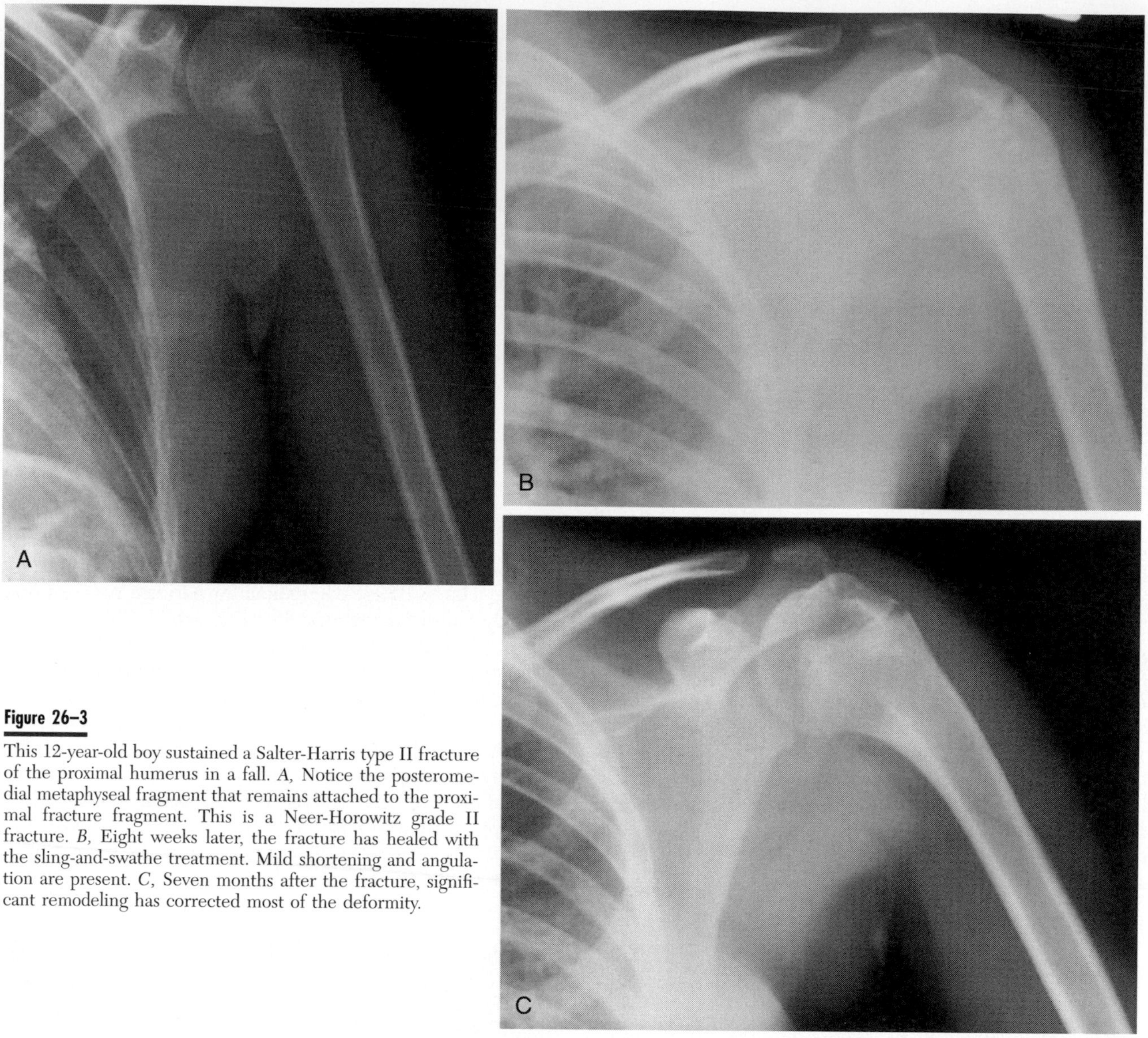

Figure 26–3

This 12-year-old boy sustained a Salter-Harris type II fracture of the proximal humerus in a fall. *A,* Notice the posteromedial metaphyseal fragment that remains attached to the proximal fracture fragment. This is a Neer-Horowitz grade II fracture. *B,* Eight weeks later, the fracture has healed with the sling-and-swathe treatment. Mild shortening and angulation are present. *C,* Seven months after the fracture, significant remodeling has corrected most of the deformity.

as discussed earlier. After reduction, proximal humeral fractures may be stable or unstable.

Displacement. Neer and Horowitz[105] classified proximal humeral physeal fractures based on the degree of displacement. Grade 1 represents up to 5 mm of displacement, grade 2 up to one third of the humeral shaft diameter, grade 3 up to two thirds of the humeral shaft diameter, and grade 4 is greater than two thirds of the shaft diameter and includes total separation. Proximal humeral fractures may be in either varus angulation, which is the most common, or valgus angulation, which is quite rare.[55]

Slipped Proximal Humeral Physis. Proximal humeral physeal slipping may occur with gymnastics with humeral weight-bearing,[32] as a complication of radiotherapy,[38] and from pituitary gigantism.[122] The epiphysis slips into a varus position and usually responds well to nonoperative treatment.

Stress Injuries. Repetitive pitching can cause physeal stress injuries that respond to temporary cessation of the pitching.[91, 154, 155]

Other Fractures. Other fractures may occur including the greater tuberosity, which has been reported in association with luxatio erecta[44, 76] or through the lesser tuberosity.[71, 125, 162]

Fracture-dislocations may be anterior associated with Salter-Harris type I, II, or III fractures,[28, 46, 52, 108] or they may be posterior[158] or inferior.[44, 76] Intrathoracic fracture dislocations have been reported in adults[56] but not in children. Fractures may be segmental involving the shaft and the neck[96, 111] or the ipsilateral forearm or elbow.[67]

Signs and Symptoms

EVALUATION OF THE NEONATAL SHOULDER

The infant who does not move the shoulder poses a diagnostic challenge. Establishment and evaluation of a differential diagnosis is the first concern. Regarding the infant's history—was the delivery normal? When was the problem noticed? Does the child move any part of the extremity? Was there a history of maternal gestational diabetes or of fetal macrosomia? Does the child nurse from each breast? A broad, useful differential diagnosis consists of clavicle fracture, proximal humeral physeal fracture, humeral shaft fracture, shoulder dislocation, brachial plexus palsy, septic shoulder, osteomyelitis, hemiplegia, and child abuse.

Observe the child initially for spontaneous motion of the upper extremity. Is there any hand or elbow motion? Are there any areas of swelling, ecchymosis, or increased warmth? Does the child move the ipsilateral lower extremity? Each area of the upper extremity should be carefully palpated. Start with the clavicle and compare it carefully with the opposite side for any change in soft tissue contour or tenderness; then examine the upper arms and shoulders. Look for any tenderness in the supraclavicular fossa. Finally, examine the spine for tenderness or swelling.

After a proximal humeral fracture, the arm generally lies in internal rotation with an obvious deformity. Patients with posterior fracture dislocation have very limited painful external rotation of the shoulder. Luxatio erecta with a greater tuberosity fracture presents as an abducted shoulder with the elbow flexed and the hand above the head with marked shoulder creases.[44] Lesser tuberosity fractures have tenderness anteriorly, limited internal rotation in adduction, and limited abduction in external rotation.[162] Impingement symptoms may occur with internal rotation.[71]

Radiographic Findings

BIRTH INJURIES

X-rays may be needed of the shoulder, clavicle, humerus, and cervical spine. Often the shoulder, clavicle, and humerus can be seen on a single anteroposterior view of both the upper extremities and the chest. An ultrasound can identify a fracture of the clavicle or the proximal humeral epiphysis, a shoulder dislocation, or a shoulder effusion. A computed tomography (CT) scan or arthrogram may be necessary. Birth injuries may be missed in children with an unossified humeral head. All that may be seen is an alteration in the scapular humeral relationship (Fig. 26–4). Although arthrograms are useful in iden-

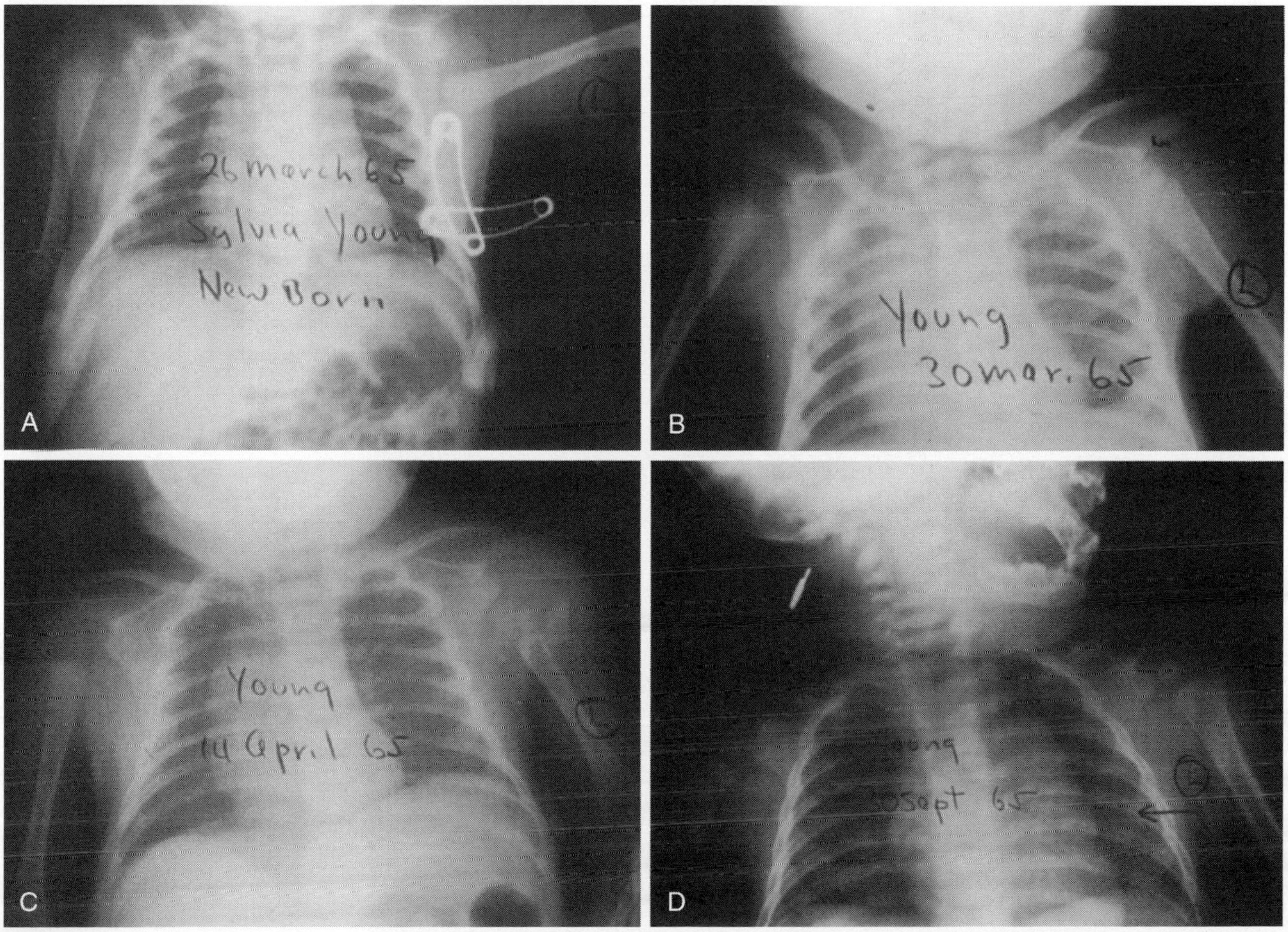

Figure 26–4

In the newborn, injury to the proximal humerus is usually a completely displaced physeal injury, the so-called pseudodislocation. *A*, Radiographs at this age are sometimes misleading owing to a lack of ossification in the proximal epiphysis. *B*, Closed manipulation can be performed by applying longitudinal traction and gentle posterior pressure over the proximal humerus. *C*, At 2 1/2 weeks, abundant callus is present and the patient is clinically asymptomatic. *D*, A 6-month follow-up radiograph shows no asymmetry compared with the opposite side.

tifying proximal humeral physeal separations,[36, 163] ultrasound is noninvasive and diagnostic.[19, 62, 156] The ultrasound is obtained with a 7.5- or 10-MHz transducer, and the baby is positioned supine with the shoulder abducted. Scaglietti[132] and Kleinman and Akins[73] described the vanishing epiphysis sign in Salter-Harris type I fractures in which the posteriorly displaced epiphysis appears to vanish on an anteroposterior radiograph compared with the opposite side. Birth fractures should have callus evident by day 10.[94] If this is not the case, child abuse should be suspected. Posterior dislocations can be missed at birth and are best seen on a CT scan.[152]

OLDER CHILDREN

The standard x-rays obtained for any shoulder injury should consist of two perpendicular x-rays to determine the glenohumeral relationship.[123, 149] The true anteroposterior view, obtained with the beam parallel to the glenohumeral joint shooting perpendicular to a line along the scapular spine, is most useful. Although an axillary lateral is preferable, it is difficult to obtain in an acutely injured shoulder necessitates a transthoracic or Y view. The apical oblique, a true anteroposterior view with a caudal tilt of 45 degrees, provides useful information about the glenoid surface and the glenohumeral joint.[35] The apical oblique and the anteroposterior x-rays together identify most injuries. When these x-rays are combined with a transcapular lateral or axillary lateral view, almost all shoulder injuries can be identified.[18] Lesser tuberosity fractures may not be visible without an axillary lateral view.[63] Radionucleotide imaging is not very useful in the proximal humerus because of the physeal uptake. Occasionally in young children, an arthrogram or ultrasound may be necessary to establish the diagnosis of a proximal humeral Salter-Harris type I physeal fracture.[99, 145] Magnetic resonance imaging (MRI) has been described showing fractures of the shoulder about the greater tuberosity and the glenoid rim and may be useful for occult fractures.[10, 127, 151] Posterior fracture dislocations can be very difficult to determine without an axillary lateral or a transscapular view and are seen best on a CT scan.[62, 152, 160]

Occasionally, an upper humeral notch is visible on the medial neck. This notch may be seen in pathologic conditions such as Gaucher's disease[88] but may also be a normal finding that probably represents the inferomedial capsular insertion.[112] Unicameral cysts, which frequently occur in the proximal humerus, were discussed earlier.

Treatment

The prognosis for birth injuries and other injuries in infants is excellent (Fig. 26–5). Gentle manipulation without general anesthesia usually reduces these fractures quite well. Ultrasound can be used during the reduction maneuver to verify the reduction. Even if reduction is not achieved, the prognosis remains good. The arm is then immobilized to the chest with a soft dressing. The fracture usually heals by 2 to 3 weeks[34, 55, 69, 85, 140, 164] and may be stable enough for the dressing to be removed after several days.[34]

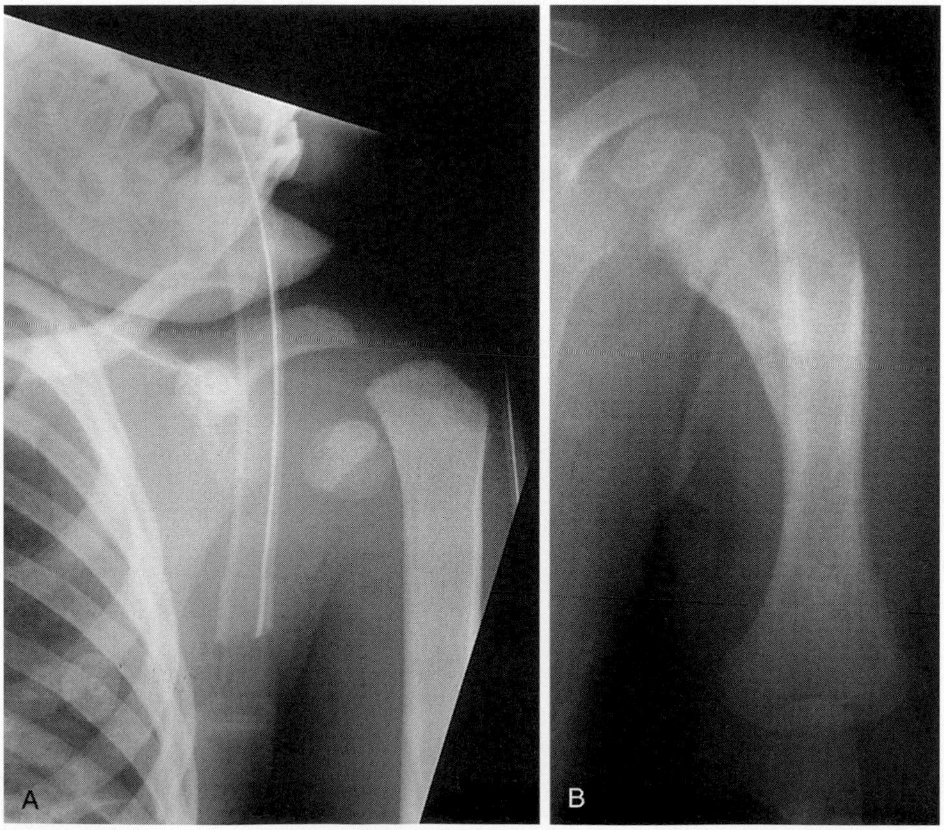

Figure 26–5

A and *B*, A proximal humeral physeal fracture from child abuse. Note the marked degree of early remodeling despite the severe displacement.

Slipped Proximal Humeral Epiphysis and Stress Fractures

A chronic *slipped proximal humeral epiphysis* is a rare disorder that is reported from gymnastics,[32] radiotherapy,[38] and hyperpituitarism.[122] *Stress injuries* from repetitive pitching are more common and usually heal well with temporary immobilization.[7, 155]

Metaphyseal Fractures

Metaphyseal fractures are almost always amenable to closed treatment. Despite their displacement, they heal and remodel quite well (Fig. 26–6).

NONOPERATIVE TREATMENT

Up to 5 years of age, proximal humeral physeal fractures are usually Salter-Harris type I, and accurate reduction of displaced fractures is not essential. The arm is manipulated with traction, abduction, and flexion similar to that of newborns.[34] Older children with minimally displaced fractures can be managed with a sling-and-swathe.

Reduction. Potential barriers to reduction include the periosteum, the capsule,[85] the shaft of the humerus protruding through a button hole tear in the capsule,[66] the periosteal cuff,[43] or the biceps tendon[83, 59] interposed between the ends of the fracture. Surgical findings include marked soft tissue damage, periosteal stripping, and a buttonholing of the shaft through the periosteum with interposition of the biceps tendon, the deltoid, and occasionally a portion of the subscapularis.[142] Neer and Horowitz[105] recommend reduction by 90 degrees of forward flexion to correct the forward displacement of the shaft, moderate abduction to correct the adduction of the shaft, and slight external rotation. Alternatively, the fracture may be reduced by longitudinal traction with the shoulder in 135 degrees of abduction, 30 degrees of forward flexion, neutral rotation, and pushing posteriorly on the shaft.[16, 69, 164] Only partial apposition is required. Williams believes that by evaluating the mechanism of injury as a combination of forced flexion, extension, medial rotation, or lateral rotation on the x-rays and by reversing the injury, a stable closed reduction can be achieved.[165]

The question becomes how aggressively to treat displaced fractures of the physis or metaphysis in older children. The displaced fracture may appear ominous on x-rays, but because of the tremendous remodeling potential, the result is often excellent if untreated. Smith notes:

> The periosteum is extremely tough; for this reason it often tightens and closes under the extruded shaft end on attempts to reduce the fracture and thus renders closed reduction difficult or impossible. If reduction is not achieved, new bone is then formed within the periosteum in the triangular space formed by the displaced epiphysis, the shaft, and the periosteum itself. Bowing of the head and upper shaft thus result in the first few months of healing. However, with time, growth, and physical activity, this bowing becomes partially corrected and the originally displaced shaft becomes absorbed.[142]

Fractures that *potentially* require reduction are most frequent after 11 years of age.[105] The results are extremely favorable in patients younger than 11 years of age, regardless of the method of treatment. Neer and Horowitz[105] recommend treating grade I and grade II fractures with a sling-and-swathe without reduction, reducing grade III fractures only if angulation is severe, and reducing grade IV fractures and applying a salute position spica cast. Dameron and Reibel[34] found that fractures with less than 20 degrees of angulation did quite well. They based treatment on the patient's age and treated displaced Salter-Harris type I fractures in patients older than 11 years of age with reduction followed by a spica cast or thoracobrachial bandage for 3 weeks while displaced Salter-Harris type II fractures were reduced and held in a thoracobrachial bandage, or, if unreducible, held in abduction, slight external rotation, and flexion with a salute position cast for 4 to 6 weeks. Larson and associates[62] evaluated 64 unoperated patients with proximal humeral physeal fractures and found that the excellent remodeling in children decreased with age. The patients with greatest angulation at follow-up had Neer and Horowitz grade IV fractures and were 11 years of age or older. They report excellent results and recommend nonoperative treatment.

Nonoperative immobilizations include the sling-and-swathe,[21] hanging arm cast,[21, 82] shoulder spica, or statue of liberty cast[55] and traction. Because these fractures can generally be reduced with traction rather than by abduction, a shoulder spica or statue of liberty position is rarely necessary to maintain the position.[64] Beringer and associates[11] reviewed the Neer grade III and grade IV fractures. Only those treated operatively developed complications, whereas the results of nonoperative treatment, including a sling-and-swathe, were excellent.

OPERATIVE TREATMENT

Intramedullary Rodding. Intramedullary rodding is possible using smooth flexible 2-mm–diameter nails inserted through the lateral epicondyle and placed intramedullary into the head.[101, 137] The rods can be used to manipulate the fracture into further reduction. The Hackethal technique may also be used.[118] Rush rods have been used in older adolescents.[161]

Percutaneous Pinning. Percutaneous pinning was described by Bohler,[13, 14] and some minor modifications have been made.[70, 74, 100, 110, 113] In this technique, the patient is placed supine using an image intensifier to visualize the humeral head and neck. After closed reduction, the pins are placed either superiorly (Fig. 26–7) or inferiorly (Fig. 26–8) to avoid the axillary nerve. A Kirschner wire is placed over the shoulder anteriorly to determine the correct orientation of the pins. The pins are placed through the distal or proximal deltoid and advanced about 30 degrees to the humeral shaft. When the pins are placed from inferiorly, the retroversion of the head relative to the shaft must be compensated. If the pins have a tendency to leave the shaft before entering the head, they may be tapped with a mallet to keep them in the medullary canal. In children, one pin is often satisfactory, although two pins or more are preferable. Alternatively, the pins may be placed through the acromion,[68] although this may increase the incidence of pin breakage. The pins are

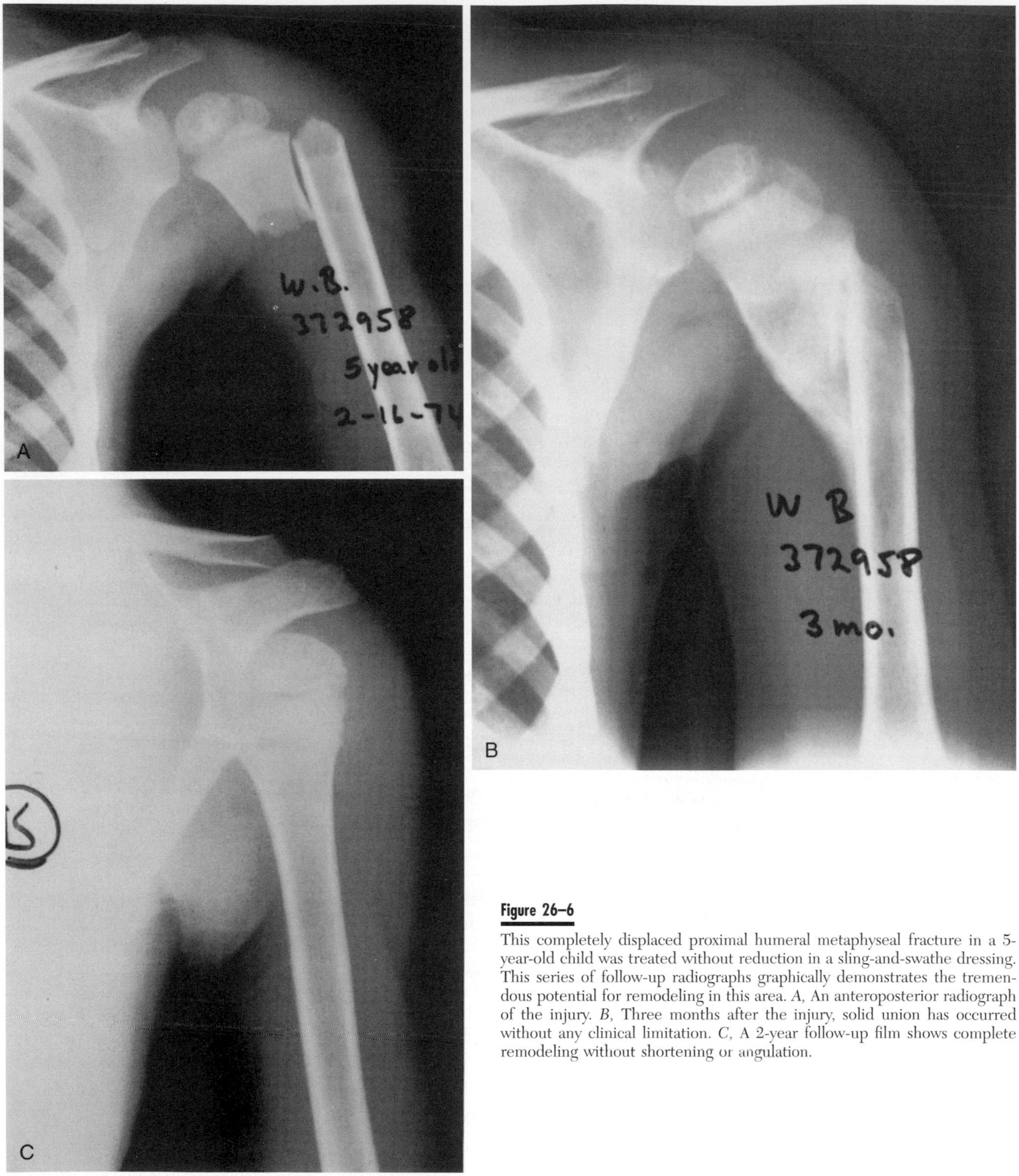

Figure 26–6

This completely displaced proximal humeral metaphyseal fracture in a 5-year-old child was treated without reduction in a sling-and-swathe dressing. This series of follow-up radiographs graphically demonstrates the tremendous potential for remodeling in this area. *A,* An anteroposterior radiograph of the injury. *B,* Three months after the injury, solid union has occurred without any clinical limitation. *C,* A 2-year follow-up film shows complete remodeling without shortening or angulation.

bent outside the skin with gauze placed between the pins and the skin to prevent excessive skin motion resulting in pain, skin irritation, and possibly infection. Open reduction and pinning have been described for severely displaced proximal humeral fractures.[45, 120] This procedure potentially may be indicated in those fracture-dislocations and Salter-Harris type III and IV fractures that cannot be adequately closed and reduced.

Open Reduction. Open reduction is performed through the deltopectoral interval. Because hypertrophic scarring occurs,[98] the approach should be made within Langer's lines and as inferiorly as possible toward the axilla.[54] The cephalic vein is reflected laterally with the deltoid upon identifying the deltopectoral interval. The fracture or fracture-dislocation can usually be identified at this point. The axillary nerve on the inferior aspect of

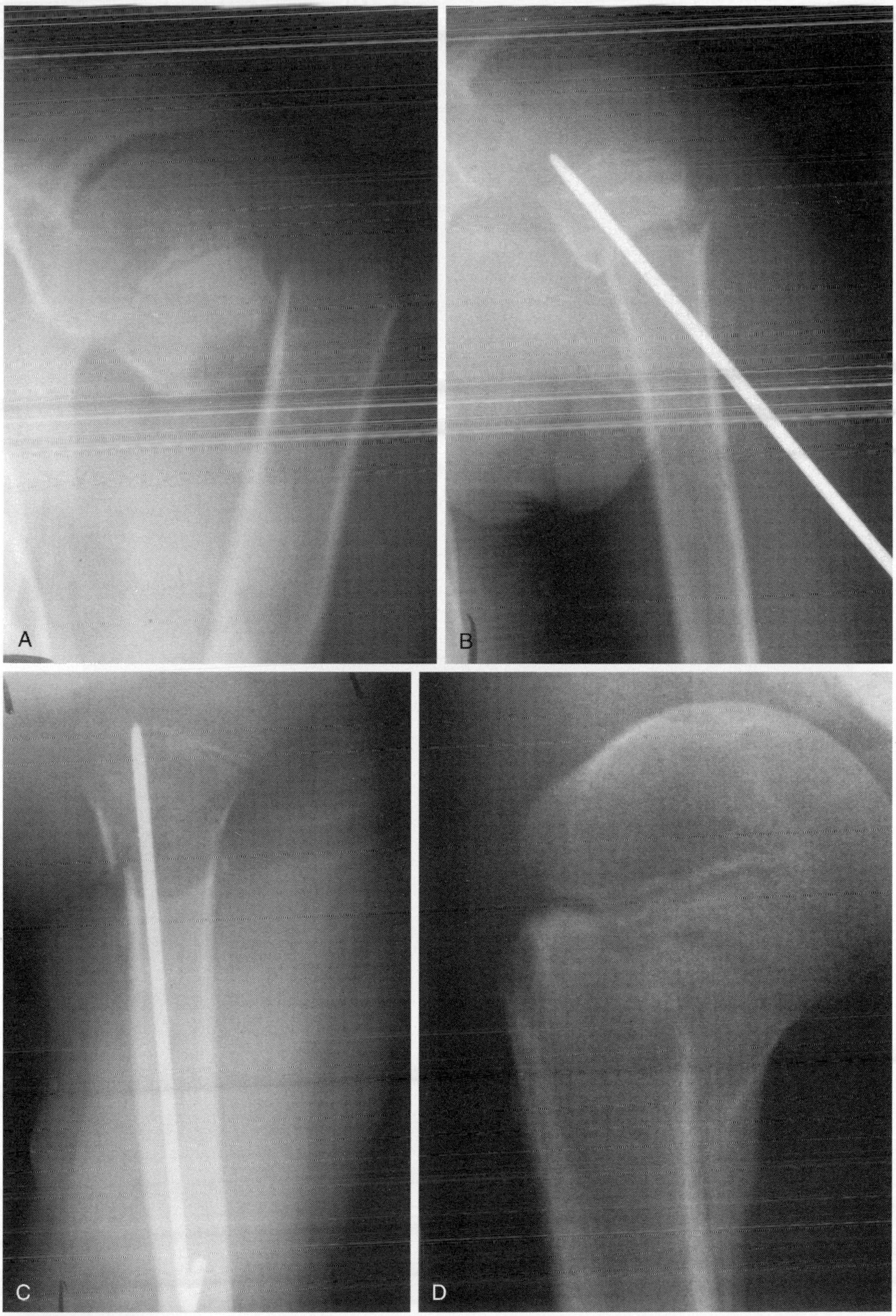

Figure 26–7

A–D, Technique of percutaneous pinning a proximal humeral metaphyseal fracture from distally to avoid the axillary nerve. Although the ultimate outcome is good, its sole advantage in the younger patient is to speed up the remodeling process. (From Rockwood CA, Wilkins KE, and Beaty J [eds]: Fractures in Children. Philadelphia: JB Lippincott, 1996.)

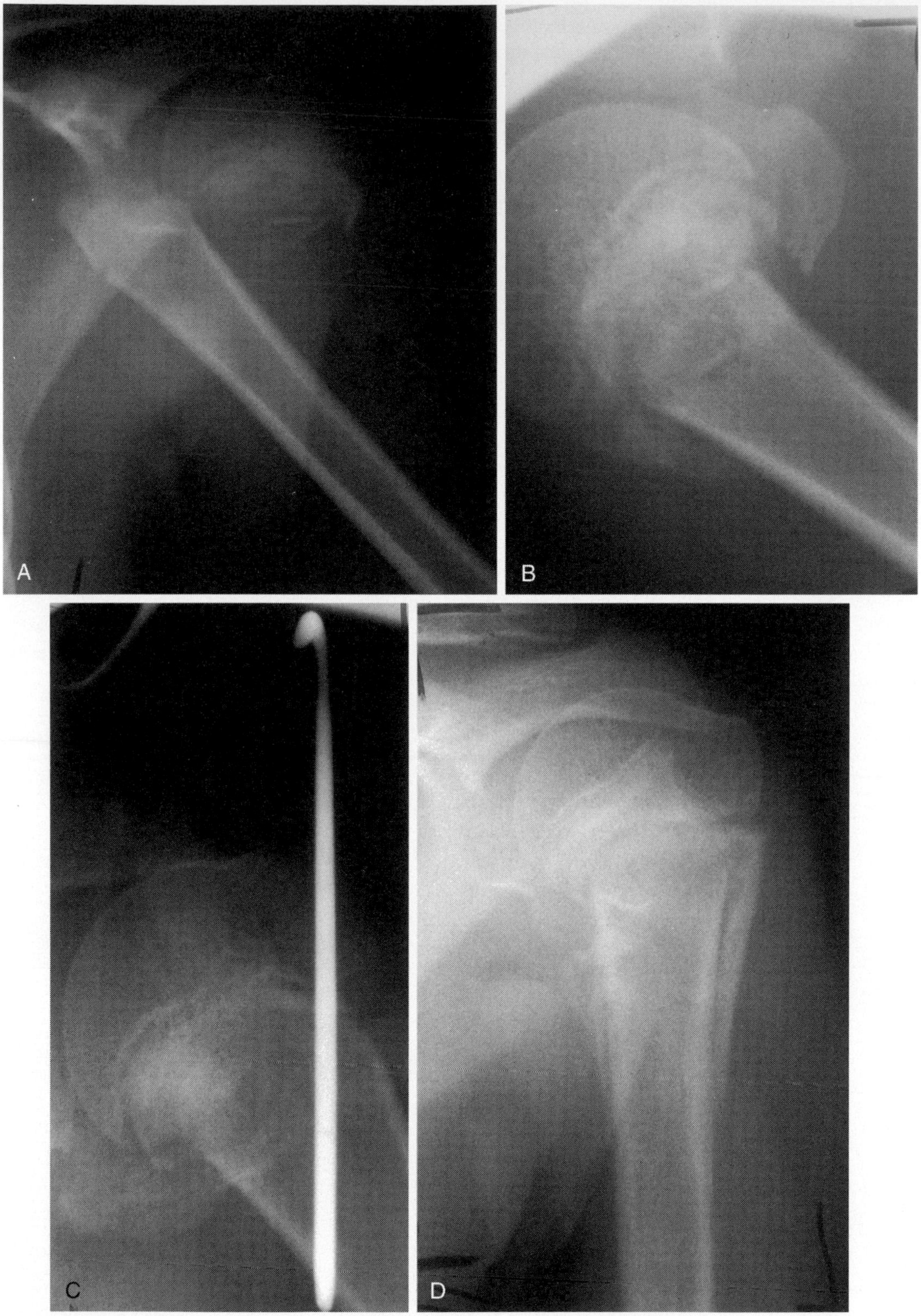

Figure 26–8

A–D, An unstable proximal humerus physeal fracture with an additional anterior lateral fragment treated by closed reduction (*B*) and pinned from proximally (*C*). Valgus angulation is rare and probably results from a fall on the abducted arm. (From Rockwood CA, Wilkins KE, and Beaty J [eds]: Fractures in Children. Philadelphia: JB Lippincott, 1996.)

the subscapularis and the anterior circumflex vessels should be identified and protected. If the fracture cannot be visualized adequately, open the subscapularis tendon and anterior capsule in layers. Reduce and hold the fracture provisionally with Kirschner wires, and place the final pins or screws (Fig. 26–9). The capsule and subscapularis tendons are repaired, and the skin is closed. The patient is placed in a soft thoracobrachial dressing or a commercial shoulder immobilizer.

Segmental fractures may be treated with open reduction and internal fixation or intramedullary pinning.[90] Alternatively, the proximal humerus fracture may be treated nonoperatively with standard treatments for the other injuries.[67, 96]

External Fixation. External fixation for fractures of the proximal humerus has been reported in adults but not in children, and external fixation has very little utility except perhaps in extensively contaminated open fractures.[78]

Fracture-Dislocations. The most important aspect of a Salter-Harris type I or II fracture-dislocation is the dislocation. The physeal fracture retains its ability to remodel.[108] Even Salter-Harris type III fractures may be treated successfully by closed reduction,[28] although they may require open reduction.[52] The mechanism of the Salter-Harris type III fracture appears to be an anterior dislocation of the shoulder with the glenoid acting as a fulcrum, causing the transepiphyseal fracture as the shoulder retracts. The labrum may be torn as well.[52] The dislocation must be reduced. The fracture is then fixed with screws or pins if the reduction is unstable.

Lesser Tuberosity Fractures. Old lesser tuberosity fractures may be treated nonoperatively.[125] The subscapularis is attached to the fracture fragment and pulled medially. In athletes with symptomatic shoulder instability, the fragments should be excised and the anterior capsule and subscapularis reconstructed.[71, 162] If the fracture is seen acutely in an athlete, it may be repaired by open reduction and internal fixation.

Greater Tuberosity Fractures. Aside from one case associated with an anterior dislocation treated by closed reduction[31] (see Fig. 26–5), the only reported greater tuberosity fractures in children occurred in association with luxatio erecta, and these fractures were treated nonoperatively. For older adolescents with greatly displaced greater tuberosity fractures, the fracture should be treated like displaced greater tuberosity fractures in adults with open reduction, internal fixation, and repair of the rotator cuff.

Operative Indications

The greatest concern in the treatment of the epiphyseal fracture of the proximal humerus is likely to be at the time of reduction when the surgeon reaches impasse in his ability to reduce the displacement of the fragments and maintain this position. Under parental pressure, expediency may supersede rationality in deciding on open reduction.

McBride and Sisler, 1965

Because of the marked remodeling potential of the proximal humerus, most fractures can be treated by a sling-and-swathe or commercial shoulder immobilizer, pain medications, and ice. Because of the initial deformity, the surgeon often feels pressed to perform a reduction. Some authors state that open reduction and internal fixation are not indicated[2, 11, 34, 142] and that nonoperative

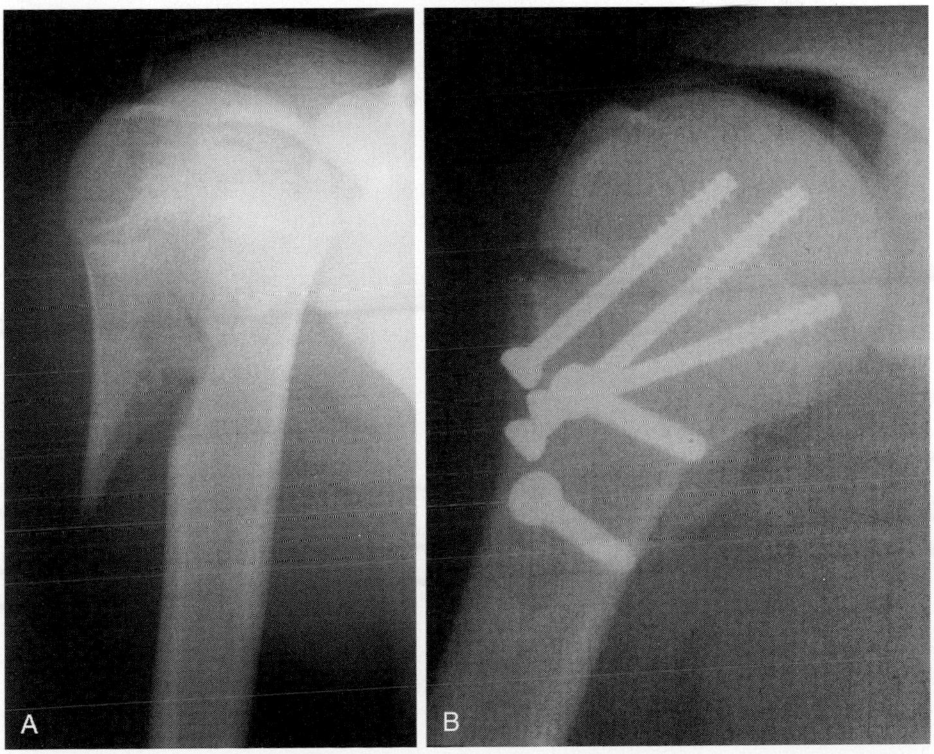

Figure 26–9

A and *B*, Proximal humerus fracture in a 14-year-old male multiple trauma victim treated with open reduction and internal fixation to facilitate early mobilization. (From Rockwood CA, Wilkins KE, and Beaty J [eds]: Fractures in Children. Philadelphia: JB Lippincott, 1996.)

treatment is appropriate, even for those with marked displacement.[11, 82] Other authors indicate that fractures in older children that cannot be adequately reduced and maintained should be reduced and pinned or openly reduced and fixed.[103, 137, 147] Bergos-Flores and associates[20] recommended a more aggressive approach in patients older than 13 years of age because of persistent deformity and limitation of motion in the older patients. Nevertheless, they noted that even these patients still function well without symptoms, despite some objective findings. Older patients who are unlikely to have marked remodeling may be considered for either open reduction and internal fixation or closed reduction and pinning. No firm guidelines exist for determining which fractures will or will not remodel sufficiently. Clinically, this is best determined by the skeletal age and by looking at the growth remaining charts, because those with little growth remaining are unlikely to remodel significant displacement.[15, 116, 117]

Multiple trauma is a potential indication for fixation to assist in patient mobilization.[93]

Open fractures that require débridment may benefit from fixation to facilitate early rehabilitation of the soft tissue injury and may be essential if the periosteum is destroyed because much of the remodeling potential is damaged.

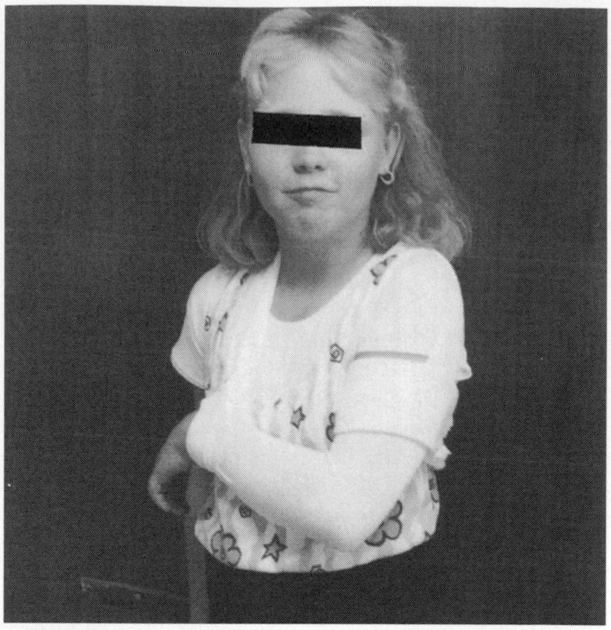

Figure 26–10

Clinical photograph of a 9-year-old girl wearing a homemade sling-and-swathe used in the treatment of proximal humerus fractures. A stockinette is padded at pressure points with cast padding and held in position with safety pins.

AUTHORS' PREFERRED TREATMENT

Nonoperative. We manage most proximal humeral physeal fractures nonoperatively even if they are displaced. We attempt a closed reduction in very displaced fractures, and then we apply a thoracobrachial dressing or occasionally a hanging arm cast in older children. We prefer Bohler's "U" plaster with a soft wrap holding the arm to the patient's chest, although a sling-and-swathe or commercial shoulder immobilizer may be satisfactory (Fig. 26–10). Metaphyseal fractures are also usually treated by the closed method. Bayonet opposition with 1 to 2 cm of overlap is quite acceptable (Fig. 26–11).

Operative. The only advantage of reduction and pinning is more rapid remodeling of the proximal humerus. This method does, however, provide a greater possibility of complications.[11] The end result without complication will probably be equivalent to leaving the fracture unreduced.

Lesser tuberosity fractures that are diagnosed acutely in athletes should be repaired. The primary goal is to restore the subscapularis tendon and anterior capsule to prevent shoulder instability. Repair is done either by using a lag screw for larger fragments or by suture through drill holes for smaller fragments.

Greater tuberosity fractures associated with dislocations should be treated with closed reduction and simple immobilization. If reduction is not satisfactory, the fracture should be openly reduced and the rotator cuff repaired.

Fracture-dislocations require reduction of the dislocation. If this cannot be obtained closed, then it must be opened. If a closed reduction of the dislocation can be obtained in Salter-Harris type I or II fractures, the fracture portion can be treated nonoperatively. Attention is focused on the dislocation rather than on the fracture. Salter-Harris type III fracture-dislocations should have an attempted closed reduction. If successful, open reduction is not required. If the fracture or the dislocation cannot be reduced closed, then open reduction is necessary.

Post Fracture Care and Rehabilitation

Birth injuries do extremely well.[39] Whereas Scaglietti[132] reported several patients with late arm length inequality and limited external rotation; in retrospect, many of these patients probably had mild brachial plexus palsies rather than proximal humeral physeal fractures.

Proximal humeral metaphyseal fractures require a slightly longer period to heal than do epiphyseal fractures. Most epiphyseal fractures are stable by 2 to 3 weeks, but 3 to 4 weeks are needed for metaphyseal fractures. If the fracture pattern is stable, then early pendulum exercises are started. However, if the fracture is unstable, exercise should be held for 3 weeks before initiating motion. After the fracture is healing well, progressive passive forward flexion, external rotation, internal rotation, and extension are begun followed by strengthening of the rotator cuff, trapezius, and deltoid. *In children,* the epiphyseal and metaphyseal fractures display marked remodeling,[4, 5, 17, 34, 43, 44, 98, 138] which may even occur in patients up to age 17.[44] Patients with a marked angular deformity may have some limitation of motion, but this is unlikely to be symptomatic.[106] Patients occasionally report some aching with weather changes[20] or discomfort with heavy lifting.[106] Bergos-Flores[20] noted that only patients with a third anterolateral fragment in association with a Salter-Harris type II fracture experienced reduced mobility and the sensation of weakness. Significant limb length inequality

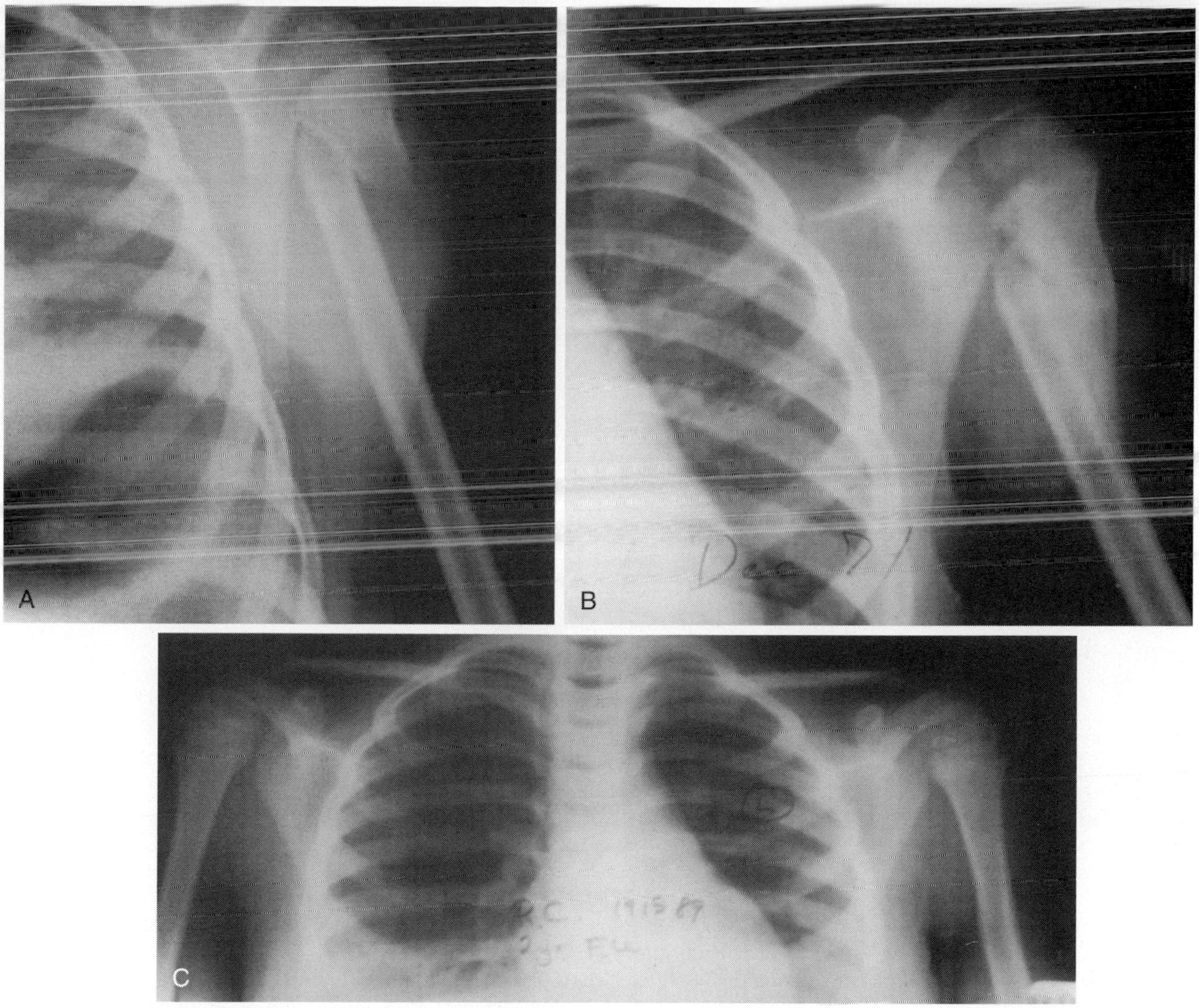

Figure 26–11

Metaphyseal fractures of the proximal humerus are common in the 6- to 10-year-old age group, with healing and remodeling being the rule. *A*, This anteroposterior initial injury radiograph demonstrates a completely displaced metaphyseal fracture of the proximal humerus in an 8 year old. *B*, Rapid healing has taken place with treatment in a sling-and-swathe. This is an 8-week follow-up x-ray. *C*, Complete remodeling is seen in this anteroposterior film taken at a 2-year follow-up.

is uncommon[8, 34] and is seldom sufficient to cause disability or poor cosmesis.

Complications

Humerus Varus. *Humerus varus* is a rare complication following childhood trauma.[37, 40, 81, 87, 153] Very few of the reported cases of humerus varus have documented neonatal trauma.[40, 81, 153] According to Ellefsen and associates[40] the injury usually occurs in the first year but may occur as late as 5 years of age. Two of their patients were victims of child abuse and suffered proximal humeral physeal fractures. The humeral neck shaft angle may decrease to 90 degrees with marked shortening (Fig. 26–12). Trueta[153] reported a similar clinical picture by experimentally damaging the proximal medial humeral physis. Functional impairment usually consists of mild to moderate limitation of glenohumeral abduction. Surgical realignment is unnecessary for most patients. Ellefsen and associates recommend that if an osteotomy is performed that it only be done to 45 degrees rather than to a complete 90 degrees. Solonen and Vastamaki[143] report good results from the osteotomy in five of seven cases operated on for limited active abduction and forward flexion.

Limb Length and Equality. Limb length inequality is rarely significant from proximal humerus fractures. It is more common in patients treated surgically than in those treated nonoperatively.[8, 34, 128]

Loss of Motion. Loss of motion is uncommon and is reported primarily from patients who are treated surgically.[8, 34, 142] Loss of motion is more common in adolescence.

Hypertrophic Scar. Hypertrophic scars from anterior reductions can be a problem with the anterior deltopectoral incision.[43, 51] This finding prompted Fraser and associates to state that "open reduction should never be done

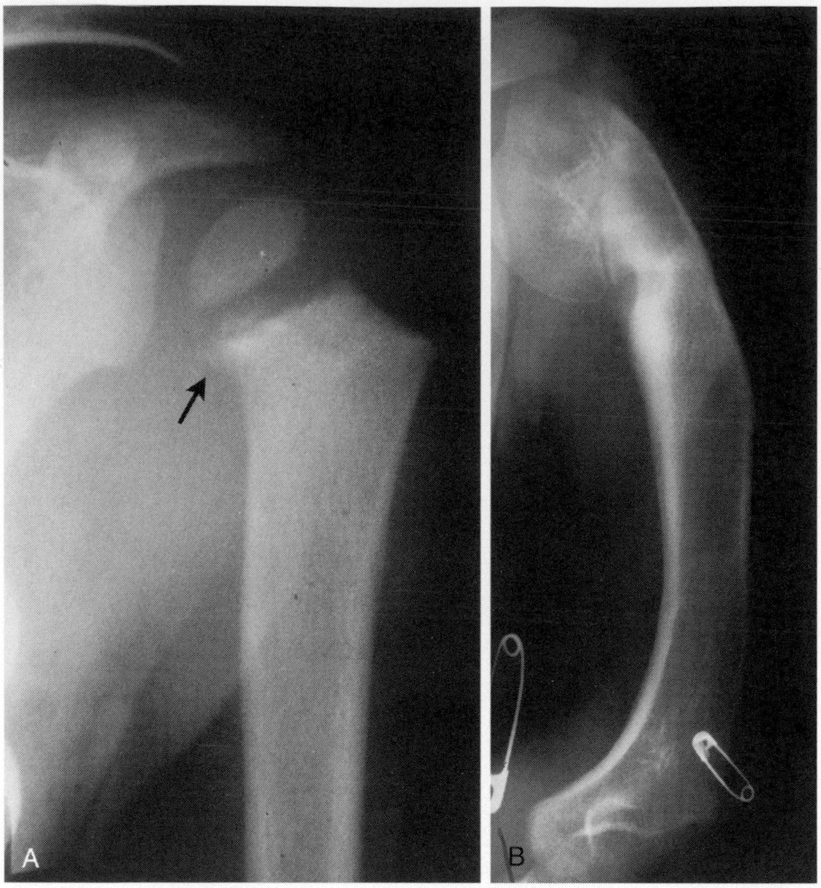

Figure 26–12

Proximal humerus varus resulting from an infection at 1½ years of age. *A,* Marked shortening; *B,* Varus. (From Rockwood CA, Wilkins KE, and Beaty J [eds]: Fractures in Children. Philadelphia: JB Lippincott, 1996.)

in girls because any benefit will be more than offset by the result of the scar."[43] An axillary approach is certainly more cosmetic than the anterior deltopectoral incision.[54, 86]

Inferior Subluxation. Inferior glenohumeral subluxation has been reported in two children with Salter-Harris type II fractures of the proximal humerus.[168] This subluxation is probably secondary to a loss of deltoid and rotator cuff tone and is best treated by a sling to support the arm and early physical therapy. The outcome is generally good.

Avascular Necrosis. Osteonecrosis has only been reported in one child and occurred after a posterior fracture-dislocation that did not undergo reduction for 2 weeks.[158] During surgery, the anterior humeral circumflex vessels and the lateral ascending branch should be avoided.

Nerve Palsy. Nerve injury may occur with fracture-dislocations.[3, 44, 158] The axillary nerve usually recovers in 4 to 6 months. If an electromyogram (EMG) does not demonstrate some recovery by this time, the nerve may be grafted. Recovery of the nerve is best from surgery within 1 year of the injury.[27] If the graft is successful, recovery is usually demonstrated in 8 to 12 months.[3]

Vascular Injury. Vascular injury, including axillary artery disruption or thrombosis[90, 136] and compartment syndromes after surgical neck fracture,[22] has been reported in adults. No reports have been made concerning children. A first rib fracture potentially indicates a subclavian artery rupture,[77] which is usually associated with signs of arterial insufficiency.

Pin Migration. Pin migration is a life-threatening problem.[89, 95] Pins should be bent outside the skin and removed after early healing. Any pins left underneath the skin must be monitored very closely with serial x-rays.

Growth Arrest. Growth arrest has been reported in a patient undergoing late open reduction of a displaced proximal humeral physeal fracture[34] and with unicameral bones cysts.[69, 102, 107]

References and Bibliography

1. Ahn JI and Park JS: Pathological fractures secondary to unicameral bone cysts. Int Orthop *18:*20–22, 1994.
2. Aitken AP: End results of fractures of the proximal humeral epiphysis. J Bone Joint Surg Am *18:*1036–1041, 1936.
3. Artico M, Salvati M, D'Andrea V, et al: Isolated lesion of the axillary nerve: Surgical treatment and outcome in 12 cases. Neurosurgery *29:*697–700, 1991.
4. Aufranc OE, Jones WN, and Bierbaum BE: Epiphyseal fracture of the proximal humerus. JAMA *207:*727–729, 1969.
5. Aufranc OE, Jones WN, and Butler JE: Epiphyseal fracture of the proximal humerus. JAMA *213:*1476–1479, 1970.
6. Baker DM: Benign unicameral bone cyst: A study of forty-five cases with long-term follow up. Clin Orthop *71:*140–151, 1970.
7. Barnett LS: Little league shoulder syndrome: Proximal humeral epiphyseolysis in adolescent baseball pitchers: A case report. J Bone Joint Surg Am *67:*495–496, 1985.
8. Baxter MP and Wiley JJ: Fractures of the proximal humeral epiphysis: Their influence on humeral growth. J Bone Joint Surg Br *68:*570–573, 1986.

9. Bengnér U, Johnell O, and Redlund-Johnell I: Changes in the incidence of fracture of the upper end of the humerus during a 30-year period: A study of 2125 fractures. Clin Orthop 231:179–182, 1988.
10. Berger PE, Ofstein RA, Jackson DW, et al: MRI demonstration of radiographically occult fractures: What have we been missing? Radiographics 9:407–436, 1989.
11. Beringer DC, Noble JS, Weiner DS, and Bell RH: Severely Displaced Proximal Humerus Fractures in Children. American Academy of Orthopaedic Surgeons, No. 168, 1994 (Abstract). (In press).
12. Blount WP: Fractures in Children. Baltimore: Williams & Wilkins, 1954, pp 9–20.
13. Bohler L: The Treatment of Fractures. New York: Grune & Stratton, 1956.
14. Bohler L: The treatment of Fractures—Supplement. New York: Grune & Stratton, 1966.
15. Bortel DT and Pritchett JW: Straight-line graphs for the predictions of growth of the upper extremities. J Bone Joint Surg Am *75*:885–892, 1993.
16. Bourdillan JF: Fracture-separation of the proximal epiphysis of the humerus. J Bone Joint Surg Br *32*:35–37, 1950.
17. Bovill EG Jr, Schneider FR, and Day L: Fracture of the proximal humerus with displacement in a child. JAMA *216*:1188–1189, 1971.
18. Broms-Dalgaard E, Davidsen E, and Sloth C: Radiographic examination of the acute shoulder. Eur J Radiol *11*:10–14, 1990.
19. Broker FHL and Burbach T: Ultrasonic diagnosis of separation of the proximal humeral epiphysis in the newborn. J Bone Joint Surg Am *72*:187–191, 1990.
20. Burgos-Flores J, Gonzalez-Herranz P, Lopez-Mondejar JA, et al: Fractures of the proximal humeral epiphysis. Int Orthop *17*:16–19, 1993.
21. Caldwell JA: Treatment of fractures in the Cincinnati General Hospital. Ann Surg *97*:161, 1933.
22. Cameron SE: Acute compartment syndrome of the triceps: A case report. Acta Orthop Scand *64*:107–108, 1993.
23. Campanacci M, De Sessa L, and Trentani C: Scaglietti's method for conservative treatment of simple bone cysts with local injections of methylprednisolone acetate. Ital J Orthop Traumatol *3*:27–36, 1977.
24. Campos OP: Treatment of bone cysts by intracavity injection of methylprednisolone acetate: A message to orthopedic surgeons. Clin Orthop *165*:43–48, 1982.
25. Camus M, Lefebvre G, Veron P, and Darbois Y: Obstetrical injuries of the newborn infant: Retrospective study a propos of 20,409 births. J Gynecol Obstet Biol Reprod (Paris) *14*:1033–1043, 1985.
26. Capanna R, Dal Monte A, Gitelis S, and Campanacci M: The natural history of unicameral bone cyst after steroid injection. Clin Orthop :204–211, 1982.
27. Coene LN and Narakas AO: Operative management of lesions of the axillary nerve, isolated or combined with other nerve lesions. Clin Neurol Neurosurg *94*(Suppl):S64–S66, 1992.
28. Cohn BT and Froimson AI: Salter 3 fracture dislocation of glenohumeral joint in a 10-year-old. Orthop Rev *15*:403–404, 1986.
29. Connolly J and Secor M: Cortisone treatment of pathologic fracture through a bone cyst. Nebr Med J *67*:286–287, 1982.
30. Croce F, Cuccurullo GD, Passaretti U, and Sadile F: Further experience in the therapy of juvenile osseous cyst using triamcinolone acetonide. Arch Putti Chir Organi Mov *31*:17–25, 1981.
31. Curtis RJJ, Dameron TB Jr, and Rockwood CA Jr: Fractures and dislocations of the shoulder in children. *In* Rockwood CAJ, Wilkins KE, and King RE(eds): Fractures in Children. Philadelphia: JB Lippincott, 1991, pp 829–919.
32. Dalldorf PG and Bryan WJ: Displaced Salter-Harris type I injury in a gymnast. A slipped capital humeral epiphysis? Orthop Rev *23*:538–541, 1994.
33. Dameron TB Jr and Grubb SA: Humeral shaft fractures in adults. South Med J *74*:1461–1467, 1981.
34. Dameron TB Jr and Reibel DB: Fractures involving the proximal humeral epiphyseal plate. J Bone Joint Surg Am *51*:289–297, 1969.
35. De Smet AA: Anterior oblique projection in radiography of the traumatized shoulder. AJR Am J Roentgenol *134*:515–518, 1980.
36. DeSimone DP and Morwessel RM: Diagnostic arthrogram of a Salter I fracture of the proximal humerus in a newborn. Orthop Rev *17*:782–785, 1988.
37. Di Filippo P, Mancini GB, and Gillio A: [Humeral fractures with paralysis of the radial nerve] [In Italian]. Arch Putti Chir Organi Mov *38*:405–409, 1990.
38. Edeiken BS, Libshitz HI, and Cohen MA: Slipped proximal humeral epiphysis: A complication of radiotherapy to the shoulder in children. Skeletal Radiol *9*:123–125, 1982.
39. Ekengren K, Bergdahl S, and Ekstrom G: Birth injuries to the epiphyseal cartilage. Acta Radiol Diagn (Stockh) *19*:197–204, 1978.
40. Ellefsen BK, Frierson MA, Raney EM, and Ogden JA: Humerus varus: A complication of neonatal, infantile, and childhood injury and infection. J Pediatr Orthop *14*:479–486, 1994.
41. Farber JM and Stanton RP: Treatment options in unicameral bone cysts. Orthopedics *13*:25–32, 1990.
42. Fernbach SK, Blumenthal DH, Poznanski AK, et al: Radiographic changes in unicameral bone cysts following direct injection of steroids: A report on 14 cases. Radiology *140*:689–695, 1981.
43. Fraser RL, Haliburton RA, and Barber JR: Displaced epiphyseal fractures of the proximal humerus. Can J Surg *10*:427–430, 1967.
44. Freundlich BD: Luxatio erecta. J Trauma *23*:434–436, 1983.
45. Frey C and Klott J: Late results of sub-capital humerus fracture in children. Z Kinderchir *44*:280–282, 1989.
46. Friedlander HL: Separation of the proximal humeral epiphysis: A case report. Clin Orthop *35*:163–170, 1964.
47. Gagnaire JC, Thoulon JM, Chappuis JP, et al: Injuries to the upper extremities in the newborn diagnosed at birth. J Gynecol Obstet Biol Reprod (Paris) *4*:245–254, 1975.
48. Galasko CS: The fate of simple bone cysts which fracture (letter). Clin Orthop *101*:302–304, 1974.
49. Gartland JJ and Cole FL: Modern concepts in the treatment of unicameral bone cysts of the proximal humerus. Orthop Clin North Am *6*:487–498, 1975.
50. Gerber C, Schneeberger AC, and Vinh TS: The arterial vascularization of the humeral head: An anatomical study. J Bone Joint Surg Am *72*:1486–1494, 1990.
51. Giebel G and Suren EG: Injuries of the proximal humeral epiphysis: Indications for surgical therapy and results [in German]. Chirurg *54*:406–410, 1983.
52. Gregg-Smith SJ and White SH: Salter-Harris III fracture-dislocation of the proximal humeral epiphysis. Injury *23*:199–200, 1992.
53. Gross SJ, Shime J, and Farine D: Shoulder dystocia: Predictors and outcome. Am J Obstet Gynecol *156*:334–336, 1987.
54. Guibert L, Allouis M, Bourdelat D, et al: Fractures and slipped epiphyses of the proximal humerus in children: Place and methods of surgical treatment. Chir Pediatr *24*:197–200, 1983.
55. Haliburton RA, Barber JR, and Fraser RL: Pseudodislocation: An unusual birth injury. Can J Surg *10*:455–462, 1967.
56. Hardcastle PH and Fisher TR: Intrathoracic displacement of the humeral head with fracture of the surgical neck. Injury *12*:313–315, 1981.
57. Harris BA: Shoulder dystocia. Clin Obstet Gynecol *27*:106–111, 1984.
58. Heim D, Herkert F, Hess P, and Regazzoni P: Surgical treatment of humeral shaft fractures—the Basel experience. J Trauma *35*:226–232, 1993.
59. Herring JA and Peterson HA: Simple bone cyst with growth arrest. J Pediatr Orthop *7*:231–235, 1987.
60. Hohl JC: Fractures of the humerus in children. Orthop Clin North Am *7*:557–571, 1976.
61. Horak J and Nilsson BE: Epidemiology of fracture of the upper end of the humerus. Clin Orthop *112*:250–253, 1975.
62. Howard CB, Shinwell E, Nyska M, and Meller I: Ultrasound diagnosis of neonatal fracture separation of the upper humeral epiphysis. J Bone Joint Surg Br *74*:471–472, 1992.
63. Howard FM and Shafer SJ: Injuries to the clavicle with neurovascular complications: A study of fourteen cases. J Bone Joint Surg Am *47*:1335–1346, 1965.
64. Howard NJ and Eloesser L: Treatment of fracture of the upper end of the humerus: An experimental and clinical study. J Bone Joint Surg Am *16*:1–29, 1934.
65. Iqbal QM: Long bone fractures among children in Malaysia. Int Surg *59*:410–415, 1974.
66. Jaberg H, Warner JJ, and Jakob RP: Percutaneous stabilization of unstable fractures of the humerus. J Bone Joint Surg Am *74*:508–515, 1992.
67. James P and Heinrich SD: Ipsilateral proximal metaphyseal and

flexion supracondylar humerus fractures with an associated olecranon avulsion fracture (Clinical Conference). Orthopedics *14:*713–716, 1991.
68. Jaschke W, Hopf G, Gerstner C, and Hiemer W: Proximal humerus fracture with dislocation in childhood: Transacromial percutaneous osteosynthesis using Kirschner wires. Zentralbl Chir *106:*618–621, 1981.
69. Jeffrey CC: Fracture separation of the upper humeral epiphysis. Surg Gynecol Obstet *96:*205–209, 1953.
70. Kapandji A: Osteosynthesis using the "palm-tree" nail technic in fractures of the surgical neck of the humerus. Ann Chir Main *8:*39–52, 1989.
71. Klasson SC, Vander Schilden JL, and Park JP: Late effect of isolated avulsion fractures of the lesser tubercle of the humerus in children: Report of two cases. J Bone Joint Surg Am *75:*1691–1694, 1993.
72. Kleiger B: Unicameral bone cyst: 15 year follow-up. Bull Hosp JT Dis *30:*53–58, 1969.
73. Kleinman PK and Akins CM: The "vanishing" epiphysis: Sign of Salter type I fracture of the proximal humerus in infancy. Br J Radiol *55:*865–867, 1982.
74. Kocialkowski A and Wallace WA: Closed percutaneous K-wire stabilization for displaced fractures of the surgical neck of the humerus. Injury *21:*209–212, 1990.
75. Kohler R and Trillaud JM: Fracture and fracture separation of the proximal humerus in children: Report of 136 cases. J Pediatr Orthop *3:*326–332, 1983.
76. Kothari K, Bernstein RM, Griffiths HJ, et al: Luxatio erecta. Skeletal Radiol *11:*47–49, 1984.
77. Kretz JG, Eisenmann B, El Badawy H, et al: Subclavian artery rupture during closed thoracobrachial injuries: Report on eleven cases (Author's translation). J Mal Vasc *6:*107–109, 1981.
78. Kristiansen B and Kofoed H: External fixation of displaced fractures of the proximal humerus: Technique and preliminary results. J Bone Joint Surg Br *69:*643–646, 1987.
79. Kuhns LR, Sherman MP, Poznanski AK, and Holt JF: Humeral head and coracoid ossification in the newborn. Radiology *107:*145–149, 1973.
80. Landin LA: Fracture patterns in children: Analysis of 8682 fractures with special reference to incidence, etiology and secular changes in Swedish urban populations. Acta Orthop Scand Suppl *54:*1–109, 1983.
81. Langenskiöld A: Adolescent humerus varus. Acta Chirurg Scand *105:*353–363, 1953.
82. Larsen CF, Kiaer T, and Lindequist S: Fractures of the proximal humerus in children: Nine-year followup of 64 unoperated on cases. Acta Orthop Scand *61:*255–257, 1990.
83. Lee HG: Operative reduction of an unusual fracture of the upper epiphyseal plate of the humerus. J Bone Joint Surg *26:*401–404, 1944.
84. Lemperg R and Liliequist B: Dislocation of the proximal epiphysis of the humerus in newborns. Acta Paediatr Scand *59:*377–380, 1970.
85. Lentz W and Meuser P: The treatment of fractures of the proximal humerus. Arch Orthop Trauma Surg *96:*283–285, 1980.
86. Leslie JT and Ryan TJ: The anterior axillary incision to approach the shoulder joint. J Bone Joint Surg Am *44:*1193–1196, 1962.
87. Levitskii FA and Al'-Masri Akhmad: Characteristics of multiple fractures of the long bones of the upper limbs and their treatment. Ortop Traumatol Protez *4:*42–45, 1989.
88. Li JK, Birch PD, and Davies AM: Proximal humeral defects in Gaucher's disease. Br J Radiol *61:*579–583, 1988.
89. Liebling G and Bartel HG: Unusual migration of a Kirschner wire following drill wire fixation of a subcapital humerus fracture. Beitr Orthop Traumatol *34:*585–587, 1987.
90. Linson MA: Axillary artery thrombosis after fracture of the humerus: A case report. J Bone Joint Surg Am *62:*1214–1215, 1980.
91. Lipscomb AB: Baseball pitching injuries in growing athletes. J Sports Med Phys Fitness *3:*25–34, 1975.
92. Lock TR and Aronson DD: Fractures in patients who have myelomeningocele. J Bone Joint Surg Am *71:*1153–1157, 1989.
93. Loder RT: Pediatric polytrauma: Orthopaedic care and hospital course. J Orthop Trauma *1:*48–54, 1987.
94. Lubrano di Diego JG, Chappuis JP, Montsegur P, et al: Apropos of 82 obstetrical astro-articular injuries of the new-born (excepting brachial plexus palsies): Limits of initial therapeutic aggression and follow-up of evolution, particularly concerning traumatic separation of upper femoral epiphysis. Chir Pediatr *19:*219–226, 1978.
95. Lyons FA and Rockwood CA: Current concepts review: Migration of pins used in operations on the shoulder. J Bone Joint Surg Am *72:*1262–1267, 1990.
96. Macfarlane I and Mushayt K: Double closed fractures of the humerus in a child: A case report. J Bone Joint Surg Am *72:* 443, 1990.
97. Madsen TE: Fractures of the extremities in the newborn. Acta Obstet Gynecol Scand *34:*41, 1955.
98. McBride ED and Sisler J: Fractures of the proximal humeral epiphysis and the juxta-epiphysial humeral shaft. Clin Orthop *38:*143–153, 1965.
99. Merten DF, Kirks DR, and Ruderman RJ: Occult humeral epiphyseal fracture in battered infants. Pediatr Radiol *10:*151–154, 1981.
100. Mestdagh H, Butruille Y, Tillie B, and Bocquet F: Results of the treatment of proximal humeral fractures by percutaneous nailing: A propos of 142 cases. Ann Chir *38:*5–13, 1984.
101. Metaizeau JP and Ligier JN: Surgical treatment of fractures of the long bones in children: Interference between osteosynthesis and the physiological processes of consolidation: Therapeutic indications. J Chir (Paris) *121:*527–537, 1984.
102. Moed BR and LaMont RL: Unicameral bone cyst complicated by growth retardation. J Bone Joint Surg Am *64:*1379–1381, 1982.
103. Müller ME, Allgöwer M, Schneider R, and Willenegger H: Manual of Internal Fixation: Techniques Recommended by the AO-ASIF Group. Berlin: Springer-Verlag, 1991.
104. Nazario AC, Tanaka CI, and Novo NF: Proximal humeral ossification center of the fetus: Time of appearance and the sensitivity and specificity of this finding. J Ultrasound Med *12:*513–515, 1993.
105. Neer CS II and Horowitz BS: Fractures of the proximal humeral epiphysial plate. Clin Orthop *41:*24–31, 1965.
106. Nilsson S and Svartholm F: Fracture of the upper end of the humerus in children: A follow-up of 44 cases. Acta Chirurg Scand *130:*433–439, 1965.
107. Norman A and Schiffman M: Simple bone cysts: Factors of age dependency. Radiology *124:*779–782, 1977.
108. Obremskey W and Routt ML Jr: Fracture-dislocation of the shoulder in a child: Case report. J Trauma *36:*137–140, 1994.
109. Ogden JA, Conlogue GJ, and Jensen P: Radiology of postnatal skeletal development: The proximal humerus. Skeletal Radiol *2:*153–160, 1978.
110. Olmeda A, Bonaga S, and Turra S: The treatment of fractures of the surgical neck of the humerus by osteosynthesis with Kirschner wires. Ital J Orthop Traumatol *15:*353–360, 1989.
111. Olszewski W and Popinski M: Fractures of the neck and shaft of the humerus as a rare form of double fractures in children [in Polish]. Chir Narzadow Ruchu Ortop Pol *39:*121–123, 1974.
112. Ozonoff MB and Ziter FM Jr: The upper humeral notch: A normal variant in children. Radiology *113:*699–701, 1974.
113. Peter RE, Hoffmeyer P, and Henley MB: Treatment of humeral diaphyseal fractures with Hackethal stacked nailing: A report of 33 cases. J Orthop Trauma *6:*14–17, 1992.
114. Peterson CA and Peterson HA: Analysis of the incidence of injuries to the epiphyseal growth plate. J Trauma *12:*275–281, 1972.
115. Peterson HA, Madhok R, Benson JT, et al: Physeal fractures. Part 1. Epidemiology in Olmsted County, Minnesota, 1979–1988. J Pediatr Orthop *14:*423–430, 1994.
116. Pritchett JW: Growth and predictions of growth in the upper extremity. J Bone Joint Surg Am *70:*520–525, 1988.
117. Pritchett JW: Growth plate activity in the upper extremity. Clin Orthop *268:*235–242, 1991.
118. Putz P, Arias C, Bremen J, et al: Treatment of epiphyseal fractures of the proximal humerus using Hackethal's bundled wires: A propos of 136 cases. Acta Orthop Belg *53:*80–87, 1987.
119. Rang M: Clavicle. *In* Children's Fractures. Philadelphia: JB Lippincott, 1983, pp 139–142.
120. Reisig VJ and Grobler B: Proximal fractures of the humerus in children. Zentralbl Chir *105:*25–31, 1980.
121. Robbins H: The treatment of unicameral or solitary bone cysts by the injection of corticosteroids. Bull Hosp Jt Dis *42:*1–16, 1982.
122. Robin GC and Kedar SS: Separation of the upper humeral epiphysis in pituitary gigantism. J Bone Joint Surg Am *44:*189–192, 1962.
123. Rockwood CA Jr, Szalay EA, Curtis RJJ, et al: X-ray evaluation of

shoulder problems. *In* Rockwood CAJ and Matsen FA III (eds). The Shoulder. Philadelphia: WB Saunders, 1990, pp 178–207.
124. Rose SH, Melton LJ, III, Morrey BF, et al: Epidemiologic features of humeral fractures. Clin Orthop *168:*24–30, 1982.
125. Ross GJ and Love MB: Isolated avulsion fracture of the lesser tuberosity of the humerus: Report of two cases. Radiology *172:*833–834, 1989.
126. Rud B, Pedersen NW, and Thomsen PB: Simple bone cysts in children treated with methylprednisolone acetate. Orthopedics *14:*185–187, 1991.
127. Runkel M, Kreitner KF, Wenda K, et al: Nuclear magnetic tomography in shoulder dislocation. Unfallchirurg *96:*124–128, 1993.
128. Sakakida K: Clinical observations on the epiphysial separation of long bones. Clin Orthop *34:*119–141, 1964.
129. Salter RB and Harris WR: Injuries involving epiphyseal plates. J Bone Joint Surg Am *45:*587–622, 1963.
130. Samilson RL: Congenital and developmental anomalies of the shoulder girdle. Orthop Clin North Am *11:*219–231, 1980.
131. Savastano AA: The treatment of bone cysts with intracyst injection of steroids: Injection of steroids will largely replace surgery in the treatment of benign bone cysts. R I Med J *62:*93–95, 1979.
132. Scaglietti O: The obstetrical shoulder trauma. Surg Gynecol Obstet *66:*868, 1938.
133. Scaglietti O, Marchetti PG, and Bartolozzi P: The effects of methylprednisolone acetate in the treatment of bone cysts: Results of three years follow-up. J Bone Joint Surg Br *61-B:*200–204, 1979.
134. Scaglietti O, Marchetti PG, and Bartolozzi P. Rizulati a distanza dell'azione topica dell'acetato de methylprednisolone in microcristalli in alcune lesioni dello scheletro. Arch Putti *30:*1, 1979.
135. Scaglietti O, Marchetti PG, and Bartolozzi P: Final results obtained in the treatment of bone cysts with methylprednisolone acetate (Depo-Medrol) and a discussion of results achieved in other bone lesions. Clin Orthop *165:*33–42, 1982.
136. Seitz J, Valdes F, and Kramer A: Acute ischemia of the upper extremity caused by axillary contused trauma: Report of 3 cases. Rev Med Chil *119:*567–571, 1991.
137. Sessa S, Lascombes P, Prevot J, et al: Centromedullary nailing in fractures of the upper end of the humerus in children and adolescents. Chir Pediatr *31:*43–46, 1990.
138. Sherk HH and Probst C: Fractures of the proximal humeral epiphysis. Orthop Clin North Am *6:*401–413, 1975.
139. Shindell R, Connolly JF, and Lippiello L: Prostaglandin levels in a unicameral bone cyst treated by corticosteroid injection. J Pediatr Orthop *7:*210–212, 1987.
140. Shulman BH and Terhune CB: Epiphyseal injuries in breech delivery. Pediatrics *8:*693–700, 1951.
141. Siegel IM: Brisement force with controlled collapse in treatment of solitary unicameral bone cyst. Arch Surg *92:*109–114, 1966.
142. Smith FM: Fracture-separation of the proximal humeral epiphysis: A study of cases seen at the Presbyterian Hospital from 1929–1953. Am J Surg *91:*627–635, 1956.
143. Solonen KA and Vastamaki M: Osteotomy of the neck of the humerus for traumatic varus deformity. Acta Orthop Scand *56:*79–80, 1985.
144. Stahl EJ and Karpman R: Normal growth and growth predictions in the upper extremity. J Hand Surg (Am) *11:*593–596, 1986.
145. Steiner GM and Sprigg A: The value of ultrasound in the assessment of bone. Br J Radiol *65:*589–593, 1992.
146. Steinhauser J: "Dislocation osteotomy" in the treatment of large juvenile bone cysts. Z Orthop Ihre Grenzgeb *119:*331–335, 1981.
147. Stewart MJ and Hundley JM: Fractures of the humerus. A comparative study in methods of treatment. J Bone Joint Surg Am *37:*681–692, 1955.
148. Struhl S, Edelson C, Pritzker H, et al: Solitary (unicameral) bone cyst: The fallen fragment sign revisited. Skeletal Radiol *18:*261–265, 1989.
149. Szalay EA and Rockwood CA Jr: Injuries of the shoulder and arm (Review). Emerg Med Clin North Am *2:*279–294, 1984.
150. Te Slaa RL and Nollen AJ: A Salter type 3 fracture of the proximal epiphysis of the humerus. Injury *18:*429–431, 1987.
151. Tirman PF, Stauffer AE, Crues JV III, et al: Saline magnetic resonance arthrography in the evaluation of glenohumeral instability. Arthroscopy *9:*550–559, 1993.
152. Troum S, Floyd WE III, and Waters PM: Posterior dislocation of the humeral head in infancy associated with obstetrical paralysis: A case report. J Bone Joint Surg Am *75:*1370–1375, 1993.
153. Trueta J. Studies of the Development and Decay of the Human Frame. Philadelphia: WB Saunders, 1968, pp 274–278.
154. Tullos HS, Erwin WD, Woods GW, et al: Unusual lesions of the pitching arm. Clin Orthop *88:*169–182, 1972.
155. Tullos HS and Fain RH: Little league shoulder: Rotational stress fracture of proximal epiphysis. J Sports Med *2:*152–153, 1974.
156. van den Broek JA and Vegter J: Echography in the diagnosis of epiphysiolysis of the proximal humerus in a newborn infant. Ned Tijdschr Geneeskd *132:*1015–1017, 1988.
157. van Vugt AB, Severijnen RV, and Festen C: Neurovascular complications in supracondylar humeral fractures in children. Arch Orthop Trauma Surg *107:*203–205, 1988.
158. Vastamaki M and Solonen KA: Posterior dislocation and fracture-dislocation of the shoulder. Acta Orthop Scand *51:*479–484, 1980.
159. Visser JD and Rietberg M: Interposition of the tendon of the long head of biceps in fracture separation of the proximal humeral epiphysis. Neth J Surg *32:*12–15, 1980.
160. Wadlington VR, Hendrix RW, and Rogers LF: Computed tomography of posterior fracture-dislocations of the shoulder. Case reports. J Trauma *32:*113–115, 1992.
161. Weseley MS, Barenfeld PA, and Eisenstein AL: Rush pin intramedullary fixation for fractures of the proximal humerus. J Trauma *17:*29–37, 1977.
162. White GM and Riley LHJ: Isolated avulsion of the subscapularis insertion in a child: A case report. J Bone Joint Surg Am *67:*635–636, 1985.
163. White SJ, Blane CE, DiPietro MA, et al: Arthrography in evaluation of birth injuries of the shoulder. Can Assoc Radiol J *38:*113–115, 1987.
164. Whitman RA: Treatment of epiphyseal displacement and fractures of the upper extremity of the humerus designed to assured deficit adjustment and fixation of the fragments. Ann Surg *47:*706–708, 1908.
165. Williams DJ: The mechanisms producing fracture-separation of the proximal humeral epiphysis. J Bone Joint Surg Br *63-B:*102–107, 1981.
166. Wong-Chung J and O'Brien T: Salter-Harris type III fracture of the proximal humeral physis. Injury *19:*453–454, 1988.
167. Worlock P and Stower M: Fracture patterns in Nottingham children. J Pediatr Orthop *6:*656–661, 1986.
168. Yosipovitch Z and Goldberg I: Inferior subluxation of the humeral head after injury to the shoulder: A brief note. J Bone Joint Surg Am *71:*751–753, 1989.
169. Yu CL, D'Astous J, and Finnegan M: Simple bone cysts: The effects of methylprednisolone on synovial cells in culture. Clin Orthop *262:*34–41, 1991.

FRACTURES OF THE CLAVICLE

The clavicle joins the thorax to the upper extremity through the sternoclavicular joint, the coracoclavicular ligaments, the acromioclavicular joint, and the muscular attachments of the deltoid, trapezius, and pectoralis major. It serves to anchor the scapula and provides a rigid base for muscular attachments that stabilize the shoulder for arm function. Without clavicular stability, the weight of the arm tends to protract the scapula, bringing it forward, medial, and downward. The clavicle also provides bony protection for the subclavian and axillary vessels and the brachial plexus.[1] Although children with hypoplastic clavicles (i.e., complete congenital absence of the clavicles from cleidocranial dysostosis) may function quite well,[1, 5, 88, 89, 96] this is not true of patients with trapezial or deltoid dysfunction from severe injury in whom the results of clavicle excision are poor.[138]

Developmental Anatomy

Embryology and Development. The clavicle is one of the first two bones, along with the mandible, to ossify.

The clavicle forms initially as membranous bone and secondarily develops growth cartilage at both ends.[42] By 7 to 8 weeks' gestation, the clavicle has already formed its adult characteristics with the typical S shape. Primary ossification starts from two separate centers, lateral and medial, either of which may have more advanced ossification.[42, 126] The area where these centers fuse corresponds with between one third to one quarter of the distance from the lateral end to the medial end at adulthood.[126] By 45 days in utero, these two ossification centers fuse to form one mass of clavicular shaft that predominates in growth to 5 years of age. Cartilaginous growth plates develop medially and laterally, and the medial physis provides approximately 80% of the longitudinal growth for the bone.[126, 129] The medial epiphysis appears between ages 11 and 19 in girls and ages 14 and 19 in boys. It fuses to the shaft between 22 to 26 years of age in men and 22 to 25 years of age in women.[76, 178] Medial clavicular epiphysiodesis is rare before 22 years of age (Fig. 26–13).[73] For this reason, many sternoclavicular dislocations are injuries through the medial physeal plate.[2, 23] Laterally, the acromioclavicular ligaments attach densely into the periosteum of the lateral clavicular epiphysis and subsequently blend into the periosteum.[127] This fact is very important in order to understand lateral clavicular injuries in children. Although a coracoclavicular joint is present in up to 10% of adults, it is not found in children.[85] Medially, the fossa for the rhomboid ligament's insertion on the inferior clavicle is visible in only 0.59% of x-rays[87] but may be histologically present bilaterally in about half the population and unilaterally in approximately 20%.[85] The lateral or acromial epiphysis is usually inapparent on x-ray and has very little longitudinal growth. It rarely develops a secondary ossification center and fuses to the clavicle by 19 years of age.

The sternoclavicular joint is a diarthrodial joint made up of the large medial end of the clavicle, the sternum, and the first rib. It is incongruous with very little bony stability in and of itself. A fibrocartilaginous disk or meniscus covers most of the articular surface. A strong series of ligaments bind the joint together. The intra-articular disk ligament is a dense fibrous structure that arises from the first rib and hemisects the joint, either completely or incompletely, attaching anteriorly and posteriorly to the strong capsular ligaments. The anterior portion of the capsular ligament is heavier and stronger than is the posterior portion. This anterior capsular ligament provides the primary support against upward and anterior displacement of the medial clavicle. The capsular ligaments attach predominantly to the epiphysis of the medial clavicle. The physis lies outside the joint capsule; therefore, in physeal injuries, the weak link is through the physis.[2, 25, 146] The joint is further protected by interclavicular and costoclavicular or rhomboid ligaments that contribute to the maintenance of "poise of the shoulder" (Fig. 26–14).[115]

The sternoclavicular joint is positioned immediately anterior to many structures exiting the mediastinum, including the innominate artery and vein, the vagus and phrenic nerves, and also the trachea and esophagus. Posteriorly displaced fractures of the medial clavicle can impinge on these structures, causing an immediate and life-threatening emergency.[1, 69, 171] The sternoclavicular joint is moveable, allowing 30 to 35 degrees of upward clavicular elevation, 35 degrees of motion in the anterior to posterior plane, and 45 to 50 degrees of rotation about the long axis of the clavicle. This articulation provides the only true articulation between the upper extremity and the axial skeleton.[1]

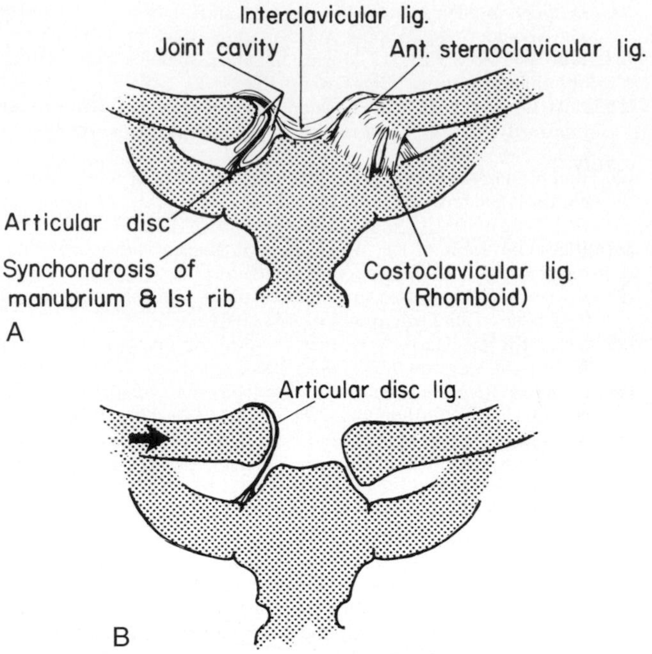

Figure 26–14

A, Schematic drawing of the anatomy of the sternoclavicular joint. Note the heavy ligamentous structure and articular disk. *B*, The articular disk ligament provides a checkrein for medial displacement of the clavicle. (From Rockwood CA and Green DP [eds]: Fractures [3 vols], 2nd ed. Philadelphia: JB Lippincott, 1984.)

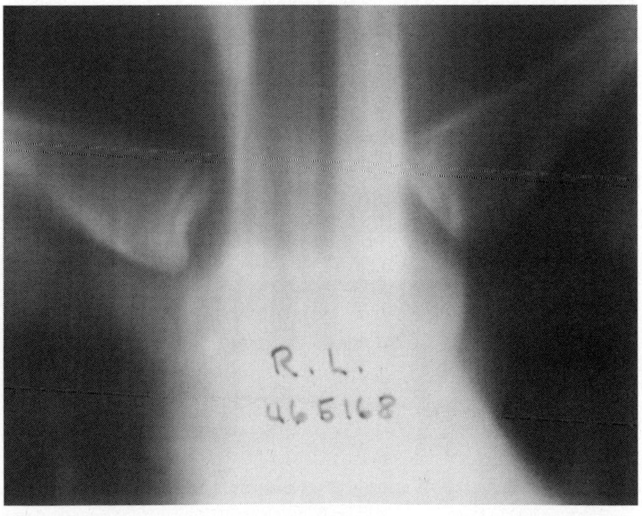

Figure 26–13

A tomogram of the medial clavicle demonstrates open epiphyses. These epiphyses do not fuse to the clavicular shaft until 22 to 25 years of age. (From Rockwood CA and Green DP [eds]: Fractures [3 vols], 2nd ed. Philadelphia: JB Lippincott, 1984.)

ACROMIOCLAVICULAR JOINT

The lateral one third of the clavicle is surrounded by an extremely thick periosteal tube that remains intact circumferentially all the way to the acromioclavicular joint. The very strong coracoclavicular ligaments attach firmly to the inferior portion of this periosteal sleeve rather than to the bone itself. At the distal extent of the clavicle, a secondary ossification center is present, although this usually remains as an unossified epiphysis. When it does become ossified, the fusion process to the shaft occurs over a very short time sequence and is rarely seen on x-ray.[41, 42] The acromioclavicular joint is a diarthrodial joint.[129] In the adult, an intra-articular disk forms to cover the distal clavicle. The joint is surrounded by a relatively weak capsule supported superiorly and inferiorly by acromioclavicular ligaments that, in a child, blend with the thick periosteum of the distal clavicle. The primary stabilizing ligaments are the strong conoid and trapezoid portions of the coracoclavicular ligaments that arise from the coracoid and attach to the undersurface of the distal clavicle and its periosteum. A fracture in this region is much more common than a dislocation. This thick periosteal tube usually remains intact inferiorly and distally along with the supporting ligamentous structures; therefore, even displaced fractures have a tremendous potential for remodeling (Fig. 26–15).[8, 25]

CLAVICULAR SHAFT

Incidence at Birth

Clavicle fractures are by far the most common skeletal injury during delivery, and reported rates range from 0.27 to 6.26%.[16, 20, 39, 47, 49, 70, 78, 80, 104, 109, 132, 148, 172, 176] In children with a birthweight greater than 4000 g, the incidence increases to more than 13%.[71] The left:right ratio is slightly less than 2:1.[104] These fractures are occasionally bilateral.[7]

Incidence in Children

In older children, the clavicle is the fourth most commonly fractured bone,[91] representing between 8 and 15.5% of all children's fractures.[66, 91, 97, 122] Nondisplaced fractures are most common in younger children, whereas displaced fractures are most common in adolescents. Almost 50% of all clavicle fractures occur in children who are 10 years of age or younger, and these fractures are more common in boys.[91, 167] The incidence is 6.3 per 1000 per 6 months.[183] In all except one study, middle third fractures are most common in children, and the incidence of lateral third fractures increases with age.[66, 122, 165, 167]

Displacement. When the clavicle is fractured, the sternocleidomastoid pulls the medial portion proximally while the distal portion is pulled inferiorly by the pectoralis minor. The overall clavicle is shortened by the pectoralis and the subclavius.[25, 128] Significant vascular injury is usually associated with direct blows.[185]

Mechanism of Injury

BIRTH

The upper clavicle is the most frequently fractured bone during delivery,[39] probably because of the pressure of the

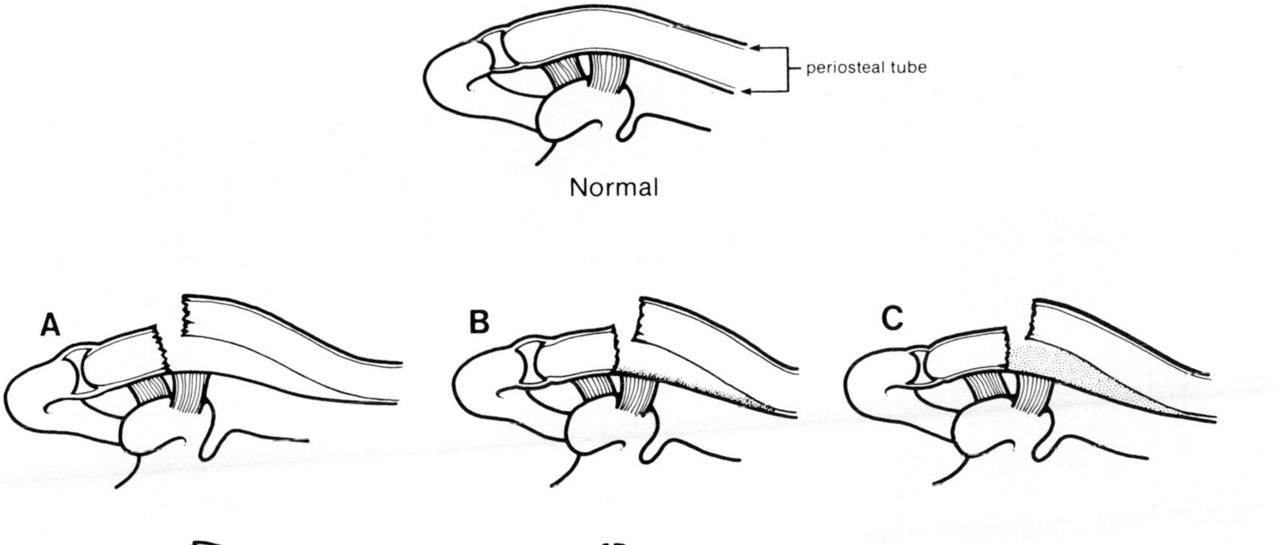

Figure 26–15

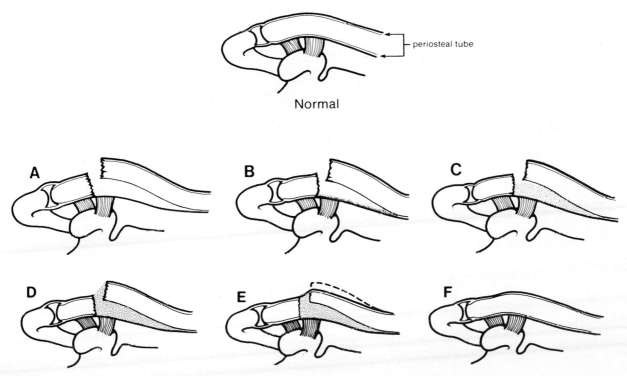

Phases of healing in fractures of the distal clavicle in children. *A,* The clavicular shaft herniates through the periosteal tube with fracture. *B,* The coracoclavicular ligaments remain in continuity with the inferior portion of the periosteal tube. *C* and *D,* Periosteal callus is formed within the tube to stabilize the fracture. *E,* Remodeling occurs with resorption of the superior prominence of the shaft fragment. *F,* Final remodeling with good stability is achieved. (From Rockwood CA and Green DP [eds]: Fractures [3 vols], 2nd ed. Philadelphia: JB Lippincott, 1984.)

anterior shoulder in the cephalic presentation against the symphysis pubis, but this fracture is occasionally caused by the obstetrician pressing on the clavicle.[104] Fractures of the clavicle are strongly associated with shoulder dystocia and heavier birthweight.[20, 39, 51, 65, 95, 104, 119, 130, 132, 172, 176] However, most fractures of the clavicle occur in uneventful deliveries,[51, 130, 172, 176] and a higher incidence of the clavicle fractures is not necessarily an indication of poor obstetric care.[20, 130, 172] A cesarean section does not completely preclude fractures of the clavicle.[118] Five to 16 kg of force are required to produce a fracture of the clavicle in stillborn infants.[104] These forces exceed those of a routine delivery.[51, 109] The incidence of concomitant brachial plexus palsies is very small,[95] although Oppenheim and associates[132] report an incidence of 5%. Whether the clavicle fracture is protective of plexus injury or portends a worse outcome is uncertain.[69]

OLDER CHILDREN

In older children, falls are the most common cause of fracture of the clavicle.[91, 122] Stanley and associates[166] analyzed the forces required to fracture the clavicle and found that indirect mechanisms such as falling on an outstretched hand are highly unlikely to result in fracture of the clavicle. Most clavicle shaft fractures occur from a direct blow either to the clavicle or to the acromion.[149, 166] Fractures of the clavicle frequently occur in sports.[91, 122] Fractures from direct blows in sports may be preventable by adequate padding.[162] Stress fractures may also occur.[134] Fractures of the clavicle may also occur with child abuse, but they are not specific.[61, 90]

Signs and Symptoms

Many fractures of the clavicle at birth are quite obvious. The most reliable clinical sign has been described as difficulty in identifying the margins of the effected clavicle when compared with the normal clavicle.[80] The child generally has an asymmetric Moro reflex.[138] Uncommonly, it has been misdiagnosed as congenital muscular torticollis.[84] If the baby does not feed from one of the mother's breasts but will feed from the other breast, a fracture of the clavicle should be suspected.[177]

In older children, the diagnosis of a clavicle injury is usually quite evident (Fig. 26–16). There is normally ecchymosis and swelling at the fracture site, which is usually quite tender. Plastic bowing, however, may not have discrete tenderness (Fig. 26–17). The most important part of the evaluation and treatment of an acute clavicle fracture is an examination to exclude injury to the underlying lungs, vascular structures, and brachial plexus.[25] Potential skin ischemia must also be evaluated.

Classification

The most common classification for fractures of the clavicle is that of Allman[2] with type I representing the middle third, type II representing those distal to the coracoclavicular ligaments, and type III representing the medial third. The type I category is generally broadened to include all fractures lateral to the sternocleidomastoid and costoclavicular or rhomboid ligament and medial to the coracoclavicular ligaments. The clavicle may be plastically bowed

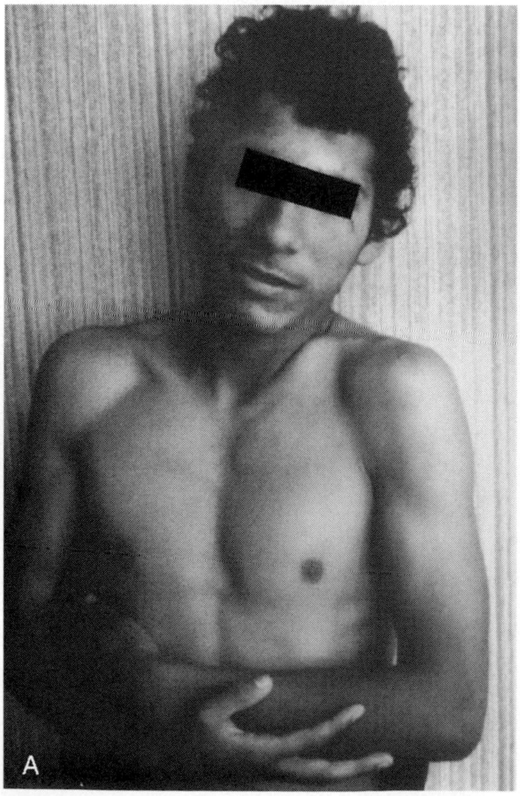

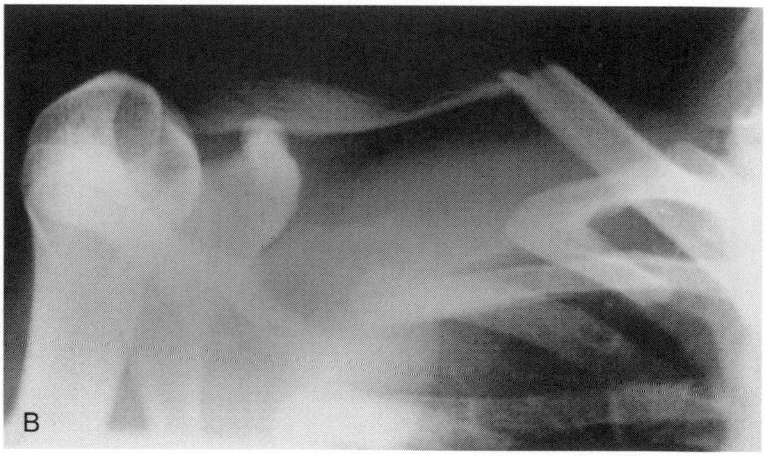

Figure 26–16

A, Clinical photograph of a young patient with a clavicle fracture. Note that the arm is supported by the good hand at the elbow and the head is tilted to the side of the fracture. *B,* The corresponding radiograph shows the clavicle fracture.

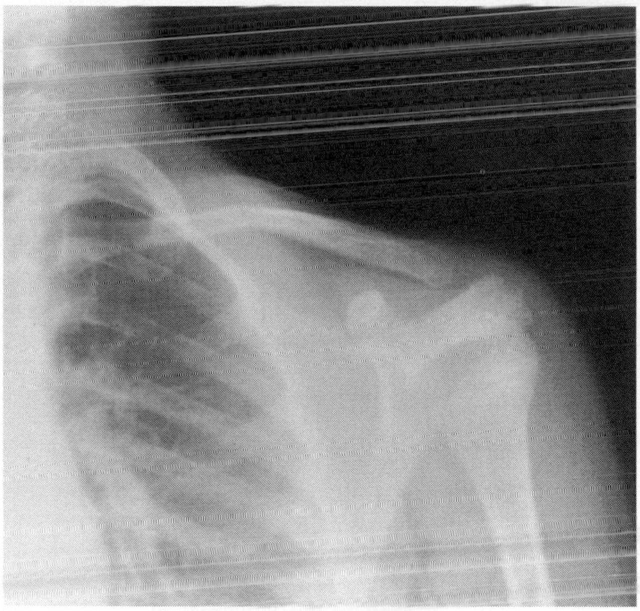

Figure 26–17

A greenstick fracture of the clavicle in an 8-year-old girl who had fallen on her outstretched arm. Note the soft tissue swelling superiorly at the fracture site. This is often a key to the diagnosis of the minimally displaced fracture.

rather than fully broken.[12] Fractures of the clavicle shaft in children may occur in association with anterior or posterior sternoclavicular injuries,[58, 61, 93] or lateral clavicular injuries,[19] or they may be segmental.[93] They may rarely be associated with scapulothoracic dislocations, or with scapular neck fractures.[95, 133, 158] The fractures are rarely bilateral and have also been reported from benign and malignant tumors.[147, 152]

Radiographic Findings

Despite the S shape of the clavicle, a single anteroposterior view is usually sufficient to diagnose a fracture. However, to determine the displacement, a cephalically directed view is helpful. Two additional radiographic views have been described. The apical oblique is obtained with the injured side angled 45 degrees toward the tube and a 20-degree cephalic tilt of the beam. This is primarily useful for detecting nondisplaced fractures of the middle third of the clavicle that are obscured by the clavicle's S shape.[179] An apical lordotic view has also been described to get an x-ray perpendicular to the anteroposterior view; however, this requires placing the shoulder in 135 degrees of abduction, which is not practical in acutely injured patients.[145] Nondisplaced fractures may show loss of soft tissue shadows compared with the opposite side.[164] Ultrasound has proved useful in the neonate[4, 84] (Fig. 26–18). It has been used successfully in a 2 year old as well,[53] although fractures at this age can usually be diagnosed by plain x-rays and by clinical examination.

Differential Diagnosis

Birth fractures usually heal promptly. The absence of the calcification in a neonate after 11 days of age should alert the physician to the possibility of child abuse.[23] Congenital pseudarthrosis is a rare, frequently asymptomatic disorder,[14, 73, 113, 175] and the pseudarthritic ends often curve and are atrophic rather than hypertrophic (Fig. 26–19). It is generally right-sided,[6, 87, 95, 106, 141] although occasionally bilateral.[15, 60] Left-sided cases are quite rare and have not been well documented except with dextrocardia.[46] The differential diagnosis is of a birth fracture or cleidocranial dysostosis.[37, 141] A birth fracture is not associated with neurofibromatosis. Proposed etiologies of the congenital pseudarthrosis include vascular pressure from the subclavian artery or failure of the two major ossification centers to unite.[6, 21, 81, 106, 141] However, the two ossification centers are always connected by areas of adjacent bone,[46] and the junction of the two ossification centers does not correspond with the site of the congenital pseudarthrosis.[126] Likewise, the clavicle is remote from the subclavian artery throughout its development.[126] This leaves the etiology of congenital pseudarthrosis still unexplained.

Clavicle Lesions. Clavicle abnormalities are numerous.[36, 163] Many lesions can be confused with or cause fractures, including benign or malignant tumors,[17, 36, 45, 137, 152, 163, 174] and erosions of the medial or lateral clavicle that occur with hyperparathyroidism and renal

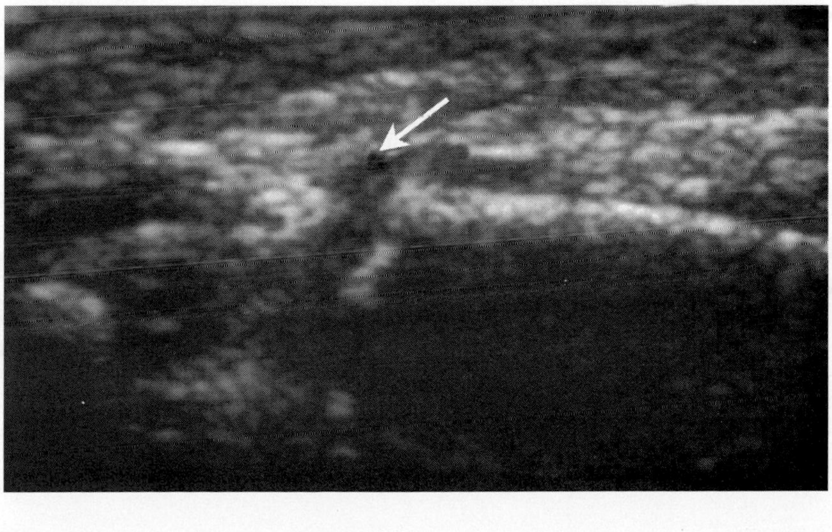

Figure 26–18

Ultrasound of a neonatal clavicle fracture demonstrating the fracture line. This is useful to determine the etiology of neonatal pseudoparalysis. (From Rockwood CA, Wilkins KE, Beaty J [eds]: Fractures in Children. Philadelphia: JB Lippincott, 1996.)

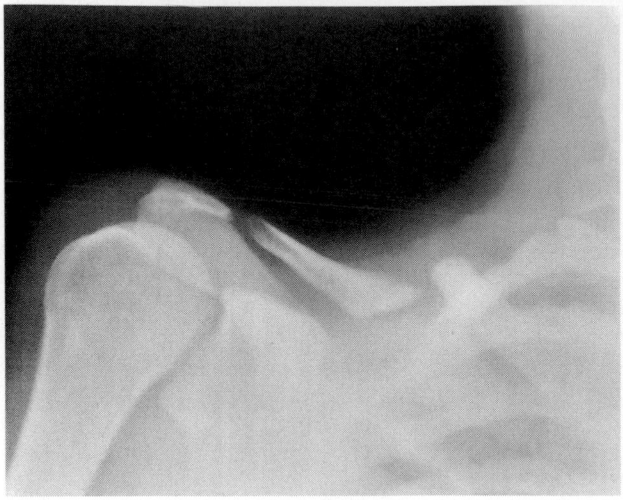

Figure 26–19

Congenital pseudarthrosis of the clavicle. This patient is asymptomatic but has a noted clinical deformity.

osteodystrophy.[54, 158, 168] Clavicular stress reactions may be difficult to distinguish from neoplasia, and the use of F-18 fluorodeoxyglucose has been described for this purpose.[134] The rhomboid fossa appears as a lucent area,[75, 170] and the coracoclavicular ligament may show some elevation of the bone surface simulating periostitis or callous formation.[170] These attachments may be confused with a tumor or a fracture. The insertion of the sternocleidomastoid in infantile muscular torticollis can also create a medial lucency.[150] A lateral clavicular hook occurs with thrombocytopenia radius aplasia syndrome, camptomelia, persistent brachial plexus palsy, and osteogenesis imperfecta,[125, 173] which must be distinguished from plastic bowing that may have a similar appearance.[12] Osteomyelitis,[44] including congenital syphilis[144] of the clavicle, is uncommon but can produce a periosteal reaction. The duration is usually longer than that of a fracture.[44, 82, 112, 114] Idiopathic hyperostosis may be quite difficult to differentiate from a low-grade infection or from a fracture of the clavicle.[28, 54, 74, 79, 103, 105] Some of the reported cases of idiopathic hyperostosis are very reminiscent of fractures occurring from child abuse.[32] Clavicular periostitis is also attributed to prostaglandin infusion[182] and to subclavian catheter insertion.[38] A branch of the supraclavicular nerve frequently passes through the clavicle and is occasionally visible.[50, 170] Gorham's disappearing bone disease[49] and Friedrich's juvenile chondrosis, which represents avascular necrosis of the medial clavicle, may occur.[33, 102, 157]

Treatment

While more than 200 methods of treatment for clavicle fractures have been described,[120] Nicoll[120] has stated:

> All that is really necessary is to support the elbow and brace the shoulders. The fractured clavicle cannot be immobilized (except perhaps by a shoulder spica incorporating the head). The usual compromise is that the patient attends daily to have his splint, strapping or bandage adjusted, thereby maintaining a reasonable degree of reduction for about a couple of hours a day, Sundays excepted.

Various splints, bandages, and dressings have been used to treat fractures of the clavicular shaft in children. Almost all clavicle shaft fractures in children can be treated nonoperatively.

Prevention. Obstetric care to prevent fractures of the clavicle can reduce the incidence by about half while maintaining the same fetal outcome.[154] Delivery of the posterior shoulder first and maneuvers are associated with a better outcome in shoulder dystocia.[56] It is generally difficult to prevent fractures of the clavicle in older children. Better pads for contact sports prevent some fractures of the clavicle by providing protection from direct blows.[162]

BIRTH INJURIES

Birth injuries rarely require treatment. Parents are instructed to lift the child by the waist rather than by the arms and to gently care for the child for about 2 weeks.[138] Parents should be instructed that a bump will appear once the fracture is healed and will take several months to fully resolve. If the child is uncomfortable, safety pinning the shirt sleeve to the shirt sufficiently prevents motion. The prognosis of *birth injuries* is excellent, and all children recover quite well.[20, 47, 100, 119, 172, 176] Preferably, the physician rather than the parents makes the diagnosis.[123] A fracture of the clavicle is no reflection on the quality of the obstetric care, and a missed fracture of the clavicle causes no harm.

PLASTIC BOWING

Bowen[12] recommends treating plasticity deformed fractures of the clavicle just like other clavicle fractures to prevent an overt fracture. Patients are followed-up and x-rayed within 2 to 4 weeks.

OLDER CHILDREN

Nonoperative Indications

Figure-of-Eight Splint. The figure-of-eight dressing is commonly used for fractures of the clavicle (Fig. 26–20). Usually these are commercial soft splints placed over the shoulders anteriorly and tied or buckled posteriorly to retract the shoulders. When used in children, it can be made out of stockinette with several sheets of cotton padding. The straps are tightened daily to remove any slackness. An additional anterior chest strap can prevent the tendency to slide laterally and exert a downward pull on the lateral clavicle.[146] Older patients should powder their arms frequently to prevent chafing.

The figure-of-eight splint does not gradually reduce the fracture.[117, 149] It can be quite uncomfortable, and if not used carefully, it can result in severe swelling, brachial plexus palsy, or compression of the neurovascular bundle.[34, 92, 117] The results are generally excellent. Ogden[128] indicates that no manipulation is needed in infants younger than 6 years of age. In children older than 6 years of age, he recommends giving a local anesthetic, retracting the shoulders over a sandbag or a knee, and tying the figure-of-eight. This treatment is supplemented

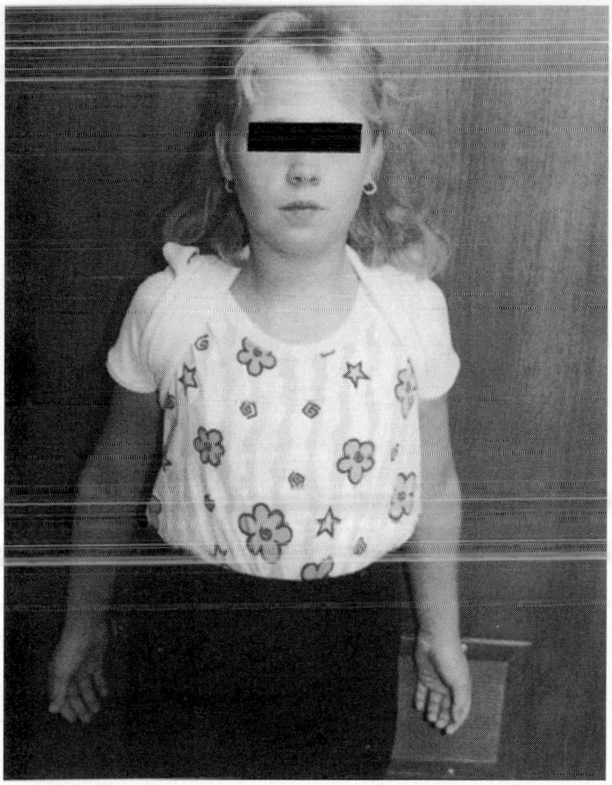

Figure 26–20

A figure-of-eight dressing applied to cause shoulder retraction. This can be uncomfortable if it pushes directly on the fracture site or irritates the lower brachial plexus.

with plaster in older patients.[128] Figure-of-eight casts have been advocated for unstable fractures with vascular injury,[111] in noncompliant teenagers,[128, 138] and in open fractures with less than optimal internal fixation.[68] Bohler[10] recommended the figure-of-eight splint for children younger than 10 years of age not because of improved results but to convince the parents that he was doing something.

Sling. Nondisplaced[138] and displaced fractures of the clavicle have good results when treated with a sling.[117, 120] Comparative studies between slings and figure-of-eight bandages show the same ultimate outcome, but the sling provides more comfort.[3, 71, 165]

Surgical. Fixation devices include suture, Kirschner wire fixation, modified Hagie pins, plate fixation, and external fixation. Intramedullary Kirschner wires result in a high incidence of pseudarthrosis with wires 2 mm in diameter or less and when causing diastasis.[160, 161] External fixation has the same indications as internal fixation with the potential advantages of no periosteal stripping and no second operation for removal.[108, 139, 155, 156, 184] Plating, with complications including superficial wound breakdown, refracture, malunion, nonunion, and difficulty in obtaining fixation in a short bone segment, has been described using the 2.7-mm ASIF dynamic compression plate (DCP),[159] 3.5-mm DCP,[136] and the low-contact DCP.[116]

Operative Indications

Potential operative indications include irreducible fractures,[11, 22, 24, 30, 159, 186] vascular injury,[135, 186] severe skin damage in open fractures,[130] marked displacement with potential skin ulceration,[128] brachial plexus palsy from clavicle compression, impingement of the clavicle upon the great vessels,[116, 186] and established symptomatic pseudarthrosis.[24, 116, 186] Severe shortening of the clavicle in adults may be associated with subjective abduction weakness[30, 129] but is unlikely to be a functional problem. Ogden describes skin ulceration from an unreduced clavicle fracture requiring subsequent débridement.[128] An irreducible clavicle in a child has been described in a 13-year-old girl who had a fracture of the clavicle and a dislocation of the sternoclavicular joint with the medial clavicle caught between the trapezius and the platysma. The girl was treated with an osseous suture and a plaster body jacket.[68] Vascular injury is not an absolute indication for internal fixation, and good results have been reported with both bed rest and open reduction with periosteal repair.[111, 171] A displaced scapular neck fracture in conjunction with a clavicle fracture may require internal fixation because of potential loss of shoulder support.[62, 94] A recent study, however, casts doubt on this.[52] Symptomatic pathologic fractures may also require fixation.[124]

In *older children,* union without permanent deformity is inevitable in children aged 10 and younger. In a series of children up to 17 years of age with head injuries and unable to have any treatment for fractures of the clavicle, all patients had excellent results with remodeling of up to 90 degrees of angulation and up to 4 cm of overlap.[180] Two patients with lateral clavicle injuries formed a double clavicle. One had complete reabsorption of the extra clavicle, whereas the other required excision later. In older teenagers and adults, shortening may be associated with some pain and subjective weakness to abduction.[31] However, this may be secondary to the surrounding soft tissue damage rather than to the injury to the clavicle itself.

AUTHORS' PREFERRED TREATMENT

Treatment of birth injuries is based on the symptoms. If the child is uncomfortable, we ask the parent to safety pin the sleeve to the shirt for a few weeks in order to keep the arm from moving into uncomfortable positions. If the child is comfortable, we inform the parents that the child will develop a bump over the fracture site. It remodels over several months and results in no long-term disability.

A number of older children present with figure-of-eight splints applied in emergency rooms and are quite uncomfortable. We usually remove the splint and replaced it with a sling, sometimes to the parent's chagrin, but to the patient's delight. We inform the parents that a bump will form over the area of the fracture, that the bone takes several months to remodel, and that it is extremely uncommon to have any subsequent difficulties. We prohibit contact sports until seeing adequate healing clinically or radiographically.

Very few indications exist for *operative treatment* of fractures of the clavicle in children. They include severe displacement with potential skin ulceration and direct impingement of the clavicle on the subclavian vessels and brachial plexus. Even these patients can sometimes be treated by closed manipulation of the fracture and by application of a figure-of-eight dressing or plaster cast. This is one of the few times that we prefer a figure-of-eight dressing to a sling. However, the figure-of-eight must be applied carefully to keep the shoulders retracted without causing lower brachial plexus irritation. Because the periosteum in children is stout, the clavicle can, if necessary, simply be placed back into the periosteal sleeve, the clavicle sutured through drill holes, and the periosteal sleeve repaired. This does not require a second operation for removal of hardware, and there is no chance of pin migration.

Complications

Malunion. *Malunion* of displaced fractures in children is inevitable.[9, 143, 167] However, as mentioned previously, children remodel quite well and have generally no long-term problems (Fig. 26–21). Other potential complications include early or late *brachial plexus palsy*.[5, 26, 27, 100] This may be caused by a figure-of-eight harness.[93, 117] If the plexus is explored, it has been suggested to correct the clavicle deformity, possibly resect the first rib, and correct any vascular lesions at the same time.[26] The *supraclavicular nerve* may be stretched;[43] however, irritation from fracture entrapment has not been reported. Reflex sympathetic dystrophy has been described in a 15-year-old boy who was hit by a football helmet.[67] *Pneumothorax* may occur in severe trauma and has been reported with birth trauma.[99] A *pseudocyst* of the clavicle has been described after a fracture; however, it is unclear what this represents.[63]

Vascular Injuries. These injuries include subclavian artery disruption, subclavian artery or vein compression, and arteriovenous fistulas.[5, 49, 64, 77, 171] Subclavian artery compression in a child can be treated with a figure-of-eight bandage and bed rest, but may require open reduction of the clavicle.[64, 171] Subclavian vein compression has been reported in a 13-year-old boy with a greenstick, posteroinferior angulated, midshaft clavicle fracture who was treated by fracture reduction using towel clips and held with a shoulder spica.[111] It is important to check the patient's pulses. Always look for evidence of vascular insufficiency, and do an angiogram if necessary.[13] Pay attention to a first rib fracture and mediastinal widening in severe trauma. Generally, vascular surgeons can do the repair through a supraclavicular approach,[151] however, a portion of the clavicle can be resected for exposure.[110]

Internal Fixation. *Internal fixation is associated with many problems* including pin migration,[35, 40, 101, 150] nonunion[36, 159, 161] refracture following plate removal[159] infection, and cosmetically unacceptable scars from both internal and external fixation.[156, 161]

Pseudarthrosis. Pseudarthrosis may result from a pathologic fracture,[124] or it may be traumatic or congenital. Traumatic pseudarthroses have been reported in children[107, 121, 140, 181] and are often, but not necessarily,[181] more symptomatic than congenital pseudarthrosis.[175] Techniques for treating traumatic pseudarthrosis were developed in adults and involve surgical intervention with compression of the site and bone grafting.[9, 18, 81, 107, 142, 181] The compression can be applied with either a dynamic compression plate or with a threaded screw such as a modified Hagie pin. Complications of pseudarthrosis repair include pneumothorax, subclavian vein damage, air embolism, and brachial plexus palsy.[30]

Congenital pseudarthrosis may be completely asymptomatic.[14] Surgery is indicated for pain or cosmesis.[15] The congenital pseudarthrosis may heal without an iliac crest bone graft.[55, 153] Because of the short fragments, it may be difficult to get good fixation with a dynamic compression plate,[29] and the repair can be complicated by brachial plexus palsy.[169] An arcuate incision over the second rib avoids the supraclavicular nerves and hides any keloid.[133]

For traumatic nonunion or pseudarthrosis, we prefer the technique of Rockwood that was reported by Boehme and associates.[9] (Fig. 26–22). In this technique, the entire extremity is draped from the base of the neck to the hand. These authors described making the incision directly over the clavicle in the lines of Langer; however, making the incision slightly inferior to the clavicle provides better cosmesis. The pseudarthrosis is exposed and débrided until bleeding bone is identified. The intramedullary canal is drilled using sequential curets and a hand drill. A modified Hagie pin* of the proper diameter is selected. One end of the pin has fine threads with a nut on it, and the other end has coarse built-up threads and a trochar

*A full set of clavicle pins and drills are produced by De Puy Orthopedic Co., Warsaw, Indiana.

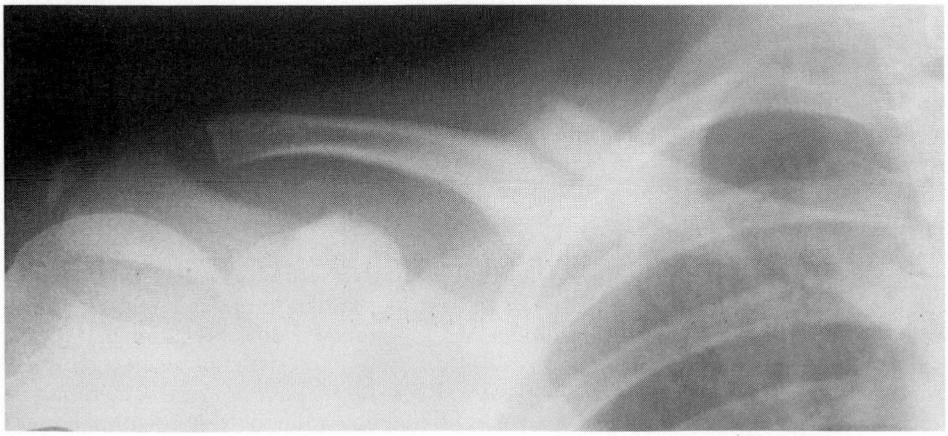

Figure 26–21

Even displaced, malunited clavicle fractures in children cause few, if any, problems. This 15 year old presented 6 weeks out from a clavicle fracture with marked shortening. He has full, painless motion and a small palpable mass. The patient was allowed to return to contact sports and has had no further difficulties. (From Rockwood CA, Wilkins KE, Beaty J [eds]: Fractures in Children. Philadelphia: JB Lippincott, 1996.)

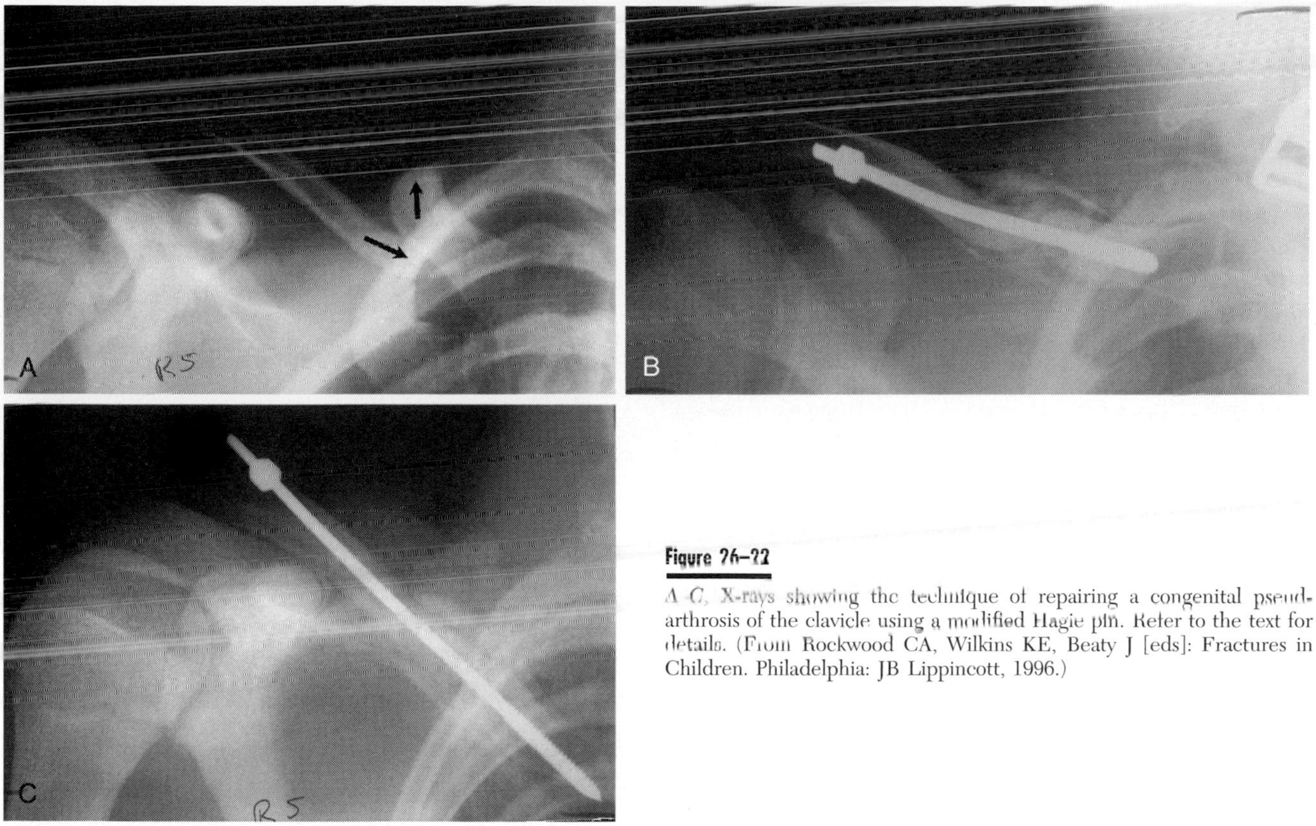

Figure 26–22

A–C, X-rays showing the technique of repairing a congenital pseudarthrosis of the clavicle using a modified Hagie pin. Refer to the text for details. (From Rockwood CA, Wilkins KE, Beaty J [eds]: Fractures in Children. Philadelphia: JB Lippincott, 1996.)

point. The end of the pin with the fine threads is drilled through the lateral fragment and enters the posterior cortex of the clavicle posterior and medial to the acromioclavicular joint. It is then drilled out to the skin through a small incision. The hand drill is then attached to the lateral end of the pin. With the pseudarthrosis held reduced, the trochar point is fed into the medullary canal and the coarse threaded end of the pin is drilled into the medial fragment. The nonthreaded portion of the pin is at the pseudarthrosis site. The nut is tightened on the pin until compression is obtained. A bone graft is placed. The pin or plate is removed once healing is complete.

References and Bibliography

1. Abbott L and Lucas D: Function of the clavicle: Its surgical significance. Ann Surg *140:*583–599, 1954.
2. Allman FL: Fractures and ligamentous injuries of the clavicle and its articulations. J Bone Joint Surg Am *49:*774, 1967.
3. Andersen K, Jensen PO, and Lauritzen J: Treatment of clavicular fractures: Figure-of-eight bandage versus a simple sling. Acta Orthop Scand *58:*71–74, 1987.
4. Bartoli E, Saporetti N, and Marchetti S: The role of echography in the diagnosis of neonatal clavicular fractures [in Italian]. Radiol Med (Torino) *77:*466–469, 1989.
5. Bateman JE: Neurovascular syndromes related to the clavicle. Clin Orthop *58:*75–82, 1968.
6. Behringer BR and Wilson FC: Congenital pseudarthrosis of the clavicle. Am J Dis Child *123:*511–517, 1972.
7. Bianchi G and Bertoni GP: Bilateral fracture of the clavicle in the newborn [in Italian]. Minerva Pediatr *19:*2226–2229, 1967.
8. Blount WP: Fractures in Children. Baltimore: Williams & Wilkins, 1954, pp 9–20.
9. Boehme D, Curtis RJ, DeHaan JT, et al: Nonunion of fractures of the midshaft of the clavicle: Treatment with a modified Hagie intramedullary pin and autogenous bonegrafting. J Bone Joint Surg Am *73:*1219–1226, 1991.
10. Bohler L: The Treatment of Fractures—Supplement. New York: Grune & Stratton, 1966.
11. Bonnet J: Fracture of the clavicle. Arch Chir Neerl *27:*143–151, 1975.
12. Bowen A: Plastic bowing of the clavicle in children: A report of two cases. J Bone Joint Surg Am *65:*403–405, 1983.
13. Bowers VD and Watkins GM: Blunt trauma to the thoracic outlet and angiography. Am Surg *49:*655–659, 1983.
14. Brooks S: Bilateral congenital pseudarthrosis of the clavicles—case report and review of the literature. Br J Clin Pract *38:*432–433, 1984.
15. Brunner C and Morger R: Congenital non-union of the clavicle [Author's translation in German]. Pediatr Padol *16:*137–141, 1981.
16. Camus M, Lefebvre G, Veron P, and Darbois Y: Obstetrical injuries of the newborn infant: Retrospective study a propos of 20,409 births. J Gynecol Obstet Biol Reprod (Paris) *14:*1033–1043, 1985.
17. Capanna R, Sudanese A, Ruggieri P, and Biagini R: Aneurysmal cyst of the clavicle. Chir Organi Mov *70:*157–161, 1985.
18. Capicotto PN, Heiple KG, and Wilbur JH: Midshaft clavicle nonunions treated with intramedullary Steinman pin fixation and onlay bone graft. J Orthop Trauma *8:*88–93, 1994.
19. Celenza M, Bertini G, De Tullio V, et al: [A case of a fracture of the clavicle associated with an acromio-clavicular luxation] [in Italian]. Minerva Med *81:*127–129, 1990.
20. Chez RA, Carlan S, Greenberg SL, and Spellacy WN: Fractured clavicle is an unavoidable event. Am J Obstet Gynecol *171:*797–798, 1994.
21. Colavita N, La Vecchia G, Book E, and Vincenzoni M: Congenital pseudarthrosis of the clavicle: Roentgenographic appearance and discussion of the aetiological and pathogenetical theories. Radiol Med (Torino) *66:*923–926, 1980.
22. Cooper SB: Fractures of the clavicle in infants and young children: ONA J *4:*187–188, 1977.
23. Cumming WA: Neonatal skeletal fractures: Birth trauma or child abuse? J Can Assoc Radiol *30:*30–33, 1979.
24. Curtis RJJ: Operative management of children's fractures of the

shoulder region (Review). Orthop Clin North Am *21:*315–324, 1990.

25. Curtis RJJ, Dameron TB Jr, and Rockwood CA Jr: Fractures and dislocations of the shoulder in children. *In* Rockwood CAJ, Wilkins KE, and King RE (eds): Fractures in Children. Philadelphia, JB Lippincott, 1991, pp 829–919.
26. Della Santa D, Narakas A, and Bonnard C: Late lesions of the brachial plexus after fracture of the clavicle. Ann Chir Main Memb Super *10:*531–540, 1991.
27. Della Santa DR and Narakas AO: Fractures of the clavicle and secondary lesions of the brachial plexus. Z Unfallchir Versicherungsmed *85:*58–65, 1992.
28. Eftekhari F, Jaffe N, Schwegel D, and Ayala A: Inflammatory metachronous hyperostosis of the clavicle and femur in children. Report of two cases, one with long-term follow-up. Skeletal Radiol *18:*9–14, 1989.
29. Engert J, Klumpp H, and Simon G: Clavicular pseudarthroses in childhood. Chirurg *50:*631–635, 1979.
30. Eskola A, Vaininonpaa S, Myllynen P, et al: Surgery for ununited clavicular fracture. Acta Orthop Scand *57:*366–367, 1986.
31. Eskola A, Vaininonpaa S, Myllynen P, et al: Outcome of clavicular fracture in 89 patients. Arch Orthop Trauma Surg *105:*337–338, 1986.
32. Finsterbush A and Husseini N: Infantile cortical hyperostosis with unusual clinical manifestations. Clin Orthop *144:*276–279, 1979.
33. Fischel RE and Bernstein D: Friedrich's disease. Br J Radiol *48:*318–319, 1975.
34. Fowler AW: Treatment of fractured clavicle. Lancet: *1:*46–47, 1968.
35. Fowler AW: Migration of a wire from the sternoclavicular joint to the pericardial cavity (Letter). Injury *13:*261–262, 1981.
36. Franklin JL, Parker JC, and King HA: Nontraumatic clavicle lesions in children. J Pediatr Orthop *7:*575–578, 1987.
37. Freedman M, Gamble J, and Lewis C: Intrauterine fracture simulating a unilateral clavicular pseudarthrosis. J Can Assoc Radiol *33:*37–38, 1982.
38. Friedman AP, Velcek FT, Haller JO, and Nagar H: Clavicular periostitis: An unusual complication of percutaneous subclavian venous catheterization. Radiology *148:*692, 1983.
39. Friedrich I, Junge WD, and Fischer B: Causes of clavicular fracture in newborns. Zentralbl Gynakol *101:*1528–1531, 1979.
40. Fueter-Tondury M: Migration of the wire after osteosynthesis. Schweiz Med Wochenschr *106:*1890–1896, 1976.
41. Gardner E: Prenatal development of the human shoulder joint. Surg Clin North Am 92:219–276, 1953.
42. Gardner E: The embryology of the clavicle. Clin Orthop *58:*9–16, 1968.
43. Gelberman RH, Verdeck WN, and Brodhead WT: Supraclavicular nerve-entrapment syndrome. J Bone Joint Surg Am *57:*119, 1975.
44. Gerscovich EO and Greenspan A: Osteomyelitis of the clavicle: Clinical, radiologic, and bacteriologic findings in ten patients. Skeletal Radiol *23:*205–210, 1994.
45. Gerscovich EO, Greenspan A, and Szabo RM.: Benign clavicular lesions that may mimic malignancy. Skeletal Radiol *20:*173–180, 1991.
46. Gibson DA and Carroll N: Congenital pseudarthrosis of the clavicle. J Bone Joint Surg Br *52:*629–643, 1970.
47. Gilbert WM and Tchabo JG: Fractured clavicle in newborns. Int Surg *73:*123–125, 1988.
48. Gitsch G and Schatten C: Incidence and potential factors in the genesis of birth injury-induced clavicular fractures. Zentralbl Gynakol *109:*909–912, 1987.
49. Glass-Royal M and Stull MA: Musculoskeletal case of the day: Gorham syndrome of the right clavicle and scapula. AJR Am J Roentgenol *154:*1335–1336, 1990.
50. Goldenberg DB and Brogdon BG: Congenital anomalies of the pectoral girdle demonstrated by chest radiography. J Can Assoc Radiol *18:*472–477, 1967.
51. Gonik B, Hollyer VL, and Allen R: Shoulder dystocia recognition: Differences in neonatal risks for injury. Am J Perinatol *8:*31–34, 1991.
52. Goodnight JM, Rockwood CA Jr, and Wirth MA: Ipsilateral fractures of the clavicle and scapula (Abstract). Submitted for Publication, 1996.
53. Graif M, Stahl-Kent V, Ben-Ami T, et al: Sonographic detection of occult bone fractures. Pediatr Radiol *18:*383–385, 1988.
54. Griffiths HJ and Ozer H: Changes in the medial half of the clavicle—new sign in renal osteodystrophy. J Can Assoc Radiol *24:*334–336, 1973.
55. Grogan DP, Love SM, Guidera KJ, and Ogden JA: Operative treatment of congenital pseudarthrosis of the clavicle. J Pediatr Orthop *11:*176–180, 1991.
56. Gross SJ, Shime J, and Farine D: Shoulder dystocia: Predictors and outcome. Am J Obstet Gynecol *156:*334–336, 1987.
57. Guidera KJ, Grogan DP, Pugh L, and Ogden JA: Hypoplastic clavicles and lateral scapular redirection. J Pediatr Orthop *11:*523–526, 1991.
58. Hardy JR: Complex clavicular injury in childhood. J Bone Joint Surg Br *74:*154, 1992.
59. Haskell L, Bloom RA, Rottem M, et al: Bilateral symmetrical clavicular periosteal reactions in a child. Diagn Imaging Clin Med *53:*310–314, 1984.
60. Herman S: Congenital bilateral pseudarthrosis of the clavicles. Clin Orthop *91:*162–163, 1973.
61. Herndon WA: Child abuse in a military population. J Pediatr Orthop *3:*73–76, 1983.
62. Herscovici D Jr, Fiennes AG, Allgower M, and Ruedi TP: The floating shoulder: Ipsilateral clavicle and scapular neck fractures. J Bone Joint Surg Br *74:*362–364, 1992.
63. Houston HE: An unusual complication of clavicular fracture. J Ky Med Assoc *75:*170–171, 1977.
64. Howard FM and Shafer SJ: Injuries to the clavicle with neurovascular complications: A study of fourteen cases. J Bone Joint Surg Am *47:*1335–1346, 1965.
65. Iffy L, Varadi V, and Jakobovits A: Common intrapartum denominators of shoulder dystocia related birth injuries. Zentralbl Gynakol *116:*33–37, 1994.
66. Iqbal QM: Long bone fractures among children in Malaysia. Int Surg *59:*410–415, 1974.
67. Ivey M, Britt M, and Johnston RV Jr: Reflex sympathetic dystrophy after clavicle fracture: Case report. J Trauma *31:*276–279, 1991.
68. Jablon M, Sutker A, and Post M: Irreducible fracture of the middle third of the clavicle: Report of a case. J Bone Joint Surg Am *61:*296–298, 1979.
69. Jackson ST, Hoffer MM, and Parrish N: Brachial-plexus palsy in the newborn. J Bone Joint Surg Am *70:*1217–1220, 1988.
70. Jelic A, Marin L, Pracny M, and Jelic N: Fractures of the clavicle in neonates. Lijec Vjesn *114:*32–35, 1992.
71. Jensen PO, Andersen K, and Lauritzen J: Treatment of midclavicular fractures: A prospective randomized trial comparing treatment with a figure-eight dressing and a simple arm sling [in Danish]. Ugeskr Laeger *147:*1986–1988, 1985.
72. Ji L, Terazawa K, Tsukamoto T, and Haga K: Estimation of age from epiphyseal union degrees of the sternal end of the clavicle. Hokkaido Igaku Zasshi *69:*104–111, 1994.
73. Jinkins WJ Jr: Congenital pseudarthrosis of the clavicle. Clin Orthop *62:*183–186, 1969.
74. Jirik FR, Stein HB, and Chalmers A: Clavicular hyperostosis with enthesopathy, hypergammaglobulinemia, and thoracic outlet syndrome. Ann Intern Med *97:*48–50, 1982.
75. Jit I and Kaur H: Rhomboid fossa in the clavicles of North Indians. Am J Phys Anthropol *70:*97–103, 1986.
76. Jit I and Kulkarni M: Times of appearance and fusion of epiphysis at the medial end of the clavicle. Indian J Med Res *64:*773–782, 1976.
77. Jojart G and Nagy G: Ultrasonographic screening of neonatal adrenal apoplexy. Int Urol Nephrol *24:*591–596, 1992.
78. Jojart G, Zubek L, and Toth G: Clavicle fracture in the newborn. Orv Hetil *132:*2655–2657, 1991.
79. Jones ET, Hensinger RN, and Holt JF: Idiopathic cortical hyperostosis. Clin Orthop *163:*210–213, 1982.
80. Joseph PR and Rosenfeld W: Clavicular fractures in neonates. Am J Dis Child *144:*165–167, 1990.
81. Jupiter JB and Leffert RD: Non-union of the clavicle: Associated complications and surgical management. J Bone Joint Surg Am *69:*753–760, 1987.
82. Jurik AG and Moller BN: Inflammatory hyperostosis and sclerosis of the clavicle. Skeletal Radiol *15:*284–290, 1986.
83. Kato T, Kanbara H, Sato S, and Tanaka I: 5 cases of clavicular fractures misdiagnosed as congenital myogenic torticollis. Seikei Geka *19:*729–732, 1968.

84. Katz R, Landman J, Dulitzky F, and Bar-Ziv J: Fracture of the clavicle in the newborn. An ultrasound diagnosis. J Ultrasound Med *7:*21–23, 1988.
85. Kaur H and Jit I: Brief communication: Coracoclavicular joint in Northwest Indians. Am J Phys Anthropol *85:*457–460, 1991.
86. Keipert JA and Campbell PE: Recurrent hyperostosis of the clavicles: An undiagnostic syndrome. Aust Paediatr J *6:*97–104, 1970.
87. Kite JH: Congenital pseudarthrosis of the clavicle. South Med J *61:*703–710, 1968.
88. Kochhar VL and Srivastava KK: Unusual lesions of the clavicle. Int Surg *61:*51–53, 1976.
89. Kochhar VL and Srivastava KK: Anatomical and functional considerations in total claviclectomy. Clin Orthop *118:*199–201, 1976.
90. Kogutt MS, Swischuk LE, and Fagan CJ: Patterns of injury and significance of uncommon fractures in the battered child syndrome. Am J Roentgenol Radium Ther Nucl Med *121:*143–149, 1974.
91. Landin LA: Fracture patterns in children: Analysis of 8682 fractures with special reference to incidence, etiology and secular changes in Swedish urban populations. Acta Orthop Scand Suppl *54:*1–109, 1983.
92. Leffert RD: Brachial-plexus injuries. N Engl J Med *291:*1059–1067, 1974.
93. Lemire L and Rosman M: Sternoclavicular epiphyseal separation with adjacent clavicular fracture. J Pediatr Orthop *4:*118–120, 1984.
94. Leung KS and Lam TP: Open reduction and internal fixation of ipsilateral fractures of the scapular neck and clavicle. J Bone Joint Surg Am *75:*1015–1018, 1993.
95. Levine MG, Holroyde J, Woods JR Jr, et al: Birth trauma: Incidence and predisposing factors. Obstet Gynecol *63:*792–795, 1984.
96. Lewis MM, Ballet FL, Kroll PG, and Bloom N: En bloc clavicular resection: Operative procedure and postoperative testing of function: Case reports. Clin Orthop *193:*214–220, 1985.
97. Lichtenberg RP: A study of 2,532 fractures in children. Am J Surg *87:*330–338, 1954.
98. Lombard JJ: Pseudarthrosis of the clavicle: A case report. S Afr Med J *66:*151–153, 1984.
99. Longo R and Ruggiero L: Left pneumothorax with subcutaneous emphysema secondary to left clavicular fracture and homolateral obstetrical paralysis of the arm in [in Italian]. Minerva Pediatr *34:*273–276, 1982.
100. Lubrano di Diego JG, Chappuis JP, Montsegur P, et al: About of 82 obstetrical astro-articular injuries of the new-born (excepting brachial plexus palsies): Limits of initial therapeutic aggression and follow-up of evolution, particularly concerning traumatic separation of upper femoral epiphysis. Chir Pediatr *19:*219–226, 1978.
101. Lyons FA and Rockwood CA: Current concepts review: Migration of pins used in operations on the shoulder. J Bone Joint Surg Am *72:*1262–1267, 1990.
102. Macule F, Ferreres A, Palliso F, et al: Aseptic necrosis of the sternal end of the clavicle Friedrich's disease. Acta Orthop Belg *56:*613–615, 1990.
103. Madsen JL: Scintigraphic detection of clavicular hyperostosis in a patient with fulminant acne. Clin Nucl Med *13:*345, 1988.
104. Madsen TE: Fractures of the extremities in the newborn. Acta Obstet Gynecol Scand *34:*41, 1955.
105. Magnus L and Sauerbrei HU: Two cases of infantile cortical hyperostosis (monostotic form). Rofo Fortschr Geb Rontgenstr Nuklearmed *128:*530–533, 1978.
106. Manashil G and Laufer S: Congenital pseudarthrosis of the clavicle: Report of three cases. AJR Am J Roentgenol *132:*678–679, 1979.
107. Manske DJ and Szabo RM: The operative treatment of mid-shaft clavicular non-unions. J Bone Joint Surg Am *67:*1367–1371, 1985.
108. Maurin X: External fixation of fractures of the clavicle. Chirurgie *101:*367–375, 1975.
109. Meghdari A, Davoodi R, and Mesbah F: Engineering analysis of shoulder dystocia in the human birth process by the finite element method. Proc Inst Mech Eng [H] *206:*243–250, 1992.
110. Meyer JP, Goldfaden D, Barrett J, et al: Subclavian and innominate artery trauma: A recent experience with nine patients. J Cardiovasc Surg (Torino) *29:*283–289, 1988.
111. Mital MA and Aufranc OE: Venous occlusion following greenstick fracture of clavicle. JAMA *206:*1301–1302, 1968.
112. Mollan RA, Craig BF, and Biggart JD: Chronic sclerosing osteomyelitis: An unusual case. J Bone Joint Surg Br *66:*583–585, 1984.
113. Morin LR, Fossey FP, Besselievre A, et al. Congenital pseudarthrosis of the clavicle. Acta Obstet Gynecol Scand *72:*120–121, 1993.
114. Mortensson W, Edeburn G, Fries M, and Nilsson R: Chronic recurrent multifocal osteomyelitis in children: A roentgenologic and scintigraphic investigation. Acta Radiol *29:*565–570, 1988.
115. Mulimba JA: Fractures of the humerus. East Afr Med J *60:*843–847, 1983.
116. Mullaji AB and Jupiter JB: Low-contact dynamic compression plating of the clavicle. Injury *25:*41–45, 1994.
117. Mullick S: Treatment of mid-clavicular fractures (Letter). Lancet *1:*499, 1967.
118. Nadas S, Gudinchet F, Capasso P, and Reinberg O: Predisposing factors in obstetrical fractures. Skeletal Radiol *22:*195–198, 1993.
119. Nadas S and Reinberg O: Obstetric fractures. Eur J Pediatr Surg *2:*165–168, 1992.
120. Nicoll EA: Annotation: Miners and mannequins. J Bone Joint Surg Br *36:*171–172, 1954.
121. Nogi J, Heckman JD, Hakala M, and Sweet DE: Non union of the clavicle in a child. A case report. Clin Orthop *110:*19–21, 1975
122. Nordqvist A and Petersson C: The incidence of fractures of the clavicle. Clin Orthop *110:*127–132, 1994.
123. O'Halloran MJ: Clavicular fractures in neonates: Frequency vs significance (Letter; comment). Am J Dis Child *145:*251, 1991.
124. O'Rourke IC and Middleton RWD: The place and efficacy of operative management of fractured clavicle. Injury *6:*236–240, 1975.
125. Oestreich AE: The lateral clavicle hook—an acquired as well as a congenital anomaly. Pediatr Radiol *11:*147–150, 1981.
126. Ogata S and Uhthoff HK: The early development and ossification of the human clavicle—an embryologic study. Acta Orthop Scand *61:*330–334, 1990.
127. Ogden JA: Distal clavicular physeal injury. Clin Orthop *188:*68–73, 1984.
128. Ogden JA: Skeletal Injury in the Child. Philadelphia: WB Saunders, 1990.
129. Ogden JA, Conlogue GJ, and Bronson ML: Radiology of postnatal skeletal development. III. The clavicle. Skeletal Radiol *4:*196–203, 1979.
130. Ohel G, Haddad S, Fischer O, and Levit A: Clavicular fracture of the neonate: Can it be predicted before birth? Am J Perinatol *10:*441–443, 1993.
131. Oni OO, Hoskinson J, and McPherson S: Closed traumatic scapulothoracic dissociation. Injury *23:*138–139, 1992.
132. Oppenheim WL, Davis A, Growdon WA et al: Clavicle fractures in the newborn. Clin Orthop *250:*176–180, 1990.
133. Owen R: Congenital pseudarthrosis of the clavicle. J Bone Joint Surg Br *52:*644–652, 1970.
134. Paul R, Ahonen A, Virtama P, et al: F-18 fluorodeoxyglucose: Its potential in differentiating between stress fracture and neoplasia. Clin Nucl Med *14:*906–908, 1989.
135. Poigenfurst J, Rappold G, and Fischer W: Plating of fresh clavicular fractures: Results of 122 operations. Injury *23:*237–241, 1992.
136. Poigenfurst J, Reiler T, and Fischer W: Plating of fresh clavicular fractures: Experience with 60 operations. Unfallchirurgie *14:*26–37, 1988.
137. Pointu J, Kehr P, Sejourne P, et al: Aneurysmal cyst of the clavicle: An uncommon lesion and a difficult diagnosis. Sem Hop *58:*1141–1143, 1982.
138. Post M: Current concepts in the treatment of fractures of the clavicle. Clin Orthop *245:*89–101, 1989.
139. Putnam MD and Walsh TM: External fixation for open fractures of the upper extremity. Hand Clin *9:*613–623, 1993.
140. Pyper JB: Non-union of fractures of the clavicle. Injury *9:*268–270, 1978.
141. Quinlan WR, Brady PG, and Regan BF: Congenital pseudarthrosis of the clavicle. Acta Orthop Scand *51:*489–492, 1980.
142. Rabenseifner L: Etiology and therapy of clavicular pseudarthrosis. Aktuel Traumatol *11:*130–132, 1981.
143. Rang M: Clavicle. *In* Rang M (ed): Children's Fractures. Philadelphia: JB Lippincott, 1983, pp 139–142.
144. Rasool MN and Govender S: Infections of the clavicle in children. Clin Orthop *265:*178–182, 1991.

145. Riemer BL, Butterfield SL, Daffner RH, and O'Keeffe RMJ: The abduction lordotic view of the clavicle: A new technique for radiographic visualization. J Orthop Trauma *5:*392–394, 1991.
146. Rowe CR: An atlas of anatomy and treatment of midclavicular fractures. Clin Orthop *58:*29–42, 1968.
147. Salam A, Eyres K, and Cleary J: Malignant Langerhans' cell histiocytosis of the clavicle: A rare pathological fracture. Br J Clin Pract *44:*652–654, 1990.
148. Salonen IS and Uusitalo R: Birth injuries: Incidence and predisposing factors. Z Kinderchir *45:*133–135, 1990.
149. Sankarankutty M and Turner BW: Fractures of the clavicle. Injury *7:*101–106, 1975.
150. Sartoris DJ, Mochizuki RM, and Parker BR: Lytic clavicular lesions in fibromatosis colli. Skeletal Radiol *10:*34–36, 1983.
151. Schaff HV and Brawley RK: Operative management of penetrating vascular injuries of the thoracic outlet. Surgery *82:*182–191, 1977.
152. Schmelzeisen H: Eosinophilic granuloma: Risk of fracture and rare site. Aktuel Traumatol *18:*(Suppl 1):67–75, 1988.
153. Schoenecker PL, Johnson GE, Howard B, and Capelli AM: Congenital pseudarthrosis. Orthop Rev *21:*855–860, 1992.
154. Schrocksnadel H, Heim K, and Dapunt O: The clavicular fracture—a questionable achievement in modern obstetrics. Geburtshilfe Frauenheilkd *49:*481–484, 1989.
155. Schuind F, Pay-Pay E, Andrianne Y, et al: Osteosynthesis of the clavicle using an external fixator. Acta Orthop Belg *55:*191–196, 1989.
156. Schuind F, Pay-Pay E, Andrianne Y, et al: External fixation of the clavicle for fracture or non-union in adults. J Bone Joint Surg Am *70:*692–695, 1988.
157. Schumacher R, Muller U, and Schuster W: Rare localization of osteochondrosis juvenilis. Radiologe *21:*165–174, 1981.
158. Schwartz EE, Lantieri R, and Teplick JG: Erosion of the inferior aspect of the clavicle in secondary hyperparathyroidism. AJR Am J Roentgenol *129:*291–295, 1977.
159. Schwarz N and Hocker K: Osteosynthesis of irreducible fractures of the clavicle with 2.7-mm ASIF plates. J Trauma *33:*179–183, 1992.
160. Schwarz N and Leixnering M: Failures of clavicular intramedullary wire fixation and their causes. Aktuel Traumatol *14:*159–163, 1984.
161. Schwarz N and Leixnering M: Technic and results of clavicular medullary wiring. Zentralbl Chir *111:*640–647, 1986.
162. Silloway KA, McLaughlin RE, Edlich RC, and Edlich RF: Clavicular fractures and acromioclavicular joint dislocations in lacrosse: Preventable injuries. J Emerg Med *3:*117–121, 1985.
163. Smith J, Yuppa F, and Watson RC: Primary tumors and tumor-like lesions of the clavicle. Skeletal Radiol *17:*235–246, 1988.
164. Snyder LA: Loss of the accompanying soft tissue shadow of the clavicle with occult fractures (Letter). South Med J *72:*243, 1979.
165. Stanley D and Norris SH: Recovery following fractures of the clavicle treated conservatively. Injury *19:*162–164, 1988.
166. Stanley D, Trowbridge EA, and Norris SH: The mechanism of clavicular fractures: A clinical and biomechanical analysis. J Bone Joint Surg *70:*461–464, 1988.
167. Taylor AR: Some observations on fractures of the clavicle. Proc R Soc Med *62:*1037–1038, 1969.
168. Teplick JG, Eftekhari F, and Haskin ME: Erosion of the sternal ends of the clavicles: A new sign of primary and secondary hyperparathyroidism. Radiology *113:*323–326, 1974.
169. Toledo LC and MacEwen GD: Severe complication of surgical treatment of congenital pseudarthrosis of the clavicle. Clin Orthop *139:*64–67, 1979.
170. Treble NJ: Normal variations in radiographs of the clavicle: Brief report. J Bone Joint Surg Br *70:*490, 1988.
171. Tse DH, Slabaugh PB, and Carlson PA: Injury to the axillary artery by a closed fracture of the clavicle: A case report. J Bone Joint Surg Am *62:*1372–1374, 1980.
172. Turnpenny PD and Nimmo A: Fractured clavicle of the newborn in a population with a high prevalence of grand-multiparity: Analysis of 78 consecutive cases. Br J Obstet Gynaecol *100:*338–341, 1993.
173. Van Goethem H and Van Goethem C: Bilateral aplasia of the radius with abnormal hooking of the claviculae and sucrose-maltose intolerance. Helv Paediatr Acta *36:*271–280, 1981.
174. Waldman RS and Powell T: Eosinophilic granuloma of the clavicle simulating primary bone neoplasm. Clin Orthop *64:*150–152, 1969.
175. Wall JJ: Congenital pseudarthrosis of the clavicle. J Bone Joint Surg Am *52:*1003–1009, 1970.
176. Walle T and Hartikainen-Sorri AL: Obstetric shoulder injury: Associated risk factors, prediction and prognosis. Acta Obstet Gynecol Scand *72:*450–454, 1993.
177. Waninger KN and Chung MK: A new clue to clavicular fracture in newborn infants (Letter)? Pediatrics *88:*657, 1991.
178. Webb PA and Suchey JM: Epiphyseal union of the anterior iliac crest and medial clavicle in a modern multiracial sample of American males and females. Am J Phys Anthropol *68:*457–466, 1985.
179. Weinberg B, Seife B, and Alonso P: The apical oblique view of the clavicle: Its usefulness in neonatal and childhood trauma. Skeletal Radiol *20:*201–203, 1991.
180. Wilkes JA and Hoffer MM: Clavicle fractures in head-injured children. J Orthop Trauma *1:*55–58, 1987.
181. Wilkins RM and Johnston RM: Ununited fractures of the clavicle. J Bone Joint Surg Am *65:*773–778, 1983.
182. Woo K, Emery J, and Peabody J: Cortical hyperostosis: A complication of prolonged prostaglandin infusion in infants awaiting cardiac transplantation. Pediatrics *93:*417–420, 1994.
183. Worlock P and Stower M: Fracture patterns in Nottingham children. J Pediatr Orthop *6:*656–661, 1986.
184. Xiao XY: Treatment of clavicular fracture patient with a percutaneous bone-embracing external clavicular microfixer. Chung Hua Wai Ko Tsa Chih *31:*657–659, 1993.
185. Yates DW: Complications of fractures of the clavicle. Injury *7:*189–193, 1976.
186. Zenni EJ Jr, Krieg JK, and Rosen MJ: Open reduction and internal fixation of clavicular fractures. J Bone Joint Surg Am *63:*147–151, 1981.

MEDIAL CLAVICLE AND STERNOCLAVICULAR INJURIES

Anatomic Considerations

The epiphysis at the medial end of the clavicle is the last epiphysis of the long bones to appear and fuses to the shaft of the clavicle at the start of the third decade (see Fig. 26–13).[13, 17, 31, 41] The anatomy of the clavicle was discussed previously. Posterior to the joint are the great vessels and mediastinal structures. The joint allows movement in three axes. It can elevate 45 degrees, depress 5 degrees, and protract and retract 15 degrees. Rotation of 45 to 50 degrees can also occur.[2, 7, 10, 27]

Incidence

The true incidence of injuries to the medial end of the clavicle in children is unknown. Knowledge of these injuries is contained in case reports and in small series that define a variety of treatments with short-term follow-up.[1, 4, 5, 9, 16, 19, 21, 38, 40, 42, 43] Rowe reports that fractures and dislocations of the medial clavicle constitute less than 6% of all injuries of the clavicle for all age groups.[35] Rang estimates that injuries to the medial clavicle comprise only 1% of all clavicle injuries in children.[33] Nordquist and Petersson found that Allman type II injuries constitute 3% of all clavicle fractures.[29]

Mechanism of Injury

Injuries to the medial clavicle may be secondary to direct or indirect trauma.[5, 16, 18, 19, 29, 32, 39] Biomechanical analysis and clinical experience suggest that most injuries to the medial clavicle are a result of direct trauma, such as a fall onto the shoulder leading to compressive loading on the clavicle. The direction of the load determines the subsequent displacement.[39]

Classification

Extraphyseal fractures of the medial clavicle in children have been reported,[14, 15] but the majority of reported injuries to this region in children are Salter Harris type I and type II injuries (Fig. 26–23).[1, 4, 9, 19, 21, 42, 43] The displacement can be anterior or posterior. Anterior displacements of sternoclavicular joint injuries occur twice as often as do posterior displacements[34, 36] in large series, but most case reports in the literature are for retrosternal displacements due to the morbidity associated with these injuries. True dislocation of the sternoclavicular joint in children is rare. Most reported cases of younger patients are part of a larger series of adults and do not exclude Salter-Harris injuries as a possibility.[16, 26, 37, 38] Painful chronic instability has been reported in a 12-year-old patient.[24]

Signs and Symptoms

Minimally displaced injuries may have few symptoms or clinical findings, and the diagnosis is often delayed. The child or parent may only notice a mass secondary to callus formation. Children with displaced injuries to the medial clavicle present with swelling and pain. They will often tilt the head toward the side of injury.[37] Initial assessment of deformity may be difficult owing to the swelling; but the contour of the chest will generally be altered (Figs. 26–24 and 26–25). Anterior dislocations are obvious on examination. Posterior dislocations can be more difficult to diagnose and may be associated with injury to the retrosternal structures. Venous congestion, choking, difficulty swallowing, diminished pulses, difficulty breathing, and neurologic complaints related to the brachial plexus have been all reported in association with these injuries and must be taken seriously.[34] These signs and symptoms may suggest underlying pneumothorax, brachial plexus injury, laceration of the superior vena cava, rupture of the esophagus, occlusion of the subclavian artery, or rupture of the trachea requiring urgent attention.

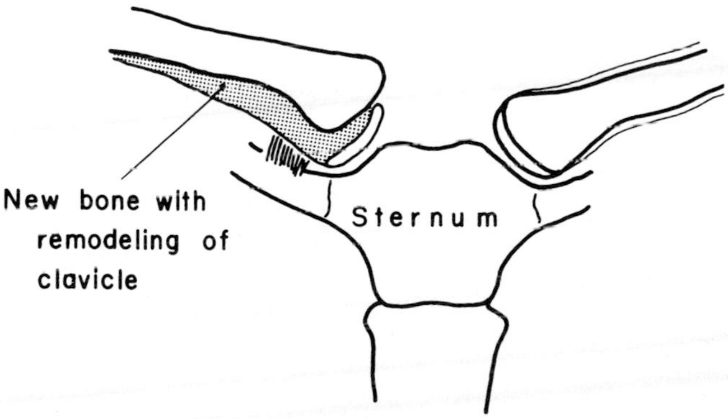

Figure 26–23

Diagram depicting a Salter-Harris type I injury to the medial clavicular physis. Healing is by periosteal new bone with significant potential for remodeling.

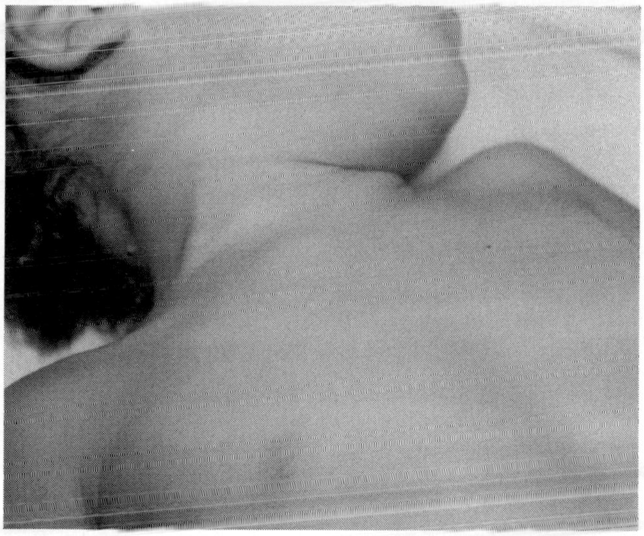

Figure 26–24

Clinical photograph of a young boy with a right anteriorly displaced medial clavicular injury.

Radiographic Findings

Several specialized radiographic techniques can aid in the imaging of fractures and dislocations of the medial clavi-

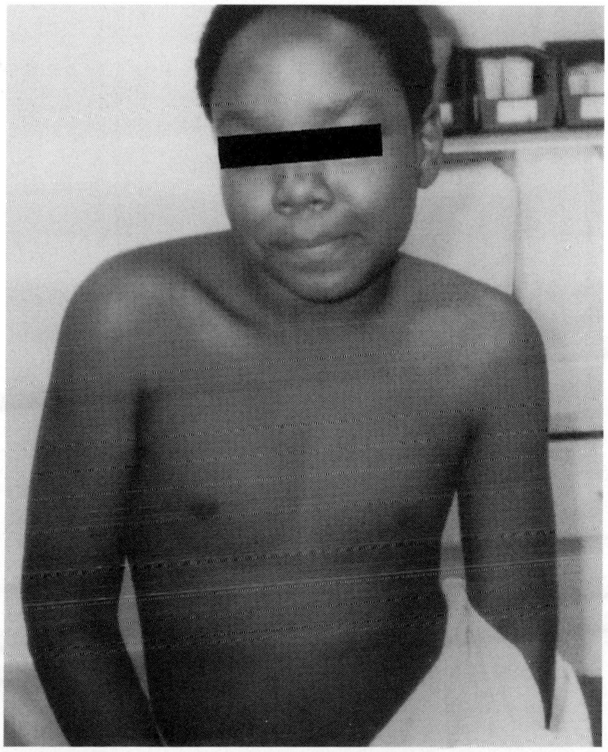

Figure 26–25

Posterior displacement of a medial clavicular injury. Notice the loss of contour of the left clavicle compared with the normal right side.

cle and sternoclavicular joint. A 40-degree cephalic tilt view (serendipity view) allows the sternoclavicular joints and medial clavicle to be seen apart from other overlapping structures[34] (Fig. 26–26). The use of plain tomography and CT scans has greatly improved the diagnosis and assessment of injuries and displacements in this anatomic region[10, 11, 20, 23] (Fig. 26–27). Ultrasound has also been useful in diagnosing and managing the reduction of retrosternal dislocations.[3]

Treatment

A child with a miminally displaced medial clavicle fracture has few symptoms or clinical findings. Only symptomatic treatment is necessary. A sling can be used for comfort with early range of motion. No reduction is necessary. The tremendous growth potential of the medial clavicular physis allows for a great deal of remodeling of malunions. Anteriorly dislocated fractures and physeal injuries that mimic anterior dislocations of the sternoclavicular joint may have a bony prominence. In the growing child, this will remodel,[34] and routine reduction of these injuries is probably not warranted. Symptomatic treatment with a sling or figure-of-eight harness for comfort yields good results.[8, 34] If a reduction is attempted, local or general anesthesia may be used. The patient is placed supine with a bolster between the shoulders. The arm is abducted 90 degrees, and longitudinal traction is applied. Posterior pressure is then gently applied over the fracture. The shoulders are held with limited immobilization (e.g., a padded figure-of-eight dressing or cast) for 3 to 4 weeks until stable.[8, 34, 36] Despite immobilization, many fractures remain unstable, tempting the surgeon to use internal fixation.[4, 9, 14] Many problems are reported with internal fixation in this area. Pin migration, which can be seen as early as 5 days post implantation,[12] can lead to pneumothorax, pericardial tamponade, and sudden death.[6, 22, 25, 28]

Physeal fractures with posterior displacement may require emergent reduction due to compromise of surrounding vital structures.[4, 5, 9, 14, 15, 19, 21, 43] Closed reduction is best attempted with a general anesthetic. The patient is placed supine with a bolster under the shoulders. Lateral traction is applied to the arm with pressure over the lateral aspect of the shoulder. The medial clavicle may be grabbed with a towel clip after sterilely preparing the area and pulling anteriorly. A palpable pop often occurs. An alternative method is to adduct the arm to the trunk with caudal traction to the arm or hand while forcing both shoulders posteriorly by direct pressure. The reduction is generally stable,[26, 34, 43] and internal fixation is not necessary. If open reduction is needed, suture fixation or repair of the periosteal tube[19, 37, 38] can hold the reduction. Limited immobilization is used for 3 to 4 weeks. Rapid healing and remodeling of the injury generally occur.[34, 43]

True sternoclavicular joint dislocation can be managed with closed reduction as described earlier. Anterior dislocations are more common than are posterior dislocations.[34] As with physeal fractures in this region, a posterior dislocation associated with symptoms for retrosternal visceral injury should undergo urgent reduction. A delay in performing closed reduction for more than 48 hours has been associated with a higher likelihood of needing to perform an open reduction.[16, 26] Clavicular osteotomy may be helpful in assisting with open reduction.[30, 37] Few problems occur with chronic anterior dislocations, but persistent pain can occur requiring late reconstruction.[24] Symptomatic, chronic dislocation of the sternoclavicular joint has been reported in a child[24] with successful late reconstruction.

AUTHORS' PREFERRED METHOD OF TREATMENT

We prefer nonoperative treatment for all true fractures and dislocations in this region. The remodeling potential of this area is great. Markedly displaced injuries in the older adolescent may merit an attempt at closed reduction under a local block. If redisplacement occurs, we do not favor operative intervention with internal fixation owing to the high incidence of complications reported. Brief immobilization of these injuries for 2 to 4 weeks should

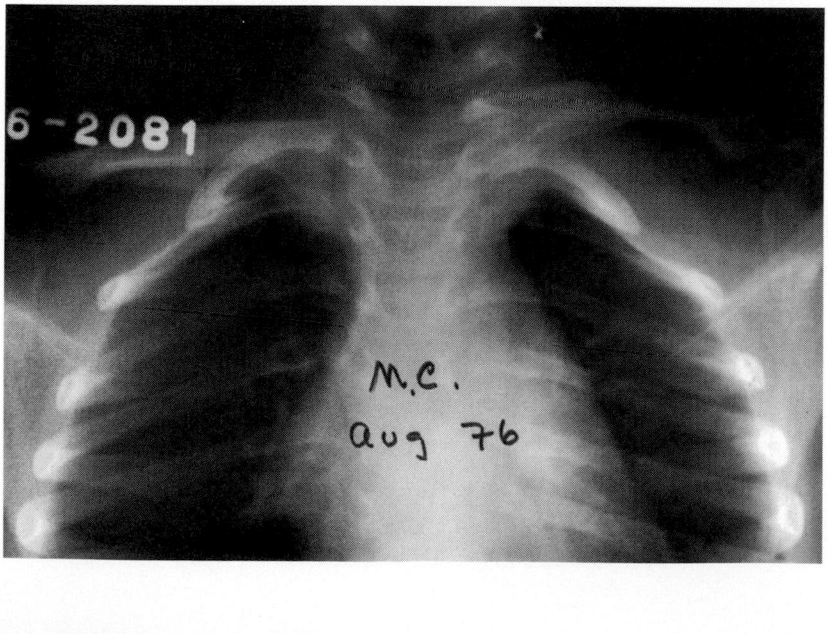

Figure 26–26

Serendipity view of the medial clavicles. This 40-degree tangential radiograph demonstrates an anterior dislocation of the left sternoclavicular joint. (From Rockwood CA and Green DP [eds]. Fractures [3 vols], 2nd ed. Philadelphia: JB Lippincott, 1984.)

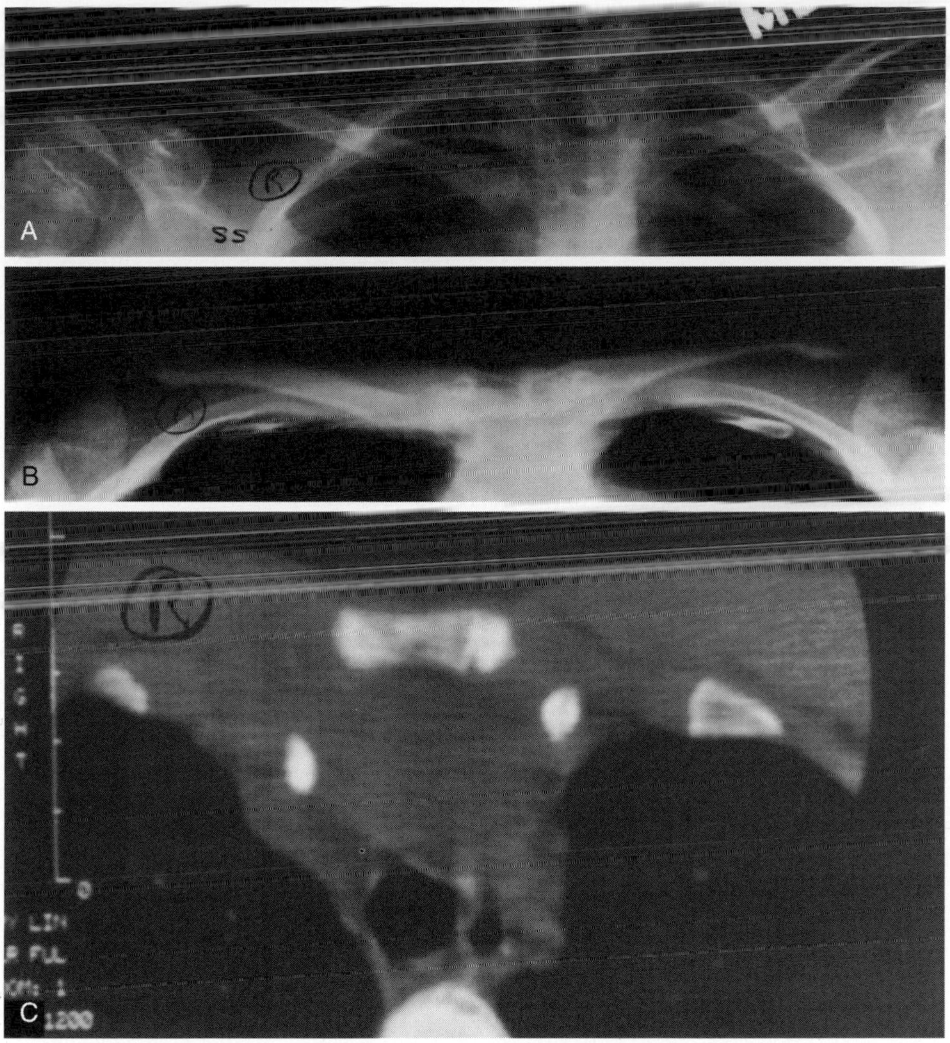

Figure 26–27

Posterior sternoclavicular dislocation of the right medial clavicle. *A,* Plain anteroposterior radiograph shows asymmetry but is difficult to interpret. *B,* Tangential view demonstrates posterior displacement. *C,* CT scan clearly demonstrates the injury as well as the relationship of the displaced medial clavicle to the mediastinal structures.

provide enough healing and stability to allow for rehabilitation. Posterior dislocations or physeal fractures with compromise of the mediastinal structures warrant urgent reduction under a general anesthetic. The method of reduction was previously described. Internal fixation is not necessary for stabilization.

References and Bibliography

1. Asher MA: Dislocations of the upper extremity in children. Orthop Clin North Am *7:*583–591, 1976.
2. Bearn JG: Direct observations on the function of the capsule of the sternoclavicular support. J Anat *101:*159–170, 1967.
3. Benson LS, Donaldson JS, and Carroll NC: Use of ultrasound in management of posterior sternoclavicular dislocation. J Ultrasound Med *10:*115–118, 1991.
4. Brooks AL and Hennisn GD: Injury to the proximal clavicular epiphysis. J Bone Joint Surg *54A:*1347, 1972.
5. Buckerfield CT and Castle ME: Acute traumatic retrosternal dislocation of the clavicle. J Bone Joint Surg *66A:*379–385, 1984.
6. Clark RL, Milgram JW, and Yawn DH: Fatal aortic perforation and cardiac tamponade due to a Kirschner wire migrating from the right sternoclavicular joint. South Med J *67:*316–318, 1974.
7. Corrigan GE: The neonatal clavicle. Biol Neonat *2:*79–92, 1959.
8. Curtis RJJ: Operative management of children's fractures of the shoulder region (Review). Orthop Clin North Am *21:*315–324, 1990.
9. Denham RH and Dingley AF: Epiphyseal separation of the medial end of the clavicle. J Bone Joint Surg *49A:*1179–1183, 1967.
10. DePalma AF: The role of the disks of the sternoclavicular and the acromioclavicular joints. Clin Orthop *13:*222–232, 1959.
11. Destouet JM, Gilula LA, Murphy WA, and Sagel SS: Computed tomography in the diagnosis of dislocations of the sternoclavicular joint. Radiology *138:*123–128, 1981.
12. Engel W: Results of stable osteosynthesis in clavicular fractures [in German]. Chirurg *41:*234–235, 1970.
13. Gardner E and Gray DJ: Prenatal development of the human shoulder and acromioclavicular joints. Am J Anat *92:*219–276, 1953.
14. Gaudernak T and Poigenfurst J: [Simultaneous dislocation-fracture of both ends of the clavicle] [in German]. Unfallchirurgie *17:*326–364, 1991.
15. Hardy JR: Complex clavicular injury in childhood. J Bone Joint Surg Br *74:*154, 1992.
16. Heinig CF: Retrosternal dislocation of the clavicle: Early recognition, x-ray diagnosis, and management. J Bone Joint Surg *50A:*830, 1968.
17. Jit I and Kulkarni M: Times of appearance and fusion of epiphysis at the medial end of the clavicle. Indian J Med Res *64:*773–782, 1976.
18. Landin LA: Fracture patterns in children: Analysis of 8682 fractures with special reference to incidence, etiology and secular changes in Swedish urban populations. Acta Orthop Scand Suppl *54:*1–109, 1983.
19. Lemire L and Rosman M: Sternoclavicular epiphyseal separation with adjacent clavicular fracture. Pediatr Orthop *4:*118–120, 1984.
20. Levisohn EM, Bunnell WP, and Yuan HA. Computed tomography in the diagnosis of dislocations of the sternoclavicular joint. Clin Orthop *140:*12–16, 1979.

21. Lewonowski K and Bassett GS: Complete posterior sternoclavicular epiphyseal separation: A case report and review of the literature. Clin Orthop *281*:84–88, 1992.
22. Longo R and Ruggiero L: Left pneumothorax with subcutaneous emphysema secondary to left clavicular fracture and homolateral obstetrical paralysis of the arm. [in Italian]. Minerva Pediatr *34*:273–276, 1982.
23. Lourie AA: Tomography in the diagnosis of posterior dislocation of the sternoclavicular joint. Acta Orthop Scand *51*:579–580, 1980.
24. Lunseth PA, Chapman KW, and Frankel VH: Surgical treatment of chronic dislocation of the sterno-clavicular joint. Bone Joint Surg Br *57*:193–196, 1975.
25. Lyons FA and Rockwood CA: Current concepts review: Migration of pins used in operations on the shoulder. J Bone Joint Surg Am *72*:1262–1267, 1990.
26. McKenzie JMM: Retrosternal dislocation of the clavicle. J Bone Joint Surg Br *45*:138–141, 1963.
27. Moseley HF: The clavicle: Its anatomy and function. Clini Orthop *58*:17–27, 1968.
28. Norback I and Markkula H: Migration of Kirschner pin from clavicle into ascending aorta. Acta Chir Scand *151*:177–179, 1985.
29. Nordquist A and Petersson C: The incidence of fractures of the clavicle. Clin Orthop *300*:127–132, 1994.
30. Omer GE Jr: Osteotomy of the clavicle in surgical reduction of anterior sternoclavicular dislocation. J Trauma *7*:584–590, 1967.
31. Owings-Webb PA: Epiphyseal union of the anterior iliac crest and medial clavicle in a modern multiracial sample of American males and females. Am J Phys Anthropol *68*:457–466, 1985.
32. Paterson DC. Retrosternal dislocation of the clavicle. J Bone Joint Surg Br *43*:90–94, 1961.
33. Rang M: Clavicle. *In* Rang M (ed): Children's Fractures. Philadelphia: JB Lippincott, 1983, pp 139–142.
34. Rockwood CA: Dislocation of the sternoclavicular joint. Instr Course Lect *24*:144–159, 1975.
35. Rowe CR: An atlas of anatomy and treatment of midclavicular fractures. Clin Orthop *58*:29–42, 1968.
36. Salvatore JE: Sternoclavicular joint dislocation. Clin Orthop *58*:51–55, 1968.
37. Selesnick FH, Jablon M, Frank C, and Post M: Retrosternal dislocation of the clavicle: Report of four cases. J Bone Joint Surg Am *66*:287–291, 1984.
38. Simurda MA: Retrosternal dislocation of the clavicle: A report of four cases and a method of repair. Can J Surg *11*:487–490, 1968.
39. Stanley D, Trowbridge EA, and Norris SH: The mechanism of clavicular fractures: A clinical and biomechanical analysis. J Bone Joint Surg *70*:461–464, 1988.
40. Thomas CB and Friedman RJ: Ipsilateral sternoclavicular dislocation and clavicle fracture. J Orthop Trauma *139*:68–69, 1989.
41. Todd TW and D'Errico J: The clavicular epiphyses. Am J Anat *41*:25–50, 1928.
42. Wheeler ME, Laaveg SJ, and Sprague BL: S-C joint disruption in an infant. Clin Orthop *139*:68–69, 1979.
43. Winter J, Sterner S, Maurer D, et al: Retrosternal epiphyseal disruption of medial clavicle: Case and review in children. Emerg Med *7*:9–13, 1989.

LATERAL CLAVICLE INJURIES

Anatomic Considerations

The anatomy of the clavicle was discussed previously.

Incidence

Rowe[22] reported 52 injuries to the lateral clavicle out of 690 clavicle fractures seen in a mixed population for an incidence of 7.5%. Nordquist and Petersson[17] found that Alman type II injuries constitute 21% of clavicle fractures in all age groups. These injuries are four to five times as common as sternoclavicular injuries,[20, 22] but the true incidence of lateral clavicular injuries in children is unknown.

Mechanism of Injury

Most injuries to the distal clavicle are due to direct shoulder trauma from falls or sports.[1, 5, 8] As the scapula is driven inferiorly, a fracture of the clavicle occurs through the lateral epiphyseal growth plate. The periosteum surrounding the distal clavicle splits, and the bone displaces leaving the coracoclavicular ligaments still attached to the inferior periosteum (Fig. 26–28).[5, 21]

Classification

True dislocation of the acromioclavicular joint can occur in older children.[5, 8, 21] These injuries are classified as in adults.[1] Most lateral clavicle injuries in children younger than 13 years of age will be Salter-Harris type I or II fractures with displacement of the medial fragment from the periosteal tube.[5, 7–9, 19, 21, 25] This fracture can be difficult to demonstrate radiographically because the distal clavicle epiphysis is often not ossified.[10, 11] Rockwood has classified injuries to the distal clavicle and acromioclavicular joint in children from reported cases in the literature[21] (Fig. 26–29).

Type I—Mild injury to acromioclavicular ligaments without disruption of the periosteal tube. The distal clavicle is stable, and x-rays are normal.

Type II—Partial disruption of the periosteal tube with mild instability of the distal clavicle. There is slight widening of the acromioclavicular joint on x-rays, and the coracoclavicular interval is normal.

Type III—A large disruption of the periosteal tube with elevation of the distal clavicle and gross instability. The coracoclavicular interval is increased 25 to 100% more than the normal shoulder.

Type IV—Similar to a type III injury, but with posterior displacement and buttonholing of the distal clavicle

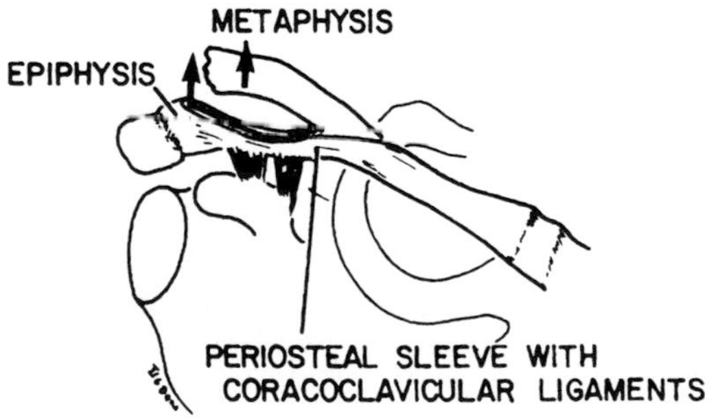

Figure 26–28

Schematic drawing of the injury pattern of the distal clavicular, showing how the clavicular metaphysis is displaced superiorly *(arrows)* through a tear in the periosteum, while the acromioclavicular joint remains intact. Similarly, the coracoclavicular ligaments, which are attaching directly into the periosteum during much of development, remain intact, so the distance between the periosteal sleeve and coracoid process remains normal. (From Ogden JA: Distal clavicular physical injury. Clin Orthop *188*:7, 1984.)

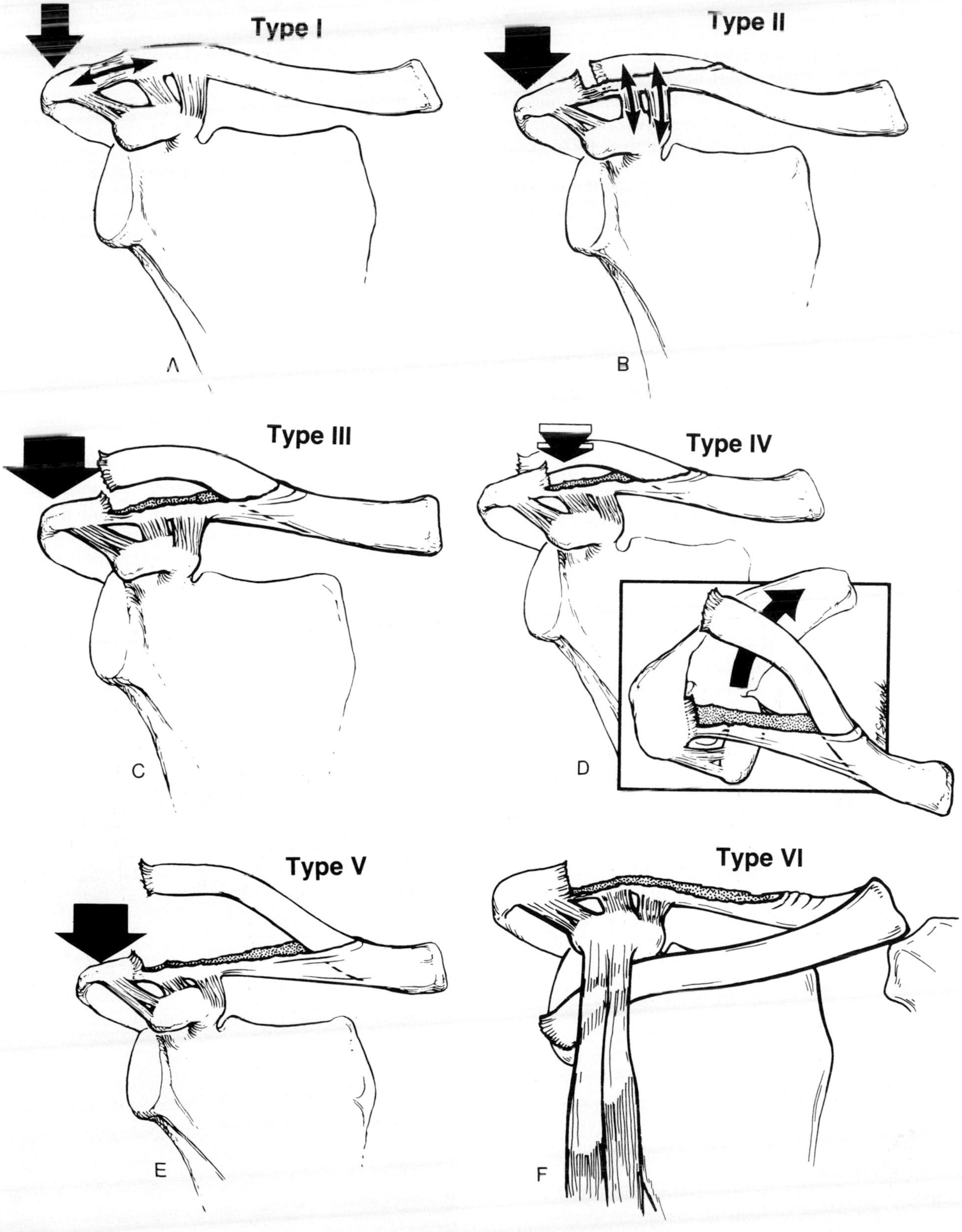

Figure 26–29

A–F, Rockwood's classification of clavicular-acromioclavicular joint injuries in children. (See text for description.) (From Rockwood CA and Green DP [eds]: Fractures [3 vols], 2nd ed. Philadelphia: JB Lippincott, 1984.)

through the trapezius muscle. There is little superior migration on an anteroposterior x-ray, but the axillary view will show posterior displacement of the clavicle relative to the acromion.[14]

Type V—Complete disruption of the periosteal tube with marked superior displacement of the clavicle into the subcutaneous tissues. The deltoid and trapezius muscle attachments to the clavicle may be disrupted. The coracoclavicular distance is increased more than 100% compared with the opposite side.

Type VI—Complete disruption of the periosteal tube with inferior dislocation of the distal clavicle to a position below the coracoid process.[13]

Since the periosteal tube remains contiguous, it will form a new clavicle while the bone displaced from the periosteal tube resorbs. During this interval, the patient will have a double clavicle.

An injury that can mimic a physeal fracture of the distal clavicle is separation of the physis at the base of the coracoid with acromioclavicular joint injury. The periosteal tube of the distal clavicle generally remains intact. This causes superior migration of the distal end of the clavicle and is a true injury of the acromioclavicular joint. These injuries have not been reported in children younger than 12 years of age.[3, 16, 23]

Signs and Symptoms

Type I and II fractures do not have significant displacement of the lateral clavicle. There will be mild swelling and tenderness with some restriction of motion due to pain. With the progressive displacement seen in type III through V injuries, there is obvious deformity with prominence of the clavicle. When these heal as a double clavicle, the old superior clavicle can become quite prominent and may occasionally be symptomatic. Swelling and pain are present with instability and tenderness of the distal clavicle.[6, 21] Type IV injuries can be easily missed owing to the posterior displacement of the clavicle.[19] There is little deformity once the swelling subsides, and radiographs look very similar to a type II injury. Type VI injuries are easily identified clinically but are rare injuries. Swelling, pain, and restricted motion are present. The acromion is prominent, and the distal end of the clavicle is not palpable. Injury to the brachial plexus and axillary vessels can occur.[13]

Radiographic Findings

Anteroposterior radiographs of this area should center the acromioclavicular joint and are best when a soft tissue technique is used. The axillary lateral view and a 20-degree cephalic tilt view help to assess the degree and direction of displacement. Stress radiographs may be helpful when injury is suspected but is not seen on routine views. Both acromioclavicular joints should be viewed simultaneously on the same x-ray plate first without and then with a light weight providing distal traction to the extremities. The coracoclavicular distance increases on the injured side if the injury is sufficient. The Stryker notch view can be very helpful to look for a fracture of the common physis of the superior glenoid and the base of the coracoid (Fig. 26–30). This radiograph is taken as an anteroposterior view of the shoulder with the patient's hand resting on top of the head.

Treatment

Since most distal clavicle injuries in children are physeal injuries without true acromioclavicular separation, there is a great potential for healing and remodeling of these injuries (Fig. 26–31). Concern about the prominence of the distal clavicle fragment with permanent deformity has been suggested as a reason for closed reduction and pin fixation in a small series of patients without long-term follow-up.[9, 15, 19] Larger reviews, however, have found that nonoperative treatment leads to predictably excellent results without any functional sequelae.[5, 8, 15] If the distal clavicle prominence leads to difficulties in the future, the prominence of the double clavicle can be excised at that time with predictably good results. For true acromioclavicular separations in older children, a series of adult patients have demonstrated that conservative treatment of complete dislocations will result in good functional and clinical outcomes.[2, 4, 18, 24] All of these data suggest that surgery for distal clavicle injuries in children is mainly for cosmetic reasons.

For the rare situation when there is marked displacement of the distal clavicle with tenting of the skin or an open fracture, open reduction and internal fixation may be necessary. In some situations, the periosteal tube can be repaired after replacing the clavicle into its periosteal

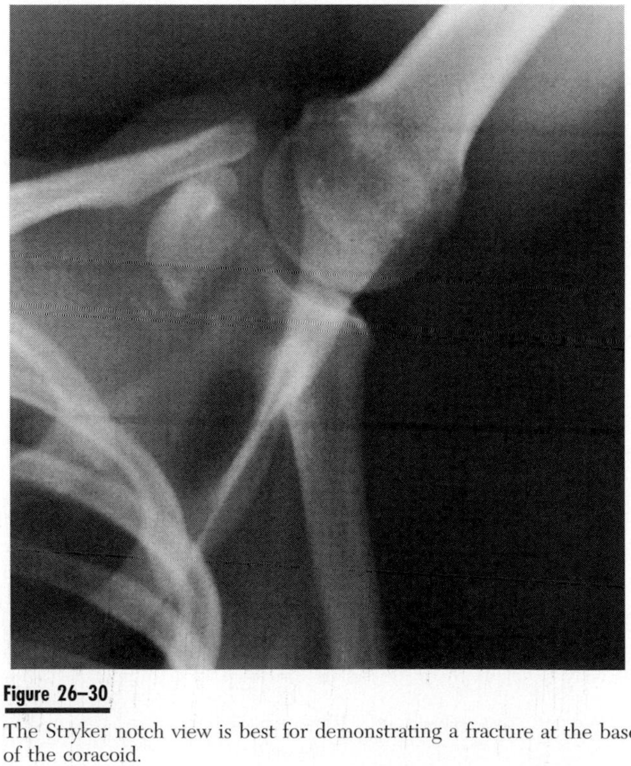

Figure 26–30

The Stryker notch view is best for demonstrating a fracture at the base of the coracoid.

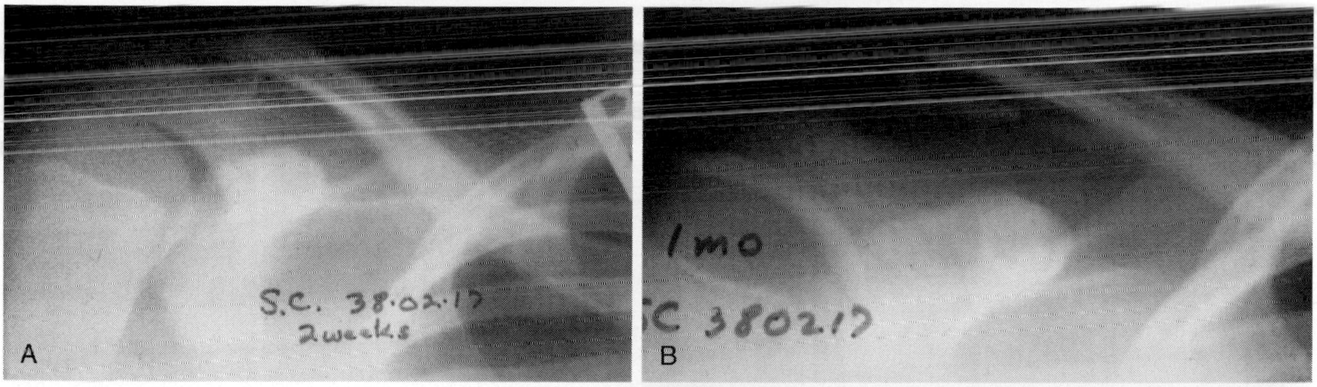

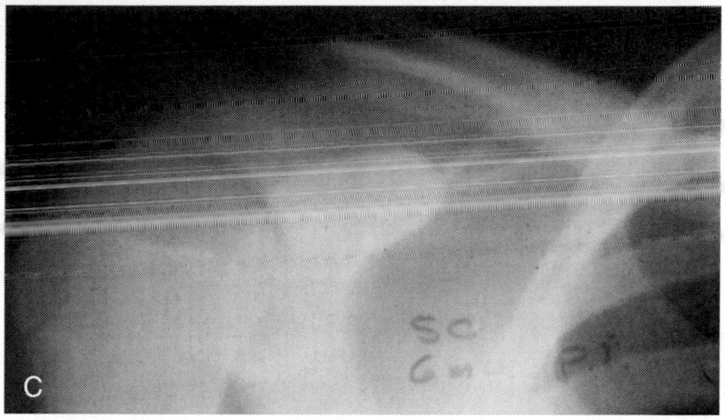

Figure 26–31

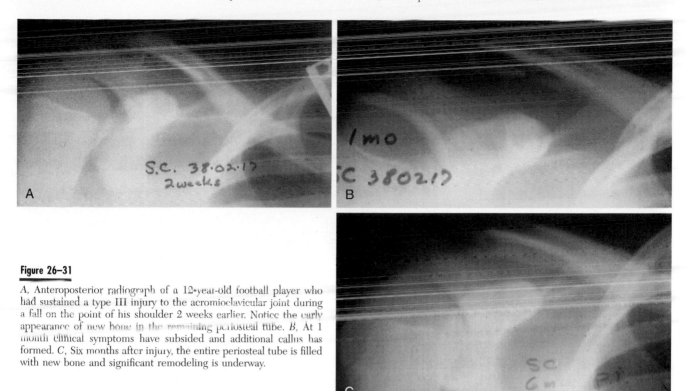

A, Anteroposterior radiograph of a 12-year-old football player who had sustained a type III injury to the acromioclavicular joint during a fall on the point of his shoulder 2 weeks earlier. Notice the early appearance of new bone in the remaining periosteal tube. *B*, At 1 month clinical symptoms have subsided and additional callus has formed. *C*, Six months after injury, the entire periosteal tube is filled with new bone and significant remodeling is underway.

bed. Temporary internal fixation with a coracoclavicular lag screw or a transacromial Kirschner wire for 4 to 6 weeks may be used.[7, 9, 12, 19]

Displaced fractures of the coracoid or glenoid physis are usually associated with an acromioclavicular joint dislocation. Open reduction and internal fixation of the coracoid fracture are recommended for these injuries. Nondisplaced fractures can be treated nonoperatively with a sling.[3, 16]

AUTHORS' PREFERRED METHOD OF TREATMENT

We prefer to treat most distal clavicle injuries in children nonoperatively. Initially, patients are placed in a sling with mild analgesics given to control early pain. Early range-of-motion and return-to-play activities are begun as soon as pain allows. Clinical healing is usually complete by 6 weeks, and resumption of full activities is allowed. For widely displaced (types IV to VI) fractures or open fractures, we recommend open reduction and temporary internal fixation by either repairing the periosteal tube or placing a coracoclavicular lag screw or Kirschner wires across the acromioclavicular joint.

Children older than 13 years of age can have true acromioclavicular dislocations. Most of these injuries have an excellent functional outcome if treated conservatively. The reader is referred to Chapter 12 on adult clavicle injuries for further references on treatment and outcome.

References and Bibliography

1. Allman FL: Fractures and ligamentous injuries of the clavicle and its articulations. J Bone Joint Surg Am *49*:774, 1967.
2. Bakalim G and Wilppula E: Surgical or conservative treatments of total dislocation of the acromioclavicular joint. Acta Chir Scand *141*:43–47, 1975.
3. Bernard TN, Brunet ME, and Haddad RJ: Fractured coracoid process in acromioclavicular dislocations: Report of four cases and review of the literature. Clin Orthop *175*:227–232, 1983.
4. Bjerneld H, Hovelius L, and Thorling J: Acromio-clavicular separations treated conservatively: A 5-year follow-up study. Acta Orthop Scand *54*:743–745, 1983.
5. Black GB, McPherson JA, and Reed MH: Traumatic pseudodislocation of the acromioclavicular joint in children: A fifteen year review. Am J Sports Med *19*:644–646, 1991.
6. Curtis RJJ: Operative management of children's fractures of the shoulder region (Review). Orthop Clin North Am *21*:315–324, 1990.
7. Edwards DJ, Kavanagh TG, and Flannery MC: Fractures of the distal clavicle: A case for fixation. Injury *23*:44–46, 1992.
8. Eidman DK, Siff SJ, and Tullos HS: Acromioclavicular lesions in children. Am J Sports Med *9*:150–154, 1981.
9. Falstie-Jensen S and Mikkelsen P: Pseudodislocation of the acromioclavicular joint. J Bone Joint Surg Br *64*:368–369, 1982.
10. Gardner E and Gray DJ: Prenatal development of the human shoulder and acromioclavicular joints. Am J Anat *92*:219–276, 1953.
11. Garn SM, Rohmann CG, and Silverman FN: Radiographic standards for postnatal ossificatin and tooth calcification. Med Radiogr Photogr *43*:45–66, 1967.
12. Gaudernak T and Poigenfurst J: [Simultaneous dislocation-fracture of both ends of the clavicle] [in German]. Unfallchirurgie *17*:362–364, 1991.
13. Gerber C and Rockwood CA Jr: Subcoracoid dislocation of the lateral end of the clavicle: A report of three cases. Bone Joint Surg Am *69*:924–927, 1987.
14. Gunther WA: Posterior dislocation of the clavicle. J Bone Joint Surg Am *31*:878, 1949.
15. Havránek P: Injuries of distal clavicular physis in children. J Pediatr Orthop *9*:213–215, 1989.
16. Montgomery SP and Loyd RD: Avulsion fracture of the coracoid epiphysis with acromioclavicular separation: Report of two cases in adolescents and review of the literature. J Bone Joint Surg Am *59*:963–965, 1977.
17. Nordquist A and Petersson C: The incidence of fractures of the clavicle. Clin Orthop *300*:127–132, 1994.

18. Nordquist A, Petersson C, and Redlund-Johnell I: The natural course of lateral clavicle fracture. 15 (11–21) year follow-up of 110 cases. Acta Orthop Scand *64*:87–91, 1993.
19. Ogden JA: Distal clavicular physeal injury. Clin Orthop *188*:68–73, 1984.
20. Rockwood CA: Dislocation of the sternoclavicular joint. Instr Course Lect *24*:144–159, 1975.
21. Rockwood CA Jr: The shoulder: Facts, confusions and myths. Int Orthop *15*:401–405, 1991.
22. Rowe CR: An atlas of anatomy and treatment of midclavicular fractures. Clin Orthop *58*:29–42, 1968.
23. Taga I, Yoneda M, and Ono K: Epiphyseal separation of the coracoid process associated with acromioclavicular sprain: A case report and review of the literature. Clin Orthop *207*:138–141, 1986.
24. Walsh WM, Peterson DA, Shelton G, and Neumann RD: Shoulder strength following acromioclavicular injury. Am J Sports Med *13*:153–158, 1985.
25. Wilkes JA and Hoffer MM: Clavicle fractures in head-injured children. J Orthop Trauma *1*:55–58, 1987.

BIPOLAR CLAVICLE INJURIES

Fractures or fracture-dislocations of both ends of the clavicle are rare injuries that are described in small series and case reports.[1–3] In adults, the injury is typically an anterior sternoclavicular dislocation and a posterior or type IV acromioclavicular dislocation. Sanders and associates recommend open reduction of the acromioclavicular dislocation in active individuals and symptomatic treatment of the acromioclavicular dislocation.[3] Beckman reported a child with a bipolar injury who was treated successfully by replacing the clavicle back into its periosteal tube without further fixation.[1]

References and Bibliography

1. Beckman T: A case of simultaneous luxation of both ends of the clavicle. Acta Chirurg Scand *56*:156–163, 1924
2. Gaudernak T and Poigenfurst J: Simultaneous dislocation-fracture of both ends of the clavicle. Unfallchirurgie *17*:362–364, 1991.
3. Sanders JO, Lyons FA, and Rockwood CA: Management of dislocations of both ends of the clavicle. J Bone Joint Surg *72A*:399–402, 1990.

FRACTURES AND DISLOCATIONS OF THE SCAPULA

Developmental Anatomy

The scapula first appears as a cartilaginous anlage at the C4 to C5 level in the fifth gestational week. During the sixth and seventh gestational weeks, it enlarges to extend from C4 to C7. During the seventh week, the shoulder joint forms and the scapula descends from the cervical area to its position overlying the first through fifth ribs. Failure of the scapula to descend results in Sprengel's deformity.[56]

Most of the scapula is formed by membranous ossification. The multiple ossification centers about the scapula can be confused with fractures (Fig. 26–32). The body's ossification center is present at birth.[53] The coracoid process ossifies from two separate centers. The first is distal and ossification closely follows the proximal humeral epiphysis but is more erratic.[37] The base of the coracoid process begins ossifying in the tenth year, forms a portion of the glenoid, and unites with the body at about age 15. Initially, the coracoid process is larger than the acromion,[42] but it gradually assumes the adult form. The acromion forms from two to five ossification centers, which appear at puberty and may fail to unite resulting in a bipartite or tripartite acromion.[13] The most anterior portion is the pre-acromion; the middle portion the mesoacromion; and the portion at the angle between the scapular spine acromion the meta-acromion separated from the base acromion. Persistence of these may be confused with an acromion fracture.[39, 42, 46] The most common os acromiale type is failure of the mesoacromion to join the meta-acromion. The junction of the os acromiale with the spine may have a distinct joint cavity and is differentiated from a fracture by round, uniform cleavage lines contrasting with a fracture's sharp, ragged edges. An os acromiale (Fig. 26–33) is rarely visible except on the axillary lateral view and is more common bilaterally than unilaterally.[42] It normally fuses to the remaining scapula at approximately age 22.[53] The glenoid forms from the ossification center at the base of the coracoid and a second horseshoe-shaped center. Centers for the vertebral border and the inferior scapula angle appear at puberty and unite with the body at about 21 years of age. Developmental anomalies of the scapula include a bipartite coracoid, coracoid duplication, absent acromion,[32] glenoid hypoplasia,[8] scapular hypoplasia, and Sprengel's anomaly.[2, 9, 13, 42, 53] Because of these numerous ossification centers, comparison radiographs and a careful clinical examination are important.

Surgical Anatomy

The scapula is a flat and triangular bone. The 17 muscular attachments control scapulothoracic motion. The scapula is highly mobile and provides approximately 60 degrees of shoulder elevation. The scapular spine divides the dorsal surface into fossae that accommodate the supraspinatus and infraspinatus muscles.

The scapula is encased in muscle and is relatively protected from trauma. Fractures and dislocations of the scapula only constitute 1% of all fractures and 5% of shoulder fractures[24, 26] and are even more uncommon in children. Fractures of the scapula are often associated with other life-threatening, severe injuries that are more important than the fracture of the scapula itself.[19, 43, 56, 58]

Classification

Several classification schemes exist for fracture of the scapula, but none are specific for children. A summary of various types of fractures is included in the following outline. The proportion of the types are 12% acromion, 11% spine, 7% coracoid, 27% neck, 10% glenoid, and 35% body.[1]

A few scapular fractures have potential pitfalls. Scapular neck fractures associated with clavicle fractures or sternoclavicular or acromioclavicular dislocations (the so-

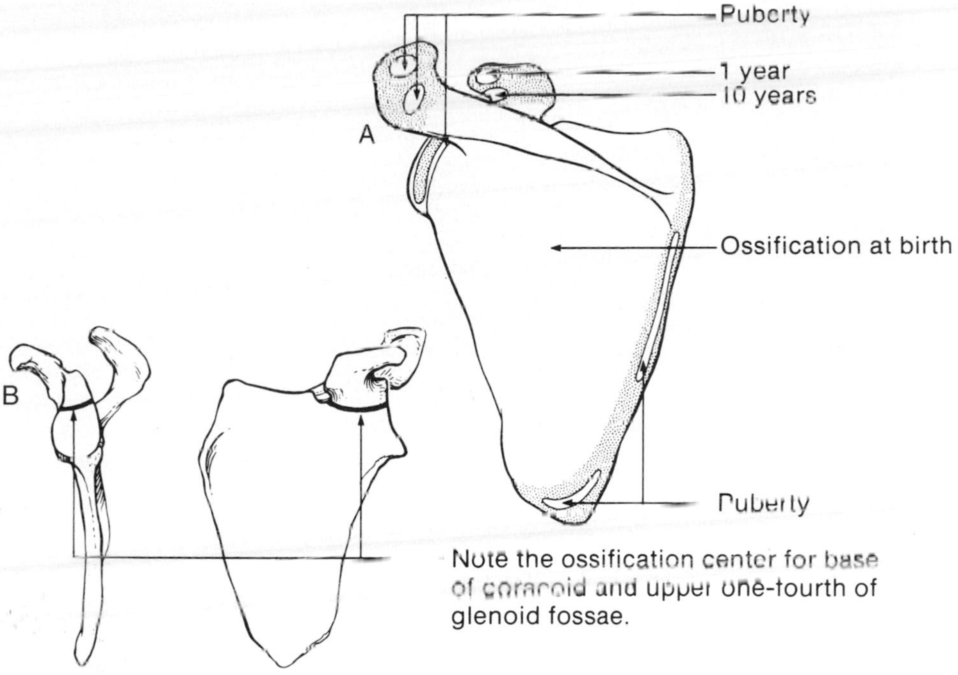

Figure 26–32

A and *B*, Multiple ossification centers of the scapula.

called floating shoulders) are potentially unstable allowing the scapular neck to displace and change the normal muscle configurations about the shoulder. Fractures through the coracoid with lateral clavicular fractures are a childhood equivalent of acromioclavicular joint dislocations[45] (Fig. 26–34). Acromial fractures with narrowing result in subacromial impingement.[36]

Scapulothoracic dissociations are classified as intrathoracic and described as the "locked scapula"[48] or as being laterally displaced.[3, 38] Open lateral dislocations are essentially incomplete forequarter amputations. The neurovascular status is at great risk. For this injury to occur, the attachment with the thorax must be broken at either the sternoclavicular joint, the acromioclavicular joint, or as a clavicle fracture. Ebraheim and associates distinguish scapulothoracic dissociation from scapulothoracic dislocation, which is a traumatic dislocation of the inferior scapulothoracic articulation with less devastating vascular and neurologic damage.[16] We find it difficult to distinguish an articulation's dissociation from its dislocation.

Ideberg classified glenoid fractures as types I to V, based on their location in the glenoid and the course of the fracture through the rest of the scapula.[28, 20] Type I or anterior avulsion fracture results from dislocations, subluxations, or direct injury and may be associated with glenohumeral instability. Large fragments with instability should be distinguished from the more common rim fractures from dislocations.[5] Type II is a transverse or oblique fracture occurring through the glenoid with an inferior free glenoid fragment that results in inferior glenohumeral subluxation. Type III fractures involve the upper third of the glenoid, including the coracoid, and are often associated with an acromial fracture, a clavicle fracture, or an acromioclavicular dislocation. A type III fracture has been reported in an adolescent.[6] A type IV fracture is a horizontal glenoid fracture extending through the body all the way to the vertebral border. Type V is a combination of type IV with a transverse fracture through the scapular neck or its inferior half with the inferior fragment floating free. Goss expanded type V to include combinations of types II, III, and IV, and Goss added a type VI that consists of a severely comminuted glenoid cavity.[22]

Goss groups scapular injuries by stability. He defined the superior shoulder suspensory complex as a bony and soft tissue ring on the end of a superior and inferior bony strut.[23, 24] The ring consists of the glenoid process, coracoid process, coracoclavicular ligaments, distal clavi-

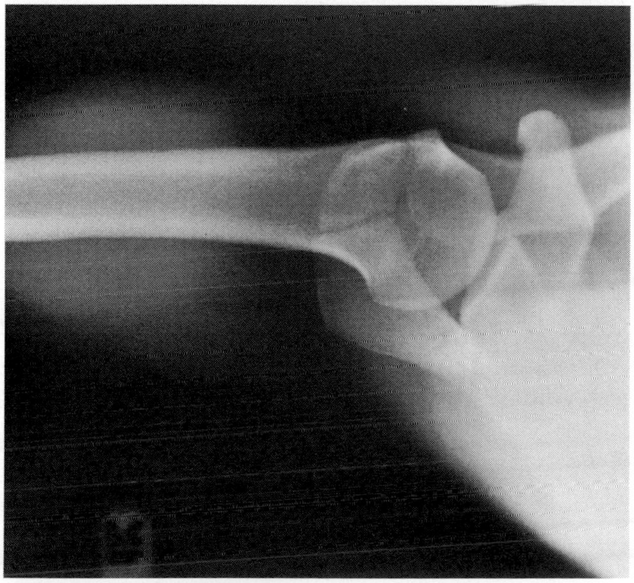

Figure 26–33

An unfused os acromiale seen on the axillary lateral view. This can be mistaken for an acute fracture of the acromion, which is a rare injury in a child.

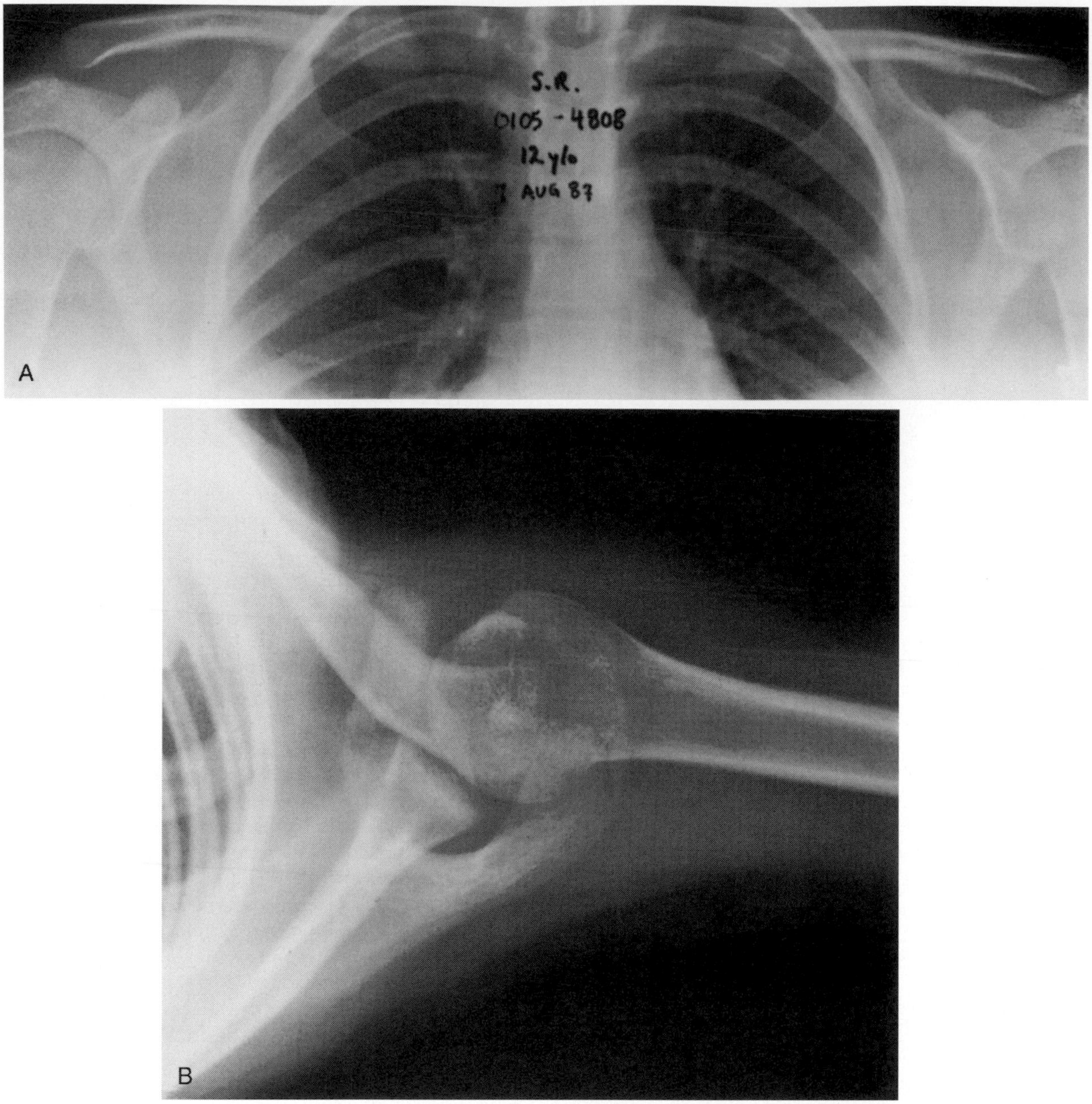

Figure 26–34

From the clinical examination, this 12-year-old boy was thought to have a distal clavicular-acromioclavicular joint injury after falling on his right shoulder. *A*, Comparison anteroposterior views of both shoulders reveal a slight depression of the right scapula but no difference in comparative coracoclavicular distances. *B*, An axillary lateral view demonstrates the condition to be a fracture of the base of the coracoid.

cle, acromial clavicular ligaments, and acromial process. The superior strut is the middle clavicle, and the inferior strut is the lateral scapular body and spine. A double disruption of this complex can result in severe displacement with potential implications for treatment.

CLASSIFICATION

Body
- Nondisplaced
- Displaced

Neck[40]
- Isolated
- Clavicular axis disrupted

Coracoid[45]
- Isolated
- Acromioclavicular joint disruption

Acromion[36]
- I—Nondisplaced; A-avulsion, B-direct trauma
- II—Displaced with no subacromial narrowing
- II—Displaced with subacromial narrowing

Glenoid fractures[28, 29]
- I—Anterior avulsion fracture
- II—Transverse with inferior free fragment
- III—Upper third including coracoid

IV—Horizontal fracture extending through body
V—Combination of II and III
VI—Extensively comminuted

Scapulothoracic dissociation[50]
- Open or closed
- Complete or incomplete amputation (traumatic forequarter amputation)
- Neurovascular status:
  - a. Intact
  - b. Partially disrupted
  - c. Completely disrupted
    - I. Intrathoracic
    - II. Lateral
      - A. Acromioclavicular joint injury
      - B. Sternoclavicular joint injury
      - C. Clavicle fracture

Mechanisms of Injury

Avulsion fractures associated with glenohumeral joint injuries are the most commonly encountered fractures of the scapula. Other fractures of the scapula generally occur after great violence.[19, 43, 56, 58] They are uncommon in infants and children but quite specific for child abuse unless a clear mechanism exists.[34] Coracoid fractures generally occur with injury to the acromioclavicular joint through the weak bone rather than the stronger ligaments.[45] Stress fractures of the acromion,[14, 25, 55, 57] coracoid,[10, 54] glenoid,[7] and at the teres minor insertion[11] are reported in adults, but the only stress fracture reported in a child is a scapular body stress fracture in a gymnast.[47]

Signs and Symptoms

Seventy-five per cent or more of patients with scapula fractures have associated injuries[1, 52] that may be life threatening.[1, 30, 52, 56] The most frequent injuries are of the head, chest, kidneys, and especially the ipsilateral lung, chest wall, and ipsilateral shoulder girdle, including the neurovascular structures.[56] Mortality in one series was 14.3%.[56]

Victims of severe trauma should be assessed and managed by the ABCs. Clinically, scapular fractures have swelling, pain, and tenderness about the scapular area if the patient is responsive. Scapular neck fractures additionally exhibit flattening of the overall shoulder contour. A careful neurovascular and chest examination is essential in all injuries to the scapula.

Imaging Studies and Differential Diagnosis

An anteroposterior view and a scapulolateral view define most scapular fractures (Fig. 26–35). Several scapular abnormalities can mimic fractures. Although acromial fractures are a strong indicator of child abuse, ossification adjacent to the tip of the acromion can be a normal finding.[33] This center is generally on the inferior portion and is anterior on the axillary view. A bone scan may be necessary to distinguish it from a fracture.[33] Os acromiale was discussed previously. Andrews and associates describe a 20-degree caudal tilt lateral with the shoulder adducted showing the lateral acromion, which may help to show an os acromiale.[4] Defects of the glenoid ossification from an ununited epiphysis, pseudoforamen of the scapula, and

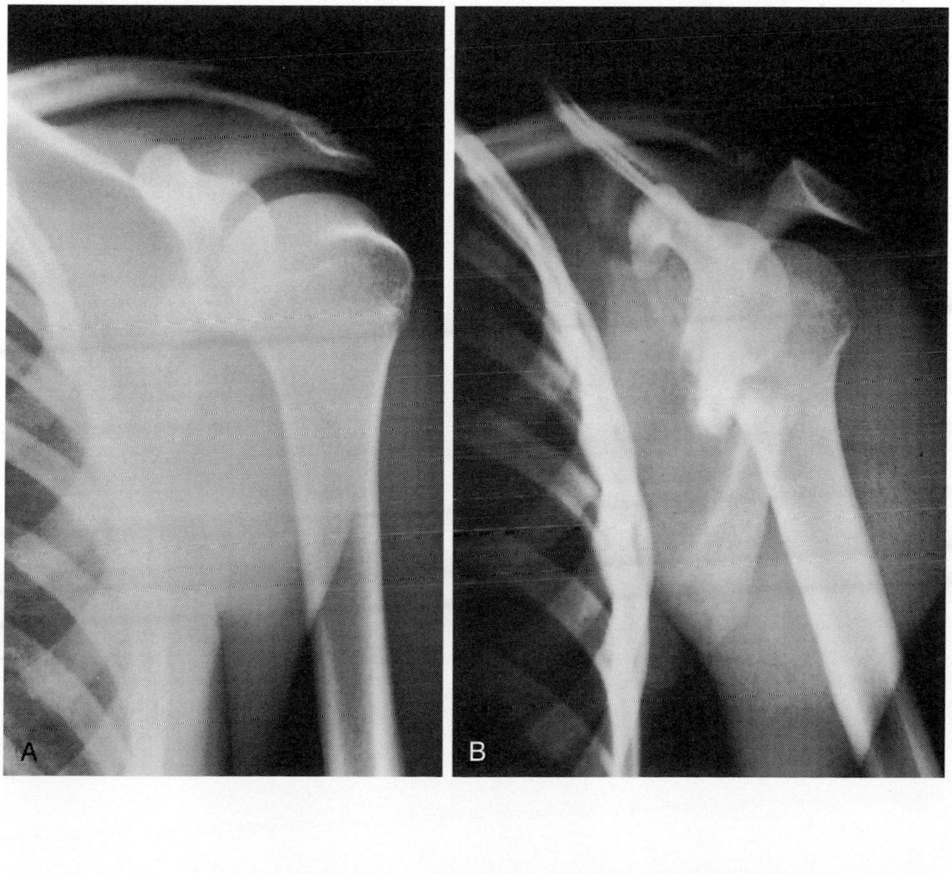

Figure 26–35

Fractures of the body of the scapula are usually associated with high-energy injuries. *A,* An anteroposterior radiograph shows a displaced body fracture. *B,* True scapular lateral view.

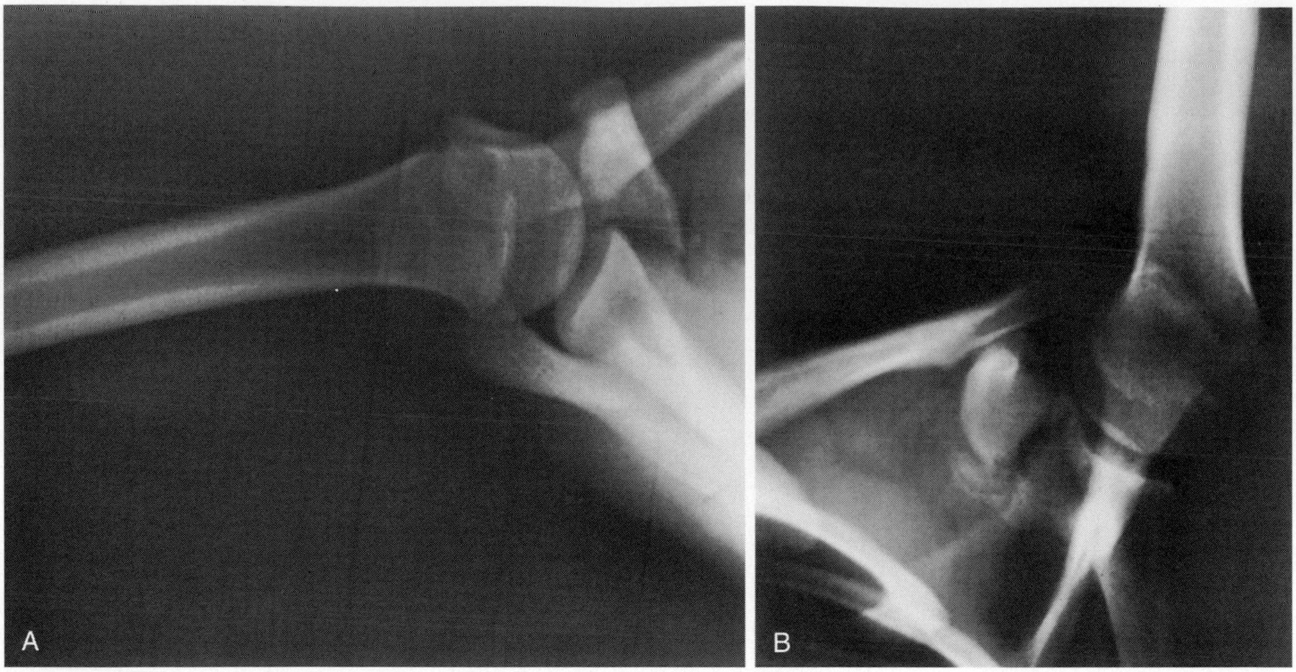

Figure 26–36

Fractures of the base of the coracoid are best seen on the Stryker notch view. *A*, Axillary lateral view of injury. *B*, Healing callus shown on the Stryker notch view.

the scapular notch must be distinguished from a fracture.[20] Coracoid fractures are best seen on a Stryker notch view (Fig. 26–36). Glenoid fractures may be difficult to visualize and are best seen on the axillary lateral view.[52] A true anteroposterior view, a West Point view, and an apical oblique view are often necessary. A CT scan is best for intra-articular fractures (Fig. 26–37), and computerized reconstructions may be needed. Scapulothoracic dislocations are best identified on a nonrotated anteroposterior chest x-ray with the medial border of the scapula displaced laterally compared with the uninjured side.[16, 31] This injury must be considered in patients with massive trauma to the upper extremity with nerve or vascular deficits and whose x-rays demonstrate lateral displacement of the scapula, a complete acromioclavicular joint separation, or a fracture of the clavicle.[51]

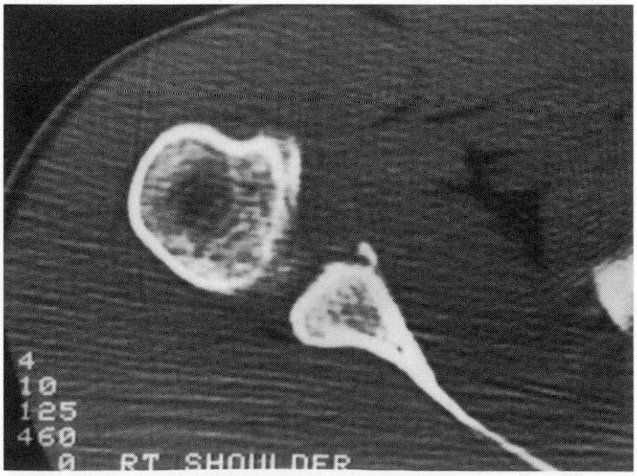

Figure 26–37

Displaced fractures of the anterior glenoid are associated with dislocations of the glenohumeral joint. A computed tomography scan is very good for assessing this lesion.

Treatment

The scapula is very flexible in children. As rare as scapular fractures are in adults, they are extremely uncommon in children, and treatments must be based on those that are found most useful in adults.

Body. Most scapular body fractures respond to conservative treatment.[17, 30, 52, 58] The muscles around the scapula tend to keep the fragments in reasonable proximity with good healing potential. In the few fractures that fail to unite, partial body fragments can be excised. Treatment of scapula body fractures is usually defined by the associated injuries.[18]

Scapula Neck. Nondisplaced fractures of the scapular neck that are not associated with fractures of the clavicle can be treated expectantly. If they are displaced significantly, closed reduction and application of a thoracobrachial cast may be sufficient. If the clavicle or its joints are disrupted, Herscovici and associates recommend open reduction of the clavicle to preserve the suspensory function of the coracoclavicular ligaments, but they leave the scapula alone.[27] Leung and Lam recommend fixing both the scapular neck fracture and the clavicle fracture.[40] Skeletal traction is an acceptable alternative.[15] A recent review casts doubt on the need for fixing these fractures.[21] In children with their stout periosteum and remodeling potential, it is doubtful that this injury would require fixation.

Coracoid Fractures. Coracoid fractures, which are nondisplaced, can be simply treated with a sling. Displaced fractures are usually associated with an acromioclavicular joint or lateral clavicular injury. These fractures should be treated by open reduction and internal fixation.[45, 52]

Acromial Fractures. Nondisplaced acromial fractures are treated with a sling. Only nondisplaced acromial fractures are reported in children.[36] Displaced acromial fractures with subacromial impingement should be reduced and stabilized with pins, screws, or a small plate.[26, 30] Nonunion is reported in adults but not in children.[44]

Glenoid Fractures. The majority of glenoid fractures, except those associated with shoulder instability, are rarely symptomatic when they heal, and these fractures can be treated closed.[59] Large fractures involving a large portion of the glenoid fossa associated with glenohumeral instability should be fixed.[35] For glenoid fractures that do not involve the anterior rim or the superior half of the glenoid, a posterior approach is easier.[41, 49, 52] Ideberg[28, 29] suggests open reduction for persistent subluxation or an unstable reduction. While he reports patients as young as 6 years,[29] the youngest patient treated surgically was 30 years of age.[28] Type II fractures associated with glenohumeral instability or inferior subluxation may require open reduction, although the approach and fixation may be quite difficult. This finding has been reported in a 16 year old who appears to have an open proximal humeral physis that was successfully treated with open reduction and internal fixation through a deltopectoral approach.[6] If there is no subluxation, it can be treated with shoulder rehabilitation. The type III fractures occur through the junction between the ossification centers of the glenoid and are often accompanied by a fractured acromion, clavicle, or acromioclavicular separation. Early motion tends to improve the position.[12, 28, 29] Type IV, V, and VI fractures are not reported in children and can be extremely difficult to treat by open reduction because the scapula has very little bone for good fixation.[22, 28, 29] In children who can tolerate prolonged immobilization, skeletal traction followed by protected motion may be satisfactory treatment.

Scapulothoracic Dislocations and Dissociation. Intrathoracic dislocation is rare. The medial border is caught between the ribs of either the third and fourth ribs or the fourth and fifth ribs. It can usually be reduced closed. DePalma[15] described reduction by hyperabduction and manually manipulating the axillary border to rotate the scapula forward while at the same time pushing it back into location. The reduction is usually stable. The patient may be more comfortable with some immobilization such as strapping or a collar and cuff. Nettrour and associates describe an open reduction of this injury in an 11-year-old boy. The rhomboid muscle is typically torn.[48] Late reduction may require soft tissue reattachment to maintain stability.

Lateral scapulothoracic dissociation is potentially life threatening.[16] Initially, the patient should be stabilized using the ABCs of trauma care. It is important to do a detailed neurovascular examination. There is generally massive injury to the entire extremity. Arteriography can help plan the vascular reconstruction if time allows. In a massive injury with a brachial plexus avulsion, amputation should be considered.[51] If any of the plexus remains intact, it is best to salvage the limb.[51] Salvage may require shoulder arthrodesis and above-elbow amputation. A successful muscular repair is reported in a child and should be considered in patients with an intact brachial plexus after the artery has been repaired.

References and Bibliography

1. Ada JR and Miller ME: Scapular fractures: Analysis of 113 cases. Clin Orthop *269:*174–180, 1991.
2. Ahn JI and Park JS: Pathological fractures secondary to unicameral bone cysts. Int Orthop *18:*20–22, 1994.
3. An HS, Vonderbrink JP, Ebraheim NA, et al: Open scapulothoracic dissociation with intact neurovascular status in a child. J Orthop Trauma *2:*36–38, 1988.
4. Andrews JR, Byrd JW, Kupferman SP, and Angelo RL: The profile view of the acromion. Clin Orthop *263:*142–146, 1991.
5. Aston JW and Gregory CF: Dislocation of the shoulder with significant fracture of the glenoid. J Bone Joint Surg Am *55:*1531–1533, 1973.
6. Aulicino PL, Reinert C, Kornberg M, and Williamson S: Displaced intra-articular glenoid fractures treated by open reduction and internal fixation. J Trauma *26:*1137–1141, 1986.
7. Bennett GE: Shoulder and elbow lesions of the professional baseball pitcher. JAMA *117:*510–514, 1941.
8. Borenstein ZC, Mink J, Oppenheim W, et al: Case report 655: Congenital glenoid dysplasia (congenital hypoplasia of the glenoid neck and fossa of the scapula, with accompanied deformity of humeral head, coracoid process, and acromion). Skeletal Radiol *20:*134–136, 1991.
9. Bostman O, Makela EA, Sodergard J, et al: Absorbable polyglycolide pins in internal fixation of fractures in children. J Pediatr Orthop *13:*242–245, 1993.
10. Boyer DW Jr: Trapshooter's shoulder: Stress fracture of the coracoid process: Case report. J Bone Joint Surg Am *57:*862, 1975.
11. Brower AC, Neff JR, and Tellema DA: An unusual scapular stress fracture. Am J Roentgenol Radium Ther Nucl Med *129:*519–520, 1977.
12. Butters KP: Fractures and dislocations of the scapula. *In* Rockwood CAJ, Green DP, and Bucholz RW (eds): Fractures in Adults. Philadelphia: JB Lippincott, 1991, pp 990–1019.
13. Chung SMK and Nissenbaum MM: Congenital and developmental defects of the shoulder (Review). Orthop Clin North Am *6:*381–392, 1975.
14. Dennis DA, Ferlic DC, and Clayton ML: Acromial stress fractures associated with cuff-tear arthropathy: A report of three cases. J Bone Joint Surg Am *68:*937–940, 1986.
15. DePalma AF: Surgery o the Shoulder. Philadelphia: JB Lippincott, 1983.
16. Ebraheim NA, An HS, Jackson WT, et al: Scapulothoracic dissociation. J Bone Joint Surg Am *70:*428–432, 1988.
17. Eskola A, Vainionpaa S, Patiala H, and Rokkanen P: Outcome of operative treatment in fresh lateral clavicular fracture. Ann Chir Gynaecol *76:*167–169, 1987.
18. Findlay RT: Fractures of the scapula. Ann Surg *93:*1001–1008, 1931.
19. Gelberman RH, Verdeck WN, and Brodhead WT: Supraclavicular nerve-entrapment syndrome. J Bone Joint Surg Am *57:*119, 1975.
20. Goldenberg DB and Brogdon BG: Congenital anomalies of the pectoral girdle demonstrated by chest radiography. J Can Assoc Radiol *18:*472–477, 1967.
21. Goodnight JM, Rockwood CA Jr, and Wirth MA: Ipsilateral fractures of the clavicle and scapula (Abstract). Submitted for Publication, 1996.
22. Goss TP: Current concepts review: Fractures of the glenoid cavity. J Bone Joint Surg Am *72:*299–305, 1992.
23. Goss TP: Double disruptions of the superior shoulder suspensory complex. J Orthop Trauma *7:*99–106, 1993.
24. Goss TP: Scapular fractures and dislocations: Diagnosis and treatment. J Am Acad Orthop Surg *3:*22–33, 1995.
25. Hall RJ and Calvert PT: Stress fracture of the acromion: An unusual mechanism and review of the literature. J Bone Joint Surg Br *77:*153–154, 1995.

26. Hardegger FH, Simpson LA, and Weber BG: The operative treatment of scapular fractures. J Bone Joint Surg Br *66*:725–731, 1984.
27. Herscovici D Jr, Fiennes AG, Allgower M, and Ruedi TP: The floating shoulder: Ipsilateral clavicle and scapular neck fractures [see comments]. J Bone Joint Surg Br *74*:362–364, 1992.
28. Ideberg R: Fractures of the scapula involving the glenoid fossa. *In* Bateman JE and Walsh RD (eds): Surgery of the Shoulder. Toronto: BC Decker, 1984, pp 63–66.
29. Ideberg R: Unusual glenoid fractures. Acta Orthop Scand *58*:191–192, 1987.
30. Imatani RJ: Fractures of the scapulae: A review of 53 fractures. J Trauma *15*:473–478, 1975.
31. Kelbel JM, Jardon OM, and Huurman WW: Scapulothoracic dislocation. Clin Orthop *209*:210–214, 1986.
32. Kim SJ and Min BH: Congenital bilateral absence of the acromion: A case report. Clin Orthop *263*:117–119, 1994.
33. Kleinman PK and Spevak MR: Variations in acromial ossification simulating infant abuse in victims of sudden infant death syndrome. Radiology *180*:185–187, 1991.
34. Kogutt MS, Swischuk LE, and Fagan CJ: Patterns of injury and significance of uncommon fractures in the battered child syndrome. Am J Roentgenol Radium Ther Nucl Med *121*:143–149, 1974.
35. Kreitner KF, Runkel M, Grebe P, et al: [MR tomography versus CT arthrography in glenohumeral instabilities] [in German]. Rofo Fortschr Geb Rontgenstr Neuen Bildgeb Verfahr *157*:37–42, 1992.
36. Kuhn JE, Blasier RB, and Carpenter JE: Fractures of the acromion process: A proposed classification system [see comments]. J Orthop Trauma *8*:6–13, 1994.
37. Kuhns LR, Sherman MP, Poznanski AK, and Holt JF: Humeral head and coracoid ossification in the newborn. Radiology *107*:145–149, 1973.
38. Lange RH and Noel SH: Traumatic lateral scapular displacement: An expanded spectrum of associated neurovascular injury. J Orthop Trauma *7*:361–366, 1993.
39. Leslie JT and Ryan TJ: The anterior axillary incision to approach the shoulder joint. J Bone Joint Surg Am *44*:1193–1196, 1962.
40. Leung KS and Lam TP: Open reduction and internal fixation of ipsilateral fractures of the scapular neck and clavicle. J Bone Joint Surg Am *75*:1015–1018, 1993.
41. Leung KS, Lam TP, and Poon KM: Operative treatment of displaced intra-articular glenoid fractures. Injury *24*:324–328, 1993.
42. McClure JG and Raney RB: Anomalies of the scapula. Clin Orthop *110*:22–31, 1975.
43. McGahan JP, Rab GT, and Dublin A: Fractures of the scapula. J Trauma *20*:880–883, 1980.
44. Mick CA and Weiland AJ: Pseudoarthrosis of a fracture of the acromion. J Trauma *23*:248–249, 1983.
45. Montgomery SP and Loyd RD: Avulsion fracture of the coracoid epiphysis with acromioclavicular separation: Report of two cases in adolescents and review of the literature. J Bone Joint Surg Am *59*:963–965, 1977.
46. Mudge MK, Wood VE, and Frykman GK: Rotator cuff tears associated with as acromiale. J Bone Joint Surg Am *66*:427–429, 1984.
47. Nagle CE and Freitas JE: Radionuclide imaging of musculoskeletal injuries in athletes with negative radiographs. Physician Sportsmed *15*:147–155, 1987.
48. Nettrour LF, Krufky EL, Mueller RE, and Raycroft JF: Locked scapula: Intrathoracic dislocation of the inferior angle. J Bone Joint Surg Am *54*:413–416, 1972.
49. Norwood LA, Matiko JA, and Terry GC: Posterior shoulder approach. Clin Orthop *201*:167–172, 1985.
50. Oni OO, Hoskinson J, and McPherson S: Closed traumatic scapulothoracic dissociation. Injury *23*:138–139, 1992.
51. Oreck SL, Burgess A, and Levine AM: Traumatic lateral displacement of the scapula: A radiographic sign of neurovascular disease. J Bone Joint Surg Am *66*:758–763, 1984.
52. Rowe CR: Fractures of the scapula. Surg Clin North Am *43*:1565–1571, 1963.
53. Samilson RL: Congenital and developmental anomalies of the shoulder girdle (Review). Orthop Clin North Am *11*:219–231, 1980.
54. Sandrock AR: Another sports fatigue fracture. Radiology *117*:274, 1975.
55. Schils JP, Freed HA, Richmond BJ, et al: Stress fracture of the acromion (Letter). AJR Am J Roentgenol *155*:1140–1141, 1990.
56. Thompson DA, Flynn TC, Miller PW, and Fischer RP: The significance of scapular fractures. J Trauma *25*:974–977, 1985.
57. Ward WG, Bergfeld JA, and Carson WG Jr: Stress fracture of the base of the acromial process. Am J Sports Med *22*:146–147, 1994.
58. Wilber MC and Evans EB: Fractures of the scapula. J Bone Joint Surg Am *59*:358–362, 1977.
59. Zdravkovic D and Damholt VV: Comminuted and severely displaced fractures of the scapula. Acta Orthop Scand *45*:60–65, 1974.

GLENOHUMERAL SUBLUXATION AND DISLOCATION IN CHILDREN

The diagnosis and management of glenohumeral dislocations in adults and adolescents is covered extensively in chapters in Chapter 14. This section focuses on special considerations for shoulder dislocations in the younger child and infant.

Anatomic Considerations

In children, the humeral attachment of the glenohumeral joint capsule is along the anatomic neck, making the capsular attachment epiphyseal except for the medial portion, which is metaphyseal. The proximal humeral epiphysis develops from three ossification centers. Union of these centers occurs at approximately 7 years of age with union of the humeral head to the humeral shaft at age 14 to 17 in girls and age 16 to 18 in boys.[12] The strong capsular attachments to the epiphysis make failure of the physis a more common injury than dislocations among children with open growth plates.

Incidence

Shoulder dislocations in children younger than 12 years of age are uncommon injuries. The incidence is reported to be 2.5 to 4.7% of all shoulder dislocations.[48, 56] Atraumatic dislocations appear to be more common in younger patients, and the incidence of traumatic dislocations rises as children enter and pass adolescence. Several authors have reported on traumatic and atraumatic dislocations in adolescents with open physes, but the ages of the patients are generally not reported.[1, 26, 27, 36, 48, 50, 55]

Classification

Classification schemes should enable a clinician to identify the etiology of the injury, give a prognosis for the natural history of the problem, and define the treatment. The rarity of dislocations in younger children makes this difficult, and no universally accepted classification scheme exists. Curtis and associates defined a classification scheme based on the etiology of dislocation that has been useful for children.[12] This classification can be further subdivided into the direction of dislocation.

- Traumatic
  - Anterior
  - Posterior
  - Inferior (luxatio erecta)
- Atraumatic

Congenital
Developmental
  Infection, neurologic
Joint laxity problems
  Ehlers-Danlos
Emotional and psychiatric problems

Mechanism of Injury

Traumatic dislocations in children, as in adults, are most commonly anterior dislocations associated with significant trauma from contact sports, falls, and motor vehicle accidents.[1, 2, 23, 36, 48, 56] There is typically a longitudinal force applied to an outstretched arm that forces the arm into an abducted, externally rotated position levering the humeral head out of the glenoid anteriorly. These injuries may be associated with physeal fractures of the proximal humerus[10, 20, 42, 43] and must be differentiated from true physeal fractures that can mimic dislocations in infants and neonates.[10, 18, 22, 33] Posterior traumatic dislocation has also been reported in children secondary to trauma and severe spasticity but is very uncommon.[17, 19, 39] Inferior dislocation with luxatio erecta of the shoulder is also rare but has been reported in association with forced manipulation of an infant with a brachial plexus injury.[32]

Atraumatic dislocations occur without a history of significant trauma. There is often bilateral involvement with multidirectional or posterior instability and an association with generalized ligamentous laxity.[4, 37, 40] The dislocations may be voluntary or involuntary.[39, 50] In voluntary dislocations, suppression of supraspinatus and infraspinatus muscle activity with firing of the pectoralis major and deltoid while positioning the arm in a vulnerable position will produce a dislocation. Congenital dysplasia of the glenoid, excessive retroversion of the glenoid, and developmental abnormalities of the proximal humerus have also been associated with recurrent dislocations.[9, 45, 57] Dislocation and subluxation of the glenohumeral joint in children have also been reported to be secondary to brachial plexus injuries, septic arthritis, Apert's syndrome, and arthrogryposis[3, 9, 11, 15, 29, 35, 46, 52] Three cases of congenital dislocation of the shoulder have also been reported with reference to several other cases in which there was no history of trauma during birth and a true dislocation without fracture at birth.[24, 30, 44]

Signs and Symptoms

A child with a traumatic anterior dislocation has presenting signs and symptoms identical to those seen in dislocations in adults.[36] There is pain and swelling with an obvious loss of normal shoulder contours due to displacement of the humeral head. As in adults, neurologic injury can occur but may be difficult to document in the younger child. In infants and neonates, physeal fractures of the proximal humerus may be indistinguishable clinically from true dislocation of the glenohumeral joint at initial presentation. The arm will be held abducted and externally rotated.[3, 13, 22, 33, 51]

Traumatic posterior dislocations of the glenohumeral joint are as rare in children as they are in adults. There is marked limitation of shoulder external rotation. There is also loss of the normal contour of the humeral head anteriorly.[17, 39]

Atraumatic dislocations do not have much pain associated with the dislocation. There are often clinical findings of generalized joint laxity and multidirectional instability.[7, 40, 47, 50] Dislocations associated with congenital anomalies or with brachial plexus injuries are also generally not painful in childhood.[3, 9, 11, 15, 52]

Radiographic Findings

The x-ray findings of traumatic dislocations in children are similar to those seen in adults. An anteroposterior film with an axillary lateral and West Point lateral view may demonstrate an associated Hill-Sachs lesion (Fig. 26–38), fracture of the glenoid rim, and congenital abnormalities of the glenoid or proximal humerus.[12] The view is useful for identifying anteroinferior bony abnormalities.[11] The use of CT scans with an arthrogram can be useful in defining the anatomy. Recent studies using MRI have compared it to CT arthrograms and show significant promise for this technique in evaluating the pathology associated with shoulder dislocations.[8, 41, 54] Retroversion of the glenoid can be demonstrated in recurrent posterior dislocators by CT scans.[57] Radiographs for atraumatic dislocations are often normal,[6, 7, 40, 50] but stress views may demonstrate inferior instability (Fig. 26–39).

Treatment

All acute traumatic shoulder dislocations should be reduced.[2, 12] Many closed methods have been described in the section on adult shoulder dislocations. The use of intra-articular lidocaine has been popular because it avoids the need for sedation and has been shown to be effective.[38] Closed reduction of a shoulder dislocation associated with a proximal humeral fracture is best attempted under a general anesthetic; however, the result is often unsuccessful and requires open reduction.[10, 20, 42, 43] Immobilization is for comfort with a sling or sling-and-swathe. The period of immobilization has not been shown to affect the rate of recurrent dislocations in younger patients.[25, 26, 36]

The rate of recurrence of shoulder dislocations in adolescents and young adults has been reported to be from 25 to 100% within 2 years of the initial dislocation, and most authors have reported a high rate of redislocation.[1, 7, 16, 25–27, 36, 47, 49, 55, 56] The presence of an associated tuberosity fracture is associated with a lower rate of redislocation.[26, 27] The lowest rates of recurrence have been found in series emphasizing an early and aggressive rotator cuff strengthening program, although the series has involved older teenagers.[1, 7]

The rarity of acute traumatic shoulder dislocations in children and adolescents along with the uncertainty of the natural history of recurrence leaves surgical indications for this disorder poorly defined. A wide variety of surgical techniques have been used successfully for repair of recurrent dislocations in adults. These techniques are

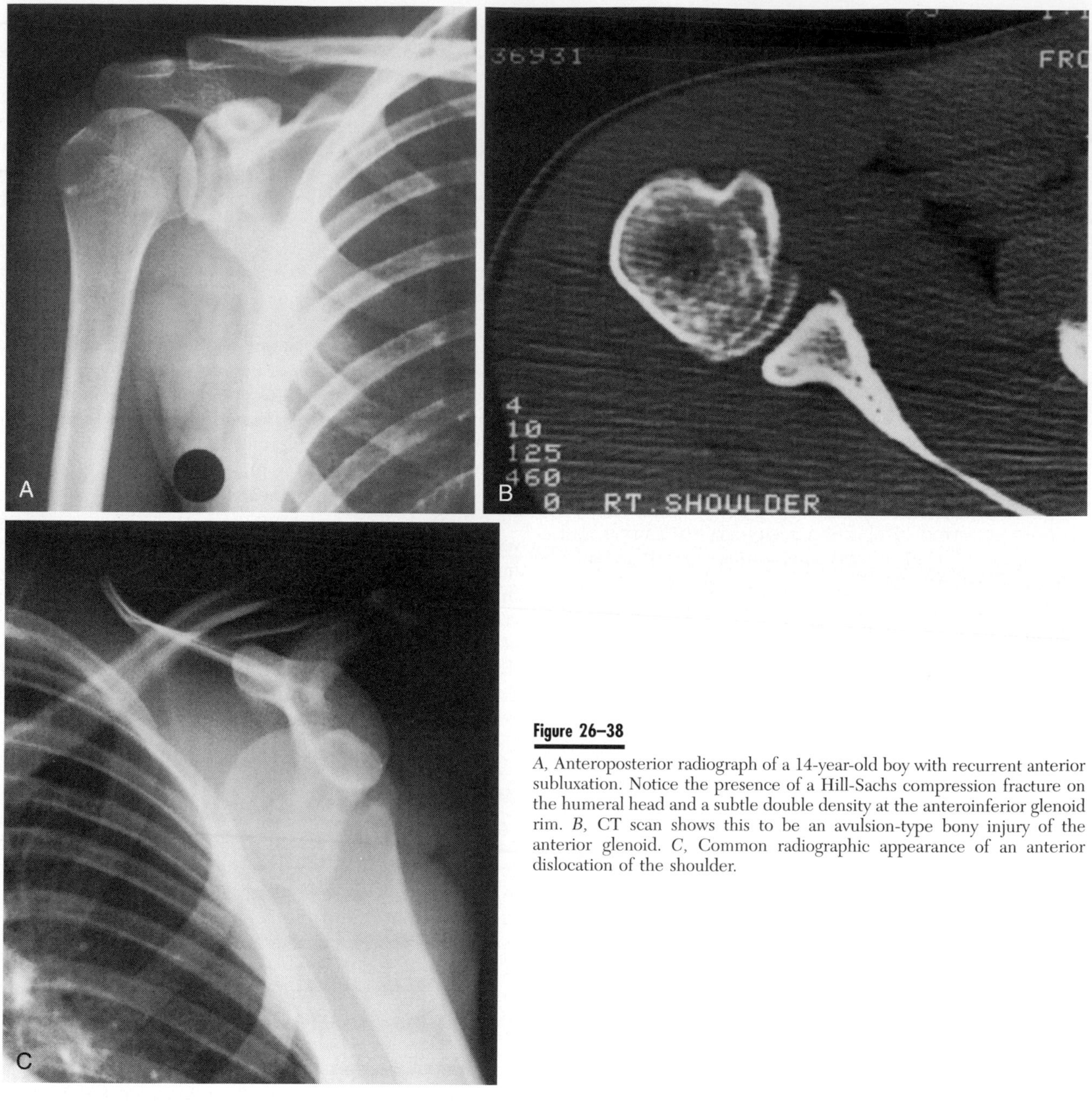

Figure 26–38

A, Anteroposterior radiograph of a 14-year-old boy with recurrent anterior subluxation. Notice the presence of a Hill-Sachs compression fracture on the humeral head and a subtle double density at the anteroinferior glenoid rim. *B,* CT scan shows this to be an avulsion-type bony injury of the anterior glenoid. *C,* Common radiographic appearance of an anterior dislocation of the shoulder.

described in Chapter 14 on glenohumeral instability in adults. Most series report young adults and adolescents within their patients but do not report the results of their younger patients separate from the overall series. The use of a coracoid bone block technique and an arthroscopically assisted labral repair in adolescents has been reported.[5, 18] In our review of the literature, no series has detailed results of the operative management of recurrent dislocations in children younger than 12 years of age.

The initial management of an atraumatic dislocation is a careful history and physical examination followed by reduction of the dislocation. It is important to be certain that the dislocation was truly atraumatic and to search for anatomic, neurologic, behavioral, or connective tissue abnormalities that may have contributed to the dislocation.[2, 7, 9, 11, 40, 45, 50, 57] Reduction of the dislocation is generally easily accomplished. Rapid institution of a vigorous rehabilitation program is generally recommended and has been successful in improving shoulder stability when psychiatric problems are not present.[7, 39, 40, 50] The management of atraumatic recurrent dislocations can be difficult. Habitual dislocators have not been found to have degenerative joint disease or pain over time unless they have had surgery to the shoulder.[28, 39, 50] Patients with involuntary dislocations may develop pain with recurrent dislocations. The instability can be unidirectional or multidirectional. Successful results have been recorded using the inferior capsular shift as described by Neer and Foster and detailed in the section on glenohumeral instability in Chapter 14.[6, 40] Recurrent posterior dislocation may benefit from the combination of posterior soft tissue and bony procedure.[34]

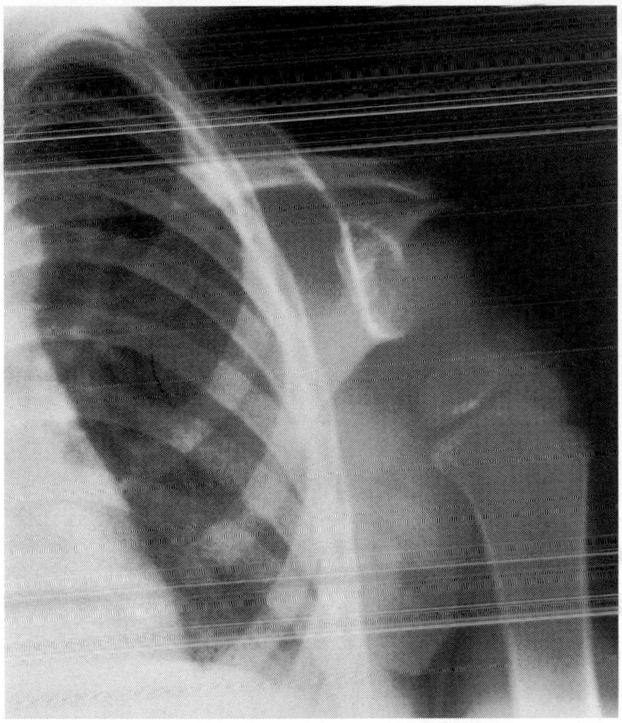

Figure 26–39

Dramatic demonstration of inferior subluxation of the glenohumeral joint in a patient with multidirectional instability. The clinical correlate is the "sulcus sign."

Reduction of chronic shoulder dislocations associated with brachial plexus injuries or obstetric trauma is unlikely to be achieved by closed methods. Open reduction via an anterior approach has been used successfully with capsulorrhaphy and release of the deltoid insertion.[3, 15, 19, 31, 32] A combined anterior/posterior approach has also been described.[53] To our knowledge, the natural history of untreated dislocations in these patients is not documented.

The natural history of shoulder instability associated with congenital abnormalities or other musculoskeletal abnormalities such as Apert's syndrome is unknown.[11, 21, 29] Correction of bony abnormalities is recommended if surgical reconstruction is undertaken, but the long-term outcomes of these procedures have not been reported.[9, 57]

Heilbronner reported on the management of a case of true congenital dislocation of the shoulder in a small newborn delivered by cesarean section with no radiographic evidence of fracture.[24, 30, 44] Treatment with adduction and internal rotation resulted in a stable and normally functioning shoulder and arm by 6 weeks.

AUTHORS' PREFERRED METHOD OF TREATMENT

For young children or adolescents with a traumatic shoulder dislocation, a gentle closed reduction should be done after a careful physical examination and history. Intra-articular lidocaine with chloral hydrate or intravenous midazolam (Versed) provide excellent analgesia for a closed reduction in children. Alternatively, a more conventional traction/countertraction method under intravenous sedation can be performed. If the child has an associated proximal humeral shaft fracture, the reduction maneuver is done under a general anesthetic, because the likelihood of needing an open reduction is high. Immobilization is used for 3 to 4 weeks until the child is comfortable and a rehabilitation program emphasizing rotater cuff and deltoid strengthening is instituted. If recurrent anterior dislocations occur, surgical intervention is indicated. We prefer an anterior approach with repair of a Bankart lesion if encountered and capsular advancement to reduce any redundancy found at the time of repair. The techniques for this are described in Chapter 14 on glenohumeral instability in adults. Immobilization with a sling is maintained for 6 weeks with early pendulum shoulder motion and elbow range of motion in the first month. Resisted external rotation exercises are avoided until 3 months. Progressive strengthening exercises are begun at 3 months and continued until 6 months after surgery. Stiffness and contractures about the shoulder are not generally encountered.

Children with atraumatic dislocations need reduction after an acute dislocation. This is generally easily accomplished. Habitual dislocation should be discouraged. We prefer to manage these children with a rehabilitation program with emphasis on rotator cuff strengthening and behavior modification to discourage voluntary dislocations. If involuntary dislocations persist after 6 to 12 months of supervised rehabilitation in patients with multidirectional instability, we proceed with the capsular procedure described by Neer.[24–26] Habitual dislocators are treated with rehabilitation and skilful neglect.

We prefer to reduce chronic shoulder dislocations associated with brachial plexus injury or birth trauma. This is done by way of an anterior approach and is accompanied by a capsulorrhaphy. The supraspinatous and deltoid muscles are generally contracted and may need release or lengthening distally to achieve reduction. In very young children, immobilization of the arm by the side for 6 weeks can stretch these muscles sufficiently so that winging of the scapula does not persist.

Children with congenital anomalies or with shoulder subluxation associated with other musculoskeletal deformities should be carefully assessed for their overall function before embarking on reconstructive surgical procedures to reduce the shoulder. Clearly defined functional goals should guide surgical efforts. There are no reported surgical series to guide reconstructive efforts.

References and Bibliography

1. Aronen JG and Regan K: Decreasing the incidence of recurrence of first time anterior shoulder dislocations with rehabilitation. Am J Sports Med *12*:382–391, 1984.
2. Asher MA: Dislocations of the upper extremity in children. Orthop Clin North Am 7:583–591, 1976.
3. Babbitt DP and Cassidy RH: Obstetrical paralysis and dislocation of the shoulder in infancy. J Bone Joint Surg Am *50*:1447–1452, 1968.
4. Banas MP, Dalldorf PG, Sebastianelli WJ, and DeHaven KE: Long-term followup of the modified Bristow procedure. Am J Sports Med *21*:666–671, 1993.
5. Barry TP, Lombardo SJ, Kerlan RD, et al: The coracoid transfer

for recurrent anterior instability of the shoulder in adolescents. J Bone Joint Surg Am *67:*383–387, 1985.
6. Bigliani LU, Pollock RG, McIlveen SJ, et al: Shift of the posteroinferior aspect of the capsule for recurrent posterior glenohumeral instability. J Bone Joint Surg Am *77:*1011–1020, 1995.
7. Burkhead WZ Jr and Rockwood CA Jr: Treatment of instability of the shoulder with an exercise program. J Bone Joint Surg Am *74:*890–896, 1992.
8. Chandnani VP, Yeager TD, Deberardino T, et al: Glenoid labral tears: Prospective evaluation with MR imaging, MR arthrography, and CT arthrography. Am J Radiol *161:*1229–1235, 1993.
9. Chung SMK and Nissenbaum MM: Congenital and developmental defects of the shoulder (Review). Orthop Clin North Am *6:*381–392, 1975.
10. Cohn BT and Froimson AI: Salter 3 fracture dislocation of glenohumeral joint in a 10-year-old. Orthop Rev *15:*403–404, 1986.
11. Cozen L: Congenital dislocation of the shoulder and other anomalies. Arch Surg *35:*956–966, 1937.
12. Curtis RJJ, Dameron TB Jr, and Rockwood CA Jr: Fractures and dislocations of the shoulder in children. *In* Rockwood CAJ, Wilkins KE, and King RE (eds): Fractures in Children. Philadelphia: JB Lippincott, 1991, pp 829–919.
13. Dameron TB Jr and Reibel DB: Fractures involving the proximal humeral epiphyseal plate. J Bone Joint Surg Am *51:*289–297, 1969.
14. De Smet AA: Anterior oblique projection in radiography of the traumatized shoulder. AJR Am J Roentgenol *134:*515–518, 1980.
15. Dunkerton MC: Posterior dislocation of the shoulder associated with obstetric brachial plexus palsy. J Bone Joint Surg Br *71:*764–766, 1989.
16. Elbaum R, Parent H, Zeller R, and Seringe R: Traumatic scapulohumeral dislocation in children and adolescents: A propos of 9 patients. Acta Orthop Belg *60:*204–209, 1994.
17. Foster WS, Ford TB, and Drez D Jr: Isolated posterior shoulder dislocation in a child: A case report. Am J Sports Med *13:*198–200, 1985.
18. Golberg BJ, Nerschl RP, McConnell JP, and Pettrone FA: Arthroscopic transglenoid suture capsulolabral repairs: Preliminary results. Am J Sports Med *21:*656–665, 1993.
19. Green NE and Wheelhouse WW: Anterior subglenoid dislocation of the shoulder in an infant following pneumococcal meningitis. Clin Orthop *135:*125–127, 1978.
20. Gregg-Smith SJ and White SH: Salter-Harris III fracture-dislocation of the proximal humeral epiphysis. Injury *23:*199–200, 1992.
21. Grieg DM: True congenital dislocation of the shoulder. Edinburgh Med J *30:*157–175, 1923.
22. Haliburton RA, Barber JR, and Fraser RL: Pseudodislocation: An unusual birth injury. Can J Surg *10:*455–462, 1967.
23. Heck CC: Anterior dislocation of the glenohumeral joint in a child. J Trauma *21:*174–175, 1981.
24. Heilbronner DM: True congenital dislocation of the shoulder. J Pediatr Orthop *10:*408–410, 1990.
25. Henry JH and Genung JA: Natural history of glenohumeral dislocation—revisited. Am J Sports Med *10:*135–137, 1982.
26. Heolen MA, Burgers AM, and Rozing PM: Prognosis of primary anterior shoulder dislocation in young adults. Arch Orthop Trauma Surg *110:*51–54, 1990.
27. Hovelius L: Anterior dislocation of the shoulder in teenagers and young adults: Five-year prognosis. J Bone Joint Surg Am *69:*393–399, 1987.
28. Huber H and Gerber C: Voluntary subluxation of the shoulder in children: A long-term follow-up study of 36 shoulders. J Bone Joint Surg Br *76:*118–122, 1994.
29. Kasser J and Upton J: The shoulder, elbow, and forearm in Apert syndrome. Clin Plast Surg *18:*381–389, 1991.
30. Kelly SW: Surgical Diseases of Children. St Louis: CV Mosby, 1924.
31. Kuhn D and Rosman M: Traumatic, nonparalytic dislocation of the shoulder in a newborn infant. J Pediatr Orthop *4:*121–122, 1984.
32. Laskin RS and Sedlin ED: Luxatio erecta in infancy. Clin Orthop *80:*126–129, 1971.
33. Lemperg R and Liliequist B: Dislocation of the proximal epiphysis of the humerus in newborns. Acta Paediatr Scand *59:*377–380, 1970.
34. Letts M: Posterior habitual dislocation of the shoulder (Abstract). Pediatric Orthopaedic Society of North America, Phoenix, 1996, p 92.
35. Lev-Toaff AS, Karasick D, and Rao VM: "Drooping shoulder"—nontraumatic causes of glenohumeral subluxation. Skeletal Radio *12:*34–36, 1984.
36. Marans HJ, Angel KR, Schemitsch EH, and Wedge JH: The fate of traumatic anterior dislocation of the shoulder in children. J Bone Joint Surg Am *74:*1242–1244, 1992.
37. Matsen FA, Thomas SC, and Rockwood CA: Glenohumeral instability. *In* Rockwood CAJ and Matsen FA (eds): The Shoulder. Philadelphia: WB Saunders, 1990, pp 526–622.
38. Matthews DE and Roberts T: Intraarticular lidocaine versus intravenous analgesic for reduction of acute anterior shoulder dislocations: A prospective randomized study. Am J Sports Med *10:*135–137, 1995.
39. May VR Jr: Posterior dislocation of the shoulder: Habitual, traumatic, and obstetrical (Review). Orthop Clin North Am *11:*271–285, 1980.
40. Neer CS and Foster CR: Inferior capsular shift for involuntary inferior and multidirectional instability of the shoulder: A preliminary report. J Bone Joint Surg Am *62:*897–908, 1980.
41. Neumann CH, Petersen SA, Jahnke AH Jr, et al: MRI in the evaluation of patients with suspected instability of the shoulder joint including a comparison with CT arthrography. Rofo Fortschr Geb Rontgenstr Neuen Bildgeb Verfahr *154:*593–600, 1991.
42. Nicastro JF and Adair DM: Fracture-dislocation of the shoulder in a 32-month-old child. J Pediatr Orthop *2:*427–429, 1982.
43. Obremskey W and Routt ML Jr: Fracture-dislocation of the shoulder in a child: Case report. J Trauma *36:*137–140, 1994.
44. Peckham FE: Two cases of congenital dislocation of the shoulder. Arch Pediatr *2:*509–511, 1904.
45. Pettersson H: Bilateral dysplasia of the neck of the scapula and associated anomalies. Acta Radiol Diagn *22:*81–84, 1981.
46. Resnik CS: Septic arthritis: A rare cause of drooping shoulder. Skeletal Radiol *21:*307–309, 1992.
47. Rockwood CA Jr: The shoulder: Facts, confusions and myths. Int Orthop *15:*401–405, 1991.
48. Rowe CR: Prognosis in dislocations of the shoulder. J Bone Joint Surg Am *38:*957–977, 1956.
49. Rowe CR: Anterior dislocations of the shoulder: Prognosis and treatment. Surg Clin North Am *43:*1609–1614, 1963.
50. Rowe CR, Pierce DS, and Clark JG: Voluntary dislocation of the shoulder: A preliminary report on a clinical, electromyographic, and psychiatric study of twenty-six patients. J Bone Joint Surg Am *55:*445–460, 1973.
51. Scaglietti O: The obstetrical shoulder trauma. Surg Gynecol Obstet *66:*868, 1938.
52. Travlos J, Goldberg I, and Boome RS: Brachial plexus lesions associated with dislocated shoulders. J Bone Joint Surg Br *72:*68–71, 1990.
53. Troum S, Floyd WE 3d, and Waters PM: Posterior dislocation of the humeral head in infancy associated with obstetrical paralysis: A case report. J Bone Joint Surg Am *75:*1370–1375, 1993.
54. Uri DS, Kneeland B, and Dalinka MK: Update in shoulder magnetic resonance imaging. Magn Reson *11:*21–44, 1995.
55. Vermeiren J, Handelberg F, Casteleyn PP, and Opdecam P: The rate of recurrence of traumatic anterior dislocation of the shoulder: A study of 154 cases and a review of the literature. Int Orthop *17:*337–341, 1993.
56. Wagner KT Jr and Lyne ED: Adolescent traumatic dislocations of the shoulder with open epiphyses. J Pediatr Orthop *3:*61–62, 1983.
57. Wirth MA, Lyons FR, and Rockwood CA Jr: Hypoplasia of the glenoid: A review of sixteen patients (Review). J Bone Joint Surg Am *75:*1175–1184, 1993.

BRACHIAL PLEXUS PALSY IN CHILDREN

While occasionally resulting from trauma, congenital masses, and viral or Parsonage-Turner syndrome, most brachial plexus palsies in children occur at the time of delivery.[3, 12, 29, 35, 42, 44, 45, 55, 66, 69] Although early examiners saw a number of late cases and had difficulty discerning subsequent deformity from etiology,[53] both experimental[11, 42, 55] and clinical[7, 11] evidence strongly implicates a traction injury (Fig. 26–40). The incidence of the birth palsy ranges from 0.5 to 2.5%[1, 12, 25, 28, 64, 65, 70] and is

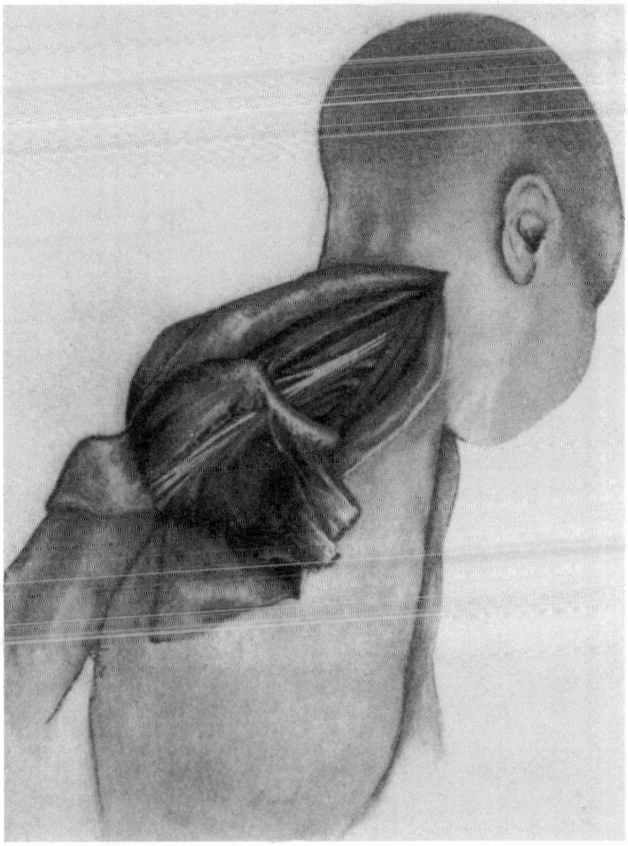

Figure 26–40

When the head and neck are separated, considerable tension is applied to the junction of the fifth and sixth cervical roots. (From Sever JW: Obstetric paralysis. Am J Dis Child *12*:541–578, 1916.)

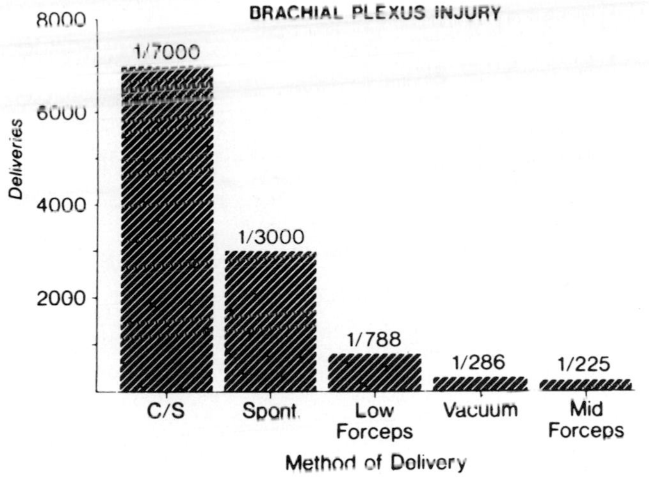

Figure 26–41

The incidence of Erb's palsy by method of delivery. (From The American College of Obstetricians and Gynecologists. McFarland LV, Raskin M, Daling JR, and Benedetti TJ: Erb/Duchenne's palsy: A consequence of fetal macrosomia and method of delivery. Obstet Gynecol *68*:784–788, 1986.)

higher in children over 4000 g, particularly in those with shoulder dystocia.[35, 64, 66] The more difficult the delivery, the greater is the likelihood of a plexus injury[7, 29, 42] (Fig. 26–41). Occasionally, however, the problem may occur without noticeable delivery problems.[30]

Smellie[58] initially described upper root injuries in 1764, whereas Duchenne,[14] in 1861, described the entity in detail. In 1874, Erb,[17] using electrical studies, showed that paralysis at the junction of the fifth and sixth roots, Erb's point, produces the typical palsy. Flaubert[18] described the characteristic lower plexus palsy in 1827, but Klumpke's later description associated her name with this.[32] Newborn plexus palsies are almost always supraclavicular. The upper plexus is more susceptible to traction within the roots and trunk, whereas the lower plexus is less susceptible to traction injuries but more susceptible to avulsion.

An accurate description of a brachial plexus injury requires anatomic localization and a description of the degree and type of disruption (Figs. 26–42 to 26–45). Typical proximal C5 and C6 injuries produce weak shoulder external rotation, abduction, and elbow flexion (Fig. 26–46). The loss of the extensor carpi radialis brevis and longus cause weak wrist dorsiflexion and radial deviation. The triceps pulls the elbow out into full extension. Upper plexus palsies may also have diaphragmatic involvement via the C4 phrenic roots. If C7 is also involved, the triceps will be weak, and the elbow positions in slight flexion. A weak triceps also implies a weak latissimus dorsi, making later transfers less predictable. Further weakness of wrist dorsiflexion and radial deviation occurs. Lower plexus

Figure 26–42

Semidiagrammatic scheme of the brachial plexus demonstrating the nerve supply to the muscles of the upper extremities. (From Taylor AS: Conclusions derived from further experience in the surgical treatment of brachial birth palsy. Am J Med Sci *146*:836–856, 1913.)

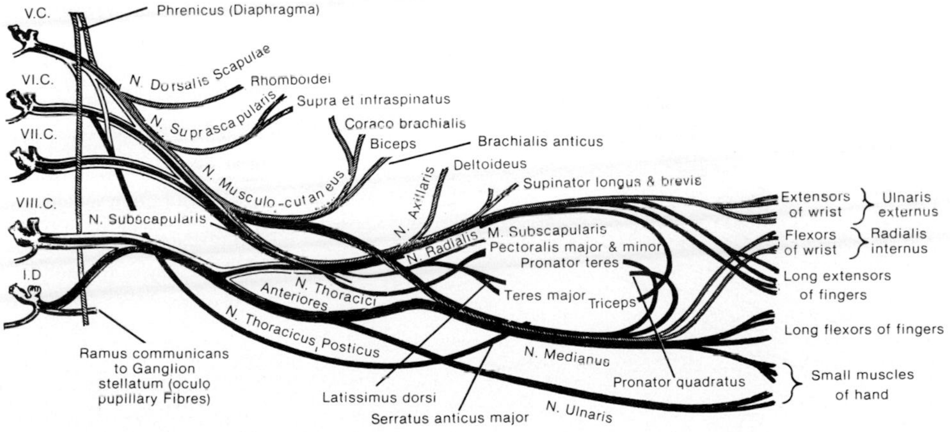

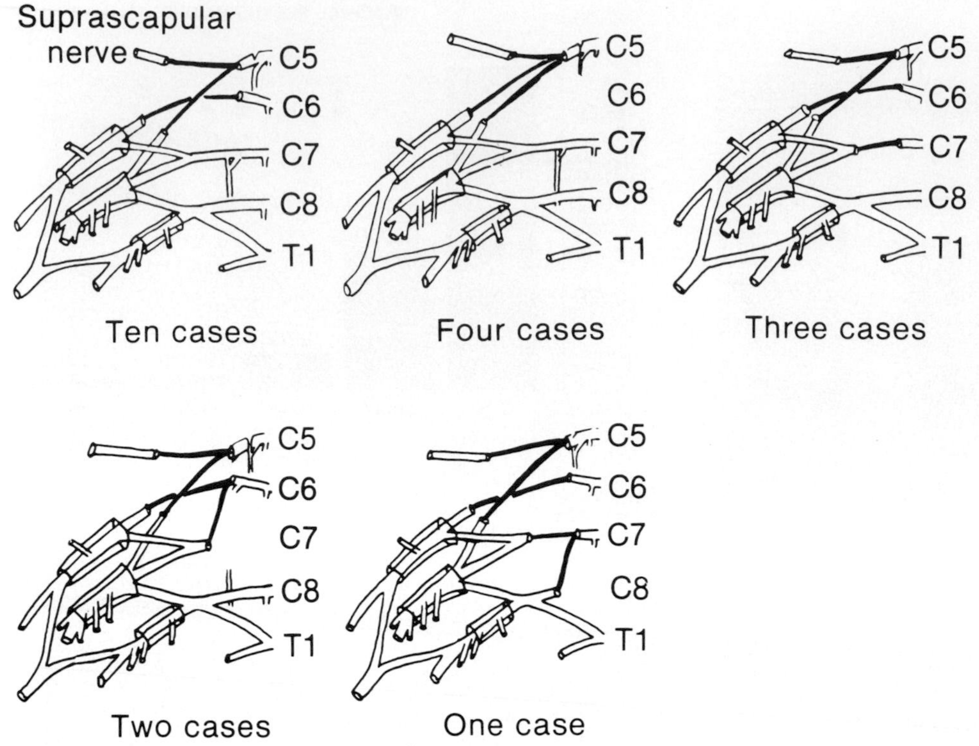

Figure 26–43

Patterns of placement of the sural nerve grafts in 20 patients. Absence of the nerve roots indicates those that were avulsed. (From Boome RS and Kaye JC: Obstetrical traction injuries of the brachial plexus. J Bone Joint Surg *70B*:571–576, 1988.)

palsies (C8, T1) have weakness of wrist flexors, particularly the flexor carpi ulnaris, and weak forearm pronation, finger flexion, extension, and intrinsics. The forearm is held in supination, and the fingers are partially flexed (Fig. 26–47). Total plexus palsies create a flail arm. Zancolli and Zancolli[71] usefully group palsies into proximal, distal, posterior cord,[3] and flaccid. Pure lower plexus or Klumpke's palsies are quite rare.[5]

Although the severity of a nerve injury may be classified according to Seddon and associates' neuropraxia,[54] neurotmesis, or axonotmesis or according to the more detailed Sunderland classification of grades 1 to 5,[60] determination of the grade of injury clinically is difficult. Examination of the newborn can also be quite difficult. Gilbert and associates recommend a repeat examination after 48 hours when the examination is easier.[21, 22, 24] The examination focuses on an asymmetric Moro reflex, the asymmetric tonic neck reflex, the resting posture of the extremity, and any evidence of a cord injury (e.g., no leg function). Other causes of an asymmetric Moro reflex should also be sought, such as a fracture of the clavicle or humerus. Once the infant is a little older, play is useful to examine for active motor function. Particular functions to watch for are active elbow flexion, shoulder abduction, hand opening, and grasp. The typical contracture of an upper plexus palsy is shoulder internal rotation, adduction, and forearm pronation (Fig. 26–48). A severe internal rotation contracture can be a functional problem (Figs. 26–49 and 26–50). Rarely, the shoulder is contracted in abduction or external rotation, but this is usually secondary to excessively vigorous splinting. A shoulder contracture can be visualized by Putti's sign[70] (Fig. 26–51)—a contracted glenohumeral joint causes the scapula to wing away from the thorax when the arm is manipulated. With lower plexus palsies, the forearm may be stuck in supination. Once the child is about 3 years of age, a more detailed

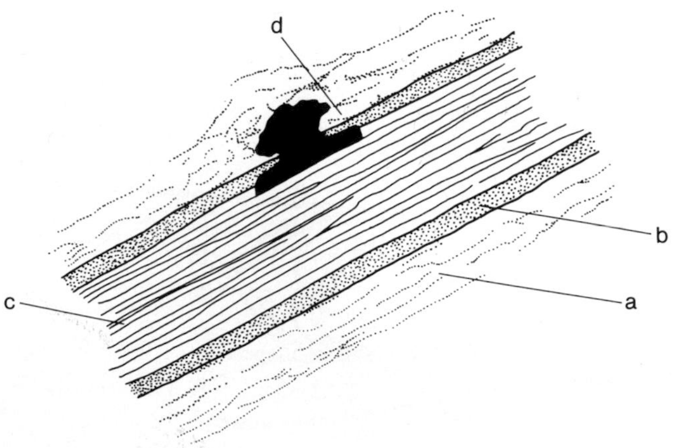

Figure 26–44

A schematic representation of the pathology in the incomplete lesions. Initial rupture of the perineural sheath produces a hematoma (d) involving the epineurium (a), perineurium (b), and nerve bundles (c). (From Clark LP, Taylor AS, and Prout TP: A study of brachial birth palsy. Am J Med Sci *130*:670–707, 1905.)

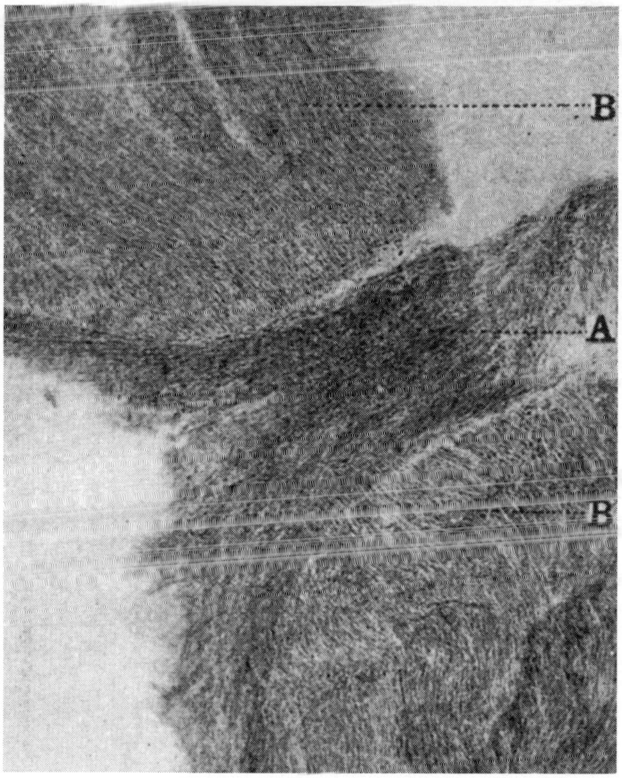

Figure 26–45

Photomicrograph demonstrating the constricting fibrous tissue *(A)* across the torn nerve fibers *(B)* (From Clark LP, Taylor As, and Prout TP: A study of brachial birth palsy. Am J Med Sci *130*:670–707, 1905.)

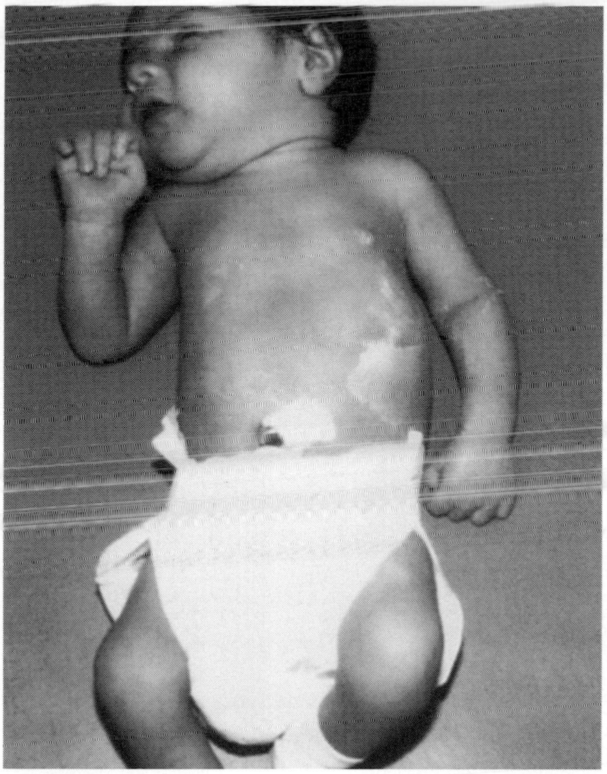

Figure 26–46

The typical posture of the upper extremity in the newborn with an upper root injury.

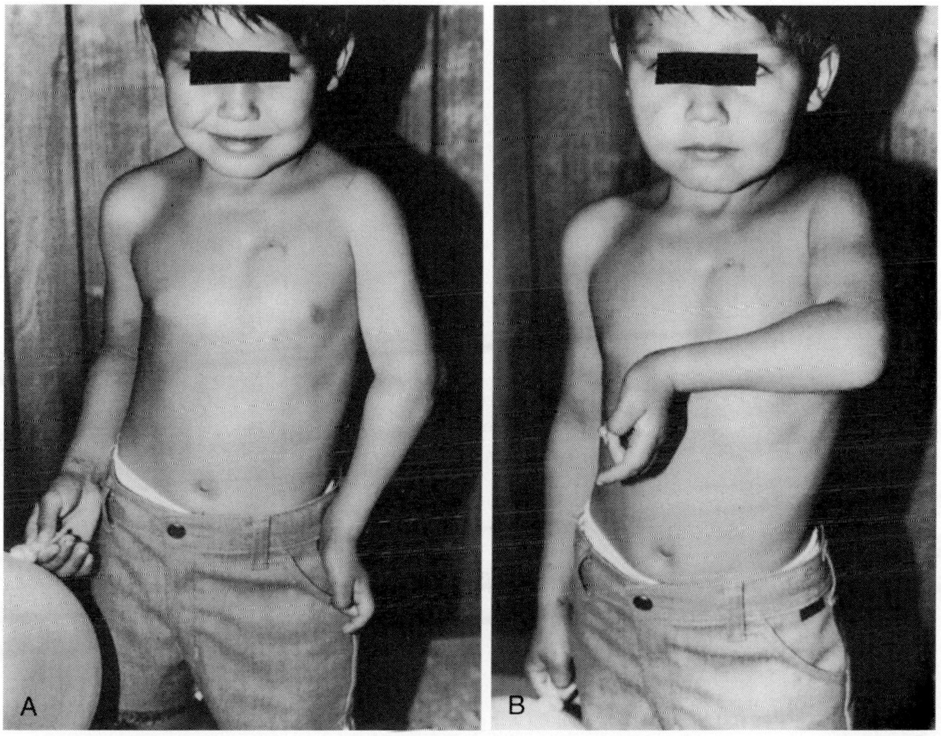

Figure 26–47

The usual posture of the arm with a lower root lesion with the elbow extended *(A)* and flexed *(B)*.

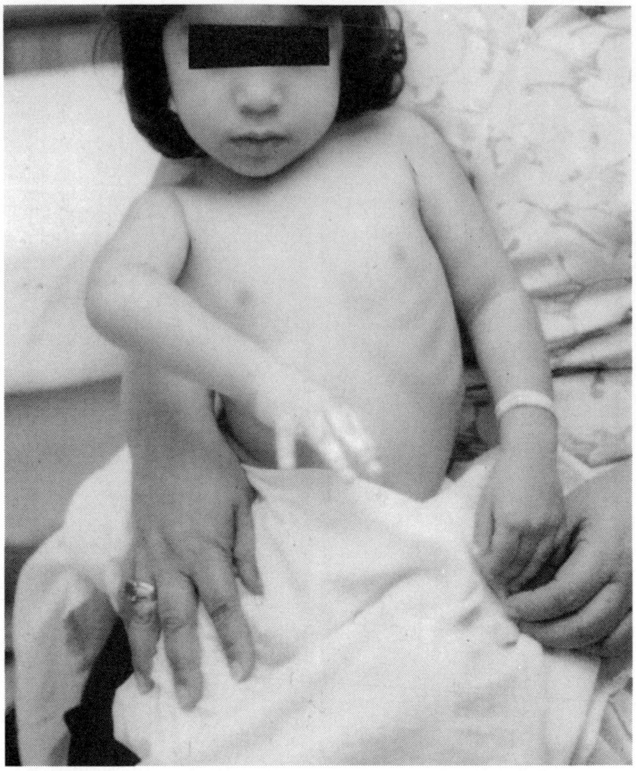

Figure 26–48

Even though this patient has shoulder abduction to 75 degrees, she is unable to put her hand to her mouth because of a 45-degree internal rotation contracture.

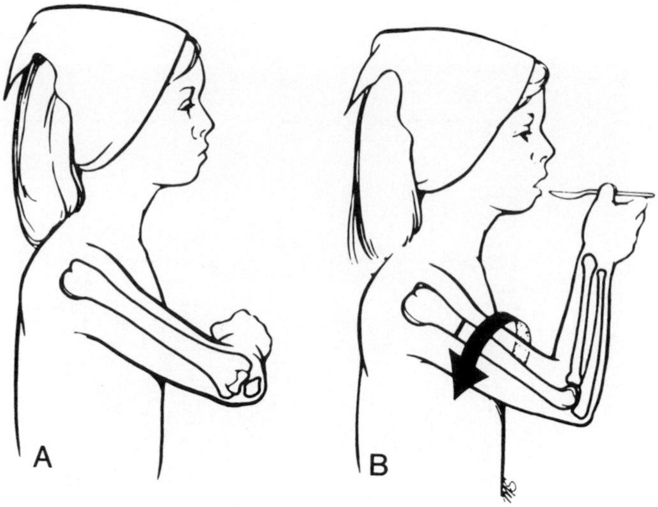

Figure 26–50

A, With limited abduction and forward flexion, the internal rotation contracture prevents the forearm and hand from reaching the face. *B*, Derotating the humerus approximately 90 degrees enables the hand to be brought to the head and face. (From Blount WP: Osteoclasis of the upper extremity in children. Acta Orthop Scand 32:374–382, 1962.)

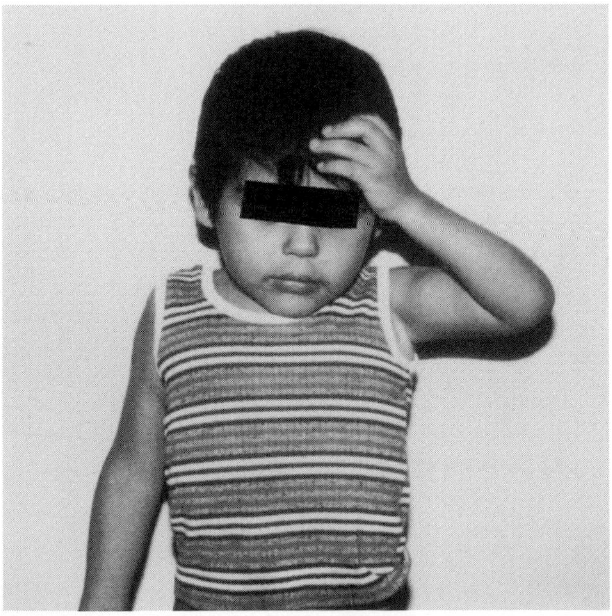

Figure 26–49

The goal in recovery is to enable the patient to reach the hand to the head or mouth.

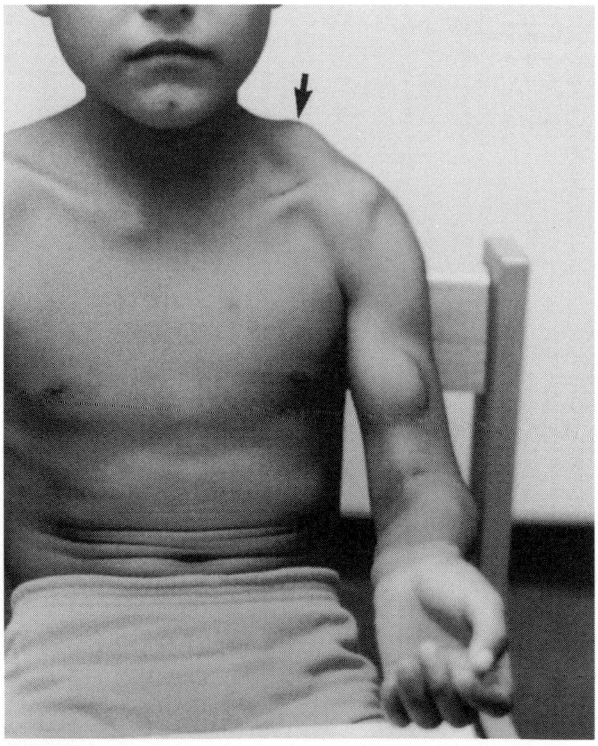

Figure 26–51

Clinical picture demonstrating the elevation of the superior border of the scapula *(arrow)* with external rotation of the humerus and abduction of the arm—the "scapular sign of Putti."

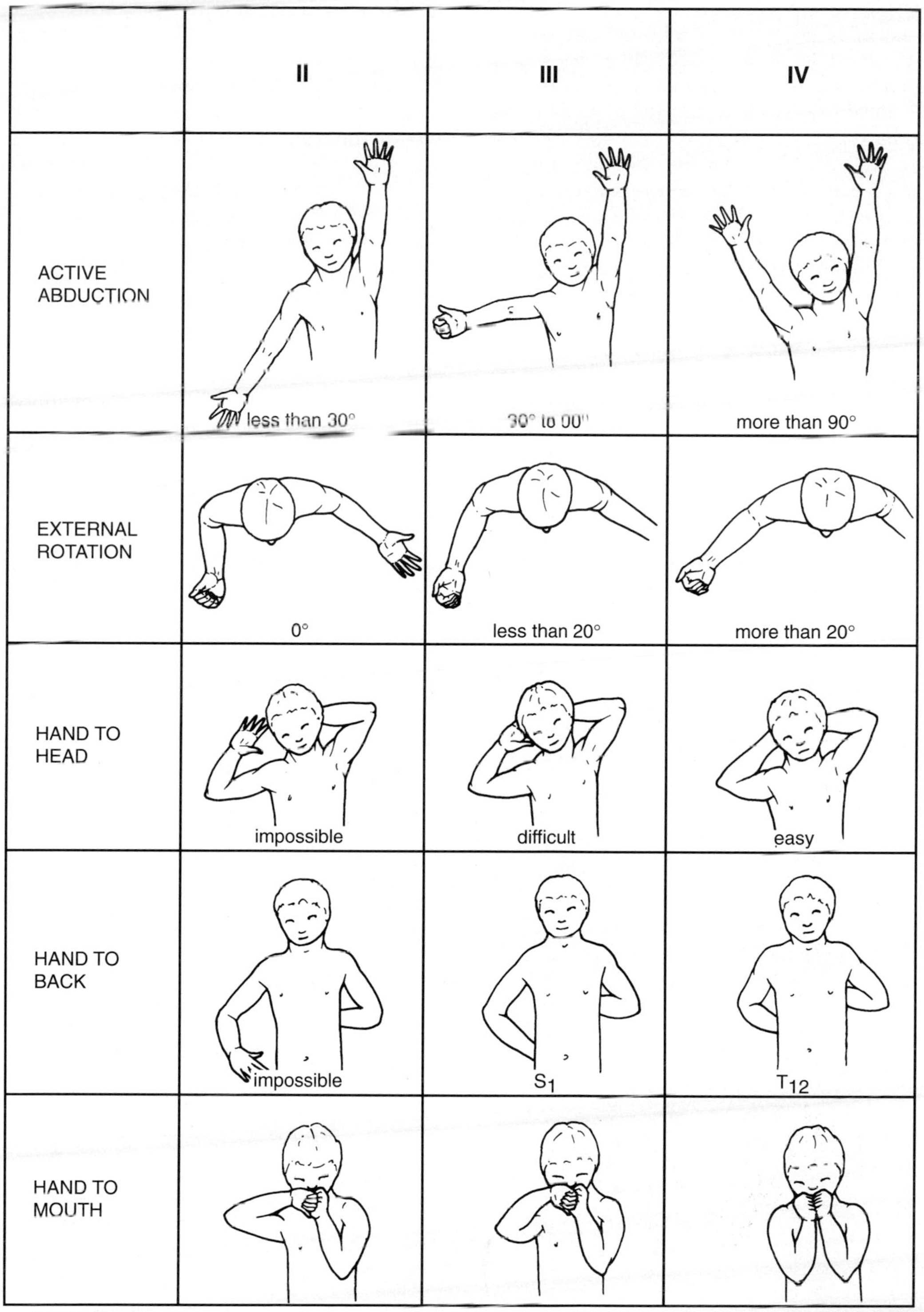
II
III
IV
ACTIVE ABDUCTION
less than 30°
30° to 90°
more than 90°
EXTERNAL ROTATION
0°
less than 20°
more than 20°
HAND TO HEAD
impossible
difficult
easy
HAND TO BACK
impossible
S_1
T_{12}
HAND TO MOUTH

Figure 26–52

Mallet classification of end results from brachial plexus palsy in newborns. (Adapted from Mallet J: Parakysie obstétricale du plexus brachial. Traitement des séquelles. Primauté du traitement de l'épaule. Méthode d'expression des résultats. Rev Chir Orthop 58[Suppl 1]:115, 1972.)

motor and sensory examination is possible. The involved limb is shorter than the normal side and may have contractures. Once contractures develop, it is difficult to examine a muscle's strength.

In general, nerve recovery to a bulky muscle like the deltoid is better than to finer muscles like the rotator cuff. Motor nerves such as the musculocutaneous recover better than do mixed nerves like the ulnar. Upper root stretch injuries have a better prognosis than do lower root stretch injuries, and infraclavicular injuries have a better prognosis than do supraclavicular injuries. Factors that indicate a worse prognosis are lower or total plexus palsy, a slow recovery indicating a more severe disruption, and evidence of root avulsion such as scapular winging (the long thoracic nerve has a very high takeoff), a Horner syndrome (primarily T1 root), and lower extremity spasticity or a phrenic nerve palsy. A lot of shoulder bruising or a physeal separation portends a poor prognosis because of the degree of trauma. The prognostic value of a fracture of the clavicle is less certain.[4] It may decompress the plexus leading to a better prognosis, or the degree of trauma may portend a worse prognosis. Myelograms, CT myelograms, or MRI can show traumatic meningoceles in root avulsions but can be misleading.[27, 40, 43, 45] MRI can be misleading, although further advances may make it useful.[19] EMGs may lead to an overly optimistic prognosis in that only minimal nerve regrowth is necessary for reinervation potentials.[57]

Treatment is made more difficult because of a lack of consensus regarding the prognosis for injuries. Some authors report a very low incidence of recovery, whereas others report more than 95% with full recovery.[8, 12, 25, 28, 35, 44, 70] Early treatment should concentrate on range of motion to prevent contractures, defining the rapidity of recovery and the level of the lesion. Splinting, which was attempted vigorously in the past, can result in debilitating shoulder abduction contractures, luxatio erecta, and radial head dislocations and is rarely done now except on a limited basis for elbow flexion contractures and perioperatively. There is little role for bracing except for rare, specific functions. Children find the braces cumbersome. The braces provide little benefit, and children usually discard them. After a while even range-of-motion exercises tend to be abandoned.

Early complications that can be overlooked are posterior shoulder dislocation[6, 15, 36, 38, 41, 62, 63, 69] and infection.[20, 67] To be certain that there is no shoulder dislocation, children with a brachial plexus palsy and limited shoulder external rotation should have an axillary lateral x-ray. This problem can be treated with open reduction through an anterior or a combined anterior and posterior approach. A neonatal septic shoulder can also present as

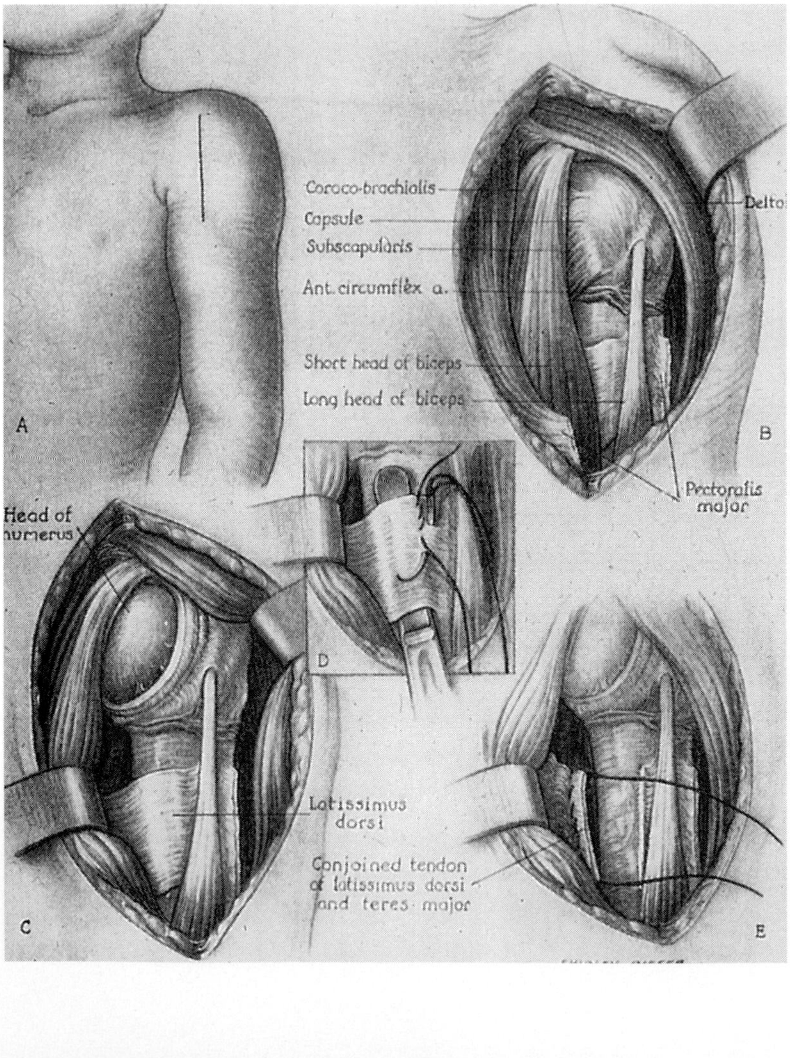

Figure 26–53

The anterior approach for the L'Episcopo procedure. *A*, The incision. *B*, The deep anterior structures after the pectoralis major has been cut. *C*, In the original description both the anterior capsule and subscapularis were cut, exposing the head of the humerus. *D*, Presuturing the conjoined tendon of the latissimus dorsi and teres major. *E*, Release of the conjoined tendon. (Reprinted by permission from the *New York State Journal of Medicine*, copyright by the Medical Society of the State of New York. From L'Episcopo JB: Restoration of muscle balance in the treatment of obstetrical paralysis. NY State J Med *39*:357–363, 1939.)

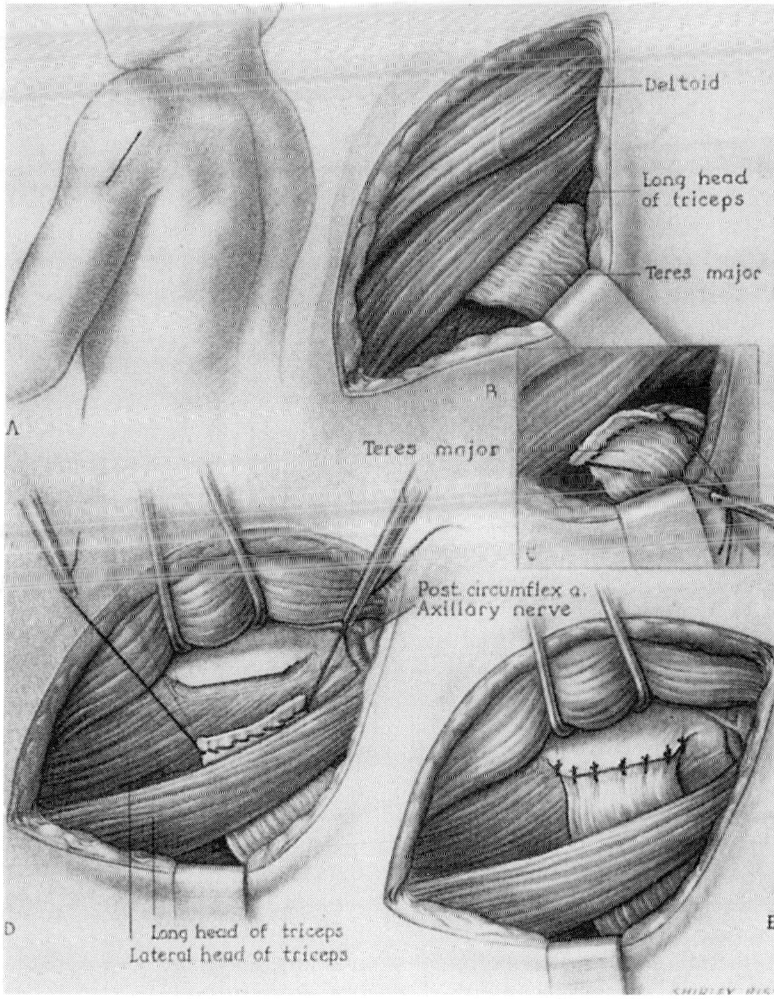

Figure 26–54

The posterior approach for the L'Episcopo procedure. *A*, Posterior incision parallel to the posterior deltoid. *B*, Exposure of the relaxed teres major posterior to the long head of the triceps. *C*, The conjoined tendons of the teres major and latissimus dorsi are pulled out of the posterior incision by their sutures. *D*, The conjoined tendons are passed under the long head of the triceps. *E*, The tendons are sutured to an anterior periosteal flap. (Reprinted by permission from the *New York State Journal of Medicine*, copyright by the Medical Society of the State of New York. From L'Episcopo JB: Restoration of muscle balance in the treatment of obstetrical paralysis. N Y State J Med *39*:357–363, 1939.)

a brachial plexus palsy.[20, 67] Typically, the shoulder and elbow move after birth and stop moving a few days later. This part of the history is extremely important, because infants may not exhibit fever and early x-rays are usually normal. Any discomfort of the shoulder should bring this diagnosis to mind. Although some literature advocates aspiration and intravenous antibiotics for this,[37] we strongly recommend open drainage through a posterior approach and intravenous antibiotics. In our experience, it still takes several weeks for the "brachial plexus palsy" to resolve.

The last decade has emphasized early exploration and nerve grafting, and the most aggressive approach has been advocated by Gilbert and associates.[21, 22, 24] Mallet[39] graded end-results based on the degree of active motion possible at the shoulder and elbow (Fig. 26–52). Using this scale, Tassin's and Gilbert's review[24] indicated that all patients without return of deltoid and biceps function by 3 months of age had poor results; therefore, if there is no biceps function (it is easier to see than deltoid function) by 3 months of age, the patient is scheduled for surgery. Part of the reason for the aggressive scheduling is the worry that some function will return during the next month and that the parents will refuse the operation. A supraclavicular incision explores the upper plexus, and a continued transclavicular incision explores the lower plexus if needed. With both complete sural nerves harvested, any questionable areas of the plexus are excised, grafted, and held with fibrin glue. Gilbert reports that the surgery improves the natural history by one Mallet grade. Full recovery cannot be ascertained before 4 years.[56]

Only recently have good comparative studies been presented from other centers. Waters[68] reviewed patients at Boston Children's Hospital with brachial plexus palsies. He found that children who recovered biceps function by 1 month of age had essentially normal function. Those who had recovery of biceps function by 3 months of age did better than did those grafted by 6 months of age. However, children observed beyond 6 months did worse than did those grafted at the same time. It appears from Waters' study that if no biceps recovery is made by 6 months, nerve exploration is justified. What remains uncertain is whether exploration between 3 and 6 months of age would improve the results. Likewise, these studies utilized the Mallet grade to determine the outcome, and its utility and observer error have not been quantified.

Some surgeons try to restore elbow flexion by grafting into the musculocutaneous nerve.[47, 71] Neurotization can be done using the intercostals, the spinal accessory, the phrenic, or any other cervical motor nerve.[26, 31, 34, 46, 51, 52] It is more successful to bulk muscles such as the deltoid or biceps than to bulk smaller muscles.[10, 59] It has been used successfully to restore shoulder abduction by grafting into the suprascapular and axillary nerves.[10]

In older children, contracture release may allow better muscle function from moderately functional muscles that are unable to overpower the contracture. The mainstay of shoulder contracture release has been the subscapularis release of Sever.[55] This has been modified by others to prevent anterior subluxation of the humerus. Zancolli and Zancolli lengthen the posterior cuff to allow the subluxation to reduce.[71] An increasingly popular operation is release of the subscapularis origin as described by Carloiz and Brahimi[9] at an early age. We have done this procedure in patients younger than 2 years of age and found it quite useful. The approach is made in a virtually bloodless plane between the latissimus dorsi and the teres minor posteriorly. The small latissimus insertion on the inferior angle of the scapula is released. This provides direct access to the anterior scapula. The scapula is then held with a towel clip or a strong suture on the inferior angle to allow manipulation. The subscapularis origin is released, and the muscle is elevated extraperiosteally until the contracture is freed. The patient is then held in a shoulder spica for 4 weeks with the shoulder in external rotation with subsequent physical therapy. This procedure must be done while the glenohumeral joint remains congruous. Transfer of the latissimus can be done at the same time or later on. Incidentally, we learned this approach from Mary Beth Ezaki and have made it our utilitarian approach to the anterior scapula for surgeries such as removing benign tumors like osteochondromas.

Numerous tendon transfers are described to restore motion.[13, 16, 23, 48, 50] L'Episcopo[33] released the shoulder contracture and transferred the latissimus dorsi and teres major to the posterior humerus to restore active external rotation (Figs. 26–53 and 26–54). Numerous variations of this operation are described. Weakness of internal rotation after this procedure prompted Tachdjian to lengthen the pectoralis major rather than to resect it.[61] Zancolli and Zancolli[71] lengthen the latissimus dorsi and circle part of it around the posterior humerus, suturing it back on itself, and transfer the pectoralis major to the distal subscapularis to restore internal rotation (Fig. 26–55). Hoffer transfers the latissimus to the posterior superior rotator cuff to restore active abduction as well as external rotation.[40] Some authors, such as Gilbert and associates,[23] have modified the Mayer operation using the trapezius to restore abduction but have not found this to be a very satisfactory operation.

Once deformity is fully established, the humeral head becomes flattened and retroverted and may subluxate or dislocate posteriorly. The entire extremity including the clavicle and scapula are smaller with a dysplastic, flattened glenoid. The coracoid process becomes lengthened. In the presence of a deformed humeral head, transfers alone are contraindicated. A humeral osteotomy to relieve the internal rotation contracture can be quite helpful for these patients. It has also been described with some additional flexion to assist forward elevation,[2] although we have no experience with this modification. We make a deltopectoral approach and expose the proximal humerus. The pectoralis major tendon is step-cut for lengthening. A four-hole plate is used, and the proximal screws are placed. The plate is removed, and the osteotomy is made. The arm is externally rotated until the hand can be placed at the hip and on top of the head then slightly externally rotated beyond this point to account for some recurrence. The patient is then placed in a shoulder spica cast. Although this operation does not change the patient's range of motion, it can place the shoulder in a much more functional position.

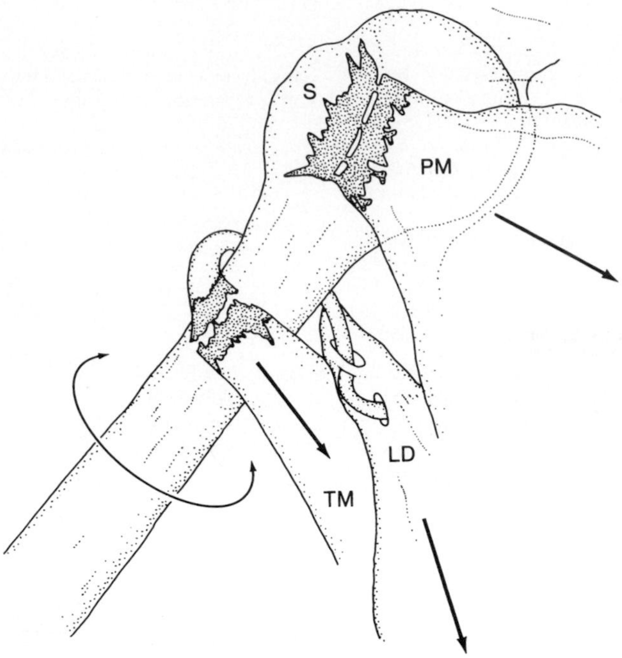

Figure 26–55

Zancolli's modification of the L'Episcopo procedure. The teres major (TM) is left intact. The distal portion of the Z-plasty of the latissimus dorsi (LD) has been passed posteriorly around the shaft of the humerus and sutured to the proximal portion. The pectoralis major (PM) is sutured to the insertion of the subscapularis (S). (From Zancolli EA: Classification and management of the shoulder in birth palsy. Orthop Clin North Am *12:*433–457, 1981.)

References and Bibliography

1. Adler JB and Patterson RL: Erb's palsy. J Bone Joint Surg Am *49:*1052–1064, 1967.
2. al Zahrani S: Modified rotational osteotomy of the humerus for Erb's palsy. Int Orthop *17:*202–204, 1993.
3. al-Qattan MM and Clarke HM: A new type of brachial plexus lesion to be added to the classical types (Letter). J Hand Surg Br *19:*673, 1994.
4. al-Qattan MM, Clarke HM, and Curtis CG: The prognostic value of concurrent clavicular fractures in newborns with obstetric brachial plexus palsy. J Hand Surg Br *19:*729–730, 1994.
5. al-Qattan MM, Clarke HM, and Curtis CG: Klumpke's birth palsy. Does it really exist (Review)? J Hand Surg Br *20:*19–23, 1995.
6. Babbitt DP and Cassidy RH: Obstetrical paralysis and dislocation of the shoulder in infancy. J Bone Joint Surg Am *50:*1447–1452, 1968.
7. Baskett TF and Allen AC: Perinatal implications of shoulder dystocia. Obstet Gynecol *86:*14–17, 1995.
8. Bodensteiner JB, Rich KM, and Landau WM: Early infantile surgery for birth-related brachial plexus injuries: Justification requires a prospective controlled study (Editorial; comment). J Child Neurol *9:*109–110, 1994.
9. Carlioz H and Brahimi L: La place de la désinsertion interne du sous-scapulaire dans le traitement de la paralysie obstétricale du

membre supérieur chez l'enfant. Ann Chirurg Infantile Paris *12*:159–168, 1971.
10. Chuang DC, Lee GW, Hashem F, and Wei FC: Restoration of shoulder abduction by nerve transfer in avulsed brachial plexus injury: Evaluation of 99 patients with various nerve transfers. Plast Reconstr Surg *96*:122–128, 1995.
11. Clark LP, Taylor AS, and Prout TP: A study of brachial plexus palsy. Am J Med Sci *130*:670–674, 1905.
12. Clarke HM and Curtis CG: An approach to obstetrical brachial plexus injuries. Hand Clin *11*:563–580, 1995.
13. Comtet JJ, Herzberg G, and Nassan AI: Biomechanical basis of transfers for shoulder paralysis. Hand Clin *5*:10, 1989.
14. Duchenne G: De l'eléctrisation localisée et de son application à la pathologie et á la Thérapeutique. Paris: JB Baillière, 1861.
15. Dunkerton MC: Posterior dislocation of the shoulder associated with obstetric brachial plexus palsy. J Bone Joint Surg Br *71*:764–766, 1989.
16. Egloff DV, Raffoul W, Bonnard C, and Stalder J: Palliative surgical procedures to restore shoulder function in obstetric brachial palsy: Critical analysis of Narakas' series. Hand Clin *11*:597–606, 1995.
17. Erb W: Uber eine eigenthumliche Localisation von Lahmungen im Plexus Brachialis. Verh Naturhistorische Midizin Heidelberg *2*:130–136, 1874.
18. Flaubert: 1827. Referenced in Clark LP, Taylor AS and Prout TP: A study of brachial plexus palsy. Am J Med Sci *130*:670–674, 1905.
19. Francel PC, Koby M, Park TS, et al: Fast spin-echo magnetic resonance imaging for radiological assessment of neonatal brachial plexus injury. J Neurosurg *83*:461–466, 1995.
20. Gabriel SR, Thometz JG, and Jaradeh S: Septic arthritis associated with brachial plexus neuropathy: A case report. J Bone Joint Surg Am *78*:103–105, 1996.
21. Gilbert A: Long-term evaluation of brachial plexus surgery in obstetrical palsy. Hand Clin *11*:583–594, 1995.
22. Gilbert A, Razaboni R, and Amar-Khodja S: Indication and results of brachial blexus surgery in obstetric palsy. Orthop Clin North Am *19*:91–105, 1988.
23. Gilbert A, Romana C, and Ayatti R: Tendon transfers for shoulder paralysis in children. Hand Clin *4*:633–642, 1988.
24. Gilbert A and Tassin JL: Réparation chirurgicale du plexus brachial dans la paralysie obstétricale. Chirurgie *110*:70, 1984.
25. Greenwald AG, Shute PC, and Shiveley JL: Brachial plexus birth palsy: A 10-year report on the incidence and prognosis. J Pediatr Orthop *4*:689–692, 1984.
26. Gu YD, Zhang GM, Chen DS, et al: Seventh-cervical nerve root transfer from the contralateral healthy side for treatment of brachial plexus root avulsion [see comments]. J Hand Surg Br *17*:518–521, 1992.
27. Gudinchet F, Maeder P, Oberson JC, and Schnyder P: Magnetic resonance imaging of the shoulder in children with brachial plexus birth palsy. Pediatr Radiol 25(Suppl) *1*:S125–8, 1995.
28. Hardy AE: Birth injuries of the brachial plexus: Incidence and prognosis. J Bone Joint Surg Br *63*:98–101, 1981.
29. Iffy L, Varadi V, and Jakobovits A: Common intrapartum denominators of shoulder dystocia related birth injuries. Zentralbl Gynakol *116*:33–37, 1994.
30. Jennett RJ, Tarby TJ, and Kreinick CJ: Brachial plexus palsy: An old problem revisited Am J Obstet Gynecol *166*:1673–1676, 1992.
31. Kawabata H, Kawai H, Masatomi T, and Yasui N: Accessory nerve neurotization in infants with brachial plexus birth palsy. Microsurgery *15*:768–772, 1994.
32. Klumpke A: Contribution à l'étude des paralysie radicularies du plexus brachial. Rev Med (Paris) *5*:591–593, 1885.
33. L'Episcopo JB: Tendon transplantation in obstetrical paralysis. Am J Surg *25*:122–125, 1934.
34. Laurent JP, Lee R, Shenaq S, et al: Neurosurgical correction of upper brachial plexus birth injuries. J Neurosurg *79*:197–203, 1993.
35. Laurent JP and Lee RT: Birth-related upper brachial plexus injuries in infants: Operative and nonoperative approaches. J Child Neurol *9*:111–117, 1994.
36. Leibolt FL and Furey JG: Obstetric paralysis with dislocation of the shoulder—a case report. J Bone Joint Surg Am *35*:227–230, 1953.
37. Lejman T, Strong M, Michno P, and Hayman M: Septic arthritis of the shoulder during the first 18 months of life. J Pediatr Orthop *15*:172–175, 1995.
38. Lichtblau PD: Shoulder dislocation in the infant: Case report and discussion. J Fla Med Assoc *64*:313–320, 1977.
39. Mallet J: Parakysie obstétricale du plexus brachial. Traitement des séquelles. Primauté du traitement de l'épaule Méthode d'expression des résultats. Rev Chir Orthop 58(Suppl 1).115, 1972.
40. Mancias P, Slopis JM, Yeakley JW, and Vriesendorp FJ: Combined brachial plexus injury and root avulsion after complicated delivery. Muscle Nerve *17*:1237–1238, 1994.
41. May VR Jr: Posterior dislocation of the shoulder: Habitual, traumatic, and obstetrical. Orthop Clin North Am *11*:271–285, 1980.
42. Meghdari A, Davoodi R, and Mesbah F: Engineering analysis of shoulder dystocia in the human birth process by the finite element method. Proc Inst Mech Eng Part 4:243–250, 1994.
43. Mehta VS, Banerji AK, and Tripathi RP: Surgical treatment of brachial plexus injuries. Br J Neurosurg *7*:491–500, 1993.
44. Michelow BJ, Clarke HM, Curtis CG, et al: The natural history of obstetrical brachial plexus palsy. Plast Reconstr Surg *93*:675–680, 1994.
45 Miller SF, Glasier CM, Griebel ML, and Boop FA: Brachial plexopathy in infants after traumatic delivery: Evaluation with MR imaging. Radiology *189*:481–484, 1993.
46. Nagano A, Yamamoto S, and Mikami Y: Intercostal nerve transfer to restore upper extremity functions after brachial plexus injury. Ann Acad Med Singapore 24(Suppl):42–45, 1995.
47. Narakas A: Surgical treatment of traction injuries of the brachial plexus. Clin Orthop *133*:71–90, 1978.
48. Narakas AO: Paralytic disorders of the shoulder girdle. Hand Clin *4*:619–632, 1988.
49. Phipps GJ and Hoffer MM: Latissimus dorsi and teres major transfer to rotator cuff for Erb's palsy. J Shoulder Elbow Surg *4*:124–129, 1995.
50. Price AE and Grossman JA: A management approach for secondary shoulder and forearm deformities following obstetrical brachial plexus injury. Hand Clin *11*:607–617, 1995.
51. Rutowski R: Neurotizations by means of the cervical plexus in over 100 patients with from one to five root avulsions of the brachial plexus. Microsurgery *14*:285–288, 1993.
52. Samardzic M, Grujicic D, and Antunovic V: Nerve transfer in brachial plexus traction injuries. J Neurosurg *76*:191–197, 1992.
53. Scaglietti O: The obstetrical shoulder trauma. Surg Gynecol Obstet *66*:868, 1938.
54. Seddon HJ, Medawar PB, and Smith H: Rate of regeneration of peripheral nerves in man. J Physiol (Paris) *102*:191–215, 1943.
55. Sever JW: Obstetric paralysis: Its etiology, pathology, clinical aspects and treatment, with a report of four hundred and seventy cases. Am J Dis Child *12*:541–578, 1916.
56. Slooff AC: Obstetric brachial plexus lesions and their neurosurgical treatment. Clin Neurol Neurosurg 95(Suppl):S73–7, 1993.
57. Slooff AC: Obstetric brachial plexus lesions and their neurosurgical treatment. Microsurgery *16*:30–34, 1995.
58. Smellie W: A Collection of Cases Preternatural and Observations in Midwifery. London: Wilson and Durham, 1764.
59. Songcharoen P: Brachial plexus injury in Thailand: A report of 520 cases. Microsurgery *16*:35–39, 1995.
60. Sunderland S: Rate of regeneration in human peripheral nerves. Arch Neurol Psych *58*:251–295, 1947.
61. Tachdjian MO: Pediatric Orthopedics. Philadelphia: WB Saunders, 1990, pp 2009–2082.
62. Travlos J, Goldberg I, and Boome RS: Brachial plexus lesions associated with dislocated shoulders. J Bone Joint Surg Br *72*:68–71, 1990.
63. Troum S, Floyd WE 3d, and Waters PM: Posterior dislocation of the humeral head in infancy associated with obstetrical paralysis: A case report. J Bone Joint Surg Am *75*:1370–1375, 1993.
64. Ubachs JM, Slooff AC, and Peeters LL: Obstetric antecedents of surgically treated obstetric brachial plexus injuries. Br J Obstet Gynaecol *102*:813–817, 1995.
65. Vassalos E, Prevedorakis C, and Paraschpoulou P: Brachial plexus palsy on the newborn. Am J Obstet Gynecol *11*:554–556, 1968.
66. Walle T and Hartikainen-Sorri AL: Obstetric shoulder injury: Associated risk factors, prediction and prognosis. Acta Obstet Gynecol Scand *72*:450–454, 1993.
67. Wang YC, Lin FK, Hung KL, and Wu DY: Brachial plexus neuropathy secondary to septic arthritis and osteomyelitis: Report of two cases. Acta Paediatr Sin *35*:449–454, 1994.
68. Waters PM: Is biceps recovery a reliable prognosticator for brachial plexus birth palsy (Abstract)? Pediatr Orthop Soc North Am Phoenix, 1996.

69. Wickstrom J: Birth injuries of the brachial plexus: Treatment of defects of the shoulder. Clin Orthop 23:196, 1962.
70. Wilkins KE: Special problems with the child's shoulder. *In* Rockwood CAJ and Matsen FA III (eds): The Shoulder. Philadelphia: WB Saunders, 1990, pp 1033–1087.
71. Zancolli EA and Zancolli ER Jr: Palliative surgical procedures in sequelae of obstetrical palsy. Hand Clin 4:643–669, 1988.

ARTHROGRYPOSIS

Arthrogryposis is a descriptive term that encompasses a wide range of pathologic conditions in which there is failure of muscle development.[10] More than 150 different types of disorders in which multiple joint contractures are a manifestation have been classified as a type of arthrogryposis.[9] The syndrome is classically grouped into two major types: a neurogenic form and a myopathic form. A high percentage of infants who die in the perinatal period of arthrogryposis will be found to have the neurogenic forms.[3] The more classic myopathic form is often called "amyoplasia" and is the type typically seen in orthopedic clinics. It accounts for up to 40% of patients with arthrogryposis in clinical surveys.[2]

The etiology of this disorder is as yet unknown. Many authors believe the myopathic form represents a type of congenital muscular dystrophy.[5, 8, 12] Abnormalities or absence of anterior horn cells have been found in autopsy specimens.[7] Distal arthrogryposis (type I) appears to have an autosomal dominant pattern of inheritance and has been mapped to the pericentromeric region of chromosome 9.[1, 6]

The pattern of involvement varies greatly. Forty-six per cent of patients have four-extremity involvement; 11% have only upper extremity involvement; and 43% have only lower extremity involvement.[11] Generally, the involvement is bilateral and symmetric. When the upper extremity is involved, there is typically internal rotation of the shoulders, extension contractures of the elbows, and flexion contractures of the wrists and fingers (Fig. 26–56).

Treatment

The management of upper extremity deformities in arthrogryposis depends on the motor function of the upper extremity, the degree of contracture present, and the functional needs of the patient.[3, 5, 9, 13] Functionally, the upper extremities should be able to assist in feeding and toileting and should be able to oppose each other.[3, 5] Surgical intervention is probably best delayed until after independent ambulation is achieved. Individuals with arthrogryposis demonstrate remarkable compensatory strategies, and a delay in treatment allows for a better evaluation of the overall function of the extremity. The goals of treatment should be to enhance function and not just to create a different appearance. Apparently severe contractures may not limit the individual, and repositioning the extremity may worsen function. Careful assessment by an experienced occupational therapist is important before intervention is considered.[3, 5, 9, 12, 13]

NONOPERATIVE TREATMENT

Stretching has not been shown to be beneficial in the management of shoulder deformities in arthrogryposis.[12, 13] Patients often use compensatory strategies involving the trunk and back to make up for absent actions.[3, 13] Special adaptive equipment for activities of daily living and clothing can help a great deal to facilitate independence. Most patients with arthrogryposis function well in adult life, but a high percentage remain partially dependent on others. The degree of dependence has been linked more to nonphysical factors than to physical deformity, underscoring the need for providing coping skills for these individuals.[4]

OPERATIVE TREATMENT

The shoulder is involved in the majority of individuals with arthrogryposis, but surgical intervention is rarely required. Adduction contractures have not been found to be a major problem for most patients. Occasionally, internal rotation contracture of the shoulder limits access to the face and mouth. Furthermore, if the hands cannot be brought together, manipulation of objects can be difficult, particularly if the hands are severely involved. Tenotomy of the pectoralis major and subscapularis advancement have not been found to be helpful in the management of

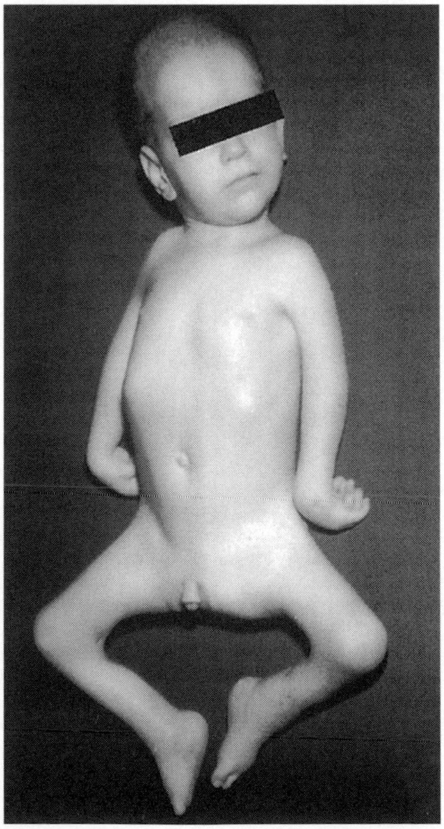

Figure 26–56

A photograph of a young child with arthrogryposis involving all four extremities. The upper extremities demonstrate the typical internal rotation of the shoulders, extension of the elbows, and flexion of the wrists and fingers.

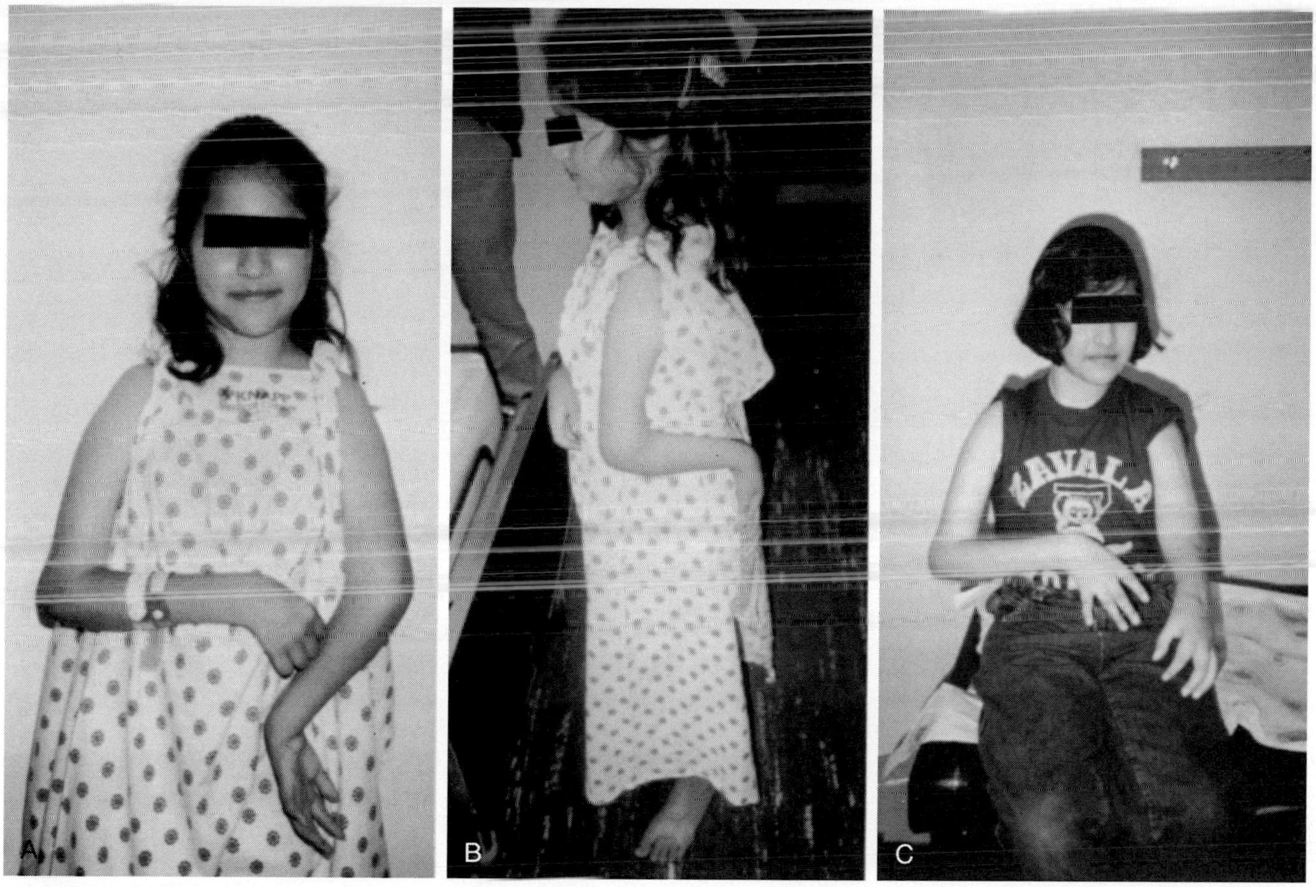

Figure 26–57

A, A preoperative view of a young teenager who has upper arthrogryposis primarily involving the upper extremities. The severe internal rotation of the shoulder limits the ability of the hand to reach the face. *B,* Photograph demonstrating the extreme internal rotation of the left upper extremity. *C,* Postoperative view after humeral derotation osteotomy and wrist fusion. The hand can now be brought to a much more functional position.

this problem.[5] Derotational osteotomy of the humerus may be indicated in some situations to allow enough external rotation so that the hand can reach the face and mouth or enough internal rotation so that it may oppose the opposite hand [3, 8, 9] (Fig. 26–57). Postoperative immobilization should be with a cast or custom orthosis in the optimal position for function.[8]

AUTHORS' PREFERRED METHOD OF TREATMENT

Surgery of the shoulder is rarely needed. Wrist, finger, and elbow function are much more important and should be addressed first. If there is severe internal or external rotation, a derotational osteotomy may be indicated. A proximal osteotomy with pin or plate fixation and postoperative immobilization in a shoulder spica cast or custom orthosis in the position of optimal function are recommended.

References and Bibliography

1. Bamshad M, Watkins WS, Zeager RK, et al: A gene for distal arthrogryposis type I maps to the percentromeric region of chromosome 9. Am J Hum Genet *55:*1153–1158, 1994.
2. Banker BQ: Neuropathologic aspects of arthrogryposis multiplex congenita. Clin Orthop *194:*30–43, 1985.
3. Bennett JB, Hansen PE, Granberry WM, and Cain TE: Surgical management of arthrogryposis in the upper extremity. J Pediatr Orthop *5:*281–286, 1985.
4. Carlson WO, Speck GJ, Vicari V, and Wager DR: Arthrogryposis multiplex congenita: A long term follow-up study. Clin Orthop *194:*115–123, 1985.
5. Drummond DS, Siller TN, and Cruess RL: Management of arthrogryposis multiplex congenita. Instr Course Lect *23:*79–95, 1974.
6. Kasai T, Oki T, Osuga T, and Nogami H: Familial arthrogryposis with distal involvement of the limbs. Clin Orthop *166:*182–184, 1982.
7. Krugliak L, Gadoth N, and Behar AJ: Neuropathic form of arthrogryposis multiplex congenita: Report of 3 cases with complete necropsy, including the first reported case of agenesis of muscle spindles. Neurol Sci *37:*179–185, 1978.
8. Lloyd-Roberts GC and Lettin AWF: Arthrogryposis multiplex congenita. J Bone Joint Surg Br *52:*494–508, 1970.
9. Shapiro F and Specht L: Current concepts review: The diagnosis and orthopaedic treatment of childhood spinal muscular atrophy, peripheral neuropathy, Friedreich ataxia, and arthrogryposis. J Bone Joint Surg Am *75:*1699–1715, 1993.
10. Stern WG: Arthrogryposis multiplex congenita. JAMA *81:*1507, 1923.
11. Swinyard CA and Mayer V: Multiple congenital contractures. JAMA *183:*23, 1963.
12. Williams P: The management of arthrogryposis. Orthop Clin North Am *9:*67–88, 1978.
13. Williams PF: Management of upper limb problems in arthrogryposis. Clin Orthop *194:*60–67, 1985.

CHAPTER

27

JOSEPH D. ZUCKERMAN, M.D.
ANDREW S. ROKITO, M.D.
FRANCES CUOMO, M.D.
MAUREEN A. GALLAGHER, PH.D.

Occupational Shoulder Disorders

In recent years there has been growing interest in work-related shoulder disorders. The number of reported cases of occupational shoulder problems has increased significantly during the past several decades.[123] This may be due either to increased automation and computerization or simply to a heightened awareness of such problems by workers and health care professionals. In either case, occupational shoulder disorders have become an extremely costly public health issue.

Several terms have been coined to describe occupational neck and shoulder pain. These terms include: occupational cervicobrachial disorder (OCD), repetitive stress injury, repetitive motion injury, and cumulative trauma disorder. In general, all of these terms refer to disorders that affect primarily the soft tissues, including the muscles, tendons, and nerves.[19, 26] They are thought to be the result of prolonged static loading of neck and shoulder girdle muscles that is required to position the arm so that repetitive tasks can be performed.

In this chapter, the epidemiology, etiology, and suggested treatment of OCD are reviewed. The chapter also covers shoulder tendinitis and its specific association with shoulder pain in the industrial setting. The relationship of glenohumeral arthritis with occupational factors is also explored. The workers' compensation system has been implicated as a major contributing factor in the sharp increase in the incidence of reported OCDs. The influence of workers' compensation on the outcome of treatment is examined. Finally, the current systems for assessing upper extremity disability and impairment are also discussed.

OCCUPATIONAL CERVICOBRACHIAL DISORDER

The term OCD refers to a symptom complex that is characterized by vague pain about the shoulder girdle, including the paracervical, parascapular, and glenohumeral musculature.[9, 47, 64, 107, 175] It may also be associated with pain that radiates into the region of the upper arm.[8] OCD is thought to be the result of cumulative trauma associated with high repetition of certain tasks in the work environment.[15, 177, 179] Several risk factors for the development of OCD have been identified, including awkward or static postures,[1, 3, 38, 40, 42, 180] repetitive arm movements, working with hands above shoulder height, and lack of rest. This syndrome has been called repetitive stress injury,[25, 111, 154] and it is considered to be part of the cumulative trauma disorders.[109]

Epidemiology

Most of the epidemiologic studies have found that OCD is particularly common among office and light assembly line workers. These jobs involve repetitive rapid movements of the hands often with the neck and shoulders in a static posture. In a review of the Japanese literature, O'Hara and co-workers found that the prevalence of OCD ranged from 2.4 to 28% for several types of occupations.[124] In a study of 339 Japanese cash register operators, 81% were found to have shoulder stiffness, and 49% had shoulder pain.[124] Other symptoms included neck pain in 31%, wrist pain in 13%, and hand and finger pain in 19% and 13%, respectively. In a study in 1979, Luopajarvi and co-workers reported a 16 to 28% prevalence of OCD among keypunch operators.[108] Cash register operators were found to have an incidence of 11 to 16%, light assembly workers 16%, typists 13%, and calculator operators 10%. In an Australian survey in 1981, Taylor and Pitcher found a 78% incidence of OCD among data-processing workers.[161] In 1985, Punnett and associates found that the prevalence of persistent shoulder discomfort in garment workers was 19.6%.[133] Burt and associates found the prevalence of discomfort and pain in the shoulder region of newspaper employees composing and editing on computer terminals to be 11%.[27] McDermott reported a significant rise in the incidence of OCD in Australia, from 2% in 1975 to 11% in 1981.[111] In 1990, the Bureau of Labor Statistics in their Annual Survey of Occupational Injuries and Illnesses reported a 100% increase in the number of cases of cumulative trauma illnesses from 1987 to 1989.[167] Shoulder region pain ranked second only to low back and neck pain in frequency. Fry found a 75% incidence of symptoms of OCD among a group of 279 musicians.[49]

Several investigators have found an exceptionally high rate of OCD among dentists.[113, 114, 136–138, 145] This is considered to be secondary to maintaining an awkward working posture for extended periods of time (Fig. 27–1). Kamwendo and co-workers found a 62% incidence of shoulder pain among a group of 420 medical secretaries.[87] Within this group, women had a significantly higher incidence of absence from work compared with men. In a study of 24 female computer operators with occipital headaches as well as neck and shoulder pain, LaBan and Meerschaert identified several predisposing factors for OCD, including impairment of visual acuity, cervical radiculopathy, prolonged cervical hyperextension, repetitive head rotation, undue elevation of the computer screen, prolonged copying of laterally displaced hard copies, the wearing of bifocals, as well as seating that is either excessively soft or that pitches the operator forward.[97]

Various constitutional symptoms have been found to be associated with OCD. O'Hara and co-workers found that generalized fatigue is as common as shoulder stiffness among cash register operators.[124] Other constitutional symptoms including headaches, insomnia, and low back pain were found to be significantly more common in cash register operators than in other office machine operators and other office workers. Westerling and Johnson, in a study of 2537 workers in Sweden, found that people with pain in the neck-shoulder region had a higher incidence of sick leave for illnesses of all types compared with job matched controls.[176] Within this same group, women had a significantly higher incidence of absence from work compared with men.

OCD is more prevalent among individuals who engage in light static occupations than those involved in heavy labor. The latter group seems to be more susceptible to rotator cuff disease. Veiersted and co-workers found a high incidence of work-related trapezius myalgia among female workers who perform light repetitive manual work.[173]

In a study comparing a group of female garment workers whose jobs involved repetitive hand motion with a group of hospital employees, Punnett and co-workers found that the prevalence of persistent shoulder, wrist, and hand pain was significantly greater among the garment workers.[133] Several studies have implicated thoracic outlet syndrome as a component of OCD. Sallstrom and Schmidt found that 32% of cash register operators and 10% of office workers with OCD also had findings consistent with thoracic outlet syndrome.[142] The diagnosis of thoracic outlet syndrome, however, was merely based on a history of numbness and paresthesias with a positive abduction-external rotation test. In general, thoracic outlet syndrome should be considered to be an entity separate from that of OCD.

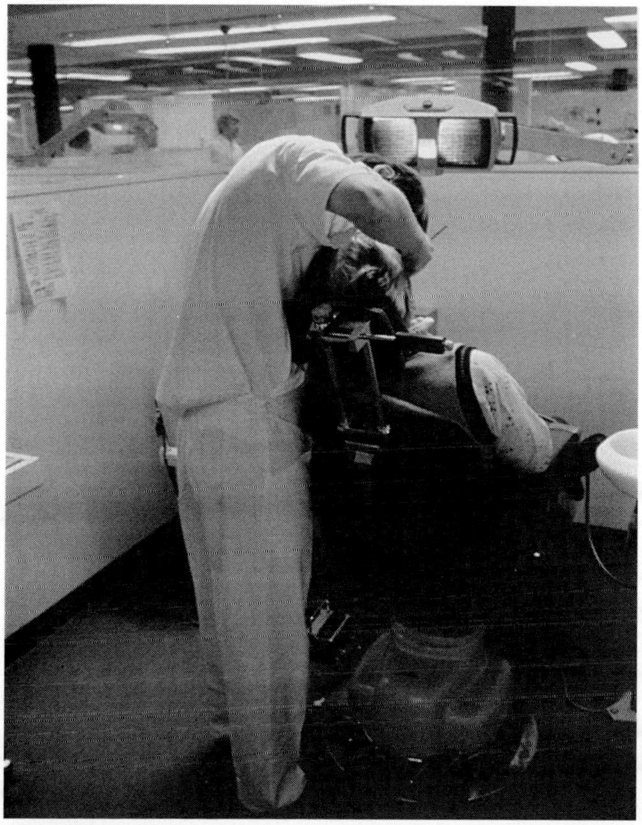

Figure 27–1

The exceptionally high rate of occupational cervicobrachial disorder among dentists is thought to be secondary to maintaining an awkward posture for extended periods of time.

Etiology

Two theories have been postulated to explain the etiology of OCD.[107] The *organic* or *physiologic* theory is based on the premise that shoulder pain is secondary to overuse caused by static overload. This theory attributes the increased incidence of OCD to be the result of increased automation and computerization.[10, 156, 173] By holding their shoulders in a position of slight abduction and forward flexion for prolonged periods, keyboard operators are particularly susceptible to OCD (Fig. 27–2). The muscle pain that develops around the shoulder girdle is in response to prolonged static loading.

The *psychosocial* theory[17, 18, 77, 78, 169, 178] attributes emotional stress to be an etiologic factor in the development of OCD. The proponents of this theory contend that OCD occurs in jobs that do not involve excessive muscle strain and consequently is not related to overuse but is more a result of psychosocial factors.[46, 166] Linton and Kamwendo surveyed 420 secretaries at a large medical center.[106] They found a higher frequency of neck and shoulder pain among secretaries in a "poor" psychological work environment compared with those in a "good" psychological work environment. The latter involves an increased awareness that shoulder pain is abnormal and may, in fact, be a symptom of a serious disease rather than normal fatigue. In a study of 607 metal industry workers, depressive and distress symptoms were found to be predictors of low back pain, neck-shoulder pain, and other musculoskeletal complaints.[104] Workers may also fear that if they ignore their symptoms, they may progress and become permanently disabling. Finally, the workers'

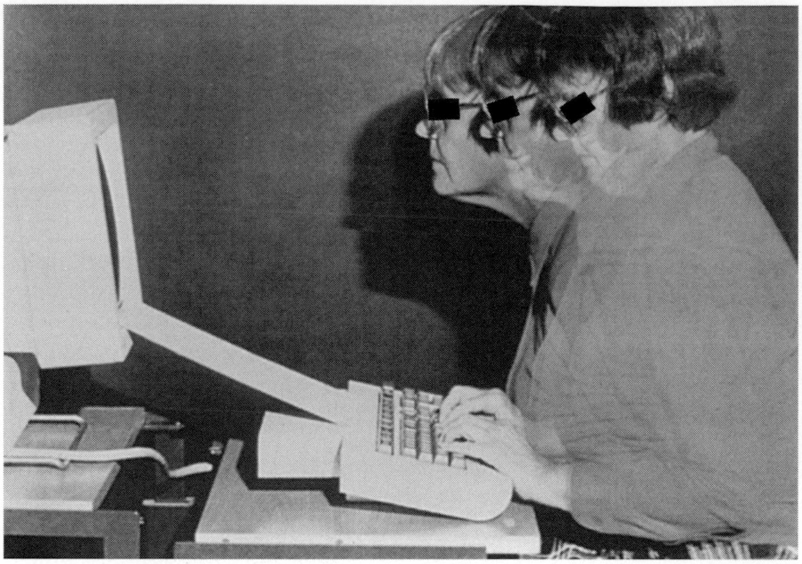

Figure 27–2

The prolonged static loading that occurs from holding the shoulders in a position of slight abduction and forward flexion makes keyboard operators particularly susceptible to occupational cervicobrachial disorder.

compensation system can contribute to this problem by awarding benefits based on the recognition that cumulative trauma can cause significant disability. Tait and associates, in a study of 201 patients with chronic pain, found that patients with litigation claims reported having pain of significant longer duration and had significantly more disability compared with nonlitigating patients.[158] Bongers and associates found a causal relationship between monotonous work, high perceived workload, and time pressure with musculoskeletal symptoms.[24]

In an effort to address the complex, multifactorial nature of OCD, Armstrong and colleagues proposed a model that incorporates both the organic and psychosocial theories.[11] In this model, *exposure* refers to the external factors such as the work requirements that produce an internal *dose* which, in turn, disturbs the internal state of the individual. Such disturbances may be mechanical, physiologic, or psychological, and these disturbances, in turn, evoke a certain *response* that includes the mechanical and metabolic changes that occur at the tissue level of the individual. Finally, *capacity*, which can be either physical or psychological, refers to the ability of the individual to resist destabilization due to various doses. This model attempts to provide a framework to explain the relationship between work exposure factors and the different responses, both psychological and physiologic, that occur.

Much research has been performed to provide objective evidence in support of the organic or physiologic theory. Such studies have involved the use of electromyography (EMG), muscle biopsies, and serum enzyme analyses.

The level of activity at which a static or continuous unchanged isometric contraction of shoulder muscles that can be sustained without injury is not known.[168] Several researchers have attempted to identify the endurance limit, defined as the highest force possible to maintain for an "unlimited" period of time. Jonsson has suggested that the static load level should always be below 5% of the maximum voluntary contraction (MVC).[83–85] In further support of this, Sjogaard and co-workers have shown that muscle fatigue occurs at 5% of MVC after 1 hour.[149]

Christensen used surface EMG to study electronics assembly line workers.[32] No significant difference was found between morning and afternoon values during an 8-hour work day, indicating that the muscles did not change their response to a sustained contraction. About half the subjects of the study complained of both neck and shoulder pain. The static contraction levels recorded were found to exceed the recommended levels of 2 to 5% of the MVC. Such recommended levels, however, are empiric, not physiologic. Hagberg and Kvarnstrom evaluated muscle endurance, or fatiguability, using EMG in 10 workers whose jobs involved high repetition with static shoulder activity.[57] All 10 workers complained of pain in the shoulder and neck regions, and the only objective finding was local tenderness. With a standardized work station position simulated, fatigue was found to occur significantly faster on the painful side than on the unaffected side. In a similar study, Johansson and colleagues, using surface EMG, found a significantly shorter endurance time for a group of 11 women in industrial work performing repetitive tasks who were diagnosed with neck and shoulder disorders than for a group performing similar work, however, without neck and shoulder disorders.[82]

In a study of 14 secretaries, surface EMG was used to measure the mean electrical activity of the trapezius.[43] The eight symptomatic patients had significantly higher electrical activity than did the asymptomatic group, and furthermore, within the symptomatic group, higher values were found on the painful side compared with the asymptomatic contralateral side. In an EMG study of 12 dentists, Milerad and associates found a relatively high muscular load on both the trapezius and the dominant extensor carpi radialis muscles.[144]

Several theories have been proposed in an attempt to explain this EMG data. It has been suggested that interstitial myofibrositis can cause reduced blood flow which, in turn, may lead to muscle ischemia and fatigue.[12] Muscle biopsy studies have demonstrated degenerated mitochondria and increased glycogen deposits.[44] Larsson and associates performed bilateral open biopsies of the trapezius muscle in 17 patients with chronic myalgia related to static load during repetitive assembly work.[98–100] Pathologic muscle fibers were identified and found to be related to the presence of myalgia. Such changes were thought to be secondary to mitochondrial dysfunction secondary to reduced local blood flow. Disuse and overprotection of the symptomatic extremity have also been suggested to account for the easy fatiguability found in the EMG studies.[36]

The trapezius muscle in particular has been found to be affected by fatigue in several different jobs, including electronics assembly,[53, 84] floor mopping,[65, 182] coffee serving,[181] meat cutting,[60] forwarder operating,[83] pillar drilling,[32] typewriting,[22] and sawing, hammering, and nailing.[81] Keyboard work position of the shoulder and arms has been theorized to explain the high static loads on the trapezius. Work position, alone, however, is probably not solely accountable for the high observed loads. Hagberg and Sundelin have suggested that excessive scapular elevation due to stress may also contribute to the increased trapezius load.[58] In a prospective study of 30 female assembly-line workers, Veiersted and associates found pre-employment EMG evaluation to be a good predictor for the later development of trapezius myalgia.[171]

In a study of 41 keyboard operators, Onishi and coworkers using EMG measured very high static loads of the trapezius.[127] They found that in most cases the keyboards were too high, resulting in increased scapular elevation or shoulder abduction.

In a study of 20 assembly line workers with neck and shoulder pain, Bjelle and colleagues found significantly high levels of muscle enzymes, including creatinine phosphokinase and aldolase in eight workers, without any underlying pathology.[20, 21] The elevated muscle enzyme levels were found to diminish after 2 to 8 weeks of sick leave. Elevated serum creatinine kinase levels have been found in welders, cash register operators, and assembly line workers.[61] Such high levels have not been observed in controllers and forklift drivers. The sustained high load necessary for light, static work has been theorized to cause severe adenosine triphosphate depletion, increased permeability, and resultant release of muscle enzymes.[59]

Edwards has proposed that muscle fatigue results from an imbalance between recruitment and relaxation.[39] An alteration in central motor control apparently leads to an imbalance in the use of muscles for static activity compared with their use in dynamic work. This theory may explain how mental stress may play a role in causing these disorders.

Using video analysis, Melin studied telephone industry workers and found significantly higher loading in subjects with OCD.[112] He theorized that this was due to observed excessive forward and outward arm movements.

Treatment

Once the diagnosis of OCD has been made, successful treatment requires not only an understanding of the basic pathophysiology of the condition but also knowledge of the specific workplace, ergonomics, and any psychosocial and economic aspects that would have an impact on patient management. Feuerstein and associates suggested the use of a multidisciplinary approach that focuses on the physical, ergonomic, and psychological factors that may contribute to prolonged disability.[45] In their study there is a significantly higher return to work rate for patients treated with a multidisciplinary approach compared with patients treated with usual care. Before making a diagnosis of OCD, it is important to consider and rule out other organic conditions that may be associated with, or predispose a worker to, OCD. Sikorski and associates, in a prospective study of 204 workers with occupationally related upper limb or neck pain, found that in the majority (58%) of cases a discrete musculoskeletal disorder existed.[147] Neurologic and vascular conditions such as cervical radiculopathy, thoracic outlet syndrome, and Raynaud's phenomenon can all be associated with OCD. Congenital or developmental deformities of the shoulder or cervical spine can also predispose a worker to OCD. Musculoskeletal neoplasms, both benign (e.g., osteochondromas) and malignant can be found about the shoulder girdle and should be considered. Referred sources of pain from other organ systems including cardiac, pulmonary, and gastrointestinal should also be ruled out.

Several classifications of OCD have been proposed. Such systems have been used for the development of treatment protocols. A five-grade classification system was developed by the OCD committee of the Japan Association of Industrial Health (Table 27–1). This system includes tendinitis as well as several neurologic and vascular symptoms that often accompany occupational shoulder pain.

A simplified three-stage system was developed by the Occupational Repetition Strain Advisory Committee in Australia. This system is based on symptom persistence and interference with work (Table 27–2).

Luck and Andersson[107] have proposed a pathophysiologic grading system that is a modification of the Australian classification (Table 27–3). This system focuses on myogenic pain.

The treatment of grade I OCD is based on the assumption that pain is due to metabolic changes from sustained static load, which resolve overnight.[62, 63] Treatment would involve shoulder girdle strengthening exercises and muscle relaxation training. The latter involves making the worker aware of static muscle tension so that he or she may change position and, thus, relax the involved muscles. Ergonomic modifications should also be done when treating grade I OCD. These modifications include modifying the work position by adjusting chair height and keyboard position and instituting more frequent rest breaks or job rotation.

In grade II, OCD pain persists for several days and is thought to be secondary to muscle inflammation and early interstitial fibrosis. Patients with grade II OCD often require a period of rest and time off from work. As in grade I OCD, treatment involves stretching and strengthening exercises and muscle relaxation training. In addition, nonsteroidal anti-inflammatory medications and trig-

Table 27–1 JAPANESE GRADING SYSTEM

			GRADE IV		
GRADE I	**GRADE II**	**GRADE III**	**Type 1**	**Type 2**	**GRADE V**
Subjective complaints without clinical findings	Subjective complaints with induration and tenderness of the neck, shoulder, and arm muscles	Includes grade II and any of the following: (1) Increased tenderness or enlargement of affected muscles (2) Positive neurologic tests (3) Paresthesia (4) Decrease in muscle strength (5) Tenderness of spinous processes of the vertebrae (6) Tenderness of the paravertebral muscles (7) Tenderness of the nerve plexus (8) Tremor of the hand or eyelid (9) Cinesalgia of the neck, shoulder, and upper extremity (10) Functional disturbance of the peripheral circulation (11) Severe pain or subjective complaints of the neck, shoulder, or upper extremity	Severe type of grade III	Direct development from grade II without passing through grade III, but having specific findings as follows: (a) Orthopedic diagnosis of the neck-shoulder-arm syndrome (b) Organic disturbances such as tendinitis or tenosynovitis (c) Autonomic nervous disturbances such as Raynaud's phenomenon, passive hyperemia, or disequilibrium (d) Mental disturbance such as anxiety, sleeplessness, thinking dysfunction, hysteria, or depression	Disturbances not only at work but also in daily life

ger point injections may provide relief. An ergonomic evaluation with modifications including changes in work position, rest breaks, job rotation, reduction in noise level, and lighting should also be performed.

With grade III OCD, patients have symptoms with multiple areas of tenderness. These patients are found to have a rapid rate of fatigue as evidenced by EMG studies. The underlying pathophysiology is assumed to be one of severe myopathy with interstitial fibrosis.[44] Therapy for this group of patients may include enrollment in a pain management program and the use of antidepressants. Ergonomic modifications usually involve vocational retraining, because these patients should be placed in a job in which static load of the shoulder girdle is minimal. Jobs that involve dynamic loads may be better tolerated by this patient population.

Stress in the workplace can be external, internal, and physiologic. All these factors can contribute to the development of OCD. External stress resulting from personal issues outside of the workplace has been found to increase baseline shoulder girdle muscle tension and reduce the ability to relax these muscles. This is especially true during high-repetition, static load positions.

Internal stress results from factors in the workplace that increase the worker's stress level. Such factors include poor lighting, high background noise, cramped working conditions, inadequate work breaks, job dissatisfaction, and excess productivity demands.

Physiologic stress will result from the muscle pain itself. Such muscles are difficult to relax and consequently, a vicious cycle is established in which sustained static load

Table 27–2 AUSTRALIAN STAGING SYSTEM

Stage I	Aching and tiredness of the affected limb that occurs during the work shift but subsides overnight and during days off work. There is no significant reduction in work performance, and there are no physical signs. This condition can persist for months and is reversible.
Stage II	Symptoms fail to settle overnight, cause a sleep disturbance, and are associated with a reduced capacity for repetitive work. Physical signs may be present. The condition usually persists for months.
Stage III	Symptoms persist at rest. Sleep is disturbed, and pain occurs with nonrepetitive movement. The person is unable to perform light duties and has difficulty with nonoccupational tasks. Physical signs are present. The condition may persist for months to years.

Table 27–3 PATHOPHYSIOLOGIC GRADING SYSTEM

Grade I (mild)	Shoulder girdle muscle pain that occurs during work or similar activities and resolves a few hours later; no findings on physical examination
Grade II (moderate)	Shoulder girdle muscle pain that persists for several days after work; muscle belly and insertional tenderness on examination
Grade III (severe)	Shoulder girdle muscle pain that is constant for weeks or longer; multiple tender areas; palpable induration indicative of muscle fibrosis; muscle belly contracture; reduced range of motion of myogenic origin

levels and their duration are increased. This, in turn, may interfere with a worker's concentration, performance, and productivity. Persistent pain may eventually interrupt the worker's sleep, which further increases the stress level.

Case Example

A 41-year-old right-hand–dominant secretary at a large investment banking corporation presents with a chief complaint of right shoulder pain. She describes the gradual onset of pain that began approximately 1 year prior to presentation. She describes diffuse, poorly localized pain about the right side of her neck and right shoulder region. Her pain is intermittent and varies in terms of severity. In general, however, her pain worsens with work and is alleviated with rest. Those specific work activities that exacerbate her symptoms include typing on a keyboard and writing. She spends approximately 9 hours a day in front of a video display terminal. Initially, her pain occurred solely during work and seemed to resolve at night.

Over the past few months, however, her pain has lingered into the evening and occasionally persists into the first part of the weekend. She has been evaluated previously by several physicians.

She has had a rheumatologic work-up for inflammatory disease, and the result was negative. She has undergone electrophysiologic studies, and the results were also negative. Her physical examination was negative other than the finding of diffuse right trapezius muscle belly tenderness. The results of x-rays of the cervical spine and shoulder were negative.

She was diagnosed as having OCD and started on a course of physical therapy that included shoulder and neck range-of-motion and stretching exercises. She was instructed in muscle relaxation techniques, counseled with regard to limiting the number of hours spent at the computer keyboard as well as on the value of rest breaks during her work day.

A work station evaluation was performed by an ergonomist, and several modifications were implemented. These modifications included the procurement of a chair with height adjustment, a wider computer keyboard, and an adjustable stand for holding hard copy that is being transcribed.

After 6 months her symptoms were much improved and by 1 year she had only minor discomfort that occurred exclusively during her work day and responded to basic stretching maneuvers.

SHOULDER TENDINITIS

Tendinitis about the shoulder, seen most commonly in the form of rotator cuff impingement, has also been reported with increasing frequency in the literature.[41, 54, 59, 62, 66, 71, 72, 103] In contrast with OCD, this diagnosis is relatively more straightforward with rather typical history and physical findings. Patients generally present with complaints of pain in front of the shoulder in the overhead, abducted, or internally rotated position. Symptoms may be alleviated with rest depending on the severity of the condition and exacerbated with repetitive arm motions in the same positions. Physical findings include rotator cuff tenderness, a positive impingement sign as described by Neer,[112] pain on resisted external rotation, and a painful arc of motion. A positive result on a subacromial lidocaine injection test demonstrates near if not complete immediate pain relief and confirms the diagnosis. Further diagnostic testing in the form of plain radiography, magnetic resonance imaging, arthrography, and ultrasound may be necessary to determine the extent of tendon injury because impingement is seen as a spectrum of pathology from inflammation and hemorrhage to full-thickness rotator cuff tear.[122] Progressive degenerative changes in the rotator cuff associated with repetitive microtrauma are most commonly believed to be caused by impingement or a rubbing of the tendon under the coracoacromial arch,[120] but other mechanisms such as chronic inflammation, hypovascularity, and direct compression from the humeral head have been described.[122, 134]

Despite their frequency and relative diagnostic simplicity, shoulder lesions are still incompletely diagnosed and classified. This may be due to several factors, including poorly defined diagnoses and broad categorization of varying shoulder disorders, the multifactorial nature of their etiology, and the paucity of prospective investigations elucidating potential risk factors.[151] The key to alleviation of this major problem involves education of not only medical personnel in the areas of early diagnosis and management but also the education of workers and supervisors in order to increase the awareness in the area of prevention. With such an approach, if early reversible disease does occur, the process can be interrupted and prevented from progressing to chronic disability, unemployment, and financial loss.

Epidemiology

Epidemiologic reports of occupational shoulder disorders may be categorized into either observational studies or field and laboratory studies. In observational studies, risk factors are often categorized as job characteristics or as job titles. Exposure to risk factors classified by job characteristics include awkward postures, static postures, heavy work, repetitive arm movement, working at the shoulder level, and lack of sufficient rest.[71] Studies have linked shoulder tendinitis to each of these categories.

Static postures characterize tasks that require workers to sustain positions for protracted periods. The onset of supraspinatus tendinitis in shipyard welders was compared with plate workers in the same company in a study performed by Herberts and associates in 1981.[72] Although the prevalence of tendinitis was similar in the two groups (18.3% and 16.2% respectively), the mean age of the welders suffering from tendinitis was 6 years less than that of the plate workers. Both jobs were rated high in physical workload, but the difference and contributing factor was considered to be the static nature of welding compared with plate work, which was classified as a dynamic task. In this same study, the prevalence of tendinitis was compared between the aforementioned two groups and clerical office workers. Although the clerks were older than the welders and plate workers, the prevalence of supraspinatus tendinitis was only 2% in the clerks compared with 27% in the other two groups. This yielded an odds ratio of approximately 9, which is a strong indicator of the strength of association between heavy work and rotator cuff tendinitis.

Repetitive arm movements and working at the shoulder level were examined by Hagberg and Wegman by surveying the results of several epidemiologic studies on exposure factors related to the incidence of rotator cuff disorders.[62] Odds ratios determined higher prevalence of shoulder disorders in groups exposed to both factors. Specifically, an odds ratio of 11 was calculated for the prevalence of rotator cuff tendinitis for work at shoulder height compared with work below that level.

Epidemiologic studies examining exposure classified by job title, although generally not as useful as information on job characteristics, can provide specific information regarding particular jobs that may be helpful in prevention. Most commonly, they are categorized as industrial, retail, or office work; however, with expanding research, it is becoming clear that almost every occupation is at some risk.

Etiology

Shoulder tendinitis is believed to be caused by several mechanisms, but the most widely held belief is that impingement of the tendon occurs beneath the coracoacromial arch as described by Neer.[120] Impingement is thought to occur as a spectrum or a continuum of pathology presenting in its earliest stage I with edema and hemorrhage, fibrosis and tendinitis in stage II, and full-thickness rotator cuff tears in stage III. Neer emphasized that both the supraspinatus tendon insertion into the greater tuberosity and the bicipital groove lie anterior to the coracoacromial arch with the shoulder in neutral position and with forward flexion of the shoulder. These structures must pass beneath the arch, providing the opportunity for impingement. Requirements common to many of the occupations afflicted with increased shoulder pathology include frequent overhead activity and the use of hand tools. These two factors increase shoulder muscle loads—especially in the rotator cuff, which accentuates the impingement process. Increased load can cause pain by energy depletion; ultrastructural rupture and tendon ischemia sustained strain reduces blood flow to the portion of the supraspinatus tendon that lies beneath the coracoacromial arch.[71]

Vascular implications were proposed by Lindbolm[105] who reported that the rotator cuff is hypovascular or avascular near the supraspinatus attachment to the greater tuberosity, known as "the critical zone"[133] where many cuff lesions occur. A vascular etiology is also suggested by the work of Rathbun and Macnab, who found areas of relative avascularity in the supraspinatus tendon that interestingly coincide with the location of impingement lesion. They reported tendon microrupture and degeneration in these avascular sites.[134] Chronic strain and inflammation in these low-flow areas reduce the strength of the tendon and therefore increase the risk of rupture over time. Activities that contribute to vascular depletion and strain over periods of time have the potential to accelerate the degenerative process, especially when combined with inadequate periods of rest during the activity. Ischemic effects are most notably associated with constant tension on the supraspinatus tendon with the arms in a flexed or abducted position.[70] As the greater tuberosity is brought into contact with the undersurface of the acromion, direct compression of the rotator cuff occurs and is accentuated by particular acromial morphology (i.e., increase curvature or hooked appearance), subacromial spurs, or distally pointing acromioclavicular osteophytes.[33, 35]

Two mechanisms for compromise of supraspinatus blood flow have been proposed: (1) Rathbun and Macnab[134] found that glenohumeral adduction puts the supraspinatus tendon under tension and "wrings out" its vessels; (2) Sigholm and associates[146] measured the effect of active shoulder flexion on subacromial pressure and reported that the normal resting pressure of 8 mm Hg was elevated to 39 mm Hg by flexion to 45 degrees and to 56 mm Hg by the addition of a 1-kg weight to the hand in the elevated position. If sustained, these pressures are sufficiently high enough to reduce the tendon microcirculation.[110]

Local muscular forces are also believed to be involved in the development and aggravation of the impingement process. As one would expect, the anterior deltoid is very active in forward flexion with the middle deltoid firing mainly in abduction. As the deltoid force is directed upward in the presence of a weakened cuff mechanism, contraction of the deltoid causes upward displacement of the humeral head so that it squeezes the remaining cuff against the coracoacromial arch, thus enhancing the impingement process. Prolonged overhead activity and the associated force generated by the deltoid toward the acromion is therefore believed to be a contributing factor (Fig. 27–3).

Sigholm and co-workers used EMG to determine the muscle forces about the glenohumeral joint.[145] The supraspinatus and infraspinatus muscles behave similarly in flexion and abduction. Both of these cuff muscles increase in activity with increasing flexion and abduction up to 45 degrees, and then the muscles reach a plateau. Higher flexion angles did not appear to increase shoulder muscle activity, and the addition of hand loads increased activity in the infraspinatus alone. It was, therefore, concluded that shoulder muscle strain could best be reduced by keeping the upper arm as close to the side of the body as possible and by reducing the weight of hand tools (Fig. 27–4).

The type of work performed also plays a role in the development of impingement. Herberts and colleagues performed an EMG study evaluating muscle strain and fatigue.[72] Muscle fatigue was found to be associated with lower muscle fiber firing frequency. Further investigation examined welders with shoulder pain categorized by age and experience.[71, 72] Inexperienced workers exhibited fatigue more frequently than did the more experienced counterparts, which indicated learning effects versus bet-

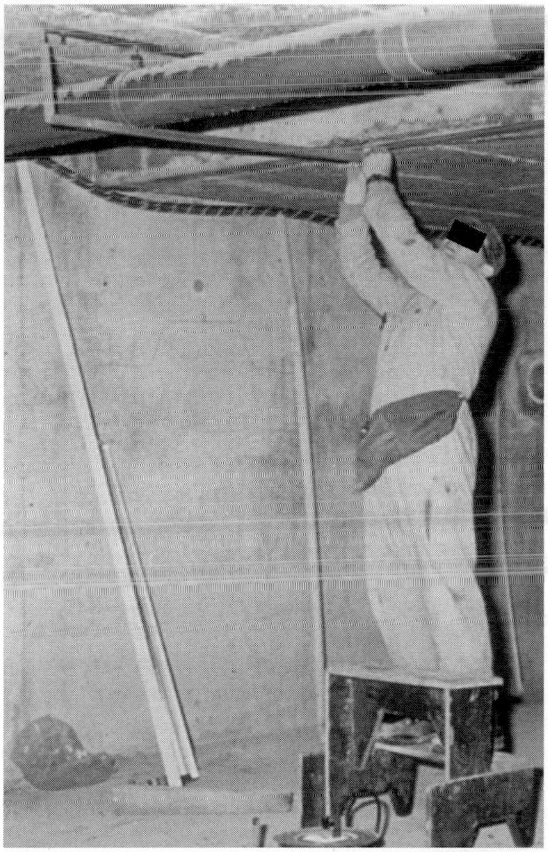

Figure 27–3

Prolonged overhead activity and the associated force generated by the deltoid toward the acromion is believed to be a contributing factor in the development of the impingement process.

ter conditioning. There was no evidence of fatigue when the tasks were performed with the hand at shoulder level with the arm in less than 30 degrees of flexion. Impingement problems became more apparent when the shoulder was placed in a greater degree of flexion. Welders who worked with the shoulder in more static or sustained positions were found to develop supraspinatus tendinitis earlier than did those whose work was more dynamic.

Other muscles about the shoulder girdle may be affected in chronic overuse situations, including the deltoid, trapezius, and biceps tendon, although much less commonly. The long head of the biceps tendon is often involved in impingement of the rotator cuff as it traverses within the rotator interval beneath the coracoacromial arch. Bicipital tendinitis is rarely seen as a primary entity that is separate and distinct from the impingement syndrome but may result from rubbing of the synovial sheath against the lesser tuberosity or from osteoarthritic spurs within the intertubular groove.

Evaluation and Treatment

The evaluation and management of shoulder tendinitis are discussed at length elsewhere in the manuscript, but points specifically related to occupational injuries necessitate emphasis. The evaluation of tendinitis about the glenohumeral joint begins, as in all areas of medicine, with a thorough history. The history includes not only the clinical symptoms and chief complaint but also questions the work environment, specific tasks performed, and the length of time that they are performed, as well as provision for adequate break periods.

How long the symptoms last and what measures are required to relieve the complaint are valuable pieces of information regarding chronicity and severity. Once the inciting event or task has been identified, the diagnosis confirmed, and the degree of severity established, the process of management may then be undertaken.

Management is often broken down into the categories of nonoperative and operative. A third and probably most important category should be added to this regimen—the category of prevention. Nonoperative treatment includes rest or avoidance of the offending task, nonsteroidal anti-inflammatory medications, and a general shoulder rehabilitation program that should be aimed initially at relieving stiffness in the shoulder and restoring normal range of motion and should slowly progress to strengthening when pain from inflammation has subsided. The benefits of judicial use of subacromial steroid injections have also been reported if the aforementioned less invasive regimen fails.[23]

Special attention toward modification of the workplace and improving or altering task techniques once the shoul-

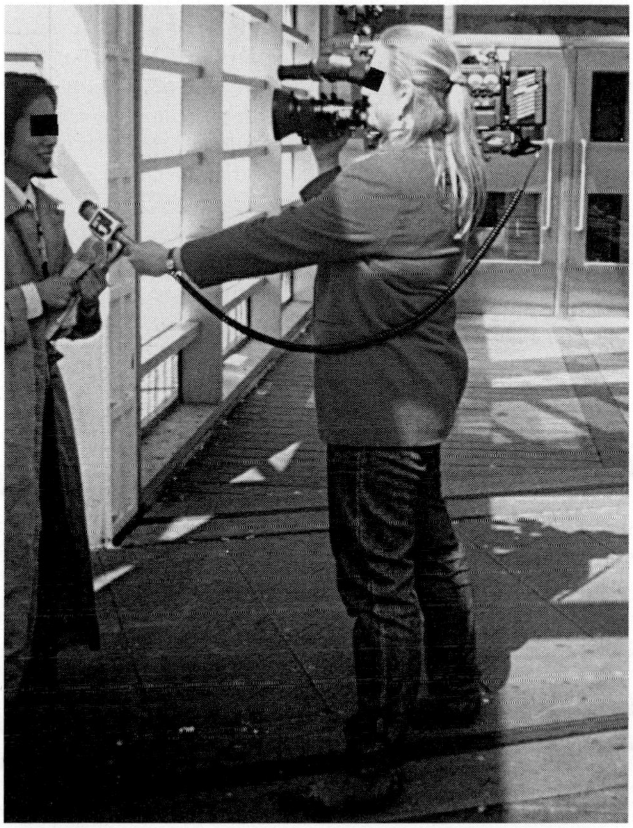

Figure 27–4

The weight of hand tools and their use at flexion and abduction angles above 30 degrees produces increased strain on muscles about the glenohumeral joint.

der has been rehabilitated is crucial in order to prevent or at least minimize a recurrence.

Operative intervention is warranted in cases involving persistent pain and disability despite compliance with an adequate nonoperative program. Subacromial decompression, whether it is arthroscopic or open, remains the procedure of choice for these resistant cases. In 1983 Neer[122] reported that the indications for acromioplasty included: (1) a positive arthrogram; (2) patients older than 40 years of age with negative arthrograms but persistent disability for 1 year, despite an adequate nonoperative program, provided that pain can be temporarily eliminated by subacromial lidocaine injection; (3) select patients younger than 40 years of age with stage II impingement; and (4) patients undergoing other procedures in which impingement is likely (e.g., shoulder arthroplasty for an old fracture). In all cases, the purpose of acromioplasty is to relieve mechanical impingement, thus preventing further rotator cuff wear.

DEGENERATIVE JOINT DISEASE

While the relationship between cumulative trauma and injury to the soft tissues about the shoulder girdle has been delineated, the association of glenohumeral arthritis with occupational factors is less clear.[7, 31, 101, 160, 164, 185] Unlike the hip and the knee, the shoulder is not a weight-bearing joint. As such, degenerative arthritis of the glenohumeral joint is relatively uncommon.

Degenerative arthritis of the glenohumeral joint has traditionally been classified as either primary (idiopathic) or secondary (post-traumatic), such as following a fracture.[121] Patients with degenerative arthritis of the glenohumeral joint commonly present with a gradual onset of anterior or posterior shoulder pain and stiffness. Symptoms are typically exacerbated with motion and tend to worsen during the day. On physical examination there may be disuse atrophy of the deltoid and rotator cuff muscles, restricted range of motion (both active and passive), and crepitus. Acromioclavicular arthritis commonly occurs concurrently with glenohumeral degenerative joint disease. This may be evidenced by tenderness to palpation over the acromioclavicular joint and pain with cross-chest adduction. Radiographs typically show joint space narrowing, subchondral sclerosis, and peripheral osteophyte formation involving the glenohumeral joint and possibly the acromioclavicular joint.

A few studies have investigated the association of glenohumeral arthritis with various occupations. Although some of these studies have reported a relationship between certain occupations and osteoarthritis of the shoulder, a direct association has not been found. Kellegren and Lawrence[89] and later Lawrence[102] found that the prevalence of glenohumeral arthritis in men was influenced by occupation. Waldron and Cox studied the skeletons of 367 workers buried in London between 1729 and 1869 and found no significant relationship between occupation and osteoarthritis of the shoulder.[174] Similarly, in a study that included 151 shoulder dissections, Petersson did not find any convincing evidence to support the notion that occupation is a factor in the development of osteoarthritis of the shoulder.[130]

As with OCD, dentists seem to be susceptible to the development of glenohumeral arthritis. Once again, this has been hypothesized to be the result of sustained static loads while maintaining the shoulder in a position of flexion and abduction with scapular elevation. In a Finnish study that included 40 dentists, Katevuo and associates found that 46% had radiographic evidence of osteoarthritis and 44% had bilateral disease.[87] In contrast, only 11 of 83 farmers in the study had findings consistent with osteoarthritis. As with OCD, individuals engaged in occupations that involve repetitive, light static loads seem to be more susceptible compared with those exposed to the high dynamic loads of heavy manual work.

It has been speculated that pneumatic drilling may predispose the worker to degenerative arthritis. In order to examine the effect of vibration exposure on the shoulder, Bovenzi and co-workers compared 67 foundry workers who used vibratory tools with 46 heavy manual laborers.[25] They found no significant difference between the two groups in the prevalence of radiographic changes in the shoulder. In general, it has been difficult to differentiate degenerative changes due to vibration from those that can simply be attributed to heavy manual work.

Degeneration of the acromioclavicular joint is more common than glenohumeral arthritis. As with glenohumeral arthritis, however, no distinct relationship with occupation has been found. In a cadaveric study, De Palma found degenerative changes in almost all subjects after age 50.[37] Petersson often identified degeneration in 30- to 50-year-old people and regularly in individuals older than 60 years.[130, 131] Because degeneration occurred with equal frequency in men and women and was of the same severity in right and left shoulders, the occupation did not appear to be a contributing factor. In a retrospective study that included 83 patients who underwent resection of the distal clavicle for arthritis, Worcester and Green found no relation to occupation.[183]

In summary, glenohumeral arthritis does not appear to be the result of overuse. Although there has been some subtle evidence to suggest that long-term repetitive trauma leads to arthritis, degenerative disorders are more difficult to attribute to work-related causes because of their insidious onset. Although it has been shown that overhead elevation of the upper extremity results in increased joint contract area, there has been no definite evidence to suggest that prolonged activity in this position leads to accelerated degeneration of the glenohumeral joint.

PREVENTION

Four basic approaches to the prevention of occupational shoulder disorders have been proposed. These approaches include workplace design, work method design, worker selection, and worker training.[95] While workplace and work method design involve intervention on the part of industry, worker selection and worker training involve fitting the worker to the job and, therefore, are not as easily attainable.[13, 117] Himmelstein and associates suggested that in addition to medical management more aggressive approaches to obtain control, avoidance of unnecessary surgery, helping patients to manage residual pain and stress, and attention to employer-employee conflicts are all important in preventing the prolonged work disabilities secondary to upper extremity disorders.[74]

Workplace Design

The overall design of the workplace can have a significant influence with regard to the stresses placed on the worker's shoulder.[45, 75, 76, 91, 94] The specific dimensions and space requirements of the workplace can dictate the amount of load that is placed on the shoulder. Shoulder loads are influenced by arm position,[29, 119] the external load that is being handled, and the specific movements of the arm. Chaffin calculated the average time that the arm can be held in various positions of flexion, abduction, and forward-reach.[30] He found that the larger the flexion or abduction angle or forward-reach position, the higher is the load moment and, consequently, the earlier fatigue will develop.

Any load that is held in the worker's hand will increase the moment acting on the shoulder proportional to the weight of the object and the distance that is held from the shoulder joint. Arm and forearm positions are affected by the orientation of the hand. The supinated hand requires the arm to be adducted and close to the trunk, whereas, with a pronated hand, the arm will be more abducted and elevated.

The degree of shoulder abduction is often determined by the vertical height of the work surface. Shoulder abduction can, in turn, lead to rotator cuff disease. Adjustable tables can help to limit the degree of shoulder abduction. In a study by Tichauer, it was found that the metabolic expenditure of grocery packing increased when the arm abduction angle exceeded 20 degrees.[162, 163]

Arm movements influence shoulder load as muscle contractions are needed to accomplish them. In general, the larger the movement, the faster it is, and the farther away from the shoulder the center of mass is, the greater the load placed upon the shoulder.

Several methods have been proposed to reduce the load placed on the shoulder in the work environment of keysorting. These methods can be divided into two groups: those that reduce the moment arm and those that reduce the external load. In order to reduce the moment arm, several things can be done including making the work station closer, standing or sitting close to the work station, sloping the work surface, adjusting the table height, and adjusting the chair height. The external load can be reduced by dividing it into several individual loads, choosing lighter tools, and providing arm supports by using arm rests and balance slings. It is also important to recognize that there is an area of joint-reach limits. It has been suggested that the work station be designed so that the reach target is below the shoulder height of a small woman. In this way, most cases of severe shoulder flexion and abduction can be avoided.

Work Method Design

Two techniques for reducing static load on the shoulder by altering the work method have been proposed: (1) the introduction of rest breaks, and (2) job rotation.[16]

Many studies have attempted to find the optimum rest break frequency, duration, and content in order to prevent shoulder disorders from static, repetitive work. Many of the studies have focused on video display terminal work. The National Institute of Occupational Safety and Health (NIOSH) has recommended a 15-minute rest break after 1 to 2 hours of video display terminal work.[157] Similarly, the Swedish National Board of Occupational Safety and Health has recommended an upper limit of 1 to 2 hours of continuous video terminal work.[157]

Although rest breaks have been found to increase productivity, too frequent breaks may affect work rhythms. Regularly scheduled rest breaks seem to be more effective than sporadic or irregularly scheduled rest periods. Optimum break frequency and break length will depend mainly on the type of work that is being performed and on the length of time that it can be sustained or the posture or static load that is held. A break length totaling 5 to 10% of the work day that is broken up into several short breaks has been suggested. Furthermore, breaks that are active can counteract stress that occurs from the work activity and seem to be more effective compared with those that involve complete rest.

By rotating from one job to another, static loading of the shoulders can be avoided. While this technique is more easily accomplished with assembly line workers, it is difficult to achieve in office workers when there is not enough job variation for this to be done.

In summary, regularly scheduled active rest breaks and rotation of a worker's individual duties can have a significant impact with regard to prevention of occupational shoulder disorders.

Worker Selection

Screening workers for job placement has been advocated as a method to prevent occupational shoulder disorders. The effectiveness of this technique, however, has not been established.[52, 96, 159] The basic physical capabilities of a worker to meet the demands of a specific job should be assessed.

Risk factors for the development of OCD have been established.[125, 126, 129, 135, 148, 153, 155] Kitayama established the following criteria that render a worker "absolutely unsuitable" for a job: a history of OCD, whiplash syndrome, uncorrectable visual acuity problems, and upper extremity functional disorders. "Relatively unsuitable" categories include: mental conditions resulting in high external stress, extremely cold fingers and hands, and loose jointedness.[93]

Worker Training

Worker training has proved to be very successful in the prevention of low back injuries. Shoulder school programs have been established; however, their effectiveness has not yet been determined. Workers should be instructed with regard to basic biomechanical principles,[67] including the use of both hands, holding loads close to the body, avoiding excessive abduction and flexion, refraining from excessive and fast arm movements, taking frequent rest breaks, and supporting the arms and tools as much as possible to avoid shoulder injuries.

Toivanen and associates found relaxation training to significantly diminish neck and shoulder pain in a group of hospital cleaners.[165] Studies are currently being performed to examine the effectiveness of prevention. Preliminary data would suggest that prevention does, indeed, work with significant reductions in complaints and sick leave for musculoskeletal disorders. Further studies are needed to develop absolute guidelines for preventing OCD.

OUTCOMES OF TREATMENT — COMPENSATION VERSUS NONCOMPENSATION

Although conflicting results and opinions have been reported in the literature, most studies find that patients with workers' compensation do not respond to surgery with the same success as do other patients.[14, 50, 68, 69, 132, 140] The potential for secondary gain is believed to complicate the recovery for these patients in many cases.[55, 56] On behalf of the compensation patient, one study has been reported by Freiman and Fenlin in which the effect of litigation and workers' compensation claims on the outcome of anterior acromioplasty in patients with chronic inflammation of the supraspinatus tendon caused by impingement syndrome was examined.[48] A comparison of three groups consisting of workers' compensation, litigation, and those with no apparent financial gain revealed a significantly longer time to return to work (an average of 14.2 weeks versus 4.7 weeks versus 2.5 weeks, respectively), although the patients in the compensation group were involved in heavy labor demanding a more complete return of shoulder endurance. Overall satisfactory pain relief and return to preinjury work activities was achieved with 91% of employed patients returning to full employment despite the potential for secondary gain.

Much more prevalent in the literature is a less optimistic outlook upon the postoperative outcome of the compensation patient. Misamore and associates reported a comparison of results in two populations of patients undergoing primary repair of the rotator cuff.[116] Twenty-four patients were receiving workers' compensation and seventy-nine patients were not. The two groups were comparable with regard to age, sex, size of the tear, and preoperative strength, pain, and active range of motion. At a mean follow-up of 45 months, only 54% of the compensation group was rated as good or excellent, compared with 92% of the noncompensation patients. Similarly, 42% of the compensation group returned to full activity as opposed to 94% of their counterparts in the study. There were no significant differences between the two groups with regard to the amount of time required to return to work, although fewer of the compensation patients returned to full activities. The average return to work in this study was 6 months, which concurs with previous reports.[14] These authors also noted that most of the unsatisfactory results were due to subjective criteria such as pain, function, and strength. The most objective measurement—active range of motion—revealed similar results in both groups, although fewer than half of the patients who were receiving compensation returned to full work activities. After repair of the rotator cuff, those who did return to work were able to do so just as quickly as patients who were not receiving compensation.

Hawkins and associates reported similar unsuccessful results in the compensation population after anterior acromioplasty for chronic impingement syndrome with an intact rotator cuff.[68] Of 108 patients, 87% were graded as satisfactory at an average follow-up of 5.2 years. Several factors influenced the results of a 13% failure rate. Most significantly was the comparison of patients claiming workers' compensation with those who did not. There were no differences in the preoperative profiles or operative findings; however, there were 22.9% unsatisfactory results in the compensation group compared with 9.2% in the noncompensation group.

UPPER EXTREMITY DISABILITY AND IMPAIRMENT EVALUATION

Expenditures related to disability and employment have escalated dramatically over the last few decades. Estimated costs of occupational illness and injury vary in the literature depending on the information source. The Bureau of Labor Statistics, the National Center for Health Statistics, and Workers' Compensation Awards are primary sources of estimates for occupational illness and injury data. At the present time there is no comprehensive national system to keep track of work-related illness and injury in the United States. The Bureau of Labor Statistics has the largest databank and does an annual survey that randomly samples OSHA logs to base estimates of incidence rates. In 1992 they reported that there were approximately 6.8 million job-related illnesses and injuries, which is an increase of 453,700 additional job-related injuries than they reported in the previous year.[152]

Disorders of the musculoskeletal system are among the most frequently reported impairments and causes of disability. The upper extremity ranks third in being most frequently affected.[90] Federal, state, and local government expenditures for workers' compensation totaled almost $21 billion in 1993. Under Social Security, $2.6 billion in benefits was paid to almost 4 million disabled workers in 1994.[152]

Disability Versus Impairment

An individual is disabled if he or she has an incapacity to perform a required activity or task. If the individual is able to compensate by either a modification in work technique or by use of an assistive device, he or she is not considered to be disabled as defined by the Americans with Disabilities Act of 1992.[80] The determination of disability is an administrative process, of which the orthopedist plays a key role in the evaluation of medical impairment.[25] When a disability determining agency requests that a form be filled out or that an examination be performed, usually an assessment of impairment is being sought. The determination of the impact of an individual's impairment on their functioning in society, or more specifically their employment, is usually performed by the determining agency. The complicated infrastructure of disability determination by which the inability to work is based not only on medical impairment, but also on the interplay of educational level, work experience, available job opportunities, psychological factors, age, and socioeconomic background. Judgments that are based on such a wide range of factors are open to some degree of variation and subjectivity.[7, 34, 108, 141, 170] A major source of difficulty in the determination of disability is that medical evaluations are relied on to make decisions regarding work capacity. This may very well be done in the absence of an actual assessment of work-related functional capacities.

Medical impairment encompasses both physical and mental entities, of which the orthopedic surgeon evaluates anatomic or physiologic defects that interfere with an individual's ability to perform certain functions in a standard fashion. Upper extremity impairments are usually expressed in terms of physical signs, such as joint range of motion.[2] Several agencies request that impairment be expressed as a percentage in relation to the whole body. Compensation agencies frequently ask the orthopedist to determine work restrictions based on the medical evaluation so they can match abilities and disabilities to specific jobs.

The orthopedist is frequently called on to provide an objective medical evaluation of impairment in the process of determination of disability. This specialist may be asked to play different roles as advisors, objective third-party examiners, patient advocates, or adjudicators according to different agencies' needs within the various disability programs. In addition, the orthopedist may be asked to determine and document medical restrictions based on a worker's illness or injury. It is, therefore, essential that there is a clear understanding of exactly what information the requesting agency wants to know. It should be recognized that in a "gatekeeping" role, the doctor-patient relationship may be directly affected.

The orthopedist should be knowledgeable and have current information regarding federal and state regulations, as well as employers' work rules. Knowledge of the workplace is an essential component when evaluating a person's disability and return to work. The orthopedist should have a clear understanding of the factors leading to work-related injuries and disorders. A review of work tasks is essential when determining work-relatedness as well as contributing factors from prior work experience. A comprehensive assessment should include information about non–work-related activities as well, such as spare-time and sports activities.

One of the most challenging tasks is to ascertain if the illness or injury is work related. This can be somewhat complex, because not only can there be variations in diagnostic criteria and definitions but also the same disorder may be considered work related in one case and not in another. The orthopedist usually has little formal training specific to the workplace. A consensus by an international expert group, at the request of the Quebec Research Institute on Occupational Health and Safety, has created a database that can be referred to on work-related musculoskeletal disorders that includes the upper extremity.

CURRENT SYSTEMS OF ASSESSING DISABILITY

Workers' Compensation

Workers' compensation is a no fault insurance system for work-related accidental injury and occupational disease for federal and state workers. Federal government employees receive benefits under the Federal Employees' Compensation Act, and state employees are provided for by separate legislation in state workers' compensation laws enacted by each state. Worker compensation laws share many characteristics but also have important differences among the federal and state systems. To further complicate the issue of what is compensable under workers' compensation, compensable conditions can vary from one state to the next, as well as benefit amounts, processing of claims, and the settlement of disputes.[73] It is important that the orthopedist understand the requirements of the state workers' compensation system. Under workers' compensation, employers must provide medical treatment and compensation benefits to employees for work-related illness or injury. Employers must demonstrate their ability to pay for workers' compensation costs by obtaining insurance coverage through a state fund, a private carrier, or by self-insurance. Four categories of compensable disabilities may be provided for under state workers' compensation: temporary total disability, temporary partial disability, permanent total disability, and permanent partial disability. The largest number of workers' compensation cases are for temporary disability and account for about three fourths of compensable claims. In addition to paying medical expenses and compensating workers for lost wages, state workers' compensation provides for survivors' benefits and vocational rehabilitation. In a study conducted by the Minnesota Blue Cross, workers' compensation costs were found to be almost twice the cost for similar conditions when compared with general liability claims.

In order to qualify for an award, a worker has to demonstrate that the injury ocurred as the result of and in the course of employment. Satisfaction of criteria for a compensation claim is not an issue in the case of overt external force-induced injuries; however, in the absence of trauma, assertions of work relatedness may be more difficult to establish. Most states require that the employee be unable to perform his or her level of work or to obtain employment that is suitable to his or her qualifications and training.

The American Medical Association's *Guides to the Evaluation of Permanent Impairment* provides a standard framework and method of analysis through which physicians can evaluate, report on, and communicate information about shoulder impairment.[6, 51] It is either recommended or mandated by law in workers' compensation cases in 38 states and two territories in the United States. The most current edition should be referred to.

Under workers' compensation, impairment is a medical issue and is defined as an alteration of an individual's health status that interferes with the activities of daily living. When using the American Medical Association's guidelines, the orthopedist can represent to what degree an individual's capacity to carry out daily activities has been diminished. Permanent impairment is defined as one that has become static or stabilized during a period of time sufficient to allow optimal tissue repair, and one that is unlikely to change despite further medical or surgical therapy.

Under workers' compensation, the evaluation or rating of a disability is a nonmedical assessment. Disability is defined as a decrease in, or the loss or absence of, the capacity of an individual to meet personal, social, or occupational demands or to meet statutory or regulatory requirements because of an impairment. A disability refers to a task that an individual cannot do; it arises out of the interaction between impairment and external requirements, with emphasis on the person's occupation. It logically follows that an "impaired" individual is not necessarily "disabled" with regard to his or her occupation. An impaired individual is considered handicapped if there are obstacles to accomplishing basic activities that can be overcome by compensating in some way for the effects of impairment. The most common cause of a dispute over compensation claims is the determination of the extent of the disability. A physician's expert opinion is then requested, and a hearing is held before the workers' compensation agency.

Railroad and Maritime Workers' Compensation

The Federal Employer's Liability Act (FELA) supersedes state compensation laws and provides for a comprehensive injury compensation system for railroad workers. Unlike the state compensation laws there are no limits on awards, and consequently the system is expensive. Although the physician determines the magnitude of impairment, under FELA a jury decides the degree of the injured worker's disability. The Jones Act provides compensation for maritime workers and provides the same rights and remedies as FELA.

Social Security

There are two disability compensation programs administered by the Social Security Administration. Workers with a recent work history in Social Security covered employment are eligible for the Social Security Disability Insurance program. Those individuals who have no recent work history but who meet a financial needs test receive benefits under the disability portion of the Supplemental Security Income Program. Both programs use the same definition of disability and the same regulations for determining disability. Disability under the Social Security Program is defined in economic terms and in terms of the person's ability to work.[79] An individual is considered disabled if the impairment is of such a severity that he or she is unable to do the work previously performed and is not able to be engaged in any other kind of substantial gainful work considering the person's age, education, and occupational experience. To be considered for benefits, a worker must be unable to work for a least 6 months. The definition of disability is more restrictive than other agencies in that the medically determined physical or mental impairment is expected to result in death or to last for at least 12 months. The impairment must have demonstrable anatomic, physiologic, or psychological abnormalities demonstrated by medically accepted clinical and laboratory diagnostic techniques. There are established medical criteria referred to as the "listing of impairments" that define disorders and the level of severity that supposedly prevents a person from working. Unlike Workers' Compensation, recipients under Social Security are subject to periodic review to determine continued eligibility.

Approximately two thirds of the initial disability claims are denied by Social Security. A claimant's eligibility is made by a team of examiners based on a review of the records. If a person is denied benefits, there is an appeal process whereby the case is reconsidered by another team of examiners. If benefits are still denied, the claimant is seen in person by a decision-maker and the claim may go to the Appeals Council of the Social Security Administration and ultimately to the federal courts.

The orthopedist is required to furnish sufficient medical evidence to Social Security, including medical history; clinical findings; laboratory findings; diagnosis based on signs and symptoms; prescribed treatment and prognosis; and a medical source statement describing what the patient can do despite his or her impairment (i.e., work-related activities such as sitting, walking, lifting, or carrying).

Private Insurance Companies

Individual disability income policies pay a fixed monetary amount of coverage and may be integrated with other public disability programs. They are provided on both an individual or a group basis. In general, benefits may be provided either for a stated period of time or to the attainment of a specific age. Most policies require that the beneficiary be re-examined by a physician designated by the insurance company to ensure continuation of benefits. Disability is defined in various ways, and requirements of coverage are determined by each company individually.

Private agencies may request that the orthopedic surgeon determine either short-term or permanent ability to work. The calculation of time off from employment is often determined by the orthopedist's past experience with a similar diagnosis. Good communication and candor are necessary to achieve the desired goal of return to work between the orthopedist, the patient, and the insurance company.

Guidelines for Degree of Impairment

The following sources are useful references that the orthopedist can utilize to evaluate impairment.

- The American Academy of Orthopaedic Surgeons' publication, *The Clinical Measurement of Joint Motion,*[5] provides a standardized, reproducible, and efficient method for the assessment of joint motion. Considerable emphasis is based on range of motion when evaluating shoulder impairment. Thus, when the various agencies request an assessment of impairment, the orthopedist can accurately assess shoulder impairment based on range of joint motion on the unaffected side, or he or she can refer to the normal comparative data provided in this publication. Normal joint kinesiology, the range of normal joint motion, and the change in joint motion with age are also discussed.
- The American Academy of Orthopaedic Surgeons also has a *Manual for Orthopaedic Surgeons in Evaluating Permanent Physical Impairment.*[4] This publication was an attempt to address the problem of inconsistencies that the orthopedist might face when formulating an opinion on impairment in relation to workers' compensation and personal injury litigation. A scoring system is proposed for the shoulder that can be used as a guide in calculating the percentage of permanent impairment and loss of function in relation to the whole arm.
- The American Medical Association has updated their *Guides to the Evaluation of Permanent Impairment.* The fourth edition was published in 1993. A format is specified in which information is acquired to analyze, record, and report information about the impairment. The medical evaluation is based on three components. First, the nature of the impairment and its consequences are documented. Second, protocols are provided to evaluate specific organ systems. The musculoskeletal section contains a protocol that can be used to systematically evaluate upper extremity impairment. Third, tables are provided that relate to the evaluation protocols. For the upper extremity, the range of active motion is rounded to the nearest 10 degrees, and a table is provided to calculate the relationship of impairment of the upper extremity to impairment of the whole person.
- The Minnesota Medical Association has developed a *Revised Temporary Disability Duration Guide*[115] to evaluate a disability that lasts for less than 52 weeks. Impairment is based primarily on the diagnosis, supported by medical history, physical findings, and diagnostics.

References and Bibliography

1. Aaras A, Westgaard RH, and Stranden E: Postural angles as an indictor of postural load and muscular injury in occupational work situations. Ergonomics *31*:915–933, 1988.
2. Abreu BC (ed): Physical Disability Manual. New York: Raven Press, 1981.
3. Alund M, Larsson SE, and Lewin T: Work-related persistent neck impairment: A study on former steelworks grinders. Ergonomics *37*:1253–1260, 1994.
4. American Academy of Orthopaedic Surgeons: Manual for Orthopaedic Surgeons in Evaluating Permanent Physical Impairment. Chicago: AAOS, 1975.
5. American Academy of Orthopaedic Surgeons: The Clinical Measurement of Joint Motion. Chicago: AAOS, 1994.
6. American Medical Association: Guides to the Evaluation of Permanent Impairment, 4th ed. Chicago: AMA, 1993.
7. Anderson JAD: Industrial rheumatology and the shoulder. Br J Rheumatol *26*:326–328, 1987.
8. Anderson JAD: Shoulder pain and tension neck and their relation to work. Scand J Work Environ Health *10*:435–442, 1984.
9. Andersson GBJ: Epidemiology of occupational neck and shoulder disorders. *In* Repetitive Motion Disorders of the Upper Extremity. Chicago: AAOS, 1995.
10. Aoyama H, O'Hara H, Oze Y, and Itani T: Recent trends in research on occupational cervicobrachial disorder. J Hum Ergol (Tokyo) *8*:39–45, 1979.
11. Armstrong T, Buckle P, Fine L, et al: A conceptual model for work-related neck and upper limb musculoskeletal disorders. Scand J Work Environ Health *19*:73–84, 1993.
12. Awad EA: Interstitial myfibrosis: Hypothesis of mechanism. Arch Phys Med Rehabil *54*:449–453, 1973.
13. Backman AL: Health survey of professional drivers. Scand J Work Environ Health *9*:30–35, 1983.
14. Bakalim G and Pasila M: Surgical treatment of rupture of the rotator cuff tendon. Acta Orthop Scand *46*:751–757, 1975.
15. Barton NJ, Hooper G, Noble J, and WM Steel: Occupational causes of disorders in the upper limb. BMJ *304*:309–311.
16. Bengt J: Electromyographic studies of job rotation. Scand J Work Environ Health Suppl *1*:108–109, 1988.
17. Bergenudd H and Johnell O: Somatic versus nonsomatic shoulder and back pain experience in middle age in relation to body build, physical fitness, bone mineral content, gamma-glutamyltransferase, occupational workload, and psychosocial factors. Spine *16*:1051–1055, 1991.
18. Bergenudd H, Lindgarde F, Nilsson B, and Petersson CJ: Shoulder pain in middle age: A study of prevalence and relation to occupational work load and psychosocial factors. Clin Orthop *231*:234–238, 1988.
19. Biundo J, Mipro RC, and Djuric V: Peripheral nerve entrapment, occupation-related syndromes, sports injuries, bursitis, and soft tissue problems of the shoulder. Curr Opin Rheumatol *7*:151–155, 1995.
20. Bjelle A, Hagberg M, and Michaelson G: Occupational and individual factors in acute shoulder-neck disorders among industrial workers. Br J Ind Med *38*:356–363, 1981.
21. Bjelle A, Hagberg M, and Michaelson G: Work-related shoulder-neck complaints in industry: A pilot study. Br J Rheumatol *26*:365–369, 1987.
22. Bjorksten M, Itani T, Jonsson B, and Hoshizawa M: Evaluation of muscular load in shoulder and forearm muscles among medical secretaries during occupational typing and some non-occupational activities. *In* Jonsson B (ed): Biomechanics, Vol X. Baltimore: University Park Press, 1987.
23. Blair B, Rokito A, Cuomo F, et al: An Analysis of the Efficacy of Corticosteroid Injection for the Treatment of Subacromial Impingement Syndrome. Presented at the 62nd Annual Meeting of the American Academy of Orthopaedic Surgeons, Orlando, Florida, February, 1995.
24. Bongers P, deWinter C, Kompier M, and Hildebrandt V: Psychosocial factors at work and musculoskeletal disease. Scand J Work Environ Health *19*:297–312, 1993.
25. Bovenzi M, Fiorito A, and Volpe C: Bone and joint disorders in the upper extremities of chipping and grinding operators. Int Arch Occup Environ Health *59*:189–198, 1987.
26. Browne CD, Nolan B, and Faithfull D: Occupational repetition strain injuries: Guidelines for diagnosis and management. Med J Aust *140*:329–332, 1984.
27. Burt S, Hornung R, and Fine LJ: Health Hazard Evaluation Report. National Institute of Occupational Safety and Health. HETA *89*:250, 1990.
28. Carey TS and Hadler NM: The role of the primary physician in disability determination for social security insurance and workers' compensation. Ann Intern Med *104*:706–710, 1986.

29. Chaffin DB and Andersson GBJ: Occupational Biomechanics. New York: John Wiley, 1984.
30. Chaffin DB: Localized muscle fatigue—definitions and measurement. J Occup Med *15*:346–354, 1973.
31. Chakravarty K and Webley M: Shoulder joint movement and its relationship to disability in the elderly. J Rheumatol *20*:1359–1361, 1993.
32. Christensen H: Muscle activity and fatigue in the shoulder muscles of assembly-plant employees. Scand J Work Environ Health *12*:582–587, 1986.
33. Codman EA: The shoulder: Rupture of the supraspinatus tendon and other lesions in or about the subacromial bursa. Florida: Krieger, 1984.
34. Croft P, Pope D, Zonca M, et al: Measurement of shoulder related disability: Results of a validation study. Ann Rheum Dis *53*:525–528, 1994.
35. Cuomo F, Kummer FJ, Zuckerman JD, et al: The Influence of Acromioclavicular Joint Morphology on Rotator Cuff Tears. Presented at the Ninth Open Meeting of the American Shoulder and Elbow Surgeons. San Francisco, February 21, 1993.
36. Danneskiold-Samsoe B, Christiansen E, Lund B, and Andersen R: Regional muscle tension and pain ("fibrosis"). Scand J Rehabil Med *15*:17–20, 1983.
37. De Palma AF: Degenerative Changes in the Sternoclavicular and Acromioclavicular Joints in Various Decades. Springfield, IL: Charles C Thomas, 1957.
38. Dimberg L, Olafsson A, Stefansson E, et al: The correlation between work environment and the occurrence of cervicobrachial symptoms. J Occup Med *31*:447–453, 1989.
39. Edwards RHT: Hypothesis of peripheral and central mechanisms underlying occupational muscle pain and injury. Eur J Appl Physiol *57*:275–281, 1988.
40. Ekberg K, Karlsson M, Axelson O, et al: Cross-sectional study of risk factors for symptoms in the neck and shoulder area. Ergonomics *38*:971–980, 1995.
41. Ekholm J: Impairments, disabilities and handicaps of patients with neck and shoulder pain: How are these consequences of disease classified? Scand J Rehabil Med Suppl 32:47–56, 1995.
42. English CJ, MacLaren WM, Court-Brown C, et al: Relations between upper limb soft tissue disorders and repetitive movements at work. Am J Ind Med *27*:75–90, 1995.
43. Erdelyi A, Sihvonen T, Helin P, and Hanninen O: Shoulder strain in keyboard workers and its alleviation by arm supports. Int Arch Occup Environ Health *60*:119–124, 1988.
44. Fassbender H and Wegner K: Morphologic and Pathogenese des Weichteirheumatimus. Z Rheumaforsch *32*:355–374, 1973.
45. Feuerstein M and Hickey PF: Ergonomic approaches in the clinical assessment of occupational musculoskeletal disorders. *In* Turk DC and Melzack R (eds): Handbook of Pain Assessment. New York: The Gilford Press, 1992, pp 71–99.
46. Flodmark BT and Aase G: Musculoskeletal symptoms and type A behaviour in blue collar workers. Br J Ind Med *49*:683–687, 1992.
47. Friedenberg ZB and Miller WT: Degenerative disc disease of the cervical spine. J Bone Joint Surg *45A*:1171–1178, 1963.
48. Frieman BG and Fenlin JM: Anterior acromioplasty: Effect of litigation and worker's compensation. J Shoulder Elbow Surg *4*:175–181, 1995.
49. Fry HJH: Overuse injury in musicians—pathology, treatment, and prevention. *In* The Arts Health Advisory Committee of the Victorian Ministry of the Arts: Proceedings of a Seminar of Repetition Strain Injury and Musicians, Melbourne, Australia, May 11, 1985.
50. Gartsman GM: Arthroscopic acromioplasty for lesions of the rotator cuff. J Bone Joint Surg *72A*:169–197, 1990.
51. Gloss DS and Wardle MG: Reliability and validity of American Medical Association's guide to ratings of permanent impairment. JAMA *248*:2292–2296, 1982.
52. Gore DR, Sepic SB, and Gardner GM: Roentgenographic findings of the cervical spine in asymptomatic people. Spine *11*:521–524, 1986.
53. Granstrom B, Kvarnstrom S, and Tiefenbacher F: Electromyography as an aid in the prevention of excessive muscle strain. Appl Ergonomics *16*:49–54, 1985.
54. Guidotti TL: Occupational repetitive strain injury. Am Fam Physician *45*:585–592, 1992.
55. Hadler NM: Occupational illness: The issue of causality. J Occup Med *26*:587–593, 1984.
56. Hadler NM: Occupational Musculoskeletal Disorders. New York: Raven Press, 1993.
57. Hagberg M and Kvarnstrom S: Muscular endurance and electromyographic fatigue in myofascial shoulder pain. Arch Phys Med Rehabil *65*:522–525, 1984.
58. Hagberg M and Sundelin G: Discomfort and load on the upper trapezius muscle when operating a word processor. Ergonomics *29*:1637–1645, 1986.
59. Hagberg M and Wegman DH: Prevalence rates and odds ratios of shoulder-neck diseases in different occupational groups. Br J Ind Med *44*:602–610, 1987.
60. Hagberg M, Jonsson B, Brundin L, et al: Musculoskeletal pain in butchers: An epidemiologic, ergonomic and electromyographic study [In Swedish]. Work and Health *12*:6–52, 1983.
61. Hagberg M, Michaelson G, and Ortelius A: Serum creatinine kinase as an indicator of local muscular strain in experimental and occupational work. Int Arch Occup Environ Health *50*:377–386, 1982.
62. Hagberg M: Occupational musculoskeletal stress and disorders of the neck and shoulder: A review of possible pathophysiology. Int Arch Occup Environ Health *53*:269–278, 1984.
63. Hagberg M: Work load and fatigue in repetitive arm elevations. Ergonomics *24*:543–555, 1981.
64. Hagg GM and Suurkula J: Zero crossing rate of electromyograms during occupational work and endurance tests as predictors for work related myalgia in the shoulder/neck region. Eur J Appl Physiol *62*:436–444, 1991.
65. Hagner IM, Hagberg M, Hammerstrom U, et al: Physical load when cleaning floors using different techniques [In Swedish]. Work and Health *29*:7–27, 1986.
66. Hammond G, Torgerson WR Jr, Dotter WE, and Leach RE: The painful shoulder. Instr Course Lect *20*:83–90, 1971.
67. Harms-Ringdahl K, Schuldt K, and Ekholm J: Principles of prevention of neck and shoulder pain. Scand J Rehabil Med Suppl *32*:87–96, 1995.
68. Hawkins RJ, Brock RM, Abrams JS, and Hobeika P: Acromioplasty for impingement with an intact rotator cuff. J Bone Joint Surg *70B*:795–797, 1988.
69. Hawkins RJ, Misamore GW, and Hobeika PE: Surgery for full thickness rotator cuff tears. J Bone Joint Surg *67A*:1349–1355, 1985.
70. Herberts P and Kadeforr R: A study of painful shoulder in welders. Acta Orthop Scand *47*:381–387, 1976.
71. Herberts P, Kadeforr R, Hogforr C, and Sigholm G: Shoulder pain and heavy manual labor. Clin Orthop *191*:166–178, 1984.
72. Herberts P, Kadefors R, Andersson G, and Petersen I: Shoulder pain in industry: An epidemiological study on welders. Acta Orthop Scand *52*:299–306, 1981.
73. Herington TN and Morse LH: Occupational Injuries: Evaluation, Management, and Prevention. St. Louis: CV Mosby, 1995.
74. Himmelstein JS, Feuerstein M, Stanek EJ, et al: Work-related upper extremity disorders and work disability: Clinical and psychosocial presentation. JOEM *37*:1278–1286, 1995.
75. Hinnen U, Laubli T, Guggenbuhl U, and Krueger M: Design of check-out systems including laser scanners for sitting work posture. Scand J Work Environ Health *18*:86–94, 1992.
76. Ho SF and Lee HS: An investigation into complaints of wrist pain and swelling among workers at a factory manufacturing motors for refrigerators. Singapore Med J *35*:274–276, 1994.
77. Holstrom EB, Lindell J, and Moritz U: Low back and neck/shoulder pain in construction workers: Occupational workload and psychosocial risk factors. Part 1. Relationship to low back pain. Spine *17*:663–671, 1992.
78. Holmstrom EB, Lindell J, and Moritz U: Low back and neck/shoulder pain in construction workers: Occupational workload and psychosocial risk factors. Part 2. Relationship to neck and shoulder pain. Spine *17*:672–677, 1992.
79. International Labour Organization: ILO Encyclopaedia of Occupational Health and Safety. Geneva, Switzerland: International Labour Organization, 1983.
80. Isernhagen SJ (ed): The Comprehensive Guide to Work Injury Management. Queenstown, MD: Aspen Publishers, 1995.
81. Itani T, Yoshizawa M, and Jonsson B: Electromyographic evaluation and subjective estimation of the muscular load in shoulder and forearm muscles during some leisure activities. *In* Johnson B

(ed): Biomechanics X-A. Champaign, IL: Human Kinetics Publishers, 1987, pp 241–247.
82. Johansson JA and Rubenowitz S: Risk indicators in the psychosocial and physical work environment for work related neck, shoulder and low back symptoms: A study among blue- and white-collar workers in eight companies. Scand J Rehabil Med *26*:131–142, 1994.
83. Jonsson B, Brundin L, Hagner IM, et al: Operating a forwarder: An electromyographic study. *In* Winter DA, Nouman RW, Wells RP, et al (eds): Biomechanics IX-B. Champaign, IL: Human Kinetics Publishers, 1985, pp 21–26.
84. Jonsson B, Hagberg M, and Sima S: Vocational electromyography in shoulder muscles in an electronics plant. *In* Morecki A, Fidelus K, Kedzior K, and Wit A (eds): Biomechanics VII, B. Baltimore: University Park Press, 1981, pp 10–15.
85. Jonsson B: The static load component in muscle work. Eur J Appl Physiol *57*:305–310, 1988.
86. Kamwendo K, Linton SJ, and Moritz U: Neck and shoulder disorders in medical secretaries. Part I. Pain prevalence and risk factors. Scand J Rehabil Med *23*:127–133, 1991.
87. Katevuo K, Aitasalo K, Lehtinen R, and Pietila J: Skeletal changes in dentists and farmers in Finland. Commun Dent Oral Epidemiol *13*:23–25, 1985.
88. Katsuyoshi M, Noriaki H, and Takamatsu M: Factor analysis of complaints of occupational cervicobrachial disorder in assembly lines of a cigarette factory. Kurume Med J *27*:253–261, 1980.
89. Kellgren JH and Lawrence JS: Rheumatism in miners. Part II. X-ray study. Br J Indust Med *9*:197–207, 1952.
90. Kelsey J: Epidemiology of Musculoskeletal Disorders. Oxford: Oxford University Press, 1982.
91. Keyserling WM, Punnett L, and Fine LJ: Postural stress of the trunk and shoulders: Identification and control of occupational risk factors. *In* Ergonomic Interventions to Prevent Musculoskeletal Injuries in Industry. Chelsea, MI: Lewis Publishers, 1987, pp 11–26.
92. Keyserling WM: Postural analysis of the trunk and shoulders in simulated real time, Ergonomics *29*:569–583, 1986.
93. Kitayama T: Health care relating to the occupational cervicobrachial disorder. J Hum Ergol (Tokyo) *11*:119–124, 1982.
94. Kluth K, Bohlemann J, and Strasser H: Rapid communication: A system for a strain-oriented analysis of the layout of assembly workplaces. Ergonomics *37*:1441–1448, 1994.
95. Kuorinka I and Forcier L (eds): Work Related Musculoskeletal Disorders: WMSDs: A Reference Book for Prevention. London, England: Taylor Francis, 1995.
96. Kuorinka I and Vikari-Juntura E: Prevalence of neck and upper limb disorders (NLD) and work load in different occupational groups: Problems in classification and diagnosis. J Hum Ergol (Tokyo) *11*:65–72, 1982.
97. LaBan MM and Meerschaert JR: Computer-generated headache: Brachiocephalgia at first byte. Am J Phys Med Rehabil *68*:183–185, 1989.
98. Larsson B, Libelius R, and Ohlsson K: Trapezius muscle changes unrelated to static work load: Chemical and morphologic controlled studies of 22 women with and without neck pain. Acta Orthop Scand *63*:203–206, 1992.
99. Larsson SE, Bengtsson A, Bodegard L, et al: Muscle changes in work-related chronic myalgia. Acta Orthop Scand *59*:552–556, 1988.
100. Larsson SE, Bodegard L, Henriksson KG, and Oberg PA: Chronic trapezius myalgia: Morphology and blood flow studied in seventeen patients. Acta Orthop Scand *61*:394–398, 1990.
101. Lawrence JS, Bremner JM, and Bier F: Osteoarthrosis: Prevalence in the population and relationship between symptoms and x-ray changes. Ann Rheum Dis *25*:1–24, 1966.
102. Lawrence JS: Rheumatism in cotton operatives. Br J Indust Med *18*:270–276, 1961.
103. Leffert RD: Disorders of the neck and shoulder. *In* Millender LH, Louis DS, and Simms BP (eds): Occupational Disorders of the Upper Extremity. New York: Churchill Livingstone, 1992.
104. Leino P and Magni G: Depressive and Distress Symptoms as Predictors of Low Back Pain, Neck-Shoulder Pain, and Other Musculoskeletal Morbidity: A 10-year Follow-up of Metal Industry Employees. Pain *53*:89–94, 1993.
105. Lindbolm K: On pathogenesis of ruptures of the tendon aponeurosis of the shoulder joint. Acta Radiol *20*:563, 1939.
106. Linton SJ and Kamwendo K: Risk factors in the psychosocial work environment for neck and shoulder pain in secretaries. J Occup Med *31*:609–613, 1989.
107. Luck JV and Andersson GBJ: Occupational shoulder disorders. *In* Rockwood CA Jr and Matsen FA III (eds): The Shoulder. Philadelphia: WB Saunders, 1990, pp 1088–1108.
108. Luopajarvi T, Kuorinka I, Virolai M, and Holmberg M: Prevalence of tenosynovitis and other injuries of the upper extremities in repetitive work. Scand J Work Environ Health *5* (Suppl 3): 48–55, 1979.
109. Mallory M and Bradford H: An invisible work place hazard getting harder to ignore. Business Week Jan. 30, 1989, pp 92–93.
110. Matsen FA III: Compartmental Syndromes. San Francisco: Grune & Stratton, 1980.
111. McDermott F: Repetition strain injury: A review of current understanding. Med J Aust *144*:196–200, 1986.
112. Melin E: Neck-shoulder loading characteristics and work technique. Ergonomics *30*:281–285, 1987.
113. Milerad E and Ekenvali L: Symptoms of the neck and upper extremities in dentists. Scand J Work Environ Health *16*:129–134, 1990.
114. Milerad E, Ericson MO, Nisell R, and Kilbom A: An electromyographic study of dental work. Ergonomics *34*:953–962, 1991.
115. Minnesota Medical Association: Worker's Compensation Permanent Partial Disability Schedule. Minneapolis: Minnesota Medical Association, 1984.
116. Misamore GW, Ziegler DW, and Rushton JC: Repair of the rotator cuff: A comparison of results of two populations of patients. J Bone Joint Surg *77A*:1335–1339, 1995.
117. Mortiz U: Conclusions and consensus statements presented by the chairmen responsible for the workshops. Scand J Rehab Med Suppl *32*:123–127, 1995.
118. National Institute of Occupational Safety and Health: Potential Health Hazards of Video Display Terminals. DHSS Publication No. 81-129. Cincinnati, OH: National Institute of Occupational Safety and Health, 1981.
119. Nayha S, Anttonen H, and Hassi J: Snowmobile driving and symptoms of the locomotive organs. Arctic Med Res Suppl *3*:41–44, 1994.
120. Neer CS: Anterior acromioplasty for the chronic impingement syndrome of the shoulder. J Bone Joint Surg *54A*:41–50, 1972.
121. Neer CS: Degenerative lesions of the proximal humeral articular surface. Clin Orthop *20*:116–124, 1961.
122. Neer CS: Impingement lesions. Clin Orthop *173*:70–77, 1983.
123. Nygren A, Berglund A, and von Koch M: Neck and shoulder pain, an increasing problem: Strategies for using insurance material to follow trends. Scand J Rehabil Med Suppl *32*:107–112, 1995.
124. O'Hara H, Aoyama H, and Itani T: Health hazard among cash register operators and the effects of improved working conditions. J Hum Ergol (Tokyo) *5*:31–40, 1976.
125. Ohlsson K, Attewell R, and Skerfving S: Self-reported symptoms in the neck and upper limbs of female assembly workers. Scand J Work Environ Health *15*:75–80, 1989.
126. Ohlsson K, Hansson GA, Balogh I, et al: Disorders of the neck and upper limbs in women in the fish processing industry. Occup Environ Med *51*:326–832, 1994.
127. Onishi N, Sakai K, and Kogi K: Arm and shoulder muscle load in various keyboard operating jobs of women. J Hum Ergol (Tokyo) *11*:89–97, 1982.
128. Osterweis M, Kleinman A, and Mechanic D (eds): Pain and Disability, Behavioral and Public Policy Perspectives. Washington, DC: National Academy Press, 1982.
129. Patterson PK, Eubanks TL, and Ramseyer R: Back discomfort prevalence and associated factors among bus drivers. Am Assoc Occup Nurs J *34*:481–484, 1986.
130. Petersson CJ: Degeneration of the acromioclavicular joint: A morphological study. Acta Orthop Scand *54*:434–438, 1983.
131. Petersson CJ: Degeneration of the glenohumeral joint: An anatomical study. Acta Orthop Scand *54*:277–283, 1983.
132. Post M and Cohen J: Impingement syndrome: A review of late stage II and early stage III lesions. Clin Orthop *207*:126–132, 1986.
133. Punnett L, Robins JM, Wegman DH, and Keyserling WM: Soft tissue disorders in the upper limbs of female garment workers. Scand J Work Environ Health *11*:417–425, 1985.
134. Rathbun J and Macnab I: The microvascular pattern of the rotator cuff. J Bone Joint Surg *52B*:548–553, 1970.

135. Rohmert W, Wos H, Norlander S, and Helbig R: Effects of vibration on arm and shoulder muscles in three body postures. Eur J Appl Physiol *58*:243–248, 1989.
136. Rundcrantz BL, Johnsson B, and Moritz U: Cervical pain and discomfort among dentists: Epidemiological, clinical and therapeutic aspects. Swed Dent *14*:71–80, 1990.
137. Rundcrantz BL, Johnsson B, and Moritz U: Occupational cervicobrachial disorders among dentists. Swed Dent J *15*:105–115, 1991.
138. Rundcrantz BL, Johnsson B, and Moritz U: Pain and discomfort in the musculoskeletal system among dentists. Swed Dent J *15*:219–228, 1991.
139. Ryan GA and Bampton M: Comparison of data process operators with and without upper limb symptoms. Community Health Studies *12*:63–68, 1988.
140. Saddemi S, Hawkins R, Morr J, and Hawkins A: Arthroscopic Subacromial Decompression: Two- to Four-Year Follow-up Study. Presented at the Ninth Open Meeting of the American Shoulder and Elbow Surgeons, San Francisco, California, February 1993.
141. Salen BA, Spangfort EV, Lygren AL, and Nordenar R: The disability rating index: An instrument for the assessment of disability in clinical settings. J Clin Epidemiol *47*:1423–1434, 1994.
142. Sallstrom J and Schmidt H: Cervicobrachial disorders in certain occupations with special reference to compression in the thoracic outlet. Am J Ind Med *6*:45–52, 1984.
143. Schierhout GH, Meyers JE, and Bridger RS: Work related musculoskeletal disorders and ergonomic stressors in the South African workforce. Occup Environ Med *52*:46–50, 1995.
144. Shugars HA, Miller D, Williams D, et al: Musculoskeletal pain among general dentists. General Dentistry *35*:272–276, 1987.
145. Sigholm G, Herberts P, Almstrom C, and Kadeforr R: Electromyographic analysis of shoulder muscle load. J Orthop Res *1*:379–386, 1984.
146. Sigholm G, Styf J, Korner L, and Herberts P: Pressure recording in the subacromial bursa. J Orthop Res *6*:123–128, 1988.
147. Sikorski J, Molan R, and Askin G: Orthopaedic basis for occupationally related arm and neck pain. Aust N Z J Surg *59*:471–478, 1989.
148. Silverstein, BA and Fine LJ: Cumulative trauma disorders of the upper extremity: A preventive strategy is needed. J Occup Med *33*:642–645, 1991.
149. Sjogaard G, Kiens B, Jorgensen K, and Saltin B: Intramuscular pressure: EMG and blood flow during low-level prolonged static contraction in man. Acta Physiol Scand *128*:475–484, 1996.
150. Social Security Administration, Social Security Bulletin, Spring 1995.
151. Sommerich CM, McGlothlin JD, and Marras WS: Occupational risk factors associated with soft tissue disorders of the shoulder: A review of recent investigations in the literature. Ergonomics *36*:697–717, 1993.
152. Health Insurance Association of America: Source Book of Health Insurance Data. New York: Health Insurance Association of America, 1995.
153. Stock SR: Workplace ergonomic factors and the development of musculoskeletal disorders of the neck and upper limbs: A meta-analysis. Am J Ind Med *19*:87–107, 1991.
154. Stone WE: Repetitive strain injuries. Med J Aust *2*:616–618, 1983.
155. Stubbs D and Peter B: Back and upper limb disorders. Practitioner *236*:34–38, 1992.
156. Suurkula J and Hagg GM: Relations between shoulder/neck disorders and EMG zero crossing shifts in female assembly workers using the test contraction method. Ergonomics *30*:1553–1564, 1987.
157. Swedish National Board of Occupational Safety and Health: Ordinance. *In* ASF 12: Concerning work with visual display units (VDUS), Stockholm, 1985.
158. Tait R, Chibnall J, and Richardson W: Litigation and employment status: Effects on patients with chronic pain. Pain *43*:37–46, 1990.
159. Takala EP, Viikari-Juntura E, Moneta GB, et al: Seasonal variation in neck and shoulder symptoms. Scand J Work Environ Health *18*:257–261, 1992.
160. Takala J, Sievers K, and Klaukka T: Rheumatic symptoms in the middle-aged population in southwestern Finland. Scand J Rheumatol Suppl *47*:15–29, 1982.
161. Taylor R and Pitcher M: Medical and ergonomic aspects of an industrial dispute concerning occupational related conditions in data process operators. Community Health Stud *13*:172–180, 1984.
162. Tichauer ER: Potential of biomechanics for solving specific hazard problems. *In* Proceedings of ASSE 1968 Conference. Park Ridge, IL: American Society of Safety Engineers, 1968, pp 149–187.
163. Tichauer ER: The Biomechanical Basis of Ergonomics: Anatomy Applied to the Design of Work Situations. New York: Wiley-Interscience, 1978.
164. Tiddia F, Cherchi GB, Pacifico L, and Chiesa C: *Yersinia enterocolitica* causing suppurative arthritis of the shoulder. J Clin Pathol *47*:760–761, 1994.
165. Toivanen H, Helin P, and Hanninen O: Impact of regular relaxation training and psychosocial working factors on neck-shoulder tension and absenteeism in hospital cleaners. J Occup Med *35*:1123–1130, 1993.
166. Tola S, Riihimaki H, Videman T, et al: Neck and shoulder symptoms among men in machine operating, dynamic physical work and sedentary work. Scand J Work Environ Health *14*:299–305, 1988.
167. US Department of Labor, Bureau of Labor Statistics: Survey of Occupational Injuries and Illnesses. Washington, DC: US Department of Labor, 1994.
168. Vasseljen O and Westgaard RH: A case-control study of trapezius muscle activity in office and manual workers with shoulder and neck pain and symptom-free controls. Int Arch Occup Environ Health *67*:11–18, 1995.
169. Vasseljen O, Westgaard RH, and Larsen S: A case-control study of psychological and psychological risk factors for shoulder and neck pain at the workplace. Int Arch Occup Environ Health *66*:375–382, 1995.
170. Vasudevan SV: Impairment, disability, and functional capacity assessment. *In* Turk DC and Melzack R (eds): Handbook of Pain Assessment. New York: The Gilford Press, 1992.
171. Veiersted K, Westgaard R, and Andersen P: Electromyographic evaluation of muscular work pattern as a predictor of trapezius myalgia. Scand J Work Environ Health *19*:284–290, 1993.
172. Veiersted KB, Westgaard RH, and Anderson P: Pattern of muscle activity during stereotyped work and its relation to muscle pain. Int Arch Occup Environ Health *62*:31–41, 1990.
173. Viikari-Juntura E: Neck and upper limb disorders among slaughterhouse workers: An epidemiologic and clinical study. Scand J Work Environ Health *9*:283–290, 1983.
174. Waldron HA and Cox M: Occupational arthropathy: Evidence from the past. Br J Ind Med *46*:420–422, 1989.
175. Waris P: Occupational cervicobrachial syndromes: A review. Scand J Work Environ Health *6* (Suppl 3):3–14, 1980.
176. Westerling D and Jonsson B: Pain from the neck-shoulder region and sick leave. Scand J Soc Med *8*:131–136, 1980.
177. Westgaard RH and Jansen T: Individual and work-related factors associated with symptoms of musculoskeletal complaints. II. Different risk factors among sewing machine operators. Br J Ind Med *49*:154–162, 1992.
178. Westgaard RH, Jensen C, and Hansen K: Individual and work-related factors associated with symptoms of musculoskeletal complaints. Int Arch Occup Environ Health *64*:405–413, 1993.
179. Westgaard RH, Jensen C, and Nilsen K: Muscle coordination and choice-reaction time tests as indicators of occupational muscle load and shoulder-neck complaints. Eur J Appl Physiol *67*:106–114, 1993.
180. Wiker SF, Chaffin DB, and Langolf GD: Shoulder posture and localized muscle fatigue and discomfort. Ergonomics *32*:211–237, 1989.
181. Winkel J, Ekblom B, and Tillberg B: Ergonomics and medical factors in shoulder/arm pain among cabin attendants as a basis for job redesign. *In* Malsvi H and Kobayashi K (eds): Biomechanics VIII-A. Champaign, IL: Human Kinetics Publishers, 1983, pp 563–567.
182. Winkel J, Ekblom B, Hagberg M, and Jonsson B: The working environment of cleaners: Evaluation of physical strain in mopping and swabbing as a basis for job redesign. *In* Ergonomics of Workstation Design. London: Butterworths, 1983, pp 35–44.
183. Worcester JN and Green DP: Osteoarthritis of the acromioclavicular joint. Clin Orthop *58*:69–73, 1968.
184. Yood RA and Goldenberg DJ: Sterno-clavicular joint arthritis. Arthritis Rheum *23*:232–239, 1980.
185. Zenz C: Occupational Medicine: Principles and Practical Applications: Chicago: Year Book Medical Publishers, 1988.

CHAPTER

28

FREDERICK A. MATSEN III, M.D.
KEVIN L. SMITH, M.D.

Effectiveness Evaluation and the Shoulder

"which was merely the common-sense notion that every hospital should follow *every* patient it treats, long enough to determine whether or not the treatment has been successful, and then to inquire 'if not, why not?' with a view to preventing similar failures in future."

E. A. CODMAN 1934

Outcomes research has seen an explosion of interest in recent years across all fields of medicine.[24, 33, 44] This growth has been driven by a number of factors that include increasing health care costs, inadequacies of research methodology, and regional variations in practice without apparent reason.[102] It has piqued the interest of groups including epidemiologists, academic physicians, third-party payers, health care systems, and patients. It is now apparent that individual practicing physicians can document their results with specific treatment programs. This is best done in terms of variables that are directly relevant to the quality of life of the patient.[4]

HISTORY

In the past, clinical studies in orthopedics were mainly investigations of small groups of patients reviewed retrospectively using parameters assessed by health care professions. We might call these variables "medical metrics," including examples such as fracture union, deformity, recurrence, strength, and range of motion. Occasionally, when patient perceptions were reported, such as pain relief and overall satisfaction, they would recommend similar treatment to others, and they would agree to the same procedure if necessary in the future, and whether they were better, the same, or worse. Results were often divided into categories of relative success, such as poor, fair, good, and excellent. Many studies lacked statistical rigor, strict inclusion or exclusion criteria, standardization of treatment methods, and consistent measures of comfort and function before and after treatment. Scores were proposed that arbitrarily attached a relative weight to various elements of the examination.[70] Most clinical studies have been reported by specialists in the procedure of interest, rather than by individuals in the general practice of orthopedics where the preponderance of care is rendered. Thus, the degree to which the reported results are relevant to the bulk of practice in the United States is uncertain.

The concept of systematically documenting the results of treatment was formalized when Codman proposed his "end result" idea in Boston just after the turn of the century.[21] He advocated critically evaluating the results of each patient's treatment over time in order to identify and understand treatment failures. It is obvious from the quote at the beginning of this chapter that Codman was an advocate of quality control for all treatment rendered, rather than only considering the results of specialists. Donabedian was the first to use the term outcome in expressing Codman's end result idea.[29] In addition, he defined two other major dimensions of quality of care, namely structure and process. Structural factors include the number of hospital beds in an institution and the quality control practices of its laboratory. These factors are easy to quantify and measure and were an early focus of the Joint Commission. Process indicators monitor the steps and actions involved in patient care and include variables such as who gives medications, how specimens are handled, and conformity with set protocols of care. Proximate outcomes relate specifically to the steps in the overall process of care. For example, the radiology department may consider the final, accurate report as its outcome. Lastly, ultimate outcome measures what exactly happens to the patient as a result of the entire course of action, including patient satisfaction, morbidity, and mortality. This is closely linked to the process of care and is the current focus of outcome study.

Karnofsky introduced the use of surveys for evaluating the success of cancer treatment in the 1940s.[50] The patient-oriented approach to evaluation of results was advocated by Lembcke.[66] Katz utilized activity of daily living scales to measure outcomes in elderly patients;[53] Bradburn looked at psychological well-being and its effect on patients;[15] Breslow introduced methods of measuring physical, mental, and social well-being;[16] and Bush developed the Health Status Index and the Quality of Well-Being (QWB) Scale.[19] These milestones set the stage for current understanding and methodology of result measurement using self-assessment questionnaires.

In the 1970s, Wennberg and Gittelsohn's epidemiologic study documented that health care utilization varied widely from one region to another.[113] This compelling finding was the catalyst that sparked much of the current interest in outcomes research. The methodology used, termed small area analysis, demonstrated large variations in the rate of tonsillectomy, hysterectomy, prostatectomy, and other procedures between regions, despite controlling for variations in population demographics.[115] A patient living in New Haven, for instance, was found to be twice as likely to undergo spine surgery for degenerative disk disease than one living in Boston, yet the latter was twice as likely to undergo total hip replacement than the former.[114] Whatever the explanation of this phenomenon, it posed the key question regarding what information is needed to justify a specified treatment.

Starting with the shoulder surgeon, Codman, orthopedics has been a leader in outcome research.[58, 59] The American Academy of Orthopaedic Surgeons has promoted this kind of investigation that provides specific outcome measurement instruments.[1, 2] Keller has advocated a terminology for different aspects of outcome research.[57] ***Efficacy*** indicates whether a procedure or technology works in the hands of select individuals in a specific setting. ***Effectiveness*** indicates that an efficacious procedure works when utilized throughout the general medical community. An *efficacious* procedure may indeed prove to be *ineffective* when used by general practitioners. Finally, ***appropriateness*** indicates that a treatment is indicated in the patients receiving it. An improperly utilized procedure may lead to better or worse results than expected, thus clouding the understanding of its value. Some studies have applied the emerging methodologies to measure the effectiveness of various orthopedic treatments.[6, 14, 20, 26, 43, 47, 48, 54, 62, 67, 74, 84, 91, 98] When considering these studies, it becomes apparent that effectiveness measurement of management methods for musculoskeletal conditions is more complex than measuring the effectiveness of an antihypertensive medication for lowering blood pressure. In the treatment of hypertension, the inclusion criteria can be simply defined; the evaluation tool is straightforward; and the person administering the treatment as well as the technique utilized are relatively unimportant. The nature of the treatment can be from the patient and the evaluator, thus permitting double-blind side-by-side comparisons of the effectiveness of treatment. None of these statements is true when we try to compare the effectiveness of surgical management of rotator cuff disease with nonoperative treatment, for example.

The literature on acromioplasty illustrates the challenges and difficulties with outcome measurement in orthopedics.[70] In each study, different inclusion criteria were applied. Distinct evaluation tools were used, many based principally on medical metrics (i.e., change in acromial shape on x-ray). The evaluation methods often were not used before and after treatment so that the success or failure of treatment could be quantified. Different definitions of "success" were used. As a result, it is difficult to compare and contrast the results and to define the indications for this most commonly performed shoulder procedure.[3, 30, 34, 45, 85, 86, 93]

Some research has been based on large databases, such as Medicare claims data.[115] Although these have the advantage of being applicable to the broad range of practice in the United States, results from these sources do not reflect change in comfort, function, or health status. Other studies involve meta-analysis of all related literature for a given area, looking for rigorous evidence to support the use of a particular treatment.[26, 64, 72] While much research has been retrospective, an increasing number use prospectively designed protocols[7, 12, 13, 18] Some authors promote the use of treatment algorithms and practice guidelines to facilitate analysis of results and to minimize practice variability noted through small area analysis.[11]

Another important concept is that of ***cost-effectiveness***.[19, 31, 40, 41, 46, 65, 89, 101] The current medical cost climate dictates that health care should not only be effective and appropriate but also worthy of the expenditures related to it.

Although effectiveness, appropriateness, and cost-effectiveness are straightforward in concept, they are challenging to measure in a clinical context:

- How is effectiveness measured and by whom?
- What does the "general medical community" mean?
- How can an "indication" be rigorously defined?
- How can the full "cost" of a treatment be determined?

EVALUATION OF INSTRUMENTS

It has been proposed that outcome instruments be judged in terms of their *validity*, *reproducibility*, *internal consistency*, and *responsiveness to change*.[107] The term *validity* is used to describe whether a given instrument actually measures what it is purported to measure. *Reproducibility* refers to the ability of a tool to yield the same result when administered on separate occasions. This is commonly referred to as test-retest reliability. The *internal consistency* of a tool implies that it is able to adequately measure a single concept irrespective of extraneous effectors. Thus, an internally consistent assessment of shoulder function should not be affected by problems with the elbow, wrist, or hand. Finally, in order to be of value, a tool must show *responsiveness to change*. If purported to measure knee function, a tool should be able to demonstrate a difference before and after knee arthroplasty, for example.

TYPES OF OUTCOME MEASUREMENTS

Medical metrics uses factors observed by health care professionals, including physical examination findings (e.g., range of motion, strength), radiographic analysis (e.g., union, loosening), and the incidence of complications, such as deep venous thrombosis and infection.[38, 43]

By contrast, *patient assessments* include documentation of parameters evident to the individual, such as mental health, social well-being, role function (as worker, parent, spouse), physical function, and ability to carry out activities of daily living (ADLs).[18, 49, 50, 58, 59] These patient assessments are most practically obtained by self-assessment questionnaires, because they are *inexpensive* to use compared with measurements of strength or range, *convenient* (they can be completed without the patient having to return to the physician's office), and *free from variability* due to differences among medical observers.

The ideal approach enables every practitioner to comply with Codman's admonition to follow every patient treated, long enough to determine whether or not the treatment has been successful, and then to inquire if not, why not? A plan can then be made to prevent similar failures in the future. From this admonition we can derive the characteristics of the desired results assessment tool:

- *Every practitioner* requires that the tool be inexpensive and easy to administer and record, such that all can use it.
- *Follow every patient* necessitates that the tool be applicable to as many different conditions as possible, simple to complete, and achievable without requiring the patient's return to the office (e.g., otherwise patients who are poor or who live a long distance away may be systematically excluded).
- *Long enough* implies that the tool enable follow-up for many years after the treatment.
- *Determine whether or not the treatment has been successful* proposes that the tool measure factors that are important to the patient (e.g., comfort and function) and that the same tool be applied before and after treatment, so that success or failure can be meaningfully defined rigorously and quantitatively in terms of a change in the results.
- *"If not, why not?"* makes it imperative that differences between the pre- and post-treatment results from the tool reliably reveal every patient who has improved and those who have worsened after implementing the treatment.
- *Preventing similar failures in the future* means that results need to be available to the specific provider such that appropriate changes can be made, because failures are often due to the individual provider's patient selection, technique, or postoperative management rather than solely to the type of operation or implant used.

It is evident that existing methods using hospital discharge data, meta analysis, or studies confined to largely specialized practices do not provide the individualized quality control advocated by Codman.

SHOULDER ASSESSMENT INSTRUMENTS

The different shoulder assessment tools currently available can be evaluated against Codman's criteria. The following include a sampling of the various types utilized, from general to specific. Beaton and associates prospectively compared the validity of five self-assessment questionnaires that measure shoulder function.[5] All performed similarly in describing patients' shoulder function and in discriminating relative severity. In light of these similarities, they proposed that one might choose a questionnaire for practical reasons, such as ease of administration or scoring.

Simple Shoulder Test

The Simple Shoulder Test (SST) is a short and simple shoulder-specific self-assessment tool that has proved to be practical within the context of busy practices.[69, 78–81] The SST consists of a set of 12 "yes" or "no" questions derived from the common complaints of patients presenting to the University of Washington Shoulder Service for evaluation. These 12 questions are listed in Table 28–1. The SST has been shown to (1) be reproducible on test-retest,[69, 79] (2) practical in a busy practice setting,[69, 79] (3) sensitive to a wide variety of shoulder disorders,[5, 69, 79] and (4) able to quantitate the change in shoulder function resulting from treatment and to permit the identification of treatment failures.[78]

Normal subjects have been shown to be able to perform essentially all of the SST functions. Conversely, the SST is sensitive to the shoulder disabilities perceived by patients presenting for evaluation and management of a wide range of shoulder disorders.[5, 69, 79]

The SST can be viewed as a minimal data set of functional information that can be collected on all patients at the time of presentation. If additional functional

Table 28–1 SIMPLE SHOULDER TEST*

1.	Is your shoulder comfortable with your arm at rest by your side?	Yes	No
2.	Does your shoulder allow you to sleep comfortably?	Yes	No
3.	Can you reach the small of your back to tuck in your shirt with your hand?	Yes	No
4.	Can you place your hand behind your head with the elbow straight out to the side?	Yes	No
5.	Can you place a coin on a shelf at the level of your shoulder without bending your elbow?	Yes	No
6.	Can you lift 1 lb (a full pint container) to the level of your shoulder without bending your elbow?	Yes	No
7.	Can you lift 8 lb (a full gallon container) to the level of the top of your head without bending your elbow?	Yes	No
8.	Can you carry 20 lb (a bag of potatoes) at your side with the affected extremity?	Yes	No
9.	Do you think you can toss a softball underhand 10 yards with the affected extremity?	Yes	No
10.	Do you think you can throw a softball overhand 20 yards with the affected extremity?	Yes	No
11.	Can you wash the back of your opposite shoulder with the affected extremity?	Yes	No
12.	Would your shoulder allow you to work full-time at your regular job?	Yes	No

*The Simple Shoulder Test (SST) is used for patient self-assessment of general shoulder function. (From Lippitt SB, Harryman DT II, and Matsen FA III: A practical tool for evaluation function: the simple shoulder test. *In* Matsen FA III, Fu FH, and Hawkins RJ [eds]: The Shoulder: A Balance of Mobility and Stability. Rosemont, IL: American Academy of Orthopaedic Surgeons, 1993, pp 501–518.)

data are needed to make the questionnaire more sensitive, questions can be added to the original 12, while keeping the minimal data set intact. For example, when studying high performance athletes, one could add questions such as: "Does your shoulder allow you to pitch (or serve) with your usual speed and control?"; "Does your shoulder allow you to swim your normal work-out?"; or "Does your shoulder allow you to compete at the varsity level in your sport?"

The simplicity of this test allows the characterization of the shoulder function of an individual patient or of a group of patients meeting specified inclusion criteria. The effectiveness of a management program can be easily characterized in terms of the change in the patient's assessment and his or her ability to perform the different functions before and after the treatment.

Rowes' Rating Sheet for Bankart Repair

One of the earliest attempts at standardizing the evaluation of shoulder function was Rowes' rating of the results of Bankart repair (Table 28–2).[97] It includes a maximum potential score of 100 points, which are subdivided into stability (50 points), motion (20 points), and function (30 points). This disease-specific instrument provides a measure of the relative success of instability surgery. The rating scale is heavily weighted to the recurrence of insta-

Table 28–2 ROWE SCORING SYSTEM

SCORING SYSTEM	UNITS	EXCELLENT (100–90)	GOOD (89–75)	FAIR (74–51)	POOR (50 or less)
Stability, no recurrence, subluxation, or apprehension	50	No recurrences	No recurrences	No recurrences	Recurrence of dislocation
Apprehension when placing arm in certain positions	30	No apprehension when placing arm in complete elevation and external rotation	Mild apprehension when placing the arm in elevation and external rotation	Moderate apprehension during elevation and external rotation	Marked apprehension during elevation and extension
Subluxation (not requiring reduction)	10	No subluxation	No subluxation	No subluxation	
Motion 100% of normal external rotation, internal rotation, and elevation	20	100% of normal external rotation, internal rotation, and complete elevation	75% of normal external rotation, internal rotation, and complete elevation	50% of normal external rotation, 75% of internal rotation and elevation	No external rotation; 50% of elevation (can get hand only to face) and 50% of internal rotation
75% of normal external rotation, and normal elevation and internal rotation	15				
50% of normal external rotation, 75% of internal rotation and elevation	5				
50% of normal external and internal rotation; no elevation	0				
Function: No limitation in work or sports; little or no discomfort	30	Performs all work and sports; no limitation in overhead activities; shoulder strong in lifting, swimming, tennis, throwing; no discomfort	Mild limitation in work and sports; shoulder strong; minimum discomfort	Moderate limitation doing overhead work and heavy lifting; unable to throw, serve hard in tennis, or swim; moderate disabling pain	Marked limitation; unable to perform overhead work and lifting; cannot throw, play tennis, or swim; chronic discomfort
Mild limitation in work or sports; little or no discomfort	25				
Moderate limitation and discomfort	10				
Marked limitation and pain	0				
Total units possible	100				

*The Rowe scoring system is used for evaluating the results of Bankart repairs. (From Rowe CR, Patel D, and Southmayd WW: The Bankart procedure: A long-term end-result study. J Bone Joint Surg *60A*:1–16, 1978.)

Table 28–3 UCLA SCORING SYSTEM*†

FUNCTION/REACTION MEASURED	POINTS
Pain	
Present all of the time and unbearable; strong medication frequently	1
Present all of the time but bearable; strong medication occasionally	2
None or little at rest, present during light activities, salicylates frequently	4
Present during heavy or particular activities only; salicylates occasionally	6
Occasional and slight	8
None	10
Function	
Unable to use limb	1
Only light activities possible	2
Able to do light housework or most activities of daily living	4
Most housework, shopping, and driving possible; able to fix hair and dress and undress, including fastening brassiere	6
Slight restriction only; able to work above shoulder level	8
Normal activities	10
Active Forward Flexion	
150 degrees or more	5
120 to 150 degrees	4
90 to 120 degrees	3
45 to 90 degrees	2
30 to 45 degrees	1
Less than 30 degrees	0
Strength of Forward Flexion (Manual Muscle Testing)	
Grade 5 (normal)	5
Grade 4 (good)	4
Grade 3 (fair)	3
Grade 2 (poor)	2
Grade I (muscle contraction)	1
Grade 0 (nothing)	0
Satisfaction of the Patient	
Satisfied and better	5
Not satisfied and worse	0

*The University of California–Los Angeles (UCLA) scoring system is used for evaluating shoulder function and patient satisfaction. (From Ellman H, Hanker G, and Bayer M: Repair of the rotator cuff: End-result study of factors influencing reconstruction. J Bone Joint Surg *68A*:1136–1144, 1986.)
†Maximum score of 35 points.

bility (50 points) but does not include the evaluation of ADLs, ability to sleep, and pain. It includes medical metrics, thus it requires that the patient return to the office for serial examination.

UCLA Shoulder Scoring System

The UCLA scale has been widely used since Ellman introduced it in 1986 (Table 28–3).[30] It utilizes a total score of 35 points with pain and function each allotted 1 to 10 points, and active forward flexion, strength of forward flexion, and patient satisfaction each totaling 1 to 5 points. The overall score is then classified as excellent (34 to 35 points), good (29 to 33 points), or poor (<29 points). The weighting of the questions has interesting consequences; for example, if a patient is unable to internally rotate to T-8 (e.g., to fasten brassiere), she loses 4 points and can only have a good result at best. This score includes medical metrics; therefore, it requires the patient to return to the office for serial examination.

Hospital for Special Surgery Shoulder-Rating Score Sheet

Altchek and associates proposed a scoring system based on a maximal possible score of 100 points for a normal shoulder (Table 28–4).[3] Pain accounts for 30 points, functional assessment for 28 points, tenderness for 5 points, impingement maneuvers for 32 points, and range of motion for 5 points. Pain was given the most weight because it is the primary symptom of concern to these authors. They developed an overall results rating scale defining excellent results as those scoring 90 to 100 points, good scoring 70 to 89 points, fair scoring 50 to 69 points, and

Table 28–4 HOSPITAL FOR SPECIAL SURGERY SCORING SYSTEM*

	NO. OF POINTS
Pain (30 points)	
None = 6 points, mild = 3, moderate = 2, severe = 0 during:	
1. Sports	______
2. Non-sports overhead reaching	______
3. Activities of daily living	______
4. Sitting at rest	______
5. Sleeping	______
Total	______
Functional limitation (28 points)	
None = 7 points, mild = 4, moderate = 2, severe = 0 during:	
1. Sports with hand overhead	______
2. Sports not involving use of the shoulder	______
3. Reaching overhead	______
4. Nonspecific activities of daily living	______
Total	______
Tenderness (5 points)	
None = 5 points, at one or two sites = 3, at more than two sites = 0	
Total	______
Impingement maneuvers (32 points)	
Indicated numbers of points are assigned for each maneuver in an all-or-none fashion, 0 points being assigned if the maneuver is:	
1. Impingement sign (15)	______
2. Abduction sign (12)	______
3. Adduction sign (5)	______
Total	______
Range of motion (5 points)	
One point is assigned for each 20-degree loss of motion in any plane, to a maximum of 5 points	
Total	______

*The Hospital for Special Surgery (HSS) scoring system is used for evaluating the results of acromioplasty. (From Altchek DW, Warren RF, Wickiewicz TL, et al: Arthroscopic acromioplasty: Technique and results. J Bone Joint Surg 72A:1198–1207, 1990.)

poor with less than 50 points. The Hospital for Special Surgery Shoulder-Rating Scale relies heavily on medical metrics, thus it requires the patient to return to the office for serial examination.

Constant Scoring System

In 1987, Constant and Murley presented their approach for measuring shoulder function (Table 28–5).[23] It involves a numeric estimation of the patient's function and evaluates the patient's pain. Point allocation includes 15 points for pain, 20 points for ADLs, 40 points for range of motion, and 35 points for strength. The Constant score gives 75% of the points based on medical metrics; it requires the patient to return to the office for serial examination.

American Shoulder and Elbow Surgeons' Form

This form includes both a patient self-evaluation section and medical metrics.[95] The patient self-evaluation section takes approximately 3 minutes to complete, requires no assistance, and includes an ADL section measured on a 4-point ordinal scale and visual analog scales to measure pain and instability. A shoulder score can be derived from the pain scales (50%) and a cumulative (ADL) score (50%). The medical metrics section includes demographic data and assessments of range of motion, physical signs, strength, and stability.

A modified version of this form is now available that reflects dysfunction of the entire upper extremity, including hand, wrist, elbow, and shoulder (Table 28–6). It is based on the premise that the arm is a kinematic chain

Table 28–5 CONSTANT SCORING SYSTEM*

PAIN	***POINTS***		
None	15		
Mild	10		
Moderate	5		
Severe	0		
ACTIVITIES OF DAILY LIVING			
Activity Level	***Points***	***Positioning***	***Points***
Full work	4	Up to waist	2
Full recreation/sport	4	Up to xiphoid	4
Unaffected sleep	2	Up to neck	6
		Up to top of head	8
		Above head	10
Total for activities of daily living: 20			
POINTS FOR FORWARD AND LATERAL ELEVATION			
Elevation (Degrees)	***Points***		
0–30	0		
31–60	2		
61–90	4		
91–120	6		
121–150	8		
151–180	10		
EXTERNAL ROTATION SCORING			
Position	***Points***		
Hand behind head with elbow held forward	2		
Hand behind head with elbow held back	2		
Hand on top of head with elbow held forward	2		
Hand on top of head with elbow held back	2		
Full elevation from on top of head	2		
Total: 10			
INTERNAL ROTATION SCORING			
Position	***Points***		
Dorsum of hand to lateral thigh	0		
Dorsum of hand to buttock	2		
Dorsum of hand to lumbosacral junction	4		
Dorsum of hand to waist (3rd lumbar vertebra)	6		
Dorsum of hand to 12th dorsal vertebra	8		
Dorsum of hand to interscapular region (DV 7)	10		

*The Constant scoring system is used for evaluating general shoulder function both objectively and subjectively. (From Constant CR and Murley AHG: A clinical method of functional assessment of the shoulder. Clin Orthop *214*:160–164, 1987.)

Table 28–6 ASES SCORING SYSTEM*

ASES PATIENT SELF-EVALUATION: INSTABILITY QUESTIONNAIRE

Does your shoulder feel unstable (as if it is going to dislocate)?	YES	NO
How unstable is your shoulder (mark line)? 0 (Very Stable) ———————————— 10 (Very Unstable)		

ASES PATIENT SELF-EVALUATION: ACTIVITY OF DAILY LIVING QUESTIONNAIRE

Circle the number in the box that indicates your ability to do the following activities:
0 = unable to do; 1 = very difficult to do; 2 = somewhat difficult; 3 = not difficult

Activity	***Right Arm***	***Left Arm***
1. Put on a coat	0 1 2 3	0 1 2 3
2. Sleep on your painful or affected side	0 1 2 3	0 1 2 3
3. Wash back or do up bra in back	0 1 2 3	0 1 2 3
4. Manage toileting	0 1 2 3	0 1 2 3
5. Comb hair	0 1 2 3	0 1 2 3
6. Reach a high shelf	0 1 2 3	0 1 2 3
7. Lift 10 lb above the shoulder	0 1 2 3	0 1 2 3
8. Throw a ball overhand	0 1 2 3	0 1 2 3
9. Do usual work—list:	0 1 2 3	0 1 2 3
10. Do usual sport—list:	0 1 2 3	0 1 2 3

ASES PHYSICIAN ASSESSMENT: RANGE OF MOTION

Range of Motion	***Right***		***Left***	
Total shoulder motion; goniometer preferred	Active	Passive	Active	Passive
Forward elevation (maximum arm-trunk angle)				
External rotation (arm comfortably at side)				
External rotation (arm at 90 degrees of abduction)				
Internal rotation (highest posterior anatomy reached with the thumb)				
Cross-body adduction (antecubital fossa to the opposite acromion)				

ASES PHYSICIAN ASSESSMENT: SIGNS

0 = none; 1 = mild; 2 = moderate; 3 = severe

Sign	***Right***	***Left***
Supraspinatus/greater tuberosity tenderness	0 1 2 3	0 1 2 3
Acromioclavicular joint tenderness	0 1 2 3	0 1 2 3
Biceps tendon tenderness (or rupture)	0 1 2 3	0 1 2 3
Other tenderness—list:	0 1 2 3	0 1 2 3
Impingement I (passive forward elevation in slight internal rotation)	Y N	Y N
Impingement II (passive internal rotation with 90 degrees of flexion)	Y N	Y N
Impingement III (90 degrees of active abduction—classic painful arc)	Y N	Y N
Subacromial crepitus	Y N	Y N
Scars—location:	Y N	Y N
Atrophy—location:	Y N	Y N
Deformity—describe:	Y N	Y N

Table continued on following page

Table 28–6 ASES SCORING SYSTEM* *(Continued)*

ASES PHYSICIAN ASSESSMENT: STRENGTH (RECORD MRC GRADE)
0 = no contraction; 1 = flicker; 2 = movement with gravity eliminated;
3 = movement against gravity; 4 = movement against some resistance; 5 = normal power

	Right	***Left***
Testing affected by pain?	Y N	Y N
Forward elevation	0 1 2 3 4 5	0 1 2 3 4 5
Abduction	0 1 2 3 4 5	0 1 2 3 4 5
External rotation (arm comfortably at side)	0 1 2 3 4 5	0 1 2 3 4 5
Internal rotation (arm comfortably at side)	0 1 2 3 4 5	0 1 2 3 4 5

ASES PHYSICIAN ASSESSMENT: INSTABILITY
0 = none; 1 = mild (0–1 cm translation)
2 = moderate (1–2 cm translation or translates to glenoid rim)
3 = severe (>2 cm translation or over rim of glenoid)

Anterior translation	0 1 2 3	0 1 2 3
Posterior translation	0 1 2 3	0 1 2 3
Interior translation (sulcus sign)	0 1 2 3	0 1 2 3
Anterior apprehension	0 1 2 3	0 1 2 3
Reproduces symptoms?	Y N	Y N
Voluntary instability?	Y N	Y N
Relocation test positive?	Y N	Y N
Generalized ligamentous laxity?	Y N	
Other physical findings:		
Examiner's name:		Date

*The American Shoulder and Elbow Surgeons (ASES) scoring system is used for evaluating general shoulder function both objectively and subjectively. (From Richards RR, An K-N, Bigliani LU, et al: A standardized method for assessment of shoulder function. J Shoulder Elbow Surg *3*:347–352, 1994.)

that acts in concert, because they all are important in positioning the hand for grasp and manipulation of the environment.

Shoulder Severity Index

Conceived by Patte, this tool seeks to assess chronically painful shoulder disabilities (Table 28–7).[90] It takes approximately 7 minutes to complete and evaluates pain in different situations of daily life, functional activities, strength, and daily handicap. It includes seven questions concerning pain, 20 for function, and one each for strength, handicap, and satisfaction.[5]

Other Tools

Many groups have altered the aforementioned scoring systems to suit various specific clinical conditions. Kay and associates revised the UCLA score to apply specifically to hemiarthroplasty results.[55] This modified, treatment-specific version is shown in Table 28–8.

Other assessment tools are very disease-specific. One example is the form proposed by Poigenfurst to evaluate specifically the results of acromioclavicular separation and its management (Table 28–9).[92]

Specific patient groups are the focus of other questionnaires. Tibone and associates proposed a scoring system

Table 28–7 SHOULDER SEVERITY SCORING SYSTEM*

ALGOFUNCTIONAL INDEX OF PATTE FOR SHOULDERS

Family name: ____________ First name: ____________ Date: ____________

Shoulder: *Right/Left*

File Number: ____________ Documented: ____________

Diagnosis: ____________

Pain (P)

Choose the figure that most appropriately describes your pain:
- 0: No pain
- 1: Mild pain
- 2: Moderate pain
- 3: Severe pain
- 4: Unbearable pain

Place this figure in each column and then multiply by the coefficient:

When resting with the arm hanging or bent	________	X	2	=	________
As soon as you try to raise your arm	________	X	1.5	=	________
Only when you repeat the movement	________	X	1	=	________
During a sudden movement	________	X	0.5	=	________
If you can't sleep on the affected shoulder, add 1 point:			+1	=	________
If you have the feeling that something "blocks" when you raise the arm:					
Forward, add 2 points			+2	=	________
Sideways, add 1 point			+1	=	________
If you take painkillers					
All the time: add 4 points			+4	=	________
From time to time: add 2 points			+2	=	________

Points = [ ] /30*

Functional Index (I)

Movements must be performed with the affected shoulder, even if these are unusual movements, and **without the help of the other hand** and without "cheating" in using the head or the trunk.

Please reply to each question using the following point system:
- 0: Without difficulty
- 1: With difficulty/0.5/1.5
- 2: Impossible

Can you:

1. Hygiene

Wash your forehead or apply make-up yourself	=	________
Wash your hair completely (even behind)	=	________
Wash under the armpit on the opposite side	=	________
Wash your opposite scapula (from in front)	=	________
Wipe yourself (after going to the toilet)	=	________
		............./10

2. Dressing

Put tight trousers on and buckle the belt	=	________
Put a pullover on or off by passing it over your head	=	________
Put a jacket on, finishing with the affected shoulder	=	________
Put your shirt into skirt or trousers (including behind)	=	________
		............./8

3. Eating: sitting at a table

Eat your soup using a spoon (elbow is not on the table)	=	________
Lift a full bottle (1 L) with your arm outstretched	=	________
Pour yourself a drink from this bottle	=	________
		............./6

Table continued on following page

Table 28–7 SHOULDER SEVERITY SCORING SYSTEM* *(Continued)*

4. Daily gestures (try to do them even if they are not usual)
   - Knitting, ironing, planing = ______
   - Military salute = ______
   - Open and close a window (or shelve light things):
     - At eye level = ______
     - Above your head = ______
   - Change an electric light bulb on the ceiling = ______
   - Clean the window panes above the level of your head = ______
   - Push open a door with your arm stretched sideways = ______
   - Change gears in a car (put into reverse gear) = ______

.............../16

I = ☐ /40

TOTAL FUNCTIONAL INDEX

Muscle Strength (MS)

How much lifting strength do you think you have lost when lifting an object (2 kg) with the arm stretched out horizontally?

- Normal strength = 0
- Less than normal strength with fatigability = 3 to 5
- Half of usual strength = 6 to 10
- No lifting strength = 15

MS = ☐ /15

Daily Handicap (H)

Rate your handicap between 0 and 100%

0% |—|—|—|—|—|—|—|—|—|—|—|—|—|—|—| 100%
(No handicap) (Unbearable handicap)

(The figure to be noted is that marked in centimeters by the patient.)
Total = (P + I + MS + H)
The algofunctional index (AF)† for functional value of the shoulder examined is:
100—total AF + = %

H = ☐ /15

Evaluation of the Result

	Favorable			*Unfavorable*		
	TB 1	B 2	M +3	M −4	E 5	1
Algofunctional index (postoperative)	>90%	>75%	>66%	>50%	<50%	2 3
Comparison of preoperative and postoperative algofunctional index			>25%	<25%		4 5

Adjustments

- Painful chronic shoulder: pain must be <5 for favorable result
- Active patient: muscular strength must be multiplied by 2 — MS × 2
- Elderly patient with limited activity or prosthetic replacement: Muscular strength must be divided by 2 — MS / 2

Subjective Result — Very pleased ☐ Pleased ☐ Dissatisfied ☐

*The Shoulder Severity scoring system was developed by Patte for patient self-assessment of painful or chronically disabled shoulders. (From Patte D: Directions for the Use of the Index Severity for Painful and/or Chronically Disabled Shoulders. Abstracts of the First Open Congress of the European Society of Surgery of the Shoulder and Elbow [SECEC], Paris, 1987, pp 36–41.)

†This algofunctional index can be used only if the pain (P) is less than 15. Otherwise, the index must be calculated again once the painful episode is over.

Table 28–8 UCLA SCORING SYSTEM—MODIFICATION FOR HEMIARTHROPLASTY*

	SCORE	FINDINGS
Pain	1	Constant, unbearable; strong medication frequently
	2	Constant, but bearable; strong medications occasionally
	4	None or little at rest; occurs with light activity; salicylates frequently
	5	With heavy or particular activities only; salicylates occasionally
	8	Occasional and slight
	10	No pain
Function	1	Unable to use arm
	2	Very light activity only
	4	Light housework or most daily living activities
	5	Most housework; washing hair; putting on brassiere; shopping; driving
	8	Slight restrictions only; able to work above shoulder level
	10	Normal activities
Muscle Power and Motion	1	Ankylosis with deformity
	2	Ankylosis with good functional position
	4	Muscle power poor to fair; elevation less than 60 degrees; internal rotation less than 45 degrees
	5	Muscle power fair to good; elevation of 90 degrees; internal rotation of 90 degrees
	8	Muscle power good or normal; elevation of 140 degrees; external rotation of 20 degrees
	10	Normal muscle power; motion near normal

*A modification of the UCLA scoring system is used for evaluating the results of shoulder hemiarthroplasty. (From Kay SP and Amstutz HC: Shoulder hemiarthroplasty at UCLA. Clin Orthop *228*:42–44, 1988.)

whose goal was the assessment of athletic shoulder problems and results.[104] This form is shown in Table 28–10.

Dawson and colleagues published their questionnaire for evaluating patients' perceptions before and after shoulder surgery.[27] This 12-item questionnaire was created specifically to measure the outcome of operations on the shoulder, excluding stabilization procedures (Table 28–11).

Others have used batteries of questions aimed at documenting the patient's history and functional status as well as postoperative results. For example, the Hughston Clinic and Steadman-Hawkins Clinic use the inventories as shown in Tables 28–12 and 28–13.

The Academy of Orthopaedic Surgeons has developed a questionnaire to evaluate upper extremity function, including the hand, wrist, elbow, and shoulder. This is part of their thrust toward a specialty wide outcomes evaluation system for essentially all musculoskeletal systems.[2] These questionnaires also include an overall health status portion. The upper extremity specific portion is shown in Table 28–14.

In 1991, a group of rheumatologists presented their approach to shoulder evaluation, the Shoulder Pain and Disability Index.[96] It includes five visual analog scales that test pain and eight scales that test function. The index requires 3 to 5 minutes for patients to complete and is moderately easy to score. This also aims at overall shoulder function and pain.

The Subjective Shoulder Rating Scale, presented in 1992, utilizes multiple choice questions that are weighted by response.[63] It takes less than 3 minutes to fill out and is easy to score. This form is oriented to a determination of impairment and deals more with overall shoulder function.[5]

Investigators in Canada have sought to develop disease-specific quality of life instruments of both instability and rotator cuff disease to use in studies of these two problems as an outcome measure.[60, 61]

HEALTH STATUS INSTRUMENTS

Shoulder disorders do not exist in isolation but rather in the context of the overall health of the individual. Health status self-assessment tests have been developed to document the patient's perception of his or her overall health and function. Shoulder-specific instruments perform differently than health status instruments (e.g., Short Form-36 [SF-36]), confirming the need for both disease-specific and overall health status measures in the complete evaluation of patients with shoulder problems.[5]

History

Health status assessments and psychological indicators have been utilized extensively throughout medicine, in-

Table 28–9 AC SEPARATION SCORING SYSTEM*

RATING CRITERIA ACCORDING TO POIGENFORST ET AL (1987)

Excellent

Maximum limitation of mobility compared with the contralateral side of no more than 10 degrees
No complaints (except sensitivity to changes in the weather)
Full athletic fitness (no paresthesia)
Radiographic findings: no dislocation or subluxation

Good

Limitation of mobility as compared with the contralateral side ranging between 1 and 20 degrees
Minor complaints during load
Full athletic fitness (minor paresthesia lateral from the scar)
Radiographic findings: no dislocation; subluxation as much as half of the clavicular diameter

Poor

Limitation of mobility compared with the contralateral side of more than 20 degrees
Complaints during normal activities or even at rest
Obvious reduction of athletic fitness (paresthesia lateral from the scar)
Radiographic findings: dislocation

*The scoring system was developed by Poigenfurst and associates specifically for evaluating results following AC separation. (From Poigenfurst J, Orthner E, and Hoffman J: Technik und ergebnisse der koraklavikularen verschraubung bei frischen akromioklavikularzerreissungen. Acta Chir Austriaca *1*:11–16, 1987.)

Table 28–10 ATHLETIC SHOULDER OUTCOME SCORING SYSTEM*

Name ____________ Age ______ Sex ______

Dominant Hand (R) ______ (L) ______ (Ambidextrous) ______

Type of Sport ____________

Position Played ____________

Years Played ____________

Prior Injury ____________

Activity Level

1. Professional (Major League)
2. Professional (Minor League)
3. College
4. High school
5. Recreational (full time)
6. Recreational (part time)

Diagnosis

1. Anterior instability
2. Posterior instability
3. Multidirectional instability
4. Recurrent dislocations
5. Impingement syndrome
6. Acromioclavicular syndrome
7. Acromioclavicular arthrosis
8. Rotator cuff repair (partial)
9. Rotator cuff repair (complete)
10. Biceps tendon rupture
11. Calcific tendinitis
12. Fracture

SUBJECTIVE (90 POINTS)

I. Pain	***Points***
No pain with competition	10
Pain after competing only	8
Pain while competing	6
Pain preventing competing	4
Pain with activities of daily living (ADLs)	2
Pain at rest	0
II. Strength/Endurance	
No weakness; normal competition fatigue	10
Weakness after competition; early competition fatigue	8
Weakness during competition; abnormal competition fatigue	6
Weakness or fatigue preventing competition	4
Weakness or fatigue with ADLs	2
Weakness or fatigue preventing ADLs	0
III. Stability	
No looseness during competition	10
Recurrent subluxations while competing	8
Dead arm syndrome while competing	6
Recurrent subluxations prevent competition	4
Recurrent subluxations during ADLs	2
Dislocations	0
IV. Intensity	
Preinjury versus postinjury hours of competition (100%)	10
Preinjury versus postinjury hours of competition (<75%)	8
Preinjury versus postinjury hours of competition (<50%)	6
Preinjury versus postinjury hours of competition (<25%)	4
Preinjury versus postinjury hours of ADLs (100%)	2
Preinjury versus postinjury hours of ADLs (<50%)	0
V. Performance	
At the same level, same proficiency	50
At the same level, decreased proficiency	40
At the same level, decreased proficiency, not acceptable to an athlete	30
Decreased level with acceptable proficiency at that level	20
Decreased level, unacceptable proficiency	10
Cannot compete, had to switch sport	0
OBJECTIVE (10 POINTS)	
Range of Motion	
Normal external rotation at 90-degree to 90-degree position; normal elevation	10
Less than 5-degree loss of external rotation; normal elevation	8
Less than 10-degree loss of external rotation; normal elevation	6
Less than 15-degree loss of external rotation; normal elevation	4
Less than 20-degree loss of external rotation; normal elevation	2
Greater than 20-degree loss of external rotation; or any loss of elevation	0

Overall Results

Excellent	90–100	Points
Good	70–89	Points
Fair	50–69	Points
Poor	<50	Points

*The Athletic Shoulder Outcome scoring system is used for evaluating general shoulder function specifically in athletes. (From Tibone JE and Bradley J: Evaluation of treatment outcomes for the athlete's shoulder. *In* Matsen FA III, Fu FH, and Hawkins RJ [eds]; Rosemont, IL: The Shoulder: A Balance of Mobility and Stability. American Academy of Orthopaedic Surgeons, 1993, pp 526–527.)

Table 28-11 SHOULDER SURGERY SCORING SYSTEM*

ITEM	SCORING CATEGORIES
During the Past 4 Weeks	
1. How would you describe the worst pain you had from your shoulder?	1 None 2 Mild 3 Moderate 4 Severe 5 Unbearable
2. Have you had any trouble dressing yourself because of your shoulder?	1 No trouble at all 2 Little trouble 3 Moderate trouble 4 Extreme difficulty 5 Impossible to do
3. Have you had any trouble getting in and out of a car or using public transportation because of your shoulder (whichever you tend to use)?	1 No trouble at all 2 Little trouble 3 Moderate trouble 4 Extreme difficulty 5 Impossible to do
4. Have you been able to use a knife and fork at the same time?	1 Yes, easily 2 With little difficulty 3 With moderate difficulty 4 With extreme difficulty 5 No, impossible
5. Could you do the household shopping on your own?	1 Yes, easily 2 With little difficulty 3 With moderate difficulty 4 With extreme difficulty 5 No, impossible
6. Could you carry a tray containing a plate of food across a room?	1 Yes, easily 2 With little difficulty 3 With moderate difficulty 4 With extreme difficulty 5 No, impossible
7. Could you brush or comb your hair with the affected arm?	1 Yes, easily 2 With little difficulty 3 With moderate difficulty 4 With extreme difficulty 5 No, impossible
8. How would you describe the pain that you usually had from your shoulder?	1 None 2 Mild 3 Moderate 4 Severe 5 Unbearable
9. Could you hang your clothes up in a wardrobe, using the affected arm?	1 Yes, easily 2 With little difficulty 3 With moderate difficulty 4 With extreme difficulty 5 No, impossible
10. Have you been able to wash and dry yourself under both arms?	1 Yes, easily 2 With little difficulty 3 With moderate difficulty 4 With extreme difficulty 5 No, impossible
11. How much has pain from your shoulder interfered with your usual work (including housework)?	1 Not at all 2 A little bit 3 Moderately 4 Greatly 5 Totally
12. Have you been troubled by pain from your shoulder in bed at night?	1 No nights 2 Only 1 or 2 nights 3 Some nights 4 Most nights 5 Every night

*The Shoulder Surgery scoring system was developed by Dawson and associates for patient self-assessment of general shoulder function after surgery. (From Dawson J, Fitzpatrick R, and Carr A: Questionnaire on the perceptions of patients about shoulder surgery. J Bone Joint Surg Br *78B*:593–600, 1996.)

cluding an evaluation of low back pain.[12, 17, 28, 37, 103, 106, 117] Similarly, problems of the shoulder are not without influences other than joint-specific. The importance of overall health status in disorders of the shoulder is not a new idea. Even Codman noted the impact of various psychological and medical issues on the patient with shoulder complaints.[22] Lorenz and associates and Coventry noted the effect of health variables on conditions of the shoulder in the 1950s.[25, 71] Several subsequent studies evaluated the characteristics of patients with frozen shoulders, once again looking at factors other than those related to the shoulder itself.[18, 36, 88] Most recently, Green and associates presented data examining the effect of psychological and psychiatric factors on failed shoulder surgery.[42]

The four most widely used and evaluated scales that are appropriate for use in musculoskeletal disease/injury are the SF-36, the QWB that forms the backbone of the Quality-Adjusted Life Years (QALYs) methodology, the Nottingham Health Profile, and the Sickness Impact Profile (SIP). These scales share the common goal of assessing many characteristics of human activity, including physical, psychological, social, and role functioning. Additionally, they share the characteristic of assessing the patient as a whole (from the patient's perspective) and not as an organ system, disease, or limb. They are internally consistent, and reproducible and can discriminate between clinical conditions of different severity. The scales are also sensitive to change in health status over time. There are additional benefits derived from the fact that they are not administered by a physician, which increases their reliability.

Self-assessments of health status have been in wide clinical use; some include evaluation of anxiety and depression, pain scales, and symptom inventories.[35, 87, 91]

Brief descriptions of these instruments follow.

Short Form-36

The SF-36 is a widely used general health status questionnaire that has been used to demonstrate the health status of control populations and populations with defined medical and psychological conditions, including the effectiveness of orthopedic management.[4, 14, 48, 51, 52, 99, 100, 103, 107–111] This form is shown in Table 28–15.

Using a standard algorithm, the responses to the questions are used to calculate eight SF-36 parameters. The maximum score for each parameter is 100.[111] The variables evaluated include "physical role function," "comfort (pain)," "physical function," "emotional role function," "social function," "vitality (energy/fatigue)," "mental health," and "general health."

Radosevich and associates have collected reference data from large populations using this instrument.[94] The control data for the SF36 were derived from three separate population-based health status surveys. These reference data cohorts did not exclude individuals with chronic back pain, arthritis, and other chronic conditions; thus, these control data represent a population cross-section and not the health status of "normal" individuals. As

Text continued on page 1331

Table 28–12 HUGHSTON SPORTS MEDICINE FOUNDATION FOLLOW-UP SHOULDER HISTORY*

1. How often does your shoulder hurt?	0	1	2	3	4	5	6	7	8	9	10	
	None										All the time	
2. How severe is the pain at its worst	0	1	2	3	4	5	6	7	8	9	10	
	None										Excruciating, requiring pain pills	
3. Does your shoulder hurt at night?	0	1	2	3	4	5	6	7	8	9	10	
	No										Severe, doesn't allow me to sleep	
4. Does the pain in your shoulder radiate to your neck or down your arm?	0	1	2	3	4	5	6	7	8	9	10	
	Never										All the time	
5. Do you feel popping when your shoulder moves?	0	1	2	3	4	5	6	7	8	9	10	
	None										Severe, all the time	
6. Does your shoulder catch when you move it?	0	1	2	3	4	5	6	7	8	9	10	
	None										Severe, all the time	
7. Does your shoulder slip when you move it?	0	1	2	3	4	5	6	7	8	9	10	
	No										Severe, all the time	
8. Is your shoulder stiff?	0	1	2	3	4	5	6	7	8	9	10	
	No										Cannot move my shoulder	
9. Do you have the feeling of your arm "going dead" with certain activities?	0	1	2	3	4	5	6	7	8	9	10	
	No										Every time I perform that activity	
10. How would you grade the strength of your shoulder compared to your normal shoulder?	0	1	2	3	4	5	6	7	8	9	10	
	Same										No strength	
11. Are you able to push objects?	0	1	2	3	4	5	6	7	8	9	10	
	No problem										Unable	
12. Are you able to pull objects?	0	1	2	3	4	5	6	7	8	9	10	
	No problem										Unable	
13. Are you able to throw objects?	0	1	2	3	4	5	6	7	8	9	10	
	No problem										Unable	
14. Are you able to lift objects (up to 10 to 15 lb)?	0	1	2	3	4	5	6	7	8	9	10	
	No problem										Unable	
15. Are you able to carry objects (10 to 15 lb) with your arms at your side?	0	1	2	3	4	5	6	7	8	9	10	
	No problem										Unable	
16. Are you able to comb your hair?	0	1	2	3	4	5	6	7	8	9	10	
	No problem										Unable	
17. Are you able to eat with utensils?	0	1	2	3	4	5	6	7	8	9	10	
	No problem										Unable	
18. Are you able to sleep on the involved side?	0	1	2	3	4	5	6	7	8	9	10	
	No problem										Unable	
19. Are you able to wash the opposite underarm?	0	1	2	3	4	5	6	7	8	9	10	
	No problem										Unable	
20. Are you able to use the involved hand for toilet care?	0	1	2	3	4	5	6	7	8	9	10	
	No problem										Unable	
21. Are you able to reach your back pocket or fasten your bra?	0	1	2	3	4	5	6	7	8	9	10	
	No problem										Unable	
22. Are you able to dress?	0	1	2	3	4	5	6	7	8	9	10	
	No problem										Unable	
23. Are you able to use your involved hand at shoulder level?	0	1	2	3	4	5	6	7	8	9	10	
	No problem										Unable	
24. Are you able to use your involved hand over your head?	0	1	2	3	4	5	6	7	8	9	10	
	No problem										Unable	
25. Are you able to perform your usual work?	0	1	2	3	4	5	6	7	8	9	10	
	No problem										Unable	
26. Are you able to perform your usual sport?	0	1	2	3	4	5	6	7	8	9	10	
	No problem										Unable	
27. Has your lifestyle changed because of your shoulder?	0	1	2	3	4	5	6	7	8	9	10	
	Not at all										Dramatically	
28. Are you satisfied with your shoulder function since surgery?	0	1	2	3	4	5	6	7	8	9	10	
	Yes										No	

COMMENTS:

*The Hughston Sports Medicine Foundation follow-up shoulder history form is used for patient self-assessment of general shoulder function and satisfaction. (From J. C. Hughston, Hughston Sports Medicine Clinic, Columbus, GA.)

Table 28–13 HAWKINS SHOULDER EVALUATION FORM*

PAIN ASSESSMENT POSTOPERATIVELY

1. Is your overall pain better than it was before surgery? Y N
2. How bad is your pain today? (Mark line)

No pain at all — Pain as bad as it can be

3. Is your pain . . . (Circle one):
   Improving Staying the same Getting worse
4. Do you require pain medications? Y N
5. Do you require narcotic analgesics? Y N
6. If yes, how many per day? (Average) # ___ Pills

FUNCTION

Circle the number that indicates your ability to do the following activities:

0 = Unable; 1 = very difficult; 2 = somewhat difficult; 3 = not difficult

Activity	*Right Arm*				*Left Arm*			
Put on a coat	0	1	2	3	0	1	2	3
Sleep on your side	0	1	2	3	0	1	2	3
Wash back/hook brassiere	0	1	2	3	0	1	2	3
Manage toileting	0	1	2	3	0	1	2	3
Comb hair	0	1	2	3	0	1	2	3
Reach a high shelf	0	1	2	3	0	1	2	3
Lift 10 lb above shoulder	0	1	2	3	0	1	2	3
Throw a ball overhead	0	1	2	3	0	1	2	3
Do usual work (List):	0	1	2	3	0	1	2	3
Do modified work (List):	0	1	2	3	0	1	2	3
Do usual sport (List):	0	1	2	3	0	1	2	3
Do modified sport (List):	0	1	2	3	0	1	2	3

At what level can you participate in sports? (Check one)

_______ 1. Significantly below my preinjury level

_______ 2. Slightly below my preinjury level

_______ 3. Equal to my preinjury

_______ 4. Above my preinjury level

OVERALL SATISFACTION

Very satisfied — Unsatisfied

*The Hawkins shoulder evaluation form is used for patient self-assessment of general shoulder function and satisfaction. (From R. J. Hawkins, Steadman Hawkins Clinic, Vail, CO.)

Table 28–14 AAOS UPPER EXTREMITY SCORING SYSTEM*

	NO DIFFICULTY	MILD DIFFICULTY	MODERATE DIFFICULTY	SEVERE DIFFICULTY	UNABLE
Open a tight or new jar	1	2	3	4	5
Write	1	2	3	4	5
Turn a key	1	2	3	4	5
Prepare a meal	1	2	3	4	5
Push open a heavy door	1	2	3	4	5
Place an object on a shelf above your head	1	2	3	4	5
Do heavy household chores (e.g., wash walls, wash floors)	1	2	3	4	5
Garden or do yardwork	1	2	3	4	5
Make a bed	1	2	3	4	5
Carry a shopping bag or briefcase	1	2	3	4	5
Carry a heavy object (over 10 lb)	1	2	3	4	5
Change a lightbulb overhead	1	2	3	4	5
Wash or blow dry your hair	1	2	3	4	5
Wash your back	1	2	3	4	5
Put on a pullover sweater	1	2	3	4	5
Use a knife to cut food	1	2	3	4	5
Recreational activities which require little effort (e.g., card playing, knitting, etc.)	1	2	3	4	5
Recreational activities in which you take some force or impact through your arm, shoulder, or hand (e.g., golf, hammering, tennis)	1	2	3	4	5
Recreational activities in which you move your arm freely (e.g., playing frisbee, badminton)	1	2	3	4	5
Manage transportation needs (getting from one place to another)					
Sexual activities	1	2	3	4	5

	NOT AT ALL	SLIGHTLY	MODERATELY	QUITE A BIT	EXTREMELY
During the **past week, to what extent** has your arm, shoulder, or hand problem interfered with your normal social activities with family, friends, neighbors, or groups? (Circle number.)	1	2	3	4	5

	NOT LIMITED AT ALL	SLIGHTLY LIMITED	MODERATELY LIMITED	VERY LIMITED	UNABLE
During the **past week** were you limited in your work or other regular daily activities as a result of your arm, shoulder, or hand problem? (Circle number.)	1	2	3	4	5

Table 28–14 AAOS UPPER EXTREMITY SCORING SYSTEM* *(Continued)*

Please rate the severity of the following symptoms in the **last week**. (Circle number).

	NONE	MILD	MODERATE	SEVERE	EXTREME
Arm, shoulder, or hand pain	1	2	3	4	5
Arm, shoulder, or hand pain when you performed any specific activity	1	2	3	4	5
Tingling (pins and needles) in your arm, shoulder, or hand	1	2	3	4	5
Weakness in your arm, shoulder, or hand	1	2	3	4	5
Stiffness in your arm, shoulder, or hand					

	NO DIFFICULTY	MILD DIFFICULTY	MODERATE DIFFICULTY	SEVERE DIFFICULTY	SO MUCH DIFFICULTY THAT I CAN'T SLEEP
During the **past week**, how much difficulty have you had sleeping because of the pain in your arm, shoulder, or hand? (Circle number.)	1	2	3	4	5

	STRONGLY DISAGREE	DISAGREE	NEITHER AGREE OR DISAGREE	AGREE	STRONGLY AGREE
I feel less capable, less confident, or less useful because of my arm, shoulder, or hand problem. (Circle number)	1	2	3	4	5

The following questions relate to the impact of your arm, shoulder, or hand problem on **playing your musical instrument or sport or both**.
If you play more than one sport or instrument (or play both), please answer with respect to the activity that is most important to you.
Please indicate the sport or instrument that is most important to you:

Please circle the number that best describes your physical ability in the past week. Did you have any difficulty:

	NO DIFFICULTY	MILD DIFFICULTY	MODERATE DIFFICULTY	SEVERE DIFFICULTY	UNABLE
Using your usual technique for playing your instrument or sport?	1	2	3	4	5
Playing your musical instrument or sport because of arm, shoulder, or hand pain?	1	2	3	4	5
Playing your musical instrument or sport as well as you would like?	1	2	3	4	5
Spending your usual amount of time practicing or playing your instrument or sport?	1	2	3	4	5

The following questions relate to the impact of your arm, shoulder or hand problem on **your work**.

Please circle the number that best describes your physical ability in the *past week*. Did you have any difficulty:

	NO DIFFICULTY	MILD DIFFICULTY	MODERATE DIFFICULTY	SEVERE DIFFICULTY	UNABLE
Using your usual technique for your work?	1	2	3	4	5
Doing your usual work because of arm, shoulder, or hand pain?	1	2	3	4	5
Doing your work as well as you would like?	1	2	3	4	5
Spending your usual amount of time doing your work?	1	2	3	4	5

*The American Academy of Orthopaedic Surgeons (AAOS) upper extremity portion of their scoring system is used for patient self-assessment of general upper extremity function. (From the American Academy of Orthopaedic Surgeons/Council of Musculoskeletal Specialty Societies/Institute for Work and Health Outcomes Data Collection Package. Version 2.0. May 1997.)

Table 28–15 HEALTH STATUS QUESTIONNAIRE (SF-36©)*

This survey asks for your views about your health. Please answer every question by circling the appropriate number: 1, 2, 3, etc. If you are unsure about how to answer a question, please give it the best answer you can and make a comment in the left margin, or on the back. Thank You.

1. In general, would you say your health is (circle one number):

Excellent	1
Very good	2
Good	3
Fair	4
Poor	5

2. Compared to one year ago, how would you rate your health in general now? (Circle one number.)

Much better now than 1 year ago	1
Somewhat better now than 1 year ago	2
About the same	3
Somewhat worse now than 1 year ago	4
Much worse now than 1 year ago	5

3. The following questions are about activities you might do during a typical day. Does your health limit you in these activities? If so, how much? (Circle 1, 2, or 3 on each line.)

	Yes, Limited a Lot	*Yes, Limited a Little*	*No, Not Limited At All*
a. Vigorous activities, such as running, lifting heavy objects, participating in strenuous sports	1	2	3
b. Moderate activities, such as moving a table, pushing a vacuum cleaner, bowling, or playing golf	1	2	3
c. Lifting or carrying groceries	1	2	3
d. Climbing several flights of stairs	1	2	3
e. Climbing one flight of stairs	1	2	3
f. Bending, kneeling, or stooping	1	2	3
g. Walking more than 1 mile	1	2	3
h. Walking several blocks	1	2	3
i. Walking one block	1	2	3
j. Bathing and dressing yourself	1	2	3

4. During the past 4 weeks, have you had any of the following problems with your work or other regular daily activities as a result of your physical health?
(Please answer YES or NO for each question by circling 1 or 2 on each line.)

	Yes	*No*
a. Cut down on the amount of time you spent on work or other activities	1	2
b. Accomplished less than you would like	1	2
c. Were limited in the kind of work or other activities	1	2
d. Had difficulty performing the work or other activities (e.g., it took extra effort)	1	2

5. During the past 4 weeks, have you had any of the following problems with your work or other regular daily activities as a result of any emotional problems (e.g., feeling depressed or anxious)?
(Please answer YES or NO for each question by circling 1 or 2 on each line.)

	Yes	*No*
a. Cut down on the amount of time you spent on work or other activities	1	2
b. Accomplished less than you would like	1	2
c. Didn't do work or other activities as carefully as usual	1	2

6. During the past 4 weeks to what extent have your physical health or emotional problems interfered with your normal social activities with family, friends, neighbors, or groups? (Circle one number.)

Not at all	1
Slightly	2
Moderately	3
Quite a bit	4
Extremely	5

7. How much body pain have you had during the past 4 weeks? (Circle one number.)

None	1
Very mild	2
Mild	3
Moderate	4
Severe	5
Very severe	6

8. During the past 4 weeks, how much did pain interfere with your normal work (including work both outside the home and housework)? (Circle one number.)

Not at all	1
A litle	2
Moderately	3
Quite a bit	4
Extremely	5

Table 28–15 HEALTH STATUS QUESTIONNAIRE (SF-36©)* (Continued)

9. These questions are about how you feel and how things have been with you during the past month. For each question, please indicate the one answer that comes closest to the way you have been feeling.

How much of the time during the past month	All of the Time	Most of the Time	A Good Bit of the Time	Some of the Time	A Little of the Time	None of the Time
a. Did you feel full of pep?	1	2	3	4	5	6
b. Have you been a very nervous person?	1	2	3	4	5	6
c. Have you felt so down in the dumps nothing could cheer you up?	1	2	3	4	5	6
d. Have you felt calm and peaceful?	1	2	3	4	5	6
e. Did you have a lot of energy?	1	2	3	4	5	6
f. Have you felt downhearted and blue?	1	2	3	4	5	6
g. Did you feel worn out?	1	2	3	4	5	6
h. Have you been a happy person?	1	2	3	4	5	6
i. Did you feel tired?	1	2	3	4	5	6
j. Has your health limited your social activities (like visiting your friends or close relatives)?	1	2	3	4	5	6

10. Please choose the answer that best describes how true or false each of the following statements is for you. (Circle one number on each line.)

	Definitely True	Mostly True	Not Sure	Mostly False	Definitely False
a. I seem to get sick a little easier than other people	1	2	3	4	5
b. I am as healthy as anybody I know	1	2	3	4	5
c. I expect my health to get worse	1	2	3	4	5
d. My health is excellent	1	2	3	4	5

11. Please answer YES or NO for each question by circling 1 or 2 on each line.

	Yes	No
a. In the past year, have you had 2 weeks or more during which you felt sad, blue, or depressed; or when you lost all interest or pleasure in things you usually care about or enjoyed?	1	2
b. Have you had 2 years or more in your life when you felt depressed or sad most days, even if you felt okay sometimes?	1	2
c. Have you felt depressed or sad much of the time in the past year?	1	2

*The Health Status Questionnaire (SF-36©) form is used for patient self-assessment of overall health status. (From Ware JE and Sherbourne CD: The MOS 36 item short-form health survey [SF-36]. I. Conceptual framework and item selection. Med Care *30[6]*:473–481, 1992.)

shown in the following figures (Figs. 28–1 to 28–8), the results from population-based controls decrease with age. Thus, if patients from different age groups are to be compared, it is useful to normalize the patients' scores using the average of control patients of similar age.[94]

The SF-36 demonstrates face validity; for instance, among 1200 randomly selected subjects completing the questionnaire, patients with arthritis had the second worst body pain score and the second most limited physical role function score. They also had the second best emotional role function score and the best mental health score out of all the chronic conditions investigated. For social function, vitality, and general health perceptions, individuals with arthritis scored in the middle of the group.[73]

The SF-36 has been validated to be reliable as self-administered (by the patient), by interviewer, by telephone, and by mail, and the form only takes 5 to 7 minutes to complete. These features make its use appealing; it is the most practical for use in a busy office or clinic setting. This instrument, however, may well have a

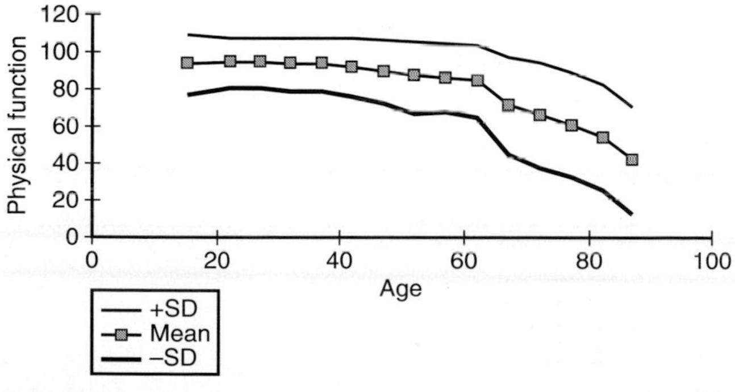

Figure 28–1

Population-based control data demonstrating change in SF-36 physical function score with age.

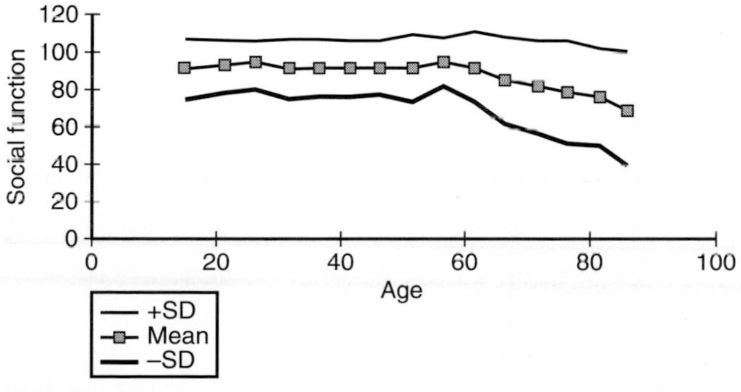

Figure 28–2

Population-based control data demonstrating change in SF-36 social function score with age.

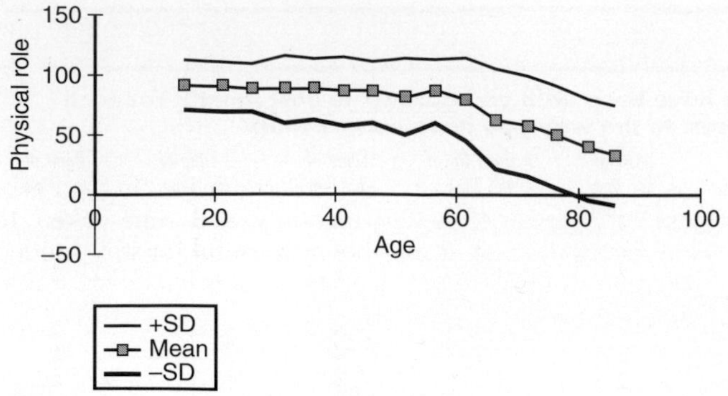

Figure 28–3

Population-based control data demonstrating change in SF-36 physical role score with age.

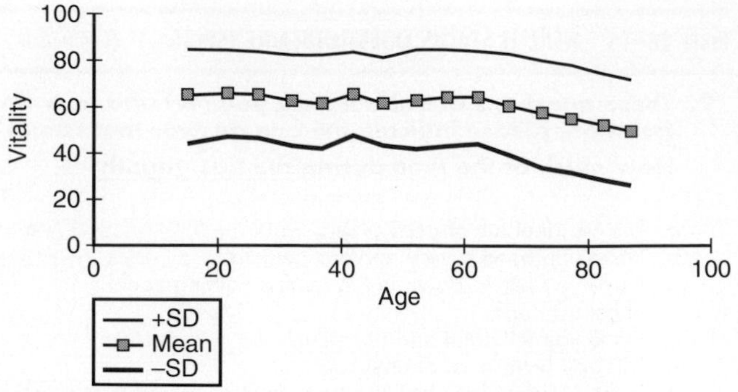

Figure 28–6

Population-based control data demonstrating change in SF-36 vitality score with age.

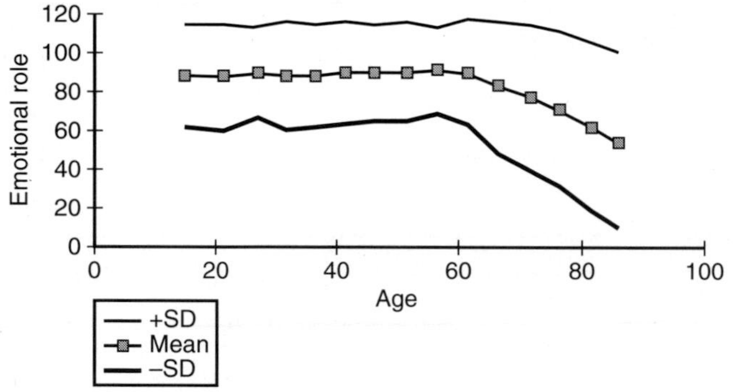

Figure 28–4

Population-based control data demonstrating change in SF-36 emotional role score with age.

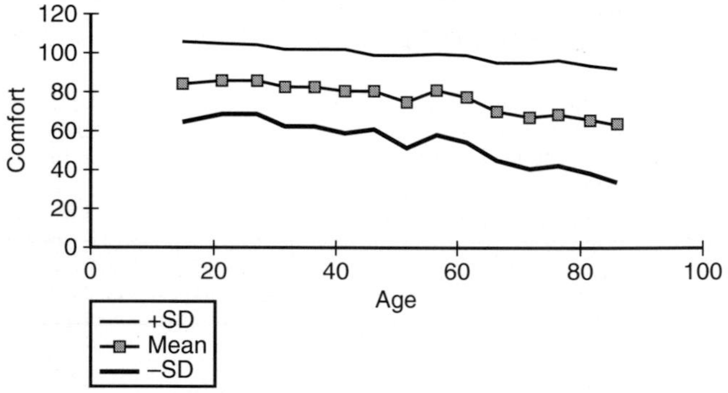

Figure 28–7

Population-based control data demonstrating change in SF-36 comfort score with age.

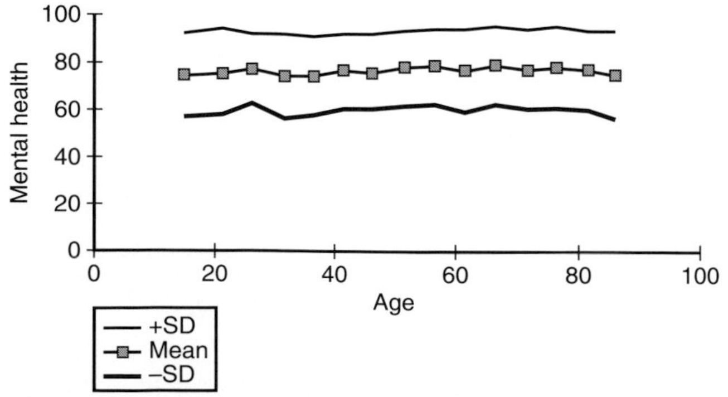

Figure 28–5

Population-based control data demonstrating change in SF-36 mental health score with age.

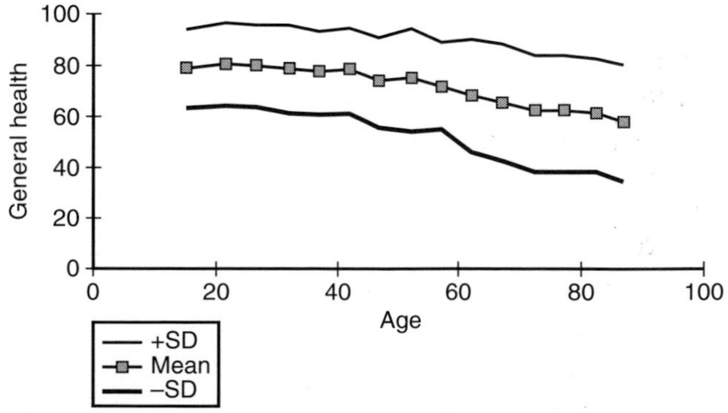

Figure 28–8

Population-based control data demonstrating change in SF-36 general health score with age.

"floor effect" for musculoskeletal conditions. This means that patients with musculoskeletal problems may "bottom out" on the scale, so that it does not differentiate different degrees of impairment. Our experience in administering the SF-36 shows that some patients with musculoskeletal disease or injury misinterpret the questions on general health as being exclusive of their musculoskeletal disease. The SF-36 also emphasizes lower extremity function rather than upper extremity function.[32, 77] Various groups have begun to develop an algorithm yielding a composite score for mental and physical overall function.

The SF-36 is helpful in responding to Codman's admonition. The form documents health status from the standpoint of the patient; it is practical and easy to complete, and it has been shown to be sensitive to musculoskeletal disease and to orthopedic treatment.

Quality of Well-Being Scale

Quality of life data are becoming increasingly important for evaluating the cost utility or cost-effectiveness of various health care programs. The QWB forms the basis for QALYs[112] and was designed to be used as an effectiveness measure for policy analysis and resource allocation. Patients respond to questions from an interviewer regarding their level of physical activity (three levels), mobility (three levels), social activity (five levels), and concerning the one symptom or problem that bothers them the most on the day when the questionnaire is administered (choice of 22 symptom complexes). Almost 80% of the population reports at least one symptom during any given 6-day period. The QWB is then calculated by factoring in preference weights, which were derived from responses to a household survey that queried respondents concerning their preferences for various health states on a scale of 1 to 10 ranging from death to perfect health. QWB scores are calculated separately for each of the 6 days preceding the interview, and the final score is the average of these six scores. Scores range from zero implying death to one denoting perfect health. Using data from large populations multiplied by years of life expectancy and cost per intervention, the QALY is obtained; cost per year of well life expectancy. QALYs provide a method for making decisions regarding resource allocation. When orthopedic interventions such as hip arthroplasty and hip fracture fixation have been studied using this methodology, they have faired well.[89, 116] The QWB physical function scale likely suffers from the floor effect in which lesser degrees of musculoskeletal function are detected.

Sickness Impact Profile

The SIP includes 136 endorsable statements developed by Bergner and associates at the University of Washington. It is best administered by trained interviewers and takes 25 to 35 minutes to complete.[8–10] Its 12 domains are addressed by simple yes or no questions. These 12 areas are scored independently and combined into a physical and a psychosocial subscale, as well as one aggregate score. Its scoring scale is 0 to 100 points with high scores denoting severe disability and low scores implying minimal deficit. Scores in excess of the mid-30s bring serious quality of life issues into question. It has been used in multiple health conditions that make comparisons of the impact of various diseases on health possible. It has been used in musculoskeletal trauma with good success.[75, 76] Because of the difficulty and time taken to administer the test, it may be most useful for well-funded outcome studies or controlled trials. It is likely that it also suffers from the floor effect.

Nottingham Health Profile

The Nottingham Health Profile is administered via an interview and has been used to assess functional outcomes of limb salvage versus early amputation.[39, 82, 83] It has been shown to be valid in other studies in Great Britain and Sweden. Part I of the profile measures subjective health status using 38 weighted questions that assess impairments in sleep, emotional reaction, mobility, energy level, pain, and social isolation. For each variable a score of 100 points represents maximal disability, whereas 0 points indicates no limitations. Part II includes seven yes or no statements that measure the influence of health problems on job, home, family life, sexual function, recreation, and enjoyment of holidays. Responses to both portions of the profile can be compared with average scores for the general population, taking into consideration such demographic factors as age and sex distributions.

The aforementioned examples are general health status instruments that have broad acceptance and lend the ability to compare the functional impact of various diseases. Disease or condition-specific instruments offer increased sensitivity and maximum limitation of floor and ceiling effects.[67]

RESULTS

Self-assessment tools reflect differences among diagnoses. The application of self-assessment tools to conditions of the shoulder is relatively recent. The authors now have a 4-year experience in applying the combination of the SF-36 and the SST to shoulder self-assessment.[80] Two previous investigations combined with the results presented here indicate that the patient's self-assessment can document and call attention to important aspects of the patient's condition that might not otherwise be detected.[78, 81]

The authors evaluated the compromise in general health status of 777 patients with nine well-characterized conditions of the shoulder by comparing them with age-matched population controls using the SF-36.[68] These patients met the necessary and sufficient criteria for one of nine shoulder diagnoses (number of patients/average age of patients): traumatic instability (TUBS, 90/30), frozen shoulder (FS, 74/56), degenerative joint disease (DJD, 160/63), partial-thickness cuff lesion (PTCL, 102/46), atraumatic instability (AMBRII, 65/27), full-thickness cuff tear (RCT, 132/60), secondary DJD (second-degree DJD, 42/54), post-traumatic stiff shoulder (PTSS, 76/45), and rheumatoid arthritis (RA, 36/56). For each patient, each of the SF-36 scores (Physical Role [PR], Comfort [C], Physical Function [PF], Social Function [SF], Emotional Role [ER], Vitality [V], General Health [GH] and Mental Health [MH]) was expressed as a percentage of the average for the age-matched control population.[94] The data are summarized here (Fig. 28–9) as the means of these percentages.

The SF-36 data from this large series of shoulder patients indicate that the physical role and comfort scores were less than 60% of age-matched controls for all nine diagnoses. Although the mental health for all groups was high, the physical function, vitality, and general health scores were particularly low for patients with rheumatoid arthritis. Self-assessment data enable orthopedic surgeons to document the compromise in health status associated with musculoskeletal conditions and the rationale for treating them. In that a goal of treatment is to restore these parameters to 100% of the population-based values, these data also provide a benchmark against which treatment effectiveness can be determined.[80] Within this highly selected population, standardized self-assessment indicated substantial, yet variable compromise of shoulder function and overall health status. Patients with rheumatoid arthritis showed major and significantly worse health status deficits than did those with osteoarthritis. These differences may be important considerations when selecting the approaches for management of patients with shoulder arthritis. For example, patients with severely limited vitality or social function scores may warrant different treatment than individuals with high scores for these parameters. Other examples of how similar data can be displayed in an understandable manner are shown in Figures 28–10 and 28–11.

Finally, the application of this methodology before and after treatment is extremely compelling. The authors have used it to evaluate the results of total shoulder arthroplasty for degenerative arthritis of the shoulder.[78] The following are the SF-36 and SST data of a group of 54 patients before and after joint replacement (Figs. 28–12 and 28–13). We have been able to document a significant improvement in many of the variables examined, thus exemplifying its effectiveness as a management scheme for shoulder arthritis in some patients.

SELF-ASSESSMENT TOOLS IN THE MEASUREMENT OF COST-EFFECTIVENESS

Measuring cost-effectiveness is challenging. The cost of various treatment methods varies substantially. Compare, for example, the cost of nonoperative and operative management of rotator cuff tears. To initiate a method by which cost-effectiveness might be compared among treatment methods, the authors conducted a preliminary study of 67 unmatched patients presenting for treatment of documented, symptomatic, full-thickness tears. Based on our clinical assessment and the desires of the patient, one of three treatment methods was selected for each patient: nonoperative management, subacromial smoothing without repair, and surgical repair. The number of patients, average age, gender, and length of follow-up for the patients in each of the three groups are shown in Table 28–16.

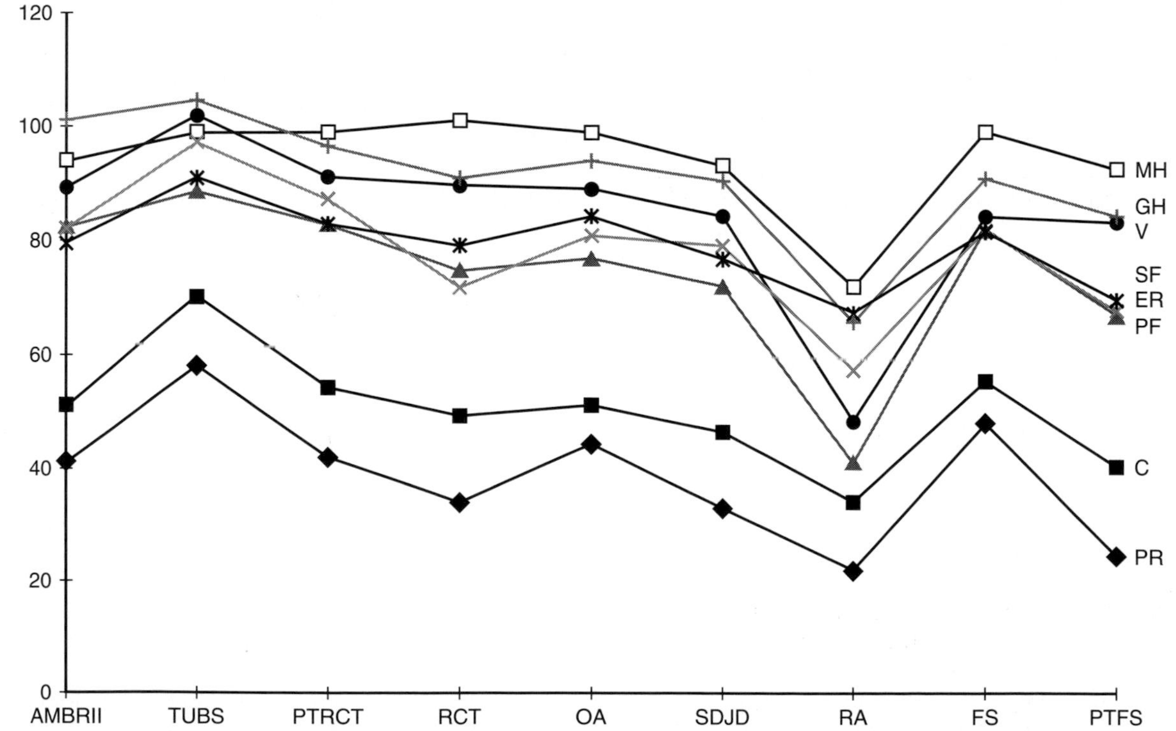

Figure 28–9

Relative compromise in general health status for patients with various shoulder conditions demonstrated by SF-36 scores as a percentage of the average for the age-matched control population.

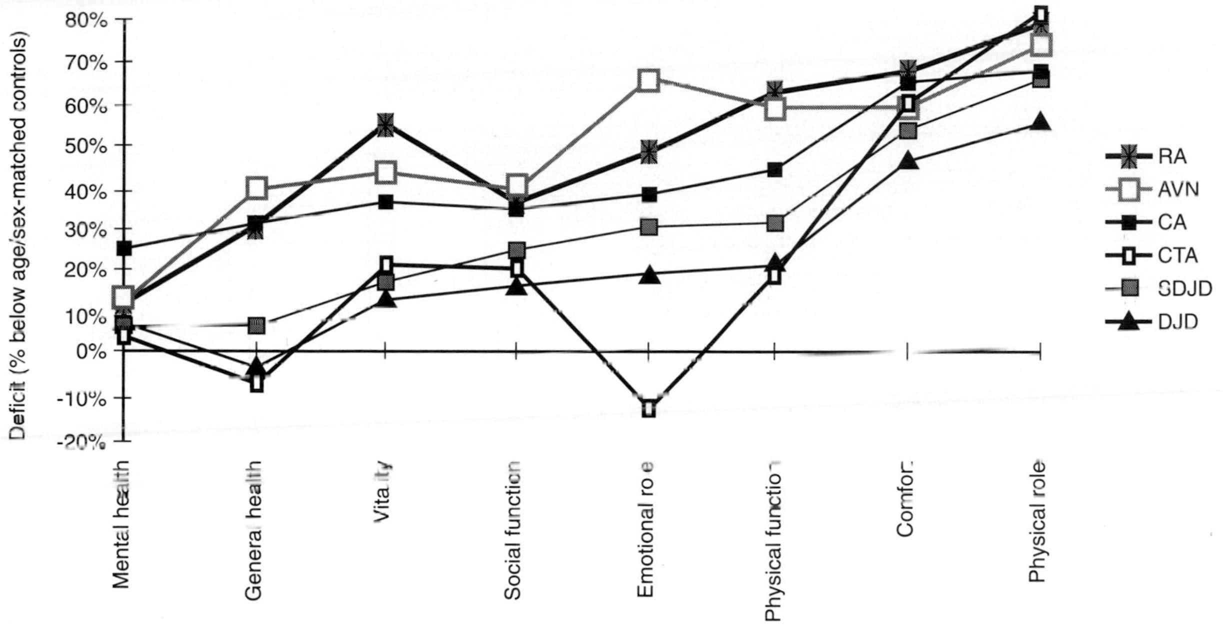

Figure 28–10

Relative compromise in general health status for patients with various shoulder conditions demonstrated by SF-36 scores as a percentage deficit versus the age-matched control population.

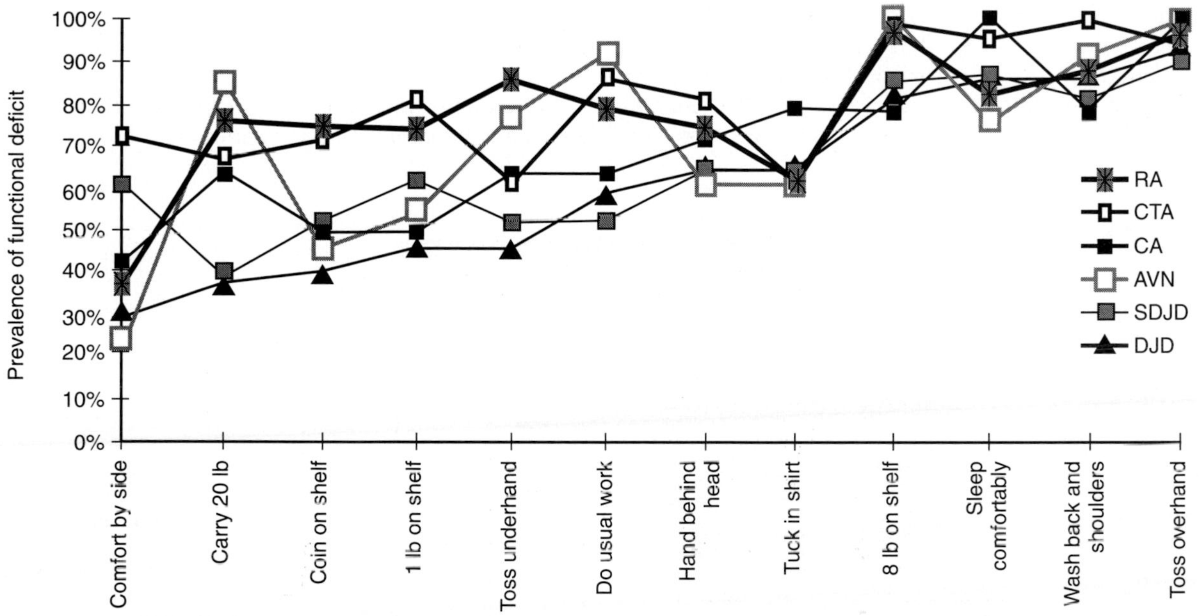

Figure 28–11

Relative compromise in shoulder function for patients with various shoulder conditions demonstrated by percentages of patients perceiving deficits on the Simple Shoulder Test (SST).

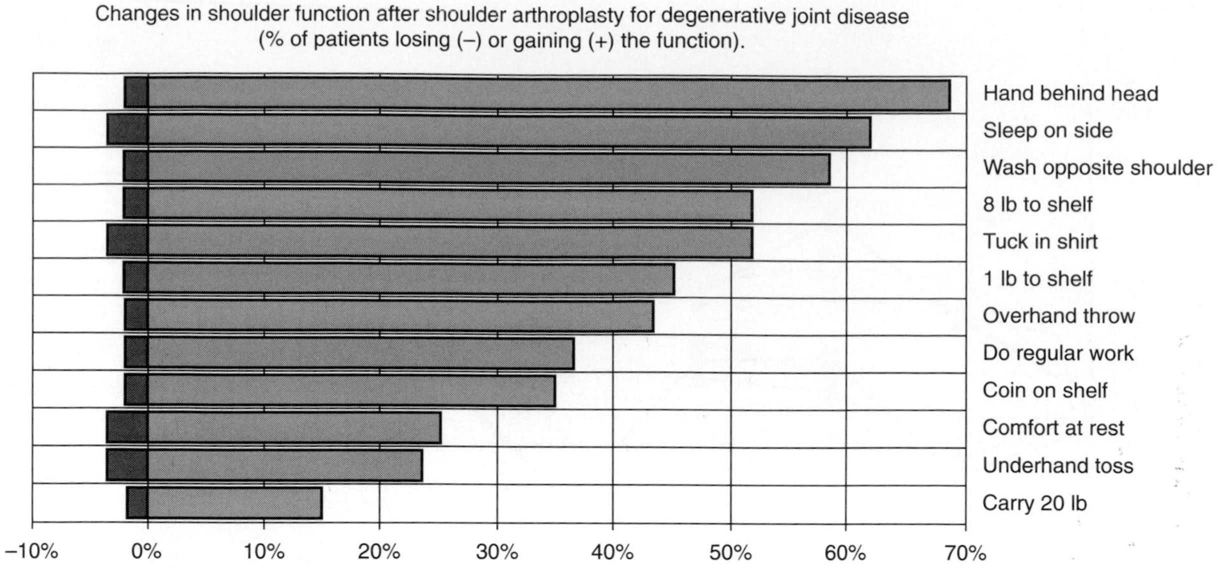

Figure 28–12

Changes in patients' perceived Simple Shoulder Test (SST) deficits before and after shoulder arthroplasty.

All patients completed SSTs measuring shoulder function and SF-36 health status questionnaires preoperatively and at follow-up. The effectiveness of treatment was measured in terms of the postoperative—preoperative change in the number of "yes" responses on the SST and the postoperative—preoperative change in the SF-36 comfort score. This analysis indicated that the greatest improvement was found in the group that had surgical repair. The changes in SST and SF-36 comfort score results for each patient were then divided by the total charges for the treatment to yield the average change/$1000 charge. In this analysis, nonoperative treatment was associated with the greatest change per unit charge (Figs. 28–14 and 28–15).

Although no conclusions can be drawn from these preliminary results, it is hoped that further studies of this type will help to determine the value of different treatment methods.

CONCLUSION

The examples presented earlier indicate that patient self-assessments of health status and shoulder function allow

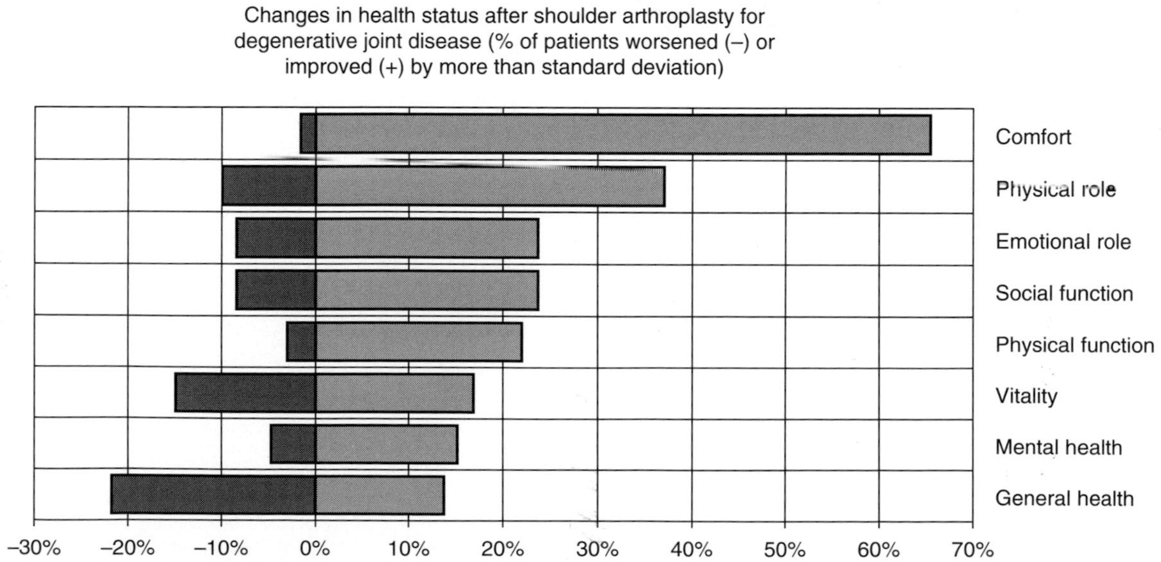

Figure 28–13

Changes in patients' perceived Health Status Questionnaire (SF-36) deficits before and after shoulder arthroplasty.

Table 28–16 PATIENT CHARACTERISTICS FOR THREE GROUPS OF ROTATOR CUFF TEAR TREATMENT*

	NO. OF PATIENTS	AVERAGE AGE	PERCENT FEMALE	AVERAGE FOLLOW-UP (yrs)
Nonoperative	36	62.4	36	1.7
Subacromial smoothing	11	67.8	45	1.7
Cuff repair	20	60.3	10	2.0

*Patient characteristics for three groups of rotator cuff tear treatments.

each physician to fulfill Codman's admonition. They provide practical, standardized, and meaningful characterization of the status of the patient at the time of presentation, which we refer to as the ingo as well as the patient's status after treatment, which is the outcome. The difference between the outcome and the ingo is the effectiveness of the treatment for the patient. Patients for whom the difference between outcome and ingo is not positive call up Codman's question–if not, why not? What is it about the disease, the patient, the treatment, or the doctor that has given rise to the failure? What are the predictors of success and failure? Dividing the effectiveness by the cost of the treatment yields a tangible measure of cost-effectiveness.

Use of standardized tools across practices will permit the combination of data in a statistically valid way so that we can better understand the factors contributing to the success and value of treatment. By using patient self-assessment as the cornerstone of these analyses, we keep our focus on the persons submitting themselves to the risks, benefits, and costs of treatment, rather than exclusively on medical metrics. In the end, the results of the analyses are easy for the individual physician to communicate to those who need to know how they are likely to benefit if this treatment is performed.

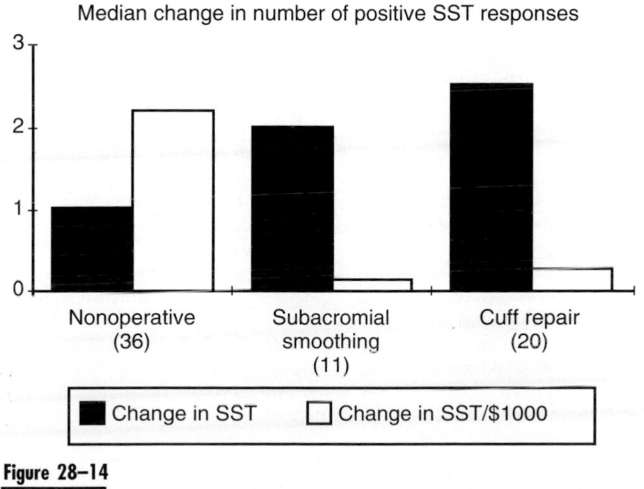

Figure 28–14

Change in the number of positive Simple Shoulder Test (SST) responses regarding shoulder function relative to the cost for three treatments of rotator cuff tears.

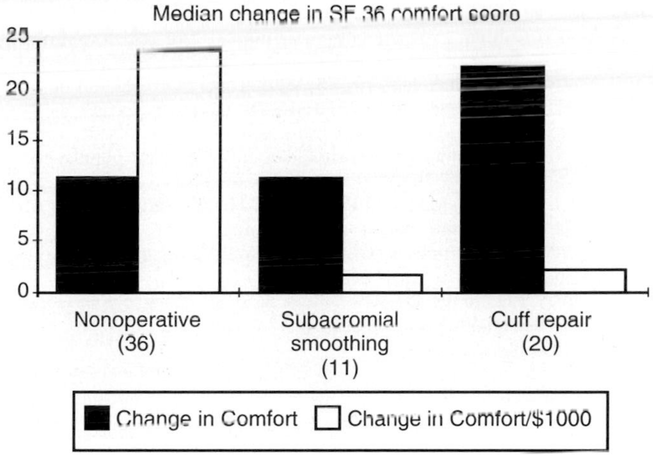

Figure 28–15

Change in the Health Status Questionnaire (SF-36) comfort score relative to the cost for three treatments of rotator cuff tears.

References and Bibliography

1. Academy plans data collection system. AAOS Bull *43*:24, 1995.
2. Academy proceeds on outcomes database. AAOS Bull *44*:29–30, 1996.
3. Altchek DW, Warren RF, Wickiewicz TL, et al: Arthroscopic acromioplasty: Technique and results. J Bone Joint Surg *72A*:1198–1207, 1990.
4. Bayley KB, London MR, Grunkemeier GL, et al: Measuring the success of treatment in patient terms. Med Care *33*(Suppl 4):AS226–AS235, 1995.
5. Beaton DE and Richards RR: Measuring function of the shoulder. J Bone Joint Surg *78A*:882–890, 1996.
6. Bellamy N, Buchanan WW, Goldsmith CH, et al: Validation study of WOMAC: A health status instrument for measuring clinically important patient relevant outcomes following total hip or knee arthroplasty in osteoarthritis. J Orthop Rheumatol *1*:95–108, 1988.
7. Benirschke SK, Melder I, Henley MB, et al: Closed interlocking nailing of femoral shaft fractures: assessment of technical complications and functional outcomes by comparison of a prospective database with retrospective review. J Orthop Trauma *7*:118–122, 1993.
8. Bergner M, Bobbitt RA, Carter WB, et al: The sickness impact profile: Development and final revision of a health status measure. Med Care *19*:787–805, 1981.
9. Bergner M, Bobbitt RA, Kressel S, et al: The sickness impact profile: Conceptual formulation and methodological development of a health status index. Int J Health Services *6*:393–415, 1976.
10. Bergner M, Bobbitt RA, Pollaro WE, et al: The sickness impact profile: Validation of a health status measure. Med Care *14*:57–67, 1976.
11. Bigos SJ: The practitioner's guide to the industrial back problem. Part II. Helping the patient with the return to work predicament. Semin Spine Surg *4*:55–63, 1992.
12. Bigos SJ, Battie MC, Fisher LD, et al: A longitudinal, prospective study of industrial back injury reporting. Clin Orthop *279*:21–34, 1992.
13. Binder AI, Bulgen DY, Hazleman BL, et al: Frozen shoulder: A long-term prospective study. Ann Rheum Dis *43*:361–364, 1984.
14. Bombardier C, Melfi CA, Paul J, et al: Comparison of a generic and a disease-specific measure of pain and physical function after knee replacement surgery. Med Care *33*(Suppl 4):AS131–44, 1995.
15. Bradburn NM: The Structure of Psychological Well-Being. Chicago: Aldine Publishing, 1969.

16. Breslow L: A quantitative approach to the World Health Organization definition of health; physical, mental and social well-being. Int J Epidemiol *1*:347–355, 1972.
17. Brown T, Nemiah JC, Barr JS, et al: Psychologic factors in low-back pain. N Engl J Med *251*:123–128, 1954.
18. Bruckner FE and Nye CJS: A prospective study of adhesive capsulitis of the shoulder (frozen shoulder) in a high risk population. Q J Med *198*:191–204, 1981.
19. Bush JW, Chen MM, and Patrick DL: Health status index in cost-effectiveness and analysis of PKU program. *In* Berg RL (ed): Health Status Indexes. Chicago: Hospital Research and Educational Trust, 1973, pp 172–208.
20. Cleary PD, Reilly DT, Greenfield S, et al: Using patient reports to assess health-related quality of life after total hip replacement. Q Life Res *2*:3–11, 1993.
21. Codman EA: The product of a hospital. Surg Gynecol Obstet *18*:491–496, 1914.
22. Codman EA: Hysteria, neurasthenia, neurosis, traumatic neuritis, malingering. *In* The Shoulder. Malaber, FL: Krieger Publishing Co., 1934, pp 400–410.
23. Constant CR and Murley AHG: A clinical method of functional assessment of the shoulder. Clin Orthop *214*:160–164, 1987.
24. Cotton P: Orthopedics research now asks, "does it work?" rather than just, "how is the procedure performed?" JAMA *265*:2164–2165, 1991.
25. Coventry MB: Problem of painful shoulder. JAMA *151*:177–185, 1953.
26. Crandell D, Richmond J, Lau J, et al: A Meta-analysis of the Treatment of Injuries of the Anterior Cruciate Ligament. Presented at the Annual Meeting, American Orthopaedic Society for Sports Medicine, Palm Springs, 1994.
27. Dawson J, Fitzpatrick R, and Carr A: Questionnaire on the perceptions of patients about shoulder surgery. J Bone Joint Surg Br *78B*:593–600, 1996.
28. Deyo RA, Andersson G, Bombardier C, et al: Outcome measures for studying patients with low back pain. Spine *19* (18S):2032S–2036S, 1994.
29. Donabedian A: Evaluating the product of medical care. Milbank Q *44*:166–203, 1966.
30. Ellman H, Hanker G, and Bayer M: Repair of the rotator cuff: end-result study of factors influencing reconstruction. J Bone Joint Surg *68A*:1136–1144, 1986.
31. Emery DD and Schneiderman LJ: Cost-effectiveness analysis in health care. Hastings Cent Rep *19*:8–13, 1989.
32. Engelberg R, Martin DP, Agel J, et al: The musculoskeletal functional assessment instrument: criterion and construct validity. J Orthop Res *14*:182–192, 1996.
33. Epstein A: The outcomes movement—will it get us where we want to go. N Engl J Med *373*:266–270, 1990.
34. Esch J, Ozerkis L, Helgager J, et al: Arthroscopic subacromial decompression: results according to the degree of rotator cuff tear. Arthroscopy *4*:241–249, 1988.
35. Fitzpatrick R, Ziebland S, Jenkinson C, et al: The social dimension of health status measures in rheumatoid arthritis. Int Dis Stud *13*:34–37, 1991.
36. Fleming A, Dodman S, Beer TC, et al: Personality in frozen shoulder. Ann Rheum Dis *35*:456–457, 1976.
37. Frymoyer JW, Rosen JC, Clements J, et al: Psychologic factors in low-back pain disability. Clin Orthop *195*:178–184, 1985.
38. Gartland JJ: Orthopaedic clinical research: Deficiencies in experimental design and determination of outcome. J Bone Joint Surg *70A*:1357–1364, 1988.
39. Georgiadis GM, Behrens FF, Joyce MJ, et al: Open tibial fractures with severe soft tissue loss-limb salvage compared with below knee amputation. J Bone Joint Surg *75A*:1431–1441, 1993.
40. Gillespie WJ and Daellenbach HG: Assessing cost-effectiveness in orthopaedic outcome studies. Orthopaedics *15*:1275–1277, 1992.
41. Gordon TA, Burleyson GP, Tielsch JM, et al: The effects of regionalization on cost and outcome for one general high-risk surgical procedure. Ann Surg *221*:43–49, 1995.
42. Green A, Norris TR, Becker GE, et al: Failed Shoulder Surgery: Psychological and Psychiatric Considerations. Presented at Specialty Day, American Shoulder and Elbow Surgeons, Atlanta, Georgia, 1996.
43. Gross M: A critique of the methodologies used in clinical studies of hip joint arthroplasty published in the English literature. J Bone Joint Surg *70A*:1364–1371, 1988.
44. Guadagnoli E and McNeil BJ: Outcomes research: Hope for the future or the latest rage? Inquiry *31*:14–24, 1994.
45. Hawkins RJ, Brock R, Abrams J, et al: Acromioplasty for impingement with an intact rotator cuff. J Bone Joint Surg *70B*:795–797, 1988.
46. Jensen I, Nygren A, Gamberale F, et al: The role of the psychologist in multidisciplinary treatments for chronic neck and shoulder pain: A controlled cost-effectiveness study. Scand J Rehabil Med *27*:19–26, 1995.
47. Johanson NA, Charlson ME, Szatrowski TP, et al: A self administered hip-rating questionnaire for the assessment of outcome after total hip replacement. J Bone Joint Surg *74A*:587–597, 1992.
48. Kantz ME, Harris WJ, Levitsky K, et al: Methods for assessing condition-specific and generic functional status outcomes after total knee replacement. Med Care *30(5 Suppl)*:MS240–252, 1990.
49. Kaplan RM and Bush JW: Health-related quality of life measurement for evaluation research and policy analysis. Health Psych *1*:61–80, 1982.
50. Karnofsky DA and Burchenal JH: The clinical evaluation of chemotherapeutic drugs. *In* MacLeod CM (ed): Evaluation of Chemotherapeutic Agents. New York: Columbia University Press, 1949, pp 191–194.
51. Katz JN, Harris TM, Larson MG, et al: Predictors of functional outcomes after arthroscopic partial meniscectomy. J Rheumatol *19*:1938–1942, 1992.
52. Katz JN, Larson MG, Phillips CB, et al: Comparative measurement sensitivity of short and longer health status instruments. Med Care *30*:917–925, 1992.
53. Katz S, Ford AB, Moskowitz RW, et al: Studies of illness in the aged. JAMA *185*:914–919, 1963.
54. Kay A, Davison B, Badley E, et al: Hip arthroplasty: patient satisfaction. Br J Rheumatol *22*:243–249, 1983.
55. Kay SP and Amstutz HC: Shoulder hemiarthroplasty at UCLA. Clin Orthop *228*:42–44, 1988.
56. Keller R, Soule DN, Wennberg JE, et al: Dealing with geographic variations in the use of hospitals: the experience of the Maine medical assessment foundation orthopaedic study group. J Bone Joint Surg *72A*:1286–1293, 1990.
57. Keller RB: How outcomes research should be done. *In* Matsen FA, III, Fu FH, and Hawkins RJ (eds): The Shoulder: A Balance of Mobility and Stability. Rosemont, IL: American Academy of Orthopaedic Surgeons, 1993, pp 487–499.
58. Keller RB: Outcomes research in orthopaedics. J Am Acad Orthop Surg *1*:122–129, 1993.
59. Keller RB, Rudicel SA, and Liang MH: Outcomes research in orthopaedics. J Bone Joint Surg *75A*:1562–1574, 1993.
60. Kirkley A: Western Ontario Rotator Cuff (WORC) Index. 1996.
61. Kirkley A: Western Ontario Shoulder Instability (WOSI) Index. 1996.
62. Kirwan JR, Currey HL, Freeman MA, et al: Overall long-term impact of total hip and knee joint replacement surgery on patients with osteoarthritis and rheumatoid arthritis. Br J Rheumatol *33*:357–360, 1990.
63. Kohn D, Geyer M, and Wulker N: The Subjective Shoulder Rating Scale (SSRS): An Examiner-Independent Scoring System. Presented at the International Congress on Surgery of the Shoulder, Paris, 1992.
64. L'Abbe KA, Detsky AS, and O'Rourke K: Meta-analysis in clinical research. Ann Intern Med *107*:224–233, 1987.
65. Lavernia CJ, Guzman JF, Gachupin-Garcia A, et al: Cost effectiveness and quality of life in arthroplasty surgery. 1996.
66. Lembcke PA: Measuring the quality of medical care through vital statistics based on hospital service areas: A comparative study of appendectomy rates. Am J Health *42*:276–286, 1952.
67. Levine DW, Simmons BP, Koris MJ, et al: A self-administered questionnaire for the assessment of severity of symptoms and functional status in carpal tunnel syndrome. J Bone Joint Surg *75A*:1585–1592, 1993.
68. Levinsohn DG and Matsen FA III: Evaluation of Nine Common Mechanical Shoulder Disorders with the SF-36 Health Status Instrument. Presented at the 64th Annual Meeting of the American Academy of Orthopaedic Surgeons, San Francisco, CA, 1997.
69. Lippitt SB, Harryman DT II, and Matsen FA III: A Practical Tool

for Evaluating Function: The Simple Shoulder Test. *In* Matsen FA III, Fu FH, and Hawkins RJ (eds): The Shoulder: A Balance of Mobility and Stability. Rosemont, IL: American Academy of Orthopaedic Surgeons, 1993, pp 501–518.
70. Lirette R, Morin F, and Kinnard P: The difficulties in assessment of results of anterior acromioplasty. Clin Orthop *278*:14–16, 1992.
71. Lorenz TH and Musser MJ: Life stress, emotions and painful stiff shoulder. Ann Intern Med *37*:1232–1244, 1952.
72. Lu-Yao GL, Keller RB, Littenberg B, et al: A meta-analysis of 106 published reports. J Bone Joint Surg *76A*:15–25, 1994.
73. Lyons RA, Lo SV, and Littlepage BNC: Comparative health status of patients with 11 common illnesses in Wales. J Epidemiol Community Health *48*:388–390, 1994.
74. Lysholm J and Gillquist J: Evaluation of knee ligament surgery results with special emphasis on use of a scoring scale. Am J Sports Med *10*:150–154, 1982.
75. MacKenzie EJ, Burgess AR, McAndrew MP, et al: Patient-oriented functional outcome after unilateral lower extremity fracture. J Orthop Trauma 7:393–401, 1993.
76. MacKenzie EJ, Cushing BM, Jurkovich GJ, et al: Physical impairment and functional outcomes six months after severe lower extremity fractures. J Trauma *34*:528–539, 1993.
77. Martin D, Engelberg R, Agel J, et al: Development of the musculoskeletal functional assessment instrument. J Orthop Res *14*:173–181, 1996.
78. Matsen FA III: Early effectiveness of shoulder arthroplasty for patients who have primary glenohumeral degenerative joint disease. J Bone Joint Surg *78A*:260–264, 1996.
79. Matsen FA III, Lippitt SB, Sidles JA, and Harryman DT II: Practical Evaluation and Management of the Shoulder. Philadelphia: WB Saunders, 1994.
80. Matsen FA III, Smith KL, DeBartolo SE, et al: A comparison of patients with late-stage rheumatoid arthritis and osteoarthritis of the shoulder using self-assessed shoulder function and health status. Arthritis Care Res *10*:43–47, 1997.
81. Matsen FA III, Ziegler DW, and DeBartolo SE: Patient self-assessment of health status in glenohumeral degenerative joint disease. J Shoulder Elbow Surg *4*:345–351, 1995.
82. McDowell I and Newell C: Measuring Health: A Guide to Rating Scales and Questionnaires. New York: Oxford University Press, 1987, pp 125–133.
83. McEwen J: The Nottingham Health Profile: A measure of perceived health. *In* Teeling-Smith G (ed): Measuring the Social Benefits of Medicine. London: Office of Health Economics, 1983, pp 75–84.
84. Mohtadi GH and Nicholas GH: Quality of life assessment as an outcome in anterior cruciate ligament reconstruction surgery. *In* Jackson DW, et al (eds): The Anterior Cruciate Ligament: Current and Future Concepts. New York: Raven Press, 1993.
85. Neer CS II: Anterior acromioplasty for the chronic impingement syndrome in the shoulder: A preliminary report. J Bone Joint Surg *54A*:41–50, 1972.
86. Neer CS II: Impingement lesions. Clin Orthop *173*:70–77, 1983.
87. Nerenz DR, Repasky DP, Whitehouse FW, et al: Ongoing assessment of health status in patients with diabetes mellitus. Med Care *30*:MS112–MS124, 1992.
88. Oesterreicher W and Van Dam G: Social psychological researches into brachialgia and periarthritis. Arthritis Rheumatol 7:670–683, 1964.
89. Parker MJ, Myles JW, Anand JK, et al: Cost-benefit analysis of hip fracture treatment. J Bone Joint Surg *74B*:261–264, 1992.
90. Patte D: Directions for the Use of the Index Severity for Painful and/or Chronically Disabled Shoulders. Paris: 1987.
91. Pitson D, Bhaskaran V, Bond H, et al: Effectiveness of knee replacement surgery in arthritis. Int J Nurs Stud *31*:49–56, 1994.
92. Poigenfurst J, Orthner E, and Hoffman J: Technik und ergebnisse der koraklavikularen verschraubung bei frischen akromioklavikularzerreissungen. Acta Chir Austriaca *1*:11–16, 1987.
93. Post M and Cohen J: Impingement syndrome: A review of late stage II and early stage III lesions. Clin Orthop *207*:126–132, 1986.
94. Radosevich DM, Wetzler H, and Wilson SM: Health Status Questionnaire (HSQ) 2.0: Scoring Comparisons and Reference Data. Bloomington, MN. Health Outcomes Institute, 1994.
95. Richards RR, An K-N, Bigliani LU, et al: A standardized method for assessment of shoulder function. J Shoulder Elbow Surg *3*:347–352, 1994.
96. Roach KE, Budiman-Mak E, Songsiridej N, et al: Development of a shoulder pain and disability index. Arthritis Care Res *4*:143–149, 1991.
97. Rowe CR, Patel D, and Southmayd WW: The Bankart procedure: A long-term end-result study. J Bone Joint Surg *60A*:1–16, 1978.
98. Shapiro ET, Rockett SE, Richmond JC, et al: Use of a Patient-Based Health Assessment for Evaluation of ACL Patients. Presented at the Annual Meeting, American Orthopaedic Society for Sports Medicine, Palm Springs, 1994.
99. Stewart AL, Hays RD, and Ware JE: The MOS short form general health survey; reliability and validity in a patient population. Med Care *26*:724–735, 1988.
100. Stewart AL, Ware JE, Brook RH, et al: Conceptualization and Measurement of Health for Adults in the Health Insurance Study. Vol II. Physical Health in Terms of Functioning. Santa Monica, CA: The Rand Corp, 1978.
101. Swiontkowski MF and Chapman JR: Cost and effectiveness issues in care of injured patients. Clin Orthop *318*:17–24, 1995.
102. Tarlov AR: Multiple influences propel outcomes field. Med Outcomes Trust Bull 3:5, 1995.
103. Tarlov AR, Ware JE, Greenfield S, et al. The medical outcomes study: An application of methods for monitoring the results of medical care. JAMA *262*:925–930, 1989.
104. Tibone JE and Bradley JP: Evaluation of treatment outcomes for the athlete's shoulder. *In* Matsen FA III, Fu FH, and Hawkins RJ (eds): The Shoulder: A Balance of Mobility and Stability. Rosemont, IL: American Academy of Orthopaedic Surgeons, 1993, pp 519–529.
105. Troup JDG, Foreman TK, Baxter CE, et al: The perception of back pain and the role of psychophysical tests of lifting capacity. 1987 Volvo Award in Clinical Sciences. Spine *12*:645–657, 1987.
106. Waddell G, McCulloch JA, Kummel E, et al: Non-organic physical signs in low back pain. Spine *5*:117–125, 1980.
107. Ware JE: Methodological considerations in the selection of health status assessment procedures. *In* Wenger NK, et al (eds): Assessment of Quality of Life in Clinical Trials of Cardiovascular Therapies. New York: Le Jac, 1984, pp 87–111.
108. Ware JE, Johnston SA, Davies-Avery A, et al: Conceptualization and measurement of health for adults in the Health Insurance Study. Vol III. Mental Health. Santa Monica, CA: Rand Corp, 1979.
109. Ware JE and Sherbourne CD: The MOS 36 item short-form health survey (SF-36). I. Conceptual framework and item selection. Med Care *30*:473–481, 1992.
110. Ware JE, Sherbourne CD, and Davies AR: Developing and testing the MOS 20-item short-form health survey: A general population application. *In* Stewart AL and Ware JE (eds): Measuring Function and Well-Being: The Medical Outcomes Study Approach. Durham, NC: Duke University Press, 1992, pp 277–290.
111. Ware JE Jr, Snow KK, Kosinski M, et al: SF-36 Health Survey, Manual and Interpretation Guide. Boston, MA: The Health Institute, New England Medical Center, 1993.
112. Weinstein MC and Stason WB: Hypertension: A Policy Perspective. Cambridge, MA: Harvard University Press, 1976.
113. Wennberg J and Gittelsohn A: Small area variations in health care delivery. Science *182*:1102–1108, 1973.
114. Wennberg JE, Freeman JL, and Culp WJ: Are hospital services rationed in New Haven or over-utilised in Boston? Lancet *1*:1185–1188, 1987.
115. Wennberg JE and Gittelsohn A: Variations in medical care among small areas. Sci Am *246*:120–134, 1987.
116. Williams A: Setting priorities in health care: An economist's view. J Bone Joint Surg *73B*:365–367, 1991.
117. Wiltsie LL and Rocchio PD: Preoperative psychological tests as predictors of success of chemonucleolysis in the treatment of the low back syndrome. J Bone Joint Surg 57A:478–484, 1975.

APPENDIX

Shoulder Function and Health Status Forms

TEST	METHOD OF ADMINISTRATION	POPULATION DESIGNED FOR	CONDITIONS USED FOR	HOW/WHERE TO GET
Health Status Questionnaire Short Form 36 (SF-36)	Self or interviewer	All	Overall health status/quality of life	Medical Outcomes Trust 20 Park Plaza, Suite 1014 Boston, MA 02116-4313
Sickness Impact Profile (SIP)	Self or interviewer	All	Overall health status/quality of life	Ann Skinner 624 N Broadway Baltimore, MD 21205
Nottingham Health Profile	Self	All	Overall health status/quality of life	Jim McEwan Department of Public Health University of Glasgow Glasgow, Scotland
Quality of Well-Being Scale (QWB)	Trained interviewer	All	Overall health status/quality of life	Holly Teetzel Department of Family and Preventative Medicine—HOAP Box 0807 UCSD, 9500 Gilman Drive La Jolla, CA 92093-0807
American Academy of Orthopaedic Surgeons (AAOS) Instruments (Upper Extremity)	Self or interviewer	Patients with upper extremity disease	Quality of life with upper extremity disease	Chad Munger Director of Research and Scientific Affairs AAOS, 6300 N River Road Rosemont, IL 60018
Simple Shoulder Test (SST)	Self	Patients with shoulder conditions	Shoulder conditions	Frederick A. Matsen III, M.D. Dept. of Orthopaedics Box 356500, UWMC 1959 NE Pacific Street Seattle, WA 98195-6500
Rowe Scale	Physician	Patients with shoulder conditions	Shoulder conditions	Carter Rowe, M.D. 1108 Princess Anne Street Fredericksburg, VA 22401-3808
Hospital for Special Surgery Scale (HSS)	Physician	Patients with shoulder conditions	Shoulder conditions	David Altchek, M.D. Hospital for Special Surgery 535 E. 70th Street New York, NY 10021
University of California–Los Angeles Score (UCLA)	Physician	Patients with shoulder conditions	Shoulder conditions	Harvard Ellman, M.D. 4 Privateer Street Marina del Rey, CA 90292-6770
American Shoulder and Elbow Surgeons Scale (ASES)	Physician	Patients with shoulder conditions	Shoulder conditions	Robin Richards, M.D. 55 Queen Street East, #800 Toronto, ON Canada M5C 1R6
Constant Score	Physician	Patients with shoulder conditions	Shoulder conditions	C. R. Constant, M.D. Department of Orthopaedic Surgery Addenbrooke's Hospital Cambridge, England

Index

Page numbers in *italics* refer to illustrations; numbers followed by t indicate tables.

C

D

H

J

K

L

P

S

T

U

V

W

X

Y

Z